CURRENT MEDICAL DIAGNOSIS & TREATMENT

From inability to let well alone; from too much zeal for the new and contempt for what is old; from putting knowledge before wisdom, Science before Art and cleverness before common sense; from treating patients as cases, from making the cure of the disease more grievous than the endurance of the same, Good Lord deliver us.

—Sir Robert Hutchison

current
MEDICAL
DIAGNOSIS
& TREATMENT

By

MARCUS A. KRUPP, MD

Clinical Professor of Medicine
Stanford University School of Medicine (Stanford)
Director of Research, Palo Alto Medical Research Foundation
Director of Laboratories, Palo Alto Medical Clinic

MILTON J. CHATTON, MD

Clinical Professor of Medicine
Stanford University School of Medicine (Stanford)
Senior Attending Physician
Santa Clara Valley Medical Center (San Jose)
Research Associate, Palo Alto Medical
Research Foundation (Palo Alto)

And Associate Authors

Lange Medical Publications

LOS ALTOS, CALIFORNIA

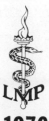

LMP

1976

A Concise Medical Library for Practitioner and Student

Current Medical Diagnosis & Treatment 1976 $14.00

Current Pediatric Diagnosis & Treatment, 4th ed. Edited by C.H. Kempe, H.K. Silver, and D. O'Brien. About 1030 pp, *illus.*	1976
Current Surgical Diagnosis & Treatment, 2nd ed. Edited by J.E. Dunphy and L.W. Way. 1123 pp, *illus.*	1975
Review of Physiological Chemistry, 15th ed. H.A. Harper. 570 pp, *illus.*	1975
Review of Medical Physiology, 7th ed. W.F. Ganong. 587 pp, *illus.*	1975
Review of Medical Microbiology, 11th ed. E. Jawetz, J.L. Melnick, and E.A. Adelberg. 528 pp, *illus.*	1974
Review of Medical Pharmacology, 4th ed. F.H. Meyers, E. Jawetz, and A. Goldfien. 721 pp, *illus.*	1974
Basic Histology. L.C. Junqueira, J. Carneiro, and A.N. Contopoulos. 453 pp, *illus.*	1975
General Urology, 8th ed. D.R. Smith. 492 pp, *illus.*	1975
General Ophthalmology, 7th ed. D. Vaughan and T. Asbury. 334 pp, *illus.*	1974
Correlative Neuroanatomy & Functional Neurology, 15th ed. J.G. Chusid. 429 pp, *illus.*	1973
Principles of Clinical Electrocardiography, 8th ed. M.J. Goldman. 400 pp, *illus.*	1973
Handbook of Psychiatry, 3rd ed. Edited by P. Solomon and V.D. Patch. 706 pp.	1974
Handbook of Surgery, 5th ed. Edited by J.L. Wilson. 877 pp, *illus.*	1973
Handbook of Obstetrics & Gynecology, 5th ed. R.C. Benson. 770 pp, *illus.*	1974
Physician's Handbook, 18th ed. M.A. Krupp, N.J. Sweet, E. Jawetz, E.G. Biglieri, and R.L. Roe. About 750 pp, *illus.*	1976
Handbook of Medical Treatment, 14th ed. Edited by M.J. Chatton. 640 pp.	1974
Handbook of Pediatrics, 11th ed. H.K. Silver, C.H. Kempe, and H.B. Bruyn. 710 pp, *illus.*	1975
Handbook of Poisoning: Diagnosis & Treatment, 8th ed. R.H. Dreisbach. 517 pp.	1974

Table of Contents

Preface vii

Authors ix

1. General Symptoms 1
   Milton J. Chatton

2. Fluid & Electrolyte Disorders 15
   Marcus A. Krupp

3. Skin & Appendages 32
   Rees B. Rees, Jr.

4. Eye 75
   Daniel Vaughan

5. Ear, Nose, & Throat 88
   Wayne W. Deatsch

6. Respiratory Tract & Mediastinum 106
   R. Morton Manson

7. Heart & Great Vessels 152
   Maurice Sokolow

8. Blood Vessels & Lymphatics 243
   John M. Erskine

9. Blood 273
   Ralph O. Wallerstein

10. Gastrointestinal Tract & Liver 321
    John V. Carbone, Lloyd L. Brandborg, & Sol Silverman, Jr.

11. Diseases of the Breast 399
    John L. Wilson

12. Gynecology & Obstetrics 415
    Ralph C. Benson

13. Arthritis & Allied Rheumatic Disorders 477
    Ephraim P. Engleman

14. Bone & Joint Diseases 502
    Floyd H. Jergesen

15. Genitourinary Tract 521
                        Marcus A. Krupp

16. Nervous System 553
                        Joseph G. Chusid

17. Psychiatric Disorders 594
                        James J. Brophy

18. Endocrine Disorders 645
                        Felix O. Kolb

19. Diabetes Mellitus, Hypoglycemia, & Lipid Disorders 727
                        John H. Karam

20. Nutrition; Nutritional & Metabolic Disorders 754
                 Milton J. Chatton & Phyllis M. Ullman

21. Introduction to Infectious Diseases 783
                 Ernest Jawetz & Moses Grossman

22. Infectious Diseases: Viral & Rickettsial 791
                 Moses Grossman & Ernest Jawetz

23. Infectious Diseases: Bacterial 814
                 Moses Grossman & Ernest Jawetz

24. Infectious Diseases: Spirochetal 841
                        Harold E. Varmus

25. Infectious Diseases: Protozoal 850
                      Robert S. Goldsmith

26. Infectious Diseases: Metazoal 863
                      Robert S. Goldsmith

27. Infectious Diseases: Mycotic 883
                        Carlyn Halde

28. Anti-infective Chemotherapeutic & Antibiotic Agents 891
                        Ernest Jawetz

29. Disorders Due to Physical Agents 914
                      Milton J. Chatton

30. Poisons 928
                      Robert H. Dreisbach

31. Medical Genetics 957
                      Margaret S. Kosek

32. Malignant Disorders 973
                      Sydney E. Salmon

33. Immunologic Disorders 987
             Samuel Strober & Hugh O. McDevitt

Appendix 999

Index 1029

Preface

This book is intended to serve the practicing physician as a useful desk reference on widely accepted technics currently available for medical diagnosis and treatment. It is not intended to be used as a textbook of medicine. Specific current references to the clinical literature and general bibliographies are included as a guide to further study.

The wide acceptance of the thirteen annual revisions of this book since its first appearance in 1962 has been most gratifying. The evaluation of new medical concepts and advances in diagnosis and treatment has been a constant challenge. Particularly difficult are the editorial decisions to delete familiar or traditional methods in favor of the new. Medical progress and space limitations are the deciding factors.

Enthusiasm for new methods has had to be weighed carefully against pragmatic considerations such as availability, feasibility, and safety. Priority of emphasis has been given to conservative diagnostic and treatment methods which have survived critical analysis. It is beyond the scope of this volume to fully discuss some of the interesting current controversial aspects of diagnosis and treatment.

Although we have dealt primarily with internal medical disorders, discussions of additional disorders commonly encountered in certain other specialties are also included. Special chapters on medical genetics, cancer chemotherapy, and immunologic disorders are intended to serve as medically oriented introductory discussions of these fields with important clinical implications for the future of patient care.

The widespread dissemination of this book overseas both in translation and in its English language editions has been a continuing source of satisfaction to all of us who have worked on it over the years. A Spanish edition is available from El Manual Moderno (Mexico City), an Italian edition from Piccin Editore (Padua), a Serbo-Croation edition from Savremena Administracija (Belgrade), a Portuguese edition from Atheneu Editora (São Paulo), a German edition from Springer-Verlag (Heidelberg), and a Japanese edition from the Maruzen Company (Tokyo). An English edition for distribution in Asia is now printed in Tokyo by Maruzen. With the appearance of the 1976 edition we are pleased to be able to announce that a Middle East edition (in English) will hereafter be available under the imprint of Librairie du Liban.

The editors wish to express their sincere thanks to their associate authors for participating so effectively in this venture, and to the many students and physicians who have contributed suggestions and criticisms for this and previous editions.

Marcus A. Krupp
Milton J. Chatton

January, 1976

The Authors

Ralph C. Benson, MD
Professor of Obstetrics & Gynecology and Chairman, Department of Obstetrics & Gynecology, University of Oregon Health Sciences Center (Portland).

Lloyd L. Brandborg, MD
Chief, Gastroenterology, Veterans Administration Hospital (San Francisco); Clinical Professor of Medicine, University of California School of Medicine (San Francisco).

James J. Brophy, MD
Associate Clinical Professor of Psychiatry, University of California School of Medicine (San Diego); Staff Psychiatrist, San Diego County Mental Health Services.

John V. Carbone, MD
Professor of Medicine, University of California School of Medicine (San Francisco).

Milton J. Chatton, MD
Clinical Professor of Medicine, Stanford University School of Medicine (Stanford); Senior Attending Physician, Santa Clara Valley Medical Center (San Jose); Research Associate, Palo Alto Medical Research Foundation (Palo Alto).

Joseph G. Chusid, MD
Associate Clinical Professor of Neurology, College of Physicians & Surgeons, Columbia University (New York City); Director of Department of Neurology, St. Vincent's Hospital and Medical Center (New York City); Associate Attending Neurologist, Columbia-Presbyterian Medical Center (New York City).

Wayne W. Deatsch, MD
Associate Clinical Professor of Otorhinolaryngology, University of California School of Medicine (San Francisco).

Robert H. Dreisbach, MD
Clinical Professor, Department of Environmental Health, University of Washington (Seattle).

Ephraim P. Engleman, MD, FACP
Clinical Professor of Medicine; Head, Rheumatic Disease Group, Department of Medicine, University of California School of Medicine (San Francisco).

John M. Erskine, MD
Associate Clinical Professor of Surgery, University of California School of Medicine (San Francisco); Associate in Surgery, Stanford University School of Medicine (Stanford).

Robert S. Goldsmith, MD, DTM&H
Associate Professor of Tropical Medicine & Epidemiology, University of California School of Medicine (San Francisco).

Moses Grossman, MD
Professor of Pediatrics, University of California School of Medicine (San Francisco); Chief of Pediatrics and Isolation Services, San Francisco General Hospital.

Carlyn Halde, PhD
Associate Professor, Department of Microbiology, University of California School of Medicine (San Francisco).

Ernest Jawetz, PhD, MD
Professor of Microbiology & Chairman, Department of Microbiology; Professor of Medicine, Lecturer in Pediatrics, University of California School of Medicine (San Francisco).

Floyd H. Jergesen, MD
Clinical Professor of Orthopedic Surgery, University of California School of Medicine (San Francisco).

John H. Karam, MD
Associate Professor of Medicine, Chief, Diabetes Clinic, and Associate Director, Metabolic Research Unit, University of California School of Medicine (San Francisco).

Felix O. Kolb, MD

Clinical Professor of Medicine, Research Physician and Associate Director, Metabolic Research Unit, University of California School of Medicine (San Francisco); Chairman, Division of Endocrinology and Metabolism, Mount Zion Hospital (San Francisco).

Margaret S. Kosek, MD

Research Associate, Palo Alto Medical Research Foundation.

Marcus A. Krupp, MD

Clinical Professor of Medicine, Stanford University School of Medicine (Stanford); Director of Research, Palo Alto Medical Research Foundation; Director of Laboratories, Palo Alto Medical Clinic.

R. Morton Manson, MD

Director, Clinical Services, Santa Clara Valley Medical Center (San Jose); Clinical Associate Professor of Medicine, Stanford University School of Medicine (Stanford).

Hugh O. McDevitt, MD

Professor of Medicine, Stanford University School of Medicine (Stanford).

Rees B. Rees, Jr., MD

Clinical Professor of Dermatology, University of California School of Medicine (San Francisco).

Sydney E. Salmon, MD

Professor of Medicine and Head, Division of Hematology and Oncology, University of Arizona College of Medicine (Tucson).

Sol Silverman, Jr., DDS

Professor of Oral Biology (Chairman of the Division), University of California School of Dentistry (San Francisco).

Maurice Sokolow, MD

Professor of Medicine, University of California School of Medicine (San Francisco).

Samuel Strober, MD

Assistant Professor of Medicine, Stanford University School of Medicine (Stanford).

Stephen Telatnik, MD

Assistant Clinical Professor, Stanford University School of Medicine (Stanford); Medical Director of Respiratory Therapy, O'Connor Hospital (San Jose).

Phyllis M. Ullman, MA

Registered Dietitian, Stanford Heart Disease Prevention Program, Stanford University Department of Medicine (Stanford).

Harold E. Varmus, MD

Associate Professor of Microbiology, University of California School of Medicine (San Francisco).

Daniel Vaughan, MD

Clinical Professor of Ophthalmology, University of California School of Medicine (San Francisco).

Ralph O. Wallerstein, MD

Clinical Professor of Medicine, University of California School of Medicine (San Francisco).

John L. Wilson, MD

Professor of Surgery, Stanford University School of Medicine (Stanford).

1...
General Symptoms

Milton J. Chatton

FEVER

Fever was well known to the ancients as an important manifestation of illness, but it remained for the development of modern medical science to provide a better understanding of the significance of body temperature variations in health and in disease. As the large number of specific causes of fever were being identified over the past century, interest also turned toward the pathophysiology of fever. Although many questions about fever remain unanswered, it is now known that the thermoregulatory center is in the hypothalamus, which, in disease, is acted upon by fever-producing (pyrogenic) substances of either exogenous (eg, microbial) or endogenous (host tissue) origin. In turn, blood warmed by the fever triggers the hypothalamus to dissipate heat by peripheral (cutaneous) dilatation and sweating and by control of the shivering mechanism.

The body temperature is normally subject to individual variation as well as to fluctuation due to physiologic factors. Exercise, digestion, sudden increase in environmental temperature, and excitement (eg, medical examination) may cause a mild transient increase in temperature. There is a slight sustained temperature rise following ovulation during the menstrual cycle and in the first trimester of pregnancy. The normal diurnal variation may be as much as 2° F, being lowest in the early morning and highest in the late afternoon.

Careful readings with a reliable thermometer will prevent errors in clinical interpretation. Oral temperatures may be unreliable in "mouth-breathers" or in patients who are uncooperative, debilitated, or in shock. Rectal or vaginal temperatures are taken in these circumstances. Tympanic thermometers, when available, are even more reliable for measuring body temperature than rectal determinations.

The average normal oral body temperature is 37° C (range 35.9–37.2° C), or 98.6° F (range 96.8–99.3° F). The normal rectal or vaginal temperature is 0.5° C (1° F) higher than the oral temperature, and the normal axillary temperature is correspondingly lower.

It is not known if fever plays any beneficial role in the body defense mechanism. In the preantibiotic era, fever was employed with limited success as nonspecific therapy for chronic infections. Markedly elevated or prolonged fevers may result in profound metabolic disturbances. Fever per se may also alter the metabolism and disposition of drugs used for the treatment of the diverse diseases associated with fever. Prolonged elevation of rectal temperature over 41° C (106° F) may result in permanent brain damage; when the rectal temperature is over 43° C (109° F), heat stroke occurs and death is common.

The characteristics of the temperature pattern (graphic record), especially when viewed in the light of other clinical findings, may be of diagnostic and prognostic value and may serve as a guide to the effectiveness of therapy.

Diagnostic Considerations

The outline below illustrates the wide variety of clinical disorders which may cause fever. Most febrile illnesses are short-lived or relatively easy to diagnose. In certain instances, however, the origin of the fever may remain obscure ("fever of undetermined origin," FUO) after the usual careful preliminary examination.

Prolonged undiagnosed fever may be arbitrarily defined as illness of unknown cause with temperatures exceeding 35.5° C (101.3° F) on several occasions for more than 3 weeks. In the USA, prolonged fevers of undetermined origin are most frequently due to infectious diseases. Increased travel, including the movement of large numbers of people, has resulted in the appearance or spread of infectious diseases which are relatively unknown to physicians not familiar with the epidemiology of diseases of remote areas. This may present problems in differential diagnosis, especially since the mode of transmission of some of these diseases is uncertain and since they frequently have highly variable incubation or latent periods. This is the case with malaria, a disease which until recently was almost extinct in the USA but increased in incidence about 20-fold between 1965 and 1970. The necessity for obtaining a travel history from all patients with FUO should be apparent.

In about 40% of cases, the cause of FUO is infectious disease. About 20% of cases of FUO are due to neoplastic disease; about 15% are due to connective tissue disease; and the remainder are due to miscellaneous causes. In 5–10% of cases the diagnosis is never established and the patients apparently recover spontaneously.

Meticulous history taking, extensive laboratory and x-ray studies, and even exploratory surgical procedures may be required (see Chapter 21).

Use of the so-called therapeutic test for the diagnosis of a fever is justified only when a specific disease is strongly suspected (eg, chloroquine for malaria). Hasty, empirical use of polypharmaceutical measures (eg, multiple antimicrobials, corticosteroids, antipyretics, analgesics) may seriously interfere with rational diagnosis and therapy and may actually be hazardous. Although mild fevers may be of psychogenic origin, this diagnosis should be made with extreme caution and should be based upon positive psychiatric criteria after careful exclusion of the possibility of organic disease.

Clinical Classification of Causes of Fever (With Examples)

(1) **Infections:** Viral, rickettsial, bacterial, fungal, and parasitic infections are the commonest causes of fever. (a) Generalized infections without localizing signs (eg, septicemia). (b) Generalized infections with localizing signs (eg, pharyngitis, scarlet fever). (c) Localized infections (eg, pyelonephritis).

(2) **Diseases of undetermined etiology:** (a) Collagen diseases (eg, systemic lupus erythematosus, polyarteritis nodosa, dermatomyositis, rheumatoid arthritis, rheumatic fever). (b) Other miscellaneous disease (eg, sarcoidosis, amyloidosis).

(3) **Central nervous system disease:** Cerebrovascular accidents, head injuries, brain and spinal cord tumors, degenerative CNS disease (eg, multiple sclerosis), spinal cord injuries.

(4) **Malignant neoplastic disease:** Primary neoplasms (eg, of thyroid, lung, liver, pancreas, and genitourinary tract). Secondary neoplasms, carcinoid.

(5) **Hematologic disease:** Lymphomas, leukemias, multiple myeloma, pernicious anemia, hemolytic anemias, hemorrhagic disease (eg, hemophilia).

(6) **Cardiovascular disease:** Myocardial infarction, thromboembolic diseases, bacterial endocarditis, congestive heart failure, paroxysmal tachycardias.

(7) **Gastrointestinal disease:** Inflammatory bowel disease, necrotic phase of hepatic cirrhosis.

(8) **Endocrine disease:** Hyperthyroidism, pheochromocytoma.

(9) **Diseases due to physical agents:** Heat stroke, radiation sickness, trauma (eg, surgery), crushing injuries.

(10) **Diseases due to chemical agents:** Drug reactions, anesthesia, anaphylactic reactions, serum sickness, chemical poisoning, pyrogen reactions (following intravenous fluids).

(11) **Disorders of fluid balance:** Dehydration, acidosis.

(12) **Psychogenic fever.**

(13) **Factitious or "false" fever.**

(14) **Unknown causes.**

Treatment

A. Removal of the Specific Cause of the Fever: The principal problem is to determine and eradicate the cause of the fever. Symptomatic measures directed solely toward depression of elevated body temperature are usually not indicated except for high, prolonged fevers.

Prevention of the serious "malignant hyperpyrexia" which may follow certain types of general anesthesia can best be accomplished by recognizing the hereditarily predisposed patient (history or evidence of myopathy; past personal or family history of difficult anesthesia) and by proper choice of anesthetic agent, with temperature monitoring during anesthesia.

B. Reduction of the Fever by Nonspecific Means: When the body temperature is greater than 40° C (104° F), particularly if prolonged, symptomatic treatment of fever may be necessary.

Oral or parenteral fluids must be administered in amounts sufficient to compensate for the extra fluid losses from perspiration and all other causes. Alcohol sponges, cold sponges, tepid baths, and ice bags may reduce fever and provide physical comfort.

Antipyretic drugs are quite effective in reducing fever and have a simultaneous analgesic effect. They may, however, obscure the clinical picture, and may cause undesirable side-effects such as sweating, nausea and vomiting, and, rarely, skin eruptions and hematologic changes. Such drugs, therefore, are to be employed cautiously in fevers due to infectious diseases and are preferably not used in the enteric fevers (eg, typhoid fever). Aspirin, 0.3—0.6 gm every 4 hours as needed, is most commonly used. Other antipyretic analgesic drugs are listed on p 9.

For reduction of very high fever (over 41.1° C [106° F]), see Heat Stroke (p 916).

Atkins E, Bodel P: Fever. New England J Med 286:27, 1972.

Beisel WR: Metabolic response to infection. Ann Rev Med 26:9, 1975.

Britt BA: Malignant hyperthermia: A pharmacogenetic disease of skeletal and cardiac muscle. New England J Med 290:1140, 1974.

Elin RJ, Vesell ES, Wolff SM: Effects of etiocholanolone-induced fever on plasma antipyrine half-lives and metabolic clearance. Clin Pharmacol Therap 17:447, 1975.

Herzberg JH, Wolff SM: Chronic factitious fever in puberty and adolescence. Psychosom Med 3:205, 1972.

Howard PH Jr, Hardin WJ: The role of surgery in fever of unknown origin. S Clin North America 52:397, 1972.

Jacoby GA, Swartz MN: Fever of undetermined origin. New England J Med 289:1407, 1973.

Wolff SM, Fauci AS, Dale DC: Unusual etiologies of fever and their evaluation. Ann Rev Med 26:277, 1975.

SHOCK SYNDROME
(Circulatory Shock)

"Shock" is a complex and incompletely understood syndrome which defies precise definition because of its heterologous origins. It is practical, however, to consider shock as a disturbance of circulation resulting in ineffective perfusion or critical reduction of perfusion of vital tissues and a wide range of systemic effects. The term is descriptive of a "classical" but highly variable pattern of signs and symptoms which usually includes systemic arterial hypotension, ashen pallor, cold and moist skin, collapse of superficial veins of the extremities, rapid and weak pulse, air hunger, thirst, oliguria, and a tendency to steadily progress toward a refractory and so-called "irreversible" phase. Recognition of early shock may be obscured by factors such as anxiety, complicating medical problems, and surrounding circumstances. The "classical" signs of shock may appear suddenly and often represent fully developed shock.

In so-called "warm shock," such as is seen in some patients with endotoxin septic shock, the skin is dry, pink, and warm and the urine volume is adequate despite the arterial hypotension and peripheral pooling.

Numerous pathophysiologic mechanisms are involved in the production of shock, such as lack of effective blood volume, reduction of cardiac output, altered peripheral vascular tone, increased capillary permeability, decreased urine output, acidosis, elevated blood lactate, and other alterations of the physicochemical characteristics of the blood. The 3 major pathophysiologic mechanisms, perhaps, are cardiac insufficiency (pump failure), altered peripheral resistance (vasoconstriction or vasodilatation), and hypovolemia. Alteration of one or more of these factors may result in altered microcirculatory flow. It is the adaptation or failure of adaptation of the microcirculation that is responsible for the arteriovenous shunting, fluid loss from the capillaries, sludging of red blood cells, and stagnant tissue hypoxia with cellular dysfunction and possible cell death which result in the shock syndrome. Little is known regarding the actual mechanisms of the metabolic vicious cycle leading to "irreversible" shock.

Debility, malnutrition, senility, temperature extremes, alcoholism, hypotensive drugs, anesthetics, autonomic disorders, diabetes, and adrenocorticoid disorders are factors which can predispose to shock.

Factors which unfavorably influence the prognosis in shock states include coma, acidosis (pH $<$ 7.30), $Pa_{CO_2} > 45$ mm Hg, serum lactate $>$ 2mM/liter, severe sepsis, anuria, heart disease, hepatic disease, and advanced age ($>$ 70 years).

Classification

No classification of shock is completely satisfactory, but one which is based upon the predominant hemodynamic changes in the various types of shock is clinically the most useful (Table 1–1). It should be apparent that in a given patient with shock several hemodynamic mechanisms are at work simultaneously so that continuous monitoring of multiple parameters of cardiovascular function is required. For example, hypovolemia and altered peripheral resistance may be significant factors in cardiogenic shock, and pump

Table 1–1. Classification of shock.

I. **Hypovolemic shock (decreased effective blood volume)**
  A. Exogenous (external) loss of fluid
    1. Whole blood (eg, hemorrhage)
    2. Plasma (eg, burns)
    3. Fluid and electrolytes (eg, vomiting, diarrhea)
  B. Endogenous (internal) loss of fluid
    1. Exudative (eg, peritonitis)
    2. Traumatic (eg, hematoma)
II. **Cardiogenic shock (pump failure)**
  A. Intrinsic myocardial disorders (eg, decreased myocardial contractility)
    1. Focal damage (eg, myocardial infarction)
    2. Generalized disorder (eg, dysrhythmia, myocarditis)
  B. Extrinsic disorders
    1. Cardiac tamponade (eg, pericardial disease)
    2. Obstruction of major blood channels (eg, pulmonary embolism)
III. **Vascular (vasomotor, distributive, low-resistance) shock (altered vascular resistance and capacity)**
  A. Increased venous capacitance (pooling) (eg, bacterial endotoxin)
  B. Decreased arteriolar resistance (eg, fright, pain, vasodilative drugs)

failure may be an important feature of hypovolemic shock. Therapeutically, this implies a real hazard in focussing on only a single deranged mechanism in treating a so-called specific type of shock.

A. Hypovolemic Shock (Oligemic, Hemorrhagic, Traumatic, Burn, or Surgical Shock): In this form of shock there is a true diminution of blood volume due to loss of whole blood or plasma from the circulation. Compensatory vasoconstriction temporarily reduces the size of the vascular bed and may temporarily maintain the blood pressure, but if fluid is not replaced immediately hypotension occurs, peripheral resistance increases, capillary and venous beds collapse, and the tissues become progressively more hypoxic. Since the vascular space is the smallest of the body fluid compartments, even a moderate sudden loss of circulating fluids can result in severe and sometimes irreversible damage to vital centers. Rapid loss of 50% of blood volume is usually fatal.

Hypovolemic shock may result from (1) loss of whole blood by hemorrhage due to external or internal injuries, (2) loss of whole blood through nontraumatic internal hemorrhage (eg, bleeding peptic ulcer, ruptured varices), (3) loss of blood and plasma in extensive fractures and crushing injuries, (4) loss of plasma and hemolysis of red cells in extensive burns, (5) loss of plasma into serous body cavities (eg, peritonitis), (6) loss of plasma due to nephrotic syndrome, or (7) loss of fluid and electrolytes (eg, vomiting, diarrhea, endocrine disturbances).

B. Cardiogenic Shock: Shock due to inability of the left ventricle to perform effectively as a pump in maintaining an adequate cardiac output occurs most frequently following myocardial infarction, but it also occurs in serious cardiac arrhythmias, pulmonary embolism, cardiac tamponade, terminal congestive failure, or as a complication of other forms of severe shock. Shock associated with myocardial infarction or other serious cardiac disease carries a very high mortality rate (75–80%) despite therapy.

Clinical findings are of limited value in predicting the course or prognosis of cardiogenic shock. Major myocardial infarction as determined by ECG, enzyme studies, and sophisticated indices of cardiovascular function may provide reasonably reliable evidence of impending shock.

C. Vascular Shock (Vasomotor, Distributive, Low-Resistance Shock): In this type of shock the available circulating volume of blood may be unaltered, but the blood volume is inadequate because the capacity of the vascular system is expanded. The increased vascular capacity may result from widespread dilatation of arteries and arterioles, arteriovenous shunting, or from venous pooling. The venous pressure is often normal.

The most common form of vascular or low-resistance shock is that due to gram-negative bacillemia, so-called septic shock. The toxemia of overwhelming infection is characterized by an initial short period of vasoconstriction followed by vasodilatation, with venous pooling of blood in the microcirculation. There is often a direct toxic action on the heart and adrenals. The mortality rate is high (40–80%). Septic shock is most commonly caused by infection due to gram-negative organisms (*Escherichia coli,* klebsiella, proteus, pseudomonas, meningococci). Gram-negative anaerobes (eg, bacteroides) are increasingly recognized as a cause of septic shock. Septic shock occurs more often in the very young and the very old, in diabetes, hematologic malignancies, diseases of the genitourinary, hepatobiliary, and intestinal tracts, in meningitis or pneumonia, and with corticosteroid, immunosuppressive, or radiation therapy. Immediate precipitating factors may be urinary, biliary, or gynecologic manipulations. Septic shock may be obscured by ineffective antibiotic therapy.

Septic shock should always be suspected when a febrile patient has chills associated with hypotension. Early, the skin may be warm and the pulse full. Hyperventilation may occur and result in respiratory alkalosis. The sensorium and urinary output are often initially normal. The classical signs of shock are manifest later. The symptoms and signs of the inciting infection are not invariably present. (See Chapter 23.)

Neurogenic or psychogenic factors, eg, spinal cord injury, pain, trauma, fright, or vasodilator drugs may also cause vascular shock. Sudden autonomic overactivity results in vasodilatation or inhibition of constriction of the arterioles and rapid peripheral and splanchnic pooling of blood. Following a period of anxiety and signs of epinephrine release (tachycardia, tremors, and pallor), there is a sudden reflex vagal stimulation with decreased cardiac output, hypotension, and decreased cerebral blood flow. In the absence of spinal cord injury or other complicating factors, the patient usually revives promptly in the recumbent position or following the administration of simple forms of treatment (eg, spirits of ammonia, physical stimuli), but observation is necessary to prevent recurrence and possible progression.

Vascular shock may also be due to anaphylaxis, histamine response, ganglionic blockade, and hypnotic drug intoxication.

Treatment

It is of vital importance to determine the specific cause or causes, contributing factors (eg, age, prior physical status, complications), severity, and duration of shock. Prompt, calculated, and decisive action is essential. Prevention or early recognition of shock is simpler and considerably more effective than the treatment of established shock. Observe and record vital signs (pulse, temperature, respiration, and blood pressure), color and texture of skin, and level of consciousness.

A. General Measures:

1. Position—Place the patient with the head and torso in the horizontal or slightly elevated position with moderate (30 degree) elevation of the legs. Avoid the so-called shock position. Simple elevation of the legs is considered to be more desirable since it is less apt to interfere with cerebral blood flow, although this too should be avoided if dyspnea is present.

2. Oxygen—Clear the airway of obstructions and secretions and, if necessary, insert an oropharyngeal or endotracheal airway. Ensure adequate ventilation by mouth-to-mouth breathing if necessary. Start oxygen by mask or nasal catheter as soon as possible. Frequent monitoring of blood gases is of the greatest importance. If arterial P_{O_2} (Pa_{O_2}) is below 60 mm Hg or if dyspnea or cyanosis is present, increased oxygen is usually required. If Pa_{O_2} fails to show a prompt rise, suspect the possibility of pulmonary shunting or so-called "shock lung" (see p 134). Mechanical respirators may be required to maintain adequate oxygen exchange.

3. Temperature—Keep the patient comfortably warm. Avoid chilling (to prevent heat loss) and excessive externally applied heat, which will further dilate the peripheral vessels.

4. Analgesics—Control severe pain promptly by the use of appropriate first aid measures and analgesic drugs. Give morphine sulfate, 8–15 mg subcut, for pain. Since subcutaneous absorption is poor in patients in shock, morphine sulfate, 10–15 mg slowly IV, may be used for severe pain. *Caution:* Do not give morphine to unconscious patients, to patients who have head injuries, or to those with respiratory depression.

5. Laboratory studies—Determine blood hemoglobin, hematocrit, and red cell count immediately for baseline and follow-up values. Obtain blood for typing and cross-matching. Laboratory studies for rapid serial determination of serum electrolytes, pH, Pa_{O_2}, and Pa_{CO_2} may be invaluable. Blood volume studies are useful in special circumstances but are not of general

practical value.

6. **Urine flow**—Urine output is a reliable indication of vital organ perfusion. Insert an indwelling catheter to monitor urine flow (which should be kept above 50 ml/hour). Urine flow less than 25 ml/hour indicates inadequate renal circulation which, if not corrected, can cause renal tubular necrosis.

7. **Central venous pressure (CVP)**—Monitor central venous pressure continuously in all shock patients. CVP determination is a simple and relatively reliable measure of adequacy of vascular volume and of the pumping action of the heart. It is not as reliable as determination of the pulmonary artery wedge pressure (by the Swan-Ganz catheter technic), which better reflects left ventricular function. In simple CVP determination, a catheter is inserted percutaneously (or by cutdown) through the antecubital or external jugular vein near or into the right atrium and is connected to a manometer. Normal values range from 5–8 cm of water. A low CVP is suggestive of low blood volume and need for fluid replacement, whereas a high CVP (above 15–17 cm) suggests either insufficient cardiac output or fluid overload. The CVP may be normal in left ventricular failure due to myocardial infarction and neurogenic shock. CVP changes in response to appropriate, cautious administration of intravenous fluids may increase the value of CVP as an indicator of blood volume and cardiac efficiency.

8. **Parenteral fluid therapy**—*Replace and maintain adequate blood volume.* Initial or emergency needs may be determined by the history, general appearance, vital signs and other physical findings, hemoglobin, and hematocrit, although these are not reliable guides for volume replacement. Under ordinary clinical conditions, determination of effective blood volume may be difficult and is subject to considerable variation. There is no simple technic or rule by which to accurately judge the fluid requirements. Continuous CVP monitoring (normal: 5–8 cm of water) may be useful for the evaluation of shock and as a guide to safe fluid replacement. Response to therapy—particularly the effect of carefully administered, gradually increasing amounts of intravenous fluids on the CVP—is a valuable index. Selection of the replacement fluid which is most appropriate for the individual case is based upon consideration of what type of fluid has been lost (whole blood, plasma, water and electrolytes), the availability of the various solutions, laboratory facilities, and, to a lesser extent, expense. Whole blood is usually the most effective replacement fluid in case of gross hemorrhage if the hematocrit is < 35%, but other readily available parenteral fluids should be given immediately pending preliminary laboratory work and the procurement of whole blood. Frozen, thawed, and washed red cells in salt solution have been used with favorable results in patients with hemorrhagic shock. If the CVP is low and the hematocrit is > 35% and there is no clinical evidence to suggest otherwise, replace blood volume with saline, dextrose, serum albumin, plasma, or plasma expanders.

(1) **Saline or dextrose solutions**—Give immediately 500–2000 ml of sodium chloride injection (physiologic saline), Ringer's injection, Ringer's bicarbonate (Ringer's injection with sodium bicarbonate added), or 5% dextrose in saline rapidly intravenously, under CVP monitoring, while making preparations for plasma expanders, plasma, serum albumin, or whole blood. The latter exert a more sustained increase in blood volume through their colloidal osmotic pressure effects than do dextrose and electrolyte solutions, although the electrolyte solutions are remarkably effective when given in adequate doses. There is little evidence that judicious saline resuscitation induces pulmonary edema in patients with prior normal cardiac and renal function. When large volumes of crystalloids are given, however, patients should be examined frequently for evidence of pulmonary edema.

(2) **Whole blood (See above.)**—Whole blood, used appropriately, may be of value in the treatment of severe or refractory shock even in the face of an apparently good hematocrit figure; this is because of the misleading effect of hemoconcentration. For **advanced shock**, especially with the suspicion of associated occult blood loss, administer 500 ml whole blood immediately and repeat with 500 ml every half hour up to a total of 2 liters or more, depending upon the presence of continued hemorrhage, clinical course, and hematocrit and CVP findings.

(3) **Plasma or serum albumin**—Various plasma preparations (such as lyophilized or reconstituted plasma) or serum albumin may be employed. Plasma is usually readily procurable for emergencies, may be rapidly set up for administration, and does not require preliminary blood typing. The quantity of plasma to be given depends upon the stage of shock and the response to therapy. The incidence of hepatitis following the use of plasma, especially of pooled commercial plasma, is a significant deterrent to its routine use in shock.

(4) **Dextrans**—Dextrans are fairly effective plasma "substitutes" for the emergency treatment of shock, but they cannot replace treatment with whole blood (or its derivatives) when the latter is necessary. The dextrans have high molecular weights, high oncotic pressures, and the necessary viscosity, but they have not proved to be as useful as plasma and their use, furthermore, is not without hazard. They have the advantages of ready availability, of compatibility with other preparations used in intravenous solutions, and of not causing infectious hepatitis.

Clinical dextran of high molecular weight (70,000) is an effective colloid because of its prolonged action, but it may interfere with blood coagulation. **Dextran 40**, a low molecular weight dextran, is available as a 10% solution in either isotonic saline or 5% dextrose in water for intravenous use. It decreases blood viscosity and possibly improves the microcirculation. Rapid initial infusion of approximately 100–150 ml within the first hour is followed by slow maintenance for a total of 10–15 ml/kg/24 hours (preferably less than 1 liter/day).

Use dextrans cautiously in patients with cardiac

disease, renal insufficiency, or marked dehydration to avoid pulmonary edema, congestive heart failure, or renal shutdown. Side-effects may be fatal. Observe for possible anaphylactoid reactions. Prolongations of bleeding time have been reported. Use with caution in patients with thrombocytopenia. Obtain blood for typing and cross-matching before dextran therapy since dextran may interfere with these tests.

9. **Vasoactive drugs**—Because of their remarkable ability to raise the blood pressure, several of the adrenergic drugs (sympathomimetic amines) have been used extensively, on a largely empiric basis, for the treatment of all types of shock. It is now known that simple blood pressure elevation produced by the vasopressor drugs has little beneficial effect on the underlying disturbances, and there is good evidence that in many instances that effect may be detrimental. Their routine use in all cases of shock is to be deplored.

Although the pharmacologic effects of the various adrenergic drugs cannot always be clearly explained and although their action in different disease states is not always predictable, certain of the known pharmacologic effects of available agents can be selectively utilized in the adjunctive therapy of shock (Table 1–2). The selection of the proper agent will obviously depend upon the carefully determined particular pathophysiologic derangement in any given patient. *The adrenergic drugs should not be considered to be a primary form of therapy in shock.* Immediate restoration of blood volume, correction of hypoxia, fluid and electrolyte disturbances, and search for treatable causes deserve first consideration. Continuous monitoring of vital signs, sensorium, central venous pressure (or pulmonary wedge pressure), and urinary output is essential to determine if, when, by how much, and for how long the adrenergic drugs are to be used.

The purely alpha-adrenergic stimulating drugs have little or no value in the treatment of shock. The mixed alpha- and beta-adrenergic agents are used most frequently, depending upon the need for adequate tissue perfusion pressure. Currently, dopamine is enjoying widespread use because of a uniquely favorable effect on renal and splanchnic blood flow, but its ultimate relative value in the treatment of shock remains to be determined. Epinephrine, of course, has a favored place among the adrenergic drugs because of its great value in the treatment of anaphylaxis, but its use is not recommended in other forms of shock. The beta-adrenergic stimulating agent isoproterenol has some value as a potent vasodilator and inotropic agent, but it is particularly apt to cause serious dysrhythmias. The alpha- and beta-adrenergic blocking agents have been largely limited to investigational use for the treatment of shock.

The principal vasoactive drugs used for shock are the following:

(1) Levarterenol bitartrate (norepinephrine) is a mixed alpha- and beta-mimetic agent, a powerful vasopressor, and a potent inotropic drug. Give 4–8 mg (4–8 ml of 0.2% solution) in 1 liter of dextrose in water IV. Avoid extravasation (may cause tissue necrosis and gangrene). With concentrations greater than 8 mg/liter, an inlying polyethylene catheter is required.

(2) Metaraminol bitartrate is both an alpha- and a beta-mimetic agent with cardiotonic as well as vasopressor effects. Give 2–10 mg IM, or 0.5–5 mg cautiously IV, or 15–100 mg by slow infusion in 250–500 ml of 5% dextrose solution IV.

(3) Isoproterenol, a beta-adrenergic stimulator, increases cardiac output by its action on the myocardial contraction mechanism and produces peripheral vasodilatation. Give 1–2 mg in 500 ml 5% dextrose in water IV. Because of its inotropic effect, an increased incidence of cardiac arrhythmias precludes its use if the cardiac rate is greater than 120/minute.

(4) Dopamine hydrochloride (Intropin) is a recently introduced endogenous catecholamine which has an added advantage over other adrenergic drugs

Table 1–2. Adrenergic drugs used in hypotensive states.
(Effects graded on a scale of 0–5.)

Drug	Vasomotor Effect		Cardiac Stimulant (Inotropic Effect)	Cardiac Output	Renal and Splanchnic Blood Flow
	Vaso-constriction	Vaso-dilatation			
Alpha-adrenergic					
Phenylephrine (Neo-Synephrine)	5	0	0	Reduced	Reduced
Mixed alpha- and beta-adrenergic					
Norepinephrine (Levophed)	4	0	2	Reduced	Reduced
Metaraminol (Aramine)	3	2	1	Reduced	Reduced
Epinephrine (Adrenalin)	4	3	4	Increased	Reduced
Dopamine (Intropin)*	2	2	2	Usually increased	Increased
Beta-adrenergic					
Isoproterenol (many trade names)	0	5	4	Increased	Usually reduced

*Claimed to have a special (dopaminergic) receptor.

because it has a beneficial effect on renal blood flow and also increases cardiac output and blood pressure. Dopamine hydrochloride, 200 mg in 500 ml sodium chloride injection USP (400 μg/ml), is given initially at a rate of 2.5 μg/kg/minute. These doses stimulate both the dopaminergic receptors, which increase the renal blood flow and urinary output; and the beta-adrenergic cardiac receptors, which increase the cardiac output. Higher levels stimulate alpha receptors to cause systemic vasoconstriction, and doses above 20 μg/kg/minute reverse the vasodilatation of the renal vessels achieved at lower levels. After an effective dosage level has been reached, the infusion rate should be adjusted periodically at the lowest point necessary to maintain adequate organ perfusion. Dopamine alone may fail to maintain adequate perfusion pressure or to relieve intense vasoconstriction, and it may sometimes be necessary to use it in combination with another appropriate adrenergic drug. Ventricular arrhythmias and anginal pain may develop during treatment.

10. Corticosteroids—The beneficial effects of large doses of corticosteroids in shock are not completely understood, and their efficacy in the many types of shock syndromes is controversial. They may be related to improved cardiac efficiency or to increased blood flow and volume to vital tissues. In the case of septic shock they may decrease sensitivity to endotoxin, but it is questionable whether adrenocorticosteroids should be used for that condition since they enhance susceptibility to infection and increase the likelihood that bacteremia will develop from a site infected with gram-negative rods (eg, urinary tract infections).

Those who express enthusiasm for corticosteroid therapy in the management of shock have suggested that corticosteroids should be administered as soon as shock is suspected—making it difficult to appraise the real value of the treatment. Dosage recommendations vary widely. Massive doses have been employed by some, (eg, methylprednisolone, 30 mg/kg IV). Treatment should be discontinued immediately if there is any evidence of gastrointestinal bleeding.

11. Diuretics—The cautious early administration of mannitol as a 10—25% solution in 500—1000 ml of normal saline or Ringer's injection has been recommended (in association with other treatment measures) in selected patients in whom oliguria is present or impending. Furosemide, 20 mg IV, has also been recommended for this purpose. Urine flow and CVP must be carefully monitored. The effectiveness of these agents in shock is still unknown.

B. Specific Measures:

1. Hemorrhage and anemia—Although crystalloids, plasma, or other volume expanders may be given as an emergency measure in shock complicating hemorrhage, severe anemia must be corrected by replacement with type-specific whole blood or packed red cells to prevent hypoxia. It is the hemorrhage, not simply the blood pressure, that requires treatment. The quantity of blood to be given will depend upon clinical response, hematocrit, and, when available, blood volume studies.

2. Hypoxia—The need for and type of oxygen therapy must be based upon clinical circumstances and arterial blood O_2 and CO_2 determinations. Oxygen is indicated for hypoxia.

3. Dehydration—Administer 500—200 ml of sodium chloride injection or 5% dextrose injection IV as needed. As soon as the patient can swallow, give fluids by mouth.

4. Acid-base balance—Abnormalities of electrolyte and acid-base balance should be corrected. If acidosis fails to respond to adequate fluid replacement as evidenced by an arterial blood pH of less than 7.35, give sodium bicarbonate, 40—100 mEq IV cautiously initially, and gauge further therapy by serial arterial pH determinations. Avoid alkalosis.

5. Adrenocortical failure—Although corticosteroid treatment is most specifically applicable to shock of Addison's crisis, it may also be of spectacular value in certain acute allergic emergencies. Corticosteroids are usually less effective but may be employed in treating cardiogenic shock, septic shock, and overwhelming intoxications.

6. Cardiac disorders—Digitalis is indicated only for those patients with preexisting or presenting evidence of cardiac failure, increased CVP, digitalis responsive arrhythmias, and, controversially, in myocardial infarction. Digitalis is of no value in shock due to other causes. Atropine may be of value in treating selected postmyocardial infarction bradycardias associated with hemodynamic abnormalities predisposing to cardiogenic shock. Parenteral fluid for volume expansion may be necessary if there is evidence of hypovolemia as suggested by a low CVP but should be given cautiously (especially sodium-containing solutions). Phlebotomy is sometimes useful in case of cardiac failure. The use of vasopressor drugs in myocardial infarction is controversial; if there is evidence of clinical shock (not merely mild hypotension), many physicians feel that mortality can be reduced by maintaining the blood pressure at levels of approximately 85 mm Hg (no more than 100 mm Hg). Continuous cardiac monitoring is highly desirable (especially when using beta-mimetic adrenergic drugs). The use of parenteral corticosteroids needs further evaluation.

Following myocardial infarction, mechanical circulatory assistance which reduces myocardial work and increases coronary perfusion—utilizing intra-aortic balloon counterpulsation on an emergency basis—may be temporarily helpful, though the effects on overall survival are not known. Emergency coronary bypass operations, infarctectomies, and repair of ventricular aneurysms, chordae, and septal defects following myocardial infarctions offer hope for some patients. It is difficult to assess the true value of these procedures at this time. (See Chapter 7.)

7. Infection—Immediate measures should be taken to combat infection, if present. Early recognition of incipient shock is critical since death often occurs in less than 48 hours. The mortality rate in gram-negative shock remains at about 50% despite advances in treatment. Initiate bacteriologic studies immediately

and before therapy, if possible. If there are any indications of shock, institute preliminary broad-spectrum antibiotic therapy until bacteriologic studies reveal the identity of the organism. "Prophylactic" antibiotics, when there is no evidence of infection, are of doubtful value and may even be harmful except when the hazard of infection is great (eg, extensive burns).

C. Evaluation of Therapy: Constant observation of the patient is imperative. The vital signs, CVP, urinary output, and laboratory studies must be monitored at appropriate intervals until the patient's condition has stabilized.

Campbell CD, Carey LC: Shock: Differential diagnosis and immediate treatment. Postgrad Med 55:85, 1974.

Cohen LS: Treatment of cardiogenic shock. California Med 118:74 (Jan), 69 (March), 1973.

Data JL, Nies AS: Dextran 40. Ann Int Med 81:500, 1974.

Goldberg LI: Dopamine: Uses of an endogenous catecholamine. New England J Med 291:707, 1974.

Gorbach SL, Bartlett JC: Anaerobic infections. (3 parts.) New England J Med 290:1177, 1237, 1289, 1974.

Guyton AC, Jones CE: Central venous pressure: Physiologic significance and clinical implications. Am Heart J 86:431, 1973.

Karliner JS: Dopamine for cardiogenic shock. JAMA 226:1217, 1973.

Melby JC: Systemic corticosteroid therapy: Pharmacology and endocrinologic considerations. Ann Int Med 81:505, 1974.

Moss GS: Traumatic shock in man. New England J Med 290:724, 1974.

Powers SR Jr: Shock and metabolism. Surg Gynec Obst 140:211, 1975.

Reichgott MJ, Melmon KL: Should corticosteroids be used in shock? M Clin North America 57:1211, 1973.

Scheidt S & others: Intra-aortic balloon counterpulsation in cardiogenic shock. New England J Med 288:979, 1973.

Schumer W, Erve PR, Miller B: Biochemical monitoring of the surgical patient. S Clin North America 55:11, 1975.

Shires GT, Carrico CJ, Canizaro PC: *Shock*. Saunders, 1973.

Stein L & others: Pulmonary edema during fluid infusion in the absence of heart failure. JAMA 229:65, 1974.

Tarazi RC: Sympathomimetic agents in the treatment of shock. Ann Int Med 81:364, 1974.

Weil MH, Shubin H: Treatment of shock caused by bacterial infections. California Med 119:7, Nov 1973.

Weil MH, Shubin H, Carlson R: Treatment of circulatory shock: Use of sympathomimetic and related vasoactive agents. JAMA 231:1280, 1975.

Willerson JT & others: Intraaortic balloon counterpulsation in patients in cardiogenic shock. Am J Med 58:183, 1975.

Winslow EJ & others: Hemodynamic studies and results of therapy in 50 patients with bacteremic shock. Am J Med 54:421, 1973.

Wolff SM, Bennett JV: Gram-negative rod bacteremia. New England J Med 291:733, 1974.

PAIN

Pain is a very important symptom, not only because it is often the primary complaint for which the patient seeks relief but also because it provides the clinician with critical diagnostic information. In taking a history from the patient with pain, there should be a careful elicitation of characteristics such as chronology, nature, location, radiation, and aggravating and alleviating factors which influence the pain.

The reaction to pain, a function of the higher centers, is extremely variable and influenced by many factors depending upon the individual patient and the situation. It is essential to determine, whenever possible, the primary cause (eg, infection, toxins) and the pathogenesis (eg, inflammation, ulceration, distention, anoxia, spasm) of pain.

The relief of pain is achieved by removal of the primary cause (eg, cure of infection), neutralization of the effect of the stimulus (eg, antacids for hyperacidity of peptic ulcer), and, when these are not feasible, by dulling or obliteration of the sense of pain (eg, palliative narcotics for terminal cancer).

The hazards of administering analgesics without first attempting to establish a diagnosis cannot be overemphasized (eg, acute abdominal pain). Analgesics, particularly narcotics, may mask the symptoms of serious acute or chronic illness.

Pain may be treated nonspecifically with drugs, physical measures (eg, heat, cold, immobilization), or surgery (eg, nerve resection, chordotomy). Acupuncture as a means of providing pain relief and even anesthesia, used in the Orient for centuries, is currently being evaluated extensively in the USA. Dramatic reports of pain relief by acupuncture, particularly of chronic pain, require further objective scrutiny.

Because psychic or emotional factors may greatly influence the pain threshold, it is important to consider the "placebo" role of all therapeutic measures for the control of pain. Pharmacologically inactive drugs may be surprisingly effective in alleviating the pain of organic as well as functional disorders—hence the hazard in the use of the placebo for differentiation of organic from functional (psychologic) pain. Reassurance and explanation are, therefore, important factors in relieving pain, with or without analgesic drugs.

Current concern about the widespread use of addictive and abused drugs—and the inconvenience resulting from official restrictions placed upon their medicinal use—may sometimes lead to reluctance to prescribe narcotic analgesics when they are needed for pain relief. It must not be assumed that the average patient is addiction prone. Although the various narcotics may have different addictive potentials, it is unreasonable to believe that addiction can be circumvented by substituting less effective but nonetheless addicting synthetic narcotic analgesics. Simply stated, it is a good rule to give the lowest effective dose of the appropriate agent for the given clinical circumstance to provide adequate symptomatic relief only as long as is necessary. Obviously, measures directed at correcting the cause of pain deserve first consideration. It may be necessary to give the narcotic on a one or 2 time or interim basis. When pain is severe and intractable, however, as in the case of terminal malignancy, it is inhumane to permit unnecessary suffering. It does not suffice that the clinician alone be aware of these general concepts or attitudes; they should be known to all individuals (eg, house officers, nurses, relatives) responsible for the administration of narcotic drugs.

Nonnarcotic Analgesics

A. Salicylates: The salicylate drugs are analgesic, antirheumatic, uricosuric, and antipyretic. They are useful in relieving myalgias, neuralgias, arthralgias, headaches, and dysmenorrhea. Untoward reactions are usually mild, consisting of dizziness and dyspepsia, but large doses may cause tinnitus, deafness, blurring of vision, nausea and vomiting, diarrhea, diaphoresis, headache, and delirium. In sensitive patients, salicylates may cause urticarias, asthma, and acute laryngeal edema.

1. Aspirin, plain, buffered, or enteric-coated, 0.3 gm tablets. Ordinary dosage is 0.3–0.6 gm with plenty of water every 4 hours as needed. Gastrointestinal irritation may sometimes be reduced by administration of the drug on a full stomach or with ½–1 tsp of baking soda or other antacid. Buffered aspirin usually available contains only small amounts of antacid, and the incidence of side-effects and the blood levels achieved are probably not appreciably different than with ordinary aspirin. The enteric-coated preparation is slower acting, but it prevents gastric irritation and is also useful for those patients who might be skeptical of the analgesic value of "ordinary aspirin." Some enteric-coated preparations, however, go through the gastrointestinal tract without being absorbed.

Aspirin can cause gastric irritation and increased microscopic blood loss from the gut in otherwise healthy individuals, and is an occasional but infrequent cause of massive gastrointestinal hemorrhage. In patients with acute or chronic gastrointestinal problems—especially gastrointestinal bleeding—or active hepatic disease, aspirin should not be used. Decision to withhold aspirin otherwise from patients who might benefit greatly from the drug must be arrived at on an individual basis.

Hypersensitivity or intolerance to aspirin, although uncommon in view of the widespread use of the drug, does occur, and in rare instances may be very serious. Aspirin intolerance may be due to allergy but is more frequently due to an unexplained primary connective tissue disorder of the susceptible patient. Intolerance to aspirin often develops spontaneously in young or middle-aged adults who were formerly able to take aspirin without difficulty. Intolerance may be manifested by rhinorrhea, nasal polyposis, asthma, prolonged bleeding time, and anaphylactic shock. The possibility that such symptoms may be caused by aspirin must always be considered, since further use of the drug is contraindicated in intolerant patients. The incidence of true aspirin allergy (ie, with an immunochemical basis) is probably less than 0.1%, although it may be higher in known asthmatic patients (2–5%).

Aspirin may interact adversely with the anticoagulant drugs and with phenylbutazone, probenecid,

and spironolactone; patients who are taking these drugs should be advised against the use of aspirin in all forms.

Aspirin ingestion increases the bleeding tendency in patients with a wide variety of bleeding problems (eg, anticoagulant therapy, von Willebrand's disease). Because of temporary impairment of platelet function by aspirin, blood donors should avoid aspirin for 48–72 hours before giving blood.

2. Other salicylate preparations—Aspirin is widely employed in combination with caffeine or with caffeine and phenacetin (APC) for so-called synergistic effects. It is very doubtful if there are any pharmacologically significant advantages of these combinations over ordinary aspirin. The large amounts of phenacetin ingested by habitual users of some of these combinations may cause serious renal damage, although the current literature throws some doubt on the role of phenacetin by itself as the cause of kidney injury.

Sodium salicylate, enteric-coated, 0.3–0.6 gm every 4 hours, may be used by patients with gastric intolerance to aspirin.

Salicylamide is a relatively weak, short-acting, salicylate-related drug which is found in numerous proprietary analgesic drug combinations. It is not hydrolyzed to salicylates in the body and so is excreted as the amide. It has doubtful advantages over aspirin except for patients with gastric intolerance or bleeding tendencies.

B. Acetaminophen, 325–650 mg orally 3–4 times daily, has analgesic potency comparable to aspirin for many painful conditions. It is the substance into which phenacetin is rapidly converted. It is less effective than aspirin in rheumatoid arthritis and other inflammatory disorders. Its antipyretic action is comparable to that of aspirin. Acetaminophen may be especially useful as a mild analgesic and antipyretic in aspirin allergy and in patients with gout. It apparently does not produce coagulation defects, it does not cause gastric irritation and mucosal bleeding, and it does not interfere with the tubular excretion of uric acid.

C. Colchicine: The "analgesic" properties of colchicine are probably due to its anti-inflammatory effects. It is used clinically almost exclusively for gouty arthritis, but it has also been reported to be effective in sarcoid arthritis.

D. Phenylbutazone and its metabolite or para-hydroxy analogue, **oxyphenbutazone,** exert a potent "analgesic" effect in painful disorders associated with inflammatory diseases. Although useful in a variety of acute rheumatic conditions, they are most effective in the treatment of acute gouty arthritis and active rheumatoid spondylitis. Because of their relatively high potential for toxicity, they should be reserved for patients who do not respond to salicylates and other simple therapeutic measures. They should be used cautiously within the recommended dosage range, usually 300–400 mg/day, or less, in divided doses. Follow the manufacturer's directions carefully. If, after a trial period of 1 week, the drugs fail to produce a favorable response, therapy should be discontinued. Toxic reactions include skin rash, hypersensitivity reaction of the serum sickness type, nausea, vomiting, stomatitis, peptic ulceration, sodium retention, blood dyscrasias, and prothrombin depression (when the drugs are used concurrently with anticoagulants of the coumarin type). As a precaution, blood counts are recommended twice weekly for the first month, weekly for the second month, and monthly thereafter. In general, the drugs should not be used in patients with gastrointestinal, renal, cardiac, or hematopoietic disease or in those receiving anticoagulant therapy. They should not be given for prolonged periods, and all patients should be observed frequently for evidence of toxicity.

E. Propoxyphene, 30—65 mg orally, and the pharmacologically similar but more stable **propoxyphene napsylate,** 100 mg every 6 hours as needed. Although related chemically to the narcotics, propoxyphene is considerably less potent in all respects. Cases of propoxyphene abuse have been reported. Side-effects are uncommon (dizziness, epigastric pain, nausea). The problem of addiction is minimal, but addiction may occur nevertheless. The claim that their analgesic potency is equal to that of codeine is questionable. Their principal use is in patients who are allergic to or who cannot tolerate aspirin or codeine. Many cases of suicide with propoxyphene have been reported. Recently, propoxyphene has been employed experimentally with some success for the alleviation of heroin withdrawal reactions.

F. Indomethacin: This analgesic and anti-inflammatory agent is said to be useful in the rheumatic disorders, although its advantages over aspirin, if any, remain controversial. It appears to be most effective in ankylosing spondylitis and in osteoarthritis of the hip. The usual dose is 25 mg 2—4 times daily, increasing the dosage, if tolerated, up to no more than 200 mg daily. Untoward effects include headache, dizziness, lightheadedness, tinnitus, psychiatric disturbances (including depression and psychosis), drug rash, stomatitis, anorexia, dyspepsia, nausea, vomiting, peptic ulceration, gastrointestinal bleeding, and diarrhea. Hematologic or hepatotoxic effects are relatively uncommon. Because of the above side-effects and toxicity, patients under treatment should be observed carefully for any evidence of toxicity. Indomethacin should not be used as a "routine" mild analgesic (eg, instead of aspirin).

G. Ibuprofen: Ibuprofen (Brufen, Motrin) is an antipyretic, anti-inflammatory analgesic recently introduced into the USA for the treatment of degenerative joint disease and rheumatoid arthritis. It is reported to cause less gastric irritation than aspirin, but its advantages in this and other respects—if any—are unclear. The recommended dosage is 300—400 mg 3 or 4 times daily. Reported side-effects include gastrointestinal disturbances, skin rashes, headaches, dizziness, and visual disturbances. It should not be used concomitantly with aspirin, nor should it be used in patients who have nasal polyps, angioedema, or bronchospasm associated with aspirin. Its use in pregnancy is not recommended.

H. Carbamazepine: This tricyclic compound, which is chemically related to imipramine, is remarkably effective in relieving pain in many patients (about 75%) with trigeminal neuralgia for prolonged periods and in some cases may induce prolonged remission of pain (see p 585). Pain relief may occur within 48 hours. Attempts are made periodically to withdraw the drug to determine if the patient has a spontaneous remission and resumed if the pain recurs. Carbamazepine has also been used unpredictably and less effectively in other severe neuralgias, in pain due to tabes dorsalis, and in trigeminal neuralgia occurring as a manifestation of multiple sclerosis. Some patients who do not respond to carbamazepine require the addition of diphenylhydantoin or surgical treatment.

I. Pentazocine: Pentazocine is a weak narcotic antagonist of the benzomorphan series which has both morphine-like and nalorphine-like characteristics. A dose of 30 mg subcut approaches the analgesic effectiveness of 10 mg of morphine sulfate and produces similar side-effects except for a slightly higher incidence and severity of drowsiness. Respiratory depression may occur. Pentazocine will not suppress abstinence symptoms in morphine-dependent subjects and can actually precipitate withdrawal in narcotic addicts. Side-effects, including respiratory depression, are similar to those of the narcotic group. A dose of 50 mg orally is approximately equivalent to 60 mg of codeine in analgesic effect, with a slightly more rapid onset and a slightly shorter duration of action. Adverse effects are somewhat comparable to but more marked than those of codeine. Dizziness and impaired thinking may occur. Pentazocine tolerance can develop. It may cause addiction and is subject to drug abuse. Withdrawal symptoms are less marked than is the case with the opiates. Caution should be exercised in administration of this drug to addiction-prone individuals, patients with severe hepatic impairment, pregnant women, and children under 12 years of age. Future legislative control may be required.

Narcotic Analgesics

The narcotic analgesics alter the perception of pain by their effects on the CNS. They are indicated for the relief of pain which is too intense to be controlled with nonnarcotic drugs or when pain is of a type not relieved by the salicylates (eg, visceral pain).

The narcotics are also mildly sedative in small doses; larger doses produce sleep, stupor, and respiratory depression. They are addictive and should be used cautiously and with careful attention to federal and state laws. Except for codeine, they should not be used for chronic illnesses except when necessary for the control of otherwise intractable pain in terminal illness.

Addiction and withdrawal are discussed in Chapter 17.

The specific treatment of intoxication with these drugs is discussed in Chapter 30.

Note: Always use the least potent narcotic drug which will control the pain, eg, codeine is preferable to meperidine, and meperidine to morphine.

A. Morphine: This drug is the most valuable of the potent narcotics for general clinical use. It causes CNS depression which results in powerful analgesia associated with sedation, euphoria, and hypnosis; selective respiratory center depression, and dulling or abolition of the cough reflex. It increases intracranial pressure. Morphine is useful for relief of acute severe pain. It is also valuable in the treatment of severe cardiac dyspnea (eg, pulmonary edema or cardiac asthma of left ventricular failure). It is a commonly used and valuable preoperative drug. Morphine is contraindicated in morphine sensitivity, bronchial asthma, undiagnosed surgical abdominal disease, hepatic insufficiency, hypothyroidism, morphinism, head injury, Addison's disease, and whenever the possibility of vomiting may be dangerous. Untoward reactions include hypnosis (may be undesirable), respiratory depression, nausea and vomiting, severe constipation, urticaria, and pruritus. The addiction tendency is great, especially in addiction-prone individuals.

1. Morphine sulfate, 8—15 mg orally or subcut. In cases of severe agonizing pain, especially pain associated with impending neurogenic shock (eg, acute pancreatitis), it may be given slowly in 5 ml physiologic saline intravenously. It is probable that only increased duration of effect is gained by increasing the dose above 10 mg.

2. Morphine adjuncts—Belladonna alkaloids, such as atropine and scopolamine, in dosages of 0.3—0.6 mg subcut administered simultaneously with morphine, may reduce some of the untoward effects of morphine. The phenothiazine tranquilizers may enhance the sedative effect of morphine, making it possible to give the latter in smaller doses.

B. Morphine Congeners: A number of drugs equivalent to morphine but offering no advantages are available. Claims of fewer side-effects should be regarded with skepticism.

The following subcutaneous doses are equivalent to 10 mg of morphine: hydromorphone, 2 mg; levorphanol, 2 mg; oxymorphone, 1 mg; phenazocine, 1 mg; piminodine, 7.5 mg.

C. Methadone: Methadone, 5—10 mg subcut, provides analgesia similar to that achieved with morphine. It is only half as effective when given orally. The onset is slower and the effect is more prolonged. It has powerful addictive properties. The only situation in which methadone is preferred is in the authorized treatment of addiction; withdrawal symptoms are ameliorated if methadone is first substituted for heroin or other opiate (see Chapter 17).

D. Meperidine: 75—150 mg orally or IM (not subcut) every 3—4 hours provides analgesia and causes less intense side-effects than morphine. It is also less addictive than morphine, but addiction to meperidine is nevertheless very common.

E. Meperidine Congeners: Alphaprodine, 60 mg subcut, and anileridine, 50 mg subcut, are equivalent to meperidine, 100 mg, except that their duration of action is shorter.

F. Oxycodone: Usually given in dosages of 3—5 mg, this drug is available only in combinations with other ingredients in analgesic and cough mixtures (Percodan, etc). It is frequently misused because the name suggests a similarity to codeine. It is more potent and more addictive than codeine.

G. Codeine: Codeine is pharmacologically similar to morphine but is less potent. Codeine diminishes the cough reflex and decreases bowel motility (constipating). It is preferred to morphine for relief of moderate degrees of pain because it is much less habit-forming and causes fewer untoward reactions (urticaria, nausea and vomiting, pruritus, dermatitis, anaphylactoid reactions).

1. Codeine phosphate, 8—65 mg orally or subcut every 3—4 hours as needed. If 65 mg is ineffective, use stronger narcotics, since larger doses of codeine are attended by increasing side reactions without increasing analgesia.

2. Codeine in dosages ranging from 8—65 mg is often used in combination with aspirin or ASA compound to produce an additive analgesic effect. The dosage is 1 tablet orally 3—4 times daily as necessary. In such mixtures codeine is the active ingredient; the aspirin is added for convenience in prescribing.

Blechman WJ & others: Ibuprofen or aspirin in rheumatoid arthritis therapy. JAMA 233:336, 1975.

Bonica JJ: *The Management of Pain,* 2nd ed. Lea & Febiger, 1974.

Bonica JJ (editor): *Recent Advances on Pain: Pathophysiology and Clinical Aspects.* Thomas, 1974.

Crill WE: Carbamazepine. Ann Int Med 79:844, 1973.

Dalkos GK: Propoxyphene jaundice. JAMA 232:835, 1975.

Forrest WH: Oral pentazocine. Ann Int Med 81:644, 1974.

Ingelfinger FJ: The side-effects of aspirin. New England J Med 290:1196, 1974.

Lee PK: Treatment of chronic pain with acupuncture. JAMA 232:1133, 1975.

Leist ER, Banwell JG: Products containing aspirin. New England J Med 291:710, 1974.

Leonards JR, Levy G, Niemczura R: Gastrointestinal blood loss during prolonged aspirin administration. New England J Med 289:1020, 1974.

Lewin AJ: Acupuncture and its role in modern medicine. Western J Med 120:27, 1974.

Lewis JR: Evaluation of ibuprofen (Motrin). A new antirheumatic agent. JAMA 233:364, 1975.

Lewis JR: Misprescribing analgesics. JAMA 228:1155, 1974.

Lockey RF & others: Familial occurrence of asthma, nasal polyps and aspirin intolerance. Ann Int Med 78:57, 1973.

Mann F & others: Treatment of intractable pain by acupuncture. Lancet 2:57, 1973.

Mills JA: Non-steroidal anti-inflammatory drugs. (2 parts.) New England J Med 290:781, 1002, 1974.

Samter M: Intolerance to aspirin. Hosp Practice 8:85, 1973.

Tennant FS: Complications of propoxyphene abuse. Arch Int Med 132:191, 1973.

Vandam LD: Analgetic drugs: The mild analgetics. New England J Med 286:20, 1972.

Vandam LD: Analgetic drugs: The potent analgetics. New England J Med 286:249, 1972.

Zimmerman HJ: Aspirin-induced hepatic injury. Ann Int Med 80:103, 1974.

SYSTEMIC ALLERGIC REACTIONS

Allergic or hypersensitivity disorders may be manifested by generalized systemic reactions as well as by localized reactions in any organ system of the body. The reactions may be acute, subacute, or chronic, immediate or delayed, and may be caused by an endless variety of offending agents (antigens)—pollens, molds, dusts, feathers, fur, venoms, food, drugs, etc.

A true allergic reaction is one which is immunologically mediated (ie, by an antibody following reexposure to an antigen). This is to be distinguished from a simple chemical reaction in an individual with an altered, damaged, or otherwise abnormal chemoreceptor system. It is particularly to be differentiated from unfavorable responses such as are produced by psychologic dislikes, overindulgence, overexposure, and—in the case of drugs—overdosages, side-reactions, and known adverse pharmacologic effects.

Several of the immunologic factors which underly hypersensitivity reactions have been identified. IgE is a unique humoral immunoglobulin which contains the reaginic antibody that plays a role in mediating many allergic reactions of the "immediate" hypersensitivity type (eg, Prausnitz-Küstner reaction, asthma, acute urticaria, hay fever, anaphylaxis). The immunologic availability of IgE results in the secretion of chemical mediators such as histamine, slow-reacting substance of anaphylaxis, and eosinophil chemotactic factor of anaphylaxis—responsible for the clinical manifestations of allergy. The antibody (IgE)-mediated response plays a primary role in immediate hypersensitivity reactions, but there is evidence that other protective body mechanisms are at work such as cellular immunity, the inflammatory response, other immunoglobulins (IgG, IgA, IgM), and the complement system. A useful classification of allergic reactions which embodies the immunopathologic mechanisms in the various allergic disorders is shown in Table 1–3.

"Delayed" hypersensitivity reactions—based upon a longer interval for the reaction to occur following a challenging antigen dose—are due largely to cell-mediated immunity and include most immunologic responses not dependent upon circulating IgE (and possibly other immune globulins). The tuberculin response and the various types of contact dermatitis are examples of the delayed reactions, which usually take hours or days to occur. Anergy, primarily a deficiency in the lymphocyte-mediated response, may be of importance in skin testing, viral infections, malignant disease, organ transplantation, and immunosuppressive therapy.

Allergic reactions may occur in otherwise nonallergic ("normal") individuals through contact with an antigen which is more or less apparent. There is no evident hereditary predisposition. The diagnosis may be confirmed by careful history, appropriate skin testing, or therapeutic trial *(caution)*. Examples are serum sickness, drug anaphylaxis, and dermatitis venenata.

Atopic, "natural or spontaneous" allergies occur

Table 1–3. Classification of allergic diseases. (After Coombs and Gell.)

Type	Mechanism	Principal Antibody	Examples
I	Anaphylaxis (immediate; antigen-induced, antibody-mediated)	IgE	Anaphylaxis (allergic), bronchial asthma, allergic rhinitis
II	Cytotoxic (antimembrane)	IgG (IgM)	Membranous glomerulonephrosis, Goodpasture's syndrome, allergic hemolytic reaction
III	Immune complex (serum sickness-like)	IgG (IgA, IgM)	Serum sickness, systemic lupus erythematosus, other vasculitides, acute viral hepatitis (?)
IV	Cell-mediated (delayed)	. . .	Contact dermatitis, infectious granulomas (tuberculosis, mycoses), reaction to parasites, chronic hepatitis

in about 10% of the population, often with a family history of similar disorders. Antigenic etiology is much more obscure than in the case of the "normal" allergies. Determination of the allergens is much more difficult since complete reliance cannot be placed upon clinical history, skin tests, or elimination diets. Positive skin tests to multiple antigens are found frequently in atopic individuals. Eosinophilia and increased serum IgE levels are characteristic but not pathognomonic of atopic disorders. The serum IgE levels do not necessarily parallel the clinical degree of allergic response. The atopic disorders include hay fever (allergic rhinitis), atopic dermatitis, allergic eczema, allergic asthma, and anaphylactic reactions. An allergic basis for some of the so-called atopic disorders has been questioned.

Feingold BF: *Introduction to Clinical Allergy.* Thomas, 1973.

Gell PGH, Coombs RRA: *Clinical Aspects of Immunology,* 3rd ed. Davis, 1973.

Norman PA: Immunotherapy (desensitization) in allergic disease. Ann Rev Med 26:337, 1975.

Samter M (editor): *Immunologic Diseases,* 2nd ed. Little, Brown, 1971.

Samter M (editor): Symposium on allergy in adults. M Clin North America 58:1, 1974.

1. ANAPHYLACTIC REACTIONS
(Anaphylactic Shock)

Anaphylactic reactions are the immediate shock-like and frequently fatal reactions which occur within minutes after administration of foreign sera or drugs. Although there is occasionally no history of exposure to the foreign substance, these acute reactions usually represent obscure induced hypersensitivity. Anaphylactic reactions may occur following the injection of sera, penicillin and other antibiotics, and practically all repeatedly administered parenteral diagnostic and therapeutic agents. Anaphylaxis may rarely occur following orally administered foods and drugs. *Note:* For this reason alone, drugs having a relatively high sensitizing risk (see below) should not be administered indiscriminately by oral, topical, or parenteral routes. Emergency drugs should be available whenever injections are given.

Symptoms of anaphylaxis include apprehension, paresthesias, generalized urticaria or edema, choking, cyanosis, wheezing, cough, incontinence, shock, fever, dilatation of pupils, loss of consciousness, and convulsions. Death may occur within 5—10 minutes.

Emergency Treatment

(1) Epinephrine solution, 0.4—1 ml of 1:1000 solution (0.4—1 mg) IM, repeated in 5—10 minutes and later as needed. If the patient does not respond immediately, give 0.1—0.2 ml of 1:1000 solution diluted in 10 ml saline *slowly* IV.

(2) Place in recumbent position. Elevate legs.

(3) Maintain adequate airway with oral airway or endotracheal tube. Emergency tracheostomy may be necessary for laryngeal edema.

(4) Diphenhydramine hydrochloride, aqueous, 5—20 mg IV, after epinephrine if necessary.

(5) Oxygen at 4—6 liters per minute.

(6) Aminophylline injection, 250—500 mg in 10—20 ml of saline *slowly* IV, for severe asthma (without shock).

(7) Intravenous fluids may be used to correct hypovolemia. If arterial hypotension is severe, vasopressor agents (eg, levarterenol, 4 mg in 1 liter dextrose in water) may be given by infusion.

(8) Hydrocortisone sodium succinate, 100—250 mg in water or saline IV over a period of 30 seconds, after epinephrine or diphenhydramine, to prevent prolonged reactions.

Prevention

A. **Precautions:** Be aware of the danger. Do not use potentially dangerous drugs unless there is a definite need. Use special precautions in giving drugs to patients with a history of hay fever, asthma, or other allergic disorders. Whenever possible, determine by inquiry whether the patient previously has been given the drug he is about to receive. If there is a report of any allergic reaction or prior administration, the hazard of giving the drug, *either orally or by injection,* must be carefully considered. Scratch or conjunctival tests with dilute solutions of the test substance and intradermal tests are unreliable and not without hazard.

One of the commoner forms of drug anaphylaxis reported is that due to penicillin. Avoidance of use of penicillin is the only sure method of avoiding allergic reactions. Semisynthetic penicillins and related compounds are, in varying degree, cross-allergenic with natural penicillins. Specific penicillin antigen tests are generally unsatisfactory and are not as reliable as the patient's history of previous reactions. A negative history or a negative skin test does not always imply safety. Conversely, a history of "allergy" or a positive skin test does not necessarily establish intolerance. If penicillin must be given as a lifesaving measure to a patient suspected for good reason of having penicillin allergy, the patient must be under close observation and provision must be made for emergency treatment of anaphylaxis.

Other drugs besides penicillin which are likely to induce anaphylaxis are immune antisera (eg, tetanus, snake antivenin), protein drugs (eg, chymotrypsin, penicillinase), dehydrocholate sodium, demecolocycline, nitrofurantoin, sulfobromophthalein (BSP), streptomycin, water-soluble iodine radiographic contrast media for parenteral use, and, rarely vaccines.

Patients who are known to be sensitive to insect bites should avoid areas where such insects are apt to be present. Protective garments (eg, gloves, netting, full-length clothing) may be necessary. Sensitized patients should always carry an insect-sting first aid kit containing a preloaded syringe of epinephrine, 1:1000, ephedrine sulfate tablet (25 mg), antihistamine tablets, and a tourniquet, and should be familiar with its use.

Individuals with known sensitivity to drugs and stings should wear a medical identification bracelet or tag (Medi-Alert) or carry an identification card.

B. **Prior Administration of Antihistaminic Drugs (Selected Patients):** Reduction of frequency and severity of anaphylactic reactions by means of the antihistaminic drugs has been reported, but they do not guarantee safety against anaphylaxis.

C. **Corticotropin and Corticosteroids:** Cautious administration of corticotropin and corticosteroids before administration of drugs to which the individual may be sensitive has been employed, but the results are unpredictable and hazardous.

D. **Densensitization:** (See p 1003.) Hypersensitivity to insect allergens may be extreme, and desensitization of suspected insect-sensitive patients, although quite effective, may be hazardous and is best performed by experienced allergists.

Busse WW & others: Immunotherapy in bee-sting anaphylaxis. JAMA 231:1154, 1975.

Kelly JF, Patterson R: Anaphylaxis: Course, mechanisms and treatment. JAMA 227:1431, 1974.

Lockey RF, Bukantz SC: Allergic emergencies. M Clin North America 58:147, 1974.

Parker CW: Drug allergy. (3 parts.) New England J Med 292:511, 732, 957, 1975.

Tests for penicillin allergy. Med Lett Drugs Ther 17:53, 1975.

2. SERUM SICKNESS-LIKE REACTIONS

"Serum sickness" is a systemic allergic reaction which occurs within 1—2 weeks after injection of any foreign serum (eg, tetanus antitoxin), and even more frequently as a result of administration of many widely prescribed drugs. It is characterized by malaise, fever, urticaria, patchy or generalized rash, lymphadenopathy, musculoskeletal aches and pains, nausea and vomiting, and abdominal pain. It is usually mild and lasts about 2–3 days. Serious neuropathy, vasculitis, and glomerulonephritis occur very rarely. In previously sensitized individuals the reaction may be severe or even fatal; the onset may occur immediately or after a latent period of hours to days.

Prevention

A. Diagnosis: Recognition of individual hypersensitivity is based upon a history of allergic diathesis or previous drug or serum reactions and warrants special preliminary testing for sensitivity and careful precautions in administering immunizing sera.

B. Desensitization: If there is any evidence of sensitivity (see p 1003) by either the conjunctival or intradermal sensitivity testing technics, it is imperative that the patient be desensitized with graded doses of the serum to be employed.

Treatment

Antihistamines (eg, tripelennamine or diphenhydramine), 25–50 mg every 4 hours as needed, or salicylates as needed for mild reactions. Antihistamines, epinephrine, ephedrine, or the corticosteroids may be required for moderate or prolonged reactions. Severe reactions should be treated as for anaphylaxis.

Primer on rheumatic diseases: Serum sickness and drug reactions. JAMA 224:726, 1973.

. . .

DRUGS USED IN ALLERGIC DISORDERS

Many manifestations of allergic reactions are due to the liberation of histamine from storage sites in the body. The treatment of allergies may thus consist of drugs which (1) prevent the effects of histamine (antihistamines—see below); (2) stabilize the membrane of mast cells at storage sites, preventing release of histamine (cromolyn—see p 113); (3) reverse the effects of histamine (epinephrine, ephedrine, and related sympathomimetic drugs—see p 112); or (4) suppress the allergic inflammatory reaction (corticosteroids—see p 112 and Table 18–16).

The Antihistamines

The antihistaminic drugs do not prevent the release of histamine caused by the antigen-antibody reaction but they do, to a limited extent, prevent the histamine from acting on blood vessels, bronchioles, and other end organs.

The antihistamines are most effective in urticaria, angioneurotic edema, hay fever, and serum sickness. They are less predictably useful in vasomotor rhinitis and contact dermatitis, and are least apt to be effective in atopic dermatitis.

The most common side-effect is sedation of the type produced by the tranquilizers; this effect may be useful but is often regarded as unpleasant by the patient. Patients receiving antihistaminic drugs should be cautioned against driving motor vehicles or piloting aircraft. Other side-effects are feelings of weakness, dizziness, various gastrointestinal complaints, atropine-like effects such as dry mouth or blurred vision, and photodermatosis. Larger doses cause excitement, ie, insomnia and tremulousness progressing to confusion and convulsions.

The antihistamines should not be used topically since they are not locally effective and are common sensitizers.

In a given patient, the choice of preparation depends upon trial and error and a decision about whether sedation is desired or not.

The sedative antihistamines have been used widely in proprietary sleep preparations.

Some commonly used antihistaminic drugs and their usual dosages are as follows:

A. Sedation Infrequent:
  *Chlorpheniramine, 4 mg 4 times daily.
  *Brompheniramine, parabromdylamine, 4 mg 4 times daily.

B. Sedation Often Prominent:
  *Diphenhydramine, 25–50 mg 4 times daily.
  *Tripelennamine, 25 mg 4 times daily.
  Pyrilamine, (contained in many combinations and brands), 50 mg 4 times daily.
  *Promethazine, 12.5–25 mg twice daily. Give twice daily only.
  Methapyrilene, 25–50 mg 4 times daily. (Used in proprietary "sleeping tablets.")
  Thonzylamine, 50–100 mg 4 times daily.

C. Other Antihistamines (Long-Acting):
  Triprolidine, 2.5 mg twice daily.
  Pyrrobutamine, 15 mg twice daily.

Kilpatrick CH: Steroid therapy for allergic diseases. M Clin North America 57:1309, 1973.

Tempero KF, Hunninghake DB: Antihistamines. Postgrad Med 48:149, 1970.

Teutsch G: Hypnotic efficacy of diphenhydramine, methapyrilene and pentobarbital. Clin Pharmacol Therap 17:195, 1975.

*Parenteral preparation available.

2...
Fluid & Electrolyte Disorders

Marcus A. Krupp

Normally, the body fluids have a specific chemical composition and are distributed in discrete anatomic compartments of relatively fixed volumes. Disease produces associated or independent abnormalities in the amounts, distribution, and solute concentrations of the body fluids. Correct diagnosis and treatment of fluid and electrolyte disorders depends upon an understanding of the chemical laws and physiologic processes which control volume, distribution, and composition. In addition, the pharmacologic or physiologic action of some components of body fluids must be considered.

Table 2–1. TBW (as percentage of body weight) in relation to age and sex.*

Age	Male	Female
10–18	59%	57%
18–40	61%	51%
40–60	55%	47%
Over 60	52%	46%

*Modified and reproduced, with permission, from Edelman & Liebman: Anatomy of body water and electrolytes. Am J Med 27:256, 1959.

BASIC CONSIDERATIONS

VOLUME & DISTRIBUTION OF BODY WATER

The volume of body water in an individual is quite constant with intake (food, water consumed, and water produced by combustion) balanced by output (respiratory water vapor, perspiration, urine). Body water content among individuals differs inversely with obesity. Since fat cells contain very little water and lean tissue is rich in water, it follows that bodies heavy with fat will contain a smaller ratio of water/body weight than lean bodies. After childhood, females usually have a higher ratio of fat/lean tissue. As humans age, they tend to gain proportionately more fat. In the average well nourished population of the United States, total body water varies as shown in Table 2–1.

The distribution of water among the body fluid compartments is dependent upon the distribution and content of solute. The ability of membranes and cells to restrict movement of solute into and from capillaries, interstitial fluid, and cells results in compartmentalization of solute with resultant distribution of water by osmosis to sustain (1) equal osmolal concentrations of solute in compartments and (2) equal concentrations of water in compartments. Differences in composition of solute in various compartments exist, but osmolality (concentration in compartment water) is equal on both sides of the membrane separating 2 compartments.

Solute concentration is expressed in terms of osmols. The term osmol refers to the relationship between molar concentration and osmotic activity of a substance in solution. The osmolarity of a substance in solution is calculated by multiplying the molar concentration by the number of particles per mol provided by ionization. Glucose in solution provides 1 particle per molecule; NaCl in solution—for all practical purposes—totally dissociates into Na^+ and Cl^-, yielding 2 particles per molecule. One mol of glucose in solution thus yields 1 osmol; 1 mol of NaCl, 2 osmols. As with electrolyte concentrations, the milliunit is more convenient. Osmols-per-kilogram-of-water is termed osmolal; osmols-per-liter-of-solution is termed osmolar. The normal osmolarity of body fluids is 285–293 mOsm/liter.

In all problems of altered osmolality, the alteration exists in all body compartments, and the excess or deficit of solute or of water must be calculated on the basis of total body water (TBW).

ELECTROLYTES

In clinical medicine, the measurement of concentrations of electrolyte in body fluids is expressed in milliequivalents per liter of the fluid. Salts in solution dissociate into ions with positive charges (cations) and with negative charges (anions). The numbers of positive and negative charges are equal, ie, a divalent cation

Table 2–2. Molar and milliequivalent weights.

	Valence	Molar Weights (gm)	Milliequivalent Weights (mg)
Cations			
Na^+	1	23	23
K^+	1	39	39
Ca^{++}	2	40	20
Mg^{++}	2	24	12
Anions			
Cl^-	1	35.5	35.5
HCO_3^-	1	61	61
$H_2PO_4^-$ $\}$ $HPO_4^=$ $\}$	$\{$ 1 $\}$ $\{$ 2 $\}$	31 (as P)	
$SO_4^=$	2	96	48

Table 2–3. Body water distribution in an average normal young adult male.*

	ml/kg† Body Weight	% of Total Body Water
Total extracellular fluid	270	45
Plasma	45	7.5
Interstitial fluid	120	20
Connective tissue and bone	90	15
Transcellular fluid	15	2.5
Total intracellular fluid	330	55
Total body water	600	100

*Modified from Edelman & Liebman: Anatomy of water and electrolytes. Am J Med 27:256, 1959.

†$\frac{ml/kg}{10}$ = %, eg, 45 ml/kg = 4.5% body weight.

(++) will be balanced by 2 monovalent anions or 1 divalent anion (- -).

One mol (gram-molecule) of a substance is the molecular weight of the substance expressed in grams. One mol of a substance contains 6.023×10^{23} molecules of that substance. If the substance can exist in ionized form, its combining capacity with a substance of opposite charge will be determined by its valence, ie, the number of charges per atom or molecule. One mol of a monovalent ion is defined as an equivalent. Thus, 1 mol of a divalent ion will yield 2 equivalents, or, to put it otherwise, 1 equivalent of a divalent ion will be provided by one-half mol of the substance. The term equivalent, therefore, is an expression of concentration in terms of electrical charge. The concentrations of ions in body fluids are small and better expressed in terms of 0.001 equivalents or milliequivalents per liter. Dissociation of some complex ions such as phosphate and protein varies with pH, thus precluding the assignment of a specific valence. (At pH 7.4, the normal pH of plasma, phosphate exists as a buffer mixture of $H_2PO_4^-$ and $HPO_4^=$ to yield an effective valence of 1.8.)

BODY FLUID COMPARTMENTS

The principal fluid compartments include plasma and interstitial fluid, which comprise the extracellular fluid, and intracellular fluid. Body fluids also are distributed to dense connective tissue, bone, and "transcellular" spaces (gut lumen, CSF, intraocular fluid), but these are relatively inaccessible and usually do not enter into clinical situations involving body fluid abnormalities.

The clinical simplification of considering body water or fluid as intracellular (ICW) or extracellular (ECW) is justified by the fact that sodium salts constitute the bulk of osmotically active solute in ECW whereas potassium salts constitute the bulk of osmotically active solute in ICW. Furthermore, almost all other

solutes present in body water can be considered to be either freely diffusible between ICW and ECW (such as urea) or osmotically inactive (such as ICW magnesium, which is largely bound to protein) and consequently are not osmotically active in either compartment, ie, they do not produce an osmotic gradient because their osmolar concentration is equal in both compartments.

The composition of the body fluids differs among the compartments. Characteristics of the electrolyte concentrations within the compartments are shown in Table 2–4.

Interstitial fluids are not readily available for assay. Clinically, one relies on determinations on plasma or serum which will provide adequate information to assess water and electrolyte derangements in the light of the clinical situation.

PHYSIOLOGY OF WATER & ELECTROLYTE & TREATMENT OF ABNORMAL STATES

In keeping with the basic considerations reviewed above, it is useful to describe the role of body fluids in support of homeostasis in terms of 3 closely related factors: volume, concentration, and pharmacologic activity. The ensuing discussion will consider the following:

Water Volume

(1) Extracellular fluid: Plasma, interstitial fluid, transcellular fluid (CSF, intraluminal intestinal fluid, ocular fluid).

(2) Intracellular fluid.

Table 2–4. Concentrations of cations and anions present in plasma, interstitial water (ISW), and intracellular water (ICW). (n.d. = Not determined.)

	Plasma, mEq/liter		ISW, mEq/liter*	ICW, mEq/liter
	Average	Range	Average	Average
Na^+	140	138–145	144	10
K^+	4	3.5–4.5	4	155
Ca^{++}	5	4.8–5.65	n.d.	3
Mg^{++}	2	1.8–2.3	n.d.	26
Total	151		*	194
Cl^-	103	97–105	114	3
HCO_3^-	27	26–30	30	10
$Protein^-$	16	14–18	n.d.	55
$HPO_4^=$	2	1.2–2.3	n.d.	95
$SO_4^=$	1	n.d.	n.d.	20
Undetermined anions	2	n.d.	n.d.	n.d.
Total	151		*	183+

*Concentrations derived by converting plasma concentrations to mEq/liter of serum water and applying Donnan factors of 0.95 for cations and 1.05 for anions.

Concentration

(1) Osmolality: Total solute concentration.

(2) Concentration of individual electrolytes.

Pharmacologic Activity

(1) Concentration of hydrogen ion (pH).

(2) Concentration of electrolytes which exert pharmacologic actions.

WATER VOLUME

"Volume" and "water" are substantially interchangeable in the context of this discussion. Volume of body water is maintained by a balance between intake and excretion. Water as such, in foods and as a product of combustion, is excreted by the kidneys, skin, and lungs. Electrolytes important in maintaining volume and distribution include the cations sodium for extracellular fluid and potassium and magnesium for intracellular fluid, and the anions chloride and bicarbonate for extracellular fluid and phosphate and protein for intracellular fluid.

Loss of water or excess of water results in corresponding change in volume in both extra- and intracellular compartments. Loss of sodium (with accompanying anion) or excess of sodium results in decrease or increase, respectively, of the volume of extracellular fluid, with water moving out of the extracellular compartment with sodium loss and into the extracellular compartment with sodium retention.

In response to changes in volume, appropriate servo or feedback mechanisms come into play. The principal elements in regulation are antidiuretic hormone for water, aldosterone and other corticosteroids for sodium (and potassium), vascular responses affecting glomerular filtration rate for water and sodium,

and, perhaps, a natriuretic hormone ("third factor") originating in the kidney.

The average adult requires at least 800–1300 ml of water per day to cover obligatory water needs. A normal adult on an ordinary diet requires 500 ml of water for renal excretion of solute in a maximally concentrated urine plus an additional amount of water to replace that lost via the skin and respiratory tract.

Fluid losses most often include electrolyte as well as water. Sweat, gastrointestinal fluids, urine, and fluid escaping from wounds contain significant quantities of electrolyte. In order to ascertain deficits of water and electrolytes, one must consider the history, change in body weight, clinical state, and appropriate determinations in plasma of concentration of each of the electrolytes, osmolality, protein, and pH. Assessment of renal function is required before repair and maintenance requirements can be determined and prescribed. Fig 2–1 indicates the variation in water required to excrete different loads of solute. The capacity of the kidney to excrete a concentrated or a dilute urine sets the limits of water requirement.

1. WATER DEFICIT

Water deficit results in a decrease in volume of both extracellular and intracellular fluids with a corresponding increase in concentration of both extracellular and intracellular solute in these fluids. In the blood, the loss of body water is reflected in an increased plasma osmolality as concentrations of plasma electrolyte and protein rise. With decreased blood volume, renal blood flow is reduced and excretion of urea falls, resulting in an elevation of urea in body fluids. Antidiuretic hormone secretion is stimulated, providing some protection from water loss by the kidney.

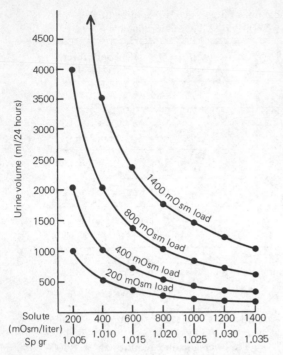

Figure 2—1. Total solute excretion and urine volume per given sp gr. (Redrawn and reproduced, with permission, from John H. Bland: *Clinical Recognition and Management of Disturbances of Body Fluids.* Saunders, 1956.)

Water deficit results from reduced intake or unusual losses. Reduced intake is likely when the patient is unconscious, disabled, unable to ingest water because of esophageal or pyloric obstruction, or receives inadequate fluids to meet maintenance and replacement needs. Fever or a hot environment increases loss from the lungs and skin. The kidney fails to conserve water when there is inadequate ADH (diabetes insipidus) or insensitivity to ADH (nephrogenic diabetes insipidus), osmotic diuresis in diabetes mellitus, inadequate tubule function due to renal disease, and impaired capacity to reabsorb water secondary to potassium depletion, hypercalcemia, correction of obstructive uropathy, or from intensive diuretic therapy.

Water deficit is characterized by thirst, flushed skin, acute weight loss, "dehydrated" appearance, dry mucous membranes, tachycardia, and oliguria. As dehydration increases, hallucinations and delirium, hyperpnea, and coma ensue.

Treatment

An essential guideline for treatment is acute change in weight, which is directly related to change in fluid volume.

Water may be provided with or without electrolyte. If water alone is needed, 2.5% dextrose solution may be given intravenously; the dextrose is oxidized to yield water.

In the presence of normal renal function, 2000–3000 ml of water per day (1500 ml/sq meter of body surface) will provide a liberal maintenance ration. If dehydration is present with increased serum sodium concentration and osmolality, extra water replacement can be estimated on the basis of restoring normal osmolality for the total body fluid volume. The need for intracellular water is reflected in the extracellular fluid with which it is in osmotic equilibrium; therefore, any correction of deviation in osmolality must be considered on the basis of the total volume of body water.

The water requirement is increased in the presence of fever as a result of increased loss via the skin and lungs.

2. WATER EXCESS

Water excess (overhydration, dilution syndrome) results in expansion of the volume of body fluid and decreased concentration (dilution) of plasma electrolyte and protein, with reduced osmolality of plasma. Similar dilutions occur intracellularly. Normally, ADH secretion is inhibited, enabling the kidneys to excrete the excess water. Water excess results from intake in excess of capacity for excretion, usually from too large a water ration during parenteral administration; or from impaired excretion due to acute or chronic renal insufficiency, renal functional changes (lowered glomerular filtration and increased water reabsorption) accompanying heart failure, liver disease with ascites, or administration of ADH or inappropriate secretion of "ADH-like" substance by neoplasms or in complex endocrine disturbances.

Water excess, particularly if severe or if it develops acutely, produces the syndrome of water intoxication, characterized by headache, nausea, vomiting, abdominal cramps, weakness, stupor, coma, and convulsions.

Treatment

The basic treatment consists of water restriction. If a real deficit of sodium exists as well, saline solutions should be employed. In the presence of severe water intoxication, administration of hypertonic saline solution may be useful to promote movement of excess intracellular water to the extracellular space, ie, to increase osmolarity and diminish intracellular water volume.

CONCENTRATION

The total concentration of solute (osmolarity) is apparently the same in intracellular and extracellular water. In the intracellular compartment, protein concentration plays a more important osmolar role than in the plasma. The protein content of interstitial fluid is small, and osmolar effects are therefore negligible. The most accessible and best index of osmolarity is the measurement of the solute concentration in the plasma by ascertaining the depression of the freezing point. An indirect and useful measurement is that of plasma sodium concentration, provided due attention is paid to hyperglycemia and high urea concentrations, which cause a significant increase in osmolality; and lipidemia and hyperproteinemia, which provide a nonaqueous addition to plasma volume. In the latter situations, sodium concentration determinations yield low values which must be interpreted with consideration of the concentration of the other constituents, ie, in terms of plasma or serum water rather than of the plasma specimen per se.

1. HYPERNATREMIA

Increased concentration of sodium in extracellular fluid and hyperosmolality may result from water loss without equivalent sodium loss (pure water volume deficit) or from excessive sodium administration with inadequate water replacement. Hypernatremia may be due to inappropriate regulation of osmolality, occasionally present with intracranial tumors.

Hypernatremia is not an index of total body content of sodium. Increased total body sodium is usually due to retention of sodium with heart failure, cirrhosis

of the liver, and nephrosis. In these states, sodium concentration in extracellular fluid is usually normal or low as a result of expansion of the total volume of body fluid.

Treatment

Treatment must be based on accurate appraisal of the significance of the alteration of the plasma sodium concentration. The clinical history and examination and corroborating laboratory data provide a guide for therapy. Hypernatremia due to water deficit is treated by replenishing water deficit (see above). If treatment with excessive quantities of sodium salts produces hypernatremia, withholding sodium may suffice. Natriuretic drugs (diuretics) may be employed to hasten excretion of the excess sodium; attention must be paid to replacement of water when diuretics are so employed.

2. HYPONATREMIA

A decreased concentration of sodium in extracellular fluid may result from loss of sodium or from dilution by retention of water. Sodium loss occurs with adrenocortical insufficiency, vigorous diuretic

Table 2–5. Relationship of serum sodium to total body sodium in various clinical states.*

Serum Sodium	Total Body Sodium	Clinical States	Fluid and Electrolyte Therapy
Low (hyponatremia) < 130 mEq/liter	High	Edematous states (eg, nephrosis, cirrhosis, cardiac disease). May also occur after severe burns and in the immediate postoperative period.	Not indicated to raise serum sodium.
	Normal	Patients on low sodium intake retaining water as a metabolic response to trauma or surgery, particularly if given excess water (dilution syndrome; water intoxication). May also occur in cirrhotic patients after paracentesis.	Mild: Restrict fluids. Severe: Hypertonic (3–5%) sodium chloride solution may be needed.
	Low	Addison's disease; salt-wasting nephritis; gastrointestinal fluid and electrolyte losses; prolonged sweating with free access to water; perhaps in prolonged use of diuretic agents and on salt-free diets.	Isotonic sodium chloride solution.
Normal 135–145 mEq/liter	High	Renal, cardiac, or hepatic disease; also carcinoma involving pleural or peritoneal cavities. Caused by renal retention of water and salt in the same osmotic ratio.	
	Low	In the early stages of rapid salt depletion from gastrointestinal losses, renal excretion of a dilute urine preserves osmolarity of body fluids. A similar situation prevails in diabetic acidosis.	
High (hypernatremia) > 150 mEq/liter	High	Excess administration of sodium salts.	Water by mouth or dextrose and water intravenously. Withhold electrolytes.
	Normal	Simple dehydration due to deprivation of water; diabetes insipidus (congenital, or acquired, as in the diuretic phase of acute renal insufficiency or after cerebral trauma).	
	Low	Prolonged sweating without access to water.	Hypotonic sodium chloride solution.

*Reproduced, with permission, from Harper HA in: *Handbook of Surgery,* 5th ed. Wilson JL (editor). Lange, 1973.

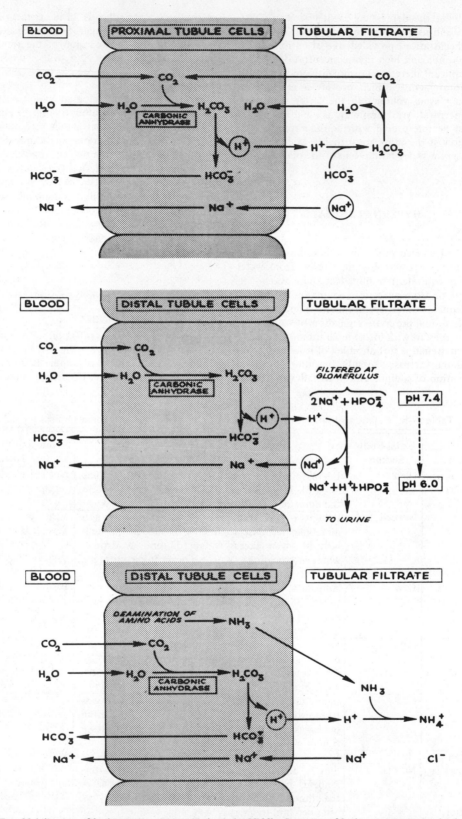

Figure 2—2. *Top:* Mobilization of hydrogen ions in proximal tubule. *Middle:* Secretion of hydrogen ions in distal tubule. *Bottom:* Production of ammonia in distal tubule. (Reproduced, with permission, from Harper HA: *Review of Physiological Chemistry,* 15th ed. Lange, 1975.)

therapy, unusual losses of gastrointestinal secretions, renal insufficiency, and severe sweating. When the deficit of water is replaced with inadequate sodium replacement, hyponatremia ensues. Increased body water volume may follow high water intake or excessive ADH secretion. Inappropriate secretion of ADH may be stimulated by drugs (clofibrate, cyclophosphamide, vincristine), pulmonary disease (tuberculosis, aspergillosis), and CNS disease (encephalitis, trauma, tumor), or it may be associated with malignant tumors (carcinoma of lung, prostate, or pancreas; thymoma). In edematous states such as congestive heart failure, hepatic cirrhosis, nephrotic syndrome, and hypoproteinemia, a decreased circulating blood volume stimulates ADH secretion. These states produce dilution syndromes characterized by hyponatremia (dilutional hyponatremia) and usually normal or high total body sodium.

Treatment

If there is a deficit of sodium, sodium chloride with or without sodium bicarbonate may be used for replacement. For replacement of moderate deficits, 0.9% sodium chloride (155 mEq of Na^+ and Cl^- per liter), or Ringer's solution with or without lactate, may be employed. For severe sodium deficit, 3% sodium chloride (513 mEq/liter) or 5% sodium chloride (855 mEq/liter) may be used with caution. More comprehensive texts on water and electrolyte metabolism must be consulted for specific information on treatment.

Dilutional hyponatremia from water retention should be treated by restriction of intake of water. In dilutional hyponatremia, total body sodium is elevated or normal and, therefore, sodium should not be administered. Fluid restriction is slow to correct the water excess and often fails to have a significant effect. Recently, furosemide has been used to produce a diuresis, which often, in this setting, yields a hypotonic urine. Electrolyte lost in the course of diuresis can be replaced as needed as hypertonic solution.

The concentrations of other electrolytes in extracellular fluids have insignificant osmolar effects.

PHARMACOLOGIC ACTIVITY OF FLUIDS & ELECTROLYTES

HYDROGEN ION CONCENTRATION

The hydrogen ion concentration (H^+) of body fluids is closely regulated with intracellular concentrations of 10^{-7} molar (pH 7.0) and extracellular fluid concentrations of 4×10^{-8} molar (pH 7.4). In spite of accumulation or loss of H^+, these concentrations are maintained at nearly normal by buffer substances

which remove or release H^+. The capacity of buffers is limited, however, and regulation is accomplished principally by the lungs and kidneys. The principal buffer substances include proteins, the oxyhemoglobin-reduced hemoglobin system, primary and secondary phosphate ions, some intracellular phosphate esters, and the carbonic acid-sodium bicarbonate system.

Most of the food used for energy is completely utilized, with production of water, CO_2, and urea. Sulfate and, to a limited extent, phosphate end-products are strong acid anions which must be "neutralized" by cation such as sodium. In the utilization of fat and carbohydrate, intermediate products include the strong acids acetoacetic acid and lactic acid. Buffers provide cation and remove H^+, which is ultimately excreted by the kidneys as acid or as ammonium ion and by the lung as CO_2 and H_2O, equivalent to carbonic acid. The anions of strong acids with cation such as sodium and ammonium are eliminated by the kidney.

The role of the lung and kidney in removal of H^+ and in regulation of H^+ concentration can be viewed as,

$$\frac{[H^+]\ [HCO_3^-]}{[B^+]\ [HCO_3^-]} \rightleftharpoons P_{CO_2} \qquad \frac{lung}{kidney}$$

Respiratory control of the partial pressure of CO_2 (P_{CO_2}) in the pulmonary alveoli and therefore in the arterial plasma determines the H_2CO_3 concentration in body fluids:

$$CO_2 + H_2O \rightleftharpoons H_2CO_3$$

The elimination of CO_2 via the lung in effect removes carbonic acid. The kidney is responsible for $BHCO_3$ concentration in body fluids, which, with H_2CO_3, constitutes one of the buffer systems for regulation of pH.

The kidney tubule cells produce carbonic acid for metabolic CO_2 and water by the following reaction:

$$CO_2 + H_2O \underset{\boxed{\text{Carbonic anhydrase}}}{\rightleftharpoons} H_2CO_3$$

The carbonic acid serves as a source of H^+ which can be exchanged for Na^+ in the tubular urine so that H^+ is excreted and Na^+ reabsorbed. The exchange affects anions of weak acids: H^+ is excreted by the tubule cell into the tubular urine, and Na^+ is reabsorbed. The H^+ in the presence of HCO_3^- in the tubular urine forms H_2CO_3, which $\rightarrow H_2O$ and CO_2, which are reabsorbed. Similarly, H^+ is exchanged for 1 Na^+ of 2 $Na^+HPO_4^=$ to $\rightarrow Na^+H_2PO_4^-$. (See Fig 2–2.)

Although the pH of urine cannot be lowered below pH 4.5, additional H^+ ion can be excreted by combination with NH_3, generated principally from glutamine within the tubule cell. NH_3 diffuses from the tubule cell into the urine within the tubule where it combines with $H^+ \rightarrow NH_4^+$, providing cation for excretion with anions of strong acids with no increase in H^+ concentration (no lowering of pH). These exchanges in the renal tubule involve active transport systems capable of maintaining a gradient in concentration of extracellular fluid H^+ of 4×10^{-8} molar (pH 7.4) against a tubular urine H^+ of 32×10^{-6} molar (pH 4.5), an 800-fold increase in H^+ concentration. (See Fig 2—2.)

CLINICAL STATES OF ALTERED H^+ CONCENTRATION

The clinical term acidosis signifies a decrease in pH (increase in H^+) of extracellular fluid; the term alkalosis signifies an increase in pH (decrease in H^+) of extracellular fluid. The change in H^+ concentration may be the result of metabolic or respiratory abnormalities.

1. RESPIRATORY ACIDOSIS

Respiratory acidosis follows ventilatory abnormalities resulting in CO_2 retention and elevation of P_{CO_2} in alveoli and arterial blood (hypercapnia). Inadequate ventilation during anesthesia, following suppression of the respiratory center by CNS disease or drugs or resulting from respiratory muscle weakness or paralysis, produces CO_2 retention. Anatomic changes in structure of the lung (emphysema) or pulmonary circulation and abnormal thoracic structure (kyphoscoliosis) may alter alveolar-capillary blood exchange or diminish effective ventilation to prevent CO_2 excretion. In association with impaired O_2 excretion, there may be impaired O_2 exchange with low alveolar and arterial P_{O_2} (hypoxia). In the presence of CO_2 retention and the resultant increase in H_2CO_3 concentration, compensatory reabsorption of HCO_3^- by the kidney provides buffer to reduce H^+ concentration, but this protection cannot be accomplished rapidly and is effective only in chronic situations that develop slowly.

The hazard of acute hypercapnia cannot be overemphasized. Buffer protection is severely limited, and renal response is very slow. Thus, an increase in P_{CO_2} can quickly produce sharp increases in H^+ concentration (decrease in pH) to levels incompatible with life. Respiratory inadequacy resulting in sudden increase in P_{CO_2} will usually result in a severe decrease in P_{O_2}, compounding the threat to life. It is apparent that periods of hypoventilation constitute a serious and often lethal complication in the immediate postoperative state, in thoracic surgery, in severe illness or shock accompanied by obtunded consciousness, in trauma to the CNS, and in the presence of heart failure, cardiac arrhythmias, and myocardial infarction.

Treatment
Treatment is directed toward improving ventilation with mechanical aids, bronchodilators, correction of heart failure, and antidotes for anesthetics or drugs suppressing the respiratory center. Tracheostomy or tracheal intubation is often required. Close monitoring of P_{CO_2}, P_{O_2}, and pH of arterial blood is essential. The respiratory center is readily rendered unresponsive by high P_{CO_2} (hypercapnia), and recovery may be very slow. In the presence of hypercapnia, relief of hypoxia with oxygen therapy may deprive the patient of the only remaining stimulus to the respiratory center and produce more severe hypoventilation with resultant CO_2 narcosis and death. Assistance with respiration is required until the respiratory center becomes normally responsive to altered CO_2 concentrations.

2. RESPIRATORY ALKALOSIS

Respiratory alkalosis is a result of hyperventilation which produces lowered P_{CO_2} and elevated pH of extracellular fluid. Anxiety is the usual cause. Hyperventilation during anesthesia or from incorrectly used mechanical ventilatory devices occurs more commonly than is generally appreciated. Renal compensation by excretion of HCO_3^- (with Na^+ predominantly) is too slow a response to be effective, and elevation of pH may reach a point at which asterixis, tetany, and increased neuromuscular irritability appear.

Treatment
Treatment of spontaneous hyperventilation consists of reducing anxiety by drugs or psychotherapy. Tetany may be alleviated by rebreathing exhaled air, which will increase P_{CO_2} and lower blood pH. Regulation of devices used in assisting with ventilation should be guided by measurement of the P_{CO_2} and pH of arterial blood.

3. METABOLIC ACIDOSIS

Metabolic acidosis occurs with starvation, uncontrolled diabetes mellitus with ketosis, electrolyte (including bicarbonate) and water loss with diarrhea or enteric fistulas, and renal insufficiency or tubular defect producing inadequate H^+ excretion. Cation loss (Na^+, K^+, Ca^{++}) and organic acid anion retention occur with starvation and uncontrolled diabetes mellitus. In the presence of renal insufficiency, phosphate and sulfate are retained and cation (especially Na^+) is lost because of limited H^+ secretion for exchange with cation in the renal tubule. A rare cause of metabolic acidosis is the ingestion of acid salts such as NH_4Cl or mandelic acid or acid precursors such as methyl alcohol; these are particularly likely to produce acidosis in the presence of renal insufficiency. Respiratory compensation for metabolic acidosis by hyperventilation reduces P_{CO_2} and thereby reduces H_2CO_3 concentration in extracellular fluid.

Treatment

Treatment is directed toward correcting the metabolic defect (eg, insulin for control of diabetes) and replenishment of water and of deficits of Na^+, K^+, HCO_3^-, and other electrolytes. Anion replacement should include bicarbonate or lactate (bicarbonate equivalent), but large quantities of bicarbonate are needed only in unusual and threatening states. The "maintenance" solution described above is adequate for most needs; lactated Ringer's solution may be preferred if larger quantities of Na^+ are required. A mixture of half 0.9% saline and half 1/6 molar sodium lactate (or bicarbonate) provides an even greater fraction of HCO_3^-. Renal insufficiency requires careful replacement of water and electrolyte deficit and closely controlled rations of water, sodium, potassium, calcium, chloride, and bicarbonate to maintain normal extracellular fluid concentrations; the elevated serum phosphate may be lowered by interfering with phosphate absorption from the gut by oral administration of aluminum hydroxide preparations. In the presence of renal insufficiency, elevated extracellular K^+ concentrations may be reduced by either oral or rectal administration of ion exchange resins which bind K^+, either ingested or secreted, and prevent absorption in the intestine (see Hyperkalemia, below), or by hemodialysis or peritoneal dialysis.

Lactic Acidosis

A rare and serious form of acidosis is that due to large quantities of lactic acid. It is presumed that severe tissue anoxia (eg, in shock) leads to anaerobic glucose metabolism with production of lactic acid. Acidosis develops abruptly and is usually severe and highly resistant to therapy with HCO_3^-. Plasma lactate concentration may rise to 8 mM/liter.

Lactic acidosis must be considered in anoxic states, hypovolemic or endotoxin shock, severe pulmonary insufficiency or pulmonary edema, heart failure, severe hepatic failure, nonketotic diabetic acidosis, following phenformin therapy, and following poisoning with paraldehyde or salicylates. Diagnosis is confirmed in states of overt acidosis by actual lactate levels or by demonstrating that a large amount of unidentified anion is present in the serum (ie, not Cl^-, HCO_3^-, $HPO_4^=$, or ketone bodies).

Shock with inadequate tissue perfusion must be corrected or treatment will be ineffectual. The primary and contributing causes must be treated vigorously and sodium bicarbonate administered in large quantities despite the dangers of sodium overload.

4. METABOLIC ALKALOSIS

Metabolic alkalosis results from loss of gastric juice rich in HCl and occurs also in association with K^+ deficit (diuretics, adrenocortical excess, abrupt correction of hypercapnia) which is characteristically accompanied by increased urinary excretion of H^+. All of these result in renal retention of HCO_3^-, producing elevated extracellular fluid bicarbonate. Respiratory compensation by hypoventilation produces an elevation in P_{CO_2}, increasing the H_2CO_3 fraction of the bicarbonate buffer system.

Treatment

Alkalosis of metabolic origin requires adequate water, K^+, and Na^+. The anion should be exclusively Cl^- to replace the HCO_3^- excess and Cl^- deficit; no lactate or bicarbonate should be employed until normal blood pH and bicarbonate levels are obtained.

POTASSIUM

Potassium is one of the major intracellular cations, occupying a role that is parallel to that of sodium in extracellular fluid. Physiologic actions of potassium are related primarily to concentration of the cation in extracellular fluid, although the intracellular concentration may have some influence. Potassium plays an important part in muscular contraction, conduction of nerve impulses, enzyme action, and cell membrane function.

Cardiac muscle excitability, conduction, and rhythm are markedly affected by changes in concentration of K^+ in extracellular fluid. Both an increase and a decrease of extracellular K^+ concentration diminish excitability and conduction rate. Higher than normal concentrations produce a marked depression of conductivity with cardiac arrest in diastole; in the presence of very low concentrations, cardiac arrest occurs in systole. The effects of abnormal K^+ concentrations in extracellular fluid upon cell membrane potential of cardiac muscle and upon depolarization and repolarization are manifested in the ECG.

Membrane potential and excitability of skeletal and smooth muscle are profoundly affected by the concentrations of K^+, Ca^{++}, and Mg^{++}, with H^+ and Na^+ also involved. Conduction across the myoneural junction is under the influence of these cations as well. At both extremes of abnormal concentration of K^+ in extracellular fluid, muscle contractility is impaired and flaccid paralysis ensues.

Potassium concentration of extracellular fluid is closely regulated between 3.5–5 mEq/liter. Excretion of the 35–100 mEq of potassium contained in the daily diet of the average adult is predominantly via the kidney. There is good evidence that the potassium in glomerular filtrate is reabsorbed in the proximal tubule and that active secretion of potassium into the tubular fluid occurs in the distal portion of the tubule.

1. HYPERKALEMIA

Causes of increased extracellular K^+ concentration include failure of the kidney to excrete ingested potassium (acute and chronic renal failure, severe oliguria due to severe dehydration or trauma); unusual release of intracellular potassium in burns, crushing injuries, or severe infections; and overtreatment with potassium salts. In metabolic acidosis, extracellular K^+ concentration is increased as K^+ shifts from cells.

The elevated K^+ concentration interferes with normal neuromuscular function to produce weakness and paralysis; abdominal distention and diarrhea may occur. As extracellular concentration of K^+ increases, the ECG reflects impaired conduction by peaked T waves of increased amplitude, atrial arrest, spread in the QRS, biphasic QRS–T complexes, and finally ventricular fibrillation and cardiac arrest.

Treatment

Treatment consists of withholding potassium and employing cation exchange resins by mouth or enema. Kayexalate, a sodium cycle sulfonic polystyrene exchange resin, 40–80 gm/day in divided doses, is usually effective. In an emergency, insulin may be employed to deposit K^+ with glycogen in the liver, and Ca^{++} may be given intravenously as an antagonist ion. Sodium bicarbonate can be given intravenously as an emergency measure in severe hyperkalemia; the increase in pH so induced results in a shift of K^+ into cells. Hemodialysis or peritoneal dialysis may be required to remove K^+ in the presence of protracted renal insufficiency.

2. HYPOKALEMIA

Potassium deficit may or may not be accompanied by lowered extracellular fluid K^+ concentration; however, when hypokalemia is present, total potassium deficit is usually profound. Exceptions to this common circumstance include the hypokalemia of alkalosis and that following administration of insulin. Causes of potassium deficit include reduced intake due to starvation or upper gastrointestinal obstruction; poor absorption in steatorrhea, short bowel syndrome, and regional enteritis; loss via the gastrointestinal tract due to emesis, diarrhea, and suction; loss via the kidney due to congenital tubule malfunction, diuresis resulting from diabetes or diuretics, accompanying metabolic alkalosis, and following excessive treatment with saline solutions containing little or no potassium; loss of interstitial fluid with burns or freezing; loss of K^+ due to adrenocortical hormone (cortisol or aldosterone) excess; and intracellular shifts in bouts of familial periodic paralysis. A low concentration of K^+ in extracellular fluid results in impaired neuromuscular function with profound weakness of skeletal muscle, leading to impaired ventilation, and of smooth muscle, producing ileus. The ECG shows decreased amplitude and broadening of T waves, prominent U waves, sagging ST segments, atrioventricular block, and, finally, cardiac arrest. Metabolic alkalosis with elevated plasma pH and bicarbonate concentration develops as a result of po-

tassium deficit which is accompanied by renal excretion of H^+ and reabsorption of bicarbonate and by movement of Na^+ and H^+ from extracellular fluid into cells as K^+ is lost. A defect of water reabsorption by the renal tubule also occurs, producing polyuria and hyposthenuria; this is only slowly ameliorated following treatment.

Treatment

Treatment requires replacement of potassium orally or parenterally. Because of the toxicity of potassium, it must be administered cautiously to prevent hyperkalemia. Furthermore, confirmation of adequate renal function is important when potassium is administered since the principal route of excretion is via the kidney. KCl in a total dose of 1–3 mEq/kg/24 hours may be given parenterally in glucose or saline solutions (or both) at a rate that will not produce hyperkalemia. Except in an emergency in which serum K^+ is extremely low and cardiac muscle and respiratory muscle activity seriously impaired, the administration of K^+ should be at a rate of 10–20 mEq per hour or less. Cl^- is always needed to relieve the hypochloremia that is associated with the accompanying metabolic alkalosis.

CALCIUM

Calcium constitutes about 2% of body weight, but only about 1% of the total body calcium is in solution in body fluid. In the plasma, calcium is present as a nondiffusible complex with protein (33%); as a diffusible but undissociated complex with anions such as citrate, bicarbonate, and phosphate (12%); and as Ca^{++} (55%). The normal total plasma (or serum) calcium concentration is 4.5–5.5 mEq/liter (9–11 mg/100 ml). The serum calcium level is responsive to 2 hormones: parathyroid hormone elevates and calcitonin lowers the concentration. Bone serves as a reservoir of calcium available to body fluids. Excretion of Ca^{++} is via the kidney.

Calcium functions as an essential ion for many enzymes. It is an important constituent of mucoproteins and mucopolysaccharides, and is essential in blood coagulation.

Along with other cations, calcium exerts an important effect on cell membrane potential and permeability manifested prominently in neuromuscular function. It plays a central role in muscle contraction as it is released from the sarcolemma to enter into the ATP-ADP reaction. During muscle relaxation, the calcium is actively transferred back to the sarcolemma and sarcoplasmic reticulum.

Neural function is sensitive to Ca^{++} concentration of interstitial fluid. Excitability is diminished by high Ca^{++} concentration and increased by low concentration. Signs of elevated Ca^{++} concentration include dulling of consciousness and stupor and muscular flaccidity and weakness. Low Ca^{++} concentration increases excitability to produce hyperirritability of muscle, tetany, and convulsions.

Cardiac muscle responds to elevated Ca^{++} concentration with increased contractility, ventricular extrasystoles, and idioventricular rhythm. These responses are accentuated in the presence of digitalis. With severe calcium toxicity, cardiac arrest in systole may occur. Low concentration of Ca^{++} produces diminished contractility of the heart and a lengthening of the Q–T interval of the ECG by prolonging the ST segment.

1. HYPERCALCEMIA

Hypercalcemia results from hyperparathyroidism, invasion of bone by neoplasm (lung, breast, kidney, thyroid), production of a parathyroid-like hormone by isolated neoplasms (ovary, kidney, lung), sarcoidosis, multiple myeloma, milk-alkali syndrome, and vitamin D intoxication.

Hypercalcemia affects neuromuscular function to produce weakness, and causes polyuria, dehydration, thirst, anorexia, vomiting, and constipation. Stupor, coma, and azotemia ensue.

Treatment

Treatment consists of control of the primary disease. Symptomatic hypercalcemia is associated with a high mortality rate; treatment must be promptly instituted. Until the primary disease can be brought under control, renal excretion of calcium with resultant decrease in serum Ca^{++} concentration can be promoted with a variety of agents. Excretion of Na^+ is accompanied by excretion of Ca^{++}; therefore, inducing natriuresis by giving Na^+ salts intravenously and by adjunctive use of diuretics is the emergency treatment of choice. Sodium chloride or sodium sulfate in large quantities (70–80 mEq/hour) with or without diuretics (furosemide) for 12–48 hours may be required. Replacement of water and of K^+ and Mg^{++} is usually necessary. The use of phosphate is hazardous and should be reserved for unusual cases refractory to saline therapy. When elevated Ca^{++} concentrations result from sarcoidosis or neoplasm, corticosteroids such as prednisone may be effective. Mithramycin is useful if elevated Ca^{++} is the result of neoplasm metastatic to bone.

2. HYPOCALCEMIA

Hypocalcemia results from hypoparathyroidism (idiopathic or postoperative), chronic renal insufficiency, rickets and osteomalacia, and malabsorption syndromes. Serum Ca^{++} concentration is reduced in association with decreased serum albumin concentrations (a physiologic relationship).

Hypocalcemia affects neuromuscular function to produce muscle cramps and tetany, convulsions, stridor and dyspnea, diplopia, abdominal cramps, and urinary frequency. Personality changes may occur. In chronic hypoparathyroidism and pseudohypoparathyroidism, cataracts may appear and calcification of basal ganglia of the brain may occur. Mental retardation and stunted growth are common in childhood.

Treatment

Treatment depends on the primary disease. Treatment of hypoparathyroidism with vitamin D and calcium is discussed in Chapter 18. For tetany due to hypocalcemia, calcium gluconate, 1–2 gm, may be given IV. A continuous infusion to sustain plasma calcium concentration may be required. Oral medication with the chloride, gluconate, levulinate, lactate, or carbonate salts of calcium will usually control milder symptoms or latent tetany. The low serum Ca^{++} associated with low serum albumin concentration does not require replacement therapy.

MAGNESIUM

About 50% of total body magnesium exists in the insoluble state in bone. Only 5% is present as extracellular cation; the remaining 45% is contained in cells as intracellular cation. The normal plasma concentration is 1.5–2.5 mEq/liter, with about one-third bound to protein and two-thirds as free cation. Excretion of magnesium ion is via the kidney, with no evidence of active tubule secretion.

Magnesium is an important prosthetic or activator ion, participating in the function of many enzymes involved in phosphate transfer reactions, including those requiring ATP or other nucleotide triphosphate as coenzymes.

Magnesium exerts physiologic effects on the nervous system resembling those of calcium. Elevated Mg^{++} concentration of interstitial fluid produces sedation and central and peripheral nervous system depression. Low concentrations produce increased irritability, disorientation, and convulsions.

Magnesium acts directly upon the myoneural junction. Elevated levels produce blockage by decreasing acetylcholine release, reducing the effect of acetylcholine on depolarization, and diminishing excitability of the muscle cell. Calcium ion exerts an antagonistic action. Low levels of magnesium increase neuromuscular irritability and contractility by increasing acetylcholine released per impulse, by increasing the sensitivity of the myoneural junction to acetylcholine, by diminishing the threshold of excitation of the motor nerve, and by enhancing the force of contraction of the myofibril. Tetany and convulsions may occur.

Cardiac muscle is affected by large increases in magnesium concentration in the range of 10–15 mEq/liter. Conduction time is increased, with lengthened duration of P–R and QRS components of the ECG. As the concentration of Mg^{++} increases further, cardiac arrest in diastole occurs.

Elevated magnesium concentrations produce vasodilatation and a drop in blood pressure by blockade of sympathetic ganglia as well as a direct effect on smooth muscle.

1. HYPERMAGNESEMIA

Magnesium excess is almost always the result of renal insufficiency and inability to excrete what has been absorbed from food or infused. Occasionally, with the use of magnesium sulfate as a cathartic, enough magnesium is absorbed to produce toxicity, particularly in the presence of impaired renal function. Manifestations of hypermagnesemia include muscle weakness, fall in blood pressure, and sedation and confusion. The ECG shows increased P–R interval, broadened QRS complexes, and elevated T waves. Death usually results from respiratory muscle paralysis.

Treatment

Treatment is directed toward alleviating renal insufficiency. Calcium acts as an antagonist to Mg^{++} and may be employed parenterally for temporary benefit. Extracorporeal or peritoneal dialysis may be indicated.

2. HYPOMAGNESEMIA

Magnesium deficit may be encountered in chronic alcoholism in association with delirium tremens, cirrhosis, pancreatitis, diabetic acidosis, starvation, diarrhea, malabsorption, prolonged gastrointestinal suction, vigorous diuresis, primary hyperaldosteronism, and hypoparathyroidism, particularly after parathyroidectomy for hyperparathyroidism and when large doses of vitamin D and calcium are consumed.

Magnesium deficit is characterized by neuromuscular and CNS hyperirritability with athetoid movements; jerking, coarse, and flapping tremors; positive Babinski response, nystagmus, tachycardia and ventricular arrhythmias, hypertension, and vasomotor changes. Confusion, disorientation, and restlessness may be prominent.

Treatment

Treatment consists of the use of parenteral fluids containing magnesium as chloride or sulfate, 10–40 mEq/day during the period of severe deficit followed by 10 mEq/day for maintenance. Magnesium sulfate may also be given IM, 4–8 gm (66–133 mEq) daily in 4 divided doses. Serum levels must be monitored to prevent the concentration from rising above 5–5.5 mEq/liter.

THE APPROACH TO DIAGNOSIS & TREATMENT OF WATER, ELECTROLYTE, & ACID-BASE DISTURBANCES

In the diagnosis and treatment of water and electrolyte derangements, one must rely upon clinical appraisal of the patient, including details of the history, the presenting disease and its complications, recent and abrupt change in weight, the physical examination, and the laboratory data bearing upon altered volume, osmolarity, distribution, and physiologic manifestations. Although a thorough knowledge of the physiologic principles of water and electrolyte metabolism and of renal function is essential to sound management and direction of therapy, the science of therapy is far from exact, and the physician must always consider and be grateful for the homeostatic resources of the patient. If renal function is reasonably good, the range between acceptable lower and upper limits of amounts of water and electrolytes is broad and the achievement of "balance" not difficult. In the presence of renal insufficiency, some endocrinopathies influencing water and electrolyte metabolism, shock, heart failure, hepatic insufficiency, severe gastrointestinal fluid loss, pulmonary insufficiency, and some rarer diseases, the patient is deprived of his homeostatic resources and the physician is called upon to substitute as best he can with close observation and meticulous quantitative therapy.

Some general principles will be included here. For difficult and complicated problems, more specialized and more complete texts must be consulted.

MAINTENANCE

Most of those who require water and electrolyte intravenously are relatively normal people who cannot take orally what they require for maintenance. It is apparent from Table 2–6 that the range of tolerance for water and electrolytes (homeostatic limits) permits reasonable latitude in therapy provided normal renal function exists to accomplish the final regulation of volume and concentration.

An average adult whose entire intake is parenteral

Table 2–6. Daily maintenance rations for patients requiring parenteral fluids.

	Per sq M Body Surface	Average Adult (60–100 kg)
Glucose	60–75 gm	100–200 gm
Na^+	50–70 mEq	80–120 mEq
K^+	50–70 mEq	80–120 mEq
Water	1500 ml	2500 ml

would receive his maintenance ration in 2500–3000 ml of 5% or 10% dextrose in 0.2% saline solution (34 mEq Na^+ + Cl^-/liter). To each liter, 30 mEq KCl could be added. In 3 liters, the total chloride intake would be 192 mEq, which is easily tolerated. An alternative would be to eliminate the KCl if parenteral fluids would be required for only 2–3 days. After 3 days of potassium-free parenteral fluids, total potassium loss may become significant and replacement is desirable. Other solutions available for maintenance therapy contain electrolyte mixtures designed to meet average adult requirements: in one example, each liter contains dextrose, 50 gm; Na^+, 40 mEq; K^+, 35 mEq; Cl^-, 40 mEq; HCO_3^- equivalent, 20 mEq; and $PO_4^\equiv$, 15 mEq. The daily administration of 2500–3000 ml satisfies the needs listed in Table 2–6.

In situations requiring maintenance or maintenance plus replacement of fluid and electrolyte by parenteral infusion, the total daily ration should be administered continuously over the 24-hour period in order to ensure the best utilization by the patient. Periodic large infusions result in responsive excretion by the kidney, reducing the opportunity for precise regulation by the kidney. Continuous infusion is desirable, particularly when losses are large and the total volume of the daily infusion is correspondingly large. With modern technics for continuous infusions, around-the-clock administration imposes little discomfort or hardship on the patient.

DEFICITS

To the maintenance ration one must add water and appropriate electrolyte for replacement of losses previously incurred and water and electrolytes to replace current losses. The amounts of water and electrolytes are dictated by clinical evaluation of deficits of each, and a further choice of anion would be dictated by the presence of metabolic acidosis or alkalosis and in some instances of respiratory acidosis.

The severity of dehydration (volume depletion) is assessed by means of the history, the magnitude of acute weight loss, and, on physical examination, the loss of elasticity of the skin and subcutaneous tissues, dry mucous membranes, tachycardia and hypotension, lethargy, and weakness. As dehydration becomes more severe, the decrease in plasma volume results in progression of hypotension and shock. Hemoconcentration progresses with loss of plasma water; electrolyte concentrations differ according to the losses incident to the primary disease; an increase in BUN reflects the decrease in glomerular filtration rate incident to circulatory changes associated with low blood volume.

Effective extracellular fluid volume and circulating blood volume accompany acutely occurring redistribution of fluid following burns, bowel obstruction, peritonitis, venous obstruction, and, rarely, lymphatic obstruction.

Treatment consists of replacement of water deficit with appropriate electrolyte replacement according to serum osmolarity (Na^+ concentration), blood pH, and serum K^+ concentration. In the presence of hyperosmolarity (hypernatremia), electrolyte-free or hypotonic solutions should be employed; if serum Na^+ concentration is normal, repletion can be accomplished with isotonic solutions. If hypo-osmolarity (hyponatremia) exists due to sodium loss, hypertonic (3–5%) NaCl solutions or hypertonic $NaHCO_3$ solutions may be required. In addition to replacement needs, maintenance requirements must be met, requiring correlation of volume, electrolyte concentration, and rate of administration to effect a normal state.

One should aim for total replacement in 48–72 hours. Time is required for circulation, diffusion, equilibration, renal response, and restoration of normal homeostatic mechanisms; a general rule is to provide daily maintenance needs plus half the deficit in the first 24 hours and a quarter of the deficit daily for 2 days thereafter to complete restitution in 72 hours. To this must be added the equivalent of continuing losses.

Common situations in which deficits may be large are discussed below. Other less common derangements are beyond the scope of this chapter. For therapeutic guidance, consult more detailed texts and specific treatises.

1. DIABETIC KETOSIS

Characterized by significant losses of water, sodium, and potassium in addition to retention of ketone body acids and a decrease in bicarbonate and pH in the extracellular fluid. Therapy is outlined in Chapter 18.

2. GASTROINTESTINAL DISEASE

Often accompanied by large losses of water, sodium, and potassium. Loss of chloride or bicarbonate is related to site of the disease or obstruction, eg, in pyloric obstruction with loss of HCl; small bowel fluid losses with loss of bicarbonate. (See Table 2–7.) Following intubation, the collected secretions should be assayed to determine the volume and losses of electrolyte that must be replaced.

3. BURNS

Edema accompanying the trauma to tissue results in sequestration of fluids in tissues beneath the burns with consequent decrease in circulating plasma volume and circulatory collapse. Therapy is described in Chapter 29.

Table 2–7. Volume and electrolyte content of gastrointestinal fluid losses.*

	Na⁺ (mEq/liter)	K⁺ (mEq/liter)	Cl⁻ (mEq/liter)	HCO₃⁻ (mEq/liter)	Volume (ml)
Gastric juice, high in acid	20 (10–30)	10 (5–40)	120 (80–150)	0	1000–9000
Gastric juice, low in acid	80 (70–140)	15 (5–40)	90 (40–120)	5–25	1000–2500
Pancreatic juice	140 (115–180)	5 (3–8)	75 (55–95)	80 (60–110)	500–1000
Bile	148 (130–160)	5 (3–12)	100 (90–120)	35 (30–40)	300–1000
Small bowel drainage	110 (80–150)	5 (2–8)	105 (60–125)	30 (20–40)	1000–3000
Distal ileum and cecum drainage	80 (40–135)	8 (5–30)	45 (20–90)	30 (20–40)	1000–3000
Diarrheal stools	120 (20–160)	25 (10–40)	90 (30–120)	45 (30–50)	500–17,000

*Average values/24 hours with range in parentheses.

4. PERITONITIS

Inflammation may produce a large collection of fluid in the peritoneal cavity. Prompt restoration of plasma volume and extracellular fluid is essential.

5. ASCITES

The association of liver disease with ascites and the consequences of therapy with diuretics may produce complex alterations of fluid distribution and electrolyte concentrations. (See Chapter 10.)

• • •

SUMMARY OF CLINICAL APPROACH

The following outline summarizes an approach to therapy with water and electrolytes. Listed are factors essential to an assessment of the state of the patient, of the urgency for treatment, and of the choice of the therapeutic agents and the quantities to be administered. This outline has been useful in planning the therapeutic attack and averting the omission of essential elements of treatment.

Problems
1. Simple maintenance.
2. Repair of deficit plus maintenance.
3. Repair plus replacement of continuing losses plus maintenance.
4. Replacement of continuing losses plus maintenance.

Situations: Acute or Chronic
   A. Acute:
   1. Respiratory—P_{CO_2} and pH. Often overlooked. H⁺ concentration can change rapidly to life-threatening levels.
   2. Organic ion acidosis (lactate, ketones), "anion gap." Normally, $Cl^- + CO_2 + 12 = Na^+$ in mEq/liter, or $Cl^- + \frac{1}{2} CO_2 + 25 = Na^+$ in mEq/liter.
   3. Plasma K⁺ concentration deficit or excess.
   4. Hyper- or hypo-osmolality, often iatrogenic.
   5. Explosive gastrointestinal loss, Addison's disease in crisis.
   6. Acute renal shutdown.
   B. Chronic:
   1. Renal insufficiency.
   2. Pulmonary insufficiency.
   3. Chronic gastrointestinal disease (gut, liver).
   4. Endocrine abnormality, especially myxedema.

Determinants in Establishing Therapy
   Sex: Females are usually fatter and, therefore, have lower total body water ratios (per kg) than males.
   Size: Fat or lean; more fat means lower ratios of total body water/kg.
   Renal and pulmonary function.
   Cause of abnormal state, ie, shock, gastrointestinal obstruction, third space sequestration, diabetes or other endocrine abnormality, malnutrition, induced by drug effect or therapeutic error.

Observations
   Weight.
   Intake, output, and loss record.
   Serum electrolytes, osmolality, urea or creatinine, protein, glucose.
   Arterial blood P_{CO_2}, pH, P_{O_2} as indicated.
   Urine specific gravity, osmolality, volume.

• • •

Tables 2–8, 2–9, 2–10, and 2–11 indicate the wide choices open to the physician in planning the restoration of water and electrolyte in the variety of clinical problems that may occur. A sound understanding of the physiologic mechanisms discussed above enables the physician to direct therapy rationally and with considerable skill. If renal and pulmonary function are compromised, the task becomes difficult and hazardous for even the best informed clinicians.

Table 2—8. Examples of solutions for parenteral infusion.

	Electrolyte Content in mEq/liter								Glucose (gm/liter)
	Na^+	K^+	Ca^{++}	Mg^{++}	NH_4^+	Cl^-	HCO_3^- Equiv*	$PO_4^{\equiv}$	
5% glucose in water									50
10% glucose in water									100
Isotonic saline (0.9%)	155					155			
Sodium chloride (5%)	855					855			
Ringer's solution	147	4	4			155			
Ringer's lactate (Hartmann's)	130	4	3			109	28		
Darrow's solution (KNL)	121	35				103	53		
Potassium chloride									
0.2% in dextrose 5%		27				27			50
0.3% in dextrose 5%		40				40			50
"Modified duodenal solution"									
with dextrose, 10%	80	36	5	3		64	60		100
"Gastric solution" with									
dextrose, 10%	63	17			70	150			100
Ammonium chloride, 0.9%					170	170			
Sodium lactate, 1/6 molar	167						167		
Sodium bicarbonate, 1/6 molar	167						167		
Examples of "maintenance solutions":									
Pediatric electrolyte									
"No. 48" with dextrose 5%	25	20		3		22	23	3	50
Maintenance electrolyte									
"No. 75" with dextrose 5%	40	35				40	20	15	50
Levulose and dextrose with									
electrolyte (Butler's II)	58	25		6		51	25	13	100
5% dextrose in 0.2% saline	34					34			50
10% dextrose in 0.45% saline	77					77			100

*HCO_3^- equivalent may be bicarbonate, lactate, acetate, gluconate or citrate, or combinations of these.
A variety of modifications of multiple electrolyte solutions are commercially available.

Table 2—9. Examples of electrolyte concentrates.

	Ampule Volume	Electrolyte Content in mEq per Ampule								
		Na^+	K^+	Ca^{++}	Mg^{++}	NH_4^+	Cl^-	HCO_3^-	Lactate	$PO_4^{\equiv}$
Potassium chloride*	10 ml		20				20			
KMC*	10 ml		25	10	10		45			
Potassium phosphate*	20 ml		40							40
Calcium gluconate, 10%	10 ml			4.5					4.5 (gluconate)	
Sodium bicarbonate, 7.5%†	50 ml	45						45		
Sodium lactate, molar†	40 ml	40							40	
Ammonium chloride*	30 ml					120	120			
Magnesium sulfate, 50%	—				8‡					

Note: The physician should always check the contents of the ampule as listed by the manufacturer.
*Dilute to 1 liter or more.
†Dilute as indicated by the manufacturer.
‡8 mEq/ml.

Table 2–10. Examples of oral electrolyte preparations.

Preparation	Supplied As	Electrolyte Content*					
		Na$^+$	K$^+$	NH$_4^+$	Ca^{++}	Cl$^-$	HCO$_3^-$
NaCl	Salt	17				17	
NaHCO$_3$	Salt	12					12
KCl	Salt		14			14	
K-triplex	Elixir		15 mEq/ 5 ml				
K gluconate (Kaon)	Elixir		7 mEq/ 5 ml				
Ca gluconate	Salt				4.5		
Ca lactate	Salt				10		
NH$_4$Cl (acidifying salt)	Salt			19†		19	
Kayexalate (ion-exchange resins)	Salt	1‡	‡				

*mEq/gm unless otherwise specified.
†NH$_4^+$ is converted to H$^+$ in the body, mEq for mEq.
‡1 gm resin removes 1 mEq K$^+$ and contributes 3 mEq Na$^+$ to patient.

Table 2–11. Equivalent values of salts
used for therapy.*

Salt	gm	mEq of Cation per Amount Stated
IV or oral		
NaCl	9	155
NaCl	5.8	100
NaCl	1	17
NaHCO$_3$	8.4	100
Na lactate	11.2	100
KCl	1.8	25
K acetate	2.5	25
K$_2$HPO$_4$	1.84	25
KH$_2$PO$_4$	0.4	
CaCl$_2$	0.5	10
Ca gluconate	2	10
MgCl$_2$	0.5	10
Oral		
K citrate	3	25
K tartrate	5	27

*Reproduced, with permission, from Krupp MA & others: *Physician's Handbook,* 18th ed. Lange, 1976.

● ● ●

Bibliography

General

Buckalew VM Jr & others: (1) Potassium balance: Walking the mEq tightrope. (2) Assessing the risks of hypokalemia. (3) Repleting the patient's potassium. (Round table discussion.) Patient Care 9:20–69, Jan 15, 1975.

Buckalew VM Jr & others: (1) Potassium balance: Walking the mEq tightrope (cont'd). (2) Hyperkalemia: Who is at risk? (3) Lowering serum K and keeping it normal. (Round table discussion.) Patient Care 9:124–155, Feb 1, 1975.

Buckalew VM Jr & others: (1) Balancing sodium on the mEq tightrope. (2) The patient threatened by hyponatremia. (3) Repleting salt in everyday practice. (4) Evaluating and treating hypernatremia. (Round table discussion.) Patient Care 10:20–58, Feb 15, 1975.

Fisch C: Relation of electrolyte disturbances to cardiac arrhythmias. Circulation 47:408, 1973.

Hutchin P: Metabolic response to surgery in relation to caloric, fluid and electrolyte intake. Curr Probl Surg, April 1971.

Lindeman RD, Papper S: Therapy of fluid and electrolyte disorders. Ann Int Med 82:64, 1975. [See also editorial note, p 114, and comments and corrections, pp 844, 845, and 846.]

Maxwell M, Kleeman CR (editors): *Clinical Disorders of Fluid and Electrolyte Metabolism*, 2nd ed. McGraw-Hill, 1972.

Pitts RF: *Physiology of the Kidney and Body Fluids*, 3rd ed. Year Book, 1974.

Schwartz AB: Diuretic-induced hypokalemia. Am Family Physician 11:101–104, 1975. [See also editor's note, p 57.]

Share L & others: Regulation of body fluids. Ann Rev Physiol 34:235, 1972.

Vidt DG: Use and abuse of intravenous solutions. JAMA 232:533, 1975. [See also editorial comment, p 516.]

Weiner M & others: Signs and symptoms of electrolyte disorders. Yale J Biol Med 43:76, 1970.

Fluid Volume & Sodium

Bricker NS, Klahr S: The physiologic basis of sodium excretion and diuresis. Advances Int Med 16:17, 1970.

Earley LE, Daugharty TM: Sodium metabolism. New England J Med 281:72, 1969.

Hantman D & others: Rapid correction of hyponatremia in the syndrome of inappropriate secretion of antidiuretic hormone. Ann Int Med 78:870, 1973.

Kleeman CR, Fichman MP: The clinical physiology of water metabolism. New England J Med 277:1300, 1967.

Loeb JN: The hyperosmolar state. New England J Med 290:1184, 1974.

Nolph KD & others: Sodium, potassium and water metabolism in the syndrome of inappropriate antidiuretic hormone secretion. Am J Med 49:534, 1970.

Schrier RW, Berl T: Hyponatremia and related disorders. The Kidney, vol 7, Jan 1974.

Hydrogen Ion

Albert MS, Dell RB, Winters RB: Quantitative displacement of acid-base equilibrium in metabolic acidosis. Ann Int Med 66:312, 1967.

Garella S & others: Severity of metabolic acidosis as a determinant of bicarbonate requirements. New England J Med 289:121, 1973.

Kassirer JP: Serious acid-base disorders. New England J Med 291:773, 1974.

Lubowitz H & others: Lactic acidosis. Arch Int Med 134:148, 1974.

Manfredi F: Effects of hypocapnia and hypercapnia on intracellular acid-base equilibrium in man. J Lab Clin Med 69:304, 1967.

Pitts RF: The role of ammonia production and excretion in the regulation of acid-base balance. New England J Med 284:32, 1971.

Seldin DW, Rector FC Jr: The generation and maintenance of metabolic alkalosis. Kidney Internat 1:306, 1972.

Simpson DP: Control of hydrogen ion homeostasis and renal acidosis. Medicine 50:503, 1971.

Statement of acid-base terminology. Ann Int Med 63:885, 1965; Anesthesiology 27:7, 1966; Ann New York Acad Sc 133:251, 1966.

Steinmetz PR: Excretion of acid by the kidney: Functional organization and cellular aspects of acidification. New England J Med 278:1102, 1968.

Tranquada RE, Grant WJ, Peterson CR: Lactic acidosis. Arch Int Med 117:192, 1966.

Van Ypersele de Strihou C, Brasseur L, McConinck J: The "carbon-dioxide response curve" for chronic hypercapnia in man. New England J Med 275:117, 1966.

Potassium

Katsikas JL & others: Disorders of potassium metabolism. M Clin North America 55:503, 1971.

Kosman ME: Management of potassium problems during long-term diuretic therapy. JAMA 230:743, 1974.

Rovner DR: Use of pharmacologic agents in the treatment of hypokalemia and hyperkalemia. Ration Drug Ther 6:1, Feb 1972.

Schwartz WB & others: Role of anions in metabolic alkalosis and potassium deficiency. New England J Med 279:630, 1968.

Surawicz B: Electrolytes and the electrocardiogram. Am J Cardiol 12:656, 1964.

Weatherall M: Ions and the actions of digitalis. Brit Heart J 28:497, 1966.

Calcium

Breuer RI, LeBauer L: Caution in the use of phosphates in the treatment of severe hypercalcemia. J Clin Endocrinol 27:695, 1967.

Foster GV: Calcitonin (thyrocalcitonin). New England J Med 279:349, 1968.

Goldsmith RS, Ingbar SH: Inorganic phosphate treatment of hypercalcemia of diverse etiologies. (2 parts.) New England J Med 274:1, 284, 1966.

Kleeman CR & others: The clinical physiology of calcium homeostasis, parathyroid hormone, and calcitonin. (2 parts.) California Med 114:16 (March), 19 (April), 1971.

Perlia CP & others: Mithramycin treatment of hypercalcemia. Cancer 25:389, 1970.

Rasmussen H: Ionic and hormonal control of calcium homeostasis. Am J Med 50:567, 1971.

Singer FR & others: Mithramycin treatment of intractable hypercalcemia due to parathyroid carcinoma. New England J Med 283:634, 1970.

Suki WN & others: Acute treatment of hypercalcemia with furosemide. New England J Med 283:836, 1970.

Magnesium

Flink EB, Jones JE (editors): The pathogenesis and clinical significance of magnesium deficiency. Ann New York Acad Sc (Article 2, entire issue), 1969.

Gitelman HJ, Welt LG: Magnesium deficiency. Ann Rev Med 20:233, 1969.

Hall RCW, Joffe JR: Hypomagnesemia: Physical and psychiatric symptoms. JAMA 224:1749, 1973.

Iseri LT, Freed J, Bures AR: Magnesium deficiency and cardiac disorders. Am J Med 58:837, 1975.

Wacker WEC, Parisi AF: Magnesium metabolism. New England J Med 278:772, 1968.

3...
Skin & Appendages

Rees B. Rees, Jr.

Diagnosis of Skin Disorders

Take a thorough case history from every patient with a skin disease. Do not neglect the role of constitutional factors in production or aggravation of skin diseases (eg, internal disease, emotional factors, dietary aberrations). Inquire about systemic and topical medications. Examine the entire body surface in good (preferably natural) light.

Planning the Treatment

Many topical agents are available for the treatment of dermatologic disorders. In general, it is better to be thoroughly familiar with a few drugs and treatment methods than to attempt to use a great many.

In planning the treatment it is necessary to consider the individual character of the patient's skin. Dry skins usually require lubricating or softening agents; moist or oily skins usually require greaseless drying agents.

Begin treatment with mild, simple remedies. In general, acute, inflamed lesions are best treated with soothing, nonirritating agents; chronic, thickened lesions with stimulating or keratolytic agents. When appropriate, apply a small amount of drug to a small area and observe for several hours for skin sensitivity.

Do not change remedies before the agent has had time to demonstrate its effectiveness. However, discontinue the drug immediately if an untoward local reaction develops.

Instruct the patient carefully on how to apply medicaments.

When in doubt about the proper method of treatment, *undertreat* rather than overtreat.

Note: Prescription numbers in the text refer to Tables 3–1 to 3–6 at the end of the chapter.

General Rules Governing Choice of Topical Treatment of Various Stages of Dermatoses

Note: The choice of treatment will vary with the individual case depending upon the characteristics of the dermatosis, the extent of the lesions, the general character of the patient's skin, previous medication and drug allergies, and other factors.

A. Acute Lesions: (Recent onset, red, burning, swollen, itching, blistering, or oozing.) Use wet preparations (Table 3–1), such as soaks, for lesions localized to extremities; cool wet dressings for localized lesions of the head, neck, trunk, or extremities; or baths for generalized lesions (see below under Pruritus).

B. Subacute Lesions: (Intermediate duration, subsiding lesions, and lesions which are less angry in appearance.) Use wet preparations as outlined above, shake lotions (Table 3–3), or both.

C. Chronic Lesions: (Longer duration, quiescent, thickened, encrusted, fissured, scaly.) Use wet preparations or shake lotions (or both) as outlined above, or any of the following: emulsions (Table 3–3); hydrophilic ointments (Table 3–4); pastes (high powder content) (Table 3–4); creams such as cold cream and vanishing creams (Table 3–4); or greasy ointments (Table 3–5).

Prevention of Complications

The most common complications of skin diseases are pyoderma, local or systemic spread of infection, overtreatment dermatitis, drug sensitivity reactions, and cosmetic disfiguration.

A. Pyoderma: Infected, inflamed, or denuded areas of skin are receptive environments for pyogenic organisms introduced by scratching, rubbing, or squeezing of skin lesions. Patients should be instructed to wash their hands frequently and to avoid manipulation of infected areas. Medications should be kept in closed containers and applied with sterile applicators, which should be discarded after use. Crusts and scabs should not be removed except by the physician. If an infection occurs in a hairy portion of the body, special care should be taken in cleansing and shaving the area.

B. Local or Systemic Spread of Infection: Almost any skin infection may spread by extension or through blood vascular or lymphatic channels. In most cases this complication is a much greater threat to the patient's health and life than the primary skin infection. A most striking and serious example is the extension of staphylococcal infections of the face to the cavernous sinuses. Lymphangitis, lymphadenitis, septicemia, renal carbuncle, bladder infections, and glomerulonephritis may occur as sequelae to primary skin infection. For these reasons it is important to institute vigorous local and systemic measures for the control of skin infections. Systemic antibiotics, selected on the basis of bacteriologic studies if time permits, should be used promptly for potentially serious infections or those associated with systemic reactions.

C. Overtreatment Dermatitis: This may be avoided if the physician and the patient are aware that undertreatment is preferable to overtreatment and if the patient is warned to avoid overenthusiastic application of topical remedies (either too much or too long). Fluorinated topical corticosteroids may induce acne-like processes on the face and atrophic striae in body folds, and in cirrhotics may induce acute adrenocortical insufficiency and aseptic bone necrosis.

D. Exfoliative Dermatitis: This complication cannot always be anticipated or avoided, but it may be minimized if a careful history of drug sensitivity is obtained before institution of drug therapy. In allergic individuals it is important to apply a small amount of topical medication in order to determine hypersensitivity. Drugs which may be required for systemic use (eg, sulfonamides, antibiotics, or antihistamines) should preferably not be used in topical preparations. Sodium sulfacetamide and erythromycin appear to be safe for topical use. Neomycin, because of its high sensitizing potential, is not the antibiotic of first choice for topical use.

E. Cosmetic Disfiguration: Disfiguration due to skin disorders may be avoided by early, careful treatment of skin lesions and by appropriate dermatologic operative technics. Self-manipulation of skin lesions, especially on the face and exposed skin areas, should be avoided.

Domonkos A: *Andrews' Diseases of the Skin.* Saunders, 1971.

PRURITUS
(Itching)

"Pruritus is that disagreeable sensation that excites the desire to scratch." (Haffenreffer.) It is the commonest presenting symptom in dermatology, and includes localized or generalized itching, stinging, crawling, and burning sensations. Pruritus is far less well tolerated than pain.

Itching is a modified form of pain, carried on slow afferent fibers.

Transient, mild pruritus may be physiologic. Pruritus may be a symptom of specific dermatologic disorders; may be idiopathic; or may foreshadow or accompany serious disease of internal origin (lymphomas and other neoplasms—especially Hodgkin's disease—hepatic or biliary disease, diabetes mellitus [generalized itching in an undiagnosed case is rare], nephritis, or drug intoxication or habituation). Perhaps the most common cause of generalized pruritus is excessive dryness of the skin, as in overbathing (especially in the elderly), borderline forms of ichthyosis, senile degeneration complicated by irritation with soaps, and low humidity due to artificial heating and cold weather. Other causes are pressure and chafing; chemical irritants (including drugs); contact and other allergies; and emotional factors.

Treatment

A. General Measures: Foods should be simple; avoid rich and spicy foods. Test diets or elimination diets are indicated for suspected food allergies. If pruritus is believed to be primarily a manifestation of an emotional disorder, direct therapy accordingly. External irritants (eg, rough clothing, occupational contactants) should be avoided. Soaps and detergents should not be used by persons with dry or irritated skin. Baths containing a small amount of bath oil may be used. Nails should be kept trimmed and clean. Avoid scratching, if possible. Unnecessary medications should be discontinued since medication itself often produces pruritus.

B. Specific Measures: Remove or treat specific causes whenever possible.

C. Local Measures:

1. Shake lotions, emulsions, and ointments, incorporating the volatile analgesics and antipruritics listed in Table 3–1, may be of value in relieving itching.

2. If the skin is too dry, an excellent principle is to wet it, as in a bath (to hydrate the keratin), and then apply petrolatum to the wet skin to trap the moisture.

3. If the skin is too moist, drying agents may afford relief, eg, wet dressings, soaks (R 1–5, R 7); shake lotions (R 13–15); and powders (R 8–11) (especially if the process is acute).

4. Tub baths—Generalized pruritus may often be effectively controlled by lukewarm baths, 15 minutes 2–3 times daily. Elderly patients with dry skin should bathe as infrequently as possible. After bathing, the skin should be blotted (not rubbed) dry. (*Caution:* Avoid excessive drying of skin by overbathing, prolonged bathing periods, and exposure to drafts after bathing.) Useful bath formulations are as follows: (1) Tar bath: Dissolve 50–100 ml of coal tar solution USP in 1 tubful (50 gallons) of warm water. (Watch for sensitivity.) (2) Bath oils: 5–25 ml in 1 tubful (50 gallons) of warm water (Alpha-Keri, Nivea skin oil, Lubath, Domol, and many others). Bubble baths should be avoided.

D. Potentiation of Topical Corticosteroid Creams: By covering selected lesions of psoriasis, lichen planus, and localized eczemas each night, first with the corticosteroid, then with a thin plastic pliable film (eg, Saran Wrap), between 1–2% of the medicament may be absorbed. Complications include miliaria, striae, pyoderma, heat stroke, adrenal cortical suppression, local skin atrophy, malodor, fungal infection, and urticarial erythema.

E. Systemic Antipruritic Drugs:

1. Antihistaminic and "antiserotonin" drugs may be tried in certain cases of pruritus of allergic or undetermined cause. There is no "preferred" antihistamine, although chlorpheniramine, 4 mg 2–4 times daily, is cheap and less likely to cause drowsiness than others.

2. Epinephrine injection, 0.25–1 ml of 1:1000 solution every 4 hours, may be of value in acute urticaria.

3. Phenobarbital, 15—30 mg 2—4 times daily, may provide useful sedation in agitated or distracted patients. Barbiturates themselves may rarely produce dermatitis.

4. Corticotropin or the corticosteroids (see Chapter 18).

Prognosis

Elimination of external factors and irritating agents is often successful in giving complete relief of pruritus. Pruritus accompanying specific skin disease will subside when the disease is brought under control. Idiopathic pruritus and that accompanying serious internal disease may not respond to any type of therapy.

Blank H & others: Symposium on corticosteroids in cutaneous diseases. 2. Weighing the risks and benefits of steroid use. Mod Med 42:45, 1974. 4. Side effects, topical preparations, and occlusion. Mod Med 43:46, 1974.

Burton JL & others: Complications of topical corticosteroid therapy in patients with liver disease. Brit J Dermat 91 (Suppl 10):22, 1974.

Chernosky M: Dry skin and its consequences. J Am Med Wom Assoc 27:133, 1972.

Fine R: Physiologic effects of systemic corticosteroids in dermatology. Cutis 11:217, 1973.

Loder JS: Treatment of jellyfish stings. JAMA 226:1228, 1973.

Mikhail GR, Sweet LC, Mellinger RC: Parenteral long-acting corticosteroids: Effect on hypothalamic-pituitary-adrenal function. Ann Allergy 31:337, 1973.

Munro DD, Clift DC: Pituitary-adrenal function after prolonged use of topical corticosteroids. Brit J Dermat 88:381, 1973.

Wilson L, Williams DI, Marsh SD: Plasma corticosteroid levels in outpatients treated with topical steroids. Brit J Dermat 88:373, 1973.

Zaynoun ST, Salti S: The effect of intracutaneous glucocorticoids on plasma cortisol levels. Brit J Dermat 88:151, 1973.

COMMON DERMATOSES

CONTACT DERMATITIS
(Dermatitis Venenata)

Essentials of Diagnosis

- Erythema and edema, often followed by vesicles and bullae in area of contact with suspected agent.
- Later weeping, crusting, and secondary infection.
- Often a history of previous reaction to suspected contactant.
- Patch test with agent usually positive in the allergic form.

General Considerations

Contact dermatitis is an acute or chronic dermatitis which results from direct skin contact with chemicals or other irritants (eg, poison ivy). Lesions are most often on exposed parts. Four-fifths of such disturbances are due to excessive exposure to or additive effects of primary or universal irritants (eg, soaps, detergents, organic solvents). Others are due to actual contact allergy. The most common allergies to dermatologic agents include antimicrobials (especially neomycin), antihistamines, anesthetics, and preservatives.

Clinical Findings

A. Symptoms and Signs: Itching, burning, and stinging are often extremely severe, distributed on exposed parts or in bizarre asymmetric patterns. The lesions consist of erythematous macules, papules, and vesicles. The affected area is often hot and swollen, with exudation, crusting, and secondary infection. The pattern of the eruption may be diagnostic (eg, typical linear streaked vesicles on the extremities and erythema and swelling of the genitals in poison oak dermatitis). The location will often suggest the cause: scalp involvement suggests hair tints, lacquer, shampoos, or tonics; face involvement, creams, soaps, shaving materials; neck involvement, jewelry, fingernail polish; etc.

B. Laboratory Findings: The patch test may be useful but has serious limitations. In the event of a positive reaction, a control test must be done on another individual to rule out primary irritation. Photopatch tests may be necessary in the case of suspected photosensitivity contact dermatitis. These are done by exposing the traditional patch test site to sunlight after 24 hours.

Differential Diagnosis

Asymmetric distribution and a history of contact help distinguish contact dermatitis from other skin lesions. Eruptions may be due to primary irritation from chemicals or allergic sensitization to contactants. The commonest sensitizers are poison oak and ivy, rubber antioxidants and accelerators, nickel, mercury, and chromium salts, formalin, ethylenediamine, turpentine, and halogenated salicylanilide antiseptics. Differentiation may be difficult if the area of involvement is consistent with that seen in other types of skin disorders such as scabies, dermatophytid, atopic dermatitis, and other eczemas.

Prevention

Prevent reexposure to irritants. Avoid soaps and detergents. Use unscented cosmetics or eliminate cosmetics entirely. Protective rubber gloves may be used. In such cases an inner cotton glove must be used. Protective (barrier) creams are almost useless. It may be necessary to change occupation or duties if occupational exposure is otherwise unavoidable.

Plant irritants (especially Rhus species, eg, poison ivy) should be destroyed by manual removal or by chemical means (2,4-D or dichlorophenoxyacetic acid) near dwellings and in frequented areas.

Prompt and thorough removal of irritants by prolonged washing or by removal with solvents or other chemical agents may be effective if done very shortly after exposure. In the case of Rhus toxin, thorough washing with soap and water must be done within a few minutes if it is to be of any value.

Most well-controlled studies indicate that injection or ingestion of Rhus antigen is of no practical clinical value.

Treatment

A. General Measures: For acute severe cases, one may give prednisone, 35 mg immediately, then 30, 25, 20, 15, 10, and 5 mg on successive days. Triamcinolone (Kenalog) IM, 40 mg once intragluteally, may be used instead. (See Chapter 18.)

B. Local Measures: Treat the stage and type of dermatitis (see p 32).

1. Acute weeping dermatitis—Do not scrub lesions with soap and water. Apply solutions (Table 3–1). Shake lotions (R 13–15) may be indicated instead of wet dressings or in intervals between wet dressings, especially for involvement of intertriginous areas or when oozing is not marked. Lesions on the extremities may be bandaged with wet dressings. Hydrocortisone and related preparations in lotion, cream, or ointment applied sparingly 2–4 times daily may be very helpful. Corticosteroid sprays may be best (avoid the eyes and genitalia).

2. Subacute dermatitis (subsiding)—Use shake lotions.

3. Chronic dermatitis (dry and lichenified)—Treat with hydrophilic, greasy ointments or creams. Tars are perhaps most useful in this stage of the dermatitis.

Prognosis

Contact dermatitis is self-limited if reexposure is prevented. Spontaneous desensitization may occur. Increasing sensitivity to industrial irritants may necessitate a change of occupation.

Baer RL & others: The most common contact allergens. Arch Dermat 108:74, 1973.

Maibach HI: Patch testing: An objective tool. Cutis 13:613, 1974.

Routine Patch Test Series (1974): Recommendation by the International Contact Dermatitis Research Group. Brit J Dermat 89:437, 1973.

Rudner EJ & others: Epidemiology of contact dermatitis in North America: 1972. Arch Dermat 108:537, 1973.

ERYTHEMA NODOSUM

Essentials of Diagnosis

- Painful red nodules on anterior aspects of legs.
- No ulceration seen.
- Slow regression over several weeks to resemble contusions.
- Some cases associated with infection or drug sensitivity.
- Women are predominantly affected.

General Considerations

Erythema nodosum is a symptom complex characterized by tender, erythematous nodules which appear most commonly on the extensor surfaces of the legs. It usually lasts about 6 weeks, and may be recurrent. It may be associated with various infections (primary coccidioidomycosis, other deep fungal infections, primary tuberculosis, streptococcosis, rheumatic fever, or syphilis) or may be due to drug sensitivity (penicillin, phenacetin, progestins). It may accompany leukemia, sarcoidosis, and ulcerative colitis. Infections with unusual organisms such as *Pasteurella (Yersinia) pseudotuberculosis* may be responsible. Erythema nodosum may be associated with pregnancy.

Clinical Findings

A. Symptoms and Signs: The swellings are exquisitely tender, and are usually preceded by fever, malaise, and arthralgia. The nodules are most often located on the anterior surfaces of the legs below the knees but may occur (rarely) on the arms, trunk, and face. The lesions, 1–10 cm in diameter, are at first pink to red; with regression, all the various hues seen in a contusion can be observed. The nodules occasionally become fluctuant, but they do not suppurate.

B. Laboratory Findings: The histologic finding of fat replacement atrophy in the corium or dermis is strongly suggestive of erythema nodosum. Hilar adenopathy is often seen on chest x-ray. Antistreptolysin titer may be elevated, and the throat culture may be positive in cases caused by streptococci.

Differential Diagnosis

Erythema induratum is seen on the posterior surfaces of the legs and shows ulceration. Nodular vasculitis is usually on the calves and is associated with phlebitis. Erythema multiforme occurs in generalized distribution. In the late stages, erythema nodosum must be distinguished from simple bruises and contusions.

Treatment

A. General Measures: Eliminate or treat the "specific" cause, eg, systemic infection and exogenous toxins. Rest in the hospital may be advisable. Focal infections should be treated, although this does not appear to influence the course of the disease. Systemic therapy directed against the lesions themselves may include tetracycline drugs, 250 mg 4 times daily for several days; or corticosteroid therapy (see Chapter 18) unless it is contraindicated (tuberculosis must be ruled out).

B. Local Treatment: This is usually not necessary. Hot or cold compresses may help.

Prognosis

The lesions usually disappear after about 6 weeks,

but they may recur. The prognosis depends in part on that of the primary disease.

Editorial: Nodose erythema. Tr St Johns Hosp Dermat Soc 58:103, 1972.

Forstrom L, Winkelmann RK: Granulomatous panniculitis in erythema nodosum. Arch Dermat 111:335, 1975.

ERYTHEMA MULTIFORME

Essentials of Diagnosis

- Sudden onset of symmetric erythematous skin lesions with history of recurrence.
- May be macular, papular, urticarial, bullous, or purpuric.
- "Target" lesions with clear centers and concentric erythematous rings may be noted.
- Mostly on extensor surfaces; may be on palms, soles, or mucous membranes.
- History of herpes simplex, systemic infection or disease, and drug reactions may be associated.

General Considerations

Erythema multiforme is an acute inflammatory, polymorphic skin disease of multiple or undetermined origin. It may occur as a primary skin disorder or as a skin manifestation of systemic infection, malignant or chronic disease of the internal organs (including chronic ulcerative colitis, rheumatoid state, lupus erythematosus, and dermatomyositis), or as a reaction to an ingested drug or injected serum. Herpes simplex virus and infestations such as ascariasis have also been implicated. The lesions occur predominantly in the spring and fall, and are most common in young people. Unfortunately, very little is known about the pathogenesis.

Clinical Findings

A. Symptoms and Signs: The onset is sudden, often accompanied by burning sensations. There may be soreness of the oral, ocular, and genital mucous membranes. Several lesions may be present with relatively little discomfort. Slight to severe headache, backache, and malaise may occur, and slight to moderate fever.

The principal sign is the symmetric distribution of grouped or isolated crops of violaceous, edematous papules, macules, or nodules, 0.5–1 cm in diameter, with dome-shaped surfaces. The lesions enlarge and become purplish. The term "multiforme" signifies that the lesions may have many varieties. In addition to those just listed, there may be vesicles, bullae, pustules, urticarial lesions, and hemorrhagic alterations. The bullae may resemble those of pemphigus, but usually are surrounded by an erythematous halo. A rather characteristic lesion is the erythema iris (herpes iris), the "bull's eye" pattern formed by an erythematous papule with central clearing. Lesions are usually on the extensor surfaces but may appear anywhere, such as the palms and soles. Mucous membrane ulcerations (aphthae) are frequent. The tracheobronchial mucosa may be involved in severe cases (Stevens-Johnson variant), causing bronchitis and atelectasis. A rare type, erythema perstans, may be present for months or years.

B. Laboratory Findings: There are no characteristic laboratory findings. Histologic changes may be suggestive but are not pathognomonic.

Differential Diagnosis

Secondary syphilis, urticaria, drug eruptions, and toxic epidermal necrolysis must be ruled out. The bullous variety of erythema multiforme is more severe and should be differentiated from dermatitis herpetiformis, pemphigus, and pemphigoid. In erythema multiforme there is usually some constitutional reaction, including fever.

Complications

Erythema multiforme may be complicated by visceral lesions (eg, pneumonitis, myocarditis, nephritis).

Prevention

Avoid all unnecessary medications in patients with a history of erythema multiforme.

Treatment

A. General Measures: Bed rest and good nursing care when fever is present.

B. Specific Measures: Eliminate causative factors such as chronic systemic infections (eg, tuberculosis), focal infections, and sensitizing drugs. Tetracycline, 250 mg 4 times daily for several days, may be useful. Corticosteroids may be tried, as for erythema nodosum. Sulfapyridine, 0.5 gm 4 times daily, may succeed where other measures fail.

C. Local Measures: Treat the stage and type of dermatitis (see p 32). For acute lesions, employ simple wet dressings and soaks or soothing lotions. (For treatment of buccal lesions, see Aphthous Ulcer in Chapter 10.) Subacute lesions require soothing lotions.

Prognosis

The illness usually lasts 2–6 weeks and may recur. The Stevens-Johnson syndrome, a variant of this process (with associated visceral involvement), may be serious or even fatal. The prognosis depends in part on that of the primary disease.

Ackerman AB: Dermal and epidermal types of erythema multiforme. (Correspondence.) Arch Dermat 111:795, 1975.

Orfanos CE, Schaumburg-Lever G, Lever WF: Dermal and epidermal types of erythema multiforme. Arch Dermat 109:682, 1974.

PEMPHIGUS

Essentials of Diagnosis
- Relapsing crops of bullae appearing on normal skin.
- Often preceded by mucous membrane bullae, erosions, and ulcerations.
- Nikolsky's sign (superficial detachment of skin after pressure or trauma) variably present.
- Acantholysis (Tzanck test) presumably is diagnostic.

General Considerations
Pemphigus is an uncommon skin disease of unknown etiology which is always fatal within 2 months to 5 years if untreated. The bullae appear spontaneously and are relatively asymptomatic, but the complications of the disease lead to great toxicity and debility. There is a surprising lack of pathologic internal medical findings; no primary lesions are found in internal organs at biopsy. The disease occurs almost exclusively in adults, and occurs in all races and ethnic groups. Studies have demonstrated the presence of circulating autoantibodies to intercellular substances. Pemphigus can present with atypical features, and repeated reevaluation of clinical features, immunofluorescent changes, and histopathology may be necessary.

Clinical Findings
A. Symptoms and Signs: Pemphigus is characterized by an insidious onset of bullae in crops or waves. The lesions may appear first on the mucous membranes, and these rapidly become erosive. Toxemia and a "mousy" odor may occur soon. Rubbing the thumb on the surface of uninvolved skin may cause easy separation of the epidermis (Nikolsky's sign).

B. Laboratory Findings: On a smear taken from the base of a bulla and stained with Giemsa's stain (Tzanck test) one may see a unique histologic picture of disruption of the epidermal intercellular connections, called acantholysis. There may be leukocytosis and eosinophilia. As the disease progresses, low serum protein levels may be found as well as serum electrolyte changes. The sedimentation rate may be elevated, and anemia may be present. Intercellular antibody may be detected by the indirect immunofluorescence test on the patient's serum.

Differential Diagnosis
Acantholysis is not seen in other bullous eruptions such as erythema multiforme, drug eruptions, contact dermatitis, or bullous impetigo, or in the less common dermatitis herpetiformis and pemphigoid. All of these diseases have gross clinical characteristics and different immunofluorescence test results which distinguish them from pemphigus.

Complications
Secondary infection commonly occurs, often causing extreme debility. Terminally there may be shock, septicemia, disturbances of electrolyte balance, cachexia, toxemia, and pneumonia.

Treatment
A. General Measures: Hospitalize the patient at bed rest and provide antibiotics, blood transfusions, and intravenous feedings as indicated. Anesthetic troches may be used before eating to ease painful oral lesions.

B. Specific Measures: Begin therapy with large initial doses of corticosteroids, eg, 120–150 mg or more of prednisone (or equivalent) to suppress blistering within 3 or 4 days. Maintain with corticosteroids by mouth, and reduce dosage as rapidly as possible to a daily minimum maintenance level sufficient to control local or systemic manifestations. Then switch to alternate day dosage. Methotrexate, azathioprine, and cyclophosphamide are being used investigationally with some success. The chief indication for these immunosuppressive drugs is intolerance to large doses of corticosteroids. They are no less hazardous. Control of the condition must be obtained with corticosteroids first. Lower doses of corticosteroids and antitumor drugs may be achieved by using them in combination.

C. Local Measures: Skin and mucous membrane lesions should be treated as for vesicular, bullous, and ulcerative lesions due to any cause (see p 32). Complicating infection requires appropriate systemic and local antibiotic therapy.

Prognosis
Pemphigus was at one time invariably fatal, but the disease can now be controlled indefinitely in many cases. Therapy may induce a complete and permanent remission, in which case maintenance therapy can be discontinued. One-half of all deaths are now related to the complications of therapy.

Cram DL: Atypical forms of pemphigus and pemphigoid. Cutis 15:202, 1975.

Glickman FS, Silvers SH: Pemphigus vulgaris treated with cyclophosphamide. Arch Dermat 107:467, 1973.

Roenigk HH Jr, Deodhar S: Pemphigus treatment with azathioprine. Arch Dermat 107:353, 1973.

Tuffanelli DL: Cutaneous immunopathology for the practitioner. Cutis 15:179, 1975.

ATOPIC DERMATITIS
(Eczema)

Essentials of Diagnosis
- Pruritic, exudative, or lichenified eruption on face, neck, upper trunk, wrists, and hands and in the folds of knees and elbows.
- Personal or family history of allergic manifestations (eg, asthma, allergic rhinitis, eczema).
- Tendency to recur, with remission from age 2 to early youth and beyond.

General Considerations

Atopic dermatitis is a chronic superficial inflammation of the skin due to a genetic predisposition. These individuals often react to allergens (notably wool and animal epidermals). It is part of the triad of hay fever-asthma-eczema. The disease usually appears in infancy, disappears at the age of 2 or 3 years, recurs in early youth, and thereafter tends to come and go. Personal or family histories of allergic disease are usually obtained. Resistance to contact sensitization suggests a defect in the cell-mediated immune system.

Clinical Findings

A. Symptoms and Signs: Itching may be extremely severe and prolonged, leading often to emotional disturbances which have been erroneously interpreted by some as being causative. The distribution of the lesions is characteristic, with involvement of the face, neck, and upper trunk ("monk's cowl"). The bends of the elbows and knees are involved. An abortive form may involve the hands alone (in which case the history of atopy is all-important). In infants the eruption usually begins on the cheeks and is often vesicular and exudative. In children (and later) it is dry, leathery, and lichenified, although intraepidermal vesicles are occasionally present histologically. Adults generally have dry, leathery, hyperpigmented or hypopigmented lesions in typical distribution.

B. Laboratory Findings: Scratch and intradermal tests are disappointing. Eosinophilia may be present. The delayed-blanch reaction to methacholine may help in diagnosing atypical atopic dermatitis. Serum immunoglobulin E may be elevated in exacerbations.

Differential Diagnosis

Distinguish from seborrheic dermatitis (frequent scalp and face involvement, greasy and scaly lesions, and quick response to therapy), contact dermatitis (especially that due to weeds), and lichen simplex chronicus (flat, more circumscribed, less extensive lesions).

Complications

Kaposi's varicelliform eruption, which includes superimposed skin infection with herpes simplex virus (eczema herpeticum) or the vaccine virus (eczema vaccinatum) may be serious. The patient should be protected from these viruses if possible.

Treatment

A. General Measures: Corticotropin or the corticosteroids may provide spectacular improvement in severe or fulminant eczema (see Chapter 18). Triamcinolone acetonide suspension, 20–30 mg IM every 3 weeks (or less often), may exert control *(caution)*. The Scholtz regimen includes cleansing with Cetaphil lotion (no soap), avoidance of wool and other irritants, 0.01% fluocinolone acetonide solution topically, water-soluble vitamin A, 100,000 units daily by mouth *(caution)*, oral antihistamines, and small doses of thyroid. Sojourns in areas with equable climate and high elevation may help (eg, Tucson or El Paso in the USA).

High doses of hydroxyzine or diphenhydramine may be useful, but the dosage must be increased gradually to avoid extreme drowsiness.

B. Specific Measures: Avoidance of temperature changes and stress may help to minimize abnormal cutaneous vascular and sweat responses.

The diet should be adequate and well balanced. There is no evidence that standardized or routine dietary restrictions are of value, especially in adults.

Attempts at desensitization to various allergens by graded injections are disappointing, and may cause severe flares.

An attempt should be made to identify and treat emotional disturbances, but this is of little practical value in the management of the dermatitis.

C. Local Treatment: Avoid all unnecessary local irritations to the skin, such as may occur from excessive bathing or as a result of exposure to irritating drugs, chemicals, greases, and soaps. Soapless detergents are not advisable. Clear up skin infections promptly (particularly those with exudates) by appropriate measures (see Chapter 28). Corticosteroids in lotion, cream, or ointment form applied sparingly twice daily may be very helpful. Grenz ray therapy (by a specialist) may be used effectively, if only temporarily.

Treat the clinical type and stage of the dermatitis:

1. For acute weeping lesions use the solutions listed in Table 3–1 as soothing or astringent soaks, baths, or wet dressings for 30 minutes 3 or 4 times daily. Shake lotions (R 13, 14) may be employed at night or when wet dressings are not desirable. Lesions on extremities, particularly, may be bandaged for protection at night.

2. Subacute or subsiding lesions may be treated with shake lotions, which may incorporate mild antipruritic or mild stimulating agents. Shake lotions are usually preferred for widespread lesions. Ointments (Table 3–5) containing mild tar may be used.

3. Chronic, dry, lichenified lesions are best treated with ointments, creams, and pastes (Table 3–4) containing lubricating, keratolytic, antipruritic, and mild keratoplastic agents as indicated. Topical corticosteroids and tars are the most popular agents in chronic eczema. Useful corticosteroids are fluocinolone acetonide, triamcinolone acetonide, and betamethasone valerate in creams, ointments, lotions, solutions, and sprays. Fluorinated topical steroids may cause rosacea, striae, and skin atrophy. Coal tar is available as 2–5% ointment, creams, and pastes. Iodochlorhydroxyquin, 3%, ointment or cream may be used in hairy areas or if there is an idiosyncrasy to tar.

Prognosis

The disease runs a chronic course, often with a tendency to disappear and recur.

Jones HE & others: Atopic disease and serum immunoglobulin-E. Brit J Dermat 92:17, 1975.

Leyden JL & others: *Staphylococcus aureus* in the lesions of atopic dermatitis. Brit J Dermat 90:525, 1974.

Medansky RS, Handler RM: Management of atopic dermatitis: Modified Scholtz technique. Cutis 12:622, 1973.
Rajka G: *Atopic Dermatitis.* Saunders, 1975.

CIRCULATORY OR STASIS DERMATITIS

Essentials of Diagnosis

- Pruritic red, weeping, swollen areas of eczema and ulceration on the lower legs.
- Older persons with history or evidence of varicose veins, arterial insufficiency, trauma, or episodes of thrombophlebitis.
- Atrophic pigmented skin with scars of old ulcerations.

General Considerations

Eczema of the legs, also called gravitational or hemostatic eczema, is common in older persons, especially men. Most cases are due to impaired circulation, as in varicose veins and arterial disorders, but the disease may be initiated or made worse by the slightest injury, excessive exposure to soap, medication, cold, low humidity, and even malnutrition. After an injury or reaction to medication in a patch of stasis dermatitis, a generalized pruritic vesicular eruption may occur (autosensitization, "toxic absorption phenomenon"). The reaction may occur spontaneously also. It is considered to be due to reaction with a heat-labile, complement-dependent, 7S γ-globulin specific for epidermal cells. Autoimmune diseases may cause leg ulcers.

Postphlebitic syndrome may cause stasis dermatitis and ulcers at any age.

Clinical Findings

Severe itching is the only symptom. Red, oozing, swollen patches of eczema are present on the backs or outer surfaces of one or both legs (often over the malleoli). Ulcers in the centers of the patches of eczema are rounded and sharply circumscribed, with dirty gray bases and thickened borders. There may be considerable edema. A variant is the hypertensive ischemic ulcer, which may be surprisingly painful.

Differential Diagnosis

Differentiate from other causes of leg ulcers such as sickle cell anemia, hypertension, erythema induratum, and the syphilitic ulcers of late syphilis. The eczema itself must be distinguished from that due to contact dermatitis (such as from overtreatment).

Treatment

A. General Measures and Prevention: Maintain general health (by proper diet, rest, and sleep) and good skin hygiene. Avoid prolonged sitting, standing, or walking, and constricting garters. Wear properly fitted shoes and stockings. Protect from trauma.

B. Specific Measures: Treat the underlying specific disease, eg, varicose veins, obstructive arterial disease

amenable to surgery, thrombophlebitis, and congestive heart failure and hypertension. Autosensitization reaction may be treated with internal and topical corticosteroids.

C. Local Measures: For acute weeping dermatitis use continuous cool wet dressings (Table 3–1). Avoid sensitizing or irritating topical medicaments. For infected eczema or ulcers use topical antibiotic (tetracycline) powders. Combinations of topical corticosteroids with antibiotics in the form of creams, lotions, and ointments may be useful for more chronic processes.

Painting indolent ulcers with Castellani's solution, 1% aqueous gentian violet, or 10% silver nitrate solution may hasten healing.

Pressure dressings with foam rubber pads and the use of support stockings may be vital in the healing of indolent stasis ulcers and stubborn stasis dermatitis. Some authors favor the use of the Unna paste boot for pressure dressings.

Dressing ulcers or eczema daily with 1% iodochlorhydroxyquin (Vioform) in Lassar's paste on Telfa pads may be very helpful.

Prognosis

The prognosis depends in great part upon the improvement of the circulation to the limb (eg, repair of varicose veins) and adequacy of treatment. There is a great tendency toward chronicity and recurrence.

Berube L: Unna's paste in leg disorders. Cutis 8:387, 1971.
Fisher AA: Topical medications in management of stasis ulcers. Angiology 22:206, 1971.
Rosewater F: Lower extremity signs of systemic disease. Cutis 13:737, 1974.

LICHEN SIMPLEX CHRONICUS
(Localized Neurodermatitis)

Essentials of Diagnosis

- Chronic itching associated with pigmented lichenified skin lesions.
- Exaggerated skin lines overlying a thickened, well circumscribed scaly plaque.
- Predilection for nape of neck, wrists, external surfaces of forearms, inner thighs, genitalia, postpopliteal and antecubital areas.

General Considerations

Lichen simplex chronicus is a persistent, usually well localized plaque several cm in diameter, commonly located on the side of the neck, the flexor aspect of the wrist, or the ankle. A "scratch-itch" cycle is a prominent feature. The lesions may arise out of normal skin, or the disease may occur as a complication of contact dermatitis or any irritative dermatitis. It is particularly common in persons of Oriental extraction living in the USA, but is said to be rare in their countries of origin. It is more common in women over 40 years of age. Only one person in 5 is born with skin which has the ability to lichenify following chronic manipulation or scratching. Atopic subjects develop it more readily than others.

Clinical Findings
Intermittent itching incites the patient to manipulate the lesions. Dry, leathery, hypertrophic, lichenified plaques appear on the neck, wrist, perineum, thigh, or almost anywhere. The patches are well localized and rectangular, with sharp borders, and are thickened and pigmented. The lines of the skin are exaggerated and divide the lesion into rectangular plaques.

Differential Diagnosis
Differentiate from other plaque-like lesions such as psoriasis, lichen planus, seborrheic dermatitis, and nummular dermatitis.

Treatment
The area should be protected and the patient encouraged to avoid stressful and emotionally charged situations if possible. Topical corticosteroids give relief. The injection of dilute triamcinolone acetonide suspension into the lesion may occasionally be curative. Application of triamcinolone acetonide, 0.1%, fluocinolone, 0.025%, or betamethasone valerate, 0.1%, cream nightly with Saran Wrap covering may be helpful. Roentgen or grenz radiation may be used conservatively by an expert in the technic.

Prognosis
The disease tends to be chronic, and will disappear in one area only to appear in another. Itching may be so intense as to interfere with sleep.

Marks R, Wells GC: Lichen simplex: Morphodynamic correlates. Brit J Dermat 88:249, 1973.
Robertson IM, Jordan JM, Whitlock FA: Emotions and skin. 2. The conditioning of scratch responses in cases of lichen simplex. Brit J Dermat 92:407, 1975.

DERMATITIS MEDICAMENTOSA
(Drug Eruption)

Essentials of Diagnosis
- Usually abrupt onset of widespread, symmetric erythematous eruption.
- May mimic any inflammatory skin condition.
- Constitutional symptoms (malaise, arthralgia, headache, and fever) may be present.

General Considerations
Dermatitis medicamentosa is an acute or chronic inflammatory skin reaction to a drug. Almost any drug, whether ingested, injected, inhaled, or absorbed,

may cause almost any type of skin reaction in any given individual at any given time. This entity does not include dermatitis caused by a drug acting locally (contact dermatitis). The eruption usually recurs upon reexposure to the same or a related drug, although identical reactions may be produced by unrelated drugs and the same drug may produce different types of reactions in different individuals. Reexposure to a suspected drug may be hazardous, although mere suspicion does not necessarily preclude the use of some essential or even lifesaving drug in a hospital setting with emergency treatment facilities available.

Clinical Findings
A. Symptoms and Signs: The onset is usually abrupt, with bright erythema and often severe itching, but may be delayed (penicillin, serum). Fever and other constitutional symptoms may be present. The skin reaction usually occurs in symmetric distribution. In a given situation the physician may suspect one specific drug (or one of several) and must therefore inquire specifically whether it has been used or not.

Drug eruptions may be briefly classified, with examples, as follows: (1) erythematous (bismuth, arsenicals, barbiturates, sulfonamides, antihistamines, atropine), (2) eczematoid or lichenoid (gold, quinacrine), (3) acneiform or pyodermic (corticotropin, iodides, corticosteroids, bromides), (4) urticarial (penicillin, antibiotics, sera), (5) bullous (iodides), (6) fixed (phenolphthalein, barbiturates), (7) exfoliative (arsenicals, gold), (8) nodose (sulfathiazole, salicylates). (9) Exanthematous eruptions may be caused by many drugs. Ampicillin for infectious mononucleosis causes a morbilliform eruption. (10) Photosensitization may also occur (phenothiazines, chlorothiazides, demeclocycline, griseofulvin, oral hypoglycemic agents).

B. Laboratory Findings: The complete blood count may show leukopenia, agranulocytosis, or evidence of aplastic anemia. Patch tests made with the suspect drug, although they are not routinely useful, may detect a drug offender when contact sensitivity is also present.

Differential Diagnosis
Distinguish from other eruptions usually by history and subsidence after drug withdrawal, although fading may be slow.

Complications
Blood dyscrasias, anaphylaxis, laryngeal edema, photosensitivity, and hepatic, renal, ocular, CNS, and other complications may occur.

Prevention
People who have had dermatitis medicamentosa should avoid analogues of known chemical "allergens" as well as known offenders. The physician should pay careful attention to a history of drug reaction.

Treatment
A. General Measures: Treat systemic manifesta-

tions as they arise (eg, anemia, icterus, purpura). Antihistamines may be of value in urticarial and angioneurotic reactions (see p 47), but use epinephrine, 1:1000, 0.5–1 ml IV or IM, as an emergency measure. Corticosteroids (see Chapter 18) may be used as for acute contact dermatitis in severe cases. Dialysis may speed drug elimination in certain cases.

B. Specific Measures: Stop all drugs, if possible, and hasten elimination from the body by increasing fluid intake. Dimercaprol (BAL) or other chelating agents such as EDTA may be tried in cases due to heavy metals (eg, arsenic, mercury, gold) (see Chapter 30). Sodium chloride, 5–10 gm daily orally, may hasten elimination of bromides and iodides in cases due to those drugs (see Chapter 30).

C. Local Measures: Treat the varieties and stages of dermatitis according to the major dermatitis which is simulated. Watch for sensitivity.

Prognosis
Drug rash usually disappears upon withdrawal of the drug and proper treatment. If systemic involvement is severe, the outcome may be fatal. It has been estimated that 100–300 deaths from penicillin occur each year in the USA.

Abel R: Fixed drug eruption of the penis from tetracycline. Cutis 12:254, 1973.

Almeyda J, Levantine A: Adverse cutaneous reactions to the penicillins: Ampicillin rashes. Brit J Dermat 87:293, 1972.

Fellner MJ & others: The usefulness of immediate skin tests to haptenes derived from penicillin. Arch Dermat 103:371, 1971.

Harber LC, Baer RL: Pathogenic mechanism of drug-induced photosensitivity. J Invest Dermat 58:327, 1972.

EXFOLIATIVE DERMATITIS

Essentials of Diagnosis
- Scaling and erythema over large area of body.
- Itching, malaise, fever, weight loss.
- Primary disease or exposure to toxic agent (contact, oral, parenteral) may be evident.

General Considerations
Exfoliative dermatitis, a disorder in which a considerable portion of the skin is reddened and covered with lamellated scales which exfoliate freely, may be due to leukemia, lymphoma, or other internal malignancy; may occur as a sequel to dermatitis medicamentosa, preexisting dermatosis, or contact dermatitis; or may be idiopathic (most cases).

Variants of ichthyosis may resemble exfoliative dermatitis.

Clinical Findings
A. Symptoms and Signs: Symptoms include itch-

ing, weakness, malaise, fever, and weight loss. Exfoliation may be generalized or universal, and sometimes includes loss of hair and nails. Generalized lymphadenopathy may be due to lymphoma or leukemia or may be part of the clinical picture of the skin disease (dermatopathic lymphadenitis). There may be mucosal sloughs.

B. Laboratory Findings: Blood and bone marrow studies and lymph node biopsy may show evidence of leukemia or lymphoma. Skin biopsy may show evidence of mycosis fungoides or a specific dermatosis (ie, psoriasis or lichen planus). Hypoproteinemia (a grave sign) and anemia may be present.

Differential Diagnosis
Differentiate from other scaling eruptions such as psoriasis, lichen planus, severe seborrheic dermatitis, and dermatitis medicamentosa, which may themselves develop into exfoliative dermatitis.

Complications
Septicemia, debility (protein loss), pneumonia, high output cardiac failure, masking of fever, hypermetabolism, thermoregulatory disorders, and anemia.

Prevention
Patients receiving sensitizing drugs should be watched carefully for the development of skin reactions of all types. The drug should be withheld until the nature of the skin reaction is determined. Proved sensitization should be considered an absolute contraindication to further administration of the drug. Dermatitis or dermatoses should not be overtreated.

Treatment
A. General Measures: Hospitalize the patient at bed rest with talc on bed sheets. Keep room at warm, constant temperature, and avoid drafts. Transfusions of whole blood or plasma may be required. Avoid all unnecessary medication.

Systemic corticosteroids may provide spectacular improvement in severe or fulminant exfoliative dermatitis, but long-term therapy should be avoided if possible (see Chapter 18). Suitable antibiotic drugs should be given when there is evidence of bacterial infection; pyoderma is a common complication of exfoliative dermatitis.

B. Specific Measures: Stop all drugs, if possible, and hasten elimination of offending drug by all means, eg, by increasing fluid intake. Dimercaprol (BAL) may lessen the severity or duration of reactions due to arsenic or gold (see Chapter 30).

C. Local Measures: Observe careful skin hygiene and avoid irritating local applications. Treat skin as for acute extensive dermatitis first with wet dressings, soothing baths (see p 33), powders (Table 3–2), and shake lotions (Table 3–3); and later with soothing oily lotions (Table 3–3) and ointments (Table 3–4).

Topical anti-infective drugs (eg, oxytetracycline, erythromycin, or polymyxin B ointment) should be used when necessary.

Prognosis

The prognosis is variable, depending often upon the prognosis of the primary disease (eg, lymphoma). Idiopathic exfoliative dermatitis is unpredictable in its duration and recurrence.

Abrahams I: Dermatitis, exfoliative, and erythroderma. Pages 82–83 in: *Current Dermatologic Management.* Maddin S (editor). Mosby, 1970.

Shuster S, Marks J: *Systemic Effects of Skin Disease.* Heinemann, 1970.

PHOTODERMATITIS
(Dermatitis Actinica, Erythema Solare or Sunburn, Polymorphous Light Sensitivity, Contact Photodermatitis)

Essentials of Diagnosis

- Painful erythema, edema, and vesiculation on sun-exposed surfaces.
- Fever, gastrointestinal symptoms, malaise, or prostration may occur.
- Proteinuria, casts, and hematuria may occur.

General Considerations

Photodermatitis is an acute or chronic inflammatory skin reaction due to overexposure or hypersensitivity to sunlight or other sources of actinic rays (cold or hot quartz), photosensitization of the skin by certain drugs, or idiosyncrasy to actinic light as seen in some constitutional disorders including the porphyrias and many hereditary disorders (phenylketonuria, xeroderma pigmentosum, and others). Contact photosensitivity may occur with perfumes, antiseptics, and other chemicals.

Clinical Findings

A. Symptoms and Signs: The acute inflammatory skin reaction is accompanied by pain, fever, gastrointestinal symptoms, malaise, and even prostration. Signs include erythema, edema, and possibly vesiculation and oozing on exposed surfaces. Exfoliation and pigmentary changes often result.

B. Laboratory Findings: Proteinuria, casts, hematuria, and hemoconcentration may be present. Look for porphyrins in urine and stool, protoporphyrins in blood, and findings in other inborn errors of metabolism. Elaborate testing for photosensitivity may be performed by experts.

Differential Diagnosis

Differentiate from contact dermatitis which may develop from one of the many substances in suntan lotions and oils. Sensitivity to actinic rays may also be part of a more serious condition such as porphyria, erythropoietic protoporphyria, lupus erythematosus, or pellagra. Phenothiazines, sulfones, chlorothiazides, griseofulvin, oral antidiabetic agents, and antibiotics may photosensitize the skin. Polymorphous light eruption appears to be an idiopathic photodermatosis which affects females predominantly, frequently starts in childhood, and lasts into late adult life. The action spectrum frequently lies in both the long (320–400 nm) and short (below 320 nm) ultraviolet wavelengths. Contact photodermatitis may be caused by halogenated salicylanilides (weak antiseptics in soaps, creams, etc).

Complications

Delayed cumulative effects in fair-skinned people include keratoses and epitheliomas. Some individuals become chronic light-reactors even when they apparently are not longer exposed to photosensitizing or phototoxic drugs.

Prevention

Persons with very fair, sensitive skins should avoid prolonged exposure to strong sun or ultraviolet radiation. Preliminary conditioning by graded exposure is advisable.

Protective agents should be applied before exposure. The best of these is 5% para-aminobenzoic acid in 50% ethyl alcohol (℞ 50).

The use of psoralens orally is controversial. For persistent light reactors and polymorphous light eruption, sunshades should be tried.

In those photodermatoses in which the action spectrum involves wavelengths outside the short ultraviolet range (ie 320 nm), sunshades must be used which contain titanium dioxide (A-Fil, Reflecta). RVPaque, which contains zinc oxide, may also be used.

Treatment

A. General Measures: Treat constitutional symptoms by appropriate supportive measures. Control pain, fever, and gastrointestinal and other symptoms as they arise. Aspirin may have some specific value. Corticosteroids, both systemically and topically, may be required for severe reactions. Beta-carotene, 50 mg daily by mouth, is effective treatment for erythropoietic protoporphyria.

B. Local Measures: Treat as for any acute dermatitis (see p 32). First use cooling and soothing wet dressings (Table 3–1), and follow with lotions (Table 3–3). Greases must be avoided because of the occlusive effect.

Prognosis

Dermatitis actinica is usually benign and self-limiting unless the burn is severe or when it occurs as an associated finding in a more serious disorder.

Castrow FE, Owens DW: Secreening for photosensitivity. Cutis 10:709, 1972.

Frain-Bell W & others: The action spectrum in polymorphic light eruption. Brit J Dermat 89:243, 1973.

Fusaro RM, Runge WJ, Johnson JA: Protection against light sensitivity with dihydroxyacetone/naphthoquinone. Internat J Dermat 11:67, 1972.

Macleod TM, Frain-Bell W: A study of chemical light screening agents. Brit J Dermat 92:417, 1975.

Mathews-Roth MM & others: Beta-carotene as an oral photoprotective agent in erythropoietic protoporphyria. JAMA 228:1004, 1974.

Rudner EJ, Mehregan AH: The cutaneous and histopathologic features of porphyria and polymorphous light eruptions. Cutis 12:354, 1973.

Wechsler HL: Porphyria cutanea tarda: Multiple blood transfusions and iron-loading. Cutis 13:434, 1974.

LICHEN PLANUS

Essentials of Diagnosis

- Pruritic, violaceous, flat-topped papules with fine white streaks and symmetric distribution.
- Commonly seen along linear scratch mark (Koebner phenomenon).
- Anterior wrists, sacral region, penis, legs, mucous membranes.
- Usually occurs in an otherwise healthy but emotionally tense person.
- Histopathology is diagnostic.

General Considerations

Lichen planus is a chronic inflammatory disease associated with emotional tension or stress. It is more common after the second decade of life and is rare in children. The cause is unknown, but there appears to be a mixture of continuous damage to the basal zone of the epidermis with persistent attempts at repopulation of the area by migrating keratinocytes. Colloid bodies appear in the upper dermis and may contain IgM as well as small amounts of IgG. Fibrin may be found in the upper dermis. These findings are not highly specific.

Clinical Findings

Itching is mild to severe. The lesions are violaceous, flat-topped, angulated papules, discrete or in clusters, on the flexor surfaces of the wrists and on the penis, lips, tongue, and buccal and vaginal mucous membranes. The papules may become bullous or ulcerated. The disease may be generalized. Mucous membrane lesions have a lacy white network overlying them which is often confused with leukoplakia. Papules are 1–4 mm in diameter, with white streaks on the surface (Wickham's striae).

Differential Diagnosis

Distinguish from similar lesions produced by quinacrine or bismuth sensitivity and other papular lesions such as psoriasis, papular eczema, and syphiloderm. Lichen planus on the mucous membranes must be differentiated from leukoplakia. Certain photo-developing or duplicating solutions may produce eruptions which mimic lichen planus.

Treatment

A. General Measures: Patients with lichen planus are often "high-strung" or tense and nervous, and episodes of dermatitis may be temporally related to emotional crises. Measures should be directed at relieving anxiety, eg, with phenobarbital, 15–30 mg 2–4 times daily orally for 1 month. Corticosteroids (see Chapter 18) may be required in severe cases. Griseofulvin (micronized), 500 mg daily by mouth, may be tried.

B. Local Measures: Use shake lotions containing tar (R 16). X-ray or grenz ray therapy (by a specialist) may be used when involvement is particularly severe. Intralesional injection of triamcinolone acetonide is useful for localized forms. Corticosteroid cream or ointment may be used nightly under thin pliable plastic film.

Prognosis

Lichen planus is a benign disease, but it may persist for months or years and may be recurrent. Oral lesions tend to be especially persistent, and neoplastic degeneration has been described.

Gunther SH: Vitamin A acid in treatment of oral lichen planus. Arch Dermat 107:277, 1973.

Michel B, Sy EK: Tissue-fixed immunoglobulins in lichen planus. In: *Immunopathology of the Skin*. Beutner EH & others (editors). Dowden, Hutchinson, & Ross, 1973.

Pinkus H: Lichenoid tissue reactions. Arch Dermat 107:840, 1973.

Sehgal VN, Rege VL: Lichen planus: Appraisal of 147 patients. Indian J Dermatol Venereol 40:104, 1974.

Sehgal VN & others: Griseofulvin therapy in lichen planus: A double-blind controlled trial. Brit J Dermat 87:383, 1972.

PSORIASIS

Essentials of Diagnosis

- Silvery scales on bright red plaques, usually on the knees, elbows, and scalp.
- Stippled nails.
- Itching is mild unless psoriasis is eruptive or occurs in body folds.
- Psoriatic arthritis may be present.
- Histopathology is specific.

General Considerations

Psoriasis is a common benign, acute or chronic, inflammatory skin disease which apparently is based upon genetic predisposition. A genetic error in the mitotic control system has been postulated. Nearly 50% of patients with psoriasis are HL-A 17 positive. The significance of this is not known. Injury or irritation of a psoriatic skin tends to provoke lesions of psoriasis in the site. Psoriasis occasionally is eruptive, particularly in periods of stress. Grave, life-threatening forms may occur.

Clinical Findings

There are usually no symptoms. Eruptive psoriasis may itch, and psoriasis in body folds itches severely (inverse psoriasis). The lesions are bright red, sharply outlined plaques covered with silvery scales. The elbows, knees, and scalp are the most common sites. Nail involvement may resemble onychomycosis. Fine stippling in the nails is pathognomonic. There may be associated arthritis which resembles the rheumatoid variety.

Differential Diagnosis

Differentiate in the scalp from seborrheic dermatitis; in body folds from intertrigo and candidasis; and in the nails from onychomycosis.

Treatment

A. **General Measures:** Warm climates seem to exert a favorable effect. Severe psoriasis calls for treatment in the hospital or a day care center with the Goeckerman or Ingram routine.

Corticotropin or corticosteroids may be necessary to give relief in fulminating cases. Methotrexate and azaribine (Triazure) are available for severe psoriasis. FDA guidelines must be followed.

Reassurance is important since these patients are apt to be discouraged by the difficulties of treatment. An attempt should be made to relieve anxieties.

B. **Local Measures:**

1. **Acute psoriasis**—Avoid irritating or stimulating drugs. Begin with a shake lotion (R 13, 14) or bland ointment (Table 3–4) containing 5% detergent solution of coal tar. As the lesions become less acute, gradually incorporate mild keratoplastic agents into lotions (Table 3–3) and hydrophilic ointments (Table 3–4).

2. **Subacute psoriasis**—Give warm baths daily, scrubbing the lesions thoroughly with a brush, soap, and water. Apply increasing concentrations of keratoplastic or stimulating agents incorporated in lotions (Table 3–3) and hydrophilic ointments (Table 3–4). Solar or ultraviolet irradiations may be applied in gradually increasing doses.

3. **Chronic psoriasis**—Administer the following ultraviolet irradiation and tar regimen daily as needed (modified from Goeckerman): Smear 2–5% coal tar ointment thickly on the skin and leave for 12–24 hours. Wipe off ointment with mineral oil, leaving a light stain. Follow with gradually increasing suberythema doses of ultraviolet light as tolerated.

Anthralin, in the form of Lasan paste (in 3 strengths) for the body, or Lasan pomade for the scalp, may be helpful. It tends to be irritating, however, and it discolors white or gray hair. It should not be used near the eyes.

Recent work suggests that exposure to sunlamps plus blacklight lamps, without systemic or topical therapy, may benefit chronic psoriasis.

Simple application twice daily of commercial tar lotions may be as effective as comparable use of potent topical corticosteroids.

For localized lesions, triamcinolone acetonide suspension, 2.5 mg/ml, may be injected intralesionally. Apply triamcinolone acetonide, 0.1%, or fluocinolone, 0.025%, cream nightly and cover with Saran Wrap. Bethamethasone valerate, 0.1% lotion, may be superior for scalp lesions. The entire body may be treated with a plastic exercise suit over a corticosteroid cream. This "Aid-to-Psoriasis" suit is obtainable from the Slim-Ez Suit Co., P.O. Box 3193, Chattanooga, Tennessee 37404, and comes in 5 sizes.

Prognosis

The course tends to be chronic and unpredictable, and the disease may be refractory to treatment.

Baden HP: Treatment of hyperkeratotic dermatitis of the palms: Sequential treatment with a keratolytic gel and corticosteroid ointment. Arch Dermat 110:737, 1974.

Bailin PL, Roenigk HH Jr, Steck W: Hospital management of psoriasis. Cutis 14:201, 1974.

Benjamin RP, Tindall JP: Plastic exercise suit occlusion. Cutis 9:493, 1972.

Farber EM, Harris DR: Hospital treatment of psoriasis. Arch Dermat 101:381, 1970. [Ingram routine.]

Leavell UW Jr, Mersack IP, Smith C: Survey of the treatment of psoriasis with hydroxyurea. Arch Dermat 107:467, 1973.

Milstein HG, Cornell RC, Stoughton RB: Azaribine in the treatment of psoriasis. Arch Dermat 108:43, 1973.

Parrish JA & others: Photochemotherapy of psoriasis with oral methoxsalen and longwave ultraviolet light. New England J Med 291:1207, 1974.

Rees RB: Psoriasis. Mod Med 40:95, 1972.

Rees RB: Psoriasis: Topical therapy. Cutis 13:53, 1974.

Stein KM & others: Hydroxyurea in the treatment of pustular psoriasis. Brit J Dermat 85:81, 1971.

Weber G: Combined 8-methoxypsoralen and black light therapy of psoriasis. Brit J Dermat 90:317, 1974.

Witten VH: A folding ultraviolet light box. Arch Dermat 107:716, 1973.

PITYRIASIS ROSEA

Essentials of Diagnosis

- Oval, fawn-colored, scaly eruption following cleavage lines of trunk.
- Herald patch commonly precedes eruption by 1–2 weeks.
- Occasional pruritus.

General Considerations

Pityriasis rosea is a common mild, noncontagious, acute inflammatory skin disease of unknown etiology. It behaves like an infectious exanthem in that it runs a definite course (usually 6 weeks) and confers a solid "immunity" (second attacks are rare). It occurs usually during the spring or fall. A chronic form of the disease occurs rarely. A good tan suppresses the eruption (in the tanned areas only).

Clinical Findings

Occasionally there is severe itching. The lesions

consist of oval, fawn-colored macules 4–5 mm in diameter following cleavage lines on the trunk. Exfoliation of the lesions causes a crinkly scale which begins in the center. The proximal portions of the extremities are involved. A "herald patch" is usually evident. This is the initial lesion, which usually precedes the later efflorescence by 1–2 weeks.

Differential Diagnosis

Differentiate from secondary syphilis, especially when lesions are numerous or smaller than usual. Tinea corporis, seborrheic dermatitis, tinea versicolor, and drug eruptions may simulate pityriasis rosea.

Treatment

Acute irritated lesions (uncommon) should be treated as for acute dermatitis with wet dressings (Table 3–1) or shake lotions (R 13–16). Apply coal tar solution, 5% in starch lotion, twice daily. Ultraviolet light is helpful.

Prognosis

Pityriasis rosea is usually an acute self-limiting illness which disappears in about 6 weeks.

Merchant M, Hammond R: Controlled study of ultraviolet light for pityriasis rosea. Cutis 14:548, 1974.

SEBORRHEIC DERMATITIS

Essentials of Diagnosis

- Dry scales or dry yellowish dandruff with or without underlying erythema.
- Scalp, central face, presternal, interscapular areas, umbilicus, and body folds.

General Considerations

Seborrheic dermatitis is an acute or chronic papulosquamous dermatitis. It is based upon a genetic predisposition mediated by an interplay of such factors as hormones, nutrition, infection, and emotional stress. The role of Pityrosporum organisms is unclear in a causative, contributory, common, or even occasional sense.

Clinical Findings

Pruritus may be present but is an inconstant finding. The scalp, face, chest, back, umbilicus, and body folds may be oily or dry, with dry scales or oily yellowish scurf. Erythema, fissuring, and secondary infection may be present.

Differential Diagnosis

Distinguish from other skin diseases of the same areas such as intertrigo and fungal infections; and from psoriasis (location).

Treatment

A. General Measures: Prescribe a well-balanced, adequate diet and restrict excess sweets, spices, hot drinks, and alcoholic beverages. Regular working hours, recreation, sleep, and simple cleanliness are recommended. Treat aggravating systemic factors such as infections, overwork, emotional stress, constipation, and dietary abnormalities.

B. Local Measures:

1. Acute, subacute, or chronic eczematous lesions—Treat as for dermatitis or eczema (see p 37). An emulsion base containing 0.5% hydrocortisone and 10% sodium sulfacetamide is useful for all forms and stages. Corticosteroid creams, lotions, or solution may be used in all stages (R 20, 39, 40). Potent fluorinated corticosteroids used regularly on the face may produce steroid rosacea.

2. Seborrhea of the scalp—Use one of the following: (1) Selsun (selenium sulfide) suspension or Capsebon once a week after shampoo. Fostex cream (containing soapless cleansers, wetting agents, sulfur, and salicylic acid) may be used as a weekly shampoo for oily seborrhea. (2) Sebulex is similar to Fostex and is also effective. Sebizon lotion (sodium sulfacetamide) may be applied once daily. (3) Sebical shampoo, containing tar and allantoin, may succeed where others fail. (4) Betamethasone valerate (Valisone), 0.1% lotion, is excellent.

3. Seborrhea of nonhairy areas—Mild stimulating lotion (R 16), ointment (R 35), or 3–5% sulfur in hydrophilic ointment (Table 3–5) may be used. (The addition of 1% salicylic acid aids in removing scales.)

4. Seborrhea of intertriginous areas—Avoid greasy ointments. Apply astringent wet dressings (R 1–5, 7) followed by 3% iodochlorhydroxyquin and 1% hydrocortisone in an emulsion base.

Prognosis

The tendency is to lifelong recurrences. Individual outbreaks may last weeks, months, or years.

Leyden JJ, Thew M, Kligman AM: Steroid rosacea. Arch Dermat 110:619, 1974.

Rees RB: Seborrheic dermatitis. Page 575 in: *Current Therapy.* Conn HF (editor). Saunders, 1975.

ACNE VULGARIS

Essentials of Diagnosis

- Pimples (papules or pustules) over the face, back, and shoulders occurring at puberty.
- Cyst formation, slow resolution, scarring.
- The most common of all skin conditions.

General Considerations

Acne vulgaris is a common inflammatory skin disease of unknown etiology apparently caused by a genetic predisposition and activated by androgens. It may occur at any time from puberty through the period of sex hormone activity. Eunuchs are spared, and the disease may be provoked by giving androgens to a predisposed individual. Identical involvement may occur in identical twins.

The disease is more common in males. Contrary to popular belief, it does not always clear spontaneously when maturity is reached. If untreated, it may persist into the 4th and even 6th decade of life. The skin lesions are the result of sebaceous overactivity, retention of sebum, overgrowth of the acne bacillus (*Corynebacterium acnes*) in incarcerated sebum, irritancy of fatty acids, and foreign body reaction to extrafollicular sebum. The role of antibiotics in controlling acne is not clearly understood, although they reduce lipases which produce irritating free fatty acids. (Topical occlusive corticosteroids may produce acne.)

Clinical Findings

There may be mild soreness, pain, or itching; inflammatory papules, pustules, ectatic pores, acne cysts, and scarring. The lesions occur mainly over the face, neck, upper chest, back, and shoulders. Comedones are common.

Self-consciousness, embarrassment, and shame may be the most disturbing symptoms.

Differential Diagnosis

Distinguish from acneiform lesions caused by bromides, iodides, and contact with chlorinated naphthalenes and diphenyls.

Complications

Cyst formation, severe scarring, and psychic trauma.

Treatment

A. **General Measures:**

1. **Education of the patient**—It should be explained that treatment is essential not only to produce an acceptable cosmetic result while the condition is active but also to prevent permanent scarring.

2. **Diet**—The diet should be adequate and well balanced. One may forbid chocolate, nuts (including peanut butter), fatty or fried foods, seafoods, alcoholic beverages, spicy foods, and excess carbohydrates, but foods are less important than formerly thought in causing acne.

3. Eliminate all possible medication, especially bromides or iodides.

4. Avoid exposure to oils and greases.

5. Treat anemia, malnutrition, infection, gastrointestinal disorders, or other factors which may aggravate acne.

6. Aggravating or complicating emotional disturbances must be taken into consideration and treated appropriately.

7. **Antibiotics**—Tetracycline, 250 mg orally every day, may exert better long-term control than any other treatment in some cases. Tetracycline may permanently discolor growing teeth.

Blood counts, blood chemistries, and urinalyses gave essentially normal findings in persons on long-term low-dose tetracycline or erythromycin therapy for acne. Gram-negative folliculitis supervening in acne during broad-spectrum antibiotic therapy will respond to stopping the antibiotic and using penicillin by mouth for a week or two. Chloramphenicol should not be used internally for acne. Minocycline, 50–200 mg daily by mouth, is advocated as adjunctive therapy in severe acne.

8. **Oral contraceptives** are said to help some young women with acne. Apparently it is the mestranol contained in them which is beneficial. Hyperpigmentation (melasma) is an occasional complication.

B. **Local Measures:** Ordinary soap is adequate for cleansing. Avoid greasy cleansing creams and other cosmetics. Shampoo the scalp 1–2 times a week (℞ 48). Extract blackheads with a comedo extractor. Incise and drain fluctuant cystic lesions with a small sharp scalpel.

1. **Keratoplastic and keratolytic agents**—Acne lotion (sulfur-zinc lotion, ℞ 18) may be applied locally to the skin at bedtime and washed off in the morning. Retin A (tretinoin) lotion or cream has been recommended for comedo acne.

2. **Keratolytic ointments and pastes**—Begin with weak preparations and increase strength as tolerated. Apply one of the following at bedtime and remove in the morning: (1) Sulfur, 2–10% in hydrophilic ointment. (2) Quinolor compound ointment.

3. **Commercial preparations** for acne include Fostex cream and cake, Fostril Hc cream, Cort-Acne lotion, Rezamid lotion, Acne-Dome cleanser, cream, and lotion, Resulin lotion, Sulforcin cream and lotion, Clantis lotion, Vanoxide lotion, Panoxyl gel, Desquam-X gel, and Benzagel. All of these gels contain benzoyl peroxide.

4. **Dermabrasion**—Cosmetic improvement may be achieved by abrasion of inactive acne lesions, particularly flat, superficial scars. The skin is first frozen and anesthetized with ethyl chloride or Freon and then carefully abraded with fine sandpaper or special motor-driven abrasive brushes. The technic is not without untoward effects, since hyperpigmentation, grooving, and scarring have been known to occur. Dark-skinned individuals do poorly.

Gentle daily abrasion may be accomplished with abrasive particles incorporated in a suitable vehicle (Pernox, Brasivol).

5. **Irradiation**—Simple exposure to sunlight in graded doses is often beneficial. Ultraviolet irradiation may be used as an adjunct to other treatment measures. Use suberythema doses in graded intervals up to the point of mild erythema and scaling. X-ray radiation (by a specialist) should be reserved for the most severe cases after other measures have failed.

6. **Liquid nitrogen spray** is useful for blanching cysts and papules.

Prognosis

Untreated acne vulgaris may persist throughout adulthood and may lead to severe scarring. The disease is chronic and tends to recur in spite of treatment.

Barranco VP: Effect of androgen-dominant and estrogen-dominant oral contraceptives on acne. Cutis 14:384, 1974.

Becker FT: Treatment of tetracycline-resistant acne vulgaris. Cutis 14:610, 1974.

Coskey RJ: Side effects of antibiotic therapy in acne vulgaris. Cutis 15:710, 1975.

Fulton JE Jr, Pablo G: Topical antibacterial therapy for acne. Arch Dermat 110:83, 1974.

Kligman AM, Mills OH Jr: "Acne cosmetica." Arch Dermat 106:843, 1972.

Leyden JJ & others: Gram-negative folliculitis: A complication of antibiotic therapy in acne vulgaris. Brit J Dermat 88:533, 1973.

Mandy SH: The art of tretinoin therapy in acne. Cutis 14:855, 1974.

Questions and answers: Are there risks in long-term, low-dose tetracycline therapy of acne vulgaris? JAMA 228:899, 1974.

Rees RB: Acne. Cutis 11:637, 1973.

Sulzberger MB: Systemic antibiotics in acne: A dermatologic viewpoint. JAMA 224:1184, 1973.

URTICARIA (HIVES) & ANGIONEUROTIC EDEMA (GIANT HIVES)

Essentials of Diagnosis

- Wheals with marked itching.
- Fever, malaise, and nausea may occur.
- History of exposure to sensitizing foods or drugs in some cases.

General Considerations

Hives is an acute or chronic inflammatory skin reaction of allergic origin. Most acute forms are caused by ingestion of foods or drugs to which the patient is sensitive. Acute urticaria is of less than 6 weeks' duration. Chronic urticaria requires the same sort of exhaustive investigation indicated for a long-continued unexplained fever. Common causes are foods (shellfish, pork, strawberries, wheat, eggs, milk, tomatoes, chocolate), drugs (antibiotics, especially penicillin, salicylates, tartrazine and amaranth (yellow and red food dyes), belladonna, iodides, bromides, serum, vaccines, phenolphthalein, opium derivatives), molds and bacteria, insect bites, parasitic infestation, and emotional disturbances. In chronic urticaria, the cause will rarely be found. There is an association between urticaria, HB Ag, and hepatitis. Contributing and aggravating factors may include cold, physical pressure, atopy, and genetic predisposition.

Clinical Findings

A. Symptoms and Signs: In addition to intolerable itching, there may also be malaise and slight fever. Nausea may result from involvement of the gastrointestinal mucosa. The wheals vary greatly in size, shape, and amount of swelling. The wheals of cholinergic urticaria are tiny, with erythematous halos. Giant hives occur in angioedema.

B. Laboratory Findings: There may be transient eosinophilia. In chronic urticaria, extensive laboratory investigations may be required in the search for occult foci of infection, food and drug sensitivity, and other possible causes. ECG abnormalities have been reported in a few cases.

Differential Diagnosis

Distinguish from contact dermatitis, poison oak, and dermographia, which is a different disease.

Complications

Laryngeal obstruction is the most important complication, especially in the angioedema variant of urticaria. Hereditary angioneurotic edema due to lack of $C'1^a$ esterase inhibitor is frequently fatal.

Prevention

Avoid reexposure to sensitizing drugs or foods and aggravating physical, systemic, or emotional factors. In the penicillin-sensitive patient exposure to occult sources of penicillin may occur, eg, in milk and other foods.

Treatment

A. General Measures: Initial castor oil purgation to remove possible antigenic substances has been recommended in acute cases. Stools may be examined for parasites. During the acute phase the diet should be simple and free of such common offenders as yeast, wheat, milk, eggs, pork, fish, shellfish, tomatoes, strawberries, and chocolate. The past history, food diaries, trial diets, and elimination diets may be helpful in determining offending foods. The patient should not remain on a restricted diet unless food sensitivity can be demonstrated. Avoid unnecessary medication. (Suspect *all* drugs.) Look for foci of infection and for systemic illness.

1. Antihistaminic drugs often give prompt and sustained symptomatic relief. Hydroxyzine may have special value.

2. Epinephrine injection, 0.3–1 ml of 1:1000 solution, subcut, for acute lesions when laryngeal edema is suspected or present, when urticaria is intense, or when antihistaminic drugs have failed to give relief.

3. Ephedrine sulfate, 25 mg orally 4 times daily, or ephedrine-sedative mixtures.

4. Systemic corticosteroids (see Chapter 18) may provide spectacular improvement in severe or fulminant angioneurotic edema. These drugs should be used only if it is apparent that the patient will not respond to more conservative measures.

5. Fresh plasma may be lifesaving during an acute attack of hereditary angioneurotic edema. Methyltestosterone Linguets, 10 mg once or twice daily, may reduce the episodes. Aminocaproic acid (Amicar) and its analogue, tranexamic acid, may help.

6. For possible parasitic causes, give a therapeutic trial of diiodohydroxyquin, 0.65 gm 3 times daily for 1 week, or a therapeutic trial with thiabendazole.

B. Local Measures: Topical antipruritic preparations are frequently of benefit (see p 33 and Table 3–2).

Prognosis

The disease is usually self-limited and lasts only a few days. The chronic form may persist for years.

Greaves MW, Yamamoto S: Urticaria. Clin Pharmacol Therap 16 (5 Part 2):895, 1974.
Hubbard RD: Urticaria due to food dyes. Cutis 14:748, 1974.
Noid HE, Schulze TW, Winkelmann RK: Diet plan for patients with salicylate-induced urticaria. Arch Dermat 109:866, 1974.
Warin RP, Champion RH: *Urticaria.* Saunders, 1974.

INTERTRIGO

Intertrigo is caused by the macerating effect of heat, moisture, and friction. It is especially likely to occur in obese persons and in humid climates. Poor hygiene is an important etiologic factor. There is often a history of seborrheic dermatitis. The symptoms are itching, stinging, and burning. The body folds develop fissures, erythema, and sodden epidermis, with superifical denudation. Urine and blood examination may reveal diabetes mellitus, and the skin examination may reveal candidiasis. A direct smear may show abundant cocci.

Treatment is as for tinea cruris (see p 58), but fungicidal agents should not be used. Recurrences are common.

MILIARIA
(Heat Rash)

Essentials of Diagnosis

- Burning, itching, superficial aggregated small vesicles or papules on covered areas of the skin.
- Hot moist climate.
- May have fever and even heat prostration.

General Considerations

Miliaria is an acute dermatitis which occurs most commonly on the upper extremities, trunk, and intertriginous areas. A hot, moist environment is the most frequent cause, but individual susceptibility is important and obese persons are most often affected. Plugging of the ostia of sweat ducts occurs, with consequent ballooning and ultimate rupture of the sweat duct, producing an irritating, stinging reaction.

Clinical Findings

The usual symptoms are burning and itching.

Fever, heat prostration, and even death may result in severe forms. The lesions consist of small superficial, reddened, thin-walled, discrete but closely aggregated vesicles, papules, or vesicopapules. The reaction occurs most commonly on covered areas of the skin.

Differential Diagnosis

Distinguish from similar skin manifestations occurring in drug rash.

Prevention

Provide optimal working conditions when possible, ie, controlled temperature, ventilation, and humidity. Avoid overbathing and the use of strong, irritating soaps. Graded exposure to sunlight or ultraviolet light may benefit persons who will later be subjected to a hot, moist atmosphere. Susceptible persons should avoid exposure to adverse atmospheric conditions.

Treatment

An antipruritic cooling lotion such as the following should be applied 2–4 times daily:

R	Menthol	1.0
	Phenol	2.0
	Glycerin	15.0
	Alcohol, qs ad	240.0

Alternative measures which have been employed with varying success are drying shake lotions (R 13 with 1% phenol, or R 14) and antipruritic powders or other dusting powders. Treat secondary infections (superficial pyoderma) with potassium permanganate soaks, compresses, or baths (Table 3–1). Tannic acid, 10% in 70% alcohol, applied locally twice daily, serves to toughen the skin. Anticholinergic drugs given by mouth may be very helpful in severe cases, eg, glycopyrrolate, 1 mg twice daily.

Prognosis

Miliaria is usually a mild disorder, but death may result in the severe forms (tropical anhidrosis and asthenia) as a result of interference with the heat-regulating mechanism. The process may also be irreversible to some extent, requiring permanent removal of the individual from the humid or hot climate.

Gordon BI: "No sweat." Cutis 15:401, 1975.
Sulzberger MB, Harris DR: Miliaria and anhidrosis. Arch Dermat 105:845, 1972.

PRURITUS ANI & VULVAE

Essentials of Diagnosis

- Itching, chiefly nocturnal, of the anogenital area.
- There may be no skin reactions; or inflammation of any degree may occur up to lichenification.

General Considerations

Most cases have no obvious cause, but multiple specific causes have been identified. Anogenital pruritus may be due to the same causes as intertrigo, lichen simplex chronicus, seborrheic dermatitis, contact dermatitis (from soap, colognes, douches, contraceptives), or may be due to irritating secretions, as in diarrhea, leukorrhea, trichomoniasis, or local disease (candidiasis, dermatophytosis). Diabetes mellitus must be ruled out. Psoriasis or seborrheic dermatitis may be present. Uncleanliness may be at fault.

Clinical Findings

A. Symptoms and Signs: The only symptom is itching, which is chiefly nocturnal. Physical findings are usually not present, but there may be erythema, fissuring, maceration, lichenification, excoriations, or changes suggestive of candidiasis or tinea.

B. Laboratory Findings: Urinalysis and blood sugar determination may reveal diabetes mellitus. Direct microscopic examination or culture of tissue scrapings may reveal yeasts, fungi, or parasites. Stool examination may show intestinal parasites.

Differential Diagnosis

Distinguish among the various causes of this condition, such as Candida organisms, parasites, local irritation from contact with drugs and irritants, and other primary skin disorders of the genital area such as psoriasis, seborrhea, or intertrigo.

Prevention

Treat all possible systemic or local causes. Instruct the patient in proper anogenital hygiene.

Treatment (See also Pruritus, p 33.)

A. General Measures: Avoid "hot," spicy foods, and drugs which can irritate the anal mucosa. Treat constipation if present (see p 322). Instruct the patient to use very soft or moistened tissue or cotton after a bowel movement and to clean thoroughly. Women should apply the same precautions after urinating. Anal douching is the best cleansing method for all types of pruritus ani. Instruct the patient regarding the harmful and pruritus-inducing effects of scratching.

B. Local Measures: Corticosteroid (see R 40) or Vioform-hydrocortisone creams are quite useful. Potent fluorinated topical corticosteroids may lead to atrophy and striae. Sitz baths twice daily are of value if the area is acutely inflamed and oozing, using silver nitrate, 1:10,000–1:200; potassium permanganate, 1:10,000; or aluminum subacetate solution, 1:20. Underclothing should be changed daily. Paint fissured or ulcerated areas with Castellani's solution.

Grenz ray therapy (by a specialist) may be used.

Prognosis

Although usually benign, anogenital pruritus may be persistent and recurrent.

Tio H: Pruritus ani. Cutis 15:689, 1975.

CALLOSITIES & CORNS (OF FEET OR TOES)

Callosities and corns are caused by pressure and friction due to faulty weight-bearing, orthopedic deformities, or improperly fitting shoes. Some persons are hereditarily predisposed to excessive and abnormal callus formation.

Tenderness on pressure and "after-pain" are the only symptoms. The hyperkeratotic well-localized overgrowths always occur at pressure points. On paring, a glassy core is found (which differentiates these disorders from plantar warts, with multiple bleeding points upon cutting across capillaries). A soft corn often occurs laterally on the proximal portion of the fourth toe as a result of pressure against the bony structure of the interphalangeal joint of the fifth toe.

Treatment consists of correcting mechanical abnormalities which cause friction and pressure. Shoes must be properly fitted, and orthopedic deformities corrected. Callosities may be removed by careful paring of the callus after a warm water soak, or with keratolytic agents, eg, Keralyt Gel (Westwood), which contains 6% salicylic acid in a gel containing propylene glycol (60%) and ethyl alcohol (19.4%). Apply locally to callus every night and cover with a polyethylene plastic film (Saran Wrap); remove in the morning. Repeat until the corn or callus is removed.

Extensive and severe palmar and plantar hyperkeratosis can be treated successfully by applying equal parts of propylene glycol and water nightly and covering with thin polyethylene plastic film (Baggies).

A metatarsal leather bar, one-half inch wide and one-fourth inch high, may be placed on the outside of the shoe just behind the weight-bearing surface of the sole. "Ripple-sole" shoes may be effective.

Women who tend to form calluses and corns should not wear confining footgear.

Murray Space-Shoes (expensive) may be specially fitted. For those who cannot afford them, Ripple Sole shoes may be used.

Baden HP, Goldsmith LA, Lee LD: A new keratolytic gel for the management of hyperkeratosis. Cutis 12:787, 1973.

CHRONIC DISCOID LUPUS ERYTHEMATOSUS

Essentials of Diagnosis

- Red, asymptomatic, localized plaques, usually on the face, often in butterfly distribution.
- Scaling, follicular plugging, atrophy, and telangiectasia of involved areas.
- Histology distinctive.

General Considerations

Lupus erythematosus is a superficial, localized

discoid inflammation of the skin occurring most frequently in areas exposed to solar or ultraviolet irradiation. The cause is not known. The disseminated type is discussed in Chapter 13.

Clinical Findings

A. Symptoms and Signs: There are usually no symptoms. The lesions consist of dusky red, well localized, single or multiple plaques, 5–20 mm in diameter, usually on the face and often in a "butterfly pattern" over the nose and cheeks. There is atrophy, telangiectasia, and follicular plugging. The lesion is usually covered by dry, horny, adherent scales.

Where indicated, a complete medical study should be made to rule out systemic lupus erythematosus.

B. Laboratory Findings: There are usually no significant laboratory findings in the chronic discoid type. If there is leukopenia or proteinuria, with or without casts, one must suspect the disseminated or systemic form of the disease. Histologic changes are distinctive. The antinuclear antibody test is perhaps best for ruling out systemic lupus erythematosus. A direct immunofluorescent test reveals basement membrane antibody.

Paramyxovirus-like structures have been found in skin lesions of polymyositis, lupus erythematosus, and dermatomyositis. Their significance is not known.

Differential Diagnosis

The scales are dry and "tack-like," and can thus be distinguished from those of seborrheic dermatitis. Differentiate also from the morphea type of basal cell epithelioma and, by absence of nodules and ulceration, from lupus vulgaris.

Complications

Dissemination may occur. There may be scarring.

Treatment

A. General Measures: Treat chronic infections. Provide protection from sunlight and all other powerful radiation. *Caution:* Do not use any form of radiation therapy.

Maintain optimal general health by well balanced diet with supplementary vitamins and iron as indicated. D-Alpha tocopherol acetate (vitamin E) may be tried in doses of 400–2000 IU daily by mouth. Vitamin E is inactivated by iron and may potentiate the effect of insulin and digitalis. Ensure adequate rest, and prescribe bed rest when the patient is febrile.

B. Medical Treatment: (For discoid type only.) *Caution:* The following drugs may cause serious eye changes. If the medication is continued, ophthalmologic examination should be done every 3 months. Wherever possible, chronic discoid lupus erythematosus should be considered a cosmetic defect only and should be treated topically or with camouflaging agents.

1. Chloroquine phosphate, 0.25 gm daily for 1 week, then 0.25 gm twice weekly. Watch for signs of toxicity.

2. Hydroxychloroquine sulfate, 0.2 gm orally daily, then twice weekly, may occasionally be effective when chloroquine is not tolerated.

C. Local Infiltration: Triamcinolone acetonide suspension, 2.5 mg/ml, may be injected into the lesions once a week or once a month. This should be tried before internal treatment (see above).

D. Corticosteroids: Corticosteroid creams applied each night and covered with airtight, thin, pliable plastic film may be useful.

Prognosis

The disease is persistent but not life-endangering unless it turns into the disseminated variety.

Epstein JH: Photobiology of lupus erythematosus. Cutis 15:212, 1975.

Rees RB, Arnold HL Jr: Vitamin E and thee. Cutis 13:761, 1974.

Tuffanelli DL: Lupus erythematosus. Arch Dermat 106:553, 1972.

VIRAL INFECTIONS
OF THE SKIN

HERPES SIMPLEX
(Cold or Fever Sore)

Essentials of Diagnosis

- Recurrent small grouped vesicles on an erythematous base, especially around oral and genital areas.
- May follow minor infections, trauma, stress, or sun exposure.
- Regional lymph nodes may be swollen and tender.
- Tzanck smear is positive for large multinucleated epithelial giant cells surrounded by acantholytic balloon cells.

General Considerations

Herpes simplex is an acute viral infection. Clinical outbreaks, which may be recurrent in the same location for years, are provoked by fever, sunburn, indigestion, fatigue, windburn, menstruation, or nervous tension.

Chronic virus multiplication, rather than latency, may account for recurrent herpes simplex.

The alleged oncogenic effect of herpesvirus II (genital) infections is causing increased concern.

Clinical Findings

The principal symptoms are burning and stinging. Neuralgia may precede and accompany attacks. The lesions consist of small, grouped vesicles which can occur anywhere but which most often occur on the lips, mouth, and genitals. Regional lymph nodes may be swollen and tender.

Differential Diagnosis

Distinguish from other vesicular lesions, especially herpes zoster and impetigo. In the genital area, differentiate from syphilis, lymphogranuloma venereum, and chancroid.

Vesicle scrapings stained with Giemsa stain gave a positive Tzanck test, which is also positive in herpes zoster, varicella, and vaccinia, which have different clinical pictures.

Complications

Pyoderma, Kaposi's varicelliform eruption (eczema herpeticum or disseminated herpes simplex), encephalitis, keratitis, and possible cervical cancer and other malignancies.

Treatment

For persistent or severe, recurrent herpes:

A. General Measures: Eliminate precipitating agents when possible.

B. Local Measures: Apply a moistened styptic pencil several times daily to abort lesions. Dust vesicles twice daily with bismuth formic iodide (BFI) powder or use shake lotions (R 13, 14); camphor spirit locally twice daily; or epinephrine, 1:100 locally twice daily. Topical corticosteroids are listed as contraindicated, but a small amount of betamethasone suspension, 0.6 mg/ml injected intralesionally, works well. Treatment of dendritic keratitis is discussed on p 78.

If there is associated cellulitis and lymphadenitis, apply cool compresses. Treat stomatitis with mild (saline) mouth washes. X-ray or grenz ray therapy (by a specialist) may be indicated in selected cases.

Some viruses can be inactivated if exposed to one of several dyes and then irradiated with ordinary white light. Heterotricyclic dyes such as proflavine have an affinity for the guanine base portions of DNA and are bound firmly to the DNA of some viruses. Exposure to light then leads to inactivation of the virus by producing breaks in the viral DNA. Application of 0.1% aqueous proflavine dye to the lesion, followed by a 15-minute exposure to any reading lamp, is effective treatment. The suggestion of carcinogenicity of dye plus light for herpes has cast doubt on the advisability of this treatment; there may be greater carcinogenicity from spontaneous mutations of untreated virus.

Idoxuridine, 5% in DMSO (not available in the USA), is reported to be effective topically.

Prognosis

Individual attacks last 1−2 weeks. Recurrences are common.

Bockstahler LE, Lytle CD, Hellman KB: *A Review of Photodynamic Therapy for Herpes Simplex: Benefits and Potential Risks.* J Publication No. (FDA) 75−8013. Department of Health, Education, & Welfare, Nov 1974.

Gibbs RC: Locally applied adrenocorticoids in treatment of herpes simplex. (Correspondence.) Arch Dermat 110:811, 1974.

Higgins PG: Recurrent herpes simplex virus infections. Brit J Dermat 91:111, 1974.

Kint A, Verlinden L: Levamisole for recurrent herpes labialis. (Correspondence.) New England J Med 291:308, 1974.

HERPES ZOSTER
(Shingles)

Essentials of Diagnosis

- Pain along course of a nerve followed by painful grouped vesicular lesions.
- Involvement is unilateral. Lesions are usually on face and trunk.
- Swelling of regional lymph nodes (inconstant).

General Considerations

Herpes zoster is an acute vesicular eruption due to a virus that is morphologically identical with the virus of varicella. It usually occurs in adults with or without a history of chickenpox during childhood and is probably a reactivation of a varicella virus infection that has been occult for many years. With rare exceptions, one attack of zoster confers lifelong immunity. Persons in anergic states (Hodgkin's disease, lymphomas, or those taking immunosuppressive drugs) are at greater risk, and generalized, life-threatening dissemination (varicella) may occur.

Clinical Findings

Pain usually precedes the eruption by 48 hours or more and may persist and actually increase in intensity after the lesions have disappeared. The lesions consist of grouped, tense, deep-seated vesicles distributed unilaterally along the neural pathways of the trunk. The commonest distributions are on the trunk or face. Regional lymph glands may be tender and swollen.

Differential Diagnosis

Since poison oak and poison ivy dermatitis may be produced unilaterally and in a streak by a single brush with the plant, it must be differentiated at times from herpes zoster. Differentiate also from similar lesions of herpes simplex, which is usually less painful.

Complications

Persistent neuralgia, anesthesia of the affected area following healing, facial or other nerve paralysis, and encephalitis may occur.

Treatment

A. General Measures: Barbiturates may help control tension and nervousness associated with neuralgia. Aspirin or APC compound with or without codeine phosphate, 30 mg, usually controls pain. A single intragluteal injection of triamcinolone acetonide suspension, 40 mg, may give prompt relief. Prednisone, 40 mg daily for 4 days and continued then in declining doses, may help. Ophthalmologic consultation should be considered for supraorbital involvement to avoid serious ocular complications. Hospitalization may be necessary in serious cases. Zoster has developed despite normal varicella-zoster antibody levels, indicating that cell-mediated immunity is more important in preventing zoster than circulating antibodies. For this reason, despite the fact that it has not been studied adequately, zoster immune globulin (ZIG) is unlikely to be beneficial in preventing or treating herpes zoster.

B. Local Measures: Calamine lotion or other shake lotions (Table 3–3) are often of value. Apply the lotion liberally and cover with a protective layer of cotton. Do not use greases. Idoxuridine, 40% in DMSO (not available in the USA), is said to relieve the deep pain of zoster when used topically.

C. Post-zoster Neuralgia: Infiltration of involved skin with triamcinolone acetonide suspension and lidocaine has been disappointing. Vitamin E, 800 units daily, should be tried.

Prognosis

The eruption persists 2–3 weeks and does not recur. Motor involvement may lead to temporary palsy. Post-zoster neuralgia, which usually occurs in elderly individuals in supraorbital distribution, is extraordinarily persistent and devastating and does not respond to treatment. Ocular involvement may lead to blindness.

Ayres S Jr, Mihan R: Post-herpes zoster neuralgia: Response to vitamin E therapy. Arch Dermat 108:855, 1973.

Brunell PA, Gershon AA: Passive immunization against varicella-zoster infections and other modes of therapy. J Infect Dis 127:415, 1973.

Izumi AK, Edwards J Jr: Herpes zoster with neurogenic bladder dysfunction. Arch Dermat 109:692, 1974.

Nuss DD: Herpes zoster: Its complications and treatment. Bull A Mil Dermat 22:43, 1974.

WARTS

Essentials of Diagnosis

- Warty elevation anywhere on skin or mucous membranes, usually no larger than 0.5 cm in diameter.
- Prolonged incubation period (average 2–18 months).
- Spontaneous "cures" are frequent (50%), but warts are often unresponsive to any treatment.
- "Recurrences" (new lesions) are frequent.

General Considerations

Warts are usually seen as solitary or clustered lesions, all presumably due to the same virus, most often on the exposed parts such as the fingers or hands. The incubation period is 2–18 months. No age group is exempt, but warts are perhaps more commonly seen in children and young adults. The virus is intranuclear, arranged in icosahedron symmetry, and 40–55 nm in diameter. It has not yet been grown in the laboratory.

Clinical Findings

There are usually no symptoms. Tenderness on pressure occurs with plantar warts; itching with anogenital warts. Occasionally a wart will produce mechanical obstruction (eg, nostril, ear canal).

Warts vary widely in shape, size, and appearance. Flat warts are most evident under oblique illumination. Subungual warts may be dry, fissured, and hyperkeratotic, and may resemble hangnails or other nonspecific changes. Plantar warts resemble plantar corns or calluses.

Prevention

Avoid contact with warts. A person with flat warts should be admonished not to scratch the areas. Occasionally an electric shaver will prevent the spread of warts in razor scratches. Anogenital warts may be transmitted venereally.

Treatment

A. Removal: Remove the warts whenever possible by one of the following means:

1. Surgical excision—Inject a small amount of local anesthetic into the base and then remove the wart with a dermal curet or scissors or by shaving off at the base of the wart with a scalpel. Trichloroacetic acid or Monsel's solution on a tightly wound cotton-tipped applicator may be painted on the wound, or electrocautery may be applied.

2. Liquid nitrogen applied with a cotton-tipped applicator until the wart is thoroughly blanched causes after-pain, but large numbers of warts may be so treated bloodlessly.

3. Keratolytic agents—Either of the following may be used:

R̶	Salicylic acid	2.5
	Lactic acid	2.5
	Flexible collodion, qs ad	15.0

Sig: Paint on warts each night with glass rod.

R̶	Salicylic acid	3.6
	Alcohol, 40%, qs ad	120.0

Sig: Paint on *flat* warts with cotton swab daily.

4. Anogenital warts are best treated by painting them weekly with 25% podophyllin in compound tincture of benzoin *(caution)*.

5. Plantar warts may be treated by applying 10% aqueous formalin, then 40% salicylic acid plaster, covered with clear plastic tape; or the warts may be filed with an emery board daily, soaked for 5 minutes in water, and then treated with 1 part each of salicylic acid and lactic acid in flexible collodion (see prescription above).

B. Immunotherapy: Warts have been shown to disappear after the individual has been sensitized to dinitrochlorobenzene and then treated topically with it *(caution)*.

Prognosis

There is a striking tendency to the development of new lesions. Warts may disappear spontaneously or may be unresponsive to treatment.

Lewis HM: Topical immunotherapy of refractory warts. Cutis 12:863, 1973.
Morison WL: In vitro assay of cell-mediated immunity to human wart antigen. Brit J Dermat 90:525, 1974.
Oriel JD: New light on warts. Dermat Digest 12:39, 1973.

BACTERIAL INFECTIONS OF THE SKIN

IMPETIGO

Impetigo is a contagious and auto-inoculable infection of the skin caused by staphylococci or streptococci or both. The infected material may be transmitted to the skin by dirty fingernails. In children, the source of infection is often another infected child.

Itching is the only symptom. The lesions consist of macules, vesicles, pustules, and honey-colored gummy crusts which when removed leave denuded red areas. The face and other exposed parts are most often involved

Impetigo must be distinguished from other vesicular and pustular lesions such as herpes simplex, varicella, and contact dermatitis (dermatitis venenata).

Treatment is as for folliculitis. Response to systemic antibiotics is usually good. The question of whether there is a place for topical antibiotics alone awaits an answer. Systemic treatment should be given if there is fever or unresponsiveness. The nephritis which occasionally develops may be fatal (particularly in infants). Erythromycin may be preferable to the penicillins for impetigo.

Bassett DCJ: Streptococcal pyoderma and acute nephritis in Trinidad. Brit J Dermat 86 (Suppl 8):55, 1972.
Noble WC & others: Prevalence of streptococci and staphylococci in lesions of impetigo. Brit J Dermat 91:209, 1974.
Taplin D, Allen AM: Bacterial pyodermas. Clin Pharmacol Therap 16 (5 Part 2):905, 1974.

ECTHYMA

Ecthyma is a deeper form of impetigo, with ulceration. It occurs frequently on the legs and other covered areas, often as a complication of debility and infestations.

Kelly C & others: Streptococcal ecthyma: Treatment with benzathine penicillin G. Arch Dermat 103:306, 1971.

BOCKHART'S IMPETIGO

Bockhart's impetigo is a staphylococcal infection which produces tense, globular painful pustules at the follicular orifices. It is a form of folliculitis (see below).

IMPETIGO NEONATORUM

Impetigo neonatorum is a highly contagious, potentially serious form of impetigo occurring in infants. It requires prompt systemic treatment and protection of other infants (isolation, exclusion from the nursery of personnel with pyoderma, etc). The lesions are bullous and massive, and accompanied by systemic toxicity. Death may occur.

Houck PW: Prevention of infection of the newborn: The question of hexachlorophene. Drug Therapy 2:90, 1972.

FOLLICULITIS
(Including Sycosis Vulgaris or Barber's Itch)

Essentials of Diagnosis
- Itching and burning in hairy areas.
- Pustules in the hair follicles.
- In sycosis, inflammation of surrounding skin area.

General Considerations

Folliculitis is caused by staphylococcal infection of a hair follicle. When the lesion is deep-seated, chronic, and recalcitrant, it is called sycosis. Sycosis is usually propagated by the auto-inoculation and trauma of shaving. The upper lip is particularly susceptible to involvement in men who suffer with chronic nasal discharge from sinusitis or hay fever.

Clinical Findings

The symptoms are slight burning and itching, and pain on manipulation of the hair. The lesions consist of pustules of the hair follicles. In sycosis the surrounding skin becomes involved also and so resembles eczema, with redness and crusting.

Differential Diagnosis

Differentiate from acne vulgaris and infections of the skin, such as impetigo.

Complications

Abscess formation.

Prevention

Correct precipitating or aggravating factors: systemic (eg, diabetes mellitus) or local causes (eg, mechanical or chemical skin irritations, discharges).

Treatment

A. Specific Measures: Systemic anti-infectives may be tried if the skin infection is resistant to local treatment; if it is extensive or severe and accompanied by a febrile reaction; if it is complicated; or if it involves the so-called "danger areas" (upper lip, nose, and eyes).

Local anti-infective agents are of presumed value and should be tried in sequence until a favorable response is obtained (allowing 3–4 days for evaluation). They should be applied initially at night and protected by dressings; soaks should be applied during the day. After the area has cleared, any of the following preparations may be applied 2–4 times daily: (1) Iodochlorhydroxyquin, 3% in cream or ointment form, locally twice daily. (2) Antibiotics, alone or in combination, as ointments locally 2–4 times daily. These include polymyxin B in combination with bacitracin or oxytetracycline, chloramphenicol, and erythromycin.

Penicillin and sulfonamides should not be used topically, with the sole exception of sodium sulfacetamide.

Povidine-iodine (Betadine) ointment, containing organic iodine, is said to be excellent topical therapy, but it stains skin and hair.

B. Local Measures: Cleanse the area gently with a weak soap solution and apply soaks or compresses to the involved area for 15 minutes twice daily (Table 3–1). When skin is softened, gently open the larger pustules and trim away necrotic tissue.

Prognosis

Folliculitis is often stubborn and persistent, lasting for months and even years.

Maibach HI, Hutton RD: Bacterial infections of the skin. Mod Med 40:82, 1972.

FURUNCULOSIS (BOILS) & CARBUNCLES

Essentials of Diagnosis

- Extremely painful inflammatory swelling of a hair follicle which forms an abscess.
- Primary predisposing debilitating disease sometimes present.
- Antibiotic-resistant strains of "hospital staph" are responsible for an increasing percentage of cases.

General Considerations

A furuncle (boil) is a deep-seated infection (abscess) involving the entire hair follicle and adjacent subcutaneous tissue. The most common sites of occurrence are the hairy parts exposed to irritation and friction, pressure, or moisture, or to the plugging action of petroleum products. Because the lesions are autoinoculable, they are often multiple. Thorough investigation usually fails to uncover a predisposing cause, although an occasional patient may have uncontrolled diabetes mellitus, nephritis, or other debilitating disease.

A carbuncle is several furuncles developing in adjoining hair follicles and coalescing to form a conglomerate, deeply situated mass with multiple drainage points.

Clinical Findings

A. Symptoms and Signs: The extreme tenderness and pain are due to pressure on nerve endings, particularly in areas where there is little room for swelling of underlying structures. The pain, fever, and malaise are more severe in carbuncles than with furuncles. The follicular abscess is either rounded or conical. It gradually enlarges, becomes fluctuant, and then softens and opens spontaneously after a few days to 1–2 weeks to discharge a core of necrotic tissue and pus. The inflammation occasionally subsides before necrosis occurs.

A carbuncle is much larger than a boil. Instead of having only one core it has 2 or more.

B. Laboratory Findings: There may be slight leukocytosis.

Differential Diagnosis

Differentiate from deep mycotic infections such as sporotrichosis and blastomycosis; from other bacterial infections such as anthrax and tularemia; and from acne cysts.

Complications

Serious and sometimes fatal cerebral thrombophlebitis may occur as a complication of a manipulated furuncle on the central portion of the upper lip or near the nasolabial folds. Perinephric abscess, osteomyelitis, and other hematogenous staphylococcal infections may also occur.

Treatment

A. Specific Measures:

1. Systemic anti-infective agents are indicated (chosen on the basis of cultures and sensitivity tests if possible). Sodium cloxacillin or erythromycin, 1 gm daily by mouth, is usually effective.

2. Bacterial recolonization with a harmless staphylococcus may be tried for recurrent furunculosis.

B. Local Measures: Immobilize the part and avoid overmanipulation of inflamed areas. Use moist heat to help larger lesions "localize." Use proper surgical incision, epilation, or debridement **after** the lesions are "mature." Do not incise deeply. Apply anti-infective ointment and bandage the area loosely during drainage.

Prognosis

Recurrent crops may harass the patient for months or years. Carbunculosis is more severe and more hazardous than furunculosis.

Kagan BM, Fannin SL, Baidie F: Spotlight on antimicrobial agents—1973. JAMA 226: 306, 1973.
Shinefield HR & others: Bacterial interference between strains of *Staphylococcus aureus,* 1960 to 1970. Am J Dis Child 121:148, 1971.

ERYSIPELAS

Essentials of Diagnosis
- Edematous, spreading, circumscribed, hot, erythematous area, with or without vesicle or bulla formation.
- Pain, malaise, chills and fever.
- Leukocytosis, increased sedimentation rate.

General Considerations

Erysipelas is an acute inflammation of the skin and subcutaneous tissue caused by infection with beta-hemolytic streptococci. It occurs classically on the cheek.

Clinical Findings

A. Symptoms and Signs: The symptoms are pain, malaise, chills, and moderate fever. A bright red spot appears first, very often near a fissure at the angle of the nose. This spreads to form a tense, sharply demarcated, glistening, smooth, hot area. The margin characteristically makes noticeable advances from day to day. The patch is somewhat edematous and can be pitted slightly with the finger. Vesicles or bullae occasionally develop on the surface. The patch does not usually become pustular or gangrenous, and heals without scar formation. The disease may complicate any break in the skin which provides a portal of entry for the organism.

B. Laboratory Findings: Leukocytosis and increased sedimentation rate almost invariably occur.

Differential Diagnosis

Distinguish from cellulitis, with its less definite margin and involvement of deeper tissues, and from erysipeloid, a benign bacillary infection producing redness of the skin of the fingers or the backs of the hands in fishermen and meat handlers.

Complications

Unless erysipelas is promptly treated, death may result from extension of the process and systemic toxicity, particularly in the very young and in the aged.

Treatment

Place the patient at bed rest with the head of his bed elevated, apply hot packs, and give aspirin for pain and fever. Penicillin is specific for beta-hemolytic streptococcus infections. Erythromycin is a good alternative.

Prognosis

Erysipelas formerly was very dangerous to life, particularly in the very young and in the aged. With antibiotic therapy the disease can now usually be quickly controlled. Prompt and adequate treatment usually will limit it to one attack.

Markowitz M, Taranta A: Managing streptococcal infections. Drug Ther Bull 3:20, 1973.

CELLULITIS

Cellulitis, a diffuse spreading infection of the skin, must be differentiated from erysipelas (a superficial form of cellulitis) because the 2 conditions are quite similar. Cellulitis involves deeper tissues and may be due to one of several organisms, usually cocci. The lesion is hot and red but has a more diffuse border than does erysipelas. Cellulitis usually occurs after a break in the skin. Recurrent attacks may sometimes affect lymphatic vessels, producing a permanent swelling called "solid edema."

The response to systemic, anti-infective measures (penicillin or broad-spectrum antibiotics) is usually prompt and satisfactory.

ERYSIPELOID

Erysipelothrix rhusiopathiae infection must be differentiated from erysipelas and cellulitis. It is usually a benign infection commonly seen in fishermen and meat handlers, which is characterized by redness of the skin, most often of a finger or the back of the hand, and which gradually extends over a period of several days. Systemic involvement which occurs rarely, is manifested by reversal of the albumin-globulin ratio and other serious changes. Endocarditis may occur.

Penicillin is usually promptly curative. Broad-spectrum antibiotics may be used instead.

DECUBITUS ULCERS
(Bedsores)

Bedsores (pressure sores) are a special type of ulcer caused by impaired blood supply and tissue nutrition due to prolonged pressure over bony or cartilaginous prominences. The skin overlying the sacrum and hips is most commonly involved, but bedsores may also be seen over the occiput, ears, elbows, heels, and ankles. They occur most readily in aged, paralyzed, and debilitated patients in whom an adequate underlying fat pad is lacking. Low-grade infection may occur.

Good nursing care and nutrition and maintenance of skin hygiene are important preventive measures. The skin and the bed linens should be kept clean and dry. Bedfast, paralyzed, moribund, or listless patients who are candidates for the development of decubiti must be turned **frequently** (at least every hour) and must be examined at pressure points for the appearance of small areas of redness and tenderness. Inflated rubber rings, rubber pillows, and an alternating pressure mattress, all of which are essential in the treatment of early lesions, are of value also in prevention.

Early lesions should also be treated with topical antibiotic powders and adhesive absorbent bandage (Gelfoam). Established lesions require surgical consultation and care. A spongy pad called "Feathersoft" may be placed under the patient and may work best in some cases. It may be laundered often. A water bed would be very useful, except when miliaria is present. A continuous dressing with 1% iodochlorhydroxyquin (Vioform) in Lassar's paste may be effective.

Schlappner OLA, Shelley WB: Polyethylene mesh: A new treatment for decubital dermatitis. JAMA 223:430, 1973.

FUNGAL INFECTIONS
OF THE SKIN

Mycotic infections are traditionally divided into 2 principal groups: superficial and deep. In this chapter we will discuss only the superficial infections: tinea capitis, tinea corporis, and tinea cruris; dermatophytosis of the feet and dermatophytid of the hands; tinea unguium (onychomycosis, or fungal infection of the nails); and tinea versicolor. Candidiasis belongs in an intermediate group but will be considered here as well as with the deep mycoses.

The diagnosis of fungal infections of the skin is usually based on the location and characteristics of the lesions and on the following laboratory examinations: (1) Direct demonstration of fungi in 10% potassium hydroxide preparations of scrapings from suspected lesions. (2) Cultures of organisms. Dermatophytes responsive to griseofulvin are easily detectable, with color change from yellow to red on dermatophyte test medium (DTM). (3) Skin tests, eg, trichophytin (not reliable) for superficial mycoses. (This test has exclusion value in suspected dermatophytid.) (4) Examination with Wood's light (an ultraviolet light with a spe-

cial filter), which causes hairs to fluoresce a brilliant green when they are infected by microsporum organisms (cause of about 90% of cases of tinea capitis in some areas of the USA). The lamp is also invaluable in following the progress of treatment. Ringworm of the scalp may be totally unsuspected yet discovered easily with Wood's light in mass surveys of school children. Trichophyton-infected hairs do not fluoresce. (5) Histologic sections stained with periodic acid-Schiff (Hotchkiss-McManus) technic. Fungal elements stain red and are easily found.

Serologic tests are of no value in the diagnosis of superficial fungal infections.

Delayed sensitivity to intradermal trichophytin appears to be a correlate of immunity, whereas immediate trichophytin reactivity is associated with chronic tinea infections.

Principles of Local Treatment

Treat acute active fungal infections initially as for any acute dermatitis (see p 32). *Note:* It may be necessary to treat the dermatitis before applying topical fungicidal medication.

Many topical fungicidal agents are strong skin irritants. *It is easy to overtreat.*

General Measures & Prevention

Keep the skin dry, since moist skin favors the growth of fungi. A cool climate is preferred. Reduce exercise and activities to prevent excessive perspiration. Dry the skin carefully after bathing or after perspiring heavily. Socks and other clothing should be changed often. Sandals or open-toed shoes should be worn. Skin secretions should be controlled with talc or other drying powders or with drying soaks (Table 3–1). Sedatives (eg, phenobarbital) may be effective in reducing skin secretions in tense, nervous people. Toughen the skin with graded daily sunbaths or with a quartz lamp.

Clayton YM: Therapy of fungal infections. Brit J Dermat 89:423, 1973.

Griseofulvin

Griseofulvin is an antibiotic obtained by fermentation of several species of penicillia. It is water-soluble and thermostable, and is not related chemically to any other antibiotic in current use. Cross-sensitization with other antibiotics has not been a problem. The drug is deposited in keratinous structures and apparently acts by interfering with reproduction of the fungal elements.

Griseofulvin is employed in oral dosage against dermatophyte or "ringworm" fungal infections. It is most effective for ringworm infections of the scalp and quite effective for involvement of the face, neck, and trunk; reasonably effective against ringworm of the groin; and less effective for involvement of hands and feet. Nail infections are least responsive to griseofulvin therapy.

The drug is supplied in microcrystalline forms

which are available in 250 mg capsules and 500 mg tablets. The average daily dose is 1 gm orally for adults and comparably less for children. A new form of griseofulvin with ultramicrosize particles in the tablet (Gris-Peg) is said to be effective in half the usual dose and is available as 250 mg tablets. Taking griseofulvin with a fatty meal adds nothing to therapy. Prolonged treatment may be required for onychomycosis.

Toxic reactions include headache, urticaria, dizziness, drowsiness, morbilliform and hemorrhagic eruptions, gastrointestinal distress, and loose stools, as well as photosensitivity and interference with the action of dicumarol. Although severe reactions are occasionally reported, hematologic studies and assays of kidney and liver function have shown the drug to be essentially free of severe side reactions.

Epstein WL, Shah V, Riegelman S: Dermatopharmacology of griseofulvin. Cutis 15:271, 1975.

Jones HE & others: Acquired immunity to dermatophytes. Arch Dermat 109:840, 1974.

Mandy SJ, Garrott TC: Miconazole treatment for severe dermatophytoses. JAMA 230:72, 1974.

Miconazole: A new topical antifungal drug. Med Lett Drugs Ther 16:97, 1974.

Oberste-Lehn H: Ideal properties of modern antifungal agent: Therapy of mycoses with clotrimazole. Postgrad MJ 50 (Suppl 1):51, 1974.

Warin RP: Antifungal agents. Practitioner 213:494, 1974.

TINEA CAPITIS
(Ringworm of Scalp)

Essentials of Diagnosis

- Round, gray, scaly "bald" patches on the scalp.
- Usually in prepuberal children.
- Often fluorescent under Wood's lamp.
- Microscopic examination or culture identifies the fungus.

General Considerations

This persistent, contagious, and sometimes epidemic infection occurs almost exclusively in children and disappears spontaneously at puberty. Two genera (Microsporum and Trichophyton) cause ringworm infections of the scalp. Microsporum accounts for many of the infections, and hairs infected with this genus fluoresce brilliantly under Wood's light. Trichophyton species account for some of the very resistant infections, which may persist into adulthood.

Clinical Findings

A. Symptoms and Signs: There are usually no symptoms, although there may be slight itching. The lesions are round, gray, scaly, apparently bald patches on the scalp. (The hairs are broken off and the patches are not actually bald.) Scalp ringworm may be undetectable with the naked eye, becoming visible only under the Wood light, in which case the hairs exhibit a brilliant green fluorescence extending down into the hair follicle.

B. Laboratory Findings: Microscopic or culture demonstration of the organisms in the hairs may be necessary.

Differential Diagnosis

Differentiate from other diseases of scalp hair such as pediculosis capitis, pyoderma, alopecia areata, and trichotillomania (voluntary pulling out of one's own hair).

Prevention

Exchange of headgear must be avoided, and infected individuals or household pets must be vigorously treated and reexamined for determination of cure. The scalp should be washed after haircuts.

Complications

Kerion (a nodular, exudative pustule), possibly followed by scarring, is the only complication.

Treatment

Microcrystalline griseofulvin, 0.25–0.5 gm by mouth daily or twice daily for 2 weeks, will cure most cases. Two percent miconazole cream or 1% clotrimazole cream or lotion may be rubbed in twice daily.

Prognosis

Tinea capitis may be very persistent, but usually clears spontaneously at puberty. Most ringworm infections of the scalp will clear spontaneously in 1–2 years even if not treated.

TINEA CORPORIS OR TINEA CIRCINATA
(Body Ringworm)

Essentials of Diagnosis

- Pruritic, ringed, scaling, centrally clearing lesions; small vesicles in a peripherally advancing border.
- On exposed skin surfaces.
- History of exposure to infected domestic animal.
- Laboratory examination by microscope or culture confirms diagnosis.

General Considerations

The lesions are often on exposed areas of the body such as the face and arms. A history of exposure to an infected cat may be obtained. All species of dermatophytes may cause this disease, but some are more common than others.

Clinical Findings

A. Symptoms and Signs: Itching is usually intense, which serves to distinguish the disease from other ringed lesions. The lesions consist of rings of vesicles with central clearing, grouped in clusters and distributed asymmetrically, usually on an exposed surface.

B. Laboratory Findings: Hyphae can be demonstrated readily by removing the cap of a vesicle and examining it microscopically in a drop of 10% potassium hydroxide. The diagnosis may be confirmed by culture.

Differential Diagnosis

Itching distinguishes tinea corporis from other skin lesions with annular configuration, such as the annular lesions of psoriasis, erythema multiforme, and pityriasis rosea.

Complications

Complications include extension of the disease to the scalp hair or nails (in which case it becomes much more difficult to cure), overtreatment dermatitis, pyoderma, and dermatophytid.

Prevention (See also p 56.)

Avoid contact with infected household pets and avoid exchange of clothing without adequate laundering.

Treatment

A. Specific Measures: Griseofulvin (microcrystalline), 0.5 gm orally daily for children and 1 gm orally daily for adults.

B. Local Measures: One percent salicylic acid and 3% precipitated sulfur in hydrophilic ointment may be rubbed into lesions twice daily. *Caution:* Do not overtreat.

Compound undecylenic acid ointment may be used in the less chronic and nonthickened lesions.

Tolnaftate (Tinactin) solution (℞ 21) or cream applied topically is effective against dermatophyte infections other than of the nails. Haloprogin, 1% cream or solution, may be used. Miconazole (MicaTin), 2% cream (℞ 38), is the most effective topical antitineal agent currently available in the USA. Clotrimazole, an imidazole similar to miconazole, has become available as a 1% liquid or cream.

Prognosis

Body ringworm usually responds promptly to griseofulvin by mouth or to conservative topical therapy.

Fulton JE Jr: Miconazole therapy for endemic fungal disease. Arch Dermat 111:596, 1975.

TINEA CRURIS
(Jock Itch)

Essentials of Diagnosis

- Marked itching in intertriginous areas.

- Peripherally spreading, sharply demarcated, centrally clearing erythematous macular lesions, with or without vesicle formation.
- May have associated tinea infection of feet.
- Laboratory examination with microscope or culture confirms diagnosis.

General Considerations

Tinea cruris lesions are confined to the groin and gluteal cleft and are as a rule more indolent than those of tinea corporis and tinea circinata. The disease often occurs in athletes as well as in persons who are obese or who perspire a great deal. Any of the dermatophytes may cause tinea cruris, and it may be transmitted to the groin from active dermatophytosis of the foot. Intractable pruritus ani may occasionally be caused by tineal infection.

Clinical Findings

A. Symptoms and Signs: Itching is usually more severe than that which occurs in seborrheic dermatitis or intertrigo. Inverse psoriasis, however, may itch even more than tinea cruris. The lesions consist of erythematous macules with sharp margins, cleared centers, and active, spreading peripheries in intertriginous areas. There may be vesicle formation at the borders, and satellite vesicular lesions are sometimes present.

B. Laboratory Findings: Hyphae can be demonstrated microscopically in 10% potassium hydroxide preparations. The organism may be cultured readily.

Differential Diagnosis

Differentiate from other lesions involving the intertriginous areas, such as candidiasis, seborrheic dermatitis, intertrigo, and psoriasis of body folds ("inverse psoriasis").

Treatment

A. General Measures: (See also p 32.) Drying powder (Table 3–2) should be dusted into the involved area 2–3 times a day, especially when perspiration is excessive. Keep the area clean and dry but avoid overbathing. Prevent intertrigo or chafing by avoiding overtreatment, which predisposes to further infection and complications. Rough-textured clothing should be avoided.

B. Specific Measures: Griseofulvin (see p 56) is indicated for severe cases. Give 1 gm orally daily for 1–2 weeks.

C. Local Measures: Treat the stage of dermatosis (see p 32). Secondarily infected or inflamed lesions are best treated with soothing and drying solutions, with the patient at bed rest. Use wet compresses of potassium permanganate, 1:10,000 (or 1:20 aluminum acetate solution), or, in case of anogenital infection, sitz baths.

Fungicidal preparations: Any of the following may be used: (1) Weak solutions of iodine (not more than 1% tincture) twice daily. (2) Carbolfuchsin solution (Castellani's paint), one-third strength, once a day. (3) Compound undecylenic acid ointment twice daily.

(4) Sulfur-salicylic acid ointment (R 35). (5) Tolnaftate (Tinactin) solution (R 21) or cream. (6) Haloprogin (Halotex), 1% cream or solution. (7) Miconazole (MicaTin), 2% cream (R 38). (8) Clotrimazole, 1% liquid or cream.

Prognosis

Tinea cruris usually responds promptly to topical or systemic treatment.

Clayton YM, Connor BL: Comparison of clotrimazole cream, Whitfield's ointment and nystatin ointment for the topical treatment of ringworm infections, pityriasis versicolor, erythrasma and candidiasis. Brit J Dermat 89:297, 1973.

TINEA MANUUM & TINEA PEDUM
(Dermatophytosis,
Tinea of Palms & Soles, "Athlete's Foot")

Essentials of Diagnosis

- Itching, burning, and stinging of interdigital webs, palms, and soles.
- Deep vesicles in acute stage.
- Exfoliation, fissuring, and maceration in subacute or chronic stages.
- Skin scrapings examined microscopically or by culture may reveal fungus.

General Considerations

Tinea of the feet is an extremely common acute or chronic dermatosis. It is possible that the causative organisms are present on the feet of most adults at all times. Certain individuals appear to be more susceptible than others. Most infections are caused by Trichophyton and Epidermophyton species.

Clinical Findings

A. Symptoms and Signs: The presenting symptom is usually itching. However, there may be burning, stinging, and other sensations, or frank pain from secondary infection with complicating cellulitis, lymphangitis, and lymphadenitis. Tinea pedum often appears as a fissuring of the toe webs, perhaps with denudation and sodden maceration. However, there may also be grouped vesicles distributed anywhere on the soles or the palms, a generalized exfoliation of the skin of the soles, or destructive nail involvement in the form of discoloration and hypertrophy of the nail substance with pithy changes. Acute reddened, weeping vesicular lesions are seen on the skin in the acute stages.

B. Laboratory Findings: Hyphae can often be demonstrated microscopically in skin scales treated with 10% potassium hydroxide. Culture with Sabouraud's medium is simple and often informative, but does not always demonstrate pathogenic fungi.

Differential Diagnosis

Differentiate from other skin conditions involving the same areas such as interdigital intertrigo, candidiasis, psoriasis, contact dermatitis (from shoes, powders, nail polish), atopic eczema, and scabies.

Prevention

The essential factor in prevention is personal hygiene. Rubber or wooden sandals should be used in community showers and bathing places. Open-toed shoes and sandals are best for general wear. Careful drying between the toes after showering is recommended. Socks should be changed frequently. Apply dusting and drying powders as necessary (Table 3–2), and place small wads of cotton between the toes at night.

Treatment

A. Specific Measures: Griseofulvin (see p 56) has been disappointing in the treatment of dermatophytosis of the feet and should be used only for severe cases or those which are recalcitrant to topical therapy.

B. Local Measures: *Caution:* Do not overtreat.

1. **Acute stage** (lasts 1–10 days)—Give aluminum subacetate solution soaks (R 4) for 20 minutes 2–3 times daily. If secondary infection is present, use soaks of 1:10,000 potassium permanganate. If secondary infection is severe or complicated, treat as described on p 32.

2. **Subacute stage**—Any of the following may be used: (1) 2% miconazole cream. (2) 1% clotrimazole cream or lotion. (3) Solution of coal tar, 5% in starch lotion, or R 16. (4) Coat tar, 1–2% in Lassar's paste.

3. **Chronic stage**—Use any of the following: (1) Sulfur-salicylic acid ointment (R 35) or cream. (2) Whitfield's ointment, one-fourth to one-half strength (R 33). (3) Compound undecylenic acid ointment twice daily. (4) Alcoholic Whitfield's solution (R 46). (5) Carbolfuchsin solution (Castellani's paint). (6) Tolnaftate (Tinactin) solution (R 21) or cream. (7) Haloprogin, 1% cream or solution. (8) Miconazole (MicaTin), 2% cream (R 38). (9) Clotrimazole (Lotrimin), 1% cream or lotion

C. Mechanical Measures: Carefully remove or debride dead or thickened tissues after soaks or baths.

D. X-Ray or Grenz Ray: Radiation therapy (by a specialist) may be of value to reduce chronic thickened eczematized lesions when other measures fail.

Prognosis

Tinea of the hands and feet usually responds well to treatment, but recurrences are common in strongly predisposed persons.

Hanifin JM, Ray LF, Lobitz WC Jr: Immunological reactivity in dermatophytosis. Brit J Dermat 90:1, 1974.
Knight AG: Human models for in vivo and in vitro assessment of topical antifungal compounds. Brit J Dermat 89:509, 1973.

DERMATOPHYTID
(Allergy or Sensitivity to Fungi)

Essentials of Diagnosis

- Pruritic, grouped vesicular lesions involving the sides and flexor aspects of the fingers and the palms.
- Fungal infection elsewhere on body, usually the feet.
- Trichophytin skin test positive. No fungus demonstrable in lesions.

General Considerations

Dermatophytid is a sensitivity reaction to an active focus of dermatophytosis elsewhere on the body, usually the feet. Fungi are present in the primary lesion but are not present in the lesions of dermatophytid. The hands are most often affected, but dermatophytid may occur on other areas of the body also.

Clinical Findings

A. Symptoms and Signs: Itching is the only symptom. The lesions consist of grouped vesicles, often involving the thenar and hypothenar eminences. Lesions are round, up to 15 mm in diameter, and may be present on the side and flexor aspects of the fingers. Lesions occasionally involve the backs of the hands or may even be generalized.

B. Laboratory Findings: The trichophyton skin test is positive, but it may also be positive with other disorders. A negative trichophytin test rules out dermatophytid. Repeated negative microscopic examinations of material taken from the lesions is necessary before the diagnosis of dermatophytid can be established. Culture from the primary site tends to reveal *Trichophyton mentagrophytes* organisms rather than *T rubrum*. There appears to be selective anergy in patients with chronic *T rubrum* infections.

Differential Diagnosis

Differentiate from all diseases causing vesicular eruptions of the hands, especially contact dermatitis, dyshidrosis, and localized forms of atopic dermatitis.

Prevention

Treat fungal infections early and adequately, and prevent recurrences (see p 56).

Treatment

General measures are as outlined on p 32. The lesions should be treated according to type of dermatitis. The primary focus should be treated with griseofulvin (see p 56) or by local measures as described for dermatophytosis (see above). A single injection of triamcinolone acetonide suspension, 30 mg intragluteally, may suppress the eruption until the causative focus is controlled.

Prognosis

Dermatophytid may occur in an explosive series of episodes, and recurrences are not uncommon; however, it clears with adequate treatment of the primary infection elsewhere on the body.

TINEA UNGUIUM
& CANDIDAL ONYCHOMYCOSIS

Essentials of Diagnosis

- Lusterless, brittle, hypertrophic, friable nails.
- Fungus demonstrated in nail section or nail dust by microscope or culture.

General Considerations

Tinea unguium is a destructive trichophyton or epidermophyton infection of one or more (but rarely all) fingernails or toenails. The species most commonly found are *Trichophyton mentagrophytes*, *T rubrum*, and *Epidermophyton floccosum. Candida albicans* causes candidal onychomycosis. "Saprophytic" fungi may cause onychomycosis.

Clinical Findings

A. Symptoms and Signs: There are usually no symptoms. The nails are lusterless, brittle, and hypertrophic, and the substance of the nail is friable and even pithy. Irregular segments of the diseased nail may be broken.

B. Laboratory Findings: Laboratory diagnosis is mandatory. Portions of the nail should be cleared with 10% potassium hydroxide and examined under the microscope for branching hyphae or collections of spores. Fungi may also be cultured, using Sabouraud's medium. Periodic acid-Schiff stain of a histologic section will also demonstrate the fungus readily.

Differential Diagnosis

Distinguish from nail changes caused by contact with strong alkalies and certain other chemicals and from those due to psoriasis, lichen planus, and candidiasis.

Treatment

A. General Measures: See p 32.

B. Specific Measures: Griseofulvin (see p 56) in full dosages daily for 3–8 months may be necessary for tinea unguium, and even this rarely cures. Candida or dermatophyte infection may be treated specifically with miconazole or clotrimazole.

C. Local Measures: Sandpaper or file the nails daily (down to nail bed if necessary). Surgical avulsion of the nail may be required.

Fungicidal agents: Apply one of the following twice daily on affected nails: (1) Miconazole (MicaTin), 2% cream (R 38). (2) Clotrimazole (Lotrimin), 1% cream or lotion.

Prognosis

Cure is difficult, even with microcrystalline griseofulvin by mouth in a dose of 1—2 gm daily for months, or with miconazole or clotrimazole.

English MP, Atkinson R: An improved method for the isolation of fungi in onychomycosis. Brit J Dermat 88:237, 1973.
Zaias N: Onychomycosis. Arch Dermat 105:263, 1972.

TINEA VERSICOLOR

Essentials of Diagnosis
- Pale macules which will not tan.
- Velvety, chamois-colored macules which scale with scraping.
- Trunk distribution the most frequent site.
- Fungus on microscopic examination of scales.

General Considerations
Tinea versicolor is a mild, superficial *Malassezia furfur* infection of the skin (usually of the trunk). The eruption is called to the patient's attention by the fact that the involved areas will not tan, and the resulting pseudoachromia may be mistaken for vitiligo. The disease is not particularly contagious and is apt to occur more frequently in those who wear heavy clothing and who perspire a great deal.

Clinical Findings
A. Symptoms and Signs: There may be mild itching. The lesions are velvety, chamois-colored macules which vary from 4—5 mm in diameter to large confluent areas. Scales may be readily obtained by scraping the area with the fingernail. Lesions may appear on the trunk, upper arms, neck, and face.

B. Laboratory Findings: Large, blunt hyphae and thick-walled budding spores may be seen under the low power objective when skin scales have been cleared in 10% potassium hydroxide. *M furfur* is difficult to culture.

Differential Diagnosis
Distinguish from vitiligo on basis of appearance. Differentiate also from seborrheic dermatitis of the same areas.

Treatment & Prognosis
Encourage good skin hygiene. Tinea versicolor responds readily to selenium sulfide suspension (Selsun), lathered on daily. Relapses are frequent. Newer topical treatments include tolnaftate (Tinactin) solution (℞ 21) and acrisorcin (Akrinol) cream.

Sulfur-salicylic acid soap (marketed by Stiefel) used on a continuing basis may be the best treatment.

Bamford JTM: Tinea versicolor treatment. (Correspondence.) Arch Dermat 110:956, 1974.

CUTANEOUS CANDIDIASIS
(Moniliasis)

Essentials of Diagnosis
- Severe pruritus of vulva, anus, or body folds.
- Superficial, denuded, beefy red areas with or without satellite vesicopustules.
- Whitish curd-like concretions on the surface.
- Fungus on microscopic examination of scales or curd.

General Considerations
Cutaneous candidiasis is a superficial fungal infection which may involve almost any cutaneous or mucous surface of the body. It is particularly likely to occur in diabetics, during pregnancy, and in obese persons who perspire freely. Antibiotics and oral contraceptive agents may be contributory. Hypoparathyroidism may be complicated by candidiasis. In the chronic forms there is often a defect in cell-mediated immunity. There probably is a range of disordered immunologic function. Latent iron deficiency may play a role, as may hypothyroidism, lymphoreticular malignancy, or thymic malformation. Idiopathic forms occur. *Candida albicans* infection may thus serve as a marker of internal disease and should alert the clinician to the need for diagnostic investigations—repeatedly if necessary.

Clinical Findings
A. Symptoms and Signs: Itching may be intense. Burning sensations are sometimes reported, particularly around the vulva and anus. The lesions consist of superficially denuded, beefy red areas in the depths of the body folds such as in the groin and the intergluteal cleft, beneath the breasts, at the angles of the mouth, and in the umbilicus. The peripheries of these denuded lesions are superficially undermined, and there may be satellite vesicopustules. Whitish, curd-like concretions may be present on the surface of the lesions (particularly in the oral and vaginal mucous membranes). Paronychia and interdigital erosions may occur.

B. Laboratory Findings: Clusters of budding cells and short hyphae can be seen under the high power lens when skin scales or curd-like lesions have been cleared in 10% potassium hydroxide. The organism may be isolated on Sabouraud's medium.

Differential Diagnosis
Differentiate from intertrigo, seborrheic dermatitis, and tinea cruris involving the same areas.

Complications
Candidiasis may spread from the skin or mucous membranes to the bladder, lungs, and other internal organs. Fungemia may cause shock and coma without mucocutaneous lesions.

Treatment
A. General Measures: Treat associated diabetes, obesity, or hyperhidrosis. Keep the parts dry and ex-

posed to air as much as possible. If possible, discontinue systemic antibiotics; if not, give nystatin by mouth concomitantly in a dose of 1.5 million units 3 times daily. Transfer factor (investigational) has helped some chronic cases, possibly by correcting defective production of migration inhibition factor. Correcting iron deficiency and giving pyridoxine and vitamin A may help also.

B. Local Measures:

1. Nails and skin—Apply nystatin cream, 100,000 units/gm, or amphotericin B lotion, 3—4 times daily. Gentian violet, 1%, or carbolfuchsin paint (Castellani's paint) may be applied 1—2 times weekly as an alternative. Miconazole (MicaTin), 2% cream, has been reported to be effective in mucocutaneous candidiasis.

2. Vulva, anal mucous membranes—Insert 1 nystatin vaginal tablet (100,000 units) nightly for 2 weeks, or apply nystatin dusting powder (100,000 units/gm) once or twice daily onto moist mucous membrane areas. Amphotericin B, gentian violet, or carbolfuchsin (see above) can also be used. Miconazole (Monistat) cream may be used intravaginally.

Prognosis

Cutaneous candidiasis may be intractable and prolonged, particularly in children, in whom the disturbance may take the form of a granuloma which resists all attempts at treatment.

Higgs JM, Wells RS: Chronic mucocutaneous candidiasis: New approaches to treatment. Brit J Dermat 89:179, 1973.

Montes LF, Herman HW: Topical use of haloprogin for candidiasis. Arch Dermat 107:773, 1973.

Rebora A & others: Experimental infection with *Candida albicans.* Arch Dermat 108:69, 1973.

Richman RA & others: Candidiasis and multiple endocrinopathy. Arch Dermat 111:625, 1975.

PARASITIC INFESTATIONS OF THE SKIN

SCABIES

Essentials of Diagnosis

- Nocturnal itching.
- Pruritic vesicles and pustules in "runs" or "galleries," especially on the sides of the fingers and the heels of the palms.
- Mites, ova, and black clots of feces visible microscopically.

General Considerations

Scabies is a common dermatitis caused by infestation with *Sarcoptes scabiei.* An entire family may be affected. The infestation usually spares the head and neck (although even these areas may be involved in infants). The mite is barely visible with the naked eye as a white dot. Scabies is usually acquired by sleeping or other close contact with an infested individual. This infestation is on the increase worldwide.

Clinical Findings

A. Symptoms and Signs: Itching occurs almost exclusively at night. The lesions consist of more or less generalized excoriations with small pruritic vesicles, pustules, and "runs" or "galleries" on the sides of the fingers and the heels of the palms. The run or gallery appears as a short irregular mark (perhaps 2—3 mm long), as if made by a sharp pencil. Characteristic lesions may occur on the nipples in females and as pruritic papules on the scrotum in males. Pruritic papules may be seen over the buttocks. Pyoderma is often the presenting sign.

B. Laboratory Findings: The adult female mite may be demonstrated by probing the fresh end of a run or gallery with a pointed scalpel. The mite tends to cling to the tip of the blade. One may shave off the entire run or gallery (or, in the scrotum, a papule) and demonstrate the female mite, her ova, and small black dots of feces. The diagnosis should be confirmed by microscopic demonstration of the organism, ova, or feces after mounting the specimen on glycerin or mineral oil.

Differential Diagnosis

Distinguish from the various forms of pediculosis and from other causes of pruritus.

Treatment & Prognosis

Unless the lesions are complicated by severe secondary pyoderma (see p 32), treatment consists primarily of disinfestation. If secondary pyoderma is present it should be treated with systemic and topical antibiotics.

Disinfestation with gamma benzene hexachloride (lindane, Gexane, Kwell), 1% in cream base, applied each night for 3 nights, has been the treatment of choice. This preparation can be used before secondary infection is controlled. Some recent evidence indicates that strains of *Sarcoptes scabiei* resistant to this drug may be developing. An alternative very effective drug is crotamiton (Eurax) cream or lotion, which may be applied in the same way as gamma benzene hexachloride.

Unless treatment is aimed at all infected persons in a family, reinfestations will probably occur.

Resistant forms are appearing, requiring multiple forms of treatment.

Carslaw RW & others: Mites in the environment of cases of Norwegian scabies. Brit J Dermat 92:333, 1975.

Downham TF II, Dieteman DR, Botvinick I: The natural history of scabies. Cutis 12:349, 1973.

Muller GV & others: Scraping for human scabies. Arch Dermat 107:70, 1973.

PEDICULOSIS

Essentials of Diagnosis

- Pruritus with excoriation.
- Nits on hair shafts; lice on skin or clothes.
- Occasionally sky-blue macules (maculae caeruleae) on the inner thighs or lower abdomen in pubic louse infestation.

General Considerations

Pediculosis is a parasitic infestation of the skin of the scalp, trunk, or pubic areas. It usually occurs among people who live in overcrowded dwellings with inadequate hygiene facilities, although pubic lice may be acquired by anyone who sits on an infested toilet seat. There are 3 different varieties: (1) Pediculosis pubis caused by *Phthirus pubis* (pubic louse, "crabs"); (2) pediculosis corporis, by *Pediculus humanus* var *corporis* (body louse); (3) pediculosis capitis, by *P humanus* var *capitis* (head louse).

Head and body lice are similar in appearance, 3–4 mm long. Head louse infestations may be transmitted by shared use of hats or combs. The body louse can seldom be found on the body, as the insect comes on the skin only to feed, and must be looked for in the seams of the underclothing.

Trench fever, relapsing fever, and typhus may be transmitted by the body louse.

Clinical Findings

Itching may be very intense in body louse infestations, and scratching may result in deep excoriations over the affected area. The clinical appearance is of gross excoriation. Pyoderma may be present and may be the presenting sign in any of these infestations. Head lice can be found on the scalp or may be manifested as small nits resembling pussy-willow buds on the scalp hairs close to the skin. They are easiest to see above the ears and at the nape of the neck. Body lice may deposit visible nits on the lanugo hair of the body. Pubic louse infestations are occasionally generalized, particularly in a hairy individual; the lice may even be found on the eyelashes and in the scalp.

Differential Diagnosis

Distinguish head louse infestation from seborrheic dermatitis, body louse infestation from scabies, and pubic louse infestation from anogenital pruritus and eczema.

Treatment

One may use the same remedies described for scabies (see above).

Prognosis

Pediculosis responds promptly to topical treatment.

Duffy DM: Ectoparasitic infections. Cutis 7:161, 1971.

SKIN LESIONS
DUE TO OTHER ARTHROPODS

Essentials of Diagnosis

- Localized rash with pruritus.
- Furuncle-like lesions containing live arthropods.
- Tender erythematous patches which migrate ("larva migrans").
- Generalized urticaria or erythema multiforme.

General Considerations

Some arthropods (eg, most pest mosquitos and biting flies) are readily detected as they bite. Many others are not, eg, because they are too small, there is no immediate reaction, or they bite during sleep. Reactions may be delayed for many hours; many severe reactions are allergic. Patients are most apt to consult a physician when the lesions are multiple and pruritus is intense. Severe attacks may be accompanied by insomnia, restlessness, fever, and faintness or even collapse. Rashes may sometimes cover the body.

Many persons will react severely only to their earliest contacts with an arthropod, thus presenting pruritic lesions when traveling, moving into new quarters, etc. Body lice, fleas, bedbugs, and local mosquitos should be borne in mind. Spiders are often incorrectly believed to be the source of bites; they rarely attack man, although the brown spider (Loxosceles) may cause severe necrotic reactions and death due to intravascular hemolysis, and the black widow spider (*Latrodectus mactans*) may cause severe systemic symptoms and death.

In addition to arthropod bites, the most common lesions are venomous stings (wasps, hornets, bees, ants, scorpions) or bites (centipedes), dermatitis due to urticating hairs of caterpillars, dermatitis due to vesicating furuncle-like lesions due to fly maggots or sand fleas in the skin, and a linear creeping eruption due to a migrating larva.

Clinical Findings

The diagnosis may be difficult when the patient has not noticed the initial attack but suffers a delayed reaction. Individual bites are frequently in clusters and tend to occur either on exposed parts (eg, midges and gnats) or under clothing, especially around the waist or at flexures (eg, small mites or insects in bedding or clothing). The reaction is often delayed for 1–24 hours or more. Pruritus is almost always present, and may be all but intolerable once the patient starts to scratch. Secondary infection, sometimes with serious consequences, may follow scratching. Allergic manifestations, including urticarial wheals, are common. Papules may become vesicular. The diagnosis is greatly aided by searching for possible exposure to arthropods and by considering the occupation and recent activities of the patient. The principal arthropods are as follows:

(1) **Bedbugs:** In crevices of beds or furniture;

bites tend to occur in lines or clusters. The closely related kissing bug has been reported with increasing frequency as attacking man.

(2) **Fleas:** In beds and floors. Rat fleas may attack the legs. Stick-tight fleas from poultry in the southern United States may be found actually attached to the skin. Tunga or chigoe fleas in South America and Africa burrow into the skin and swell, and secondary infection occurs readily following maltreatment.

(3) **Ticks:** Usually picked up by brushing against low vegetation. Larval ticks may attack in large numbers and cause much distress; in Africa and India they have been confused with chiggers. Ascending paralysis may occasionally be traced to a tick bite, and removal of the embedded tick is essential.

(4) **Chiggers or red-bugs** are larvas of trombiculid mites. A few species confined to particular countries and usually to restricted and locally recognized habitats (eg, berry patches, woodland edge, lawns, brush turkey mounds in Australia, poultry farms) attack man, often around the waist, on the ankles, or in flexures, raising intensely itching erythematous papules after a delay of many hours. The red chiggers may sometimes be seen in the center of papules which have not yet been scratched. Chiggers are the commonest cause of distressing multiple lesions due to arthropods.

(5) **Bird mites:** Larger than chiggers, infesting chicken houses, pigeon lofts, or nests of birds in eaves. Bites are multiple anywhere on the body, although poultry handlers are most often attacked on the hands and forearms. Room air conditioning units may suck in bird mites and infest the inhabitants of the room.

Rodent mites from mice or rats may cause similar effects. In the case of bird mites and rodent mites the diagnosis may readily be overlooked and the patient treated for other dermatoses or for psychogenic dermatosis. Intractable "acarophobia" may result from early neglect or misdiagnosis.

(6) **Mites in stored products:** These are white and almost invisible, and infest products such as copra ("copra itch"), vanilla pods ("vanillism"), sugar, straw, cotton seeds, and cereals. Persons who handle these products may be attacked, especially on the hands and forearms and sometimes on the feet. Infested bedding may occasionally lead to generalized dermatitis.

(7) **Caterpillars of moths with urticating hairs:** The hairs are blown from cocoons or carried by emergent moths, causing severe and often seasonally recurrent outbreaks after mass emergence, eg, in some southern states of the USA.

(8) **Tungiasis** is due to the burrowing flea known as *Tunga penetrans* (also known as chigoe, jigger; not the same as chigger) found in Africa, the West Indies, and South America. The female burrows under the skin, sucks blood, swells to the size of 0.5 cm, and then ejects her eggs onto the ground. Ulceration, lymphangitis, gangrene, and septicemia may result, possibly with fatality. Chloroform or ether on a cotton pledget will kill the insect when applied to the lesion, and disinfestation may be accomplished with insecticide applied to the terrain.

Differential Diagnosis

Arthropods should be considered in the differential diagnosis of skin lesions showing any of the above symptoms.

Prevention

Arthropod infestations are best prevented by avoidance of contaminated areas, personal cleanliness, and disinfection of clothing, bed clothes, and furniture as indicated. Lice, chiggers, red-bugs, and mites can be killed by lindane applied to the head and clothing. (It is not necessary to remove clothing.) Benzyl benzoate and dimethylphthalate are excellent acaricides; clothing should be impregnated by spray or by dipping in a soapy emulsion.

Treatment

Caution: Avoid local overtreatment.

Living arthropods should be removed carefully with tweezers after application of alcohol. Preserve in alcohol for identification. (*Caution:* In endemic Rocky Mountain spotted fever areas, do not remove ticks with the bare fingers for fear of becoming infected.) Children in particular should be prevented from scratching.

Apply corticosteroid lotions or creams. If they are not available, crotamiton (Eurax) cream or lotion may be used; it is a miticide as well as an antipruritic. Calamine lotion or a cool wet dressing is always appropriate. Antibiotic creams, lotions, or powders may be applied if secondary infection is suspected.

Localized persistent lesions may be treated with intralesional corticosteroids. Avoid exercise and excessive warmth. Codeine may be given for pain. Creams containing local anesthetics are not very effective and may be sensitizing. (See also Myiasis in Chapter 26.)

Stings produced by many arthropods may be alleviated by applying papain powder (Adolph's meat tenderizer) mixed with water.

Frazier CA: Biting insects. Arch Dermat 107:400, 1973.
Goodman RS: Insect bite reactions: Some unusual histopathologic changes. Cutis 15:393, 1975.
Loder JS: Treatment of jellyfish stings. JAMA 226:1228, 1973.
Maibach HI, Khan AA, Akers W: Use of insect repellents for maximum efficiency. Arch Dermat 109:32, 1974.

TUMORS OF THE SKIN

General Considerations

Areas exposed to chronic irritation (sun, chemicals, friction) are especially susceptible to neoplastic disease. The blue-eyed, sandy-complexioned person living under conditions of excessive sun exposure is a most likely candidate for skin cancer, especially of the squamous cell or basal cell variety. In the southwestern United States skin cancer is the commonest skin problem, being even more common than acne vulgaris.

Classification

The following classification is admittedly oversimplified; almost any tumor arising from embryonal cells in the various stages of their development can be found in the skin.

A. Malignant:

1. Squamous cell carcinoma and senile keratoses usually occur on exposed parts in blue-eyed, sandy-complexioned persons. Squamous cell carcinoma may develop very rapidly, attaining a diameter of 1 cm within 2 weeks. It appears as a small red, conical, hard nodule which quickly ulcerates. Metastasis may occur early. Keratoacanthomas are benign growths which resemble squamous cell carcinoma.

2. Basal cell carcinomas also occur mostly on exposed parts. They grow slowly, attaining a size of 1–2 cm in diameter only after a year's growth. They present a waxy appearance, with telangiectatic vessels easily visible. Metastases almost never occur.

3. Paget's disease, considered by some to be a manifestation of apocrine sweat gland carcinoma, may occur around the nipple, resembling chronic eczema, or may involve apocrine areas such as the genitalia.

4. Malignant melanoma is the most malignant of all skin cancers, with an overall salvage rate of about 25%. Prognosis varies with the depth of invasion, the most superficial type—Hutchinson's freckle—being histologically malignant but clinically relatively benign. True melanomas vary from macules to nodules, with a surprising play of colors from flesh tint to pitch black and a frequent admixture of white, blue, purple, and red. The border tends to be irregular, and growth may be rapid. Treatment consists of wide excision, with lymph node dissection varying with the depth of the lesion, the location, and the background of the surgeon.

B. Premalignant: Keratoses and leukoplakia have a marked tendency to be malignant. Actinic keratoses occur on exposed parts of the body in persons of fair complexion, and nonactinic keratoses may be provoked by exposure to arsenic systemically or occupational irritants such as tars. In keratoses the cells are atypical and similar to those seen in squamous cell epitheliomas, but these changes are well contained by an intact epidermal-dermal junction. Leukoplakia is the counterpart of keratoses occurring on mucous membranes. One sees similar changes microscopically, plus the development of granular and horny layers which are not seen normally in mucous membranes or transitional epithelium. Leukoplakia may occur on the basis of individual predisposition or may be provoked by exposure to irritants such as excessive sunlight (lower lip), associated disease (eg, syphilitic glossitis), excessive pipe smoking, and chewing tobacco.

C. Benign:

1. Seborrheic warts, considered by some to be nevoid, consist of benign overgrowths of epithelium which have a pigmented velvety or warty surface. They are extremely common, both on exposed and covered parts, and are commonly mistaken for melanomas or other types of cutaneous neoplasms.

2. Bowen's disease (intraepidermal squamous cell epithelioma) is relatively uncommon and resembles a plaque of psoriasis. The course is relatively benign, but malignant progression may occur.

D. Nevi:

1. Nevus cell nevi are almost always benign, and almost everyone has at least a few of these lesions. They usually appear in childhood, and tend to spontaneous fibrosis during the declining years.

2. Junctional nevi, which consist of clear nevus cells and usually some melanin, have nevus cells on both sides of the epidermal junction. They are possible forerunners of malignant melanoma. If a nevus grows rapidly, darkens, or bleeds, the possibility of melanomatous degeneration should be considered.

3. Compound nevi, composed of junctional elements as well as clear nevus cells in the dermis, may also tend to develop into malignant melanoma. Dermal cellular nevi are quite benign.

4. Blue nevi are benign, although they give rise occasionally to malignant melanoma. They are small, slightly elevated, and blue-black.

5. Epithelial nevi include several types of verrucous epithelial overgrowths, usually in linear distribution. Microscopically, cells found normally in the epidermis are present. Such lesions rarely degenerate into squamous or basal cell carcinomas.

6. Freckles consist of excess amounts of melanin in the melanocytes in the basal layer of the epidermis. Ephelides, or juvenile freckles, may be evanescent; lentigines, or senile freckles, are usually larger and more persistent.

7. Hemangiomas are malformations and overgrowths of blood vessels. Many should be merely observed, not treated. Surgical intervention may be necessary in special situations.

Clinical Findings

A. Symptoms and Signs: The very absence of symptoms such as itching should lead one to suspect skin neoplasm when a growth is present. Soreness or pain (from ulceration or rapid growth) is occasionally reported.

Tumors of the skin consist of small nodules of varying rates of growth. The more rapid the growth, the more urgent the diagnosis. Any change in the texture or appearance of the skin should at least make the physician think of premalignant or malignant change. Whitish patches on mucous membranes, especially if their surfaces are rough, may suggest leukoplakia. Ulceration, crusting, or bleeding of any swollen area may point to cutaneous malignancy.

B. Laboratory Findings: Microscopic examination of biopsied or excised tissue usually is diagnostic for any of the lesions listed above. When malignant melanoma is suspected, the biopsy incision should include the entire lesion and a wide margin of normal skin.

Complications

Squamous cell carcinoma is particularly likely to metastasize to regional lymph glands and then to distant sites. Basal cell carcinomas, if neglected, may cause extensive local destruction; or occult spread may occur. Death may eventually take place with these "locally malignant" tumors as a result of invasion of vital structures. Melanomas spread similarly to the way in which squamous cell carcinomas do, and frequently spread hematogenously also.

Treatment

A. Surgical Measures: Both benign and malignant tumors of the skin may be removed surgically by any of the following technics. All removed nevus cell nevi should be examined histopathologically.

1. Electrosurgery—Curettage with a dermal curet followed by electrodesiccation; removal with a cutting current; or electrocoagulation.

2. Scalpel surgery.

3. Chemosurgery (Mohs technic)—In this microscopically controlled technic the tissues are fixed with zinc chloride, dissected bloodlessly, and then examined histologically. Tissue sites in which malignant cells persist are re-treated until tumor-free. A newer modification eliminates the fixation with zinc chloride. This method should be considered when other methods of treatment have failed.

4. Cryosurgery, using liquid nitrogen spray or probes, has proved of value for selected premalignant and malignant skin lesions.

B. Radiation: (By a specialist.)

1. X-ray therapy is successful for squamous cell and basal cell carcinomas. In general, malignant melanomas are unresponsive.

2. Radium and its products used interstitially or in contact may give excellent results.

C. Topical Chemotherapy: Application of 5-fluorouracil, 1% in propylene glycol, to keratoses nightly for one month, is effective. Protect the eyes. Treat complicating dermatitis with topical corticosteroids.

Prognosis

Cancer of the skin accounts for about 2% of all cancer fatalities in the United States. All cases are potentially curable if treated early. However, even with the best care, a 100% cure rate has never been attained. The outlook with malignant melanoma is more serious.

Premalignant lesions such as senile, arsenical, and occupational keratoses and leukoplakia have a favorable prognosis if treated early. Arsenical keratoses and leukoplakia sometimes progress to squamous cell carcinoma and death despite the best of care.

Only one in 0.1–1 million cellular nevi develops into a malignant melanoma.

Epstein WL & others: Halo nevi and melanoma. JAMA 225:353, 1973.
Freeman RG, Duncan WC: Recurrent skin cancer. Arch Dermat 107:395, 1973.
Mandel SL: Leukoplakia: The white spectre. Cutis 13:225, 1974.
Mihm MC Jr & others: Early detection of primary cutaneous malignant melanoma: A color atlas. New England J Med 289:989, 1973.
Simmonds WL: Double-blind investigation comparing a 1%-vs-5% 5-fluorouracil topical cream in patients with multiple actinic keratoses. Cutis 12:615, 1973.
Torre D: Dermatological cryosurgery: A progress report. Cutis 11:782, 1973.
Tromovitch TA, Stegman SJ: Microscopically controlled excision of skin tumors. Arch Dermat 110:231, 1974.
Walton RG: The management of pigmented nevi. Cutis 10:611, 1972.

MISCELLANEOUS SKIN, HAIR, & NAIL DISORDERS

PIGMENTARY DISORDERS

Melanin is formed in the melanocytes in the basal layer of the epidermis. Its precursor, the amino acid tyrosine, is slowly converted to dihydroxyphenylalanine (dopa) by tyrosinase, and there are many further chemical steps to the ultimate formation of melanin. This system may be affected by external influences such as exposure to sun, heat, trauma, ionizing radiation, heavy metals, and changes in oxygen potential. These influences may result in hyperpigmentation, hypopigmentation, or both. Local trauma may destroy melanocytes temporarily or permanently, causing hypopigmentation, sometimes with surrounding hyperpigmentation as in eczema and dermatitis. Internal influences include melanocyte-stimulating hormone (MSH) from the pituitary gland, which is increased in pregnancy and in states in which there is an inadequate normal output of hydrocortisone by the adrenal cortex. Melatonin, a pineal hormone, regulates pigment dispersion and aggregation.

Other pigmentary disorders include those resulting from exposure to exogenous pigments such as carotenemia, argyria, deposition of other metals, and tattooing. Other endogenous pigmentary disorders are attributable to metabolic substances, including hemosiderin (iron), in purpuric processes and in hemochromatosis; mercaptans, homogentisic acid (ochronosis), bile pigments, and carotenes.

Classification

Pigmentary disorders may be classified as primary or secondary and as hyperpigmentary or hypopigmentary.

A. Primary Pigmentary Disorders: These are nevoid or congenital, and include pigmented nevi, Mongolian spots, and incontinentia pigmenti, vitiligo, albinism, and piebaldism. Vitiligo is a genetically determined lack of pigmentation in which melanocytes which lack tyrosinase are present in involved areas. Vitiligo, found in approximately 1% of the population, may be associated with hyperthyroidism and hypothyroidism, pernicious anemia, diabetes mellitus, addisonism, and carcinoma of the stomach. Albinism, partial or total, occurs as a genetically determined recessive trait. Piebaldism, a localized hypomelanosis, is an autosomal dominant trait.

B. Secondary Pigmentary Disorders: Hyper- or hypopigmentation may occur following overexposure to sunlight or heat or as a result of excoriation or direct physical injury. Hyperpigmentation occurs in arsenical melanosis or in association with Addison's disease (due to lack of the inhibitory influence of hydrocortisone on the production of MSH by the pituitary gland). Several disorders of clinical importance are as follows:

1. Chloasma (melasma)—This is essentially a nevoid disorder occurring as patterned hyperpigmentation of the face. It is often associated with exaggeration of normal pigmentation elsewhere, such as in the axillas, the linea alba, the groins, and around the nipples. It is common during pregnancy as a result of the stimulus of MSH and tends to fade following each pregnancy. Oral progestins (contraceptive) may cause chloasma.

2. Berlock hyperpigmentation can be provoked by hypersensitivity to essential oils in perfumes, and these should be excluded wherever possible.

3. Leukoderma or secondary depigmentation may complicate atopic dermatitis, lichen planus, psoriasis, alopecia areata, lichen simplex chronicus, and such systemic conditions as myxedema, thyrotoxicosis, syphilis, and toxemias. It may follow local skin trauma of various sorts, or may complicate dermatitis due to exposure to gold or arsenic. Antioxidants in rubber goods, such as monobenzyl ether of hydroquinone, can cause leukoderma from the wearing of gauntlet gloves, rubber pads in brassieres, etc. This is most likely to occur in blacks.

4. Ephelides (juvenile freckles) and **lentigines** (senile freckles).

5. Drugs—Pigmentation may be produced by chloroquine and chlorpromazine.

Differential Diagnosis

One must distinguish true lack of pigment from pseudoachromia such as occurs in tinea versicolor, pityriasis simplex, and seborrheic dermatitis. It may be difficult to differentiate true vitiligo from leukoderma and even from partial albinism.

Complications

The development of solar keratoses and epitheliomas is more likely to occur in persons with vitiligo and albinism. Vitiligo tends to create pruritus in anogenital folds. There may be severe emotional trauma in extensive vitiligo and other types of hypo- and hyperpigmentations, particularly in naturally dark-skinned persons.

Treatment & Prognosis

There is no increase of pigment in partial or total albinism; return of pigment is rare in vitiligo; in leukoderma, repigmentation may occur spontaneously. The only effective treatment for vitiligo (with some response in 10—15% of patients only) is topical or systemic therapy with methoxsalen (Oxsoralen), available as 10 mg capsules or 1% lotion. The topical preparation should be used in no greater than 1:10,000 concentration, as it may cause severe phototoxic effects and blisters. (It can be cut 100 times with a mixture of ether, alcohol, and propylene glycol, or isopropyl alcohol may be used.) Methoxsalen is given in a dosage of 20 mg orally each morning (2—4 hours before exposure to sunlight) for weeks or months, and in combination with judicious exposure to sunlight may bring about repigmentation in vitiligo. Liver function tests are not necessary. Trioxsalen (Trisoralen) may be given by mouth in one-half the dosage of methoxsalen.

Localized ephelides and lentigines may be destroyed by careful application of a saturated solution of liquid phenol on a tightly wound cotton applicator. Chloasma and other forms of hyperpigmentation may be treated by protecting the skin from the sun and with cosmetics such as Covermark (Lydia O'Leary Company) or A-Fil (Texas Pharmacal Company). Cosmetics containing perfumes should not be used.

Bleaching preparations generally contain hydroquinone or its derivatives. This is not without hazard, and it is best to start with the weakest preparation offered by the manufacturer. The use of this kind of bleach may result in unexpected hypopigmentation, particularly with prolonged use.

Treatment of other pigmentary disorders should be directed toward avoidance of the causative agent if possible (as in carotenemia) or treatment of the underlying disorder. A new formula for treating melasma, ephelides, and postinflammatory hyperpigmentation is hydrophilic ointment containing 0.1% tretinoin, 5% hydroquinone, and 0.1% dexamethasone, plus an alcoholic sunscreen containing 5% para-aminobenzoic acid. Senile lentigines are resistant.

Kaidbey KH, Kligman AM: Photopigmentation with trioxsalen. Arch Dermat 109:674, 1974.
Kandil E: Treatment of vitiligo with 0.1% betamethasone 17-valerate in isopropyl alcohol—a double-blind trial. Brit J Dermat 91:457, 1974.
Kligman AM, Willis, I: A new formula for depigmenting human skin. Arch Dermat 111:40, 1975.
McGregor BC & others: Vitiligo and multiple glandular insufficiencies. JAMA 219:724, 1972.
Sehgal VN: Trioxsalen therapy for vitiligo. Arch Dermat 109:578, 1974.
Stewart TW, Savage D: Cosmetic camouflage in dermatology. Brit J Dermat 86:530, 1972.

BALDNESS
(Alopecia)

Baldness Due to Scarring

Cicatricial baldness may occur following chemical or physical trauma, lichen planopilaris, severe bacterial or fungal infections, severe herpes zoster, chronic discoid lupus erythematosus, scleroderma, and excessive ionizing radiation. The specific cause is often suggested by the history, the distribution of hair loss, and the appearance of the skin, as in lupus erythematosus and other infections. Biopsy may be necessary to differentiate lupus from the others.

Scarring alopecias are irreversible and permanent. There is no treatment, except for surgical hair transplants.

Baldness Not Due to Scarring

Noncicatricial baldness may be classified according to distribution as alopecia universalis (generalized but not total hair loss), alopecia totalis (complete hair loss), and alopecia areata (patchy baldness).

Nonscarring alopecia may occur in association with various **systemic diseases** such as disseminated lupus erythematosus, cachexia, lymphomas, uncontrolled diabetes, severe thyroid or pituitary hypofunction, and dermatomyositis. The only treatment necessary is prompt and adequate control of the underlying disorder, in which case hair loss may be reversible.

Male pattern baldness, the most common form of alopecia, is of genetic predetermination. The earliest changes occur at the anterior portions of the calvarium on either side of the "widow's peak." Associated seborrhea is common, and is evident as excessive oiliness and erythema of the scalp, with scaling. Premature loss of hair in a young adult male may give rise to a severe neurotic reaction. The extent of hair loss is variable and unpredictable. There is no treatment except surgical transplants, and the patient should be cautioned not to spend money on advertised lotions or massage devices. Seborrhea may be treated as described on p 45.

Diffuse idiopathic alopecia of women only seems to be increasing in incidence. The cause is not known but is considered by some to be the counterpart of male baldness ("androgenetic alopecia"). The disease may not be apparent until about 80% of the hair is lost, and is then manifest as a diffuse thinning of the hair over the entire scalp (especially over the calvarium). Testosterone excretion has been shown to be elevated in some cases. These women may develop a neurotic reaction comparable in severity to cancerophobia. Associated seborrhea should be controlled. Estrogens internally and topically may be tried, as may low-dose interrupted courses of corticosteroids. Deficiency of iron storage may play a role. There is some evidence that an inhibitor of lipid auto-oxidation (possibly D,a-tocopheryl by mouth) might be of value in reducing hair loss.

Telogen effluvium may be the cause of temporary hair loss in some women. A transitory increase occurs in the number of hairs in the telogen (resting) phase of the hair growth cycle. This may occur spontaneously, may appear at the termination of pregnancy, or may be provoked by hormonal contraceptives, especially the monophasic contraceptives. If an abnormally high proportion of telogen hairs is present before taking the contraceptive, lasting improvement in hair growth may be expected. In one study, the only cause of telogen effluvium was found to be iron deficiency, and the hair counts bore a clear relationship to the serum iron levels.

Alopecia areata is of unknown cause. Histopathologically, there are numerous small anagen hairs and a lymphocytic infiltrate. The bare patches may be perfectly smooth, or a few hairs may remain. Severe forms may be treated by injection of triamcinolone acetonide suspension into the patches or by judicious use of systemic corticosteroid therapy, although systemic therapy is rarely justified unless the disease is of serious emotional or economic significance.

Systemic corticosteroids have also been used in the treatment of generalized and total alopecia. Prednisone, 20 mg orally every other morning, may be given for several months with the usual precautions. Alopecia areata is usually self-limiting, with complete regrowth of hair, but some mild cases are permanent and the extensive forms are usually permanent, as are the totalis and universalis types also.

Cataracts may complicate extensive alopecia areata.

In **trichotillomania** (the pulling out of one's own hair), the patches of hair loss are irregular and growing hairs are always present since they cannot be pulled out until they are long enough.

Drug-induced alopecia is becoming increasingly important. Such drugs include thallium, excessive and prolonged use of vitamin A, antimitotic agents, anticoagulants, clofibrate (rarely), antithyroid drugs, oral contraceptives, trimethadione, allopurinol, amphetamines, salicylates, gentamicin, and levodopa.

Abel E, Munro DD: Intralesional treatment of alopecia areata with triamcinolone acetonide by jet injector. Brit J Dermat 88:55, 1973.

Kern F & others: Alopecia areata: Immunologic studies and treatment with prednisone. Arch Dermat 107:407, 1973.

Levantine A, Almeyda J: Drug induced alopecia. Brit J Dermat 89:549, 1973.

Muller SA, Winkelmann R: Trichotillomania. Arch Dermat 105:535, 1972.

Price VH: Office diagnosis of structural hair anomalies. Cutis 15:231, 1975.

Thiele FAJ: Chemical aspects of hair loss and its cosmetological significance. Brit J Dermat 92:355, 1975.

Verbov J: Steroid solution treatment of alopecia areata. Arch Dermat 108:135, 1973.

Vickers CFH: Iron deficiency and the skin. Brit J Dermat 89 (Suppl 9):10, 1973.

HIRSUTISM

Hirsutism may be diffuse or localized, acquired or congenital. Essential hirsutism of women is most clearly manifested in the bearded area and on the upper lip, but it may be present on the chest and around the nipples as well. Endocrinologic studies may be necessary to rule out excessive androgen secretion. Suppression of androgenic adrenocortical output by the inhibitory pituitary action of small doses of oral corticosteroids may be indicated in some cases. If hirsutism is due to excessive androgen excretion, extirpation of the offending gland may be followed by disappearance of excessive hair. Wax depilation of unwanted hair may be satisfactory for some women. Papillary damage thereby may discourage hair growth.

Dalla Pria S & others: Antiandrogen in acne and idiopathic hirsutism. J Invest Dermat 52:348, 1969.
Ridley CM: A critical evaluation of the procedures available for the treatment of hirsutism. Brit J Dermat 81:146, 1969.

KELOIDS & HYPERTROPHIC SCARS

Keloids are tumors consisting of actively growing fibrous tissue which occur as a result of trauma or irritation in predisposed persons, especially those of dark-skinned races. The trauma may be relatively trivial, such as an acne lesion. Keloids behave as neoplasms, although they are not malignant. Spontaneous digitations may project from the central growth, and the tumors may become large and disfiguring. There may be itching and burning sensations with both types of tumor.

Hypertrophic scars, usually seen following surgery or accidental trauma, tend to be raised, red, and indurated. After a few months or longer they lose their redness and become soft and flat. Removal should not be attempted until all induration has subsided.

Intralesional injection of a corticosteroid suspension is effective against hypertrophic scars. The treatment of keloids is less satisfactory; surgical excision, x-ray therapy, and freezing with solid CO_2 or liquid nitrogen are used, as well as injection of corticosteroid suspensions into the lesions. They tend to involute in older age groups.

Sheard C: Removal of keloids. Cutis 11:865, 1973.

NAIL DISORDERS

Nail changes are never pathognomonic of a specific systemic or cutaneous disease. All of the nail manifestations of systemic disorders may be seen also in the absence of any systemic illness.

Nail dystrophies cannot usually be related to changes in thyroid function, hypovitaminosis, nutritional disturbances, or generalized allergic reactions.

Classification

Nail disorders may be classified as (1) local, (2) congenital or genetic, and (3) those associated with systemic or generalized skin diseases.

A. Local Nail Disorders:

1. Onycholysis (distal separation of the nails, usually of the fingers) is caused by excess exposure to water, soaps, detergents, alkalies, and industrial keratolytic agents. Nail hardeners and demethylchlortetracycline may cause onycholysis. Hypothyroidism is said to play a part.

2. Distortion of the nail occurs as a result of chronic inflammation of the nail matrix underlying the eponychial fold.

3. Discoloration and pithy changes, accompanied by a musty odor, are seen in ringworm infection.

4. Grooving and other changes may be caused by warts, nevi, etc impinging on the nail matrix.

5. Allergic reactions (to formaldehyde and resins in undercoats and polishes) involving the nail bed or matrix formerly caused hemorrhagic streaking of the nails, accumulation of keratin under the free margins of the nails, and great tenderness of the nail beds.

6. Beau's lines (transverse furrows) may be due to faulty manicuring.

B. Congenital and Genetic Nail Disorders:

1. A longitudinal single nail groove may occur as a result of a genetic or traumatic defect in the nail matrix underlying the eponychial fold.

2. Nail atrophy may be congenital.

3. Hippocratic nails (club fingers) may be congenital.

C. Nail Changes Associated With Systemic or Generalized Skin Diseases:

1. Beau's lines (transverse furrows) may follow any serious systemic illness.

2. Atrophy of the nails may be related to trauma or vascular or neurologic disease.

3. Hippocratic nails (club fingers) are occasionally related to prolonged anoxemia brought about by cardiopulmonary disorders.

4. Spoon nails are often seen in patients with anemia.

5. Stippling of the nails is seen in psoriasis.

6. Nail changes may be seen also with alopecia areata, lichen planus, and keratosis follicularis.

Differential Diagnosis

It is important to distinguish congenital and genetic disorders from those caused by trauma and environmental disorders. Nail changes due to ringworm or dermatophyte fungi may be difficult to differentiate from onychia due to candida infections. Direct microscopic examination of a specimen cleared with 10% potassium hydroxide, or culture on Sabouraud's medium, may be diagnostic. Ringworm of the nails may be closely similar to the changes seen in psoriasis and lichen planus, in which case careful observation of more characteristic lesions elsewhere on the body is essential to the diagnosis of the nail disorders.

Complications

Secondary bacterial infection occasionally occurs

in onychódystrophies, and leads to considerable pain and disability and possibly more serious consequences if circulation or innervation is impaired. Toenail changes may lead to ingrown nail, in turn often complicated by bacterial infection and occasionally by exuberant granulation tissue. Poor manicuring and poorly fitting shoes may contribute to this complication. Cellulitis may result.

Treatment & Prognosis

Treatment consists usually of careful debridement and manicuring and, above all, reduction of exposure to irritants (soaps, detergents, alkali, bleaches, solvents, etc). Antifungal measures may be used in the case of onychomycosis and candidal onychia, antibacterial measures may be used for bacterial complications. When nail changes are associated with specific diseases, such as psoriasis and lichen planus, one may use appropriate measures, but the nail changes are usually very slow to reverse themselves. Congenital or genetic nail disorders are usually uncorrectable. Longitudinal grooving due to temporary lesions of the matrix, such as warts, synovial cysts, and other impingements, may be cured by removal of the offending lesion. Intradermal triamcinolone acetonide suspension, 2.5 mg/ml, may be injected in the area of the nail matrix at intervals of 2—4 weeks for the successful management of various types of nail dystrophies (psoriasis, lichen planus, onycholysis, longitudinal splitting, grooving from synovial cysts, and others).

Abell E, Samman PD: Intradermal triamcinolone treatment of nail dystrophies. Brit J Dermat 89:191, 1973.

Bean WB: Nail growth: 30 years of observation. Arch Int Med 134:497, 1974.

Fredriksson T: Topically applied fluorouracil in treatment of psoriatic nails. Arch Dermat 110:735, 1974.

Table 3—1. Simple solutions: For soaks and wet dressings.

Indications: For acute, red, swollen, itching, infected, weeping, or vesicular lesions.

Technic: Solutions must be applied cool (hot for infections).

(1) Basin soaks (2—5 quarts of solution) for hands and feet, 15 minutes twice daily.

(2) Wet dressings (for localized lesions). Use Turkish towel; keep saturated with solution.

(a) Open dressings for very acute lesions and when marked cleansing and soothing action is desired. Frequent applications are necessary (eg, 30 minutes 2—3 times daily).

(b) Covered dressings should not be used.

Agent	Action*	Range of Concentrations Used	Most Common Strength Used	Preparation of Solution of Most Commonly Employed Strength
Plain tap water	*	—	—	
R 1 Sodium chloride	*	6:1000—15:1000 (0.6—1.5%)	0.9%	2 tsp to 1 liter of water.
R 2 Sodium bicarbonate	Antipruritic	1:50—1:20 (2—5%)	3%	8 tsp to 1 liter of water.
R 3 Magnesium sulfate	Antipruritic	1:50—1:25 (2—4%)	3%	8 tsp to 1 liter of water.
R 4 Aluminum subacetate solution	Astringent	1:200—1:10 (0.5—10%)	5%	Domeboro powder, 2 tsp, or 50 ml Burow's solution to 1 liter of water.
R 5 Silver nitrate	Astringent, antiseptic, stains the skin	1:10,000—1:200 (0.01—0.5%)	1:400 0.25%	10 ml of 25% AgNO$_3$ solution or 2.5 gm AgNO$_3$ to 1 liter of water.
R 6 Neomycin, 0.1% solution	Antibacterial		0.1%	0.1%. As wet dressings for exudative pyodermas. May sensitize.
R 7 Potassium permanganate	Antipruritic, oxidizing, antiseptic, astringent, stains the skin	1:10,000—1:400 (0.01—0.25%)	1:10,000 0.01%	One 0.3 gm tablet to 3 liters of water or 0.1 gm tablet to 1 liter of water.

*All of the solutions listed have a drying, soothing, and cleansing action also.

Table 3—2. Powders.

Name	Prescription	Instructions and Remarks
R 8 Absorbable gelatin sponge (nonsterile)	Gelfoam powder, 10 gm	For leg ulcers and other indolent ulcers. It is absorbable hemostatic gelatin. Apply twice daily. Use antibiotic topical powder also.
R 9 Talc		Simple dusting powder.
R 10 Antibiotic powder, topical	Oxytetracycline (Terramycin), neomycin-polymyxin-bacitracin (Neosporin), or tetracycline (Achromycin) topical powder	For pyodermas. Dust on lesions twice daily.
R 11 Nystatin (Mycostatin)	R Nystatin, 100,000 U/gm dusting powder, 15 gm	Dusting powder twice daily for candidiasis.

Table 3—3. Lotions and emulsions.

Liquid mixtures containing medicaments in solution or suspension are useful in a wide variety of localized and generalized skin lesions because they are easy to apply and remove. They often have a marked drying effect and must not be used if this effect is undesirable. The following are some useful, well-known lotions.

Lotion and Action	Prescription		Instructions and Remarks
℞ 12 Topocide lotion	Benzyl benzoate lotion		For generalized application. Scabicide and lousicide.
℞ 13 Calamine lotion (soothing, drying)	℞ Prepared calamine Zinc oxide Glycerin Magma of bentonite Lime water, qs ad	8.0 8.0 2.0 25.0 100.0	Apply locally 3—4 times daily or as needed. Use for acute dermatitis. Avoid excessive drying by prolonged use of this lotion (as with other nonoily lotions). Add 1% phenol for antipruritic effect.
℞ 14 Starch lotion (antipruritic, soothing, drying)	℞ Starch, corn Zinc oxide Glycerin Lime water, qs ad	24.0 24.0 12.0 120.0	Apply locally twice daily and as needed. Use for acute dermatitis. Useful basic lotion to which other agents may be added.
℞ 15 Oily lotion (soothing, drying, lubricating)	℞ Zinc oxide Olive oil Lime water, $\overline{aa}$ qs ad	10.0 120.0	Apply locally 3—4 times daily or as needed. Use for acute dermatitis. Less drying than ℞ 13 and 14.
℞ 16 Coal tar lotion (soothing, drying, keratoplastic)	℞ Solution of coal tar Zinc oxide Starch Glycerin Water, qs ad	12.0 24.0 24.0 36.0 120.0	Apply locally at night. Scrub in a.m. Use for subacute dermatitis. Useful mild stimulating lotion. Do not use on hairy or infected areas.
℞ 17 Sun screen emulsion (protective)	℞ PABA Emulsion base, qs ad	3.0 30.0	Apply locally to skin before each exposure to the sun.
℞ 18 Acne lotion	℞ Sulfur, ppt Zinc sulfate $\overline{aa}$ Sodium borate Zinc oxide $\overline{aa}$ Acetone Camphor water Rose water, $\overline{aa}$ qs ad	 3.6 6.0 30.0 120.0	Apply locally at night for acne.
℞ 19 Amphotericin B (Fungizone)	℞ Fungizone lotion	30.0	Apply twice daily and as needed for mucocutaneous candidiasis.
℞ 20 Fluocinolone acetonide, 0.01% solution, or betamethasone valerate, 0.1% lotion	Synalar solution Valisone lotion	30.0 20.0	Apply twice daily for scalp dermatitis and atopic dermatitis. Avoid eyes and genitalia. Apply to scalp nightly and cover with plastic shower cap for seborrheic dermatitis or psoriasis.
℞ 21 Tolnaftate solution	Tinactin solution	10.0	Apply twice daily for dermatophyte (tinea) fungal infections. Ineffective for onychomycosis.
℞ 22 Underarm lotion (antiperspirant)	℞ Aluminum chloride Glycerin Distilled water, qs ad	60.0 30.0 240.0	Apply small quantity to underarms each morning. Useful antiperspirant.

Table 3—4. Ointment bases.

Indications:
1. To trap moisture in a dry skin.
2. To provide mechanical protection to the underlying lesions.
3. To help absorb or imbibe transudates from underlying lesions. (This holds true only for the hydrophilic preparations.)

4. To apply active medicinal agents to the skin.
Contraindications:
1. Acute, inflamed, oozing lesions.
2. Hairy areas (except the hydrophilic preparations).

Preparation	Prescription	Properties
Ointments		
℞ 23 Petrolatum, white		Chemically inert. Retards penetration of incorporated medicaments in some cases.
℞ 24 Petrolatum, hydrophilic	3% cholesterol in petrolatum, white wax, and stearyl alcohol.	Favors penetration of incorporated medicaments. Imbibes water (hydrophilic).
℞ 25 Wool fat, hydrous (lanolin)		Adheres well to skin; stable; favors penetration. Watch for sensitization.
℞ 26 Wool fat (anhydrous lanolin)		Imbibes water. Favors penetration. Watch for sensitization.
℞ 27 Zinc oxide ointment	20% zinc oxide in liquid petrolatum, wool fat, wax, and white petrolatum.	Mechanical protection; imbibes water; stiffens ointment (gives "body" to ointment) and makes it adhere to skin.
℞ 28 Theobroma oil (cocoa butter)		Melts at body temperature.
Creams		
(Contain water; more softening and soothing than ointments.)		
℞ 29 Hydrophilic ointment	℞ Methylparaben 0.025 Propylparaben 0.015 Stearyl alcohol 25.0 White petrolatum 25.0 Propylene glycol 12.0 Polyoxyl 40 stearate 5.0 Purified water, qs ad 100.0	Favors penetration, imbibes water; good vehicle for water-soluble medicaments. Parabens may sensitize the skin (rarely).
℞ 30 Rose-water ointment	℞ Spermaceti 12.5 White wax 12.0 Expressed almond oil 56.0 Sodium borate 0.5 Rose water 5.0 Distilled water 14.0 Rose oil 0.02	"Cold cream" (water in oil); cooling and soothing effect.
℞ 31 Emulsion base	℞ Duponal C 1.6 Cetyl alcohol 7.0 Stearyl alcohol 7.0 White petrolatum 20.0 Heavy liquid petrolatum 2.0 Butoben 0.05 Distilled water, qs ad 100.0	Nonheating and nonirritating. Less messy than other creams and ointments.
Pastes		
(High powder content. Promote evaporation and cooling; decrease vesiculation.)		
℞ 32 Zinc oxide paste (Lassar's paste)	℞ Zinc oxide 25.0 Starch 25.0 Petrolatum, white, qs ad 100.0	Mechanical protective. Increases adhesion but decreases penetration of medicaments.*

*Add 2% cholesterol or 5% acetyl alcohol to increase water-imbibing power.

Table 3—5. Ointments and creams: Miscellaneous standard prescriptions.

Common Name	Prescriptions	Instructions and Remarks
℞ 33 Ointment of benzoic and salicylic acid (Whitfield's)	℞ Benzoic acid　　　　6.0 Salicylic acid　　　　3.0 Polyethylene glycol 　ointment, qs ad　　100.0	Apply locally at bedtime. Fungicide. Often prescribed in one-half to one-fourth strength. Not for acute or subacute lesions.
℞ 34 Aluminum acetate ointment ("1-2-3")	℞ Aluminum 　acetate solution　　10.0 Wool fat　　　　　　20.0 Zinc oxide paste　　30.0	Apply locally to skin as needed. Valuable on receding inflammatory processes.
℞ 35 Sulfur-salicylic acid ointment	℞ Sulfur　　　　　1.0–3.0 Salicylic acid　　1.0–3.0 Petrolatum, qs ad　　100.0	Apply locally as needed. Potent fungicide. *Note:* Not for acute or subacute lesions.
℞ 36 Acrisorcin cream	Akrinol cream　　　50.0	Apply twice daily for tinea versicolor. Avoid eyes and genitalia.
℞ 37 Desonide cream 0.05%	Tridesilon cream　　15.0	Apply to face twice daily for seborrheic dermatitis and rosacea. Use Quinolor compound ointment every other night
℞ 38 Miconazole nitrate, 2% cream, or Clotrimazole, 1% cream	MicaTin cream or Monistat cream Lotrimin cream　　30.0	Apply twice daily for "athlete's foot," "ringworm," or candidiasis. Same as for miconazole
℞ 39 Hydrocortisone ointment or cream	Available as 0.25, 1.5, 1, and 2.5% ointment in 5 gm to 120 gm quantities.	Apply a thin film twice daily. Combined with tar, antibiotics, or iodochlorhydroxyquin. Do not use in dendritic keratitis.
℞ 40 Triamcinolone (0.025 or 0.1%), fluocinolone (0.01 or 0.25%), betamethasone valerate (0.1%), fluocinonide (0.05%), desonide (0.05%), or halcinonide (0.1%)	℞ Ointment or cream　15.0–60.0	Apply each night and cover with thin plastic film (Saran Wrap) for localized eczema or psoriasis. May be used overnight under a plastic suit for generalized psoriasis. *(Caution.)* Or: Rub in a thin film twice daily for any noninfected dermatitis or eczema. Avoid the eyes.

Table 3—6. Solutions, tinctures, and paints.

℞ 41 Gentian violet	1% aqueous solution.	Antiseptic (gram-positive organisms) and fungicide (candida).
℞ 42 Sodium thiosulfate	10% aqueous solution.	Fungicide (especially for tinea versicolor).
℞ 43 Silver nitrate	1–10% aqueous solution.	Cauterizing and astringent for fissures and ulcers.
℞ 44 Chrysarobin	4% in chloroform.	For candidal paronychia.
℞ 45 Nitromersol	0.5% (1:200 tincture) (Metaphen)	Bacteriostatic and germicidal.
℞ 46 Alcoholic "Whitfield's" solution	℞ Salicylic acid　　　　2.0 Benzoic acid　　　　4.0 Alcohol 40% qs ad　　120.0	Apply locally. Fungistat combination. May substitute bay rum for alcohol.
℞ 47 Benzoin, compound tr		Full strength.
℞ 48 Soft soap liniment	65% soap.	Useful detergent
℞ 49 Antiseborrheic shampoo	Selsun, Fostex, Sebulex, Capsebon, Alvinine, Sebical, Ionil T, Vanseb-T, Sebutone, Iocon	Contains detergents, salicylic acid, sulfur compounds, tar and allantoin, or quinoline. Some may cause excess oiliness.
℞ 50 Sun-screening tr	℞ 5% PABA in 50% ethanol	More effective than most sunscreens.
℞ 51 Clotrimazole, 1% in polyethylene glycol 400	℞ Lotrimin solution	Apply twice daily for dermatophyte or candidal infections.

Table 3—7. Gels

℞ 52 Betamethasone benzoate gel, 0.025%, or fluocinonide, 0.05% gel	Benisone 　or Flurobate gel 　or Topsyn gel	Especially valuable in hairy areas. (All are corticosteroids.)

4...
Eye

Daniel Vaughan

NONSPECIFIC MANIFESTATIONS OF EYE DISEASES

Pain

The 2 most serious eye disorders which cause pain are iritis and acute glaucoma. If neither is present, look for a corneal abrasion or foreign body, or a foreign body concealed beneath the upper eyelid.

Blurred Vision

The most important causes of blurred vision are refractive error, corneal opacities, cataract, vitreous clouding, retinal detachment, macular degeneration, central retinal vein thrombosis, central retinal artery occlusion, optic neuritis, and optic atrophy.

Conjunctival Discharge

Discharge is usually caused by bacterial or viral conjunctivitis.

"Eyestrain"

This is a common ocular complaint which usually means eye discomfort associated with prolonged reading or close work. Significant refractive error, early presbyopia, inadequate illumination, or phoria (usually exophoria with poor convergence) should be ruled out.

Photophobia

Photophobia suggests iritis, keratitis, corneal ulcer, or ocular albinism.

"Spots"

"Spots before the eyes" are vitreous opacities which usually have no clinical significance; in unusual instances they signify impending retinal detachment or posterior uveitis.

Headache

Headache is only occasionally due to ocular disorders. The causes of ocular headache are in general the same as for "eyestrain" (above).

Table 4—1. Differential diagnosis of common causes of inflamed eye.

	Acute Conjunctivitis	Acute Iritis*	Acute Glaucoma†	Corneal Trauma or Infection
Incidence	Extremely common	Common	Uncommon	Common
Discharge	Moderate to copious	None	None	Watery or purulent
Vision	No effect on vision	Slightly blurred	Markedly blurred	Usually blurred
Pain	None	Moderate	Severe	Moderate to severe
Conjunctival injection	Diffuse; more toward fornices	Mainly circumcorneal	Diffuse	Diffuse
Cornea	Clear	Usually clear	Steamy	Clarity change related to cause
Pupil size	Normal	Small	Moderately dilated and fixed	Normal
Pupillary light response	Normal	Poor	None	Normal
Intraocular pressure	Normal	Normal	Elevated	Normal
Smear	Causative organisms	No organisms	No organisms	Organisms found only in corneal ulcers due to infection

*Acute anterior uveitis.
†Angle closure glaucoma.

Diplopia

Double vision is due to muscle imbalance or to paralysis of an extraocular muscle as a result of inflammation (including thyroid myopathy), hemorrhage, trauma, tumefaction, or infection of the 3rd, 4th, or 6th nerves. The 6th nerve is most commonly affected.

OCULAR EMERGENCIES

ACUTE (ANGLE-CLOSURE) GLAUCOMA

Acute glaucoma can occur only with the closure of a preexisting narrow anterior chamber angle. If the pupil dilates spontaneously or is dilated with a mydriatic or cycloplegic, the angle will close and an attack of acute glaucoma is precipitated; for this reason it is a wise precaution to examine the anterior chamber angle before instilling these drugs. About 1% of people over age 35 have narrow anterior chamber angles, but many of these never develop acute glaucoma.

A quiet eye with a narrow anterior chamber angle may convert spontaneously to angle-closure glaucoma. The process can be precipitated by anything that will dilate the pupil, eg, indiscriminate use of mydriatics or cycloplegics by the patient or the physician. The cycloplegic can be administered in the form of eyedrops or systemically, eg, by the anesthetist ordering scopolamine or atropine prior to a cholecystectomy, or in the form of "cold medications" containing atropine-like drugs. Increased circulating epinephrine in times of stress can also dilate the pupil and cause acute glaucoma. Sitting in a darkened movie theater can have the same effect.

Patients with acute glaucoma seek treatment immediately because of extreme pain and blurring of vision. The eye is red, the cornea is steamy, and the pupil is moderately dilated and does not react to light. Intraocular pressure is elevated (tonometry).

Acute glaucoma must be differentiated from conjunctivitis and acute iritis and from corneal abrasion—especially after a general anesthetic.

Peripheral iridectomy within 12–48 hours after onset of symptoms will usually result in a permanent cure. Untreated acute glaucoma results in complete and permanent blindness within 2–5 days after onset of symptoms. Before surgery, the intraocular pressure must be lowered by means of miotics instilled locally and osmotic agents and carbonic anhydrase inhibitors administered systemically.

Three different osmotic agents (urea, mannitol, and glycerol) are available for lowering intraocular pressure preoperatively in angle-closure glaucoma. Urea and mannitol are administered intravenously. Glycerol is gaining popularity because it is given orally. The dosage of all 3 of these osmotic drugs is about 1.5 gm/kg.

Armaly MF: Glaucoma: Annual review. Arch Ophth 93:146, 1975.

Bietti G: Intraocular pressure and glaucoma. Am J Ophth 73:475, 1972.

Hetherington J: Symposium: Glaucoma. Tr Am Acad Ophth 78:239, 1974.

Hyams SW, Friedman Z, Keroub C: Fellow eye in angle-closure glaucoma. Brit J Ophth 59:207, 1975.

Watson PG (editor): Glaucoma. (Perrers Taylor Memorial.) Brit J Ophth 56:146, 1972. [Many articles. Entire issue devoted to subject.]

FOREIGN BODIES

If a patient complains of "something in my eye" and gives a consistent history, he usually has a foreign body even though it may not be readily visible. Almost all foreign bodies, however, can be seen under oblique illumination with the aid of a hand flashlight and loupe.

Note the time, place, and other circumstances of the accident. Test visual acuity before treatment is instituted as a basis for comparison in the event of complications.

Conjunctival Foreign Body

Foreign body of the upper tarsal conjunctiva is suggested by pain and blepharospasm of sudden onset in the presence of a clear cornea and by less pain on blinking when the eye is turned (right or left) so that the cornea is away from the foreign body location. After instilling a local anesthetic, evert the lid by grasping the lashes gently and exerting pressure on the midportion of the outer surface of the upper lid with an applicator. If a foreign body is present, it can be easily removed by passing a sterile wet cotton applicator across the conjunctival surface.

Corneal Foreign Body

When a corneal foreign body is suspected but is not apparent on simple inspection, instill fluorescein into the conjunctival sac and examine the cornea with the aid of a magnifying device and strong illumination. The foreign body may then be removed with a sterile wet cotton applicator. An antibiotic should be instilled, eg, polymyxin-bacitracin ointment. It is not necessary to patch the eye, but the patient must be examined in 24 hours for secondary infection of the crater. If it is not possible to remove the corneal foreign body in this manner, it should be removed by an ophthalmologist. Steel foreign bodies usually leave a diffuse rust ring. This requires excision of the affected tissue and is best done under local anesthesia using a slitlamp. *Caution:* Anesthetic drops should not be given to the patient for his use. If there is no infection, a layer of corneal epithelial cells will line the crater within 24 hours. It should be emphasized that the intact corneal epithelium forms an effective barrier to infection. Once the corneal epithelium is disturbed, the cornea becomes extremely susceptible to infection.

Early infection is manifested by a white necrotic area around the crater and a small amount of gray exudate. These patients should be referred immediately to an ophthalmologist.

Untreated corneal infection may lead to severe corneal ulceration, panophthalmitis, and loss of the eye.

Intraocular Foreign Body

A patient with an intraocular foreign body should be referred immediately to an ophthalmologist. With delay the ocular media become progressively more cloudy, and a foreign body visible shortly after the injury may not be visible several hours later. The foreign body can often be removed through the point of entry, or through an incision in the sclera near its location, with a magnet.

The visual prognosis is generally poor.

Percival SPB: A decade of intraocular foreign bodies. Brit J Ophth 56:454, 1972.
Rosenthal AR, Appleton B: Intraocular copper foreign bodies. Am J Ophth 79:613, 1975.

CORNEAL ABRASIONS

A patient with a corneal abrasion complains of severe pain, especially with movement of the lid over the cornea.

Record the history and visual acuity. Examine the cornea and conjunctiva with a light and loupe to rule out a foreign body. If an abrasion is suspected but cannot be seen, instill sterile fluorescein into the conjunctival sac; the area of corneal abrasion will stain a deeper green than the surrounding cornea.

Instill polymyxin-bacitracin (Polysporin) ophthalmic ointment and apply a bandage with firm pressure to prevent movement of the lid. The patient should rest at home, keeping the fellow eye closed, and should be observed on the following day to be certain that the cornea has healed. Recurrent corneal erosion is common following corneal abrasions, and all such cases should be referred to an ophthalmologist.

Lemp MA: Cornea and sclera: Annual review. Arch Ophth 92:158, 1974.

CONTUSIONS

Contusion injuries of the eye and surrounding structures may cause ecchymosis ("black eye"), sub-

conjunctival hemorrhage, edema or rupture of the cornea, hemorrhage into the anterior chamber (hyphema), rupture of the root of the iris (iridodialysis), paralysis of the pupillary sphincter, paralysis of the muscles of accommodation, cataract, subluxation or luxation of the lens, vitreous hemorrhage, retinal hemorrhage and retinal edema (most common in the macular area), detachment of the retina, rupture of the choroid, fracture of the orbital floor ("blowout fracture"), and optic nerve injury. Many of these injuries are immediately apparent; others may not become apparent for days or weeks. Patients with moderate to severe contusions should be seen by an ophthalmologist.

Any injury severe enough to cause hyphema involves the danger of secondary hemorrhage which may cause intractable glaucoma with permanent visual loss. Any patient with traumatic hyphema should be put at bed rest for 6—7 days with both eyes bandaged to lessen the chance of secondary hemorrhage. Secondary hemorrhage rarely occurs after this time.

Eagling EM: Ocular damage after blunt trauma to the eye. Brit J Ophth 58:126, 1974.
Paton D, Goldberg MF: *Injuries of the Eye, the Lids, and the Orbit: Diagnosis and Management.* Saunders, 1970.
Rumelt MB, Terry EJ: Blowout fractures. Am J Ophth 73:451, 1972.
Yasuna E: Management of traumatic hyphema. Arch Ophth 91:190, 1974.

ULTRAVIOLET KERATITIS
(Actinic Keratitis)

Ultraviolet burns of the cornea are usually caused by exposure to a welding arc or to the sun when skiing ("snow blindness"). There are no immediate symptoms, but about 12 hours later the patient complains of agonizing pain and severe photophobia. Slitlamp examination after instillation of sterile fluorescein shows diffuse punctate staining of both corneas.

Treatment consists of local steroid therapy, systemic analgesics, and sedatives as indicated. All patients recover within 24—48 hours without complications. Local anesthetics should not be prescribed.

See reference under Corneal Abrasions, above.

CORNEAL ULCER

Corneal ulcers constitute a medical emergency. The typical gray, necrotic corneal ulcer is preceded by trauma, usually a corneal foreign body. The eye is red with lacrimation and conjunctival discharge, and the patient complains of blurred vision, pain, and photophobia.

Prompt treatment is essential to help prevent complications. Visual impairment may occur due to corneal scarring or infection.

Corneal ulcers have many causes including bacterial, viral, fungal, and allergic. Only the most serious types will be discussed here.

Pneumococcal ("Acute Serpiginous") Ulcer

Diplococcus pneumoniae is a common bacterial cause of corneal ulcer. The early ulcer is gray and fairly well circumscribed.

Since the pneumococcus is sensitive to both sulfonamides and antibiotics, local therapy is usually effective. If untreated, the cornea may perforate. Concurrent dacryocystitis, if present, should also be treated.

Pseudomonas Ulcer

A less common but much more virulent cause of corneal ulcer is *Pseudomonas aeruginosa*. The ulceration characteristically starts in a traumatized area and spreads rapidly, frequently causing perforation of the cornea and loss of the eye within 48 hours. *Pseudomonas aeruginosa* usually produces a pathognomonic bluish-green pigment.

Early diagnosis and vigorous treatment with gentamicin locally are essential to help save the eye.

Herpes Simplex (Dendritic) Keratitis

Corneal ulceration caused by herpes simplex virus is more common than any bacterial ulcer. It is almost always unilateral, and may affect any age group of either sex. It is often preceded by upper respiratory tract infection with fever and facial "cold sores."

The commonest finding is of one or more dendritic ulcers (superficial branching gray areas) on the corneal surface. These are composed of clear vesicles in the corneal epithelium; when the vesicles rupture, the area stains green with fluorescein. Although the dendritic figure is its most characteristic manifestation, herpes simplex keratitis may appear in a number of other configurations.

Treatment consists of removing the virus-containing corneal epithelium without disturbing Bowman's membrane or the corneal stroma. This is best done by an ophthalmologist. *Caution:* Do not give local corticosteroids, as they enhance the activity of the virus by impairing the natural inflammatory response. This may lead to perforation of the cornea and loss of the eye.

Idoxuridine (IUDR; 5-iodo-2-deoxyuridine) is quite effective against herpes simplex keratitis. It is instilled locally as 0.1% solution, 2 drops in the affected eye every hour day and night for about 3 days; if improvement is noted after that time, give the drug approximately every 2 hours for 2 days and then gradually withdraw over a period of 3 more days.

Many ophthalmologists still prefer to remove the affected corneal epithelium mechanically and apply a pressure bandage for a few days until the epithelium regenerates.

Brightbill FS: Central corneal ulcers. Ann Ophth 4:331, 1972.

Burns RP: *Pseudomonas aeruginosa* keratitis: Mixed infections of the eye. Am J Ophth 67:257, 1969.

Gasset AR, Kaufman HE: Hydrophilic lens therapy of superficial corneal ulcers. Ann Ophth 5:139, 1973.

Lemp MA: Corneal and sclera: Annual review. Arch Ophth 92:158, 1974.

Smolin G, Okumoto M: Herpes simplex keratitis. Arch Ophth 83:746, 1970.

Smolin G, Tabbara K, Okumoto M: Guinea pig herpes simplex keratitis treated with a lymphocyte extract. Am J Ophth 78:921, 1974.

Thygeson P, Okumoto M: Keratomycosis: A preventable disease. Tr Am Acad Ophth 78:433, 1974.

CHEMICAL CONJUNCTIVITIS & KERATITIS

Chemical burns are treated by irrigation of the eyes with saline solution or plain water as soon as possible after exposure. Do **not** neutralize an acid with an alkali or vice versa, as the heat generated by the reaction may cause further damage. Alkali injuries require prolonged irrigation since alkalies are not precipitated by the proteins of the eye as are acids. The pupil should be dilated with 0.2% scopolamine or 2% atropine. A combination corticosteroid and antibiotic solution or ointment is instilled frequently. Complications include symblepharon, corneal scarring, tear duct obstruction, and secondary infection.

Brown SI & others: Alkali-burned cornea. Am J Ophth 77:538, 1974.

GONOCOCCAL CONJUNCTIVITIS

Gonococcal conjunctivitis, which may cause corneal ulceration, is manifested by a copious purulent discharge. The diagnosis may be confirmed by a stained smear and culture of the discharge. Prompt treatment with local and systemic penicillin is required.

SYMPATHETIC OPHTHALMIA
(Sympathetic Uveitis)

Sympathetic ophthalmia is a rare, severe bilateral granulomatous uveitis. The cause is not known, but the disease may occur at any time from 1 week to many years after a penetrating injury through the ciliary body. The injured (exciting) eye becomes inflamed first and the fellow (sympathizing) eye second. Symptoms and signs include blurred vision with light sensitivity and redness.

The best treatment of sympathetic ophthalmia is prevention by removing the damaged eye. Any severely injured eye (eg, one with perforation of the sclera and ciliary body, with loss of vitreous and retinal damage) can incite sympathetic uveitis. Early enucleation may prevent this. The decision about when and if enucleation should be performed is controversial and requires the most careful consideration. In established cases of sympathetic ophthalmia, systemic corticosteroid therapy may be helpful. Without treatment, the disease progresses gradually to bilateral blindness.

Kay ML, Yanoff M, Katowitz JA: Sympathetic uveitis. Am J Ophth 78:90, 1974.
Morse PH, Duke JR: Sympathetic ophthalmitis. Am J Ophth 68:508, 1968.

LACERATIONS

Lids

If the lid margin is lacerated, the patient should be referred for specialized care since permanent notching may result. Lacerations of the lower eyelid near the inner canthus often sever the lower canaliculus. These require specialized care to attempt to restore the function of the torn canaliculus. Lid lacerations not involving the margin may be sutured just as any other skin laceration.

Conjunctiva

In superficial lacerations of the conjunctiva, sutures are not necessary. In order to prevent infection, instill a broad-spectrum antibiotic ointment into the eye 2–3 times a day until the laceration is healed.

Cornea or Sclera

Keep examination and manipulation at an absolute minimum, since pressure may result in extrusion of the intraocular contents. Bandage the eye lightly and cover with a metal shield which rests on the orbital bones above and below. Instruct the patient not to squeeze his eyes shut and to remain as quiet as possible. Transfer him to an ophthalmologist for further care.

Tredici TJ: Management of ophthalmic casualties in Southeast Asia. Mil Med 133:355, 1968.

ORBITAL CELLULITIS

Orbital cellulitis is manifested by an abrupt onset of fever, proptosis, and swelling and redness of the lids. It is usually caused by a pyogenic organism. Immediate treatment with systemic antibiotics is indicated to prevent brain abscess. The response to antibiotics is usually excellent.

Trokel SL: The orbit: Annual review. Arch Ophth 89:152, 1973.

VITREOUS HEMORRHAGE

Hemorrhage into the vitreous body may obscure a retinal detachment. Treatment by an ophthalmologist is indicated.

Jaffe NS: The vitreous: Annual review. Arch Ophth 90:69, 1973.

COMMON OCULAR DISORDERS

CONJUNCTIVITIS

Conjunctivitis is the most common eye disease in the Western Hemisphere. It may be acute or chronic. Most cases are exogenous and due to bacterial, viral, or chlamydial infection, though endogenous inflammation may occur (eg, phlyctenular conjunctivitis, a delayed hypersensitivity response to circulating tuberculoprotein). Other causes are allergy, chemical irritations, and fungal or parasitic infection. The mode of transmission of infectious conjunctivitis is usually direct contact, ie, via fingers, towels, or handkerchiefs, to the opposite eye or to other persons.

Conjunctivitis must be differentiated from iritis, glaucoma, corneal trauma, and keratitis.

Bacterial Conjunctivitis

The organisms found most commonly in bacterial conjunctivitis are *Diplococcus pneumoniae, Staphylococcus aureus,* Koch-Weeks bacillus, and Morax-Axenfeld bacillus. All produce a copious, purulent discharge. There is no pain or blurring of vision. The disease is usually self-limited, lasting about 10–14 days if untreated. A sulfonamide or antibiotic ointment instilled locally 3 times daily will usually clear the infection in 2–3 days. Do not use antibiotic-corticosteroid combinations.

Viral Conjunctivitis

One of the commonest causes of viral conjunctivitis is adenovirus type 3, which is usually associated with pharyngitis, fever, malaise, and preauricular adenopathy. Locally, the palpebral conjunctivas are red and there is a copious watery discharge and scanty exudate. Children are more often affected than adults, and contaminated swimming pools are frequently the source of the virus. There is no specific treatment, although local sulfonamide therapy may prevent secondary bacterial infection. The disease usually lasts about 10 days.

Chlamydial Conjunctivitis

A. Trachoma: Trachoma is one of the major causes of blindness in the world. In endemic areas, the disease is contracted in childhood. In children, trachoma is usually insidious, with minimal symptoms. In adults, the disease is acute and is manifested by redness, itching, tearing, and minimal discharge. The clinical picture consists of bilateral follicular conjunctivitis, epithelial keratitis, and corneal vascularization (pannus). Cicatrization of the conjunctiva occurs in the later stages of trachoma and usually follows necrosis of the conjunctival follicles. Scarring of the tarsal conjunctiva may result in entropion and trichiasis. Scarring of the limbal follicles results in round peripheral depressions with a clear central epithelium known as Herbert's pits. Superficial vascularization and scarring of the cornea cause decrease in vision. In endemic areas, superimposed bacterial conjunctivitis may aggravate the disease process.

The specific diagnosis can be made in Giemsa-stained conjunctival scrapings by the presence of typical cytoplasmic inclusions in epithelial cells. In active trachoma, the smear may also include polymorphonuclear leukocytes, plasma cells, and debris-filled macrophages (Leber cells).

Trachoma is transmitted from eye to eye by contact with contaminated fingers, towels, eye cosmetics, or other objects.

Treatment should be started on the basis of clinical findings without waiting for laboratory confirmation. Medical treatment consists of oral tetracycline given in full doses for 3–5 weeks. Local treatment is not necessary. *Caution:* Do not give tetracyclines during pregnancy or to young children, and do not use old preparations.

Hygienic measures are of great importance both in prevention and treatment.

Corneal scarring may require corneal transplantation. Entropion and trichiasis require plastic surgery to evert the lids. Dacryocystorhinostomy may be required in nasolacrimal duct obstruction.

B. Inclusion Conjunctivitis: This is a venereal infection that causes subclinical cervicitis in the female and urethritis in the male. About 40% of nongonorrheal urethritis in men is caused by chlamydiae. The agent is transmitted by sexual intercourse, and the eye is occasionally infected by contact with genital secretions. The newborn contracts the disease by passage through the infected birth canal. In the past, the disease had been transmitted by exposure of the eyes to contaminated water in swimming pools, and for this reason it was referred to as "swimming pool conjunctivitis." Adequate chlorination of swimming pools has eliminated this mode of transmission.

Inclusion conjunctivitis (blenorrhea) of the newborn usually occurs about 5–12 days after birth. The disease is characterized by bilateral redness, a mucopurulent exudate, and papillary hypertrophy. If pseudomembranes occur, the disease may result in fine scars of the conjunctiva.

In babies, 1% tetracycline drops in oil instilled 5–6 times daily for 2–3 weeks is very effective.

Adult inclusion conjunctivitis occurs most frequently in sexually active young adults. The disease starts with acute redness, discharge, and irritation. The eye findings consist of follicular conjunctivitis with mild keratitis. A nontender preauricular lymph node can often be palpated. Healing leaves no sequelae. The cytology of the conjunctival scrapings is similar to that of trachoma, but cytoplasmic inclusions are found more frequently.

In adults, the 1% tetracycline drops in oil should be supplemented by tetracycline, 1–1.5 gm daily orally for 2–3 weeks.

Allergic Conjunctivitis

Allergic conjunctivitis is common, and is most often associated with hay fever. It causes bilateral tearing, itching, and redness, and a minimal stringy discharge. It is usually chronic and recurrent. Short-term local corticosteroid therapy is often effective. Allergy is the usual cause of the alarming sudden painless chemosis seen in children.

Fungal & Parasitic Conjunctivitis

Fungal and parasitic conjunctivitides are rare in most parts of the world, and are usually unilateral. They often present with a localized inflammatory granuloma. A more common example is leptothrix conjunctivitis, which occurs in persons in close contact with cats.

Ophthalmia Neonatorum

Ophthalmia neonatorum is any infection of the conjunctiva in the newborn. Common types are chemical (silver nitrate), bacterial (staphylococcal, pneumococcal, gonococcal), *Escherichia coli,* and chlamydial (inclusion blennorrhea).

The diagnosis can often be made by knowing the date of onset of symptoms. Silver nitrate conjunctivitis occurs within 24 hours after birth, bacterial conjunctivitis within 2–5 days, and inclusion blennorrhea within 5–10 days. The diagnosis is confirmed by cultures and by microscopic examination of a smear of the conjunctival scrapings.

Silver nitrate conjunctivitis will clear in a few days without treatment. Bacterial conjunctivitis and inclusion blennorrhea respond well to specific antibiotic or sulfonamide therapy.

Gonococcal conjunctivitis in newborn infants may be prevented by instilling silver nitrate solution, 1%, or penicillin ointment, 100,000 units/gm, into the conjunctival sac of each eye immediately after birth. More concentrated silver nitrate solutions will cause permanent corneal scarring, and even 1% solution frequently causes chemical conjunctivitis; many ophthalmologists therefore recommend that penicillin be substituted. The disadvantage of penicillin prophylaxis is that it may favor the emergence of penicillin-resistant strains of staphylococci in the nursery. In most states of the USA some form of prophylaxis is required, usually either silver nitrate or penicillin.

Boniuk M: Eyelids, lacrimal apparatus, and conjunctiva: Annual review. Arch Ophth 90:239, 1973.

Conference on trachoma and allied diseases. Am J Ophth 63:1027, 1967.

Dawson CR: Epidemic Koch-Weeks conjunctivitis and trachoma in the Coachella Valley of California. Am J Ophth 49:801, 1960.

Jarudi N & others: Bacterial conjunctivitis. Am J Ophth 79:790, 1975.

Thygeson P: Follicular conjunctivitis. Chap 2, pp 31–44, in: *Contemporary Ophthalmology Honoring Sir Stewart Duke-Elder.* Bellows JG (editor). Williams & Wilkins, 1972.

Thygeson P, Dawson CR: Trachoma and follicular conjunctivitis in children. Arch Ophth 75:3, 1966.

Yoneda C & others: Cytology as a guide to the presence of chlamydial inclusions in Giemsa-stained conjunctival smears in severe endemic trachoma. Brit J Ophth 59:116, 1975.

PINGUECULA

Pinguecula is a yellow nodule of hyaline and elastic tissue on either side of the cornea (more commonly on the nasal side) in the area of the lid fissure. The nodules rarely grow, but inflammation is common. No treatment is indicated. Pinguecula is common in persons over 35 years of age.

PTERYGIUM

Pterygium is a fleshy, bilateral, triangular encroachment of a pinguecula onto the nasal side of the cornea and is usually associated with constant exposure to wind and dust. Excision is indicated if the growth threatens vision by approaching the pupillary area or if severe symptoms of burning or photophobia are present. Pterygium occurs most commonly in people who are frequently exposed to a combination of wind, sun, sand, and dust. For these reasons it is fairly common in southwestern USA.

UVEITIS
(Iritis, Iridocyclytis)

Uveitis is any inflammation of the uveal tract (iris, ciliary body, and choroid). Inflammation of the iris primarily is called anterior uveitis, iridocyclitis, or iritis; inflammation of the choroid (and usually the retina as well) is called posterior uveitis or chorioretinitis.

Uveitis may be either granulomatous (exogenous) or nongranulomatous (endogenous); the latter is more common. The disease is usually unilateral, and signs and symptoms are similar in both types, varying only in intensity. Early diagnosis and treatment are important to prevent the formation of posterior synechias.

Uveitis must be differentiated from conjunctivitis, acute glaucoma, and corneal ulcer.

Nongranulomatous Uveitis (Endogenous)

Most cases of nongranulomatous uveitis are of apparently spontaneous onset, but there is a fairly close correlation with Marie-Strümpell ankylosing spondylitis. The iris and ciliary body are primarily affected, but occasional foci are found in the choroid. Exacerbations parallel the rheumatic process.

The onset is acute, with marked pain, redness, photophobia, and blurred vision. A circumcorneal flush, caused by dilated limbal blood vessels, is present. Fine white keratic precipitates (KP) on the posterior surface of the cornea can be seen with the slitlamp or with a loupe. The pupil is small, and there may be a collection of fibrin with cells in the anterior chamber. If posterior synechias are present, the pupil will be irregular and the light reflex will be absent.

Local and systemic corticosteroid therapy tends to shorten the course. Warm compresses will decrease pain. Atropine, 2%, 2 drops into the affected eye twice daily, will prevent posterior synechia formation and alleviate photophobia. Recurrences are common, but the prognosis is good.

Granulomatous Uveitis (Exogenous)

Granulomatous uveitis usually follows invasion by the causative organism, eg, *Mycobacterium tuberculosis* or *Toxoplasma gondii*, although these pathogens are rarely recovered. Any or all parts of the uveal tract may be affected, but there is a predilection for the choroid.

Granulomatous uveitis is more subtle than nongranulomatous uveitis in that there is usually less pain and redness, but the permanent eye damage is relatively devastating. The onset is usually slow, and the affected eye may be only slightly and diffusely red. Because of vitreous haze and retinal involvement, vision may be more blurred than would be expected in view of the apparent mildness of the process. Pain is minimal or absent and photophobia is slight. The pupil may be normal or, if posterior synechias are present, slightly smaller than normal and irregular. Large gray "mutton fat" keratic precipitates on the posterior surface of the cornea may be seen with the slitlamp or loupe. The anterior chamber may be cloudy. Iris nodules are commonly present, and there may be vitreous haze. Fresh lesions of the choroid appear yellow when viewed with the ophthalmoscope.

Treatment is usually unsatisfactory since the causative agent is rarely identified. The pupil should be kept dilated with atropine and associated systemic disease treated as indicated. The visual prognosis is fair.

Maumenee AE: Clinical entities in "uveitis": An approach to the study of intraocular inflammation. Am J Ophth 69:1, 1970.

O'Connor GR: The uvea: Annual review. Arch Ophth 91:401, 1974.

HORDEOLUM

Hordeolum is a common staphylococcal abscess which is characterized by a localized red, swollen, acutely tender area on the upper or lower lid. Internal hordeolum is a meibomian gland abscess which points to the skin or to the conjunctival side of the lid; external hordeolum or sty (infection of the glands of Moll or Zeis) is smaller and on the margin.

The primary symptom is pain, the intensity of which is directly related to the amount of swelling.

Warm compresses are helpful. Incision is indicated if resolution does not begin within 48 hours. An antibiotic or sulfonamide instilled into the conjunctival sac every 3 hours may be beneficial during the acute stage. Internal hordeolum may lead to generalized cellulitis of the lid.

CHALAZION

Chalazion is a common granulomatous inflammation of a meibomian gland, characterized by a hard, nontender swelling on the upper or lower lid. It may be preceded by a sty. The majority point toward the conjunctival side.

If the chalazion is large enough to impress the cornea, vision will be distorted. The conjunctiva in the region of the chalazion is red and elevated.

Treatment consists of excision by an ophthalmologist.

Boniuk M: Eyelids, lacrimal apparatus, and conjunctiva: Annual review. Arch Ophth 90:239, 1973.

TUMORS

Verrucae and papillomas of the skin of the lids can usually be excised by the general physician. Malignancy should be ruled out by microscopic examination of the excised material.

BLEPHARITIS
(Granulated Eyelids)

Blepharitis is a common chronic, bilateral inflammation of the lid margins. It may be ulcerative *(Staphylococcus aureus)* or nonulcerative (seborrheic). The latter type may be caused by *Pityrosporum ovale,* although the relationship is not definite. Both types are usually present. Seborrhea of the scalp, brows, and frequently of the ears is almost always associated with seborrheic blepharitis.

Symptoms are irritation, burning, and itching. The eyes are "red-rimmed," and scales or "granulations" can be seen clinging to the lashes. In the staphylococcal type, the scales are dry, the lid margins are red and ulcerated, and the lashes tend to fall out; in the seborrheic type the scales are greasy, ulceration is absent, and the lid margins are less red. In the more common mixed type, both dry and greasy scales are present, and the lid margins are red and may be ulcerated.

Cleanliness of the scalp, eyebrows, and lid margins is essential to effective local therapy. Scales must be removed from the lids daily with a damp cotton applicator.

An antistaphylococcal antibiotic or sulfonamide eye ointment is applied with a cotton applicator once daily to the lid margins. The treatment of both types is similar except that in severe staphylococcal blepharitis antibiotic sensitivity studies may be required.

Thygeson P: Complications of staphylococcic blepharitis. Am J Ophth 68:446, 1969.

See also Boniuk reference, above.

ENTROPION & ECTROPION

Entropion (inward turning of the lid, usually the lower) occurs occasionally in older people as a result of degeneration of the lid fascia. Surgery is indicated if the lashes rub on the cornea.

Ectropion (outward turning of the lower lid) is fairly common in elderly people. Surgery is indicated if ectropion causes excessive tearing, exposure keratitis, or a cosmetic problem.

DACRYOCYSTITIS

Dacryocystitis is a common infection of the lacrimal sac. It may be acute or chronic and occurs most often in infants and in persons over 40. It is usually unilateral.

Adult Dacryocystitis

The cause of obstruction is usually unknown, but

a history of trauma to the nose may be obtained. In acute dacryocystitis the usual infectious agent is *Staphylococcus aureus* or *Streptococcus pyogenes;* in the chronic form, *Diplococcus pneumoniae* or, occasionally, *Haemophilus influenzae* is found. Mixed infections do not occur.

Acute dacryocystitis is characterized by pain, swelling, tenderness, and redness in the tear sac area; purulent material may be expressed. In chronic dacryocystitis tearing and discharge are the principal signs. Mucus or pus may be expressed from the tear sac.

Acute dacryocystitis responds well to systemic antibiotic therapy, but recurrences are common if the obstruction is not surgically removed. The chronic form may be kept latent by using antibiotic eye drops, but relief of the obstruction is the only cure.

Infantile Dacryocystitis

Normally the nasolacrimal ducts open spontaneously during the first month of life. Occasionally one of the ducts fails to canalize and a secondary pneumococcal dacryocystitis develops. When this happens, forceful massage of the tear sac is indicated, and antibiotic or sulfonamide drops should be instilled in the conjunctival sac 4—5 times daily. If this is not successful after a few weeks, probing of the nasolacrimal duct is indicated regardless of the infant's age. To minimize spread of the infection, penicillin is sometimes given intramuscularly 2 days before probing; the tear sac is irrigated freely just before probing. One probing is effective in about 75% of cases; in the remainder cure can almost always be achieved by repeated probings.

See Boniuk reference, above.

CHRONIC (OPEN-ANGLE) GLAUCOMA

Essentials of Diagnosis

- Insidious onset in older age groups.
- No symptoms in early stages.
- Gradual loss of peripheral vision over a period of years.
- Persistent elevation of intraocular pressure associated with pathologic cupping of the optic disks.
- *Note:* "Halos around lights" are not present unless the intraocular tension is markedly elevated.

General Considerations

In chronic glaucoma the intraocular pressure is consistently elevated. Over a period of months or years this results in optic atrophy with loss of vision varying from a slight constriction of the upper nasal peripheral visual fields to complete blindness.

The cause of the decreased rate of aqueous outflow in chronic glaucoma has not been clearly demonstrated. The disease is bilateral and is genetically determined, most likely as an autosomal recessive trait which is so common that it is easily confused with dominant inheritance (pseudo-dominant). Infantile glaucoma usually has an autosomal recessive mode of inheritance.

In the USA it is estimated that there are 2 million people with glaucoma; about half of these cases are undetected. About 90% of all cases of glaucoma are of the chronic open-angle type.

Clinical Findings

Patients with chronic glaucoma have no symptoms initially. There may be slight cupping of the optic disk. The visual fields gradually constrict, but central vision remains good until late in the disease.

Tonometry, ophthalmoscopic visualization of the optic nerve, and central visual field testing are the 3 prime tests for the diagnosis and continued clinical evaluation of glaucoma. The normal intraocular pressure is about 10—25 mm Hg. Except in acute glaucoma, however, the diagnosis is never made on the basis of one tonometric measurement, since various factors can influence the pressure (eg, diurnal variation). Transient elevations of intraocular pressure do not constitute glaucoma (for the same reason that periodic elevations of blood pressure do not constitute hypertensive disease).

Prevention

All persons over age 20 should have tonometric and ophthalmoscopic examinations every 3—5 years. They may be done by the general physician, internist, or ophthalmologist. If there is a family history of glaucoma, annual examination is indicated. Mydriatic and cycloplegic drugs should not be used in any patient with glaucoma until the anterior chamber angle has been evaluated by gonioscopy.

Treatment

Most patients can be controlled with miotics, eg, pilocarpine, 1—2%, 3—4 times daily. Pilocarpine increases the rate of outflow of aqueous. Carbonic anhydrase inhibitors—eg, acetazolamide, ethoxzolamide—decrease the rate of aqueous production. Epinephrine eyedrops, 0.5—2%, decrease aqueous production and increase outflow. (*Caution:* Epinephrine is contraindicated if the anterior chamber angle is narrow.) Treatment must be continued through life.

Prognosis

Untreated chronic glaucoma which begins at age 40—45 will probably cause complete blindness by age 60—65. Early diagnosis and treatment will preserve useful vision throughout life in most cases.

Armaly MF: Glaucoma: Annual review. Arch Ophth 93:146, 1975.
Bietti G: Intraocular pressure and glaucoma. Am J Ophth 73:475, 1972.
Hetherington J: Symposium: Glaucoma. Tr Am Acad Ophth

78:239, 1974.

Kronfeld PC: Functional characteristics of surgically produced outflow channels. Am J Ophth 67:451, 1969.

Lazenby GW, Reed JW, Grant WM: Short-term tests of anticholinergic medication in open-angle glaucoma. Arch Ophth 80:443, 1968.

Morgan RW, Drance SM: Chronic open-angle glaucoma and ocular hypertension. Brit J Ophth 59:211, 1975.

Watson PG (editor): Glaucoma. (Perrers Taylor Memorial.) Brit J Ophth 56:146, 1972. [Entire issue.]

RETINAL DETACHMENT

Essentials of Diagnosis

- Blurred vision in one eye becoming progressively worse. ("A curtain came down over one of my eyes.")
- No pain or redness.
- Visible detachment ophthalmoscopically.

General Considerations

Detachment of the retina is usually spontaneous but may be secondary to trauma. Spontaneous detachment occurs most frequently in persons over 50 years old. Predisposing causes such as aphakia and myopia are common.

Clinical Findings

As soon as the retina is torn, a transudate from the choroidal vessels, mixed with vitreous, combines with abnormal vitreous traction on the retina and the force of gravity to strip the retina from the choroid. The superior temporal area is the most common site of detachment. The area of detachment rapidly increases, causing corresponding progressive visual loss. Central vision remains intact until the macula becomes detached.

On ophthalmoscopic examination the retina is seen hanging in the vitreous like a gray cloud. One or more retinal tears, usually crescent-shaped and red or orange, are always present, and can be seen by an experienced examiner.

Differential Diagnosis

Sudden partial loss of vision in one eye may also be due to retinal or vitreous hemorrhage.

Treatment

All cases of retinal detachment should be referred immediately to an ophthalmologist. If the patient must be transported a long distance, his head should be positioned so that the detached portion of the retina will recede with the aid of gravity. For example, a patient with a superior temporal retinal detachment in the right eye should lie on his back with his head turned to the right. Position is less important for a short trip.

Treatment consists of drainage of the subretinal fluid and closure of the retinal tears by diathermy or scleral buckling (or both). This produces an inflammatory reaction which causes the retina to adhere to the choroid. Photocoagulation is of value in a limited number of cases of minimal detachment. It consists of focusing a strong light ("burning glass") through the pupil to create an artificial inflammation between the choroid and the retina.

The **laser** (light amplification by stimulated emission of radiation) is occasionally used in the same manner as the photocoagulator.

The main use of the photocoagulator and laser is in the prevention of detachment by sealing small retinal tears before detachment occurs.

Cryosurgery is also being used effectively in the treatment of retinal detachment. A supercooled probe is applied to the sclera to cause a chorioretinal scar with minimal scleral damage. This decreased scleral damage (as compared with diathermy) makes the operation less hazardous and, because scar formation is minimal, greatly facilitates reoperation. Cryosurgery may eventually replace diathermy completely.

Prognosis

About 80% of uncomplicated cases can be cured with one operation; an additional 10% will need repeated operations; the remainder never reattach. The prognosis is worse if the macula is detached, if there are many vitreous strands, or if the detachment is of long duration. Without treatment, retinal detachment almost always becomes total in 1–6 months. Spontaneous detachments are ultimately bilateral in 20–25% of cases.

Brockhurst RJ, Criswick VG: Retinal detachment. Arch Ophth 82:641, 1969.

Robertson DM, Norton EWD: Long-term follow-up of treated retinal breaks. Am J Ophth 75:395, 1973.

Tasman W: The retina and optic nerve: Annual review. Arch Ophth 92:71, 1974.

CATARACT

Essentials of Diagnosis

- Blurred vision, progressive over months or years.
- No pain or redness.
- Lens opacities, which may be grossly visible.

General Considerations

A cataract is a lens opacity. Cataracts are usually bilateral. They may be congenital or may occur as a result of trauma or, less commonly, systemic disease. Senile cataract is by far the most common type; most persons over 60 have some degree of lens opacity.

Clinical Findings

Even in its early stages a cataract can be seen through a dilated pupil with an ophthalmoscope, a slitlamp, or an ordinary hand illuminator. As the cataract matures the retina will become increasingly difficult to visualize, until finally the fundus reflection is absent. At this point the pupil is white and the cataract is mature.

The degree of visual loss corresponds to the density of the cataract.

Treatment

Only a small percentage of senile cataracts require surgical removal. Degree of visual impairment is the prime surgical criterion; other factors include age, general health, and occupation. Treatment of senile cataract consists of removal of the entire lens followed by refractive correction with a spectacle cataract lens. Contact lenses are replacing the heavy cataract lenses mainly in younger patients and patients of any age requiring surgery in one eye only.

Cryoextraction, using a supercooled metal probe, is the commonest method now being employed for surgical removal of senile cataracts. Phacoemulsification and phacofragmentation are still undergoing extensive clinical trials, particularly in people under 45 years of age (softer cataracts). Compared with the standard technic, both of these procedures offer the advantages of requiring a smaller incision and shorter recovery period.

Prognosis

If surgery is indicated, lens extraction improves visual acuity in 95% of cases. The remainder either have preexisting retinal damage or develop postoperative complications such as glaucoma, hemorrhage, retinal detachment, or infection.

DeVoe AG & others: Symposium: Phaecoemulsification. Tr Am Acad Ophth 78:op3, 1974.
Kelman C: Phaco-emulsification and aspiration. Am J Ophth 75:764, 1973.
Kirsch RE: The lens: Annual review. Arch Ophth 93:284, 1975.
Maumenee AE: Cataract extraction with the cryoprobe. Tr Am Acad Ophth 73:1044, 1969.
Shock JP: Phacofragmentation and irrigation of cataracts: A preliminary report. Am J Ophth 74:187, 1972.

STRABISMUS

Essentials of Diagnosis

- History of eyes deviating.
- Demonstration of deviation by corneal reflection and cover tests.
- Reduced visual acuity in the deviating eye.

General Considerations

About 5% of children are born with or develop a malfunction of binocular coordination known as strabismus. In descending order of frequency, the eyes may deviate inward (esotropia), outward (exotropia),

upward (hypertropia), or downward (hypotropia). The cause is not known, but fusion is lacking in almost all cases. If a child is born with straight eyes but has inherited "weak fusion," he may develop strabismus.

Clinical Findings

Children with frank strabismus first develop diplopia. They soon learn to suppress the image from the deviating eye and the vision in that eye therefore fails to develop. This is the first stage of amblyopia ex anopsia.

Most cases of strabismus are obvious, but if the angle of deviation is small or if the strabismus is intermittent, the diagnosis may be obscure. The best method for detecting strabismus is to direct a light toward each pupil from a distance of 1–2 feet. If the corneal reflection is seen in the center of each pupil, the eyes can be presumed to be straight at that moment.

As a further diagnostic test ("cover test"), cover the right eye with an opaque object ("cover") and instruct the patient to fix his gaze on the examining light with the left eye. If fusion is weak, covering the right eye will disturb the fusion process sufficiently to allow the right eye to deviate, and this can be observed behind the cover. The right eye may swing back into alignment when the cover is removed (phoria). In obvious strabismus, the covered eye will maintain the deviated position after the cover is removed (tropia). Ask the patient to follow the examining light with both eyes to the right, left, up, and down to rule out extraocular muscle paralysis. If there is a history of deviation but it cannot be demonstrated, the patient should be reexamined in 6 months.

Prevention

Amblyopia due to strabismus can be detected by routine visual acuity examination of all **preschool** children. Visual acuity testing is best done with an illiterate E card close to the fourth birthday by the child's mother but is often performed in the physician's office as a routine procedure. Treatment by occlusion of the good eye is simple and effective.

The prevention of blindness by these simple diagnostic and treatment procedures is one of the most rewarding experiences in medical practice.

Treatment

The objectives in the treatment of strabismus are (1) good visual acuity in each eye; (2) straight eyes, for cosmetic purposes; and (3) coordinate function of both eyes.

The best time to initiate treatment is around the age of 6 months. If treatment is delayed beyond this time the child will favor the straight eye and suppress the image in the other eye; this results in failure of visual development (amblyopia ex anopsia) in the deviating eye.

If the child is under 7 years of age and has an amblyopic eye, the amblyopia can be cured by occluding the good eye. At 1 year of age, patching may be successful within 1 week; at 6 years it may take a

year to achieve the same result, ie, to equalize the
visual acuity in both eyes. Prolonged patching seldom
impairs vision in the good eye.

Surgery is usually performed after the visual acuity has been equalized. If the visual acuity is the same
in both eyes and the eyes can be made reasonably
straight through surgery (or with glasses, as in the case
of accommodative esotropia), eye exercises (orthop-
tics) may assist the patient in learning to use his eyes
together (fusion).

Prognosis

The prognosis is more favorable for strabismus
which has its onset at age 1–4 than for strabismus
which is present at birth; better for divergent (outward
deviation) than for convergent strabismus; and better
for intermittent than for constant strabismus.

Burian HM: Pathophysiological basis of amblyopia and its treat-
    ment. Am J Ophth 67:1, 1969.
Reinecke RD: Strabismus: Annual review. Arch Ophth 91:501,
    1974.
Von Noorden GK & others: Surgical treatment of congenital
    esotropia. Tr Am Acad Ophth 76:1465, 1972.
Watson PG (editor): Strabismus: Cambridge Ophthalmological
    Symposium. Brit J Ophth 58:157, 1974.

.   .   .

PRINCIPLES OF TREATMENT
OF OCULAR INFECTIONS

Identification of Pathogen

Before one can determine the drug of choice, the
causative organism must be identified. For example, a
pneumococcal corneal ulcer will respond to treatment
with a sulfonamide, penicillin, or any broad-spectrum
antibiotic, but this is not true in the case of corneal
ulcer due to *Pseudomonas aeruginosa,* which requires
vigorous treatment with polymyxin or gentamicin.
Another example is staphylococcal dacryocystitis,
which, if it does not respond to penicillin, is most
likely to respond to erythromycin.

Choice of Alternative Drugs

In the treatment of infectious eye disease, eg,
conjunctivitis, one should always use the drug which is
the most effective, the least likely to cause complications, and the least expensive. It is also preferable to
use a drug which is not usually given systemically, eg,
sulfacetamide or bacitracin. Of the available antibacterial agents, the sulfonamides come closest to meeting
these specifications. Two reliable sulfonamides for
ophthalmic use are sulfisoxazole and sodium sulfacetamide. The sulfonamides have the added advantages of
low allergenicity and effectiveness against the chlamydial group of organisms. They are available in ointment or solution form.

Two of the most effective broad-spectrum antibiotics for ophthalmic use are gentamicin and neomycin. Both of these drugs have some effect against gram-
negative as well as gram-positive organisms; allergic
reactions to neomycin are common. Other antibiotics
frequently used are erythromycin, the tetracyclines,
bacitracin, and polymyxin. Combined bacitracin-
polymyxin ointment is often used prophylactically
after corneal foreign body removal for the protection
it affords against both gram-positive and gram-negative
organisms.

Method of Administration

Most ocular anti-infective drugs are administered
locally. Systemic administration as well is required for
all intraocular infections, corneal ulcer, orbital cellulitis, dacryocystitis, and any severe external infection
which does not respond to local treatment.

Ointment vs Liquid Medications

Ointments have greater therapeutic effectiveness
than solutions since contact can be maintained longer.
However, they do cause blurring of vision; if this must
be avoided, solutions should be used.

Havener WH: *Ocular Pharmacology,* 3rd ed. Mosby, 1974.
Leopold IH (editor): *Symposium on Ocular Therapy.* Vol 6.
    Mosby, 1973.
Richardson KT: Pharmacology and toxicology: Annual review.
    Arch Ophth 89:65, 1973.

TECHNICS USED IN THE TREATMENT
OF OCULAR DISORDERS

Instilling Medications

Place the patient in a chair with his head tilted
back, both eyes open, and looking up. Retract the
lower lid slightly and instill 2 drops of liquid into the
lower cul-de-sac. Have the patient look down while
finger contact on the lower lid is maintained. Do not
let him squeeze his eye shut.

Ointments are instilled in the same general manner.

Self-Medication

The same technics are used as described above,
except that drops are usually better instilled with the
patient lying down.

Eye Bandage

Most eye bandages should be applied firmly
enough to hold the lid securely against the cornea. An
ordinary patch consisting of gauze-covered cotton is
usually sufficient. Tape is applied from the cheek to
the forehead. If more pressure is desired, use 2 or 3
bandages. The black eye patch is difficult to sterilize
and therefore is seldom used in modern medical practice.

Warm Compresses

A clean towel or washcloth soaked in warm tap water is applied to the affected eye 2—4 times a day for 10—15 minutes.

Removal of a Superficial Corneal Foreign Body

Record the patient's visual acuity, if possible, and instill sterile local anesthetic drops. With the patient sitting or lying down, an assistant should direct a strong light into the eye so that the rays strike the cornea obliquely. Using either a loupe or a slitlamp the physician locates the foreign body on the corneal surface. He may remove it with a sterile wet cotton applicator or, if this fails, with a spud, holding the lids apart with the other hand to prevent blinking. An antibacterial ointment (eg, polymyxin-bacitracin) is instilled after the foreign body has been removed. It is preferable not to patch the eye, but the patient must be seen on the following day to make certain healing is under way.

PRECAUTIONS IN THE MANAGEMENT OF OCULAR DISORDERS

Use of Local Anesthetics

Unsupervised self-administration of local anesthetics is dangerous because the patient may further injure an anesthetized eye without knowing it. The drug may also prevent the normal healing process. An abrasion expected to heal in 24 hours may still be present a month or more under "treatment" with a local anesthetic.

Pupillary Dilation

Cycloplegics and mydriatics should be used with caution. Dilating the pupil can precipitate an attack of acute glaucoma if the patient has a narrow anterior chamber angle.

Local Corticosteroid Therapy

Repeated use of local corticosteroids presents several serious hazards: herpes simplex (dendritic) keratitis, fungal overgrowth, open-angle glaucoma, and cataract formation. Furthermore, perforation of the cornea may occur when the corticosteroids are used for herpes simplex keratitis.

Contaminated Eye Medications

Ophthalmic solutions must be prepared with the same degree of care as fluids intended for intravenous administration.

Tetracaine, proparacaine, physostigmine, and fluorescein are most likely to become contaminated. The most dangerous is fluorescein, as this solution is frequently contaminated with *Pseudomonas aeruginosa,* an organism which can rapidly destroy the eye. Sterile fluorescein filter paper strips are now available and are recommended in place of fluorescein solutions.

The following rules should be observed in handling eye medications for use in the diagnostic examination of uninjured eyes: (1) Obtain solutions in small amounts from the pharmacy. (2) Be certain that the solution is sterile as prepared and that it contains an effective antibacterial agent. (3) Date the bottle at the time it is procured.

Plastic dropper bottles are becoming more popular each year. Solutions from these bottles are safe to use in uninjured eyes. Whether in plastic or glass containers, eye solutions should not be used for long periods of time after the bottle is first opened. Two weeks is a reasonable time to use a solution before discarding.

If the eye has been injured accidentally or by surgical trauma, it is of the greatest importance to use sterile medications supplied in sterile, disposable, single use eye-dropper units.

Fungal Overgrowth

Since antibiotics, like corticosteroids, when used over a prolonged period of time in bacterial corneal ulcers, favor the development of secondary fungal corneal infection, the sulfonamides should be used whenever they are adequate for the purpose.

Sensitization

A significant portion of a soluble substance instilled in the eye may pass into the blood stream. This suggests that an antibiotic instilled into the eye can sensitize the patient to that drug and cause a hypersensitivity reaction upon subsequent systemic administration.

5...
Ear, Nose, & Throat

Wayne W. Deatsch

DISEASES OF THE EAR

HEARING LOSS

Classification

A. **Sensorineural (Nerve, Perceptive) Deafness:**
1. Receptor end organ (cochlea).
2. Neural pathways.
3. Central (auditory cortex). Cortical lesions are bilateral.

B. **Conductive Deafness:** Disturbances of the external or middle ear preventing normal sound transmission.

C. **Mixed Deafness:** Combined sensorineural and conduction deafness.

D. **Functional Deafness:** No organic lesion can be detected.

General Considerations

Five to 10% of people have a hearing defect, temporarily or permanently, which is severe enough to impair their normal function. Hearing loss may occur at any age and produces disability depending upon the degree of loss, the age at which it occurs (interference with language and speech development), and whether one or both ears are affected.

Sensorineural hearing loss may be congenital, due to birth trauma, maternal rubella, erythroblastosis fetalis, or malformations of the inner ear; or it may be due to traumatic injury to the inner ear or 8th nerve, vascular disorders with hemorrhage or thrombosis in the inner ear, ototoxic agents (Table 5–1), bacterial and viral infections (meningitis, encephalitis, mumps, etc), severe febrile illnesses, Ménière's disease, posterior fossa tumors, multiple sclerosis, presbyacusis, and prolonged or repeated exposure to loud sound.

Conductive hearing loss may also be congenital, due to malformations of the external or middle ear. Trauma may produce perforation of the eardrum or disruption of the ossicular chain. Inflammatory middle ear disease may produce serous otitis media, acute or chronic purulent otitis media, or adhesive otitis media. Otosclerosis, a common familial conductive hearing loss with onset in middle life, produces ankylosis of the stapes by overgrowth of new spongy bone; the cause is not known.

Clinical Findings

The older patient will usually be aware of hearing loss of significant degree, and an accurate history is of importance to determine etiology. All the causes of hearing loss listed above must be investigated. In particular, the age at onset, degree of loss, progression, associated tinnitus or vertigo, exposure to head trauma, sound trauma, ototoxic drugs, previous infection, and severe febrile illnesses must be checked.

In infants and young children the diagnosis is often suggested by failure of speech development, lack of cooperation, inability to concentrate, and slow progress in learning.

A complete ear, nose, and throat examination is essential in all patients with hearing loss. Most important is examination of the ear canal, eardrum, and middle ear with the magnifying otoscope to detect even slight abnormalities. Attention must be given to obstructing or infected adenoid and tonsils, nasal and sinus infection, and evidences of other cranial nerve disturbance.

Special tests of value are as follows:

(1) Whispered and spoken voice test: In a quiet room, with the other ear covered, the tested normal ear should be able to accurately perceive the spoken voice at 20 feet and the whispered voice at 15 feet.

(2) Tuning fork tests: The 500 and 1000 cps forks are the most important. These tests detect lateralization of the sounds of the fork and demonstrate comparative disturbances of air conduction and bone conduction (to distinguish conductive loss and nerve type loss).

(3) Audiometric tests (pure tone, speech tests, and other highly specialized audiometric tests) provide quantitative measurements of the degree of hearing loss. Audiometry is invaluable in following the progress of patients with ear disorders and hearing impairment and for the proper fitting and evaluation of hearing aids.

(4) Labyrinthine tests give valuable objective evidence of inner ear function. An absent or altered labyrinthine response is quite significant. The test is done by irrigating the ear canals with hot or cold water to produce nystagmus and vertigo. The response in each

Table 5—1. Ototoxic drugs.*

Drug	Auditory Disturbance	Vestibular Disturbance	Remarks
Antibiotics			
Capreomycin	+	+	Rare.
Dihydrostrep-tomycin	++	±	Frequent, severe, irreversible.
Gentamicin	+	++	Frequent.
Kanamycin	++	±	Occasional. Onset may be delayed.
Neomycin	++	±	Occasional. Any route of administration.
Paromomycin	++	±	Occasional.
Streptomycin	++	++	Frequent.
Vancomycin	++	+	Occasional.
Viomycin	++	++	Frequent.
Diuretics			
Ethacrynic acid	++	+	Occasional. Usually transient.
Furosemide	++	+	Following intravenous use. Usually transient.
Salicylates	+	++	Tinnitus. Tone decay. Usually reversible.
Antimalarials			
Chloroquine	++	+	Rare. Progressive, irreversible.
Quinine (and quinidine)	+	++	Tinnitus. Usually reversible, transitory deafness (rare).

*Ototoxicity of offending drugs may be enhanced by (1) impaired renal function due to renal damage, shock, dehydration, etc; (2) high dosages of drug, such as salicylates in rheumatoid arthritis; and (3) perhaps by potentiation by other drugs (eg, diuretics). ¶Other drugs reported to be ototoxic include medroxyprogesterone, mumps vaccine, mechlorethamine, nortriptyline, and propylthiouracil.

Table 5—2. Differentiation of sensorineural and conductive deafness.

	Conductive Deafness	Sensorineural Deafness
Patient's voice	Speaks softly	Speaks loudly
Effect of noisy environment	Hears best	Hears poorly
Speech discrimination	Good	Poor
Hearing on telephone	Good	Poor
Weber test lateralization	To diseased ear	To good ear
Rinne test	Negative (AC = BC)	Positive (AC > BC)

AC = Air conduction. BC = Bone conduction.

ear should be equal.

(5) The electronystagmogram (ENG) may be of value in the identification, recording, and interpretation of nystagmus, especially in response to labyrinthine tests.

Treatment

A. Hearing Loss in Children:

1. Nerve deafness—Although there is usually little that can be done medically or surgically to restore nerve function in most types of sensorineural deafness, preventive measures, early diagnosis, auditory rehabilitation, and education are essential for total treatment. Prompt treatment of bacterial infections of the CNS (meningitis, etc) and the prompt treatment of severe febrile illnesses may prevent some development of nerve deafness. During treatment with known ototoxic drugs, hearing should be checked regularly and the drug discontinued if hearing begins to be impaired. If other equally effective drugs are available, ototoxic drugs should not be used. Management consists of rehabilitation and education. A hearing aid is valuable if there is residual hearing. Speech reading and speech training must be incorporated into the educational program.

2. Conductive deafness—Acute suppurative otitis media with eardrum bulging should be treated with myringotomy in addition to medical management. Acute otitis media may be treated medically, but the patient must be carefully followed to ensure that the infection completely resolves. Otherwise, residual fluid in the middle ear may produce a conductive hearing loss due to persistent serous otitis media, glue ear, or adhesive otitis media. Antibiotics in adequate doses and nasal decongestants should be administered for at least 7 days and often longer. This is necessary to prevent smoldering, partially eradicated infections that may recur in a few days without antibiotic-resistant organisms. Paracentesis and aspiration may be necessary.

Serous otitis media is common in children as well as in adults. Vigorous early treatment will usually reverse the hearing loss. Investigation and treatment of contributing nasal allergy or infection combined with aspiration of fluid from the middle ear is effective. Removal of obstructing or infected tonsils and adenoidal tissue may be necessary. In protracted and recurrent cases, repeat adenoidectomy or myringotomy and insertion of indwelling ventilating tubes may be necessary. Follow-up eustachian tube inflations are often required. The progress of each case must be carefully followed by audiometric testing.

Chronic otitis media in childhood should be treated vigorously to attempt to cure the disease and preserve or restore hearing. Many cases respond to cleansing followed by instillation of powders (eg, chloramphenicol and boric acid) or antibiotic solutions. Attention must again be directed to underlying nasal or sinus disease and infected or obstructing tonsils and adenoid. Other cases require surgery of the middle ear or mastoid (or both). Bilateral congenital anomalies of the external ear canal and middle ear can sometimes be corrected surgically. This should be done before plastic repair of the external ear is made. Small central perforations of the eardrum can be closed by patching with a paper or other membrane as an office procedure. Larger central perforations may be closed with a vein graft or skin graft. Marginal perforations usually require skin grafting and mastoid exploration.

The patient should be evaluated for a hearing aid by a competent otolaryngologist and audiologist.

B. Hearing Loss in Adults:

1. Nerve deafness—Nerve loss due to acoustic trauma will sometimes improve over a period of 6 months if the patient can avoid exposure to loud noise. The best treatment is prevention of exposure to loud noise either by avoiding the sources of noise (industry, recreation, military) or by wearing suitable protective ear plugs or other noise attenuators. Recent observations of hearing loss after exposure to highly amplified "rock" music should be noted. The nerve loss of Ménière's disease often improves with treatment and between attacks. There is no medical or surgical treatment for actual nerve damage in other forms of sensorineural deafness except as mentioned above. Prompt treatment of bacterial CNS infections and severe febrile illnesses, and the avoidance (if possible) or discontinuance of ototoxic drug administration if hearing loss begins to develop, are of the utmost importance. A hearing aid should not be recommended for a patient with deafness unless audiometric testing (pure tone and speech) indicates that the patient will probably learn to use the instrument satisfactorily. The learning of speech reading (lip reading) as well as auditory training by a hard-of-hearing patient is of definite value in rehabilitation.

2. Conductive deafness—Important advances have been made recently in the surgical treatment of middle ear deafness. Otosclerosis may be treated successfully by a direct operation on the fixed stapes through the ear canal and middle ear. The most recent technics involve removal of the stapes and replacement of the foot plate with a graft (vein, fat, or gelfoam) and replacement of the stapes crura with a prosthesis (wire or plastic strut).

Perforations of the eardrum can be repaired by vein, fascia, or skin grafting (myringoplasty).

Mastoid and middle ear operations have been designed for the treatment of suppuration and the removal of cholesteatoma and to preserve or improve hearing by skin grafting and by replacing or realigning the ossicular chain (tympanoplasty).

Serous otitis media in adults is treated in the same manner as in children.

Nerve deafness due to Ménière's disease will sometimes respond to early, adequate, and prolonged treatment. A fluctuating loss has a more favorable prognosis than a sudden severe loss. The basis of medical management is sodium restriction (1 gm sodium diet), antihistamines (eg, diphenhydramine or dimenhydrinate 4 times daily for 1–2 months), potassium substitution for sodium (KCl, 1 gm 3 times daily for 1–2 weeks),

vasodilators (nicotinic acid in flushing doses 4 times daily), and reassurance.

The advisability of hearing aids should be determined by competent otolaryngologic and audiologic consultants.

Bess FH, Poynor RE: Snowmobile engine noise and hearing. Arch Otol 95:164, 1972.

Boston Collaborative Drug Surveillance Program: Drug-induced deafness—a cooperative study. JAMA 224:515, 1973.

Fredrikson HM: Noise exposure: Legal viewpoint. Tr Am Acad Ophth 75:1272, 1971.

Handbook of antimicrobial therapy: Principal adverse effects of antimicrobial drugs. Med Lett Drugs Ther, 1974.

House HP & others: Symposium on stapes surgery. Laryngoscope 80:1256, 1970.

Konigsmark BW: Hereditary deafness in man. (3 parts.) New England J Med 281:713, 774, 827, 1969.

McConnell F: A new approach to the management of childhood deafness. P Clin North America 17:347, 1970.

Nilges TC & others: Iatrogenic ototoxicity. Ann Surg 173:281, 1971.

Rupp RR: Understanding the problems of presbyacusis: An overview on hearing loss associated with aging. Geriatrics 25:100, 1970.

Sheehy JL, Gardner G Jr, Hambley WM: Tuning fork tests in modern otology. Arch Otol 94:132, 1971.

DISEASES OF THE EXTERNAL EAR

1. IMPACTED CERUMEN

Cerumen is the normal secretion of the cartilaginous part of the ear canal which serves a protective function. Normally it dries and falls out of the ear canal, but it may accumulate within the canal because of dryness or scaling of the skin, narrowing or tortuosity of the ear canal, or excess hair in the ear canal. It may be packed in deeper by repeated unskilled attempts to remove it. There are usually no symptoms until the canal becomes completely occluded, when a feeling of fullness, deafness or tinnitus, or a cough due to reflex stimulation of the vagus nerve may occur. Otoscopy reveals the mass of yellow, brown, or black wax which may be sticky and soft or waxy, or stony hard.

If the mass is firm and movable, it may be removed through the speculum with a dull ring curette or a cotton applicator. If this is painful, the impaction may be removed by irrigation with water at body temperature, directing the stream of water from a large syringe at the wall of the ear canal and catching the solution in a basin held beneath the ear. If the impaction is very hard and adherent and cannot be readily removed by irrigation, it must be softened by repeated instillations of oily (baby oil) ear drops, glycerin (70% by volume), or peroxide (3%), and irrigated again in 2–3 days.

2. EXTERNAL OTITIS

External otitis may vary in severity from a diffuse mild eczematoid dermatitis to cellulitis or even furunculosis of the ear canal. It is frequently referred to as a fungal infection of the ear, although in many cases there is no infection and the reaction is a contact dermatitis (earphones, earrings) or a variant of seborrheic dermatitis. Infections of the ear canal are usually bacterial (staphylococcal and gram-negative rods), although a few are caused by fungi (aspergillus, mucor, penicillium). Predisposing factors are moisture in the ear canal in a warm, moist climate or due to swimming or bathing, trauma due to attempts to clean or scratch the itching ear, and seborrheic and allergic dermatitis.

Clinical Findings

A. Symptoms and Signs: Itching and pain in the dry, scaling ear canal are the chief symptoms. There may be a watery or purulent discharge and intermittent deafness. Pain may become extreme when the ear canal becomes completely occluded with edematous skin and debris. Preauricular, postauricular, or cervical adenopathy or fever indicate increasing severity of infection.

Examination shows crusting, scaling, erythema, edema, and pustule formation. Cerumen is absent. There may be evidence of seborrheic dermatitis elsewhere.

B. Laboratory Findings: The white count may be normal or elevated.

C. Special Examinations: After the canal is cleansed so that the eardrum is visible, otitis media can often be excluded if tuning fork tests indicate normal or nearly normal hearing.

Differential Diagnosis

Diffuse eczematoid dermatitis of the ear canal, diffuse infected dermatitis, and furuncle of the ear canal must be distinguished from dermatitis due to contact with foreign objects (hearing aids, earphones) or infected material draining from the middle ear through a perforated eardrum.

Treatment

A. Systemic Treatment: If there is evidence of extension of infection beyond the skin of the ear canal (lymphadenopathy or fever), systemic antibiotics may be necessary. Systemic analgesics are required for pain.

B. Local Treatment: The objectives of local treatment are to keep the ear canal clean and dry and to protect it from trauma. Debris may be removed from the canal by gently wiping it with a cotton applicator or with suction or, occasionally, irrigation. The use of Debrox (carbamide peroxide in anhydrous glycerol) 3 times daily often helps to remove debris.

Topical antibiotic ointments and ear drops (eg, neomycin polymyxin, bacitracin) applied to the ear canal with a cotton wick for 24 hours followed by the use of ear drops twice daily help to control infection.

Topical corticosteroids aid in decreasing inflammatory edema and controlling the often underlying dermatitis. Many antifungal and antimicrobial agents may be used topically, but some must be used with caution because of the possibility of local sensitivity reactions. Compresses of Burow's solution or 0.5% acetic acid are sometimes effective against acute weeping infected eczema when other measures fail. Seventy percent alcohol frequently controls itching in the dry, scaling ear canal.

Severe (malignant) otitis externa, as in diabetes, may require vigorous treatment including hospitalization.

Prognosis

Depending upon the cause, external otitis may be refractory to treatment, and recurrences are frequent.

Worgan D: Treatment of otitis externa. Practitioner 202:817, 1969.

DISEASES OF THE MIDDLE EAR

1. ACUTE OTITIS MEDIA

Essentials of Diagnosis

- Ear pain, a sensation of fullness in the ear, and hearing loss; aural discharge.
- Onset following an upper respiratory infection.
- Fever and chills.

General Considerations

Acute otitis media most commonly occurs in infants and children, but it may occur at any age. Suppuration of the middle ear usually occurs following or accompanying disease of the upper respiratory tract. Beta-hemolytic streptococci, staphylococci, pneumococci, and *Haemophilus influenzae* are the usual infecting organisms. The acute inflammation of the middle ear mucosa is followed by acute suppuration and then a more severe suppuration with perforation of the tympanic membrane and occasionally with necrosis of the middle ear mucosa and eardrum.

Clinical Findings

A. Symptoms and Signs: The principal symptoms are ear pain, deafness, fever, chills, and a feeling of fullness and pressure in the ear. The eardrum at first shows dilatation of the blood vessels on the malleus and at the annulus; this is followed by diffuse dullness and hyperemia of the eardrum and loss of normal landmarks (short process of malleus) and bulging of the drum as the pressure of retained secretions increases in the middle ear. If the eardrum ruptures, discharge is found in the ear canal; the discharge may be pulsating. Fever is usually present.

B. Laboratory Findings: The white count is usually increased. Culture of the drainage will reveal the infecting organism.

C. Special Examinations: Hearing tests will show a conductive hearing loss.

Differential Diagnosis

Acute otitis media with bulging of the eardrum must be distinguished from myringitis bullosa, usually by the presence of more than one bleb in the ear canal and the absence of marked hearing loss. Acute otitis media with drainage must be distinguished from acute external otitis. The history of a preceding upper respiratory tract infection and hearing loss confirm the diagnosis of otitis media. Acute exacerbation of chronic otitis media is diagnosed by a history of otorrhea and hearing loss and by finding scar tissue on the eardrum. Reflex otalgia (pharyngitis, laryngitis, dental disease, temporomandibular joint disease) is present if there are no acute inflammatory changes in the ear canal or eardrum and no fever.

Complications

Acute mastoiditis, labyrinthitis, or meningitis may occur as complications.

Treatment

A. Systemic Treatment: Bed rest, analgesics, and systemic antibiotics are usually required. Penicillin or a broad-spectrum antibiotic is usually the drug of choice, and should be continued for at least 7–10 days to minimize the likelihood of recurrence of an incompletely resolved infection after a latent period. Nasal decongestants, topical and systemic, help restore eustachian tube function.

B. Local Treatment: Ear drops are of limited value except in the mildest cases. Local heat may hasten resolution. Local cold applications relieve pain occasionally. The most important aspect of treatment is myringotomy when the infection does not resolve promptly or when bulging of the eardrum indicates that a discharge is present and is under pressure. Myringotomy should also be promptly performed if there is continued pain or fever, increasing hearing loss, or vertigo.

Prognosis

Acute otitis media adequately treated with antibiotics and myringotomy if indicated resolves with rare exceptions. Complicating mastoiditis occurs most commonly following inadequate or no treatment. Persistent conductive hearing loss with or without middle ear fluid may occur following incomplete resolution of the infection. It is imperative to examine the ears and to test the hearing after otitis media to prevent persistent conductive hearing loss with serous otitis media or "glue ear."

Beales PH: Acute otitis media. Practitioner 199:752, 1967.
DeSanto LW, Stickler GB: Acute otitis media in children. Postgrad Med 45:210, 1969.

Hambley WM: External otitis versus otitis media. GP 34:136, Oct 1966.
Hemenway WG, Smith RO: Treating acute otitis media. (2 parts.) Postgrad Med 47:110, 135, 1970.
Palmer BW: Hemorrhagic bullous myringitis: Recent concepts of etiology and complications. Eye Ear Nose Throat Month 47:562, 1968.

2. CHRONIC OTITIS MEDIA

Chronic inflammation of the middle ear is nearly always associated with perforation of the eardrum. It is important to distinguish the relatively benign chronic otitis associated with eustachian tube disease—characterized by central perforation of the eardrum and often mucoid otorrhea occurring with an upper respiratory tract infection—from the chronic otitis associated with mastoid disease that is potentially much more dangerous; the latter is characterized by perforation of Shrapnell's membrane or posterior marginal perforation of the eardrum, often with foul-smelling drainage and cholesteatoma formation. Drainage from the ear and impaired hearing are frequent symptoms.

Treatment of the chronic "tubal ear" should be directed at improving eustachian tube function by correcting nasal or sinus infection or treating infected or hypertrophied tonsils or adenoids, nasal polyps, deviated nasal septum, and nasal allergy. Ear drops (antibiotic solutions) or dusting powders (iodine, boric acid, or antibiotics) and frequent cleansing of the ear are of value. Systemic antibiotics are often of value. If there is evidence of continued suppuration or if mastoiditis or other complications occur, radical or modified radical mastoidectomy should be done. In some cases of chronic otitis media where hearing loss has occurred—and if the middle ear infection is quiescent and eustachian tube function is adequate—reconstructive middle ear operations (tympanoplasty) can be attempted to improve the hearing.

Diamant M: Chronic middle ear discharge. Eye Ear Nose Throat Month 44:77, 1965.
Goodwin MR: Acute mastoiditis and acute labyrinthitis without mastoidectomy. Laryngoscope 78:227, 1968.
Hill FT: Comprehensive care in the treatment of chronic suppurative otitis media. Laryngoscope 71:587, 1961.
Juers AL, Patterson CN, Farrior JB: Symposium on tympanoplasty. I. Office closure of tympanic perforations—passé. II. Silastic sponge implants in tympanoplasty. III. Tympanoplasty: The anterior atticotympanotomy. Surgery of the posterior tympanic recesses. Laryngoscope 78:756, 1968.
Macbeth R: Chronically discharging ear. Practitioner 199:735, 1967.
Ruggles RL, Koconis CA: Tympanic perforations: Safe or not? Laryngoscope 77:337, 1967.
Thomas GL: Cholesteatoma of the ear. California Med 108:205, 1968.

3. SEROUS OTITIS MEDIA

Serous otitis media may occur at any age. It is characterized by the accumulation of sterile fluid (serous or mucoid) in the middle ear, producing symptoms of hearing loss, a full, plugged feeling in the ear, and an unnatural reverberation of the patient's voice. It may be caused by (1) an obstruction of the eustachian tube which prevents normal ventilation of the middle ear and subsequent transudation of serous fluid; (2) an incompletely resolved exudate of purulent otitis media; or (3) an allergic exudate of serous fluid into the middle ear.

Examination shows a conductive hearing loss and a retracted eardrum, often with a characteristic "ground glass" amber discoloration and impaired mobility of the eardrum with the pneumatic otoscope. Air-fluid bubbles or a fluid level can sometimes be seen through the eardrum.

The absence of fever, pain, and toxic symptoms distinguish serous otitis media from acute otitis media. Cancer of the nasopharynx must be ruled out in persistent unilateral serous otitis media in an adult.

Local treatment consists of eustachian tube inflations, paracentesis of the eardrum with aspiration of the middle ear contents, and nasal decongestants (0.25% phenylephrine nasal spray or phenylpropanolamine, 25—50 orally 3 times daily). Antihistamines should be given if there is any suggestion of contributing nasal allergy. Underlying factors must be corrected by control of nasal allergy and treatment of nasal or sinus infection. Tonsillectomy and adenoidectomy may sometimes be necessary. Indwelling plastic ventilating tubes after myringotomy and local or systemic use of corticosteroids may help in persistent cases.

Chan JCM, Logan GB, McBean JB: Serous otitis media and allergy. Am J Dis Child 114:684, 1967.
Draper WL: Secretory otitis media in children: A study of 540 children. Laryngoscope 77:636, 1967.
Oppenheimer RP, Siegel JR: Treatment of serous otitis in children. GP 35:105, March 1967.
Thomas GL: Management of chronic middle ear effusion. California Med 110:300, 1969.

4. MASTOIDITIS

Acute mastoiditis is a complication of acute suppurative otitis media. Bony necrosis of the mastoid process and breakdown of the bony intercellular structures occur in the second to third week. When this occurs there is evidence of continued drainage from the middle ear, mastoid tenderness, systemic manifestations of sepsis (fever, headache), and x-ray evidence of bone destruction.

If suppurative mastoiditis develops in spite of antibiotic therapy, mastoidectomy must be done.

Acute mastoiditis is rarely seen since chemotherapeutic and antibiotic therapy has become available for the treatment of acute suppurative otitis media.

Chronic mastoiditis is a complication of chronic otitis media. If the disease occurs in infancy the mastoid bone does not develop cellular structure but becomes dense and sclerotic. Infection is usually limited to the antral area. However, x-ray findings of a sclerotic mastoid does not necessarily mean that a chronic infection is present, only that an infection was present in infancy and that as a result the mastoid air cells are not well developed. The presence of infection must be determined by clinical findings. In some cases of marginal perforation or Shrapnell's membrane perforation (attic perforation) of the eardrum, cholesteatomas develop. Cholesteatoma is produced by the ingrowth of squamous epithelium from the skin of the external ear canal into the middle ear or mastoid, forming an epithelial cyst. Desquamation and laminated growth of the cyst may produce erosion of adjacent bone or soft tissue.

Antibiotic drugs are usually of limited usefulness in clearing the infection in chronic mastoiditis, but they may be effective in the treatment of complications. Some cases of chronic otitis media and mastoiditis can be managed by local cleansing of the ear and instillation of antibiotic powders or solutions. Other cases may require radical or modified radical mastoidectomy or tympanoplasty.

Schukenecht HF, Applebaum EL: Surgery for hearing loss. New England J Med 280:1154, 1969.
Schwartzman JA, Pulec JL, Linthicum FH Jr: Uncommon granulomatous diseases of the ear: Differential diagnosis. Ann Otol Rhin Laryng 81:389, 1972.
Sheehy JL: Tympanoplasty with mastoidectomy: A re-evaluation. Laryngoscope 80:1212, 1970.
Zoller H: Acute mastoiditis and its complications: Changing trend. South MJ 65:477, 1972.

COMPLICATIONS OF MIDDLE EAR INFECTIONS

Following Acute Suppurative Otitis Media & Mastoiditis

A. Subperiosteal abscess following acute otitis media and mastoiditis is infrequent. Simple mastoidectomy is required.

B. Facial nerve paralysis developing in the first few hours or days after the onset of acute otitis media is due to edema of the nerve in the bony facial canal. Conservative treatment is usually indicated (antibiotics, myringotomy, supportive measures).

C. Meningitis, epidural, subdural, and brain abscess, and sigmoid sinus thrombosis are serious complications of suppurative otitis media and mastoiditis which may be masked by antibiotic drugs. Surgical treatment of the mastoid disease and its complications is required.

D. Conductive Deafness: See p 90.

Following Chronic Otitis Media

A. Acute exacerbations of chronic otitis media and mastoiditis may lead to meningitis, epidural, subdural, and brain abscess, and sigmoid sinus thrombosis, requiring antibiotic therapy and surgery.

B. Facial nerve paralysis is usually the result of direct pressure on the nerve by cholesteatoma or granulation tissue. Mastoidectomy and decompression of the facial nerve are necessary.

C. Conductive Deafness: See p 90.

Beeden AG & others: Intracranial complications of middle ear disease and mastoid surgery. J Neurol Sc 9:261, 1969.

Brydoy B, Ellekjaer EF: Otogenic meningitis: Five-year study. J Laryng 86:871, 1972.

Juselius H, Kaltiokallio K: Complications of acute and chronic otitis media in the antibiotic era. Acta oto-laryng 74:445, 1972.

Ritter FN: Chronic suppurative otitis media and the pathologic labyrinthine fistula. Laryngoscope 80:1025, 1970.

DISEASES OF THE INNER EAR

1. MÉNIÈRE'S DISEASE
(Paroxysmal Labyrinthine Vertigo)

Essentials of Diagnosis

- Intermittent attacks of vertigo, nausea, vomiting, profuse sweating.
- Progressive, often unilateral nerve type hearing loss and continuous tinnitus.

General Considerations

Ménière's syndrome is characterized by recurrent episodes of severe vertigo associated with deafness and tinnitus. It is encountered most often in men in the age group from 40–60. The cause is not known, but "endolymphatic hydrops" with marked dilatation of the cochlear duct is the pathologic finding. Ménière's syndrome may follow head trauma or middle ear infection, but many cases develop without apparent damage to the nervous system or ear.

Clinical Findings

Intermittent severe vertigo, which may appear to throw the subject to the ground, is the principal symptom. Brief loss of consciousness occasionally occurs in an attack. "Spinning" of surrounding objects is often noted. Nausea, vomiting, and profuse perspiration are often associated. The attacks may last from a few minutes to several hours. The frequency of attacks varies considerably even in the same patient. Headache, nerve type hearing loss, and tinnitus occur during and persist between attacks. Hearing loss is apt to be progressive, and is unilateral in 90% of cases. Nystagmus may occur during attacks of vertigo. An altered labyrinthine response is often demonstrated by means of the caloric or Bárány test. There is increased sensitivity to loud sounds. Audiometric tests show recruitment, decreased speech discrimination, and a nerve type hearing loss.

Differential Diagnosis

Distinguish the vertigo from that produced by posterior fossa tumors (other findings such as papilledema, increased CSF pressure and protein, and brain stem signs). Differentiate dizziness and lightheadedness from those seen in some systemic diseases, brain stem vascular disease, and psychiatric disorders. Special diagnostic audiometry, electronystagmography, and x-rays of the internal auditory canals are often necessary for differential diagnosis.

Treatment

Reassurance is important, since many of these patients have a marked psychic overlay. A salt-free diet and ammonium chloride, 1–2 gm 4 times daily, may be helpful. Diuretics such as acetazolamide (Diamox) and chlorothiazide (Diuril) may also be used. Nicotinic acid, 50–100 mg IV 2–3 times daily, or 100 mg orally 5–6 times daily, has been found useful. The antihistamines, especially diphenhydramine hydrochloride (Benadryl) and dimenhydrinate (Dramamine), in doses of 50–100 mg 3–4 times daily, appear to be of benefit to some patients. Parenteral diphenhydramine or dimenhydrinate–or atropine sulfate, 0.6 mg–may stop the acute attack.

Destructive surgery on the labyrinth or vestibular nerve may be necessary in a few severe cases which do not respond to medical measures.

Prognosis

Ménière's syndrome is a chronic recurrent disease which persists for several years. Remission or improvement of vertigo after treatment is often noted; however, tinnitus and deafness usually are unaffected and permanent. Progression is slow and sometimes stops before complete deafness occurs.

Cessation of attacks of vertigo may follow complete loss of hearing.

Procedures which destroy or interrupt an affected vestibular portion of acoustic nerve (such as destruction of the labyrinth or section of the acoustic nerve) may prevent further attacks of vertigo.

Lindsay JR, Kohut RI, Sciarra PA: Ménière's disease: Pathology and manifestations. Ann Otol Rhin Laryng 76:5, 1967.

McCabe BF: Clinical aspects of the differential diagnosis of end-organ vertigo. Ann Otol Rhin Laryng 77:193, 1968.

Proud GO: Practical testing methods for vestibular disorders: Office tests. Ann Otol Rhin Laryng 77:199, 1968.

Pulec JL: Symposium on Ménière's disease. Laryngoscope 82:1703, 1972.

Simonton KM: Ménière's disease and medical treatment of vertigo. Mayo Clin Proc 44:81, 1969.

Symposium on vertigo. Arch Otolaryng 85:497, 1967.

2. TINNITUS

Tinnitus is a sensation of noise in the ears or head that may be objective (heard by the examiner) or subjective. Objective tinnitus is uncommon, and is usually caused by transmitted vascular vibrations in the blood vessels of the head and neck or by rhythmic rapid contractions of the muscles of the soft palate or middle ear. The examiner can often hear the sound through a stethoscope placed over the ear or can see movements of the eardrum or palate.

Subjective tinnitus usually accompanies hearing loss or other disorders of the external, middle, or inner ear. Although the etiology is unknown, it is presumed to be due to irritation of nerve endings in the cochlea by degenerative vascular or vasomotor disease. Most patients state that the noise is bearable during the day but is much louder and more disturbing at night when the masking effect of environmental sounds is not present.

If possible, treatment is directed at the underlying cause. If the etiology cannot be determined, reassurance may be all that is necessary. An air conduction hearing aid during the day and a pillow speaker for music or other masking sound during the night may be necessary in severe cases. Sedation may be used sparingly. Difficult cases may require the close cooperation of an otolaryngologist, internist, neurologist, and psychiatrist.

Fowler EP: Subjective head noises (tinnitus aurium)—genesis and differential diagnostic significance: A few facts and several speculations. Laryngoscope 75:1610, 1965.
Parkin JL: Tinnitus evaluation. Am Family Physician 8:151, 1973.

3. ACUTE NONSUPPURATIVE LABYRINTHITIS

Acute inflammation of the inner ear characteristically follows respiratory tract infections and is manifested by intense vertigo, usually with marked tinnitus, a staggering gait, and nystagmus. Hearing loss is often not present.

Bed rest, preferably in a darkened room, is indicated until severe symptoms subside. Antibiotics are of little value unless there is associated infection of the middle ear or mastoid bone. Antihistamine drugs (as for motion sickness) may be of value. Sedation is generally helpful. Give phenobarbital, 15–60 mg 3–4 times daily. Chlorpromazine hydrochloride (Thorazine), 50 mg IM (or other phenothiazine derivative), is useful in the acute early phase.

Attacks of labyrinthitis may last for several days. Recovery is usually complete.

Sheehy JL: The dizzy patient. Arch Otolaryng 86:18, 1967.

Smith JL: Evaluation of the dizzy patient. Eye Ear Nose Throat Month 45:58, 1966.
Symposium on vertigo. Arch Otolaryng 85:497, 1967.

4. ACUTE SUPPURATIVE LABYRINTHITIS

Acute suppurative labyrinthitis is an infection of the intralabyrinthine structures. It may occur following acute otitis media and mastoiditis, acute exacerbations of chronic otitis media and mastoiditis, or meningitis unrelated to ear diseases. There is usually total destruction of labyrinthine function in the affected area and complete unilateral deafness.

Antibiotics and surgical drainage are indicated.

5. CHRONIC LABYRINTHITIS

Chronic labyrinthitis is secondary to erosion of the bony labyrinthine capsule (usually the lateral semicircular canal) by cholesteatoma. The patient has chronic episodes of vertigo, and attacks of vertigo can be reproduced by increasing the air pressure in the ear canal with a pneumatic otoscope (positive fistula test).

Mastoidectomy and removal of the cholesteatoma are required.

DISEASES OF THE NOSE

NASAL VESTIBULITIS

Inflammation of the nasal vestibule may occur as a dermatitis of the skin of the nose, often as a result of irritation from a nasal discharge; as a fissure resulting from chronic dermatitis or the trauma of picking or wiping the nose; or as a furuncle, usually after pulling hairs from the nose. Symptoms vary from scaling and weeping to edema, hyperemia, intense pain, and abscess formation. Fissures usually occur at the junction of the columella with the ala or with the floor of the nose. Careful cleansing of nasal discharge, avoidance of pulling nasal hairs, and protection with petrolatum or boric acid ointment may prevent these problems and the grave complications of cavernous sinus thrombosis.

The application of soothing, protective, and antimicrobial ointments (eg, 5% ammoniated mercury, 3% iodochlorhydroxyquin cream, neomycin, polymyxin, or bacitracin ointments) several times daily for several days after symptoms disappear is usually adequate treatment. For more severe infections, systemic antibiotics, local heat, and general supportive measures may be necessary.

NASAL SEPTAL HEMATOMA & ABSCESS

Septal hematoma occurs following trauma to the nose. The swollen septum produces nasal obstruction and frontal headache. Septal abscess usually is the result of an infected septal hematoma. It may occur following a furuncle in the vestibule, and produces nasal obstruction, headache, fever, malaise, pain in the nose, and tenderness over the nasal dorsum.

Septal hematoma may be treated conservatively by observation for possible infection; it should resolve in 4–6 weeks. It may also be relieved by aspiration with a large-bore needle or by incision and drainage, in both cases taking extreme precautions to prevent infection.

Septal abscess must be drained by wide incision of one side of the septum and suction. Necrotic pieces of cartilage may be cautiously removed. The incision must be wide enough to prevent early closure or must be spread open daily. Nasal packing may be necessary to control bleeding. Systemic antibiotic therapy is required.

Destruction of cartilage causes saddle deformity.

Fearon B, McKendry JB, Parker J: Abscess of the nasal septum in children. Arch Otolaryng 74:408, 1961.

"COMMON RESPIRATORY DISEASE"
(Common Cold, Grippe, Acute Bronchitis, Tracheobronchitis)

This group of diseases includes the numerous self-limited, usually viral infections of the upper respiratory tract. Children 1–5 years old are most susceptible, and adults from 25–35 next most susceptible. The incidence is lowest during the summer months. Exposure to cold, chilling, and dampness are probably of little etiologic significance.

Known agents which may cause this syndrome include the rhinoviruses (30 different serologic types), adenovirus, echoviruses, coxsackievirus, influenza viruses, parainfluenza viruses, and mycoplasmal organisms. This great diversity probably explains the frequent recurrence of "colds" in many individuals.

Clinical Findings

A. Symptoms and Signs: The patient complains of malaise, "feverishness" with usually little or no fever, and headache. Nasal discomfort (burning, fullness, itching) is a prominent feature, with watery discharge and sneezing followed shortly by mucoid to purulent discharge and nasal obstruction. Throat symptoms include "dryness," mild to moderate "soreness" rather than actual pain, hoarseness, and "tickling." Cough with scanty sputum and substernal aching may occur. Serious obstruction may occur in infants and young children or in adults with underlying bronchopulmonary disease (eg, emphysema).

The nasal mucosa is reddened and edematous. The external nares are red. The pharynx and tonsils usually show mild to moderate injection without edema or exudate. Cases of pharyngitis with considerable injection and exudate which fail to yield beta-hemolytic streptococci on repeated culture should probably be included in this group.

Cervical lymph nodes may be enlarged and slightly tender. Herpes labialis is common.

B. Laboratory Findings: The white count may be slightly elevated, but in most cases this is due to secondary bacterial infection.

Differential Diagnosis

Many specific infectious diseases present initial manifestations indistinguishable from those of common respiratory disease. Vigilance is required to avoid diagnostic errors of omission (eg, meningococcal infection, diphtheria).

Influenza is recognized by its epidemic occurrence and by serologic confirmation.

Exanthematous diseases (especially measles and chickenpox) may simulate common respiratory disease in their preeruptive phase.

In the initial phase, beta-hemolytic streptococcal pharyngitis may be clinically indistinguishable from acute nonstreptococcal exudative pharyngitis. Cultures make the diagnosis.

Complications

Complications result from secondary bacterial infections, often aided by the obstruction of respiration passages (eg, sinus ostia, bronchioles). They include purulent sinusitis, otitis media, bacterial pneumonia, and tonsillitis.

Treatment

No specific treatment is available. Antibiotics are used only to prevent secondary infection in patients with low pulmonary and cardiac reserves and to treat complicating secondary infections.

General measures consist of rest, sufficient fluids to prevent dehydration, and a light, palatable, well balanced diet. Aspirin may be given for headache, sore throat, muscle soreness, and fever. Vasoconstrictors give temporary relief of nasal obstruction and rhinorrhea. Phenylephrine hydrochloride (Neo-Synephrine), 0.25%, several drops in each nostril every 2–3 hours; or phenylpropanolamine hydrochloride (Propadrine), 25–50 mg every 4–6 hours, is satisfactory for this purpose. Antihistamines may relieve the early symptoms of mucous membrane inflammation. Cough may be reduced by inhaling steam or with codeine phosphate, 8–15 mg orally every 2–4 hours. Application of heat to the area of the sinuses may relieve nasal obstruction.

The use of large doses of vitamin C (1 gm or more daily), although advocated by some, remains of unproved value.

Johnson HE & others: Viral infections and the common cold (panel discussion). Dis Chest 45:46, 1964.

Tyrrell DAJ: *Common Colds and Related Diseases*. Williams & Wilkins, 1966.

Vitamin C: Were the trials well controlled and are large doses safe? Med Lett Drugs Ther 13:46, 1971.

Wilson CWM, Loh HS: Common cold and vitamin C. Lancet 1:638, 1973.

ALLERGIC RHINITIS
(Hay Fever)

Essentials of Diagnosis

- Watery nasal discharge, sneezing, itching eyes and nose.
- Pale, boggy mucous membranes.
- Eosinophilia of nasal secretions and blood.

General Considerations

See discussion under Bronchial Asthma.

Clinical Findings

A. Symptoms and Signs: The principal symptoms are nasal congestion, a profuse, watery nasal discharge, itching of the nasal mucosa leading to paroxysms of violent sneezing, conjunctival itching and burning, and lacrimation. The nasal mucosa are pale blue and boggy. Polyps may be present. The conjunctivas are often reddened and swollen.

B. Laboratory Findings: A smear of the nasal secretions reveals increased numbers of eosinophils. (In infections, neutrophils predominate.) The peripheral blood may reveal mild (5–10%) or occasionally marked (30–40%) eosinophilia, even between clinical episodes.

Skin tests may be of aid in the detection of the allergens but must be correlated with the clinical picture to determine their significance.

Differential Diagnosis

A history of an allergy aids in distinguishing allergic rhinitis from the common upper respiratory infections; hay fever should be suspected in young children as the real cause of repeated "colds."

Treatment

A. Specific Measures: There is no true specific treatment. Hyposensitization or desensitization is sometimes beneficial and consists of administering the allergen (usually pollen) in gradually increasing doses to induce an "immunity." For best results, therapy should be started 3–6 months before the beginning of the hay fever season.

B. General Measures:

1. Antihistamines give relief in 60–80% of patients, but their effectiveness often wanes as the season continues.

2. Sympathomimetic drugs such as ephedrine and phenylpropanolamine are effective by themselves or in combination with the antihistamines.

3. Sedation may be of value for tense or nervous patients.

4. The corticosteroids are useful in severe hay fever which cannot be controlled by the agents mentioned above. Prednisone, 20–40 mg by mouth daily in divided doses, may be used for several days until symptoms are controlled. Dosage should then be reduced gradually (over a period of 7–10 days) to the smallest daily dose that will suppress symptoms. Discontinue steroid therapy as soon as possible.

5. Maintenance of an allergen-free atmosphere and the use of dust-proof respirator masks and room air filters are often of value during the pollen season if the patient must remain in the area. When dust is the offending agent, prepare a dust-free bedroom as follows: Cover the mattress and pillow with an air-tight nonantigenic material (plastic or sheet rubber). Remove all carpets, drapes, bedspreads, and other lint-producing materials, and all ornate furniture or other objects which are not easily dusted. Blankets should be of synthetic material if possible.

Household pets must be considered possible sources of allergens.

Prognosis

Allergic rhinitis is a self-limited though recurrent disorder with mild morbidity and no mortality.

Criep LH: Nasal allergy: An interdisciplinary problem. Eye Ear Nose Throat Month 44:70, 1965.

Stroh JE: Allergic rhinitis. Postgrad Med 45:151, 1969.

Williams RI: Modern concepts in clinical management of allergy in otolaryngology. Laryngoscope 76:1389, 1966.

SINUS INFECTION

Essentials of Diagnosis

Acute:

- History of acute upper respiratory infection, dental infection, or nasal allergy.
- Pain, tenderness, redness, swelling over the involved sinus.
- Nasal congestion and purulent nasal discharge.
- Clouding of sinuses on x-ray or transillumination.
- Fever, chills, malaise, headache.
- Teeth hurt or feel "long" (maxillary sinusitis), or swelling occurs near the nasal canthus of eye (ethmoid sinusitis).

Chronic:

- Nasal obstruction.
- Postnasal discharge.
- Clouding of sinus on x-ray or transillumination.
- Pain is not a common finding.

General Considerations

Acute sinus infection usually follows an acute upper respiratory infection, swimming or diving, dental abscess or extractions, or nasal allergies, or occurs as an exacerbation of a chronic sinus infection. Isolated acute frontal sinus infection is rare. Acute ethmoiditis is most common in infants and children. Chronic pyogenic infections of single sinuses do occur, but this is less common than pansinusitis.

Clinical Findings

A. Symptoms and Signs:

1. Acute sinusitis–The symptoms resemble those of acute rhinitis but are more severe. There is headache and facial pain, tenderness and swelling with nasal obstruction, and a purulent nasal and postnasal discharge, sometimes causing sore throat and cough. The headache typically is worse during the day and subsides in the evening. Acute maxillary sinusitis may cause pain in the teeth and a feeling of "long teeth." Acute ethmoiditis causes headache between and behind the eyes, and eye motion increases the pain. Tenderness medially in the roof of the orbit occurs with frontal sinusitis. Fever and systemic symptoms vary with the severity of the infection.

2. Chronic sinusitis–Chronic sinus infection may produce no symptoms. A mild postnasal discharge and a musty odor or nonproductive cough may be the only symptoms. Nasal obstruction and sometimes profuse purulent nasal and postnasal discharge may also occur.

B. Laboratory Findings: In acute sinusitis the white count may be elevated, and culture of nasal discharge usually shows the pyogenic organisms.

C. Other Examinations: X-ray and transillumination show clouding of the involved sinuses.

Differential Diagnosis

Acute dental infection usually produces greater facial swelling lower in the face with more marked tenderness of the involved tooth than does maxillary sinusitis. The more localized swelling and tenderness and greater involvement of the eyelids with absence of nasal discharge distinguishes an infected tear sac from ethmoiditis. X-ray examination gives more definite evidence of sinus involvement.

An isolated chronic maxillary sinusitis without obvious underlying cause suggests dental disease or neoplasm.

Complications

Chronic sinusitis is the commonest complication of acute sinusitis. Orbital cellulitis and abscess may follow ethmoiditis or frontal sinusitis. Frontal sinusitis may be complicated by meningitis or extradural, subdural, or brain abscess. Osteomyelitis of the facial or frontal bones may occur.

Treatment

A. Acute Sinusitis: Place the patient at bed rest and give sedatives, analgesics, a light diet, and fluids. Oral nasal decongestants (eg, phenylpropanolamine,

25–50 mg 3 times daily) and systemic antibiotics frequently produce prompt resolution of the infection. Broad-spectrum antibiotics appear to be most beneficial, but nearly all antibiotics have been effective.

Local heat, topical nasal decongestants (eg, 0.25% phenylephrine), and gentle spot suctioning of the nasal discharge are helpful.

The sinuses must not be manipulated during the acute infection. Antrum irrigation is of value after the acute inflammation has subsided. Acute frontal sinusitis is treated medically and conservatively; cannulation is rarely warranted. Trephining of the sinus floor may occasionally be indicated in acute fulminating infections. Acute ethmoid infections respond to medical management; if external fluctuation develops incision and drainage is indicated.

B. Chronic Sinusitis: When the infecting organism has been identified the suitable antibiotic is given systemically. Irrigation of the antra or Proetz displacement may help drainage. Conservative surgery to promote drainage is of value (removal of polyps, submucous resection of an obstructing septum, intranasal antrotomy). If conservative treatment is not effective, more radical sinus surgery by the external approach may be considered.

C. Treatment of Complications:

1. Osteomyelitis, meningitis, abscess–Give supportive measures and antibiotics. Remove necrotic bone and drain abscesses as required.

2. Orbital fistulas–Treat the underlying sinus disease and close the tract surgically.

3. Oroantral fistula–Remove underlying sinus infection by the Caldwell-Luc operation and close the tract.

4. Mucoceles (mucopyoceles)–Surgical excision.

Prognosis

Acute infections usually respond to medical management and irrigation.

Chronic infections often require surgical correction. Chronic frontal sinusitis is especially likely to persist or recur.

Axelsson A & others: Treatment of acute maxillary sinusitis. Ann Otol Rhin Laryng 82:186, 1973.

Axelsson A & others: Treatment of acute maxillary sinusitis. Acta oto-laryng 70:71, 1970.

Bryant FL: Conservative surgery for chronic maxillary sinusitis. Laryngoscope 77:575, 1967.

Davison FW: Chronic sinus disease: Differential diagnosis. Laryngoscope 78:1738, 1968.

Harner SG, Newell RC: Treatment of frontal osteomyelitis. Laryngoscope 79:1281, 1969.

Haynes RE, Cramblett HG: Acute ethmoiditis. Am J Dis Child 114:261, 1967.

McCabe BF: "I've got sinus." GP 32:135, Sept 1965.

Wassermann D: Acute paranasal sinusitis and cavernous sinus thrombosis. Arch Otolaryng 86:205, 1967.

NASAL TUMORS

Benign Tumors

Angioma, fibroma, papilloma, chondroma, and osteoma are the most common types of benign neoplasms of the nose and sinuses. Nasal tumors produce obstruction and nasal discharge when they become large enough. Severe epistaxis occurs with angioma. Secondary infection may occur. Pressure atrophy of surrounding structures, widening of the nasal bridge, and displacement of the eye may occur. X-rays and biopsy usually establish the diagnosis.

Treatment consists of complete removal with permanent intranasal drainage of involved sinuses.

Malignant Tumors

Many nasal malignancies originate in the sinuses and extend into the nose. Sarcoma and carcinoma occur. Symptoms and signs may not occur until late; the most common are obstruction, discharge, epistaxis, pain, swelling of the face, and diplopia. X-ray shows clouding of the sinuses that may suggest infection; secondary infection is frequently present. Bony destruction may show on x-rays. Cytologic smears of antrum irrigation fluid and "cell buttons" may rarely show malignant cells. Biopsy is diagnostic.

Surgical excision is usually the treatment of choice. Some cases may be treated by biopsy followed by x-ray therapy or, occasionally, surgery plus irradiation or cautery.

Chiang T-C, Griem ML: Nasopharyngeal cancer. S Clin North America 53:121, 1973.

Harrison DFN: Management of malignant tumors affecting maxillary and ethmoidal sinuses. J Laryng 87:749, 1973.

Matz GJ, Conner JH: Nasopharyngeal cancer. Laryngoscope 78:763, 1968.

Oliver P: Cancer of the nose and paranasal sinuses. S Clin North America 47:595, 1967.

EPISTAXIS
(Nosebleed)

The most common sites of nasal bleeding are the mucosal vessels over the cartilaginous nasal septum (Kiesselbach's area or Little's area) and the anterior tip of the inferior turbinate. Bleeding is usually due to external trauma to the nose, nasal infection (especially with vigorous nose-blowing), or drying of the nasal mucosa when humidity is low. Minor trauma such as nose-picking may lead to ulcerations of the nasal septum and subsequent hemorrhage. Up to 5% of nosebleeds originate posteriorly in the nose where the bleeding site cannot be seen; these can cause great problems in management.

Nosebleed may escape diagnosis if the blood drains into the pharynx and is swallowed. In these cases bloody or "coffee-ground" vomitus may be the first clue.

Underlying causes of nosebleed such as blood dyscrasias, hypertension, hemorrhagic disease, nasal tumors, and certain infectious diseases (measles or rheumatic fever) must be considered in any case of recurrent or profuse nosebleed without obvious cause.

Treatment

A. Specific Measures: Treatment of the underlying disease depends upon an adequate examination to detect cardiovascular, renal, or liver disease, blood dyscrasias, coagulation defects, or other systemic disorders contributing to the nosebleed. Give transfusions as necessary if blood loss is excessive.

B. Local Measures: Have the patient sit up and forward with his head tipped downward to prevent swallowing and aspiration of blood. Good illumination (with a head mirror or headlight) is essential to proper examination and treatment.

1. Anterior epistaxis—Pressure over the area (pinching the nose) for 5 minutes is often sufficient to stop bleeding. This may be combined with packing the bleeding nostril with a pledget of cotton moistened with hydrogen peroxide, 0.25% phenylephrine, or 1:1000 epinephrine solution.

After active bleeding has stopped (or if pressure fails to stop bleeding), a cotton pledget moistened with a topical anesthetic (1% tetracaine or 5% cocaine) applied to the bleeding area will provide anesthesia for cauterization with a chromic acid bead, trichloroacetic acid, or an electrocautery. After cauterization, lubrication with petrolatum helps prevent crusting. A second cauterization is infrequently necessary.

If the source of bleeding is not accessible to cauterization (beneath the inferior turbinate, behind septal spurs, or high in the vault) or is not controlled by cauterization, the nasal cavity must be packed. After maximum shrinkage of the mucosa has been achieved with a suitable decongestant (0.25% phenylephrine or 2% ephedrine) and topical anesthesia, the nasal cavity can be tightly packed with half-inch gauze lubricated with petrolatum or cod liver oil. Pack the gauze into the nose in layers, starting either in the vault or on the floor of the nasal cavity. The packing may be left in place as long as 5—6 days if the patient is given adequate analgesics for pain and antibiotic medication to help prevent suppurative otitis media and sinusitis.

2. Posterior epistaxis—Posterior bleeding can sometimes be controlled only by means of a posterior nasal pack. This accomplishes 2 things: it compresses and controls bleeding sites in the nasopharynx or posterior choana, and it provides a "backstop" for very firm anterior packing that might otherwise be dislodged into the pharynx.

The postnasal pack is prepared as follows: (1) Sew 3 strings (No. 1 braided silk) through and through the center of a rolled 4 × 4 gauze sponge. (2) Pass a soft rubber catheter through the bleeding nostril into the pharynx and out through the mouth. (3) Attach 2 of the strings to the catheter tip and draw them through the mouth and out through the bleeding nostril. (4) Guide the gauze pack with a finger into the nasopharynx and posterior choana, taking care not to roll the uvula upward beneath the pack. (5) Anchor the 2 strings over a gauze bolster at the anterior nares. (6) Allow the third string to remain in the mouth and tape it to the face, or cut it about 4 inches long and allow it to dangle in the pharynx; it is used later to remove the pack.

The pack should not be left in place more than 4 days. The patient's ears should be examined daily for evidence of acute otitis media. Bleeding may recur when the pack is removed, or may even continue with the packing in place. If this occurs, the pack must usually be changed or reinserted under general anesthesia.

If the bleeding persists beneath or behind an inaccessible nasal septal spur, submucous resection of the septum may be necessary to relieve traction on the mucosal vessels and to permit more effective packing.

If bleeding persists from a site low in the nasal cavity, external carotid artery ligation in the neck or internal maxillary artery ligation in the pterygomaxillary fossa must be considered. Uncontrolled bleeding from high in the vault of the nose may necessitate ligation of the anterior or posterior ethmoidal artery (or both) as it passes from the orbit into the ethmoidal labyrinth.

Prognosis

Most anterior nosebleeds are easily treated as an office procedure; complicated nosebleed or posterior nosebleed may require hospitalization for 2–3 weeks.

Severe nosebleed in cirrhotics or patients with borderline coronary arterial insufficiency may produce severe complications.

Call WH: Control of epistaxis. S Clin North America 49:1235, 1969.
McDevitt TJ, Goh AS, Acquarelli MJ: Epistaxis: Management and prevention. Laryngoscope 77:1109, 1967.
Middleton P: Surgery for epistaxis. Laryngoscope 77:1011, 1967.
Rosnagle RS & others: Specific vessel ligation for epistaxis. Laryngoscope 83:517, 1973.

DISEASES OF THE PHARYNX

SIMPLE PHARYNGITIS

Acute simple (catarrhal) pharyngitis is an acute inflammation of the mucosa of the pharynx which to some extent involves the lymphatic structures also. It usually occurs as part of an upper respiratory tract disorder which may also affect the nose, sinuses, larynx, and trachea. The most common causes are bacterial or viral infection; rarely, it is due to inhalation of irritant gases or ingestion of irritant liquids. Pharyngitis may occur as part of the syndrome of an acute specific infection (eg, measles, scarlet fever, whooping cough).

The inflammation may be diffuse or localized (lateral pharyngitis). Drying of the mucosa occurs in pharyngitis sicca.

In acute pharyngitis the throat is dry and sore. Systemic symptoms are fever and malaise. The pharyngeal mucosa is red and slightly swollen, with thick, sticky mucus. The disease lasts only a few days.

Chronic pharyngitis may produce few symptoms, eg, throat dryness with thick mucus and cough; or recurrent acute episodes of more severe throat pain, dull hyperemia and mild swelling of the mucosa (especially the tonsil pillars), and thick tenacious mucus often in the hypopharynx.

The treatment of acute pharyngitis is symptomatic: rest, light diet, analgesics, and warm, nonirritating gargles or throat irrigations. Antibiotics may be used for initial or complicating bacterial infection.

Chronic pharyngitis is treated by removing underlying causes such as infections of the nose, sinuses, or tonsils and by restricting irritants such as alcohol, spicy foods, and tobacco. Local removal of the tenacious secretion with suction or saline irrigation and application of 2% silver nitrate are helpful.

ACUTE TONSILLITIS

Acute tonsillitis is nearly always a bacterial infection, often due to streptococci. It is a contagious airborne or food-borne infection which can occur in any age group but is more common in children. Associated adenoidal infection in children is usual.

The onset is sudden, with sore throat, fever, chills, headache, anorexia, and malaise. The tonsils are swollen and red; the tonsillar pillars and pharynx are red, and pus or exudate is present on the tonsils or in the crypts. The cervical lymph nodes frequently are tender and enlarged. The white count may be elevated, and throat cultures will show the infecting organism.

Other causes of sore throat and fever which must be distinguished from acute tonsillitis include simple pharyngitis, infectious mononucleosis, Vincent's angina, diphtheria, agranulocytosis, and mycotic infections. Smear and culture from the throat identify the bacterial and mycotic infections. The white count helps distinguish viral infections and blood dyscrasias. The white count and heterophil antibody titer will make the diagnosis of infectious mononucleosis.

The complications of local extension are chronic tonsillitis, acute otitis media, acute rhinitis and sinusitis, peritonsillar abscess or other deep neck abscess, and cervical lymph node abscess. Nephritis, osteomyelitis, rheumatic fever, or pneumonia may follow streptococcal tonsillitis.

Treatment consists of bed rest, fluids, a light diet, analgesics, and antibiotics as required. Local relief of pain may be obtained with frequent gargles or throat irrigations using hot, nonirritating solutions (eg, saline, 30% glucose, aspirin).

Spontaneous resolution usually occurs after 5–7 days. Vigorous treatment may shorten the course, prevents many complications, and makes the patient more comfortable.

Gau DW & others: Streptococcic tonsillitis in general practice: Comparison of cephalexin and penicillin therapy. Practitioner 208:276, 1972.
Malcomson KG: Tonsillitis: Acute and chronic. Practitioner 199:777, 1967.

CHRONIC TONSILLITIS

Chronic tonsillitis usually results from repeated or unresolved acute infection. It is manifested by persistent dull hyperemia. Mild edema and scarring of the tonsils and tonsillar pillars may occur, and the crypts may contain abnormal secretions. Other symptoms and signs may range from a mild scratching sensation in the throat to cough, fetid breath, and a pharyngeal exudate. An enlarged cervical lymph node is common. The size of the tonsils is of little significance in determining the presence of chronic infection. Chronic infection may predispose to recurrent acute infections.

The treatment of significant chronic tonsillar infection is surgical excision (see below). Intercurrent acute infections and chronic infections in people who are poor operative risks (because of advanced age or severe systemic or hemorrhagic diseases) are treated medically as outlined above for acute infections. Chronic infection can rarely be eradicated by conservative treatment.

Adenotonsillectomy (T & A)

The value of adenotonsillectomy, the indications for and the contraindications to the operation, and the optimal time for the operation when it is indicated have been the subject of much controversy. Most surgeons agree that there are occasions when the operation is of definite benefit to the patient and that there are circumstances in which it is definitely contraindicated. Even when a strong indication for surgery is present, however, the decision to operate must not be made until all pertinent restraining factors (eg, medical, psychologic, social) have been evaluated.

Surgery is contraindicated during episodes of acute tonsillar infection.

A. Strong Indications: Whenever the infected or hypertrophied tonsils and adenoid are almost certainly the underlying or only cause of the disease, or when the tonsils are malignant.

1. Recurrent acute infection or chronic infection of tonsils and adenoid.

2. Recurrent acute ear infections.

3. Peritonsillar abscess.

B. Equivocal Indications: When the infected or hypertrophied tonsils are likely to be the cause of the disease or are contributing to or aggravating the disease: (Other possible contributing factors must first be investigated and ruled out or treated.)

1. Snoring and mouth breathing.

2. Large tonsils.

3. Poor eating habits in a frail, often anemic child.

4. Allergic rhinitis and asthma.

5. Systemic disease, eg, nephritis, rheumatic or congenital heart disease, rheumatic fever (considered a strong indication by some, even in the absence of local disease).

6. Frequent upper respiratory tract infections.

C. Relative Contraindications: When the operation may do more harm than good unless special precautions are taken:

1. Cleft palate—Further speech impairment can occur following adenotonsillectomy. The lateral adenoidal masses only should be removed.

2. The mere presence of tonsils and adenoid.

3. Systemic disease, eg, uncontrolled diabetes, tuberculosis, heart disease.

4. Intercurrent infection.

5. Hemorrhagic disease (eg, hemophilia).

D. Absolute Contraindications: When the operation will certainly do more harm than good.

Boyle WF: Adenotonsillectomy in children: Modern indications and preparation. Postgrad Med 40:489, 1966.
Fox JM: Indications for tonsillectomy and adenoidectomy. Postgrad Med 48:96, 1970.
Paradise JL: Why T & A remains moot. Pediatrics 49:648, 1972.
Poydhouse N: A controlled study of adenotonsillectomy. Arch Otol 92:611, 1970.

PERITONSILLAR ABSCESS
(Quinsy)

Peritonsillar abscess is a complication of acute tonsillitis which occurs when the infection spreads to the potential peritonsillar space deep to the tonsil between the tonsillar capsule and the constrictor pharyngis muscle. Mixed pyogenic organisms (streptococci, staphylococci, pneumococci) are usually obtained upon culture. The sore throat of tonsillitis suddenly becomes more severe on one side when the infection breaks through the tonsillar capsule; dysphagia increases, trismus may be present, and one-sided swelling pushes the tonsil and tonsillar pillar toward or across the midline. The swelling extends to the soft palate, and the uvula is displaced. Fluctuation develops between the 3rd and 5th days.

Symptomatic care and antibiotic therapy are indicated. After the abscess becomes fluctuant, it must be incised and drained. The walls of the abscess should be spread daily to prevent re-formation of the abscess. After the infection subsides, tonsillectomy should be done to prevent recurrences.

Hora JF: Deep-neck infections. Arch Otolaryng 77:129, 1963.

LUDWIG'S ANGINA
(Cellulitis of the Floor of the Mouth)

Ludwig's angina is a severe pyogenic infection of the sublingual and submaxillary spaces of the floor of the mouth and the anterior neck. A rapidly spreading diffuse cellulitis or abscess formation pushes the tongue upward against the roof of the mouth, limiting its motion and causing pain. The airway may become obstructed, or the infection may spread downward in the neck.

Supportive treatment and large doses of antibiotics are necessary. If abscess occurs, external incision and drainage should be performed. Local anesthesia avoids the danger of immediate obstruction of the airway, which may occur if general anesthesia is used. Because of the diffuse nature of the infection, large quantities of free pus are seldom obtained. Incision must be adequate and the fascial spaces above and below the hyoglossus muscle must be opened by blunt dissection. A tracheostomy may be necessary.

RETROPHARYNGEAL ABSCESS

Retropharyngeal abscess is a pyogenic infection which occurs most often in infants and children. Suppuration occurs in the fascial space between the posterior pharyngeal wall and the prevertebral fascia as a result of suppurative lymph node infection, usually following tonsillar, nasal, or sinus infection. The symptoms are difficulty in swallowing and breathing, and fever. The posterior pharyngeal wall is tender and swollen.

Early treatment (antibiotics, hydration) may produce resolution. If fluctuation occurs incision and drainage are required, with the patient in full Trendelenburg position, adequate lighting, and suction equipment at hand. General anesthesia is avoided because of the danger of laryngeal obstruction and aspiration. Tracheostomy may be necessary.

Hora JF: Deep-neck infections. Arch Otolaryng 77:129, 1963.

PARAPHARYNGEAL ABSCESS

Parapharyngeal abscess is a pyogenic infection which occurs as a complication of acute tonsillitis,

peritonsillar abscess, dental infection, or acute pharyngitis. It is localized in the fascial space outside the constrictor pharyngis muscle and deep to the investing cervical fascia, in close relationship to the carotid sheath and the stylopharyngeus and stylohyoid muscles. Infection can spread along the carotid sheath into the mediastinum. There are signs and symptoms of sepsis, bulging of the lateral pharyngeal wall, and trismus. The veins of the neck and scalp may be distended as a consequence of pressure upon the jugular vein. Brawny swelling and redness may develop later in the neck below the angle of the mandible.

Early treatment consists of hydration and antibiotics in large doses. Intraoral incision and drainage should be done only by a surgeon familiar with this area because of the danger of hemorrhage from large blood vessels. External incision and drainage at the angle of the jaw and upper neck can be done if pus is sought deep in the neck by blunt dissection.

Caution is required in giving general anesthesia because of the hazard of airway obstruction. Local anesthesia or a tracheostomy for general anesthesia should be considered.

Alexander DW, Leonard JR, Trail ML: Vascular complications of deep neck abscesses: A report of four cases. Otolaryngology 78:361, 1968.

DISEASES OF THE LARYNX

ACUTE LARYNGITIS

Acute inflammation of the laryngeal mucosa due to bacterial or viral infection may occur singly or in association with acute rhinitis, pharyngitis, or tracheitis. It may also occur with influenza, measles, or diphtheria, or as a result of inhalation of irritants. Hoarseness is the chief symptom. Pain and cough are often present. Stridor and dyspnea may occur if edema is marked. Examination of the larynx shows redness of the mucosa and edema with or without exudate. The acute inflammation may extend into the bronchi and lungs, and slight hemoptysis may occur if coughing ruptures small blood vessels.

Treatment consists of voice rest, decreased smoking, control of underlying nasal, sinus, or throat infections, and control of cough. Steam inhalations and local cold or heat to the neck may provide relief. Systemic antibiotics are helpful in bacterial infections. If marked edema produces dyspnea and stridor, parenteral steroids may decrease the edema sufficiently so that tracheostomy can be withheld.

Hawkins DB & others: Acute epiglottiditis in adults. Laryngoscope 83:1211, 1973.
Ross JA: Special problems in acute laryngotracheobronchitis.

Laryngoscope 79:1218, 1969.

Tos M: Nasotracheal intubation in acute epiglottitis. Arch Otol 97:373, 1973.

CHRONIC LARYNGITIS

Chronic inflammation of the laryngeal mucosa may be due to many causes, including repeated acute laryngitis, chronic vocal abuse, chronic inhalation of irritants (including smoking), chronic sinus and throat infection, syphilis and tuberculosis (rare today), allergy, and hypometabolic states. Chronic hoarseness is the chief symptom. Cough, expectoration of tenacious secretions, and a feeling of dryness in the throat are often present. Examination shows signs of chronic inflammation; a thickened, dull, edematous mucosa of the vocal cords; and polypoid changes, whitish plaques, and thickened secretions. Ulceration is occasionally seen.

Chest x-ray and other tests for signs of tuberculosis, serologic tests for syphilis, and biopsy to rule out carcinoma may be required.

Treatment consists of correcting the underlying cause, if any; antibiotics for sinus and throat infections; antiallergenic measures when indicated; decreased smoking, and voice rest.

Norris CM: Treatment of laryngitis. Mod Treat 2:1208, 1965.

TUMORS OF THE LARYNX

Essentials of Diagnosis

- Hoarseness is the principal symptom.
- Respiratory obstruction.
- Sore throat, "sticking" sensation in throat, pain referred to the ear.
- Cough or hemoptysis.
- Dysphagia.

General Considerations

Tumors of the larynx may be benign or malignant. Both produce similar symptoms and may be considered together. The symptoms depend upon the size and location of the tumor.

Benign laryngeal tumors may be neoplastic (eg, papilloma, fibroma), may be due to allergy or metabolic disturbance (polyps), or may be due to extrinsic or intrinsic trauma (singer's nodules, intubation granuloma). Ninety-five percent of malignant laryngeal tumors are squamous cell carcinomas, but sarcoma, adenocarcinoma, and others occur.

Clinical Findings

Hoarseness is the earliest and principal manifestation of vocal cord tumor. As the tumor enlarges, stridor and dyspnea may occur, usually late. With tumors elsewhere in the larynx (false cord, epiglottis, arytenoepiglottic fold, piriform sinus), voice change may be a late symptom and minor throat discomfort (sometimes referred to the ear), dysphagia, or mild cough may be the only early symptoms. Laryngeal examination usually shows a mass or ulceration at the tumor site. Submucosal tumors may be manifested only as a fullness or swelling of the affected area. Biopsy examination establishes the diagnosis.

Differential Diagnosis

Tumors of the larynx must be distinguished from chronic laryngitis, tuberculosis, syphilis, contact ulcer, granulomas, and laryngeal paralysis. Laryngeal symptoms lasting longer than 2–3 weeks must be investigated. Direct or indirect laryngoscopy is often diagnostic. Chest x-ray and other tests for tuberculosis, serologic tests for syphilis, laryngeal biopsy, and bacteriologic cultures usually establish a firm diagnosis.

Treatment & Prognosis

Almost all of the technics involved in intralaryngeal manipulation and surgery require the skills of an otolaryngologist.

Small, asymptomatic benign tumors may require no treatment other than diagnosis to rule out malignancy. Vocal cord polyps or ulcers due to metabolic disturbances (allergy or hypothyroidism) or to vocal misuse or other trauma may improve when the underlying problem is treated. Small benign tumors of the vocal cord producing hoarseness may be locally excised under direct or indirect laryngoscopy. Direct laryngoscopy with use of the operating microscope with microlaryngeal instruments has made possible greater precision in laryngeal surgery. Larger benign tumors—especially papillomas, which have a great tendency to recur—may require laryngotomy for adequate excision.

Malignant tumors are treated by external irradiation or surgical excision. Irradiation is suitable for superficial malignancies confined to the vocal cord which show no evidence of invasion of muscle or cartilage. More extensive tumors require surgical excision and often en bloc neck node dissection. At times, combined planned preoperative irradiation followed by surgical excision can provide better control of malignancy.

Goldman JL & others: Combined therapy for cancer of the laryngopharynx. Arch Otol 92:221, 1970.

Matz GJ, Marks JE, Lowry LD: Carcinoma of the larynx. S Clin North America 53:159, 1973.

Peres CA & others: Irradiation of early carcinoma of the larynx. Arch Otol 93:465, 1971.

Shaw HJ: Cancer of the larynx. Practitioner 199:785, 1967.

Work WP, Boyle WF: Cancer of the larynx. Laryngoscope 71:830, 1961.

TRACHEOSTOMY

There are 4 indications for tracheostomy: (1) respiratory obstruction at the level of the larynx or above; (2) inability to clear tracheobronchial secretions; (3) for administration of anesthesia; and (4) to place the larynx at rest.

The causes of airway obstruction at or above the larynx include infections (laryngotracheobronchitis, epiglottitis, and diphtheria), tumors, edema (allergic, infectious, post-irradiation), trauma, and foreign bodies. Upper airway obstruction produces suprasternal, intercostal, and epigastric retraction and signs of hypoxia, including restlessness, increasing pulse, and, as a late finding, cyanosis. Disorders which interfere with normal sphincter action of the larynx, permit aspiration of pharyngeal secretions, and prevent effective cough include loss of consciousness and organic muscular paresis due to poisoning, cerebrovascular accidents, postoperative state, poliomyelitis, and organic CNS disease. There are some surgical situations, especially in surgery of the head or neck, where an endotracheal tube cannot be introduced through the nose or mouth but can be introduced through a tracheostomy. Intralaryngeal disease rarely may require tracheostomy to place the larynx at rest.

Two kinds of tracheostomies are performed: emergency and elective. **Emergency tracheostomy** must be done immediately even if proper equipment and assistance is not available. In these circumstances, **cricothyrotomy** is a safe procedure which can be performed rapidly as follows: With a scissors or knife the skin is cut vertically over the cricothyroid membrane (the part of the airway nearest the skin), a transverse incision is made in this membrane, and the wound is spread with the knife handle or other dilator. It is essential to stay in the midline and to promptly replace this emergency airway with a proper tracheostomy. If a laryngoscope and endotracheal tube or a bronchoscope are available, the airway may be established with one of these devices and a deliberate tracheostomy then performed.

Elective tracheostomy is done under general or local anesthesia while the patient's airway is still adequate or has been reestablished with an endotracheal tube or bronchoscope. The precise surgical technic may vary, eg, with midline or horizontal incision, blunt or sharp dissection, retraction or division of the thyroid isthmus; but the principles are the same in all: (1) avoid trauma to the cricoid cartilage, (2) stay in the midline to avoid trauma to lateral neck structures, and (3) do not close the incision tightly, thus minimizing subcutaneous emphysema.

Post-tracheostomy care must include humidifying the inspired air to keep secretions loose and prevent the formation of mucus plugs and crusts, frequent cleaning (every 2–4 hours) of the inner tube, avoidance of heavy sedation, and constant attention during the first 24–48 hours. Uninterrupted observation may not be necessary with some adults, but with small children it is absolutely necessary that a nurse, hospital attendant, or member of the family be in constant attendance as long as the tracheostomy is maintained.

The use of cuffed tracheostomy tubes facilitates positive pressure assisted or controlled respiration. The cuff must be deflated intermittently because prolonged inflation may result in tracheal mucosal ulceration and granuloma formation or tracheal stenosis.

Beatrous WP: Tracheostomy (tracheotomy)—its expanded indications and its present status: Based on an analysis of 1,000 consecutive operations and a review of the recent literature. Laryngoscope 78:3, 1968.

Bryant LR, Trinkle JK, Dubilien L: Reappraisal of tracheal injury from cuffed tracheostomy tubes. JAMA 215:625, 1971.

Chew JY, Cantrell RW: Tracheostomy: Complications and their management. Arch Otol 96:538, 1972.

Taillens J-P: Modern indications for tracheotomy in cases of acute and chronic asphyxia. Advances Otol-Rhino-Laryng 15:1, 1968.

FOREIGN BODIES IN THE AIR & FOOD PASSAGES

Foreign bodies may lodge in the larynx, bronchi, or esophagus, usually while eating, following sudden inspiration caused by surprise, as a result of simple carelessness while holding something in the mouth, or while unconscious. Eighty percent of cases of inhaled or swallowed foreign bodies occur in children under 15 years of age. In adults most foreign bodies are large boluses of food or bones lodged in the esophagus as a result of hasty eating or full dentures which impair normal sensation in the mouth.

Esophageal foreign bodies are usually found at the thoracic inlet, less commonly at the cardia or midesophagus. If laryngeal foreign bodies completely block the airway, asphyxia is imminent. A foreign body small enough to pass the glottis will seldom lodge in the trachea but will be found in the bronchi. The relatively sharp angle of the left bronchus and the straight right bronchus cause most bronchial foreign bodies to be found in the right side. Nearly all foreign bodies that enter food or air passages through the mouth and do not enter the stomach can be removed by the same route.

Laryngeal Foreign Bodies

Laryngeal foreign bodies may produce hoarseness, stridor, cough, and gagging; may obstruct the airway partially or completely and cause dyspnea, stridor, or asphyxia; and may produce inflammatory symptoms of fever, pain, tenderness, and swelling. They can be removed with a grasping forceps through a direct laryngoscope under topical or general anesthesia. The patient should be in the Trendelenburg position to prevent the foreign body from entering the trachea or esophagus, and a bronchoscope and esophagoscope of proper size should be available in case this happens.

A small laryngeal foreign body may become lodged in the bronchi (see below).

Bronchial Foreign Bodies

Bronchial foreign bodies usually produce an initial episode of coughing followed by an asymptomatic ("silent") period varying from a few hours (some vegetable foreign bodies) to months or years (less irritating nonvegetable foreign bodies) before obstructive and inflammatory symptoms occur (cough, wheezing, atelectasis, and pulmonary infection). If the foreign body lodges in such a way as to create a valve effect, obstructive emphysema of a pulmonary segment or lobe may be present. Recurrent episodes of cough and pulmonary infection, especially if unilateral, are suggestive of foreign body. X-rays will show a foreign body if it is radiopaque. Nonradiopaque foreign bodies will be revealed on x-ray only by the signs of bronchial obstruction and infection. Vegetable foreign bodies produce earlier and more severe inflammatory symptoms than nonvegetable objects.

In the differential diagnosis it is necessary to consider pneumonia, bronchiectasis, lung abscess, and tuberculosis.

Bronchial foreign bodies are removed through a bronchoscope with suitable forceps by a skilled endoscopist. General anesthesia is usually employed. In the case of very small radiopaque foreign bodies (eg, straight pins) in the periphery of the lung which cannot be located with the bronchoscope alone, a biplane fluoroscope can sometimes be used. Thoracotomy is occasionally necessary to remove foreign bodies in the periphery of the lung.

Unrecognized bronchial foreign bodies may produce severe and progressive pulmonary infection, with pneumonia, abscess, and empyema. In children, bronchoscopic manipulation may produce laryngeal edema severe enough to require tracheostomy.

Esophageal Foreign Bodies

Esophageal foreign bodies usually produce immediate symptoms of coughing and gagging; pain in the neck at the level of the thyroid cartilage, with a sensation of something "stuck in the throat"; and difficulty in swallowing or inability to swallow food or saliva. Occasionally, however, especially in children, weeks or months may pass before symptoms of infection or obstruction occur. Pooling of saliva in the pyriform sinuses is suggestive of esophageal obstruction. X-rays will show opaque objects, but often will not show a bolus of meat or a bone. Fluoroscopic observation as the patient swallows a capsule filled with barium sulfate or a wisp of cotton impregnated with barium sulfate is a useful means of locating suspected foreign bodies, since the radiopaque test object will be delayed by the foreign body in its transit through the esophagus.

Esophageal foreign bodies near the cardia may produce pain in the interscapular area.

Esophageal foreign bodies should be removed through the esophagoscope by a skilled endoscopist. Only rarely does an esophageal foreign body constitute an emergency, and so the delay involved in referral is not usually hazardous. Blind probing in an effort to dislodge a foreign body is extremely hazardous.

Perforation of the esophagus by an esophageal foreign body or during endoscopic removal may lead to mediastinal infection (fatal in 50% of cases) or, rarely, severe hemorrhage.

Goff WF: What to do when foreign bodies are inhaled or ingested. Postgrad Med 44:135, 1968.

Kallay F, Hirschberg J, Csermely G: Treatment of airways with foreign bodies in infants. Arch Otolaryng 88:303, 1968.

6...
Respiratory Tract & Mediastinum

R. Morton Manson

NONSPECIFIC MANIFESTATIONS

Cough

Cough is probably the most common symptom of respiratory disease. It may be produced by disturbances anywhere from the oropharynx to the terminal bronchioles. Cough may also occur in diseases not primarily respiratory in nature, eg, congestive heart failure, mitral valve disease, otitis media, or subdiaphragmatic irritation. Patients often overlook or minimize a chronic cough, and detailed interrogation is sometimes necessary. Cough may be dry or may be accompanied by sputum. Paroxysmal cough suggests bronchial obstruction.

Dyspnea

Exertional dyspnea may appear with impaired ventilation (eg, restrictive or obstructive defects), inefficient mechanics of breathing, or with diffusion defects.

Dyspnea at rest is more characteristic of congestive heart failure than of chronic pulmonary disease, but it does appear in diffuse pulmonary diseases causing a diffusion defect and when secondary factors are superimposed on a low pulmonary reserve (eg, bronchitis in an emphysematous patient). Acute illnesses (pneumonia, spontaneous pneumothorax, bronchial asthma, massive atelectasis) can produce marked dyspnea at rest.

Orthopnea is usually considered to be presumptive evidence of congestive heart failure, but some pulmonary patients breathe more easily in a sitting position (bronchial asthma).

Expectoration

The characteristics of the sputum must not be neglected. Mucoid sputum is seen in tracheobronchitis and asthma. A yellow or greenish sputum suggests bacterial infection. Foul-smelling sputum suggests anaerobic infection (eg, putrid lung abscess). Pink, frothy sputum is seen in pulmonary edema. "Rusty" sputum is typical of pneumococcal pneumonia. Copious sputum separating into layers is characteristic of bronchiectasis.

The production of large amounts of sputum with a change of posture (eg, upon arising in the morning) occurs when dependent cavities or bronchiectatic spaces suddenly empty into the bronchial tree.

Wheezing

Wheezing is the characteristic manifestation of bronchial narrowing. It occurs during expiration. Forced expiration may elicit wheezing that is absent during normal breathing. In bronchial asthma, it is paroxysmal and diffuse. Acute left ventricular failure may produce diffuse wheezing which is differentiated from asthma and bronchitis by associated signs of congestive failure and prolonged arm-to-tongue circulation time. A persistent localized wheeze is evidence of local bronchial obstruction (eg, carcinoma, inflammatory stenosis, foreign body).

Chest Pain

Pain due to lung disease is usually due to involvement of the parietal pleura (the visceral pleura is insensitive to pain) or the chest wall, including its bony and cartilaginous structures. Pleural pain is usually unilateral and aggravated by changes in intrathoracic pressure (cough, sneeze, deep breathing). Diaphragmatic irritation may cause pain referred to the anterior shoulder (central irritation) or to the upper abdomen (peripheral irritation). Involvement of the chest wall structures is usually accompanied by tenderness, and pain from this location is more constant and less affected by breathing and coughing.

Localized swelling, pain, and tenderness of one or more costosternal cartilages, caused by a nonspecific inflammation, occurs occasionally (Tietze's syndrome) and may be mistaken for cardiac or pulmonary disease.

Cardiac pain is usually substernal and frequently radiates to the neck, jaw, left shoulder, or arm. Such pain produced by exercise and relieved by rest is almost always due to myocardial ischemia. Pericardial inflammation produces substernal or precordial pain that is aggravated by deep breathing. Pain from esophageal irritation or spasm is deep and central and is altered by swallowing. Deep, persistent, aching chest pain may be caused by localized neoplasms.

A careful history is essential to the identification of chest pain.

Hemoptysis

Spitting or coughing of blood may occur in many bronchopulmonary diseases. Bronchitis, tuberculosis, carcinoma, and bronchiectasis are the most common causes. Bleeding of more than a few ounces is uncommon. Fatal hemorrhage is rare. Bleeding from the nose or pharynx may lead to a history of blood-spitting. Collateral circulation between the bronchial and pulmonary veins may cause hemoptysis in mitral stenosis. When associated with chest pain and shock, hemoptysis suggests pulmonary infarction.

Cyanosis

Cyanosis represents increased concentration of reduced hemoglobin in the blood (> 5 gm/100 ml), which can result from a number of defects of function in pulmonary disease: (1) impaired diffusion from alveoli to capillaries; (2) inadequate gross ventilation of alveoli; and (3) disturbed perfusion/ventilation relationships (increased intrapulmonary "shunts"). Cyanosis is less evident or does not occur in patients with hypoxia due to anemia or histotoxic hypoxia. It is more marked if the patient is cold.

Reduced hemoglobin in the blood may not be manifested as frank cyanosis even when present to a significant degree.

Polycythemia

Increase in the total erythrocyte mass may be very striking as a compensatory response to the chronic anoxemia of pulmonary insufficiency. Primary polycythemia (erythremia) is usually associated with a normal arterial oxygen saturation, but differentiation from the secondary variety is not always easy on this or any other basis.

Polycythemia is discussed in Chapter 9.

Pulmonary Osteoarthropathy

Pulmonary hypertrophic osteoarthropathy refers to those changes in the bones and soft tissues of the extremities seen in some patients with chronic pulmonary disease. These include clubbing of the fingers and toes, subperiosteal proliferation in the long bones, arthralgia, polyarthritis, and nonpitting edema of the skin. The pathogenesis of pulmonary osteoarthropathy is not understood.

Clubbing is frequently seen in bronchiectasis, bronchial carcinoma, and lung abscess; it is unusual in tuberculosis. It may also be caused by such diverse nonpulmonary disorders as congenital heart disease and hepatic cirrhosis; and it may occur as a congenital trait.

Such manifestations have been known to disappear with correction of the pulmonary disorder (eg, resection of a localized bronchial carcinoma).

Rodman GP (editor): Primer in rheumatic diseases, 7th ed. JAMA 224 (Suppl):662, 1973.

Holling HE, Bradley RS: Hypertrophic osteoarthropathy. JAMA 178:977, 1961.

DISORDERS OF THE BRONCHI

BRONCHITIS

Bronchitis or inflammation of the bronchi due to infection or irritation may occur as a primary disorder or may be a prominent finding in many pulmonary diseases (eg, tuberculosis, bronchiectasis, emphysema), but its clinical importance, unfortunately, is often underemphasized.

Acute bronchitis is characterized by fever, productive (mucopurulent to purulent) cough, and absence of x-ray findings. On examination, musical rhonchi are commonly heard, and wheezing is occasionally present. Acute bronchitis is common in viral infections and in the healthy adult is rarely serious, but in infants and small children respiratory obstruction may be severe and life-threatening. In the adult with chronic pulmonary insufficiency (especially emphysema), superimposed acute bronchitis may lead to critical impairment of ventilation and death. Sputum cultures usually yield the common mouth organisms. Occasionally, specific pathogens such as pneumococci or beta-hemolytic streptococci are found. *Haemophilus influenzae* may cause bronchitis in children.

Chronic bronchitis is characterized by a productive cough of long duration without a clear prodrome of acute upper respiratory infection. Very commonly, in older patients there is coexisting emphysema; and the terms emphysema and bronchitis have been used to designate the same clinical entity. The term chronic obstructive bronchopulmonary disease has been used for these patients, although they may at times be free of airway obstruction.

Sputum cultures are usually not helpful and contain only a mixture of mouth organisms.

Earlier enthusiasm for determination of the "closing volume" as a reliable indicator of early, reversible disease of the small airways (2 mm diameter or less) has been tempered by conflicting reports regarding the specificity of this test. The older and simpler determination of the forced expiratory volume in 1 second (FEV_1) remains the most practical test for screening purposes (Table 6–1).

Treatment

A. Acute Bronchitis: Bed rest is advisable, and smoking should be prohibited. Sufficient fluids should be provided to prevent dehydration. Steam or mist inhalation is usually helpful in relieving cough. An antihistamine may help relieve bronchial inflammation. Severe cough may be controlled with an antitussive agent such as codeine phosphate, 15–30 mg every 3–4 hours. Ephedrine, 25 mg orally, or a similar bronchodilator, is helpful if bronchospasm is present. Aspirin will help reduce fever and make the patient more comfortable. Antibiotics should be used in an attempt to prevent secondary infection in patients with impaired

Table 6–1. Pulmonary function tests most useful to the clinician.

Test	Clinical Significance	Normal Values
Vital capacity (VC) Maximum volume that can be expelled after a maximum inspiration. No time limit.	Repeated abnormal values (more or less than 20% of predicted) may be significant. Main value is in following course of cardiopulmonary or respiratory disease with serial tests.	Male: VC = (27.63 − [0.112 × age in years]) × height in cm; Female: VC = (21.78 − [0.101 × age in years]) × height in cm
Forced expiratory volume (FEV) "Timed vital capacity." Maximum volume expelled in a timed interval, usually 1 or 3 seconds.	A reduced timed volume usually indicates obstructive bronchopulmonary disease. Improvement after a bronchodilator indicates some degree of reversibility.	FEV_1 sec = 83% of actual VC; FEV_3 sec = 97% of actual VC
Maximal expiratory flow rate (MEFR) Measurement of maximal flow rate of a single expelled breath, expressed in liters/minute.	A reduced flow rate has the same significance as a reduced FEV. The test requires little effort, and several types of small, portable instruments are available. Suitable for screening tests.	Adult male = > 400 liters/minute; Adult female = > 300 liters/minute
Maximal voluntary ventilation (MVV) "Maximal breathing capacity." Maximal volume expelled in 12–15 seconds of forced breathing, expressed in liters/minute.	Measures essentially the same function as FEV and MEFR. An additional confirmation test of FEV and MEFR. Requires sustained effort and a greater degree of cooperation of the patient.	There is a wide variation of normal values depending upon age, size, and sex. The following formulas can be used as a guide for predicted values. Male = (86.5 − [0.522 × age in years]) × sq m body surface; Female = (71.3 − [0.474 × age in years]) × sq m body surface

When low values are obtained, the above tests should be repeated after administration of a bronchodilator.

Test	Clinical Significance	Normal Values
O_2 tension (arterial) (Pa_{O_2})	Hypoxemia which is not apparent clinically can be detected. This and the determinations listed below are readily available in most hospital laboratories and are essential in the diagnosis of respiratory insufficiency and the management of oxygen and ventilation therapy.	Arterial O_2 tension (Pa_{O_2}) = 90–100 mm Hg
CO_2 tension (arterial) (Pa_{CO_2}) Plasma bicarbonate (HCO_3) pH of arterial blood	Important values in the diagnosis and management of respiratory acidosis due to CO_2 retention.	Pa_{CO_2}, 40 mm Hg; Plasma HCO_3^-, 24 mEq/liter; pH, 7.40

respiratory or cardiac function or debility from other illness, and in infants and children with severe symptoms. Sputum cultures are not usually helpful. Although not routinely used, when an antibiotic is indicated, use penicillin procaine G, 600,000 units IM twice daily; penicillin G tablets, 400,000 units or 250 mg 4 times daily; one of the tetracycline drugs, 250–500 mg 4 times daily; or ampicillin, 250–500 mg 4 times daily.

B. Chronic Bronchitis: The possibility that the "bronchitis" is secondary to some serious underlying disease must always be kept in mind. Sources of possible chronic irritation should be avoided (eg, smoking, allergenic agents, fumes or other irritants). A change of climate to a dry, temperate area may sometimes be warranted. Nonproductive cough should be suppressed with codeine phosphate, 15–30 mg every 3–4 hours, or a comparable antitussive agent. Thick sputum should be liquefied by adequate fluid intake and cool or heated mist inhalations. Bronchial spasm (frequently present with paroxysmal coughing) should be relieved with ephedrine sulfate, 8–25 mg, or related drugs, orally every 4 hours, or isoproterenol hydrochloride, 1:200 solution by nebulization every 2–4 hours. Sometimes ephedrine and isoproterenol may be used together advantageously. Bronchial inflammation due to allergy may be reduced by the use of antihistamine drugs; in severe, intractable cases, the use of corticosteroid drugs such as prednisone is justified. Prednisone is given orally in an initial dosage of 5–10 mg 4 times daily for 3–4 days and then gradually reduced to the smallest possible maintenance dose or, preferably, eliminated over the next 7 days.

Antibiotics are indicated if the sputum is purulent. Penicillin, one of the tetracyclines, or ampicillin given orally may be used. (See treatment of acute bronchitis for dosage.) If improvement does not occur in several days, sputum culture to determine the predominating organisms and antibiotic sensitivities may be helpful. After control of cough and sputum are achieved, prolonged maintenance treatment with half the usual dosage may be necessary to prevent relapse. The use of maintenance antibiotic therapy may decrease the severity and duration, but not the frequency, of intercurrent acute respiratory infections. This is especially so where pneumococci are repeatedly recovered during acute episodes.

For treatment of acute and chronic respiratory failure, see p 137.

Bates DV: Chronic bronchitis and emphysema. (2 parts.) New England J Med 278:546, 600, 1968.

Fletcher CM: Recent clinical and epidemiological studies of chronic bronchitis. Scandinav J Resp Dis 48:285, 1967.

Holdaway D, Romer AC, Gardner PS: The diagnosis and management of bronchiolitis. Pediatrics 39:924, 1967.

Macklem PT: Small airway disease. Am J Med 52:721, 1972.

Macklem PT & others: Workshop on screening programs for early diagnosis of airway obstruction. Am Rev Resp Dis 109:567, 1974.

Malone DN, Gould JC, Grant IWB: A comparative study of ampicillin, tetracycline hydrochloride, and methacycline hydrochloride in acute exacerbations of chronic bronchitis. Lancet 2:594, 1968.

McCarthy DS & others: Measurement of "closing volume" as a simple and sensitive test for early detection of small airway disease. Am J Med 52:747, 1972.

McFadden ER Jr, Linden DA: A reduction in maximum midexpiratory flow rate, a spirographic manifestation of small airway disease. Am J Med 52:725, 1972.

Stuart-Harris CH: Pulmonary hypertension and chronic obstructive bronchitis. Am Rev Resp Dis 97:9, 1968.

Tager I, Speizer FE: Role of infection in chronic bronchitis. New England J Med 292:563, 1975.

BRONCHIECTASIS

Essentials of Diagnosis

- Chronic cough with expectoration of large amounts of purulent sputum, hemoptysis.
- Rales and rhonchi over lower lobes.
- X-ray of chest reveals little; bronchograms show characteristic dilatations.

General Considerations

Bronchiectasis is a dilatation of the medium-size bronchi with destruction of bronchial elastic and muscular elements. It may be caused by pulmonary infections (eg, pneumonia, pertussis, or tuberculosis), or by bronchial obstruction (eg, due to foreign bodies or extrinsic pressure). Atelectasis due to bronchial wall destruction and congenital defects in children (eg, situs inversus, pulmonary cysts, absent frontal sinuses) are commonly associated with bronchiectasis. The incidence of the disease has been greatly reduced by the improved treatment of pulmonary infections with antibiotics.

In many patients, a history of onset following a single episode of pulmonary disease (usually in childhood) is obtained. Sinusitis is present in many patients, but its relation to the bronchial disease is not well understood.

Since infection and bronchial obstruction, however, do not regularly produce significant bronchiectasis, unknown intrinsic factors are presumed to play a role.

Delayed resolution of pneumonia should always suggest underlying bronchial disease.

Clinical Findings

A. Symptoms and Signs: Symptoms arise as a result of impaired bronchial function (ie, loss of expansile and ciliary function) and stasis, which permits secretions to accumulate in the dilated segments. The patient gives a history of a chronic productive cough and "bronchitis-like" symptoms associated with repeated bouts of pneumonia. Chronic cough and expectoration are characteristic. Large amounts of purulent sputum, which often separates into 3 layers (sediment, fluid, foam) on standing, are produced. Expectoration is greatest with changes of posture (allowing sudden drainage of bronchiectatic segments) such as arising from bed.

Hemoptysis occurs in about 50% of cases; it is occasionally severe but rarely fatal. This may be the only symptom. Even in tuberculosis, secondary bronchiectasis may be the main source of bleeding.

Weight loss, asthenia, night sweats, and fever are the result of chronic and acutely exacerbating pulmonary infection.

Pulmonary insufficiency may result from recurrent destruction of pulmonary tissue with resulting fibrosis and emphysema.

Rales and rhonchi over the lower lobes are the most prominent physical findings, and if they are persistently absent the diagnosis of bronchiectasis is questionable. They are more frequently elicited if the examination is carried out before and after postural drainage with coughing (head-down position). Retraction of the chest wall, diminished thoracic excursion, and mediastinal shift toward the side of major involvement will be noted in long-standing disease with loss of lung tissue. Signs of pneumonia may be present during acute infection.

Emaciation, cyanosis, and clubbing of the fingers are seen in advanced cases.

B. Laboratory Findings: Not characteristic. Polycythemia, secondary to pulmonary insufficiency, may be present in advanced disease. Sputum smears and cultures help to rule out active tuberculosis (especially important in bronchiectasis of the upper lobe). Pneumococci are found in some cases. Pseudomonas and enterobacter strains may become established after repeated use of antibiotics.

C. X-Ray Findings: Plain chest films are at times helpful. Increased pulmonary markings at the lung bases together with multiple radiolucencies strongly suggest the diagnosis. Patches of chronic inflammation may be present.

Selective instillation of iodized contrast media into the bronchial tree (bronchograms) reveals sacculated, cylindric, or fusiform dilatations with loss of the normal "tree-in-full-bloom" pattern of the terminal bronchi.

Caution: Bronchographic examination is contraindicated during acute infections and in patients who are sensitive to iodine.

The use of barium or tantalum as a contrast medium has not yet had wide application.

D. Instrumental Examination: Although bronchoscopy does not allow visualization of the bronchiectatic areas, it may reveal bronchial obstruction as the underlying pathology, may identify pulmonary segments giving rise to sputum, and can be utilized for bronchography.

Differential Diagnosis

Differentiate from chronic bronchitis, tuberculosis (which also may cause bronchiectasis), and lung abscess; other causes of hemoptysis such as carcinoma and adenoma.

Complications

Recurrent infection in poorly drained pulmonary segments leads to chronic suppuration and pulmonary insufficiency. Complications include severe or fatal hemoptysis, progressive pulmonary insufficiency, chronic cor pulmonale, and amyloidosis.

Treatment

  A. General Measures:
  1. Environment—
    a. A warm, dry climate may be beneficial.
    b. Avoidance of smoke, fumes, and dusts.
    c. Smoking should be stopped.
  2. Control of bronchial secretions (improved drainage)—
    a. Postural drainage is an effective measure for relieving symptoms in many patients and should always be tried. The patient should assume the position that gives maximum drainage (usually lying on the bed in the prone, supine, or either lateral position with the hips elevated on several pillows with no pillow under the head) and maintain any effective position for 10 minutes 2—4 times daily. The first drainage is upon awakening and the last at bedtime.
    b. Liquefaction of thick sputum is promoted by inhalations of warm or cold mist. Mucolytic agents such as acetylcysteine given by aerosol may also be helpful.
    c. Bed position—Elevation of the foot of the bed on 4-inch blocks may enhance drainage.
  3. Control of respiratory infections—
    a. Acute respiratory infections should be minimized by avoiding exposure where possible. Broad spectrum antibiotics should be used promptly in such infections in an attempt to prevent secondary bacterial invasion. Annual immunization for influenza may be beneficial.
    b. Chronic sinus infections should be treated and, if possible, eliminated.
  B. Specific Measures: Antibiotic therapy reduces cough, sputum, and other symptoms, especially during acute exacerbations, but these benefits may be transient. The antibiotics are therefore best used intermittently as exacerbations occur. Prolonged use of antibiotics in maintenance dosage (usually half the regular dose) is sometimes indicated.
    1. Penicillin may be used parenterally (best for attacks of acute pneumonia; see below) or orally. Give 250 mg (400,000 units) penicillin G 4 times daily.
    2. Tetracycline drugs, 250 mg 4 times daily.
    3. The use of other antibiotics should be guided by sensitivity studies.
    4. Aerosolized antibiotics (penicillin, streptomycin) are of no value.
    5. Bronchoscopic drainage—This is of value initially to determine the origin of the secretions and to identify bronchial stenosis or obstruction. Dilatation or removal of the obstruction can sometimes be accomplished.
  C. Surgical Treatment: Pulmonary resection is indicated (1) for younger patients in otherwise good

health with recurring symptoms, and (2) for patients with severe symptoms (especially recurrent hemorrhage) due to localized unilateral disease who are otherwise good surgical risks. The results after adequate resection may be good.

When a large sputum volume is present and resectional surgery is not feasible, a permanent tracheostomy or tracheal fistula may permit better drainage by allowing frequent catheter aspiration.

Prognosis

The judicious use of antibiotics and surgery has greatly improved the prognosis in bronchiectasis.

Borrie J, Lichter I: Surgical treatment of bronchiectasis: A ten-year survey. Brit MJ 2:908, 1965.

Bradford JK, DeCamp PT: Bronchiectasis. S Clin North America 46:1485, 1966.

Crofton J: Prognosis and treatment of bronchiectasis. (2 parts.) Brit MJ 1:721, 783, 1966.

Ferguson TB, Burford TH: The changing pattern of pulmonary suppuration: Surgical implications. Dis Chest 53:396, 1968.

Sealey WC, Bradham RR, Young WC Jr: The surgical treatment of multisegmental and localized bronchiectasis. Surg Gynec Obst 123:80, 1966.

DISORDERS OF THE LUNGS

LUNG DISEASES DUE TO IMMUNOLOGIC REACTIONS

Within the past decade, progress in immunology has resulted in greater understanding of the pathogenetic mechanisms underlying a large group of what were at one time regarded as unrelated bronchopulmonary diseases. It is now possible to categorize certain diseases of the lung as being hypersensitivity manifestations of one of the 4 types of allergic reactions described and classified by Gell and Coombs (Table 1−1):

Type I: Immediate, IgE-mediated
   Bronchial asthma (atopic)
Type II: Cytotoxic
   Silicosis and other pneumoconioses
   Goodpasture's syndrome
Type III: Immune complex disease
   Pulmonary vasculitis (SLE and other vasculitides)
   Extrinsic allergic alveolitis
Type IV: Delayed type, cell-mediated
   PIE, delayed type (helminthic)

Callerame ML & others: Immunologic reactions of bronchial tissues in asthma. New England J Med 284:459, 1971.

Coombs RRA, Gell PGH: Classification of allergic reactions responsible for clinical hypersensitivity and disease. Pages 575−596 in: *Clinical Aspects of Immunology,* 2nd ed. Gell PGH, Coombs RRA (editors). Oxford Univ Press, 1968.

McCombs RP: Diseases due to immunologic reactions in the lungs. (2 parts.) New England J Med 286:1186, 1245, 1972.

Scadding JG: Eosinophilic infiltrations of the lungs in asthmatics. Proc Roy Soc Med 64:381, 1971.

Solberg CO: Glomerulonephritis with initial lung purpura (Goodpasture's syndrome): Survival of two patients out of four. Acta med scandinav 186:401, 1969.

1. ASTHMA

Essentials of Diagnosis

- Recurrent acute attacks of wheezing, dyspnea, cough, and mucoid sputum.
- Prolonged expiration with generalized wheezing and musical rales.

General Considerations

Asthma is a bronchial hypersensitivity disorder characterized by reversible airway obstruction produced by a combination of mucosal edema, constriction of the bronchial musculature, and excessive secretion of viscid mucus, causing mucous plugs.

Atopic or "extrinsic" asthma has been thought to result from sensitization of the bronchial mucosa by tissue-specific antibodies. The antibodies produced are specific immunoglobulins of the IgE (type I) class. Exposure to the appropriate allergens by inhalation results in an antigen-antibody reaction which releases vasoactive bronchoconstrictive chemical mediators, causing the characteristic tissue changes. More recent work suggests that reflex stimulation of the parasympathetic nervous system, possibly via irritant receptors in the bronchial mucosa, may be equally important in the pathogenesis.

Approximately 50% of asthmatics are of the non-atopic ("intrinsic") type in which the bronchial reaction occurs in response to nonimmunologic stimuli such as infection, irritating inhalants, cold air, exercise, and emotional upset. Here it appears that reflex stimulation of the parasympathetic nervous system in susceptible individuals is the major mechanism. These patients do not demonstrate elevated IgE antibodies in their serum, and the history does not suggest hypersensitivity to specific allergens.

Clinical Findings

A. Signs and Symptoms: Asthma is characterized by recurrent attacks of wheezing, dyspnea, cough, and expectoration of tenacious mucoid sputum. Symptoms may be mild and occur only in association with respiratory infection, or they may occur in various degrees of severity to the point of being life-threatening. Classical allergic (atopic) asthma usually begins in childhood and becomes progressively more severe throughout life, although spontaneous remissions may occur in adulthood. Hay fever often accompanies atopic asthma. Other forms of asthma with similar symptoms usually occur in later life.

The acute attack is characterized by dyspnea associated with expiratory wheezing which may be heard without a stethoscope. Cough may be present but is usually not the predominant symptom.

When asthma becomes prolonged, with severe intractable wheezing, it is known as status asthmaticus.

B. Laboratory Findings: The sputum is characteristically tenacious and mucoid, containing "plugs" and "spirals." Eosinophils are seen microscopically. The differential blood count may show eosinophilia. In severe, acute bronchospasm, arterial hypoxemia may be present due to disturbed perfusion/ventilation relationships, alveolar hypoventilation, or functional right-to-left shunts. Most patients with allergic asthma (and a few with "intrinsic" asthma) have elevated serum levels of immunoglobulin E (IgE). IgE determinations are not generally available.

C. X-Ray Findings: Chest films usually show no abnormalities. Reversible hyperexpansion may occur in severe paroxysms, or hyperexpansion may persist (emphysema) in long-standing cases. Transient, migratory pulmonary infiltrations have been reported. It is possible that pneumothorax will complicate severe attacks.

Differential Diagnosis

Distinguish wheezing from that due to bronchitis, obstructive emphysema, and congestive heart failure.

Complications

Chronic bronchial asthma may lead to such complications as chronic pulmonary emphysema and chronic cor pulmonale. Other complications may include atelectasis, pulmonary infection, and pneumothorax.

Treatment

The treatment may be divided into 2 phases: (1) treatment of the acute attack and (2) interim therapy, which is aimed at preventing further attacks. Epinephrine and intravenous aminophylline are the drugs of choice for the emergency management of acute bronchial asthma. However, for status asthmaticus or for acute attacks in epinephrine-resistant patients, the adrenal corticosteroids are usually necessary. Intravenous hydrocortisone and methylprednisolone are the preparations of choice. *Note:* Epinephrine must be used cautiously in patients with "cardiac asthma," hypertension, or angina.

A. Treatment of the Acute Attack: Eliminate known allergens from the patient's environment. Maintain adequate rest and relieve apprehension by reassurance and sedatives. Treat respiratory infections vigorously with antibiotics. Give fluids orally or parenterally as necessary to prevent dehydration and liquefy secretions. Inhalation of water mist, either cool or heated, may help loosen tenacious secretions.

1. Drugs—

a. Epinephrine (1:1000), 0.2–0.5 ml subcut, is the initial drug of choice. It may be repeated every 1–2 hours.

b. Aminophylline, 0.25 gm in 10–20 ml saline *slowly* IV, can be used if epinephrine is not effective. Both can be given initially in moderately severe attacks.

c. Nebulized drugs—Most useful in mild attacks.

(1) Isoproterenol, 1:200, 1–2 inhalations from a hand nebulizer every 30–60 minutes, or 0.5 ml in 2.5–3 ml saline by compressed air nebulizer or IPPB every 4 hours.

(2) Isoetharine with phenylephrine (Bronkosol) may be used in the same manner as isoproterenol, 1:200.

(3) Epinephrine (1:100) (for inhalation only), 1–2 inhalations from hand nebulizer. Do not use for prolonged nebulization.

d. Corticosteroid drugs—Most effective in severe attacks which do not respond satisfactorily to the above bronchodilators. Use prednisone, 40–60 mg/day in divided doses, and gradually reduce to zero over 7–10 days. In moderate to severe attacks, hydrocortisone sodium succinate, 100–200 mg IV, may be given simultaneously with the first dose of oral corticosteroid.

e. Other drugs—

(1) Methylxanthines, ephedrine, and similar agents given orally are of limited value in stopping an asthmatic attack (see below).

(2) Sedation should be avoided in severe asthma. In mild to moderate symptoms, phenobarbital, 30 mg, or diazepam, 5 mg 3–4 times daily, may be helpful in counteracting the CNS stimulant effects of sympathomimetic bronchodilator drugs.

f. Fluids—Patients with persistent symptoms who require hospitalization generally need supplemental intravenous fluids to help liquefy secretions.

g. Oxygen by nasal prongs or mask or by IPPB (mask or mouthpiece) is indicated in the presence of moderate to severe symptoms.

2. Status asthmaticus—When severe wheezing persists after use of the measures listed above, hospitalization is required. If arterial blood gases can be measured, a P_{O_2} of less than 50 mm Hg in the presence of a normal (40 mm Hg) or elevated P_{CO_2} is an indication for hospitalization.

The principal drugs for the treatment of the hospitalized patient are the following:

a. **Aminophylline**—Give an initial dose of 5.6 mg/kg (reduce if the drug has been given just prior to hospitalization) and follow with a continuous intravenous infusion of 0.9 mg/kg/hour. Serum theophylline levels are available in many hospitals and are helpful in assuring adequate dosage and avoiding toxicity. Levels of 10–20 μg/ml are necessary for optimum treatment. Levels above 20 μg/ml are usually toxic.

b. **Corticosteroids**—The drugs of choice are either hydrocortisone sodium succinate (Solu-Cortef), 100 mg IV every hour, or methylprednisolone sodium succinate (Solu-Medrol), 80 mg IV every hour, until improvement is established. Prednisone, 20 mg orally 4 times daily, or methylprednisolone (Medrol), 16 mg orally 4 times daily, can be started at the same time and continued after the intravenous steroids are no longer needed.

B. Other Measures: Oxygen by nasal prongs or mask should be given in sufficient concentration to relieve hypoxemia.

Intravenous fluids—up to 4 liters of 5% dextrose in water—should be given in the first 24 hours to liquefy secretions. Electrolytes should be monitored as fluid administration is continued.

IPPB by mouthpiece or mask with nebulized isoproterenol or isoetharine with phenylephrine (Bronkosol), 0.5 ml in 3 ml of 0.5 N saline, may be used intermittently or continuously. The addition of chest percussion and postural drainage every 2—4 hours will usually aid in clearing tenacious secretions.

Arterial blood gases should be monitored every 30—60 minutes initially. Unrelieved hypoxemia or a rising P_{CO_2} or, if blood gas measurements are not available, clinical deterioration of the patient is an indication for intubation and assisted or controlled respiration. After intubation, sedation with small doses of diazepam or morphine intravenously may be necessary to permit ventilatory control by the respirator.

When control of wheezing or removal of secretions cannot be accomplished with the above measures, general anesthesia with fluothane (Halothane) together with bronchoscopy for aspiration and saline lavage of secretions may be lifesaving.

C. Interim Therapy: Attempt to identify the offending allergens. Emotional disturbances should be eliminated if possible. Patients with "intrinsic" asthma (usually associated with bronchitis) may be helped by antibiotic therapy.

Oral aminophylline in doses sufficient to produce therapeutic blood levels (see above) is usually helpful. Various combinations of ephedrine or hydroxyzine, aminophylline, and a barbiturate, available in tablets and capsules, are less effective.

Nebulized isoproterenol, 1:200, or isoetharine, from a hand nebulizer, is useful in controlling mild symptoms and preventing more severe episodes.

Two newer catecholamines—salbutamol and terbutaline (Brethine)—have been used extensively in Europe and appear to be superior bronchodilators with fewer side-effects. The latter drug is now available in the USA.

Antihistamines may give relief in some patients, but their use in bronchial asthma has generally been disappointing.

Patients who are not helped by other measures may be treated on a long-term basis with prednisone or a similar corticosteroid. The dosage employed should be just sufficient to keep the patient comfortable and relatively free of symptoms. Begin with 5 mg 3—4 times daily.

Cromolyn sodium (Aarane, Intal) is useful mainly in atopic asthma. It acts to specifically inhibit the liberation of mediators of anaphylaxis initiated by the antigen-antibody reaction. It is effective only during remissions to prevent recurrent attacks and to reduce the requirement for corticosteroids. It is administered as a micronized powder by inhalation. Occasional pharyngeal and tracheal irritation has been noted, but no systemic side-effects have been reported.

Prognosis

Most patients with bronchial asthma adjust well to the necessity for continued medical treatment throughout life. Inadequate control or persistent aggravation by unmodified environmental conditions favors the development of incapacitating or even life-threatening complications.

Dulfarro MJ: Bronchodilators, pulmonary function, and asthma. Ann Int Med 68:955, 1968.

Fitch KD, Morton AR: Specificity of exercise in exercise-induced asthma. Brit MJ 4:577, 1971.

Franklin W: Treatment of severe asthma. New England J Med 290:1469, 1974.

Freedman BJ, Meisner P, Hill GB: A comparison of different bronchodilators in asthma. Thorax 23:590, 1968.

Irani FA & others: Evaluation of disodium cromoglycate in intrinsic and extrinsic asthma. Am Rev Resp Dis 106:179, 1972.

Johnstone DE: A study of the natural history of bronchial asthma in children. Am J Dis Child 115:213, 1968.

Mannsell K, Pearson RSB, Livingstone JL: Long-term corticosteroid treatment of asthma. Brit MJ 1:661, 1968.

Mathison DA & others: Cromolyn treatment of asthma. JAMA 216:1454, 1971.

McFadden ER Jr: Exertional dyspnea and cough as preludes to acute attacks of bronchial asthma. New England J Med 292:555, 1975.

Mitenko PA, Ogilvie RI: Rational intravenous doses of theophylline. New England J Med 289:600, 1973.

O'Loughlin JM: A nonallergist's guide to bronchial asthma. Drug Therapy 4:23, 1974.

Reed CE: The pathogenesis of asthma. M Clin North America 58:53, 1974.

Richerson HB: Symptomatic treatment of adults with bronchial asthma. M Clin North America 58:135, 1974.

Stevenson DD & others: Provoking factors in bronchial asthma. Arch Int Med 135:777, 1975.

Weinberger M & others: Interaction of ephedrine and theophylline. Clin Pharmacol Therap 17:585, 1975.

Zwillich CW & others: Theophylline-induced seizures in adults. Ann Int Med 82:784, 1975.

2. PULMONARY INFILTRATIONS WITH EOSINOPHILIA
(PIE Syndrome)

This relatively uncommon syndrome is characterized by migratory multiple pulmonary infiltrates and eosinophilia (up to 80%) in the peripheral blood. Fever, dyspnea, and cough are inconstant.

This syndrome results from a type I immediate hypersensitivity reaction to certain fungi *(Aspergillus*

Table 6—2. Pneumoconioses.*

Disease and Occupation	Causative Particle and Pathology	Clinical Features	X-Ray Findings
Silicosis† (mining, drilling, blasting, grinding, abrasive manufacture; various other processes exposing silica to high temperatures, such as iron moulding or ceramic manufacture)	Free silica, crystobalite, and tridymite (toxic isomers produced by exposure of silica to high temperatures) cause immunologic tissue reactions producing nodules, fibrosis, lymphatic blockage, emphysema, and hilar adenopathy.	Required exposure is 2—20 years. Dyspnea on exertion, dry cough. Frequent infections, especially tuberculosis. Pulmonary insufficiency, chronic cor pulmonale.	Hilar adenopathy; peripheral ("eggshell") calcification of hilar nodes; nodules (inner, midlung fields), overall increased radiolucency, fibrosis. Signs of associated tuberculosis.
Asbestosis (asbestos mining and processing)	Magnesium silicate (particle size 20—200 μm), rod-shaped bodies visible in tissue sections and sputum, causing obstruction of bronchioles, distal atelectasis, fibrosis (little nodulation).	Required exposure 2—8 years. Dyspnea early. Productive cough. Pulmonary insufficiency. "Corns" on skin of extremities (imbedded particles). Possible increased incidence of bronchogenic carcinoma and malignant mesothelioma.	Fine reticular markings in lower lung fields. Thickening of pleura ("ground glass" appearance), obliteration of costophrenic angles. Bilateral pleural calcifications.
Berylliosis (beryllium production, manufacture of fluorescent powders)	Beryllium particles. **Acute:** Patchy infiltrations, resembling bronchial pneumonia. **Chronic:** Alveolar septal granuloma causing fine nodules. Fibrosis not prominent. Elastic tissue damaged, causing emphysema. No hilar adenopathy.	**Acute:** After a few weeks of exposure, upper respiratory symptoms; "bronchitis," "pneumonia" later. **Chronic:** Required exposure 6—18 months. Dyspnea, cough, weight loss, cyanosis, skin lesions, pulmonary insufficiency, cor pulmonale.	**Acute:** Clear at first, then patchy infiltrations. **Chronic:** Scattered minute ("sandpaper") nodules. Later, larger nodules, diffuse reticular markings. No hilar adenopathy.
Bauxite pneumoconiosis (Shaver's disease; aluminosis)	May be due to other toxic contaminants rather than aluminum dust per se, causing fibrosis, hilar adenopathy, atelectasis.	Required exposure is several months to 2 years. Dyspnea (marked pulmonary insufficiency). Attacks of spontaneous pneumothorax.	Hilar and mediastinal adenopathy, irregularity of diaphragms, fibrosis, emphysema.
Anthracosis (rarely dissociated from silicosis) (mining, city dwellers)	Coal dust, causing black discoloration of lungs, nodes, distant organs (nodules rare).	Progressive disease (fibrosis, emphysema) reported in Welsh soft-coal workers. Silica may be an important factor.	"Reticulation," fine nodules. Coal dust may produce large densities by deposition without fibrosis.
Siderosis (iron ore processing, metal drilling, electric arc welding)	Iron oxides, metallic iron, causing "red" (oxides) and "black" (metallic) discoloration of lung. "Red" type leads to fibrosis. "Black" type associated with silicosis.	Symptoms are those of associated silicosis.	Dependent mainly on associated silicosis.

*Actual exposure is rarely to one dust alone.
†Silicosis is discussed more fully on p 115.

fumigatus, Candida albicans) and bacterial enzymes *(Bacillus subtilis)*. It also results from immediate (type I) and delayed (type IV) hypersensitivity reactions to systemic helminth infestations (ascariasis and schistosomiasis) which have a pulmonary cycle.

Eosinophilic pulmonary infiltrations developing in patients with nonallergic "intrinsic" asthma present a different syndrome. Blood eosinophilia is generally greater, and the densities seen in the chest x-ray tend to be more bizarre and unrelated to bronchopulmonary segments. The pulmonary lesions also show a more striking tendency to wax and wane and to "migrate."

Treatment is largely symptomatic. Pulmonary manifestations may be controlled by corticosteroids and, when indicated, anthelmintic agents. Antifungal agents are not effective.

Carrington CB & others: Chronic eosinophilia pneumonia. New England J Med 280:787, 1969.

Ford RM: Transient pulmonary eosinophilia and asthma: A review of 20 cases occurring in 5702 asthma sufferers. Am Rev Resp Dis 93:797, 1966.

McCombs RP: Disease due to immunologic reactions in the lungs. (2 parts.) New England J Med 286:1186, 1245, 1972.

Robertson CL & others: Chronic eosinophilic pneumonia. Radiology 101:57, 1971.

3. SILICOSIS

Essentials of Diagnosis

- History of exposure to dust containing silicon dioxide (eg, hard-rock mining, sandblasting).
- Characteristic x-ray changes: Bilateral nodules, fibrosis, hilar lymphadenopathy.
- Recurrent respiratory infections.
- *Note:* Tuberculosis is a common complication.

General Considerations

Silicosis is one of the chronic fibrotic pulmonary diseases caused by inhalation of inorganic occupational dusts, the pneumoconioses (Table 6–2). In the case of silicosis, free silica (silicon dioxide) is by far the most common offender. Prolonged exposure is usually required. Immunoglobulins of the type II (cytotoxic) class (IgG and IgM) have been demonstrated in silicotic tissue, and it appears that further study of the immunologic mechanism will clarify the pathogenesis of this unusual disease.

Clinical Findings

A. Symptoms and Signs: Symptoms may be absent or may consist only of unusual susceptibility to upper respiratory tract infections, "bronchitis," and pneumonia. Dyspnea on exertion is the most common presenting complaint. It may progress slowly for years.

Cough usually develops and is dry initially but later becomes productive, frequently with blood-streaked sputum. Severe and, occasionally, fatal hemoptysis may occur.

Physical findings may be absent in patients with advanced silicosis.

B. Laboratory Findings: Sputum studies for acid-fast bacilli are indicated to rule out silicotuberculosis. Lung biopsy is occasionally indicated to establish the diagnosis for compensation purposes.

C. X-Ray Findings: Chest x-rays are not diagnostic but often strongly suggest the diagnosis. Abnormalities are usually bilateral, symmetric, and predominant in the inner midlung fields. Small nodules tend to be of uniform size and density. Enlargement of hilar nodes is a relatively early finding. Peripheral calcification of the nodes, giving an "eggshell" appearance, may occur later. Fibrosis is manifested by fine linear markings and reticulation. Coalescence of nodules produces larger densities. Associated emphysema gives an x-ray picture of increased radiolucency, often quite striking at the lung bases.

Treatment

No specific treatment is available. Symptomatic treatment is indicated for chronic cough and wheezing. When tuberculosis occurs (a not uncommon complication), antituberculous drugs must be given as for the treatment of advanced tuberculosis (see p 126). In the presence of a positive tuberculin skin test and no other evidence of active tuberculosis, isoniazid, 300 mg daily, should be given for 2 years.

Prognosis

Gradually progressive dyspnea may be present for years. The development of complications, especially tuberculosis, markedly worsens the prognosis.

Gaensler EA, Addington WW: Current concepts: Asbestos or ferruginous bodies. New England J Med 280:488, 1969.

Gaensler EA & others: Graphite pneumoconiosis of electrotypers. Am J Med 41:864, 1966.

Miller A & others: Pulmonary fibrosis: Association with asbestos fibers. New England J Med 292:41, 1975.

Schepers GWH: Lung disease caused by inorganic and organic dust. Dis Chest 44:133, 1963.

Therdos PA: Lung biopsy in the diagnosis of the pneumoconioses. Dis Chest 53:271, 1968.

Whipple HE (editor): Biological effects of asbestos. Ann New York Acad Sc 132: Article 1, Dec 1965.

4. PNEUMOCONIOSES OTHER THAN SILICOSIS

(See Table 6–2.)

The following substances, when inhaled, cause varying degrees of pulmonary inflammation, fibrosis, emphysema, and disability, usually to a lesser degree than silicon dioxide: coal dust, bauxite (aluminum and silicon), asbestos (dehydrated calcium-magnesium silicate), mica dust (aluminum silicates), talc (hydrous magnesium silicate), graphite (crystallized carbon plus silicon dioxide), beryllium, and diatomaceous earth. The latter is almost pure silicon dioxide but produces effects essentially like those of silicosis only when heated (flux calcined) in the manufacture of abrasives.

Identification of these pulmonary dust diseases depends upon a careful inquiry into possible occupational or casual exposure.

Treatment is symptomatic.

See references under Silicosis, above.

5. GOODPASTURE'S SYNDROME

This disease consists of chronic, relapsing pulmonary hemosiderosis, often in association with fatal glomerulonephritis. Recent elucidation of a type II immunologic mechanism indicates that the same antibody affects both the alveolar and glomerular basement membranes.

Clinical features include cough with recurrent hemoptysis, dyspnea, pulmonary infiltrates, and hypochromic iron deficiency anemia due to large amounts of hemoglobin broken down and deposited as hemosiderin in the lungs. Evidence of glomerulonephritis and progressive renal failure is common.

The prognosis is generally poor, although milder forms do occur and treatment with corticosteroids or immunosuppressive drugs may be helpful. A few patients with terminal glomerulonephritis have been treated with bilateral nephrectomy and transplantation of one kidney. When this has been successful, the pulmonary lesions have resolved.

Nowakowski A & others: Goodpasture's syndrome: Recovery from severe pulmonary hemorrhage after bilateral nephrectomy. Ann Int Med 75:243, 1971.
Proskey AJ & others: Goodpasture's syndrome: A report of five cases and review of the literature. Am J Med 48:162, 1970.

6. PULMONARY VASCULITIS

This is a group of hypersensitivity diseases in which pulmonary vasculitis is a manifestation of a systemic disease. The immunologic mechanism seems also to involve type III antibody formation in response to various antigens such as heterologous serum, RNA, DNA, streptococci, and certain drugs such as sulfonamides, hexamethonium, and nitrofurantoin. Serum sickness, polyarteritis nodosa, systemic lupus erythematosus, and interstitial pneumonitis are manifestations of this type of reaction. (See Chapter 13.)

Wegener's granulomatosis is a variant characterized by both granuloma formation and necrotizing angiitis, often in association with glomerular involvement and necrotizing lesions in the nasal sinuses. Pathologic changes in the lungs include vascular necrosis, hemorrhage, granuloma formation, and interstitial pneumonitis.

Corticosteroids and immunosuppressive agents have been used with variable success to suppress the inflammatory and granulomatous reactions in this disorder. The offending antigen, if known, should be removed.

7. EXTRINSIC ALLERGIC ALVEOLITIS

Extrinsic allergic alveolitis results from type III (immune complex) antigen-antibody reactions. This is caused by exposure to moldy dusts containing various fungi. Also included are the thermophilic actinomycetes responsible for the hypersensitivity pneumonitis caused by contaminated air conditioning systems. Other clinical manifestations of these hypersensitivity states are referred to as farmer's lung (due to inhalation of moldy hay), bagassosis (moldy sugar cane), maple bark disease (moldy bark), and byssinosis (cotton dust).

The clinical picture is that of an acute pneumonia beginning within hours after exposure to one of these antigens in a person sensitized by previous exposures. A history of exposure is of paramount importance in the diagnosis.

Treatment consists of cessation of exposure and, if symptoms are severe, a course of corticosteroid treatment. Pulmonary fibrosis may result from severe or repeated episodes.

Hapke EJ & others: Farmer's lung: A clinical, radiographic, functional, and serologic correlation of acute and chronic stages. Thorax 23:451, 1968.
Nicholson DP: Bagasse worker's lung. Am Rev Resp Dis 97:546, 1968.
Rankin J & others: Pulmonary granulomatoses due to inhaled organic antigens. M Clin North America 51:459, 1967.

INFECTIONS OF THE LUNG*

Pneumonia due to infection may be caused by a wide variety of organisms, mostly bacterial or viral. For proper treatment, it is crucial to identify the

*By Ernest Jawetz, PhD, MD.

causative agent by sputum examination with stained smear and culture and by blood cultures. Transtracheal aspiration and even lung puncture (by one who is experienced in this technic) may be required.

PNEUMOCOCCAL PNEUMONIA

Essentials of Diagnosis
- Sudden onset of shaking chills, fever, chest pain, and cough with rust-colored sputum.
- X-rays show infiltration, often lobar in distribution.
- Pneumococci are present in the sputum and often in the blood.
- Leukocytosis.

General Considerations
Pneumonia is an inflammatory process in lung parenchyma most commonly caused by infection. The consolidation of pneumonia must be differentiated from pulmonary infarction, atelectasis with bronchial obstruction, and congestive heart failure, but it may coexist with any of these conditions. The pneumococcus accounts for 60–80% of primary bacterial pneumonias; types I–VIII are most commonly found in adults, whereas type XIV is common in children. These pathogenic organisms are frequently present among the normal flora of the respiratory tract. The development of pneumonia must therefore usually be attributed to an impairment of natural resistance. Conditions leading to aspiration of secretions include obliteration of the cough or epiglottal reflex, impairment of upward migration of mucous sheets (propelled by cilia), and impairment of alveolar phagocyte function. Among conditions which predispose to pneumonia are viral respiratory diseases, malnutrition, exposure to cold, noxious gases, alcohol intoxication, depression of cerebral functions by drugs, and cardiac failure. Pneumonic consolidation may be in one or more lobes, or patchy in distribution.

Clinical Findings
A. Symptoms and Signs: The onset is usually sudden, with shaking chills, "stabbing" chest pain (exaggerated by respiration but sometimes referred to the shoulder, abdomen, or flank), high fever, cough and "rusty" sputum, and occasionally vomiting. A history of recent respiratory illness can often be elicited.

The patient appears severely ill, with marked tachypnea (30–40/minute) but no orthopnea. Respirations are grunting, nares flaring, and the patient often lies on the affected side in an attempt to splint the chest. Herpes simplex lesions are often present.

Initially, chest excursion is diminished on the involved side, breath sounds are suppressed, and fine inspiratory rales are heard. Later, the classical signs (absent breath sounds, dullness, etc) of consolidation appear. A pleural friction rub or abdominal distention

may be present. During resolution of the pneumonia, the signs of consolidation are replaced by rales. Physical findings are often inconclusive, and repeated x-ray examination is helpful.

B. Laboratory Findings: Blood cultures are positive for pneumococci in 15–25% of cases early in the disease. In peripheral blood, leukocytosis (20–35 thousand/cu mm) is the rule, and a low white count carries a poorer prognosis.

Expectorated sputum must be examined by Gram's stain and by culture. In the smears, the presence of many squamous epithelial cells suggests heavy contamination with saliva and nasopharyngeal secretions, and such specimens are of doubtful value. Typical sputum from pneumococcal pneumonia contains many red and white cells and many pneumococci. If good sputum specimens are not obtainable, a transtracheal aspirate may reveal the etiologic agent, but this procedure is not without risk. A microscopic "quellung" reaction with pooled antiserum most rapidly identifies pneumococci in sputum.

C. X-Ray Findings: Initially, there may be no findings or a vague haziness across the involved part of the lung field. Later, typical consolidation is well defined either in lobar or in patchy distribution. Fluid shadows in the costophrenic angles may appear before pleural exudate can be detected by physical examination. During resolution of the consolidation, areas of radiolucency may appear, suggesting "pseudocavitation."

Treatment
A blood culture and a good sputum specimen for smear and culture should always be obtained before treatment is started. The dosage and route of administration of antimicrobial drugs are influenced to some extent by the clinical severity of the disease, the presence of unfavorable prognostic signs (see below), and the presence of complications.

A. Antibacterial Therapy: Penicillin G is the drug of choice. It is given parenterally at first in dosages ranging from procaine penicillin, 600,000 units every 12 hours IM for moderate illness, to aqueous penicillin G, 1 million units given every 4 hours rapidly into an IV infusion in the most severe cases. Only after there has been a definite response to treatment should oral penicillin V (400,000 units every 4–6 hours) be considered. All pneumococci are susceptible to penicillin at present. Some strains resistant to tetracyclines, erythromycin, or lincomycin have been encountered. Therefore, these alternatives to penicillin (eg, in patients with documented hypersensitivity) may fail, but they (or cephalexin, 0.5 gm every 4–6 hours) can be tried orally in mildly ill patients. In more severely ill persons, cefazolin, 4 gm IV or IM daily, is a reasonable alternative. Treatment with an effective drug should be continued for 3 days after defervescence.

Sulfonamides are not in favor now because the therapeutic response is slower than with penicillin. However, sulfisoxazole diolamine or sodium sulfadiazine, 4–6 gm IV, followed by maintenance doses IV or orally, is adequate (if not optimal) treatment for many cases of pneumococcal pneumonia. Sulfonamide precautions (see Chapter 28) must be observed.

B. General Supportive Treatment:

1. Ventilation and oxygenation—An adequate airway must be maintained—if necessary, by tracheal suction, endotracheal tube, or tracheostomy. Oxygen must be supplied to any patient with severe pneumonia, cyanosis, or marked dyspnea; this will also help to prevent pulmonary edema. Oxygen may be supplied by nasal catheter, soft rubber mask, or oxygen tent. With masks, a 95% oxygen concentration can be maintained, whereas with nasal tubes or tents the concentration will reach only 40–50%. However, masks are difficult to tolerate because of cough and expectoration. Oxygen must be humidified to prevent drying of secretions.

2. Shock and pulmonary edema—These are the most frequent causes of death in pneumonia. Oxygen administration tends to prevent pulmonary edema; impending right heart failure must be managed, and digitalization is urgent. Treat shock as outlined in Chapter 1.

3. Toxic delirium—This occurs in any severe pneumonia and may be particularly difficult to manage in alcoholics. It must be controlled to prevent exhaustion and circulatory failure. This is best done by means of a phenothiazine (eg, promazine, 50–100 mg IM) or paraldehyde (8–12 ml orally, repeated as necessary every 4 hours; or 5 ml IM, repeated in 30 minutes if necessary). Anxiety and restlessness during waking hours may also be treated with phenobarbital, 15–30 mg every 4 hours. Pentobarbital, 0.1 gm, or flurazepam (Dalmane), 30 mg, at bedtime, helps to ensure adequate rest. While administering sedatives or tranquilizers, it is helpful to check the patient's sensorium frequently for any change suggestive of pneumococcal meningitis, which would make a diagnostic lumbar puncture mandatory.

4. Fluids—Patients with pneumococcal pneumonia may perspire profusely and lose much fluid and salt. Sufficient fluid must be given to maintain a daily urinary output of at least 1500 ml. Electrolytes must be kept in balance.

5. Diet—Initially, the dyspneic patient will be anorexic, and a liquid diet will be preferred. With improvement, a normal diet will be tolerated. If complications suggest a long illness, a high-protein, high-caloric diet with vitamin supplementation is indicated.

6. Cough—If cough interferes with sleep and rest, it may be suppressed with codeine phosphate, 15–30 mg every 3–4 hours subcut or orally; or by elixir of terpin hydrate with codeine, 1 tsp every 3–4 hours as necessary.

7. Pleuritic pain—For mild pain, spray ethyl chloride over the area of greatest pain for about 1 minute, and then along the long axis of the body through the entire area of pain, so that a line of frost about 1 inch wide is formed. This gives relief for 1–10 hours in the great majority of patients. Codeine phosphate, 15–30 mg, may be given as necessary for pain. For very severe

pain, use meperidine, 50–100 mg, or morphine sulfate, 10–15 mg, or procaine hydrochloride solution, 0.5–1% subcut, in a series of injections passing through the area of greatest pain and 5 cm higher and lower.

8. Abdominal distention—Abdominal distention is usually due to air swallowing in severe dyspnea, and is a frequent problem in patients with pneumonia. Breathing oxygen in high concentrations (90–100%) is useful because oxygen is rapidly absorbed from the intestines. Neostigmine methylsulfate, 1:2000, 1 ml subcut, and insertion of a rectal tube will usually produce rapid initial decompression. Gastric dilatation can be relieved by suction through a nasal tube passed into the stomach.

9. Congestive failure—(Distinguish from shock and pulmonary edema.) In elderly patients or patients with preexisting heart disease, congestive failure may be precipitated by pneumonia. Rapid digitalization is indicated.

10. Cardiac arrhythmias—Extrasystoles usually require no treatment. If atrial fibrillation or flutter develops, rapid failure may be precipitated. Rapid digitalization is usually indicated in these cases.

C. Evaluation of Treatment: With proper selection of antimicrobial drugs, there should be marked improvement and defervescence in 72 hours or less. If this fails to occur, one must consider 3 main possibilities: (1) the presence of a serious complication such as empyema, pulmonary suppuration associated with bronchial obstruction, endocarditis, or meningitis; (2) infection by an organism other than the pneumococcus and resistant to the drug used; and (3) possible drug fever or other associated disease. If there is evidence of pleural fluid, it must be aspirated promptly, smeared, and cultured to detect infection or empyema which requires drainage. If an organism other than the pneumococcus is shown by laboratory examination to be the probable etiologic agent, treatment must be directed against it.

Complications

Complications of pneumococcal pneumonia occur with the following approximate frequencies: sterile pleural effusion (4–8%), empyema (0.5–2%), endocarditis and meningitis (0.1–0.3%), and pericarditis (0.1%). Other complications, eg, pneumococcal arthritis, are even more rare. Fibrous organization of the pneumonia (in place of resolution) occurs sometimes but rarely causes disability. All pleural fluid collections must be aspirated and examined by smear and culture to permit early treatment of empyema.

Prognosis

Untreated pneumococcal pneumonia has a mortality rate of 20–40%. The following are unfavorable prognostic signs: age over 45 years, presence of other disease (eg, heart failure, cirrhosis), pregnancy, absence of leukocytosis, bacteremia, marked proteinuria, pulmonary edema, and shock.

With early and adequate penicillin treatment, the

fatality rate is about 5%, but in bacteremic pneumonia it is 17%. Most fatalities occur in the age groups under 2 years and over 45 years. In untreated, uncomplicated cases, resolution by crisis (or more gradually) occurs 7–10 days after onset. Experimental vaccines of 12 types are in trial.

Austrian R: Random gleanings from a life with the pneumococcus. J Infect Dis 131:474, 1975.

Brewin A & others: High dose penicillin therapy in pneumococcal pneumonia. JAMA 230:409, 1974.

Sullivan RJ & others: Adult pneumonia in a general hospital: Etiology and risk factors. Arch Int Med 129:935, 1972.

Turck M: Current therapy of bacterial pneumonias. M Clin North America 51:541, 1967.

OTHER BACTERIAL PNEUMONIAS

Primary bacterial pneumonias caused by single bacterial species other than the pneumococcus may account for up to 15% of all bacterial pneumonias at present. All of these pneumonias may have somewhat similar physical findings and x-ray evidence of pulmonary infiltration or consolidation. For proper treatment it is crucial to identify the etiologic agent by blood culture and by sputum examination with stained smear and culture. Transtracheal aspiration or even lung puncture may be needed for specific diagnosis and treatment.

Klebsiella Pneumonia

Klebsiella pneumoniae (Friedländer's bacillus) occurs as a member of the normal bacterial flora in the respiratory tract or gut of 5–20% of the population. Primary pneumonia due to this organism occurs mainly in persons 40–60 years of age with a history of alcoholism, malnutrition, or debilitating diseases. Klebsiella pneumonia is also a frequent type of superinfection in persons hospitalized for serious disease, including other types of pneumonia treated with antimicrobial drugs.

The onset is usually sudden, with chills, fever, dyspnea, cyanosis, and profound toxicity. The sputum is often red ("currant jelly"), mucoid, sticky, and difficult to expectorate. Physical findings and white counts are variable. The disease may be fulminating and progress rapidly to a fatal outcome. In subacute forms, there is a tendency to necrosis of lung tissue and abscess formation.

The diagnosis is based on finding short, encapsulated gram-negative bacteria as the predominant organism in sputum smears (in poorly stained smears they may be mistaken for pneumococci) and klebsiellae in blood and sputum cultures. Immediate intensive antimicrobial treatment is essential. Kanamycin, 0.5 gm, is injected IM every 6–8 hours (15 mg/kg/day); and cephalothin, 6–10 gm IV, is sometimes given in addition. When drug-resistant klebsiella infections occur in a hospital environment, gentamicin, 5–8

mg/kg/day, may be injected IM in 3 equal doses. Antimicrobial treatment may have to be continued for more than 2 weeks to avoid relapses. General supportive treatment is the same as for pneumococcal pneumonia.

The fatality rate in untreated klebsiella pneumonia is 40–60%. Even with apparently adequate treatment, the fatality rate may be near 30%.

Pierce AK, Sanford, JP: Aerobic gram-negative pneumonias. Am Rev Resp Dis 110:647, 1974.

Haemophilus Influenzae Pneumonia

This is a rare form of primary bacterial pneumonia in adults. It has occurred in the presence of cardiac disease, hypogammaglobulinemia, and chronic lung disease. Symptoms and signs do not distinguish this from other bacterial pneumonias. The sputum may be bloody, but gram-stained smears may be misinterpreted. The diagnosis ultimately rests on the results of cultures of blood and sputum.

Treatment with ampicillin, 1–1.5 gm orally every 6 hours or 150 mg/kg/day IV, may be expected to cure the infection. An alternative method of treatment is with chloramphenicol, 0.5 gm orally every 6 hours. General measures are the same as for pneumococcal pneumonia.

Johnson WD & others: *Hemophilus Influenzae* pneumonia in adults: Report of five cases and review of the literature. Am Rev Resp Dis 97:1112, 1968.

Pseudomonas, Proteus, & Serratia Pneumonia

Pneumonias caused by various species of proteus, pseudomonas, and serratia occur with increasing frequency in debilitated persons with chronic lung or heart disease and alcoholism, or as superinfections in patients who have required inhalation therapy or tracheal suction and have received antimicrobial drugs. Contaminated equipment may be an important etiologic factor.

These pneumonias are associated with early delirium, massive consolidation often proceeding to necrosis and multiple abscess formation, and a high fatality rate. Gentamicin, 3–5 mg/kg/day IM in 3 divided doses, plus carbenicillin, 18–30 gm/day by IV infusion, appears to be a possible method of treatment. With renal failure, the dosage must be adjusted downward to prevent nephrotoxicity.

Meltz DJ, Grieco MH: *Serratia marcescens* pneumonia. Arch Int Med 132:359, 1973.

Pennington JE & others: Pseudomonas pneumonia. Am J Med 55:155, 1973.

Tillotson JR, Lerner AM: Characteristics of pneumonias caused by *B proteus.* Ann Int Med 68:287, 1968.

Streptococcal Pneumonia

Pneumonia due to hemolytic streptococci occurs usually as a sequel to viral infection of the respiratory tract, especially influenza or measles, or in persons with underlying pulmonary disease. The patients are usually severely toxic and cyanotic. Pleural effusion develops frequently and early and progresses to empyema in one-third of untreated patients. The diagnosis rests on finding large numbers of streptococci in smears of sputum and culturing hemolytic streptococci from blood and sputum.

The treatment of choice is with penicillin G in a dosage similar to that for pneumococcal pneumonia (see above). If treatment is started early, the prognosis is good.

Staphylococcal Pneumonia

Pneumonia caused by *Staphylococcus aureus* occurs as a sequel to viral infections of the respiratory tract (eg, influenza) and in debilitated (eg, postsurgical) patients or hospitalized infants, especially after antimicrobial drug administration. There is often a history of a mild illness with headache, cough, and generalized aches which abruptly changes to a very severe illness with high fever, chills, and exaggerated cough with purulent or blood-streaked sputum and deep cyanosis. There may be early signs of pleural effusion, empyema, or tension pneumothorax. X-ray examination reveals lung consolidation, pneumatoceles, abscesses, empyema, and pneumothorax. The demonstration of pyopneumothorax and of cavities with air-fluid levels by x-ray is highly suggestive of staphylococcal pneumonia. The diagnosis must be made by examination of sputum by smear (masses of white cells and gram-positive cocci, many intracellular), culture (predominantly *S aureus*), pleural fluid culture, and blood culture. The white count is elevated, usually to more than 20,000/cu mm.

Initial therapy (based on sputum smear) consists of full systemic doses of a cephalosporin, a penicillinase-resistant penicillin, or vancomycin. The dosages are as follows: cephalothin, 8–14 gm/day IV; methicillin, 8–16 gm/day IV; vancomycin, 2 gm/day IV; nafcillin, 6–12 gm/day IV. If the staphylococcus proves to be penicillin-sensitive by laboratory test, penicillin G, 20–60 million units/day IV, is the antibiotic of choice. If empyema develops, drainage must be established. If pneumothorax develops, it is treated as described on p 148.

The prognosis varies with the underlying condition of the patient and the drug susceptibility of the organism.

Cattaneo SM, Kilman JW: Surgical therapy of empyema. Arch Surg 106:564, 1973.

Bacteroides Pneumonia

Pneumonias caused by anaerobic Bacteroides species occur as complications of abdominal or pelvic bacteroides infections and in patients with chronic lung disease. Pleural effusions and empyema develop early and are a main feature of the disease, which is often subacute or chronic. The diagnosis is based on the foul odor of the empyema and the demonstration of pleomorphic gram-negative anaerobes. Drainage of empyema must be combined with intensive penicillin or clindamycin treatment.

Bartlett JG & others: Percutaneous transtracheal aspiration in the diagnosis of anaerobic pulmonary infection. Ann Int Med 79:535, 1973.

Tillotson JR, Lerner AM: Bacteroides pneumonias: Character of cases with empyema. Ann Int Med 68:308, 1968.

Pneumocystis Carinii Pneumonia

This is a rare disorder which occurs in debilitated children or in patients who are immunosuppressed or suffer from leukemia. The diagnosis can be made by lung biopsy and the demonstration of typical cysts of the parasite *P carinii* in impression smears from lung tissue stained with methenamine-silver. Pentamidine isethionate, 4 mg/kg/day IM, may be curative.

Gentry LO & others: *Pneumocystis carinii* pneumonia. California Med 116:6, April 1972.

Walzer PD & others: *Pneumocystis carinii* pneumonia in the United States. Ann Int Med 80:83, 1974.

"MIXED" BACTERIAL PNEUMONIAS
(Hypostatic Pneumonia, "Terminal" Pneumonia, Bronchopneumonia)

Essentials of Diagnosis

- Variable onset of fever, cough, dyspnea, expectoration.
- Symptoms and signs often masked by primary (debilitating) disease.
- Greenish-yellow sputum (purulent) with mixed flora.
- Leukocytosis (often absent in aged and debilitated).
- Patchy infiltration on chest x-ray.

General Considerations

Mixed bacterial pneumonias include those in which culture and smear reveal several organisms, not one of which can clearly be identified as the etiologic agent. They usually appear as complications of surgery or other trauma, various chronic illnesses (cardiac failure, advanced carcinoma, uremia), and certain acute illnesses (eg, measles, influenza). They are common complications of chronic pulmonary diseases such as bronchiectasis and emphysema. Old people are most commonly affected ("terminal" pneumonia). Patients treated with intermittent positive pressure breathing apparatus or immunosuppressive drugs may develop pneumonia due to gram-negative rods.

The following findings in a debilitated, chronically ill, or aged person suggest a complicating pneumonia: (1) worsening of cough, dyspnea, cyanosis; (2) low-grade, irregular fever; (3) purulent sputum; and (4) patchy basal densities on a chest film (in addition to previously noted densities caused by a primary underlying disease, if any).

Clinical Findings

A. Symptoms and Signs: The onset is usually insidious, with low-grade fever, cough, expectoration, and dyspnea which may become marked and lead to cyanosis. The physical findings are extremely variable and may not be impressive against a background of chronic cardiac or pulmonary disease. Those signs listed under other bacterial pneumonias may also be present with this type.

B. Laboratory Findings: The appearance of a greenish or yellowish (purulent) sputum should suggest a complicating pneumonia. Smears and cultures reveal a mixed flora, often including anaerobes. Predominant types should be noted. Leukocytosis is often absent in the aged and debilitated patient.

C. X-Ray Findings: X-ray shows patchy, irregular infiltrations, most commonly posterior and basal (in bedridden patients). Abscess formation may be observed. Careful interpretation is necessary in order to avoid confusion with shadows due to preexisting heart or lung disease.

Differential Diagnosis

Mixed bacterial pneumonias must be differentiated from tuberculosis, carcinoma, and other specific mycotic, bacterial, and viral pulmonary infections (to which they may be secondary).

Treatment

Where no specific microorganisms are present in the sputum, broad-spectrum antibiotics can be used. Give ampicillin, 1–1.5 gm, or tetracycline, 0.5 gm, every 6 hours orally. If staphylococci are present in the sputum in large numbers, treat as for staphylococcal pneumonia. If gram-negative rods are prevalent, their identification and drug sensitivity guide treatment.

If anaerobes, especially bacteroides, play a significant part, penicillin (for *Bacteroides melaninogenicus*) or clindamycin (for *B fragilis*) may have to be given.

Prognosis

The prognosis depends upon the nature and severity of the underlying pulmonary disease and varies with the predominating organism.

Gorbach SL, Bartlett JG: Anaerobic infections. New England J Med 290:1177, 1974.

Graybill JR & others: Nosocomial pneumonia. Am Rev Resp Dis 108:1130, 1973.

Hahn HH: Beaty HN: Transtracheal aspiration in the evaluation of patients with pneumonia. Ann Int Med 72:183, 1970.

Klein JO: Diagnostic lung puncture in the pneumonias of children. Pediatrics 44:486, 1969.

ASPIRATION PNEUMONIA

Aspiration pneumonia is an especially severe type of pneumonia with a high mortality rate. It results from the aspiration of gastric contents. Important predisposing factors include impairment of the swallowing mechanism (eg, esophageal disease), inadequate cough reflex (eg, anesthesia, postoperative state, CNS disease, drug abuse), and impaired gastric emptying (eg, pyloric obstruction). Pulmonary injury is due in large part to the low pH (< 2.5) of gastric secretions.

Scattered areas of pulmonary edema and bronchospasm occur, and the x-ray appearance may be confused with that of pulmonary emboli, atelectasis, bronchopneumonia, and congestive heart failure.

Treatment is as for "mixed" bacterial pneumonias. The use of corticosteroids in full doses seems to be of value in reducing the severity of the inflammatory reaction (eg, hydrocortisone, 200 mg IM initially and 50 mg IM every 6 hours for 2 days; then 25 mg IM every 6 hours for the next 2 days).

Bronchoscopic aspiration may be attempted, but it may be possible to remove only a small amount of the aspirated fluids. The mortality rate is over 60%.

Bartlett JG, Gorbach SL, Finegold SM: The bacteriology of aspiration pneumonia. Am J Med 56:202, 1974.

Cameron JL, Zuidema GD: Aspiration pneumonia. JAMA 219:1194, 1972.

Ribaudo CA, Grace WJ: Pulmonary aspiration. Am J Med 50:510, 1971.

Vandam LD: Aspiration of gastric contents in the operative period. New England J Med 273:1206, 1965.

PRIMARY ATYPICAL PNEUMONIA
(Viral or Mycoplasmal Pneumonia)

Essentials of Diagnosis

- Gradually increasing cough with scanty sputum and fever.
- Minimal physical signs on chest examination.
- X-ray evidence of infiltration.
- White blood count in normal range or low.

General Considerations

The PAP syndrome may be caused by a variety of viral and mycoplasmal agents. It must be differentiated from specific bacterial, mycobacterial, and fungal pneumonias and from neoplastic diseases. An attempt should be made to diagnose the specific agent causing the infection by means of appropriate laboratory tests and epidemiologic investigations. Prominent causative agents include adenoviruses (especially types 4, 7, and 14 in military personnel), influenza viruses, and *Mycoplasma pneumoniae*. Viral and mycoplasmal pneumonias are transmitted by droplets from person to person. Only 10–20% of *M pneumoniae* infections produce pneumonia; the others are asymptomatic or present as upper respiratory disease. However, mycoplasmal pneumonia is probably the most common type of pneumonia encountered in otherwise healthy young adults (eg, university students).

Clinical Findings

A. Symptoms and Signs: The clinical picture varies widely, both in the spontaneous and experimentally induced forms. Symptoms may be mild, as in the "common cold" or "flu"; hence the likelihood that many diseases previously diagnosed as "upper respiratory infection" were in fact pneumonias. Occasional severe cases occur which may be fatal.

The disease often begins as a mild upper respiratory tract infection proceeding to a dry cough which grows worse, increasing fever, hoarseness, headache, and generalized aching. Extreme fatigue is common. Pleuritic pain and effusion are uncommon.

Physical findings are frequently sparse and sometimes completely absent in the face of a surprising degree of infiltration as seen on x-ray. Rales are usually heard. Diminished breath sounds over the involved areas may be noted in early cases.

B. Laboratory Findings: The sputum is scanty, rarely blood-tinged. Smear and culture show only the usual flora of the mouth. The white count may be normal or may show mild to severe leukopenia. Mild leukocytosis may appear later in the course of the disease.

Autohemagglutinins for human type O erythrocytes (cold agglutinins) appear in the convalescent phase of mycoplasmal pneumonia (seldom before the second week) in about 50% of cases. To be significant, a rise in titer must be $> 1:10$ during the second week.

Specific antibodies to mycoplasma may be demonstrated. *M pneumoniae* can be grown from respiratory secretions on special media.

C. X-Ray Findings: Linear infiltrates tend to appear first at hilar areas, extending later into the middle and basal portions of both lungs. The initial appearance of these changes may be delayed, and clearing on x-ray usually occurs within 3 weeks. There is considerable variation in the x-ray pattern, and no configuration is diagnostic.

Complications

Pleural effusions occur in 5–20% of cases. Atelectasis, pneumothorax, pericarditis, myocarditis, secondary bacterial pneumonia, and acute hemolytic anemia may occur. Bronchiectasis also has been seen as a late complication.

Treatment

General measures are as for pneumococcal pneumonia.

In mild cases of mycoplasmal pneumonia antimicrobial drugs are not indicated. Severe cases may be treated with erythromycin (0.5 gm orally every 6 hours) or tetracycline (0.5 gm orally every 6–8 hours). Rarely is it necessary to administer these drugs intravenously.

Prognosis

Mortality in untreated cases is low. Fever usually disappears by the 10th day, although x-ray abnormalities persist for longer periods.

Alexander ER & others: Pneumonia due to *Mycoplasma pneumoniae*. New England J Med 275:131, 1966.
See also references under Pneumococcal Pneumonia.

LIPOID PNEUMONIA

This disease is an aspiration pneumonia associated with the use of oily medications. Fibrosis and the presence of macrophages containing oil droplets are the histologic features.

Symptoms and signs vary widely, at times resembling those of acute pneumonia (fever, productive cough) or chronic lung disease (weight loss, night sweats). There may be no symptoms but striking x-ray densities. Patients must be carefully questioned about the use of mineral oil, oily nose drops, or ointments used in the nose. Physical signs vary accordingly and are not diagnostic. Peribronchial infiltrations, diffuse lobar densities, scattered discrete densities, and even central cavitation have all been described on x-ray. Leukocytosis may occur with acute symptoms. Proper examination of the sputum for oil droplet-laden macrophages will often establish the diagnosis.

Treatment is nonspecific and symptomatic. Use of the oil-containing preparation should be discontinued. When this is done, further progression of the disease usually does not occur and the prognosis is good. Large solitary masses may require resection.

Hinshaw HC, Garland LH: *Diseases of the Chest*, 3rd ed. Saunders, 1969.
Schwindt WD, Barbee RA, Jones RJ: Lipoid pneumonia. Arch Surg 95:652; 1967.

PNEUMONIAS DUE TO SPECIFIC VIRUSES, RICKETTSIAE, & CHLAMYDIAE

The important specific viral, rickettsial, and chlamydial (bedsonial) infections which may produce pneumonia include influenza, Q fever, Rocky Mountain spotted fever, typhus, and psittacosis (ornithosis). The exanthematous viral diseases (rubeola, varicella, variola, and vaccinia) all give rise occasionally to specific pneumonias.

These pneumonias are indistinguishable from primary atypical pneumonia on the basis of pulmonary physical and x-ray findings. Diagnosis depends upon recognition of the specific systemic disease by extrapulmonary features (eg, rash), a history of exposure to vectors (eg, parrots, ticks), epidemiologic information, and demonstration of a significant rise in specific antibody titers. Bacterial superinfection in viral disease may be difficult to rule out.

The treatment of viral pneumonia is symptomatic. Anti-infective chemotherapy for chlamydial diseases is discussed in Chapter 23. Treat rickettsial pneumonias as outlined in the discussion of rickettsioses.

See references under Pneumococcal Pneumonia.

LUNG ABSCESS

Essentials of Diagnosis
- Development of pulmonary symptoms about 1–2 weeks after possible aspiration, bronchial obstruction, or previous pneumonia.
- Septic fever and sweats, periodic sudden expectoration of large amounts of purulent, foul-smelling, or "musty" sputum. Hemoptysis may occur.
- X-ray density with central radiolucency and fluid level.

General Considerations
Lung abscess is an inflammatory lesion which is the result of necrosis of lung tissue. It is characterized by the onset of pulmonary symptoms 10–14 days after disruptions of bronchopulmonary function or alteration of bronchopulmonary structure by any of the following means: (1) Aspiration of infected material (eg, during oral surgery). (2) Suppression of cough reflex (eg, in coma or with drugs). (3) Bronchial obstruction (eg, postoperative atelectasis, foreign bodies, neoplasms). (4) Pneumonias, especially bacterial. (5) Ischemia (eg, following pulmonary infarction). (6) Septicemia (especially staphylococcal). Infection with pyogenic or anaerobic bacteria in any of these situations causes lung abscess. The usual location is the superior segment of the lower lobe or the lower portion of the upper lobe of the right lung. Pleuritis and—at times—rupture into the pleural space, with bronchopleural fistula (empyema, pyopneumothorax), may occur.

If inadequately treated, lung abscess usually becomes chronic.

Clinical Findings
A. Symptoms and Signs: Onset may be abrupt or gradual. Symptoms include fever (septic type), sweats, cough, and chest pain. Cough is often nonproductive at onset. Expectoration of foul-smelling brown or gray sputum (mixed infection with anaerobic organisms) or green or yellow "musty" sputum without an offensive odor (infection with a single pyogenic organism), often suddenly in large quantities, is common in lung abscess. Blood-streaked sputum is also common.

Pleural pain, especially with coughing, is common because the abscess is often subpleural.

Weight loss, anemia, and pulmonary osteoarthropathy may appear when the abscess becomes chronic (8–12 weeks after onset).

Physical findings may be minimal. Consolidation due to pneumonitis surrounding the abscess is the most frequent finding. Rupture into the pleural space produces signs of fluid or pneumothorax.

B. Laboratory Findings: Sputum cultures are usually inadequate in determining the bacterial cause of a lung abscess. Transtracheal aspirates (see Ries reference) should be obtained with the proper technic employed to culture anaerobic organisms in addition to the usual aerobic cultures. Special media and methods of transporting specimens are required for anaerobic organisms.

Smear and cultures for the tubercle bacilli are required, especially in lesions of the upper lobe and in chronic abscess.

C. X-Ray Findings: A dense shadow is the initial finding. A central radiolucency, often with a visible fluid level, appears as surrounding densities subside. Tomograms (section films) may be necessary to demonstrate cavitation.

Chest films may also reveal associated primary lesions (eg, bronchogenic carcinoma); allow assessment of response to therapy; provide anatomic localization where surgery is contemplated; and give information on pleural complications.

D. Instrumental Examination: Bronchoscopy should be performed routinely to obtain specimens for examination and to improve drainage and remove possible foreign bodies. Up to 10% of lung abscesses may be secondary to bronchogenic carcinoma.

Differential Diagnosis
Differentiate from other causes of pulmonary cavitation: tuberculosis, bronchogenic carcinoma, mycotic infections, and staphylococcal pneumonia.

Treatment
Postural drainage and bronchoscopy are important to promote drainage of secretions.

A. Acute Abscess: Intensive antibacterial therapy is necessary to prevent further destruction of lung tissue. While the results of cultures and sensitivity tests are pending, treatment can be started with penicillin, 600,000 units every 6 hours (erythromycin, 500 mg every 6 hours, can be used in patients with a history of penicillin allergy), and tetracycline, 500 mg every 6 hours. If the patient improves, long-term treatment (1–2 months) is necessary to assure a cure. If the patient fails to respond significantly to the initial treatment, surgery may be indicated without delay. Failure of fever to subside after 2 weeks of therapy, abscess diameter of more than 6 cm, and very thick cavity walls are all factors which lessen the likelihood of success with nonsurgical treatment alone.

B. Chronic Abscess: After acute systemic manifestations have subsided, the abscess may persist. Although many of these patients with chronic lung abscess can be cured with long-term treatment with appropriate antibacterial agents, surgery is occasionally required.

Complications
Rupture of pus into the pleural space (empyema)

causes severe symptoms: increase in fever, marked pleural pain, and sweating; the patient becomes "toxic" in appearance. In chronic abscess, severe and even fatal hemorrhage may occur. Metastatic brain abscess is a well-recognized complication. Bronchiectasis may occur as a sequel to lung abscess even when the abscess itself is cured. Amyloidosis may occur if suppuration has continued for a long time.

Prognosis

The prognosis is excellent in acute abscess with prompt and intensive antibiotic therapy. The incidence of chronic abscess is consequently low. In chronic cases, surgery is curative.

Barnett TB, Herring CL: Lung abscess. Arch Int Med 127:217, 1971.
Bartlett JG, Rosenblatt JE, Finegold SM: Percutaneous transtracheal aspiration in the diagnosis of anaerobic pulmonary infection. Ann Int Med 79:535, 1973.
Bartlett JG & others: Bacteriology and treatment of primary lung abscess. Ann Rev Resp Dis 109:510, 1974.
Perlman LV, Lerner E, D'Esopo N: Clinical classification and analysis of 97 cases of lung abscess. Am Rev Resp Dis 99:390, 1969.
Ries K & others: Transtracheal aspiration in pulmonary infection. Arch Int Med 133:453, 1974.

PULMONARY TUBERCULOSIS

Essentials of Diagnosis

- Presenting signs and symptoms are usually minimal: malaise, lassitude, easy fatigability, anorexia, mild weight loss, afternoon fever, cough, apical rales, hemoptysis.
- Symptoms and signs may be entirely absent.
- Positive tuberculin skin test; especially a recent change from negative to positive.
- Apical or subapical infiltrates, often with cavities.
- *Mycobacterium tuberculosis* in sputum or in gastric or tracheal washings.

General Considerations

Pulmonary tuberculosis is a specific pulmonary infection caused by the acid-fast organism *M tuberculosis,* and characterized by the formation of tubercles in the lung. The first or primary infection is usually a self-limited disease in children which escapes detection. A few develop progressive primary tuberculosis. Another small percentage of patients, after a latency period of months to years, develop progressive pulmonary disease of the adult type. Primary infection occurring in adults may evolve into adult type disease without developing the characteristic changes of primary disease seen in children. While most people who are infected at any age never develop the disease, it is not always possible to predict which ones are at risk. Malnutrition, diabetes, measles, chronic corticosteroid administration, silicosis, and general debility may predispose to the progression of infection to disease. Once primary infection has occurred, the person's future risk is from those same tubercle bacilli. Superinfection ("exogenous reinfection") occurs rarely if at all.

Clinical Findings

A. Symptoms and Signs: Symptoms may be absent—or mild and nonspecific—in the presence of active disease. When present, the most frequent symptoms are cough, malaise, easy fatigability, weight loss, low-grade afternoon fever, night sweats, and pleuritic pain. Cough, when present, has no specific characteristics. Blood in the sputum is strongly suggestive of tuberculosis. Patients with pulmonary tuberculosis occasionally present with symptoms due to extrapulmonary complications such as laryngeal, renal, or CNS involvement.

Pulmonary signs may be difficult to elicit even in the presence of active disease. Fine persistent rales over the upper lobes may be found. These are best heard during inspiration after a slight cough. Advanced disease may lead to retraction of the chest wall, deviation of the trachea, wheezes, rales, and signs of pneumonic consolidation. Signs of cavitation are unreliable.

Pulmonary tuberculosis cannot be ruled out by physical examination alone. A chest x-ray is the minimum requirement.

B. Skin Testing:

1. Tuberculin skin test—This test is based on skin hypersensitivity to a specific bacterial protein antigen. Tuberculin may be administered intracutaneously (Mantoux) and by multiple puncture methods (eg, tine test, Heaf test). The intracutaneous method employing purified protein derivative (PPD-S) in the intermediate strength (5 tuberculin units) is the most reliable, and current recommendations are that a much more stable, standardized liquid PPD containing Tween-80 be used rather than the dissolved tablets, which quickly lose their potency once in solution. The patch test (Vollmer) should not be used.

a. Positive reaction—A positive reaction (induration 10 mm or more in diameter) indicates past or present infection. The skin test becomes positive 2–8 weeks after infection with the tubercle bacillus. The incidence of positive reactions varies with population groups and is higher among disadvantaged segments in all countries. False-positive reactions may occur as a result of cross-sensitivity to atypical mycobacteria (see below).

b. Negative reaction—A negative reaction (induration less than 5 mm in diameter), for all practical purposes, rules out tuberculous etiology of pulmonary disease. Anergy (disappearance or marked decrease in the tuberculin reaction in the presence of a tuberculous infection) is a rare phenomenon which occurs with overwhelming tuberculosis, exanthematous diseases, corticosteroid treatment, sarcoidosis, debility, and occasionally with increased age. The possibility of defective testing material must also be considered.

c. Doubtful reaction—A doubtful reaction (induration of 5–9 mm) may be due to a very recent infection, cross-sensitivity to nontuberculous mycobacteria, or partial anergy due to one of the causes listed above. If no disease is seen in the chest x-ray, repeat the skin test in 1 month. If it is still "doubtful," repeat the test again in 3 months, and if it is still in question repeat the chest x-ray. In the presence of x-ray lesions and a "doubtful" reaction, the diagnosis should be pursued with bacteriologic studies.

d. Conversion reaction—A conversion reaction is a positive reaction that has developed within a year after a known negative reaction. It implies recent infection and is an important finding because the risk of developing disease is greatest during the first 1–2 years after infection.

2. Bacteriologic studies—Recovery of the tubercle bacillus from sputum or gastric or tracheal washings is the only incontrovertible diagnostic finding. Pleural effusion fluid or biopsy material, tracheal wash with saline, or sputum induction by inhalation of a heated aerosol (5% saline) produces a more reliable specimen for bacteriologic examination if there is no spontaneous sputum production.

a. Sputum—Direct smears are positive when the bacterial count is high. Positive smears should always be confirmed by culture, although treatment is usually started before culture results are completed. Sensitivities to the major antituberculosis drugs should be determined for organisms obtained by culture.

Fresh sputum should be obtained for culture, although tubercle bacilli will usually survive several days in specimens transmitted by mail.

Culture is more sensitive than smear examination, but the time required for growth of organisms (4–6 weeks) is a disadvantage. Certain atypical acid-fast organisms may cause confusion. Newer bacteriologic methods usually permit the differentiation of *M tuberculosis* from atypical mycobacteria as well as differentiation of the several groups of the latter (see below).

b. Gastric washings—Stained smears of gastric washings are of no value because of the occurrence of nontuberculous acid-fast organisms. Culture of gastric contents is especially useful for patients who cannot cooperate (eg, children, senile patients).

3. Biopsies—Enlarged lymph nodes in supraclavicular or cervical areas should be searched for carefully, since they may reveal an extension of the underlying pulmonary disease easily accessible by biopsy. In addition to histologic examination, excised nodes should always be cultured for tubercle bacilli and fungi. Pleural and pulmonary biopsy may also give valuable diagnostic information.

C. X-Ray Findings: Chest films disclose disease in almost all cases. Failures occur where lesions are hidden behind ribs, cardiovascular structures, and the diaphragm. A single film is usually insufficient for diagnosis. Although many features suggest the likelihood of tuberculosis (see below), there is no pathognomonic x-ray pattern.

Hilar lymph node enlargement associated with a small parenchymal lesion which heals with calcification is the usual picture of primary infection. Many "primaries" (proved by change of tuberculin skin test from negative to positive) do not present x-ray abnormalities. Very large nodes are unusual in adults, in whom "primary" infection cannot be distinguished from postprimary progression by x-ray findings.

Apical and subapical infiltrations are the usual presenting x-ray features of "adult" (postprimary progression) tuberculosis. Lordotic views may be required to reveal such lesions where uncertainty exists in the posteroanterior projection.

Cavitation is presumptive evidence of tuberculous activity. Tomograms are occasionally necessary for the demonstration of cavities.

Fibrotic disease, with dense, well delineated strands, may dominate the picture. The physician should not assume that these lesions are inactive.

Solitary nodules, miliary lesions, and lobar consolidation (acute caseous pneumonia) present difficult problems in differential diagnosis.

Lower lung field tuberculosis in the absence of upper lobe lesions is uncommon (about 3% of all cases).

Serial films are often crucial in the establishment of activity and are indispensable in the selection and evaluation of therapy.

Differential Diagnosis

Tuberculosis can mimic nearly any pulmonary disease. Important diseases to be considered are bacterial and viral pneumonias, lung abscess, pulmonary mycoses, bronchogenic carcinoma, sarcoidosis, pneumoconioses, and "atypical" (nontuberculous) mycobacterial infections.

Recovery of tubercle bacilli by culture establishes the diagnosis of tuberculosis. A negative tuberculin skin test makes the diagnosis of tuberculosis very unlikely. If carcinoma is suspected and cannot be promptly excluded, early tissue diagnosis by thoracotomy may be indicated without waiting for culture results.

Prevention

A. Isolation Precautions: Persons in contact with patients with active tuberculosis who are newly diagnosed or suspected of having the disease should wear masks, although the protection afforded is questionable. Patients must be taught to effectively cover the mouth and nose with disposable tissue during coughing. The patient should wear a mask when hospital personnel are present or when he leaves his room.

Patients with previously untreated disease who are cooperative, who have no cough (or cover their mouths when coughing), and who have been on antituberculosis drug treatment for at least 2 weeks are not hazardous to be around even without special precautions. Hospital personnel with negative tuberculin skin tests who are in contact with tuberculosis patients should have repeat skin tests twice a year.

B. Examination of Contacts: Close contacts must

be examined by skin test when an active case is discovered. Those with positive tests should have a chest x-ray. Those who have negative skin tests should be retested 2 months after contact with the active case has been broken. Those with positive skin tests and negative x-rays should receive preventive treatment with isoniazid (see ¶ D, below). Some authorities recommend giving all close contacts (with negative x-rays) isoniazid for 1 year whether the skin test is positive or negative.

C. BCG Vaccination: Although it is generally agreed that BCG vaccination offers some protection to tuberculin-negative persons, several factors limit its usefulness. In most parts of the world, the risk of developing tuberculosis is slight among tuberculin-negative persons. Converting tuberculin-negative people to positive reactors by vaccination deprives the clinician of an important tuberculosis control measure, ie, the discovery of early infection by skin testing and treatment of converters with isoniazid. For these reasons, BCG vaccination is recommended only where exposure to tuberculosis is great and the usual tuberculosis control measures are not possible.

D. Treatment of Tuberculin Reactors (Without Other Evidence of Active Disease): Certain tuberculin reactors should be given preventive treatment with isoniazid. These include the following:

(1) Close contacts of recently diagnosed tuberculosis patients with active disease. Infants and children who have had such exposure should be given isoniazid even if the tuberculin test is negative. If they are still negative 3 months after exposure has been discontinued, treatment may be stopped. Adult contacts who are initially negative to tuberculin should be retested in 3 months and treated if the test has become positive.

(2) Persons with positive skin tests and x-ray findings compatible with nonprogressive tuberculosis.

(3) Those who have had a conversion from a negative to a positive skin test within 2 years.

(4) Persons with special risk factors such as prolonged corticosteroid treatment for other disease, immunosuppressive therapy, hematologic and reticuloendothelial disorders such as Hodgkin's disease and leukemia, diabetes mellitus, silicosis, and postgastrectomy patients.

(5) All patients under age 35 should be considered for preventive treatment in the absence of the conditions listed above. Children up to age 6 should be treated.

Preventive treatment for the above groups consists of isoniazid, 300 mg daily (10 mg/kg/day for children) for 1 year.

Prior to treatment, the presence of possible contraindications should be determined:

(1) A history of adverse reaction to isoniazid.

(2) Evidence or strong suspicion of progressive tuberculosis. (These patients should be treated as outlined below for active disease.)

(3) A previous course of adequate treatment with isoniazid.

(4) The presence of active liver disease.

(5) Pregnancy. Because of potential risk to the fetus, preventive treatment should be postponed until the postpartum period.

Because of the known—although low—incidence of isoniazid-induced liver damage, patients receiving preventive treatment should be cautioned regarding the symptoms of isoniazid toxity (unexplained fever, rash, gastroentestinal symptoms) and advised to stop the drug and report to the physician if such symptoms appear. Routine liver function testing of patients without a history of liver disease is not useful. Patients with a history of liver disease for whom preventive treatment is strongly indicated should be investigated before treatment and monitored periodically during treatment.

Treatment

A. Drug Therapy: (See Table 6–3.) Drug treatment is the most important single measure in the management of tuberculosis and is indicated in all cases of active disease.

Bed rest is advisable if there are symptoms such as fever, hemoptysis, or severe cough, and usually is needed only for a few weeks. In general, return to normal physical activity is permitted following a brief period of observation after an effective drug regimen has been established. Patients with positive sputum must be isolated until effective treatment has been given for at least 2 weeks.

The present recommendation is for prolonged administration of combinations of the major drugs listed below. Many patients seem to benefit from prolonged treatment even after moderate resistance of the organisms to the drugs has been shown by sensitivity tests. Most authorities advise a minimum of 12 months of drug treatment after the "inactive" status has been attained (x-ray lesions stable, no cavitation, and cultures negative—all for at least 6 months).

The principal drugs currently used in the treatment of pulmonary tuberculosis are isoniazid (INH), rifampin, streptomycin, and ethambutol. Experience accumulated to date with the 2 newest major drugs, rifampin and ethambutol, suggests that 3-drug regimens may no longer be necessary for initial treatment or for retreatment. For initial treatment, rifampin-isoniazid is probably the most effective and least toxic regimen. Isoniazid-ethambutol is also a very effective combination. It is suggested that, when possible, rifampin-isoniazid be given for the first 3–4 months and that isoniazid-ethambutol then be substituted for the duration of treatment. When rifampin is not used, streptomycin should be added in the treatment of far-advanced disease.

For retreatment, when neither drug has been previously used, rifampin-ethambutol is the combination of choice.

Sensitivity tests on tubercle bacilli recovered by culture should be started, using the major drugs, before treatment is initiated. When the results of these studies are obtained (4–6 weeks later), it may be necessary to modify the drug regimen.

Table 6—3. Primary antituberculosis drugs.

Drug	Adult Dose	Remarks
Isoniazid (INH)	5—10 mg/kg/day orally*	With the sole exception of isoniazid treatment
Rifampin	600 mg/day orally†	of tuberculin reactors, these drugs should not
Streptomycin	1 gm IM daily or twice weekly	be used singly in tuberculosis (see text).
Ethambutol‡	15 mg/kg/day orally in a single dose	
Aminosalicylic acid (PAS)	4—5 gm orally 3 times daily after meals	Use as a second drug only when ethambutol is not available.
Combined therapy (initial treatment)		
Isoniazid and	As above	Preferred regimen, at least for the first 3—4 months; then change to isoniazid-ethambutol.
rifampin	As above	
Isoniazid and	As above	Alternative regimen: Use all 3 initially, stopping streptomycin after cultures are negative. Use
ethambutol and	As above	streptomycin daily for first 2 weeks.
streptomycin	As above	

*May be given in a single dose. When 10 mg/kg/day are used, give also pyridoxine, 25—50 mg/day orally.
†In children, 15—20 mg/kg daily, 600 mg maximum.
‡Monitor visual acuity (see text).

1. Isoniazid (INH)—This is the most effective drug currently available. However, when used alone its effectiveness is decreased by the early emergence of bacterial resistance.

Isoniazid is indicated for any active tuberculosis lesion, including primary tuberculosis in children. It is of particular value in miliary tuberculosis, tuberculous meningitis, and other forms of extrapulmonary tuberculosis. Adverse reactions to the drug are infrequent with the usual dose of 5 mg/kg/day. Hepatitis (apparently due to isoniazid) has been reported more frequently in the past few years. Caution should be used in prescribing the drug for patients with liver dysfunction. All patients should be advised to stop the drug and report to their physician if any signs or symptoms appear that could be due to the medicine. Hypersensitivity reactions may occur. With large doses, peripheral neuropathy and, rarely, CNS irritability may occur. The latter are related to pyridoxine depletion. Supplementary doses of pyridoxine (25—50 mg/day orally) should be given.

2. Rifampin—Rifampin is a semisynthetic derivative of rifamycin. It is given orally and is well tolerated except for occasional gastrointestinal irritation and rare hypersensitivity reactions. Its teratogenic potential when used in pregnant women is not yet known. Its use with one or more of the major drugs, preferably including isoniazid, can be recommended for the initial treatment or the retreatment of tuberculosis. It is still expensive.

The adult dose is 600 mg daily orally in one dose; for children, give 10—20 mg/kg/day orally, not to exceed 600 mg/day.

3. Streptomycin sulfate—The indications for this drug are the same as for isoniazid except that it is less effective than isoniazid in advanced tuberculosis. It must be given in combination with other drugs. Streptomycin may cause 8th nerve damage (vertigo and, rarely, deafness), especially with prolonged daily use. This may become irreversible if the drug is continued.

Toxic reactions to streptomycin are few when the drug is given twice weekly, which gives an adequate therapeutic response except in the more serious forms of the disease, where daily dosage may be necessary. Generalized dermatitis occasionally occurs, in which case the drug must be discontinued. Perioral numbness often appears shortly after injection and may last for several hours. By itself it can be ignored.

4. Ethambutol—At present, the principal indication for use of ethambutol is as a replacement for aminosalicylic acid. Ethambutol is given orally, 15 mg/kg/day. The daily amount should be rounded off to the nearest 100 mg and given as a single dose.

Ethambutol is relatively free of side-effects. Retrobulbar neuritis has been noted, but when the drug is used in the recommended dosage this has been a minor and reversible complication. Visual acuity should be determined before and monthly during treatment; the drug should be stopped if a decrease in visual acuity occurs. Its use should be avoided in infants and young children in whom visual acuity cannot be monitored.

5. Aminosalicylic acid (PAS)—This drug has a low level of antituberculosis activity but when used with other drugs delays the emergence of resistant organisms. Toxic reactions are frequent. When fever, dermatitis, or hepatitis due to PAS toxicity occurs, the drug must be stopped. Diarrhea and nausea and vomiting may sometimes be overcome by using a different form of the drug or by stopping the drug for several days and then resuming it in small doses and gradually increasing it to the usual dose.

6. Other antituberculosis drugs—These are more

toxic and less effective than those described above. They are used in various combinations in the treatment of disease resistant to the primary drugs. Retreatment in the presence of resistant organisms should be guided by drug sensitivity tests. The addition of a single effective drug to a failing regimen is usually fruitless. A planned program using at least 3 carefully selected drugs simultaneously is recommended. The second line drugs ethionamide, cycloserine, pyrazinamide, and viomycin are discussed in Chapter 28.

7. **Corticosteroids**—The corticosteroids are used occasionally in conjunction with antituberculosis drug treatment in certain extrapulmonary forms of tuberculosis. Their use in pulmonary tuberculosis is beneficial only in extensive disease with severe toxic symptoms.

B. Collapse Therapy (Pneumothorax, Pneumoperitoneum): This type of treatment is no longer used in the treatment of tuberculosis.

C. Surgery:

1. **Pulmonary resection**—Resection is an important mode of treatment in selected cases, although very few patients now require surgery for pulmonary tuberculosis. Pulmonary resection is indicated in any of the following circumstances: (1) When there is a localized pulmonary nodule and the possibility of cancer cannot be excluded. (2) For bronchial stenosis. (3) For any localized chronic focus which has not improved substantially after 3–6 months of adequate drug therapy, and where tubercle bacilli persist in the sputum.

2. **Thoracoplasty**—This operation is no longer used as a primary treatment measure. It is occasionally used (1) to reduce the pleural "dead space" after a large pulmonary resection and thus minimize distention of the remaining lung, or (2) to close a chronic empyema space.

D. Diet: No special diets have been shown to be of benefit in tuberculosis. Normal weight should be maintained.

E. Climate: There is little evidence that climate is of any significance in the management of tuberculosis. The availability of good medical care is far more important.

F. Symptomatic Treatment: The patient should be reassured that his symptoms will disappear as the illness is brought under control.

1. **Cough**—In general, cough in tuberculosis should not be abolished with drugs. Productive cough should be encouraged, and the patient should be taught to cover his mouth and cough with minimal effort. If it becomes necessary to suppress exhausting cough, codeine phosphate, 8–15 mg orally every 4–6 hours as necessary, may be helpful. Patients with large cavities who produce copious sputum may be helped by postural drainage. When secondary infection is present, penicillin or broad-spectrum antibiotics may be indicated.

2. **Hemorrhage**—The chief danger of hemorrhage in tuberculosis is not sudden death but aspiration of the infected blood and spread of the disease to other parts of the lungs. Observe the patient for shock (see Chapter 1). Reassurance is most important in allaying apprehension. Phenobarbital sodium, 60–120 mg subcut, may be of value in quieting the apprehensive patient. Use cough inhibitors carefully in the treatment of hemorrhage. Codeine phosphate, 8–15 mg every 4–6 hours, should be given to suppress (but not to abolish) cough. *Caution:* Do not give morphine.

Continued severe bleeding can sometimes be controlled with posterior pituitary injection, 1 ml (10 IU) *slowly* IV in 10 ml of normal saline.

Bed rest is essential during periods of hemorrhage. Instruct the patient in the proper method of coughing (see above).

G. Response to Treatment: A favorable symptomatic response to treatment is usually reported within 2–3 weeks; improvement can usually be observed on x-rays within 4 weeks; and positive sputum usually becomes negative within 2 months. There is good evidence that most patients with previously untreated tuberculosis who are on a good drug regimen do not transmit the disease after 2–3 weeks of treatment even though tubercle bacilli may still be present in the sputum. Repeated x-ray examination and sputum tests, preferably cultures, should be done at monthly intervals during the first few months of treatment. When improvement is established, the interval between x-rays can be lengthened. When sputum becomes negative on culture and surgery is not indicated, a rapid return to normal activities can be permitted (see below). If there is no x-ray improvement or sputum conversion within 3 months, the treatment program should be reevaluated. Tuberculosis is considered "inactive" when the following criteria (National Tuberculosis Association Diagnostic Standards) have been satisfied for at least 6 months: (1) no symptoms; (2) x-ray appearance stable, without evidence of cavitation; and (3) sputum (or gastric or bronchial washings) negative for tubercle bacilli by culture. It should be emphasized that patients who are on a good chemotherapy regimen and are asymptomatic may resume their normal physical activities before the criteria for "inactive" disease have been met. This, of course, presumes that arrangements for continuation of proper treatment are made and followed.

Prognosis

Very few people die of pulmonary tuberculosis when modern treatment methods are used before the disease reaches a very advanced stage. Most patients, including those with advanced disease, can be restored to a normal state of health within 12 months (although, as noted above, drug treatment is continued for a longer period).

A good treatment program should result in a 95% cure rate in all cases of initially treated disease. Of those who remain inactive 2 years after cessation of proper treatment, less than 1% can be expected to relapse. Prolonged follow-up of this group of patients is unnecessary. Inadequately treated patients should have regular follow-up examinations indefinitely.

Bobrowitz ID: Ethambutol-isoniazid versus streptomycin-ethambutol-isoniazid in original treatment of cavitary tuberculosis. Am Rev Resp Dis 109:548, 1974.

Committee on Preventive Therapy of Tuberculous Infection, American Thoracic Society. Am Rev Resp Dis 110:371, 1974.

Committee on Revision of Diagnostic Standards, American Thoracic Society: *Diagnostic Standards and Classification of Tuberculosis.* National Tuberculosis and Respiratory Diseases Association, 1969.

Committee on Therapy, American Thoracic Society: Adrenal corticosteroids and tuberculosis. Am Rev Resp Dis 97:484, 1968.

Crofton J: The chemotherapy of bacterial respiratory infections. Am Rev Resp Dis 101:841, 1970.

Crofton J: Problems of drug resistance in tuberculosis: The newer antituberculosis drugs. Postgrad MJ 47:748, 1971.

Cryer PE, Kissane J (editors): Miliary tuberculosis. Am J Med 58:847, 1975.

Holden M & others: Frequency of negative intermediate-strength tuberculin sensitivity in patients with active tuberculosis. New England J Med 285:1506, 1971.

Ihm HJ & others: Pneumothorax associated with pulmonary tuberculosis. J Thoracic Cardiovas Surg 64:211, 1972.

Lefrak SS & others: Chemoprophylaxis of tuberculosis. Arch Int Med 135:606, 1975.

Newman R & others: Rifampin in initial treatment of pulmonary tuberculosis. A USPHS tuberculosis therapy trial. Am Rev Resp Dis 103:461, 1971.

Noganna K: Some of the BCG trials and certain aspects involved in them. Am Rev Resp Dis 109:497, 1974.

Oseasohn R: Current use of BCG. Am Rev Resp Dis 109:500, 1974.

Radner D: Toxicologic and pharmacologic aspects of rifampin. Chest 64:213, 1973.

Rifampin in the treatment of pulmonary tuberculosis. Dis Chest 61:517, June 1972. [Special issue.]

Stead WW: The clinical spectrum of primary tuberculosis in adults: Confusion with reinfection in the pathogenesis of chronic tuberculosis. Ann Int Med 68:731, 1968.

Vall-Spinosa A, Lester TW: Rifampin: Characteristics and role in the chemotherapy of tuberculosis. Ann Int Med 74:758, 1971.

PULMONARY DISEASE DUE TO OTHER ("ATYPICAL") MYCOBACTERIA

Certain mycobacteria other than the tubercle bacillus, which are ordinarily saprophytic and occur widely distributed in nature, under certain circumstances produce chronic progressive pulmonary disease that is clinically similar to pulmonary tuberculosis. Cervical lymphadenitis is now more commonly due to these organisms (in the USA) than to tuberculosis, and is very similar clinically.

These organisms are identical with tubercle bacilli microscopically and are differentiated by certain cultural characteristics. The atypical mycobacteria are divided into 4 groups, designated groups I, II, III, and IV. Group I mycobacteria are photochromogens, ie, when cultured in vitro they develop a yellow color on exposure to light. The best known group I mycobacteria are *M kansasii* and *M marinum.* Group II mycobacteria are scotochromogens, characterized by the appearance of yellow-orange coloration in in vitro culture even if grown in the dark. One of the species of this group is *M scrofulaceum,* known to cause cervical adenitis. Group III mycobacteria are nonphotochromogens. Like *M tuberculosis,* they generally remain a buff color when cultured in vitro. The best known member of this group is *M intracellulare* (the Battey organism). Group IV mycobacteria are distinguished by a relatively rapid rate of growth (days instead of weeks) and hence are designated "rapid growers." This group is seldom pathogenic and often appears as a contaminant. *M fortuitum,* however, can cause disease in humans.

Groups I and III and, more rarely, group II organisms may produce pulmonary disease which is clinically similar to "typical" tuberculosis but can be distinguished from it by bacterial culture technics. Because atypical acid-fast bacilli may exist as nonpathogenic saprophytes in man, care must be taken to identify them as the cause of disease.

Infection with atypical mycobacteria and subsequent delayed hypersensitivity to them may result in cross-sensitivity to the tuberculin skin test antigen (PPD-S). The size of the reaction to PPD-S in these infections is considerably less than that due to tuberculosis. Further clarification may be obtained by dual testing with PPD-S and PPD-B (antigen derived from the Battey bacillus, or type III atypical mycobacteria).

Skin test antigens from atypical mycobacteria are available. However, their use to precisely identify the specific organism is very limited, and reliance on bacteriologic results is preferred.

Transmission of atypical disease from man to man has not been reported, so that spread of infection among humans need not be feared. Atypical mycobacterial infection is more frequently seen in people with chronic pulmonary and systemic diseases.

Drug resistance of mycobacteria organisms from a suspected tuberculosis patient who has never been treated with antituberculosis drugs suggests that they are atypical mycobacteria. In spite of the in vitro drug resistance, patients with atypical mycobacteriosis may show marked response to these drugs. This is especially true of *M kansasii;* more than 80% of patients with this infection may expect cure on the triple drug regimen of isoniazid, ethambutol, and streptomycin. Group III disease responds less favorably, but with the use of additional drugs a high rate of success may be achieved.

Treatment with the chemotherapeutic agents which are effective in tuberculosis has been generally less predictable, and surgery may be required.

Goldman KP: Treatment of mycobacterial infection of the lungs. Thorax 23:94, 1968.

Johanson WG Jr, Nicholson DP: Pulmonary disease due to *Mycobacterium kansasii:* An analysis of some factors affecting prognosis. Am Rev Resp Dis 99:73, 1969.

Palmer CE, Edwards LB: Identifying the tuberculous infected: The dual-test technique. JAMA 205:167, 1968.

BRONCHOGENIC CARCINOMA

Essentials of Diagnosis

- Insidious onset with cough, localized wheeze, or hemoptysis; often asymptomatic.
- May present as an unresolved pneumonia, atelectasis, or pleurisy with effusion (often bloody), or as a pulmonary nodule seen on x-ray.
- Metastases to other organs may produce initial symptoms.
- Endocrine, biochemical, and neuromuscular disorders (see below) may be the presenting features of bronchogenic carcinoma.

General Considerations

Cancer arising in the mucosa of the bronchial tree is the most common intrathoracic malignancy. It occurs predominantly in men (8:1) and may appear at any age, but most cases occur in the cancer age group (over 40).

The importance of genetic and environmental factors in the etiology of bronchogenic carcinoma is not known. However, the disease is relatively rare in nonsmokers. Local invasion of ribs, mediastinal structures, and nerve plexuses and distant metastases to the liver, adrenals, kidneys, and brain are common.

Clinical Findings

A. Symptoms and Signs: Persistent, nonproductive cough, hemoptysis, and localized persistent wheeze are the major symptoms produced by bronchial irritation, erosion, and partial obstruction (although there may be no symptoms). These are often attributed to "cigarette cough" or "chronic bronchitis."

Pulmonary infections (pneumonitis, lung abscess) occurring distal to a bronchial obstruction frequently dominate the clinical picture and mask an underlying neoplasm. Any atypical pulmonary infection (persisting, recurring, or responding incompletely to therapy) should suggest carcinoma.

Metastases frequently give rise to the first symptoms, eg, bone or chest pain in osseous or pleural involvement; neurologic symptoms due to brain involvement.

In general, pulmonary signs result from the sequelae of bronchial erosion, bronchial obstruction, pleural involvement, and mediastinal invasion. When a solitary small lesion does not produce hemoptysis, significant bronchial obstruction, or pleural involvement, there are no clinical findings. If the lesion is large enough, there may be physical (and x-ray) signs of partial or complete bronchial obstruction with associated atelectasis and infection.

Clubbing of the fingers, nonpitting edema of the extremities, and periosteal overgrowth (seen on x-ray) may appear rapidly (and have been known to precede chest x-ray signs) with a localized carcinoma and may regress spectacularly following surgical removal.

Local spread is characterized by pleural fluid (bloody effusion is commonly present), signs of mediastinal invasion (pericardial effusion, hoarseness and brassy cough, stridor, dysphagia), and signs of regional metastases. Bronchogenic carcinoma in the upper part of the lung may produce Pancoast's syndrome (ipsilateral Horner's syndrome and shoulder-arm pain).

Particular attention must be paid to involvement of scalene nodes and the development of liver nodules as sites of metastases. Careful neurologic examination must be performed for evidence of brain metastases.

Uncommon metabolic manifestations of bronchogenic carcinoma have been recognized: myasthenic symptoms resembling myasthenia gravis; peripheral neuritis involving both sensory and motor components; clubbing of the digits; Cushing's syndrome; carcinoid syndrome (hyperserotoninemia), even when the tissue is not carcinoid; hypercalcemia not due to osseous metastases; and hyponatremia due to inappropriate excessive secretion of antidiuretic hormone (ADH). These manifestations may disappear when the tumor is removed and do not necessarily signify a grave prognosis.

B. Laboratory Findings: (The definitive stage of diagnosis.)

1. Sputum cytology—A positive diagnosis of bronchogenic carcinoma can be made in 60—70% of cases on the basis of sputum cytology by qualified cytologists. Several fresh specimens should be studied.

2. Bronchoscopy—Visualization and biopsy by forceps or brush is possible in 75—80% of cases, especially with the flexible fiberoptic bronchoscope. The collection of washings for cytology is also more productive with this instrument.

3. Biopsy of the scalene fat pad may reveal lymph nodes containing metastatic carcinoma. This procedure is indicated in the presence of possible hilar or mediastinal node involvement.

4. Mediastinoscopy is an extension of the scalene node biopsy concept by which tissue from deeper nodes (and therefore of greater diagnostic value) is obtained. In experienced hands, it is a valuable procedure.

5. Needle aspiration biopsy of localized lesions under careful fluoroscopic control with an image amplifier appears to be a useful and safe procedure.

6. Exploratory thoracotomy may be the only way to establish the nature of a mass when other studies are negative.

C. X-Ray Findings: The chest film offers the greatest possibility of early diagnosis and cure. Solitary nodules which do not cause symptoms or signs can be detected only by this method. Thirty to 60% of these "coin" lesions have proved to be carcinomas at thoracotomy.

The varied x-ray patterns with which bronchogenic carcinoma may present include perihilar mass (34—36%), atelectasis (segmental or lobar) (21—23%), pleural effusion (5—15%), and mediastinal lymph node enlargement (5—15%).

The follow-up investigation of a pulmonary infection should include search for evidence of delayed or incomplete resolution, associated masses, and hilar or mediastinal lymph node enlargement. The latter can best be demonstrated with barium in the esophagus. Chest films at weekly intervals are recommended for pneumonias not responding satisfactorily to therapy, especially in high-risk individuals.

Treatment

Early detection and surgical removal before metastases occur offer the only hope of cure. For this reason, a routine chest x-ray once a year for all men over 40 who are smokers has been strongly recommended despite the small yield in terms of curable disease. Pulmonary function should be carefully evaluated prior to thoracotomy.

Symptoms due to inoperable lesions may be temporarily controlled by nonoperative means. The coordination of radiation therapy with the available chemotherapeutic agents used in combinations of smaller, less toxic doses administered over a longer period of time seems to offer some hope of improved palliation and, rarely, a cure.

Prognosis

Early diagnosis is important if the lesion is to be found in an operable stage. At present only about 8% of all patients are alive 5 years after diagnosis. Undifferentiated tumors have a poorer prognosis than those which are differentiated. Carcinomas of the main stem bronchi have a very poor prognosis.

Adams WF: Current concepts of surgical management of carcinoma of the lung. Dis Chest 51:233, 1967.

Albertini RE & others: Arterial hypoxemia induced by fiberoptic bronchoscopy. JAMA 230:1666, 1974.

Boucot KR, Weiss W: Lung cancer detected by semi-annual screening. JAMA 224:1361, 1973.

Caldwell WL, Bagshaw MA: Indications for and results of irradiation of carcinoma of the lung. Cancer 22:999, 1968.

Carbone PP & others; Lung cancer: Perspectives and prospects. Ann Int Med 73:1003, 1970.

Flynn JR, Rossi NP, Lawton RL: Mediastinoscopy in carcinoma of the lung. Arch Surg 94:243, 1967.

Green N & others: Cancer of the lung: An in-depth analysis of prognostic factors. Cancer 28:229, 1971.

Hodgkin JE: Evaluation before thoracotomy. Western J Med 122:104, 1975.

LeRoux BT: Bronchial carcinoma. Thorax 23:136, 1968.

Nathan MH: Management of the solitary pulmonary nodule. JAMA 227:1141, 1974.

Paulson DL: Carcinoma of the lung. Curr Probl Surg, Nov 1967.

Pearson FG: An evaluation of mediastinoscopy in the management of presumably operable bronchogenic carcinoma. J Thoracic Cardiovas Surg 53:617, 1968.

Remington J: Smoking, sputum and lung cancer. Brit MJ 1:732, 1968.

Solomon DA & others: Cytology in fiberoptic bronchoscopy. Chest 65:616, 1974.

Stevens GM & others: Needle aspiration biopsy of localized pulmonary lesions. California Med 106:92, 1967.

Stoloff IL: The prognostic value of bronchoscopy in primary lung cancer. JAMA 227:299, 1974.

Valaitis J & others: Bronchogenic carcinoma in situ in asymptomatic high-risk population of smokers. J Thoracic Cardiovas Surg 57:325, 1969.

Watson WL: *Lung Cancer: A Study of 5000 Memorial Hospital Cases.* Mosby, 1968.

Weiss W & others: Risk of lung cancer. JAMA 222:799, 1972.

Yrigoyen E, Fujikawa YF: Flexible fiberoptic bronchoscopy: Anesthesia, technique and results. Western J Med 122:117, 1975.

BRONCHIAL ADENOMA

Bronchial adenoma (neoplasm arising in the glandular structures of the bronchial mucous membranes) is the most common (80%) "benign" bronchopulmonary neoplasm. Sex distribution is equal; age incidence is somewhat lower than that of bronchogenic carcinoma. It is locally invasive.

The great majority of bronchial adenomas arise in the proximal bronchi. The onset is insidious. Cough and localized wheeze are similar to those of bronchogenic carcinoma. These tumors are quite vascular; hemoptysis is common, occurring in 25–30% of cases.

Since bronchial adenoma does not tend to exfoliate, sputum examination is not helpful. Differentiation from bronchogenic carcinoma thus depends upon bronchoscopic biopsy or exploratory thoracotomy.

In many cases bronchial adenoma can be distinguished from bronchogenic carcinoma only by histologic and cytologic study. Distinguish also from other benign obstructions, eg, foreign body, tuberculous bronchial stenosis.

Treatment

It is usually necessary to remove the neoplasm by lobectomy. Occasionally, pedunculated noninvasive adenomas may be removed by bronchoscopy, but serious bleeding can occur in such cases (even with biopsy alone).

The prognosis is good. The tumor tends to be locally invasive, but 5–10% metastasize slowly. Fatalities are not usually due to metastases but are associated with bronchiectasis, pneumonitis, hemorrhages, the complications of surgery, or asphyxiation secondary to obstruction by the tumor.

Baldwin JN, Grimes OF: Bronchial adenomas. Surg Gynec Obst 124:813, 1967.

Batson JF, Gale JW, Hickey RC: Bronchial adenomata. Arch Surg 92:623, 1966.

Donahue JK, Weichert RF, Ochsner JL: Bronchial adenoma. Ann Surg 167:873, 1968.

Tolis GA & others: Bronchial adenomas. Surg Gynec Obst 134:605, 1972.

BRONCHIOLAR CARCINOMA
(Alveolar Cell Carcinoma, Pulmonary Adenomatosis)

Bronchiolar carcinoma is a relatively uncommon pulmonary malignancy (3–5% of lung cancers) which grows slowly and metastasizes late. In contrast to bronchogenic carcinoma, it is often bilateral. The neoplastic cells line the alveoli and bronchioles. Sex distribution is equal. Most cases occur in the age group from 50–60.

Since this neoplasm originates in the bronchiolar or alveolar lining, the major bronchi are not involved and symptoms develop late. Chest pain and cough are the most frequent symptoms. Copious watery or mucoid sputum sometimes occurs with diffuse disease and, when present, is almost pathognomonic. With widespread lung involvement, dyspnea, cyanosis, dullness to percussion, clubbing, and cor pulmonale develop.

Cytologic examination of sputum is valuable since this tumor commonly exfoliates.

The usual x-ray picture is of bilateral multiple lung nodules or areas of consolidation, but solitary nodules may be present (approximately 25%) and calcification may occur.

There are usually no diagnostic features that distinguish this from other types of lung cancer. Bilateral lesions, either discrete or diffuse, are more common. Solitary lesions may partly calcify and resemble granulomas.

The tumor metastasizes by bronchogenic spread of exfoliated cells and also by lymphatic and hematogenous routes.

Treatment

If involvement is unilateral and localized and there is no evidence of extrapulmonary extension, surgical excision is warranted.

Prognosis

Widespread pulmonary involvement is the usual cause of death. Metastases occur in 50% of cases (25% are lymphatic or hematogenous). With resection of solitary lesions, 25–35% 5-year survival rates have been reported.

Delarue NC & others: Bronchiolo-alveolar carcinoma: A reappraisal after 24 years. Cancer 29:90, 1972.

Hewlett TH & others: Bronchiolar carcinoma of the lung: Review of 39 patients. J Thoracic Cardiovas Surg 48:614, 1964.

Knudson RJ & others: Unusual cancer of the lung. II. Bronchiolar carcinoma of the lung. Dis Chest 48:628, 1965.

Kress MB, Allan WB: Bronchiolo-alveolar tumors of the lung. Bull Johns Hopkins Hosp 112:115, 1963.

Ludington LG & others: Bronchiolar carcinoma (alveolar cell), another great imitator: A review of 41 cases. Chest 61:622, 1972.

ALVEOLAR PROTEINOSIS

Alveolar proteinosis is a chronic, progressive, often fatal disease of unknown cause (and unrecognized before 1958) characterized by progressive dyspnea, cough, intermittent fever, pulmonary infiltrations on x-ray, and pulmonary insufficiency of the alveolar-capillary block syndrome type. The diagnosis is based on the histologic findings (at biopsy or autopsy) of striking replacement of the alveolar air spaces with a granular, amorphous material which stains characteristically with periodic acid-Schiff stain. The chemical similarity between this material, which appears to be a phospholipid (palmitoyl lecithin), and the surface-active agent normally secreted by the alveolar epithelium suggests the possibility of an abnormal hypersecretion of this substance. These patients seem to be prone to the development of nocardiosis and other fungus infections.

Methods have been described for irrigating the involved lung with saline or heparin solutions via endobronchial catheter. Large quantities of the proteinaceous material can thus be removed, and this results in clearing by x-ray and temporary or prolonged improvement in pulmonary function.

Gerard has reported one case that was treated successfully with intensive IPPB and nebulized proteolytic enzyme.

Gerard FP, Sabety AM, Lurie W: Pulmonary alveolar proteinosis: Practical management. J Thoracic Cardiovas Surg 57:273, 1969.

Ramirez-R J: Alveolar proteinosis: Importance of pulmonary lavage. Am Rev Resp Dis 103:666, 1971.

Ramirez-R J: Pulmonary alveolar proteinosis. Arch Int Med 119:147, 1967.

SILO-FILLER'S DISEASE

Silo-filler's disease is an agricultural industrial pulmonary disease caused by inhalation of nitrogen dioxide fumes emanating from silos which have been freshly filled (eg, with corn or alfalfa). The toxic inhalant causes increased capillary permeability resulting in a form of pulmonary edema.

The initial phase, appearing promptly after exposure, consists of cough, dyspnea, and weakness. This is followed by a quiescent phase, with some persistence of dyspnea and weakness, followed by a second acute phase with fever, chills, malaise, increasing cough and dyspnea, tachypnea and tachycardia, and diffuse rales and rhonchi. Extensive miliary infiltrates are present on x-ray. Death may occur within 2–3 weeks after onset, or there may be gradual recovery over a period of 1–2 months.

Oxygen, intermittent positive pressure breathing, antibiotics, and corticosteroids have been used in treatment.

Preventive measures include avoiding entry into silos if fumes are present and assuring good ventilation of silos by any means necessary.

Donoghue FE, Schmidt HW: Farmer's lung and silo-filler's disease. M Clin North America 48:903, 1964.

PULMONARY ATELECTASIS

Essentials of Diagnosis

- Acute: sudden marked symptoms of dyspnea, cyanosis, fever, even if area is small.
- Chronic: almost no symptoms even if area is large.
- Homogeneous density on x-ray.
- Mediastinal shift toward involved side, diaphragm up, narrowing of intercostal spaces.

General Considerations

Pulmonary atelectasis is collapse and nonaeration of lung segments distal to complete bronchial obstruction produced by a wide variety of diseases (eg, pneumonia, asthma). A clinical history consistent with retention of secretions, aspiration of a foreign body, or bronchial infection can usually be obtained.

Postoperative atelectasis is the most common variety (occurs in 2–5% of patients after major surgery). The onset is usually 24–72 hours after operation.

Bronchial obstruction prevents entry of air into the distal segment lobe or even the entire lung.

Compensatory changes occur to "fill in the space" previously occupied by the collapsed lung: (1) shift of the mediastinum toward the side of collapse, (2) upward displacement of the diaphragm on the involved side, and (3) overexpansion of remaining lung tissue on both sides ("compensatory emphysema").

Compression of the lung from without (eg, pleural effusion) is of far less physiologic significance than atelectasis due to obstruction.

Clinical Findings

A. Symptoms and Signs: The severity of symptoms depends upon the site of obstruction and the rate at which it develops, and the presence or absence of infection in the atelectatic area. The more acute the onset (eg, postoperative atelectasis), the more marked the symptoms. Massive collapse in acute atelectasis causes marked dyspnea, cyanosis, tachycardia, chest pain, and fever. Lesser degrees of collapse produce variable symptoms, but even a small acute atelectasis may produce symptoms.

Symptoms, eg, wheezing and cough, are often due to the obstruction itself or to infection distal to the block.

The physical findings in acute atelectasis include tachycardia (often out of proportion to the amount of fever), decrease of chest motion on the affected side, with narrowing of intercostal spaces; displacement of the mediastinum to the involved side, as shown by the shift of the trachea, cardiac apex, and dullness; percussion dullness; and decreased to absent vocal fremitus, breath sounds, and voice sounds. Bronchial breath sounds are occasionally present over the atelectatic area and may alternate with diminished breath sounds.

In chronic atelectasis, displacement of the mediastinum is modified by the slowness of compensatory changes, rigidity of the mediastinum due to the underlying disease, and changes of the elasticity of the surrounding diseased lung.

B. X-Ray Findings: The collapsed segment is visible as a homogeneous "ground glass" density. The atelectatic portion of lung is denser than a comparable area of consolidation because no air is present with the fluid. The volume of the collapsed lobe diminishes markedly. The diaphragm is displaced upward on the side of the collapse. Mediastinal shift to the involved side is a major diagnostic feature. Pleural fluid is not infrequently noted on the affected side, but it fails to displace the mediastinum back to the midline and the fluid line is seen to run downward and laterally from the midline instead of upward and laterally (as in fluid without atelectasis).

C. Instrumental Examination: Bronchoscopy is very helpful in diagnosis and treatment.

Differential Diagnosis

Pulmonary atelectasis must be distinguished from lobar pneumonia, other pulmonary infections, pulmonary infarction, and pleural effusion.

Complications

The sequelae of unrelieved obstruction with atelectasis are infection, destruction of lung tissue with fibrosis, and bronchiectasis.

Treatment

A. Postoperative Atelectasis: Force the patient to cough and to hyperventilate. In patients who are unable to cooperate, a small plastic tube (Intracath) can be introduced transtracheally and taped in place. Through this, 1–2 ml of saline can be introduced every hour to stimulate coughing. Bronchodilatation by aerosol with an intermittent positive pressure apparatus (eg, Bennett, Bird, or other machines) has been demonstrated to resolve many cases of postoperative atelectasis. The addition of a mucolytic agent such as acetylcysteine may help dissolve plugs of mucus. The apparatus should be used for 30 minutes every 2–3 hours for 24 hours before deciding that other measures are necessary. The use of IPPB postoperatively in patients with chronic pulmonary disease is also effective in preventing atelectasis. Preoperative instruction is helpful.

If the above fail or atelectasis is massive, aspiration of mucus by bronchoscopy is indicated.

Give procaine penicillin G, 600,000 units IM, twice daily, or tetracycline, 250 mg orally 4 times daily.

B. Spontaneous Atelectasis: Bronchoscopy is indicated to determine the nature of the obstruction and to institute appropriate treatment.

Prognosis

Although the outlook is usually good in postoperative atelectasis, unrelieved collapse may result in death (when massive) or in prolonged morbidity (when lobar or segmental).

Thomas PA, Lynch RE, Merrigan EH: Incidence of contralateral pulmonary atelectasis after thoracotomy: An evaluation of preventive after care. Dis Chest 51:288, 1967.

ADULT RESPIRATORY DISTRESS SYNDROME
("Shock" Lung, "Pump" Lung)

Essentials of Diagnosis
- Dyspnea and cyanosis in a patient being treated for traumatic shock.
- Evidence of decreased pulmonary compliance.
- Blood gas changes.
- X-ray: Patchy infiltrates which may progress to consolidation.

General Considerations

This condition is characterized by interstitial edema and interalveolar exudation occurring in previously healthy lungs. It is being more frequently recognized, and its pathogenesis and causes are becoming clearer. It occurs after massive injury with shock, heart-lung perfusion procedures, fat embolism, aspiration pneumonia, and certain viral pneumonias. The pathogenesis appears to involve a leak in the pulmonary capillary endothelium with interstitial edema and alveolar hemorrhage and loss of surfactant, resulting in atelectasis, the formation of a hyaline membrane, and plugging of small arteries. This results in a severe diffusion defect and disturbance of the perfusion-ventilation ratio (physiologic shunting). Loss of pulmonary compliance (stiff lungs) and a decrease in functional residual capacity occur.

A common aggravating factor in the development of this disorder is overloading of the circulation with blood and fluids in the treatment of traumatic shock. Dependence on central venous pressure measurements as a guide to fluid replacement will cause this error in this situation. Urine output, state of consciousness, stable vital signs, and warm extremities are safer guides.

Clinical Findings

A. Symptoms and Signs: The principal symptoms are progressive dyspnea and cyanosis following one of the predisposing conditions listed above. Physical examination usually shows dyspnea, cyanosis, grunting respiration, intercostal retraction, and signs of progressive pulmonary consolidation. When assisted ventila-

tion is instituted, progressively higher pressures are needed to maintain an adequate tidal volume (decreased compliance).

B. Laboratory Findings: Laboratory studies typically show a reduced Pa_{O_2}, a normal or decreased Pa_{CO_2} (elevated Pa_{CO_2} is an ominous sign), and a normal or elevated arterial blood pH.

C. X-Ray Findings: Chest x-rays show patches of density initially which coalesce to form larger areas of consolidation. There is usually a 12–24 hour delay between the injury and the appearance of pulmonary infiltrations.

Treatment

A. Preventive Measures: The syndrome may be prevented in some cases by (1) prompt treatment of shock (see Chapter 1), (2) avoidance of fluid overload, (3) prevention of aspiration, (4) early use of respirators in high-risk patients, and (5) early use of corticosteroids in selected patients.

B. Avoidance of Fluid Overload: If fluid retention appears to be aggravating the pulmonary condition, the use of an intravenous diuretic (eg, furosemide) may improve pulmonary fluid overload. Fluids should be restricted to 1500–2000 ml/day. Salt restriction is also important. The Swan-Ganz catheter to measure pulmonary wedge pressure is the most accurate procedure for determining volume adequacy in terms of pumping ability of the heart.

C. Respiratory Support: The volume ventilator is capable of consistently delivering large tidal volumes (15–20 ml/kg) even at high pressures. The volume ventilator also possesses the versatility to deliver a modified respiratory flow wave. Advantageous wave modifications include positive end-expiratory pressure (PEEP) and inspiratory hold. These modifications minimize alveolar collapse and increase compliance. Sufficient concentrations of oxygen must be supplied to maintain a Pa_{O_2} of at least 55–60 mm Hg. To avoid oxygen toxicity, the concentrations of oxygen delivered (FI_{O_2}) must be kept below 55%. Adequate humidification and frequent position changes are important.

D. Corticosteroids: Hydrocortisone, 1 gm IV per 24-hour period, may be beneficial in cases of aspiration, fat embolism, septic shock, and those not responding to the above therapy.

E. Antibiotics: Antibiotics should be used only to treat invasive infections. Frequent sputum cultures and sensitivity tests permit the choice of specific antibiotics. Indiscriminate use of broad spectrum antibiotics imposes a hazard of superinfection.

Course & Prognosis

These patients may require many days of this type of support before the process is reversed. Serial x-rays and blood gas studies are the best guides to treatment. The mortality rate remains high.

Ashbaugh DG & others: Continuous positive pressure breathing (CPPB) in adult respiratory distress syndrome. J Thoracic

Cardiovas Surg 57:31, 1969.

Bredenberg CE & others: Respiratory failure in shock. Ann Surg 169:392, 1969.

Ferstenfeld JE & others: Recognition and treatment of adult respiratory distress syndrome secondary to viral interstitial pneumonia. Am J Med 58:709, 1975.

Murray JF: Shock lung. California Med 112:43, Feb 1970.

Petty TL: PEEP. Chest 61:309, 1972.

Petty TL, Ashbaugh DG: The adult respiratory distress syndrome. Chest 60:233, 1971.

CHRONIC PULMONARY EMPHYSEMA

Essentials of Diagnosis

- Insidious onset of exertional dyspnea; dyspnea at rest only in late stages.
- Prolonged expiratory phase and wheezing are common.
- Productive cough, often ineffective in clearing the bronchi.
- Barrel chest; use of accessory muscles of respiration.
- Over-aerated lung fields and flattened diaphragm on chest x-ray are frequently observed.

General Considerations

Pulmonary emphysema is characterized by diffuse distention and over-aeration of the alveoli, disruption of intra-alveolar septa, loss of pulmonary elasticity, increased lung volume, and impaired pulmonary function due to disturbed ventilation and altered gas and blood flow. Partial obstruction of smaller bronchi is often present.

Emphysema may occur (1) in the absence of a history of preceding chronic lung disease (etiology is unknown, although an inherent defect in pulmonary elastic tissue has been suggested); (2) secondary to chronic diffuse bronchial obstruction (eg, bronchitis, asthma); or (3) in association with fibrotic pulmonary disease (eg, silicosis, fibrosis). Many investigators feel that cigarette smoking is a major cause. Both heredity and smoking appear to be important in the causation of emphysema.

A familial predilection for chronic obstructive pulmonary disease has been noted. An association with a deficiency of the glycoprotein alpha₁ antitrypsin has been shown to be a genetically determined dominant trait with a high incidence of emphysema occurring, often in the 4th and 5th decades, in homozygous individuals. The gross deficiency can be determined by serum protein electrophoresis, but identification of the genetic phenotype requires a complex diffusion study of the serum. The identification and classification of younger people with this defect may permit genetic counseling in the future, and in a person with early symptoms would enable the physician to emphasize the need to interdict smoking and observe other preventive measures.

Pulmonary emphysema is the most common cause of chronic respiratory failure and chronic cor pulmonale. It is predominantly a disease of men over the age of 45.

Localized areas of emphysema occur in many pulmonary diseases and are usually of no importance. Giant bullae sometimes occur and may cause spontaneous pneumothorax.

Clinical Findings

A. Symptoms and Signs: The diagnosis of physiologically significant emphysema depends upon a history of exertional dyspnea and chronic productive cough (the most frequent presenting symptoms). Onset is usually insidious. Dyspnea at rest and orthopnea are unusual even with advanced emphysema (except with superimposed acute bronchial disease). Cough is frequently aggravated by intercurrent respiratory infections. Bouts of wheezing are not unusual. (Minor respiratory infections which would be of no consequence to patients with normal lungs can produce fatal or near-fatal disturbances of respiratory function in the patient with emphysema.)

Weakness, lethargy, anorexia, and weight loss are due to hypoxia, the increased muscular activity required for breathing, and respiratory acidosis. When ventilatory insufficiency is severe, headache, impaired sensorium, asterixis (flapping tremor), papilledema, and miosis may be encountered.

In the typical patient with advanced emphysema the chest is maintained in a fixed inspiratory position ("barrel-shaped") with increased anteroposterior diameter. The neck appears shortened. Accessory muscles of respiration (sternomastoids, pectorals, scaleni) are employed along with overuse of abdominal and upper intercostal muscles. Palpation confirms decreased costal motion, with a tendency of the entire thorax to move vertically as a unit. Diffuse hyperresonance, especially at the bases, masks the normal cardiac and hepatic dullness. Descent of diaphragms is decreased to absent. Breath sounds are diminished, with a prolonged and high-pitched expiratory phase. Scattered wheezes and rhonchi are often present.

In the absence of pulmonary function testing equipment, several simple procedures can be used during the physical examination to confirm the presence of significant ventilatory obstruction. The total vital capacity should normally be exhaled in 3 seconds with maximum effort. This can easily be timed with a stopwatch or second hand. If the emptying time is longer than 5 seconds, significant bronchial obstruction is present.

The match test is also helpful. If the patient is unable to blow out a match held 6 inches from the open mouth, severe ventilatory obstruction is usually present.

The liver is depressed by the flattened diaphragm and may be palpable 2–3 cm below the costal margin. The lips and nail beds are frequently cyanotic. The face is frequently ruddy to ruddy-cyanotic, reflecting anoxia and compensatory polycythemia. Clubbing of the digits occasionally occurs, along with other manifestations of chronic pulmonary osteoarthropathy.

Peripheral edema and venous distention occur if right heart failure (cor pulmonale) is present.

B. X-Ray Findings: Hyperinflation of lung fields is most marked at the bases and behind the sternum. The anteroposterior chest diameter is increased. Low, flat diaphragms move poorly on fluoroscopy. Bullae may appear as thin-walled translucent areas devoid of lung markings, occasionally of immense size. Scintillation scanning and pulmonary angiography are helpful in evaluating the nonaffected lung when surgical excision of large bullae is being considered.

C. Laboratory Findings: Vital capacity may be normal in emphysema even though extensive disease is present. Increased residual air volume is the most characteristic abnormality, but its determination is done in the pulmonary function laboratory. A reduction in the timed vital capacity is a simple and direct measure of obstruction and air-trapping.

Ventilatory insufficiency causes alveolar hypoxia and decreased Pa_{O_2} in the blood. If this condition persists, the Pa_{CO_2} increases as a result of the inability of the lungs to blow off CO_2. Initially, this developing acidosis is compensated for by retention of bicarbonate by the kidneys. When this mechanism fails, the pH of the blood falls and there is progressive respiratory acidosis. Measurement of these blood gases and the blood pH is readily available in most hospitals. The determinations should be done on arterial blood. Pa_{O_2} less than 50 mm Hg or a Pa_{CO_2} greater than 50 mm Hg signifies respiratory failure. The pH may remain normal in the presence of respiratory failure (elevated Pa_{CO_2}) until the compensatory mechanisms are overcome.

The red blood count and packed cell volume may be increased (secondary polycythemia), but marked polycythemia is not a frequent finding in emphysema. Absence of the usual alpha$_1$-globulin peak in the serum protein electrophoretic pattern may be a clue to the hereditary origin of the emphysema (alpha$_1$-antitrypsin deficiency).

Differential Diagnosis

The dyspnea of chronic pulmonary emphysema must be distinguished from that due to congestive heart failure, chronic bronchitis, and asthma.

Complications

Recurrent acute suppurative infections of the bronchioles are manifested by increase in dyspnea, cyanosis, fever, and the production of purulent sputum. Such infections are a grave matter in patients with poor pulmonary function since they can precipitate acute respiratory failure.

Indiscriminate prolonged administration of oxygen at ambient pressure to patients in respiratory acidosis may remove the last remaining stimulus to respiration—ie, hypoxia—resulting in hypoventilation, increasing acidosis, and coma (see below). Sedatives must be avoided.

Spontaneous pneumothorax may result from rupture of an emphysematous bleb into the pleural space.

Congestive right heart failure (cor pulmonale) may result from chronic emphysema.

Treatment

Since many patients have an associated chronic bronchitis with some elements of spasm, therapy is generally similar to that outlined for chronic bronchitis or chronic asthma. Give bronchodilators to relieve spasm and sputum liquefiers (mist inhalation, supplemental fluids) to thin tenacious secretions. Control infection with specific antibiotics (or tetracycline if bacterial sensitivity cannot be determined). Prolonged antimicrobial therapy may be necessary.

If the above methods fail to relieve bronchial obstruction, corticosteroids may give dramatic relief. For long-term use they should be given in minimum dosage with careful attention to the dangers and precautions outlined in Chapter 18. Localized giant bullae in the absence of severe generalized emphysema may require excision.

For treatment of acute and chronic respiratory failure, see next section. Chronic pulmonary heart disease is discussed in Chapter 7.

Prognosis

Emphysema is characterized by steady progression, but the rate of deterioration varies greatly among patients with this type of disease. Some degree of nonobstructive emphysema which does not lead to disability is not uncommon in the aged. When moderate to severe symptoms are present, the 5-year survival rate is reduced to 50%. Symptoms due to bronchial obstruction can often be improved, but the long-term outcome is usually not changed.

Auerbach O & others: Relation of smoking and age to emphysema: Whole-lung section study. New England J Med 286:853, 1972.

Bates DV: Chronic bronchitis and emphysema. (2 parts.) New England J Med 278:546, 600, 1968.

Bode FR & others: Reversibility of pulmonary function abnormalities in smokers: A prospective study of early diagnostic tests of small airways disease. Am J Med 59:43, 1975.

Burrows B, Earle RH: Course and prognosis in chronic obstructive lung disease. New England J Med 280:297, 1969.

Emirgil C & others: A study of the long-term effect of therapy in chronic obstructive pulmonary disease. Am J Med 47:367, 1969.

Falk GA, Briscoe WA: Alpha$_1$-antitrypsin deficiency in chronic obstructive pulmonary disease. Ann Int Med 72:427, 1970.

Filley GF: Emphysema and chronic bronchitis: Clinical manifestations and their physiologic significance. M Clin North America 51:283, 1967.

Hodgkin JE & others: Chronic obstructive airway diseases: Current concepts in diagnosis and comprehensive care. JAMA 232:1243, 1975.

Kilburn KH: New clues for the emphysemas. Am J Med 58:591, 1975.

Larson RK & others: Genetic and environmental determinants

of chronic obstructive pulmonary disease. Ann Int Med 72:627, 1970.

Lopez-Majano V & others: Pulmonary resection in bullous disease. Am Rev Resp Dis 99:554, 1969.

Murray JF & others: Early diagnosis of chronic obstructive lung disease. California Med 116:37, March 1972.

Petty TL: *Intensive and Rehabilitative Respiratory Care,* 2nd ed. Lea & Febiger, 1974.

Reid L: *The Pathology of Emphysema.* Year Book, 1967.

Schloerb RB & others: Potassium depletion in patients with chronic respiratory failure. Am Rev Resp Dis 102:53, 1970.

Stevens PM & others: Pathophysiology of hereditary emphysema. Ann Int Med 74:672, 1971.

Ziment I: Why are they saying bad things about IPPB? Resp Care 18:677, 1973.

MANAGEMENT OF ACUTE & CHRONIC ADULT RESPIRATORY FAILURE*

The diagnosis of respiratory failure is made most accurately from arterial blood gases obtained while the patient is breathing room air. A partial pressure of oxygen in arterial blood (Pa_{O_2}) of less than 50 mm Hg with or without elevated blood CO_2 (hypercapnia) is diagnostic of respiratory failure. A partial pressure of CO_2 in arterial blood (Pa_{CO_2}) of greater than 50 mm Hg is also diagnostic of respiratory failure. When hypercapnia is present, acute respiratory failure is identified by the presence of a low arterial pH (respiratory acidosis). In chronic respiratory failure, the respiratory acidosis is compensated by bicarbonate retention and a concomitant normalization of pH. Mixed respiratory and metabolic acid-base disorders may complicate the differentiation of acute and chronic failure.

Note that many conditions other than chronic obstructive lung disease are included in the following list of disorders that may be associated with respiratory failure:

(1) Airway obstruction:
Emphysema
Chronic bronchitis
Asthma
Cardiac disorders leading to massive pulmonary congestion

(2) Restrictive defects:
Interstitial fibrosis of all types
Pleural effusion
Pneumothorax
Infiltrative diseases, ie, pneumonia, atelectasis
Obesity
Abdominal distention of all types

(3) CNS depression:
Drugs
Head injury
CNS infection

*By Stephen Telatnik, MD.

(4) Chest wall abnormalities:
Congenital and acquired deformities
Trauma (flail chest)
Neuromuscular disease or blockade

Symptoms & Signs

The manifestations of acute respiratory failure are those of hypoxemia and respiratory acidosis as well as of the underlying disease. Hypoxemic findings include headache, restlessness, confusion, unconsciousness, tachycardia, hypotension, and warm extremities. Findings in respiratory acidosis include headache, dizziness, confusion, coma, miosis, papilledema, diaphoresis, tachycardia, and asterixis. The chronic manifestations of hypoxemia are principally those of polycythemia and cor pulmonale.

Treatment of Acute Respiratory Failure (ARF)

A. General Measures: The nature of the underlying disease and the clinical condition of the patient as well as the arterial blood gases determine the most appropriate treatment. Intubation may be required when ABG are normal, as in acute progressive muscular paralysis before ARF occurs. In this instance, a rapidly diminishing vital capacity would be an important objective finding. Adult respiratory distress syndrome (ARDS) with severe hypoxemia alone may require tracheal intubation if Pa_{O_2} cannot be maintained above 55 mm Hg with oxygen delivered by other means (see p 134). Asthmatics should be considered for intubation if Pa_{CO_2} rises rapidly even without hypercapnia in the face of continuing exhaustive respiratory effort (see p 112). The principal indication for intubation in chronic obstructive airway disease is increasing respiratory acidosis despite attempts to maintain adequate oxygenation ($Pa_{O_2} > 55$ mm Hg) and to improve ventilation by conservative management.

B. Conservative Management of ARF in Chronic Obstructive Lung Disease: The objective of therapy in ARF focuses on maintaining adequate oxygenation and preventing acid-base imbalance, primarily respiratory acidosis. Initially, therapy should be instituted without intubation.

1. Oxygen—Continuous oxygen is delivered at a rate of flow sufficient to maintain adequate oxygenation ($Pa_{O_2} > 55$ mm Hg) without precipitating further respiratory acidosis. Usually, 1–4 liters/minute via nasal prongs will accomplish this goal even with nasal congestion and mouth breathing. Other methods of supplying oxygen include nasal cannula, nonrebreathing masks, and masks utilizing a Venturi device to maintain a specific concentration of oxygen.

2. Relief of bronchospasm—

a. Aminophylline is given initially in a dose of 250–500 mg IV over a 10-minute period while closely monitoring the patient for tachycardia and other arrhythmias. Maintenance therapy is preferably administered as 250–500 mg IV in 50 ml of fluid over 30 minutes every 6 hours. Side-effects of nausea, vomiting, arrhythmias, convulsions, and circulatory failure may limit the effectiveness of aminophylline in the relief of bronchospasm. Effective therapy and avoidance of side-effects can be best achieved by monitoring plasma aminophylline levels when available.

b. Aerosolized bronchodilators should be administered with IPPB devices as soon as the patient can cooperate. Isoetharine with phenylephrine (Bronkosol), 0.5 ml in 3 ml of saline, and isoproterenol, 1:200, 0.5 ml in 3 ml saline, are 2 common bronchodilator solutions used. They are delivered with an IPPB device operated by compressed air during a 15-minute period. This type of treatment may be given every 30 minutes to 2 hours depending on clinical conditions. IPPB treatment given solely to overcome hypoventilation may tire the patient and increase the ventilation-perfusion abnormality.

3. Mist—Continuous aerosol generated by a Venturi or ultrasonic nebulizer helps to reduce the viscosity of secretions and aids in their clearance.

4. Coughing and deep breathing—Vigorous efforts to compel the patient to cough properly and to breathe deeply to improve ventilation are often neglected but extremely useful adjuncts.

5. Drugs—The appropriate administration of antibiotics, corticosteroids, potassium chloride, diuretics, and digitalis may be necessary for maintenance after the initial critical period.

6. Intubation—Intubation may be necessary if the above measures do not effectively improve ventilation in 1–4 hours as determined by serial ABG.

C. Management of the Ventilator-Supported Patient: Volume-controlled mechanical ventilators deliver a preset volume of gas regardless of the amount of pressure required. Pressure-controlled devices deliver volume until a preset pressure is reached; that volume is dependent upon the flow rate and compliance of the patient's lungs. In many forms of ARF, a pressure-controlled ventilator is adequate. However, if pressures greater than 35 cm water or precise volumes are required, a volume-controlled ventilator would be more suitable. Most volume-controlled ventilators are dependent upon electrical power; most pressure-controlled ventilators are not. Caution must be used with oxygen-driven pressure-controlled ventilators on air-dilution setting because concentrations of oxygen varying from 40–80% may be delivered depending upon compliance (lung stiffness). Both types may automatically breathe for the patient (controlled ventilation) or cycle with initiation of breathing by the patient (assisted ventilation). Sustained ventilation with these devices is accomplished through an endotracheal tube or tracheostomy with a low-pressure cuffed tube.

The effective management of ventilator-dependent patients can be facilitated by a physiologic evaluation of the ventilator-patient system. Accurately performed ABG are essential. Each time arterial blood is drawn, several additional parameters of ventilator functions should be measured to evaluate results of ABG in terms of adequacy of ventilatory support: (1) the fraction of inspired oxygen (F_{IO_2}); (2) the respiratory frequency per minute (f); (3) the tidal volume (V_T), which is the amount of air expired with each breath;

and (4) peak airway pressure (PAP), which is the reading of the pressure gauge at the end of inspiration. These values are necessary to make the following determinations:

, **1. Effective compliance**—This is determined by dividing the tidal volume by peak airway pressure (V_T/PAP). (Normal: 35–50 ml/cm water.) This value represents resistance to air flow in the patient-ventilator system as well as compliance of the patient's lungs and thorax. In cases of ARF with decreased effective compliance, improvement of the patient is usually accompanied by an increase in effective compliance. This measurement is most valuable in detecting changes in resistance or compliance during ventilator support. If V_T (with pressure-controlled ventilator) can be restored or a decrease in pressure (with volume-controlled ventilator) can be accomplished by decreasing flow rate, the cause of decreased effective compliance is probably increased resistance (obstruction to airflow) rather than decreased compliance (restriction to lung expansion). Causes of increased resistance include kinked ventilator tubing, obstruction of the endotracheal tube by compression from overinflation of the cuff or collection of secretions, dislodgement of the tube, and obstruction of larger bronchi by secretions or bronchospasm. For a few hours after intubation, decreased compliance may really be due to fighting the ventilator, and this requires respiratory drive suppression. Morphine, 2 mg IV every 15–20 minutes, or diazepam, 2–5 mg IV intermittently, is commonly used. After the patient becomes initially accustomed to the ventilator, other causes of decreased compliance should be suspected: abdominal distention (every patient with endotracheal intubation should have a nasogastric tube for the first 24 hours), pleural effusion, pneumothorax, pulmonary edema, endotracheal tube in right main stem bronchus, pneumonia, or atelectasis. Atelectasis usually responds to the simple maneuver of deep sighing. Therefore, several forced tidal volumes of 1500–2000 ml should be attempted early in the investigation of decreased effective compliance.

2. Minute ventilation ($\dot{V}_E$)—Minute ventilation is the number of liters of air expired per minute. It is determined by multiplying respiratory frequency and tidal volume (f × V_T) or using a spirometer on the exhalation port for a full minute. Ventilator settings initially should be adjusted to deliver 8–12 liters/minute with f = 8–12 and V_T = 800–1200 ml. Proper regulation of minute ventilation is based on the amount of CO_2 retention as indicated by Pa_{CO_2}. Hypercapnia with respiratory acidosis requires an increase of $\dot{V}_E$, whereas respiratory alkalosis requires a decrease. A progressive decrease of $\dot{V}_E$ accompanies improvement of disease processes causing respiratory acidosis because of ventilation-perfusion derangement. This results because improved matching of alveolar ventilation to capillary blood flow provides increased efficiency of gas exchange with less gas volume.

3. Alveolar-arterial oxygen gradient ($A-a_{DO_2}$)—This is the difference between estimated alveolar partial pressure of oxygen and Pa_{O_2} and represents the pulmonary shunt due primarily to ventilation-perfusion inequality. The normal range for 100% oxygen is 25–65 mm Hg. Since the alveolar partial pressure is dependent upon F_{IO_2}, an estimate of $A-aD_{O_2}$ can be made by comparing F_{IO_2} to Pa_{O_2} and is important in detecting changes in physiologic pulmonary shunt. Large gradients requiring an F_{IO_2} greater than 0.55 (55% oxygen concentration) to maintain adequate oxygenation may lead to oxygen toxicity. Oxygen toxicity may be suspected when new bilateral alveolar infiltrates are found on chest x-ray and decreasing effective compliance and increasing hypoxemia respond only temporarily to deep sighing technics. $A-aD_{O_2}$ can be dramatically improved by the use of positive end-expiratory pressure (PEEP). By maintaining 5–15 cm water pressure and not allowing the normal expiratory return to atmospheric pressure, alveolar collapse is prevented and ventilation is better matched to perfusion. This decrease in shunt effect is proposed as the mechanism for narrowing of $A-aD_{O_2}$ by the use of PEEP. Some ventilators have a built-in mechanism for employing PEEP; however, the use of a wide-bore tube from the exhalation port submerged below water to a depth sufficient to obtain the desired amount of PEEP is as effective. Employ extreme caution to avoid cardiovascular decompensation when PEEP is initially added to ventilatory support.

Other parameters should be followed which are not directly related to ventilator function but are important to the total care of the patient in ARF. Frequent determinations of hemoglobin are necessary because of an increased incidence of gastrointestinal bleeding. Accurate fluid intake and output measurements may help to identify and prevent abnormalities of fluid and electrolyte balance. Frequent serum electrolyte determinations and occasional urinary electrolytes are advisable because of the possibility of hyponatremia, hypokalemia, and hypochloremia. A high incidence of arrhythmias—especially tachyarrhythmias—justifies cardiac monitoring and periodic ECGs. Periodic sputum cultures and sensitivities detect changes in bacterial flora of preexisting infection or distressingly frequent superinfection. Daily chest x-rays may reveal infiltrates, vascular congestion, and atelectasis not apparent clinically.

In addition to the general measures described previously for the treatment of any patient with acute respiratory failure, ventilator-sustained patients require special tracheal airway care. The cuff should be inflated only to the extent that air leakage on inspiration is stopped. Newer low-pressure soft cuffs help avoid many of the tracheal complications of prolonged airway management. Deflation of the cuff need be done only at the time of suctioning with any type of cuff. Suctioning should be done with aseptic technic and disposable suction catheters of adequate length used only once. Suctioning should be done quickly in patients with severe hypoxemia and in any case should not exceed 15 seconds. Frequent regular positional changes and adequate sighing technics help prevent hypostatic pulmonary changes.

D. Weaning: The final goal in treatment is to end the patient's dependence on the ventilator. The change from assisted to spontaneous ventilation should be based on objective clinical and laboratory criteria, as follows: (1) Stabilization of vital signs, ABG, and electrolytes and correction of underlying precipitating or aggravating conditions. (2) $A-aD_{O_2}$ less than 400 mm Hg on 100% oxygen. (3) Effective compliance greater than 20 ml/cm water. (4) Adequate vital capacity, as measured by any of several measurements, eg, (a) greater than 1 liter, (b) greater than 10 ml/kg body weight, (c) twice normal tidal volume.

Weaning involves the orderly progression from controlled to assisted ventilation to delivery of oxygen and mist to the tracheal tube via T-tube connector and finally to extubation. The critical step from assisted ventilation to T-tube should be attempted every morning after at least 2 or 3 of the above criteria have been met. Adequate oxygenation and humidification must be maintained through a T-tube connector attached to the tracheal or tracheostomy tube. ABG are obtained after 30 minutes of T-tube maintenance to determine adequacy of oxygenation and the ability of the patient to avoid respiratory acidosis. The patient should be maintained on a T-tube with IPPB given every 1–4 hours, preferably for 24 hours. Adequate oxygenation and stable acid-base balance justify extubation after such an appropriate period of observation. A new weaning technic, intermittent mandatory ventilation (IMV), may replace the abrupt transition from continuous assisted ventilation to T-tube or aid in weaning difficult cases (see Downs reference, below).

E. Complications: Airway problems occur frequently and are usually due to faulty supervision. Airway disconnection, obstruction of airway by inadequately suctioned secretions, oxygen toxicity, and gross maladjustment of ventilator settings are examples of avoidable problems. However, even in well-managed patients, gram-negative pneumonias, gastrointestinal bleeding, tachyarrhythmias, neurologic abnormalities, and electrolyte disturbances occur. Complications of all organ systems may eventually be involved in protracted ventilator cases.

Treatment of Chronic Respiratory Failure (CRF)

Relief of hypoxemia and avoidance of respiratory acidosis by treatment of bronchospasm, adequate clearing of secretions, and control of infection form the basis for treatment of chronic respiratory failure. Basic therapy is modified for associated problems. Treatment of chronic respiratory failure in restrictive disease is directed at hypoxemia and its complications. Although life may not be prolonged, symptomatic relief alone justifies treatment of CRF.

A. Oxygen Therapy: Supplemental oxygen during exercise and at rest may be provided by compressed oxygen in cylinders or liquid oxygen reservoir and a walker system. The goals of treatment are (1) reduction of reversible components of pulmonary hypertension, thereby relieving right heart strain; (2) retardation of secondary polycythemia; and (3) reduction of dyspnea and increase of exercise tolerance. Maintenance of P_{aO_2} greater than 60 mm Hg usually provides sufficient oxygen content to accomplish these goals, but individual responses must be determined. Attention should be given to the worsening of hypoxemia that occurs during sleep.

B. Aerosol Therapy: Delivery of bronchodilators and mist to liquefy secretions constitutes basic aerosol therapy. Although IPPB may be necessary in some severely obstructed patients to deliver these aerosols, most patients do not need IPPB devices. In fact, serious question has been raised whether IPPB is clearly indicated other than for sustained ventilation via artificial airway (see Ziment reference, p 137).

1. Aerosolized drug therapy—Bronchodilators—most commonly isoproterenol and isoetharine with phenylephrine—and occasionally mucolytic agents such as acetylcysteine may be delivered by small or large volume nebulizers powered either by oxygen or an air compressor. These devices may be modified by a Y-connector to deliver the aerosol intermittently. Dilution of 0.25—0.5 ml of bronchodilator with 2.5—4 ml of saline may be necessary depending upon the duration of therapy and mode of delivery. Treatments usually are administered 4 times a day and as needed for wheezing.

2. Bland aerosol therapy—Water, saline, or sodium bicarbonate solution may be delivered effectively by using simple devices such as facial saunas or baby bottle warmers. Large volumes of smaller particle size are generated by heated Venturi and ultrasonic nebulizers, but these are principally for hospital use.

C. Physical Therapy: Oxygen, medication, and aerosol therapy are greatly enhanced by appropriate well-directed physical therapy, which may obviate the need for mechanical respiratory devices.

1. Chest physical therapy—Proper breathing technics, cough maneuvers, and postural drainage with vibration and percussion of the chest wall not only help to relieve dyspnea and improve ventilation but are essential to clearing of secretions loosened by bronchodilator and aerosol therapy.

2. General physical therapy—Loss of muscle strength is common in chronic respiratory failure because of inadequate oxygen reserves to sustain usual activities. Improvement of muscle tone by progressive passive and active exercises decreases oxygen demand with normal exercise. Furthermore, coordination of breathing with walking improves efficiency and decreases the disability of chronic respiratory failure.

D. Oral Bronchodilators: Xanthines and sympathomimetic amines may be important ancillary therapy. Properly used, cardiovascular, nervous system, and gastrointestinal side-effects can be minimized and the need for corticosteroids decreased. Liquid formulations such as elixir of theophylline, 15—30 ml (80—160 mg) 3 or 4 times daily, allow for variation of dose within patient tolerance. Monitor blood theophylline levels when possible.

E. Corticosteroids: Although other forms of therapy with fewer serious side-effects should be attempted, corticosteroids must not be withheld from dyspneic patients with bronchospasm. Initially, prednisone, 10 mg 4 times daily orally, may be given and increased every 24 hours until bronchospasm is completely relieved. If bronchospasm fails to respond to corticosteroid therapy, reevaluation of bronchial toilet technics and consideration of hospitalization for aggressive aerosol therapy and chest physiotherapy are advisable. After bronchospasm has been completely relieved and effective aerosol therapy instituted, gradual reduction of corticosteroid dosage every 3—7 days may be accomplished. Cessation of corticosteroids is preferred, but reduction to intermittent or small daily divided maintenance doses may be all that can be achieved.

F. Antibiotics: Aggressive use of broad spectrum antibiotics such as tetracycline and ampicillin may be required in treating respiratory infection.

G. Environmental Control: Avoidance of smoking, high air pollution, fumes, pollens, and dusts is essential but difficult to achieve. Smoking is the single most important contributing factor to deterioration of patients with chronic obstructive lung disease.

H. Miscellaneous: Phlebotomy to reduce secondary polycythemia improves circulation and decreases the possiblity of thromboembolic disease. Digitalis preparations and diuretics are necessary when heart failure occurs. Potassium replacement is required in many cases.

Burke RH, George RB: Acute respiratory failure in chronic obstructive pulmonary disease. Arch Int Med 132:865, 1973.

Downs JB & others: Intermittent mandatory ventilation: A new approach to weaning patients from mechanical ventilators. Chest 64:331, 1973.

Feeley TW, Hedley-Whyte J: Weaning from controlled ventilation and oxygen. New England J Med 292:903, 1975.

Koo KW, Sax DS, Snider GL: Arterial blood gases and pH during sleep in chronic obstructive pulmonary disease. Am J Med 58:663, 1975.

Petty TL: *Intensive and Rehabilitative Respiratory Care,* 2nd ed. Lea & Febiger, 1974.

Petty TL: Bigelow DB, Levine BE: The simplicity and safety of arterial puncture. JAMA 195:693, 1966.

Piafsky KM, Ogilvie RI: Dosage of theophylline in bronchial asthma. New England J Med 292:1218, 1975.

Pontoppidan HB & others: Acute respiratory failure in the adult. (3 parts.) New England J Med 287:690, 743, 799, 1972.

Rogers RM (editor): Symposium on cardiorespiratory intensive care. Chest 62:15—585 (Aug), 63S—118S (Nov), 1972.

•   •   •

OBESITY & HYPOVENTILATION

This syndrome has been described in extremely obese individuals who show no evidence of primary disease of the lungs or heart. It is characterized by somnolence (or sometimes insomnia), cyanosis, periodic respirations, hypoxia, hypercapnia, secondary polycythemia, right ventricular hypertrophy, and heart failure. It has been called the "Pickwickian syndrome" because of its similarity to Dickens' description of the fat boy in *The Pickwick Papers.*

Weight reduction appears to reverse the abnormalities. Oral progesterone therapy has been found effective in some patients by causing hyperventilation.

Grant JL, Arnold W Jr: Idiopathic hypoventilation. JAMA 194:119, 1965.
Lyons HA, Huang CT: Therapeutic use of progesterone in alveolar hypoventilation associated with obesity. Am J Med 44:881, 1968.
Sutton FD Jr & others: Progesterone for outpatient treatment of Pickwickian syndrome. Ann Int Med 83:476, 1975.

THE ALVEOLAR-CAPILLARY BLOCK SYNDROME

This clinical syndrome, due to impaired oxygen-diffusing capacity of the lungs, occurs in a variety of diseases which involve the alveolar-capillary interface. Prominent among these are sarcoidosis, berylliosis, scleroderma, bronchiolar carcinoma, miliary tuberculosis, mitral stenosis, and asbestosis. Recent studies suggest that decrease in the total pulmonary capillary bed, decrease in the total pulmonary diffusing surface, and disturbance in the ventilation/blood flow relationship may be more important in pathogenesis than thickening of the alveolar walls.

The principal clinical features are hyperventilation, tachypnea, dyspnea, cyanosis, and basal rales. Signs of bronchial obstruction (eg, wheezing) are usually absent. Chest films almost always reveal striking and diffuse infiltration.

The syndrome may be recognized by pulmonary function tests which reveal the following: (1) uniform reduction in lung volume with normal residual volume/ total lung capacity ratio, (2) well-preserved maximum voluntary ventilation (MVV), (3) decreased diffusing capacity, (4) hypoxemia, and (5) normal or decreased arterial CO_2 tension.

Treatment is directed at the underlying cause of the impaired oxygen diffusion. If this is reversible, improvement can be anticipated. Miliary tuberculosis and some forms of pulmonary edema are reversible with appropriate treatment. Diffuse pulmonary sarcoidosis in its acute form and some types of nonspecific granuloma respond dramatically to corticosteroid drugs. When fibrosis is well established, improvement usually does not occur.

Burrows B: Pulmonary diffusion and alveolar-capillary block. M Clin North America 51:427, 1967.

ACUTE PULMONARY EDEMA OF EXTRINSIC ORIGIN

Typical pulmonary edema in the absence of the usual underlying cardiac disease and arising de novo in previously healthy lungs has been described after the use of some drugs (nitrofurantoin, heroin), the inhalation of smoke and other toxic substances (causing altered capillary permeability), fluid overload, and after rapid ascent to altitudes exceeding 10,000 feet ("altitude pulmonary edema"). Pulmonary edema occurs in some patients after severe CNS trauma. It appears to be neurogenically mediated and may be due to adrenergic overactivity, causing a shift of blood from the systemic to the pulmonary circulation.

General measures which may be helpful in the treatment of pulmonary edema due to these causes include the following: (1) supplemental oxygen, usually administered by intermittent or continuous positive pressure technics, (2) tracheal suction, (3) intravenous diuretics, (4) intravenous aminophylline, (5) correction of respiratory or metabolic acidosis, and (6) corticosteroid drugs when increased capillary permeability is suspected (up to 1 gm of hydrocortisone IV daily).

Nicklaus JM, Snyder AB: Nitrofurantoin pulmonary reactions. Arch Int Med 121:151, 1968.
Robin ED & others: Pulmonary edema. (2 parts.) New England J Med 288:239, 292, 1973.
Simmons RL & others: Pulmonary edema following head injury. Ann Surg 170:39, 1969.
Stein L & others: Pulmonary edema during fluid infusion in the absence of heart failure. JAMA 229:65, 1974.

IDIOPATHIC INTERSTITIAL PNEUMONIA OR FIBROSIS

This is a group of pneumonias characterized by a significant cellular infiltrate in the interstitial tissue of the alveoli.

This entity was first described by Hamman and Rich in 1933. Their cases were rapidly progressive and fatal. Since then, many cases with similar pathologic findings and varying rates of progression have been described. It is now recognized that the disease is often chronic and may occasionally be reversible. Immunologic mechanisms may play a role in some instances, and rheumatoid factor is frequently present. Rheumatoid factor is a 19S macroglobulin antibody which forms immune complexes with other globulins.

All of the known causes of pulmonary fibrosis such as infection, exposure to toxic inhalants, systemic use of toxic substances, and various systemic diseases must be excluded before this diagnosis can be made. A familial form of the disease has also been reported.

Symptoms include chronic cough and progressive dyspnea. Physical findings may be absent or minimal.

Loud crackling rales eventually appear. Clubbing of the fingers may be an early finding. Signs of cor pulmonale appear in the more advanced stage of the disease. Laboratory studies are not characteristic. Pulmonary function tests show a restriction of lung volume and vital capacity with little or no bronchial obstruction. An increase in the alveolar-arterial oxygen pressure gradient occurs which appears to be due mainly to an imbalance of ventilation and perfusion rather than a reduced diffusion capacity, or "alveolar capillary block."

Chest x-rays show initially a diffuse "ground glass" density progressing to more obvious fibrotic changes ("reticular pattern," "lacework," etc) and finally to fibrocystic or honeycomb lung.

Lung biopsy is often necessary for definitive diagnosis.

Treatment with large doses of corticosteroids for several weeks followed by gradual reduction to a lower maintenance dose occasionally has a favorable effect in the early stages of pulmonary fibrosis, but the course is unpredictable.

Desquamative interstitial pneumonia is a similar but pathologically distinct entity that behaves clinically like other forms of idiopathic interstitial pneumonia. It is said to be much more responsive to corticosteroid treatment—especially in the early desquamative stage, before fibrosis has become prominent.

Gaensler EA & others: Chronic interstitial pneumonias. Clin Notes Resp Dis 10(4):3, 1972.
Patchefsky AS & others: Desquamative interstitial pneumonia. Arch Int Med 132:222, 1973.
Solliday NH & others: Familial chronic interstitial pneumonia. Am Rev Resp Dis 108:193, 1973.

SARCOIDOSIS
(Boeck's Sarcoid)

Essentials of Diagnosis

- Hilar adenopathy and nodular or fibrous infiltration of both lungs on the chest x-ray.
- Tuberculin reaction usually negative; no bacteriologic evidence of tuberculosis.
- Biopsy (most commonly the lymph nodes and skin) reveals noncaseating granuloma.
- Occasionally, the skin, bones, joints, salivary glands, and uvea are also involved.
- Black race more often affected.

General Considerations

Boeck's sarcoid is a chronic noncaseating epithelioid cell granuloma which may involve various organs but most commonly the lungs. The granulomatous tissue changes are not pathognomonic. When no specific cause can be determined, the clinical entitity is called Boeck's sarcoid or sarcoidosis. There is growing evidence that an unidentified viral agent may be involved in this "idiopathic" form. Distribution is worldwide,

but the incidence is highest in the temperate zones, especially in the southeastern USA. The incidence in the black population is 14 times that in whites. The usual age range is 20–40. Sex incidence is approximately equal.

Since the lungs are most commonly involved, sarcoidosis is an important entity in the differential diagnosis of pulmonary and mediastinal diseases.

Clinical Findings

A. Symptoms and Signs: Pulmonary symptoms and signs are commonly absent in spite of marked x-ray abnormalities. Constitutional symptoms, such as night sweats, fever, and loss of weight, are often minimal or absent. Cough and dyspnea occur late in patients with progressive pulmonary lesions, although they may occasionally occur early in the presence of an acute onset.

Skin lesions consist of nodules and diffuse infiltrations, especially of the face, ears, nose, and extensor surfaces. Atrophic scars may follow healing. Erythema nodosum may occur.

Other clinical manifestations are very uncommon. Enlargement of the tracheobronchial nodes may produce cough and dyspnea due to compression. Persistent painless enlargement of the parotid and other salivary glands may occur. There may also be lacrimal gland involvement; variable involvement of the eyes with conjunctivitis, iritis, and corneal and vitreous opacities; and involvement of the retina.

Polyarthritis may occur.

Myocardial lesions may result in arrhythmias, conduction defects, and even cardiac failure.

Paralysis of the facial muscles, soft palate, and vocal cords and peripheral neuritis may be encountered.

B. Skin Tests: Tuberculin and various fungus antigen skin tests are usually negative. Antigen prepared from sarcoid nodes and injected intracutaneously reproduces the sarcoid tubercle locally, usually after weeks or months, in most patients with sarcoidosis (Kveim reaction). The value of this test is limited because of the time required and also because positive reactions may occur in the presence of lymphadenopathy due to diverse causes.

C. Laboratory Findings: Serum globulin, calcium, and alkaline phosphatase may be elevated. Pulmonary function tests in those with parenchymal lesions usually show a restriction of the vital capacity without significant evidence of obstruction. The carbon monoxide diffusion capacity is usually decreased in the presence of parenchymal pulmonary lesions.

Biopsy is the definitive diagnostic procedure. Skin and lymph nodes are the most accessible sites. Even small, inconspicuous nodes may reveal typical lesions. Lymph nodes anterior to the scalenus anticus muscle are "connected" to the mediastinal nodes, and biopsy of these nodes reveals a high incidence of positive results (70%). When more superficial sites fail to reveal the lesion, biopsy of the mediastinal nodes by mediastinoscopy or needle biopsy of the liver (which is frequently involved) may be of value. Although lung biopsy will reveal the granuloma in the highest percentage of cases, it is usually not called for.

D. X-Ray Findings: The principal finding is hilar adenopathy, which is bilateral and striking ("potato nodes"). Paratracheal nodes also are frequently enlarged. Pulmonary infiltrates may be nodular, patchy, or linear and are usually centrally located. More advanced pulmonary changes include interstitial fibrosis, bullous emphysema, and bronchiectasis. Hilar nodes usually regress or disappear as parenchymatous lesions appear. Characteristic "punched out" areas in the small bones of the hands and feet may be seen but are uncommon.

Differential Diagnosis

The most important diseases to be differentiated are tuberculosis, the collagen diseases, mycotic infections, the malignant lymphomas (especially Hodgkin's disease), and other diseases producing x-ray patterns of hilar lymphadenopathy or miliary pulmonary nodules. The relatively asymptomatic nature of sarcoidosis in the presence of obvious clinical disease is an important differential feature.

Treatment

There is no specific treatment. Absence of symptoms and spontaneous resolution is common. When extensive pulmonary disease is present which is symptomatic or progressive, corticosteroid treatment may be helpful. Prednisone, 40 mg orally daily, should be given for at least 1 month. If no symptomatic or x-ray improvement has occurred, discontinue the drug gradually. If there has been improvement, reduce the prednisone gradually to 20 mg/day and continue as long as further clearing occurs. When stability of symptoms or x-ray lesions has been achieved, continue the corticosteroid for another 4–6 weeks in gradually decreasing doses until the drug is eliminated. Exacerbations of symptoms or x-ray lesions may indicate the need for more prolonged treatment.

Prognosis

Sarcoidosis is a relatively benign disease. The overall mortality rate is about 5%. Hilar adenopathy usually resolves without treatment. Pulmonary lesions are more likely to persist with or without treatment. Complications may include cardiac failure (due to actual myocardial involvement or cor pulmonale) and pulmonary insufficiency when pulmonary lesions are progressive. The altered diffusion capacity tends to persist even after other signs and symptoms have cleared.

Buckley CE III, Dorsey FC: A comparison of serum immuno-globulin concentrations in sarcoidosis and tuberculosis. Ann Int Med 72:37, 1970.

Deenstra H, Van Ditmars MJ: Sarcoidosis. Dis Chest 53:57, 1968.

Freundlich IM & others: Sarcoidosis: Typical and atypical thoracic manifestations. Clin Radiol 21:376, 1970.

Israel HL, Ostrow A: Sarcoidosis and aspergilloma. Am J Med 47:243, 1969.

Israel HL & others: A controlled trial of prednisone treatment of sarcoidosis. Am Rev Resp Dis 107:609, 1973.

Israel HL & others: Kveim reaction and lymphadenopathy in sarcoidosis and other diseases. New England J Med 284:345, 1971.

Mitchell DN, Scadding JG: Sarcoidosis. Am Rev Resp Dis 110:774, 1974.

Siltzbach LE & others: Course and prognosis of sarcoidosis around the world. Am J Med 57:847, 1974.

WEGENER'S GRANULOMATOSIS

This is a necrotizing granuloma of unknown etiology which involves the upper respiratory tract and the lungs and is associated with a diffuse vasculitis involving both arteries and veins. Renal failure due to glomerulitis and pulmonary failure is the usual cause of death. A limited form of the disease with pulmonary lesions and with or without upper respiratory disease and no renal or other systemic involvement has been described. Most patients with Wegener's disease do have renal involvement, and this is the determining factor in the prognosis. The sex distribution is equal, and the disease usually appears in the 4th and 5th decade in previously healthy people. The condition may be a variant of disseminated polyarteritis.

Clinical manifestations include epistaxis, severe sinusitis, hemoptysis, pulmonary consolidation, blood eosinophilia, hemorrhagic skin lesions, and progressive renal failure.

Treatment with cytotoxic agents, especially cyclophosphamide (Cytoxan) and azathioprine (Imuran), has definitely improved the prognosis in Wegener's disease, which formerly had a 2-year mortality rate of 80% when renal involvement was present. Corticosteroid treatment does not alter the prognosis but may be helpful in the presence of acute inflammatory manifestations.

Fauci AS, Wolff SM: Wegener's granulomatosis: Studies in eighteen patients and a review of the literature. Medicine 52:535, 1973.

Israel HL, Patchefsky AS: Wegener's granulomatosis of lung: Diagnosis and treatment. Ann Int Med 74:881, 1971.

Kjellstrand CM & others: Acute fulminant Wegener's granulomatosis. Arch Int Med 134:40, 1974.

Novack SN, Pearson CM: Cyclophosphamide therapy in Wegener's granulomatosis. New England J Med 284:938, 1971.

Raitt JW: Wegener's granulomatosis: Treatment with cytotoxic agents and adrenocorticoids. Ann Int Med 74:344, 1971.

PULMONARY THROMBOEMBOLISM

Essentials of Diagnosis

- Sudden onset of dyspnea and anxiety, with or without substernal pain, is characteristic of a large pulmonary embolus. Signs of acute right heart failure and circulatory collapse may follow shortly.

● Less severe dyspnea, pleuritic pain, cough, hemoptysis, and an x-ray density in the lung are characteristic of pulmonary infarction.

● Gradually developing, unexplained dyspnea with or without pulmonary x-ray densities may indicate repeated minor embolization to the lungs.

● A history or clinical findings of thrombophlebitis are common in patients with pulmonary embolism.

General Considerations

Thrombotic emboli arise from thromboses in the deep veins of the lower extremities. (Emboli of air, fat, and tumor cells are not discussed here.) This event is so common in the older, bedridden, early postpartum, or postoperative patient (especially after extensive abdominal or pelvic surgery) that any sudden appearance of pulmonary or cardiac symptoms and signs in such patients should at once suggest this diagnosis.

Clinical Findings

The clinical and laboratory manifestations of pulmonary embolism often depend on the level at which the obstruction occurs, hence on the size of the embolus. In a terminal artery, the findings may be minimal or absent until repeated embolization has occurred; in a medium-sized artery, predominantly pulmonary symptoms and signs and x-ray densities; in a large artery, predominantly cardiac signs of acute right heart failure with distention of neck veins and liver and ECG changes, progressing to shock, syncope, cyanosis, and sudden death. The latter symptoms and signs are those of the embolism per se. Hemoptysis, pleuritic pain, and infiltrates on x-ray are a result of lung infarction which appears 12–36 hours after embolism.

The source of embolus is frequently clinically "silent" (deep leg veins, pelvic veins, superficial veins).

A. Symptoms and Signs: These are characteristically sudden and episodic, interspersed with "silent" intervals. Chest pain (present in 75% of cases) may be pleuritic or anginal (not dependent upon preexisting coronary disease). Dyspnea (50% of cases) varies from mild wheezing to frank pulmonary edema. Sudden dyspnea in the absence of obvious evidence of cardiac or pulmonary disease is a characteristic of pulmonary embolism. Cough occurs in about 30% of cases, hemoptysis in about 25%. Syncope is a much more frequent symptom in pulmonary embolism than in acute myocardial infarction.

Temperature commonly rises sharply at the onset of symptoms; this may be the sole manifestation of pulmonary embolism. Shaking chills are rare.

Cardiac signs include tachycardia, accentuation of the second pulmonic sound, loud systolic murmur, protodiastolic gallop, vascular collapse ("shock"), cyanosis, and elevated central venous pressure (over 15 cm H_2O).

Pulmonary signs, which may be transient, include rales, signs of consolidation, pleural friction rub, and (occasionally) signs of pleural fluid. These are secondary to pulmonary infarction.

B. Laboratory Findings: Low arterial P_{O_2} and P_{CO_2} are characteristic. Normal P_{O_2} excludes massive embolism. Other laboratory studies are unreliable. Moderate leukocytosis occurs in 70% of cases; hyperbilirubinemia appears in about half of cases after 24 hours. The sedimentation rate is elevated. Serum LDH is usually elevated, and SGOT may or may not be elevated.

C. X-Ray Findings: X-ray changes, which are not characteristic, are usually a result of pulmonary infarction. Enlargement of the main pulmonary artery, elevation of the diaphragm, small pleural effusion, and a density in the lung, which may be delayed several days, are frequent findings.

The technic of scanning for radioactivity from a radioactive isotope injected intravenously may reveal negative defects in the lung areas distal to pulmonary artery obstruction and has been useful as a screening technic where ordinary x-rays reveal no lesions. (Negative defects may appear in many other lung diseases, but with the latter there are usually obvious associated x-ray densities.) A refinement of this examination involves a determination of the distribution of ventilation by inhalation of a radioisotope (xenon Xe 133) immediately following the perfusion test. The demonstration of normal ventilation of an area of lung in the absence of perfusion is a strong indication of pulmonary embolism.

Pulmonary angiography is the most definitive procedure for confirming the diagnosis and estimating the extent of involvement of the pulmonary vasculature.

D. ECG Findings: These are often transient, evolve rapidly in at least 10–20% of cases, and would probably be encountered oftener if more frequent tracings were obtained. Standard leads show a deep S in lead I; prominent Q with inverted T in lead III; tall P in lead II (occasionally); and right axis deviation. Precordial leads show inverted T waves in V_{1-4}; transient, incomplete right bundle branch block; prominent R waves over the right precordium; and displacement of the transitional zone to the left ("clockwise rotation").

Differential Diagnosis

Differentiate from myocardial infarction, dissecting aneurysm, acute pneumonias, atelectasis, pneumothorax, and obscure cardiac and pulmonary causes of dyspnea and chest pain.

Treatment

A. Emergency Measures:

1. Give oxygen in high concentration (preferably 100%) by mask to overcome anoxia. This also helps prevent cardiorespiratory failure.

2. Place a central venous catheter for measurement of central venous pressure, administration of drugs and fluids, and for emergency phlebotomy if needed.

3. Heparin, 10,000 units IV every 6 hours for 4 doses, has been shown to be helpful, apparently through vasodilatation and bronchodilatation. (Do not use if contraindication to anticoagulant exists.) Anticoagulation should be continued during hospitalization with heparin in the usual manner, monitored by the Lee-White coagulation time or the partial prothrombin time (PPT). Long-term anticoagulation may be continued with oral warfarin.

4. For severe pain, give meperidine, 50–100 mg subcut or IV; or morphine, 8–15 mg subcut or IV. These agents should be avoided in the presence of shock. (Intramuscular medications should not be used in heparinized patients.)

5. Treat shock, if present, with vasopressor drugs such as isoproterenol, 4 mg/liter; levarterenol bitartrate (Levophed), 4 mg/liter; or metaraminol bitartrate (Aramine, Pressonex), 15–100 mg in 500 ml 5% dextrose solution IV. Adjust the rate of infusion to maintain the systolic pressure at about 90 mm Hg.

6. Pulmonary embolectomy is feasible with modern cardiopulmonary bypass technics, and a number of successful cases have been reported. This procedure must be considered, if facilities are available, when embolization is massive. The above measures do not reverse hypotension and other life-threatening manifestations. The ultimate role of surgery and precise means of selecting candidates for this approach are now being explored.

B. Follow-Up Treatment: Observe carefully for secondary infection, and institute antibiotic treatment promptly if signs occur. If pleural effusion occurs and embarrasses respiration, remove fluid by paracentesis. Recurrence of emboli in spite of adequate anticoagulation may require vena caval interruption. Several methods of partially occluding the vena cava to avoid the adverse effects of total occlusion have been described. These appear to be less effective and offer no significant advantage over complete occlusion.

Prognosis

Pulmonary embolism is a common cause of sudden death. The prognosis is grave when acute cor pulmonale or vascular collapse (shock) occurs. Recovery from small emboli is frequent. The mortality rate rises with each episode of embolism.

Clagett GP, Salzman EW: Prevention of venous thromboembolism in surgical patients. New England J Med 290:93, 1974.

Crane C & others: The management of major pulmonary embolism. Surg Gynec Obst 128:27, 1969.

Dalen JE, Dexter L: Pulmonary embolism. JAMA 207:1505, 1969.

Eberlein TJ, Carey LC: Comparison of surgical managements for pulmonary emboli. Ann Surg 179:836, 1973.

Fleming HA, Bailey SM: Massive pulmonary embolism in healthy people. Brit MJ 1:1322, 1966.

Gray FD: *Pulmonary Embolism: Natural History and Treatment.* Lea & Febiger, 1966.

Kafer ER: Respiratory function in pulmonary thromboembolic disease. Am J Med 47:904, 1969.

Kakvan M, Masuoka S: Clinical study of pulmonary embolism. Am J Surg 121:432, 1971.

McNeil BJ, Holman L, Adelstein SJ: The scintigraphic definition of pulmonary embolism. JAMA 227:753, 1974.

Schowengerdt CG, Schreiber JT: Interruption of the vena cava in the treatment of pulmonary embolism. Surg Gynec Obst 132:645, 1971.

Secker-Walker RH: Scintillation scanning in diagnosis of pulmonary embolism. Brit MJ 1:206, 1968.

Szucs MM Jr & others: Diagnostic sensitivity of laboratory findings in acute pulmonary embolism. Ann Int Med 74:161, 1971.

DISEASES OF THE PLEURA

FIBRINOUS PLEURISY

Deposition of a fibrinous exudate on the pleural surface is the cardinal pathologic feature of fibrinous pleurisy. This is usually secondary to a pulmonary disease; pneumonia, pulmonary infarction, and neoplasm are the most frequent causes. Fibrinous pleurisy may precede the development of pleural effusion.

Chest pain is typically "pleuritic," ie, it is greatest during inspiration. Pain is minimal or absent when the breath is held or when the ribs are splinted. Referred pain may occur from the diaphragmatic pleura to the shoulder and neck (central diaphragm) or upper abdomen (peripheral diaphragm).

Pleural friction rub ("to-and-fro," "squeaky-leather," or "grating" sounds) with respirations is pathognomonic. It may occur without pleuritic pain and vice versa. Splinting of the involved chest is characteristic, with decreased motion and shallow, "grunting" respirations. The patient lies on the painful side. Other findings reflect the underlying pulmonary disease.

Treatment is aimed at the underlying disease. The treatment of the pleurisy consists only of relieving pain. Analgesics may be used as necessary. Strapping the chest with adhesive tape may give relief by restricting movement. Procaine intercostal block may be used in more severe cases.

Fibrinous pleurisy clears promptly with the resolution of the primary process. Pleural scars may remain and create minor diagnostic difficulties on future chest x-rays.

PLEURAL EFFUSION

Essentials of Diagnosis

- Dyspnea if effusion is large; may be asymptomatic.
- Pain of pleurisy often precedes the pleural effusion.

- Decreased breath sounds, flatness to percussion, egophony.
- The underlying cardiac or pulmonary disease may be the major source of symptoms and signs.
- X-ray evidence of pleural fluid.

General Considerations

Any fluid collection (transudate or exudate) in the pleural space constitutes a pleural effusion. Numerous disease processes of inflammatory, circulatory, and neoplastic origin can cause pleural effusion. Every effort should be directed toward the diagnosis of the primary disease. "Idiopathic" pleural effusion often proves to be of tuberculous origin.

Clinical Findings

A. Symptoms and Signs: There may be no symptoms. Chest or shoulder pain may be present at onset, especially when fibrinous pleurisy precedes the effusion. Dyspnea may be mild or, with large or rapidly forming effusions, severe. Cardiac failure may be associated with effusion. Fever, sweats, cough, and expectoration may occur, depending upon the underlying cause.

Physical findings include decreased motion of the chest and decreased to absent vocal fremitus on the side of the fluid, flat percussion note and decreased to absent breath sounds over the fluid, and egophony (*e*-to-*a* sound) at the upper level of the fluid. With large effusions the mediastinum shifts away from the fluid (as shown by displacement of the trachea and the cardiac apex), although underlying atelectasis may result in a shift toward the fluid. Signs resembling those of consolidation (dullness, bronchial breath sounds, bronchophony) are occasionally elicited over the fluid, presumably as a result of compression of the underlying lung by large, rapidly forming effusions.

B. X-Ray Findings: Three hundred ml or more must be present before fluid can be demonstrated by x-ray. Obliteration of the costophrenic angle is the earliest sign. Later, a homogeneous triangular density with a concave medial border extends upward to the axilla; other borders are formed by the lateral chest wall and the diaphragm. The mediastinum shifts away from the fluid (displaced heart and tracheal air shadow). The mobility of the fluid shadow, which "pours" into dependent areas of pleural space when the patient is placed on the involved side, may aid in the demonstration of small effusions. An atypical distribution of fluid along the interlobar fissures or in loculated areas may be noted.

C. Thoracentesis: This is the definitive diagnostic procedure. It demonstrates conclusively the presence of fluid and provides samples for study of physical characteristics, protein content, cells, and infectious agents. Thoracentesis should be performed carefully to avoid introducing infection and puncturing the visceral pleura.

1. Removal of fluid for examination—Remove 50–1000 ml. Use a 3-way stopcock to avoid introduc-

tion of air. Care must be exercised to avoid contaminating the pleural space.

2. Pleural fluid examination—(Specimen must be fresh.) Measurement of specific gravity or determination of protein content should be done to distinguish a transudate from an exudate (specific gravity of 1.015 and protein of 3 gm/100 ml are the approximate division points). Smear and stain for the detection of organisms and the nature of the cellular content. Collect a specimen in an anticoagulant tube for cell count. Cultures on appropriate media are indicated for all fluids from unexplained pleural effusions to demonstrate the presence of tubercle bacilli, other bacteria, or fungi. Perform pathologic examination of a centrifuged "button" if there is any suspicion of malignancy.

LDH levels have frequently been found to be increased in effusions due to malignancy. Chylous effusions usually signify an interruption of the thoracic duct by a malignancy.

D. Pleural Biopsy: This procedure has become very simple and valuable as a result of the development of better biopsy needles (eg, Abrams' needle) which permit thoracentesis and removal of one or more tissue specimens with the same needle. Pleural biopsy is indicated whenever the diagnosis is in doubt. If the tissue is not diagnostic, several more specimens should be taken.

Treatment

A. Postpneumonic and Other Sterile Effusions: Remove readily obtainable fluid by multiple thoracentesis, at daily intervals if necessary. Removal of more than 1000 ml initially is not advisable. Reexamine subsequent fluid specimens to rule out empyema if the pleuritis does not respond to treatment.

B. Tuberculous Effusion: Uncomplicated pleural effusion due to tuberculosis is treated essentially as minimal pulmonary tuberculosis. A course of isoniazid (INH) plus one of the other major antituberculosis drugs (Table 6–2) is recommended. Many patients with untreated tuberculous effusions develop pulmonary tuberculosis later, usually within 5 years.

Removal of all readily available fluid by thoracentesis is advisable to minimize later pleural fibrosis. When high fever persists for longer than 2 weeks, hematogenous dissemination should be suspected.

C. Effusions Due to Malignant Tumors: These tend to reaccumulate rapidly and require frequent removal. An attempt should be made to control the re-formation of fluid by irradiation of the hemithorax or by the use of intrapleural cytotoxic agents.

Prognosis

The prognosis is that of the underlying disease.

Committee on Therapy, American Thoracic Society: Therapy of pleural effusion. Am Rev Resp Dis 97:479, 1968.

Gaensler EA: "Idiopathic" pleural effusion. New England J Med 283:816, 1970.

Levine BW, Castleman B: Recurrent pleural effusion. New England J Med 290:152, 1974.

Maher GG, Berger HW: Massive pleural effusion: Malignant and nonmalignant causes in 46 patients. Am Rev Resp Dis 105:458, 1972.

HYDROTHORAX

The term hydrothorax generally denotes the presence of a collection of serous fluid having a specific gravity of less than 1.015 or a protein content of less than 3 gm/100 ml (transudate). The most common cause is congestive heart failure, but lymphatic obstruction and obstruction of the superior vena cava or vena azygos may also cause hydrothorax. The not unusual finding of hydrothorax in hepatic cirrhosis with ascites (6%) is explained by recent observations of ready transfer of radioiodine-labeled albumin from the peritoneal to the pleural spaces. The initial examination of the pleural fluid should be as described above.

The fluid should be removed by thoracentesis when it causes dyspnea.

The prognosis is that of the underlying disease.

HEMOTHORAX

Hemothorax (pooling of blood in a pleural space) is most commonly due to trauma but may also follow tumor, tuberculosis, and pulmonary infarction. The physical findings are the same as those of pleural effusion. Military experience has shown that early removal of all blood from the pleural space is desirable. If this cannot be accomplished by thoracentesis, an intercostal tube with water-seal drainage is indicated. If bleeding continues, thoracotomy is indicated. Great care must be taken during aspiration to avoid bacterial contamination of the pleural cavity. Surgical removal of residual blood clots may be necessary.

PLEURAL EMPYEMA
(Nontuberculous)

Acute infection of the pleural space may result from (1) direct spread from adjacent bacterial pneumonia, (2) rupture of lung abscess into the pleural space, (3) invasion from subphrenic infection, or (4) traumatic penetration. The availability of early and specific therapy for these conditions has made empyema an uncommon disease.

The clinical findings are often obscured by the primary underlying disease. Pleural pain, fever, and "toxicity" after clinical improvement of the primary disease, in association with physical and x-ray signs of pleural fluid, are characteristic. Thoracentesis reveals a frankly purulent exudate from which the etiologic organism may be cultured. Empyema, like lung ab-

scess, may become chronic, with a prolonged course and little tendency to spontaneous resorption (especially in bronchiectasis and tuberculosis).

The key to nonsurgical treatment of acute empyema is early diagnosis. Any collection of fluid occurring in the course of pulmonary inflammatory disease should be removed at once. If pus is present, a specimen should be obtained for Gram's stain and cultures, including cultures for anaerobic organisms. (Coagulase-positive *Staphylococcus aureus* and coliform organisms are the most common aerobic bacteria causing empyema; bacteroides and peptostreptococci are the most frequently encountered anaerobic organisms.) The empyema should be aspirated as completely as possible. Some early localized empyemas can be treated by thoracentesis and antibiotic therapy alone. Any large or loculated empyema should be drained immediately via an intercostal tube. In some instances, open thoracotomy may be required to ensure adequate drainage.

As soon as specimens have been obtained for culture, parenteral antibiotic treatment should be started with penicillin, 600,000 units IM every 6 hours or, alternatively, cephalothin, 8 gm IV daily. When the pus has a foul odor or the empyema is thought to be secondary to an intra-abdominal infection, chloramphenicol, 50 mg/kg/day orally, should be added to the initial treatment. The object is to obliterate the empyema space as soon as possible. Irrigations with saline through the catheter may be necessary. Chronic empyema usually results from inadequately treated acute empyema or from a bronchopleural fistula. Surgical drainage with or without decortication is usually necessary.

Emerson JD & others: Empyema. J Thoracic Cardiovas Surg 62:967, 1971.

Geha AS: Pleural empyema: Changing etiologic, bacteriologic and therapeutic aspects. J Thoracic Cardiovas Surg 61:626, 1971.

Simmons EM & others: Review of nontuberculous empyema at the University of Missouri Medical Center from 1957 to 1971. J Thoracic Cardiovas Surg 64:578, 1972.

Snider GL, Soleh SS: Empyema of the thorax in adults: Review of 105 cases. Dis Chest 54:410, 1968.

Sullivan KM & others: Anaerobic empyema thoracis. Arch Int Med 131:521, 1973.

SPONTANEOUS PNEUMOTHORAX

Essentials of Diagnosis

- Sudden onset of chest pain referred to the shoulder or arm on the involved side; associated dyspnea.
- Hyperresonance, decreased chest motion, decreased breath and voice sounds on involved side; mediastinal shift away from involved side.
- Chest x-ray revealing retraction of the lung from the parietal pleura is diagnostic.

General Considerations

The cause of spontaneous pneumothorax is unknown in 90% of cases, but it may be secondary to pulmonary disease. The idiopathic form typically occurs in healthy young males with no demonstrable pulmonary disease other than the subpleural blebs usually found on thoracotomy or (rarely) autopsy.

Entry of air into the pleural space from a rent in the visceral pleura causes partial to complete collapse of the underlying lung. Collapse usually is self-limited by rapid sealing of the tear. Occasionally a "valve effect" occurs, with progressive entry of air on inspiration and failure of exit on expiration, and with increasing intrapleural pressure (tension pneumothorax). This has a profound effect on cardiorespiratory dynamics and may be fatal if not treated promptly.

Clinical Findings

A. Symptoms and Signs: Symptoms are occasionally minimal (vague chest discomfort, dry cough) or may even be overlooked. Characteristically, however, the onset is sudden and not necessarily related to exertion, with chest pain referred to the shoulder and arm on the affected side. Pain is aggravated by physical activity and by breathing, producing dyspnea. Fever is usually not present. Shock and cyanosis occur in tension pneumothorax, where high intrapleural pressure interferes with venous return to the heart.

Physical findings consist of decreased chest motion and decreased to absent vocal fremitus and breath sounds on the affected side. (Breath sounds may be abnormally loud and harsh on the normal side.) The percussion note is hyperresonant over the involved side. With large pneumothorax, the mediastinum shifts away from the affected side and a metallic "close to" sound can be heard with the stethoscope when one coin is tapped against another held to the chest ("coin sign"). A "tapping" sound roughly synchronous with the heartbeat is occasionally heard in left-sided pneumothorax.

B. X-Ray Findings: Air in the pleural space with a visible border of retracted lung (difficult to see if the collapse is small) is best seen over the apex and in films taken in expiration. Retraction may be confined to one area of the lung (pleural adhesions in other areas). Contralateral shift of the mediastinum is demonstrated by displacement of the tracheal air shadow and cardiac apex. (Great amounts of air are present with tension pneumothorax.) Pleural fluid (bleeding from a ruptured area or torn adhesion) is occasionally visible but is seldom present in large quantity.

Differential Diagnosis

Spontaneous pneumothorax may be secondary to pulmonary disease (eg, tuberculosis, abscess, bullous emphysema) but is most commonly due to unexplained rupture of small blebs on the visceral lung surface. The cause of bleb formation and the exact mechanism of rupture in idiopathic cases are not known. Fifty percent of cases occur in the age group from 20–24; 85% in men. Onset may occur during exercise or at complete rest. Chest pain must be differentiated from that of myocardial infarction (especially when there is shoulder-arm radiation), pulmonary embolism, and acute fibrinous pleurisy.

Treatment

A. Emergency Measures for Tension Pneumothorax: *Note:* This is a medical emergency. Insert a trocar or large-bore, short-beveled needle into the anterior part of the affected chest (just into the pleural space to avoid trauma to the expanding lung). After tension has been relieved, a simple one-way valve made from a rubber glove finger, slit at the end, can be tied to the hub of the trocar or needle. As soon as possible, a catheter should be introduced into the pleural space via a trocar or by direct incision (No. 14 or No. 16 Foley catheter) and attached to a water trap with the end of the tubing under 1–2 cm of water. (A plastic catheter mounted on a disposable aluminum stylet and packaged ready to use is available. It obviates the need for a trocar and is suitable for both emergency and definitive treatment.) A suction pump (with a maximum vacuum of −30 cm of water) may be attached to the water trap.

If pain is severe, give morphine sulfate, 8–15 mg subcut. Treat shock (see Chapter 1). Follow-up treatment is as for spontaneous pneumothorax.

B. Spontaneous Pneumothorax Without Increased Intrathoracic Pressure: Bed rest is essential until the air leak has stopped. If tuberculosis is present, treat accordingly. Pleural pain should be treated with analgesics. If cough is annoying, codeine sulfate, 15–60 mg every 3–4 hours, should be used. Aspirate air if dyspnea is present or if the pneumothorax space is large enough to aspirate safely. If air leakage continues, an intercostal catheter attached to a water trap and suction pump (see above) may be necessary. Continue suction until the lung has been reexpanded for 24 hours. Administer oxygen if dyspnea is present. In some cases of spontaneous pneumothorax where the lung does not expand or if there are repeated episodes of collapse, exploratory thoracotomy may be necessary.

Prognosis

The outlook is very good in "idiopathic" cases but is more serious in secondary cases because of the danger of infection of the pleural space. Recurrence occurs in 15–20%, usually on the same side. After 2 episodes, surgical correction should be considered. Patients with a history of spontaneous pneumothorax should be advised to avoid flying in unpressurized aircraft and high altitudes. Hemothorax occurs in about 10% of cases. Empyema may occur where underlying disease, especially tuberculosis, is present. Failure of lung to reexpand, with fibrothorax, is rare in the idiopathic type.

Tension pneumothorax is a true emergency.

Fuchs HS: Idiopathic spontaneous pneumothorax and flying. Aerospace Med 38:1283, 1967.

Inouye WY, Berggreh RB, Johnson J: Spontaneous pneumo-
    thorax: Treatment and mortality. Dis Chest 51:67, 1967.
Killen DA, Gobbel WG Jr: *Spontaneous Pneumothorax*. Little,
    Brown, 1968.
Spontaneous pneumothorax. (Editorial.) Brit MJ 1:720, 1968.

TRAUMATIC PNEUMOTHORAX

Note: This is an emergency. Open chest wounds (sucking wounds) must be made airtight by any available means (eg, bandage, handkerchief, shirt, or other material) and closed surgically as soon as possible.

Traumatic pneumothorax due to lung puncture or laceration (fractured rib, bullet, etc) is managed like spontaneous pneumothorax (above). Surgery is frequently required.

DISEASES OF THE MEDIASTINUM

MEDIASTINAL TUMOR

Mediastinal masses are often clinically "silent" until they become large. They are frequently discovered on routine chest x-rays and fluoroscopy, where their position, density, and mobility are of aid in differential diagnosis. Biopsy is often the only way to make a differential diagnosis.

Because of their proximity to the heart, great vessels, esophagus, air passages, and surrounding nerves, even benign lesions are potentially serious.

The symptoms and signs are usually due to compression and distortion of surrounding structures. Pain is usually substernal. It originates in the afferent lower cervical and upper thoracic segments (may mimic "cardiac" pain), and occasionally radiates to the shoulder, neck, arms, or back. Cough suggests tracheal and bronchial involvement. Dyspnea is due to airway obstruction (which may lead to pulmonary infections). Respirations may be stertorous, with suprasternal retraction on inspiration. Hoarseness is associated with compression paralysis of the thoracic portion of the left recurrent laryngeal nerve. Dysphagia is due to extrinsic compression of the esophagus with obstruction; it varies from mild to severe.

Compression of the heart or great vessels is an unusual cause of symptoms.

Tracheal shift is due to displacement by mass. Tracheal tug is associated with adjacent aortic aneurysms with transmitted pulsations.

The superior vena cava syndrome consists of dilated neck veins, fullness of the neck and face, and

collateral veins on the thoracic wall. It is caused by compression of the superior vena cava.

Horner's syndrome (ipsilateral miosis, ptosis, and enophthalmos) is due to compression of sympathetic outflow pathways.

Chest x-rays after a swallow of barium are essential. Fluoroscopy should be done to detect pulsations. Angiography may be helpful to identify vascular stricture. Lymph node biopsy of palpable (eg, cervical, supraclavicular) or nonpalpable (anterior scalene, paratracheal) nodes may be definitive. Mediastinoscopy and mediastinotomy are being used with increasing frequency. Exploratory thoracotomy is often necessary for diagnosis and treatment.

Treatment will depend upon the primary disease. The prognosis is variable, depending upon the cause and the histologic characteristics of the mass.

Boyd DP, Midell AI: Mediastinal cysts and tumors: An analysis
    of 96 cases. S Clin North America 48:493, 1968.
Burke WA, Burford TH, Dorfman RF: Hodgkin's disease of the
    mediastinum. Ann Thoracic Surg 3:287, 1967.
Holmes-Sellors T, Thackery AC, Thomson AD: Tumours of the
    thymus: A review of 88 operational cases. Thorax 22:193,
    1967.
Rubush JL & others: Mediastinal tumors. J Cardiovas Surg
    65:216, 1973.

PNEUMOMEDIASTINUM

Essentials of Diagnosis
- Sudden onset of severe retrosternal pain.
- Crepitus on palpation of neck and chest.
- Crunching sound simultaneous with heart beat.
- X-ray is diagnostic.

General Considerations

Free air in the mediastinum may be secondary to perforation of the intrathoracic esophagus or respiratory tract or may be caused by spontaneous rupture of an alveolus into the perivascular interstitial tissues of the lung. Air may also be sucked into the mediastinum through an open neck wound or from an area of emphysema in the neck resulting from a chest wound. Spontaneous pneumomediastinum is often associated with spontaneous pneumothorax, most often of the tension type.

Clinical Findings

A. **Symptoms and Signs:** Symptoms are often minimal. Typically, the air escapes into the subcutaneous tissues of the neck and then over the rest of the body and retroperitoneally. If pneumothorax (especially tension pneumothorax) is present also, there is usually a sudden onset of severe retrosternal pain radiating to the neck, shoulders, and anus (retroperitoneal dissection).

Table 6—4. Differential diagnosis of mediastinal tumors.

Metastases may occur in any portion of the mediastinum. Among infrequent mediastinal masses are lipoma and meningocele.

Lesion	Density	Mobility (Fluoroscopy)	Clinical Features
Anterior			
Teratoma	Translucent upper area merging with denser underlying shadow. Presence of teeth or bone is pathognomonic. Tends to calcify.	May change in shape with respirations (fluid contents compressible).	Often clinically silent. Occasional rupture into bronchus with coughing up of hair and sebaceous material. May be associated with other congenital anomalies.
Lymphoma (Hodgkin's disease, lymphosarcoma)	Dense, rounded masses. Usually bilateral.	May show transmitted pulsations when close to vessels. Relatively fixed.	Prominent systemic symptoms (eg, fever, cachexia, anemia, pruritus). Lymphadenopathy in palpable areas.
Substernal thyroid	Merges with soft tissues of neck. May have hazy calcification.	Moves with swallowing. Usually displaces trachea.	Upper portion is often palpable in the neck. Signs of thyrotoxicosis may be present.
Thymus thymoma	Soft tissue density.	Usually fixed.	Physiologic in infants; usually malignant in adults. Benign enlargement is present in up to 15% of cases with myasthenia gravis.
Bronchogenic cyst	May contain air over fluid (communication with bronchus).	May be seen to rise with swallowing.	May become infected, simulating ordinary lung abscess.
Middle			
Pericardial cysts	Soft tissue.	Usually solitary; move with heart.	Asymptomatic.
Leiomyoma of the esophagus	A single circumscribed mass.	Fixed. Outline with barium in esophagus.	Usually a history of dysphagia.
Posterior			
Neurofibroma	Close relationship to thoracic spine.	Fixed.	Often "silent" when discovered. Radicular pain may be prominent. Usually not associated with generalized neurofibromatosis (Von Recklinghausen). May produce compression of spinal cord.
Ganglioneuroma	Close relationship to thoracic spine.	Usually in children.	Potentially malignant.
Neuroblastoma	Close relationship to thoracic spine.	Usually in children.	Malignant.
Aneurysm, descending aorta		Expansile.	Erosion of vertebrae may produce back pain.

Dyspnea is not usually severe. Uncommonly, high intramediastinal pressure results in compression of the heart and blood vessels with marked dyspnea, shock, and even death ("air block"); hemodynamics are similar to those of pericardial tamponade.

Subcutaneous emphysema with crepitus on palpation of the skin of the neck or upper chest is common. Air may cause grotesque puffing of the neck and face.

"Crackling" or "crunching" sounds (Hamman's sign) in the substernal and precordial areas synchronous with the heart beat are characteristic, but are occasionally due to left-sided pneumothorax.

B. X-Ray Findings: These are definitive, showing radiolucency surrounding the heart border and radiolucent streaking of the upper mediastinum; and radiolucency of the retrosternal area on a lateral film taken at full expiration and in the subcutaneous tissues of the neck and shoulder areas.

Differential Diagnosis

The pain of pneumomediastinum may simulate that of myocardial infarction.

Treatment

No treatment is usually required unless infection occurs, but a prompt search should be made for the underlying cause (eg, pneumothorax, ruptured bronchus, perforated esophagus).

Prognosis

Spontaneous recovery usually occurs if the underlying cause is corrected. If symptoms are progressive, the condition may be due to a ruptured esophagus and emergency tracheostomy may be required.

Gray JM, Hanson GC: Mediastinal emphysema: Aetiology, diagnosis, and treatment. Thorax 21:325, 1966.

ACUTE MEDIASTINITIS

Acute inflammation of the mediastinal space may be due to traumatic perforation of the esophagus or trachea (eg, during instrumentation or by lodged foreign bodies); spontaneous perforation of the esophagus (as in carcinoma); or lymphatic and direct spread from an infection of the neck or head, eg, retropharyngeal and cervical abscess.

Onset is usually within 24 hours after perforation. Findings include substernal and neck pain; progressive dysphagia, dyspnea, fever, chills, prostration, and "toxicity"; and signs of pneumomediastinum.

There may be no radiographic findings. Mediastinal widening is visible as a diffuse soft tissue density. Mediastinal mass (abscess), with or without a fluid level, may be visible.

Treatment

Treatment consists of large doses of penicillin plus chloramphenicol until organism sensitivities are determined. Surgical drainage in the cervical region is indicated when a collection of pus bulges in that area, or drainage by mediastinotomy when a widened mediastinal shadow is seen by x-ray.

Prognosis

Without treatment, the mortality rate is high; with treatment, the prognosis is markedly improved.

CHRONIC MEDIASTINITIS

Granulomatous and fibrous mediastinitis accounts for about 10% of the lesions presenting a mediastinal mass by x-ray. The most common causes are histoplasmosis, tuberculosis, and sarcoidosis (in that order).

The clinical manifestations include widening of the mediastinum by x-ray, superior vena caval obstruction, and, occasionally, partial esophageal or tracheobronchial obstruction.

Scalene or mediastinal node biopsy may establish the cause, or exploration may be necessary.

Granulomatous disease may respond to specific treatment and corticosteroids. Obstruction due to fibrosis may be amenable to surgical decompression.

Schowengerdt CG & others: Granulomatous and fibrous mediastinitis: A review and analysis of 180 cases. J Thoracic Cardiovas Surg 57:365, 1969.

7...
Heart & Great Vessels

Maurice Sokolow

The diagnosis of any cardiovascular disease consists of (1) determining the etiology, (2) identifying the structural changes, (3) defining the physiologic abnormalities, and (4) assessing the remaining functional capacity of the heart. Treatment and the estimation of prognosis are both based upon a clear understanding of these 4 factors.

Etiology is established by considering the patient's age, the history, the specific abnormalities present, and appropriate laboratory studies such as antistreptolysin O titer, serologic test for syphilis, serum thyroxine, serum cholesterol and triglycerides, serum and urine catecholamines, and serum enzymes. Abnormalities of cardiac structure and function are identified by careful physical examination combined with radiologic, echocardiographic, and ECG studies. Cardiac catheterization is needed to determine the extent of shunts and to measure the pressures in the heart chambers, aorta, or pulmonary artery. Dye-dilution tests are useful in some otherwise undetectable right-to-left or left-to-right shunts. Biplane angiography and cineangiography are of great value in outlining the anatomy of congenital and acquired abnormalities, the degree of valvular insufficiencies, and cardiac tumors as well as assessing left ventricular function by calculation of left ventricular volumes, left ventricular ejection fraction, and similar data.

Radioisotope scanning of the heart with technetium 99m pyrophosphate is a noninvasive technic that has been shown to be reliable for the early detection of myocardial infarction and for serial determination of the size of the infarct. The anatomic area of the infarction correlates well with electrocardiographic and pathologic evidence of infarction. Furthermore, the use of radioisotopes increases understanding of regional myocardial blood flow by demonstrating decreased perfusion in localized areas when myocardial ischemia is induced by exercise.

Ultrasound (echocardiography) is of considerable value in diagnosing pericardial effusion, valvular disease (especially mitral stenosis), abnormal motion of the anterior mitral leaflet in hypertrophic cardiomyopathy, and left atrial tumor. It also allows estimation of the ejection fraction and the relative sizes of the septum and the atrial and ventricular muscle walls.

NONSPECIFIC MANIFESTATIONS

The most common symptoms resulting from heart disease are dyspnea, fatigue, chest pain, and palpitation. However, because any of these symptoms may be due to noncardiac disorders (even in patients with known heart disease), the proper interpretation of their significance depends upon systematic inquiry and diagnostic studies.

Dyspnea

Dyspnea due to heart disease is almost always associated with cardiac enlargement and other structural or physiologic changes.

The most common type of dyspnea due to heart disease is **exertional dyspnea**—distinct shortness of breath upon moderate exertion which is relieved by rest.

Orthopnea is dyspnea in recumbency which is promptly relieved by sitting up.

Paroxysmal nocturnal dyspnea suddenly awakens the patient and forces him to sit on the side of the bed or stand up for relief. It may be the first symptom of left ventricular failure or tight mitral stenosis.

Noncardiac causes of exertional dyspnea include poor physical condition, obesity, debility, advanced age, chronic lung disease, anemia, and obstruction of the nasal passages. Orthopnea occurs in extreme obesity, tense ascites due to any cause, abdominal distention due to gastrointestinal disease, and in the third trimester of pregnancy. Paroxysmal nocturnal dyspnea can be simulated by bronchial asthma appearing in adult life for the first time and by airway obstruction due to paratracheal tumors.

Anxiety states and cardiac neuroses can produce any form of dyspnea, but such patients often describe sighing respirations and complain of inability to take in a satisfying breath. Psychogenic dyspnea is also associated with acute respiratory alkalosis, which causes lightheadedness or mental clouding, paresthesias of the limbs or around the mouth, and at times frank tetany, tremulousness, and apprehension.

Fatigue

Easy fatigability which is relieved by rest is common in low-output states and heart failure. It may be the chief complaint (rather than dyspnea) in congenital heart disease, cor pulmonale, or mitral stenosis complicated by pulmonary hypertension. Asthenia—chronic exhaustion and lethargy which are not improved by rest—is due to such psychologic disorders as depression, cardiac neuroses, and chronic anxiety; or may be a component of effort syndrome ("neurocirculatory asthenia"). Noncardiac organic causes of fatigue include chronic infections, anemia, endocrine and metabolic disorders, chronic poisoning, habitual use of depressant or sedative drugs, malignancy, connective tissue diseases, and any debilitating illness.

Chest Pain

Chest pain occurs in the following cardiovascular disorders: angina pectoris (in which the pain is due to intermittent ischemia of the myocardium); myocardial infarction; myopericarditis, pericardial effusion or tamponade; aortic dissection or aneurysm; and pulmonary embolism or infarction.

Chest pain is one of the most common presenting complaints in medicine. Careful evaluation includes inquiry concerning its quality, location, radiation, duration, and the factors which precipitate, aggravate, or relieve it. Serial examinations are often required, as well as laboratory tests. Exercise tests, therapeutic tests, and selective coronary cineangiography are sometimes required.

The following noncardiac disorders are often associated with chest pain which resembles or is indistinguishable from that of heart disease: (1) Arthritis or disk disease of the lower cervical and upper thoracic spine (dorsal or ventral nerve root pain). (2) Cardiac neurosis. (3) Neurocirculatory asthenia and other emotional disorders. (4) Sliding hiatus hernia, acute or chronic cholecystitis, acute pancreatitis, cardiospasm, peptic ulcer, esophageal pain. (5) Disorders causing local chest wall pain, eg, costochondritis, strain or inflammation of the pectoral and intercostal muscles and ligaments, postmyocardial infarction syndrome, "shoulder-hand" syndrome. (6) Periarthritis of the left shoulder. (7) Spontaneous pneumothorax. (8) Pleurisy, spinal cord disease, mediastinal tumor, neoplastic invasion of ribs or vertebrae. (9) Mediastinal emphysema.

Palpitation

Consciousness of rapid, forceful, or irregular beating is the most common complaint referable to the heart. In the vast majority of instances palpitation is due to increased awareness of normal heart action, either because of anxiety about the presence of heart disease or secondary to long-standing emotional disorders such as neurocirculatory asthenia. Organic causes are anemia, thyrotoxicosis, debility, and paroxysmal arrhythmias.

Two types of palpitation are most often described: **Sinus tachycardia,** a rapid, forceful pounding which may begin gradually or suddenly but invariably slows gradually, occurs normally on exertion or during excitement. **Premature ventricular systoles** cause a sen-

sation of the heart "skipping a beat" or "stopping and turning over."

Patients with true paroxysmal tachycardia describe a rapid, regular palpitation or "fluttering" sensation which begins suddenly, lasts minutes or hours, and then ceases abruptly. In younger patients there are no other symptoms unless the attacks are prolonged. In older patients paroxysmal arrhythmias may produce angina pectoris, congestive heart failure, dizziness, or syncope. Paroxysmal atrial fibrillation is felt as a rapid irregular pounding which begins and ends suddenly. Chronic atrial fibrillation and flutter are in themselves often not perceived by the patient except after exercise or excitement when the ventricular rate increases.

An ECG taken during an episode of palpitation establishes the diagnosis. However, clinical observation of the heart rate and rhythm and the effect of exercise and carotid sinus pressure, together with an assessment of the overall clinical picture (age of patient, associated heart and other diseases), permits diagnosis in the great majority of cases without electrocardiograms.

SIGNS OF HEART DISEASE

Valuable information pertaining to the etiology, nature, and extent of heart disease is often found on general physical examination, eg, Argyll Robertson pupils, splinter hemorrhages, splenomegaly, diffuse goiter, large kidneys, congenital anomalies, or epigastric bruit. Abnormal pulsations of the neck veins or precordium, height of the venous pressure, cyanosis, clubbing, and edema should be carefully noted. Careful palpation may disclose right or left ventricular hypertrophy, thrills, and diastolic movements. Close attention should be paid to the character of the left ventricular impulse, whether heaving, hyperdynamic, or normal, and whether it is displaced to the left or not.

Edema

Edema caused by heart failure appears first in the ankles and lower legs of ambulatory patients and over the sacrum, flanks, buttocks, and posterior thighs of bedridden patients.

The mere presence of edema does not establish a diagnosis of heart failure in a patient who also complains of dyspnea. Significant edema occurs often in obese patients and those with incompetent leg veins and healed thrombophlebitis. Garters, rolled or elastic-top stockings, tight girdles, prolonged sitting or standing, premenstrual fluid retention, and "idiopathic edema of women" are other common noncardiac causes. Nephrosis or terminal nephritis, cirrhosis with tense ascites, congenital or acquired lymphedema, hypoproteinemia, severe malnutrition or anemia, and obstruction of the inferior vena cava can produce dependent edema.

Cyanosis

Cyanosis is classified as central or peripheral. Central cyanosis results from low arterial oxygen saturation caused by intracardiac right-to-left shunts, pulmonary arteriovenous fistula, certain chronic lung diseases, or pneumonia. It is differentiated from peripheral cyanosis by being present also on warm mucous membranes such as the insides of the lips and cheeks and on the tongue and conjunctivas, and is established by determining the arterial oxygen tension (P_{O_2}) and saturation. Polycythemia vera may produce central cyanosis despite normal oxygen saturation since the larger numbers of red cells produce a proportionately greater increase in the amount of reduced hemoglobin. A useful means of differentiating cyanosis caused by a shunt in the heart or lung from that caused by primary lung disease is to administer 100% oxygen: Cyanosis caused by shunt will be unaffected, whereas that due to parenchymal lung disease will disappear or decrease.

Peripheral cyanosis occurs in the presence of normal arterial oxygen saturation. It only occurs on cool portions of the body, such as the fingertips, nose, ears, and cheeks. It is caused by slowed circulation through peripheral vascular beds, which allow the capillary blood to give up more than normal amounts of oxygen. Reduced cardiac output due to mitral stenosis, pulmonary stenosis, or heart failure causes peripheral cyanosis. The most common causes, however, are nervous tension with cold, clammy hands and exposure to cold.

Murmurs, Sounds, & Clicks

Auscultation permits the examiner to determine the presence of structural or functional abnormalities by noting changes in the first or second heart sounds, the presence of additional heart sounds, extracardiac sounds, systolic pulmonary or aortic ejection clicks, mid and late systolic clicks associated with mitral disease, and by analysis of murmurs. The examiner must also recognize the sounds which have no known pathologic significance: normally split first sound, normal third sound, cardiorespiratory murmurs, and the innocent heart murmurs. Accurate interpretation of murmurs is difficult in the presence of gross heart failure with very low cardiac output or rapid ventricular rates. In these situations restoration of compensation or slowing of the ventricular rate may cause prominent murmurs to decrease in intensity; previously faint or inaudible murmurs may in turn become loud. Murmurs are graded on the basis of intensity into grades I (least intense) to VI (most intense). With experience, most examiners rarely differ by more than one grade in evaluating a murmur.

A. Systolic Murmurs: A soft short systolic murmur at any valve area may be innocent if there are no other abnormalities and if it changes markedly with respiration and position. Exercise and tachycardia increase the intensity of any murmur. This so-called innocent or functional systolic murmur, usually present at the mitral or pulmonary area, is "ejection" in type (crescendo-decrescendo, ending before systole is complete, and related to the ejection of blood from the right or left ventricle into the pulmonary artery or aorta, respectively). It is most easily heard in recumbent, thin-chested individuals; full inspiration causes it to disappear or diminish markedly, whereas full expiration may accentuate it considerably. The louder a systolic murmur, the more likely it is to be organic in origin. Any systolic murmur associated with a thrill at that valve area is due to valvular or outflow tract disease unless there is gross anemia. An apical pansystolic murmur (a "regurgitant" murmur) which merges with and replaces the first sound and which is well transmitted into the left axilla or left infrascapular area is organic, ie, is due to deformity of the mitral valve or dilatation of the mitral valve ring with regurgitation. An aortic systolic murmur is "ejection" in type and midsystolic. It is transmitted into the carotids or upper interscapular area when due to organic disease of the aortic valve or to dilatation of the base of the aorta, and is often heard well at the apex of the heart.

B. Diastolic Murmurs: Diastolic murmurs may result from dilatation of the heart (acute myocarditis, severe anemia), dilatation of the aortic ring (marked hypertension), deformity of a valve, rapid diastolic flow, or intracardiac shunts. When listening for diastolic murmurs, attention should be focused only on diastole, excluding from awareness as far as possible (once one has determined the timing) the first heart sound and any systolic murmurs.

C. Systolic Time Intervals: It has been demonstrated that left ventricular function can be assessed indirectly by quantitating the ratio (PEP/LVET; preejection period/left ventricular ejection time) by simultaneous phonocardiography, indirect carotid pulse tracing, and ECG. The LVET is prolonged by impaired left ventricular function (as in patients with angina pectoris after exercise), and the ratio makes correction for heart rate unnecessary.

Braunwald E: Regulation of the circulation. New England J Med 290:1124, 1974.

Braunwald E, Swan HJC (editors): Cooperative study on cardiac catheterization. Circulation 37 (Suppl 3), 1968.

Carlsson E: *Measurement of Cardiac Chamber Volumes and Dimensions by Radiographic Methods: A Methodological Study With Some Physiological Applications.* Univ of California Press, 1970.

Craige E, Millward DK: Diastolic and continuous murmurs. Progr Cardiovas Dis 14:38, 1971.

DeSanctis RW: Diagnostic and therapeutic uses of atrial pacing. Circulation 43:748, 1971.

Feigenbaum H: New aspects of echocardiography. Circulation 47:833, 1973.

Friedberg CK: *Diseases of the Heart,* 3rd ed. Saunders, 1966.

Hurst JW, Logue RB: *The Heart, Arteries and Veins,* 3rd ed. McGraw-Hill, 1974.

Leatham AG: *Auscultation of the Heart and Phonocardiography.* Churchill, 1970.

Marshall RJ, Shepherd JT: *Cardiac Function in Health and Disease.* Saunders, 1968.

Mendel D: *A Practice of Cardiac Catheterization.* Blackwell, 1968.

Mitchell JH, Hefner LL, Monroe RG: Performance of the left ventricle. Am J Med 53:473, 1972.

Mounsey P: Praecordial pulsations in health and disease. Postgrad MJ 44:134, 1968.

Murray JA, Johnston W, Reid JM: Echocardiographic determination of left ventricular dimensions, volumes and performance. Am J Cardiol 30:252, 1972.

Patterson JA & others: Treadmill exercise in assessment of the functional capacity of patients with cardiac disease. Am J Cardiol 30:757, 1972.

Reddy PS, Shaver JA, Leonard JJ: Cardiac systole murmurs: Pathophysiology and differential diagnosis. Progr Cardiovas Dis 14:1, 1971.

Segal BL & others: Echocardiography: Current concepts and clinical application. Am J Med 57:267, 1974.

Starmer CF, McIntosh HD, Whalen RE: Electrical hazards and cardiovascular function. New England J Med 284:181, 1971.

Swan HJ & others: Catheterization of the heart in man with use of a flow-directed balloon-tipped catheter. New England J Med 283:447, 1970.

Tavel ME: *Clinical Phonocardiography and External Pulse Recording.* Year Book, 1967.

Weissler AM: Noninvasive methods for assessing left ventricular performance in man. Am J Cardiol 34:111, 1974.

Zelis R & others: The cardiovascular effects of morphine: The peripheral capacitance and resistance vessels in human subjects. J Clin Invest 54:1247, 1974.

. . .

FUNCTIONAL & THERAPEUTIC CLASSIFICATION OF HEART DISEASE*

Functional Capacity (Four classes.)

Class I: No limitation of physical activity. Ordinary physical activity does not cause undue fatigue, palpitation, dyspnea, or anginal pain.

Class II: Slight limitation of physical activity. Comfortable at rest, but ordinary physical activity results in fatigue, palpitation, dyspnea, or anginal pain.

Class III: Marked limitation of physical activity. Comfortable at rest, but less than ordinary activity causes fatigue, palpitation, dyspnea, or anginal pain.

Class IV: Unable to carry on any physical activity without discomfort. Symptoms of cardiac insufficiency, or of the anginal syndrome, may be present even at rest. If any physical activity is undertaken, discomfort is increased.

Therapeutic Classification (Five classes.)

Class A: Physical activity need not be restricted.

Class B: Ordinary physical activity need not be restricted, but unusually severe or competitive efforts should be avoided.

Class C: Ordinary physical activity should be moderately restricted, and more strenuous efforts should be discontinued.

Class D: Ordinary physical activity should be markedly restricted.

Class E: Patient should be at complete rest, confined to bed or chair.

CONGENITAL HEART DISEASES

Congenital lesions account for about 2% of all heart disease in adults.

The following classification and relative frequency of defects is based on a study by Paul Wood (Wood P: *Diseases of the Heart and Circulation,* 3rd ed. Lippincott, 1968).

Classification

  A. **Without Shunt:**
    1. **Right-sided**—Pulmonary stenosis (12%).
    2. **Left-sided**—Coarctation of aorta (9%); aortic stenosis (3%).
  B. **With Shunt:**
    1. **Acyanotic**—
      Atrial septal defect (20%).
      Patent ductus arteriosus (13%).
      Ventricular septal defect (9%).
    2. **Cyanotic**—
      Tetralogy of Fallot (11%).
      Pulmonary stenosis with reversed interatrial shunt (3%).
      Eisenmenger's syndrome (3%).
      Tricuspid atresia (1.5%).

Noncardiac congenital anomalies are present in an estimated 20% of cases. Particularly common are mongolism, Marfan's syndrome, and chromosomal abnormalities such as Turner's syndrome.

Pathogenesis of Clinical Manifestations

Congenital heart disease produces symptoms and signs by one or more of the following mechanisms:

A. Stenosis of a Valve or Vessel (A, above): Hypertrophy of the proximal ventricle occurs and there is eventual heart failure with the usual manifestations.

B. Left-to-Right Shunt (B 1, above): Shunting of blood from the left atrium or ventricle to the right atrium or ventricle increases the work of the right ventricle and the amount of pulmonary blood flow at the expense of systemic flow. In large shunts, and in smaller ones during exercise, this discrepancy is exaggerated, and dyspnea and fatigue occur. For unknown reasons, some of these shunts cause pulmonary hypertension; reversal of shunt then occurs, converting the original left-to-right shunt into a right-to-left shunt (Eisenmenger's syndrome). Hemoptysis may occur.

*Criteria Committee, New York Heart Association.

C. Right-to-Left Shunt (B 2, above): Shunting of "venous" blood from the right atrium or ventricle into the aorta, left atrium, or left ventricle, bypassing the pulmonary circulation, causes arterial unsaturation which beyond a certain point is recognizable clinically as cyanosis. Especially in tetralogy, squatting may bring relief of exertional dyspnea and fatigue. Syncope occurs when pulmonary blood flow is very low. Compensatory polycythemia results from the persistent unsaturation, and this in turn may be responsible for cerebral thrombosis in severe cases. Clubbing usually accompanies gross cyanosis.

In addition to the specific hemodynamic effects of the lesions themselves, metastatic brain abscess is a hazard in right-to-left shunts and bacterial endocarditis may develop, especially in ventricular septal defect, patent ductus arteriosus, and bicuspid aortic valve.

In addition to x-ray and ECG study, cardiac catheterization, biplane or cineangiocardiography, or dye-dilution curves are often necessary to delineate the exact nature and magnitude of existing defects.

Differential Diagnosis

A. Auscultatory Signs: A history of a murmur present in infancy, congenital anomalies elsewhere in the body, and the finding of murmurs and thrills in areas separate from those of valve lesions found in rheumatic heart disease are helpful. A thrill and murmur along the left sternal border are most often due to congenital heart disease, although acquired aortic stenosis may confuse the diagnosis. Soft to prominent apical mid-diastolic murmurs are present in septal defect and patent ductus arteriosus but none of the other characteristics of mitral stenosis are present. Venous hum over the upper parasternal area may be confused with the continuous murmur of patent ductus arteriosus or aortic-pulmonary communication, but the former is markedly diminished by recumbency.

B. Cyanosis With Clubbing: Cyanosis, clubbing, and polycythemia may also occur in chronic cor pulmonale secondary to lung disease, in congenital pulmonary arteriovenous fistula, and in hepatic disease with right-to-left shunts. When there is serious question regarding the origin of cyanosis and clubbing, measurement of response of arterial oxygen to inhalation of 100% oxygen is helpful, because the arterial oxygen saturation cannot rise to normal if a shunt is present.

C. Cyanosis Without Clubbing: Cyanosis without clubbing and polycythemia is usually due to venous stasis; it is "peripheral," secondary to reduced cardiac output, or slowed peripheral circulation. Arterial oxygen saturation is normal.

If after careful study potentially remediable congenital heart disease remains a diagnostic possibility, the patient should be referred for cardiac catheterization, angiocardiography, and dye dilution studies.

Griffiths SP, Ellis K: Differential diagnosis of cyanotic congenital heart disease. Progr Cardiovas Dis 14:93, 1971.
Keith JD, Rowe RD, Vlad P: *Heart Disease in Infancy and Childhood,* 2nd ed. Macmillan, 1967.
Moss AJ, Adams FH: *Heart Disease in Infants, Children and Adolescents.* Williams & Wilkins, 1968.
Murphy KF & others: Ultrasound in the diagnosis of congenital heart disease. Am Heart J 89:638, 1975.
Nadas AS, Fyler DC: *Pediatric Cardiology,* 3rd ed. Saunders, 1972.
Perloff JK: *The Clinical Recognition of Congenital Heart Disease.* Saunders, 1970.
Rudolph AM: *Congenital Diseases of the Heart: Clinical Physiological Considerations in Diagnosis and Management.* Year Book, 1974.
Stanger P & others: Complications of cardiac catheterization of neonates, infants, and children: A three-year study. Circulation 50:595, 1974.
Watson H (editor): *Paediatric Cardiology.* Mosby, 1968.

PURE PULMONARY STENOSIS

Stenosis of the pulmonary valve or infundibulum increases the resistance to outflow, raises the right ventricular pressure, and limits the amount of pulmonary blood flow. Since there is no shunt, arterial saturation is normal, but severe stenosis causes peripheral cyanosis by reducing cardiac output. Clubbing or polycythemia does not develop unless a patent foramen ovale or atrial septal defect is present, permitting shunting of blood from the right to the left atrium.

Clinical Findings

A. Symptoms and Signs: Mild cases (right ventricular-pulmonary artery gradient < 50 mm Hg) are asymptomatic. Moderate to severe stenosis (gradients exceeding 80 mm Hg) causes dyspnea on exertion (in the absence of heart failure), fainting, and chest pain. Right ventricular failure develops eventually in severe cases, producing edema, increased dyspnea, and fatigue.

There is a palpable right ventricular heave. A loud, harsh systolic murmur and a prominent thrill is present in the left second and third interspaces parasternally; the murmur is in the third and fourth interspaces in infundibular stenosis. The second sound is obscured by the murmur in severe cases; the pulmonic component is diminished, delayed, or absent. Both components are audible in mild cases. A presystolic gallop and a prominent *a* wave in the venous pulse are present in severe cases.

B. X-Ray Findings and Fluoroscopy: The heart size may be normal, or there may be a prominent right ventricle and atrium or gross cardiac enlargement, depending upon the severity. The pulmonary artery is dilated with weak or absent pulsations in valvular stenosis, normal in infundibular stenosis. Pulmonary vascularity is normal or (in severe cases with right-to-left shunts) diminished.

C. ECG Findings: Right axis or right ventricular hypertrophy; peaked P waves and right atrial abnormality.

D. Special Studies: Cardiac catheterization permits estimation of the gradient across the pulmonic valve, determines whether the stenosis is valvular or infundibular, and, together with dye studies, demonstrates the presence or absence of associated shunts. Angiography delineates the anatomy of the defect, including the infundibulum of the right ventricle.

Treatment

Pure pulmonic stenosis with evidence of progressive hypertrophy and resting gradients over 75—80 mm Hg is treated surgically with low operative mortality and excellent results in most cases. All lesions are corrected under direct vision; those with associated outflow tract hypertrophy are often approached through a ventriculotomy.

Prognosis

Patients with mild stenosis may have a normal life expectancy unless bacterial endocarditis occurs. Severe stenosis causes refractory heart failure in the twenties and thirties. Moderate stenosis may be asymptomatic in childhood and adolescence, but cardiac symptoms and cardiac failure occur with increasing frequency as the patient becomes older. Only 12% of patients survive past age 50. In patients with pure pulmonic stenosis, the incidence of bacterial endocarditis is about 1% per year.

Campbell M: Natural history of congenital pulmonary stenosis. Brit Heart J 31:394, 1969.

Johnson LW & others: Pulmonic stenosis in the adult. New England J Med 287:1159, 1972.

Møller I, Wennevold A, Lynborg KE: The natural history of pulmonary stenosis: Long-term follow-up with serial heart catheterizations. Cardiology 58:193, 1973.

Shem-Tov A & others: Corrected transposition of the great arteries: A modified approach to the clinical diagnosis in 30 cases. Am J Cardiol 27:99, 1971.

Tandon R, Nadas AS, Gross RE: Results of open-heart surgery in patients with pulmonic stenosis and intact ventricular septum: A report of 108 cases. Circulation 31:190, 1965.

PULMONARY STENOSIS WITH REVERSED INTERATRIAL SHUNT

The elevated pressure in the right ventricle causes right ventricular hypertrophy and decreased distensibility. Venous blood therefore passes more readily from the right atrium through the atrial defect into the left atrium. Arterial unsaturation results, and may be sufficient to produce all the consequences of "cyanotic congenital heart disease."

Clinical Findings

A. Symptoms and Signs: Exertional dyspnea and fatigue; cyanosis, clubbing, and polycythemia; a long, harsh pulmonic systolic murmur and thrill; and slight to prominent right pulmonary artery pulsation and right ventricular heave.

B. X-Ray Findings: Slight to moderate cardiac en-largement, decreased pulmonary vascularity, and a dilated pulmonary artery (in valvular stenosis).

C. ECG Findings: Right ventricular hypertrophy and prominent P waves.

D. Special Studies: Cardiac catheterization and angiocardiography are helpful in distinguishing this lesion from tetralogy.

Treatment

Correction of pulmonic stenosis decreases right ventricular pressure and permits the atrial shunt to again become left to right if it is not closed. The shunt is usually corrected at the same operation.

Prognosis

Without surgical treatment, survival beyond early adult life is rare.

COARCTATION OF THE AORTA

The adult type of coarctation of the aorta consists of localized narrowing of the aortic arch just distal to the origin of the left subclavian artery in the region of the ligamentum arteriosum. A bicuspid aortic valve is present in 25% of cases. Blood pressure is elevated in the aorta and its branches proximal to the coarctation and decreased distally. Collateral circulation between the high and low pressure aortic segments develops through the intercostal arteries and branches of the subclavian arteries. .

Clinical Findings

A. Symptoms and Signs: There are no symptoms until the hypertension produces left ventricular failure or cerebral hemorrhage. Strong arterial pulsations are seen in the neck and suprasternal notch. Hypertension is present in the arms but the pressure is normal or low in the legs. This difference is exaggerated by exercise, which is helpful in the diagnosis of doubtful cases. Femoral pulsations are absent or weak and delayed in comparison with the brachial pulse. Visible or palpable collateral arteries are present in the intercostal spaces and along the borders of the scapulas. Patients with large collaterals may have relatively small gradients but still have severe coarctation. Late systolic ejection murmurs at the base are often heard better posteriorly, especially over the spinous processes.

B. X-Ray Findings: X-ray shows scalloping of the ribs due to enlarged collateral intercostal arteries; dilatation of the left subclavian artery and poststenotic aortic dilatation ("3" sign); and left ventricular enlargement.

C. ECG Findings: The ECG shows left ventricular hypertrophy; it may be normal in mild cases.

Treatment

Resection of the coarcted site is a more difficult operative procedure than ligation of a patent ductus arteriosus, and the surgical mortality is in the neighborhood of 1%. The risks of the disease are such, however, that if a skilled heart surgeon is available all coarctations in patients up to the age of 20 years should be resected. In patients between the ages of 20 and 35, surgery is advisable if the patient is showing evidence of left ventricular strain. The mortality rises considerably in patients over 50 years of age, and surgery in this age group is of doubtful value.

Prognosis

Most patients with the adult form of coarctation die before the age of 40 from the complications of hypertension, rupture of the aorta, bacterial endocarditis, or cerebral hemorrhage (congenital aneurysms). However, 25% have a normal cardiovascular prognosis and die of causes unrelated to the coarctation.

Campbell M: Natural history of coarctation of the aorta. Brit Heart J 32:633, 1970.

Karnell J: Coarctation of the aorta. Circulation 38 (Suppl 5):35, 1968.

Simon AB, Zloto AE: Coarctation of the aorta: Longitudinal assessment of operated patients. Circulation 50:456, 1974.

ATRIAL SEPTAL DEFECT

The most common form of atrial septal defect is persistence of the ostium secundum in the mid-septum; less commonly, the ostium primum (which is low in the septum, involving the endocardial cushion) persists, in which case mitral or tricuspid abnormalities may also be present. In both instances, normally oxygenated blood from the left atrium passes into the right atrium, increasing the right ventricular output and the pulmonary blood flow. In the primum defect, mitral valve insufficiency produces, additionally, strain on the left ventricle.

Clinical Findings

A. Symptoms and Signs: Most patients with moderate secundum defects are asymptomatic. With large shunts, exertional dyspnea or cardiac failure may develop. Prominent right ventricular pulsations are readily visible and palpable. A moderately loud systolic ejection murmur can be heard in the second and third interspaces parasternally due to increased flow across the pulmonic valve, as well as an apical or xiphoid mid-diastolic soft murmur due to increased flow across the tricuspid valve, especially on inspiration. Thrills are uncommon. The second sound is widely split, and does not vary with respiration.

B. X-Ray Findings: Large pulmonary arteries with vigorous pulsations, increased pulmonary vascularity, an enlarged right atrium and ventricle, and a small aortic knob.

C. ECG Findings: Right axis or right ventricular hypertrophy may be present in ostium secundum de-

fects. Incomplete or complete right bundle branch block is present in most cases, and left superior axis deviation with counterclockwise rotation in the frontal plane in ostium primum defect.

D. Special Studies: Cardiac catheterization permits calculation of the amount of blood shunted, the intracardiac and pulmonary pressures, and the pulmonary vascular resistance. The catheter may pass through the defect into the left atrium. Angiocardiography may reveal primum defects or mitral insufficiency.

Treatment

Small atrial septal defects do not require surgery. Lesions with a large left to right shunt (more than 2 or 3 times systemic flow) with slight or no increased pulmonary arterial resistance should be operated upon. The surgical risks now are sufficiently low so that patients with a pulmonary to systemic flow rate of 2:1 should probably be operated on.

Surgery should be withheld from patients with pulmonary hypertension with reversed shunt because of the risk of acute right heart failure.

Prognosis

Patients with small shunts may live a normal life span; with larger shunts, they survive to middle or late life before pulmonary hypertension or heart failure appear. The latter is precipitated most often by atrial fibrillation, or raised pulmonary vascular resistance. Large shunts cause disability by age 40. Raised pulmonary vascular resistance secondary to pulmonary hypertension rarely occurs in childhood or young adult life in secundum defects but is more common in primum defects; after age 40, pulmonary hypertension, cardiac arrhythmia, and left ventricular failure may occur in secundum defects.

The surgical mortality with cardiac bypass is small ($< 1\%$) in patients under 45 years of age who are not in cardiac failure and have pulmonary artery pressures < 60 mm Hg. It increases to 6–10% in patients over age 40 with cardiac failure or pulmonary artery pressures > 60 mm Hg. Most of the survivors show considerable improvement.

Cohn LH, Morrow AG, Braunwald E: Operative treatment of atrial septal defect: Clinical and haemodynamic assessments in 175 patients. Brit Heart J 29:725, 1967.

Dalen JE, Haynes FW, Dexter L: Life expectancy with atrial septal defect: Influence of complicating pulmonary vascular disease. JAMA 200:112, 1967.

Dave KS & others: Atrial septal defect in adults. Am J Cardiol 31:7, 1973.

Gault JH & others: Atrial septal defect in patients over the age of 40 years: Clinical and hemodynamic studies and the effects of operation. Circulation 37:261, 1968.

Kimball KG, McIlroy MB: Pulmonary hypertension in patients with congenital heart disease. Am J Med 41:883, 1966.

Kulbertus HE, Coyne JJ, Hallidie-Smith KA: Electrocardiographic correlation of anatomical and haemodynamic data in ostium primum atrial septal defects. Brit Heart J 30:464, 1968.

Rahimtoola SH, Kirklin JW, Burchell HB: Atrial septal defect. Circulation 38 (Suppl 5):2, 1968.

Tikoff G & others: Clinical and hemodynamic observations after surgical closure of large atrial septal defect complicated by heart failure. Am J Cardiol 23:810, 1969.

PATENT DUCTUS ARTERIOSUS

The embryonic ductus arteriosus fails to close normally and persists as a shunt connecting the left pulmonary artery and aorta, usually near the origin of the left subclavian artery. Blood flows from the aorta through the ductus into the pulmonary artery continuously in systole and diastole; it is a form of arteriovenous fistula, increasing the work of the left ventricle. In some patients, obliterative changes in the pulmonary vessels cause pulmonary hypertension. Then the shunt is bidirectional or right-to-left.

Clinical Findings

A. Symptoms and Signs: There are no symptoms until or unless left ventricular failure develops. The heart is of normal size or slightly enlarged with a forceful apex beat. Pulse pressure is wide and diastolic pressure is low. A continuous, rough "machinery" murmur, accentuated in late systole at the time of S_2, is heard best in the left first and second interspaces at the sternal border. Thrills are common. Paradoxic splitting of the second sound may be present if there is considerable left ventricular hypertrophy.

B. X-Ray Findings: The heart is normal in size and contour, or there may be left ventricular and left atrial enlargement. The pulmonary artery, aorta, and left atrium are prominent.

C. ECG Findings: Normal pattern or left ventricular hypertrophy, depending upon the width of the ductus.

D. Special Studies: Cardiac catheterization establishes the presence of a left-to-right shunt. The catheter may be passed through the ductus into the aorta from the pulmonary artery, and, when combined with angiography, excludes other lesions (such as ruptured sinus of Valsalva into the right heart), which may cause a similar murmur.

Treatment

Because of the low operative mortality rate ($<$ 1%) in skilled hands, division and closure is recommended in both children and adults. The mortality rate becomes higher as the patient becomes older. This necessitates caution in recommending surgery in older adults who are asymptomatic and have no left ventricular hypertrophy. Subacute bacterial endocarditis is the major hazard in this group.

The indications for ligation or division of a patent ductus arteriosus in the presence of pulmonary hypertension are controversial, but current opinion favors ligation whenever the pulmonary vascular resistance is low or only moderately elevated and the flow through the ductus is permanently or intermittently from left to right, ie, when pulmonary blood flow is increased, and the pulmonary artery pressure is $<$ 100 mm Hg.

Prognosis

Large shunts cause a high mortality from cardiac failure early in life. Smaller shunts are compatible with long survival, congestive heart failure being the most common complication. Bacterial endocarditis may also occur. A small percentage of patients develops pulmonary hypertension and reversal of shunt, such that the lower legs, especially the toes, appear cyanotic in contrast to normally pink fingers. At this stage, the patient is inoperable.

Campbell M: Natural history of persistent ductus arteriosus. Brit Heart J 30:4, 1968.

Espino-Vela J, Cardenas N, Cruz R: Patent ductus arteriosus: With special reference to patients with pulmonary hypertension. Circulation 38 (Suppl 5):45, 1968.

Rudolph AM & others: Hemodynamic basis for clinical manifestations of patent ductus arteriosus. Am Heart J 68:447, 1964.

VENTRICULAR SEPTAL DEFECT

In this lesion a persistent opening in the upper interventricular septum due to failure of fusion with the aortic septum permits blood to pass from the high-pressure left ventricle into the low-pressure right ventricle in small or moderately large ventricular septal defects; in large ventricular septal defects, the pressures in the 2 ventricles are equal and the shunt depends on the relative pulmonary and systemic vascular resistance. In one-fourth to one-third of cases the shunt is not large enough to strain the heart. With large shunts, both left and right ventricular strain may develop.

Clinical Findings

A. Symptoms and Signs: The clinical features are dependent upon the size of the defect and the presence or absence of a raised pulmonary vascular resistance. If the latter is normal and the defect is small, the left-to-right shunt is small; if the defect is large, the resistance to flow between the ventricles is small and the left-to-right shunt is large; a rise in pulmonary vascular resistance decreases the left-to-right shunt and converts the pansystolic murmur into a "lopsided" diamond ejection murmur. A long, loud, harsh systolic murmur and thrill are found in the left 3rd and 4th interspaces along the sternum, and may be the only finding in small defects. In large shunts a right ventricular heave is palpable and a mid-diastolic "flow murmur" and a third heart sound may be heard at the apex.

B. X-Ray Findings: With large shunts the right or left ventricle (or both), the left atrium, and the pulmonary arteries are enlarged, and pulmonary vascularity is increased.

C. ECG Findings: May be normal or may show right, left, or biventricular hypertrophy, depending on the size of the defect and the pulmonary vascular resistance.

D. Special Studies: Cardiac catheterization permits a definitive diagnosis in all but the most trivial defects. Infants with cardiac failure should be studied to establish the diagnosis and determine the appropriate treatment.

Treatment

Ventricular septal defects vary in severity from trivial asymptomatic lesions with normal cardiac hemodynamics to extensive lesions causing death from cardiac failure in infancy. The former do not require surgery. The ideal case for curative repair with cardiac bypass technics is one with a large left-to-right shunt, left ventricular hypertrophy, and only moderate pulmonary hypertension. When severe pulmonary hypertension is present (pulmonary arterial pressures > 85 mm Hg) and the left-to-right shunt is small, the surgical mortality risk is at least 50%. If the shunt is reversed, surgery is contraindicated. If surgery is required because of unrelenting cardiac failure in infancy due to a large left-to-right shunt, pulmonary artery banding may decrease the shunt and tide the patient over until age 5 or 6, when definitive repair can be done. Early closure of the defect rather than banding is now the preferred procedure in some centers. It has become increasingly evident that some defects (perhaps as many as 30–50%) close spontaneously. Therefore, surgery should be deferred until late childhood unless the disability is severe or unless pulmonary hypertension is observed to progress or to develop.

Prognosis

Patients with the typical murmur as the only abnormality have a normal life expectancy except for the threat of bacterial endocarditis. With large shunts, congestive heart failure may develop early in life and survival beyond age 40 is unusual. Shunt reversal occurs in an estimated 25%, producing Eisenmenger's syndrome. Postoperative surgical studies have shown that surgery is of no benefit if the pulmonary vascular resistance exceeds one-third of the systemic vascular resistance.

Campbell M: Natural history of ventricular septal defect. Brit Heart J 33:246, 1971.

Clarkson PM & others: Prognosis for patients with ventricular septal defect and severe pulmonary vascular obstructive disease. Circulation 38:129, 1968.

Collins G & others: Ventricular septal defect: Clinical and hemodynamic changes in the first five years of life. Am Heart J 84:695, 1972.

Glasser SP & others: Thirty-two cases of interventricular septal defect and aortic insufficiency: Clinical, hemodynamic and surgical features. Am J Med 53:473, 1972.

Hallidie-Smith KA & others: Effects of surgical closure of ventricular septal defects upon pulmonary vascular disease. Brit Heart J 31:246, 1969.

Hoffman JE, Rudolph AM: The natural history of isolated ventricular septal defect with special reference to the selection of patients for surgery. Advances Pediat 17:57, 1970.

Plass R & others: Angiocardiographic diagnosis of aortic insufficiency in cases of ventricular septal defect associated with partial prolapse of the aortic valve. Cardiology 58:257, 1973.

TETRALOGY OF FALLOT

Pulmonary stenosis together with a high interventricular septal defect, which allow the right ventricle to empty into the aorta, prevent venous blood from passing normally into the pulmonary artery. Instead, blood passes from the right ventricle into the aorta and into the left ventricle. Aortic blood is therefore markedly unsaturated, and cyanosis, polycythemia, and clubbing appear early. Exercise causes cyanosis to deepen.

Clinical Findings

A. Symptoms and Signs: Physical development is retarded in severe cases. Dyspnea is common; squatting relieves fatigue and dyspnea; and syncope occasionally occurs. Prominent signs are cyanosis and clubbing, a slight right ventricular heave and absent apical impulse, and a short, harsh systolic murmur and thrill along the left sternal border. The heart is not enlarged. A single loud second sound is heard unless the lesion is mild, when the second sound is split with the pulmonary component decreased in amplitude.

B. X-Ray Findings: The lung fields are abnormally clear. The apex of the heart is blunted, with a concavity in the pulmonary artery segment (boot-shaped heart). A right aortic arch is present in 25% of cases.

C. ECG Findings: Moderate right ventricular hypertrophy is almost always present. Prominent P waves are occasionally present.

D. Special Studies: Cardiac catheterization and right ventricular angiocardiography together establish the diagnosis and define the anatomy. Aortography has been recommended as a routine procedure in patients who are being considered for radical corrective surgery to show the aortic branches and unexpected associated defects.

Treatment

Tetralogy of Fallot is treated surgically using extracorporeal circulation, and the operative mortality rate is reasonably low. Patients with underdeveloped pulmonary arteries and those weighing less than 15 kg should be given a preliminary Blalock type shunt if severe oxygen deprivation (as indicated by cyanosis) threatens survival. Propranolol (Inderal) has been used with benefit for episodes of syncope due to infundibular contraction.

Prognosis

Tetralogy is the commonest cause of cyanotic congenital heart disease in adults, and survival to adult life is not common. Severe hypoxemia is the commonest cause of death. Cerebral thromboses secondary to polycythemia are also common. The severity of the syndrome is dominated by the magnitude of the pulmonic stenosis; the greater the stenosis, the greater the right-to-left shunt and the smaller the pulmonary blood flow.

Cole RB & others: Long-term results of aortopulmonary anastomosis for tetralogy of Fallot: Morbidity and mortality, 1946–1969. Circulation 43 (Suppl 2):263, 1971.

Crawford DW, Simpson E, McIlroy MB: Cardiopulmonary function in Fallot's tetralogy after palliative shunting operations. Am Heart J 74:463, 1967.

Kirklin JW: The tetralogy of Fallot. Am J Roentgenol 102:253, 1968.

Rees S, Somerville J: Aortography in Fallot's tetralogy and variants. Brit Heart J 31:146, 1969.

EISENMENGER'S SYNDROME
(Pulmonary Hypertension in Congenital Heart Disease)

This lesion was originally defined as ventricular septal defect, right ventricular hypertrophy, and overriding of the aorta, producing cyanosis, but it is now thought of as pulmonary hypertension causing reversal of any originally left-to-right shunt. In order of frequency the defects most commonly resulting in this mechanism of shunt reversal are ventricular septal defect, patent ductus arteriosus, and atrial septal defect (rare under age 21 or in secundum defects). The cause of the pulmonary hypertension is not known; in many cases it may have been present from birth. The increased pulmonary vascular resistance causes right ventricular hypertrophy, and variable shunt reversal occurs. Blood still passes from left to right as well as from right to left.

Clinical Findings

A. **Symptoms and Signs:** Moderate to severe exertional dyspnea is common. Ventricular septal defect and atrial septal defect cause cyanosis with clubbing and polycythemia. Reversed ductus causes cyanosis of the lower legs and toes. Right ventricular and pulmonary artery pulsations are palpable; a systolic murmur can be heard along the left sternal border; and there may be an early pulmonic systolic ejection click.

B. **X-Ray Findings:** Large, actively pulsating central pulmonary arteries with reduced peripheral pulmonary vascularity are noted on fluoroscopy.

C. **ECG Findings:** Right ventricular hypertrophy with peaked P waves is the usual finding.

D. **Special Studies:** Cardiac catheterization, angiocardiography, and dye dilution studies may be necessary to establish the site of the shunt.

Treatment

No surgical treatment is effective in Eisenmenger's syndrome.

Prognosis

Most patients die of heart failure, vascular thrombosis, or endocarditis before 30 years of age.

Wood P: The Eisenmenger syndrome. (2 parts.) Brit MJ 2:701, 755, 1958.

TRICUSPID ATRESIA

Atresia of the tricuspid valve may occur (1) as an isolated lesion; (2) with stenosis of the pulmonary arteries together with atrial septal defect; or (3) in association with ventricular septal defect or patent ductus arteriosus. Blood from the right atrium passes into the left atrium and reaches the lungs by passing through a ventricular septal defect into the right ventricle or, when the right ventricle and the pulmonary artery are rudimentary, by shunting from the aorta into the pulmonary circulation through a patent ductus.

Examination reveals a strong apical impulse, a systolic murmur and thrill along the left sternal border, cyanosis, clubbing, and polycythemia. The ECG reveals left axis deviation or left ventricular hypertrophy. Angiocardiography and cardiac catheterization are necessary for definitive diagnosis. Anastomosis of the subclavian artery to the pulmonary artery (Blalock) is probably the procedure of choice if the pulmonary blood flow is low. The benefits of anastomosis of the right atrium to the pulmonary artery have not yet been established.

The prognosis for life is poor. Only an occasional patient survives to adulthood.

Campbell M: Tricuspid atresia and its prognosis with and without surgical treatment. Brit Heart J 23:699, 1961.

Ross DN, Somerville J: Surgical correction of tricuspid atresia. Lancet 1:845, 1973.

Watson H: Natural history of Ebstein's anomaly of tricuspid valve in childhood and adolescence: An international cooperative study of 505 cases. Brit Heart J 36:417, 1974.

ACQUIRED HEART DISEASES

RHEUMATIC FEVER

Criteria for Diagnosis (Modified After Jones)
    A. **Major Criteria:**
        1. Carditis.
        2. Sydenham's chorea.

3. Subcutaneous (fascial) nodules.
4. Erythema marginatum.
5. Polyarthritis.
B. **Minor Criteria:**
   1. Fever.
   2. Polyarthralgia.
   3. Prolongation of P–R interval.
   4. Increased sedimentation rate or C-reactive protein.
   5. Evidence of antecedent beta-hemolytic streptococcus infection.
   6. Verified history of previous rheumatic fever or presence of rheumatic valvular disease.

The diagnosis of rheumatic fever is almost certain when 2 or more major criteria are present. Nevertheless, rheumatoid arthritis, neurocirculatory asthenia, bacterial endocarditis, connective tissue diseases, serum sickness, penicillin reaction, and chronic infectious disease can reproduce the early manifestations of rheumatic fever.

General Considerations

Rheumatic fever is a subacute or chronic systemic disease which for unknown reasons may either be self-limiting or lead to slowly progressive valvular deformity. Rarely, it is acute and fulminant.

Rheumatic fever is the commonest cause of heart disease in people under 50 years of age. In overall incidence, it ranks third behind hypertension and atherosclerotic coronary disease. It is somewhat more common in males than in females, but chorea is seen more frequently in females. The peak incidence occurs between the ages of 5 and 15; rheumatic fever is rare before the age of 4 and after 50.

Rheumatic fever is initiated by an infection with group A hemolytic streptococci, appearing usually 1–4 weeks after tonsillitis, nasopharyngitis, or otitis.

The acute phase of rheumatic fever may involve the endocardium, myocardium, pericardium, synovial joint linings, lungs, or pleura. The characteristic lesion is a perivascular granulomatous reaction and vasculitis. The mitral valve is attacked in 75–80% of cases, the aortic valve in 30%, the tricuspid and pulmonary valve in less than 5%. Small pink granules appear on the surface of the edematous valve. Healing may be complete, or a progressive scarring due to subacute or chronic inflammation may develop over months and years.

Clinical Findings

A. **Major Criteria:**

1. **Carditis**–The presence of carditis establishes the diagnosis of rheumatic fever whenever there is (1) a definite history of rheumatic fever, or (2) valvular disease clearly of rheumatic origin, or (3) whenever a streptococcal infection of the upper respiratory tract is known to have occurred within the preceding 4 weeks. Carditis is most apt to be evident in children and adolescents; in adults, it is often best detected by serial ECG study. Any of the following establishes the presence of carditis:

a. Pericarditis–Either fibrinous (with a pleuritic type of precordial, epigastric, or left shoulder pain; friction rub; characteristic ST–T changes on the ECG) or with effusion of any degree. It is uncommon in adults and is at times diagnosed by the progressive increase in "heart shadow" on serial chest x-rays.

b. Cardiac enlargement, detected by physical signs or x-ray, indicating dilatation of a weakened, inflamed myocardium. Serial x-rays are often needed to detect the change in size.

c. Frank congestive failure, right- and left-sided–Right heart failure is more prominent in children, and painful engorgement of the liver is a valuable sign.

d. Mitral or aortic diastolic murmurs, indicative of dilatation of a valve ring or the myocardium with or without associated valvulitis.

In the absence of any of the above definite signs the diagnosis of carditis depends upon the following less specific abnormalities considered in relation to the total clinical picture.

(1) ECG changes: P–R prolongation greater than 0.04 second above the patient's normal is the most significant abnormality; changing contour of P waves or inversion of T waves is less specific.

(2) Changing quality of heart sounds.

(3) Pansystolic apical murmur which persists or becomes louder during the course of the disease and is transmitted into the axilla. The Carey Coombs short mid-diastolic murmur should be carefully sought.

(4) Gallop rhythm: Difficult to differentiate from the physiologic third sound in children and adolescents.

(5) Sinus tachycardia out of proportion to the degree of fever, persisting during sleep and markedly increased by slight activity.

(6) Arrhythmias, shifting pacemaker, ectopic beats.

2. **The 2 following signs** occur most often in association with severe carditis and so are of little value in initial diagnosis; occasionally, however, they appear before carditis is evident and constitute strong presumptive evidence of rheumatic fever.

a. Erythema marginatum (annulare)–Frequently associated with skin nodules. The lesions begin as rapidly enlarging macules which assume the shape of rings or crescents with clear centers. They may be slightly raised and confluent. The rash may be transient or may persist for long periods.

b. Subcutaneous nodules–These are uncommon except in children. The nodules may be few or many, are usually small (2 cm or less in diameter), firm, non-tender, and are attached to fascia or tendon sheaths over bony prominences such as the elbows, the dorsal surfaces of the hands, the malleoli, the vertebral spines, and the occiput. They persist for days or weeks, are usually recurrent, and are clinically indistinguishable from the nodules of rheumatoid arthritis.

3. **Sydenham's chorea** may appear suddenly as an isolated entity with no "minor criteria" or may develop in the course of overt rheumatic fever. Eventually 50% of cases have other signs of rheumatic fever. Girls

are more frequently affected, and occurrence in adults is rare. Chorea consists of continual, nonrepetitive, purposeless jerky movements of the limbs, trunk, and facial muscles. Milder forms masquerade as undue restlessness as the patient attempts to convert uncontrolled movements into seemingly purposeful movements. Facial grimaces of infinite variety are common. These movements are made worse by emotional tension and disappear entirely during sleep. The episode lasts several weeks, occasionally months.

4. **Arthritis**—The arthritis of rheumatic fever is characteristically a migratory polyarthritis of gradual or sudden onset which involves the large joints sequentially, one becoming hot, red, swollen, and tender as the inflammation in the previously involved joint subsides. The body temperature rises progressively as each successive joint becomes inflamed. In adults only a single or a small joint may be affected. The acute arthritis lasts 1–5 weeks and subsides without residual deformity. *Note:* Joint involvement is considered a major criterion only when definite effusion and signs of inflammation are present. This is in contrast to arthralgia, in which pain or stiffness is present without these objective signs. Prompt response of arthritis to therapeutic doses of salicylates is characteristic (but not diagnostic) of rheumatic fever.

With respect to arthritis, the dictum, "one major and 2 minor criteria," is a source of diagnostic confusion. Arthritis and arthralgia are common in children and young adults, often accompanied by fever and an increased sedimentation rate. Streptococcal infection or "sore throat" is also common. Coincidental association of these factors thus often leads to an unwarranted diagnosis of rheumatic fever. A definite diagnosis requires bona fide evidence of carditis or the appearance of additional rheumatic manifestations such as erythema marginatum or chorea.

B. **Minor Criteria:** The following common nonspecific manifestations of rheumatic fever are of diagnostic help only when associated with other more specific features:

1. **Fever** is always present with arthritis and carditis. In subacute or chronic phases it is low-grade and may be continuous or intermittent. Fever is important only as evidence of an inflammatory process. Certain children and even adults may have normal peak temperatures of 37.5–37.8° C (99.5–100° F), and this should not be construed erroneously as "fever."

2. **Malaise, asthenia, weight loss, and anorexia** may be the only overt effects of a smoldering rheumatic state but are also characteristic of any chronic active disease.

3. **Abdominal pain** is common. It is variable in site and severity and occasionally leads to an unnecessary laparotomy. It may result from liver engorgement, sterile rheumatic peritonitis, or rheumatic arteritis, or may be referred from the pleura or pericardium.

4. **Recurrent epistaxis** is believed by some clinicians to be an indication of "subclinical" rheumatic fever.

5. **"Growing pains"** in joints, periarticular tissues, or muscle insertions may be a symptom of rheumatic fever ("arthralgia").

C. **Laboratory Findings:** These are helpful in 3 ways:

1. As nonspecific evidence of inflammatory disease—Sedimentation rate and white count are almost always increased during active rheumatic fever except when chorea is the only clinical sign. Variable leukocytosis and normochromic anemia may appear. Slight proteinuria and microhematuria are occasionally seen and do not necessarily indicate concomitant glomerulonephritis.

2. As evidence of antecedent beta-hemolytic streptococcal infection—A high titer or increasing antistreptolysin O titer indicates recent infection but does not mean that rheumatic fever is present. Throat culture is positive for beta-hemolytic streptococci in 50% of cases of active rheumatic fever.

3. As strong evidence against the diagnosis—A low antistreptolysin O titer (50 Todd units) which does not rise on repeated tests tends to rule out rheumatic fever. A normal sedimentation rate is rare in the presence of active rheumatic fever.

Differential Diagnosis

Rheumatic fever may be confused with the following: rheumatoid arthritis, osteomyelitis, traumatic joint disease, neurocirculatory asthenia or cardiac neurosis, bacterial endocarditis, pulmonary tuberculosis, chronic meningococcemia, acute poliomyelitis, disseminated lupus erythematosus, serum sickness, drug sensitivity, leukemia, sickle cell anemia, inactive rheumatic heart disease, congenital heart disease, and "surgical abdomen."

Complications

Congestive heart failure occurs in severe cases. Other complications include cardiac arrhythmias, pericarditis with large effusion, rheumatic pneumonitis, pulmonary embolism and infarction, cardiac invalidism, and early or late development of permanent heart valve deformity.

Prevention of Recurrent Rheumatic Fever

The principles of prevention are to avoid beta-hemolytic streptococcal infections if possible and to treat streptococcal infections promptly and intensively with appropriate antibiotics.

A. **General Measures:** Avoid contact with persons who have "colds" or other upper respiratory infections. Patients with rheumatic fever do better in an equable climate, where streptococcal infections are less common.

B. **Prevention of Infection:** Two methods of prevention are now advocated:

1. **Penicillin**—The preferred method of prophylaxis is with benzathine penicillin G (Bicillin), 1.2 million units IM every 4 weeks. Oral penicillin (200–250 thousand units daily before breakfast) may be used instead but is less reliable. Prophylaxis is advocated especially for children who have had one or

more acute attacks and should be given throughout the school year. Adults should receive preventive therapy for about 5 years after an attack.

2. **Sulfonamides**—If the patient is sensitive to penicillin, give sulfadiazine, 1 gm daily throughout the year. *Caution:* Patients receiving sulfonamides should have periodic blood counts and urinalyses. If there is any tendency toward leukopenia, the drug should be stopped immediately.

C. **Treatment of Streptococcal Sore Throat:** It has been shown that prompt therapy (within 24 hours) of streptococcal infections will prevent most attacks of acute rheumatic fever. (See Chapter 23.)

Treatment

A. **Medical Treatment:**

1. **The salicylates** markedly reduce fever, relieve joint pain, and may reduce joint swelling. There is no evidence that they have any effect on the natural course of the disease. *Note:* The salicylates should be continued as long as necessary to relieve pain, swelling, or fever. If withdrawal results in a recurrence of symptoms, treatment should immediately be reinstituted.

a. Sodium salicylate is the most widely used of this group of drugs. Maximum dose is 1—2 gm every 2—4 hours orally to allay symptoms and fever; 4—6 gm/day suffices in most adults. In an occasional patient maximum doses may not be completely effective. There is no evidence that intravenous administration has any advantage over the oral route. Early toxic reactions to the salicylates include tinnitus, nausea, and vomiting. Antacids are usually given with salicylates to reduce gastric irritation. *Caution:* Never use sodium salicylate or sodium bicarbonate in patients with acute rheumatic fever who have associated cardiac failure.

b. Aspirin may be substituted for sodium salicylate, with the same dosages and precautions.

2. **Penicillin** should be employed in the treatment at any time during the course of the disease to eradicate any existing streptococcal infection.

3. **Corticosteroids**—Careful studies have shown no clear or consistent proof that cardiac damage is prevented or minimized by corticosteroids even when they are given early in large doses. Corticosteroids are effective anti-inflammatory agents for reversing the acute exudative phase of rheumatic fever and are probably more potent for this purpose than salicylates. A short course of corticosteroids usually causes rapid improvement in the acute manifestations of rheumatic fever and is indicated in severe cases. There may be prompt disappearance of fever, malaise, tachycardia, and polyarthritis. Abnormal ECG changes (prolonged P—R interval) and sedimentation rates may return to normal limits within a week.

A suggested schedule, to be started as soon as severe rheumatic fever is diagnosed, is as follows: Give prednisone, 5—10 mg orally every 6 hours for 3 weeks, and then gradually withdraw over a period of 3 weeks by reducing and then discontinuing first the nighttime, then the evening, and finally the daytime doses. In severe cases the dosage should be increased, if necessary, to levels adequate to control symptoms (see the discussion of the methods, dangers, and precautions in the use of corticosteroids in Chapter 18).

B. **General Measures:** Bed rest should be enforced until all signs of active rheumatic fever have disappeared. The criteria for this are as follows: Return of the temperature to normal with the patient at bed rest and without medications; normal sedimentation rate; normal resting pulse rate (under 100 in adults); return of ECG to normal or fixation of abnormalities. The patient may then be allowed up slowly, but several months should elapse before return to full activity unless the rheumatic fever was exceedingly mild. Maintain good nutrition.

C. **Treatment of Complications:**

1. **Congestive failure**—Treat as for congestive failure, with the following variations:

a. A low-sodium diet and diuretics are of particular value in promoting diuresis and treating failure in acute rheumatic fever.

b. Digitalis is usually not as effective in acute rheumatic fever as in most cases of congestive failure and may accentuate the myocardial irritability, producing arrhythmias which further embarrass the heart. Digitalis should be given, but with extreme care.

c. Many cases of congestive failure are due to acute myocarditis. These often respond dramatically to corticotropin (ACTH) or the corticosteroids. When sodium-retaining hormonal agents are employed, rigorous sodium restriction (< 200 mg daily) or thiazide drugs are imperative.

2. **Pericarditis**—Treat as any acute nonpurulent pericarditis. The rheumatic effusion is sterile, and antibiotics are of no value. The general principles include relief of pain, by opiates if necessary, and removal of fluid by cardiac paracentesis if tamponade develops. This, however, is rarely necessary. If paracentesis is performed it should be preceded and followed by a short course of penicillin therapy to prevent infection of the pericardium. Corticotropin (ACTH) and the corticosteroids as well as salicylates should be continued or started, as they seem to have a specific favorable effect in aiding resorption of the fluid.

Prognosis

Initial episodes of rheumatic fever last months in children and weeks in adults. Twenty percent of children have recurrences within 5 years. Recurrences are uncommon after 5 years of well-being, and rare after the age of 21. The immediate mortality is 1—2%. Persistent rheumatic activity with a greatly enlarged heart, heart failure, and pericarditis indicate a poor prognosis; 30% of children thus affected die within 10 years of the initial attack. Otherwise the prognosis for life is good. Eighty percent of all patients attain adult life, and half of these have little if any limitation of activity. Approximately one-third of young patients have detectable valvular damage after the initial episode, most commonly a combination of mitral stenosis and insufficiency. After 10 years, two-thirds of surviving patients will have detectable valvular disease. In adults, residual heart damage occurs in less than 20% and is generally less severe. Mitral insufficiency is the commonest residual, and aortic insufficiency is much more common than in children. The influence of steroids on prognosis is as yet not known. Twenty percent of patients who have chorea develop valvular deformity even after a long latent period of apparent well-being.

Combined Rheumatic Fever Study Group: A comparison of short-term, intensive prednisone and acetylsalicylic acid therapy in the treatment of acute rheumatic fever. New England J Med 272:63, 1965.

Feinstein AR, Spagnuolo M: The clinical patterns of acute rheumatic fever: A reappraisal. Medicine 41:279, 1962.

Feinstein AR, Stern EK: Clinical effects of recurrent attacks of acute rheumatic fever: A prospective epidemiologic study of 105 episodes. J Chronic Dis 20:13, 1967.

Markowitz M, Kuttner AG: *Rheumatic Fever: Diagnosis, Management and Prevention.* Saunders, 1965.

Sokolow M, Snell A: Atypical features of rheumatic fever in young adults. JAMA 133:981, 1947.

Tompkins DG, Boxerbaum B, Liebman J: Long-term prognosis of rheumatic fever patients receiving regular intramuscular benzathine penicillin. Circulation 45:543, 1972.

RHEUMATIC HEART DISEASE
(Rheumatic Valvulitis, Inactive)

Chronic rheumatic heart disease results from single or repeated attacks of rheumatic fever which produce rigidity and deformity of the cusps, fusion of the commissures, or shortening and fusion of the chordae tendineae. Stenosis or insufficiency results and both often coexist, although one or the other predominates. The mitral valve alone is affected in 50–60% of cases; combined lesions of the aortic and mitral valves occur in 20%; pure aortic lesions in 10%. Tricuspid involvement occurs only in association with mitral or aortic disease in about 10% of cases. The pulmonary valve is rarely affected.

Clinical Findings
A history of rheumatic fever is obtainable in only 60% of patients with rheumatic heart disease.

The earliest evidence of organic valvular disease is a significant murmur. The earliest evidence of hemodynamically significant valvular lesions is found on x-ray, fluoroscopy, and ECG study, since these will reveal the earliest stages of specific chamber enlargement. Careful physical examination also permits accurate diagnosis of advanced valve lesions.

The important findings in each of the major valve lesions are summarized in Table 7–1. Hemodynamic changes, symptoms, associated findings, and course are discussed below.

Management of Asymptomatic Valvular Heart Disease
A. Prevention:
1. Recurrences of acute rheumatic fever can be prevented by (1) avoiding exposure to streptococcal infections; (2) continuous antibiotic prophylaxis in selected patients under 35 (those with acute rheumatic fever in the preceding 5 years) and those who have been exposed to known hemolytic streptococcal infections; and (3) prompt and adequate treatment of infections due to hemolytic streptococci.

2. The patient should be given advice regarding dental extraction, urologic procedures, surgical procedures, etc to prevent bacteremia and possible subacute bacterial endocarditis.

B. General Measures: Vocational guidance is necessary to anticipate possible reduced exercise tolerance in later life. Follow-up observations should emphasize early recognition of disturbances of thyroid function, anemia, and arrhythmias; maintenance of general health, and avoidance of obesity and excessive physical exertion.

1. MITRAL STENOSIS

Over 75% of patients with mitral stenosis are women below the age of 45. Relatively slight degrees of narrowing are sufficient to produce the auscultatory signs. When the valve has narrowed to less than 1.5 sq cm, the left atrial pressure must rise to maintain normal flow across the valve and a normal cardiac output. This results in a pressure difference between the left atrium and left ventricle during diastole, which may be present in mild cases only during periods of rapid ventricular filling (in mid-diastole or following atrial systole) and, in more severe cases, may persist all through diastole. The pressure gradient (and the length of the diastolic murmur) reflects the severity of the mitral stenosis; they persist throughout diastole when the lesion is severe or when the ventricular rate is rapid. The duration is shorter and confined to the middle of diastole when the lesion is slight or the ventricular rate is slow. Both the flow and the pressure gradient must be known in order to compute the valve area according to Gorlin's formula. When the left atrial pressure is raised, the pulmonary venous capillary "wedge" pressure is also raised. The latter increases further as a consequence of incomplete left atrial emptying, when the heart rate increases and the duration of diastole decreases with exercise or tachycardia. In mild cases, the left atrial pressure and the cardiac output may be essentially normal and the patients asymptomatic; but in moderate stenosis, with tachycardia or exercise, dyspnea and fatigue appear as the left atrial pressure rises. With severe stenosis, the left atrial pressure is sufficiently high at rest to produce pulmonary venous congestion at rest, worsening rapidly with exercise. Recumbency at night further increases the pulmonary blood volume, causing orthopnea, paroxysmal nocturnal dyspnea, or actual transudation of fluid into the alveoli, leading to acute pulmonary edema. Severe pulmonary congestion may also be initiated by acute

Table 7–1. Differential diagnosis of rheumatic heart disease.

	Mitral Stenosis	Mitral Insufficiency	Aortic Stenosis	Aortic Insufficiency	Tricuspid Stenosis	Tricuspid Insufficiency
Inspection	Malar flush. Precordial bulge and diffuse pulsation in young patients.	Usually forceful apical impulse to left of MCL.	Localized heaving PMI. Carotid pulsations weak, exhibiting slow rise.	Generalized pallor. Strong, abrupt carotid pulsations. Forceful PMI to left of MCL and down. Capillary pulsations.	Giant a wave in jugular pulse with sinus rhythm. Often olive-colored skin (mixed jaundice and local cyanosis).	Large v wave in jugular pulse.
Palpation	"Tapping" sensation over area of expected PMI. Mid-diastolic and/or presystolic thrill at apex. Small pulse. Right ventricular pulsation left 3rd–5th ICS parasternally when pulmonary hypertension is present.	Forceful, brisk PMI; systolic thrill over PMI. Pulse normal, small, or slightly collapsing.	Powerful, heaving localized PMI to left of MCL and slightly down. Systolic thrill over aortic area (best felt with patient leaning forward, breath held in maximum expiration). Plateau pulse; small and slowly rising.	Apical impulse forceful and displaced significantly to left and down. Water-hammer pulses.	Mid-diastolic thrill between lower left sternal border and PMI. Presystolic pulsation of liver (sinus rhythm only).	Right ventricular pulsation. Occasionally systolic thrill at lower left sternal edge. Systolic pulsation of liver.
Percussion	Dullness in left 3rd ICS parasternally. ACD normal or slightly enlarged to left only.	ACD increased to left of MCL and slightly down.	ACD slightly enlarged to left and down.	Definite cardiac enlargement to left and down.		Usually cardiac enlargement to left and right.
Heart sounds, rhythm, and BP	Loud snapping M_1. Opening snap along left sternal border or at apex. Atrial fibrillation common. BP normal.	M_1 normal or buried in murmur. 3rd heart sound. Delayed opening snap occasionally present. Atrial fibrillation common. BP normal.	A_2 normal, or delayed and weak; may be absent. BP normal or systolic pressure normal with high diastolic level. Ejection click occasionally present just preceding murmur.	Sounds normal or A_2 loud. Wide pulse pressure with diastolic pressure < 60 mm Hg.	M_1 often loud.	Atrial fibrillation usually present.

MCL = Midclavicular line
PMI = Point of maximal impulse
ICS = Intercostal space
ACD = Area of cardiac disease

P_2 = Pulmonary second sound
M_1 = Mitral first sound
A_2 = Aortic second sound
BP = Blood pressure

Murmurs Location and transmission	Sharply localized at or near apex. Graham Steell murmur along lower left sternal border in severe pulmonary hypertension.	Loudest over PMI; transmitted to left axilla, left infrascapular area.	Right 2nd ICS parasternally and/or at apex; heard in carotids and occasionally in upper interscapular area.	Loudest along left sternal border in 3rd–4th interspace. Also heard over aortic area and apex.	3rd–5th ICS along left sternal border out to apex.	As for tricuspid stenosis.
Timing	Onset at opening snap ("mid-diastolic") with presystolic accentuation if in sinus rhythm. Graham Steell begins with P_2 (immediate diastolic).	Pansystolic: begins with M_1 and ends at or after A_2.	Midsystolic: begins after M_1; ends before A_2, reaches maximum intensity in midsystole.	Begins immediately after aortic 2nd sound and ends before 1st sound.	As for mitral stenosis.	As for mitral insufficiency.
Character	Low-pitched, rumbling; presystolic murmur merges with loud M1 in a "crescendo." Graham Steell highly-pitched, blowing.	Blowing, high-pitched; occasionally harsh or musical.	Harsh, rough.	Blowing, often faint.	As for mitral stenosis.	Blowing, coarse, or musical.
Optimum auscultatory conditions	After exercise, left lateral recumbency. Bell chest piece lightly applied.	After exercise; diaphragm chest piece.	Patient resting, leaning forward, breath held in full expiration. Bell chest piece, lightly applied.	Slow heart rate; patient leaning forward, breath held in full expiration. Diaphragm chest piece.	Murmur usually louder during and at peak of inspiration. Patient recumbent. Bell chest piece.	Murmur usually becomes louder during inspiration.
X-ray and fluoroscopy*	Straight left heart border. Large left atrium sharply indenting esophagus. Large right ventricle and pulmonary artery if pulmonary hypertension present.	Enlarged left ventricle and left atrium; systolic expansion of left atrium if enlargement not extreme.	Concentric left ventricular hypertrophy. Prominent ascending aorta, small knob. Calcified valve common.	Moderate to great left ventricular hypertrophy. Prominent aortic knob. Strong aortic pulsation on fluoroscopy.	Enlarged right atrium only.	Enlarged right atrium and ventricle.
ECG	Broad P waves in standard leads; broad negative phase of diphasic P in V_1. Normal axis. If pulmonary hypertension is present, tall peaked P waves, right axis deviation or right ventricular hypertrophy appear.	Left axis deviation or frank left ventricular hypertrophy. P waves broad, tall, or notched in standard leads; broad negative phase of diphasic P in V_1.	Left ventricular hypertrophy.	Left ventricular hypertrophy.	Wide, tall peaked P waves. Normal axis.	Right axis usual.

*Technetium 99m pertechnetate radioisotope scans and echocardiography are being increasingly used to augment x-ray studies.

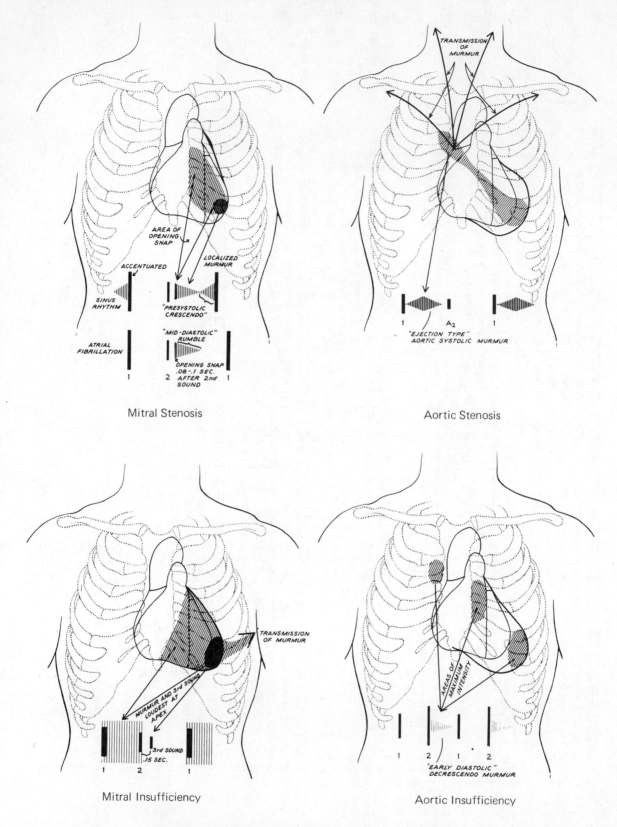

Figure 7—1. Murmurs and cardiac enlargement in common valve lesions.

bronchitis or any acute respiratory infection, by development of subacute bacterial endocarditis, or recurrence of acute rheumatic carditis. As a result of long-standing pulmonary venous hypertension, anastomoses develop between the pulmonary and bronchial veins in the form of bronchial submucosal varices. These often rupture, producing mild or severe hemoptysis.

Fifty to 80% of patients develop paroxysmal or chronic atrial fibrillation which, until the ventricular rate is controlled, may precipitate dyspnea or pulmonary edema. Twenty to 30% of these patients in turn will later have major emboli in the cerebral, visceral, or peripheral arteries as a consequence of thrombus formation in the left atrium.

In a few patients, for unknown reasons, the pulmonary arterioles become narrowed or constricted; this greatly increases the pulmonary artery pressure and the pulmonary vascular resistance, and accelerates the development of right ventricular hypertrophy and right ventricular failure. These patients have relatively little dyspnea but experience great fatigue and weakness on exertion because of the markedly reduced cardiac output.

Special diagnostic studies such as echocardiography, left ventricular angiocardiography, dye dilution, and pressure curves from the left ventricle and left atrium during left heart catheterization or left ventricular puncture may prove helpful in difficult cases. Echocardiography is particularly valuable in the diagnosis of mitral stenosis, showing a decreased closing slope of the anterior mitral valve leaflet in mid-diastole with increased reflectance due to thickness of the leaflet and chordae. The anterior and posterior leaflets are fixed and move together, rather than in opposite directions, as normally.

Treatment

Closed mitral valvulotomy is advisable only if symptoms are due to a mechanical obstruction of the mitral valve and not due to mitral insufficiency or associated aortic valve disease. Most surgeons prefer to perform all mitral valvulotomies under "open bypass," believing that a better repair is possible under direct vision. If the signs of mitral stenosis are present but there is no systolic murmur, mitral regurgitation is exceedingly unlikely. If there is a loud pansystolic murmur at the apex in association with an accentuated, often early third heart sound, a soft first sound, and no opening snap, the diagnosis of predominant mitral regurgitation is likely even if a short mid-diastolic murmur can be heard at the apex. Unless hypertension or an aortic valvular lesion is present, left ventricular hypertrophy shown on ECG should make one very cautious in recommending closed operation for mitral stenosis because in this circumstance the mitral valve is probably regurgitant. If there is a moderate systolic murmur at the apex, the diagnosis depends upon a consideration of the total findings.

Replacement of the valve is indicated when combined stenosis and insufficiency are present, or if anatomically the mitral valve is so distorted and calcified that a satisfactory fracture, even if the operation is performed "open" under cardiopulmonary bypass, is not possible (see Mitral Insufficiency). Systemic embolism probably is an indication for open operation.

Special diagnostic studies such as left ventricular angiocardiography, dye dilution, and pressure curves from the left ventricle and left atrium during left heart catheterization or left ventricular puncture may prove helpful in difficult cases.

Because the course of mitral stenosis is highly variable and because of the significant mortality (3–5%) as well as morbidity of mitral valvulotomy and the frequency of restenosis, surgery is not advised in mild cases with slight exertional dyspnea and fatigue only. Indications for surgery include the following: (1) Signs of mitral stenosis with a pliable valve (opening snap, snapping first sound). (2) Uncontrollable pulmonary edema. (3) Disabling dyspnea and occasionally pulmonary edema. (4) Evidence of pulmonary hypertension with right ventricular hypertrophy and early congestive failure. (5) Increased pulmonary arteriolar resistance, with marked dyspnea and increased P_2. These patients are apt to develop right heart failure and emboli. (6) Right heart failure or tricuspid incompetence (or both) when secondary to marked mitral valve disease.

Continuous anticoagulant therapy is required for patients treated by valve replacement.

Barnhorst DA & others: Long-term follow-up of isolated replacement of the aortic or mitral valve with the Starr-Edwards prosthesis. Am J Cardiol 35:228, 1975.

Baron MG: The angiocardiographic diagnosis of valvular stenosis. Circulation 44:143, 1971.

Brawley RK, Donahoo JS, Gott VL: Current status of the Beall, Bjork-Shiley, Braunwald-Cutter, Lillehei-Kaster and Smeloff-Cutter cardiac valve prostheses. Am J Cardiol 35:855, 1975.

Kirklin JW, Pacifico AD: Surgery for acquired valvular heart disease. New England J Med 288:133, 1973.

Rapaport E & others: Natural history of aortic and mitral valve disease. Am J Cardiol 35:221, 1975.

Roberts WC, Perloff JK: Mitral valvular disease. Ann Int Med 77:939, 1972.

Wood P: An appreciation of mitral stenosis. Brit MJ 1:1051, 1954.

2. MITRAL INSUFFICIENCY

During ventricular systole, the mitral leaflets do not close normally and blood is forced back into the atrium as well as through the aortic valve. The net effect is an increased volume of work by the left ventricle. The left atrium enlarges progressively, but the pressure in pulmonary veins and capillaries rises only transiently during exertion. Patients have exertional dyspnea and fatigue which usually progress slowly over many years. Left ventricular failure eventually develops, and orthopnea and paroxysmal dyspnea may appear, followed rapidly by the symptoms of right heart failure.

The chronic course described here is for rheumatic mitral insufficiency; the course may be different and more acute when mitral insufficiency is caused by other than rheumatic fever. (See Nonrheumatic Mitral Insufficiency, below.)

When heart failure is fully developed, the response to therapy is incomplete and the patient remains incapacitated. Mitral insufficiency, like stenosis, predisposes to atrial fibrillation; but this arrhythmia is less likely to provoke acute pulmonary congestion, and fewer than 5% of patients have peripheral arterial emboli. Mitral insufficiency especially predisposes to subacute bacterial endocarditis.

Clinically, mitral insufficiency is characterized by a pansystolic murmur maximal at the apex, radiating to the axilla and occasionally to the base; a hyperdynamic left ventricular impulse and a brisk carotid upstroke; and a prominent third heart sound. When there is slight associated mitral stenosis, a short middiastolic murmur and a late opening snap may be present. The magnitude of the left ventricular hypertrophy is usually moderate, both clinically and electrocardiographically, and most of the enlargement of the cardiac shadow seen on x-ray is due to considerable diffuse enlargement of the left atrium. Calcification of the mitral valve is common, though less common than in pure mitral stenosis. The same is true of enlargement of the main pulmonary artery on x-ray.

Hemodynamically, the most striking feature of severe rheumatic mitral insufficiency is an elevated left atrial pressure with a large v wave and a rapid y descent due to rapid filling of the left ventricle. Overwork of the left ventricle ultimately leads to left ventricular failure and reduced cardiac output, but for many years the left ventricular end-diastolic pressure and the cardiac output may be normal at rest, even with considerable increase in left ventricular volume.

Patients with rheumatic mitral insufficiency have systemic emboli and pulmonary hypertension less often—and atrial fibrillation more often—than do patients with mitral stenosis. Because of the frequency of combined mitral stenosis and insufficiency, and because of the difficulty in some patients with fixed valves to specify which is dominant, dogmatic differentiation is unwise.

When mitral insufficiency is combined with aortic stenosis or aortic insufficiency, patients may become symptomatic with lesser hemodynamic abnormalities of both valves than if the valves were diseased individually.

Nonrheumatic mitral insufficiency. Mitral insufficiency may be due to causes other than rheumatic fever and have different clinical findings and a different clinical course. The most common are those secondary to rupture of the chordae tendineae, usually secondary to infective endocarditis but occasionally occurring spontaneously or after trauma; the so-called "floppy valve syndrome" or "click" syndrome (a connective tissue disorder related to Marfan's syndrome in which a peculiar late systolic "whoop" is heard); and

mitral insufficiency secondary to infective endocarditis with perforation of a cusp. Papillary muscle dysfunction or necrosis following acute myocardial infarction is less common. When the mitral insufficiency is due to papillary dysfunction, it may subside as the infarction heals. Other causes include cardiac tumors, especially left atrial myxoma, and surgically acquired mitral insufficiency. In contrast to rheumatic mitral insufficiency, the other varieties usually develop cardiac failure more rapidly, are in sinus rhythm rather than atrial fibrillation, occur in males more often than females, have little or no enlargement of the left atrium, have no calcification of the mitral valve, have no associated mitral stenosis, and often present an angiographic appearance which may be helpful. The difference in the clinical picture may be due to the fact that nonrheumatic causes of mitral insufficiency are more acute and patients get into trouble within months or 1–2 years, whereas in rheumatic mitral insufficiency the course develops over a period of many years. Because the course of nonrheumatic mitral insufficiency may be more fulminant, surgical treatment with replacement of the valves is often a more urgent consideration.

Echocardiography is valuable in demonstrating disruption of chordal support of the mitral valve with prolapse of either or both mitral valve leaflets; the diagnostic finding is posterior prolapse of the leaflet in systole, usually associated with early diastolic anterior motion of the posterior leaflet. This is to be contrasted with the echocardiographic findings of the mid-systolic click, late systolic murmur syndrome (Barlow's syndrome), in which there is late systolic prolapse (notching of the posterior mitral valve leaflet) without the diagnostic early anterior motion seen in chordal rupture.

Treatment

Reconstructive operations on the mitral valve are infrequent today and usually performed for a perforated leaflet in bacterial endocarditis or, rarely, because of ruptured chordae. When the disability is great enough to warrant the surgical risk, open heart surgery using cardiopulmonary bypass is almost always required, with replacement of the diseased valve with a prosthetic device. Various types of prosthetic devices have been employed, the most common being the Cutter or the Starr-Edwards ball valve. Late complications have occurred, however, including degenerative changes in the Silastic ball, so that many of the ball valves are now completely covered by cloth. Alternatively, low-profile disk type valves, homografts, and heterografts are being used by some surgeons. It is still too soon to determine which is the best design and type of valve replacement, and the decision in any particular case should be left to the experienced surgeon. In addition to changes in the valve itself, late complications of valve replacement include systemic embolization, leaks of the valve, hemolytic anemia, and, occasionally, sudden death, particularly in aortic valve replacements.

Prognosis

The early and late embolic complications must be recognized, but the surgical mortality has declined with greater experience. The fate of the prosthesis over the long term is uncertain. Follow-up studies have shown considerable clinical and hemodynamic improvement in surviving patients, including reversal of pulmonary and left atrial hypertension. Usually, however, some hemodynamic abnormality persists.

Dodge HT, Kennedy JW, Petersen JL: Quantitative angiocardiographic methods in the evaluation of valvular heart disease. Progr Cardiovas Dis 16:1, 1973.

Ellis LB, Ramirez A: The clinical course of patients with severe "rheumatic" mitral insufficiency. Am Heart J 78:406, 1969.

Goodman DJ & others: Effect of nitroprusside on left ventricular dynamics in mitral regurgitation. Circulation 50:1025, 1974.

Jeresaty RM: Mitral valve prolapse-click syndrome. Progr Cardiovas Dis 15:623, 1973.

Kloster FE: Diagnosis and management of complications of prosthetic heart valves. Am J Cardiol 35:872, 1975.

O'Rourke RA & others: Prolapsing mitral valve leaflet syndrome. Western J Med 122:217, 1975.

Pocock WA, Barlow JB: Etiology and electrocardiographic features of the billowing posterior mitral leaflet syndrome. Am J Med 51:731, 1971.

Porter GA, Bennett WM, Wilson JW: Renal consequences of valvular heart disease. Am J Cardiol 35:886, 1975.

Rizzon P & others: Familial syndrome of midsystolic click and late systolic murmur. Brit Heart J 35:245, 1973.

Sanders CA & others: Etiology and differential diagnosis of acute mitral regurgitation. Progr Cardiovas Dis 14:129, 1971.

Wigle ED, Auger P: Sudden, severe mitral insufficiency. Canad MAJ 96:1493, 1967.

3. AORTIC STENOSIS

Over 80% of patients with aortic stenosis are men. Slight narrowing, roughened valves, or aortic dilatation may produce the typical murmur and thrill without causing significant hemodynamic effects. In mild to moderate cases, the characteristic signs are an ejection systolic murmur at the aortic area transmitted to the neck and apex and an ejection systolic click at the aortic area; in severe cases, a palpable left ventricular heave, often reversed splitting of the second sound, and a weak aortic second sound. The chest film reveals dilatation of the ascending aorta in valvular stenosis. When the valve area is less than one-fifth of normal, ventricular systole becomes prolonged and the typical plateau pulse develops. At this stage exertional dyspnea, fatigue, and pounding of the heart are noted. Cardiac output is ultimately markedly reduced so that patients have angina pectoris, great weakness or giddiness on exertion, or syncope. Survival beyond 3 years is uncommon if any of these appear. Many patients develop myocardial infarction, and 30% or more die suddenly. The stenosis may be valvular, subvalvular, or

supravalvular, requiring identification and differential surgical procedures.

Most patients require complete preoperative study, including right and left heart catheterization and aortic, coronary, and left ventricular angiograms to evaluate the presence and degree of associated valve regurgitation and coronary stenoses. Echocardiography is helpful in demonstrating impaired or absent aortic valve motion with increased reflectance of the valve structures, increased aortic root diameter, and increased septal and left ventricular posterior wall thickness. Ultrasound is less reliable in estimating the severity of the aortic stenosis.

Hemodynamically, the cardinal feature of valvular aortic stenosis is a systolic gradient across the aortic valve (systolic pressure difference between the left ventricle and the aorta). As the valve area narrows (can be estimated if both gradient and flow across the valve are known), the gradient increases; the elevated left ventricular systolic pressure causes considerable concentric left ventricular hypertrophy, which results in a normal cardiac output until relatively late in the course of the disease. The left ventricular end-diastolic pressure may be elevated because of decreased compliance of the ventricle, even with normal cardiac output and no or minimal symptoms. Later, left atrial pressure rises with exercise and left ventricular failure may occur, and the cardiac output is reduced, especially with exercise. At this point, the triad of syncope on unaccustomed effort, left ventricular failure, and angina pectoris all may coexist, and a critical aortic valve area of 0.6–0.7 sq cm is reached.

The arterial pulse characteristically is slow-rising, is of low amplitude, and has a well-defined anacrotic shoulder on the ascending limb—low in severe and high in mild aortic stenosis.

Aortic valvular stenosis must be distinguished from supravalvular obstruction and from outflow obstruction of the left ventricular infundibulum (muscular subaortic obstruction; idiopathic hypertrophic subaortic stenosis). The former is congenital and uncommon; surgical experience is limited, and results depend on the findings in the ascending aorta. In the latter variety, the obstruction may be intermittent, aggravated by digitalis or inotropic influences, and relieved by propranolol (Inderal) or sedation. If the patients are symptomatic, have severe obstruction to left ventricular flow, and achieve no benefit from propranolol, surgery is advised. Myotomy and limited resection of the hypertrophied muscle have produced gratifying results (see p 231).

Treatment

The indications for surgical correction of aortic stenosis are progressive left ventricular failure, attacks of syncope due to cerebral ischemia, angina pectoris when it is thought to be due to the decreased cardiac output of aortic stenosis and not to associated coronary artery disease, or hemodynamic (aortic value area < 1 sq cm) and clinical evidence of severe aortic stenosis even in patients with few symptoms. In the presence of both mitral and aortic stenosis, surgical correction or replacement of both valves can be performed at the same procedure.

The lesion must be severe before surgery can be recommended. Aortic valve replacement with a prosthetic or homograft valve is now the procedure of choice. Reconstructive procedures have proved unsatisfactory but may be necessary in severe congenital aortic stenosis when small enough prostheses are not available.

Follow-up of patients who have had valve replacement reveals an early surgical mortality of 5% and a late mortality of 10–20%. Good results occur in 85% of the surviving patients. Striking hemodynamic improvement can be documented in those judged clinically to have a good result.

In the first month following surgery, arrhythmias are the most common cause of death, whereas during 5 years following surgery the most common causes of death are sudden death and coronary disease.

Bache RJ, Wang Y, Jorgensen CR: Hemodynamic effects of exercise in isolated valvular aortic stenosis. Circulation 44:1003, 1971.

Cohen LS, Friedman WF, Braunwald E: Natural history of mild congenital aortic stenosis elucidated by serial hemodynamic studies. Am J Cardiol 30:1, 1972.

El-Said G & others: Natural hemodynamic history of congenital aortic stenosis in childhood. Am J Cardiol 30:6, 1972.

Feizi Ö, Symons C, Yacoub M: Echocardiography of the aortic valve. 1. Studies of normal aortic valve, aortic stenosis, aortic regurgitation, and mixed aortic valve disease. Brit Heart J 36:341, 1972.

Frank S, Johnson A, Ross J Jr: Natural history of valvular aortic stenosis. Brit Heart J 35:41, 1973.

Hirshfeld JW & others: Indices predicting long-term survival after valve replacement in patients with aortic regurgitation and patients with aortic stenosis. Circulation 50:1190, 1974.

Kerzacky AK & others: Combined mitral and aortic valve disease. Am J Cardiol 25:588, 1970.

Lee SJK & others: Hemodynamic changes following correction of severe aortic stenosis using the Cutter-Smeloff prosthesis. Circulation 42:719, 1970.

Oakley CM, Hallidie-Smith KA: Assessment of site and severity in congenital aortic stenosis. Brit Heart J 29:367, 1967.

Pacifico AD, Karp RB, Kirklin JW: Homografts for replacement of the aortic valve. Circulation 45 (Suppl 1):1, 1972.

Pansegrau DG & others: Supravalvular aortic stenosis in adults. Am J Cardiol 31:635, 1973.

Perloff JK: Clinical recognition of aortic stenosis: The physical signs and differential diagnosis of the various forms of obstruction to left ventricular outflow. Progr Cardiovas Dis 10:323, 1968.

Rotman M & others: Aortic valvular disease: Comparison of types and their medical and surgical management. Am J Med 51:241, 1971.

Wood P: Aortic stenosis. Am J Cardiol 1:553, 1958.

4. AORTIC INSUFFICIENCY

For many years the only sign may be a soft aortic diastolic murmur, ie, "auscultatory" aortic insufficiency, indicating regurgitation of a small amount of blood through the incompetent leaflets during diastole. As the valve deformity increases, larger and larger amounts regurgitate, diastolic blood pressure falls, the pulse wave assumes its characteristic contour, and the left ventricle progressively enlarges. This is the stage of "dynamic" aortic insufficiency. Many patients remain asymptomatic even at this point, or experience exertional dyspnea. Left ventricular failure often begins abruptly with acute pulmonary edema or recurrent paroxysmal nocturnal dyspnea and orthopnea; fatigue, weakness, and exertional dyspnea are then incapacitating. Angina pectoris, or protracted chest pain simulating angina, appears in many. The heart failure is relatively refractory to treatment and is the chief cause of death. Ten to 15% of patients with aortic insufficiency die suddenly.

Hemodynamically, because of the large volume load upon the left ventricle, patients show a large stroke output but no abnormality of the minute cardiac output or left ventricular end-diastolic pressure until late in the course of the disease. The latter (unlike aortic stenosis) remains normal until late in the disease and may abruptly rise when failure occurs and be reflected in a rise in left atrial pressure. The left ventricular volume is increased, but compliance does not decrease until late, when the combination of decreased compliance and left ventricular failure raises the left ventricular end-diastolic pressure. The arterial pulse characteristically has a rapid rise and fall (Corrigan's pulse), with an elevated systolic and lowered diastolic pressure and thus a widened pulse pressure. Echocardiography is helpful in establishing the presence of aortic valve insufficiency by demonstrating fluttering of the mitral valve leaflet during diastole. The magnitude of the aortic insufficiency is best quantified by supra-aortic cineangiography. Early closure of the mitral valve by echocardiography is a valuable sign of severe aortic insufficiency.

Nonrheumatic aortic insufficiency. Although rheumatic aortic insufficiency is the most common variety, other causes must be considered such as dissecting aneurysm of the aorta, infective endocarditis, hypertension, rheumatoid arthritis, and ruptured aneurysm of the sinus of Valsalva. When aortic insufficiency develops acutely (as in dissecting aneurysm or perforated cusp during infective endocarditis), left ventricular failure may develop rapidly and surgery may be urgently required. Differentiation of the clinical pictures of acute and chronic aortic insufficiency is as important as it is in acute and chronic mitral insufficiency. Patients with acute aortic insufficiency may not have the large dilated left ventricle that is so common in chronic aortic insufficiency, and acute left ventricular failure may occur in these individuals with great rapidity.

Treatment

Aortic insufficiency usually requires prosthetic replacement of the entire valve. The substantial surgical risk and the uncertain prognosis limit the indications to patients with class III or class IV lesions. The ideal time for replacement is uncertain because many patients survive for 5–10 years on medical treatment despite substantial insufficiency and left ventricular hypertrophy. The long-term "survival" of the prosthetic or homograft valve is not known. Emboli are less frequent than with mitral valve replacement, but require continuous anticoagulants unless a homograft has been used. The surgical risk is less with aortic insufficiency than with aortic stenosis.

Aortic insufficiency which appears or worsens after subacute infective endocarditis may lead to severe cardiac failure in weeks or months even though the infection is controlled. Surgical removal of the valve is indicated even during the infection if cardiac failure worsens despite medical treatment. Patients should be observed closely for many months after endocarditis.

Replacement of the valve may become a surgical emergency if perforation of a cusp or rupture of the sinus of Valsalva or of the subaortic valvular structure occurs, causing acute severe left ventricular failure. Great judgment is required to determine the timing of and need for physiologic studies.

Baronders JA, Sarde M: Some changing aspects of aortic regurgitation. Arch Int Med 124:600, 1969.

Botvinick EH & others: Echocardiographic demonstration of early mitral valve closure in severe aortic insufficiency: Its clinical implications. Circulation 51:836, 1975.

Eddleman EE Jr & others: Critical analysis of clinical factors in estimating severity of aortic valve disease. Am J Cardiol 31:687, 1973.

Gault JH & others: Left ventricular performance following correction of free aortic regurgitation. Circulation 42:773, 1970.

Goldschlager N & others: The natural history of aortic regurgitation. Am J Med 54:577, 1973.

Hunt D & others: Quantitative evaluation of cineaortography in the assessment of aortic regurgitation. Am J Cardiol 31:696, 1973.

Lee SJK & others: Circulatory changes in severe aortic regurgitation before and after surgical correction. Am J Cardiol 28:442, 1971.

Mennel RG & others: The preoperative assessment of aortic regurgitation: Cineaortography vs electromagnetic flowmeter. Am J Cardiol 29:360, 1972.

Paulus HE, Pearson CM, Pitts W Jr: Aortic insufficiency in five patients with Reiter's syndrome: A detailed clinical and pathologic study. Am J Med 53:464, 1972.

Scheu H, Rothlin M, Hegglin R: Aortic insufficiency. Circulation 38 (Suppl 5):77, 1968.

Shein KI & others: Combined aortic and mitral incompetence: Clinical features and surgical management. Am Heart J 76:728, 1968.

Spagnuolo M & others: Natural history of rheumatic aortic regurgitation: Criteria predictive of death, congestive heart failure, and angina in young patients. Circulation 44:368, 1971.

Wigle ED, Labrosse CJ: Sudden, severe aortic insufficiency. Circulation 32:708, 1965.

5. TRICUSPID STENOSIS

Most patients with tricuspid stenosis are women, and mitral valve disease is usually present also. Tricuspid stenosis acts as a mechanical block to the return of blood to the heart, and the systemic venous engorgement is analogous to the pulmonary venous engorgement caused by mitral stenosis. Tricuspid stenosis should be suspected when "right heart failure" appears early in the course of mitral disease, marked by hepatomegaly, ascites, and dependent edema. These are more prominent when atrial fibrillation is present. Severe fatigue is usual. Cardiac cirrhosis develops early, and patients acquire a characteristic complexion which is a blend of peripheral cyanosis and slight jaundice. Careful examination is needed to differentiate the typical diastolic rumble along the lower left sternal border from the murmur of mitral stenosis. In the presence of sinus rhythm, a presystolic liver pulsation can be found in half of the patients. In atrial fibrillation only the slow emptying of the jugular vein during diastole is noted. A giant right atrium on a chest film or angiogram is frequently found in tricuspid valve disease.

Hemodynamically, a diastolic pressure gradient of 5–15 mm Hg is found across the tricuspid valve between the right atrium and the right ventricle in conjunction with a raised pressure in the right atrium and jugular veins, with prominent *a* waves and a slow *y* descent because of slow right ventricular filling. Hepatic enlargement, ascites, and dependent edema develop when the mean right atrial pressure is about 15 mm Hg. The cardiac output is usually low, but it rises slightly with exercise.

Treatment

Congenital tricuspid stenosis is associated with an underdeveloped right ventricle and does not lend itself to valvotomy. Diversion of the superior vena caval flow into the right lung is a relatively safe closed procedure which confers a significant degree of palliation.

Acquired tricuspid stenosis may be amenable to valvotomy under direct vision, but it usually requires a prosthetic valve replacement.

Sanders CA & others: Tricuspid stenosis: A difficult diagnosis in the presence of atrial fibrillation. Circulation 33:26, 1966.

6. TRICUSPID INSUFFICIENCY

Tricuspid insufficiency affects the right ventricle just as mitral insufficiency affects the left ventricle. The symptoms and signs of organic tricuspid valve disease due to rheumatic heart disease are identical with those resulting from right ventricular failure due to any cause. The valvular lesion can be suspected in the presence of mitral disease by noting a relatively early onset of right heart failure and a harsh systolic murmur along the lower left sternal border which is separate from the mitral murmur and which often increases in intensity during and just after inspiration.

Hemodynamically, tricuspid insufficiency is characterized by a prominent regurgitant systolic (v) wave in the right atrium and jugular venous pulse, with a rapid y descent and a small or absent x descent, and by regurgitation of blood from the right ventricle to the right atrium during systole as seen in right ventricular angiography. The regurgitant wave, like the systolic murmur, is increased with inspiration, and its size depends upon the size of the right atrium. The volume of regurgitation can be estimated by right ventricular angiography.

Treatment

Replacement of the tricuspid valve is being performed with decreasing frequency in recent years. Tricuspid insufficiency secondary to severe mitral valve disease may regress when only the mitral valve is replaced.

Hansing CE, Rowe GC: Tricuspid insufficiency: A study of hemodynamics and pathogenesis. Circulation 45:793, 1972.

．　．　．

Prognosis of Rheumatic Heart Disease (Untreated)

Recurrent rheumatic fever may produce fatal heart failure at any time, and infective endocarditis is a constant threat. However, many patients may remain asymptomatic for years.

A. Mitral Stenosis: In general, patients with severe mitral stenosis die of intractable congestive failure in the 30's or 40's after a prolonged period of disability.

B. Mitral Insufficiency and Aortic Valve Lesions: These patients become symptomatic later in life, but death occurs within a few years after the onset of symptoms of congestive heart failure.

C. Aortic Stenosis: When angina, left ventricular failure, or syncope is present, death usually occurs within 3 years.

D. Tricuspid Lesions: These are usually associated with mitral valve disease. The prognosis is surprisingly good, with survival for up to 10 years after the onset of edema, but patients are incapacitated by fatigue.

INFECTIVE ENDOCARDITIS*

Essentials of Diagnosis

Subacute:
- Patient with rheumatic, congenital, or atherosclerotic heart disease or degenerative myxomatous change in the mitral valve sup-

*By Ernest Jawetz, PhD, MD.

porting structures.
- Continuous fever, weight loss, joint and muscle pains, fatigue, anemia.
- Heart murmur, splenomegaly, petechiae, embolic phenomena.
- Blood culture positive.

Acute:
- Patient with acute infection or recent history of surgery or instrumentation, or narcotic addiction.
- High fever, sudden change or appearance of new murmurs, embolic phenomena, petechiae, splenomegaly, and toxic appearance.

General Considerations

Subacute "bacterial" endocarditis (SBE) is a smoldering bacterial infection of the endocardium usually superimposed on preexisting rheumatic or calcific valvular or congenital heart disease. Bacteremia following a respiratory infection, dental work, or cystoscopy is often the initiating event, but in many instances the source of infection is not known. Streptococci, especially *Streptococcus viridans* and *S faecalis,* are the usual etiologic agents; staphylococci are occasionally responsible, but virtually any microorganism, including fungi, can cause endocarditis.

Bacteria lodge on the endocardium of valves (usually aortic and mitral) and multiply. Fibrin and platelet thrombi are deposited, forming irregular friable vegetations which break off to give emboli to the brain, peripheral arteries, or viscera. Embolic nephritis or true glomerulonephritis sometimes produces renal failure. Shedding of bacteria into the blood stream from the involved valves may produce mycotic aneurysms which, however, rarely rupture. Active rheumatic carditis may be present. SBE produces mild to moderate systemic symptoms; cerebral, renal, splenic, or mesenteric emboli; heart failure; or any combination of these. The onset usually follows bacteremia from one of the sources cited above within days or weeks.

Acute bacterial endocarditis (ABE) is a rapidly progressive infection of normal or abnormal valves, usually developing in the course of heavy bacteremia from acute infections such as staphylococcal sepsis, postabortal pelvic infection, or intravenous injection of narcotics. It may also occur as a complication of cardiac surgery, transurethral prostatectomy, or surgery on infected tissue. Hemolytic staphylococci and gram-negative coliform organisms are now the most common pathogens. Among narcotic users, staphylococci, candida, and gram-negative bacteria are prominent causes of endocarditis.

Acute endocarditis produces large, friable vegetations, severe embolic episodes with metastatic abscess formation, and rapid perforation, tearing, or destruction of the affected valves or rupture of chordae tendineae.

Clinical Findings

A. Symptoms and Signs: Fever is present in most

cases, although afebrile periods may occur, especially in the aged. Any or all of the following may occur also: night sweats, chills, malaise, fatigue, anorexia, weight loss; vague muscle aching, arthralgia, or redness and swelling of the joints; sudden visual disturbances, aphasia, or hemiplegia due to cerebral emboli; pain in the abdomen, chest, or flanks due to mesenteric, splenic, pulmonary, or renal emboli; nosebleeds, easy bruisability, and symptoms of heart failure. In ABE, the course is more fulminating and the patient is very toxic.

In SBE, evidence of rheumatic, congenital, or calcific heart disease is usually present. Findings include tachycardia, splenomegaly; petechiae of the skin, mucous membranes, and ocular fundi, or beneath the nails as "splinter hemorrhages"; clubbing of the fingers and toes; pallor or a yellowish-brown tint of the skin; neurologic residuals of cerebral emboli; and tender red nodules of the finger or toe pads. Heart murmurs may be considered "insignificant" in infection of the tricuspid and pulmonary valve, where recurrent pulmonary infarction suggesting pneumonia may be a prominent feature. The clinical picture is often atypical in older persons, since fever, chills, and leukocytosis may be absent.

ABE presents as a severe infection associated with chills, high fever, prostration, and multiple, serious embolic phenomena. These may be superimposed on the antecedent causative infection (eg, pneumonia, furunculosis, pelvic infection) or may appear abruptly following instrumentation, surgery, or self-injection of narcotics. Heart murmurs may change rapidly, and heart failure occurs early.

ABE or SBE may develop during "prophylactic" or inadequate therapeutic antibiotic administration. In these circumstances the onset is "masked" and a sudden embolic episode, the appearance of petechiae, unexplained heart failure, changing murmurs, or a rising temperature may be the first clue.

B. Laboratory Findings: In suspected SBE, take 2 blood cultures daily for 3–5 days. Within 2–7 days of incubation, 85–95% of these cultures will grow organisms and permit specific drug selection. In ABE, take 2 or 3 cultures during the emergency work-up; then begin antibiotic treatment. In the presence of repeated negative blood cultures (eg, in uremic patients), bone marrow should be cultured.

The administration of an antimicrobial drug may interfere with positive blood cultures for 7–10 days.

Normochromic anemia, a markedly elevated sedimentation rate, variable leukocytosis, microscopic hematuria, proteinuria, and casts are commonly present in SBE and ABE. Nitrogen retention may be the first clue, especially in older patients. Rheumatoid factor is demonstrable in the serum of 50–60% of cases of SBE of more than 6 weeks' standing.

Complications

The complications of ABE or SBE include peripheral arterial emboli (producing hemiplegias or aphasia; infarction of the bowel, kidney, or spleen; or acute arterial insufficiency of an arm or leg); congestive heart failure, renal failure, hemorrhagic tendency, anemia, and metastatic abscess formation (especially in ABE). Splenic abscess may cause lack of response to therapy, or relapse.

Differential Diagnosis

SBE must be differentiated from various seemingly primary disease states. Hemiplegia, intractable heart failure, anemia, a bleeding tendency, or uremia may be caused by SBE. If a patient presenting with any of these illnesses has fever or a heart murmur, blood cultures should be taken.

Specific diseases that require differentiation are the lymphomas, thrombocytopenic purpura, leukemia, acute rheumatic fever, disseminated lupus erythematosus, polyarteritis nodosa, chronic meningococcemia, brucellosis, disseminated or miliary tuberculosis, and nonbacterial thrombotic endocarditis or chronic wasting disease.

ABE masquerades as a severe systemic response to an obvious preexisting infection. It can be recognized only by noting rapid clinical deterioration, bacteremia, the appearance or sudden change of heart murmurs, heart failure, and major embolic accidents, especially to the CNS, simulating meningitis.

Prevention

A. Medical Measures: Some cases of endocarditis arise after dental procedures or surgery of the oropharynx and genitourinary tract. Patients with known cardiac anomalies who are to have any of these procedures should be prepared in one of the following ways, although failures sometimes occur:

(1) 600,000 units procaine penicillin with 600,000 units crystalline penicillin, IM, 1 hour before surgery, and then 600,000 units procaine penicillin IM daily for 2 days.

(2) 500,000 units penicillin V orally 4 times daily on the day of surgery and for 2 days after surgery.

(3) In case of penicillin sensitivity, or in persons receiving penicillin prophylaxis for rheumatic fever, give erythromycin, 250 mg orally 4 times daily on the day of surgery and for 2 days afterward, or vancomycin, 0.5 gm every 8 hours IV for 1 day.

(4) For genitourinary or gastrointestinal surgery, give kanamycin, 1 gm IM daily, or gentamicin, 120 mg IM daily, in addition to (1).

B. Surgical Measures: Surgery may be warranted for the prevention of bacterial endocarditis in selected patients with surgically correctable congenital lesions (eg, patent ductus arteriosus) or acquired lesions (eg, symptomatic aortic and mitral valvular disease). Preoperative antibiotic therapy should be instituted as above. Mycotic aneurysms also must be treated surgically.

Treatment

A. Specific Measures: The most important consideration in the treatment of bacterial endocarditis is a bactericidal concentration of antibiotics in contact with the infecting organism, which is often localized in avascular tissues or in vegetations. Penicillin, because of its high degree of bactericidal activity against the great majority of bacteria which produce bacterial endocarditis, and because of its low incidence of side reactions, is by far the most useful drug. Synergistic combinations of antibiotics have proved valuable at times. Few cases have been cured by bacteriostatic drugs used alone.

Positive blood cultures are invaluable to confirm the diagnosis and to guide treatment with tests of susceptibility of the infecting organism to various antibiotics or combinations of antibiotics. Two blood cultures should be obtained daily for 3–5 days before instituting treatment, except in desperately ill patients in whom antibiotic therapy is started after emergency work-up including 2–3 blood cultures.

Note: **Control of antimicrobial treatment.** Negative blood cultures are a minimal initial requirement of effective therapy. An assay of serum bactericidal activity is the best guide to support the selection of drugs and the daily dose, after treatment has been started. During therapy, the patient's serum diluted 1:5 or 1:10 should (at least during part of the interval between drug doses) be rapidly bactericidal in vitro under standardized laboratory conditions for the organisms initially grown from the patient's blood stream.

1. **Penicillin** is the drug of choice in a large majority of cases of bacterial endocarditis. It should be administered parenterally at first to all patients until adequate serum bactericidal activity has been established. A shift to oral administration can be considered only in patients with exquisitely susceptible infecting organisms where control over oral drug intake (about 5 times the parenteral dose) and adequacy of serum levels can be maintained.

The dosage of penicillin is a function of the susceptibility of the organism. Viridans streptococci susceptible to 0.1 unit penicillin/ml (more than 80%) can be eradicated from bacterial endocarditis by administering penicillin G, 3–5 million units daily for 3–4 weeks. This is given conveniently by IM injection of 1.2 million units procaine penicillin 3 times daily. Streptococci killed by 1 but not by 0.1 unit/ml require penicillin G (aqueous), 5–10 million units daily for 4 weeks. This can be given IM or IV. Streptococci and other organisms killed by penicillin in concentrations greater than 1 unit/ml require more than 10 million units penicillin G, usually administered in divided doses given every 4 hours as a bolus into a continuous intravenous drip in part of the daily fluid requirement of 5% glucose in water or saline. The following complications must be considered: (a) Each million units of potassium penicillin contains about 1.7 milliequivalents of potassium, which arouses concern about potassium toxicity. (b) At very high concentrations of penicillin, there is enough diffusion into the CNS to cause neurotoxicity. (c) With intravenous antibiotic therapy of long duration, there is a significant risk of superinfection; to minimize this possibility, injection sites must be changed each 48 hours and must be kept scrupulously aseptic.

If bacteremia and signs of bacterial endocarditis activity persist, the dosage can be increased (500 million units penicillin G have been given daily) until serum assay and clinical response are satisfactory. If blood cultures are negative and serum assay suggests adequate drug effect, continuing symptoms or signs may have to be attributed to causes other than active infection.

2. **Combined penicillin and aminoglycoside**—The addition of streptomycin, kanamycin, or gentamicin enhances the bactericidal activity of penicillins for many streptococci, particularly enterococci (*S faecalis*). In endocarditis due to viridans streptococci, streptomycin sulfate, 0.5 gm, can be injected IM 2 times daily for 10 days (in addition to penicillin given as above). The total time of treatment can then be reduced to 21 days (instead of 4 weeks). In endocarditis due to enterococci, streptomycin, 0.5 gm, kanamycin, 0.5 gm, or gentamicin, 80 mg, is injected every 8–12 hours while penicillin G (10–60 million units daily) or ampicillin (8–20 gm daily) is injected IV for 4–5 weeks. This combined treatment has a better record of eradicating enterococci from endocarditis than penicillin alone and represents one of the best examples of antibiotic synergism. Other drug combinations can occasionally be discovered by laboratory test to treat endocarditis caused by particularly resistant microorganisms.

3. **Cephalothin**, 6–12 gm daily IV, or cefazolin, 4 gm daily IM, has been used for streptococcal and staphylococcal endocarditis as a substitute for penicillin in allergic individuals. Hypersensitivity to cephalosporins and other untoward reactions may occur. Cephalosporins usually fail in enterococcal endocarditis.

4. **Methicillin,** 6–18 gm daily IV for 4–6 weeks, has been used in endocarditis caused by penicillinase-producing staphylococci. Alternative drugs are nafcillin, 8–16 gm IV, and oxacillin, 8–16 gm IV daily, given for the same period. Vancomycin, 2–4 gm IV daily, has been given for 2–4 weeks in staphylococcal endocarditis. All of these are best given by "push" in 20 minutes every 2–6 hours into an intravenous infusion.

5. **Tetracyclines, erythromycins, lincomycins, and similar drugs** which are mainly bacteriostatic are not drugs of choice in bacterial endocarditis. If administered to patients with fever of unknown origin, these drugs suppress bacteremia temporarily and produce symptomatic improvement. However, they generally fail to eradicate the infection, permit progression of the lesion, and interfere with specific diagnosis. In endocarditis caused by Bacteroides species, clindamycin may be the drug of choice. Dosage must be judged by serum assay and patient tolerance. Tetracyclines may be indicated in rickettsial endocarditis.

6. In endocarditis caused by gram-negative bacteria of the enteric flora, **kanamycin**, 0.5 gm IM every 6–12 hours, or **gentamicin**, 5–7 mg/kg/day IM in 3 divided doses, may be the principal drug, sometimes

combined with cephalothin, 6–12 gm/day IV, or carbenicillin, 12–30 gm/day IV, to give bactericidal combinations by laboratory test. Polymyxin B and colistin have not proved to be clinically useful in endocarditis caused by Pseudomonas species in spite of susceptibility of the organisms in vitro. Only surgical removal of the infected site (eg, patch over septal defect, prosthesis) in the cardiovascular system has led to cure of pseudomonas endocarditis. With all these drugs, constant vigilance regarding nephro-, neuro-, and ototoxicity—and serum level determinations—may be essential. Dosages must be adjusted if renal function is impaired.

7. Fungal endocarditis due to Candida species usually cannot be cured by drug treatment alone. Resection of the involved valve combined with amphotericin B, 0.5–1 mg/kg/day IV, has occasionally been successful.

8. In patients with a clinical picture typical of bacterial endocarditis but with persistently negative blood cultures, empirical treatment with **penicillin G,** 20–50 million units/day IV, plus **gentamicin,** 5 mg/kg/day IM, can be given for 4 weeks. Several of the manifestations of the disease should show marked improvement with such treatment. If there is no clinical improvement in 3–5 days, a therapeutic trial of other drugs (see above) is warranted.

9. **Follow-up and recurrences**—At the end of the established treatment period of 3–6 weeks, all antimicrobial therapy should be stopped. After 3 days, blood cultures are taken once weekly for 4 weeks while the patient is observed carefully. Most bacteriologic relapses occur during this time, but some recurrences are delayed for several months. Embolic phenomena and fever may occur both during and after successful treatment and—by themselves—are not adequate grounds for retreatment. An initial adequate course of therapy in bacteriologically proved bacterial endocarditis can result in up to 90% bacteriologic cure. If bacteriologic relapse occurs, the organism must be isolated and tested again, and a second—often longer—course of treatment administered with properly selected drugs.

In spite of bacteriologic cure, 50% of patients treated for bacterial endocarditis progress to cardiac failure in 5–10 years. This mechanical failure can be attributed in part to valvular deformities (eg, perforation of cusp, tearing of chordae) caused by the bacterial infection and in part to the healing and scarring process. Therefore, surgical correction of abnormalities in cardiovascular dynamics or possible valvular prostheses must be considered as part of the follow-up.

B. **General Measures:** Supportive treatment, as for any severe infection, must be given. Anemia, if severe, may require transfusion of blood or red cell mass. Anticoagulants (eg, heparin, bishydroxycoumarin) are not indicated in uncomplicated bacterial endocarditis and may contribute to hemorrhagic complications.

C. **Treatment of Complications:**

1. **Infarctions** of organs in the systemic circulation usually result from emboli originating in vegetations in the left heart. Emboli derived from right heart lesions may produce pulmonary infarction. Treatment is symptomatic and anticoagulants are sometimes helpful. Embolectomy can be attempted if an accessible site can be located. Fungal vegetations may produce massive arterial occlusions.

2. **Cardiac failure**—Myocarditis, which frequently accompanies infective endocarditis of long duration, and increasing deformity of heart valves may precipitate cardiac failure and require digitalization and sodium restriction. In such patients, the sodium salts of penicillins are undesirable, and potassium or calcium salts are preferred. Early valve replacement may have to be considered during antimicrobial therapy if there is evidence of progressive severe heart failure. Because of the bad prognosis of progressive aortic insufficiency developing with endocarditis, insertion of an aortic valve prosthesis may be essential after only 2–3 weeks, or less, of satisfactory antimicrobial drug therapy.

3. Many patients with bacterial endocarditis develop **nitrogen retention** due to focal embolic nephritis or glomerulonephritis. This requires adjustment of drug dosage and—rarely—temporary treatment of uremia until renal function improves during antimicrobial therapy.

Prognosis

Bacterial endocarditis is uniformly fatal unless the bacterial infection can be eradicated, but in a few cases surgical removal of an infected A-V fistula or patent ductus arteriosus has been curative. The poorest prognosis for bacteriologic cure exists in patients with consistently negative blood cultures and long delay in therapy; in those with very highly resistant organisms; and in those with an infected prosthesis. If bacteriologic cure is accomplished, the prognosis depends on the adequacy of cardiovascular function as mechanical distortions and impairment of dynamics develop during infection and healing. Only about 60% of patients with bacteriologically cured bacterial endocarditis are well 5 years after treatment. Among valve lesions, aortic insufficiency carries the worst outlook and merits the most prompt surgical consideration. Among embolic events, those to the brain have the poorest prognosis. Cerebral emboli and rupture of mycotic aneurysms may occur even after bacteriologic cure. Renal functional impairment is generally reversible during early adequate antimicrobial therapy.

Bennett WM, Singer I, Coggins CJ: A guide to drug therapy in renal failure. JAMA 230:1544, 1974.

Buchbinder NA, Roberts WC: Valvular infective endocarditis. Am J Med 53:7, 1972.

Dismukes WE & others: Prosthetic valve endocarditis: Analysis of 38 cases. Circulation 48:365, 1973.

Elster SK & others: *Hemophilus aphrophilus* endocarditis: Review of 23 cases. Am J Cardiol 35:72, 1975.

Griffin FM Jr, Jones G, Cobbs CG: Aortic insufficiency in bacterial endocarditis. Ann Int Med 76:23, 1972.

Johnson DH, Rosenthal A, Nadas AS: A forty-year review of bacterial endocarditis in infancy and childhood. Circulation 51:581, 1975.

Lachman AS & others: Infective endocarditis in the billowing mitral leaflet syndrome. Brit Heart J 37:326, 1975.

Lerner PI: Infective endocarditis: A review of selected topics. M Clin North America 58:605, 1974.

Lerner PL, Weinstein L: Infective endocarditis in the antibiotic era. (4 parts.) New England J Med 274:199, 259, 323, 388, 1966.

Menda KB, Gorbach SL: Favorable experience with bacterial endocarditis in heroin addicts. Ann Int Med 78:25, 1973.

Nastro LJ, Finegold SM: Endocarditis due to anaerobic gram-negative bacilli. Am J Med 54:481, 1973.

Weinstein L: "Modern" infective endocarditis. JAMA 233:260, 1974.

Weinstein L, Schlesinger JJ: Pathoanatomic, pathophysiologic, and clinical correlations in endocarditis. (2 parts.) New England J Med 291:832, 1122, 1974.

Wilson WR & others: Prosthetic valve endocarditis. Ann Int Med 82:751, 1975.

HYPERTENSIVE CARDIOVASCULAR DISEASE

The criteria for the diagnosis of hypertension are arbitrary, because the arterial pressure rises with age and varies from one occasion of measurement to another. Most authorities consider hypertension to be present when the diastolic pressure consistently exceeds 100 mm Hg in a person more than 60 years of age, or 90 mm Hg in a person less than 50 years of age. WHO places upper limits of normal at 160/95 mm Hg. The vascular complications of hypertension are thought to be the consequence of the raised arterial pressure and associated atherosclerosis of major arterial circuits.

Hypertension which has not demonstrably affected the heart is called "hypertensive vascular disease." When left ventricular hypertrophy, heart failure, or coronary artery disease is present, "hypertensive cardiovascular disease" is the appropriate term.

Hypertension is uncommon before age 20, although recent data suggest a higher frequency if one uses different criteria for children, such as pressure exceeding the 90th percentile for age. In young people it is commonly caused by chronic glomerulonephritis, renal artery stenosis, pyelonephritis, or coarctation of the aorta.

Transient elevation of blood pressure caused by excitement, apprehension, or exertion and the purely systolic elevation of blood pressure in elderly people caused by loss of elasticity in their major arteries do not constitute hypertensive disease.

Hypertension is an important preventable cause of cardiovascular disease; prospective studies have shown that, without treatment, hypertension greatly increases the incidence of cardiac failure, coronary heart disease with angina pectoris and myocardial infarction, hemorrhagic and thrombotic stroke, and renal failure. Epidemiologic studies have shown that only a small percentage of the population is receiving effective antihypertensive therapy; education of the physician and the patient is necessary to identify the patient with hypertension, to treat him adequately, and to reinforce the concept that treatment is a lifelong process and that compliance with the treatment program is essential to an effective result. The prevention—as well as the reversibility—of hypertensive complications by antihypertensive therapy is a major public health concern.

Etiology & Classification

A. Primary Hypertension: In about 85% of cases of hypertensive vascular or cardiovascular disease, no cause can be established. The onset of essential hypertension is usually between ages 25 and 55. The family history is usually suggestive of hypertension (stroke, "sudden death," heart failure). Women are affected more often than men. Elevations in pressure are transient early in the course of the disease but eventually become permanent. Even in established cases the blood pressure fluctuates widely in response to emotional stress, especially anger, resentment, and frustration. The resting blood pressure is lower than single casual office readings, and can be determined after several hours' rest in bed. Blood pressures taken by the patient at home or during daily activities using a portable apparatus are lower than those recorded in the office, clinic, or hospital. It is not established which readings are most reliable in estimating prognosis.

Note: All of the foregoing may be true in other forms of hypertension also. A diagnosis of essential hypertension is warranted only after repeated, thorough search for specific causes has been unsuccessful.

Primary hypertension does not always have uniform pathophysiologic features; there is evidence that subsets of patients can be identified in terms of factors that regulate the blood pressure in the normal population. These include baroreceptor activity, cardiac output, systemic vascular resistance, blood volume, activity of the sympathetic and central nervous systems, and the renin-angiotensin-aldosterone system. This last system has received intensive investigation in the past few years. **Renin,** a proteolytic enzyme, is secreted by the juxtaglomerular cells surrounding the afferent arterioles near the vascular pole of the kidney in response to a signal which is related to stretch of the afferent arteriole or to decreased volume or sodium content. The renin then acts on a substrate in the plasma, producing angiotensin I, which is then acted upon by a converting enzyme to form angiotensin II, which is the most potent pressor substance known. Angiotensin II, by an effect on the zona glomerulosa of the adrenal cortex, increases the secretion of aldosterone, which results in sodium and water retention by its characteristic action on the distal renal tubule, thus restoring blood volume; by negative feedback, the secretion of renin is then reduced until equilibrium results. Approximately 20% of hypertensive patients have low plasma renin but normal aldosterone production, and 15% have high plasma renin in the absence of the accelerated or malignant phase. These subsets may have important prognostic and therapeutic implications because it is inferred that low-renin hypertension is due to increased secretion of an as yet unknown mineralocorticoid which increases the blood volume; these patients respond very well to drugs such as thiazides, spironolactone, and other diuretics that deplete plasma and extracellular volume. The effect of the diuretics is less dramatic in high-renin hypertensives, in whom overaction of the unknown mineralocorticoid is presumably not present and arteriolar vasoconstriction is thought to be the dominant physiologic abnormality raising the systemic vascular resistance. Propranolol and other beta-adrenergic blocking agents are more effective in reducing the plasma renin activity in the high-renin group than in low-renin hypertension. Some studies, however, have failed to demonstrate parallel falls in plasma renin and arterial pressure. Laragh and his associates believe that low-renin hypertension has a better prognosis than high- or normal-renin hypertension, but other investigators disagree. Further study is required to determine whether subsets of hypertensives, as determined by their physiologic and biochemical abnormalities, respond selectively to different antihypertensive agents and whether the latter should be "tailored" to them.

B. Secondary Hypertension:

1. Renal hypertension—

a. Vascular—Narrowing of one or both renal arteries due to atherosclerosis, fibromuscular hyperplasia, or other causes has come to be recognized as perhaps the most common cause of curable hypertension. It may present in the same manner as essential hypertension but may be suspected in the following circumstances: (1) if the onset is after age 50; (2) if there are epigastric or renal artery bruits; (3) if there is atherosclerosis elsewhere; (4) if there are variations in the size and appearance, time of appearance of contrast media, or delayed hyperconcentration of contrast material in the involved kidney on the intravenous urogram; (5) if there are increased amounts (relative to the other kidney) of renin activity in renal vein blood; (6) if there is abnormal excretion of radioactive materials by renal scan; or (7) if atherosclerosis or fibromuscular hyperplasia can be demonstrated by renal artery angiogram.

The functional significance of an established lesion is determined (1) by demonstrating increased renal vein renin on the involved side as compared to the opposite side, and (2) by means of the Howard-Stamey test with decreased sodium concentration and increased osmolality in the urine on the involved side. When both tests are positive in the presence of a severely stenosed proximal renal artery lesion, reconstructive surgery offers a very good prognosis.

b. Parenchymal—Chronic glomerulonephritis and pyelonephritis have in the past accounted for the largest group of known causes of hypertension. Unilateral pyelonephritis is rare but can often be cured by surgery. Polycystic kidney disease and congenital or acquired obstructive hydronephrosis are rare causes. Acute glomerulonephritis is often associated with hypertension.

2. Endocrine—Pheochromocytoma, a tumor of the adrenal medulla or (rarely) of chromaffin tissue along a sympathetic chain, causes sustained or intermittent hypertension by releasing norepinephrine and epinephrine into the blood stream. Cushing's syndrome, primary aldosteronism, 17-hydroxylase deficiency, congenital adrenal hyperplasia with virilism, and deoxycorticosterone overtreatment of patients with adrenal insufficiency regularly cause hypertension. An eosinophilic tumor of the pituitary, producing acromegaly, may also cause hypertension.

3. Coarctation of the aorta—Congenital constriction of the arch of the aorta produces hypertension in the upper extremities and carotid arteries. Blood pressure in the legs is normal or low.

4. Miscellaneous—Hypertension of varying severity is present in toxemias of pregnancy, following use of oral contraceptive agents, increased intracranial pressure due to tumor or hematoma, overdistention of a neurogenic bladder, and in the late stages of polyarteritis nodosa, disseminated lupus erythematosus, and scleroderma.

C. Malignant Hypertension: (See Hypertensive Crises, p 184.) Any form of sustained hypertension, primary or secondary, may abruptly become accelerated, with diastolic pressure rising rapidly above 130 mm Hg and causing widespread arteriolar necroses and hyperplasia of the intima of the interlobular arteries of the kidney, in turn causing ischemic atrophy of the nephron. Without treatment, there is rapidly progressive renal failure, left ventricular failure, and stroke. The raised arterial pressure results in papilledema and hemorrhages and exudates in the retinas; these signs may precede clinical evidence of renal impairment and are the most reliable definitive clinical signs of malignant hypertension, although fibrinoid necrosis of the kidney may occur in the presence of soft exudates and hemorrhages alone. If no treatment is given, the mortality rate approaches 100% in 2 years with an 80% mortality rate in 1 year—hence the term malignant. Examination of the retinas for evidence of accelerated hypertension is necessary in all hypertensive patients, because the early stages of the malignant phase may be essentially asymptomatic although severe headache, acute visual disturbances, and gross hematuria are the usual presenting manifestations. Cardiac and renal failure may occur with great rapidity, and treatment to lower the blood pressure is urgent (see p 182).

Pathogenesis

Essential and renal hypertension are due to increased peripheral arteriolar resistance of unknown mechanism. Unless heart failure or edema is present, cardiac output and blood volume are not affected in well-established cases. Renal pressor substances may play a role in essential and renal hypertension, but this has not been demonstrated in humans.

In pheochromocytoma hypertension is due to varying combinations of increased cardiac output and peripheral resistance caused by epinephrine and norepinephrine, respectively.

The mechanism of production of hypertension by adrenal glucocorticoids, aldosterone, and deoxycorticosterone is not known. The hypertension of coarctation of the aorta is thought to result directly from the constriction, which causes the left ventricle to eject blood into a "short chamber," although the renal mechanism may be involved.

Pathology

Sustained hypertension causes the initially reversible ("functional") arteriolar narrowing to become permanent ("structural") as a result of intimal thickening, hypertrophy of the muscular coats, and hyaline degeneration. In malignant hypertension, arteriolar necrosis (especially in the renal vessels) develops rapidly and is responsible for the acute onset of renal failure. The dominant manifestations of hypertension are secondary to left ventricular hypertrophy and failure and to the widespread arteriolar and arterial lesions. Hypertension accelerates the development of coronary and cerebral artery atherosclerosis; myocardial infarction and cerebral hemorrhage or thrombosis are common sequelae.

Clinical Findings

The clinical and laboratory findings are mainly referable to the degree of vascular deterioration and involvement of the "target organs": heart, brain, kidneys, eyes, and peripheral arteries.

A. Symptoms: Mild to moderate essential hypertension is compatible with normal health and well being for many years. Vague symptoms usually appear after the patient learns he has "high blood pressure." Suboccipital headaches, characteristically occurring early in the morning and subsiding during the day, are common, but any type of headache may occur (even simulating migraine). Other common complaints are lightheadedness, tinnitus, "fullness in the head," easy fatigability, loss of energy, and palpitations. These symptoms are caused by anxiety about hypertension or by associated psychologic disturbances.

Patients with pheochromocytoma which secretes predominantly norepinephrine usually have sustained hypertension. Intermittent release of catechol causes attacks (lasting minutes to hours) of acute anxiety, palpitation, profuse perspiration, pallor, trembling, and nausea and vomiting; blood pressure is markedly elevated during the attack, and angina or acute pulmonary edema may occur. In primary aldosteronism, patients may have recurrent episodes of generalized muscular weakness or paralysis, paresthesias, polyuria, and nocturia due to associated hypokalemia.

Cardiac involvement secondary to increased work of the left ventricle, overcoming the raised systemic vascular resistance, often leads to paroxysmal nocturnal dyspnea or cardiac asthma with or without symptoms of chronic left ventricular failure. Angina pectoris or myocardial infarction may develop.

Progressive renal involvement may not produce striking symptoms, but nocturia or intermittent hematuria may ultimately occur.

Peripheral arterial disease most commonly causes intermittent claudication. When the terminal aorta is narrowed or occluded, pain in the buttocks and low back pain appear on walking and men become impotent.

Cerebral involvement causes (1) hemiplegia or aphasia due to thrombosis or (2) sudden hemorrhage from rupture of small intracerebral aneurysms (Charcot), leading to death in hours or days. In malignant hypertension (and occasionally in its absence), severe headache, confusion, coma, convulsions, blurred vision, transient neurologic signs, and nausea and vomiting may occur ("hypertensive encephalopathy"). The mechanism of their production is probably acute capillary congestion and exudation with cerebral edema. The findings are usually reversible with adequate treatment.

B. Signs: Physical findings depend upon the cause of hypertension, its duration and severity, and the degree of effect on target organs.

1. Blood pressure—The diagnosis of hypertension is not warranted in patients under the age of 50 unless the blood pressure exceeds 140/90 mm Hg on at least 3 separate occasions after the patient has rested 20 or more minutes in familiar, quiet surroundings. Casual readings (ie, those taken in the usual fashion) may be much higher than this in the absence of hypertensive disease, since with rest the pressures return to normal; this is vascular hyperreactivity, not hypertension.

2. Retinas—The Keith-Wagener (KW) classification of retinal changes in hypertension has prognostic significance and correlates well with the clinical course.

KW1 = Minimal arteriolar narrowing.

KW2 = More marked narrowing and arteriovenous nicking.

KW3 = Flame-shaped or circular hemorrhages and fluffy "cotton wool" exudates.

KW4 = Any of the above plus papilledema, ie, elevation of the optic disk, obliteration of the physiologic cup, or blurring of the disk margins. By definition, malignant hypertension is always associated with papilledema.

3. Heart and arteries—A loud aortic second sound and an early systolic ejection click may occur. Evidence of left ventricular enlargement with a left ventricular heave indicates well-established disease. With onset of left ventricular failure, pulmonary basal rales, gallop rhythm, and pulsus alternans may be noted; a presystolic gallop alone does not necessarily imply failure but may be due to decreased compliance of the left ventricle.

4. Pulses—Direct comparison should be made of both carotid, radial, femoral, popliteal, and pedal pulses, and the presence or absence of bruits over major vessels, including the abdominal aorta and iliacs, should be determined. Blood pressure should be taken in both arms and legs.

5. Cerebrum—Neurologic residuals of cerebral thrombosis or hemorrhage may be present, ranging from only a positive Babinski or Hoffman reflex to frank hemiplegia or hemianopsia.

6. Endocrine status—The signs of Cushing's disease should be noted if present: trunk obesity, hirsutism, acne, purple striae, and finely grained skin. One kidney may be displaced by an adrenal tumor. In primary aldosteronism, flaccid paralysis or muscular weakness and hypoactive or absent tendon reflexes may be noted as well as diminished or absent vasomotor circulatory reflexes.

7. Coarctation of aorta—Weak or delayed femoral pulses (in comparison with radial pulses) in younger people justify a diagnosis of coarctation of the aorta. Confirmatory signs are a basal systolic murmur transmitted to the interscapular area and palpable collateral arteries along the inferior rib margins and especially around the scapular borders.

8. Renal artery stenosis—A characteristic arterial bruit may be heard with a diaphragm stethoscope in the left or right epigastrium, transmitted from the affected renal artery. The bruit can often be traced into the flank and to the costovertebral angle.

9. Renal parenchymal disease—The patient may have a "uremic" appearance and odor. Polycystic kidneys are large and readily palpable.

C. Laboratory Findings: Routine urinalysis may disclose a low fixed specific gravity compatible with advanced renal parenchymal disease or hypokalemic nephropathy of primary aldosteronism. In both, BUN and serum creatinine are elevated and anemia due to advanced azotemia may be present. In aldosteronism, however, the serum potassium is low and the serum sodium and CO_2 elevated; the reverse is true in uremia associated with primary renal disease.

Proteinuria, granular casts, and occasionally microhematuria occur in nephrosclerosis; differentiation from chronic nephritis on this basis is impossible.

Demonstrable bacilluria in a fresh clean specimen suggests chronic pyelonephritis; white cell casts are rarely found. Pyuria is frequently absent. Quantitative culture of a clean specimen must be performed on all patients and repeated at intervals, since bacilluria in chronic pyelonephritis may be intermittent.

Quantitative determination of urinary excretion of 17-hydroxycorticosteroids or catecholamines and vanillylmandelic acid is indicated if the clinical picture suggests Cushing's disease or pheochromocytoma, respectively. Urinary aldosterone need not be determined routinely; except in very early or borderline instances, the diagnosis usually can be strongly suspected by blood chemistry.

Tests for pheochromocytoma:

(1) Determine 24-hour urinary catecholamines (see Appendix) or vanillylmandelic acid (normal: 0.7–6.8 mg/24 hours). In most centers, catechol excretion has replaced the provocation tests (histamine and phentolamine [Regitine]) as a screening method.

(2) Test in presence of sustained hypertension due to pheochromocytoma: The baseline blood pressure should be determined while the patient rests for 20 minutes. It should exceed 170/110 mm Hg. Phen-

tolamine (Regitine), 2.5–5 mg rapidly IV, best given into the tubing of an infusion during which the levels of the blood pressure have been stabilized, should produce a sustained fall of at least 35/25 mm Hg within 2–5 minutes in patients with pheochromocytoma. *Note:* Sedatives, antihypertensive drugs, and uremia may cause a false-positive test.

(3) Provocative test for a patient with normal blood pressure: Give 0.01–0.025 mg of histamine base in 0.5 ml of normal saline in a tuberculin syringe rapidly IV, leaving the needle in the vein (so that phentolamine can be given to lower excessive blood pressure rise in response to histamine). A blood pressure rise of 60/30 mm Hg or a rise greater than that following a cold pressor test occurs within 2 minutes when pheochromocytoma is present.

D. X-Ray Findings: Chest x-ray may disclose rib notching and the small aortic knob of coarctation and indicate the degree of cardiac enlargement caused by hypertension. Intravenous urograms yield valuable information on relative renal size, relative rate of appearance and disappearance of the contrast material, renal displacement, the presence of obstruction, and pyelonephritis, and are diagnostic of polycystic disease.

E. ECG Findings: ECG can estimate the degree of left ventricular hypertrophy and will show signs of coronary artery disease with conduction disturbances and significant Q waves. In aldosteronism the Q–T interval is prolonged.

F. Special Studies: Selective angiography combined with intravenous urograms and tomography is useful in visualizing adrenal tumors. If renal artery stenosis is suspected, intravenous urograms are indicated. It may also be necessary to perform transfemoral aortography with the contrast medium introduced at a level at or just below the orifices of the renal arteries; differential radioisotope excretion studies or renal vein renin determinations on the 2 kidneys; or differential urinary function studies on each kidney (differential water, electrolyte, inulin, PAH, and dye excretion measurements).

G. Physiologic and Biochemical Studies of Cardiac Output, Blood Volume, Systemic Vascular Resistance, Plasma Renin, Angiotensin, and Aldosterone: As indicated on p 178, subsets of patients with hypertension have prognostic and therapeutic significance, and new technology allows determination of these factors with precision.

H. Follow-Up Studies: If specific causes have been excluded, periodic ophthalmoscopic study and evaluation of cardiac and renal status by ECG, chest x-ray, PSP excretion, creatinine clearance, BUN, urinary specific gravity, and urine protein determinations are advised to observe the progression of the disease.

Treatment With Hypotensive Drugs

Many patients with mild hypertension, especially middle-aged women, live years in comfort without treatment. Great care should therefore be exercised before subjecting these patients to the disagreeable side-effects and potential dangers of a continuous program of drug therapy, especially if the diastolic pressure is less than 100 mm Hg.

Hypertension varies strikingly in severity in different patients; treatment at present should be varied depending upon the severity of the hypertension, the presence of complications, and the physiologic and biochemical subsets referred to earlier.

Factors which unfavorably influence the prognosis in chronic arterial hypertension and which accordingly determine the nature of drug therapy to be recommended include the following: (1) high diastolic and systolic blood pressure levels; (2) male sex (worse in men than women); (3) early age at onset; (4) black race; (5) retinal abnormalities (see p 180); (6) cardiac abnormalities (eg, ECG changes, cardiomegaly, angina); (7) cerebrovascular accidents: (8) renal abnormalities; (9) plasma renin; and (10) family history of hypertension.

Recent large-scale studies demonstrate convincingly that appropriate drug treatment of asymptomatic moderate degrees of chronic hypertension ($\geqslant 105$ mm Hg diastolic) results in significantly lower morbidity and mortality rates from cardiovascular diseases (heart failure, hemorrhagic stroke, renal failure) than are reported in untreated control patients. Current insurance data have shown that even slight increases in blood pressure decrease survival, especially by causing premature atherosclerosis.

There is considerable variation of opinion among clinicians about the preference for and the proper sequence of administration of the several drugs that are available. A certain amount of trial and error is involved in selection of the proper agents for each patient, depending upon response to treatment, tolerance of the medication, and the ability of the patient to cooperate. None of the drugs are devoid of undesirable side reactions. The least toxic drugs should be used for mild hypertension. Combinations of drugs working by different mechanisms are frequently necessary to sustain reduced blood pressure and minimize toxicity, but this may make it difficult to evaluate treatment. Fixed-dose combinations should be avoided, especially early in the course of treatment.

In mild to moderate hypertension, therapy is usually initiated with thiazides or (less frequently) other classes of diuretics. If blood pressure is not controlled by diuretics alone after a period of 1–3 weeks, the second drug may be either reserpine, hydralazine, or methyldopa. A recent report suggests that carcinoma of the breast may occur more frequently in patients receiving rauwolfia derivatives; caution must be exercised in recommending the drug until the FDA completes its analysis of the data. In moderate arterial hypertension (diastolic pressure of 110–130 mm Hg), it may be advisable to initiate treatment with a combination of thiazides and reserpine plus, if indicated, hydralazine. The combination of the vasodilator (hydralazine) and propranolol (a beta-adrenergic blocker which counteracts the increased sympathetic discharge resulting from hydralazine) has proved effective with few side-effects. In severe cases or when patients fail to respond to other agents, the combination of a thiazide and guanethidine should be used. In general, guanethidine should replace rather than be added to reserpine or methyldopa when the latter have proved to be ineffective. If hypertension is complicated by renal failure, methyldopa and hydralazine are usually the most effective agents, although newer agents not yet approved by the FDA show considerable advantages (propranolol, minoxidil).

Malignant hypertension should be treated with rapidly acting hypotensive drugs.

The monoamine oxidase inhibitors should not be used in combination with any of the antihypertensive drugs because of the possibility of provoking hypertensive crises. Amphetamines and tricyclic antidepressants (eg, amitriptyline [Elavil] block the effectiveness of guanethidine and may occasionally aggravate hypertension.

A. Indications for Hypotensive Drugs:

1. Definite indications—Hypotensive drug therapy is definitely indicated in malignant hypertension; in hypertensive cardiac failure (pulmonary edema) when "fresh" acute myocardial infarction has been excluded; for rapidly increasing diastolic blood pressure with left ventricular hypertrophy and dilatation; for hypertensive encephalopathy; when there is evidence of deterioration in the heart and fundi (exudates and hemorrhages), especially in young (particularly male and black) patients; in dissecting aneurysm in hypertensives; or when there are persistent diastolic pressures exceeding 105 mm Hg.

2. Probable indications—Hypotensive drugs are indicated in recurrent mild cerebral thrombosis with neurologic sequelae and high diastolic pressure; in intractable coronary insufficiency with high diastolic pressure; when the diastolic blood pressure varies between 100–105 mm Hg without evidence of the complications of hypertension, especially in patients under age 50; or for severe intractable hypertensive headaches (in the absence of obvious emotional stress). Younger patients, those with positive family histories of early death from cardiovascular disease, black males, and all patients with evidence of target organ damage should be treated if they have consistent diastolic pressures exceeding 90–95 mm Hg.

3. Doubtful indications—Hypotensive drug therapy is probably not indicated for mild benign essential hypertension in elderly women or for early transient hypertension in young people who present no objective evidence of vascular deterioration or complications.

B. Drugs Available: Antihypertensive agents, once begun for significant hypertension, should be continued indefinitely, especially in those with severe hypertension before treatment.

1. Oral diuretic agents—Thiazides such as chlorothiazide reduce the dose required of blocking agents to about half and are additive with other agents. Give chlorothiazide (Diuril), 0.5–1 gm/day in divided doses, with due caution for electrolyte depletion, especially in patients receiving digitalis; or hydrochlorothiazide

(Hydrodiuril, Esidrix), 50 mg 1—2 times daily. If patients respond well, the dose may be decreased to 25 mg. Other oral diuretic agents are probably as effective, but the more potent ones (ethacrynic acid [Edecrin] or furosemide [Lasix]) may lead to electrolyte and volume depletion more readily than the thiazides. To avoid hypokalemia, some authorities advise adding potassium-retaining drugs such as spironolactone (Aldactone), 25 mg 3 times daily, or triamterene (Dyrenium) when oral diuretics are used. If this is done, serum potassium must be checked frequently and potassium salts not used to avoid hyperkalemia. The potassium-retaining drugs should not be used in renal failure or oliguria. As indicated previously, diuretics (including spironolactone) are most effective in low-renin hypertension. Hyperuricemia and hyperglycemia may occur with the use of thiazides, and probenecid, allopurinol, or oral hypoglycemic agents may be necessary.

2. **Rauwolfia drugs**—Rauwolfia has a relatively slight hypotensive action but may be useful because of its mild sedative effect and its value as an adjunct when combined with hydralazine (Apresoline) or chlorothiazide. Nasal stuffiness, gastric hyperacidity, sodium retention, and severe depression may occur, in which case the drug should be withdrawn. See above for potential hazard of carcinoma of the breast. Give either of the following: (1) Reserpine, 0.1—0.25 mg daily orally. *Caution:* Do not use if there is a history of previous mental depression. Reserpine may also be given IM, 1—2.5 mg every 8—12 hours, for a short time in hypertensive emergencies. (2) Rauwolfia (Raudixin), 100—200 mg daily.

3. **Hydralazine hydrochloride (Apresoline)**—The initial dosage of this drug is 10—25 mg orally twice daily, progressively increasing to a total dosage of 200 mg/day. The results of the oral use of this drug as a sole method of therapy are often not impressive; however, because it is a vasodilator and does not decrease the renal blood flow, it is useful as an adjunct to oral postganglionic or ganglionic blocking agents as well as to the oral diuretics, especially if there is impaired renal function.

Toxic side-effects are common when large doses of hydralazine are used alone but uncommon when the drug is used in combination with chlorothiazide in doses not exceeding 200 mg/day or with rauwolfia or propranolol. The most important are headache and palpitations with tachycardia due to reflex baroreceptor response to the lowered pressure induced by vasodilatation. A syndrome resembling systemic lupus erythematosus has occurred, usually after large doses have been given for many months.

4. **Methyldopa (Aldomet)**—An initial dose of 250 mg 2 or 3 times daily orally is gradually increased at intervals of 2—3 days to a total daily dose (divided into 2—4 doses) of 0.75—2.5 gm. Both supine and standing pressures are reduced in about two-thirds of cases of moderate hypertension; the postural effect may predominate, especially in patients receiving reserpine. Concomitant thiazide therapy is desirable both to po-

tentiate the hypotensive effects of the drug and to counteract the fluid retention which (with drowsiness) is its main side-effect. As with other hypotensive agents, methyldopa should be given under close supervision by the physician until a stable dose schedule is established. A positive Coombs test and uncommon hemolytic anemia may occur. Fever is a rare toxic reaction.

5. **Postganglionic and ganglionic blocking agents**—
a. **Postganglionic blocking agents**—Guanethidine (Ismelin) acts by blocking the postganglionic adrenergic neurons; tolerance rarely occurs. The drug can be given in a single daily dose; it is effective and well tolerated; and it does not produce parasympathetic blockage. The initial dose is 10 mg orally, increasing gradually to tolerance at weekly intervals. Postural hypotension (especially in the morning on awakening and after exercise), diarrhea, muscle aching, and lack of ejaculation in men are the major symptoms of toxicity.

b. **Ganglionic blocking agents**—These agents are used very infrequently today because they block parasympathetics and have been superseded by guanethidine in most clinics. Pentolinium tartrate (Ansolysen), chlorisondamine chloride (Ecolid), and mecamylamine hydrochloride (Inversine) can be used orally or subcutaneously. The initial doses of the oral ganglionic blocking compounds are as follows: Hexamethonium (Methium), 125 mg; pentolinium tartrate (Ansolysen), 10—20 mg; chlorisondamine chloride (Ecolid), 10—20 mg. Mecamylamine (Inversine) is given in doses beginning with 1—2.5 mg once or twice daily and increased by increments of 2.5 mg per dose until a satisfactory standing pressure is achieved. The effects of these types of drugs are enhanced by concurrent thiazide administration. With the exception of mecamylamine, absorption following oral administration is small and irregular, with resultant unpredictable falls in blood pressure.

c. **Basic principles in use of the ganglionic and postganglionic drugs**—(1) Hospitalize the patient under close supervision if the elevated pressure is severe or if the patient has encephalopathy, evidence of accelerated or malignant phase, dissecting aortic aneurysm, or left ventricular failure. (2) Start with a small initial dose and increase gradually, depending upon the tolerance and response of the patient. (3) The degree of reduction of blood pressure should be only moderate in the first week or so, and no attempt should be made to reduce the pressure to normal until it has been demonstrated that the patient can tolerate systolic pressures of about 160 mm Hg without hypotensive symptoms. (4) Postural hypotension, which is greatest at the height of the effect of the drug, should be considered not only as a potential danger to the patient but also as a therapeutic weapon to prolong the hypotensive action of the drug after the peak effect has worn off. (5) Minimize the dose of blocking agent required (and thereby minimize side-effects) by prior administration of reserpine, 0.25 mg/day, or thiazide drugs (see above), or both. (6) Minimize constipation by use of laxatives or, if necessary, neostigmine by mouth. (7) Minimize diarrhea (from guanethidine) by the use of small doses of codeine. (8) Warn the patient of the effects of additional vasodilatation due to heat, including hot baths, alcohol, and immobility following exercise. The effect of these drugs should be evaluated in an ambulatory patient in the erect position. Otherwise, excessive doses will be given.

d. Determination of adequate dosage—A trial of 1–2 weeks is usually required to determine the dose necessary to lower the blood pressure to about 160/100 mm Hg. The patient may then be seen on an outpatient basis and the dose gradually increased to that level which produces the desired fall of blood pressure. Constipation is to be avoided in patients receiving oral methonium compounds because it increases the absorption of the drug; laxatives should be given to ensure a daily bowel movement.

Although determination of the proper drug dosage is difficult, it is usually considered satisfactory if standing diastolic pressures of 90–100 mm Hg or less are achieved (especially after exercise) or a systolic pressure of 150–160 mm Hg or less. Since the effectiveness of the drug cannot be determined by casual blood pressure readings in the physician's office, the following methods have been used to determine effective dosage: (1) Home blood pressure readings are recorded and shown to the physician at his regular visits. The physician may increase or decrease the dose, and the patient is instructed to decrease the dose whenever the blood pressure falls below 150/90, and not to take a dose if the blood pressure is below 130/80 in the recumbent position. (2) Motionless standing for 1 minute before taking the drug is advocated to prevent excessive hypotension. Blood pressure will then be sufficiently high so that an additional quantity can be taken without harm. This only guards against excessive dosage; it does not indicate when the dose has been inadequate. (3) Periodic hospitalization is advisable for 1–2 days to determine basal blood pressure readings. These readings are often 25–50 mm Hg less than readings obtained in the doctor's office and can be used for more accurate control of the blocking compounds. (4) Blood pressure recordings throughout the day, using portable equipment, give a more representative record of the patient's usual pressures, but the apparatus is not generally available.

e. Side-effects and hazards of ganglionic and postganglionic blocking agents—

(1) Acute hypotensive reactions are manifested by faintness, weakness, and nausea and vomiting. The patient should be instructed to lie down immediately and place his feet higher than his head. Unless the hypotensive effect is too severe, the symptoms pass rapidly with this postural assistance. If the symptoms persist, give a vasopressor drug such as phenylephrine hydrochloride (Neo-Synephrine) or methoxamine (Vasoxyl) subcutaneously, or a slow, continuous intravenous infusion of levarterenol bitartrate (Levophed), 4 mg/liter, titrated carefully, because occasional patients are unusually sensitive to some vasopressors.

(2) Acute or progressive renal failure due to decreased renal blood flow or filtration pressure may necessitate discontinuing the drug.

(3) Vascular thromboses and renal failure are hazards in older patients who suffer severe and abrupt falls of blood pressure.

(4) A low-sodium diet potentiates the action of blocking compounds. If an individual receiving fixed doses of the drug is given a low-sodium diet, hypotensive symptoms may occur. It is usually desirable to place the patient on a 2 gm sodium diet at the onset of therapy.

(5) Alcohol, hot climate, vasodilator drugs, vigorous exercise, and salt depletion potentiate the action of ganglionic and postganglionic compounds.

(6) Parasympatholytic effects due to parasympathetic blocking by the ganglionic blocking agents (but not guanethidine) will cause blurring of vision, constipation, and dryness of the mouth; these can be corrected in part by the use of neostigmine orally in doses of 7.5–15 mg. Simple laxatives should be tried initially for constipation.

6. Newer drugs—Propranolol and other beta-adrenergic blocking agents have been shown to be effective in the treatment of hypertension—especially that associated with high plasma renin—and especially when given in conjunction with oral diuretics and vasodilators such as hydralazine or the newer, more potent vasodilator minoxidil. Neither propranolol nor minoxidil has been approved as yet by the FDA for the treatment of hypertension. These and other vasodilators decrease the systemic vascular resistance and lower the arterial pressure but require the addition of a drug that decreases the baroreceptor sympathetic discharge in order to prevent tachycardia and headache.

C. Acute Hypertensive Crises: Patients with acute severe hypertension (diastolic blood pressure > 150 mm Hg) must be hospitalized and treated on an emergency basis with parenteral hypotensive drugs. The most important of the hypertensive "crises" are those of acute hypertensive encephalopathy, acute pulmonary edema associated with a marked rise in blood pressure in hypertensive patients with left ventricular failure, malignant hypertension, acute dissecting aneurysm of the aorta with a high arterial pressure, and hemorrhagic stroke with marked elevation of blood pressure.

Constant monitoring of the blood pressure, preferably in an intensive care unit, is required. The patient should be sitting up or the head of the bed should be elevated 30 degrees. BUN and serum creatinine should be determined daily if BUN is > 50 mg/100 ml. Advance preparation should be made to treat excessive pressure drop (see Chapter 1).

Several parenteral antihypertensive drugs are available, but no single agent can be classified as the drug of choice.

1. Rapidly acting agents—

a. Diazoxide (Hyperstat), 300 mg IV in a single dose, acts promptly as a vasodilator without decreasing cardiac output or renal blood flow. It has been used most extensively in toxemia of pregnancy, malignant hypertension, and acute hypertensive encephalopathy.

b. The ganglionic blocking agent trimethaphan (Arfonad), 1 ampule of 500 mg in 1 liter 5% dextrose in water, is given IV at a rate of 1–4 ml/minute with the patient sitting so as to utilize gravity if the hypotensive effect is excessive. It takes effect within a few minutes and lasts for the duration of the infusion. The objective should be to reduce the diastolic blood pressure to about 110 mm Hg over a period of about 1 hour.

c. Sodium nitroprusside (8–50 μg/minute) by constant intravenous infusion lowers the blood pressure within seconds by direct arteriolar vasodilatation. As with trimethaphan, close monitoring by nurse or physician is essential to avoid excessive fall in blood pressure.

d. An alternative rapidly acting gang025-ioplegic drug, pentolinium tartrate (Ansolysen), 1–2 mg subcut or IM, may be given every 1–2 hours, depending upon response.

2. Delayed acting agents—

a. Reserpine, 1–2.5 mg IM every 8 hours.

b. Hydralazine (Apresoline), 5–20 mg IM every 2–4 hours.

c. Methyldopa (Aldomet), 500 mg IV every 2–4 hours, takes effect more slowly than the ganglioplegics, and its effect lasts for 8–12 hours.

D. Subsequent Therapy: When the blood pressure has been brought under control, guanethidine (Ismelin) is given orally combined with thiazides or other oral antihypertensive agents and parenteral drugs are tapered off over a period of 2–3 days.

E. Other Methods of Treatment: A rigid low-sodium diet (containing 350 mg of sodium or less per day) has been made unnecessary by the introduction of chlorothiazide (Diuril); 2 gm of sodium are usually allowed.

Attempts to treat hypertensive patients with psychoanalytic methods have not been successful, although attention to the emotional needs of such patients is an important adjunct to treatment.

For nervousness, give phenobarbital, 15–30 mg 3–4 times daily, or similar mild sedatives. Tricyclic antidepressants should be avoided if guanethidine is used because they compete with guanethidine uptake and the antihypertensive effect of the latter is diminished.

F. Hypertension in the Presence of Renal Failure: In the presence of renal failure, hypertension is extremely blood volume dependent. If the blood pressure is not reduced by vigorous use of antihypertensive drugs, including furosemide (Lasix), propranolol, and minoxidil, or repeated injections of diazoxide, renal dialysis should be employed; in most instances, the blood pressure will be reduced as the patient achieves a dry weight state. Rarely—especially in those patients with high plasma renin levels—bilateral nephrectomy is necessary to control severe hypertension. The presence of renal failure is an adverse prognostic sign, but vigorous therapy often can reverse the malignant phase

which is associated with renal failure and thus prolong life. Propranolol and minoxidil are not yet approved by the FDA for treatment of hypertension but are available for research purposes.

Treatment of Complications

The cardiac, cerebral, and renal complications of hypertension are discussed under congestive failure, angina pectoris, myocardial infarction, cerebral hemorrhage, cerebral thrombosis, and renal failure.

The headache of hypertension is of unknown cause but is often of emotional origin except in the presence of accelerated or malignant hypertension. Suggestion and explanation are often helpful. Hypotensive drugs are most effective in relieving severe headache associated with the malignant or premalignant phase of hypertension.

Prognosis

Although many patients with slight elevation of blood pressure live a normal span, most patients with untreated hypertensive cardiovascular disease die of complications within 20 years of onset. Before the effective antihypertensive drugs were available, 70% of patients died of heart failure or coronary artery disease, 15% of cerebral hemorrhage, and 10% of uremia.

Antihypertensive therapy has dramatically changed the prognosis of hypertensive patients. Within the past 10 years, the mortality rate has decreased 40%; cardiac failure, renal failure, and malignant hypertension rarely occur in the well-treated patient, and the incidence of hemorrhagic stroke and dissecting aneurysm is greatly decreased. Not only are heart failure and malignant hypertension prevented by antihypertensive therapy with control of the blood pressure; in the Veterans Administration Study, they were reversed by the introduction of antihypertensive drugs when these complications occurred in a group of patients receiving placebo therapy. It is not known whether early treatment of hypertension in a younger patient will prevent the clinical manifestations of coronary heart disease, which were not prevented by antihypertensive treatment in the Veterans Administration Study.

The results of treatment are of course related to its adequacy; poor treatment has essentially the same result as no treatment. The response to treatment should therefore be monitored and the patient's compliance sought by education, prevention of long waiting times at visits, and persuasion to continue a lifelong program of drug treatment which often has some unpleasant side-effects. The benefits of antihypertensive therapy are most obvious in younger patients, before atherosclerosis has occurred, and less obvious in older patients who have other risk factors of atherosclerosis (see p 187) such as hypercholesterolemia, hypertriglyceridemia, diabetes, cigarette smoking, etc. Attention to multiple risk factors in the hypertensive patient should improve prognosis; various studies are under way throughout the world to test this hypothesis.

Axelrod J, Weinshilboum R: Catecholamines. New England J Med 287:237, 1972.

Beevers DG & others: Antihypertensive treatment and the course of established cerebral vascular disease. Lancet 1:1407, 1973.

Bengtsson U, Hogdahl AM, Hood B: Chronic non-obstructive pyelonephritis and hypertension: A long-term study. Quart J Med 37:361, 1968.

Bhatia SK, Frohlich ED: Hemodynamic comparison of agents useful in hypertensive emergencies. Am Heart J 85:367, 1973.

Bookstein JJ & others: Radiologic aspects of renovascular hypertension. JAMA 221:366, 1972.

Bravo EL, Tarazi RC, Dustan HP: β-Adrenergic blockade in diuretic-treated patients with essential hypertension. New England J Med 292:66, 1975.

Breckenridge A, Dollery CT, Parry EHO: Prognosis of treated hypertension: Changes in life expectancy and causes of death between 1952 and 1967. Quart J Med 39:411, 1970.

Brunner HR & others: Angiotensin-II blockade in man by sar[1]-ala[8]-angiotensin II for understanding and treatment of high blood pressure. Lancet 2:1045, 1973.

Cohn JN, Limas CJ, Guiha N: Hypertension and the heart. Arch Int Med 133:969, 1974.

Cole FM, Yates PO: Comparative incidence of cerebrovascular lesions in normotensive and hypertensive patients. Neurology 18:255, 1968.

Committee on Hypertension: Drug treatment of ambulatory patients with hypertension. JAMA 225:1647, 1973.

Dalen JE & others: Dissection of the thoracic aorta: Medical or surgical therapy? Am J Cardiol 34:803, 1974.

Douglas JG, Hollifield JW, Liddle GW: Treatment of low-renin essential hypertension: Comparison of spironolactone and a hydrochlorothiazide-triamterene combination. JAMA 227:518, 1974.

Dustan HP: Atherosclerosis complicating chronic hypertension. Circulation 50:871, 1974.

Eddy RL & others: Cushing's syndrome: A prospective study of diagnostic methods. Am J Med 55:621, 1973.

Finnerty FA Jr, Mattie EC, Finnerty FA III: Hypertension in the inner city: 1. Analysis of clinical dropouts. Circulation 47:73, 1973.

Frohlich ED: Hypertension 1973: Treatment—why and how. Ann Int Med 78:717, 1973.

Genest J & others: Renin in hypertension: How important as risk factor? Canad MAJ 109:475, 1973.

George JM & others: The syndrome of primary aldosteronism. Am J Med 48:343, 1970.

Goldfien A: Treatment of pheochromocytoma. Mod Treat 3:1360, 1966.

Hansson L: Beta-adrenergic blockade in essential hypertension. Acta med scandinav (Suppl) 550:1, 1973.

Humerfelt SB: An epidemiological study of high blood pressure. Acta med scandinav 175: Suppl 407, 1963.

Hunt JC & others: Renal and renovascular hypertension: A reasoned approach to diagnosis and management. Arch Int Med 133:988, 1974.

Hussain RA & others: Differential renal venous renin activity in diagnosis of renovascular hypertension: Review of 29 cases. Am J Cardiol 32:707, 1973.

Kannel WB: Role of blood pressure in cardiovascular morbidity and mortality. Progr Cardiovas Dis 17:5, 1974.

Kaplan NM: The prognostic implications of plasma renin in essential hypertension. JAMA 231:167, 1975.

Koch-Weser J: Vasodilator drugs in the treatment of hypertension. Arch Int Med 133:1017, 1974.

Kosman ME: Management of potassium problems during long-term diuretic therapy. JAMA 230:743, 1974.

Laragh JH (editor): Symposium on high blood pressure: Mechanisms and management. Am J Cardiol 32:497, 1973.

Lauper NT & others: Pheochromocytoma: Fine structural, biochemical, and clinical observations. Am J Cardiol 30:197, 1972.

Liddle GW, Shute AM: The evolution of Cushing's syndrome. Advances Int Med 15:41, 1969.

Locksley HB: Hemorrhagic strokes: Principal causes, natural history, and treatment. M Clin North America 52:1193, 1968.

Loggie JMH: Systemic hypertension in children and adolescents: Causes and treatment. P Clin North America 18:1273, 1971.

Mack TH & others: Reserpine and breast cancer in a retirement community. New England J Med 292:1366, 1975.

Mroczek WJ & others: The value of aggressive therapy in the hypertensive patient with azotemia. Circulation 40:893, 1969.

Oparil S, Haber E: The renin-angiotensin system. New England J Med 291:389, 1974.

Orth DN, Liddle GW: Results of treating Cushing's syndrome. New England J Med 285:243, 1971.

Perloff D & others: Renal vascular hypertension: Further experiences. Am Heart J 74:614, 1967.

Pickering G: Hypertension. Am J Med 52:570, 1972.

Safar ME & others: Hemodynamic study of 85 patients with borderline hypertension. Am J Cardiol 31:315, 1973.

Sandok BA, Whisnant JP: Hypertension and the brain. Arch Int Med 133:947, 1974.

Sannerstedt R, Bjure J, Varnauskas E: Correlation between electrocardiographic changes and systemic hemodynamics in human arterial hypertension. Am J Cardiol 26:117, 197z.

Schottstaedt MF, Sokolow M: The natural history and course of hypertension with papilledema (malignant hypertension). Am Heart J 45:331, 1952.

Sokolow M, Perloff D: The choice of drugs and the management of essential hypertension. Progr Cardiovas Dis 8:253, 1965.

Sokolow M, Perloff D: The prognosis of essential hypertension treated conservatively. Circulation 23:697, 1961.

Sokolow M & others: Relationship between level of blood pressure measured casually and by portable recorders and severity of complications in essential hypertension. Circulation 34:279, 1966.

Spittel JA Jr: Differential diagnosis of dissecting aneurysm. Progr Cardiovas Dis 14:225, 1971.

Symposium on hypertension mechanisms and management. Am J Med 52:565, 1972.

Veterans Administration Cooperative Study Group on Antihypertensive Agents. 1. Effects of treatment on morbidity in hypertension. 2 Results in patients with diastolic pressure averaging 90 through 114 mm Hg. JAMA 202:1028, 1967; 213:1143, 1970.

Veterans Administration Cooperative Study Group on Antihypertensive agents. 3. Influence of age, diastolic pressure and prior cardiovascular disease; further analysis of side-effects. Circulation 45:991, 1972.

Veterans Administration Cooperative Study Group on Antihypertensive Agents. Return of elevated blood pressure after withdrawal of antihypertensive drugs. Circulation 51:1107, 1975.

Wheat MW Jr & others: Acute dissecting aneurysms of the aorta: Treatment and results in 64 patients. J Thoracic Cardiovas Surg 58:344, 1969.

ARTERIOSCLEROTIC HEART DISEASE
(Arteriosclerotic Coronary Artery Disease; Ischemic Heart Disease)

Arteriosclerotic heart disease, or obliterative atherosclerosis of the coronary arteries, is the commonest underlying cause of cardiovascular disability and death. A disorder of lipid metabolism is thought to be responsible for the localized subintimal accumulations of fatty and fibrous tissue which progressively obstruct the epicardial portions of the coronary arteries and their main branches.

Prevention of Ischemic Heart Disease: Management of the Patient With High Risk Factors

Although it has been shown that individuals who have the risk factors listed below—especially if they are present in combination and if the patient is under age 50—have a high risk of developing clinical disease, there is little evidence that correcting them will prevent further progression of the disease once it has occurred. Emphasis should therefore be given to prevention. Hypertension and diabetes should be adequately treated; cigarette smoking should be discouraged; and optimal weight and physical fitness should be encouraged. Management of the hyperlipidemias requires a knowledge of the different types of abnormalities. Table 19—5 summarizes the most authoritative classification. Treatment, according to Fredrickson, is as follows:

Type I: Reduce fat intake to 35 gm/day.

Type II: Reduce saturated fats and cholesterol in the diet and try one of the following drugs: Cholestyramine (Cuemid), 16—32 gm daily in divided doses with meals; beta-sitosterol (Cytellin), 12—18 gm/day in divided doses before meals; clofibrate (Atromid-S), 500 mg 4 times daily. Cholestyramine binds bile acids, increasing their excretion; beta-sitosterol interferes with the absorption of cholesterol; and clofibrate interferes with the synthesis of cholesterol. Side-effects include gastrointestinal upsets. Careful follow-up by the physician for unexpected side-effects is essential.

Type III: Reduce body weight to ideal weight and prescribe a low-fat, low-cholesterol diet as for type II. Clofibrate (Atromid-S), 2 gm daily, may reduce cholesterol levels 25—50% and triglyceride levels 40—80%.

Type IV: Reduce body weight with a high-protein, low-fat, low-carbohydrate diet to ideal weight and substitute polyunsaturated fats for saturated fats. Clofibrate may be of value, but dietary treatment is more effective.

Type V: Same as for type IV.

Risk factors (established by prospective studies) which predispose to the development of ischemic heart disease include genetic predispositions, arterial hypertension, diabetes mellitus, hypercholesterolemia and hypertriglyceridemia, and cigarette smoking (more than a pack a day). Other factors of less importance include obesity and possibly physical fitness.

Men are more often affected than women by an overall ratio of 4:1; before the age of 40 the ratio is 8:1, and beyond age 70 it is 1:1. In men the peak incidence of clinical manifestations is age 50—60; in women, age 60—70. Advanced stages of atherosclerotic coronary artery disease, even complete occlusion, may remain clinically silent, being discovered incidentally after death due to other causes. At present, the only means of determining the location and extent of narrowing is coronary angiography. There is no correlation between the clinical symptoms and signs and the extent of disease.

The pathophysiology underlying the clinical manifestations of arteriosclerotic heart disease may be listed as follows:

Clinical Expression	Mechanism
1. Angina pectoris.	1. Transient, localized myocardial ischemia.
2. Acute myocardial infarction.	2. Arterial occlusion.
3. Intermediate coronary syndrome.	3. Prolonged myocardial ischemia, with or without myocardial necrosis.
4. Heart failure, acute and chronic arrhythmias, conduction disturbances, abnormal ECG.	4. Gradual fibrosis of myocardium or conduction system. May result from (2) or (3) also.
5. Sudden death.	5. Any of the above, plus ventricular arrhythmia, or Stokes-Adams attacks.

1. ANGINA PECTORIS

Essentials of Diagnosis

- Squeezing or pressure-like pain, retrosternal or slightly to the left, which appears quickly during exertion, may radiate in a set pattern, and subsides with rest.
- Seventy percent have diagnostic ECG abnormalities after mild exercise; the remaining 30% have normal tracings or nondiagnostic abnormalities.

General Considerations

Angina pectoris is usually due to arteriosclerotic heart disease, but in rare instances it may occur in the absence of significant disease of the coronary arteries as a result of severe aortic stenosis or insufficiency, syphilitic aortitis, increased metabolic demands as in hyperthyroidism or after thyroid therapy, marked anemia, or paroxysmal tachycardias with very rapid ventricular rates. The underlying mechanism is a discrepancy between the myocardial demands for oxygen and the amount delivered through the coronary arteries. Three groups of variables determine the production of relative or absolute myocardial ischemia:

(1) **Limitation of oxygen delivered by the coronary arteries:** (a) Vessel factors include atherosclerotic narrowing, lack of collateral circulation, and reflex narrowing in response to emotion, cold, upper gastrointestinal disease, or smoking. (b) Blood factors consist of anemia, hypoxemia, and polycythemia (increased viscosity). (c) Circulatory factors are fall in blood pressure due to arrhythmias, orthostatic hypotension, bleeding, and Valsalva's maneuver; and decreased filling pressure of or flow to the coronary arteries due to aortic stenosis or insufficiency.

(2) **Increased cardiac output:** Physiologic factors are exertion, excitement, digestion and metabolism following a heavy meal. Pathologic factors (high-output states) include anemia, thyrotoxicosis, arteriovenous fistula, and pheochromocytoma.

(3) **Increased myocardial demands for oxygen:** May be due to increased work of the heart, as in aortic stenosis, aortic insufficiency, and diastolic hypertension; or increased oxygen consumption due to thyrotoxicosis or in any state characterized by increased catecholamine excretion (pheochromocytoma, strong emotion, and hypoglycemia).

Physiologic changes in patients developing exercise-induced angina during cardiac catheterization have shown a rise in arterial pressure and a considerable rise in left ventricular end-diastolic pressure just before the angina and the ischemic changes in the ECG appeared. Myocardial oxygen consumption increased similarly. The changes indicate that left ventricular failure or decreased compliance coincides with the appearance of angina.

Clinical Findings

A. History: The diagnosis of angina pectoris depends almost entirely upon the history, and it is of the utmost importance that the patient be allowed to describe the symptoms in his own way, using his hands to demonstrate the location and quality of the symptom. The history should specifically include the following categories:

1. **Circumstances that precipitate and relieve angina**—Angina most commonly occurs during walking, especially up an incline or a flight of stairs. Exertion which involves straining, closing the glottis, and immobilizing the thorax precipitates an attack most rapidly. Regardless of the type of activity, angina occurs *during* exertion and subsides promptly if the patient stands or sits quietly. Patients prefer to remain upright rather than lie down. Some patients obtain relief by belching, and for this reason may attribute their distress to "stomach trouble." The amount of activity required to produce angina varies with each patient, but it is always less after meals, during excitement, or on exposure to a cold wind. Heavy meals and strong emotion can provoke an attack in the absence of exertion.

2. **Characteristics of the discomfort**—Patients often do not refer to angina as a "pain" but as a sensation of squeezing, burning, pressing, choking, aching, bursting, "gas," or tightness. It is commonly attributed to "indigestion." The distress of angina is never a sharply localized or darting pain which can be pointed to with a finger. It appears quickly during exertion, and increases rapidly in intensity until the patient is compelled to stop and rest even though the initial discomfort may not be severe.

3. **Location and radiation**—The distribution of the distress may vary widely in different patients but is always the same for each individual patient. In 80–90% of cases the discomfort is felt behind or slightly to the left of the sternum. When it begins farther to the left or, uncommonly, on the right, it characteristically moves centrally and is felt deep in the chest. Although angina may radiate to any segment from C2 to T10, it radiates most often to the left shoulder and upper arm, frequently moving down the inner volar aspect of the arm to the elbow, forearm, wrist, or 4th and 5th fingers. Radiation to the right shoulder and distally is less common, but the characteristics are the same. Occasionally angina may be referred to, or felt initially in, the lower jaw, the base or back of the neck, the interscapular area, or high in the left back.

Angina may almost certainly be excluded when the patient designates the only site of pain by pointing to the area of the apical impulse with one finger.

4. **Duration of attacks**—Angina is of clearly defined short duration, and subsides completely without residual discomfort. If the attack is precipitated by exertion and the patient promptly stops to rest, the distress of angina usually lasts less than 3 minutes (although most patients think it is longer). Attacks following a heavy meal or which are brought on by anger often last 15–20 minutes.

5. **Effect of nitroglycerin**—The diagnosis of angina pectoris is strongly supported (1) if 0.4 mg of nitroglycerin (glyceryl trinitrate) invariably shortens an attack and (2) if that amount taken immediately beforehand invariably permits greater exertion before the onset of angina or prevents angina entirely. However, this source of diagnostic information is less reliable than the characteristic history.

6. **Unrelated disorders** that intensify angina should be considered. Cholecystitis, sliding hiatus hernia, thyrotoxicosis, paroxysmal arrhythmias, orthostatic hypotension, or left ventricular failure may account for unusual variants of angina pectoris.

B. Signs: Examination during a spontaneous or induced attack frequently reveals a significant elevation in systolic and diastolic blood pressure; occasionally gallop rhythm is present during pain only. Carotid sinus massage often causes the pain to subside more quickly than usual if it slows the cardiac rate, and is a helpful maneuver in instances of "atypical angina."

It is important to detect signs of diseases that may contribute to arteriosclerotic heart disease, eg, diabetes mellitus (retinopathy or neuropathy), xanthomatosis (tuberosa, plana, or tendinosa); or disorders that intensify the angina, such as hypertension, thyrotoxicosis, orthostatic hypotension, and aortic stenosis or mitral stenosis.

The cardiovascular examination is normal in 25–40% of patients with angina. In the remainder, evidence of occlusive disease of the peripheral arteries, hypertensive retinopathy and cardiomegaly, significant murmurs, or signs of cardiac failure may be noted.

C. **Laboratory Findings:** Anemia, hypercholesterolemia, hypertriglyceridemia, diabetes mellitus, hypoglycemia, hyperthyroidism, and upper gastrointestinal diseases should be investigated as possible contributory factors. STS should be done routinely. A chest film should be taken to exclude pulmonary, cardiac, and skeletal abnormalities.

D. **ECG Findings:** The resting ECG is normal in 25% of patients with angina. In the remainder, abnormalities include atrioventricular or intraventricular conduction defects, patterns of left ventricular hypertrophy, old myocardial infarction, or nonspecific ST–T changes.

An exercise test may be warranted if the diagnosis is seriously in doubt. In order to avoid exercising a patient with acute or subacute myocardial ischemia, do not do an exercise test if the onset of the pain is of recent origin. Interpretation of the test may be difficult if the resting ECG is abnormal or if the patient has been receiving digitalis. A positive ECG exercise test consists of at least a 1 mm horizontal depression or definite sag of at least 0.08 second of the ST segment in one or more leads. Depression of the ST junction alone ("J"), flattening of T waves, or minor ST segment depression is not diagnostic. In the standardized test, significant changes occur in only 50–60% of patients with angina. The percentage is much higher when tracings are taken during a spontaneous attack or if a more extensive exercise test is used.

Patients with angina pectoris who develop ischemic changes with exercise may prove on coronary angiography to have one-, 2-, or 3-vessel disease, with corresponding differences in prognosis (see below). Almost all patients with 2- or 3-vessel disease have ischemic changes on exercise; failure to develop ST–T changes with exercise suggests single-vessel disease, often confined to the right coronary or circumflex arteries.

E. **Coronary and Left Ventricular Angiography:** In the past few years, selective coronary cineangiocardiography has been performed with increased frequency in many centers, utilizing multiple views with either the Sones or the Judkins technic. Low mortality rates in the range of 0.2% have been described by experienced operators, but morbidity varies from 1–7%. Episodes of cardiac ischemia, arrhythmias, pulmonary edema, or thrombosis of arteries used in the study prevent its use in all patients with coronary disease. The procedure demands experienced physicians and facilities for monitoring of rhythm and other vital functions, as well as resuscitation equipment. Cost is a major concern. The procedure should not be used solely for the purpose of diagnosis of angina except in rare cases.

Whereas the diagnosis of angina pectoris is made on the basis of the history, the degree and variety of coronary stenotic lesions—as well as impairment of left ventricular contractility—require anatomic visualization. There are good clinical data to indicate that the prognosis in patients with clinical coronary disease and angina pectoris is directly related to the extent of the coronary lesion (whether the stenoses affected one, 2, or all 3 coronary arteries or the main left coronary artery) and the left ventricular function and contractility; the 5-year mortality rate has been shown to be 3–6 times as great if 3 vessels—as opposed to one—are involved or if the ejection fraction is reduced or if ventricular aneurysm or its lesser manifestations of dyskinesis or asynergy are present.

Practically all patients with abnormal coronary angiograms have ischemic exercise ECGs, but about a third of patients with negative exercise tests have positive coronary angiograms. Coronary angiograms have therefore been recommended in patients with atypical chest pain thought to be anginal but with negative exercise studies.

Sones has shown that single-vessel disease occurs in 25% of patients with angina pectoris or myocardial infarction and that isolated disease of the left main or circumflex coronary artery is rare. Patients with cardiac failure, with left ventricular asynergy, or with decreased ejection fractions usually have 2- or 3-vessel disease.

Differential Diagnosis

Psychophysiologic cardiovascular reactions are a loosely defined group of disorders having in common dull aching chest pains often described as "heart pain," lasting hours or days, often aggravated by exertion but not promptly relieved by rest. Darting, knife-like pains of momentary duration at the apex or over the precordium are often present also. Emotional tension and fatigue make the pain worse. Dyspnea of the hyperventilation variety, palpitation, fatigue, and headache are also usually present. Continual exhaustion is a frequent complaint.

The "anterior chest wall syndrome" is characterized by sharply localized tenderness of intercostal muscles, pressure on which reproduces the chest pain. Sprain or inflammation of the chondrocostal junctions, which may be warm, swollen, and red (so-called Tietze's syndrome), may result in diffuse chest pain which is also reproduced by local pressure. Intercostal neuritis (herpes zoster, diabetes mellitus, etc) may confuse the diagnosis.

Xiphoid tenderness and lower sternal pain may arise from and be reproduced by pressure on the xiphoid process.

Any of the above may occur in a patient with angina.

Cervical or thoracic spine disease (degenerative disk disease, postural strain, "arthritis") involving the dorsal roots produces sudden sharp, severe chest pain similar to angina in location and "radiation" but related to specific movements of the neck or spine, recumbency, and straining or lifting. Pain due to cervical thoracic disk disease involves the outer or dorsal aspect of the arm and the thumb and index fingers rather than the ring and little fingers.

Peptic ulcer, chronic cholecystitis, cardiospasm, and functional gastrointestinal disease are often suspected because some patients indisputably obtain relief from angina by belching. In these disorders, symptoms are related to food intake rather than physical exertion. X-ray and fluoroscopic study are helpful in diagnosis. The pain is relieved by appropriate diet and drug therapy.

Hiatus hernia is characterized by lower chest and upper abdominal pain after heavy meals occurring in recumbency or upon bending over. The pain is relieved by bland diet, antacids, semi-Fowler position, and walking.

Degenerative and inflammatory lesions of the left shoulder, cervical rib, and the scalenus anticus syndrome are differentiated from angina by the fact that the pain is precipitated by movement of the arm and shoulder, paresthesias are present in the left arm, and postural exercises and pillow support to the shoulders in bed give relief.

"Tight" mitral stenosis or pulmonary hypertension resulting from chronic pulmonary disease can on occasion produce chest pain which is indistinguishable from angina pectoris, including ST segment sagging or depression. The clinical findings of mitral stenosis or of the lung disease are evident, and the ECG invariably discloses right axis deviation or frank right ventricular hypertrophy.

Spontaneous pneumothorax is a benign disorder that may cause chest pain as well as dyspnea and create confusion with angina pectoris as well as myocardial infarction.

Treatment

A. Treatment of Acute Attack:

1. Nitroglycerin is the drug of choice; it acts in about 1–2 minutes. As soon as the attack begins, place one 0.3 mg tablet under the tongue and allow it to dissolve. The dose may be increased to 0.4–0.6 mg if no relief is obtained from a smaller dose. Nitroglycerin. may be used freely whenever an attack occurs or may be used in order to prevent an attack (see below). It may cause headache and hypotension.

2. Amyl nitrite, 1 pearl crushed and inhaled, acts in about 10 seconds. This drug usually causes flushing of the face, pounding of the pulse, and sometimes dizziness and headache. These reactions may be minimized by inhaling the drug from a distance or by rapidly passing the crushed pearl before the nose. The patient soon learns how to vary the amount of drug he wishes to inhale.

3. Long-acting nitrates and other related drugs have no place in the therapy of the acute attack.

4. Alcohol—One or 2 oz of whisky or brandy may be a helpful home remedy.

5. General measures—The patient should stand still or sit or lie down as soon as the pain begins and remain quiet until the attack is over. This is the natural reaction of most patients, but some try to "work the attack off" and patients should be warned against this.

B. Prevention of Further Attacks:

1. Angina may coexist with or be aggravated by left ventricular failure, obvious or incipient. Treatment of the cardiac failure with diuretics or digitalis or both, as well as by other methods such as prolonged rest, etc, may be extremely helpful in the treatment of angina pectoris.

2. Nitroglycerin (glyceryl trinitrate), 0.3–0.6 mg under the tongue just before activity.

3. Long-acting nitrates—Pentaerythritol tetranitrate (Peritrate), 10 mg orally 3 times daily before meals; erithrityl tetranitrate (Cardilate), 10–15 mg sublingually 3 times daily; and isosorbide dinitrate (Isordil), 10 mg 4 times daily. There is no convincing evidence that these agents prolong life in patients with coronary heart disease or are better than placebos.

4. Propranolol (Inderal), 10–30 mg 3 times daily increased to tolerance, has been given with benefit to patients with angina if left ventricular failure, past or present, is absent. Care must be exercised during its use, and the precautions noted on p 241 should be observed. Combinations with long-acting nitrates such as isosorbide dinitrate have been shown to be significantly better than either drug used alone.

5. Xanthines may be of some benefit, given preferably by rectal suppository (250–500 mg).

6. The objective of production of myxedema by means of thiouracil compounds or radioactive iodine (see Chapter 18) is to reduce the work of the heart. Good results have been reported in about half of cases of intractable angina, but this method should not be used until prolonged rest and attention to the emotional needs of the patient have ruled out a transient reversible coronary insufficiency. It is rarely used today.

7. General measures—The patient must avoid all habits and activities that he knows will bring on an attack. Coexisting disorders (especially anemia) which may lead to increased cardiac ischemia must be treated. Most patients with angina do not require prolonged bed rest, but rest and relaxation are beneficial. Adequate mental rest is also important. Obese patients should be placed on a reducing diet low in animal fats and their weight brought to normal or slightly subnormal levels. Tobacco is best avoided or used in moderation because it produces tachycardia and elevation in blood pressure and because cigarette smoking has been shown to be a risk factor in coronary heart disease. Smoking may precipitate ventricular arrhythmias and sudden death in patients with coronary disease. Physical fitness resulting from a regular exercise program has been thought to be helpful, but the benefits may be mainly psychologic, ie, an improved overall sense of well-being. There is little conclusive evidence that such a program prolongs life.

8. Sedatives or tranquilizers may reduce the frequency of attacks.

9. Control hyperlipidemia—See above.

10. As an experimental procedure, some authorities advocate partial ileal bypass surgery, which reduces the serum lipids 40% over a 5-year period. This procedure has not gained widespread acceptance, however.

Prognosis

Most studies indicate that the average mortality rate of angina pectoris over a period of 5 years is approximately 3—4% per year. The percentage varies from 1—15% depending upon whether the coronary angiogram reveals one-, 2-, or 3-vessel disease; whether the ejection fraction on the left ventricular angiogram is < 50%; whether abnormal contraction patterns are present; and whether the patient has evidence of resting ischemic changes on the ECG, hypertension, or evidence of left ventricular failure at the time of the angina pectoris. Despite the variations, the course is unpredictable in the individual patient. Hypertension increases the afterload of the left ventricle, leading to myocardial hypertrophy, which contributes to the increased requirement of coronary blood flow.

The course is prolonged, with variable frequency and severity of attacks punctuated by periods of complete remission and episodes of myocardial infarction, or terminated by sudden death. The last is often unpredictable and contributes to the great anxiety caused by the disease. Diabetes mellitus, hypertension, cardiac hypertrophy, congestive failure, myocardial infarction, arrhythmias, and conduction defects (as shown on ECG) shorten the life expectancy. Onset prior to age 40 or a family history of early cardiac death is prognostically unfavorable.

Half of all patients die suddenly, and an additional third after myocardial infarction. Heart failure accounts for most of the remainder of deaths.

Bemis CE & others: Progression of coronary artery disease: A clinical arteriographic study. Circulation 47:455, 1973.

Boyle D & others: Ischaemic heart-disease in diabetics. Lancet 1:338, 1972.

Burggraf GW, Parker JO: Hemodynamic effects of amyl nitrite in coronary artery disease. Am J Cardiol 32:772, 1973.

Cannon PJ: Radioisotopic studies of the regional myocardial circulation. Circulation 51:955, 1975.

Carvalho ACA, Colman RW, Lees RS: Clofibrate reversal of platelet hypersensitivity in hyperbetalipoproteinemia. Circulation 50:570, 1974.

Chait A & others: Clinical and metabolic study of alcoholic hyperlipidaemia. Lancet 2:62, 1972.

Cohn PF & others: Diagnostic accuracy of 2-step postexercise ECG: Results in 305 subjects studied by coronary arteriography. JAMA 220:501, 1972.

The Coronary Drug Project Research Group: Clofibrate and niacin in coronary heart disease. JAMA 231:360, 1975.

Drugs for prophylaxis of angina pectoris. Med Lett Drugs Ther 17:57, 1975.

Ferguson RJ & others: Effect of physical training on treadmill exercise, capacity collateral circulation and progression of coronary disease. Am J Cardiol 34:764, 1974.

FitzGibbon GM & others: A double Master's two-step test: Clinical, angiographic and hemodynamic correlations. Ann Int Med 74:509, 1971.

Frank CW, Weinblatt E, Shapiro S: Angina pectoris in men: Prognostic significance of selected medical factors. Circulation 47:509, 1973.

Froelicher VF, Oberman A: Analysis of epidemiologic studies of physical inactivity as risk factor for coronary disease. Progr Cardiovas Dis 15:41, 1972.

Gordon T, Kannel WB: Predisposition to atherosclerosis in the head, heart, and legs: The Framingham Study. JAMA 221:661, 1972.

Goldstein JL & others: Hyperlipidemia in coronary heart disease. J Clin Invest 52:1544, 1973.

Hamby RI, Gupta MP, Young MW: Clinical and hemodynamic aspects of single vessel coronary artery disease. Am Heart J 85:458, 1973.

Havel RJ: Pathogenesis, differentiation and management of hypertriglyceridemia. Advances Int Med 15:117, 1969.

Holmberg S & others: Coronary circulation during heavy exercise in control subjects and patients with coronary heart disease. Acta med scandinav 190:465, 1971.

Kannel WB, Feinleib M: Natural history of angina pectoris in the Framingham Study: Prognosis and survival. Am J Cardiol 29:154, 1972.

Kannel WB & others: Precursors of sudden coronary death: Factors related to the incidence of sudden death. Circulation 51:606, 1975.

Klaus AP & others: Comparative evaluation of sublingual long-acting nitrates. Circulation 48:519, 1973.

Levy RI & others: Dietary and drug treatment of primary hyperlipoproteinemia. Ann Int Med 77:267, 1972.

Morgan-Jones A: The nature of the coronary problem. Brit Heart J 32.583, 1970.

Morris JN, Gardner MJ: Epidemiology of ischemic heart disease. Am J Med 46:683, 1969.

National Heart and Lung Institute Task Force on Arteriosclerosis: *Arteriosclerosis: A Report.* 2 vols. US Department of Health, Education, and Welfare, 1971. [Vol 1—$0.50. Publ No. (NIH) 72—137. Vol 2—$2.75. Publ No. (NIH) 72—219. Order from: Superintendent of Documents, Government Printing Office, Washington, DC 20402.]

Parker JO & others: Reversible cardiac failure during angina pectoris. Circulation 39:745, 1969.

Prevention of complications of coronary arteriography. (Editorial.) Circulation 49:599, 1974.

Redwood DR, Rosing DR, Epstein SE: Circulatory and symptomatic effects of physical training in patients with coronary-artery disease and angina pectoris. New England J Med 286:959, 1972.

Reeves TJ & others: Natural history of angina pectoris. Am J Cardiol 33:423, 1974.

Riseman JEF: The clinical course of angina pectoris. Am J Med Sc 252:146, 1966.

Roberts WC: Coronary arteries in fatal acute myocardial infarction. Circulation 45:215, 1972.

Ross RS: The case for prevention of coronary heart disease. Circulation 51:1, 1975.

Saltups A & others: Left ventricular hemodynamics in patients with coronary artery disease and in normal subjects. Am J Med 50:8, 1971.

Sampson JJ, Cheitlin MD: Pathophysiology and differential diagnosis of cardiac pain. Progr Cardiovas Dis 13:507, 1971.

Seltzer CC: Smoking and coronary heart disease. JAMA 203:193, 1968.

Sones FM Jr: Indications and value of coronary arteriography. Circulation 46:1155, 1972.

Vlodaver Z & others: Correlation of the antemortem coronary

arteriogram and the postmortem specimen. Circulation 47:162, 1973.

Webster JS, Moberg C, Rincon G: Natural history of severe proximal coronary artery disease as documented by coronary cineangiography. Am J Cardiol 33:195, 1974.

Wiener L, Dwyer EM Jr, Cox JW: Hemodynamic effects of nitroglycerin, propranolol and their combination in coronary heart disease. Circulation 39:623, 1969.

Willerson JT & others: Technetium stannous pyrophosphate myocardial scintigrams in patients with chest pain of varying etiology. Circulation 51:1046, 1975.

2. INTERMEDIATE CORONARY SYNDROME
(Unstable Angina)

This syndrome, called by some preinfarction angina, unstable angina, premature or impending myocardial infarction, or coronary insufficiency, refers to a syndrome intermediate between the angina pectoris of effort and acute myocardial infarction in the spectrum of clinical events that occur in coronary heart disease. It has received special attention because of the adverse prognosis and unpredictability of sudden onset of severe myocardial infarction in some of these patients. Since the mortality rate in acute myocardial infarction is greatest in the first few hours, recognition of a syndrome with increased likelihood of impending infarction requires hospitalization and monitoring in the coronary care unit to avert sudden arrhythmias and death.

The syndrome is recognized by the appearance of pain that has a different character, duration, radiation, and severity—or by pain that over a period of hours or days has a crescendo quality of increased ease of production, or of occurrence at rest or during the night. Angina that appears for the first time usually indicates occlusion of a coronary branch and may progress to myocardial infarction or gradually subside, but the same close monitoring is required.

Patients who have the clinical features described but do not develop signs of myocardial infarction such as fever, tachycardia, serial enzyme changes, or serial electrocardiographic changes are considered to be in precarious balance between coronary supply and demand and should be treated as though they have had a small myocardial infarction. Some authorities believe that the mortality rate is 20–40% over a 6-month period; others are more sanguine and cite a 15% mortality over a period of 1–2 years. Because of the uncertain course and the desire to prevent myocardial infarction, there is a wave of enthusiasm for coronary angiography during the acute phase, with coronary bypass surgery (see below) if severe localized lesions with good peripheral run-off are seen in the angiographic study.

The difference of opinion between those who advocate immediate operation and those who prefer to manage patients medically cannot be resolved until more definitive studies become available.

Follow-up shows that patients who entered the coronary care unit because of acceleration of the clinical coronary syndrome suggesting infarction, but in whom infarction was not demonstrated, have a higher death rate over a 1–2 year period than ordinary angina pectoris patients and so need close supervision.

Armstrong A & others: Natural history of acute coronary heart attacks. Brit Heart J 34:67, 1972.

Cannom DS, Harrison DC, Schroeder JS: Hemodynamic observations in patients with unstable angina pectoris. Am J Cardiol 33:17, 1974.

Conti CR & others: Unstable angina pectoris: Morbidity and mortality in 57 consecutive patients evaluated angiographically. Am J Cardiol 32:745, 1973.

Cosby RS & others: Clinicoarteriographic correlations in angina pectoris with and without myocardial infarction. Am J Cardiol 30:472, 1972.

Fulton M & others: Natural history of unstable angina. Lancet 1:860, 1972.

Gazes PC & others: Preinfarctional (unstable) angina—A prospective study—Ten year follow-up: Prognostic significance of electrocardiographic changes. Circulation 48:331, 1973.

Krauss KR, Hutter AW Jr, DeSanctis RW: Acute coronary insufficiency: Course and follow-up. Circulation 45 (Suppl 1):1, 1972.

Lown B, Wolf M: Approaches to sudden death from coronary heart disease. Circulation 44:130, 1971.

McCans JL, Parker JO: Left ventricular pressure-volume relationships during myocardial ischemia in man. Circulation 48:775, 1973.

Sampson JJ, Hyatt KH: Management of the patient with severe angina pectoris: An internist's point of view. Circulation 46:1885, 1972.

Symposium on angina pectoris. Circulation 46:1035, 1972.

Weintraub RM & others: Treatment of preinfarction angina with intraaortic balloon counterpulsation and surgery. Am J Cardiol 34:809, 1974.

SURGERY FOR CORONARY HEART DISEASE

In the past 3 years, considerable progress has been made in the indications and modifications of bypass procedures for coronary artery stenosis. The procedure most commonly used is anastomosis of a graft of the saphenous vein from the aorta to the distal portion of the obstructed coronary artery, beyond the stenosis. Single, double, or even triple bypass grafts have been made in the same patient, and the initial results are most promising. The data show that in some patients there is improvement of left ventricular function, increased cardiac output, improved cardiac contraction, and relief of angina pectoris. The grafts have remained patent in about 70% of the patients, but the period of observation has been short and it remains to be seen how long the grafts will remain patent. Furthermore, apart from a surgical mortality rate of about 5% and an incidence of late closure of the bypass graft of about 20%, the major complication of coronary bypass surgery in 10–20% of patients is the development of a new myocardial infarction. In one study, two-thirds of patients, following surgery, had at least one new occlusion of a previously patent coronary artery as studied by coronary angiography. Further study of the incidence of postoperative myocardial infarction is essential in order to put the indications for the procedure into proper perspective.

The indications for bypass surgery include major stenosis (at least 50–70%) of the proximal segment of a coronary artery, combined with a distal segment without significant disease and with a circumference of more than 4 mm that permits a satisfactory anastomosis in a patient with angina pectoris difficult to control by medical means. The preoperative determination of whether the distal portion of an artery is suitable for bypass requires coronary angiograms of high quality.

The availability of this new surgical procedure, which shows considerable promise in the treatment of coronary heart disease, has sharpened and broadened the indications for **coronary angiography**. The most common indication is severe angina pectoris, unimproved by restricted activity and nitroglycerin. Most recently, the indications for coronary angiograms and possible bypass surgery have been extended to include preinfarction angina and possibly angina which follows a myocardial infarction. Because of the frequent coexistence of dyskinesia or aneurysm of the left ventricle, dysfunction of the papillary muscle, or ventricular septal defect, patients studied by coronary angiography should have concurrent left ventricular cineangiography to determine localized areas of dyskinesia or mitral insufficiency. Some surgeons have done infarctectomies if the patient following an acute myocardial infarction has shock or pump failure, but the mortality rate is very high and these operations must be considered experimental. The same can be said of doing bypass surgery in the presence of apparent extension of an acute myocardial infarction.

Ventricular aneurysms and areas of dyskinesia and akinesia have been found to occur more frequently than previously thought, primarily because they were not obvious on a plain film of the chest but could be seen in a left ventricular cineangiogram. At present it is not considered wise to resect the aneurysm unless the patient is in cardiac failure and there is well-demarcated paradoxic motion. Patients with left ventricular failure of undetermined cause should have a coronary angiogram and a left ventricular cineangiogram to exclude left ventricular aneurysm or localized areas of impaired contraction secondary to coronary heart disease.

Implantation of the internal mammary arteries into the myocardium, the so-called Vineberg procedure, is being performed less and less often as the results have been shown to be inadequate; in many institutions, the procedure has been abandoned in favor of bypass surgery.

Adams DF, Fraser DB, Abrams HL: The complications of coronary arteriography. Circulation 48:609, 1973.

Anderson RP & others: The prognosis of patients with coronary artery disease after coronary bypass operations: Time-related progress of 532 patients with disabling angina pectoris. Circulation 50:274, 1974.

Arbogast R, Solignac A, Bourassa MG: Influence of aortocoronary saphenous vein bypass surgery on left ventricular volumes and ejection fraction: Comparison before and one year after surgery in 51 patients. Am J Med 54:290, 1973.

Cannom DS & others: The long-term follow-up of patients undergoing saphenous vein bypass surgery. Circulation 49:77, 1974.

Dunkman WB & others: Medical perspectives in coronary artery surgery: A caveat. Ann Int Med 81:817, 1974.

Gott VL: Outlook for patients after coronary artery revascularization. Am J Cardiol 33:431, 1974.

Graber JD & others: Ventricular aneurysm: An appraisal of diagnosis and surgical treatment. Brit Heart J 34:830, 1972.

Kouchoukos NT, Kirklin JW, Oberman A: An appraisal of coronary bypass grafting. Circulation 50:11, 1974.

Kouchoukos NT & others: Surgical versus medical treatment of occlusive disease confined to the left anterior descending coronary artery. Am J Cardiol 35:866, 1975.

Manley JC, Johnson WD: Effects of surgery on angina (pre- and postinfarction) and myocardial function (failure). Circulation 46:1208, 1972.

Maurer BJ & others: Changes in grafted and nongrafted coronary arteries following saphenous vein bypass grafting. Circulation 50:293, 1974.

Rose MR & others: Electrocardiographic and serum enzyme changes of myocardial infarction after coronary artery bypass surgery. Am J Cardiol 33:215, 1974.

Sheldon WC & others: Vein graft surgery for coronary artery disease: Survival and angiographic results in 1,000 patients. Suppl 3 to Circulation 47 and 48, July 1973.

Swan HJC & others: Myocardial revascularization for acute and chronic coronary heart disease. Ann Int Med 79:851, 1973.

3. ACUTE MYOCARDIAL INFARCTION

Essentials of Diagnosis

- Sudden but not instantaneous development of pressing anterior chest pain which may produce arrhythmias, hypotension, shock, or cardiac failure.

- Rarely painless, masquerading as acute congestive heart failure, syncope, cerebral thrombosis, or "unexplained" shock.

- Fever, leukocytosis, rising sedimentation rate, elevated SGOT and LDH within 24–48 hours.

- ECG: Abnormal Q waves, elevated ST; later, symmetric inversion of T waves.

General Considerations

Myocardial infarction is ischemic necrosis of a localized area of the myocardium due to occlusion of a coronary artery by thrombus formation or subintimal hemorrhage at the site of atheromatous narrowing. Less often, complete occlusion by proliferation of the intimal plaques or by hemorrhage into a plaque is responsible. Infarction may occur in the absence of complete occlusion if coronary blood flow is temporarily reduced, as in postoperative or traumatic shock, gastrointestinal bleeding or hypotension due to any cause, or dehydration. Rarely, embolic occlusion, syphilitic aortitis, or acute vasculitis cause infarction.

The location and extent of infarction depend upon the anatomic distribution of the vessel, the site of current and previous occlusions, and the adequacy of collateral circulation. Thrombosis occurs most commonly in the anterior descending branch of the left coronary artery, resulting in infarction of the anterior left ventricle. Occlusion of the left circumflex artery produces anterolateral infarction. Right coronary thrombosis leads to infarction of the posteroinferior portion of the left ventricle.

The hemodynamic findings are related directly to the extent of necrosis or scarring of the myocardium. In mild infarction, the hemodynamics may be normal. With more severe disease, there may be a raised left ventricular end-diastolic pressure with associated increase in the pulmonary artery diastolic pressure, decreased cardiac output, and decreased ejection fraction in the left ventricular angiogram. When the patient is hypotensive or in shock, the cardiac output is considerably reduced in conjunction with evidences of left ventricular failure and a high left ventricular filling pressure. The "wedge" and left ventricular diastolic pressure may be raised, with no abnormality in the right ventricular diastolic pressure or in the right atrial pressure; thus, the superior vena cava or right atrial pressures are often misleading because they do not reflect left ventricular events. They are, however, valuable if the pressures are very low, indicating the possibility of hypovolemia; the response to volume loads may be helpful in producing an increased cardiac output. The presence of a large V wave in the right ventricular pressure pulse is helpful in diagnosing acute mitral insufficiency due to papillary muscle dysfunction in patients who abruptly worsen, with development of cardiac failure. Similarly, raised oxygen content in the right ventricle under similar circumstances helps in diagnosis of perforated ventricular septum.

Clinical Findings

A. Symptoms:

1. **Premonitory pain**—Over one-third of patients give a history of alteration in the pattern of angina, sudden onset of atypical angina, or unusual "indigestion" felt in the chest.

2. **Pain of infarction**—This may begin during rest (even in sleep) or activity. It is similar to angina in location and radiation but is more severe, does not subside with rest, and builds up rapidly or in waves to maximum intensity in the space of a few minutes or longer. Nitroglycerin has no effect. The pain may last for hours if unrelieved by narcotics, and is often unbearable. The patient breaks out in a cold sweat, feels weak and apprehensive, and moves about, seeking a position of comfort. He prefers not to lie quietly. Lightheadedness, syncope, dyspnea, orthopnea, cough, wheezing, nausea and vomiting, or abdominal bloating may also be present, singly or in any combination.

3. **Painless infarction**—In 5—15% of cases, pain is absent or minor and is overshadowed by the immediate complications, notably acute pulmonary edema or rapidly developing heart failure, profound weakness, shock, syncope, or cerebral thrombosis.

B. Signs:
Physical findings are highly variable; the presence of rales, gallop rhythm, tachycardia, and hypotension correlate well with hemodynamic and clinical evidences of the severity of the attack and the extent of the necrosed myocardium.

1. **Shock**—Shock may be described as a systolic blood pressure below 80 mm Hg (or slightly higher with prior hypertension) along with gray facial color, mental dullness, cold clammy skin, peripheral cyanosis, decreased urine output, tachycardia or bradycardia, and weak pulse. Shock is present only in severe attacks (incidence about 8—14%). Shock may be caused primarily by the pain rather than the hemodynamic effects of the infarction; if so, distinct improvement occurs within 30—60 minutes after relief of pain and administration of oxygen.

2. **Cardiac effects**—In the severe attack, the first and second heart sounds are faint, often indistinguishable on auscultation, and assume the so-called "tic-tac" quality. Gallop rhythm, distended neck veins, and basal rales are often present. Acute pulmonary edema or rapidly progressive congestive failure may dominate the picture. In less severe attacks, examination is normal or there may be diminished intensity of the first sound or low systolic blood pressure. Pericardial friction rub appears in 20—30% of cases between the second and fifth days; it is often transient or intermittent.

3. **Fever**—Fever is absent at the onset (in contrast to acute pericarditis) and during prolonged shock. It usually rises to 37.8—39.4° C (100—103° F)—rarely to 40.6° C (105° F)—within 24 hours and persists for 3—7 days (rarely longer).

C. Laboratory Findings:
Leukocytosis of 10—20 thousand cells/cu mm usually develops on the second day and disappears in 1 week. The sedimentation rate is normal at onset, rises on the second or third day, and remains elevated for 1—3 weeks. SGOT activity increases in 6—12 hours, reaches a peak in 24—48 hours, and returns to normal in 3—5 days. Serum lactic acid dehydrogenase may remain elevated for 5—7 days. Serial determinations are helpful in equivocal instances. Creatine phosphokinase (CPK) isoenzyme activity may increase earliest, and, when determined every 2 hours, gives an estimate of the magnitude of the infarction.

D. ECG Findings:
ECG changes do not correlate well with the clinical severity of the infarction. The characteristic pattern consists of specific changes which undergo a stereotyped "evolution" over a matter of weeks in the average case. At the onset there is elevation of ST segment and T wave and abnormal Q waves; the ST segment progressively returns to the baselines as T waves become symmetrically inverted. An unequivocal ECG diagnosis of infarction can only be made in the presence of all 3 abnormalities. Serial

ST—T changes alone are compatible with but not diagnostic of infarction. The characteristic changes are not seen in the presence of left bundle branch block or when a previous infarct has permanently altered the ECG. Even in these instances an ECG taken early in an attack often shows ST segment displacement.

E. Sudden Death: Sudden death may be the first manifestation of coronary heart disease in about 20% of cases, and, as shown in the cases in which an ECG has been done, is usually due to ventricular fibrillation. After resuscitation, no clear evidence of myocardial infarction can be found on ECG or serial enzyme studies in about 50% of cases, but the incidence of prior heart disease, angina, hypertension, or diabetes is high in this group of patients. Approximately 50—60% of all coronary deaths are sudden. Most patients who die suddenly as a result of coronary atherosclerosis do so within 1—2 hours; have had some prodromal symptoms within the previous 2 weeks; and at autopsy have hypertrophied hearts and diffuse coronary disease. Even in the absence of apparent clinical disease, severe coronary atherosclerosis is usually found in patients who die suddenly. Considerable study is under way to better define those circumstances that favor sudden death, especially in patients with angina pectoris, previous myocardial infarction, hypertension, or diabetes. Ventricular premature beats in a healthy population do not increase the relative risk of sudden death, but they do increase the risk in patients with known coronary disease.

Differential Diagnosis

In acute pericarditis, fever often precedes the onset of pain, which is predominantly pleuritic and is significantly relieved by breath-holding and specific body positions. The friction rub appears early, is louder, is heard over a greater area, and is more persistent than in infarction, and a pleuropericardial rub is often present. There are no QRS changes, and T wave inversion is more widespread without reciprocal changes (except in aVR). SGOT and LDH are rarely elevated.

Dissecting aneurysm causes violent chest pain which is often of maximum severity at onset. It typically spreads up or down the chest and back over a period of hours. Changes in pulses, changing aortic murmurs, and left pleural effusion or cardiac tamponade are distinctive features. Blood pressure does not fall early. Syncope or neurologic abnormalities are common. ECG changes are not diagnostic of infarction unless the coronary ostia are involved in the proximal dissection.

Acute pulmonary embolism may cause chest pain indistinguishable from myocardial infarction as well as hypotension, dyspnea, and distended neck veins, but the ECG, regardless of coronary-like changes, will usually show right axis deviation or right ventricular conduction defect early in the course of the acute process. SGOT, CPK, and LDH are often elevated, as in myocardial infarction. If the attack is not fatal, pulmonary infarction follows, frequently causing pleuritic pain, hemoptysis, and localized lung findings. Thrombophlebitis is often found on careful examination of the legs, groins, and lower abdomen.

Cervical or thoracic spine disease produces sudden, severe chest pain similar to myocardial infarction; but orthopedic measures give relief and the ECG is normal.

Hiatus hernia may simulate the pain of infarction, and the T waves may be flat or even inverted during the attack, but there is no hypotension or subsequent fever, leukocytosis, or increase in sedimentation rate, SGOT, or LDH.

Acute pancreatitis and acute cholecystitis may superficially mimic infarction. A past history of gastrointestinal symptoms, present findings in the abdomen, jaundice, elevated serum amylase, and x-ray findings differentiate these. Most helpful is the absence of diagnostic serial ECG changes.

Spontaneous pneumothorax, mediastinal emphysema, preeruptive herpes zoster, and severe psychophysiologic cardiovascular reactions are other disorders that may have to be differentiated from myocardial infarction.

Complications

Congestive heart failure and shock may be present at onset of infarction or may develop insidiously or abruptly following an arrhythmia or pulmonary embolization. Sedation and weakness may mask the presence of dyspnea and orthopnea. Distention of neck veins, persistent basal rales, gallop rhythm, the appearance of the murmur of mitral insufficiency, abnormal cardiac pulsations, an enlarging tender liver, and sacral edema should be sought daily. Portal chest x-ray films to recognize pulmonary venous congestion are desirable.

If anticoagulants are not given, pulmonary embolism secondary to phlebitis of the leg or pelvic veins occurs in 10—20% of patients during the acute and convalescent stage.

Arrhythmias occur commonly after myocardial infarction and are thought to be the cause of death in about 40% of patients. The mechanism is either cardiac arrest or ventricular fibrillation; the former occurs following shock or heart failure, and the latter is more apt to be a primary event (although it can be secondary). Continuous monitoring has revealed a higher incidence of ventricular tachycardia, complete AV block, and other less serious arrhythmias than was formerly suspected. Ventricular premature beats often precede more serious arrhythmias in late or secondary but not in early or primary ventricular fibrillation. Atrial arrhythmias are less common and often transient, as is the case with atrial fibrillation. The prompt recognition of arrhythmias is essential in order to initiate treatment.

Cerebrovascular accident may result from a fall in blood pressure associated with myocardial infarction or from embolism secondary to a mural thrombus. It is advisable to take an ECG in all patients with "cerebrovascular accident."

Recurrent myocardial infarction or extension of

the infarction occurs in about 5% of patients during recovery from the initial attack.

Rupture of the heart is uncommon. When it occurs, it is usually in the first week.

Perforation of the ventricular septum is rare, characterized by the sudden appearance of a loud, harsh systolic murmur and thrill over the lower left parasternal area or apex and acute heart failure. This must be distinguished from mitral insufficiency caused by papillary muscle infarction or dysfunction. The diagnosis may sometimes be made by passing (at the bedside) a pulmonary artery flow-directed catheter and noting the size of the v wave in the wedged position and the O_2 content in the right ventricle. Both lesions may precipitate cardiac failure and require cardiac surgery when the patient's condition has stabilized in weeks or months and right and left heart catheterization reveals a significant hemodynamic lesion. Emergency surgical repair is sometimes required but has a high mortality rate. An effort should be made to delay surgery for at least a month.

Ventricular aneurysm and peripheral arterial embolism may occur early or not for months after recovery. The spectrum of ventricular aneurysm is now recognized to extend from frank outpocketing of an area of myocardium with well-demarcated paradoxic pulsations to localized poor contraction or irregular pulsation seen on cineangiography. Approximately 20% of patients develop some form of aneurysm or left ventricular hypokinesis, recognized clinically by abnormal paradoxic precordial pulsations and proved by cinefluoroscopy or left ventricular cineangiography. Some of these patients develop refractory cardiac failure and benefit from surgical excision.

The shoulder-hand syndrome is a rare preventable disorder caused by prolonged immobilization of the arms and shoulders, possibly due to "reflex sympathetic dystrophy." Early pain and tenderness over the affected shoulder is followed by pain and swelling and weakness of the hand, with excessive or deficient sweating.

Oliguria, anuria, or, rarely, tubular necrosis may result if shock persists.

Treatment

A. Immediate Treatment: There is convincing evidence that patients are treated best in a special coronary care unit equipped with continuous monitoring, alarm, recording, pacemaker, and resuscitation equipment, and with specially trained nurses and physicians. It is now clear that the risk of ventricular fibrillation and sudden death is much greater in the first few hours after the onset of the myocardial infarction. Every effort should be made to admit these patients to the coronary care unit as soon as possible to decrease the incidence of death outside the hospital. Some cities (notably Belfast, Ireland) are using specially equipped coronary ambulances to minimize the fatalities by providing "precoronary unit care." Prophylactic antiarrhythmia programs are also undergoing research study and trial.

1. Rest—Attempt to allay apprehension and anxiety. Physical and mental rest in the most comfortable position is essential during the first 2–3 weeks, when rupture of the heart is most apt to occur. The patient should not be allowed to feed or care for himself during the first few days unless the attack is mild, without shock or other complications. Special nursing care is highly desirable. A bedside toilet probably requires less effort than the use of a bedpan.

Adequate sleep is as vital in patients with myocardial infarction as it is with those suffering from cardiac failure. Sedatives should be used as necessary to provide sufficient sleep, and morphine derivatives should not be withheld in the first few days if they are indicated.

2. Analgesia—When pain is severe, give morphine sulfate, 5–10 mg slowly IV. If the pain is not relieved in 15 minutes, repeat this dosage. Further injections can be given subcut, 5–10 mg as necessary for continued relief. The subcutaneous route is used unless the attack is severe or the patient is in shock. If the patient is in shock with severe pain, slow intravenous administration may be necessary. *Caution:* Do not give a second dose of morphine if respirations are below 12/minute. Morphine may cause venous pooling and decreased cardiac output with fainting if the patient is allowed to sit or stand or if he is transported with his head up.

Meperidine and hydromorphone are preferred by some because they are said to produce less nausea and vomiting. The dosage of hydromorphone is 4 mg IM or IV. The dosage of meperidine is 50–100 mg IM as needed or smaller doses IV.

Aminophylline, 0.5 gm IV very slowly (1–2 ml per minute), may be helpful if the pain is not relieved by opiates or oxygen (see below).

3. Oxygen is often useful and sometimes necessary for the relief of dyspnea, cyanosis, pulmonary edema, shock, and chest pain. Positive pressure breathing often induces struggling and decreased venous return and may aggravate myocardial ischemia.

4. Anticoagulant therapy is a controversial matter in the milder cases (rapid relief of pain, minimal signs of myocardial necrosis, absence of shock or cardiac failure). In severe cases of myocardial infarction, anticoagulants are generally recommended.

B. Follow-Up: Alert clinical observation for evidence of extension of the infarction, new infarction, the appearance of complications, or symptoms requiring treatment is essential. Recurrent pain days or weeks after the initial pain has subsided suggests extension of the myocardial necrosis; confirmation should be sought in the ECG and in other clinical features. The same methods of treatment are used as for the first infarction, but a further period of rest is required. Preventive methods to decrease the risk of progressive coronary disease (unproved) are discussed on p 187.

C. Treatment of Complications:

1. Cardiac failure and cardiogenic shock—Left ventricular performance suffers in all patients with acute myocardial infarction. The degree of failure depends upon the magnitude of the new infarction and the state of the myocardium as modified by previous episodes of myocardial ischemia, myocardial infarction, or left ventricular disease due to hypertension or to other cardiac diseases. A small first myocardial infarction in a patient with no underlying cardiac disease usually produces no or minimal evidence of impaired left ventricular performance as judged by symptoms and signs and by hemodynamic monitoring of cardiac output, left ventricular filling pressure, and arterial pressure. If the myocardial infarction is large and occurs in a patient who has had previous infarctions with large areas of scar and borderline compensation, the patient may rapidly go into severe cardiac failure. When hypotension and impaired perfusion of the vital organs are present, cardiogenic shock may occur. The range of possibilities, then, is from no evidence of impaired cardiac function to gross cardiogenic shock with a high mortality rate. It is appropriate, then, to discuss the subject as a continuum, with treatment adjusted according to the degree of severity.

Some degree of cardiac failure, usually left ventricular, can be detected in 20–50% of patients with acute myocardial infarction unless the attack is mild. The findings are usually not overt. The patient may or may not complain of dyspnea; clinical examination may reveal pulmonary rales, diastolic gallop rhythm with a third heart sound, an accentuated pulmonary second sound, pulsus alternans, and pulmonary venous congestion by radiologic examination. The typical central congestion with bat wing densities does not occur unless the patient develops acute pulmonary edema. The development of Kerley B lines occurs later, with chronic failure, and may not be present even though the pulmonary venous wedge pressure is elevated. The increased pulmonary congestion in the upper lobes is usually part of a generalized pulmonary venous congestion at this phase, but if the process continues there may be reversal of the normal flow pattern with upper lobe congestion and lower lobe oligemia as pulmonary arterial constriction occurs in the lower lobes. The radiologic findings may be out of phase with the clinical findings because they take somewhat longer to develop and to regress. It is valuable to obtain serial portable chest films to check for the presence of unsuspected pulmonary venous congestion. In patients who are being monitored by a bedside Swan-Ganz catheter, a raised pulmonary venous wedge pressure can be found in the absence of the radiologic findings.

If the evidence of left ventricular failure is minimal or subclinical, treatment can be conservative, consisting of oral diuretics such as hydrochlorothiazide, 50–100 mg, oxygen to relieve hypoxemia, and avoidance of sodium-containing fluids.

With more severe left ventricular failure that is not promptly relieved by diuretic therapy, more aggressive therapy should be considered—preceded by hemodynamic monitoring of the arterial pressure, of the pulmonary venous wedge pressure (left ventricular filling pressure), and of the cardiac output. Stroke work index can be computed from these measure-

ments, and rational therapy can be given on the basis of the specific hemodynamic abnormality found. It is hazardous to continue to use potent therapeutic agents unless hemodynamic monitoring is available so that the results of the intervention can be observed and the dose of the various drugs adjusted.

Hypotension is often the first sign that cardiac failure may be more severe than is suggested by slight dyspnea and pulmonary rales, especially if it persists after pain is relieved. When monitoring reveals that the left ventricular filling pressure is low (< 12 mm Hg) and the cardiac output is normal, despite the low arterial pressure, hypovolemia is the most probable cause and should be treated by increments of volume replacement beginning with 100 ml of saline or salt-poor albumin or other similar fluids (eg, dextran). Increments of volume repletion can be given every 5–10 minutes until the left ventricular filling pressure rises. If the cardiac output does not increase as the left ventricular filling pressure increases to 15–20 mm Hg, further volume replacement should be stopped to prevent pulmonary edema, which may occur quite abruptly. If the only hemodynamic abnormality is a raised left ventricular filling pressure, with blood pressure and output normally maintained, more vigorous diuresis can be attempted with larger doses of furosemide. Excessive diuresis must be avoided because the patient may then become dehydrated and, although the filling pressure may fall, the blood pressure may also fall and the patient will need further volume repletion. Some patients with acute myocardial infarction have hypotension with impaired tissue perfusion primarily from failure of compensatory peripheral vasoconstriction without a substantial change in filling pressure or cardiac output; these patients often respond with a rise in arterial pressure to sympathomimetic amines (norepinephrine and dopamine) which stimulate the beta-adrenergic receptors. Both drugs should be infused at a slow rate to avoid tachycardia, marked increases in blood pressure, and ventricular arrhythmias. The physician's aim is to maintain the blood pressure but also to prevent arrhythmias. When the cardiac dysfunction is more severe, with reduced cardiac output, increased left ventricular filling pressure (above 20 mm Hg), and arterial blood pressure at or above 90 mm Hg, vasodilator therapy can be cautiously begun while the hemodynamic result is monitored. Drugs such as sodium nitroprusside, phentolamine, or nitroglycerin, given by intravenous drip, decrease the impedance to left ventricular ejection, reduce left ventricular volume and filling pressure, may improve the left ventricular stroke work index, decrease the myocardial oxygen consumption (MVO_2), and improve perfusion to the brain, kidney, and heart. Striking changes have been observed by Parmley and Chatterjee, and temporary improvement is often considerable and may tide the patient over a critical period. Vasodilator therapy cannot be used if there is considerable reduction in arterial pressure because further reduction by the vasodilator therapy may aggravate the situation, making the patient worse. Efforts, therefore, must be made to raise the arterial pressure to about 100 mm Hg before vasodilator therapy can be used. If this is not possible with vasopressors without worsening the left ventricular filling pressure and aggravating the cardiac failure, aortic balloon counter-pulsation may be used as a dramatic temporary circulatory assist to raise the arterial pressure and to make vasodilator therapy possible. Counter-pulsation removes blood from the aorta during systole and returns it in diastole. Its removal during systole decreases impedance to left ventricular ejection, reducing the afterload and the work of the left ventricle, and results in fall in left ventricular filling pressure similar to that achieved by vasodilators. However, blood is returned during diastole, raising the diastolic blood pressure, increasing coronary perfusion, and improving left ventricular function by decreasing myocardial ischemia. Parmley and Chatterjee found that the combination of external counter-pulsation followed by vasodilator therapy with sodium nitroprusside significantly improved left ventricular "pump" function in acute myocardial infarction with cardiogenic shock and consequently reduced mortality. External counter-pulsation increased the mean diastolic pressure 7 mm Hg, with a peak increase of 20 mm Hg and an increase in cardiac index of 14%. External counter-pulsation was followed by infusion of nitroprusside, 60–200 μg/minute, and phentolamine, 0.1 to 2 mg/minute. The use of these 2 new procedures reduced the mortality rate in cardiogenic shock about 50% and allowed patients to leave the hospital even though they continued to show some evidences of left ventricular failure The long-term prognosis in patients who have been successfully treated by balloon assist for cardiogenic shock is still poor (approximately 10% survival in 1 year) because of the extensive underlying disease inferred from the presence of cardiogenic shock.

Invasive balloon counter-pulsation as well as the noninvasive external counter-pulsation can be used as a temporary measure to tide the patient over acute "power failure" and gain time to consider the desirability of performing coronary angiograms as well as the feasibility of coronary bypass surgery if the lesions are shown to be amenable to surgery because of strategically located sites of severe stenosis. The surgical mortality rate in patients recovering from cardiogenic shock is high, and more data are required before a definite conclusion can be reached about the feasibility of bypass surgery in such cases.

The poor response to medical as well as surgical therapy in patients with cardiogenic shock following myocardial infarction can be appreciated when one considers that at least 50% of the left ventricle has been shown to be damaged in autopsy studies of such patients. The left ventricular filling pressure is usually considerably more than 20 mm Hg. The left ventricular stroke work is usually less than 20 gram meters per square meter (gm m/m^2) and often less than 15 gm m/m^2, and hypoxemia with a P_{O_2} of less than 40–50 mm Hg is frequently found. The high wedge pressure (left ventricular filling pressure) induces dyspnea; impaired peripheral perfusion resulting from the decreased cardiac output is recognized clinically by cold, pale, clammy skin, cerebral obtundation, low urine output, and evidences of venous constriction.

Monitoring of the hemodynamic parameters mentioned above is valuable in prognosis. Patients with left ventricular filling pressures less than 15 mm Hg and stroke work indices of more than 35 or 40 gm m/m^2 have an excellent prognosis, whereas if the filling pressure exceeds 20 mm Hg and the stroke work index is less than 20 gm m/m^2 or especially if it is 15 gm m/m^2, a poor outcome is likely. It is in patients with a poor prognosis that aggressive therapy is warranted before severe deterioration of the patient has occurred. The various drugs and forms of therapy discussed should be considered as therapeutic trials; the physician should begin, vary, and stop various types of therapy depending upon the hemodynamic response. One cannot be dogmatic in advance about doses and preferences for certain drugs over others; adjustments are necessary as treatment proceeds.

Digitalis, the time-honored inotropic agent, is infrequently used today in the treatment of cardiac failure in the setting of acute myocardial infarction, primarily because of its tendency to produce ventricular arrhythmias and its relative ineffectiveness in the setting of severe left ventricular pump failure. When cardiac failure is severe, requiring inotropic agents, digitalis should certainly be given a trial. However, in milder varieties of cardiac failure the drug should probably be withheld, primarily because the development of ventricular arrhythmias places the physician in the dilemma of deciding whether they are the result of the digitalis therapy or a natural consequence of the myocardial ischemia. Digitalis should still be used if the patient has atrial fibrillation with a rapid ventricular rate.

2. Arrhythmias—Ventricular premature beats are common. They indicate increased irritability of the damaged myocardium and may presage ventricular tachycardia or fibrillation. Lidocaine (Xylocaine), 50–100 mg IV, followed by an intravenous infusion at a rate of 1–2 mg/minute, is the drug of choice. Alternatives are procainamide, quinidine sulfate, or, if digitalis is thought to be responsible for the arrhythmia, potassium salts. Aggressive treatment of ventricular arrhythmias may prevent ventricular fibrillation and cardiac arrest, although these severe arrhythmias may occur without warning, especially early in the course of the disease.

Ventricular tachycardia is an emergency (see p 207). Ventricular fibrillation should be instantly recognized on the alarm system at the nursing station, and defibrillation should be accomplished within 30 seconds. In most coronary care units, defibrillation is performed by specially trained nurses if a skilled physician is not immediately available. Lidocaine (Xylocaine) should be given by intravenous infusion (1–2 mg/minute) to prevent recurrence.

Atrial fibrillation is usually transient. If this persists, if the patient tolerates it poorly, or if congestive heart failure occurs, digitalize with care or treat by cardioversion.

Recurrent ventricular arrhythmias, when they occur following myocardial infarction—especially if associated with ventricular aneurysm and cardiac failure—may respond to surgical resection of the aneurysm and bypass surgery which should be considered whenever the arrhythmias are life-threatening and difficult to control with drugs.

3. Stokes-Adams attack with heart block—(See p 211.) *This is an emergency.* Complete heart block complicates acute myocardial infarction in 6–10% of cases. It has a high mortality, usually lasts less than a week, and often can be treated by artificial pacing through a transvenous catheter placed in the right ventricle. Pacing at a rate of 70–80 may greatly improve the cardiac output and tissue perfusion and prevent Stokes-Adams attacks. Stokes-Adams attacks with fatal syncope are rare in the presence of inferior myocardial infarction because the AV conduction damage is nodal and due to transient ischemia from occlusion of a branch of the right coronary artery. When AV conduction defects occur in anterior infarction, they usually represent widespread necrosis of the septum and the conduction system, involving the bundle of His or the bundle branches, usually with decreased left ventricular function and ventricular asynergy. Complete heart block may occur rapidly, and a temporary artificial demand pacemaker should therefore be introduced if AV conduction delay occurs in anterior infarction. It is still an open question whether a prophylactic pacemaker should be inserted when right bundle branch block and left anterior hemiblock develop acutely in the presence of anterior infarction (see section on AV conduction system defects). Demand pacemakers are preferred over fixed rate pacemakers because the AV conduction defects are usually transient and subside within a week, and ventricular arrhythmias may result from competition between the artificial pacemaker and the patient's own natural pacemaker (see below). Temporary pacemakers are usually left in place for a week after the AV conduction becomes normal. Rarely, a permanent pacemaker may be required in anterior infarction.

Second degree AV block with Wenckebach pauses (see below) and narrow QRS complexes are not routinely paced if the patient has inferior infarction. His bundle recordings have demonstrated that if the conduction defect is in the AV node, above the bundle of His (as is the usual finding in inferior infarctions), Stokes-Adams attacks are uncommon even if complete block develops. This is in contrast to the AV conduction defect that occurs in anterior infarctions, in which His bundle recordings and pathologic data show that the block is usually distal to the AV node, within the bundle of His or in the bundle branches; Stokes-Adams attacks with fatalities occur if the patient is not protected by a pacemaker.

Sinus bradycardia (see p 203), especially in inferior infarction, may precede AV block and provide a setting in which ventricular arrhythmias may occur. Further, with decreased cardiac output seen in acute myocardial infarction, perfusion of the vital organs may be inadequate with a slow heart rate. Atropine, 0.25–1 mg IV, is desirable in such situations, with close observation to determine its effectiveness and side-effects since ventricular arrhythmias have resulted from atropine. If atropine is ineffective or if the bradycardia is marked or associated with block, a temporary prophylactic transvenous demand pacemaker should be inserted into the right ventricle. Asystole may occur unpredictably, so electrode catheters should be placed prophylactically in patients with anterior infarctions who have complete AV block or type II Mobitz AV block, or in inferior infarctions with complete AV block. Some question arises in anterior infarction with left anterior hemiblock with a normal P–R interval. Infusions of lidocaine should be given to prevent ventricular fibrillation if AV block subsides and competition occurs with the patient's own pacemaker. Demand rather than fixed rate pacemakers are preferable for this reason.

Ventricular fibrillation is the major hazard associated with pacing in acute myocardial infarction because of competition between the patient's own pacemaker and that of the artificial pacemaker. For this reason, patients with first degree AV block or with type I second degree AV block with Wenckebach pauses and narrow QRS complexes in inferior infarction are not routinely paced. Demand pacemaker, activated by a delay in the appearance of the QRS complex, may be preferred, so that, when AV conduction is unstable and intermittent, competition between the normal and artificial pacemaker will not occur.

4. Thromboembolic phenomena are common during the course of myocardial infarction. Anticoagulants should be administered promptly. For treatment of pulmonary embolism, see discussion in Chapter 6.

5. Oliguria, anuria, acute tubular necrosis—See Chapter 15.

6. Rupture, perforation of the interventricular septum, mitral insufficiency from papillary muscle dysfunction or rupture, and aneurysm—Surgical repair is indicated for perforated ventricular septum or mitral insufficiency after the lesion has stabilized (for 4–10 weeks, if possible), if cardiac failure has persisted. Patients with mitral insufficiency, following myocardial infarction, when associated with left ventricular failure requiring surgery, have a high incidence of raised left ventricular end-diastolic pressure (more than 15 mm Hg) or a reduced cardiac output (less than 2.5 liters/minute/sq m). The surgical mortality rate is higher than in replacement of the mitral valve in other varieties of mitral insufficiency, but the end results are often gratifying. Resection of aneurysm is recommended in the presence of unequivocal ventricular aneurysm with persistent cardiac failure but not for minor asymptomatic aneurysm or for diffuse, flabby, irregular hypokinesis and cardiac failure. No treatment is available for cardiac rupture.

7. Shoulder-hand syndrome—Best treated by preventive physical therapy instituted early.

8. Activity status in convalescence—The minimum period of rest should be at least 3 weeks in the average case; in mild cases without any complications, early careful ambulation after 7–10 days is being increasingly advised. If the infarction has been very severe, this should be increased to about 6 weeks. The program for most patients is 1 month of rest, 1 month of slowly increasing activity, and 1 month of restricted activity before returning to work. The amount of rest should be individualized according to the severity of the myocardial infarction and the response of the patient.

The patient should not be permitted to walk freely about the room for about 7–10 days after he is first allowed out of bed. Gradual resumption of activity is most important. He should remain on the same floor, with gradually increasing periods of walking, slowly and without producing chest pain, dyspnea, undue tachycardia, or fatigue. When first allowed out of doors, usually not until 1 month after the infarction, he should avoid hills and stairs for another month.

Prognosis

The overall mortality during the first month after the infarction averages 30%. Most of the deaths occur in the first 12 hours. In the mild attack clinical manifestations subside promptly and the initial mortality is less than 5%. Clinically severe myocardial infarction may require 6–12 weeks for full recovery. The mortality rises to 60–90% with prolonged shock, severe early heart failure, leukocytosis over 25,000 with eosinophilia, fever above 40° C (104° F), uncontrolled diabetes mellitus, old age, and previous definite infarction, especially if these occur in combination. Pulmonary embolism which is not treated with anticoagulants, persistent arrhythmias, and extension of the infarct superimpose a mortality of 15–20% during early convalescence.

Long-term survival is related to the availability of medical care and the presence of other chronic diseases in addition to the residuals of infarction. Complete clinical and ECG recovery is compatible with survival of 10–15 years. Patients with residual heart failure die within 1–5 years.

Various prospective studies are under way to improve the clinician's ability to predict which patients surviving myocardial infarction are apt to die prematurely. Those with findings suggesting highest risks (evidence of residual ischemia on the ECG, cardiac failure, conduction defects, and atherosclerosis elsewhere) may have 6 times the mortality rate of patients with findings suggesting lowest risks. As has been stated previously, the extent of the anatomic stenosis and the left ventricular function are the major factors in prognosis.

Studies are under way in various centers to select patients with the highest risks, to treat them vigorously, and to monitor them closely.

Aspenstrom G & others: Collaborative analysis of long-term anticoagulant administration after acute myocardial infarction. Lancet 1:203, 1970.

Assessment of short-term anticoagulant administration after cardiac infarction. Brit MJ 1:335, 1969.

Atkins JM & others: Ventricular conduction blocks and sudden death in acute myocardial infarction. New England J Med 288:281, 1973.

Baxley WA, Jones WB, Dodge HT: Left ventricular anatomical and functional abnormalities in chronic postinfarction heart failure. Ann Int Med 74:499, 1971.

Bloch A & others: Early mobilization after myocardial infarction: A controlled study. Am J Cardiol 34:152, 1974.

Chatterjee K & others: Hemodynamic and metabolic responses to vasodilator therapy in acute myocardial infarction. Circulation 48:1183, 1973.

Coronary Drug Project Research Group: Prognostic importance of premature beats following myocardial infarction. JAMA 223:1116, 1973.

Davis RW, Ebert PA: Ventricular aneurysm: A clinical-pathologic correlation. Am J Cardiol 29:1, 1972.

DeSanctis RW, Block P, Hutter AM Jr: Tachyarrhythmias in myocardial infarction. Circulation 45:681, 1972.

Epstein SE & others: The early phase of acute myocardial infarction: Pharmacologic aspects of therapy. Ann Int Med 78:918, 1973.

Erhardt LR: Clinical and pathological observations in different types of acute myocardial infarction: A study of 84 patients deceased after treatment in a coronary care unit. Acta med scandinav (Suppl 560), 1974.

Forrester JS, Chatterjee K, Swan HJC: Hemodynamic monitoring in patients with acute myocardial infarction. JAMA 226:60, 1973.

Genton E: Guidelines for heparin therapy. Ann Int Med 80:77, 1974.

Gold HK: Intraaortic balloon pumping for ventricular septal defect or mitral regurgitation complicating acute myocardial infarction. Circulation 47:1191, 1973.

Greene HL & others: Hemodynamic effects of plasma volume expansion and prognostic implications in acute myocardial infarction. Circulation 49:106, 1974.

Hamilton GW, Murray JA, Kennedy JW: Quantitative angiocardiography in ischemic heart disease: The spectrum of abnormal left ventricular function and the role of abnormally contracting segments. Circulation 45:1065, 1972.

Heikkila J: Mitral incompetence as a complication of acute myocardial infarction. Acta med scandinav 182 (Suppl 475):1, 1967.

Hutter AM Jr: Early hospital discharge after myocardial infarction. New England J Med 288:1141, 1973.

James TN: Pathogenesis of arrhythmias and acute myocardial infarction. Am J Cardiol 24:791, 1969.

Killip T: Management of arrhythmias in acute myocardial infarction. Hosp Practice 7:131, 1972.

Kostuk W & others: Correlations between the chest film and hemodynamics in acute myocardial infarction. Circulation 48:624, 1973.

Leren P: The effect of plasma cholesterol lowering diet in male survivors of myocardial infarction. Acta med scandinav 179 (Suppl 466):1, 1966.

Levine HD, Young E, Williams RA: Electrocardiogram and vectorcardiogram in myocardial infarction. Circulation 45:457, 1972.

Lown B, Klein MD, Herschberg PI: Coronary and precoronary care. Am J Med 46:705, 1969.

Lown B & others: Sensitivity to digitalis in acute myocardial infarction. Am J Cardiol 30:388, 1972.

Margolis JR & others: Clinical features of unrecognized myocardial infarction: Silent and symptomatic, 18-year follow-up: The Framingham Study. Am J Cardiol 32:1, 1973.

Moraski RE & others: Left ventricular function in patients with and without myocardial infarction and one, two or three vessel coronary artery disease. Am J Cardiol 35:1, 1975.

Moss AJ (editor): Symposium on the prehospital phase of acute myocardial infarction. Arch Int Med 129:681, 1972.

Mundth ED & others: Surgery for complications of acute myocardial infarction. Circulation 45:1279, 1972.

Norris RM, Mercer CJ: Significance of idioventricular rhythms in acute myocardial infarction. Progr Cardiovas Dis 16:455, 1974.

Parkey RW & others: A new method for radionuclide imaging of acute myocardial infarction in humans. Circulation 50:540, 1974.

Parmley WW & others: Hemodynamic effects of noninvasive systolic unloading (nitroprusside) and diastolic augmentation (external counterpulsation) in patients with acute myocardial infarction: Am J Cardiol 33:819, 1974.

Perloff JK, Talano JV, Ronan JA Jr: Noninvasive techniques in acute myocardial infarction. Progr Cardiovas Dis 13:437, 1971.

Perry LW, Scott LP: Anomalous left coronary artery from pulmonary artery: Report of 11 cases: Review of indications for and results of surgery. Circulation 41:1043, 1970.

Rahimtoola SH & others: Effects of ouabain on impaired left ventricular function in acute myocardial infarction. New England J Med 287:527, 1972.

Ratshin RA, Rackley CE, Russell RO Jr: Hemodynamic evaluation of left ventricular function in shock complicating myocardial infarction. Circulation 45:127, 1972.

Roberts WC, Buja LM: The frequency and significance of coronary arterial thrombi and other observations in fatal acute myocardial infarction: A study of 107 necropsy patients. Am J Med 52:425, 1972.

Rotman M, Wagner GS, Wallace AG: Bradyarrhythmias in acute myocardial infarction. Circulation 45:703, 1972.

Rotman M & others: Significance of high degree atrioventricular block in acute posterior myocardial infarction: The importance of clinical setting and mechanism of block. Circulation 47:257, 1973.

Sanders CA & others: Mechanical circulatory assistance: Current status and experience with combining circulatory assistance, emergency coronary angiography, and acute myocardial revascularization. Circulation 45:1292, 1972.

Scanlon PJ & others: Accelerated angina pectoris: Clinical, hemodynamic, arteriographic, and therapeutic experience in 85 patients. Circulation 47:19, 1973.

Selzer A, Gerbode F, Kerth WJ: Clinical, hemodynamic and surgical considerations of rupture of the ventricular septum after myocardial infarction. Am Heart J 78:598, 1969.

Shell WE, Sobel BE: Protection of jeopardized ischemic myocardium by reduction of ventricular afterload. New England J Med 291:481, 1974.

Simon AB, Alonzo AA: Sudden death in nonhospitalized cardiac patients: An epidemiologic study with implications for intervention technics. Arch Int Med 132:163, 1973.

Sobel BE, Shell WE: Serum enzyme determinations in the diagnosis and assessment of myocardial infarction. Circulation 45:471, 1972.

Swan HJC & others: Hemodynamic spectrum of myocardial infarction and cardiogenic shock: A conceptual model. Circulation 45:1097, 1972.

Walker JA & others: Determinants of angiographic patency of aortocoronary vein bypass grafts. Circulation 45 (Suppl 1):1, 1972.

Walsh MJ & others: Mobile coronary care. Brit Heart J 34:701, 1972.

Weber KT & others: Left ventricular dysfunction following acute myocardial infarction. Am J Med 54:697, 1973.

Weil MH, Shubin H, Carlson R: Treatment of circulatory shock: Use of sympathomimetic and related vasoactive agents. JAMA 231:1280, 1975.

Williams RA & others: Electrocardiographic, arteriographic and ventriculographic correlations in transmural myocardial infarction. Am J Cardiol 31:595, 1973.

Wolk MJ, Scheidt S, Killip T: Heart failure complicating acute myocardial infarction. Circulation 45:1125, 1972.

DISTURBANCES OF RATE & RHYTHM

The presence of a significant arrhythmia should be suspected in any of the following circumstances: (1) when there is a history of sudden onset and sudden termination of palpitation or rapid heart action; (2) when the heart rhythm is grossly irregular; (3) when the heart rate is below 40 or above 140/minute; (4) when the heart rate does not change with breath-holding or exercise; (5) when a rapid heart rate suddenly slows during carotid sinus massage; (6) when the first heart sound varies in intensity; or (7) when a patient develops sudden anginal pain, shock, congestive heart failure, or syncope.

The complete diagnosis of an arrhythmia consists of accurate identification of the site of origin of the abnormality and proper assessment of its significance. The most common arrhythmias are sinus arrhythmia, sinus tachycardia, sinus bradycardia, atrial and ventricular premature beats, and paroxysmal atrial tachycardia. These occur in normal and diseased hearts alike and have no significance except insofar as they alter circulatory dynamics. Atrial fibrillation and flutter occur most commonly in patients with arteriosclerotic or rheumatic heart disease, but thyrotoxicosis, acute infections, or trauma may precipitate them in the absence of heart disease. Ventricular tachycardia is a serious disorder of rhythm and appears most often in the presence of advanced coronary artery disease. Partial or complete heart block also results from coronary heart disease but is most commonly due to fibrosis of the conduction system. Digitalis toxicity is a frequent cause of many types of arrhythmia.

From the physiologic standpoint, arrhythmias are harmful to the extent that they reduce cardiac output, lower blood pressure, and interfere with perfusion of the vital territories of the brain, heart, and kidney. Rapid heart rates may cause any or all of these changes and, in the presence of heart disease, may precipitate acute heart failure or pulmonary edema, angina pectoris or myocardial infarction, syncope, poor cerebration with confusion, or cerebral thrombosis. Patients with otherwise normal hearts may tolerate rapid rates with no symptoms other than palpitation or fluttering, but prolonged attacks usually cause weakness, exertional dyspnea, and precordial aching. The rate at which slow heart rates produce symptoms at rest or on exertion depends upon the underlying state of the cardiac muscle and its ability to increase its stroke output. If the heart rate abruptly slows, as with the onset of complete heart block or transient standstill, syncope or convulsions may result.

If possible, elicit a history of previous attacks and precipitating factors, symptoms of heart failure, and anginal pain. Examine for cardiac enlargement, significant murmurs, signs of heart failure, and hypotension. Count the heart rate for 1 minute. If the rate is seemingly regular, repeat the count twice to determine if the rate is absolutely regular; if irregular, determine whether pulse deficit is present. If there is no severe failure, angina, or recent infarction, determine the effects of breath-holding, exercise, and change of position on the heart rate and rhythm. Massage the right and left carotid sinus successively for 30 seconds while listening to the heart; cease massage as soon as a change in rate occurs. Note whether the first heart sound varies in intensity. Examine the neck veins for abnormal pulsations or cannon waves.

The final diagnosis of arrhythmias depends upon the ECG. However, consideration of the patient's age, the type of associated heart disease, and the results of the examination permit a diagnosis in most cases before the ECG is taken.

His bundle recordings aid in the interpretation of complex arrhythmias, especially when there is a question about whether the rhythm is atrial or ventricular, by demonstrating the supraventricular or ventricular origin of wide QRS complexes. If the QRS complex follows the His bundle spike, ventricular aberrancy is present and treatment is influenced accordingly. His bundle recordings also aid in the recognition of concealed premature depolarizations, especially of the His bundle with antegrade and retrograde AV block; His bundle depolarizations affect subsequent cycles by retrograde conduction to the atrioventricular node, producing a prolonged P–R interval and nonconducted P waves (see below).

Baum RS, Alvarez H III, Cobb LA: Survival after resuscitation from out-of-hospital ventricular fibrillation. Circulation 50:1231, 1974.

Bigger JT Jr: Pharmacologic and clinical control of antiarrhythmic drugs. Am J Med 58:479, 1975.

Castellanos A Jr, Castillo CA, Agha AS: Contribution of His bundle recordings to the understanding of clinical arrhythmias. Am J Cardiol 28:499, 1971.

Cranefield PF, Wit AL, Hoffman BF: Genesis of cardiac arrhythmias. Circulation 47:190, 1973.

Damato AN, Gallagher JJ, Lau SH: Application of His bundle recordings in diagnosing conduction disorders. Progr Cardiovas Dis 14:601, 1972.

Damato AN, Lau SH: Concealed and supernormal atrioventricular conduction. Circulation 43:967, 1971.

Fisch C: Relation of electrolyte disturbances to cardiac arrhyth-

mias. Circulation 47:408, 1973.

Fisch C, Zipes DP, McHenry PL: Rate dependent aberrancy. Circulation 48:714, 1973.

Hoffman BF, Rosen MR, Wit AL: Electrophysiology and pharmacology of cardiac arrhythmias. 3. The causes and treatment of cardiac arrhythmias. Part A. Am Heart J 89:115, 1975.

James TN: Order and disorder in the rhythm of the heart. Circulation 47:362, 1973.

Jelinek MV, Lown B: Exercise stress testing for exposure of cardiac arrhythmia. Progr Cardiovas Dis 16:497, 1974.

Langendorf R, Pick A: Artificial pacing of the human heart: Its contribution to the understanding of arrhythmias. Am J Cardiol 28:516, 1971.

Massumi RA, Ali N: Accelerated isorhythmic ventricular rhythms. Am J Cardiol 26:170, 1970.

Pamintuan JC, Dreyfus LS, Watanabe Y: Comparative mechanisms of antiarrhythmic agents. Am J Cardiol 26:512, 1970.

Pick A: Mechanisms of cardiac arrhythmias: From hypothesis to physiologic fact. Am Heart J 86:249, 1973.

Pick A, Langendorf R: Recent advances in the differential diagnosis of AV junctional arrhythmia. Am Heart J 76:553, 1968.

Rodstein M, Wolloch L, Gubner RS: Mortality study of significance of extrasystoles in insured population. Circulation 44:617, 1971.

Ryan M, Lown B, Horn H: Comparison of ventricular ectopic activity during 24-hour monitoring and exercise testing in patients with coronary heart disease. New England J Med 292:224, 1975.

Samet P: Cardiac arrhythmias: Hemodynamic sequelae of cardiac arrhythmias. Circulation 47:399, 1973.

Schamroth L: How to approach an arrhythmia. Circulation 47:420, 1973.

Singer DH, Lazzara R, Hoffman BF: Interrelationships between automaticity and conduction in Purkinje fibers. Circulation Res 21:537, 1967.

Sokolow M, Perloff D: The clinical pharmacology and use of quinidine in heart disease. Progr Cardiovas Dis 3:316, 1961.

SINUS ARRHYTHMIA

Sinus arrhythmia is a cyclical increase in normal heart rate with inspiration and decrease with expiration. It results from reflex changes in vagal influence on the normal pacemaker and disappears with breath-holding or increase of heart rate due to any cause. The arrhythmia has no significance except in older persons, when it may be associated with coronary artery disease.

SINUS TACHYCARDIA

Sinus tachycardia is a heart rate faster than 100 beats/minute which is caused by rapid impulse formation by the normal pacemaker secondary to fever, exercise, emotion, anemia, shock, thyrotoxicosis, or drug effect. The rate may reach 180 beats/minute in young persons but rarely exceed 160 beats/minute. The rhythm is basically regular, but serial 1-minute counts of the heart rate indicate that it varies 5 or more beats/minute with changes in position, with breath-holding or sedation, or with correction of the underlying disorder. The rate slows gradually, but tachycardia may begin abruptly in response to sudden emotional stimuli.

SINUS BRADYCARDIA
(Sick Sinus Syndrome; Tachycardia-Bradycardia)
(See p 209.)

Sinus bradycardia is a heart rate slower than 60 beats/minute due to increased vagal influence on the normal pacemaker. The rate increases after exercise or administration of atropine. Slight degrees have no significance unless there is underlying heart disease, especially coronary heart disease or acute myocardial infarction. Elderly patients may develop weakness, confusion, or even syncope with slow heart rates. Atrial and ventricular ectopic rhythms are more apt to occur with slow ventricular rates. It may be desirable to use ephedrine or atropine in some patients to speed the heart rate. Rarely, artificial pacemakers are necessary.

In recent years a syndrome known as the "sick sinus" rhythm, or tachycardia-bradycardia syndrome, has become increasingly noted. This consists of abnormalities of the pacemaker function of the sinus node or in conduction from the sinus node to the AV node. The patients may have sinus bradycardia, sinus standstill, or SA block. In conjunction with a slow atrial rate resulting from these abnormalities, paroxysmal atrial arrhythmias and perfusion abnormalities may occur. The patient may have alternately a slow rate (which may not be adequate to perfuse the vital organs) or a rapid atrial tachycardia or atrial fibrillation which may produce symptoms as a result of the rapid ventricular rate. Treatment of the atrial arrhythmias with drugs such as quinidine or digitalis may enhance the conduction difficulties of the sinus node or the sino-atrial transmission; treatment is best effected by inserting an artificial demand pacemaker into the right ventricle to prevent sinus slowing and then using various antiarrhythmic agents (see Atrial Arrhythmias) to prevent the paroxysmal atrial arrhythmias.

In some patients, the increased heart rate resulting from the implanted artificial pacemaker may improve left ventricular function over a period of weeks or months, so that the recurrent atrial arrhythmias become less frequent and the pharmacologic treatment becomes less urgent; the patient may become asymptomatic with the use of the implanted pacemaker alone.

Chokshi DS & others: Treatment of sinoatrial rhythm disturbances with permanent cardiac pacing. Am J Cardiol 32:215, 1973.

Conde CA & others: Effectiveness of pacemaker treatment in the bradycardia-tachycardia syndrome. Am J Cardiol 32:209, 1973.

Ferrer MI: The sick sinus syndrome. Circulation 47:635, 1973.

Kaplan BM & others: Tachycardia-bradycardia syndrome (so-called "sick sinus syndrome"). Am J Cardiol 31:497, 1973.

Moss AJ, Davis RJ: Brady-tachy syndrome. Progr Cardiovas Dis 16:439, 1974.

Rokseth R, Hatle L: Prospective study on the occurrence and management of chronic sinoatrial disease, with follow-up. Brit Heart J 36:582, 1974.

Scheinman MM & others: The sick sinus and ailing atrium. Western J Med 121:473, 1974.

Sigurd B & others: Adams-Stokes syndrome caused by sinoatrial block. Brit Heart J 35:1002, 1973.

ATRIAL PREMATURE BEATS

Atrial premature beats occur when an ectopic focus in the atria fires off before the next expected impulse from the sinus node. Ventricular systole occurs prematurely, and the compensatory pause following this is only slightly longer than the normal interval between beats. Such premature beats occur with equal frequency in normal or diseased hearts and are never sufficient basis for a diagnosis of heart disease. Speeding of the heart rate by any means usually abolishes premature beats.

Strauss HC & others: Premature atrial stimulation as a key to the understanding of sinoatrial conduction in man. Circulation 47:86, 1973.

PAROXYSMAL ATRIAL TACHYCARDIA

This is the commonest paroxysmal tachycardia. It occurs more often in young patients with normal hearts. Attacks begin and end abruptly, and usually last several hours. The heart rate may be 140–240/minute (usually 170–220/minute) and is perfectly regular, ie, the rate will not vary more than 1–2 beats/minute. Exercise, change of position, and breath-holding have no effect. Carotid sinus massage or induced gagging or vomiting either have no effect or promptly abolish the attack. Patients are asymptomatic except for awareness of rapid heart action unless there is underlying heart disease, especially mitral stenosis and coronary heart disease. In prolonged attacks with rapid rates, dyspnea or tightness in the chest may be felt. Paroxysmal atrial tachycardia may result from digitalis toxicity, and then is associated with AV block so that only every second or, rarely, every third atrial impulse reaches the ventricles (so-called PAT with block).

Recent electrophysiologic studies have demonstrated that the mechanism of paroxysmal atrial tachycardia is reentry from an atrial premature beat through an AV node whose conduction has been slowed. As a result, a single premature atrial beat may precipitate tachycardia if it is appropriately timed. Similarly, a single atrial premature beat may terminate atrial tachycardia by making the reentry pathway refractory.

Prevention of Attacks

A. **Specific Measures:** Attempt to find and remove the cause, especially emotional stress, fatigue, or excessive use of alcohol or tobacco.

B. **Drugs:**

1. Quinidine sulfate, 0.2–0.6 gm 3–4 times daily, may be used to prevent frequent and troublesome attacks. Begin with small doses and increase if the attacks are not prevented and toxic effects do not occur.

2. If quinidine is not effective or not tolerated, full digitalization and maintenance may prevent or decrease the frequency of attacks.

3. Procainamide hydrochloride (Pronestyl) in a maintenance dosage of 250–500 mg 3 times daily may be tried if quinidine and digitalis are not successful.

4. Propranolol (Inderal), 10–40 mg 3–4 times daily, has been shown to prevent recurrent atrial arrhythmias even in patients refractory to quinidine and procainamide. Use *cautiously* (if at all) in patients with early heart failure, heart block, or bronchospasm.

Treatment of the Acute Attack

In the absence of heart disease, serious effects are rare. Most attacks subside spontaneously, and the physician should not use remedies that are more dangerous than the disease. Particular effort should be made to terminate the attack quickly if it persists for several days; if cardiac failure, syncope, or anginal pain develops; or if there is underlying cardiac disease.

A. **Mechanical Measures:** A variety of methods have been used to interrupt attacks, and the patient may learn to do these himself. These include Valsalva's maneuver (holding the breath and contracting the chest and abdominal muscles), stretching the arms and body, lowering the head between the knees, coughing, and breath-holding. These maneuvers, as is true also of carotid sinus pressure (see below), stimulate the vagus, increase AV conduction delay, and so block the reentry mechanism, terminating the arrhythmia.

B. **Vagal Stimulation:**

1. **Carotid sinus pressure**—With the patient relaxed in the semi-recumbent position, firm but gentle pressure and massage are applied first over one carotid sinus for 10–20 seconds and then over the other. Pressure should not be exerted on both carotid sinuses at the same time. Continuous auscultation of the heart is required so that carotid sinus pressure can be withdrawn as soon as the attack ceases. Carotid sinus pressure will interrupt about half of the attacks, especially if the patient has been digitalized or sedated.

2. **Bilateral eyeball pressure** has been recommended, but it is rarely as effective as carotid sinus pressure and involves the risk of detaching the retina.

3. **Induced vomiting** (except in cases of syncope, anginal pain, or severe cardiac disease).

C. **Drug Therapy:** If mechanical measures fail and the attack continues (particularly if the above symptoms are present), drugs should be employed. There is no unanimity of opinion about the most effective drugs, but the following are satisfactory: (1) Parasympathetic stimulating drugs such as edrophonium (Tensilon), 5–10 mg IV. This results in enhancement of the AV conduction delay, breaking the reentry mechanism. (2) Verapamil is a new drug used in England for the same purpose with conspicuous success. (3) Pressor agents. (4) Procainamide. (5) Propranolol. (6) Digitalis.

D. **Cessation of Drug Therapy:** Paroxysmal atrial tachycardia, usually with 2:1 block, may be due to digitalis toxicity (increased dosage or excessive potassium diuresis). Treatment consists of stopping digitalis and diuretics and treating the patient for digitalis toxicity with potassium.

E. **Cardioversion** (see below) may be used if the clinical situation is severe enough to warrant anesthesia and electric precordial shock. Because of the possibility of digitalis intoxication as the cause of atrial or junctional tachycardia (especially if there is associated AV block), electric shock should be used in progressively increasing amounts beginning with 10 wattseconds. If ventricular premature beats develop, use lidocaine (Xylocaine), 50–100 mg IV, and, if the premature beats disappear, one can repeat the shock. Cardioversion should be abandoned for the time being if the premature beats recur. Alternatively, rapid atrial pacing may terminate the attack and may be the preferred treatment if digitalis excess is present, and Wolff-Parkinson-White syndrome is not present. External radiofrequency stimulation of an artificial ventricular pacemaker may stop the attack by interrupting the reentry cycle through the mechanism of a beat that fortuitously enters the AV node, making it refractory to the circus pathway.

Bigger JT Jr, Goldreyer BN: Mechanism of supraventricular tachycardia. Circulation 42:673, 1973.

Goldreyer BN, Gallagher JJ, Damato AN: The electrophysiologic demonstration of atrial ectopic tachycardia in man. Am Heart J 85:205, 1973.

Pittman DE & others: Rapid atrial stimulation: Successful method of conversion of atrial flutter and atrial tachycardia. Am J Cardiol 32:700, 1973.

Rutkowski MM, Doyle EF, Cohen SN: Drug therapy of heart disease in pediatric patients. 3. The therapeutic challenge of supraventricular tachyarrhythmias in infants and children. Am Heart J 86:562, 1973.

Ticzon AR, Whalen RW: Refractory supraventricular tachycardias. Circulation 47:652, 1973.

Vergara GS & others: Conversion of supraventricular tachycardias with rapid atrial stimulation. Circulation 46:788, 1972.

ATRIAL FIBRILLATION

Atrial fibrillation is the commonest chronic arrhythmia. It occurs most frequently in rheumatic heart disease, especially mitral stenosis, and arteriosclerotic heart disease. It may appear paroxysmally before becoming the established rhythm in thyrotoxicosis. Infection, trauma, surgery, poisoning, or excessive alcohol intake may cause attacks of atrial fibrillation in patients with normal hearts. It is the only common arrhythmia in which the ventricular rate is rapid and the rhythm irregular. An ectopic atrial pacemaker fires 400–600 times/minute. The impulses pass through the atria at varying speeds and are mostly blocked at the AV node. The ventricular response is completely irregular, ranging from 80–160 beats/minute in the untreated state. Because of the varying stroke volumes induced by the varying periods of diastolic filling, not all ventricular beats result in a palpable peripheral pulse. The difference between the apical rate and pulse rate is the "pulse deficit"; this deficit is greater when the ventricular rate is high. Exercise intensifies the irregularity when the heart rate is slow. Carotid sinus massage has no or little effect.

Prevention

See Paroxysmal Atrial Tachycardia, above.

Treatment

A. Paroxysmal Atrial Fibrillation:

1. Digitalis—Digitalis is the drug of choice, especially when the arrhythmia occurs in persons with organic heart disease (particularly mitral stenosis) or with rapid ventricular rates, or when the symptoms or signs of cardiac failure have appeared. *Note:* Digitalis should not be used when atrial fibrillation occurs in Wolff-Parkinson-White syndrome; it may decrease AV conduction in the normal pathway and enhance it in the aberrant pathway, possibly resulting in very rapid ventricular rates.

In case of doubt about whether to use quinidine or digitalis first in the ordinary patient, digitalis should be given because it controls the ventricular rate by producing an AV block, which is the immediate objective of treatment. The objective of treatment with quinidine or DC cardioversion is to abolish the atrial ectopic rhythm, and it is quite safe to wait until the ventricular rate is brought under control with digitalis. Give full digitalizing doses, with the objective of slowing the ventricular rate to 70–80/minute and avoiding toxic manifestations. In paroxysmal fibrillation there is no clear evidence that the use of digitalis will result in established fibrillation.

2. Cardioversion—In cases where an attack of atrial fibrillation persists in an otherwise normal heart with a ventricular rate under 140 and with no other symptoms or signs of cardiac failure, cardioversion may be used at once to convert the rhythm to sinus rhythm. Quinidine is used rarely today to effect conversion to sinus rhythm.

B. Chronic Atrial Fibrillation: Opinion varies, but the following indications for conversion of atrial fibrillation serve as a general guide. Each case must be individualized. In general, conversion is attempted whenever it is thought that the patient will be better off with sinus rhythm than with atrial fibrillation: (1) Atrial fibrillation persisting after thyrotoxicosis has been treated surgically or by other means. (2) Atrial fibrillation of a few weeks' duration in an individual with no or only slight cardiac disease. (3) Atrial fibrillation associated with frequent embolic phenomena. (4) Refractory cardiac failure induced by the atrial fibrillation. (5) Severe palpitations due to inability to decrease the ventricular rate with digitalis; this may be obvious only on exertion. (6) Atrial fibrillation appearing for the first time postoperatively in patients with a technically successful mitral valvulotomy.

1. Digitalis—Thorough digitalization is the first step. The patient is then usually placed on maintenance digitalis indefinitely. The object of digitalization is to slow the ventricular rate and to improve myocardial efficiency, but digitalis toxicity is to be avoided and digitalis is stopped for 2 days before cardioversion.

2. Countershock—Synchronized DC countershock, 2.5 mscc, 10–400 watt-seconds, under general anesthesia, has converted many patients to sinus rhythm even when quinidine has failed or was not tolerated in adequate dosage. It is now the procedure of choice in converting chronic atrial fibrillation (or flutter). DC shock should be avoided in the presence of digitalis toxicity. Relapses have been a problem, and further work is required to determine the long-term benefits.

3. Quinidine is used to abolish the ectopic rhythm once the ventricular rate is controlled with digitalis if the countershock is not available. It is potentially hazardous and should be used only in carefully selected cases by a physician thoroughly familiar with the drug and by a method which ensures close medical supervision (preferably in the hospital), while conversion to sinus rhythm is being attempted. Maintenance doses are used following conversion with countershock to maintain sinus rhythm. *Caution:* See p 237 for dangers of quinidine therapy.

4. Propranolol (Inderal), 10–40 mg 3–4 times daily, may be used to slow the ventricular rate when this fails to occur satisfactorily with digitalis. Use *cautiously* (if at all) in the presence of cardiac failure, heart block, or bronchospasm.

Cramer G: Early and late results of conversion of atrial fibrillation with quinidine: A clinical and hemodynamic study. Acta med scandinav, Suppl 490, 1968.

Hillestad L & others: Quinidine in maintenance of sinus rhythm after electroconversion of chronic atrial fibrillation. Brit Heart J 33:518, 1971.

Hornsten TR, Bruce RA: Effects of atrial fibrillation on exercise performance in patients with cardiac disease. Circulation 37:543, 1968.

Hurst JW & others: Management of patients with atrial fibrillation. Am J Med 37:728, 1964.

Kleiger R, Lown B: Cardioversion and digitalis. 2. Clinical

studies. Circulation 33:878, 1966.

Lown B: Electrical reversion of cardiac arrhythmias. Brit Heart J 29:469, 1967.

Sokolow M, Ball RE: Factors influencing conversion of chronic atrial fibrillation with special reference to serum quinidine concentration. Circulation 14:568, 1956.

Vassaux C, Lown B: Cardioversion of supraventricular tachycardias. Circulation 39:791, 1969.

ATRIAL FLUTTER

Atrial flutter is uncommon and usually occurs in patients with rheumatic or coronary heart disease, cor pulmonale, atrial septal defect, or as a result of quinidine effect on atrial fibrillation. Ectopic impulse formation occurs at rates of 250–350, with transmission of every 2nd, 3rd, or 4th impulse through the AV node to the ventricles. The ventricular rate is usually ½ the atrial rate (2:1 block), or 150/minute. Carotid sinus massage causes sudden slowing or standstill, with rapid return of the rate to the original level on release of pressure. When the ventricular rate is 75 (4:1 block), exercise may cause sudden doubling of the rate to 150 (2:1 block). The first heart sound varies slightly in intensity from beat to beat.

Prevention

Similar to prevention of atrial tachycardia.

Treatment

A. Paroxysmal Atrial Flutter: Treatment is similar to that of paroxysmal atrial tachycardia except that digitalis is the drug of choice. The arrhythmia tends to become established more often than does atrial or nodal tachycardia.

B. Chronic Atrial Flutter:

1. Digitalis is the drug of choice. It increases the AV block and prevents a 2:1 or 1:1 conduction. In about half of cases atrial fibrillation or sinus rhythm results from full digitalization. Digitalis may be given by any of the usual methods. Oral medication is usually sufficient, although the intravenous route may be used if the situation is critical and DC cardioversion is not available. Digitalis must often be given in larger doses than are usually required for cardiac failure. When a fixed 4:1 conduction is produced by digitalis, a slightly increased dose may convert the flutter to atrial fibrillation or sinus rhythm; or DC countershock may be used.

2. Propranolol (Inderal) may be used as in atrial fibrillation to slow the ventricular rate if this is difficult with digitalis. (See Atrial Fibrillation, above).

3. DC countershock as in atrial fibrillation (see above). This is rapidly becoming the treatment of choice because of the ease and effectiveness of the procedure in restoring sinus rhythm and because the toxic effects of large doses of digitalis and quinidine can be avoided.

4. Quinidine should not as a rule be used to treat atrial flutter unless the patient is fully digitalized with a slow ventricular rate, because of the danger of producing a 1:1 conduction. If digitalis results in only a 4:1 conduction or produces atrial fibrillation which does not spontaneously convert to sinus rhythm, quinidine may be given if DC cardioversion is not available.

AV NODAL (JUNCTIONAL) RHYTHM

The AV node or the atrial-nodal junction or the nodal-His bundle junction may assume pacemaker activity for the heart, usually at a rate of 40–60 beats/minute. This may occur in normal hearts, myocarditis, coronary artery disease, or as a result of digitalis therapy. The rate responds normally to exercise, and the diagnosis is often a surprise finding on ECG. Careful examination of the jugular pulse may reveal the presence of cannon waves. Patients are often asymptomatic. Digitalis toxicity must be considered in each case.

Junctional rhythm is often an escape rhythm and may occur with sinus pauses or SA block in the so-called sick sinus syndrome (see above).

AV NODAL (JUNCTIONAL) TACHYCARDIA

This arrhythmia is due to rapid, regular impulse formation in the AV nodal junction or bundle of His with regular transmission to the ventricles. The usual rates are 140–240/minute. Nodal or junctional tachycardia may be a benign condition or may reflect serious myocardial disease; it is more common than other arrhythmias in cor pulmonale and may often be the result of digitalis toxicity, which increases the rate of impulse formation in subsidiary pacemaker cells. Aberrant conduction often makes the distinction from ventricular tachycardia difficult, especially if there is retrograde conduction to the atria. The width of the QRS complexes and the direction of the initial QRS vector in the right precordial leads are useful. In supraventricular tachycardia with aberrancy, the QRS width is often only minimally increased and the initial vector in V_1 is similar to the pattern seen normally in right bundle branch block. In ventricular tachycardia, the QRS is much wider and the initial vector in V_1 does not resemble right bundle branch block.

In the diagnosis of supraventricular arrhythmias with aberrant conduction and their differentiation from ventricular arrhythmias, His bundle electrograms may be very helpful. A bipolar or tripolar catheter can be inserted percutaneously via the femoral vein and positioned in the right ventricle in the region of the tricuspid valve. It is then possible to record impulses from the atria, bundle of His, and His-Purkinje-ventricular system. In any given arrhythmia, one can see whether the His bundle spikes precede each QRS complex, in which case the rhythm originates above the ventricles. If the ventricular complex is not preceded by a His spike or atrial activity, the ectopic focus arises distal to the bundle of His. One can determine the interval between the atrial spike and the His spike and between the His spike and the beginning of the QRS to determine where AV conduction delays occur. His bundle recordings are also valuable in atrial fibrillation to distinguish between aberrant conduction from a rapid ventricular rate and ventricular premature beats, or ventricular tachycardia. If the His spike precedes each ventricular complex in the ECG, ventricular tachycardia is excluded.

If the diagnosis can be made by clinical and routine electrocardiography, the cost and hazards of cardiac catheterization should be avoided.

Treatment is along the same lines as for atrial tachycardia.

Easley RM Jr, Goldstein S: Differentiation of ventricular tachycardia from junctional tachycardia with aberrant conduction: The use of competitive atrial pacing. Circulation 37:1015, 1968.

Konecke LL, Knoebel SB: Nonparoxysmal junctional tachycardia complicating acute myocardial infarction. Circulation 45:367, 1972.

Lindsay AE, Schamroth L: Atrioventricular junctional parasystole with concealed conduction simulating second degree atrioventricular block. Am J Cardiol 31:397, 1973.

Marriott HJL: Differential diagnosis of supraventricular and ventricular tachycardia. Geriatrics 25:91, 1970.

Rosen KM: Junctional tachycardia: Mechanisms, diagnosis, differential diagnosis and management. Circulation 47:654, 1973.

VENTRICULAR PREMATURE BEATS

Ventricular premature beats are similar to atrial premature beats in mechanism and manifestations but are much more common. Together, they are the commonest causes of a grossly irregular rhythm with a normal heart rate. Ectopic impulse formation causes ventricular contraction to occur sooner than the next expected beat. The sound of this contraction is audible and is followed by a longer than normal pause since the next expected beat does not occur (compensatory pause). The interval between the preceding normal beat and the beat following the compensatory pause is exactly twice the normal interval between beats in the case of ventricular premature beats, and slightly less than this with atrial premature beats. Single premature beats which occur after every normal beat produce bigeminy. Exercise generally abolishes premature beats, and the rhythm becomes regular.

Premature beats have no definite significance unless they arise from multiple foci, occur with rapid ventricular rates or in runs, or appear when digitalis is given. Sudden death occurs more frequently (presumably as a result of ventricular fibrillation) when ventric-

ular premature beats occur in the presence of known coronary disease but not otherwise. Often, no organic heart disease can be found.

Treatment

If no associated cardiac disease is present and if the ectopic beats are infrequent, occur late in diastole, and produce no palpitations, no specific therapy is indicated.

If ventricular premature beats are due to digitalis toxicity, withdraw digitalis and diuretics for 3–5 days or until the arrhythmia disappears and then resume medication in smaller dosage. Phenytoin (Dilantin) may be of value (see below). At times, however, patients with cardiac failure who are receiving digitalis may develop ventricular premature beats which are due not to digitalis toxicity but to inadequate digitalization and cardiac failure. If in doubt as to the cause, withdraw digitalis for several days and treat the cardiac failure with other available methods (see p 217). In these circumstances, the ventricular premature beats often disappear as the cardiac failure improves.

Potassium chloride, 1–3 gm 4 times daily, is often helpful in ventricular premature beats of digitalis origin.

Quinidine or procainamide should be used orally to abolish ventricular premature beats when they occur in runs or from several foci in patients with heart disease. For premature beats in myocardial infarction, see p 198.

Blackburn H & others: Premature ventricular complexes induced by stress testing: Their frequency and response to physical conditioning. Am J Cardiol 31:441, 1973.

Goldschlager N, Cake D, Cohn K: Exercise-induced ventricular arrhythmias in patients with coronary artery disease. Am J Cardiol 31:434, 1973.

Jelinek MV, Lohrbauer L, Lown B: Antiarrhythmic drug therapy for sporadic ventricular ectopic arrhythmias. Circulation 49:659, 1974.

Lown B & others: Sleep and ventricular premature beats. Circulation 48:691, 1973.

PAROXYSMAL VENTRICULAR TACHYCARDIA

This is an uncommon serious arrhythmia due to rapid ectopic impulse formation in the ventricles. The rate may be 160–240. It usually lasts hours but may persist for days if untreated. The rhythm is almost completely regular but is less regular than in atrial tachycardia, and the first sound may vary slightly in intensity from beat to beat. Carotid sinus massage has no effect.

Paroxysmal ventricular tachycardia usually occurs after myocardial infarction or as a result of digitalis toxicity. Pain due to myocardial ischemia, fall in blood pressure, and shock are common.

Prevention

The drugs of choice are quinidine and procainamide or, if ventricular premature beats occur during acute myocardial infarction, a constant infusion of lidocaine (Xylocaine) at a rate of 1–2 mg/minute.

Treatment

A. Average Case:

1. **DC countershock** has replaced pharmacologic methods of treatment of ventricular tachycardia in all but the mildest cases.

2. **Lidocaine (Xylocaine)**, 50–100 mg IV followed by 1–4 mg/minute IV, has largely replaced quinidine and procainamide because of its short duration of action and infrequent hypotensive effect (see below).

3. **Quinidine**, 0.4 gm orally every 2 hours for 3 doses, if the attack is well tolerated and the patient is not in shock and if DC cardioversion is not available. If the attack continues and there is no toxicity from the quinidine, increase the dose to 0.6 gm orally every 2 hours for 3 doses or use DC countershock. If countershock is not available and the larger oral dosage of quinidine is not successful, change to procainamide.

4. **Procainamide hydrochloride (Pronestyl)**, 0.5–1.5 gm orally every 4–6 hours, may be substituted for quinidine if quinidine is ineffective or produces toxic symptoms.

5. **Phenytoin (Dilantin)** 5 mg/kg IV or 100–250 mg IV very slowly, has been used with success in ventricular arrhythmias, especially when they are due to digitalis. Sinus rhythm may be induced, and digitalis-induced ventricular arrhythmias may be prevented when DC shock is given. Slow administration and careful ECG and blood pressure monitoring are necessary.

B. More Severe Case: (Or when other medication has failed.)

1. **DC countershock** (see above).

2. **Lidocaine (Xylocaine)** 50–100 mg IV, repeated if necessary.

3. **Procainamide hydrochloride (Pronestyl)**, 0.5–1 gm, may be given IM and repeated in 4 hours; or IV, 100 mg every 5 minutes.

4. **Quinidine gluconate**, 0.8 gm or 0.5 gm of quinidine base, may be given IM and repeated every 2 hours for 2–3 doses.

5. **Propranolol (Inderal)** may be given slowly IV in 1 mg doses under constant clinical ECG monitoring. The precautions noted under the atrial arrhythmias should be observed. Propranolol is rarely used in ventricular tachycardia unless cardioversion is not available.

C. Urgent Case:

1. **DC countershock,** depolarizing the entire heart, has proved of great value in patients not responding to lidocaine or procainamide, even in acute myocardial infarction. Under general anesthesia or intravenous diazepam (Valium), a DC shock, synchronized to the downstroke of the R wave of the ECG, 2.5 msec in duration, and 50–400 watt-seconds, can be given.

2. **Lidocaine (Xylocaine)**, 1 mg/kg in 1 or 2% solution (50–100 mg for an adult), given IV has proved effective. If the arrhythmia recurs, one may give an IV infusion of 50 mg/hour (1 gm diluted to 1 liter of 5% glucose) (about 1–2 mg/minute) or repeat the intravenous injection twice at 20-minute intervals.

3. **Procainamide hydrochloride (Pronestyl)**, 1 gm *slowly* IV (at a rate not to exceed 100 mg/minute). During the infusion, continuous ECG or, at least, repeated blood pressure determinations are essential. Severe hypotension may result from the medication.

4. **Quinidine** may be given IV as quinidine gluconate, 0.8 gm diluted with 50 ml of 5% glucose *slowly* (1 ml/minute), with continuous ECG and determination of blood pressure. When giving intravenous quinidine in severe cases (particularly when the previous rhythm was complete AV block), the physician should be alert to the possibility of precipitating ventricular fibrillation or asystole. (See Heart-Lung Resuscitation.)

5. **Propranolol (Inderal)** may be given as for more severe cases (above).

6. **Vasopressor drugs for shock**—If shock is present as a result of ventricular tachycardia or results from the drugs given intravenously, it can be treated with vasopressor drugs as described under the treatment of shock (see Chapter 1).

7. **Other drugs**—(1) Magnesium sulfate, 10 ml of a 20% solution, may be given *slowly* IV. Calcium salts should be readily available to counteract magnesium toxicity. (2) Intravenous morphine or meperidine (Demerol) is sometimes successful.

8. **Digitalis** is usually contraindicated in ventricular tachycardia; however, in some patients with cardiac failure in whom the above-mentioned drugs have failed to restore sinus rhythm, full digitalization, given carefully, has been successful.

9. **Temporary transvenous cardiac pacing** may capture the rhythm from the ectopic ventricular tachycardia and has been used when anti-arrhythmia drugs have failed.

Bigger JT Jr, Heissenbuttel RH: Clinical use of antiarrhythmic drugs. Postgrad Med 47:119, 1970.

Bleifer SB & others: Relation between premature ventricular complexes and development of ventricular tachycardia. Am J Cardiol 31:400, 1973.

Collinsworth KA, Kalman SM, Harrison DC: The clinical pharmacology of lidocaine as an antiarrhythmic drug. Circulation 50:1217, 1974.

Cranefield PF: Ventricular fibrillation. New England J Med 289:732, 1973.

Helfant RH & others: The clinical use of DPH (Dilantin) in the treatment and prevention of cardiac arrhythmias. Am Heart J 77:315, 1969.

Johnson RA & others: Chronic overdrive pacing in the control of refractory ventricular arrhythmias. Ann Int Med 80:380, 1974.

Kiss ZS, Smith D, Sloman G: Electrical cardiac pacing in patients without heart block. Australasian Ann Med 19:220, 1970.

Lown B, Temte JV, Arter WJ: Ventricular tachyarrhythmias: Clinical aspects. Circulation 47:1364, 1973.

Massumi RA, Tawakkol AA, Kistin AD: Reevaluation of electrocardiographic and bedside criteria for diagnosis of ventricular tachycardia. Circulation 36:628, 1967.

VENTRICULAR FLUTTER & FIBRILLATION

These arrhythmias represent more advanced stages of ventricular tachycardia in which the rate of impulse formation is more rapid and transmission becomes irregular, resulting in ineffective ventricular contractions. Diagnosis can be established only by ECG. Ventricular flutter-fibrillation is rapidly fatal unless terminated by defibrillation. It is usually associated with severe myocardial damage, but may be precipitated by epinephrine, quinidine, or digitalis.

Treatment

A. Surgical and Mechanical Measures: External cardiac massage and prompt ventilation until electric defibrillation is the treatment of choice (see Appendix). Continuous monitoring of patients with acute myocardial infarction has shown at least half of sudden expected deaths to be due to ventricular fibrillation. Prompt treatment may be lifesaving. Surgical exposure of the heart with direct cardiac massage is infrequently performed today except during cardiac operations.

B. Medical Treatment: Usually ineffective. In paroxysmal episodes, try to prevent (as in ventricular tachycardia).

Bennett MA, Pentecost BL: Warning of cardiac arrest due to ventricular fibrillation and tachycardia. Lancet 1:1351, 1972.

Liberthson RR & others: Prehospital ventricular defibrillation: Prognosis and follow-up course. New England J Med 291:317, 1974.

DISTURBANCES OF CONDUCTION

SINO-ATRIAL (SA) BLOCK
(See p 203.)

In SA block the normal pacemaker fails to initiate the depolarizing impulse at irregular or regular intervals or, rarely, in a fixed 2:1 ratio. This failure is apparently due to heightened vagal tone and is not usually related to the presence of heart disease but may be due to digitalis. Exercise and atropine therefore abolish SA block. This arrhythmia can be recognized by the fact that no sound is audible during the prolonged interval between beats (in contrast to ventricular premature beats). There are no symptoms unless the period of standstill extends over the span of several beats, in which case momentary faintness or even syncope may occur. In susceptible individuals, carotid sinus massage induces SA block. The sick sinus syndrome, in which SA block is combined with sinus arrest, sinus bradycardia, and paroxysmal atrial arrhythmia, is discussed under sinus bradycardia, above.

Treatment

In most cases no treatment is required. The causative factors, especially digitalis, should be eliminated if possible. The following drugs may be tried: (1) Atropine sulfate, 0.6 mg 4 times daily orally. (2) Ephedrine sulfate, 25 mg orally 4 times daily. In more prolonged cases, give atropine, 0.5–1 mg IV. When SA block is associated with the sick sinus syndrome with paroxysmal atrial arrhythmias, therapy requires a combination of a transvenous artificial pacemaker and antiarrhythmic drug as described under sinus bradycardia.

ATRIOVENTRICULAR CONDUCTION SYSTEM
(Bundle Branch Block)
(See p 201.)

Conduction of the cardiac impulse from the atria to the ventricles should be considered as a continuous system: the impulse originates normally in the SA node and passes via various internodal tracts to the AV node. From here, the impulse spreads via the bundle of His into a trifascicular branching system consisting of a right bundle and the left anterior superior and left posterior inferior branches of the left bundle. Conduction then continues via the Purkinje system to the ventricular myocardium. Atrioventricular block may occur anywhere between the atrioventricular node to involvement of both bundle branches. Block need not be due to disease in the AV node itself; His bundle recordings have demonstrated that the site of the block or blocks can be single or multiple and may be localized in the AV node, the bundle of His, or anywhere in the conduction system distal to the bundle of His. Bilateral bundle branch block, involving both bundles, the common bundle, or the right bundle and one of the left branches, have all been shown to be involved in some cases of AV block. Stressing the conduction system by increasing the heart rate by atrial pacing can produce AV block, usually proximal to the bundle of His.

Conduction defects may be due to drugs (such as digitalis), coronary heart disease, acute inflammatory myocarditis or rheumatic fever, or fibrosis of the conduction system of the cardiac skeleton. The last is being recognized with increasing frequency.

Prognosis and treatment may vary depending on whether the block is proximal or distal to the bundle of His. The prognosis is better when the block is proximal. The data are incomplete, and more prospective clinical studies will be required before one will be able to predict when complete AV block and Stokes-Adams attacks are likely to occur and when an artificial pacemaker should be used. His bundle recordings—in conjunction with clinical studies—have demonstrated that block is almost always in the AV node when there is only partial AV block with prolonged P—R interval or when the second degree AV block (see below) is characterized by the Wenckebach phenomenon, with partial progressive P—R delay with dropped beats, and when QRS complexes are narrow. This is the usual situation in congenital atrioventricular block and in inferior myocardial infarction. Syncope and Stokes-Adams attacks are uncommon. In contrast, the conduction defect is almost always distal to the AV node, with a greater likelihood of the development of complete AV block, syncope, and sudden death; when there is Mobitz type II or second degree AV conduction defect with dropped beats not preceded by progressive delay of previous P—R intervals; when the QRS complex is widened; and when the AV conduction defects occur in the setting of anterior myocardial infarction.

If one studies patients with right or left bundle branch blocks with His bundle technics, AV conduction defects are occasionally found when not seen in the ordinary ECG; in others, they may appear with the passage of time. A combination which is prone to AV block is right bundle branch block and left anterior hemiblock, with a frontal plane axis of approximately −45 to −60 degrees. This bifascicular block may be present for months or years without symptoms or AV conduction delay. However, about 10% of these patients subsequently develop AV block, making the block trifascicular, which is associated with an increased likelihood of Stokes-Adams attacks. Further prospective studies are needed to clarify the indications for prophylactic use of artificial demand pacemakers, which currently are used when bifascicular block occurs in anterior myocardial infarction or with symptoms of syncope.

Partial AV block. Partial AV block consists of prolongation of the conduction time of the normal impulse from the atria to the ventricles; as indicated above, this can occur distal as well as proximal to the bundle of His. AV block is classified by the degree of block: In partial AV block, the P—R interval is prolonged to 0.21 second or more (at normal heart rates), but every atrial impulse reaches the ventricles. Its presence can be suspected clinically when the first heart sound is faint in the presence of a vigorous apical impulse. There may be a presystolic gallop rhythm due to audible atrial contraction.

Second degree AV block. In second degree AV block the delay in conduction increases to the point where every sinus impulse does not reach the ventricles, resulting in failure of a ventricular contraction, ie, every so often a beat is dropped. After a beat is dropped, the AV conduction system recovers, and in 2:1 block the next P—R is usually normal. The cycle may be repeated regularly or irregularly, producing a 2:1, 3:1, or other intervals of rhythm. Dropped beats are distinguished from premature beats by the fact that during the interval between peripheral pulses there is no sound at the apex as well as no beat felt at the

wrist, whereas in premature beats there may be no beat felt at the wrist but one can hear a faint premature beat at the apex.

Second degree AV block is divided into (1) Mobitz type I with partial progressive AV block and dropped beats (Wenckebach pauses) and (2) Mobitz type II with intermittent dropped beats not preceded by a prolonged P—R interval. As indicated in the section on myocardial infarction, Mobitz type I usually occurs when the conduction defect is in the AV node— as during an inferior myocardial infarction—and infrequently leads to Stokes-Adams attacks. Type II is due to a block in or distal to the bundle of His. It is more apt to occur in anterior myocardial infarction and frequently leads to Stokes-Adams attacks with complete AV block and, therefore, requires artificial pacing.

Complete (third degree) heart block is a more advanced form of block. Complete AV block is usually due to a lesion distal to the His bundle and associated with bilateral bundle branch block; occasionally, the block is proximal to the bundle of His. In the latter, the QRS is usually (but not always) normal in width (less than 0.12 second) and the ventricular rate is faster—usually greater than 50/minute. In the former, the QRS is wide and the ventricular rate is slower, usually less than 50/minute. Inferior infarction causes ischemia of the AV node from a compromised nodal artery from the right coronary, whereas anterior infarction results in destruction of the ventricular septum with bilateral bundle branch block. Transmission of atrial impulses through the AV node is completely blocked, and a ventricular pacemaker maintains a slow, regular ventricular rate, usually less than 45 beats/minute. Exercise does not increase the rate. The first heart sound varies greatly in loudness; wide pulse pressure, changing systolic blood pressure level, and cannon venous pulsations in the neck are also present. Patients may be asymptomatic or complain of weakness or dyspnea if the rate is less than 35/minute—at times at even higher rates if the left ventricle cannot increase its stroke output. During periods of transition from partial to complete heart block, certain patients have ventricular asystole which lasts several seconds to minutes. Syncope occurs abruptly, and if the asystole is prolonged beyond a few seconds convulsive movements appear (Stokes-Adams syndrome). Asystole of 2—3 minutes is usually fatal.

Treatment

A. Prolonged Conduction and Incomplete Heart Block: In the absence of Stokes-Adams syndrome (see below), treatment of AV conduction defects is rarely successful except by elimination of drugs, if they are causative, or by the subsidence of acute myocarditis. Prolongation of the AV conduction itself usually needs no treatment (except careful observation) unless there is complete heart block (see below) or in anterior infarction, especially if the AV conduction defect is associated with left anterior hemiblock or bundle branch block. Cardiac failure or weakness may occur with slow ventricular rates. Ephedrine or isoproterenol should be given to increase the rate of the ventricular pacemaker (see below).

See p 210 for a discussion of the danger of complete AV block in patients with partial AV block and bundle branch block.

B. Complete Heart Block and Stokes-Adams Syndrome: Try to eliminate or treat the cause. The objective of treatment is to obtain an idioventricular pacemaker discharging at a rate of at least 40/minute or more, but data with artificial pacing indicate that a ventricular rate of 70 is superior.

1. Artificial transvenous or transventricular pacemaker—Implantation of myocardial electrodes with platinum wires tunneled to a zinc-cadmium battery placed subcutaneously in the abdomen has been largely replaced by transvenous introduction of the electrode catheter into the right ventricle. Dramatic improvement in cardiac failure, cerebral symptoms, and syncopal attacks has resulted in earlier use of artificial pacing in many patients. When syncopal attacks have occurred, a catheter pacemaker may be lifesaving.

Pacemakers are now introduced following a single proved Stokes-Adams attack, and are used with increasing frequency when slow ventricular rates induce cerebral or cardiac insufficiency. Follow-up of patients with pacemakers is essential to establish early the presence of faulty functioning.

When AV block is intermittent but causing syncope, a demand pacemaker is preferable because it is activated only during bradycardia, thus decreasing the likelihood of ventricular fibrillation caused by stimulation of the heart during the vulnerable period resulting from competition between the natural and artificial pacemakers.

2. Isoproterenol hydrochloride, 5—15 mg, may be given sublingually 3 or 4 times daily or oftener, or by IV infusion, 2—15 mg/500 ml.

3. Ephedrine sulfate, 25—60 mg orally 4 times daily, is often effective. The dose must be sufficient to prevent the attacks. If necessary, secobarbital sodium, 30 mg, may be given with each dose of ephedrine.

4. Epinephrine—If attacks are frequent and are not controlled with ephedrine or isoproterenol, epinephrine, 0.5 ml of 1:1000 solution, may be given every 8 hours as needed, or 0.2 ml of a 1:1000 solution may be given subcutaneously every 2 hours. Epinephrine is used less often than (1) and (2) above, but epinephrine is valuable if procedures (1) and (2) are not available.

5. Intracardiac epinephrine injection, 0.5 ml of a 1:1000 solution, may be given if cardiac standstill persists.

6. Corticosteroids occasionally reverse complete AV block if it is of recent onset.

Cannom DS, Goldreyer BN, Damato AN: Atrioventricular conduction system in left bundle-branch block with normal QRS axis. Circulation 46:129, 1972.

Castellanos A Jr, Lemberg L: Diagnosis of isolated and combined block in the bundle branches and the divisions of the left branch. Circulation 43:971, 1971.

Clarke M, Keith JD: Atrioventricular conduction in acute rheumatic fever. Brit Heart J 34:472, 1972.

Conklin EF & others: Use of the permanent transvenous pacemaker in 168 consecutive patients. Am Heart J 82:4, 1971.

Dhingra RC & others: The significance of second degree atrioventricular block and bundle branch block: Observations regarding site and type of block. Circulation 49:638, 1974.

Dhingra RC & others: Syncope in patients with chronic bifascicular block: Significance, causative mechanisms, and clinical implications. Ann Int Med 81:302, 1974.

Gallagher JJ & others: Manifest and concealed reentry: A mechanism of AV nodal Wenckebach in man. Circulation 47:752, 1973.

Gilcrest AR: Clinical aspects of high grade heart block. Scot Med J 3:53, 1958.

Harris A & others: Aetiology of chronic heart block: A clinicopathological correlation of 65 cases. Brit Heart J 31:206, 1969.

Helfant RH, Scherlag BJ: *His Bundle Electrocardiography.* Medcom Press, 1974.

Hudson REB: Surgical pathology of the conducting system of the heart. Brit Heart J 29:646, 1967.

Jensen G & others: Adams-Stokes syndrome caused by paroxysmal third-degree atrioventricular block. Brit Heart J 35:516, 1973.

Langendorf R & others: Observations on second degree atrioventricular block, including new criteria for the differential diagnosis between type I and type II block. Am J Cardiol 29:1, 1972.

Lie KI & others: Factors influencing prognosis of bundle branch block complicating acute antero-septal infarction: The value of His bundle recordings. Circulation 50:935, 1974.

Lown B, Kosowsky BD: Artificial cardiac pacemakers. (3 parts.) New England J Med 283:907, 971, 1023, 1970.

Luy G, Bahl OP, Massie E: Intermittent left bundle branch block. Am Heart J 85:332, 1973.

Medrano GA & others: Clinical electrocardiographic and vectorcardiographic diagnosis of left posterior subdivision block, isolated or associated with RBBB. Am Heart J 84:727, 1972.

Merideth J, Pruitt RD: Disturbances in cardiac conduction and their management. Circulation 47:1098, 1973.

Narula OS, Samet P: Right bundle branch block with normal, left or right axis deviation: Analysis by His bundle recordings. Am J Med 51:432, 1971.

Narula OS & others: Atrioventricular block: Localization and classification by His bundle recordings. Am J Med 50:146, 1971.

Norris RM: Heart block in posterior and anterior myocardial infarction. Brit Heart J 31:352, 1969.

Pick A, Langendorf R: The dual function of the A-V junction. Am Heart J 88:790, 1974.

Pomerantz B, O'Rourke RA: The Stokes-Adams syndrome. Am J Med 46:941, 1969.

Roberts N, Olley P: His bundle electrogram in children: Statistical correlation of the atrioventricular conduction times in children with their age and heart rate. Brit Heart J 34:1099, 1972.

Rosen KM & others: Chronic heart block in adults: Clinical and electrophysiological observations. Arch Int Med 131:663, 1973.

Rosenbaum MB: The hemiblocks: Diagnostic criteria and clinical significance. Mod Concepts Cardiovas Dis 39:141, 1970.

Scheinman M, Brenman B: Clinical and anatomic implications of intraventricular conduction blocks in acute myocardial infarction. Circulation 46:753, 1972.

Scheinman M, Weiss A, Kunkel F: His bundle recordings in patients with bundle branch block and transient neurologic symptoms. Circulation 48:322, 1973.

Siddons H, Sowton E: *Cardiac Pacemakers.* Thomas, 1967.

Smithen CS & others: Analysis of heart block and dysrhythmias by His bundle electrograms. Cardiovas Res 6:129, 1972.

Spurrell RAJ, Smithen CS, Sowton E: Study of right bundle-branch block in association with either left anterior hemiblock or left posterior hemiblock using His bundle electrograms. Brit Heart J 34:800, 1972.

Thilenius OG & others: Hemodynamic studies in children with congenital atrioventricular block. Am J Cardiol 30:13, 1972.

Titus JL: Cardiac arrhythmias. 1. Anatomy of the conduction system. Circulation 47:170, 1973.

Watanabe Y, Dreifus LS: Levels of concealment in second degree and advanced second degree AV block. Am Heart J 84:330, 1972.

See also references for Paroxysmal Ventricular Tachycardia.

ACCELERATED CONDUCTION SYNDROME
(Wolff-Parkinson-White Syndrome)
(Ventricular Preexcitation)

This condition is a form of ventricular preexcitation in which early activation of the ventricle occurs via accessory pathways that bypass the AV node, combined with normal spread of activation, producing fusion ventricular beats. The cardiac impulse is initiated (as normally) in the sinus node and then short-circuits the AV node in an anomalous fashion, usually via the lateral bundles of Kent but possibly also via the James fibers or the Mahaim fibers which spread from the bundle of His to the ventricular septum. The precise anatomy of the bypass tracks is not completely known but has been recently clarified by the use of epicardial mapping. Wolff-Parkinson-White syndrome may be constant or intermittent, the latter often brought on by a change in atrial rate.

Preexcitation has been characterized into different types depending upon the location of the accessory bypass tracks, but these are variable. Type A is from the left accessory bypass, producing an ECG pattern in V₁ of right ventricular hypertrophy or right bundle branch block; type B preexcitation results from early activation via the right lateral accessory pathway, producing an ECG pattern similar to that of left bundle branch block. In addition to the characteristic ECG changes (see below), Wolff-Parkinson-White syndrome is associated with frequent atrial paroxysmal arrhythmias, usually atrial tachycardia but occasionally atrial fibrillation. The mechanism of the atrial arrhythmia is thought to be reentry in which impulses from the atria pass through the normal AV conduction system to the ventricle and then return in retrograde fashion to the atria via the anomalous pathway. When the atria, the

atrioventricular junction, or the AV node is no longer refractory, the retrograde impulse may reexcite portions of the specialized normal AV pathway which conduct to the ventricles and so set up a self-perpetuating circuit. Recent electrophysiologic studies have shown that the circuit is antegrade through the normal AV pathway and retrograde through the anomalous pathway because the refractory period of the latter is shorter.

Clinical Findings

The diagnosis is usually made electrocardiographically, even in patients who do not have a history of paroxysmal arrhythmia. During the arrhythmia it may be difficult to see the characteristic pattern, especially if there is a rapid atrial rate. The typical findings include a short P–R interval, a wide QRS complex, and a slurred delta wave at the onset of the QRS, representing the bypass through the accessory pathway. The total P–R plus the QRS interval is essentially normal; it has been called "falsely long" bundle branch block. The delta wave is usually short—about 0.05 sec—and the P–R interval in some cases may be essentially normal. About half of patients have no symptoms, while the other half have episodes of paroxysmal atrial arrhythmia which may only be noted by 12- to 24-hour Holter monitoring. The arrhythmia may be the precipitating symptom in many patients, may last a few seconds and produce trivial or no symptoms, or may last hours and be disabling. It was formerly thought that death was rare during an attack of arrhythmia; this opinion has changed, possibly because of the very rapid ventricular rates which may occur if the patient has atrial fibrillation and the refractory period of the anomalous pathway is decreased by drugs such as digitalis.

Treatment

Asymptomatic patients in whom the condition is discovered by chance during a routine ECG should be alerted to the possibility of the development of atrial arrhythmias so that they can inform their physician—especially if the arrhythmia is atrial fibrillation, for which digitalis should not be used because it increases the block in the AV node while decreasing the refractory period of the anomalous pathway. The rapid atrial impulses may then be transmitted directly to the ventricle, and rapid ventricular rates or even ventricular fibrillation may ensue. The data on this point are incomplete, and more studies are required with respect to the use of digitalis in atrial fibrillation in patients with Wolff-Parkinson-White syndrome.

Patients who have episodes of paroxysmal atrial arrhythmias require a different approach; some authorities believe it wise to determine the refractory period of both the normal and the anomalous pathways to the ventricle so as to select drugs such as digitalis which do not decrease the refractory period of the anomalous pathway. Newer studies using His bundle recording and induced premature beats make this possible. Most cases of paroxysmal atrial tachycardia can be treated in the usual fashion by interrupting the reentry circuit by increasing the block in the AV node by maneuvers such as carotid sinus massage, by drugs that stimulate the vagus, or with digitalis if the rhythm is PAT and not atrial fibrillation (see PAT, above). Drugs that increase the block in the anomalous pathway may be helpful; of these, procainamide, propranolol, and quinidine are the most effective. Verapamil, not yet approved by the FDA, has little effect on the anomalous pathway and therefore may be particularly valuable in Wolff-Parkinson-White syndrome. Atrial pacing has been used for the reason that a random beat might by chance excite a portion of the reentrant pathway, making it refractory to the oncoming circus wave; there is a risk that atrial pacing may increase the impulses to the ventricles via the anomalous pathway and so raise the ventricular rate. DC shock (cardioversion) or procainamide or propranolol intravenously should be considered in emergency situations. If the attacks of atrial arrhythmia are frequent and are difficult to control, efforts to prevent the arrhythmia are indicated and constitute some of the recent developments in the field.

Prevention of Atrial Arrhythmias

Drugs that prevent the reentry phenomena by slowing conduction or increasing the refractory period of the AV node may all be helpful, as in PAT in the absence of Wolff-Parkinson-White syndrome. Quinidine, propranolol, and procainamide are valuable, and, if one is certain that atrial fibrillation is not the arrhythmia, digitalis may prevent the attacks. Drugs used in combination may sometimes be effective when one used singly is not. Side-effects from one may prevent it from being used to maximum effect, such as when bradycardia complicates propranolol. A ventricular pacemaker may be inserted and may be activated externally by a magnet or by radiofrequency, hoping that a chance premature beat may interrupt the reentry cycle.

Surgical resection of the anomalous pathway is being performed with increasing frequency, preceded by careful electrophysiologic studies and epicardial mapping to determine the area of earliest ventricular excitation at the time of surgery. When the anomalous pathway is clearly mapped, resection may interrupt the pathway and prevent both the delta wave and the subsequent arrhythmias. The sequence of ventricular activation varies in different patients, and new insights have been provided by Durrer, Wallace, and their groups, among others. Type B Wolff-Parkinson-White syndrome has been resected with more success because of its more accessible location, but recently type A has also been successfully resected. Observations on the accessory pathways are still being obtained, and it is now clear that Wolff-Parkinson-White syndrome is not uniform and requires careful study before surgical treatment is undertaken.

The forme fruste of Wolff-Parkinson-White syndrome, the so-called Lown-Ganong-Levine syndrome, with a short P–R and normal QRS without a delta wave, is thought to represent another variety of short-circuiting of the AV node; it also is associated with an increased frequency of paroxysmal atrial arrhythmias, but the author knows of no attempts at surgical correction. This may be because a dual pathway in the AV node rather than an accessory bypass track may be responsible for the preexcitation.

Boineau JP & others: Epicardial mapping in Wolff-Parkinson-White syndrome. Arch Int Med 135:422, 1975.

Caracta AR & others: Electrophysiologic studies in the syndrome of short P–R interval, normal QRS complex. Am J Cardiol 31:245, 1973.

Durrer D, Schuilenburg RM, Wellens HJJ: Pre-excitation revisited. Am J Cardiol 25:690, 1970.

Gallager JJ & others: Wolff-Parkinson-White syndrome: The problem, evaluation and surgical correction. Circulation 51:767, 1975.

Massumi RA, Vera Z: Patterns and mechanisms of QRS normalization in patients with Wolff-Parkinson-White syndrome. Am J Cardiol 28:541, 1971.

Moore EN, Spear JF, Boineau JP: Recent electrophysiologic studies on the Wolff-Parkinson-White syndrome. New England J Med 289:956, 1973.

Narula OS: Wolff-Parkinson-White syndrome: A review. Circulation 47:872, 1973.

Spurrell RAJ, Krikler DM, Sowton E: Effects of verapamil on electrophysiological properties of anomalous atrioventricular connexion in Wolff-Parkinson-White syndrome. Brit Heart J 36:256, 1974.

Spurrell RAJ, Krikler DM, Sowton E: Problems concerning assessment of anatomical site of accessory pathway in Wolff-Parkinson-White syndrome. Brit Heart J 37:127, 1975.

Wallace AG & others: Surgical correction of anomalous left ventricular pre-excitation: Wolff-Parkinson-White (type A). Circulation 49:206, 1974.

Wellens HJ, Durrer D: Effect of digitalis on atrioventricular conduction and circus-movement tachycardias in patients with Wolff-Parkinson-White syndrome. Circulation 47:1229, 1973.

Wellens HJ, Durrer D: Wolff-Parkinson-White syndrome and atrial fibrillation: Relation between refractory period of accessory pathway and ventricular rate during atrial fibrillation. Am J Cardiol 34:777, 1974.

CARDIAC FAILURE

Essentials of Diagnosis

Left Ventricular Failure:

- Exertional dyspnea, cough, fatigue, orthopnea, paroxysmal nocturnal dyspnea, cardiac enlargement, rales, gallop rhythm, and pulmonary venous congestion.

Right Ventricular Failure:

- Elevated venous pressure, hepatomegaly, dependent edema.

Both:

- Combination of above.

General Considerations

The function of the heart is to pump an adequate volume of blood (which it receives from the veins) to the various tissues of the body as required by their metabolic needs. Left ventricular performance is a function of preload, afterload, contractility, and heart rate. Various compensatory mechanisms are brought into play when the heart is diseased, when the work load is increased, or when the tissue demands are enhanced. When these compensatory methods fail, a clinical syndrome develops which may only be obvious when the demands on the heart are increased, as with exercise or emotion, but which may be absent at rest. Heart failure may be present, therefore, when the cardiac output is elevated, normal, or decreased with respect to the average; but regardless of the absolute level the cardiac output in cardiac failure is reduced relative to the metabolic demands of the body, assuming an adequate venous return. Markedly reduced venous return (as in hemorrhage) is peripheral vascular failure, not cardiac failure. In thyrotoxicosis with heart failure, the cardiac output may be greater than usual and yet insufficient for the increased metabolic needs occasioned by the increased secretion of thyroxine.

The left or right ventricle alone may fail initially—usually the former—but ultimately, especially after salt and water retention occurs (see below), combined failure is the rule.

Left ventricular failure is most commonly due to hypertension, coronary heart disease, or valvular heart disease, usually aortic valvular disease. Less commonly, mitral valvular disease, hypertrophic cardiomyopathy, left-to-right shunts, congenital heart lesions, and congestive cardiomyopathies are responsible. Infective endocarditis may occur de novo or may complicate other valvular diseases and aggravate left ventricular failure. Cardiac failure may also occur in various connective tissue disorders, thyrotoxicosis, severe anemia, arteriovenous fistulas, myocarditis, beriberi, and myocardial involvement by tumors or granulomas.

Right ventricular failure is most commonly due to mitral stenosis with raised pulmonary vascular resistance, pulmonary parenchymal or vascular disease, pulmonary valvular stenosis, or, less commonly, tricuspid valvular disease or infective endocarditis involving the right side of the heart. Carcinoid involving the pulmonary valve or tricuspid valve is a rare cause.

In at least half of cases, demonstrable precipitating diseases or factors which increase the work load of the heart may be present, and these factors should be sought in every patient with cardiac failure. They include arrhythmias, respiratory infection, myocardial infarction, pulmonary embolism, rheumatic carditis, thyrotoxicosis, anemia, excessive salt intake, corticosteroid administration, pregnancy, and excessive or rapid administration of parenteral fluids.

Etiology

The basic causes of ventricular failure are as follows:

A. Myocardial Weakness or Inflammation: Coronary artery disease, myocarditis.

B. Excess Work Load:

1. Increased resistance to ejection—Hypertension, stenosis of aortic or pulmonary valves, hypertrophic cardiomyopathy.

2. Increased stroke volume—Aortic insufficiency, mitral insufficiency, tricuspid insufficiency, congenital left-to-right shunts.

3. Increased body demands—Thyrotoxicosis, anemia, pregnancy, arteriovenous fistula.

Hemodynamics & Pathophysiology

The compensatory mechanisms by which the heart responds to an increased load include the following: (1) concentric hypertrophy, which provides larger contractile cells; (2) increased fiber length or dilatation, which increases the force of contraction by the Frank-Starling law; and (3) increased sympathetic nervous system activity, by which the force of contraction is increased at any fiber length without increasing the filling pressure.

Concentric hypertrophy is most apt to occur when the load placed on the heart is due to increased resistance to ejection with increased impedance, characteristically seen in aortic stenosis and hypertension; early in the course of the disease, the only abnormality of cardiac function that can be determined is left ventricular hypertrophy, recognized both clinically and by electrocardiography. The increased thickness of the left ventricle decreases its distensibility or compliance, so that the left ventricular end-diastolic pressure is raised with a normal left ventricular volume; the raised filling pressure is required to augment left ventricular output by the Starling principle. The raised left ventricular end-diastolic pressure need not indicate left ventricular failure but is seen whenever compliance is decreased, as in the cardiac states noted above or in hypertrophic cardiomyopathy or infiltrative cardiomyopathy. It also occurs early in acute myocardial infarction, when the infarcted area becomes stiff and less distensible. Later—eg, in patients with hypertension or aortic stenosis—left ventricular volume increases (because cardiac hypertrophy alone is insufficient to compensate), the left ventricular end-diastolic pressure rises even further, and left ventricular failure occurs.

When the increased cardiac load is due to increased stroke volume, typically represented by aortic insufficiency, the increased stretch increases fiber length and so increases the force of left ventricular contraction by the Frank-Starling principle. As the stretch increases, left ventricular volume increases, as can be demonstrated by enlargement of the heart on the plain film of the chest, by echocardiography, or by left ventricular angiography. In these circumstances, distensibility is not decreased, and it is common to find an increased left ventricular volume with a normal or increased cardiac output and left ventricular filling pressure. When left ventricular performance falls in the latter stages of this type of lesion (as well as in the various types of secondary cardiomyopathies, known as congestive cardiomyopathy), the ejection fraction (the difference between left ventricular diastolic and systolic volume) becomes decreased from its normal value of 60–70% as left ventricular failure occurs and may be as low as 10–20% in very severe failure. This decreased ability of the left ventricle to eject in systole correlates with other more sophisticated measures of left ventricular performance. It is best determined by left ventricular angiography, although echocardiography provides an estimate. In general, patients tolerate increased volume load better than increased resistance load even though left ventricular wall tension and myocardial oxygen consumption increase when the heart is dilated and enlarged.

Increased sympathetic stimulation can be demonstrated in patients with cardiac failure by increased concentration of catecholamines in the blood and urine and by depletion of norepinephrine in cardiac tissue, notably atrial appendages removed at surgery. Sarnoff and Braunwald, as well as other investigators, have demonstrated the importance of the sympathetic nervous system in improving cardiac contractility in cardiac failure. Beta-adrenergic blocking drugs such as propranolol, by decreasing the sympathetic drive to the heart, may worsen or precipitate left ventricular failure.

Although the pathophysiology of left ventricular failure has been described above, the same mechanisms can be visualized in right ventricular failure; pulmonary valve stenosis can be compared to aortic valve stenosis and tricuspid insufficiency can be compared to mitral insufficiency.

Early in the course of various cardiac diseases, the compensatory mechanisms are adequate to maintain a normal cardiac output and normal intracardiac pressures at rest and after exercise. Hypertrophy can be recognized on the ECG or plain chest film. This stage of compensated heart disease becomes "decompensated" as ventricular volume and filling pressures of the respective ventricles increase—although, as stated earlier, a raised filling pressure may be due to decreased compliance rather than ventricular failure early in the course of the disease. As the filling pressure increases, pulmonary venous congestion occurs as the raised left atrial pressure is transmitted backward. This leads to interstitial and then alveolar edema of the lungs, resulting in a continuum of symptoms of left ventricular failure, with dyspnea, exertional cough, orthopnea, paroxysmal nocturnal dyspnea, and pulmonary edema when the disease involves the left ventricle. Raised venous pressure, hepatomegaly, dependent edema, and ascites occur when the disease involves the right ventricle. Cardiac output may be normal at this phase— especially at rest—but may be decreased on exercise; as the cardiac output on exercise diminishes, tachycardia occurs and thus increases the minute cardiac output when the stroke volume cannot increase adequately. The AV oxygen difference widens so the tissues can extract more oxygen to compensate for the decreased cardiac output. When the ventricular filling pressure is increased—especially when compliance is decreased—

atrial hypertrophy increases the force of atrial systole and so aids filling; loss of this "atrial kick" can be devastating when atrial fibrillation occurs.

Apart from the changes in pressure, volume, compliance, and contractility just described, secondary retention of salt and water is responsible for many of the symptoms and signs of cardiac failure. When the cardiac output decreases in cardiac failure, the glomerular filtration rate falls; this is sensed by the macula densa between the afferent and efferent arterioles or by the juxtaglomerular cells surrounding the afferent arteriole of the kidney, resulting in increased secretion of renin. This proteolytic enzyme acts on renin substrate in the plasma to form angiotensin I, which is converted to angiotensin II in one passage through the lungs. Angiotensin II increases the secretion of aldosterone from the adrenal cortex, which in turn acts on the distal renal tubule to increase the reabsorption of sodium from the renal tubule. The increased sodium reabsorption leads to increased osmolality of the serum, which decreases the secretion of antidiuretic hormone from the pituitary, causing retention of an equivalent amount of water until osmolality is restored. The increased sodium and water retention leads to an increase in blood volume, which, by raising the hydrostatic pressure in the capillaries, leads first to interstitial edema and then to transudation of fluid into tissues which have decreased tissue pressure, such as the subcutaneous tissues. As a result, edema of the ankles and lower extremities occurs when the patient is ambulatory and in the sacral area when he is recumbent. Symptoms such as dyspnea and edema are aggravated by salt and water retention and are reversed by the use of diuretics and low-sodium diets.

The precise point at which "cardiac failure" occurs in the course of cardiac disease is difficult to determine, although in the overt stage cardiac failure is quite obvious.

Clinical Findings

These vary depending on whether the cardiac failure is acute or chronic, whether the increased load is on the left or right ventricle or both, and the cause.

A. Symptoms and Signs:

1. Left ventricular failure—Left ventricular failure is characterized predominantly by symptoms: exertional dyspnea, cough, fatigue, weakness, and nocturia. **Exertional dyspnea,** which is caused by pulmonary venous engorgement and increased stiffness of the lungs, resembles the normal ventilatory response to exercise but is associated with increased awareness of breathlessness and difficulty in breathing. In heart failure, the patient regularly becomes short of breath during an amount of exertion which previously caused no difficulty. As the pulmonary engorgement progresses, less and less activity brings on dyspnea until it is present even when the patient is at rest (rest dyspnea). **Orthopnea,** or shortness of breath occurring in recumbency which is promptly relieved by propping up the head or trunk, is precipitated by the further increase in pulmonary engorgement on recumbency. **Paroxysmal**

nocturnal dyspnea or cough may appear at any time and is often the first indication of left ventricular failure caused by severe hypertension, aortic stenosis or insufficiency, or myocardial infarction. It also occurs in patients with tight mitral stenosis in advanced stages. It is an exaggerated form of orthopnea, the patient awakening from sleep gasping for breath, and compelled to sit or stand up for relief. Cough is frequently present. With bronchospasm, patients may have inspiratory and expiratory wheezing (so-called cardiac asthma). The paroxysmal cough and dyspnea may pass in a few minutes to several hours, or may progress to acute pulmonary edema. Patients become pale or frankly cyanotic, sweat profusely, and complain of great air hunger. Cough productive of frothy white or pink sputum is characteristic. The attack may subside in 1 to several hours, or the left ventricle may progressively weaken, leading to shock and death.

These forms of dyspnea must be distinguished from those occurring commonly in many other conditions. Advanced age, debility, poor physical conditioning, obesity, chronic pulmonary disease, and severe anemia commonly produce exertional dyspnea. Extreme obesity (Pickwickian syndrome), ascites from any cause, abdominal distention from gastrointestinal disease, or advanced stages of pregnancy may produce orthopnea in the absence of preexisting heart disease. Bronchial asthma appearing in middle life may be symptomatically difficult to distinguish from the paroxysmal nocturnal dyspnea of left ventricular failure. Patients with neurocirculatory asthenia or anxiety states with psychophysiologic cardiovascular reactions may suffer from sighing respirations simulating dyspnea.

Exertional fatigue and weakness due to reduced cardiac output are late symptoms and disappear promptly on resting. Severe fatigue, rather than dyspnea, is the chief complaint of patients with mitral stenosis who have developed pulmonary hypertension and low cardiac output.

Nocturia occurs as a result of the excretion of edema fluid accumulated during the day and the increased renal perfusion in the recumbent position; it reflects the decreased work of the heart at rest and often the effects of diuretics given during the day.

In the absence of overt right ventricular failure, examination should disclose the following: (1) the basic cause of the left ventricular failure (hypertension, aortic or mitral valve disease, myocardial infarction); (2) left ventricular hypertrophy, in which the apical impulse is forceful or heaving, displaced to the left and downward, confirmed by ECG and chest x-ray; and (3) radiologic evidence of pulmonary venous distention such as redistribution of blood to the upper lobes, Kerley B lines, or, in acute left ventricular failure, butterfly pattern hilar congestion. Hydrothorax may be present.

The following may or may not be present and are not necessary for diagnosis: basilar parenchymal rales which do not clear on coughing, gallop rhythm, pulsus alternans, and an accentuated pulmonary component of the second sound ("P2"). The chest x-ray may reveal pulmonary venous congestion and left atrial enlargement in the case of mitral stenosis, and shows unquestioned left ventricular enlargement in the usual case, except with acute myocardial infarction or cardiac arrhythmia.

2. **Right ventricular failure**—Right ventricular failure is characterized predominantly by signs. It develops after left ventricular failure of even short duration. Mitral stenosis, pulmonary valve stenosis, cor pulmonale, tricuspid insufficiency, and such complications of congenital disease as Eisenmenger's syndrome resulting from ventricular or atrial septal defects may produce relatively pure right ventricular failure. Tricuspid stenosis produces the same systemic congestion as right ventricular failure. **Anorexia, bloating,** or **exertional right upper abdominal pains** are common, reflecting hepatic and visceral engorgement secondary to elevated venous pressure. **Oliguria** is present in the daytime, polyuria at night. Weakness and mental aberration are present in severe cases.

The venous pressure can be estimated by noting the extent of jugular filling (during normal expiration) above the level of the clavicles when the patient is propped up so that his trunk makes a 30 degree angle with the bed. A simple water manometer allows serial determinations of the venous pressure at the bedside (zero level junction of lower and middle thirds of the AP diameter of the chest is a commonly used reference point). Normal pressure is $6-10$ cm H_2O.

Right ventricular hypertrophy in pure right failure is demonstrated by lower sternal or left parasternal systolic heave independent of the apical impulse. The liver is enlarged, tender, and pulsating. Ascites is rarely prominent; when it appears early and in massive amounts, cardiac tamponade, constrictive pericarditis, or tricuspid stenosis should be considered. Dependent edema caused by heart failure usually subsides overnight initially but eventually persists and increases in extent. Pleural effusion is more common on the right side. Coolness of the extremities and peripheral cyanosis of the nail beds are due to reduced peripheral blood flow. Sinus tachycardia is present.

The ECG findings indicate pure right ventricular hypertrophy in pure right-sided failure and, usually, evidence of left ventricular hypertrophy or coronary artery disease when left-sided failure is predominant.

Right atrial and ventricular enlargement is noted on the chest film in pure right heart failure, but specific chamber enlargement is difficult to define when right heart failure is secondary to left heart failure.

Determination of systolic time intervals (see p 154) with echocardiography may provide an indirect means of assessing impaired left ventricular function prior to the development of cardiac failure. Left ventricular cineangiograms provide a direct visual picture of left ventricular contraction and ejection.

B. Laboratory Findings: Red and white cell counts, hemoglobin, packed cell volume, and sedimentation rate are normal in uncomplicated left heart failure. Polycythemia may occur in chronic cor pulmonale. Urinalysis often discloses significant proteinuria and granular casts. The BUN may be elevated because of reduced renal blood flow, but the urine specific gravity is high in the absence of primary renal disease. The serum sodium, potassium, CO_2, and chloride are within normal limits in ordinary congestive heart failure before diuretics are used. Specific tests should be made for any suspected unusual causes or complications contributing to heart failure, eg, thyrotoxicosis, infective endocarditis, syphilis, connective tissue disease, pheochromocytoma.

Differential Diagnosis

Congestive heart failure must be differentiated from pericardial effusion, constrictive pericarditis, neurocirculatory asthenia, acute and chronic pulmonary disease, bronchial asthma, cirrhosis, carcinoma of the lung, nephrosis or nephritis, mediastinal tumor, repeated pulmonary emboli, obstruction of the vena cava, and anemia.

Consideration of the history together with physical findings of organic cardiovascular disease, enlarged heart with ventricular heaves, character of the arterial pulse, gallop rhythm, pulsus alternans, elevated venous pressure in the absence of collateral venous circulation, and prolonged circulation time differentiates congestive heart failure from these conditions.

Treatment

The objectives of treatment are to remove the cause, increase the force and efficiency of myocardial contraction, and reduce the abnormal retention of sodium and water. The patient shares a significant responsibility in the management of his disease, because treatment is long-term and involves restrictions in diet and activity and the reliable use of cardiac drugs.

Potentially curable causes of congestive heart failure must be specifically considered: valvular heart disease, constrictive pericarditis, mitral stenosis, pulmonary stenosis, tricuspid stenosis, infective endocarditis, thyrotoxicosis, myxedema heart, peripheral arteriovenous fistula, beriberi, and recurrent arrhythmias.

Specific search should be made for reversible noncardiac causes of failure originating outside the heart, eg, thyrotoxicosis, anemia, myxedema, nutritional disturbances (especially vitamin B deficiency), arteriovenous fistulas, polycythemia vera, and Paget's disease.

Determine, treat, and eliminate, if possible, the factor precipitating the cardiac failure, eg, infection (especially respiratory), pulmonary infarction, overexertion, increased sodium intake, discontinuation of medication (especially digitalis); the onset of arrhythmia, particularly with rapid ventricular rates (eg, atrial fibrillation); myocardial infarction, and anemia.

A. Rest: Rest in bed or sitting in a chair decreases the work of the heart and promotes sodium diuresis. Morphine- or barbiturate-induced sleep comes as a welcome relief to a patient who has spent many sleepless, dyspneic nights with his disease. Adequate rest should be maintained until compensation has occurred and then should be replaced by progressive ambulation. Most patients can use a bedside toilet with no more effort than is required for a bedpan.

Rest should be continued as long as necessary to permit the heart to regain reserve strength, but should not be so prolonged as to cause generalized debility of the patient.

Patients are usually more comfortable in a cool room.

Cardiac patients at bed rest are prone to develop phlebitis. They should be given passive or active leg exercises and an elastic stocking to prevent phlebothrombosis.

B. Diet: (See Table 7-2.) At the onset of therapy, give frequent (4-6) small, bland, low-caloric, low-residue meals with vitamin supplements. The degree of sodium restriction depends upon the severity of the failure and the ease with which it can be controlled by other means. Even with the use of diuretics, unlimited sodium intake is unwise. Evaluation of the previous intake of sodium will provide a baseline upon which to gauge the degree of restriction required. Before drastic sodium restriction is instituted, the renal function should be evaluated to determine if the kidneys can conserve sodium. Because cardiac failure is a long-term illness, dietary and other restrictions should be modified according to the habits and preferences of the patient. The availability of potent oral diuretics usually allows the patient to have at least a 2 gm sodium diet, which usually means no added salt at the table and avoidance of highly salted foods such as ham, bacon, and potato chips. It is often helpful early in the course of treatment to see whether cardiac failure can be treated by rest and sodium restriction alone so as to avoid the side-effects of diuretic therapy. Most patients, however, find a low-sodium diet difficult to maintain, and total reliance on a strict low-sodium intake is usually inadvisable. Vitamin supplements may be indicated. Restricted diets and anorexia may lead to malnutrition and avitaminosis, with a superimposed beriberi type of failure.

C. Digitalis: (see p 233.) Digitalis increases the speed and force of cardiac contraction. Increased cardiac output, decreased cardiac volume and ventricular diastolic pressure, and a fall in right atrial and peripheral venous pressure frequently follow digitalization in patients with cardiac failure. The glycosides available are qualitatively similar. They differ in speed of action, dosage, and rate of excretion. It is advisable to become familiar with a rapid intravenous and a rapid oral method. Rapid digitalization is indicated in atrial flutter and fibrillation with fast ventricular rates and in acute pulmonary edema; otherwise, slow digitalization is preferred.

D. Removal of Sodium and Water:

1. Thiazide diuretics—(See p 239.) Sodium diuresis is most conveniently accomplished by the use of an orally active agent such as chlorothiazide (Diuril) or any of its analogues. The diuretics can be given daily or preferably intermittently depending on the need. Dietary or supplementary potassium must be adequate to prevent potassium depletion and digitalis toxicity.

Table 7—2. Dietary plan for low-sodium diet: 1800 calories.
(Adapted from: *Sodium Restricted Diets*. American Heart Association, 1969.)

Food	Average Sodium per Serving	Sodium Levels/Day		
		500 mg	1000 mg	1500–3000 mg*
Milk: whole, low-fat, nonfat	120 mg/8 oz	1 glass (8 oz) daily†	2 glasses (16 oz) daily†	2 glasses or more daily
Egg, prepared in any way without salt	57 mg/egg	1	1	1
Meat, poultry, fish, fresh or frozen; beef, lamb, veal, pork, fish, chicken, turkey‡	25 mg/oz	6 oz cooked or substitute	6 oz cooked or substitute	6 or more oz cooked (small amounts regular cheese)
Fruits, all kinds: fresh, frozen, canned, dried, or juices	2 mg/half-cup	4 or more servings daily	4 or more servings daily	4 or more servings daily
Vegetables: fresh, frozen, or dietetic canned, green or yellow	9 mg/half-cup	3 or more servings daily §	3 or more servings daily	3 or more servings daily**
Breads, enriched white or whole grain	120 mg/slice	None	None	3 or more servings daily
Breads, low-sodium	5 mg/slice	4 or more slices daily	4 or more slices daily	As desired
Cereals, regular cooked (without salt, nonenriched)	1 mg/cup	As desired	As desired	As desired
Cereals, dry, prepared (cornflakes, etc)	165–300 mg/cup	None	None	1 serving daily
Cereals: shredded wheat, puffed wheat, puffed rice	1 mg/cup	As desired	As desired	As desired
Starches: potatoes (white or sweet), corn, lima beans, peas, mixed vegetables††	5–10 mg/half-cup	1 or more servings daily	1 or more servings daily	As desired
Starches: rice, macaroni, spaghetti, noodles	1 mg/half-cup	As desired	As desired	As desired
Butter, margarine	40 mg/tsp	None	None	4 or more servings daily
Unsalted butter, margarine	0.04 mg/tsp	4 or more tsp daily	4 or more tsp daily	As desired
Oils	None	As desired	As desired	As desired
Salad dressings	80–200 mg/tsp	None	None	In moderation
Unsalted salad dressings	Up to 0.4 mg/tsp	As desired	As desired	As desired
Homemade soups, with allowed milk, meats, vegetables	Varies with the sodium content of ingredients	As desired	As desired	As desired
Sugars, syrups, jellies, honey, candies (hard sugar)	None	As desired	As desired	As desired
Desserts: homemade (salt-free) gelatin, ice cream, sherbet, meringues, puddings, pound cakes	10–50 mg/serving	As desired	As desired	As desired

Table 7–2 (cont'd). Dietary plan for low-sodium diet: 1800 calories.

Food	Average Sodium per Serving	Sodium Levels/Day		
		500 mg	1000 mg	1500–3000 mg*
Salt	2300 mg/tsp	None	None	½ tsp daily*
Monosodium glutamate (Accent, Ajino-moto)	750 mg/tsp	None	None	In place of salt
Baking soda (sodium bicarbonate)	1000 mg/tsp	None	None	Moderate use in cooking
Baking powder	370 mg/tsp	None	None	Moderate use in cooking

Avoid: Canned vegetables or vegetable juices unless low-sodium dietetic canned; canned soups, soda crackers, potato chips, pretzels, "snack foods," quick or hot breads, waffles, pancakes, olives, pickles, relishes, condiments such as ketchup, mustard, chili sauce, salted nuts, sauerkraut.

*Small amounts of salt (up to ½ tsp/day) may be used in cooking or at the table.
†Buttermilk should not be used.
‡*Avoid* salted or cured or smoked meats, fish, or chicken; ham, bacon, sausage, luncheon meats, frankfurters, sardines, canned tuna or salmon (unless without salt), shellfish, regular cottage cheese and cheddar type cheeses.
Substitutes: Low-sodium cheese or dietetic peanut butter.
§On 500 mg sodium diet, avoid the following vegetables: Artichokes, beet greens, beets, carrots, celery, chard, dandelion greens, hominy, kale, mustard greens, spinach, sauerkraut, white turnips.
**May use any fresh, frozen, or drained regular canned vegetables except sauerkraut.
††Only fresh or dietetic canned lima beans and peas. The frozen are packed with salt.

2. Mercurial diuretics—The mercurial diuretics (see p 240) are slightly more potent than the thiazide diuretics but are infrequently used today because they must be given parenterally. Because potassium depletion is less and free water clearance is increased, mercurials may be helpful in dilutional hyponatremia. They decrease the sodium and chloride reabsorption in the renal tubules but are ineffective in the presence of alkalosis, and the effects are potentiated by giving acids such as chlorides or lysine if there is associated liver disease. Mercurials should be used in small doses of 0.5–1 ml; their effect is noted in about 2 hours and lasts 10–12 hours.

3. Aldosterone antagonists—Spironolactone (Aldactone) causes sodium diuresis without potassium loss and can be combined with a thiazide to neutralize the potassium-wasting effect of thiazides. The onset of clinical effect may be delayed for 1 week. Response is variable but may be striking. The initial dosage is 25 mg 4 times daily. Drowsiness, hyperkalemia, hypovolemia, hypotension, and breast tenderness may occur. Similar potassium sparing may occur with triamterene (Dyrenium; see p 240), which may be used in combination with thiazides, ethacrynic acid, or furosemide (see below). *Caution:* Check serum potassium and avoid potassium supplements.

4. Furosemide (Lasix), 40–80 mg orally (see p 240), and **ethacrynic acid (Edecrin)**, 25–100 mg orally, are potent diuretics of short duration. They cause nausea and diarrhea more often than the thiazides, especially with regular dosage. The considerable diuresis may cause a significant fall in glomerular filtration rate and hypokalemia, and these drugs must therefore be used with considerable caution. The rapid onset of action (within 30 minutes) makes them valuable on occasion for treatment of acute pulmonary edema, but

their potency increases the hazards and the thiazides are probably preferable for the average patient with congestive failure unless there is associated renal failure. They are effective even in the presence of low glomerular filtration rates or in disturbances in acid-base balance or electrolyte metabolism.

E. Oxygen Therapy: Useful when respiratory distress or low P_{O_2} with hypoxemia is present.

F. Sympathetic and Other Inotropic Agents: Isoproterenol, dopamine, and glucagon may have a place in therapy if digitalis is contraindicated, especially in the postoperative period after open heart surgery or following acute myocardial infarction.

G. Vasodilators in the Treatment of Cardiac Failure: An important advance in cardiac therapeutics concerns the use of vasodilator therapy with drugs such as sodium nitroprusside in the treatment of severe cardiac failure responding inadequately to the usual therapy of bed rest, digitalis and diuretics, removal of precipitating factors, and application of all the other principles of therapy discussed above. Patients with congestive cardiomyopathy or ischemic cardiomyopathy often respond inadequately to digitalis; aggressive diuretic therapy, while causing improvement of symptoms, induces weakness, hypokalemia, and hypovolemia. Furthermore, cardiac failure rapidly recurs when these patients become ambulatory, and they frequently are in need of hospital care.

Hemodynamic studies in coronary care units have shown that patients with left ventricular failure and cardiogenic shock, with a low cardiac output, and a high left ventricular filling pressure (LVFP) (> 20 mm Hg), often improve when impedance to left ventricular output and afterload are reduced by vasodilator therapy. It was a natural extension of this experience to use vasodilator therapy to decrease afterload in patients with other types of severe cardiac failure, especially left ventricular failure. The results to date have been impressive, at least over short periods; Cohn and his associates in Georgetown have demonstrated a prompt, rapid reduction in left ventricular filling pressure, an increase in cardiac output, slowing of the heart rate, and almost a doubling of the forward ejection fraction and stroke volume following the use of sodium nitroprusside. Diuresis and clinical improvement accompany the hemodynamic changes. Sodium nitroprusside (Nipride) was begun at a rate of 15 μg/minute and the drip rate increased at intervals of 3–5 minutes until the pulmonary capillary wedge pressure was reduced to normal or became stable, provided the systolic blood pressure remained above 100 mm Hg. The final infusion rate averaged 40 μg/minute. Chatterjee found that vasodilator therapy in mitral regurgitation reduced the regurgitant flow, improved the systolic emptying of the left ventricle, and thus increased the forward ejection fraction. Left ventricular wall tension was reduced by the decreased impedance because of the decreased left ventricular chamber size. The resultant improved left ventricular performance has important therapeutic possibilities. Vasodilator therapy is still experimental and should only be used when patients can be monitored closely, as in the coronary care unit, when hypotension can be avoided and when serum thiocyanate levels can be monitored to avoid toxicity. Once clinical improvement has occurred following the intravenous infusion of nitroprusside, it might be possible to maintain improvement with oral vasodilator agents such as isosorbide dinitrate (Isordil), hydralazine, and minoxidil. This awaits future research.

H. **Mechanical Measures:** Paracentesis of fluid in the chest and abdomen should be undertaken if respiration is embarrassed. Since sodium retention may occur as a result of fluid collection in the chest, abdomen, and legs, diuresis may occur following the procedure. Venesection (in low-output failure in the absence of anemia), rotating tourniquets, Southey tubes, and acupuncture may be beneficial if the more conventional forms of treatment fail. Southey tubes and acupuncture are especially valuable in severe right heart failure with obstinate dependent edema. Care must be taken to avoid a severe low-sodium syndrome with hyperkalemia.

I. **Peritoneal Dialysis:** Hypertonic peritoneal dialysis is an effective method, reserved for patients with severe heart failure, dilutional hyponatremia, and renal failure. Some remissions have been dramatic; and the method should be given a greater trial.

J. **Observation During Treatment of Cardiac Failure:** Record the following at every visit:

1. Status of original symptoms.
2. New symptoms or signs.
3. Morning weight or weight with same clothes.
4. Presence of the signs of congestive failure (venous engorgement and pulsations, pulmonary rales, pleural fluid, engorgement of the liver, presence of edema).

5. Examination of the heart and blood vessels (cardiac sounds, gallop rhythm, friction rub, cardiac rhythm and apical rate, cardiac size, peripheral arterial pulsations, and status of the veins).
6. Blood pressure and presence of pulsus alternans.
7. Evidence of phlebothrombosis.

Prognosis

Without treatment, the prognosis of left ventricular failure is poor, with the 5-year mortality being approximately 50%. The availability of potent diuretics, effective antihypertensive therapy, and surgical replacement of stenotic and regurgitant cardiac valves has vastly improved the outlook for patients with these conditions. However, the prognosis is still unsatisfactory in congestive cardiomyopathy with failure, myocardial infarction with failure, and any condition not remediable by surgery or correction of the underlying pathogenetic factor. Pulmonary embolization secondary to venous thrombosis in the leg veins is common, as are pulmonary infections, cardiac cirrhosis, and peripheral arterial embolization from mural thrombi on the endocardium. In general, the speed and adequacy of response to therapy is the most reliable guide to prognosis. Detection and removal of a precipitating condition prolongs survival. The age of the patient, the degree of cardiac enlargement, the extent of myocardial damage, and the severity of underlying cardiac and associated diseases must all be considered. Survival is longer in failure due to mitral insufficiency or that precipitated by atrial fibrillation. Survival is shorter when failure is due to mitral stenosis, syphilitic aortic insufficiency, calcific aortic stenosis, myocardial infarction, chronic pulmonary disease, and severe hypertension.

See also section on digitalis and diuretics (pp 233 and 239).

Ahearn DJ, Maher JF: Heart failure as a complication of hemodialysis arteriovenous fistula. Ann Int Med 77:201, 1972.

Cairns KB & others: Clinical and hemodynamic results of peritoneal dialysis for severe cardiac failure. Am Heart J 76:227, 1968.

Dodge HT: Hemodynamic aspects of cardiac failure. Hosp Practice 6:91, Jan 1971.

Earley LE: Current concepts: Diuretics. (2 parts.) New England J Med 276:966, 1023, 1967.

Franciosa JA & others: Hemodynamic effects of orally administered isosorbide dinitrate in patients with congestive heart failure. Circulation 50:1020, 1974.

Frand UI, Shim CS, William MH Jr: Heroin-induced pulmonary edema. Ann Int Med 77:29, 1972.

Guiha NH & others: Treatment of refractory heart failure with infusion of nitroprusside. New England J Med 291:587, 1974.

Mason DT, Zelis R, Wikman-Coffelt J: Symposium on congestive heart failure: Recent advances in structure, biochemistry, physiology and pharmacology. Am J Cardiol 32:395, 1973.

McKee PA & others: Natural history of congestive heart failure: The Framingham Study. New England J Med 285:1441, 1971.

Mitchell JH, Wallace AG, Skinner NS Jr: Intrinsic effects of heart rate on left ventricular performance. Am J Physiol 205:41, 1963.

Walker WG: Indications and contraindications for diuretic therapy. Ann New York Acad Sc 139:481, 1966.

SPECIAL PROBLEMS IN THE MANAGEMENT OF CONGESTIVE HEART FAILURE

Acute Pulmonary Edema

Acute pulmonary edema is a grave emergency. Treatment may vary depending upon the cause and severity. For example, in a mild attack, morphine and rest in bed alone may suffice; in an attack due to atrial fibrillation with rapid ventricular rate, lanatoside C or digoxin given intravenously or cardioversion may be required.

The patient should be elevated to the semi-Fowler position or placed in a chair; this decreases the venous return to the heart. Morphine sulfate, 5–10 mg IV or IM, relieves anxiety, depresses pulmonary reflexes, and induces sleep. Relief from forceful respiration decreases the negative intrathoracic pressure and the venous return to the heart.

Oxygen should be administered in high concentrations by mask or (for children) by hood or tent. Moderate concentrations (40–60%) can be achieved with an oxygen tent or nasal catheter. Oxygen relieves hypoxia and dyspnea and decreases pulmonary capillary permeability.

Positive-pressure breathing for short periods may be of great value in improving ventilation. Antifoaming agents to lower the surface tension of the bronchial secretions may be helpful.

Soft rubber tourniquets or blood pressure cuffs, applied with sufficient pressure to obstruct venous but not arterial flow and rotated every 15 minutes, will effectively reduce the venous return to the heart. The tourniquets should be removed gradually as the attack subsides. About 700 ml of blood may be trapped in the extremities by this method. Venesection (300–700 ml) is the most direct way of reducing the venous return to the heart and may strikingly increase cardiac output and decrease right atrial and peripheral venous pressure in low-output cardiac failure. It is contraindicated if anemia is present.

Furosemide (Lasix; see above), 40–80 mg IV, or ethacrynic acid (Edecrin), 25–100 mg orally or 25–50 mg IV is useful because of the potent and prompt diuretic action of these drugs.

Rapid digitalization is of value. Extreme care should be taken in giving digitalis intravenously to a previously digitalized patient.

Aminophylline, 0.25–0.5 gm slowly IV, is often helpful. It increases cardiac output, renal blood flow, glomerular filtration rate, and urine output of water and sodium. Rectal aminophylline suppositories, 0.25–0.5 gm, are often helpful and are more convenient for the patient.

In the acute recurrent pulmonary edema of hypertensive heart disease and in the presence of severe hypertension, vasodilator therapy with sodium nitroprusside as outlined above (in addition to other measures outlined for acute hypertensive emergencies on p 184) may be helpful. Care must be taken not to produce hypotension.

Refractory Cardiac Failure

When the treatment measures outlined above do not result in clinical improvement, reevaluate the total situation with particular attention to the following questions:

(1) Is the diagnosis correct?

(2) Has bed rest been adequate? Is the patient receiving more sodium than ordered? Have treatment measures been carefully and properly administered? A review of the patient's activities, diet, and medications is essential.

(3) Are any of the following present or to be considered: Unrecognized recurrent pulmonary infarction, anemia, masked hyperthyroidism, vitamin deficiency, infective endocarditis, abrupt worsening or production of valvular insufficiencies, silent myocardial infarction, arrhythmias, ball valve variance, ventricular aneurysm, AV fistulas, use of corticosteroids, or uncontrolled hypertension?

(4) Have complications such as acute rheumatic myocarditis or infective endocarditis been superimposed upon a rheumatic heart?

(5) Are there electrolyte abnormalities which may have resulted from diet or diuretics? Electrolyte disturbances may lead to mercurial resistance, produce a low-sodium syndrome, or, in the case of a low potassium, enhance digitalis intoxication.

(6) Is the renal function adequate for the use of thiazides? If not, furosemide should be used.

(7) Has the patient been taking his medication regularly? If so, has there been a change in the preparation of digitalis? (See p 233 on digitalis bioavailability.)

Management of Convalescence

Provide adequate rest and exercise within tolerance. Careful attention should be paid to the treatment of noncardiac causes of cardiac failure and to the avoidance of precipitating factors.

A. Digitalization: Once digitalis is started for cardiac failure, it is usually necessary to continue it for life, unless the diagnosis is faulty or the failure is acute and secondary to paroxysmal arrhythmias, overwhelming systemic disorders, or shock due to acute myocardial infarction.

B. Low-Sodium Diet: Allow 1.5 gm sodium chloride (600 mg of sodium) per day. It is advisable to check the patient's serum sodium or urinary sodium frequently to be certain that hyponatremia and hypovolemia are not occurring. An inadequate sodium intake in the presence of severe renal impairment can precipitate fatal renal failure. If thiazide compounds are used, it is wise to allow the ambulatory patient at least 2 gm of sodium a day in his diet.

A high-sodium diet is particularly apt to maintain cardiac failure if the patient concurrently is up and about, stimulating aldosterone secretion. Dietary review often reveals that the patient is not restricting his sodium adequately.

C. Diuretics: The adequately digitalized patient on a sodium-restricted diet may still accumulate edema fluid. Diuretic drugs should be added to his regimen in the amounts necessary to prevent this accumulation.

The thiazide diuretics, because of the greater convenience of oral administration, are most widely used. Any one of the agents listed in Table 7—5 can be given (preferably intermittently) several times each week but can be given daily if necessary. Because potassium depletion is a hazard in the use of the thiazide diuretics, potassium must be added, either as potassium chloride, 1 gm 3 times daily, or by the use of fruit juices, fruits (dried apricots, dates, prunes, bananas), and vegetables. Potassium-sparing diuretics (spironolactone or triamterene) can be added instead. Do not use if renal failure or oliguria is present.

Electrocyte Disturbances in Cardiac Failure

During treatment of cardiac failure, several types of electrolyte disturbance may be seen.

A. Hypochloremic Alkalosis: This is due to chloride excretion out of proportion to sodium loss following diuresis, producing a low serum chloride and a high serum bicarbonate. Serum sodium and potassium levels may be normal or low. Symptoms of dehydration may be present: dry mucous membranes and loss of tissue turgor and a latent or manifest tetany.

Treatment is with ammonium chloride, 4—6 gm/day for 3—4 days, repeated after an interval of 3—4 days. This must be done with *caution* if there is associated severe liver disease. Potassium salts may be given if a potassium deficit exists (see below). If tetany is present, calcium salts must be given concurrently.

Low serum sodium may be dilutional and may occur in association with hypokalemic alkalosis; restriction of fluids and administration of potassium salts such as potassium chloride may be helpful. Hypokalemic and hypochloremic alkalosis may coexist.

B. Low-Sodium Syndrome: In the absence of edema, the onset of weakness, oliguria, sweating, and azotemia heralds the "low-salt syndrome." Excessive diuresis, hot weather, fever, and vomiting are additional predisposing factors. Low serum sodium may be present without alkalosis or acidosis, or it may be complicated by dehydration and acidosis. It may follow severe sodium restriction accompanied by diuresis.

In mild cases treatment consists merely of increasing the sodium intake. For severe cases, treat with intravenous hypertonic saline.

The total body sodium is usually increased when edema is present in spite of hyponatremia. In such cases sodium should not be administered, but water should be restricted to counteract the dilutional hyponatremia.

C. Hypokalemia: This may result from excessive potassium excretion due to the administration of mercurial, thiazide, or the newer potent diuretics, or acetazolamide (Diamox), or following the administration of acid or ammonia resins to patients receiving a low-sodium diet. Hypokalemia may induce digitalis intoxication.

Treatment consists of giving potassium chloride, 3—6 gm daily orally, provided renal function is adequate. *Caution:* Parenteral potassium salts should not be administered in the presence of acidosis or renal failure.

High-Output Failure

The term "high-output failure" means that, in the presence of fully developed congestive heart failure, the cardiac output is greater than normal but still insufficient for the needs of the body. It occurs characteristically when pre-existing heart disease is complicated by thyrotoxicosis, severe anemia (hemoglobin < 8 gm/100 ml), pregnancy, arteriovenous fistula, beriberi, and occasionally by Paget's disease of bone, or chronic pulmonary disease or liver disease with arterial oxygen unsaturation.

The clinical picture of congestive heart failure is present except for more marked tachycardia, overactive heart, bounding pulses, and warm hands and skin generally. The circulation time may be short or normal in the face of elevated venous pressure. This combination is never found in uncomplicated heart failure except when fever or one of the disorders listed above is present.

Treatment is directed at the failure as well as at the associated illness, eg, anemia, thyrotoxicosis.

Aberman A, Fulop M: The metabolic and respiratory acidosis of acute pulmonary edema. Ann Int Med 76:173, 1972.

Cohn JN & others: Chronic vasodilator therapy in the management of cardiogenic shock and intractable left ventricular failure. Ann Int Med 81:777, 1974.

Duberstein JL, Kaufman DM: A clinical study of an epidemic of heroin intoxication and heroin-induced pulmonary edema. Am J Med 51:704, 1971.

Friedberg CK: Prevention of heart failure. Am J Cardiol 22:190, 1968.

Hultgren HN, Flamm MD: Pulmonary edema. Mod Concepts Cardiovas Dis 38:1, 1969.

Leonard JJ, deGroot WJ: The thyroid state and the cardiovascular system. Mod Concepts Cardiovas Dis 38:23, 1969.

Scheinman M, Brown M, Rapaport E: Hemodynamic effects of ethacrynic acid in patients with refractory acute left ventricular failure. Am J Med 50:291, 1971.

Schreiner BF Jr & others: The pathophysiology of pulmonary congestion. Progr Cardiovas Dis 14:47, 1971.

See also references for Cardiac Failure on p 220.

DISEASES OF THE PERICARDIUM

ACUTE PERICARDITIS

Essentials of Diagnosis

- Pleuritic or persisting substernal or precordial pain referred to the left neck, shoulder, or back.
- Pericardial friction rub.
- ECG: Early, concordant ST elevation; late, general symmetric T inversion without Q waves or reciprocal changes except in aVR.

General Considerations

In approximate order of frequency, **infectious pericarditis** is caused by viruses, *Mycobacterium tuberculosis,* pyogenic bacteria associated with bacteremia or septicemia (pneumococcus, hemolytic streptococcus, *Staphylococcus aureus,* meningococcus, gonococcus), and brucella. **Inflammatory pericarditis** includes all diseases associated with acute vasculitis, most commonly disseminated lupus erythematosus, acute rheumatic fever, and serum sickness. A miscellaneous group includes pericarditis which occurs after pericardiectomy, myocardial infarction, or trauma; pericarditis associated with uremia, metastatic tumors, and the lymphomas; and hemorrhagic pericarditis due to dissecting aneurysm.

Acute pericarditis is traditionally classified as fibrinous or pericarditis with effusion, in which the pericardial cavity contains significant amounts of transudate, blood, exudate, or pus. Varying degrees of myocarditis accompany pericarditis and are responsible for the ECG changes in ST–T contours.

Clinical Findings

A. Symptoms and Signs: Acute viral pericarditis is more common in men 20–50 years of age and often follows a "viral" respiratory infection. The onset of pain is usually sudden; pain is precordial or substernal, pleuritic or steady (or both), and radiates to the left neck, shoulder, back, or epigastrium. It is worse in the supine position and may be accentuated by swallowing. Tachycardia and a pericardial (often pleuropericardial) friction rub are present.

Fever is 37.8–39.4° C (100–103° F) or higher in infectious pericarditis, and is determined by the febrile pattern of the underlying disease in the other varieties.

B. Laboratory Findings: Leukocytosis of 10–20 thousand is usually present in acute viral pericarditis; leukopenia may be noted in pericarditis associated with disseminated lupus erythematosus. LE cells should be sought in isolated acute pericarditis.

C. X-Ray Findings: Chest x-rays may show cardiac dilatation, pneumonitis, and pleural effusion.

D. ECG Findings: Initially, ECG changes consist only of ST–T segment elevation in all leads, with preservation of normal upward concavity. Return to the baseline in a few days is followed by T wave inversion. Reciprocal changes are absent except in aVR, and Q waves do not appear.

E. Echocardiography: Echocardiography is most valuable in the diagnosis of pericardial effusion. It can be done at the bedside, is noninvasive, and can be repeated frequently. Echocardiography reveals, in contrast to normal, an echo-free space separating the anterior wall of the right ventricle from the chest and the posterior wall of the left ventricle from the lung. The procedure is valuable in the differentiation between cardiac dilatation and pericardial effusion, especially in the presence of what may be tamponade.

Differential Diagnosis

A. Acute Myocardial Infarction: Acute viral pericarditis usually follows a respiratory infection, occurs in the age group from 20–50 years, and characteristically presents with pleuritic pain. Fever, friction rub, leukocytosis, and an elevated sedimentation rate are found at the onset rather than 24–72 hours later. ECG changes are usually distinctive. SGOT or LDH are only rarely elevated even in severe pericarditis.

B. Acute Pleurisy: Pericardial friction rub is differentiated from pleural friction rub by its persistence when the breath is held, although there may also be a pleuro-pericardial friction sound which is related to respiration. ECG changes are diagnostic of pericarditis in the absence of a rub.

C. Confusion of Rub With Murmurs: Pericardial friction rubs are differentiated by their changing character, lack of association with the usual areas of murmurs, high-pitched or "scratchy" quality, asynchrony with heart sounds, and often triple character.

Complications

Pericardial effusion is the only noteworthy complication. Cardiac dilatation accompanying acute viral pericarditis rarely produces heart failure but may cause arrhythmias.

Treatment

Treat the underlying condition and give analgesics as necessary for relief of pain. Salicylates and corticotropin (ACTH) or the corticosteroids are useful in rheumatic pericarditis. See below for pericardial effusion and tamponade.

Prognosis

The prognosis of viral pericarditis is usually excellent; recovery occurs in 2 weeks to 3 months; recurrences are uncommon but may occur; and residual pericardial thickening or persistent ECG abnormalities are rare. The promptness and adequacy of antibiotic and surgical treatment determine the outcome in tuberculous and purulent pericarditis. Other manifestations of disseminated lupus erythematosus may become apparent after an attack of presumed "viral" pericarditis. In the miscellaneous group, the basic disorder determines the prognosis.

Fowler NO, Manitsas GT: Infectious pericarditis. Progr Cardiovas Dis 16:323, 1973.

Montgomery JZ & others: Hemodynamic and diagnostic features of pericardial disease. Western J Med 122:295, 1975.

Schrire V: Pericarditis (with particular reference to tuberculous pericarditis). Australasian Ann Med 16:41, 1967.

Spodick DH: Differential diagnosis of acute pericarditis. Progr Cardiovas Dis 14:192, 1971.

PERICARDITIS WITH EFFUSION

The most common causes of pericardial effusion are uremia, tuberculosis, malignancy, postcardiac surgery, myxedema, rheumatoid arthritis, lymphoma, sarcoidosis, purulent pericarditis, and connective tissue diseases. Rare types include chylous and "chronic idiopathic" pericarditis.

The speed of accumulation determines the physiologic importance of the effusion. Massive pericardial effusions, if they accumulate slowly, may produce no symptoms. However, sudden hemorrhage into the pericardium or sudden accumulation of relatively small effusions may raise the intrapericardial pressure to the point of cardiac tamponade, in which the fluid limits venous inflow and diastolic filling of the heart. In tamponade the cardiac output falls, the pulse pressure narrows, and tachycardia and elevation of venous pressure appear as compensatory mechanisms. Shock and death may result if tamponade is not relieved.

Clinical Findings

A. Symptoms and Signs: Pain is often absent but may be present as in acute pericarditis and as a dull, diffuse, oppressive precordial or substernal distress. Dyspnea and cough cause the patient to sit up and lean forward for relief. Dysphagia is prominent. Fever and other symptoms depend upon the primary disease (eg, septicemia, empyema, malignancy).

The area of "cardiac" dullness is enlarged and the apex beat is often not palpable or is well within the lateral border of dullness. Friction rub may persist despite a large effusion. In tamponade, distended neck veins, paradoxic pulse, inspiratory distention of the neck veins, and narrow pulse pressure are present. Liver enlargement, ascites, and leg edema depend upon the degree and duration of tamponade. Acute cardiac tamponade produces the clinical picture of shock.

B. Laboratory Findings: The cause of acute effusion is determined by bacteriologic and cytologic study of aspirated fluid and by the presence of primary disease elsewhere (tuberculosis, lupus erythymatosus, malignancy, myxedema, sarcoidosis, septicemia, lymphoma, etc); of chronic effusion, by pericardial biopsy. Leukocytosis and a rapid sedimentation rate are present when the effusion is infectious or inflammatory. The arm-to-tongue circulation time is normal in the presence of large effusion without tamponade; this is often a clue to the correct interpretation of a "large heart shadow" on chest x-ray. In myxedema, pericardial effusion and prolongation of the circulation time are present without tamponade.

C. X-Ray Findings: A rapidly enlarging "cardiac" silhouette with sharply defined margins, an acute right cardiophrenic angle, clear lung fields, and pleural effusion are common. Cardiac pulsations are feeble or absent. Intravenous CO_2 administration allows estimation of the distance between the atrial cavity and the pericardial sac by x-ray, as does also the position of a catheter in the right atrium. Angiocardiography is usually helpful in establishing the diagnosis of pericardial effusion.

D. ECG Findings: The T waves are low, flat, diphasic, or inverted in all leads; the QRS voltage is uniformly low.

E. Echocardiography: See p 223.

Differential Diagnosis

Cardiac dilatation with congestive heart failure may be impossible to differentiate from pericarditis with effusion if pleural effusion is also present. Pulmonary rales, gallop rhythm, and raised jugular venous pressure may be of clinical value in assessing cardiac failure. Rapid changes in heart size as seen by x-ray, clear lung fields with normal hilar vessels, definite paradoxic pulse, and absent cardiac pulsations on fluoroscopy are rare in congestive failure. Echocardiography is often definitive in the diagnosis of pericardial effusion. In a patient with "heart failure," the absence of significant murmurs, arrhythmia, and hypertension should suggest pericarditis with effusion.

Complications

Cardiac tamponade is a serious complication. Rapidly developing pericardial effusions or hemorrhage into the pericardial sac may so impede venous return and cardiac filling that cardiac output falls and irreversible shock occurs. Anticoagulant therapy creates a serious hazard of hemorrhage.

Purulent pericarditis is usually secondary to other infection elsewhere but is at times caused by contamination of a previous pericardial tap.

Treatment

A. Emergency Treatment (Paracentesis): The indications for pericardial paracentesis are the symptoms and signs of cardiac tamponade. As the pericardial fluid increases in amount, and particularly when it increases rapidly, the venous pressure may rise toward its limit of 22–24 cm water and the cardiac output may progressively fall. When this occurs, the patient becomes weak, pale, and dyspneic, and the pulse pressure becomes very narrow and the pulse rapid and thready, ie, the patient goes into shock. Under these circumstances removal of the pericardial fluid may be lifesaving; the fluid should be removed slowly to avoid cardiac dilatation or sudden reflex changes in rate and rhythm.

1. Sites of puncture—(*Caution:* Avoid puncture of the ventricular muscle.) Puncture may be made at the left 5th or 6th interspace about 1 cm within the area of cardiac dullness or 1–2 cm inside the left heart border as localized by x-ray (roughly 7–8 cm outside the left sternal line). The needle is pushed slowly inward and slightly upward. If effusion is present, one should find fluid within 3–5 cm—at times 7–8 cm. Puncture may also be made in the epigastric area between the xiphoid process and the left sternal margin. Insert the needle upward at an angle of about 30 degrees, pointed toward the midline. The pericardium is reached at about 3–4 cm.

2. Equipment—No. 16 or 18 needle with short bevel and fitting stylet; No. 26 or 27 needle to infiltrate the skin with procaine; and a 20–30 ml syringe to remove fluid. The syringe should be connected to the needle with a 4-inch piece of rubber tubing to prevent excessive movement of the needle. A sterile ground wire is connected between the needle and the V lead of a well grounded ECG machine in order to indicate when the myocardium is entered. Proper grounding of the patient and the ECG is essential to prevent accidental induction of ventricular fibrillation.

3. Technic—Clean and sterilize skin over the area to be punctured. Drape the surrounding area with sterile towels. Infiltrate the skin with 1–2% procaine solution. Insert the needle (detached from the syringe and without a stylet) slowly into the skin, following the directions according to the site selected. When the fluid is encountered it must be withdrawn slowly. When the needle encounters the epicardium, the monitoring ECG will show a sudden upward shift of the ST segment, indicating the limit to which the needle may be advanced. This technic greatly decreases the likelihood of cardiac puncture. A small polyethylene catheter can be introduced through the needle for removal of large amounts of fluid.

After the needle is removed, a simple dressing over the needle puncture is adequate.

B. Specific Measures:

1. Tuberculous pericarditis—Treat the systemic infection with bed rest, attention to nutrition and other general factors, and intensive antituberculosis chemotherapy. If fever and signs of pericardial effusion do not rapidly subside and are still obvious in 1 month, surgical decortication of the pericardium should be considered in order to prevent chronic constrictive pericarditis. Good judgment is required to determine when the disease is progressing despite medical treatment and when signs of constriction are appearing.

2. Rheumatic pericarditis with effusion—Treat as for rheumatic fever. The salicylates may help in causing fluid resorption. Paracentesis is usually unnecessary but should be performed if tamponade occurs.

3. Hydropericardium due to heart failure—Treatment of the congestive failure is usually sufficient.

4. Hemopericardium due to rupture of adjacent structure (usually post-traumatic)—If fluid accumulation is excessive, remove fluid at once.

5. Infection—Treat infection with appropriate chemotherapeutic agents and perform paracentesis as needed to relieve pressure. When fluid is being removed

instill 50,000–150,000 units of penicillin or the equivalent topical amount of streptomycin or other indicated antibiotic into the pericardial sac, and repeat whenever a tap is performed. Chemotherapeutic agents should be continued as long as purulent effusion is present. If fluid is encapsulated or the patient is not responding to therapy, surgical drainage via pericardiotomy may be necessary.

6. Uremic pericarditis often clears clinically after beginning therapy with chronic dialysis. Severe tamponade may require pericardiectomy.

7. Myxedema—Treat with T_3 because its short half-life is protective in case angina or arrhythmia occurs; change to T_4 after 1–2 weeks.

8. Connective tissue disorders—Treat with corticosteroids.

9. Others—Treat sarcoidosis, lymphoma, and tumors with radiotherapy or chemotherapy.

Prognosis

Tuberculous pericarditis causes death in the majority of untreated cases and results in chronic constrictive pericarditis in many that survive. The mortality rate is very low with early and adequate treatment; the long-term effect on the incidence of constrictive pericarditis is not known.

Acute benign pericarditis is only rarely a fatal disorder.

Rheumatic pericarditis, if severe and protracted, is associated with myocarditis, and this determines the immediate prognosis. Residual pericardial disease of clinical significance does not occur.

Purulent pericarditis, since it is usually associated with a blood stream infection or infection elsewhere, is usually fatal if not treated; however, it responds satisfactorily to antibiotics.

Comty CM, Cohen SL, Shapiro FL: Pericarditis in chronic uremia and its sequels. Ann Int Med 75:173, 1971.

Golinko RJ & others: The mechanism of pulsus paradoxus during acute pericardial tamponade. J Clin Invest 42:249, 1963.

Gotsman MS, Schrire V: A pericardiocentesis electrode needle. Brit Heart J 28:566, 1966.

Rich LL, Lisa CP, Nasser WK: Carcinoid pericarditis. Am J Med 54:522, 1973.

Shabetai R & others: Hemodynamics, cardiac tamponade and constrictive pericarditis: Symposium on pericardial disease. Am J Cardiol 26:445, 1970.

CHRONIC CONSTRICTIVE PERICARDITIS

Essentials of Diagnosis

- Markedly elevated venous pressure.
- Slight to moderate cardiac enlargement and quiet heart action.
- Paradoxic pulse.
- Ascites out of proportion to degree of ankle edema.

General Considerations

Encasement of the myocardium by an adherent, dense fibrous pericardium may be asymptomatic or may prevent ventricular expansion during diastole. If this happens the stroke volume is low and fixed and cardiac output can be increased only by tachycardia. Venous pressure rises as in congestive heart failure, and this, together with renal retention of sodium and water, produces the peripheral signs of right heart failure.

Clinical Findings

A. Symptoms and Signs: The principal symptoms are slowly progressive dyspnea, fatigue, and weakness on exertion, abdominal distention, and leg edema. Examination shows markedly distended neck veins with weak or absent systolic pulsations but prominent diastolic retraction, a moderately enlarged heart with a quiet precordium in the presence of tachycardia, faint heart sounds, a palpable and audible pericardial knock in early diastole, a low pulse pressure with a high diastolic level, paradoxic pulse, enlarged liver, ascites, and edema of both legs and the scrotum. Atrial fibrillation is frequently present.

B. Laboratory Findings: The arm-to-tongue circulation time is prolonged. Rarely, tuberculous infection of the lungs or other organ is noted.

C. X-Ray and Fluoroscopic Findings: The "heart" is usually moderately enlarged. Its shape is not consistent with valvular or hypertensive heart disease. Pulsations are weak or absent. Lung fields are clear. Pericardial calcification is common but is not diagnostic of constrictive pericarditis. Diagnostic ultrasound may be of assistance.

D. ECG Findings: T waves are flat or inverted; low voltage of QRS complexes is variable. Atrial fibrillation is common.

Differential Diagnosis

Marked venous engorgement in the neck without systolic pulsation, slight to moderate cardiac enlargement, absence of significant murmurs or hypertension, paradoxic pulse, and ECG changes distinguish chronic constrictive pericarditis from tricuspid stenosis, congestive heart failure from any cause, especially cardiomyopathy, cirrhosis of the liver, mediastinal tumor, nephrosis, and obstruction of the vena cava.

Complications

In tuberculous cases, a miliary spread or acute flare-up of the intrapericardial infection may occur.

Thrombophlebitis of the leg veins may occur secondary to elevated venous pressure, venous stasis, and inactivity.

Treatment

Give a low-sodium diet and diuretics as in cardiac failure to combat ascites and congestive failure. Digitalis is usually of little value unless the patient has atrial fibrillation.

Surgical removal of the constricting pericardium can frequently restore a patient to normal health. If congestive phenomena are chronic or the pericarditis is progressive, surgical intervention is the only method offering possible cure. In a large London hospital, the recent surgical mortality was 4%, and 85% of patients were greatly benefited by the procedure.

Prognosis

Constrictive pericarditis known to be due to tuberculosis is usually fatal without antituberculosis drugs and surgery. Most patients with constrictive pericarditis due to any cause have increasing disability because of ascites and edema and die of mechanical "heart failure." A few patients show no progression of symptoms or signs for years. Spontaneous regression is rare.

Conti CR, Friesinger GC: Chronic constrictive pericarditis: Clinical and laboratory findings in 11 cases. Johns Hopkins Med J 120:262, 1967.

Hancock EW: Constrictive pericarditis: Clinical clues to diagnosis. JAMA 232:176, 1975.

Kloster FE & others: Hemodynamic studies following pericardiectomy for constrictive pericarditis. Circulation 32:415, 1965.

Somerville W: Constrictive pericarditis, with special reference to the change in natural history brought about by surgical intervention. Circulation 38 (Suppl 5):102, 1968.

DISEASES OF THE MYOCARDIUM

CHRONIC OR SUBACUTE PULMONARY HEART DISEASE
(Chronic or Subacute Cor Pulmonale)

Essentials of Diagnosis

- Symptoms and signs of chronic bronchitis and pulmonary emphysema.
- No significant murmurs or hypertension.
- ECG: tall, peaked P waves, right axis deviation, and right ventricular hypertrophy.
- Chest x-ray: enlarged right ventricle and pulmonary artery.

General Considerations

Cor pulmonale refers to the right ventricular hypertrophy and eventual failure resulting from pulmonary parenchymal or vascular disease. It may be acute, subacute, or, most commonly, chronic, and its clinical features depend both upon the primary disease and its effects on the heart.

Chronic cor pulmonale is most commonly caused by chronic obstructive pulmonary emphysema, often referred to as "chronic asthmatic bronchitis." Less common or rare causes include pneumoconiosis, pulmonary fibrosis, kyphoscoliosis, primary pulmonary hypertension, repeated episodes of subclinical pulmonary embolization, and obliterative pulmonary capillary infiltration from metastatic carcinoma. Emphysema and associated fibrosis result in obliteration of capillaries and disturbance of pulmonary function with resultant hypoxia. Compensatory polycythemia and increased cardiac output also appear. The combined effect of these changes is increased pulmonary artery pressure, which in turn leads to right ventricular hypertrophy and eventual failure of the "high-output" variety.

Clinical Findings

A. Symptoms and Signs: The dominant symptoms of compensated cor pulmonale are respiratory in origin: chronic productive cough, exertional dyspnea, wheezing respirations, undue fatigability, and weakness. When the pulmonary disease has advanced sufficiently to cause right ventricular failure, these symptoms are intensified. In addition, dependent edema, right upper quadrant pain, and digestive disturbances may appear. The signs of cor pulmonale include cyanosis, clubbing, distended neck veins, right ventricular heave or gallop (or both), pulmonary emphysema, prominent lower sternal or epigastric pulsations, and enlarged tender liver, and dependent edema. The heart size cannot be determined because of emphysema, but there is no evidence of valvular disease. Pulses are full and the extremities warm unless the patient is terminal or in shock.

B. Laboratory Findings: Polycythemia is usually present in cor pulmonale secondary to emphysema. The arterial oxygen saturation is below 85%; P_{CO_2} is often elevated. Venous pressure is significantly elevated in right ventricular failure, but the circulation time may be normal or only slightly prolonged. Pulmonary function studies define the nature of the pulmonary disease.

C. ECG Findings: Electrocardiography shows right axis deviation and peaked P waves. Deep S waves are present in lead V_6. Left axis deviation may be noted in patients with pulmonary emphysema. Frank right ventricular hypertrophy is uncommon except in "primary pulmonary hypertension," in which this is the rule.

D. X-Ray Findings: Chest x-ray discloses the presence or absence of parenchymal disease and a prominent or enlarged right ventricle, pulmonary conus, and artery.

E. Other Studies: Cardiac catheterization and right ventricular angiograms reveal pulmonary artery pressures and right ventricular anatomy.

Differential Diagnosis

In its early stages cor pulmonale can be diagnosed only on x-ray or ECG evidence. When frank congestive signs appear, differentiation from primary left ventricular failure is possible by considering the predominant history of respiratory complaints, the absence of orthopnea, the degree of cyanosis, bounding pulses, and warm extremities in the presence of edema. ECG

demonstration of right axis deviation, normal or only moderately prolonged circulation time, and absence of demonstrable factors pointing to left failure are helpful. Catheterization of the right heart, angiography, and pulmonary function studies will establish a definitive diagnosis.

Complications

Intercurrent respiratory infections increase dyspnea, cough, and cyanosis and may precipitate a dangerous degree of respiratory acidosis in advanced emphysema. Neurologic manifestations of CO_2 narcosis may appear: disorientation, somnolence, coma, and occasionally convulsions.

Treatment

A. Specific Measures: Give appropriate antibiotic therapy for the respiratory infection that so commonly precedes failure in this type of case. The patient may be afebrile.

B. General Measures:

1. Intermittent positive-pressure mask breathing, eg, with the Bennett, Emerson, Bird, or similar respirator, at pressure settings of +10 to +15 (inspiration) may be helpful. Patients who do not breathe spontaneously may be treated advantageously with the automatic Bird respirator; the other nonautomatic apparatuses may be operated manually. These devices provide a convenient, effective method of administering bronchial dilators, antifoaming agents, and aerosols (see Chapter 6). None of the intermittent devices controlled by the patient lower the cardiac output.

2. In cor pulmonale, intermittent positive-pressure breathing, especially when combined with effective bronchial dilators, is probably the most effective therapeutic measure. The use of mechanical devices in acute respiratory distress may not be helpful and should perhaps be postponed until other measures have improved the situation.

3. CNS depressants, especially narcotics, barbiturates, and hypnotics, are strongly *contraindicated* in the treatment of cardiac failure secondary to primary pulmonary disease (cor pulmonale) owing to their marked depressant action on the respiratory centers.

4. Treat heart failure in the usual way with bed rest, restriction of sodium, diuretics, and digitalis. Digitalis may not be effective if cardiac output is high.

5. Give acetazolamide (Diamox), 250 mg daily, after adequate ventilation has been restored, ie, when CO_2 elimination is effective.

Prognosis

Compensated cor pulmonale has the same outlook as the underlying pulmonary disease. Once congestive signs appear, the average life expectancy is 2–5 years, but survival is significantly longer when uncomplicated emphysema is the cause. Left ventricular failure secondary to coronary artery disease, hypertension, or aortic valve lesions may develop and shorten expectancy accordingly.

Alpert JS & others: Treatment of massive pulmonary embolism: The role of pulmonary embolectomy. Am Heart J 89:413, 1975.

Comroe JH Jr, Nadel JA: Screening tests of pulmonary function. New England J Med 282:1249, 1970.

Comroe JH Jr & others: *The Lung: Clinical Physiology and Pulmonary Function Tests,* 2nd ed. Year Book, 1962.

Ferrer MI: Cor pulmonale (pulmonary heart disease): Present-day status. Am Heart J 89:657, 1975.

Hougie C: Thromboembolism and oral contraceptives. Am Heart J 85:538, 1973.

McDonald IG & others: Major pulmonary embolism: A correlation of clinical findings, haemodynamics, pulmonary angiography, and pathological physiology. Brit Heart J 34: 356, 1972.

McIntyre KM, Sasahara AA, Littman D: Relation of the electrocardiogram to hemodynamic alterations in pulmonary embolism. Am J Cardiol 30:205, 1972.

McNeil BJ, Holman BL, Adelstein SJ: The scintigraphic definition of pulmonary embolism. JAMA 227:753, 1974.

Moses DC, Silver TM, Bookstein JJ: The complementary roles of chest radiography, lung scanning, and selective pulmonary angiography in the diagnosis of pulmonary embolism. Circulation 49:179, 1974.

Oakley CM, Goodwin JF: Current clinical aspects of cor pulmonale. Am J Cardiol 20:842, 1967.

Pontoppidan H, Geffin B, Lowenstein E: Acute respiratory failure in the adult. New England J Med 287:690, 1972.

Sleeper JC, Orgain ES, McIntosh HD: Primary pulmonary hypertension: Review of clinical features and pathologic physiology with a report of pulmonary hemodynamics derived from repeated catheterization. Circulation 26: 1358, 1962.

Vandenbergh E, Clement J, van de Woestijne KP: Course and prognosis of patients with advanced chronic obstructive pulmonary disease: Evaluation by means of functional indices. Am J Med 55:736, 1973.

Wilhelmsen L, Hagman M, Werko L: Recurrent pulmonary embolism: Incidence, predisposing factors and prognosis. Acta med scandinav 192:565, 1972.

SYPHILITIC CARDIOVASCULAR DISEASE

Essentials of Diagnosis

- Linear calcification or localized dilatation of the ascending aorta on x-ray.
- Aortic valvular insufficiency without stenosis or mitral valve disease.
- Aneurysm of the aorta.
- Coronary ostial stenosis.
- Evidence of syphilitic etiology: history of infection, positive STS, or presence of other forms of late syphilis.

General Considerations

Syphilitic "heart disease" may consist of aortic valvular insufficiency (most common), aortic dilatation or aneurysm, or narrowing of the coronary ostia. It comprises less than 5% of all heart disease in population groups which have ready access to effective treat-ment of syphilis. It is more common in men (3:1) and is usually diagnosed between the ages of 35 and 55 (10–20 years after the primary infection). STS are positive in about 85% of untreated cases. The ascending aorta, arch, and descending aorta are most commonly affected; the abdominal aorta is rarely involved. Aortic valve insufficiency occurs in about 10% of cases of untreated syphilitic aortitis. One or both of the coronary ostia may be partially occluded.

Clinical Findings

A. Aortitis: There are no symptoms, and physical signs are absent unless dilatation has occurred. In a man under the age of 40 without hypertension or demonstrable arteriosclerosis, a ringing or accentuated second aortic sound with or without a soft aortic systolic murmur is "suggestive" of syphilitic aortitis. Fluoroscopic evidence of increased width and pulsation of the ascending aorta, best seen in the left anterior oblique view, in the absence of elongation, is also suggestive. Linear calcification limited to the root of the aorta and arch is almost diagnostic.

B. Aortic Insufficiency: Clinical, x-ray, and ECG manifestations are as for rheumatic aortic insufficiency. Ten percent of cases are associated with saccular aneurysm. Aortic insufficiency may produce no symptoms for long periods; once heart failure develops, however, it soon becomes refractory to treatment and in most cases death occurs within 2–5 years.

C. Aortic Aneurysm: Symptoms and signs are dependent upon the site and size of the aneurysm. Aneurysm of the ascending aorta is characterized by visible pulsation or dullness of the manubrium and in the first to third interspaces parasternally; lowered blood pressure in the right arm; and an aortic systolic murmur and thrill without peripheral signs of aortic stenosis. Aneurysm of the aortic arch is characterized by cough, dyspnea, and recurrent pulmonary infections (compression of trachea or right main stem bronchus); hoarseness (compression of recurrent laryngeal nerve); edema of the face and neck, distended neck veins, and prominent veins over upper chest (compression of superior vena cava); and dysphagia (compression of the esophagus). Aneurysm of the descending aorta is usually asymptomatic; when it is large it may erode the ribs or spine, producing pain which is worse in recumbency and visible or palpable pulsations medial to the left scapula.

X-ray findings consist of saccular or sharply defined fusiform bulging of the thoracic aorta with increased pulsation. Clot formation or periaortic fibrosis may dampen the pulsations and simulate a solid tumor. Transaxillary or retrograde femoral artery injections of radiopaque contrast media differentiate the 2 by demonstrating continuity of the aorta with the lumen of the aneurysm.

D. Narrowing of the Coronary Artery Ostia: Angina pectoris is identical to that seen in coronary heart disease. Its syphilitic origin can only be inferred in the presence of one of the other manifestations of syphilitic aortitis.

Differential Diagnosis

The clinical picture can mimic rheumatic and arteriosclerotic heart disease and rheumatoid arthritis. Syphilitic aneurysms are indistinguishable clinically from those caused by arteriosclerosis.

Treatment

A. Specific Measures: Treat syphilis as outlined in Chapter 24. Several subsequent courses of penicillin are advised by some authorities at intervals of 6 months or 1 year, especially if the STS remains positive.

B. General Measures: Bed rest may be desirable during treatment with penicillin, because of the possibility of Herxheimer's reaction.

C. Surgical Measures: Surgical repair of the aneurysm has been attempted but is hazardous. Successful surgical endarterectomy for coronary ostia stenosis has been accomplished. Surgical correction of aortic insufficiency may be necessary.

Complications

A. Aortic Insufficiency: Left ventricular hypertrophy, which may progress to failure.

B. Aortic Aneurysm: Recurrent pulmonary infection, bronchiectasis, atelectasis, bronchial hemorrhage, and rupture or dissection of the aneurysm.

Prognosis

A. Aortitis: Ten to 20% of patients develop aortic insufficiency and other manifestations of syphilitic cardiovascular disease; in the remainder, life expectancy is not affected.

B. Aortic Insufficiency: If penicillin is given when the signs of aortic insufficiency are purely auscultatory, the progress of the lesion may be slowed or even arrested; this significantly improves the prognosis for survival.

C. Aortic Aneurysm: Once aneurysms have reached sufficient size to produce symptoms by compression of adjacent structures, life expectancy is measured in months. Longer survival is possible when the aneurysm is small and effective therapy for syphilis has been given. Death is usually due to rupture of the aneurysm.

D. Narrowing of the Coronary Artery Ostia: This condition tends to aggravate the heart failure due to syphilitic aortic insufficiency and predisposes to sudden death. Surgical correction has been successfully accomplished.

Beck W: Syphilitic obstruction of coronary ostia successfully treated by endarterectomy. Brit Heart J 27:911, 1965.

CARDIOMYOPATHIES
(Acute & Chronic Myocarditis & Endomyocardial Diseases)

Acute myocarditis is a focal or diffuse inflammation of the myocardium occurring during or after many viral, bacterial, rickettsial, spirochetal, fungal, and parasitic diseases or after various drugs (emetine, daunomycin). Mild forms are very common and are recognizable only by serial ECG changes. Severe myocarditis producing signs and symptoms occurs most commonly in acute rheumatic fever, diphtheria, scrub typhus, and Chagas' disease (*Trypanosoma cruzi* infection). Bacteremia, viral pneumonia and encephalitis, and trichinosis may be associated with myocarditis of varying severity.

Myocardial disease includes a wide variety of noninfectious myocardial diseases whose clinical manifestations are similar to those of myocarditis except that peripheral embolization and refractory heart failure are more common and the process is more chronic. A partial list of these includes alcoholic cardiomyopathy, Fiedler's isolated myocarditis, subendocardial fibroelastosis, idiopathic cardiac hypertrophy (congenital and adult), familial cardiomegaly, idiopathic myocardial failure in pregnancy, connective tissue diseases (scleroderma, disseminated lupus erythematosus, polyarteritis nodosa), serum sickness, and amyloidosis. Hypertrophic cardiomyopathy is discussed separately (see below) because it seems to be a different genetic disease with special characteristics.

Primary myocardial disease (cardiomyopathy) constitutes a group of diseases, often of unknown cause, that usually develops insidiously, although it may occasionally follow acute myocarditis. Various names have been given to the entity, eg, primary myocardial disease, primary cardiomyopathy, idiopathic cardiac hypertrophy. The left ventricle is usually dominantly involved, although in some cases the right ventricle as well as the septum may be involved.

Patients with primary cardiomyopathy usually present with unexplained left ventricular hypertrophy or left ventricular failure which usually progresses over a period of months or a few years. Associated symptoms include embolic phenomena, cardiac arrhythmias, and clinical and hemodynamic evidence of either obstructive or restrictive left ventricular disease.

Among known causes of cardiomyopathy, ischemic and alcoholic cardiomyopathy are perhaps the most common, although opinion differs about whether alcohol directly affects the myocardial cells (producing cardiomyopathy) or whether it operates via the mechanism of thiamine deficiency (beriberi heart). The former opinion is most widespread and is perhaps supported by the best evidence. Other generalized diseases often associated with cardiomyopathy are primary amyloidosis, scleroderma, sarcoidosis, and endocardial fibrosis in Africa. Postpartum myocarditis and heart failure are thought to be variants of the cardiomyopathies, but the evidence is not clear. Glycogen storage disease and various neurologic disorders also may be associated with primary myocardial disease.

Primary cardiomyopathy is often diagnosed by eliminating all known causes and will probably continue to be so until its cause becomes known.

Clinical Findings

A. Symptoms and Signs: Mild forms of myocarditis are asymptomatic and are overshadowed by the underlying disease. Severe myocarditis may result in weakness, syncope, dizziness, dyspnea, nausea, vomiting, chest pain, and shock or sudden death. In endomyocardial diseases the course may be acute, subacute, or chronic, but the symptoms are similar. Fiedler's myocarditis, idiopathic cardiac hypertrophy, idiopathic heart failure of pregnancy, and other primary myocardial diseases are characterized by peripheral emboli and heart failure. Noncardiac manifestations of the underlying disease may be noted, as in carcinoid syndrome, Friedreich's ataxia, and the collagen diseases.

In addition to those of the underlying disease (eg, hemochromatosis, scleroderma), signs include fever, tachycardia, cardiac enlargement, faint heart sounds, changing systolic murmurs, arrhythmias, variable congestive heart failure (predominantly right-sided), with hepatomegaly, gallop rhythm, pulsus alternans, and distended neck veins; and signs of cerebral or peripheral embolization. The obstructive cardiomyopathies may present as idiopathic left ventricular failure and may simulate aortic stenosis, chronic constrictive pericarditis, beriberi heart disease, etc.

B. ECG Findings: Partial to complete atrioventricular block and intraventricular conduction defects; diffusely flat to inverted T waves; and low voltage QRS. In mild myocarditis, only transient flattening or inversion of T waves may be noted.

C. X-Ray Findings: Radiographic examination (including cardiac catheterization and left ventricular angiograms) shows increased left ventricular volume, pulmonary venous congestion, and evidences of left ventricular failure.

Differential Diagnosis

Myocarditis and endomyocardial disorders vary so much in clinical signs that they are confused with thyrotoxicosis, bacterial endocarditis, "painless" coronary artery disease, rheumatic heart disease with faint or atypical murmurs, pericardial tamponade, and neoplastic disease of the heart. Sinus tachycardia and minor ECG changes are an insufficient basis for diagnosis.

Treatment

No specific therapy is available except in the obstructive cardiomyopathies of the left ventricle. Surgical excision of the subaortic stenosis or ventricular septectomy is now feasible under cardiopulmonary bypass if propranolol is ineffective. Corticosteroids are occasionally helpful in the connective tissue group of diseases. Anticoagulant therapy may be indicated for patients with embolization. The general principles of treatment of cardiac failure and anemia should be followed as they prove to be applicable in specific individual cases.

In the presence of cardiac failure, left ventricular cineangiography and coronary angiography are frequently necessary to exclude coronary heart disease with dyskinesia and aneurysms which are amenable to surgical excision.

Prognosis

The common forms of acute myocarditis rarely produce disability or death. The overall mortality rate in diphtheritic myocarditis is 25%; the death rate approaches 100% if shock or congestive heart failure occurs and is 50–75% with complete heart block. Mortality is similarly high in Chagas' disease. Myocarditis is the chief cause of death in scrub typhus. With the exception of rheumatic fever, there are no late sequelae after recovery.

Abelmann WH: Myocarditis. New England J Med 275:832, 1966.

Alexander CS: Cobalt-beer cardiomyopathy: A clinical and pathologic study of twenty-eight cases. Am J Med 53:395, 1972.

Amyloidosis: Clinical conference. Am J Med 53:495, 1972.

Blieden LC, Moller JH: Cardiac involvement in inherited disorders of metabolism. Progr Cardiovas Dis 16:615, 1974.

Demakis JG & others: Natural course of peripartum cardiomyopathy. Circulation 44:1053, 1971.

Field BJ & others: Left ventricular function and hypertrophy in cardiomyopathy with depressed ejection fraction. Circulation 47:1022, 1973.

Fleming HA: Sarcoid heart disease. Brit Heart J 36:54, 1974.

Fowler NO: Differential diagnosis of cardiomyopathies. Progr Cardiovas Dis 14:113, 1971.

Hamm BRI & others: Primary myocardial disease: Clinical, hemodynamic, and angiographic correlates in 50 patients. Am J Cardiol 25:625, 1970.

Harvey WP, Segal JP, Gurel T: The clinical spectrum of primary myocardial disease. Progr Cardiovas Dis 7:17, 1964.

Kreulen TH, Gorlin R, Herman MV: Ventriculographic patterns and hemodynamics in primary myocardial disease. Circulation 47:299, 1973.

Liedtke AJ, DeMuth WE Jr: Nonpenetrating cardiac injuries: A collective review. Am Heart J 86:687, 1973.

Millward DK, McLaurin LP, Craige E: Echocardiographic studies of the mitral valve in patients with congestive cardiomyopathy and mitral regurgitation. Am Heart J 85:413, 1973.

Perloff JK: The cardiomyopathies: Current concepts. Circulation 44:942, 1971.

Pietras RJ & others: Cardiovascular response in hyperthyroidism: The influence of adrenergic-receptor blockade. Arch Int Med 129:426, 1972.

Rose HD: Recurrent illness following acute coxsackie B4 myocarditis. Am J Med 54:544, 1973.

Smith WG: Coxsackie B myopericarditis in adults. Am Heart J 80:34, 1970.

Sommers K & others: Hemodynamic features of severe endomyocardial fibrosis of the right ventricle, including comparison with constrictive pericarditis. Brit Heart J 30:322, 1968.

Trell E & others: Carcinoid heart disease. Am J Med 54:433, 1973.

Westermark P, Stenkvist B: A new method for the diagnosis of systemic amyloidosis. Arch Int Med 132:522, 1973.

HYPERTROPHIC CARDIOMYOPATHY
(Idiopathic Hypertrophic Subaortic Stenosis, IHSS)

Hypertrophic cardiomyopathy, a genetic disease of unknown origin, is more common than was formerly thought. It is due essentially to asymmetric hypertrophy of the septum and free wall of the left ventricle in association with variable obstruction of the left ventricular outflow tract. Hypertrophy of the right ventricle with obstruction of the right ventricular outflow tract may coexist. The degree of obstruction is highly variable and is related to the contractile force of the left ventricle, the systemic vascular resistance (the "afterload"), and the left ventricular diastolic volume. Factors which increase the force of left ventricular contraction such as inotropic agents (digitalis, isoproterenol) or the first beat following a post-extrasystolic pause cause or increase obstruction and result in a pressure difference or gradient across the left ventricular cavity below the aortic valve. Similarly, decrease in the systemic vascular resistance (such as occurs with amyl nitrite) decreases the impedance to left ventricular outflow and the pressure gradient becomes increased as obstruction develops.

The obstruction to left ventricular outflow is caused by impingement of the anterior leaflet of the mitral valve against the septum which can be recognized clearly on echocardiography, a reliable noninvasive diagnostic technic. The abnormal position of the anterior leaflet also results in mitral insufficiency with its characteristic pansystolic murmur; patients have as well a late crescendo ejection systolic murmur resulting from the left ventricular outflow tract obstruction. The carotid pulse and the left ventricular pressure pulse have a rapid upstroke time since the forceful ejection of the hypertrophied left ventricle ejects most of the blood during the initial part of systole. When the increased force of contraction results in obstruction of the outflow tract, the ejection of blood is abruptly slowed and a slower (double-humped) secondary wave then appears in both the left ventricular pressure pulse and in the carotid artery as ejection continues. The palpable fourth heart sound due to decreased compliance of the left ventricle causes a "triple-humped" pressure pulse which can be demonstrated by palpation and by the apexcardiogram.

Patients with hypertrophic cardiomyopathy demonstrate left ventricular hypertrophy electrocardiographically and radiologically. Left ventricular catheterization and angiography demonstrate the variable pressure gradient (which can be induced during the study) across the ventricular outflow tract, the narrow systolic left ventricular outflow tract with marked, irregular septal hypertrophy, and abnormalities of systolic contraction which differ from those seen in valvular aortic stenosis. The left ventricular end-diastolic pressure is almost always raised, especially after exercise, resulting from the considerably decreased compliance of the hypertrophied left ventricle. Inflow obstruction from decreased distensibility causes slow filling of the left ventricle, a large *a* wave, a slow *y* descent, and a small *v* wave in the left atrium.

The course of the disease is variable, depending on when it is first recognized, but inflow obstruction ultimately worsens and as the left ventricular end-diastolic pressure and left atrial pressure rise, dyspnea may occur; later, cardiac output falls.

The appearance of atrial fibrillation may, by further interfering with left ventricular filling, precipitate congestive failure. Systemic embolism, angina pectoris, syncope, and sudden death may also terminate the disease. Infective endocarditis may involve the mitral valve.

Treatment begins with beta-adrenergic blocking agents such as propranolol to reduce the left ventricular end-diastolic pressure induced by exercise and sympathetic stimulation; compliance is increased and left ventricular contractility is decreased, lessening the obstruction to left ventricular outflow. If the patient remains symptomatic and receives no benefit from propranolol, surgery may be advised. Myotomy and limited resection of the hypertrophied muscle have occasionally produced gratifying results.

Adelman AG & others: The clinical course in muscular subaortic stenosis. Ann Int Med 77:515, 1972.

Cooley DA, Leachman RD, Wukasch DC: Diffuse muscular subaortic stenosis: Surgical treatment. Am J Cardiol 31:1, 1973.

Glancy DL, Epstein SE: Differential diagnosis of type and severity of obstruction to left ventricular outflow. Progr Cardiovas Dis 14:153, 1971.

Goodwin JF: Hypertrophic diseases of the myocardium. Progr Cardiovas Dis 16:199, 1973.

Goodwin JF: Treatment of the cardiomyopathies. Am J Cardiol 32:341, 1973.

Hardarson T & others: Prognosis and mortality of hypertrophic obstructive cardiomyopathy. Lancet 2:1462, 1973.

Henry WL, Clark CE, Epstein SE: Asymmetric septal hypertrophy (ASH): The unifying link in the IHSS disease spectrum. Circulation 47:827, 1973.

Powell WJ Jr & others: Symptomatic prognosis in patients with idiopathic hypertrophic subaortic stenosis (IHSS). Am J Med 55:15, 1973.

Shah PM & others: Echocardiographic assessment of the effects of surgery and propranolol on the dynamics of outflow obstruction in hypertrophic subaortic stenosis. Circulation 45:616, 1972.

Stenson RE & others: Hypertrophic subaortic stenosis. Am J Cardiol 31:763, 1973.

Tajik AJ & others: Idiopathic hypertrophic subaortic stenosis: Long-term surgical follow-up. Am J Cardiol 34:815, 1974.

Whiting RB & others: Idiopathic hypertrophic subaortic stenosis in the elderly. New England J Med 285:196, 1971.

PRIMARY CARDIAC TUMORS

Primary cardiac tumors are rare and constitute only a small fraction of all tumors that involve the heart or pericardium. Metastases may appear in the myocardium or the pericardium and infrequently affect left ventricular function, although when pericardial effusion occurs the patient may show manifestations of pericardial tamponade. The most common primary malignancies of the heart are sarcomas of various types.

A cardiac tumor may obstruct the venous or arterial vessels in the region of the heart; may obstruct the superior or inferior vena cava; or may interfere with left ventricular filling or left ventricular output.

The diagnosis is suggested by bizarre outlines of the cardiac shadow on plain films; by a clinical picture of malignancy elsewhere; by the relationship of posture to symptoms of syncope or vertigo as well as to murmurs; and, in the case of pericardial effusion, by the finding of malignant cells in the fluid. Definitive diagnosis is by cineangiocardiography, which may demonstrate obstruction of any chamber. A recent patient presented with evidences of tricuspid stenosis due to angiosarcoma of the right atrium.

The most common benign tumor of the heart is myxoma—usually left atrial myxoma—although the right atrium may be involved and, more rarely, either ventricle. The patient usually presents in one of 3 ways: (1) With intermittent symptoms of syncope, vertigo, and dyspnea as well as signs suggesting mitral valve disease. There may be changing murmurs and differences of opinion among examiners. The tumor is usually on a stalk and is mobile, and the degree of mitral valve obstruction varies depending upon its position and varying hemodynamic events. The patient may therefore have a mid-diastolic murmur even with an opening snap in one position but not in another. (2) Systemic emboli (common in about a third of cases). In 2 patients, the diagnosis was made by histologic recognition of myxoma in the embolic tissue removed at surgery. (3) Systemic symptoms and signs which are thought to be immunologic in origin, consisting of fever, tachycardia, raised sedimentation rate, anemia, clubbed fingers, protein abnormalities, raised serum globulin, etc. These may, however, be absent.

The diagnosis of tumor is made by echocardiography, which shows a filling defect posterior to the anterior mitral valve leaflet in diastole, and by cineangiocardiography, in which a filling defect is demonstrated.

Dicus R: Atrial myxoma. California Med 111:200, 1969.

Edwards JE: The effects of non-malignant cardiac tumors upon the cardiovascular system. Cardiovas Clin 4:281, 1972.

Glasser ST & others: Left atrial myxoma. Am J Med 50:113, 1971.

Goodwin JF: The spectrum of cardiac tumors. Am J Cardiol 21:307, 1968.

Harbold NB, Gau GT: Echocardiographic diagnosis of right atrial myxoma. Mayo Clin Proc 48:284, 1973.

Harvey WP: Clinical aspects of cardiac tumors. Am J Cardiol 21:328, 1968.

Miller JI: Primary cardiac tumors: Surgical considerations and results of operation. Circulation 45:1134 (Suppl 1), 1972.

Nasser WK & others: Atrial myxoma. 1. Clinical and pathologic features in nine cases. Am Heart J 83:694, 1972.

Peters MN & others: The clinical syndrome of atrial myxoma. JAMA 230:695, 1974.

Pritchard RW: Tumors of the heart: A review of subject and report of 150 cases. Arch Path 51:98, 1951.

Selzer A, Sakai FJ, Popper RW: Protean clinical manifestations of primary tumors of the heart. Am J Med 52:9, 1972.

Srivastava TN, Fletcher E: The echocardiogram in left atrial myxoma. Am J Med 54:136, 1973.

Steiner RE: Radiological aspects of cardiac tumors. Am J Cardiol 21:344, 1968.

Waxler EB, Kawai N, Kasparian H: Right atrial myxoma: Echocardiographic, phonocardiographic and hemodynamic signs. Am Heart J 83:251, 1972.

THE CARDIAC PATIENT & SURGERY

Major surgery in the cardiac patient is inevitably more hazardous than in patients with normal hearts. When shock, hemorrhage, hypoxia, struggling during induction, thromboembolism, and hypoventilation occur in a patient with heart disease the danger of coronary occlusion, myocardial infarction, cardiac failure, and arrhythmias is increased.

The major cardiac lesions which increase the risks of surgery are rheumatic heart disease (especially aortic stenosis); coronary heart disease (about 5% additional hazard); and syphilitic cardiovascular disease, especially if there is involvement of the coronary ostia (as suggested by associated angina). Hypertension without cardiac or renal involvement does not usually add to the surgical risk.

If possible, surgery of important magnitude and duration in patients with recent congestive failure should be delayed 3 weeks after recovery; in patients with recent myocardial infarction a delay of 3–6 months is advisable. The patient should be brought into the best cardiac state possible before surgery with medications, diet, and vitamin supplements. Anemia should be corrected. Presurgical electrolyte management is also very important in the cardiac patient.

In inducing and maintaining anesthesia in a cardiac patient, adequate ventilation, oxygenation, and smooth induction without struggling are important.

During surgery, hypotension should be treated promptly if it occurs, anemia avoided, and fluid therapy given to maintain optimal cardiac reserve.

Improvements in anesthesia and surgical skill have reduced the risk of major surgery in recent years. The presence of cardiac disease increases the risk but should not per se deny patients the benefits of elective but necessary surgery.

The following information will assist in estimating the likelihood of cardiac failure in a pregnant woman: (1) functional class before pregnancy; (2) the age of the patient; (3) the size of the heart; (4) the structural lesion of the heart; (5) the presence of arrhythmias; (6) the patient's socioeconomic status (eg, if children are at home or if the patient must work); (7) the intelligence and cooperation of the patient; and (8) the presence of associated disease.

THE CARDIAC PATIENT & PREGNANCY

Assessment of Risk of Heart Disease in Pregnancy

A. Little or No Functional Incapacity: Almost all patients who are asymptomatic or who have only mild symptoms with ordinary activities can continue to term under close medical supervision. If the patient develops more severe symptoms with activity she should be hospitalized, treated for failure, and kept in bed until term.

B. Moderate or Marked Functional Incapacity: If the patient has pure mitral stenosis and develops acute pulmonary edema or has moderate to marked symptoms with activity, mitral valvulotomy should be considered. This has been successfully accomplished up to the 8th month. If the patient does not have an operable lesion, she should be hospitalized, treated for cardiac failure, and kept in bed until term.

C. Severe Functional Incapacity: All patients seen during the first trimester who have symptoms on little or no activity and who do not have an operable cardiac lesion should be aborted, because of the high incidence of recurrent failure and death in this group of patients. Tubal ligation should be considered.

Physiologic Load Which Pregnancy Imposes on the Heart

The work of the heart increases by about 50% at the beginning of about the third month, when the blood volume and cardiac output increase. The placenta acts as an arteriovenous fistula. Cardiac failure may occur at any time from the end of the first trimester up to 2–3 weeks before term, at which time the load for some unaccountable reason decreases.

Sodium should be restricted after the second month.

Management of Labor

Current opinion holds that vaginal delivery is to be preferred except when there is an obstetric indication for cesarean section. Coarctation of the aorta may be the only cardiac disease which contraindicates vaginal delivery because of the danger of aortic rupture.

The second stage should be made as short as possible, using forceps when possible. Ergonovine maleate (Ergotrate) should probably not be used because of the increased work of the heart which it causes.

Conradsson T, Werkö L: Management of heart disease in pregnancy. Progr Cardiovas Dis 16:407, 1974.

Gilchrist AR: Cardiological problems in younger women including those of pregnancy and the puerperium. Brit MJ 1:209, 1963.

Handin RI: Thromboembolic complications of pregnancy and oral contraceptives. Progr Cardiovas Dis 16:395, 1974.

Metcalfe J, Ueland K: Maternal cardiovascular adjustments to pregnancy. Progr Cardiovas Dis 16:363, 1974.

Sullivan JM: Blood pressure elevation in pregnancy. Progr Cardiovas Dis 16:375, 1974.

Szekely P, Snaith L: *Heart Disease and Pregnancy*. Churchill, 1974.

CARDIOVASCULAR DRUGS

DIGITALIS & DIGITALIS-LIKE PREPARATIONS*

Action of Digitalis & Digitalis-Like Preparations

The fundamental action of digitalis glycosides is to increase the force and velocity of cardiac contraction, whether or not the heart is failing. When the heart is not failing, augmentation of the contractile state of the heart can be demonstrated by the increased peak rate of change of the ventricular pressure curve even if there is no increase of cardiac output. It is not established how, at the cellular level, digitalis increases contractility, but one theory (Braunwald) proposes that it does so by potentiating excitation-contraction coupling by increasing the intracytoplasmic calcium ion concentration during activation as the sarcoplasmic reticulum releases calcium ions. Electrophysiologically, digitalis increases the automaticity of secondary pacemakers in the atrial-AV nodal junction and in the AV node-His bundle junctions, as well as in secondary pacemakers throughout the Purkinje system. Digitalis also decreases impulse conduction of the heart, which may lead to reentry phenomena and ventricular irritability. Digitalis blocks conduction through the AV node, and this action is most helpful in slowing the ventricular rate in atrial fibrillation, but it also may produce partial or complete AV block. The drug may induce junctional tachycardia or AV dissociation by enhancing the automaticity of the junctional pacemakers or may cause ventricular premature beats, ventricular tachycardia, or ventricular fibrillation.

In congestive heart failure, digitalis, by enhancing the force of contraction of the ventricle, significantly increases cardiac output, decreases right atrial pressure, decreases the venous pressure, and increases the excretion of sodium and water and so corrects some of the hemodynamic and metabolic alterations in cardiac failure. The inotropic effect of digitalis fortunately occurs

*See also p 217.

before the toxic manifestations, although the thera-
peutic-toxic ratio often is quite narrow. All of the digitalis preparations seem to be similar with respect to the
relative inotropic action as compared to the effect on
impulse formation and impulse conduction.

Principles of Administration

A. Digitalization: Traditionally, it was thought
that digitalis must be administered initially in large
doses to achieve tissue saturation and so produce a
therapeutic effect. It is now recognized that initial
large doses are necessary only when digitalization must
be carried out rapidly to reach a steady state in 1–3
days. Otherwise, digoxin, 0.25–0.5 mg daily, will permit serum digitalis levels to reach a steady state in
7–10 days–sometimes as early as 5 days–producing
an adequate therapeutic effect. The half-life of digoxin
is 36 hours; 5 such half-lives are sufficient to produce a
steady state in which the amount metabolized and excreted balances that absorbed. Unless digitalization is
required in less than 2 weeks, the slower method of
administration allows digitalization to occur with a
lesser likelihood of toxicity because the patient can be
observed frequently as the serum digitalis level is rising.

Recent work has shown marked variation in gastrointestinal absorption of various preparations of
digoxin from different manufacturers. Studies have
shown this to be due to particle size, fillers, and, most
importantly, dissolution rate. As a result, the FDA
now requires batch-by-batch approval with respect to
dissolution rate before the drug can be marketed. The
variability in bioavailability created a serious situation
in 1970 and 1971, when blood levels resulting from
equivalent dosage of digoxin from different manufacturers varied 6-fold. This caused a hazard of overdigi-
talization in some patients and underdigitalization in
others when their prescriptions were refilled. If care is
taken to demand only recently approved digitalis preparations, such marked differences in absorption can be
avoided.

B. Criteria of Adequate Digitalization: Digitalis is
administered until a therapeutic effect has been obtained (eg, relief of congestive failure or slowing of the
ventricular rate in atrial fibrillation), or until the earliest toxic effect (anorexia or arrhythmia) appears.

1. In congestive failure with normal rhythm–Digitalization is adequate if: (1) diuretic action is adequate, and edema fluid is lost; (2) cardiac size is decreased as dilatation becomes less; (3) venous pressure
and circulation time return to normal; (4) the heart
rate decreases (if increase was due to failure); (5) an
engorged tender liver becomes smaller and nontender.

2. In atrial fibrillation–When the rate is below 80
after exercise, one can usually consider the patient adequately digitalized. Exercise consists of requiring bed
patients to sit up 5 times and ambulatory patients to
hop up and down on one foot 5 times.

C. ECG Effects: The most characteristic change
which digitalis produces in the ECG is sagging of the
ST segment and displacement of the T waves in a direction opposite to that of the main deflection. Later the

P–R interval may be prolonged. The ST–T changes cannot be used as criteria of digitalis toxicity, for the
effects appear before saturation is present and persist
for 2–3 weeks after digitalis has been discontinued.
However, the ECG is often of value in determining
whether digitalis has been administered in the past 2–3
weeks and may give an idea of the amount.

D. Toxic Effects of Digitalis: There are no nontoxic digitalis preparations, and the difference between
the therapeutic and toxic level is very small.

1. Slight toxicity–Anorexia, ventricular ectopic
beats, bradycardia.

2. Moderate toxicity–Nausea and vomiting, headache, malaise, ventricular premature beats.

3. Severe toxicity–Diarrhea, blurring of vision,
confusion, disorientation, junctional (nodal) tachycardia, AV dissociation, paroxysmal atrial tachycardia
with block, atrial fibrillation, ventricular tachycardia,
SA or AV block.

4. Extreme toxicity–High-degree conduction
blocks and ventricular fibrillation.

Because many arrhythmias occur in the absence
as well as in the presence of digitalis toxicity, it is
often difficult for the physician to know whether the
drug has caused the arrhythmia. A high degree of probability exists with respect to multifocal ventricular
beats, junctional AV nodal tachycardia, AV dissociation not associated with AV block, and paroxysmal atrial tachycardia with block. Ventricular tachycardia is common in acute myocardial infarction but
may be due to digitalis toxicity. When digitalis is continued despite the presence of the above arrhythmias
(thought likely as an index of digitalis toxicity), the
mortality is very high.

In the past several years, quantitative methods for
determining digitalis in the serum or plasma have been
perfected. The most promising technic seems to be
radioimmunoassay. Although there is an overlap in the
serum concentrations of digoxin as determined by
radioimmunoassay, Smith found that the serum levels
in patients considered to be digitalis toxic averaged 2
(± 1.5) ng/ml, as compared to 1 (± 0.7) in patients
judged to be nontoxic. Serum levels may prove helpful
in the case of doubtful digitalis toxicity but must be
interpreted in the light of factors other than toxicity
that influence serum levels.

E. Relationship of Digitalis to Potassium Ion:
There is an antagonism between potassium and digitalis, and digitalis toxicity is more likely to occur in
any clinical situation in which potassium is decreased
in the cells or serum, eg, as a result of potassium diuresis due to mercurial or thiazide diuretics, or following
corticosteroid therapy. In these circumstances, potassium ion should be given.

F. Treatment of Severe Digitalis Toxicity: Withhold digitalis and diuretics until the manifestations of
toxicity have subsided, and treat the cardiac failure, if
present, with other means. Give potassium salts, 4–8
gm orally per day in divided doses, or, depending upon
the clinical urgency, well-diluted intravenous potas-

sium salts slowly (not more than 20–30 mEq/hour). In emergency circumstances, potassium may be given more rapidly under ECG control. Do not give potassium salts intravenously in the presence of high-grade AV block or renal failure. One can treat premonitory ventricular arrhythmias with lidocaine, diphenylhydantoin, propranolol, or procainamide. *Caution:* Cardioversion should be used with great caution if digitalis toxicity is suspected. It may precipitate digitalis-induced arrhythmias or be followed by more serious arrhythmias such as ventricular tachycardia. If essential, administer electrical cardioversion in small graded increments or use atrial pacing.

The differentiation of digitalis toxicity and inadequate digitalization is sometimes quite difficult, but serum digitalis levels may be helpful. The only safe procedure, if uncertain, is to withhold digitalis and diuretics and treat the cardiac failure with restriction of sodium and other means to improve cardiac function. Nausea, vomiting, and arrhythmias which are in fact due to digitalis toxicity will subside in 2–3 days. *Caution:* Do not give rapid-acting intravenous digitalis preparations to a patient taking digitalis who is apparently in failure unless it is certain that the manifestations observed are not due to digitalis toxicity.

G. Choice of Digitalis Preparation: (See Table 7–3.) All of the cardiac glycosides have similar pharmacologic properties, differing only in dose, absorption, speed of onset of action, and duration of action. With digitalis leaf and digitoxin there is a long latent period before maximal effect is achieved (half-life, 4–6 days), and the duration of effect is long. Digoxin (Lanoxin), lanatoside C (Cedilanid), and deslanoside (Cedilanid-D) have a much more rapid onset of action and briefer duration of effect (half-life, 36 hours). Acetyldigitoxin (Acylanid) is recommended only for oral administration and is equivalent to digoxin. Gitalin (Gitaligin) has properties intermediate between those of digitoxin and digoxin. Ouabain exerts its effect within a few minutes, but it is rarely used in the USA because other parenteral glycosides are available.

Indications for Administration of Digitalis

(1) Cardiac failure (left, right, or combined), with sinus rhythm or atrial fibrillation.

(2) Atrial fibrillation or flutter with a rapid ventricular rate.

(3) Supraventricular paroxysmal tachycardia.

(4) Prevention of paroxysmal atrial arrhythmias in patients in whom quinidine has failed or cannot be tolerated.

Routes of Administration of Digitalis

A. Parenteral Administration:

1. Emergency digitalization—(1) Acute pulmonary edema or other severe failure. Caution should be used in giving the full digitalizing dose in a single injection intravenously under these circumstances. The drug should be given slowly, in divided doses. (2) Treatment of atrial arrhythmias when the need for control of the ventricular rate is urgent.

2. Inability to take digitalis orally, eg, in nausea and vomiting due to any cause, in coma, and postoperatively.

B. Oral Administration: Oral administration is used unless parenteral administration is indicated (Table 7–4).

Methods of Digitalization

A. Untreated Cases: (When the patient has received no digitalis in the preceding 2 weeks.)

1. **Parenteral digitalization—***Caution:* Never administer a full digitalizing dose intravenously unless it is certain that no digitalis has been given in the preceding 2 weeks. Always give intravenous preparations slowly.

Select the drug on the basis of the rapidity of effect needed. Except in extreme emergencies do not give the entire average digitalizing dose in a single dose. A good general rule is to give one-half to two-thirds of the average digitalizing dose immediately and then give increments of one-fourth at intervals of 2–4 hours until the desired effect occurs. Observe carefully for digitalis toxicity. When the initial dose is given parenterally, it is advisable to give also an average maintenance dose of a digitalis preparation if the patient is able to swallow. Optimal digitalization can thus be achieved and maintained from the start. It is not necessary to give the same glycoside orally that was used for the initial medication (eg, may digitalize with intravenous lanatoside C and give digitalis leaf for maintenance).

A history of digitalis therapy is often difficult to obtain, and digitalis toxicity has occurred in patients who have denied or were unaware of having received the drug. This is another reason for not giving a full digitalizing dose in a single injection as well as for determining digitalis blood levels.

Individualize the dosage schedule for each patient.

2. **Rapid oral digitalization (within 24 hours)**—It is usually unwise to attempt to digitalize with a single oral dose, since nausea and vomiting are common and make it very difficult to estimate the degree of digitalization. Multiple oral doses are usually adequate for initial digitalization. Close medical observation is required before each dose is given, and further doses should be withdrawn at the first sign or symptom of toxicity.

3. **Slow digitalization**—At times it is desirable to digitalize slowly over the course of a week, especially if the patient cannot be closely observed during this period. Any of the digitalis preparations can be given in daily doses 2 or 3 times the average maintenance dose for 5–7 days. The total digitalizing dose may be somewhat greater than when digitalization is rapid. As soon as toxic symptoms appear the drug should be stopped for 1 day and the patient given the average maintenance dose.

B. Partially Treated Cases: If a digitalis preparation has been taken within 2 weeks, give one-fourth of the estimated digitalizing dose and then give additional

Table 7–3. Digitalis and digitalis-like preparations.*

Glycoside and Preparations Available	Dose		Rapid Method of Administration	Speed; Maximum Action and duration
	Digitalizing	Maintenance		
Parenteral preparations				
Ouabain, 1 and 2 ml ampules, 0.25 mg	0.25–0.5 mg	Not used for maintenance	0.25–0.5 mg (1–2 ml) diluted in 10 ml saline slowly IV; follow with another drug (see below).	½–1½ hours; duration, 2–4 days.
Deslanoside (Cedilanid-D), 2 and 4 ml ampules, 0.4 and 0.8 mg	8 ml (1.6 mg)	0.2–0.4 mg (1–2 ml)	1.2 mg (6 ml) IV or IM and follow with 0.2–0.4 mg (1–2 ml) IV or IM every 3–4 hours until effect is obtained.	1–2 hours; duration, 3–6 days.
Digitoxin (dilute before use), 1 and 2 ml ampules, 0.2 and 0.4 mg	1.2 mg (6 ml)	0.05–0.2 mg	0.6 mg (3 ml) IV or IM followed by 0.2–0.4 mg every 4–6 hours until 1.2 mg has been given.	3–8 hours; duration, 14–21 days.
Digoxin (Lanoxin), 2 ml ampules, 0.25 mg/ml	1.5 mg (6 ml)	0.25–0.75 mg (1–3 ml)	0.5–1 mg (2–4 ml) IV and 0.25–0.5 mg (1–2 ml) in 3–4 hours; then 0.25 mg (1 ml) every 3–4 hours until effect is obtained.	1–2 hours; duration, 3–6 days.
Oral preparations				
Digitalis, 0.03, 0.06, and 0.1 gm tablets	1–1.5 gm	0.05–0.2 gm	0.6 gm at once; 0.4 gm in 6–8 hours; 0.2 gm every 6 hours for 2–3 doses; then 0.1 gm twice daily until effect is obtained.	6–8 hours; duration, 18–21 days.
Digitoxin, 0.1, 0.15, and 0.2 mg tablets	1.2 mg	0.05–0.2 mg	0.6 mg at once and repeat in 12 hours and then 0.2 mg twice daily until effect is obtained.	6–8 hours; duration, 14–21 days.
Digoxin, 0.25 and 0.5 mg tablets	1.5–3 mg	0.15–0.5 mg	1 mg at once, and then 0.25–0.5 mg every 6 hours. Total, 3 mg.	4–6 hours; duration, 2–6 days.
Lanatoside C (Cedilanid), 0.5 mg tablets	7.5 mg	0.5–1.5 mg	2 mg at once, and then 0.5–0.75 mg every 6 hours until effect is obtained.	
Acetyldigitoxin (Acylanid), 0.1 and 0.2 mg tablets	1.6–2.4 mg	0.1–0.2 mg	1.6 mg in 24 hours or 0.6–1 mg daily until effect is obtained.	4–6 hours; duration, 14–21 days.
Gitalin (Gitaligin), 0.5 mg tablets	4–6 mg	0.5 mg	1 mg 3 times first day followed by 0.5 mg every 6 hours until effect is obtained.	4–6 hours; duration, 8–14 days.

*Check manufacturers' descriptive literature. Dosage sizes of tablets and ampules change from time to time.

digitalis cautiously, observing the response at intervals of 6–12 hours.

Maintenance Doses & Methods

The oral route is preferred in maintaining digitalization. The exact maintenance dose must be determined clinically for each patient.

Cohn K & others: Variability of hemodynamic responses to acute digitalization in chronic cardiac failure due to cardiomyopathy and coronary artery disease. Am J Cardiol 35:461, 1975.

Doherty JE: Digitalis glycosides: Pharmacokinetics and their clinical implications. Ann Int Med 79:229, 1973.

Fisch C: Treatment of arrhythmias due to digitalis. J Indiana MA 60:146, 1967.

Greenspan K, Lord TJ: Digitalis and vagal stimulation during atrial fibrillation: Effects on atrioventricular conduction and ventricular arrhythmias. Cardiovas Res 7:241, 1973.

Jacobs D, Donoso E, Friedberg C: A-V dissociation: A relatively frequent arrhythmia. Medicine 40:101, 1961.

Kastor JA: Digitalis intoxication in patients with atrial fibrillation. Circulation 47:888, 1973.

Lown B, Wittenberg S: Cardioversion and digitalis. 3. Effect of change in serum potassium concentration. Am J Cardiol

Table 7—4. Oral administration of the digitalis drugs.

Urgency	Drug	Dosage
Moderate	Digitalis	0.4 gm every 8 hours for 3 doses.
	Digitoxin	0.4 mg every 8 hours for 3 doses.
	Digoxin	0.5 mg every 8 hours for 3 doses.
Interme- diate	Digitalis	0.2 gm 3 times daily for 2 days, or 0.1 gm 4 times daily for 3 days.
	Digitoxin	0.2 mg 3 times daily for 2 days.
	Digoxin	0.5 mg twice daily for 2 days, or 0.25 mg 3 times daily for 3 days.
Least	Digitalis	0.1 gm 3 times daily for 4—5 days.
	Digitoxin	0.1 mg 3 times daily for 4—6 days.
	Digoxin	0.25—0.5 mg twice daily for 4—6 days.

21:513, 1968.

Marcus FI: Digitalis pharmacokinetics and metabolism. Am J Med 58:452, 1975.

Rosen MR & others: Mechanisms of digitalis toxicity: Effects of ouabain on phase four of canine Purkinje fiber transmembrane potentials. Circulation 47:681, 1973.

Smith TW: Digitalis toxicity: Epidemiology and clinical use of serum concentration measurements. Am J Med 58:470, 1975.

Smith TW, Haber E: Digitalis (4 parts.) New England J Med 289:945, 1010, 1063, 1125, 1973.

QUINIDINE*

Quinidine is a valuable drug in the management of most cardiac arrhythmias. It increases the effective refractory period of cardiac muscle; slows the rate of atrial and ventricular conduction; decreases the excitability of the myocardium; reduces vagal tone; and has a general depressant action on smooth muscle, causing vasodilatation. As far as conversion of atrial fibrillation is concerned, several of these pharmacologic actions oppose each other; the clinical effect depends upon which action predominates.

Quinidine can be given orally, intramuscularly, or intravenously, as occasion demands. The intravenous route should be used only in urgent situations by physicians experienced in the use of the drug. Quinidine is rapidly absorbed following oral administration,

*Quinine may be used, but it is only about 30% as effective as quinidine. Only quinidine will be discussed here.

reaches a peak level of effectiveness in about 2 hours, and is excreted slowly; about 30% of the peak level remains after 12 hours. Only 10—20% of orally administered quinidine is excreted in the urine; the remainder is metabolized in the body.

After 5 or 6 doses have been given at 2-hour intervals, no significant rise in blood level occurs with further doses at the same interval. When a fixed dose of quinidine is given 4 times a day, as in a maintenance schedule, the blood level rises progressively but more slowly, reaching a maximum in about 48—72 hours. The midday blood levels then reach a steady state as long as this same schedule is maintained. If higher blood levels are desired, the individual dose must be increased or the interval between doses shortened. Because 30—40% of the peak blood level of quinidine is still present in the serum 12 hours after the last of a series of repeated doses of quinidine, a fixed dosage schedule such as 0.4 gm every 2 hours for 5 doses can be repeated for several days to produce increasing concentrations of quinidine in the blood.

Long-acting quinidine preparations are available and permit 2 or 3 rather than 4 daily doses of quinidine sulfate to obtain the desired effect. They should be used only to prevent recurrence and not for conversion of chronic arrhythmias.

Indications & Contraindications

Conflicting opinions have been expressed by cardiologists on the indications, dosages, and dangers in the use of quinidine. It must be remembered that patients taking quinidine have organic cardiac disease; unpredictable accidents occur even when quinidine is not given.

A. Indications: The use of quinidine as the primary agent to convert established atrial and ventricular arrhythmias has been superseded by the use of DC cardioversion because of its greater effectiveness and safety. If DC conversion is not available or is contraindicated for any reason, one should recall that quinidine can be used for the conversion of established atrial fibrillation, atrial flutter, and ventricular and junctional tachycardia. Quinidine is valuable in the prevention of recurrent paroxysmal arrhythmias and the suppression of frequent premature beats, especially following myocardial infarction, after surgery, and in similar clinical situations.

B. Contraindications: Quinidine idiosyncrasy and complete heart block are absolute contraindications to the use of quinidine. Relative contraindications are bundle branch block, thyrotoxicosis, acute rheumatic fever, and infective endocarditis.

Preparations & Routes of Administration

(1) Quinidine sulfate should be given orally except when parenteral quinidine is specifically indicated.

(2) The intramuscular preparation can be used if the patient is unable to take the medication orally and the situation is not critical. Quinidine gluconate, 0.8 gm in 10 ml ampules, is available.

(3) An intravenous preparation should be used only when great urgency requires it and only by a physician familiar with the use of the drug. Quinidine gluconate, 0.8 gm in 10 ml ampules, can be diluted with 50–100 ml of 5% glucose and given slowly IV at a rate of 1 ml/minute.

Toxicity

A. **Myocardial Toxicity**: The myocardial toxicity is the most important and should be specifically looked for when quinidine is used. The earliest effects are seen on ECG: prolongation of the Q–T interval and QRS interval, and ventricular premature beats or ventricular tachycardia.

B. **Nausea, vomiting, and diarrhea** may be sufficiently severe to require cessation of the drug.

C. **Cinchonism**: Tinnitus, vertigo, and headache may be severe enough to necessitate withdrawal of the drug. *Caution:* When the QRS interval becomes more than half again as wide as before treatment, or when runs of ventricular premature beats or ventricular tachycardia occur, quinidine should be stopped immediately. In rare instances ventricular tachycardia may progress to ventricular fibrillation and sudden death.

In patients with atrial fibrillation who are converted with quinidine, transient sino-atrial block may occur at the time of conversion and junctional rhythm may be temporarily noted. This has no clinical significance. Transient prolongation of the P–R interval occasionally occurs when sinus rhythm follows quinidine conversion of atrial fibrillation; this usually subsides spontaneously with smaller maintenance doses.

D. **Other Cardiovascular Effects**:

1. Hypotension may occur when large doses of quinidine are used or if the drug is given parenterally. It rarely is significant with ordinary oral doses.

2. Emboli occur in about 1% of patients with chronic atrial fibrillation converted with quinidine. The prevalence is higher in untreated atrial fibrillation; in fact, atrial fibrillation with frequent emboli is an important reason for attempting to convert to sinus rhythm. Anticoagulants are advised for 2 weeks before conversion to prevent the development of new thrombi in the atria in patients with a history of recent emboli.

E. **Idiosyncrasy**: Fever, purpura, rash, or severe hypotension following a test dose of 0.1 gm.

Conversion to Sinus Rhythm

Cardioversion is preferable to quinidine for this purpose (see above). If cardioversion is not available or is contraindicated, quinidine may be used.

The patient should be under constant observation, preferably in a hospital. Give a test dose of 0.1 gm and wait 2 hours to exclude the possibility of idiosyncrasy.

If the patient has atrial fibrillation or atrial flutter, complete digitalization is advised to slow the ventricular rate and to improve cardiac function. If digitalis is not used, the altered atrioventricular conduction resulting from quinidine may cause a rise in ventricular rate of 30–50 beats per minute and may force cessation of quinidine therapy.

For a patient with chronic arrhythmia in cardiac failure in whom immediate conversion is not essential, additional measures (eg, sodium restriction, diuretics) are indicated before quinidine is given. The patient should be ambulatory for 2 weeks to decrease the likelihood of venous thrombosis. Two weeks of anticoagulant therapy may be desirable, but the data are incomplete regarding its value.

In elective cases, 0.2–0.4 gm every 6 hours can be given for 2–3 days, increasing the dose if no toxic effects have occurred and the arrhythmia persists. If reversion to sinus rhythm is required more quickly, give 0.4 gm every 2 hours for 5–6 doses on the first day; this produces an average blood level of 6–7 mg/liter. Each succeeding dose produces a smaller increment in the blood level, and if conversion does not occur after 5–6 doses larger amounts must be given. In urgent circumstances, begin immediately after the 5th dose; otherwise it is best to wait until the next morning and begin again with 0.6 gm every 2 hours. Giving the drug more frequently than every 2 hours is not warranted since it takes that long for the peak effect of the preceding dose to be reached. In most cases 0.6 gm every 2 hours for 5 doses will convert the arrhythmia to sinus rhythm. If it does not, higher doses can be used if no toxicity• has been encountered and it is urgent to convert the arrhythmia. Eighty percent of the successful conversions occur with daily doses of 3 gm or less.

Increasing quinidine effect can be roughly estimated by serial determinations of blood quinidine levels; by determining the atrial rate of fibrillation; and by measurement of the Q–T and QRS intervals. Rate of fibrillation is best determined on V_1, the right precordial lead in the ECG. The atrial rate is slowed markedly in atrial fibrillation; as the rate approaches 200–250/minute, conversion is near. As Q–T and QRS widen up to 25–30% above the initial values, significant quinidine effects can be predicted.

Bloomfield SS & others: Natural history of cardiac arrhythmias and their prevention with quinidine in patients with acute coronary insufficiency. Circulation 47:967, 1973.

Goldstein A, Aronow L, Kalman SM: *Principles of Drug Action: The Basis of Pharmacology.* Harper, 1968.

Sokolow M, Perloff DB: The clinical pharmacology and use of quinidine in heart disease. Progr Cardiovas Dis 3:316, 1961.

Wallace AG & others: Electrophysiologic effects of quinidine. Circulation Res 19:960, 1966.

NITRITES & NITRATES

The nitrites are smooth muscle relaxants. Whether diseased coronary arteries are able to dilate in response to nitrite administration has recently been questioned.

The relief of angina is probably due to a decrease in cardiac work resulting from a decrease in venous return and subsequent cardiac output secondary to venous pooling due to relaxation of the capacitance vessels.

Rapid-Acting

The rapid-acting preparations (nitroglycerin and amyl nitrite) are useful in terminating an episode of angina or in preventing it if given just before exercise.

A. Nitroglycerin (Glyceryl Trinitrate) Tablets: Place 1 tablet (0.3–0.6 mg) under the tongue as necessary. Effective in 1–2 minutes; effect lasts 15–40 minutes.

B. Amyl Nitrite "Pearl": Break pearl (contains 0.2 ml) in cloth and inhale as necessary. Effective in 10 seconds; effect lasts 5–10 minutes.

Long-Acting Nitrates

The usefulness of these preparations has not been clearly established. The onset of their effect after single doses is delayed for 15–60 minutes but persists for 1–3 hours. Repeated doses may lead to tolerance, and the results of clinical trials are, at best, conflicting.

The following organic nitrates are administered orally or sublingually 4 times a day. (1) Pentaerythritol tetranitrate (Peritrate), 10–20 mg. (2) Erythrityl tetranitrate (Cardilate), 15 mg (sublingually). (3) Mannitol hexanitrate (Nitranitol), 15–60 mg. (4) Trolnitrate phosphate (Metamine, Nitretamin), 2–4 mg. (5) Isosorbide dinitrate (Isordil), 10 mg.

The effect of concurrently administered propranolol is enhanced by the nitrates.

XANTHINES

Cardiac catheterization and metabolic balance studies have demonstrated that intravenous xanthines increase the cardiac output, increase renal blood flow and glomerular filtration rate, and enhance the excretion of sodium and water; they therefore may be valuable in the treatment of cardiac failure. They have also been shown to increase the coronary blood flow when used in large doses, and may on occasion be helpful in angina pectoris.

Preparations

Oral preparations are not useful.

A. Parenteral: Aminophylline injection, 0.25–0.5 gm IV slowly over a 5-minute period, or IM; may repeat in 2–4 hours.

B. Rectal: Rectal suppositories containing aminophylline, 0.3–0.5 gm, may be valuable in an impending attack of cardiac asthma or in nocturnal angina pectoris.

DIURETICS

Diuretics are drugs which suppress renal tubular reabsorption of sodium. They are used in the treatment of diseases associated with excess sodium retention and consequent fluid accumulation (edema), eg, congestive heart failure. The orally active diuretics (Table 7–5) have also been used in the treatment of hypertension, since sodium and volume depletion (as well as other mechanisms) potentiates the effects of hypotensive drugs.

Thiazide (Thiodiazine, Disulfonamide) Diuretics

Drugs of this class have the great advantage of being effective in oral form. The marked sodium loss which they cause is accompanied by potassium diuresis of a potentially toxic degree, especially if digitalis is being given concurrently. These sulfonamide derivatives have only a slight carbonic anhydrase inhibiting effect.

The thiazide diuretics are useful in potentiating the effect of hypotensive drugs and in the treatment of edema due to congestive heart failure, renal disease, cirrhosis, and other sodium retention states. They also may be used in the treatment of diabetes insipidus.

The thiazides are contraindicated in acute renal failure and must be used in smaller doses and with careful observation in cirrhotic patients and in patients receiving digitalis.

Potassium depletion is the principal side-effect, and is most likely to occur early in the use of these drugs when diuresis is most marked. If the diet is deficient in fresh fruits and vegetables, potassium chloride, 1 gm 3–4 times daily, should be given. Intermittent

Table 7–5. Useful oral diuretics.

	Daily Dose
Bendroflumethiazide (Benuron, Naturetin)	5–10 mg
Benzthiazide (Exna)	25–100 mg
Chlorothiazide (Diuril)	250–1000 mg
Chlorthalidone (Hygroton)	50–200 mg
Cyclothiazide (Anhydron)	1–2 mg
Ethacrynic acid (Edecrin)	100–200 mg
Flumethiazide (Ademol)	250–1000 mg
Furosemide (Lasix)	40–80 mg
Hydrochlorothiazide (Esidrix, Hydrodiuril, Oretic)	25–100 mg
Hydroflumethiazide (Di-Ademil, Saluron)	25–100 mg
Methyclothiazide (Enduron)	2.5–10 mg
Polythiazide (Renese)	1–4 mg
Quinethazone (Hydromox)	50–100 mg
Spironolactone (Aldactone)	50–100 mg
Triamterene (Dyrenium)	100–200 mg
Trichlormethiazide (Metahydrin, Naqua)	2–8 mg

diuretic therapy or the use of potassium-sparing diuretics may prevent hypokalemia. The possibility of precipitating digitalis toxicity by potassium diuresis must be considered in patients receiving digitalis.

Other untoward effects are allergic reactions such as skin rashes, pruritus, and, rarely, bone marrow depression; gastrointestinal disturbances; photosensitization; elevated serum uric acid, with the precipitation of gout; impaired glucose tolerance; and raised BUN.

It is agreed that the amount of sodium in the diet should be kept reasonably constant. One can restrict sodium in order to reduce the dose of the diuretic.

The available thiazides are listed below. Chlorthalidone (Hygroton) is not a thiodiazine but a sulfonamide which is otherwise similar to the other drugs listed. In treating edema a large dose may be used initially if necessary, but the dose should be decreased rapidly and doses given at longer than daily intervals if "dry" weight is maintained.

If potassium supplements are used because of K$^+$ loss, use liquid or nonenteric-coated potassium salts.

Ethacrynic Acid (Edecrin) & Furosemide (Lasix)

Ethacrynic acid is a new potent diuretic, a derivative of aryloxyacetic acid, which can be used for the same indications as the thiazides (see above). It is more potent, more rapid in action (30–60 minutes), and causes a greater depletion of sodium and potassium and hence a danger of hyponatremia, hypovolemia, and hypokalemic alkalosis. Intermittent therapy is advised, beginning with small doses (25–50 mg) with caution in patients with impaired renal function and those receiving digitalis.

Similar rapid, potent effects can be obtained with furosemide, a nonthiazide, nonmercurial diuretic which can be given orally or intravenously. It has the advantage, apart from its rapid action, of not affecting carbohydrate metabolism. The initial daily dosage is 20–40 mg. *Caution:* Observe patient for hearing impairment and discontinue ethacrynic acid if there is any evidence of hearing loss. Both drugs—unlike the thiazides—are effective in renal failure with a low glomerular filtration rate.

Mercurial Diuretics

Intramuscularly or subcutaneously administered mercurial diuretics, which were standard drugs for many years, are slightly more potent than the thiazide diuretics. They cause less potassium diuresis, but are more often responsible for sodium depletion. No satisfactory oral preparations are available. The mercurial diuretics are now used only for an occasional difficult patient with congestive heart failure and usually only after a trial with an oral diuretic.

The dose of each of the following mercurial diuretics is 0.5–2 ml of the prepared solution given no oftener than once daily: chlormerodrin (Neohydrin), meralluride (Mercuhydrin), mercaptomerin (Thiomerin), mercurophylline (Mercuzanthin), mercumatilin (Cumertilin), merethoxylline procaine (Dicurin Procaine), and mersalyl (Salyrgan).

Carbonic Anhydrase Inhibitors

These drugs, exemplified by acetazolamide (Diamox), are sulfonamide derivatives which depress the renal tubular reabsorption of bicarbonate. This action leads to only a transient and minor sodium diuresis but a persistent decrease of plasma bicarbonate concentrations and increase of plasma chloride concentration. Administered once or twice a week, these drugs are sometimes useful in the treatment of congestive failure associated with cor pulmonale or to potentiate the action of mercurial diuretics.

Carbonic anhydrase inhibitors may cause drowsiness, paresthesias, and minor allergic reactions.

For diuresis, acetazolamide is given in doses of 250–500 mg 2–3 times per week. Ethoxzolamide (Cardrase) is used in 62.5–125 mg doses. Experience with dichlorphenamide (Daranide) and methazolamide (Neptazane) is limited to their use in glaucoma.

Aldosterone Antagonist

Spironolactone (Aldactone) is an antagonist to aldosterone, the adrenal steroid which controls renal tubular reabsorption of sodium. It therefore causes sodium diuresis without potassium loss. It can be combined with a thiazide to neutralize the potassium-wasting effect of the latter drug. The onset of effect may be delayed for as long as a week. The response of patients with congestive failure and primary aldosteronism has been variable. The drug should be regarded as a promising supplementary diuretic in the resistant edema of cirrhosis and nephrosis, but it is expensive and may cause hyperkalemia. Serial serum potassium determinations and ECG observation is advised. Initial dosage is 25 mg 4 times daily. Drowsiness, breast tenderness, hyponatremia, hyperkalemia, and hypotension may occur. *Caution:* Avoid using potassium supplementation, and do not use in renal failure to prevent hyperkalemia.

Triamterene (Dyrenium)

Like spironolactone, triamterene may be valuable when combined with the thiazides to prevent hypokalemia as well as to provide a slightly additive diuretic effect. It may be added to the mercurial diuretics in the same way. The BUN as well as the serum potassium may rise following triamterene administration, and these components should be monitored during treatment. Mild gastrointestinal side-effects may occur. The usual dose is 100 mg twice daily after meals initially, followed by 50–100 mg daily as a maintenance dose depending upon response. *Caution:* As for spironolactone (above).

PROCAINAMIDE HYDROCHLORIDE

Procainamide (Pronestyl) depresses ectopic pacemakers, prevents arrhythmias under cyclopropane anesthesia following epinephrine, and is useful in the treatment of junctional and ventricular arrhythmias. To a lesser degree, it can be used to prevent these arrhythmias. It has a much less potent effect on the atrial than on the ventricular arrhythmias. Whether procainamide or quinidine is the drug of choice in the ventricular arrhythmias has not been settled.

Dosage & Administration

A. Oral Preparations: Supplied as 250 mg capsules. 0.25–1 gm orally every 4–6 hours is the recommended dose.

B. Intramuscular Preparations: Supplied as 1 gm ampules in 10 ml diluent. The peak effect occurs within 15–60 minutes, and a significant blood level is still present after 6 hours. The blood level is higher and the decrease is slower in patients with congestive failure and renal insufficiency. Hypotension is infrequent with intramuscular use of the drug in the above dosage.

C. Intravenous Preparations: Supplied as 1 gm ampules in 10 ml diluent. Can be used for ventricular tachycardia of a severe or urgent nature. The drug should be given very slowly, 50–100 mg/minute up to a dose of 1 gm with continuous blood pressure and, if possible, ECG control.

Toxicity

The toxicity of procainamide is the same as that of quinidine (with the exception of cinchonism).

(1) Severe hypotension is noted, particularly with the parenteral use of procainamide, and may be severe enough to require withdrawal of the drug or the use of concurrent pressor therapy. This is why frequent blood pressure determinations are necessary.

(2) Prolongation of the QRS interval and ventricular arrhythmias may occur, as with quinidine.

(3) Systemic lupus erythematosus may be initiated or aggravated by procainamide and makes prolonged oral therapy often impractical.

Giardina EV, Heissenbuttel RH, Bigger JT Jr: Intermittent intravenous procaine amide to treat ventricular arrhythmias: Correlation of plasma concentration with effect on arrhythmia, electrocardiogram, and blood pressure. Ann Int Med 78:183, 1973.
Koch-Weser J, Klein SW: Procainamide dosage schedules, plasma concentrations, and clinical effects. JAMA 215:1454, 1971.
Rosen MR, Gelband H, Hoffman BF: Canine electrocardiographic and cardiac electrophysiologic changes induced by procainamide. Circulation 46:528, 1972.

ADRENERGIC BETA RECEPTOR BLOCKADE

Norepinephrine, the specific neurotransmitter liberated at the sympathetic nerve terminals, as well as other drugs and hormones, exert their effects via effector sites known as receptors. The concept of alpha and beta receptor sites was conceived by Ahlquist to explain differing effector responses to different chemical agents, although no anatomic or chemical structure has been identified which is a receptor. Adrenergic receptors are those parts of effector cells which allow them to detect and respond to norepinephrine and related compounds. They can be described only in terms of the effector response to drug application. Ahlquist showed that beta receptors are associated with cardiac stimulation, vasodilatation, and relaxation of smooth muscle in the bronchi, myometrium, and intestine. Alpha receptors are associated with vasoconstriction, relaxation of the intestinal muscle, and contraction of the dilator muscles of the pupil. The specific agonist for alpha receptors is phenylephrine; adrenergic alpha receptor blocking agents are substances that specifically block responses to phenylephrine. The specific agonist for beta receptors is isoproterenol; beta-adrenergic blockers block the responses to isoproterenol but have no effect on the response to phenylephrine. There may be a third or other receptors to explain some of the responses observed in man.

Chemical agents that interfere with the action of sympathetic amines at the receptor site have been found to have therapeutic use in conditions in which adrenergic beta receptor activity is excessive or undesirable. The adrenergic beta receptor blocking agent utilized most frequently today is propranolol (Inderal), which competitively and specifically blocks the responses of the beta receptor to isoproterenol and other sympathomimetic amines.

Administration

Propranolol (Inderal) can be used orally, 10 mg 4 times daily, increasing to 180–200 mg/day with close follow-up; or intravenously, 1–5 mg, 1 mg/minute, with careful ECG monitoring. *Caution:* Because sympathetic activity is important for left ventricular function, particularly in the failing heart, beta blockers may be hazardous in the presence of cardiac failure and should be used with great caution or not at all if incipient or actual failure is present. Beta blockers prolong AV conduction and may aggravate high-grade AV block; the presence of AV block should be considered a contraindication. Beta blockers may produce bronchospasm by blocking the bronchial relaxation of the catecholamines and should be used with great caution in patients who have a tendency to bronchial asthma. Do not use if patients are receiving MAO inhibitors.

Clinical Use of Propranolol

A. Anti-Arrhythmic Activity: There is good evidence that propranolol converts some atrial and ventricular arrhythmias to normal and may prevent the recurrence of paroxysmal atrial and ventricular arrhythmias, especially when they are caused by digitalis. Because of its negative chronotropic action, propranolol may slow the ventricular rate in patients with atrial fibrillation and flutter whose ventricular rate cannot be slowed with digitalis. The negative inotropic action of propranolol should be appreciated even when the heart rate is controlled. The drug does not replace other established anti-arrhythmic agents.

B. Angina Pectoris: Propranolol may increase exercise tolerance, reduce the frequency of attacks, and prevent the ischemic ECG changes with exercise because it reduces cardiac work and myocardial oxygen consumption as well as slowing the heart after exercise and preventing ventricular premature beats. The beneficial effect may be enhanced when propranolol is combined with long-acting nitrates. Treatment of angina pectoris is a controversial subject because of the subjective nature of the symptom and the frequent improvement resulting from the use of placebos.

C. Hypertrophic Cardiomyopathy: Propranolol reduces the obstructive gradient caused by endogenous and exogenous catecholamines, producing clinical improvement in many patients and thus avoiding the necessity of surgical treatment; surgical treatment should be delayed until the response to propranolol is determined.

D. Hypertension: Propranolol has a moderate antihypertensive action, especially when plasma renin is high and when diuretics and vasodilators are also used; patients may require large doses of the drug.

E. Pheochromocytoma: Although alpha adrenergic blocking drugs—phentolamine (Regitine) or phenoxybenzamine (Dibenzyline)—restore the blood volume and diminish the risk of abrupt rises in pressure before and during surgical treatment, they do not prevent the tachycardia produced by the release of catecholamines. Therefore, propranolol is a useful adjunct in the preparation of patients with pheochromocytoma for surgery.

F. Tetralogy of Fallot: Spells of increased cyanosis and of syncope may be due to increased contraction of the infundibulum of the right ventricle, presumably from sympathetic impulses. Propranolol has been helpful in relaxing the infundibulum, decreasing the frequency of these serious episodes.

Ahlquist RP: Agents which block adrenergic β-receptors. Ann Rev Pharmacol 8:259, 1968.

Battock DJ, Alvarez H, Chidsey CA: Effects of propranolol and isosorbide dinitrate on exercise performance and adrenergic activity in patients with angina pectoris. Circulation 39:157, 1969.

Cullhed I, Parrow A: Acute hemodynamic changes following beta-adrenergic blockade in hyperthyroidism. Acta med scandinav 184:235, 1968.

Current status of propranolol hydrochloride (Inderal). JAMA 225:1380, 1973.

Dwyer EM Jr, Wiener L, Cox JW: Effects of beta-adrenergic blockade (propranolol) on left ventricular hemodynamics and the electrocardiogram during exercise-induced angina pectoris. Circulation 38:250, 1968.

Epstein SE, Braunwald E: Inhibition of the adrenergic nervous system in the treatment of angina pectoris. M Clin North America 52:1031, 1968.

Gibson D, Sowton E: The use of beta-adrenergic receptor blocking drugs in dysrhythmias. Progr Cardiovas Dis 12:16, 1969.

Lewis CM, Brink AJ: Beta-adrenergic blockade: Hemodynamics and myocardial energy metabolism in patients with ischemic heart disease. Am J Cardiol 21:846, 1968.

Mason DT: Autonomic nervous system and regulation of cardiovascular performance. Anesthesiology 29:724, 1968.

Nicotero JA & others: Effects of propranolol on the pressor response to noxious stimuli in hypertensive patients. Am J Cardiol 22:657, 1968.

Parker JO, West RO, DiGiorgi S: Hemodynamic effects of propranolol in coronary heart disease. Am J Cardiol 21:11, 1968.

Seides SF & others: The electrophysiology of propranolol in man. Am Heart J 88:733, 1974.

Symposium on catecholamines in cardiovascular physiology and disease. Circulation Res 21, Suppl 3, 1967.

Whalen RE, Morris JJ Jr, McIntosh HB: Hemodynamic effects of beta-adrenergic blockade at controlled ventricular rates. Am Heart J 76:775, 1968.

Williams EMV, Bagwell EE, Singh BN: Cardiospecificity of beta-receptor blockade. Cardiovas Res 7:226, 1973.

ACIDIFYING SALTS
(Chlorides)

Chlorides alone are rarely effective diuretics, but they enhance the action of mercurial diuretics, especially when the patient becomes refractory to repeated injections of mercurials. It is thought that chlorides act by producing acidosis and by serving as anions to enhance the excretion of sodium ions. Ammonium chloride, 2 gm 3 times daily, may be given 2–4 days before a mercurial injection and then omitted for 3–4 days before repeating the drug in cyclic fashion. Other chlorides are equally effective, and if the patient has hepatic disease—in which case ammonium ions are potentially toxic—one can give lysine monohydrochloride in similar cyclic fashion. It is given in powder form, 5–10 gm 3–4 times daily for 2–5 days, dissolved in any palatable fluid. Each gram of lysine monohydrochloride provides about 5 mEq of chloride.

The chlorides in large doses and if continued may produce hyperchloremic acidosis with severe dyspnea and gastrointestinal symptoms. Because of the hazard of acidosis, chlorides should not be used in the presence of impaired renal function and the ammonium ion should not be used in hepatic disease.

8...
Blood Vessels & Lymphatics

John M. Erskine

DEGENERATIVE & INFLAMMATORY ARTERIAL DISEASES

Arteriosclerosis accounts for most of the forms of degenerative arterial disease. Its incidence increases with age; although manifestations of the disease may appear in the 4th decade, people over 40 (particularly men) are most commonly affected. Diseases which predispose to arteriosclerosis include the hyperlipidemic states, diabetes mellitus, and hypertension. Arteriosclerosis tends to be a generalized disease with some degree of involvement of all major arteries, but it produces its major clinical manifestations by critical involvement of one essential artery at a time. Gradual narrowing and ultimate occlusion of the artery is the most common course of the disease, but weakening of the arterial wall with aneurysmal dilatation of the arterial segment also occurs.

Less common forms of degenerative and inflammatory arterial disease which must be considered are cystic medial necrosis of the aorta, syphilitic aortitis and arteritis, arteritis of both large and small arteries of undetermined cause, thromboangiitis obliterans (Buerger's disease), and fibrodysplasia of visceral arteries.

DISEASES OF THE AORTA

ANEURYSMS OF THE THORACIC AORTA

Antibiotic therapy has reduced the incidence of syphilitic aneurysms; most thoracic aneurysms are now due to arteriosclerosis. Very rapid deceleration, as in an automobile or airplane accident, can result in a tear of the thoracic aorta just beyond the origin of the left subclavian artery with the formation of an aneurysm in those that survive the initial injury. Cystic medial necrosis, a poorly understood degenerative condition of the aorta, may lead to a thoracic aneurysm in rela-

tively young people. Only one-sixth of aortic aneurysms are thoracic.

Clinical Findings

Manifestations depend largely on the size and position of the aneurysm and its rate of growth.

A. Symptoms and Signs: There may be no symptoms. Substernal, back, or neck pain may occur, as well as symptoms and signs due to pressure on (1) the trachea (dyspnea, stridor, a brassy cough), (2) the esophagus (dysphagia), (3) the left recurrent laryngeal nerve (hoarseness), or (4) the superior vena cava (edema in the neck and arms; distended neck veins). The findings of regurgitation at the aortic valve may be present.

B. Laboratory Findings: The serology may be positive if the aneurysm is syphilitic.

C. X-Ray Findings: In addition to routine chest x-rays, aortography is necessary to substantiate the diagnosis and to delineate the precise location and extent of the aneurysm and its relation to the vessels arising from the arch. An esophagogram may be of value.

Differential Diagnosis

It may be difficult to determine whether a mass in the mediastinum is an aneurysm, a neoplasm, or a cyst. Aortography will distinguish an aneurysm from the other masses in that area and should be performed if there is any question regarding the nature of a mass. Ultrasonic studies may also be of value.

Treatment

Aneurysms of the thoracic aorta often progress with increasing symptoms and finally rupture. Resection of aneurysms is now considered the treatment of choice if technically feasible and if the patient's general condition is such that the major surgical procedure usually required can be done with an acceptable risk. This is especially true if an aneurysm is large, associated with symptoms and signs, and limited to the ascending or descending aorta. Small, asymptomatic aneurysms, especially in poor risk patients, are perhaps better followed and treated only if progressive enlargement occurs. In these individuals, hypertension—if present—should be controlled.

Saccular aneurysms with narrow necks can often

be excised without occluding the aorta. Fusiform aortic aneurysms require resection and grafting of the aortic defect, usually with the patient on partial or complete cardiac bypass. If the aortic valve is involved, an aortic valve replacement may be necessary. Paraplegia is a dreaded complication of excision and graft replacement of aneurysms involving the descending thoracic aorta.

Prognosis

Small aneurysms and those discovered months or years following an episode of rapid deceleration may change very little over a period of years, and death may result from causes other than rupture in many cases. If the aneurysm is large—and (especially) if it is symptomatic and associated with hypertension or arteriosclerotic cardiovascular disease—the prognosis is poor. In general, one-third will be dead in 3 years, one-half in 5 years, and two-thirds in 10 years, but only about one-third of all deaths will result from rupture. Saccular aneurysms, those distal to the left subclavian artery, and even those limited to the ascending aorta can now be removed with an acceptable mortality rate. Resection of aneurysms of the arch carries a very high mortality.

Bennett DE, Cherry JK: The natural history of traumatic aneurysms of the aorta. Surgery 61:516, 1967.

Björk VO, Björk L: Surgical treatment of aneurysms of the descending thoracic aorta. J Cardiovas Surg 7:50, 1966.

Crisler C, Bahnson HT: Aneurysms of the aorta. Curr Probl Surg Dec, 1972.

Joyce JW & others: Aneurysms of the thoracic aorta: A clinical study with special reference to prognosis. Circulation 29:176, 1964.

Kahn AM, Joseph WK, Hughes RK: Traumatic aneurysms of the thoracic aorta. Ann Thoracic Surg 4:175, 1967.

DISSECTING ANEURYSMS
OF THE AORTA
(Acute Aortic Dissection)

Essentials of Diagnosis

- Sudden severe chest pain with radiation to the back, abdomen, and hips.
- Shock may be present, though often not until the later stages.
- CNS changes may occur.
- A history of hypertension is usually present.
- Dissection occurs most frequently in males.

General Considerations

Most aortas in which aortic dissection occurs have evidence of a degenerative process primarily in the media; two-thirds have cystic medial necrosis, one-fifth have degeneration of smooth muscle and elastic tissue in that layer, and the rest are arteriosclerotic or occasionally syphilitic in origin. Most dissections occur

after age 50, and hypertension is generally present; when they occur before age 40, Marfan's syndrome, pregnancy, or congenital heart disease is usually present. The origin of the dissection is in the ascending aorta in two-thirds of patients (types I and II); just beyond the left subclavian artery is the next most frequent site (type III). The initial intimal tear probably results from the constant movement of the ascending and proximal descending aorta, related to the pulsatile flow of blood from the heart; when degenerative changes in the media are present, dissection will start. Both hypertension and a forceful pulse wave are important in the propagation of the dissection, which may extend from the ascending aorta distally to the abdominal aorta or beyond (type I), though sometimes it remains limited to the ascending aorta and the aortic valve area (type II). Death, which may occur after hours, days, or weeks, is usually due to rupture of the aorta into the pericardial sac (cardiac tamponade) or into the left pleural cavity or the retroperitoneal tissue. The dissection may occasionally decompress itself by rupturing back into the aortic lumen (recanalization), and blood may then flow through both the true and false lumens; spontaneous cure and long-term survival can thus occur.

Clinical Findings

A. Symptoms and Signs: Severe, persistent pain of sudden onset is usually present, most often in the anterior chest or in the middorsal area, and may later progress to the abdominal and hip areas. Radiation into the neck and down the arms (so frequent in myocardial infarction) generally does not occur. Usually there is only a mild decrease in the prerupture hypertensive levels; if shock is present, it may respond to relatively small amounts of transfused blood. Partial or complete occlusion of the arteries arising from the aortic arch or of the intercostal and lumbar arteries may lead to such CNS findings as convulsions, hemiplegia, or paralysis of the lower extremities. Peripheral pulses and blood pressures may be diminished or unequal. Murmurs may appear over arteries along with signs of acute arterial insufficiency. An aortic diastolic murmur may develop as a result of dissection close to the aortic valve, causing secondary valvular insufficiency. Fever is often present.

B. Laboratory Findings: Leukocytosis is usually present. Acute ECG changes may not develop unless the dissection involves the coronary ostium or unless cardiac failure develops from acute aortic valvular insufficiency or from cardiac tamponade as a result of leakage into the pericardial sac.

C. X-Ray Findings: Chest x-rays may show widening of the mediastinum or of the aorta, with changes in the configuration and thickness of the aortic wall in successive films. There may be findings of pleural or pericardial effusion. The diagnosis can usually be confirmed or ruled out by an aortogram. Positive findings include an aortic wall greater than 1 cm in thickness with or without an open intimal tear and a false channel. Survival is better in those without a free communication between the aortic lumen and the false dissection channel.

Differential Diagnosis

Dissecting aneurysm is most commonly confused with myocardial infarction. Patients with dissecting aneurysm may also have heart disease with old or recent ECG changes.

Treatment

A. Medical Treatment: A combined and detailed program of intensive medical and surgical monitoring should be established promptly and continued after the diagnosis has been established and a total commitment to pharmacologic treatment initiated. This generally includes the simultaneous reduction of the systolic blood pressure to 100–120 mm Hg and reduction of the pulsatile aortic flow by means of the following: (1) Start trimethaphan (Arfonad), 1–2 mg/ml as intravenous drip, with the flow rate regulated to maintain the desired blood pressure. This drug is used only for 28–48 hours, by which time the other agents should be effective. (2) At the same time, start (a) reserpine, 1–2 mg IM every 4–6 hours, or propranolol (Inderal), 1 mg IM every 4–6 hours (these drugs can be used in combination); and (b) guanethidine (Ismelin), 25–50 mg orally every 12 hours. Elevate the head of the bed 30–45 degrees and follow ECG, blood pressure, central venous pressure, and hourly recording of urine output. If the state of consciousness worsens or urine output decreases significantly, allow the blood pressure to rise somewhat; if the chest and back pain does not diminish promptly, consider lowering the blood pressure to 70–80 mm Hg. Maintain urine output at 25–30 ml/hour. Follow with daily chest films. An aortogram that offers a full and detailed examination of the entire aorta should be obtained within hours of admission. If hypertension is not present, the pulsatile flow should still be reduced with reserpine (at least 0.5 mg/day) or propranolol (60–120 mg/day) and the drug should be continued for long-term therapy.

B. Surgical Treatment: Surgery is indicated in the acute, subacute, or chronic phase if a team trained in cardiovascular surgery is available and if (1) progressive, severe aortic valvular insufficiency develops, (2) chest pain is not relieved or reappears, (3) a saccular aneurysm appears, (4) significant compromise or occlusion of a major branch of the aorta develops, or (5) progressive enlargement with impending rupture or leaking from the aneurysm occurs. When possible, the origin of the dissection should be removed and the false lumen obliterated; an aortic graft is usually necessary, and occasionally an aortic valve will also be needed. If flow to vital organs is through the false lumen, the establishment of a reentry channel into the true lumen may arrest progressive dissection.

Prognosis

Without treatment, the mortality rate at 3 months is 90%, but only 3% die immediately; 21% are dead in 24 hours, and 60% in 2 weeks. Survival without treatment, usually by recanalization, does occasionally occur, and intensive pharmacologic methods to lower the pulse wave and blood pressure will lead to healing of the dissected aorta in 85% of patients with an acute dissection and will convert others to a subacute or chronic form. Surgery in carefully selected patients in this group may yield a mortality rate well below the overall rate of > 40% generally encountered in the acute dissections that are operated on as the initial form of therapy.

Cooley DA & others: Surgical treatment of aneurysm of the ascending aorta. Arch Surg 101:734, 1970.

Gore I, Hirst AE Jr: Dissecting aneurysm of the aorta. Progr Cardiovas Dis 16:103, 1973.

Lindsay J Jr, Hurst JW: Clinical features and prognosis in dissecting aneurysm of the aorta: A reappraisal. Circulation 35:880, 1967.

Shuford WH & others: Problems in the aortographic diagnosis of dissecting aneurysms of the aorta. New England J Med 280:225, 1969.

Shumway NE & others: Management of acute aortic disections. Ann Thoracic Surg 10:237, 1970.

Wheat MW Jr: Treatment of dissecting aneurysms of the aorta: Current status. Progr Cardiovas Dis 16:87, 1973.

Wheat MW Jr, Palmer RF: Dissecting aneurysms of the aorta. Curr Probl Surg, July 1971.

ANEURYSMS OF THE ABDOMINAL AORTA

The vast majority of aneurysms of the abdominal aorta are below the origin of the renal arteries and generally involve the bifurcation of the aorta and thus the proximal end of the common iliac arteries. Aneurysms of the upper abdominal aorta are rare. Most aneurysms of the distal aorta are arteriosclerotic in origin and fusiform in shape. Eighty percent of aortic aneurysms are in the distal aorta.

Clinical Findings

A. Symptoms and Signs: Three phases can be recognized:

1. Asymptomatic—A pulsating mid and upper abdominal mass may be discovered on a routine physical examination, most frequently in men over 50. The calcification which frequently exists in the wall of the aneurysm may be discovered at the time of an abdominal x-ray examination. As a general rule, surgical resection should be advised even for an asymptomatic aneurysm, particularly if it is large. Although small aneurysms (< 7 cm) also rupture, surgery may occasionally be withheld if the patient is a poor operative risk and especially if he has significant cardiac, renal, pulmonary, or distal peripheral obliterative vascular disease. If hypertension is present, it should be controlled by medication. If the aneurysm later increases in size as determined by repeated physical and ultrasonic examinations or if it becomes symptomatic, operative treatment should be reconsidered.

2. Symptomatic—Pain varies from mild midabdominal or lumbar discomfort to more severe constant or intermittent abdominal and back pain requiring narcotics for relief. Intermittent pain may be associated with a phase of enlargement or intramural dissection. Pain is an unfavorable prognostic sign which usually justifies surgery. Peripheral emboli and thrombosis, which commonly complicate the most distal aneurysms, are infrequent in abdominal lesions.

3. Rupture—Rupture of an aneurysm almost always causes death in a few hours and is therefore an indication for immediate surgical intervention. Pain is usually severe and sudden in onset. Because the dissection is most often into the retroperitoneal tissues, which offer some resistance, shock and other manifestations of blood loss may at first be mild or absent; but free uncontrolled bleeding inevitably follows, resulting in death. There is an expanding, pulsating abdominal and flank mass, and subcutaneous ecchymosis is occasionally present in the flank or groin. About half of such patients can be saved by emergency surgery.

B. Laboratory Findings: Cardiac and renal function should be evaluated by means of ECG, urinalysis, and BUN determination. Ultrasonic studies may be of value, particularly in obese individuals.

C. X-Ray Findings: Calcification in the wall of the aneurysm usually outlines the lesion on anteroposterior and lateral plain films of the abdomen. In some cases the position of the aneurysm in relation to the renal arteries can be identified by intravenous urograms, but more often the examination is inconclusive. Bony erosion of the vertebrae does not occur in abdominal aneurysms. Translumbar aortograms are seldom employed; the aneurysm may be ruptured by the procedure, and the information gained regarding the upper limits of the lesion may be inaccurate since a solid thrombus generally occupies most of the aneurysm, except for a central channel through which the blood flows. If distal occlusive disease or renovascular hypertension is suspected, an aortogram may be indicated to study the extent of the distal disease or the condition of the renal arteries.

Treatment

Surgical excision and grafting of the defect is indicated on all aneurysms of the distal aorta except when the lesion is very small and asymptomatic or when the general condition of the patient is so poor that the surgical risk is greater than the risk of rupture.

Prognosis

The mortality rate following elective surgical resection is 5–10%; of those that survive surgery, approximately 50% are alive 5 years later. Among unoperated patients, approximately 20–30% survive 5 years, and many die of causes other than aneurysm rupture. In general, a patient with an aortic aneurysm has a 3-fold greater chance of dying as a consequence of rupture of the aneurysm than of dying from surgical resection.

Bergan & others: Modern management of abdominal aortic aneurysms. S Clin North America 54:175, 1974.

Campbell GS: Physiological and technical factors in the surgical treatment of abdominal aortic aneurysms. Surgery 62: 789, 1967.

Haimovici H: Abdominal aortic aneurysm: A critical clinical reappraisal. J Cardiovas Surg 8:181, 1967.

Schatz IJ, Fairbairn JF, Juergens JL: Abdominal aortic aneurysms: Reappraisal. Circulation 26:200, 1962.

Scott HW Jr & others: Comparative study of elective resection and expectant treatment of abdominal aortic aneurysm. Surg Gynec Obst 129:1, 1969.

Szilagy DE & others: Clinical fate of the patient with asymptomatic abdominal aortic aneurysm and unfit for surgical treatment. Arch Surg 104:600, 1972.

•   •   •

FEMORAL & POPLITEAL ANEURYSMS

Aneurysms of the femoral or popliteal arteries are not uncommon. They are usually arteriosclerotic in origin, in which case they may be multiple and are often bilateral. They may also be due to trauma. Syphilitic or mycotic aneurysms occur occasionally, the latter after an episode of bacteremia or, more often, from a septic embolus.

The diagnosis is usually not difficult, although a lesion in the popliteal area may go unnoticed until attention is focused on the area by a complication of the aneurysm. The cardinal finding is a firm, pulsating mass in the femoral or popliteal area, often associated with a bruit. Pulsation may not be present if thrombosis has already taken place. The distal circulation may be impaired, especially if the gelatinous thrombus which so frequently fills most of the aneurysm has partially or completely occluded the central lumen or if emboli from this thrombus have blocked one or more of the distal vessels. Arteriography may be helpful in outlining the extent of the aneurysm and the status of the peripheral vessels.

Rupture can occur, and it may result in death or loss of the limb. Complete thrombosis causes distal gangrene in about one-third of popliteal aneurysms. Emboli to the distal vessels from the thrombus lining the wall of the aneurysm often cause ischemic changes or gangrene. Thrombophlebitis can occur as a result of pressure obstruction of a neighboring vein. Pressure on the tibial or peroneal nerves may produce pain in the lower leg. Arterial insufficiency with or without gangrene distal to the aneurysm may occur, leading to amputation.

Surgical excision of the aneurysm with grafting of the defect is the treatment of choice in the larger femoral and popliteal aneurysms, particularly if there is evidence of progressive enlargement or developing complications. Bypassing a popliteal aneurysm by means of a vein graft with proximal and distal ligation of the aneurysm is another and perhaps a more satisfactory approach. The incidence of loss of limb following resection and grafting is low. Thrombophlebitis may occur postoperatively from manipulation or damage of the neighboring veins.

Baird RJ & others: Popliteal aneurysms: A review and analysis of 61 cases. Surgery 59:911, 1966.
Cutler BS, Darling RC: Surgical management of arteriosclerotic femoral aneurysms. Surgery 74:764, 1973.
Edwards WS: Exclusion and saphenous vein bypass of popliteal aneurysms. Surg Gynec Obst 128:829, 1969.
Howell JF & others: Surgical treatment of peripheral arteriosclerotic aneurysm. S Clin North America 46:979, 1966.

ARTERIOSCLEROTIC OCCLUSIVE DISEASE

OCCLUSIVE DISEASE OF THE AORTA & ILIAC ARTERIES

Occlusive disease of the aorta and the iliac arteries begins most frequently just proximal to the bifurcation of the common iliac arteries and at or just distal to the bifurcation of the aorta. Atherosclerotic changes occur in the intima and media, often with associated perivascular inflammation and calcified plaques in the media. Progression involves the complete occlusion of one or both common iliac arteries and then the abdominal aorta up to the segment just below the renal vessels. Although atherosclerosis is a generalized disease, occlusion tends to be segmental in distribution, and when the involvement is in the aorto-iliac vessels there may be minimal atherosclerosis in the more distal external iliac and femoral arteries. The best candidates for direct arterial surgery are those with localized occlusions at or just beyond the aortic bifurcation with relatively normal vessels proximally and distally.

Men age 50 and older are most commonly affected. Many are smokers or have coronary artery disease or hypertension.

Clinical Findings

Intermittent claudication is almost always present in the calf muscles and is usually present in the thighs and buttocks also. It is most often bilateral and progressive, so that by the time the patient seeks help the pain may be produced by walking a block or less. Difficulty in having or sustaining an erection is a common complaint in men. Coldness of the feet may be present; rest pain is infrequent.

Femoral pulses are absent or very weak. Pulses distal to the femoral area are usually absent. A pulsation in the abdominal aorta is usually present. A bruit may be heard over the aorta or the iliac or femoral arteries. Atrophic changes of the skin, subcutaneous tissues, and muscles of the distal leg are usually minimal or absent, and dependent rubor and coolness of the skin of the foot are minimal unless distal arterial disease is also present.

If surgery is being seriously considered, a translumbar aortogram is indicated and will usually give valuable information regarding the level and extent of the occlusion and the condition of the vessels distal to the block.

Treatment

Surgical treatment is indicated if claudication interferes appreciably with the patient's essential activities or work. It is generally not advisable if the condition alters the individual's activities in only minor ways. The objective of treatment is reestablishment of blood flow through the narrowed or occluded aorto-iliac segment. This can be achieved by arterial prosthesis or thrombo-endarterectomy.

A. Arterial Graft (Prosthesis): An arterial prosthesis, bypassing the occluded segment, is the treatment of choice in the more extensive aorto-iliac occlusions, and in general the bifurcation graft extends from the abdominal aorta to the distal external iliac or common femoral arteries.

B. Thrombo-endarterectomy: This procedure, which avoids the use of a prosthesis, is generally used when the occlusion is limited to the common iliac arteries and when the external iliac and common femoral arteries are free of significant occlusive disease.

C. Sympathectomy: A bilateral lumbar sympathectomy should be added to the direct arterial procedure in most cases, except in men who are still sexually active.

Prognosis

The operative mortality rate is relatively low, and the immediate and long-term benefits are often impressive. Improvement is both subjective and objective, with relief of all or most of the claudication and in many cases return of all of the pulses in the extremities.

Barker WE & others: Aortoiliac endarterectomy case series followed 10 years or more. Surgery 67:5, 1970.
Garrett HE & others: Surgical considerations in the treatment of aorto-iliac occlusive disease. S Clin North America 46:949, 1966.
Humphries AW & others: Experiences with aortoiliac and femoropopliteal endarterectomy. Surgery 65:48, 1969.
Kouchoukos NT & others: Operative therapy for aortoiliac arterial occlusive disease. Arch Surg 96:628, 1968.
Linton RR & others: Aortoiliofemoral atherosclerotic occlusive disease: Comparative results of endarterectomy and Dacron bypass grafts. Surgery 70:974, 1971.

OCCLUSIVE DISEASE OF THE
FEMORAL & POPLITEAL ARTERIES

In the region of the thigh and knee, the vessels most frequently blocked by occlusive disease are the superficial femoral artery and the popliteal artery. Atherosclerotic changes usually appear first at the most distal point of the superficial femoral artery where it passes through the adductor magnus tendon into the popliteal space. In time, the whole superficial femoral artery and the proximal popliteal artery may become occluded. The common femoral and deep femoral arteries are usually patent and relatively free of disease, though the origin of the profunda femoris is sometimes narrowed. The distal popliteal and its 3 terminal branches may also be relatively free of occlusive disease.

Clinical Findings

As a rule, the changes are initially more advanced in one extremity than the other, although similar changes often appear later in the opposite extremity.

A. Symptoms and Signs: Intermittent claudication, which often appears upon as little exertion as walking ½–1 block, is confined to the calf and foot. Atrophic changes in the lower leg and foot may be quite definite, with loss of hair, thinning of the skin and subcutaneous tissues, and diminution in the size of the muscles. Dependent rubor and blanching on elevation of the foot are usually present. When the leg is lowered after elevation, venous filling on the dorsal aspect of the foot may be slowed to 15–20 seconds or more. The foot is usually cool or cold. If these findings are marked or if rest pain is present, significant occlusive disease in the aorto-iliac or lower leg vessels should also be suspected. The common femoral pulsations are usually of fair or good quality, though a bruit may be heard and no popliteal or pedal pulses can be felt.

B. X-Ray Findings: X-rays of the thigh and leg may show calcification of superficial femoral and popliteal vessels. A femoral arteriogram will show the location and extent of the block as well as the status of the distal vessels, and lateral or oblique views will reveal whether the origin of the profunda femoris is narrow. Often it is important to know the condition of the aorto-iliac vessels also since a relatively normal inflow as well as an adequate distal "run-off" is important in determining the likelihood of success of an arterial procedure. A translumbar aortogram should be done rather than a femoral arteriogram if there is any question that significant aorto-iliac disease also exists.

Treatment

Surgery is indicated (1) if intermittent claudication interferes significantly with the patient's essential physical activities such as his ability to earn a living or (2) if pregangrenous or gangrenous lesions appear on the foot and it is hoped that a major amputation can be avoided.

A. Arterial Graft: An autogenous vein graft using a reversed segment of the great saphenous vein can be placed, bypassing the occluded segment. Synthetic arterial prostheses have not proved to be very satisfactory in this area because of the relatively high incidence of early or late thrombosis.

B. Thrombo-endarterectomy: Thrombo-endarterectomy with removal of the central occluding core may be successful, particularly if the occluded and stenotic segment is very short.

When significant aorto-iliac or common femoral occlusive disease exists as well as superficial femoral and popliteal occlusions, it is usually better to relieve the obstructions in the larger, proximal arteries and deliver more blood flow to the profunda femoris than to operate on the smaller distal vessels where the chances of success are less favorable.

C. Sympathectomy: Lumbar sympathectomy may be used as an adjunct to grafting or endarterectomy or as the only operation if an arterial procedure is thought inadvisable. It can be done a few days before or at the same time as an artery procedure; the vasodilator effect of sympathectomy may improve the circulation to the skin of the lower leg and foot, especially if there is considerable arterial disease in the vessels in those areas.

Prognosis

Thrombosis of the "bypass" graft or of the endarterectomized vessel either in the immediate postoperative period or months or years later is relatively frequent in the superficial femoral-popliteal area. This is particularly true if one or more of the 3 terminal branches of the distal popliteal artery are occluded or badly diseased or if endarterectomy or a synthetic prosthesis is used. For this reason, operation is usually not recommended for mild or moderate claudication, and many of these patients will go for years without much progression of their symptoms or the development of ischemia or gangrene. Some may improve as collateral circulation develops. The chances of success are even less in patients with ischemia or early gangrene, but the procedure is often justified because some limbs can be saved from amputation. Failure of the graft or the endarterectomy may make the condition of the limb worse than it was before the procedure. The long-term overall patency rate for the saphenous vein bypass grafts—the procedure of choice in most cases—is in the range of 60–70%.

Dale WA: Autogenous vein grafts for femoropopliteal arterial repair. Surg Gynec Obst 123:1282, 1966.

Darling RC & others: Saphenous vein bypass grafts for femoropopliteal occlusive disease. Surgery 61:31, 1967.

Linton RR, Wilde WL: Modifications in the technique for femoropopliteal saphenous vein bypass autografts. Surgery 67:234, 1970.

Rob CG & others: Femoropopliteal bypass grafts utilizing autogenous veins. Circulation 37 & 38 (Suppl 2):37, 1968.

OCCLUSIVE DISEASE OF THE ARTERIES IN THE LOWER LEG & FOOT

Occlusive processes in the lower leg and foot may involve, in order of incidence, the tibial and common peroneal arteries and their branches to the muscles, the pedal vessels, and occasionally the small digital vessels. Symptoms depend upon the vessels that are narrowed or thrombosed, the suddenness and extent of the occlusion, and the status of the proximal and collateral vessels. The clinical picture may thus vary from a rather 'stable form of vascular insufficiency to a slowly progressive form which over months or years may ultimately result in atrophy, ischemic pain, and finally gangrene. A rapidly progressive and extensive thrombosis will result in acute ischemia and often gangrene.

Clinical Findings

Although all of the possible manifestations of vascular disease in the lower leg and foot cannot be described here, there are certain significant clinical aspects which enter into the evaluation of these patients.

A. Symptoms:

1. Claudication—Intermittent claudication is the commonest presenting symptom. Aching fatigue during exertion usually appears first in the calf muscles; in more severe cases a constant or cramping pain may be brought on by walking only a short distance. Less commonly, the feet are the site of most of the pain. Pain that lasts longer than 10 minutes after rest suggests some other disease, such as arthritis. The distance that the patient can walk before pain becomes severe enough to necessitate a few minutes' rest gives a rough estimate of circulatory inadequacy: 2 blocks (400–500 yards) or more is mild, 1 block is moderate, and one-half block or less is severe.

2. Rest pain—Rest pain may be due to sepsis or ischemia. The former is usually throbbing, whereas ischemia usually produces a persistent, gnawing ache with occasional spasms of sharp pain. Rest pain often comes on in bed at night when the cardiac output is less. Some relief is often obtained by uncovering the foot and placing it in a dependent position. In more advanced stages, the pain may be constant and so severe that even narcotics may not relieve it. Ischemic neuropathy is an important factor in this condition. The patient may request amputation.

3. Muscle cramps—Sudden painful contractions that last only a few minutes but leave a soreness for minutes or days in a pulseless leg are usually related to the arterial disease.

B. Signs:

1. Absence of pulsations—Careful palpation over the femoral, popliteal, dorsalis pedis, and posterior tibial arteries should be done to determine which pulsations are present. Although the popliteal pulse may be present, both pedal pulses are usually absent. Exercise in certain patients with arterial disease may make pedal pulses disappear. If a popliteal pulse is present, a direct surgical approach on the vessels of the lower extremity is not likely to be of value.

2. Color changes in the feet—Defective blood supply causes anoxic paralysis of the capillaries and a bluish-red skin (rubor). The rate of return of color following blanching induced by local pressure is an inaccurate index of circulatory adequacy because the blood that returns on release of the pressure does not necessarily represent true circulation.

a. Pallor upon elevation—If pallor appears rapidly upon elevation of the foot from the horizontal—or if it appears when the leg is only slightly raised—the circulatory status is poor.

b. Flushing time—Color normally returns in a few seconds to a foot placed in a dependent position after 1–2 minutes of elevation of the entire lower extremity. The poorer the collateral circulation, the longer the interval before flushing begins to appear in the toes. If flushing time is over 20 seconds—and especially if it appears only after 45–60 seconds—the arterial disease is extensive.

c. Dependent rubor—Beefy redness of the toes or foot on dependency is frequently present in occlusive disease, but it may not reach its full extent until a minute or more after the leg has been placed in the dependent position. Dependent rubor implies moderate or severe arterial occlusive disease.

d. Rubor of stasis—When almost complete stasis in the distal vessels occurs, with venous as well as arterial thrombosis and extravasation of red blood cells, redness of the toes and forefoot may develop which may not completely disappear on elevation of the leg. Usually, however, there is pallor of the skin surrounding the red area in the elevated leg. This disorder is often associated with severe pain and is more commonly noted in thromboangiitis obliterans than in atherosclerosis.

e. Patchy cyanosis and pallor indicate a severe degree of ischemia; it is seen frequently following acute thrombosis or recent embolus.

3. Venous filling time—If the valves in the saphenous system are competent, venous filling is a valuable gauge of collateral circulation of the foot. If the veins on the dorsum of the foot begin to fill in 30 seconds or more when the leg is placed in a dependent position after having been elevated for a minute, the circulatory impairment in the leg is severe.

4. Local tissue changes—Diminished arterial flow causes wasting of the subcutaneous tissues of the foot and lower leg. Hair is lost over these areas, the skin becomes smooth and shiny, and the nails become thickened and deformed. Infections are common following minor injuries or even without injury at the edge of a nail or under a thick callus. Once established, infection may become indolent and chronic with the formation of an ischemic ulcer which is often located over a pressure point of the foot; or the infection may lead to localized or progressive gangrene. Local heat should not be used in the treatment of such an infection.

5. Skin temperature—If arterial circulation is inadequate, the leg will feel quite cool, especially if there is considerable vasoconstrictor activity or if significant ischemia is present.

6. Sweating—Sweating is under the control of the sympathetic nervous system and is therefore an index of the degree of autonomic activity in the extremity. If a patient with occlusive disease still notes sweating of the feet, some degree of sympathetic activity is present and lumbar sympathectomy may be of benefit.

C. X-Ray Findings: Films of the lower leg and foot may show calcification of the vessels and thinning of the bones. If there is a draining sinus or an ulcer close to a bone or joint, osteomyelitis may be apparent on the film. If fairly strong popliteal pulses can be felt, arteriography is not likely to be of much value as a guide to surgical treatment; sometimes, however, the status of the femoral or popliteal arteries must be evaluated in this way.

D. Physiologic Testing: Pressure and blood flow measurements may now be done in an extremity distal to occlusive disease utilizing electronic equipment of various types which make use of ultrasonic beams, radioactive isotope clearance, and plethysmography. Such measurements are useful in the initial evaluation and also in following the progress of the vascular disease or evaluating the results of treatment.

E. Arterial Disease in Diabetic Patients: Atherosclerosis develops more often and earlier in patients with diabetes mellitus, especially if the disease has been poorly controlled over a period of years. Either the large or small vessels may be involved, but occlusion of the smaller vessels is relatively more frequent than in the nondiabetic, and thus they more often have the form of the disease that may not be suitable for arterial surgery. The resistance to infection is less. Anesthesia of the toes and distal foot (due to diabetic neuropathy) develops in some and predisposes to injury and secondary ulcers. In patients with such neurogenic ulcers, pain may be minimal and the peripheral circulation may be adequate, so that local healing may take place at a relatively normal rate. Recurrent trouble is frequent, however, and because of the sensory deficit, injury and secondary infection may be advanced before the condition is noted. Poor vision due to diabetic retinopathy makes care of the feet more difficult and injuries more likely (see p 736).

Ulcers and gangrene, when present, are more likely to be moist and infected and progress more rapidly, often with a more generalized inflammatory response.

Treatment

A. Intermittent Claudication: The patient should be instructed to walk slowly, take short steps, avoid stairs and hills, and to stop for brief rests to avoid pain. Walking, however, is the most effective way to develop collateral circulation, and walking up to the point of claudication followed by a 3-minute rest should be done at least 8 times a day.

B. Circulatory Insufficiency in the Foot and Toes: Sympathectomy may be indicated even when the femoral pulse is absent or when pregangrenous changes are present in the toes. Moderate or marked rest pain usually implies such advanced changes that the procedure will often be of little or no benefit. The operation usually results in a dry, warmer foot, and is of value for patients whose marginally adequate circulation becomes dangerously reduced by vasoconstrictive reflexes. The additional collateral flow serves to protect the leg should further vascular occlusions occur. Vasodilator drugs are usually of little or no value and may actually be harmful, since blood flow studies show a decrease in the blood supply to the ischemic limb of the elderly arteriosclerotic patient at the height of systemic vasodilatation due to drugs. Other measures as outlined under Instructions in the Care of the Feet should also be employed (see p 736).

C. Infections, Ulcers, and Gangrene of the Toes or Foot:

1. Early treatment of acute infections—Place the patient at complete bed rest with the leg in a horizontal or slightly depressed position. An open or discharging lesion should be covered with a light gauze dressing, but tape should not be used on the skin. Culture and sensitivity studies should be obtained if there is any purulent discharge, but if advancing infection is present an appropriate antibiotic should be started immediately. Purulent pockets should be drained.

Ulcerations covered with necrotic tissue can often be prepared for spontaneous healing or grafting with wet dressings of sterile saline changed 3—4 times a day. Petrolatum or Xeroform gauze and a bacitracin-neomycin ointment may also help soften crusted infected areas and aid drainage.

Treat diabetes and anemia, if present.

2. Early management of established gangrene—In most instances an area of gangrene will progress to a point where the circulation provided by the inflammatory reaction is sufficient to prevent progressive tissue death. The process will at least temporarily demarcate at that level. This can be encouraged by measures similar to those outlined in the preceding section on the treatment of acute infection. If the skin is intact and the gangrene is dry and due only to arterial occlusion, antibiotics should be withheld. If infection is present or if the gangrene is moist, antibiotics should be used in an effort to limit the process and prevent septicemia.

If the gangrene involves only a segment of skin and the underlying superficial tissue, sympathectomy and, if possible, an artery graft may reverse the process. The necrotic tissue can then be removed and the ulcer grafted or allowed to heal as outlined above in the section on ulcers. If the hoped-for healing does not occur and amputation is required, it can sometimes be carried out at a more distal level because of those procedures.

3. Amputations for gangrene—

a. A toe which is gangrenous to its base can sometimes be amputated through the necrotic tissue and left open; this procedure may be employed to establish adequate drainage when there is active infection with undrained pus in addition to the gangrene.

b. When the distal part of the toe is gangrenous

and there is sufficient circulation in the proximal toe, a closed amputation can be carried out after the area has become well demarcated and inflammation has subsided.

c. Transmetatarsal amputation can be considered if the gangrene involves one or more toes down to but not into the foot and if the circulation in the distal foot seems adequate to support healing.

d. Below the knee is the amputation level of choice when gangrene or ischemia in the foot is so distributed that local amputation (as outlined above) is not possible. The preservation of the knee and proximal part of the lower leg is most important in that a more useful prosthesis can then be applied and the patient can walk with greater ease than he can with the prosthesis made for the above-knee stump. Indeed, very few of those with the proximal amputation ever walk again, and generally spend the rest of their lives confined to a wheel chair and bed. Turning in bed is more difficult for the individual with the higher amputation. Even when the circulation below the knee is quite poor, successful healing of the stump is often achieved by the use of a longer posterior flap, meticulous and gentle technic, and often a rigid cast to support a well padded stump dressing. Amputation below the knee should be attempted provided there is a chance of success.

e. Amputation above the knee (through the distal thigh in the supracondylar area) is indicated in patients with very advanced peripheral vascular disease requiring amputation because of gangrene, particularly if the leg as well as the foot is extensively involved with gangrene and infection. It is also employed if an attempted below-knee amputation has failed to heal. Even if the femoral artery is obliterated, there will be sufficient collateral circulation to allow healing provided gentle technic with good hemostasis is used.

f. Guillotine amputation—Infection with bacteremia or septicemia occasionally develops secondary to gangrene of the lower extremity. This usually requires emergency amputation above or below the knee. In such a situation, it is often wise to leave the stump open so that it can heal by secondary intention or be revised or reamputated when the infection has been controlled.

Burgess EM, Romano RL: The management of lower extremity amputees using immediate postsurgery prosthesis. Clin Orthop 57:137, 1968.

Crawford ES & others: Occlusive disease of the femoral artery and its branches. S Clin North America 46:991, 1966.

Moore WS & others: Below knee amputation for vascular insufficiency. Arch Surg 97:886, 1968.

Myers KA, Irvine WT: Objective study of lumbar sympathectomy. Brit MJ 1:879, 1966.

Shaw RS, Austen WG, Stipa S: A ten year study of the effect of lumbar sympathectomy on the peripheral circulation of patients with arteriosclerotic occlusive disease. Surg Gynec Obst 119:486, 1964.

Sizer JS, Wheelock FC Jr: Digital amputations in diabetic patients. Surgery 72:980, 1972.

Szilagyi DE & others: Lumbar sympathectomy: Current role in treatment of arteriosclerotic occlusive disease. Arch Surg 95:753, 1967.

OCCLUSIVE CEREBROVASCULAR DISEASE

Although gradual mental deterioration, episodes of weakness or dizzy spells, blurred vision, or sudden complete hemiplegia may be due to a variety of causes, arteriosclerotic occlusive or ulcerative disease accounts for many of these problems (see pp 566–572). The lesion is often located in the extracranial arteries in segmental distribution. The areas most often involved are (1) the common carotid bifurcation, including the origins of the internal and external carotid arteries; (2) the origin of the vertebral artery; and (3) the intrathoracic segments of the aortic arch branches (though these vessels may occasionally be occluded as a result of a nonspecific arteritis). Because more than one vessel may be involved, complete evaluation of symptoms thought to be due to cerebral or brain stem ischemia on the basis of reduction of total blood flow to the brain below a critical point should include studies of the entire brachiocephalic system.

Clinical Findings

A. Symptoms: There is no completely consistent correlation between the clinical findings and the degree and location of the occlusive arterial processes. In insufficiency related primarily to the carotid vessels, the symptoms are primarily contralateral to the side of the clinically significant stenosis and are usually those of supratentorial involvement: weakness of the extremities or face, anesthesia, aphasia, mental confusion, memory deterioration, personality changes, hemiplegia, and coma.

Insufficiency related primarily to the vertebral and basilar vessels results in subtentorial symptoms such as vertigo (especially on standing up), unsteady gait, and diplopia or bilateral blurring of vision.

Transient episodes of altered vision may occur from microemboli of fibrin, platelet thrombi, or fragments of arteriosclerotic material which may arise from arteriosclerotic ulcers in the carotid artery, and the emboli may be noted in the retinal arteries on the same side as the diseased (but not necessarily stenotic) carotid artery. Visual alterations may also result from insufficient blood flow to the brain as a consequence of significant occlusive arterial lesions on the same side.

Neurologic symptoms without infarction, often manifested by transient ischemic attacks (TIA), may arise either from periods of temporary reduction of cerebral blood flow or from embolization of small fragments of clot or atheromatous material from ulcerated areas of proximal arterial disease (microemboli) to the cerebral cortex or to retinal arteries. Momentary weakness or numbness of the contralateral arm or leg and temporary partial or complete loss of vision of the ipsilateral eye or both eyes (amaurosis fugax) are common though not specific manifestations.

The **subclavian steal syndrome** is due to complete occlusion of the proximal left subclavian or of the innominate artery, with the result that some of the collateral blood flow to the arm is through the vertebral artery on the involved side as a retrograde flow, causing reduction of the total blood supply to the brain. Exercise of the arm may thus be associated not only with claudication but also occasionally with CNS symptoms. These symptoms usually disappear in time without specific treatment.

B. Signs: Bruits, diminished or absent pulsations, and a blood pressure difference in the 2 arms of more than 10 mm Hg are indications of occlusive disease in the brachiocephalic arteries. The most significant bruit is one that is sharply localized high in the lateral neck close to the angle of the jaw overlying the common carotid bifurcation. The murmur of aortic stenosis may be heard as a bruit over the subclavian and carotid arteries; when there are no such heart murmurs, the bruit generally denotes disease in these arteries. Bruits and angiographic lesions have a clear relationship, whether or not the patient has symptoms; the absence of a bruit does not exclude the possibility of carotid artery stenosis, and microemboli can arise from ulcerations of arteries without much stenosis or bruit. Only the common carotid and the superficial temporal pulses can be felt with accuracy; the internal carotid pulses cannot usually be palpated. Disease in the subclavian artery may be manifested by a diminished axillary pulse.

The Doppler ultrasound technic may be used to detect stenoses in the carotid arteries; the vertebral and the supraorbital arteries may also be examined by this method. The collateral blood flow to the brain that develops through the external carotid artery in the presence of complete occlusion of the internal carotid artery may be detected by this means.

C. X-Ray Findings: Arteriographic visualization of the brachiocephalic arteries is of great value in defining the location and degree of stenoses, the presence of symptomatic or asymptomatic arterial occlusions, and the nature of the collateral flow to the brain in the presence of significant stenoses or thromboses. The study may also help to differentiate an arterial lesion from other CNS problems such as brain tumor. Arteriograms are indicated whenever it is suspected that operation might be required. The ideal study includes the carotid vessels with their intracranial branches and the vertebral-basilar system, usually by means of transfemoral percutaneous catheterization of the aortic arch and its branches (Seldinger technic).

Treatment

A. Medical Treatment: Both acute stroke and major neurologic deficits are treated by medical means as discussed in the section on cerebrovascular accidents in Chapter 16.

B. Surgical Treatment: Operative treatment may be indicated for extracranial arterial stenosis or ulceration associated with intermittent or transient symptoms or mental deterioration.

Endarterectomy is generally employed to treat occlusive or ulcerative lesions of the bifurcation of the common carotid. There is evidence that the vessel can be clamped with relative safety—and without maintaining blood flow through an internal shunt—while the arterial procedure is in progress if the pressure in the internal carotid artery is 50 mm Hg or more. Great care should be taken to avoid hypotension in these patients; general anesthesia is usually used.

Occlusions at or close to the aortic arch can generally be treated without opening the chest by employing bypass grafts in the neck connecting a subclavian artery to the ipsilateral carotid artery. In the case of occlusion of the origin of the vertebral artery, anastomosis of that artery to the common carotid has been used. If both carotid and vertebral artery stenoses exist, the carotid lesion should be selected for treatment. When the internal carotid is completely occluded, microsurgical technic may be used to anastomose the superficial temporal artery to a suitable artery on the surface of the brain.

Prognosis

The prognosis and results of therapy are related to the number of vessels involved, the degree of stenosis in each, the collateral flow in the circle of Willis, and the specific effects of the occlusive disease on the function of the brain. Although surgery can be done in carefully selected patients with an acceptable mortality of 1–2% or less and with few long-term complications, it still has not been proved statistically that life is prolonged in patients treated surgically as compared to those treated by nonsurgical means. Transient ischemic attacks can often be eliminated by surgery, and although future strokes can occur in such patients, other arterial lesions are generally responsible for the later problems.

Egan RW, Upson JF: Carotid artery surgery for cerebral vascular insufficiency. Angiology 16:698, 1965.

Fields WS & others: Joint study of extracranial arterial occlusion. JAMA 211:1993, 1970; 224:985, 1973.

Gillespie JA (editor): *Extracranial Cerebrovascular Disease and Its Management.* Appleton-Century-Crofts, 1969.

Hohf RP: The clinical evaluation and surgery of internal carotid insufficiency. S Clin North America 47:71, 1967.

Santschi DR & others: The subclavian steal syndrome: Clinical and angiographic considerations in 74 cases in adults. J Thoracic Cardiovas Surg 51:103, 1966.

Thompson JE: *Surgery for Cerebrovascular Insufficiency.* Thomas, 1968.

Wylie EJ, Ehrenfeld WK: *Extracranial Occlusive Cerebrovascular Disease: Diagnosis and Management.* Saunders, 1970.

RENOVASCULAR HYPERTENSION

Stenosis (or occlusion) in a renal artery or one of its branches with reduction of blood flow to the tissue supplied by that vessel may cause increased production of renin from the ischemic kidney tissue and hypertension may develop as a result. The most common cause of this condition is arteriosclerosis, which characteristically is associated with stenosis at the origin of one or both of the renal arteries. It generally develops in individuals over 50, usually men; is often associated with other manifestations of arteriosclerosis and may coexist with essential hypertension. Fibromuscular dysplasia of one or both renal arteries, a relatively common form of renal artery stenosis, generally develops in individuals between 20 and 40, mostly women, and usually involves fibrous thickening of the media of the artery (though intimal and subadventitial fibrodysplasia also may occur). These conditions are progressive. The process may involve not only the main renal artery (usually the middle and distal thirds) but also the branches. Other forms of the disease are secondary to congenital arterial defects (hypoplasia, aneurysms) which may result in very severe hypertension in children. Renal artery emboli and kidney infarcts may result in hypertension of sudden onset. Blunt trauma to the kidney with specific injury to a renal artery may lead to hypertension; early repair of the injured artery will prevent such a development.

Clinical Findings

A. **Symptoms and Signs:** The history and physical examination are usually not helpful in differentiating renovascular hypertension from essential hypertension. The most significant finding in patients with renovascular hypertension is a bruit in the upper abdomen (present in about 50% of cases). Children under 10 with normal femoral pulses and hypertension are very likely to have renovascular hypertension and should be studied and, if possible, treated surgically, since the hypertension in such cases is a particularly severe and destructive form of the disease. Persons under age 50 with hypertension of sudden onset without other explanation should undergo diagnostic evaluation for renovascular hypertension. About one-fourth of patients over age 60 with hypertension have arteriosclerotic occlusive disease in the renal arteries.

B. **Laboratory and X-Ray Findings:** Routine urine and blood chemical determinations are not helpful; the diagnosis of renovascular hypertension depends on special diagnostic procedures. Of these, assay of the renal vein renin content is most helpful.

1. Renal vein renin determinations (from blood samples obtained by catheterization of the renal veins) that show a greater renin content on one side are highly suggestive of a stenotic arterial lesion on the side with the higher renin level. A renal vein renin ratio greater than 1.5:1 is considered significant. In the case of bilateral renal artery disease, there will be no significant difference in renin concentration on one side as compared to the other. This study has proved to be diagnostically reliable in about three-fourths of patients studied.

2. Renal arteriography is not indicated in mildly hypertensive patients or those who are unacceptable operative risks, but in patients with significant hypertension—especially those under age 50—it is important in demonstrating renal artery stenosis and sometimes increased collateral vessels provided selective and oblique films are obtained.

3. Rapid sequence intravenous urography is a fairly good screening study. False-negative results are often reported, especially in patients with bilateral renal artery stenosis. A difference of more than 1 cm in the length of the 2 kidneys or a difference in the time required for the nephrogram or urogram to be completed may be important findings. This study is reliably positive in 50–60% of patients.

4. Split renal function studies are of value, but only if done with great care.

Treatment

In carefully selected cases of renovascular hypertension, removal or, preferably, saphenous vein bypass of the arterial stenosis will result in a satisfactory long-term blood pressure response in 85–95% of children and those with fibromuscular dysplasia but in only 25–50% of those with arteriosclerosis. In patients over age 50, antihypertensive drug therapy is probably the treatment of choice. Nephrectomy should not be employed as the primary mode of therapy because the other kidney may later become involved with the same lesion. It relieves hypertension in only one-fourth of cases and thus should be employed only for urologic indications. Patients with bilateral renal artery stenosis present additional problems in diagnosis and management.

Biglieri EG & others: Renal vein renin in various forms of renal hypertension. Lancet 1:1194, 1972.

Foster JH, Dean RH: Changing concepts in renovascular hypertension. S Clin North America 54:257, 1974.

Foster JH & others: Ten years' experience with the surgical management of renovascular hypertension. Ann Surg 177:755, 1973.

Fry WJ & others: Autogenous saphenous vein aortorenal grafts: Ten years' experience. Arch Surg 105:855, 1972.

CELIAC & SUPERIOR MESENTERIC ARTERY DISEASE

Aneurysms or occlusive disease occasionally occur in the visceral branches of the abdominal aorta. Fibromuscular dysplasia of these visceral arteries and compression of the celiac artery by adjoining diaphragmatic ligamentous attachments are also suspected of compromising blood flow to the gut. Chronic arterial insufficiency to the intestine is generally manifested by postprandial pain and malabsorption leading to weight loss. A bruit is usually present. A common pattern of symptoms, signs, and laboratory findings is hard to define, and, because of the variability of symptoms, the condition should be considered in all older patients with atypical or unexplained abdominal complaints. Catheter angiography (lateral and anteroposterior views) may reveal the location and extent of the occlusive disease and show whether arterial surgery is indicated. Although endarterectomy has been employed, bypass graft from the aorta to a point in the visceral artery distal to the stenosis is favored now. Compression of the celiac artery by the median arcuate ligament of the diaphragm may be treated by division of the ligament with relief of symptoms in half of cases. Thrombosis of the superior mesenteric artery or embolism generally results in infarction of the bowel. (See Mesenteric Vascular Occlusion in Chapter 10.)

Bergan JJ & others: Intestinal ischemic syndromes. Ann Surg 169:120, 1969.
Rob C: Surgical diseases of the celiac and mesenteric arteries. Arch Surg 93:21, 1966.
Stoney RJ, Wylie EJ: Recognition and surgical management of visceral ischemic syndromes. Ann Surg 164:714, 1966.
Szilagyi DE & others: The celiac artery compression syndrome: Does it exist? Surgery 72:849, 1972.

ACUTE ARTERIAL OCCLUSION

Essentials of Diagnosis

- Symptoms and signs depend on the artery occluded, the organ or region supplied by the artery, and the adequacy of the collateral circulation to the area primarily involved.
- Occlusion in an extremity usually results in pain, numbness, tingling, weakness, and coldness. There is pallor or mottling; motor, reflex, and sensory alteration or loss; and collapsed superficial veins. Pulsations in arteries distal to the occlusion are absent.
- Occlusions in other areas result in such conditions as cerebral vascular accidents, intestinal ischemia and gangrene, and renal or splenic infarcts.

Differential Diagnosis

The primary diagnosis is between arterial embolism and thrombosis. In an older individual with both arteriosclerotic vascular disease and cardiac disease, the differentiation may be very difficult. Acute thrombophlebitis with arterial spasm can be distinguished on the basis of a normal or elevated skin temperature, distended veins, and edema.

1. ARTERIAL EMBOLISM

Arterial embolism occurs as a complication of atrial fibrillation secondary to rheumatic heart disease (36%) and arteriosclerotic heart disease without myocardial infarction (25%) and with infarction (12%). Myocardial infarction without fibrillation accounts for 14%. Unusual sources (aneurysm, left atrial myxoma, or arterial thrombus) or undetermined sources each account for approximately 6% of emboli.

Emboli tend to lodge at the bifurcation of major arteries, with over half going to the aortic bifurcation or the vessels in the lower extremities; the carotid system is involved in 20%, the upper extremity in 16%, and the mesenteric arteries in 5%. Emboli from arterial ulcerations are usually small, giving rise to transient symptoms in the toes or brain.

Clinical Findings

In an extremity, the initial symptoms are usually pain (sudden or gradual in onset), numbness, coldness, and tingling. Signs include absence of pulsations in the arteries distal to the block, coldness, pallor or mottling, hypesthesia or anesthesia, and weakness or paralysis of the involved muscles. The superficial veins are collapsed. Later, blebs and skin necrosis may appear, and gangrene may occur.

Treatment

Immediate embolectomy is the treatment of choice in almost all early cases. It should be done within 12 hours of the embolic episode if possible. If a longer delay has occurred or if there is clinical evidence of tissue necrosis, embolectomy may be associated with too high a mortality; in such circumstances, nonoperative measures (as outlined below) should be depended upon, accepting amputation at a later date in some of these cases.

A. Emergency Preoperative Care:

1. Heparin—Heparin sodium, 5000 units IV, should be given as soon as the diagnosis is made or suspected in an effort to prevent distal thrombosis. The effect of this dose will usually be dissipated by the time the patient has been moved to surgery. If a 4–5 hour delay is anticipated, 3000–4000 units should also be given IM.

2. Sympathetic block—A sympathetic block should not be attempted once heparin has been given, and it is better to emphasize heparin treatment and surgery at the earliest moment rather than to risk the delay involved in a blocking procedure. If the patient is considered inoperable, a sympathetic block may occasionally be tried before heparin is given.

3. Protect the part—Keep the extremity at or below the horizontal plane. Do not apply heat or cold to the involved extremity (but heat to an uninvolved extremity may help produce reflex vasodilatation). Protect from hard surfaces and overlying bedclothes.

4. Vasodilators—Papaverine, 60 mg IV every 2–3 hours, may be given. Whisky, 1½ oz 4 times daily, or nicotinic acid, 50 mg 4 times daily, may also be tried if surgery is not considered possible.

5. Analgesics—Pain should be relieved with an analgesic.

6. Arteriography—Arteriography is often of value either before or during surgery. There may be more than one embolus in an extremity; x-ray studies may help locate a distal embolus or determine the extent of the thrombosis.

B. Surgical Treatment: Local anesthesia is generally used if the occlusion is in an artery to an extremity. After removing the embolus through the arteriotomy, the proximal and distal artery should be explored for additional emboli or secondary thrombi by means of a specially designed catheter with a small inflatable balloon at the tip (Fogarty catheter). An embolus at the aortic bifurcation or in the iliac artery can often be removed under local anesthesia through common femoral arteriotomies with the use of these same catheters. Heparinization for a week or more postoperatively is indicated, and prolonged anticoagulation with warfarin is often indicated after that.

Delayed embolectomy carried out more than 12 hours following the embolus—and particularly when there is also evidence of muscle swelling or necrosis—involves a high risk of acute respiratory distress syndrome or acute renal shutdown; rapid deterioration and death may result. Anticoagulation rather than surgery may be the safer approach under such circumstances or in any case where it appears that significant tissue necrosis has already taken place even though amputation may become necessary later.

Prognosis

Arterial embolism is a threat not only to the limb (5–25% amputation rate) but also to the life of the patient (15–40% mortality rate). Emergency surgery is poorly tolerated by patients with advanced cardiac disease. Hospital mortality is high; over 60% die of heart disease and others of pulmonary emboli.

The mortality rate increases with the size and location of the embolus; aortic and iliac emboli are the most dangerous. Concomitant cerebral or mesenteric embolism may occur, as well as progressive cardiac failure. Emboli associated with hypertensive or arteriosclerotic heart disease have a poorer prognosis than those arising from rheumatic valvular disease in younger patients. Emboli recur in almost half of the entire group of patients and in over half of those with atrial fibrillation.

In patients with atrial fibrillation an attempt should be made to restore normal rhythm with quinidine or cardioversion, although restoration of normal rhythm tends to be permanent only in patients with recent or transitory fibrillation. Long-term anticoagulant therapy may diminish the danger of further emboli. Correction of mitral stenosis is indicated in selected individuals. Heart surgery done in the earlier stages of mitral stenosis diminishes the chance of later embolic complications.

2. ACUTE ARTERIAL THROMBOSIS

Acute arterial thrombosis generally occurs in an artery extensively involved with arteriosclerosis, resulting in almost complete obliteration of the channel. Blood flowing through such a narrow, irregular, or ulcerated lumen may clot, leading to a sudden, complete occlusion of the narrow segment. The thrombosis may then propagate either up or down the artery to a point where the blood is flowing rapidly through a somewhat less diseased artery (usually to a significant arterial branch proximally or one or more functioning collateral vessels distally). Occasionally the thrombosis is precipitated when the blood stream dissects up and displaces an arteriosclerotic plaque, blocking the lumen; trauma to the artery may precipitate a similar event. Inflammatory involvement of the arterial wall, with narrowing of the channel as in thromboangiitis obliterans, will also lead to acute thrombosis. Chronic mechanical irritation of the subclavian artery compressed by a cervical rib may also lead to a complete occlusion. Thrombosis in a diseased artery may be secondary to an episode of hypotension or cardiac failure. Polycythemia and dehydration also increase the chance of thrombosis.

Chronic, incomplete arterial obstruction usually results in the establishment of some collateral flow, and further flow will develop relatively rapidly through the collaterals once complete occlusion has developed. The extremity may go through an extremely critical period of hours or days, however, while the additional collateral circulation develops around the block. The survival of the tissue distal to the block depends on the development of adequate collateral circulation, which in turn depends on the location and length of the arterial thrombosis and whether undesirable conditions such as shock, heart failure, anemia, or hemoconcentration can be corrected promptly.

Clinical Findings

The local findings in the extremity are usually very similar to those described in the section on arterial embolus. The following differential points should be checked: (1) Are there manifestations of advanced occlusive arterial disease in other areas, especially the opposite extremity (bruit, absent pulses, secondary changes) as described on p 246? Is there a history of intermittent claudication? These clinical manifestations are suggestive but not diagnostic of thrombosis. (2) Is there a history or are there findings of a recent episode of atrial fibrillation or myocardial infarction? If so, an embolus is more likely than a thrombosis. (3) ECG and serum enzyme studies may give added information regarding the presence of a silent myocardial infarction and its likelihood as a source of an embolus. (4) An emergency arteriogram may be of value in making a more accurate differential diagnosis and in planning the therapy.

Treatment

Whereas emergency embolectomy is the usual approach in the case of an early occlusion from an embolus, a nonoperative approach is frequently used in the case of thrombosis for 2 reasons: (1) The segment of thrombosed artery may be quite long, requiring rather extensive and difficult surgery (thromboendarterectomy or artery graft). The removal of a single embolus in a normal or nearly normal artery is, by comparison, relatively easy and quick. (2) The extremity is more likely to survive without development of gangrene because some collateral circulation has usually formed during the stenotic phase before acute thrombosis. With an embolus, this is not usually the case; the block is most often at a major arterial bifurcation, occluding both branches, and the associated arterial spasm is usually more acute.

Treatment is therefore as outlined under emergency preoperative care for the arterial embolus (see above), with observation for hours or days. Gradual improvement in the circulation of the distal areas of the extremity is usually noted. If this does not occur and if tissue necrosis seems likely, emergency surgery may be considered, particularly if an arteriogram reveals that the thrombosis is not too extensive and that the vessel distal to the thrombosis is relatively normal and free of disease. Sympathectomy may occasionally tip the balance in a borderline situation and save an extremity not considered amenable to direct arterial surgery.

Prognosis

Limb survival usually occurs with acute thrombosis of the iliac or superficial femoral arteries; gangrene is more likely if the popliteal is suddenly occluded, especially if the period between occlusion and treatment is long or if there is considerable arterial spasm or proximal arterial occlusive disease. If the limb does survive the acute occlusion, a period of observation and evaluation will usually be possible and the late treatment and prognosis is outlined above in the section on occlusive disease of the iliac, femoral, and popliteal arteries.

Darling RC & others: Arterial embolism. Surg Gynec Obst 124:106, 1967.
Deterling RA Jr: Acute arterial occlusion. S Clin North America 46:587, 1966.
Fogarty TJ: Catheter technic for arterial embolectomy. J Cardiovas Surg 8:22, 1967.
Hallman GL & others: Surgical considerations in arterial embolism. S Clin North America 46:1013, 1966.
Thompson JE & others: Arterial embolectomy. Surgery 67:212, 1970.
Wessler S & others: Studies in peripheral arterial occlusive disease. III. Acute arterial occlusion. Circulation 17:512, 1958.

* * *

THROMBOANGIITIS OBLITERANS (TAO)
(Buerger's Disease)

Essentials of Diagnosis

- Almost always in young men who smoke.
- Extremities involved with inflammatory occlusions of the more distal arteries, with circulatory insufficiency of the toes or fingers.
- Thromboses of superficial veins may also occur.
- Course is intermittent and amputation may be necessary, especially if smoking is not stopped.

General Considerations

Buerger's disease is an episodic and segmental inflammatory and thrombotic process of the arteries and veins, principally in the limbs. It is seen most commonly in men between the ages of 25 and 35. The effects of the disease are almost solely due to occlusion of the arteries. The symptoms are primarily due to ischemia, complicated in the later stages by infection and tissue necrosis. The inflammatory process is intermittent, with quiescent periods lasting weeks, months, or years.

The clinical differential diagnosis between Buerger's disease and atherosclerotic peripheral vascular disease may be difficult or impossible.

The arteries of the legs are most commonly affected. The plantar and digital vessels and those in the lower leg (especially the posterior tibial artery) are most frequently involved. Occlusion of the femoral-popliteal arteries does not often occur. In the upper extremity, the distal arteries are most commonly affected. Different arterial segments may become occluded in successive episodes; a certain amount of recanalization occurs during quiescent periods.

Superficial migratory thrombophletitis is a common early indication of the disease.

The cause is not known, but alteration in the collagen in the vessels suggests that it may be a collagen disorder. A history of smoking is almost always obtained, and little or no progress can be made in treatment if the patient continues to smoke.

Clinical Findings

The signs and symptoms are primarily those of arterial insufficiency, and the differentiation from arteriosclerotic peripheral vascular disease may be difficult; however, the following findings suggest Buerger's disease:

(1) The patient is a man between the ages of 20 and 40 who smokes.

(2) There is a history or finding of small, red, tender cords resulting from migratory superficial segmental thrombophlebitis, usually in the saphenous tributaries rather than the main vessel. A biopsy of such a vein often gives microscopic proof of Buerger's disease.

(3) Intermittent claudication is common and is frequently noted in the palm of the hand or arch of

the foot. Instep claudication is common with Buerger's disease and is unusual in patients with arteriosclerotic occlusive disease. Rest pain is common and, when present, is persistent. It takes the form of gnawing or aching, often interferes with sleeping and eating, and tends to be more pronounced than in the patient with atherosclerosis. Numbness, diminished sensation, and pricking and burning pains may be present as a result of ischemic neuropathy.

(4) The digit or the entire distal portion of the foot may be pale and cold or there may be rubor which may remain relatively unchanged by posture; the skin may not blanch on elevation, and on dependency the intensity of the rubor is often more pronounced than that seen in the atherosclerotic group. The distal vascular changes are often asymmetric, so that not all of the toes are affected to the same degree. Absence or impairment of pulsations in the dorsalis pedis, posterior tibial, ulnar, or radial artery is frequent.

(5) Trophic changes may be present, often with painful indolent ulcerations along the nail margins.

(6) There is usually evidence of disease in both legs and possibly also in the hands and lower arms. There may be a history or findings of Raynaud's phenomenon in the finger or distal foot.

(7) The course is usually intermittent, with acute and often dramatic episodes followed by rather definite remissions. When the collateral vessels as well as the main channels have become occluded, an exacerbation is more likely to lead to gangrene and amputation. The course in the patient with atherosclerosis tends to be less dramatic and more persistent.

Differential Diagnosis

Arteriosclerosis obliterans occurs in a somewhat older age group, sometimes with associated hyperlipidemia and vessel calcification and without associated phlebitis.

Scleroderma causes characteristic skin changes prior to definite vascular findings.

Raynaud's disease causes symmetric bilateral color changes, primarily in young women. There is no impairment of arterial pulsations.

Livedo reticularis and acrocyanosis are vasospastic diseases which do not affect peripheral pulsations.

Frostbite may produce superficial gangrene. Pulsations proximal to the region of gangrene are not impaired, and there is a history of exposure to cold. Nonvascular trophic ulcers may occur in tabes dorsalis, syringomyelia, and other diseases associated with sensory loss. In these disorders pulsations are present and there are no postural color changes.

Among the neuromuscular conditions, the lesions most commonly confused with Buerger's disease are protruded intervertebral disks, metatarsalgia, and ther mechanical foot derangements. None of these cause typical claudication or changes in peripheral pulsations.

Treatment

The principles of therapy are the same as those outlined for atherosclerotic peripheral vascular disease, but the long-range outlook is better in patients with Buerger's disease, so that when possible the approach should be more conservative and tissue loss kept to a minimum.

A. General Measures: Smoking must be given up; the physician should be emphatic and insistent on this point. The disease is almost sure to progress if this advice is not heeded.

See the discussion of instructions in the care of the feet on p 736.

B. Surgical Treatment:

1. Sympathectomy—Sympathectomy is useful in eliminating the vasospastic manifestations of the disease and aiding in the establishment of collateral circulation. It may also relieve the milder or moderate forms of intermittent claudication and rest pain. If amputation of a digit is necessary, sympathectomy should precede amputation for it may aid in the healing of the surgical wound.

2. Arterial grafts—Arterial grafting procedures are seldom indicated in patients with Buerger's disease because they do not usually have a complete block in the ileofemoral region.

3. Amputation—The indications for amputation are similar in many respects to those outlined for the atherosclerotic group (see above), although the approach should be more conservative from the point of view of the preservation of tissue. Most patients with Buerger's disease who are managed carefully and stop smoking do not require amputation of the fingers or toes. It is almost never necessary to amputate the entire hand.

If there is evidence of both large and small vessel disease, the results of conservative management are poor and amputation is frequently necessary. Pain may become so severe that the conservative approach must be discarded.

Prognosis

Except in the case of the rapidly progressive form of the disease—and provided the patient stops smoking and takes good care of his feet—the prognosis for survival of the extremities is good. Buerger's disease rarely results in death.

Abramson DI & others: Thromboangiitis obliterans: A true clinical entity. Am J Cardiol 12:107, 1963.

Brown H & others: Thromboangiitis obliterans. Brit J Surg 56:59, 1969.

Eadie DGA & others: Buerger's disease. Brit J Surg 55:452, 1968.

Schatz IJ, Fine G, Eyler WR: Thromboangiitis obliterans. Brit Heart J 28:84, 1966.

IDIOPATHIC ARTERITIS OF TAKAYASU
("Pulseless Disease")

Pulseless disease, most frequent in young women, is a polyarteritis of unknown etiology, with particular predilection for the branches of the aortic arch. It occurs particularly in Orientals. Manifestations, depending upon the vessel or vessels involved, may include evidence of cerebrovascular insufficiency, with dizzy spells and visual disturbances; and absent pulses in the arms, with a rich collateral flow in the shoulder, chest, and neck areas.

Pulseless disease must be differentiated from lupus erythematosus and from vascular lesions of the aortic arch due to syphilis and atherosclerosis.

The arteritis leads to progressive occlusion of the proximal carotid, innominate, or subclavian arteries and, unless treated by bypass grafts of the involved vessels, can lead to blindness and hemiplegia.

Austen WG, Shaw RS: Surgical treatment of pulseless (Takayasu's) disease. New England J Med 270:1228, 1964.
Johnson CD, Ziakle TJ, Smith LL: Occlusive disease of the vessels of the aortic arch: Diagnosis and management. California Med 108:20, 1968.

TEMPORAL ARTERITIS
(Giant Cell Arteritis)

Temporal arteritis is a disease of unknown cause that occurs in the elderly. Because the characteristic giant cells are frequently present not only in the temporal arteries but in the aorta and its branches as well, the condition is frequently called giant cell arteritis. The arterial manifestations may be preceded by musculoskeletal symptomatology identical to that of polymyalgia rheumatica, and the 2 conditions presumably represent different clinical manifestations of the same disease.

Clinical Findings

A. Symptoms and Signs: Prodromal symptoms consisting of aches and pains of joints or muscles and malaise may exist for several years. A low-grade fever, anorexia, fatigue, and weight loss may also precede the development of localizing symptoms by weeks or months. Severe throbbing frontal or occipital headaches may then appear and persist for some time. Intermittent claudication of the jaw is common. Ocular complications consisting of sudden or gradual loss of vision in one or both eyes (50% bilateral) may then appear as a result of involvement of the central retinal artery. Systemic complications from arterial lesions in the cerebral or coronary vessels or the aorta may lead to a cerebral or myocardial infarction or aortic dissection.

The involved temporal or occipital arteries are firm, tender cords which may be nodular and are usually pulseless. Erythema in the same region is usually present. Vascular abnormalities may be present in the retinas.

B. Laboratory Findings: Mild anemia, leukocytosis, and a markedly elevated sedimentation rate are usually present. Liver function tests may be abnormal. Biopsy of the involved temporal artery will yield a microscopic diagnosis (though occasionally the temporal artery is not involved even in advanced cases).

C. X-Ray Findings: Temporal arteriography may be useful as a screening procedure and may also help to determine the proper biopsy site.

Treatment

Smoking should be discontinued.

A. Analgesia: Relief of pain with analgesics is indicated, but the stronger narcotics should not be used because of the danger of addiction in chronic cases. Local infiltration with lidocaine may be of value.

B. Corticosteroid Therapy: Corticosteroid therapy should be begun as soon as the diagnosis is made. The prodromal symptoms and headaches respond promptly to this therapy, and the ocular complications can be prevented. Large doses should be used initially (300 mg of cortisone daily or comparable amounts of the newer analogues). Maintain on 200 mg of cortisone (or equivalent) until symptoms are controlled (usually 2–5 weeks) and then reduce the dosage gradually but maintain on 25–75 mg of cortisone (or equivalent) until the disease has run its course. Symptoms can reappear after therapy has been diminished or discontinued, so continued observation is necessary.

Prognosis

Temporal arteritis is often a self-limited disease which may persist for 2 months to 2 years. If diagnosed and treated early, the ocular and grave systemic complications can be prevented. Blindness and death may result if the disease is not diagnosed and treated.

Andrews JM: Giant-cell ("temporal") arteritis: A disease with variable clinical manifestations. Neurology 16:963, 1966.
Bevan AT, Dunnill MS, Harrison MJG: Clinical and biopsy findings in temporal arteritis. Ann Rheumat Dis 27:271, 1968.
Birkhead NC, Wagener HP, Shick RM: Treatment of temporal arteritis with adrenal corticosteroids: Results in fifty-five cases in which lesion was proved at biopsy. JAMA 163:821, 1957.
Goodman JA: Polymyalgia rheumatica. California Med 111:484, 1969.
Hamilton CR Jr & others: Giant cell arteritis: including temporal arteritis and polymyalgia rheumatia. Medicine 50:1, 1971.
Harrison MJG, Bevan AT: Early symptoms of temporal arteritis. Lancet 2:638, 1967.

VASOSPASTIC DISORDERS

RAYNAUD'S DISEASE & RAYNAUD'S PHENOMENON

Essentials of Diagnosis

- Paroxysmal bilateral symmetrical pallor and cyanosis followed by rubor of the skin of the digits.
- Precipitated by cold or emotional upset; relieved by warmth.
- Gangrene absent or minimal.
- Primarily a disorder of young women.

General Considerations

Raynaud's disease is the primary or idiopathic form of paroxysmal digital cyanosis. Raynaud's phenomenon, which is more common than Raynaud's disease, may be due to a number of regional or systemic disorders.

In Raynaud's disease the digital arteries respond excessively to vasospastic stimuli. The cause is not known, but some abnormality of the sympathetic nervous system seems to be active in this entity. The disease occurs primarily in females between puberty and age 40, and a family history of a vasospastic phenomenon can often be obtained.

Clinical Findings

Raynaud's disease and Raynaud's phenomenon are characterized by intermittent attacks of pallor or cyanosis—or pallor followed by cyanosis—in the fingers (and rarely the toes), precipitated by cold or occasionally by emotional upsets. Early in the course of the disease, only 1–2 fingertips may be affected; as the disease progresses, all the fingers down to the distal palm may be involved. The thumbs are rarely affected. General as well as local body cooling is usually necessary. Recovery usually begins near the base of the fingers as a bright red return of color to the cyanotic or pale digit. During recovery there may be intense rubor, throbbing, paresthesia, and slight swelling. Attacks usually terminate spontaneously or upon returning to a warm room or putting the extremity in warm water. Between attacks there may be no abnormal findings. Sensory changes which often accompany vasomotor manifestations include numbness, stiffness, diminished sensation, and aching pain. The condition may progress to atrophy of the terminal fat pads and the digital skin, and gangrenous ulcers may appear near the fingertips which heal during warm weather.

Raynaud's disease appears first between the ages of 15 and 45, almost always in women. It tends to be progressive, and, unlike Raynaud's phenomenon (which may be unilateral and may involve only 1–2 fingers), symmetric involvement of the fingers of both hands is ultimately the rule. Spasm gradually becomes more frequent and prolonged. Gangrene of the whole finger is rare, and the peripheral pulses are normal.

Differential Diagnosis

Differentiation must be made between Raynaud's disease and the numerous disorders which may be associated with Raynaud's phenomenon. These include thromboangiitis obliterans, arteriosclerosis obliterans, thoracic outlet syndromes, collagen diseases, and cryoglobulinemia.

The differentiation from thromboangiitis obliterans is usually not difficult since thromboangiitis obliterans is generally a disease of men; peripheral pulses are often diminished or absent; and, when Raynaud's phenomenon occurs in association with thromboangiitis obliterans, it is usually in only 1–2 digits.

Raynaud's phenomenon may occur in patients with the thoracic outlet syndromes (including cervical rib and scalenus anticus problems). The symptoms in these disorders are generally unilateral, and brachial plexus compression symptoms tend to dominate the clinical picture. The various maneuvers and tests helpful in diagnosing these conditions should be performed on any patient with unilateral Raynaud's phenomenon.

It may be difficult to differentiate the skin thickening in Raynaud's disease from the early stages of scleroderma with Raynaud's phenomenon. If Raynaud's phenomenon has been present for some years but sclerodermatous changes are minimal, the diagnosis of Raynaud's disease is more likely. The skin of the face, neck, and chest is involved in the later stages of scleroderma, and esophageal involvement is manifested by dysphagia. '

Raynaud's phenomenon is occasionally the presenting complaint in systemic lupus erythematosus.

Cryoglobulins (abnormal proteins which are precipitated on exposure to cold) cause a disorder simulating Raynaud's disease. They are usually found in serious systemic diseases, and the diagnosis is not difficult. Testing for cryoglobulins may be worthwhile in atypical cases of Raynaud's phenomenon.

In acrocyanosis, cyanosis of the hands is permanent and diffuse.

Frostbite may lead to chronic changes with Raynaud's phenomenon. Ergot poisoning, particularly the prolonged or excessive use of ergotamine, must also be considered.

Treatment

A. General Measures: The body should be kept warm, and the hands especially should be protected from exposure to cold; gloves should be worn when out in the cold. The hands should be protected from injury at all times; wounds heal slowly, and infections are hard to control. Softening and lubricating lotion to control the fissured dry skin should be applied to the hands frequently. Smoking should be stopped.

B. Vasodilators: Vasodilator drugs are of limited value but may be of some benefit when there is peripheral vasoconstriction without significant organic vascular disease. In the relatively large doses used, side-effects are troublesome. Reserpine, methyldopa, nitroglycerin (or a longer-acting nitrate), nicotinic acid, and papaverine have been used.

C. Surgical Treatment: Sympathectomy may be indicated when attacks have become frequent and severe, interfering with work and well-being—and particularly if trophic changes have developed. In the lower extremities, complete relief usually results, whereas bilateral dorsal sympathectomies generally result in improvement though a vascular tone (not sympathetic) often ultimately develops. The symptoms which may thus reappear in 2–5 years are usually milder and less frequent. The results are better if a bilateral Horner's syndrome results (entire stellate ganglion removed). Sympathectomies are of limited value in very advanced cases.

Prognosis

Raynaud's disease is usually benign, causing mild discomfort on exposure to cold and progressing very slightly over the years. In a few cases rapid progression does occur, so that the slightest change in temperature may precipitate color changes. It is in this situation that sclerodactylia and small areas of gangrene may be noted, and such patients may become quite disabled by severe pain, limitation of motion, and secondary fixation of distal joints.

Gifford RW Jr: The clinical significance of Raynaud's phenomenon and Raynaud's disease. M Clin North America 42:963, 1958.
Kirtley JA & others: Cervicothoracic sympathectomy in neurovascular abnormalities of the upper extremities. Ann Surg 165:869, 1967.
Kontos HA & others: Effect of reserpine in Raynaud's phenomenon. Circulation 39:259, 1969.
Varad DP, Lawrence AM: Suppression of Raynaud's phenomenon by methyldopa. Arch Int Med 124:13, 1969.
See also reference under Acrocyanosis, below.

LIVEDO RETICULARIS

Livedo reticularis is a vasospastic disorder of unknown cause which results in constant mottled discoloration on large areas of the extremities, generally in a fishnet pattern with reticulated cyanotic areas surrounding a paler central core. It occurs primarily in young women. It may be associated with occult malignancy.

Livedo reticularis is most apparent on the thighs and forearms and occasionally on the lower abdomen, and is most pronounced in cold weather. The color may change to a reddish hue in warm weather but never entirely disappears spontaneously. A few patients complain of paresthesias, coldness, or numbness in the involved areas. Recurrent ulcerations in the lower extremities may occur in severe cases.

Bluish mottling of the extremities is diagnostic. The peripheral pulses are normal. The extremity may be cold, with increased perspiration.

Livedo reticularis must be differentiated from acrocyanosis, Raynaud's disease, and organic occlusive diseases.

Treatment consists of protection from exposure to cold, and use of vasodilators (see above) in more severe cases. If ulceration or gangrene is present, bed rest, compresses, vasodilators, and occasionally sympathectomy may be indicated.

In most instances, livedo reticularis is entirely benign. The rare patient who develops ulcerations or gangrene should be studied for underlying systemic disease.

Barker NW, Hines EA, Craig W McK: Livedo reticularis: A peripheral arterial disease. Am Heart J 21:592, 1941.
See also reference under Acrocyanosis, below.

ACROCYANOSIS

Acrocyanosis is an uncommon symmetrical condition which involves the skin of the hands and feet and, to a lesser degree, the forearms and legs. It is associated with arteriolar vasoconstriction and dilatation of the subpapillary venous plexus of the skin through which deoxygenated blood slowly circulates. It is worse in cold weather but does not completely disappear during the warm season. It occurs in either sex, is most common in the teens and 20s, and usually improves with advancing age or during pregnancy. It is characterized by coldness, sweating, slight edema, and cyanotic discoloration of the involved areas. Pain, trophic lesions, and disability do not occur, and the peripheral pulses are present. The individual may thus be reassured and encouraged to dress warmly in cold weather.

Gifford RW Jr: Arteriospastic disorders of extremities. Circulation 27:970, 1963.

• • •

ERYTHROMELALGIA
(Erythermalgia)

Erythromelalgia is a paroxysmal bilateral vasodilative disorder of unknown etiology. Idiopathic (primary) erythromelalgia occurs in otherwise healthy persons, rarely in children, and affects men and women equally. A secondary type is occasionally seen in patients with polycythemia vera, hypertension, gout, and organic neurologic diseases.

The chief symptom is bilateral burning distress which lasts minutes to hours, first involving circumscribed areas on the soles or palms (or both) and, as the disease progresses, the entire extremity. The attack occurs in response to stimuli producing vasodilatation (eg, exercise, warm environment), especially at night when the extremities are warmed under bedclothes. Reddening or cyanosis as well as heat may be noted. Relief may be obtained by cooling the affected part and by elevation.

No findings are generally present between attacks. On induction of the syndrome, heat and redness are noted in association with the typical pain. Skin temperature and arterial pulsations are increased, and the involved areas may sweat profusely.

Erythromelalgia must be differentiated from peripheral neuritis and organic occlusive diseases as well as from acrocyanosis.

In primary erythromelalgia, aspirin may give excellent relief. The patient should avoid warm environments. In severe cases, if medical measures fail, section or crushing of peripheral nerves may be necessary to relieve pain.

Primary idiopathic erythromelalgia is uniformly benign. The prognosis in secondary erythromelalgia depends upon the underlying disease.

Babb RR & others: Erythermalgia: Review of 51 cases. Circulation 29:136, 1964.

Pepper H: Primary erythermalgia: Report of a patient treated with methysergide maleate. JAMA 203:1066, 1968.

VASOMOTOR DISORDERS ASSOCIATED WITH TRAUMA

POST-TRAUMATIC SYMPATHETIC DYSTROPHY
(Causalgia)

Essentials of Diagnosis

- Burning or aching pain following trauma to an extremity of a severity which is greater than that expected from the initiating injury.
- Manifestations of vasomotor instability are generally present and include temperature, color, and texture alterations of the skin of the involved extremity.

General Considerations

Pain—usually burning or aching—in an injured extremity is the single most common finding, and the disparity between the severity of the inciting injury and the degree of pain experienced is the most characteristic feature. Crushing injuries with lacerations and soft tissue destruction are the most common causes, but closed fractures, simple lacerations, burns (especially electric), and elective operative procedures are also responsible for this syndrome. It is rare in children. The manifestations of pain and the associated objective changes may be relatively mild or quite severe, and the initial manifestations often change if the condition proceeds to a chronic stage.

Clinical Findings

In the early stages, the pain, tenderness, and hyperesthesia may be strictly localized to the injured area and the extremity may be warm, dry, swollen, and red or slightly cyanotic. The involved extremity is held in a splinted position by the muscles, and the nails may become ridged and the hair long. In advanced stages, the pain is more diffuse and worse at night; the extremity becomes cool and clammy and intolerant of temperature changes (particularly cold); and the skin becomes glossy and atrophic. The joints become stiff, generally in a position that makes the extremity useless. The dominant concern of the patient may become avoidance of the slightest stimuli to the extremity and especially to the trigger points that may develop. The bones become osteoporotic.

Prevention

During operations on an extremity, peripheral nerves should be handled only when absolutely necessary and then with utmost gentleness. Splinting of an injured extremity for an adequate period during the early, painful phase of recovery, together with adequate analgesics, may help prevent this condition.

Treatment & Prognosis

A. **Conservative Treatment:** It is most important that the condition be recognized and treated in the early stages, when the manifestations are most easily reversed and major secondary changes have not yet developed. In mild, early cases with minimal skin and joint changes, physical therapy involving active and passive exercises combined with trifluoperazine, 1 or 2 mg twice daily, or diazepam, 2 mg twice daily, may relieve symptoms. Protecting the extremity from irritating stimuli is important, and the use of nonaddicting analgesics may be necessary.

B. **Surgical Treatment:** If the condition fails to respond to conservative treatment or if there are more severe or advanced objective findings, sympathetic blocks (stellate ganglion or lumbar) are indicated, usually in a series on consecutive days. Intensive physical therapy may be used during the pain-free periods following effective blocks. Patients who achieve significant temporary relief of symptoms after sympathetic blocks but fail to obtain permanent relief are often cured by sympathectomy. In the advanced forms—particularly in association with major local changes and emotional reactions—the prognosis for a useful life is poor. The newer neurosurgical approaches using implantable electronic biostimulator devices to block pain impulses in the cervical spinal cord have met with some success.

Kleinert HE & others: Post-traumatic sympathetic dystrophy. Orthop Clin North America 4:917, 1973.

SUDECK'S ATROPHY

Sudeck's atrophy is an acute atrophy of the bones of an extremity which usually develops after minor injury, especially to the ankle or wrist. Symptoms and signs of vasomotor hyperactivity include pain of a burning type made worse by movement, edema, local heat, and swelling. The limb may ultimately become cold, cyanotic, and wasted, with stiffness of the joints, and this may be referred to as post-traumatic vasomotor dystrophy. Secondary fractures occasionally occur in the atrophic bones.

Prophylaxis consists of adequate early treatment of sprains and other similar injuries. The early manifestations are usually treated by physical therapy: mild heat, light massage, and gentle movement of the joints. A walking type of plaster cast for the foot and ankle region may be of value.

In severe and chronic forms, sympathectomy may give relief.

DEGENERATIVE & INFLAMMATORY VENOUS DISEASE

VARICOSE VEINS

Essentials of Diagnosis

- Dilated, tortuous superficial veins in the lower extremities.
- May be asymptomatic or may be associated with fatigue, aching discomfort, or pain.
- Edema, pigmentation, and ulceration of the skin of the distal leg may develop.

General Considerations

Varicose veins develop predominantly in the lower extremities. They consist of abnormally dilated, elongated, and tortuous alterations in the saphenous veins and their tributaries. These vessels lie immediately beneath the skin and superficial to the deep fascia; they therefore do not have as adequate support as the veins deep in the leg, which are surrounded by muscles. In many cases there is an inherited abnormality of the vein wall allowing increased distensibility, incompetence of the valves, and formation of varicosities. Other contributory factors are prolonged standing over a number of years, pregnancy, obesity, and, perhaps, aging.

Secondary varicosities can develop as a result of obstructive changes and valve damage in the deep venous system following thrombophlebitis, or occasionally as a result of proximal venous occlusion due to neo-plasm. Congenital or acquired arteriovenous fistulas are also associated with varicosities.

The long saphenous vein and its tributaries are most commonly involved, but the short saphenous vein may also be affected. There may be one or many incompetent perforating veins in the thigh and lower leg, so that blood can reflux into the varicosities not only from above, by way of the saphenofemoral junction, but also from the deep system of veins through the incompetent perforators. Largely because of these valvular defects, venous pressure in the superficial veins does not fall appreciably on walking; over the years, the veins progressively enlarge and the surrounding tissue and skin develop secondary changes such as fibrosis, chronic edema, and skin pigmentation and atrophy.

Clinical Findings

A. Symptoms: The severity of the symptoms caused by varicose veins is not necessarily correlated with the number and size of the varicosities; extensive varicose veins may produce no subjective symptoms, whereas minimal varicosities may produce many symptoms. Aching or burning discomfort, fatigue, or pain in the lower leg brought on by periods of standing are the most common complaints. Cramps may occur, but intermittent claudication and coldness of the feet are not associated with varicose veins. One must be careful to distinguish between the symptoms of arteriosclerotic peripheral vascular disease and those of venous disease, since occlusive arterial disease usually contraindicates the operative treatment of varicosities. Itching from an associated eczematoid dermatitis may occur in the region of the veins.

B. Signs: Dilated, tortuous, elongated veins beneath the skin in the thigh and leg are generally readily visible in the standing individual, although in very obese patients palpation and percussion may be necessary to detect their presence and location. Secondary tissue changes may be absent even in extensive varicosities; but if the varicosities are of long duration, brownish pigmentation and thinning of the skin above the ankle are often present. Swelling may occur, but signs of severe chronic venous stasis such as extensive swelling, fibrosis, pigmentation, and ulceration of the distal lower leg usually denote the postphlebitic state (see p 267).

C. Trendelenburg's Test: Of use in determining the competence of the valves at the proximal end of the long saphenous vein close to the saphenofemoral junction, in the long saphenous vein in the thigh and leg, and in the communicating veins between the superficial and deep vessels.

1. With the patient supine, elevate the leg. If there is no organic venous obstruction, varicosities will empty immediately.

2. Place a rubber tourniquet around the upper thigh and ask the patient to stand.

a. If the long saphenous vein remains empty for 30 seconds or more and then fills very slowly from below over a period of 1–2 minutes, the valves close to the saphenofemoral junction are incompetent, the valves in the communicating veins are competent, and the blood is flowing through them in the normal direction (superficial to deep). On release of the tourniquet, if the veins fill rapidly from above, the incompetence of the proximal valves is confirmed.

b. If the varicosities fill rapidly, the communicating veins between the deep and the superficial vessels are incompetent and blood is refluxing into the varicosed vessels. If, on release of the tourniquet, no additional filling of the varicosities occurs, the valves in the saphenous vein close to the saphenofemoral junction are competent; if, on the other hand, further distention of the varicosities occurs when the tourniquet is released, the valves at the upper end of the long saphenous vein are also incompetent. The precise site of these defective perforating veins can often be determined by repetition of this maneuver while placing the tourniquet at successively lower levels or using 2 or 3 tourniquets at different levels. If varices in the leg fill within less than 30 seconds with the tourniquet at the midthigh level but remain relatively empty with the tourniquet at the knee level, an incompetent short saphenous vein should be suspected.

Differential Diagnosis

Primary varicose veins should be differentiated from those secondary to (1) chronic venous insufficiency of the deep system of veins (see p 269), (2) retroperitoneal vein obstruction from extrinsic pressure on fibrosis, (3) arteriovenous fistula (congenital or acquired), so that a bruit is present and a thrill is often palpable; and (4) congenital venous malformation. Venography may be of value in the investigation of some of these problems. If significant occlusion of the deep venous system is suspected and extensive varicose vein surgery is being considered, phlebography of the deep system should be performed to be certain that the deep veins are patent before the superficial veins are removed.

Complications

If thin, atrophic, pigmented skin has developed at or above the ankle, secondary ulcerations may occur—often as a result of little or no trauma. An ulcer will occasionally extend into the varix, and the resulting fistula will be associated with profuse hemorrhage unless the leg is elevated and local pressure is applied to the bleeding point.

Chronic stasis dermatitis with fungal and bacterial infection may be a problem (see Chronic Venous Insufficiency, p 269).

Thrombophlebitis may develop in the varicosities, particularly in postoperative patients and pregnant or postpartum women or those taking oral contraceptives. Local trauma or prolonged periods of sitting may also lead to superficial venous thrombosis. Extension of the thrombosis into the deep venous system by way of the perforating veins or through the saphenofemoral junction may occur. (See Thrombophlebitis, below.)

Prevention

Individuals with a strong family history of varicose veins or those with early or minimal varicosities, particularly if their activities involve a great deal of standing or if pregnancy develops, should use elastic stockings to protect their veins from the chronic venous hypertension that results during long periods of sitting or standing.

Treatment

A. Nonsurgical Treatment: The use of elastic stockings (medium or heavy weight) to give external support to the veins of the proximal foot and leg up to but not including the knee is the best nonoperative approach to the management of varicose veins. When elastic stockings are worn during the hours that involve much standing or sitting and when combined with the habit of elevation of the legs when possible, reasonably good control of the varicosities can be maintained and progression of the condition and the development of complications can often be avoided. This approach may be used in elderly patients, in those that refuse or wish to defer surgery, sometimes in women with mild or moderate varicosities who are going to have more children, and in those with mild asymptomatic varicosities.

B. Surgical Treatment: The surgical treatment of varicose veins consists of interruption or removal of the varicosities and the incompetent perforating veins. Accurate delineation and division of the latter are required to prevent recurrence. The most important phase of the procedure is transection and ligation of the long saphenous vein precisely at its junction with the common femoral vein combined with ligation and division of the 5 or 6 tributaries joining the terminal 3–10 cm of this vein.

Following this initial procedure, the remaining surgery may involve the following: (1) Stripping (removal) of the long saphenous vein, usually from the ankle to the proximal end and generally with an internal stripper and general anesthesia. (2) Multiple distal ligations of the long saphenous vein and its tributaries. This procedure is usually employed in older patients, in those with minimal varicosities, or in those undergoing treatment for recurrences following previous stripping procedures. The entire procedure can be done under local anesthesia and is associated with less morbidity than stripping; however, there is a higher incidence of recurrent varicosities. (3) Subfascial ligations are sometimes employed to control multiple incompetent perforating veins in the leg. (4) Skin grafting of varicose ulcers may occasionally be necessary for those that do not heal when treated (a) with rest, elevation, and saline compresses; or (b) in the ambulatory patient, with firm compression of the lower leg and foot as afforded by Unna's boot or some other form of compression boot dressing.

C. Compression Sclerotherapy: Sclerotherapy to obliterate and produce permanent fibrosis of the collapsed veins is generally reserved for the treatment of residual small varicosities following definitive varicose vein surgery, although it is used by some who have become very competent in this technic as a primary form of treatment. Following the injection of a small amount of sclerosing solution (3% sodium tetradecyl sulfate [Sotradecol] is often used) into the vein, continuous pressure is applied to that segment of vein for 6 weeks. Multiple sites can be injected initially and others subsequently. It should not be used in allergic or pregnant individuals or those with local infection, thrombophlebitis, or arteriosclerosis.

Prognosis

Patients should be informed that even extensive and carefully performed surgery may not prevent the development of additional varicosities and that further (though usually more limited) surgery may be necessary in later years. If extensive varicosities reappear after surgery, the completeness of the high ligation should be questioned and reexploration of the saphenofemoral area may be necessary. Even after adequate treatment of varicose veins, the secondary tissue changes may not regress.

Burges CM: A practical approach to the treatment of varicose veins. S Clin North America 43:1385, 1963.

Carter BN II, Johns TNP: Recurrent varicose veins: Anatomical and physiological observations. Ann Surg 159:1017, 1964.

Dodd H, Cockett FB: *The Pathology of the Veins of the Lower Limb.* Livingstone, 1956.

Hobbs JT: Surgery and sclerotherapy in the treatment of varicose veins: A random trial. Arch Surg 109:793, 1974.

Larson HL & others: Long-term results after vein surgery: Study of 1000 cases after 10 years. Mayo Clin Proc 49:114, 1974.

Massell TB, Raphael HA: Cause and prevention of failure in varicose vein operations. California Med 118:1, May 1973.

Sherman RS: Varicose veins. S Clin North America 44:1369, 1964.

THROMBOPHLEBITIS

Venous thrombosis may arise as a complication of many different clinical conditions, and it can also develop in individuals who have been active and in good health. The thrombotic process, once established, is generally quite similar in all cases no matter what the cause, though the initiating causes may be quite variable. Common causes include traumatic exposure of subendothelial tissue to the endothelium of the vein and a variety of intravascular stimuli affecting the blood (antigen-antibody complexes, viruses, bacteria, endotoxins, etc).

Within a few days, the thrombus becomes adherent to the vein wall and secondary inflammation develops. There is less danger of an embolus at this stage, though there may still be a free-floating tail in a more proximal vein. Ultimately, the thrombus is invaded by fibroblasts, resulting in scarring of the wall of the vein and destruction of its valves. Central recanalization

may occur with restoration of blood flow, although directional control is permanently lost because valves do not regain competency. The resulting venous stasis and altered hemodynamic forces cause dependent edema and, ultimately, other distressing sequelae of the postphlebitic leg.

1. THROMBOPHLEBITIS OF THE DEEP VEINS

Essentials of Diagnosis

- Pain and swelling in the involved extremity.
- Calf tenderness and positive Homans sign.
- May be no clinical manifestations.

General Considerations

Thrombophlebitis is partial or complete occlusion of a vein by a thrombus with a secondary inflammatory reaction in the wall of the vein. It is encountered most frequently in the deep veins of the legs and pelvis in postoperative or postpartum patients during the 4th—14th days, and in patients with fractures or other trauma, cardiac disease, or stroke, especially if prolonged bed rest is involved. Radioisotope fibrinogen uptake tests reveal that small, clinically silent thrombosis takes place in the calf veins in 30—60% of those who have major surgical or medical illnesses or major injuries; propagation of the thrombosis into the popliteal and femoral veins occurs in approximately 10% of these patients. In the postoperative patient, the initial thrombosis generally occurs during the major surgical procedure or in the first 24 hours following operation (or injury).

The deep veins of the calf are most frequently involved (approximately 80%), but the thrombotic process may start in or progress to the femoral and iliac veins. The site of origin is at times in the pelvic veins or in the long saphenous vein.

Predisposing factors are aging, malignancy, shock, dehydration, anemia, obesity, and chronic infection. Perhaps the most important etiologic factors in thrombophlebitis are venous stasis and pressure changes in the endothelium of the vein wall which develop when the legs lie for hours without moving on the bed or operating table. Exposed subendothelial tissue or a variety of intravascular stimuli affecting the blood result in the release of platelet constituents; platelet aggregates form, followed by the deposition of fibrin, leukocytes, and, finally, red cells, and a thrombus results which can then propagate along the vein.

Pregnancy and the oral contraceptive drugs are associated with thrombophlebitis in some women; the medication should be permanently discontinued in those who develop phlebitis and should not be prescribed for those with a history of venous thrombosis.

Clinical Findings

In approximately half of patients with thrombophlebitis there are no symptoms or signs in the extremity in the early stages. The patient often suffers a pulmonary embolus, presumably from the leg veins, without symptoms or demonstrable abnormalities in the extremities.

A. Symptoms: The patient may complain of a dull ache, a tight feeling, or frank pain in the calf or, in more extensive cases, the whole leg, especially when walking. A feeling of anxiety is not uncommon.

B. Signs: Typical findings, though variable and unreliable and in many cases absent, are as follows: slight swelling in the involved calf, as noted by careful measurements; distention of the peripheral veins; tenderness and induration or spasm in the calf muscles, with or without pain in the calf, produced by dorsiflexion of the foot (Homans' sign); warmth of the affected leg when both legs are exposed to room temperature for a few minutes; and slight fever and tachycardia. When the femoral and iliac veins are also involved, there may be tenderness over these veins and the swelling in the extremity may be marked (phlegmasia alba dolens). The skin may be cyanotic if venous obstruction is severe (phlegmasia cerulea dolens), or pale and cool if a reflex arterial spasm is superimposed.

C. Additional Diagnostic Technics: Because of the difficulty in making a precise diagnosis by history and examination and because as accurate a diagnosis as possible is desirable before relatively prolonged and extensive therapy is initiated, new diagnostic approaches are being used with increasing frequency:

1. Phlebography, the most accurate and complete method of diagnosis thus far available, will define by x-ray means the location and extent of the thrombosis, if present (thrombi in the profunda femoris and internal iliac veins will not be demonstrated). Bilateral studies are of importance in planning therapy. Because of the time and expense involved, this test is not used as a screening study.

2. The fibrinogen uptake test (not yet available for general use) defines the presence of small thrombi in the calf and allows observation of the thrombotic process over a period of several days. Its use will undoubtedly increase in the coming years for it is the most sensitive test for developing deep venous thrombosis in the calf, popliteal, and femoral veins and the process can be followed by daily testing.

3. The ultrasound blood flow detector (or impedance plethysmography, which has similar diagnostic value) allows the major veins in an extremity to be examined for thrombosis; the accuracy of these tests is not great, but they may prove to be a safe, simple, and rapid screening procedure for detection of thrombosis in large veins in high-risk patients.

Differential Diagnosis

Calf muscle strain or contusion may be difficult to differentiate from thrombophlebitis; phlebography may be required to determine the correct diagnosis.

Cellulitis may be confused with thrombophlebitis; with infection there is usually as associated wound, and inflammation of the skin is more marked.

Obstruction of the lymphatics or the iliac vein in the retroperitoneal area from tumor or irradiation may lead to unilateral swelling, but it is usually more chronic and painless. An acute arterial occlusion is more painful, the distal pulses are absent, there is usually no swelling, and the superficial veins in the foot fill slowly when emptied.

Bilateral leg edema is more likely to be due to heart, kidney, or liver disease.

Complications

A. Pulmonary Embolism: Pulmonary embolism occurs when a thrombus becomes detached from its site of origin in a vein and is carried to the pulmonary arteries. Approximately 70% arise from the lower extremities, 20% from the pelvic veins, and the rest from other areas or the right atrium. As the inflammatory response in the vein wall to the thrombus increases, the thrombus becomes progressively more adherent to the vessel of origin and thus less likely to embolize. An unattached, free-floating extension of the thrombus may still exist, however, which can break off from the adherent thrombus and embolize.

A small or moderately large pulmonary embolism obstructing blood flow through one or more of the branches of the pulmonary artery, and sometimes leading to infarction of lung tissue, may be present without any associated pulmonary symptoms, signs, or x-ray findings. Clinical manifestations, when present, take the form of pleuritic pain (often with a transient friction rub), a dry cough (sometimes associated with hemoptysis), local rales in the area of involvement, a small amount of pleural fluid, and often x-ray evidence of pulmonary consolidation or diminished vascular markings. Fever and increased pulse and respiratory rates are often present. The LDH, bilirubin, white count, fibrin degradation products, and sedimentation rate may be elevated, and transient ECG changes may occur. The radioactive isotope lung scan may reveal a perfusion defect which, though consistent with embolism, must still be differentiated from other causes of pulmonary consolidation. This is particularly true if x-ray changes also exist. Pulmonary echography (ultrasound) may aid in diagnosis of an embolus, particularly when no infarction has occurred.

Massive pulmonary embolism is associated with shock, dyspnea, and cyanosis, and often with ECG changes characteristic of cor pulmonale. Death may occur in minutes or hours. The pulmonary artery pressure is elevated, and pulmonary angiography will demonstrate a significant obstruction of the right or left pulmonary artery or one of the major branches. (See Pulmonary Thromboembolism, p 143, for other details of diagnosis and treatment.)

B. Chronic Venous Insufficiency: Chronic venous insufficiency with or without secondary varicosities is a late complication of deep thrombophlebitis. (See Chronic Venous Insufficiency, p 269.)

Prevention

Great attention must be devoted to the effective

prevention of thrombophlebitis.

(1) The legs, well padded, should be elevated 10–20 degrees during a long operation.

(2) Patients with a history of phlebitis or with varicose veins should have elastic supports on the legs during and after operation or delivery or when an illness demands many days in bed.

(3) Predisposing conditions such as hypovolemic shock, dehydration, anemia, infection, and congestive heart failure should be recognized and treated promptly and aggressively, particularly in older patients and those with cancer. Birth control pills should be discontinued for several weeks prior to elective surgery.

(4) Postoperative exercises of the legs should be started at the close of the operative procedure while the patient is still on the operating table or in the recovery room and continued for several days. Early ambulation (but not standing or sitting) is likewise of value and should be started as soon as possible after operation or acute illness. If bed rest is necessary, passive or active bed exercises should be instituted and continued as long as the patient must remain in bed (eg, active or passive flexion of the toes, ankles, knees, and hips repeated frequently while the patient is awake). The bedclothes should be kept loose so that the legs can be moved freely and turning in bed can be done with ease. Deep breathing should be encouraged.

(5) Elevation of the foot of the bed 15–30 degrees may be of value in patients predisposed to thrombophlebitis. Venous stasis may be diminished by keeping the head of the bed near the horizontal and avoiding bed adjustments or pillows which result in prolonged flexion of the knees.

(6) Prophylactic use of anticoagulants may occasionally be indicated, particularly in patients with a fracture of the femur or tibia or in high-risk medical or surgical patients. Although the prothrombin depressant drugs were initially employed and were shown to have definite protective value, heparin in low doses (5000 units every 12 hours) has been found to reduce the incidence of thrombosis even more and can usually be used without major hemorrhagic complications even when given before surgery and resumed 10–24 hours following surgery. If anticoagulants are to be used in high-risk patients, they should be started within 1–2 days after the injury or before surgery and should be continued for at least 7 days postoperatively—probably longer following major fractures. Dextran 40 (500 ml of 6% solution IV over 6–8 hours) may also reduce the incidence of thrombophlebitis in high-risk patients. (See below.)

(7) Brief but regular periods of walking during long airplane and automobile trips should be encouraged since venous thromboses do occur during such times even in active, healthy adults.

Treatment of Acute Thrombophlebitis

A. Local Measures: The legs should be elevated 15–20 degrees; the trunk should be kept horizontal; and the head and shoulders may be supported with pillows. After 5–10 days, when the inflammatory aspects have had time to produce a more adherent thrombus (and provided the swelling and local symptoms have largely subsided), walking but not standing or sitting is permitted. The time out of bed and walking is increased each day.

Elastic bandages or stockings are applied from the toes to just below the knees as soon as the diagnosis is made and continued until the swelling tendency has disappeared, often for months. Bandages and anticoagulants initially, and intermittent elevation of the legs subsequently, help prevent postphlebitic changes. These measures are perhaps even more important if surgical ligation of the femoral vein or the vena cava has been necessary.

B. Medical Treatment (Anticoagulants): Anticoagulant therapy is considered to be definitive in most cases of deep thrombophlebitis with or without pulmonary embolism. There is evidence that the relatively high incidence of fatal pulmonary embolism secondary to venous thrombosis is significantly reduced by adequate anticoagulant therapy, and the incidence of death from additional emboli following an initial embolus is apparently reduced from approximately 20% to 1–2%. Progressive thrombosis with its associated morbidity is also reduced considerably, and the chronic secondary changes in the involved leg are probably also less severe. Heparin acts rapidly and is unsurpassed as the anticoagulant of choice for short-term therapy; but it can only be given parenterally, and this means that hospitalization is necessary. It should be used at least during the initial phase of treatment. Later, especially if a prolonged period of anticoagulant therapy is thought to be advisable, one of the longer acting oral drugs such as warfarin or dicumarol can be used. (See Surgical Measures, below, for contraindications to anticoagulants.)

The rate of subsidence of symptoms is variable, and occasional cases are quite refractory to therapy. Therapy should probably be continued for at least 12–14 days for venous thrombosis and 21–28 days for pulmonary embolism. It may have to be continued for a longer period if signs and symptoms of active or unresolved thrombosis persist or if the patient has a marked thrombotic tendency with a history of recurrent acute episodes. In the patients who were active at the time the thrombophlebitis developed (ie, those with a significant thrombotic tendency), long-term anticoagulant therapy over a period of 6 or more months is probably advisable. This is particularly true if there has been an associated pulmonary embolus.

1. Heparin—Before starting heparin therapy, a clotting time (and prothrombin time) should be determined. The therapeutic range is considered to be 1½–2 times the baseline pretreatment value. The normal activated clotting time (ACT) at 37° C is 80–130 seconds. The normal whole blood partial thromboplastin time (WBPTT or BaSon test) is 55–75 seconds. If the less precise Lee-White clotting time is to be used, the therapeutic range is 2–3 times the baseline pretreatment value, usually 6–15 minutes.

The patient's response to heparin must be observed closely by one of these laboratory determinations, usually on a daily basis, for the dose of heparin required to maintain the clotting time at a therapeutic level may vary considerably with individuals or even in the same patient at different times during the course of treatment. To be of most value in the management of the anticoagulant regimen, the test should be done just before the next scheduled dose of heparin. Several methods of administration are available.

a. **Deep subcutaneous**–Intermittent administration of sodium heparin every 6 hours, with a clotting time at least once every 24 hours done one-half hour before the next scheduled dose, is a convenient method. For the adult of average size, 7000–9000 units every 6 hours is a reasonable starting dose; after 1 or 2 days of therapy, the required dose usually drops to a range of 5000–7000 units. Small hematomas at the injection site can be expected, and these areas may be painful.

b. **Intravenous**–Intermittent intravenous injections of heparin sodium on a 4–6-hour basis may be used. The usual initial dose is 5000 units followed by an individualized dose of 5000–8000 units every 4–6 hours depending on the laboratory studies. Special needle units are available that facilitate intermittent intravenous injections without the necessity of a continuous infusion of fluid. Continuous intravenous infusion may also be used, beginning with 10,000 units in 1 liter of 5% glucose at 15–25 drops/minute and alternating the rate of flow depending on the laboratory studies done initially every few hours until the proper dosage and rate of flow have been established. Initial control is more difficult by this route, but its use is worthwhile in a patient manifesting extreme thrombotic tendencies and in those that must be anticoagulated very rapidly with a large dose, eg, the patient who has just had a massive pulmonary embolus. In such cases, the postembolic reflex bronchial constriction appears to be blocked by large doses of heparin in the range of 15,000 units initially and 80–100 thousand units in the first 24–28 hours. Furthermore, by neutralizing thrombin, it inhibits propagation of thrombosis in the pulmonary arteries and prevents platelet accretion on the embolus. In very critical situations, such high-dose therapy started the moment the diagnosis is seriously considered and before the diagnosis is established with certainty may save a life.

Many prefer to use only heparin for anticoagulation; those that shift to the prothrombin depressant drugs usually do so after the symptoms and signs of thrombosis have largely or completely subsided. Heparin may thus be used for the first 7–14 days (sometimes even longer) and withdrawn only when the prothrombin time has been depressed to the therapeutic range by means of 2–3 days of overlapping therapy, by which time all the anticoagulant effects of the drug will be active. Postmenopausal women, who have more hemorrhagic complications with heparin administration than other patients, may be shifted somewhat sooner to a prothrombin depressant.

2. **Oral anticoagulants**–Prothrombin depressant drugs include coumarin and indandione derivatives; of these warfarin sodium (Coumadin) is generally used now. The loading dose during the first 36–48 hours of therapy is usually 25–35 mg; the maintenance dose is in the range of 2.5–15 mg/day. The usual maintenance dose is 5–7.5 mg daily and must be determined for each individual patient. The approximate duration of effect of the drug is 2–3 days. A pretreatment prothrombin time should be determined, and, if prolonged as compared with the control value, less drug should be used. Smaller doses should be used in the elderly, in patients with kidney or liver disease, and in those with congestive heart failure or chronic illness. Interaction with many other drugs does occur, and the anticoagulant effect may be either potentiated or reduced; this possibility must be considered if the individual is already receiving other drugs at the time the anticoagulant is started. Careful attention to the maintenance dose is also required when a new drug which enhances or inhibits the anticoagulant effect is added or one that was in use is withdrawn. Interacting drugs should be avoided if possible.

A good therapeutic effect has been achieved when the prothrombin time is 1½–2 times the control value (28–16% of normal). Further prolongation of the prothrombin time may result in bleeding complications. At the beginning of treatment, daily prothrombin activities should be determined and the subsequent dose withheld until the report is received. In well-stabilized patients, weekly or even monthly determination may be adequate.

3. **Treatment of bleeding and overdosage**– Protamine sulfate intravenously will neutralize previously administered heparin. Phytonadione (Mephyton [oral], AquaMephyton [IV]) will counteract the effect of prothrombin depressant drugs, and if transfusion is necessary fresh blood should be used. Aspirin, if being used, should also be stopped. (See also p 936.)

4. **Thrombolytic therapy**–Thrombolytic therapy with fibrinolytic drugs such as streptokinase or urokinase may become more generally used to clear occluded veins in the legs as well as obstructing pulmonary emboli. Proteolytic enzymes that remove fibrinogen from the circulation (Arvin, Reptilase) may also prove to be clinically useful in the treatment of thromboembolism.

C. **Surgical Measures:**

1. **Vein ligation**–Ligation or plication of the inferior vena cava with a partially occluding plastic clip or, less commonly, of one or both common femoral veins is recommended when anticoagulant therapy is contraindicated. Examples are patients who are pregnant, those with peptic ulcer, hiatus hernia, significant liver or kidney disease, or known clotting defect, and those with malignant hypertension with retinopathy, a history of cerebrovascular accident or recent head trauma, or those who are 1–3 days postoperative, especially if the operation has involved extensive dissection or surgery on the brain or spinal cord. Vein ligation is also indicated if there are signs of propagation of the thrombus or if emboli continue to occur during ade-

quate anticoagulant therapy; if pulmonary hypertension has developed from multiple small emboli; after pulmonary artery embolectomy; or if septic phlebitis is present (ligate only if sepsis is present). Simultaneous ligation of the ovarian veins is advocated when pelvic vein thrombosis is present.

The chance of a second, possibly fatal pulmonary embolism is appreciably reduced after ligation or plication of the inferior vena cava, but recurrent emboli may still occur (6–36%), and the surgical mortality rate is about 14%.

Although some degree of chronic edema of the legs may develop as a result of ligation (15–30%), it can usually be minimized if anticoagulant therapy is resumed 1–2 days following surgery and if follow-up care, consisting of elastic supports to the lower legs and elevation of the legs at intervals, is continued for at least 1 year (see next section).

2. Femoral vein thrombectomy—In the rare case of massive venous occlusion (phlegmasia cerulea dolens) which has not responded to sympathetic block, elevation of the leg, heparin, and fluid and electrolyte replacement, a femoral vein thrombectomy to remove the iliofemoral thrombosis may be considered if the condition is of recent onset (1–2 days).

Prognosis

With adequate treatment the patient usually returns to normal health and activity within 3–6 weeks. The prognosis in most cases is good once the period of danger of pulmonary embolism has passed, but for the first 2–3 weeks it is guarded. Occasionally, recurrent episodes of phlebitis occur in spite of good local and anticoagulant management. Such cases may even have recurrent pulmonary emboli. Chronic venous insufficiency may result, with its associated complications.

Browse NL: Current thoughts on venous thromboembolism. S Clin North America 54:229, 1974.

Freeark RJ & others: Posttraumatic venous thrombosis. Arch Surg 95:567, 1967.

Gallus AS & others: Small subcutaneous doses of heparin in prevention of venous thrombosis. New England J Med 288:545, 1973.

Gardner AMN & others: Partial occlusion of the inferior vena cava in the prevention of pulmonary embolism. Surg Gynec Obst 138:17, 1974.

Haller JA Jr: *Deep Thrombophlebitis: Pathophysiology and Treatment.* Saunders, 1967.

Hershey FB & others: Phlebography in diagnosis and management of venous diseases of the legs. M Clin North America 51:161, 1967.

Hume M, Sevitt S, Thomas DP: *Venous Thrombosis and Pulmonary Embolism.* Harvard Univ Press, 1970.

Moser KM, Stein M: *Pulmonary Thromboembolism.* Year Book, 1973.

Mustard JF & others: Thromboembolism: A manifestation of the response of blood to injury. Circulation 42:1, 1970.

Negus D & others: I-125 labelled fibrinogen in the diagnosis of deep vein thrombosis and its correlation with phlebography. Brit J Surg 55:835, 1968.

Sevitt S, Gallagher N: Venous thrombosis and pulmonary embolism. Brit J Surg 48:475, 1961.

Sigel B & others: The epidemiology of lower extremity deep venous thrombosis in surgical patients. Ann Surg 179:278, 1974.

Skillman JJ: Postoperative deep vein thrombosis and pulmonary embolism: A selective review and personal viewpoint. Surgery 75:114, 1974.

Skinner DB & others: Anticoagulant prophylaxis in surgical patients. Surg Gynec Obst 125:741, 1967.

Spittell JA Jr: Thrombophlebitis and pulmonary embolism. Circulation 27:976, 1963.

2. THROMBOPHLEBITIS OF THE SUPERFICIAL VEINS

Essentials of Diagnosis

- Induration, redness, and tenderness along a superficial vein.
- No significant swelling of the extremity.

General Considerations

Superficial thrombophlebitis may occur spontaneously, as in pregnant or postpartum women or in individuals with varicose veins or thromboangiitis obliterans; or it may be associated with trauma, as in the case of a blow to the leg or following intravenous therapy with irritating solutions. In the migratory or recurrent form, thromboangiitis should be suspected. It may also be a manifestation of abdominal malignancy such as carcinoma of the pancreas and may be the earliest sign. The long saphenous vein is most often involved. Superficial thrombophlebitis may be associated with occult deep vein thrombosis in about 20% of cases. Pulmonary emboli are infrequent but do occur.

Short-term plastic venous catheterization of superficial arm veins is now in routine use. The catheter should be observed daily for signs of local inflammation. It should be removed if a local reaction develops in the vein, and in any case it should be removed in 48 hours. If further intravenous therapy is necessary, a new catheter may be inserted in a new vein. Serious septic complications can occur if these rules are not followed. The "butterfly" type of intravenous needle is in many ways safer because it cannot be kept in the same vein as long.

Clinical Findings

The patient usually experiences a dull pain in the region of the involved vein. Local findings consist of induration, redness, and tenderness along the course of a vein. The process may be localized, or it may involve most of the long saphenous vein and its tributaries. The inflammatory reaction generally subsides in 1–2 weeks; a firm cord may remain for a much longer period. Edema of the extremity and deep calf tenderness are absent unless deep thrombophlebitis has also developed. If chills and high fever develop, septic thrombophlebitis exists.

Differential Diagnosis

The linear rather than circular nature of the lesion and the distribution along the course of a superficial vein serve to differentiate superficial phlebitis from cellulitis, erythema nodosum, erythema induratum, panniculitis, and fibromyositis. Lymphangitis and deep thrombophlebitis must also be considered.

Treatment

If the process is well localized and not near the saphenofemoral junction, local heat and bed rest with the leg elevated are usually effective in limiting the thrombosis. Phenylbutazone, 100 mg 3 times daily for 5 days, may aid in the resolution of the inflammatory process but is contraindicated in individuals with peptic ulcer.

If the process is very extensive or shows a tendency to proceed upward toward the saphenofemoral junction, or if it is in the proximity of the saphenofemoral junction initially, ligation and division of the saphenous vein at the saphenofemoral junction is indicated. The inflammatory process usually regresses following this procedure, though removal of the involved segment of vein (stripping) may result in a more rapid recovery.

Anticoagulation therapy is usually not indicated unless there seems to be a rapid progression of the disease. It is indicated if there is extension into the deep system.

Septic thrombophlebitis requires excision of the involved vein and its infected thrombus in order to halt the continued seeding of the blood with bacteria.

Prognosis

The course is generally benign and brief, and the prognosis depends on the underlying pathology. Phlebitis of a saphenous vein occasionally extends to the deep veins, in which case pulmonary embolism may occur.

Bentley DW, Lepper MH: Septicemia related to indwelling venous catheter. JAMA 206:1749, 1968.
Stein JM, Pruitt BA Jr: Suppurative thrombophlebitis. New England J Med 282:1452, 1970.

CHRONIC VENOUS INSUFFICIENCY

Essentials of Diagnosis

- A history is often obtained of phlebitis or leg injury.
- Ankle edema is the earliest sign.
- Stasis pigmentation, dermatitis, subcutaneous induration, and often varicosities occur later.
- Ulceration at or above the ankle is common (stasis ulcer).

General Considerations

Chronic venous insufficiency generally results from changes secondary to deep thrombophlebitis although a definite history of phlebitis is often not obtainable. It can also occur as a result of neoplastic obstruction of the pelvic veins or congenital or acquired arteriovenous fistula.

When insufficiency is secondary to deep thrombophlebitis (the postphlebitic syndrome), the valves in the deep venous channels (and sometimes in the perforating veins) have been damaged or destroyed by the thrombotic process. The recanalized, valveless, irregular deep veins are functionally inadequate, and the pumping action of the contracting calf muscles does not lower the venous pressure during walking. Thus, the venous pressure remains high at all times and secondary changes eventually take place in the venules, capillaries, subcutaneous tissues, skin, and superficial veins. Primary varicose veins with no abnormalities of the deep venous system may also result in the changes of chronic venous stasis.

Clinical Findings

Chronic venous insufficiency is characterized first by progressive edema of the leg (particularly the lower leg) and later also by secondary changes in the skin and subcutaneous tissues. The usual sypmptoms are itching, a dull discomfort made worse by periods of standing, and pain if an ulceration is present. The skin is usually thin, shiny, atrophic, and cyanotic, and a brownish pigmentation often develops. Eczema is often present, and there may be large areas of superficial weeping dermatitis. The subcutaneous tissues are thick and fibrous. Recurrent ulcerations are common, usually just above the ankle, on the medial or anterior aspect of the leg; healing results in a thin scar on a fibrotic base which breaks down with minor trauma. Varicosities often appear which are associated with incompetent perforating veins.

Differential Diagnosis

Congestive heart failure and chronic renal disease may result in bilateral edema of the lower extremities, but generally there are also sacral edema and the clinical and laboratory findings of heart or kidney failure.

Lymphedema is associated with a brawny thickening in the subcutaneous tissue which does not respond readily to elevation; varicosities are absent, and there is often a history of recurrent episodes of cellulitis (see p 272).

Primary varicose veins may be difficult to differentiate from the secondary varicosities that often develop in this condition; the history of acute phlebitis or leg trauma may be helpful, but phlebography to define the condition of the deep venous system may occasionally be necessary (see p 262).

Other conditions associated with chronic ulcers of the leg include arterial insufficiency (often very painful), sickle cell anemia (positive sickle cell test), erythema induratum (bilateral and usually on the posterior aspect of the lower part of the leg), and fungal infections (cultures specific; no chronic swelling or varicosities).

Prevention

Irreversible tissue changes and associated complications in the lower legs can be minimized through early and energetic treatment of acute thrombophlebitis with anticoagulants and specific measures to avoid chronic edema in subsequent years. The latter can be done by elastic supports to the lower legs during the day and evening, intermittent periods of elevation of the legs, and elevation of the legs throughout the night.

Treatment

A. General Measures: Bed rest, with the legs elevated to diminish chronic edema, is fundamental in the treatment of the acute complications of chronic venous insufficiency. Measures to control the tendency toward edema include (1) intermittent elevation of the legs during the day and elevation of the legs at night, (2) avoidance of long periods of sitting or standing, and (3) the use of well-fitting, heavy duty elastic supports worn from the mid foot to just below the knee during the day and evening if there is any tendency for swelling to develop.

B. Stasis Dermatitis: Eczematous eruption may be acute or chronic, and the treatment varies accordingly.

1. **Acute weeping dermatitis**—(see also p 39.)

a. Wet compresses for 1 hour 4 times daily of either boric acid solution (1 tbsp/liter of water), potassium permanganate solution (100 mg/liter of water), or aluminum acetate buffered solution (Burow's solution) (2 tablets/liter of water).

b. Compresses are followed with 0.5% hydrocortisone cream in a water-soluble base. (Neomycin may be incorporated into this cream.)

c. Systemic antibiotics may be indicated if active infection is present.

2. **Subsiding or chronic dermatitis**—

a. Continue the hydrocortisone cream for 1–2 weeks or until no further improvement is noted. Cordran tape, a plastic, corticosteroid impregnated tape, is a convenient way to apply both medication and dressing.

b. Zinc oxide ointment with ichthammol (Ichthyol), 3%, 1–2 times a day, cleaned off as desired with mineral oil.

c. Carbolfuchsin (Castellani's) paint to the toes and nails 1–2 times a week may help control dermatophytosis and onychomycosis. Desenex powder, ointment, or aerosol may also be used.

3. Energetic treatment of chronic edema, as outlined in sections A and C, with almost complete bed rest during the acute phase.

C. Ulceration: Ulcerations are preferably treated with compresses of isotonic saline solution, which aid the healing of the ulcer or may help prepare the base for a skin graft. A lesion can sometimes be treated on an ambulatory basis by means of a semirigid boot applied to the leg after much of the swelling has been reduced by a period of elevation. Such a boot must be changed every 1–2 weeks, depending to some extent on the amount of drainage from the ulcer. The ulcer, tendons, and bony prominences must be adequately padded. Special ointments on the ulcer are not neces-

sary. The semirigid boot may be made with Unna's paste or with Viscopaste (a bandage impregnated with gelatin and zinc oxide) or Gauztex bandage (impregnated with a nonallergenic self-adhering compound). After the ulcer has healed, elastic stockings are used. Occasionally, the ulcer is so large and chronic that total excision of the ulcer with skin graft of the defect is the best approach. This is often combined with ligation of all incompetent perforating veins, either superficial or deep to the deep fascia.

D. Secondary Varicosities: Varicosities secondary to damage to the deep system of veins may in turn contribute to undesirable changes in the tissues of the lower leg. Varicosities should occasionally be removed and the incompetent perforators ligated, but the tendency toward edema will persist and the measures outlined above (¶ A) will be required for life. Varicosities can often be treated along with edema by elastic stockings and other nonoperative measures. If the obstructive element in the deep system is severe, it may be most undesirable to remove superficial channels which may be carrying most of the blood out of the leg. In the more complicated forms of postphlebitic conditions (and even, in certain instances, in acute phlebitis), phlebography may be of value in mapping out by means of x-rays the areas of obstruction or incompetence of the deep veins of the leg. The selection of treatment may depend on such a study.

Prognosis

Individuals with chronic venous insufficiency often have recurrent problems, particularly if measures to counteract persistent venous hypertension, edema, and secondary tissue changes are not conscientiously adhered to throughout life. Additional episodes of acute thrombophlebitis can occur.

Haller JA: Pathophysiology and management of postphlebitic venous insufficiency. South MJ 63:177, 1970.

Field P, van Boxel P: The role of the Linton flap procedure in the management of stasis dermatitis and ulceration in the lower limb. Surgery 70:920, 1971.

Haeger K: The treatment of the severe post-thrombotic state: A comparison of some surgical and conservative methods. Angiology 19:439, 1968.

SUPERIOR VENA CAVA OBSTRUCTION

Obstruction of the superior vena cava is a relatively rare condition which is usually secondary to the neoplastic or inflammatory process in the superior mediastinum. The most frequent causes are (1) neoplasms, such as lymphomas, primary malignant mediastinal tumors, or carcinoma of the lung with direct extension; (2) chronic fibrotic mediastinitis, either of unknown origin or secondary to tuberculosis or pyogenic infection; (3) thrombophlebitis, often by extension of the process from the axillary or subclavian vein into the innominate and vena cava;

(4) aneurysm of the aortic arch; and (5) constrictive pericarditis.

Clinical Findings

A. Symptoms and Signs: Initially, the cutaneous veins may be dilated and the eyelids may be edematous. Later, there may be rather general swelling of the head and arms. If the venous congestion is marked, there may be a degree of cyanosis of that area with engorged veins and even some CNS symptoms. All signs and symptoms may be exaggerated by bending over or lying down so that the patients spend their time sitting up and avoiding physical exertion.

B. Laboratory Findings: The venous pressure in the arm is elevated (often over 20 cm water) and is normal in the leg. A supraclavicular lymph node biopsy may supply a tissue diagnosis.

C. X-Ray Findings: Chest x-rays and venograms may be quite helpful in defining the nature of the primary problem.

Treatment

If the primary problem is due to a malignant neoplasm, radiation therapy or chemotherapy may relieve the pressure on the superior vena cava. Surgery is usually not indicated, though it may be necessary in order to arrive at a diagnosis. If the process results from tuberculosis, antituberculosis chemotherapy is indicated. In cases secondary to mediastinal fibrosis, excision of the fibrous tissue around the great vessels may reestablish flow; if complete thrombosis has occurred, a graft may be tried, though such grafts generally thrombose.

Prognosis

The prognosis depends upon the nature of the obstructive lesion; it is especially bad when malignancy or aortic aneurysm is the cause. Even with mediastinitis and primary thrombophlebitis, the mortality is high.

Failor HJ, Edwards JE, Hodgson CH: Etiologic factors in obstruction of the superior vena cava: A pathologic study. Proc Staff Meet Mayo Clin 33:671, 1958.

Lowenberg EL & others: The superior vena cava syndrome. Dis Chest 47:323, 1965.

DISEASES OF THE LYMPHATIC CHANNELS

LYMPHANGITIS & LYMPHADENITIS

Essentials of Diagnosis

- Red streak from wound or area of cellulitis toward regional lymph nodes, which are usually enlarged and tender.
- Chills and fever often present.

General Considerations

Lymphangitis and lymphadenitis are common manifestations of a bacterial infection which is usually caused by the hemolytic streptococcus and usually arises from an area of cellulitis, generally at the site of an infected wound. The wound may be very small or superficial or an established abscess may be present, feeding bacteria into the lymphatics. The involvement of the lymphatics is often manifested by a red streak in the skin extending in the direction of the regional lymph nodes which are, in turn, generally tender and enlarged. Systemic manifestations include fever, chills, and malaise. The infection may progress rapidly, often in a matter of hours, and may lead to bacteremia or septicemia and even death.

Clinical Findings

A. Symptoms and Signs: Throbbing pain is usually present in the area of cellulitis at the site of bacterial invasion. Malaise, anorexia, sweating, chills, and fever (37.8–40° C [100–104° F]) develop rapidly. Pain or discomfort is noted in the regional nodes. The red streak, when present, may be definite but it may be very faint and easily missed. It is not usually tender or indurated, as is the area of cellulitis. The involved regional lymph nodes may be enlarged 2–3 times and are often acutely tender. The pulse is often rapid.

B. Laboratory Findings: Leukocytosis with an increase in immature cells is usually present. Later, a blood culture may be positive. Culture and sensitivity studies on the wound exudate or pus may be helpful in treatment of the more severe or refractory infections.

Differential Diagnosis

Lymphangitis may be confused with superficial thrombophlebitis, but the erythematous reaction associated with thrombosis overlies the induration of the venous thrombus and the inflammatory reaction in and around the vein. Venous thrombosis does not result in lymphadenitis, and a wound of entrance with the associated cellulitis is generally absent. Superficial thrombophlebitis frequently arises as a result of intravenous therapy, particularly when catheters are left in place for more than 2 days; if bacteria have also been introduced, suppurative thrombophlebitis may develop.

Cat-scratch fever should be considered when multiple, superficial cat scratches are noted on the extremity and the lymphadenitis, though often very large, is relatively nontender.

Neither of these conditions is accompanied by the systemic manifestations that often occur with acute cellulitis with lymphangitis and lymphadenitis.

Treatment

A. General Measures: Rest, splinting, elevation of the area, heat, and symptomatic treatment of local pain and systemic reaction are useful.

B. Specific Measures: Antibiotic therapy should always be instituted when local infection becomes invasive, as manifested by cellulitis and lymphangitis. A culture of any purulent discharge available should be obtained (often there is nothing to culture), and antibiotic therapy should be started in full doses at once. Because the causative organism is so frequently the streptococcus, penicillin is usually the drug of choice. If the patient is allergic to penicillin, erythromycin or one of the other drugs that are effective against gram-positive bacteria may be used. (See Chapter 28.)

C. Wound Care: Drainage of pus from an infected wound should be carried out, generally after the above measures have been instituted, and only when it is clear that there is an abscess associated with the site of initial infection. An area of cellulitis should not be incised because the infection may be spread by attempted drainage when pus is not present. It is extremely important to differentiate cellulitis from soft tissue infections that require early and aggressive incision and often resection of necrotic infected tissue, eg, acute streptococcal hemolytic gangrene, necrotizing fasciitis, gram-negative anaerobic cutaneous gangrene, and progressive bacterial synergistic gangrene.

Prognosis

With proper therapy and particularly with the use of an antibiotic effective against the invading bacteria, control of the infection can usually be achieved in a few days and septicemia prevented. Delayed or inadequate therapy can still lead to overwhelming infection and death.

Baxter CR: Surgical management of soft tissue infections. S Clin North America 52:1483, 1972.
Shick RM: Recurrent lymphangitis and cellulitis of the extremities. M Clin North America 33:1089, 1949.

LYMPHEDEMA

Essentials of Diagnosis

- Painless edema of one or both lower extremities, primarily in young females.
- Initially, pitting edema, which becomes brawny and often nonpitting with time.
- Ulceration, varicosities, and stasis pigmentation do not occur.
- There may be episodes of lymphangitis and cellulitis.

General Considerations

The underlying mechanism in lymphedema is impairment of the flow of lymph from an extremity. When due to congenital developmental abnormalities of the lymphatics, it is referred to as the primary form. The secondary form results when an inflammatory or mechanical obstruction of the lymphatics occurs such as from trauma, regional lymph node resection or irradiation, or extensive involvement of regional nodes by malignant disease or filariasis. Secondary dilatation of the lymphatics that occurs in both forms leads to incompetence of the valve system, disrupting the orderly flow along the lymph vessels, and results in progressive stasis of a protein-rich fluid with secondary fibrosis. Episodes of acute and chronic inflammation may be superimposed, with further stasis and fibrosis. Hypertrophy of the limb results, with markedly thickened and fibrotic skin and subcutaneous tissue and diminution in the fatty tissue.

Lymphangiography and radioactive isotope studies are sometimes useful in defining the specific lymphatic defect.

Treatment

There is no very satisfactory treatment for lymphedema, but the following measures can be instituted: (1) The flow of lymph out of the extremity, with a consequent decrease in the degree of stasis, can be aided through intermittent elevation of the extremity, especially during the sleeping hours (foot of bed elevated 15–20 degrees, achieved by placing pillows beneath the mattress); the constant use of elastic bandages or carefully fitted heavy duty elastic stockings; and massage toward the trunk—either by hand or by means of pneumatic pressure devices designed to milk edema out of an extremity. (2) Secondary cellulitis in the extremity should be avoided by means of good hygiene and treatment of any trichophytosis of the toes. Once an infection starts, it should be treated by very adequate periods of rest, elevation, and antibiotics. Infection can be a serious and recurring problem and often difficult to control. Intermittent prophylactic antibiotics may occasionally be necessary. (3) Intermittent courses of diuretic therapy, especially in those with premenstrual or seasonal exacerbations. (4) Surgery is indicated in severe cases when conservative management fails to control the size of the limb or when recurrent attacks of infection cannot be prevented by other means. It is not indicated for cosmetic reasons since the cosmetic results are poor. In carefully selected cases, there are operative procedures that may give satisfactory functional results. Occasionally, amputation is used as a last resort in very severe forms or when lymphangiosarcoma develops in the extremity.

Battezzati M, Donini I, Marsilli E: The morphologic and physiologic basis for a new classification of lymphoedema. J Cardiovas Surg 8:52, 1967.
Dale WA: *The Swollen Leg: Current Problems in Surgery.* Year Book, 1973.
Goldsmith HS: Long-term evaluation of omental transposition for chronic lymphedema. Ann Surg 180:847, 1974.
Kinmouth JB & others: Primary lymphoedema: Clinical and lymphangiographic studies of a series of 107 patients in which the lower limbs were affected. Brit J Surg 45:1, 1958.
Thompson N: The surgical treatment of chronic lymphoedema of the extremity. S Clin North America 47:445, 1967.

9 . . .
Blood

Ralph O. Wallerstein

ANEMIAS

Diagnosis of Anemia

Anemia is a common clinical finding, and an explanation must always be sought. Extensive investigations are sometimes required to determine the cause. The answers to the following 4 fundamental questions are always relevant to a complete evaluation of the anemia patient: (1) Is there evidence of iron deficiency? (2) Is the anemia megaloblastic? (3) Is there evidence of hemolysis? (4) Is the bone marrow hypoactive?

Iron deficiency must be considered in all anemias of obscure origin—regardless of red cell morphology. Staining for marrow hemosiderin is the most reliable technic; marrow hemosiderin is always absent in iron deficiency anemia and is normal or increased in all other forms. Determination of serum iron and total iron-binding capacity is almost as useful. The combination of low serum iron and elevated total iron-binding capacity is seen only in iron deficiency anemia. If these tools are not available, recourse must be had to obtaining a history of blood loss or evidence of it by stool guaiac determination.

The diagnosis of moderately severe megaloblastic anemia (fewer than 3 million red cells/cu mm) can always be made by examination of the blood and bone marrow. The blood shows oval macrocytes and hyper-

Table 9–1. The anemias.

Type	Characteristic Findings
Iron deficiency	Low serum iron, high TIBC, absent marrow hemosiderin.
Megaloblastic	Characteristic red cell, white cell, and marrow morphology.
Hemolytic	High reticulocyte count, low or absent haptoglobin, high indirect bilirubin.
Marrow failure Absolute (eg, aplastic anemia)	Pancytopenia; normal marrow tissue replaced by fat.
Relative (eg, infection, azotemia, cancer, liver disease, myxedema)	Red cell, white cell, and serum factors often have no distinguishing characteristics. The marrow picture is not striking.

segmented granulocytes; the bone marrow contains megaloblasts.

The major hemolytic disorders, regardless of type, have in common reticulocytosis, slightly increased serum bilirubin (indirect), and an increased number of nucleated red cells in the marrow.

In hypoplastic anemia the bone marrow is fatty and contains relatively few nucleated red cells.

In any case of undiagnosed normocytic normochromic anemia which does not fall into the above 4 groups, the following causes must be considered: infection, azotemia, malignancy, myxedema, and liver disease.

IRON DEFICIENCY ANEMIA

Essentials of Diagnosis

- Pallor, lassitude.
- Hypochromia, microcytosis; red blood count less reduced than hemoglobin.
- Serum iron low; total iron-binding capacity increased.
- Bone marrow hemosiderin absent.
- Blood loss usually occult.

General Considerations

Iron deficiency anemia in the adult is almost always due to blood loss. Excessive menstrual flow and gastrointestinal bleeding (due to hiatus hernia, gastritis, peptic ulcer, previous gastrectomy, polyps, malignancy, hemorrhoids, or excessive salicylate intake) are the principal causes. Gastrointestinal bleeding is usually chronic and occult. Rare causes include hemosiderinuria, pulmonary hemosiderosis, excessive blood donation, faulty diet, and habitual starch eating.

A normal daily diet contains 12–15 mg of iron, or approximately 6 mg of iron per 1000 calories, of which 5–10% (0.6–1.5 mg) is absorbed. (More iron is absorbed in iron deficiency anemia.) Because less than 1 mg of iron is excreted normally per day, normal persons are in positive iron balance. Chronic bleeding of as little as 2–4 ml of blood per day may lead to a negative iron balance and iron deficiency anemia.

Clinical Findings

A. Symptoms and Signs: In addition to symptoms of the primary disease (if any), symptoms due to anemia may be present: easy fatigability, dyspnea, palpitation, angina, and tachycardia. Waxy pallor, brittle hair and nails, smooth tongue, cheilosis, and dysphagia are late findings.

B. Laboratory Findings: The hemoglobin may fall to as low as 3 gm/100 ml, but the red cell count is rarely below 2.5 million/cu mm and the red cells are usually microcytic and hypochromic (although in approximately 20% of adults the red cells are normocytic and nearly normochromic). Reticulocytes and platelets are normal or increased. The white count is normal. Serum iron is usually below 30 μg/100 ml (normal is 90–150 μg/100 ml); total iron-binding capacity is elevated to 350–500 μg/100 ml (normal is 250–350 μg/100 ml). Percent saturation is 10% or less.

The most critical test is the bone marrow stain for hemosiderin; stainable iron is always absent in iron deficiency anemia. The bone marrow aspirate contains increased numbers of nucleated red cells; the normoblasts have only scanty cytoplasm.

Differential Diagnosis

Iron deficiency anemia is the only anemia in which hemosiderin is absent in bone marrow; in all other types of anemia iron is present in bone marrow in normal or increased amounts. In thalassemia minor (which is also manifested by a hypochromic, microcytic anemia) the red cells are smaller and have a more abnormal appearance (for a given degree of anemia); the red count may be above normal and the hemoglobin is rarely below 9 gm/100 ml, and the bone marrow hemosiderin, serum iron, and total iron-binding capacity are normal.

Iron deficiency anemia must be differentiated from other hypochromic anemias.

A. Anemia of Infection: (See p 293.) Red cells are normocytic and mildly hypochromic. Serum iron is low, but total iron-binding capacity is also decreased. Bone marrow hemosiderin is present.

B. Sideroachrestic Anemias: See p 285.

C. Some Hemoglobinopathies: All hemoglobin abnormalities involving the thalassemia gene are microcytic and hypochromic, eg, S-thalassemia, hemoglobin C-thalassemia, and hemoglobin H disease; the red cells in hemoglobin E disease may be quite small. The diagnosis is made by hemoglobin electrophoresis.

Complications

Severe dysphagia (Plummer-Vinson syndrome) develops in some patients. Iron deficiency anemia may be the presenting finding in gastrointestinal cancer. In patients with heart disease, severe anemia may precipitate angina pectoris or congestive heart failure.

Treatment

Iron is specific for this type of anemia. It should be started as soon as an etiologic diagnosis has been made. Transfusions are rarely needed. A satisfactory response to iron therapy, whether oral or parenteral, is indicated by a rise in hemoglobin of at least 2 gm/100 ml in 3 weeks. Failure of hemoglobin levels to rise in a week or 2 does not necessarily mean failure of therapy. Reticulocytes often do not rise measurably when the baseline hemoglobin was over 7.5 gm/100 ml.

A. Oral Preparations and Dosages: The maximum absorption is considered to be about 25 mg/day. Give one of the following: (1) ferrous sulfate, 0.2 gm 3 times daily after meals; or (2) ferrous gluconate, 0.3 gm 3 times daily after meals. Oral iron should be continued for 3 months after hemoglobin values return to normal in order to replenish iron stores.

Many other iron salts and chelates, often mixed with other metals or vitamins, are promoted, but none are more useful in iron deficiency anemia than ferrous sulfate. The degree of gastrointestinal irritation and the amount absorbed are functions of the iron content of the salt or complex.

B. Parenteral Iron: The indications are intolerance to oral iron, refractoriness to oral iron (poor absorption), gastrointestinal disease precluding the use of oral iron, continued blood loss, and replacement of depleted iron stores when oral iron fails. Parenteral iron should be given only in the amounts necessary to correct the deficiency. Calculate the total dosage as follows: 250 mg for each gm of hemoglobin below normal. (Normal: men, 14–16 gm; women, 12–16 gm.)

Iron dextran injection (Imferon) for intramuscular use contains 5% metallic iron (50 mg/ml). Give 50 mg (1 ml) immediately and then 100–250 mg IM daily or every other day until the total dose has been given. Inject deeply with a 2 inch needle into the upper outer quadrant of the buttock, using the "Z" technic (pulling the skin to one side before inserting the needle) to prevent leakage of the solution and discoloration of the skin. This preparation may also be given intravenously. It is best administered in doses of 250–500 mg; a test dose of 0.5 ml should be given first; if the patient experiences no unusual reaction, the entire amount may be given over 3–5 minutes.

Prognosis

Following iron therapy all the signs and symptoms of iron deficiency anemia are reversible unless blood loss continues. Bleeding in excess of 500 ml/week over a period of weeks or months probably cannot be treated successfully by iron medication alone.

Committee on Iron Deficiency: Iron deficiency in the United States. JAMA 203:407, 1968.

Crosby WH: Iron and anemia. Disease-A-Month, Jan 1966.

Kasper CK, Whissell DYE, Wallerstein RO: Clinical aspects of iron deficiency. JAMA 191:359, 1965.

PERNICIOUS ANEMIA
(Addisonian Anemia)

Essentials of Diagnosis

- Anorexia, dyspepsia; smooth, sore tongue.
- Constant, symmetric numbness and tingling of the feet.
- Pallor and a trace of jaundice.
- Oval macrocytes, pancytopenia, hypersegmented neutrophils.
- Megaloblastic bone marrow.

General Considerations

Pernicious anemia is a conditioned vitamin B_{12} deficiency due to an absorption defect, not dietary lack. Intrinsic factor is absent. The defect is rare before age 35; it is more common in persons of Scandinavian, English, and Irish extraction, and is very rare in Orientals. Predisposition to pernicious anemia is probably inherited as a single, dominant, autosomal factor. About 40% of patients have a 7S gamma "autoantibody" with activity against intrinsic factor in their serum; approximately twice that many have antibody against parietal cells. A precipitable antibody to intrinsic factor may also be present in their gastric juice.

Intrinsic factor is secreted by the gastric mucosa; it makes possible absorption of vitamin B_{12}, mostly at the distal ileum, in the presence of calcium and at a pH of 5–7. It is probably a mucopolypeptide or mucopolysaccharide with a molecular weight of 50,000.

Total body vitamin B_{12} content is estimated to be 5 mg; daily loss is approximately 2.5 µg. Clinical and hematologic evidence of pernicious anemia appears when the body vitamin B_{12} pool has been reduced to 10% of normal.

Clinical vitamin B_{12} deficiency may also be caused by gastrectomy, regional ileitis, certain intestinal malformations involving the ileum, resection of the ileum, and fish tapeworm disease.

Clinical Findings

A. Symptoms and Signs: Patients with pernicious anemia may tolerate their disease well and have few symptoms. Anemia may cause easy fatigability, dyspnea, palpitation, angina, and tachycardia. Vitamin B_{12} deficiency may lead to glossitis, gastrointestinal symptoms such as belching, indigestion, anorexia, and diarrhea; CNS symptoms occur in approximately 10% of patients and include constant symmetric numbness and tingling of the lower extremities, ataxia, mental disturbances, and loss of vibration sense and deep reflexes; sensory symptoms usually appear before the motor symptoms and signs.

B. Laboratory Findings:

1. Blood—In addition to the characteristic large oval red cells there are a few small misshapen red cells. This poikilocytosis is a reflection of the ineffective erythropoiesis in the marrow. The white blood count is usually under 5000/cu mm. The granulocytes, which constitute less than 50% of white cells, tend to be hypersegmented. Platelets usually are reduced (40–100 thousand/cu mm). Reticulocytes range from less than 1% to 3%. The unconjugated bilirubin is increased, but rarely above 2 mg/100 ml.

2. Bone marrow—The bone marrow is hyperactive and is easily entered with the aspiration needle. The characteristic megaloblastic abnormalities are particularly evident in the more mature forms. Giant metamyelocytes are prominent. Megakaryocytes are hypersegmented and reduced in number. Hemosiderin is increased and in the form of fine granules.

3. Other laboratory tests—Patients secrete no free gastric acid and very little gastric juice. Even after injection of histamine or betazole hydrochloride, 50 mg (1 ml), the pH remains above 7.0. Serum LDH (lactate dehydrogenase) activity is excessively elevated. Haptoglobin is usually absent. Serum vitamin B_{12} concentration (normally 300–400 pg/ml) is less than 100 pg/ml. Absorption of [57]Co-labeled vitamin B_{12} is greatly impaired. This is demonstrated by the Schilling test, which involves the oral administration of a small (0.5 µg) dose of radiocobalt-labeled vitamin B_{12} followed 2 hours later by the parenteral administration of 1000 µg of unlabeled vitamin B_{12}. Less than 5% of the radioactive vitamin B_{12} is excreted in the urine in 24 hours (normal: 15–40%), but simultaneous administration of intrinsic factor increases the excretion of vitamin B_{12} 5-fold or more. Vitamin B_{12} absorption may also be measured by externally monitoring hepatic uptake after oral administration of [57]Co-labeled vitamin B_{12}. The Schilling test is useful only in (1) differentiating addisonian pernicious anemia from megaloblastic anemias due to folic acid deficiency; (2) diagnosing addisonian pernicious anemia in remission; and (3) diagnosing defective vitamin B_{12} absorption in patients with combined system disease before the onset of anemia. The Schilling test may give a false low value (decreased urinary radioactivity) in the following situations: inadequate urine collection, impaired kidney function, diarrhea, and occasionally in hypothyroidism. Low values which are not improved by simultaneous administration of intrinsic factor are characteristically seen with malabsorption involving disease of the ileum and with fish tapeworm disease (even in asymptomatic carriers).

Some patients with pernicious anemia in relapse may have intestinal malabsorption as well; their Schilling test is not improved by intrinsic factor until after several months of vitamin B_{12} therapy.

Differential Diagnosis

Pernicious anemia must be differentiated from folic acid deficiency (see below) by means of vitamin B_{12} absorption tests or serum levels of vitamin B_{12} and folic acid.

Large red cells are not seen exclusively in the megaloblastic anemias, but their oval appearance is characteristic, as are the hypersegmented white cells and the megaloblasts of the marrow.

In the various hemolytic anemias some young nucleated red cells in the marrow may resemble megaloblasts; however, there are no oval macrocytes and no hypersegmented PMNs, and the reticulocytes are above 3%.

Treatment

Pernicious anemia in relapse is treated with vitamin B_{12} (cyanocobalamin), 100 μg IM 1–3 times per week until blood values return to normal. Thereafter, 100 μg IM monthly are given. The patient must be impressed that the need for vitamin B_{12} injections will continue for the rest of his life.

Patients who have undergone total gastrectomy should receive maintenance doses of vitamin B_{12} (100 μg IM monthly).

Prognosis

Untreated pernicious anemia is fatal. With parenteral vitamin B_{12} therapy the reticulocytes begin to increase on the 4th day and reach a peak between the 6th and 10th days. The magnitude of the reticulocyte peak correlates well with the degree of anemia; with an initial red count of 1 million/cu mm, a maximum reticulocyte count of 40% may be anticipated. Normal hemoglobin values are obtained in about 6 weeks. CNS symptoms are reversible if they are of relatively short duration (less than 6 months), but may be permanent if they have existed longer. Histamine-fast achlorhydria persists; the Schilling test remains abnormal.

Castle WB: Current concepts of pernicious anemia. Am J Med 48:541, 1970.

Chanarin I: *The Megaloblastic Anemias.* Blackwell, 1969.

Heinrich HC: Metabolic basis of the diagnosis and therapy in vitamin B_{12} deficiency. Pages 199–249 in: *Seminars in Hematology.* Vol 1. Grune & Stratton, 1964.

Sullivan LW: Vitamin B_{12} metabolism and megaloblastic anemia. Seminars Hemat 7:6, 1970.

FOLIC ACID DEFICIENCY

Folic acid deficiency produces the same hematologic findings as pernicious anemia, but blood changes occur sooner because folate storage lasts for only 1–2 months. The most common cause is malnutrition, especially in association with alcoholism ("nutritional megaloblastic anemia"). Folic acid deficiency may develop in sprue and may complicate certain chronic hemolytic anemias (eg, sickle cell anemia). It is occasionally seen in epileptics receiving primidone, diphenylhydantoin, or phenobarbital, which interfere with absorption of folate; in patients following treatment with methotrexate, pyrimethamine, or triamterene, which block the reduction of folic acid to its metabolically active form, folinic acid; and in pregnancy (especially when associated with vomiting and inadequate diet, toxemia, and twins). In megaloblastic anemias due to folic acid deficiency, CNS symptoms are lacking, free gastric acid may be present, and the vitamin B_{12} absorption test (Schilling) is normal. In sprue, vitamin B_{12} absorption may be impaired even after administration of intrinsic factor. Serum folate activity is less than 3 ng/ml (normal is 7 ng/ml or more), and urine formiminoglutamic acid after histidine loading is increased.

"Pernicious" or megaloblastic anemia of pregnancy is caused by folic acid, not vitamin B_{12} deficiency. Poor nutrition is the major factor in its development. The requirement for folic acid increases markedly during pregnancy. Low serum folate levels are found in approximately 20% of pregnancies; the incidence of deficiency is much higher with twins, toxemia, or abruptio placentae. Only a small percentage of women with low levels of folic acid have megaloblastic anemia.

The diagnosis is made by finding hypersegmented polymorphonuclear leukocytes in the blood and megaloblastic maturation in the marrow. Oval macrocytes are found less consistently than in other megaloblastic anemias; the red cell MCV is not necessarily elevated.

For therapy, give folic acid, 5 mg daily orally, until hematologic remission occurs.

In megaloblastic anemia of infancy and in megaloblastic anemia due to malnutrition or antiepileptic therapy, folic acid is given only until a hematologic remission is obtained. No maintenance therapy is necessary.

A patient with sprue or malabsorption syndrome may require initial therapy with parenteral folic acid and maintenance with oral folic acid. Some of these patients have an associated vitamin B_{12} or iron deficiency and have to be treated accordingly. Others require the addition of corticosteroids for relief of symptoms.

Folic acid is available in 0.25 and 1 mg tablets for oral administration and as solution (5 and 15 mg/ml) for intramuscular use. The oral dosage is 1 mg daily.

Folinic acid (Leucovorin) should be administered in doses of 3 mg IM daily when needed. An oral tablet has been developed but is not available as yet.

Herbert V: Diagnosis and treatment of folic acid deficiency. M Clin North America 46:1365, 1962.

Streiff RR: Folic acid deficiency anemia. Seminars Hemat 7:23, 1970.

APLASTIC ANEMIA

Essentials of Diagnosis

- Lassitude, pallor, purpura, bleeding.
- Pancytopenia, fatty bone marrow.
- History of exposure to an offending drug or x-ray radiation.

General Considerations

Aplastic anemia may occur at any age. Its incidence is approximately 4 per million population. It is characterized by pancytopenia or a selective depression of red cells, white cells, or platelets. In over half of cases the etiology is not known. It may occur as a toxic reaction to many chemicals and drugs, eg, chloramphenicol, benzene, phenylbutazone, and mephenytoin. Hair dyes, plant sprays, insecticides, volatile solvents, large doses of antileukemic drugs, and excessive x-ray or ionizing radiation may also cause this disease. Rarely, an associated thymoma is found.

Clinical Findings

A. Symptoms and Signs: Anemia may cause lassitude, pallor, fatigue, tachycardia, thrombocytopenia, purpura, bleeding, neutropenia, and infections with high fever.

B. Laboratory Findings: The red cell count may be below 1 million/cu mm. The cells are usually slightly macrocytic. The reticulocyte count is often low, but may be normal or even slightly elevated. The white count may be less than 2000/cu mm and the platelet count less than 30,000/cu mm. The serum bilirubin is usually below normal. The standard chemical analyses, including serum protein, SGOT, LDH, and BUN, are normal. Bone marrow is fatty, with very few red and white cells and megakaryocytes. Hemosiderin is present.

Fixed tissue section made from the marrow aspirate or biopsy and stained with hematoxylin and eosin are best for demonstrating the characteristic architecture of an aplastic bone marrow; smears of the aspirate stained with Wright's stain are not adequate for diagnosis.

Differential Diagnosis

In hypersplenism, the marrow is hyperactive and the spleen is large.

In myelofibrosis the spleen and liver are enlarged; red cells vary in size and shape; bizarre and tear-shaped cells may be seen; leukocytosis is common; the platelet count may be low, normal, or even elevated, and giant platelets are common; the marrow is fibrotic rather than fatty and is difficult to aspirate; and evidence of extramedullary hematopoiesis may be seen in the liver and spleen.

Aleukemic leukemia, malignant lymphoma, and Hodgkin's disease may cause pancytopenia. The correct diagnosis is made by marrow biopsy.

Complications

Long-term transfusion therapy may lead to development of leukoagglutinins and hemosiderosis. Overwhelming infection secondary to the leukopenia and hemorrhage secondary to thrombocytopenia are frequently terminal events.

Some patients make a partial recovery and develop a syndrome resembling paroxysmal nocturnal hemoglobinuria.

Treatment

A. General Measures: A very thorough search for possible toxic agents must be made. All unnecessary medications must be discontinued. A detailed history of the patient's personal and work habits is essential. Patients should be specifically asked whether they have taken any agents for infection, arthritis, or convulsions and whether they have been exposed to radiation. Even after a careful search, no cause can be found in approximately half of patients.

B. Androgenic Steroids: These are the only agents currently available that are effective in stimulating the marrow to make new cells, particularly red cells. The erythrocytic response takes usually 2 months before the therapeutic trial is abandoned. The most commonly used agents are as follows: (1) Fluoxymesterone, 40–100 mg daily orally (2, 5, and 10 mg tablets). (2) Oxymetholone, 2.5 mg/kg/day orally (2.5, 5, 10, and 50 mg tablets). (3) Methandrostenolone, 40–100 mg/day orally (2.5 and 5 mg tablets). (4) Testosterone enanthate, 200–400 mg/kg/day twice weekly IM (100 and 200 mg/ml). (5) Nandrolone decanoate, 1.5–3 mg/kg/week IM (50 mg/ml or 100 mg/ml).

The first 3 agents listed are alkylated in the 17-alpha position; the other 2 are not. The adverse effects of these agents include virilization, sodium and water retention, hepatic changes, and occasionally muscle cramps. They also cause amenorrhea, and women receiving these drugs do not need oral contraceptives. All of these effects are reversible when the drug is withdrawn or the dose reduced.

The effects on the liver include jaundice, increased retention of BSP, and elevations of serum LDH, SGOT, SGPT, alkaline phosphatase, and conjugated bilirubin. The lesion is cholestatic jaundice; bile accumulates in the canaliculi, parenchyma, and Kupffer cells. To avoid jaundice, one may have to use one of the parenterally given nonalkylated androgenic steroids. If jaundice persists, a search must be made for Australia antigen in the blood.

Cobaltous chloride in doses of 100–150 mg daily orally has been reported to produce some response in red cells. An association of thymoma with aplastic anemia has also been reported, although thymoma is more commonly associated with pure red cell anemia.

Corticosteroids, iron, vitamin B_{12}, liver extract, folic acid, and pyridoxine are of no value and should not be given.

C. Transfusion: Transfusions are best given in the form of packed red cells. The blood does not have to be from the same day's procurement, but the maximum benefit for the longest duration is derived if the blood is no more than a few days old. Some patients receive 5 or 6 units given over a couple of days, once every 6 weeks; others prefer small but more frequent blood transfusions.

When platelets are needed, they are best administered as fresh whole blood. If a large number of platelets are necessary, platelet concentrates can be given. Repeat administration almost invariably leads to the development of antibodies. Tissue typing to determine histocompatibility between the donor and the recipient is sometimes used.

Complications of transfusion therapy include development of leukoagglutinins, manifested by chills and fever following transfusion. Antibody to white cells can be demonstrated by cytotoxicity studies. All subsequent transfusions should be in the form of red cells, white cell poor—ie, with the buffy coat removed.

On very rare occasions, recipients who lack IgA develop hives on the basis of antibody to IgA.

D. Splenectomy: When the patient fails to respond to the above measures—particularly when bleeding occurs as a result of thrombocytopenia or when transfused blood hemolyzes rapidly—splenectomy is sometimes considered. Occasional (usually delayed) successes have been reported, but the value of the procedure is not established and it must be considered experimental.

E. Bone Marrow Transplantation: When HL-A compatible donors are available, marrow transplants are now feasible in a few medical centers.

F. Treatment of Complications (Infections): Antibiotics should not be given prophylactically even when leukopenia is severe. When infections occur, specific antibiotics are used if possible. If the bacterial agent cannot be identified, a broad-spectrum antibacterial agent (eg, gentamicin, 1 mg/kg every 8 hours IV) and a penicillinase-resistant bactericidal agent (eg, cloxacillin, 4 gm daily orally) are used. Patients must pay meticulous attention to personal hygiene and avoid exposure to infections.

Prognosis

The mortality with severe bone marrow depression is over 50%; hemorrhage and overwhelming infection are the main causes of death. The course—from onset of anemia to death—is usually only a few months. Some patients can be maintained on transfusions for years. Partial or complete spontaneous remission may occur.

Lewis SM: Course and prognosis in aplastic anaemia. Brit MJ 1:1027, 1965.
Scott JL, Cartwright GE, Wintrobe MM: Acquired aplastic anemia: An analysis of thirty-nine cases and review of the pertinent literature. Medicine 38:119, 1959.
Van der Weyden M, Firkin BG: The management of aplastic anemia in adults. Brit J Haemat 22:1, 1972.

ANEMIA OF LEAD POISONING

The red cell indices in lead poisoning are usually normal but may show some hypochromia. Coarse basophilic stippling is characteristic; marked stippling in patients with normal or nearly normal hemoglobins is seen only in lead poisoning and thalassemia minor. Blood collected in double oxalate or calcium disodium edetate may inhibit formation of stippling. White cells and platelets are normal. Stippling is more striking in the bone marrow, but the marrow is otherwise not remarkable. Red cell ^{51}Cr survival shows moderately diminished red cell life spans (half-life 18—28 days). Red cell protoporphyrin is greatly increased. Whole blood levels of lead are above 70 μg/100 ml (normal,

20—30 μg/100 ml); urinary delta-aminolevulinic acid levels are greater than 8 mg/24 hours (normal, 3—5 mg); and urinary coproporphyrin levels are 1 mg/24 hours or more (normal, 0.1—0.3 mg).

The qualitative Watson-Ehrlich reaction is a good screening test for lead poisoning. When lead poisoning is suspected but the above values are borderline, one should measure the 24-hour urinary lead after a provocative injection of calcium disodium edetate, 0.5 gm dissolved in 10 ml of saline and given IM or IV. The test is positive when more than 0.8 mg of lead are excreted in 24 hours.

Sources of lead poisoning are paint chips ingested by children, industrial fumes inhaled by adults (eg, battery workers), radiators decorated with lead paint, and improperly glazed earthenware used as drinking vessels.

If symptoms are mild, no treatment is necessary. With fairly severe symptoms (eg, abdominal cramps), one may consider calcium disodium edetate, 0.5—1 gm IV daily; if symptoms are less severe, give penicillamine (Cuprimine), 250 mg orally 4 times daily.

Albahary C: Lead poisoning and hemopoiesis. Am J Med 52:367, 1972.
Byers RK: Lead poisoning: Review of the literature and report on 45 cases. Pediatrics 23:585, 1959.
Chisolm JJ: Disturbances in the biosynthesis of heme in lead intoxication. J Pediat 64:174, 1964.

ANEMIA OF MYXEDEMA

Some patients with very low thyroid function have a moderately severe anemia. A similar blood picture may be seen in hypopituitary disease. The red blood cell count is rarely below 3 million/cu mm and the hemoglobin is rarely less than 9 gm/100 ml. The anemia tends to be macrocytic and normochromic. However, iron deficiency, a frequent complication, especially in women with menorrhagia, will produce hypochromic microcytic anemia. Bone marrow cellularity is decreased with increase in fat spaces. Nucleated red cells are normoblastic. White cells and platelets are normal.

Thyroid medication induces a gradual return to normal hemoglobin levels and red blood count in 3—4 months.

Tudhope JR, Wilson GM: Anemia in hypothyroidism. Lancet 1:703, 1962.

PURE RED CELL APLASIA

This is a relatively rare condition (less common than aplastic anemia) characterized by moderate to severe anemia, very low reticulocyte counts, aplasia of red cell precursors, and normal white blood cells and platelets. It may occur as a congenital disorder, presenting as profound anemia in the first 3 months of life (Blackfan-Diamond syndrome).

The adult form may be secondary to several causes. Preleukemic leukemia must always be considered and the granulocytic series carefully scrutinized for abnormalities. Selective red cell hypoplasia develops in most patients with renal failure. Some cases are associated with thymoma. Some degree of red cell aplasia occasionally accompanies infections. Acute red cell aplasia may develop during the course of hemolytic anemia, eg, in hereditary spherocytosis or sickle cell anemia ("aplastic crisis"). Rarely, autoimmune hemolytic anemia may have an aplastic phase. A form of this disorder occurs in severe protein malnutrition (kwashiorkor). Under experimental conditions, riboflavin (vitamin B_2) deficiency has led to selective red cell aplasia. These disorders do not usually show the degree of red cell aplasia seen in the idiopathic cases and those that result from the toxic effects of drugs. Drugs that have been implicated on occasion as the causative agent in this anemia are chloramphenicol, diphenylhydantoin, quinacrine, sulfathiazole, benzol, and antituberculosis agents. These drugs usually produce pancytopenia and total marrow aplasia but occasionally cause only selected red cell aplasia.

The only signs and symptoms are those of anemia. The red count may be as low as 1 million/cu mm, but the red cells look normal under the microscope and have no unusual shape or inclusions. Reticulocytes are reduced to 0.1% or even less. White cells and platelets are normal in number and appearance. Serum iron may be elevated.

The marrow has a normal architecture and normal or increased iron stores, confined to histiocytes. Nucleated red cells usually total less than 100 per 1000 white cells. They are normoblastic. White cells, megakaryocytes, and stromal cells are unremarkable.

Serum creatinine and chest x-ray should be obtained. A leukocyte alkaline phosphatase and bone marrow chromosome cultured for Philadelphia chromosome may be worthwhile. Erythropoietin is usually greatly increased.

Underlying conditions must be corrected. Corticosteroids are very effective in children but are less consistently beneficial in adults. Prednisone, 10–20 mg 3–4 times daily, may be tried. Immunotherapy with cyclophosphamide and prednisone shows some promise. Testosterone is helpful in some patients. Benefits from cobalt or vitamin B_2 have been reported on occasion.

If a thymoma is found, its removal does not necessarily produce a hematologic remission.

Dameshek W & others: Pure red cell anemia and thymoma. Seminars Hemat 4:222, 1967.

Krantz SB: Pure red cell aplasia. New England J Med 291:345, 1974.

Tsai SY, Levin WC: Chronic erythrocytic hypoplasia in adults: Review of the literature and report of a case. Am J Med 22:322, 1957.

HEMOLYTIC ANEMIAS

1. ACQUIRED HEMOLYTIC ANEMIA

Essentials of Diagnosis

- Fatigue, malaise, pallor, jaundice.
- Splenomegaly.
- Persistent anemia and reticulocytosis.
- Coombs test usually positive.

General Considerations

A positive direct Coombs test (Table 9–2) means that a plasma protein, usually either IgG or complement, has become fixed abnormally and relatively irreversibly to the red cell surface. The protein is detected by the Coombs serum, which is prepared by immunizing certain laboratory animals against human immunoglobulins or complement.

When done with the usual "broad-spectrum" antiglobulin serum, a positive Coombs test indicates attachment to the red cell membrane of gamma globulin, compounds of complement, transferrin, a complex of certain drugs and gamma globulin, or possibly other globulins. A "weak" positive direct Coombs test without hemolysis may be found occasionally in a variety of unrelated clinical conditions, eg, rheumatoid arthritis, ulcerative colitis, and leukemia. Appropriate clinical information and a few serologic tests usually lead to the correct diagnosis.

Two major types of red cell coating with protein exist—the IgG type ("gamma Coombs") and the complement type ("nongamma Coombs"), often associated with a cold antibody. The former is found in lymphoma, systemic lupus erythematosus, and certain drug reactions, but in two-thirds of cases no specific cause is found. In the nongamma type, a component of com-

Table 9–2. Positive Coombs test.
(Most common examples of specific causes.)

Neoplastic	
Chronic lymphatic leukemia	G
Lymphosarcoma	G
Reticulum cell sarcoma	G and C
Hodgkin's disease	G
Collagen diseases	
Lupus erythematosus	G and C
Rheumatoid arthritis	G and C
Infectious diseases	
Cytomegalic virus disease	G
Viral pneumonia	C
Infectious mononucleosis	C
Drugs	
Penicillin	G
Methyldopa	G

Legend: G = anti-IgG
C = anticomplement

plement rather than of gamma globulin is fixed to the red cell surface; the concentration of complement in the patient's serum is correspondingly low. These antibodies may develop after viral pneumonia, with reticulum cell sarcoma, and with certain drugs; in half of cases, no cause is found.

Occasionally, auto-antibodies have Rh specificity, eg, some patients with autoimmune hemolytic anemia or a positive direct Coombs test have antibodies against a specific antigen present on their own red cells; this occurs in approximately one-third of cases and usually involves anti-E, anti-c, or anti-e antibodies.

Red cell coating in vivo as described above is always referred to as the "direct" Coombs test. In approximately half of these, the indirect Coombs test is also positive. This test measures circulating antibody in patients' serum. In the autoimmune hemolytic anemias, the indirect Coombs test is, of course, only positive when the direct Coombs test is positive, the positive indirect test merely indicating an excess of antibody.

Autoimmune hemolytic anemia may occur following exposure to certain agents. Three different mechanisms are recognized:

(1) Penicillin in large doses can produce this type of hemolytic anemia; it may act as a hapten to stimulate antibody formation. The antigen-antibody combination "coats" red cells, and a positive direct Coombs test with hemolytic anemia may develop.

(2) Several drugs can bring some immune injury to red cells, platelets, and white cells without first attaching to the cell surface. These agents stimulate antibody formation; the drug and its appropriate antibody then combine, attach to red cells, and damage them. The role of the red cells has been referred to as that of an "innocent bystander." The antibody is usually of the anticomplement or IgM type. Stibophen, quinidine, and quinine are among the drugs implicated in this type of reaction.

(3) A third mechanism for the development of a positive Coombs test has been observed with the use of the antihypertensive agent methyldopa. Approximately 20% of patients who take this drug develop a positive Coombs test, but only 1–2% of these develop hemolytic anemia. The drug, while of prime etiologic importance, does not itself participate in the ultimate reaction. It perhaps produces some subtle changes on the red cell surface, possibly by interfering with normal biosynthesis of membrane components, causing alterations which result in "new" antigens.

A positive Coombs test in a patient who has been transfused recently (within a few weeks) must be interpreted with great caution. The "coated" cells may be incompatible donor cells in a patient who has antibodies from a prior transfusion. The incompatibility occasionally leads to delayed (by 4–14 days) transfusion reactions that may simulate "autoimmune" hemolytic anemia.

Hemolysis without antibody (negative Coombs test) may develop in uremia, cirrhosis, diffuse vasculitis, cancer, and in some bacterial infections.

Clinical Findings

A. Symptoms and Signs: Manifestations of anemia (weakness, pallor, dyspnea, palpitation, dizziness) or hemolysis (fever, jaundice, splenomegaly, hepatomegaly) may be present.

B. Laboratory Findings: Acquired hemolytic anemia is usually normocytic and normochromic. Spherocytes and nucleated red cells may be seen. White cell and platelet counts are frequently elevated, but leukopenia and thrombocytopenia may occur. The reticulocyte count is usually over 10%, often very high (50% or even more), but occasionally low. The bone marrow shows marked erythroid hyperplasia and ample hemosiderin. Indirect bilirubin may be elevated to 4 mg/100 ml. There is no bile in the urine. Stool urobilinogen may be greatly increased. Haptoglobin may be low or absent. Normal donor blood has short survival.

Differential Diagnosis

The hemoglobinopathies are differentiated by electrophoresis. In hemolytic anemia associated with cirrhosis the primary disease is usually evident. In hereditary spherocytosis and in congenital nonspherocytic hemolytic anemia the Coombs test is negative. In refractory normoblastic anemia with intramedullary hemolysis, the reticulocyte count is not elevated, bone marrow shows many sideroblasts, and donor blood survives normally.

Complications

The hemolytic anemia may become acute, with shock, upper abdominal pain, and prostration. Thrombocytopenic purpura may develop.

Treatment

Treatment must often be directed against the underlying disease. Transfusions are only palliative, and their effects are dissipated rapidly since donor cells are also destroyed at an accelerated rate.

A. Medical Treatment: Prednisolone (or equivalent), 10–20 mg 4 times daily, is given orally until normal hemoglobin values are reached or undesirable side-effects develop. The dose may be reduced rapidly to 20 mg/day and then decreased by 5 mg each week until the smallest dose needed to maintain normal hemoglobin levels is being given. Occasionally, medication can then be discontinued. Patients must be reexamined every 4 weeks even when in remission because there is always a danger of sudden relapse.

B. Surgical Treatment: When corticosteroids fail or when large doses are required for maintenance, splenectomy must be considered. Preliminary ^{51}Cr red cell life span determinations and body surface counting over the spleen to determine splenic radioactivity should be done before the decision to operate is made. When this is more than twice normal, as compared to the liver, splenectomy is likely to be of value.

Prognosis

In idiopathic acquired hemolytic anemia, prolonged remissions may occur spontaneously or following splenectomy or corticosteroid therapy; some cases are fatal. Often the prognosis depends upon that of the underlying disorder.

Allgood JW, Chaplin H: Idiopathic acquired autoimmune hemolytic anemia. Am J Med 43:254, 1967.

Dacie JV: Autoimmune hemolytic anemia. Brit J Med 2:381, 1970.

Drugs and the Coombs antiglobulin test. (Editorial.) New England J Med 277:157, 1967.

Garratty G, Petz LD: Drug induced hemolytic anemia. Am J Med 58:398, 1975.

2. HEREDITARY SPHEROCYTOSIS
(Congenital Hemolytic Anemia; Congenital Hemolytic Jaundice)

Essentials of Diagnosis

- Malaise, abdominal discomfort.
- Jaundice, anemia, splenomegaly.
- Spherocytosis, increased osmotic fragility of red cells, negative Coombs test.

General Considerations

In hereditary spherocytosis, the red cells have a defective membrane which is abnormally permeable to sodium. To prevent excessive intracellular sodium accumulation, which in turn would lead to influx of water and cell rupture, increased metabolic work must be done by the cells. The necessary energy is derived from increased glycolysis. Glucose deprivation, as it occurs in the spleen—and in vitro during the performance of the autohemolysis or incubated osmotic fragility tests—leads to red cell destruction. When red cells from a patient with hereditary spherocytosis are transfused to a normal recipient, they are destroyed in the (normal) spleen. On the other hand, normal donor blood survives almost normally in a patient with hereditary spherocytosis. The disease is chronic, hereditary, and transmitted by a dominant autosomal gene; and is seen in all races. In 25% of cases no family involvement can be demonstrated. It may be first manifested in the newborn period, and may resemble hemolytic disease due to ABO incompatibility; but in some patients the disease is not discovered until after the age of 80.

Clinical Findings

A. Symptoms and Signs: There may be easy fatigability and moderate and constant jaundice; the spleen is almost always enlarged and may cause left upper quadrant fullness and discomfort. Splenic infarction may cause acute pain. The anemia may be intensified during infections, following trauma, and during pregnancy.

On rare occasions an acute "aplastic" anemia develops with profound anemia and, in some cases, fever, headache, abdominal pain, and pancytopenia with hypoactive marrow. In occasional instances there may be no clinical findings; the diagnosis is made only because the discovery of the disease in a more severely afflicted relative has led to an intensive search and laboratory testing of the blood.

B. Laboratory Findings: The red blood count is moderately decreased (3–4 million/cu mm). The red cells are small (MCB = 70–80 fl) and hyperchromic (MCHC = 36–40%). Spherocytes in varying numbers are seen on the smear. The reticulocyte count is usually increased; the white cell and platelet counts may be only moderately increased.

In the bone marrow there is marked erythroid hyperplasia; hemosiderin is present in only moderate amounts since the spleen is the main reservoir of iron in this disorder.

Indirect serum bilirubin and stool urobilinogen are usually elevated; haptoglobins often decreased or even absent. The Coombs test is negative.

Osmotic fragility is characteristically increased; hemolysis of 5–10% of cells may be observed at saline concentrations of 0.6% or even higher. The response may be normal in some patients, but a sample of defibrinated blood incubated at 37° C for 24 hours ("incubated fragility test") will show increased hemolysis when compared to normal blood similarly treated.

Autohemolysis of defibrinated blood incubated under sterile conditions for 48 hours is usually greatly increased (10–20% compared to a normal value of less than 5%).

The addition of 10% glucose prior to incubation will decrease the amount of autohemolysis.

Red cell survival studies, using the patient's own blood labeled with ^{51}Cr, will show a greatly shortened red cell life span and sequestration in the spleen.

Differential Diagnosis

Spherocytes in large numbers occur in many patients with autoimmune hemolytic anemia. Osmotic fragility and autohemolysis are similarly increased, but are less consistently improved by glucose. The positive Coombs test, negative family history, and sharply reduced survival of normal donor blood in these patients establish the diagnosis.

Spherocytes are also seen in hemoglobin C disease, in some drug-induced hemolytic anemias, in some alcoholics, and in patients with extensive burns.

Complications

Gallstones composed principally of bile pigments (reflecting increased metabolism of hemoglobin) occur in up to 85% of adults and may develop even in children. Leg ulcers are occasionally seen. During febrile illnesses, aplastic crises may occur with profound anemia and decreased white cell and platelet counts, but little jaundice.

Treatment

There is no specific medical treatment for this disorder.

A. Surgical Treatment: Splenectomy should be done in patients with an enlarged spleen, anemia, or jaundice. Preoperative transfusion is rarely necessary.

When there is associated cholelithiasis, splenectomy should precede cholecystectomy unless both procedures are done at the same time. Splenectomy is usually deferred until after the first few years of life.

B. Treatment of Aplastic Crisis: Prompt and adequate transfusion therapy is necessary to prevent cardiovascular collapse. Antibiotics may be necessary to treat precipitating infections.

Prognosis

Splenectomy eliminates anemia and jaundice, but abnormal red cell morphology and abnormal osmotic fragility persist. Red cell life span is almost normal after splenectomy.

Jacob HS: Abnormality in the physiology of the erythrocyte membrane in hereditary spherocytosis. Am J Med 41:734, 1966.

Jandl J, Cooper RA: Hereditary spherocytosis. Pages 1323–1327 in: *The Metabolic Basis of Inherited Disease,* 3rd ed. Stanbury JB, Wyngaarden JB, Fredrickson DS (editors). McGraw-Hill, 1972.

3. OVALOCYTOSIS
(Hereditary Elliptocytosis)

Ovalocytosis is inherited as an autosomal dominant trait with variable clinical expressions. It is equally common in males and females, and occurs in all ethnic groups. The determining gene is on the same chromosome that carries the Rh blood group gene. Twenty-five to 90% of the red cells may be oval. It is thought to occur in 4 out of 10,000 individuals in the USA. About 12% of subjects have moderate anemia, a palpable spleen, and slight jaundice. Reticulocyte counts are elevated. Patients may have marked poikilocytosis and some spherocytes. Incubated osmotic fragility and autohemolysis may be increased but are restored to normal by glucose. Splenectomy is usually beneficial in patients with overt hemolysis.

The disorder is usually asymptomatic, without anemia and with normal red cell indices, but red cell survival is often shortened. In some patients the red cells are more oval than elliptical; a few spherocytes may be seen.

Cutting HO & others: Autosomal dominant hemolytic anemia characterized by ovalocytosis. Am J Med 39:21, 1965.

Geerdink RA & others: Hereditary spherocytosis and hyperhemolysis. Acta med scandinav 179:715, 1966.

Greenberg LH, Tanaka RK: Hereditary elliptocytosis with hemolytic anemia: A family study of five affected members. California Med 110:389, 1969.

4. ACUTE HEMOLYTIC ANEMIA

Essentials of Diagnosis

- Sudden onset with chills, fever, nausea, vomiting, or pain in abdomen or back.
- Pallor, slight jaundice, splenomegaly.
- Red or black urine.

General Considerations

Acute hemolytic anemia may be drug-induced, especially in sensitive individuals (see Glucose-6-Phosphate Dehydrogenase Deficiency); it may be due to certain infections, eg, *Escherichia coli* infections, hemolytic streptococcal septicemia, *Clostridium welchii* infections, and malaria; it may be seen in some forms of cancer and malignant lymphomas, and in some diseases of uncertain origin, eg, lupus erythematosus and infectious mononucleosis. It is usually seen during the course of paroxysmal nocturnal hemoglobinuria, thrombotic thrombocytopenic purpura, paroxysmal cold hemoglobinuria, and when high titered cold agglutinins develop during convalescence from viral pneumonia. Sometimes the cause is not known.

Clinical Findings

A. Symptoms and Signs: The onset is fulminating, with chills, fever, abdominal pain, pallor, jaundice, weakness, and tachycardia.

B. Laboratory Findings: The anemia is usually normocytic and normochromic, but spherocytes, burr cells, microspherocytes, and nucleated red cells may be seen. The red cell count and hemoglobin are lowest several days after the onset of symptoms. The white count may reach 50,000/cu mm and the platelet count 1 million/cu mm, but occasionally both are decreased. A blood smear stained with methyl violet may show Heinz bodies (small granules in red cells), which are not visible with Wright's stain. Reticulocytes may be greatly increased. The Coombs test is usually negative.

The bone marrow is hyperplastic, with a predominance of nucleated red cells. There may be hemoglobinemia lasting a few hours, followed by methemalbuminemia (manifested by a brown discoloration of the serum) for a few days and usually a moderately elevated indirect bilirubin value. Haptoglobin, a glycoprotein migrating electrophoretically with alpha$_2$ globulin, which can normally bind 50–150 mg/100 ml of free hemoglobin, disappears from the serum.

The urine may contain hemoglobin and hemosiderin; urobilinogen may be elevated, but not bile. Stool urobilinogen is increased. Red cell enzyme studies may show a deficiency of glucose-6-phosphate dehydrogenase; cold agglutinins may be found in atypical pneumonia; slightly acid serum may hemolyze the cells in paroxysmal nocturnal hemoglobinuria (Ham's test); and a circulating hemolysin may be found in paroxysmal cold hemoglobinuria (Donath-Landsteiner test).

Differential Diagnosis

The fulminant onset of acute hemolytic anemia,

with chills and fever, may simulate an infection. The abdominal pain may suggest surgical illness; the profound anemia suggests blood loss. In acute hemolytic anemia, however, the serum is invariably pigmented as a result of the products of hemolysis. A pink serum indicates free hemoglobin; a brown serum, methemalbumin; and a yellow serum, bilirubin.

Complications

Shock may occur if the development of anemia is sufficiently abrupt or severe. Acute tubular necrosis secondary to profound ischemia and precipitated hemoglobin in the renal tubules may lead to acute renal failure.

Treatment

Acute hemolytic anemia may be a medical emergency. The patient should be hospitalized, all medications discontinued, and possible causes investigated.

Spontaneous remission frequently occurs. Even patients who are not critically ill are observed for a few days for a gradual decline of reticulocytosis, followed by a hemoglobin rise of 1–2 gm/100 ml/week. Under these circumstances only supportive therapy need be given.

A. **General Measures**: Since acute renal failure is a potential hazard, serum electrolytes and BUN are determined and strict attention is paid to fluid intake and output and electrolyte administration.

B. **Transfusions**: Transfusions are used only to combat shock or anoxia; packed red cells are preferable to whole blood. Rarely is it necessary or desirable to raise the hemoglobin level above 8 gm/100 ml with transfusions.

C. **Corticosteroids**: If reticulocytosis persists and hemoglobin levels do not rise, if there is a continuous drop in hemoglobin, or if the patient is severely ill, give prednisolone (or equivalent), 10–20 mg 4 times daily. Corticosteroids are continued until serum and urine are clear of hemolytic products and the hemoglobin level is normal. The dose may be reduced rapidly at first to 20 mg/day and then decreased by 5 mg each week. Splenectomy is rarely if ever indicated in acute hemolytic anemia.

Prognosis

Acute hemolytic anemia usually remits spontaneously, either because the offending agent is removed or because only a portion of the patient's red cells, usually the older ones, are sensitive to the toxin. Hemolytic anemias secondary to serious underlying disorders such as metastatic cancer, thrombotic thrombocytopenic purpura, or *Clostridium welchii* infection (as seen with induced abortion) are often rapidly fatal.

Wallerstein RO, Aggeler PM: Acute hemolytic anemia. Am J Med 37:92, 1964.

5. PAROXYSMAL NOCTURNAL HEMOGLOBINURIA

Paroxysmal nocturnal hemoglobinuria is a chronic hemolytic anemia of variable severity, characterized by rather constant hemoglobinemia and hemosiderinuria and recurrent episodes of acute hemolysis with chills, fever, pain, and hemoglobinuria.

The basic disorder is an unknown intracellular defect; hemolysis is produced by interaction between the abnormal cells and several factors present in normal serum: magnesium, properdin, and complement-like components.

The onset is usually in adult life, and the disease is not familial. Spleen and liver may be slightly enlarged. White cell and platelet counts are often decreased; the reticulocyte count is increased. The bone marrow is usually hyperactive but may be hypoplastic; aplastic anemia occasionally precedes the clinical development of this disorder.

The indirect serum bilirubin is elevated. Hemoglobinemia and methemalbuminemia are often present. Haptoglobins are absent, LDH markedly elevated, the red cell acetylcholinesterase level is low. The intrinsic red cell defect is demonstrated by finding hemolysis on incubation of the patient's red cells in normal acidified serum (Ham's test). The sucrose hemolysis test is excellent for screening. Hemoglobin electrophoresis, osmotic fragility, and the Coombs test are normal.

Complications consist of overwhelming infection, aplastic crises, and thromboses. After years of hemosiderinuria, iron deficiency may develop.

Transfusion reactions occur where the donor blood (plasma) hemolyzes the patient's red cells.

Transfusions are given for severe anemia or complications such as trauma, infections, thromboses, or leg ulcers. The administration of 1 liter of 6% dextran solution, preferably of relatively high molecular weight (150,000), before transfusion may prevent hemolysis of the patient's own cells by donor serum.

Crosby WH: Paroxysmal nocturnal hemoglobinuria. Relation of the clinical manifestations to underlying pathogenic mechanisms. Blood 8:769, 1953.

Hartman RC, Jenkins DE: The sugar-water test for paroxysmal nocturnal hemoglobinuria. New England J Med 275:155, 1966.

6. HEREDITARY NONSPHEROCYTIC HEMOLYTIC ANEMIA

Essentials of Diagnosis

- Moderate anemia.
- Familial and congenital.
- Spleen slightly enlarged.
- No spherocytes; osmotic fragility normal.
- High reticulocyte count.

General Considerations

This is a heterogeneous group of congenital hemolytic anemias caused by intrinsic red cell defects. Specific enzyme deficiencies have been found for most of them. These disorders are usually inherited as an autosomal recessive trait. Some involve the Embden-Meyerhof (anaerobic) pathway. Pyruvate kinase deficiency, which is usually found in northern Europeans, is the most common; the rest are quite rare. Others involve the hexose monophosphate (pentose phosphate) shunt, but, with the exception of glucose-6-phosphate dehydrogenase (G6PD) deficiency, which is described in more detail below, they are quite rare.

Clinical Findings

A. Symptoms and Signs: Anemia and jaundice are usually discovered in early childhood. The clinical spectrum in pyruvate kinase deficiency varies from severe neonatal jaundice, requiring exchange transfusions, to fully compensated hemolysis, but in general it is more severe than hereditary spherocytosis.

B. Laboratory Findings: Hemoglobin levels vary from 6–12 gm/100 ml. The red cells may be slightly large, and spiculed, contracted, and oval cells may be seen; reticulocyte counts are relatively high, especially after splenectomy. In all of these conditions, Howell-Jolly bodies (nuclear remnants in red cells) and Pappenheimer bodies (iron particle inclusions visible with Wright's stain) may be prominent, especially after splenectomy. White cells and platelets are normal. The marrow shows marked erythroid hyperplasia. Osmotic fragility is normal. In general, autohemolysis is clearly increased after 48 hours and not reduced by glucose (Dacie type II).

A fluorescent spot screening test for pyruvate kinase deficiency is available. The other rare abnormalities can be discovered only by relatively sophisticated biochemical technics.

Differential Diagnosis

In hereditary spherocytosis the red cells are small and round, osmotic fragility is increased, and jaundice is often prominent.

In acquired hemolytic anemia the Coombs test is positive. In refractory normoblastic anemia the reticulocyte count is low and the spleen is not palpable. In the hemoglobinopathies the diagnosis is made by hemoglobin electrophoresis.

In the newborn this condition may be very difficult to differentiate from hemolytic anemia due to ABO incompatibility.

Complications

There may be associated cholelithiasis and cholecystitis.

Treatment

Whole blood transfusions may be necessary. Splenectomy is not curative but may ameliorate some of these conditions, especially pyruvate kinase deficiency.

DeGruchy GC, Grimes AJ: The non-spherocytic congenital hemolytic anemias. Brit J Haemat 23 (Suppl), 1972.

Valentine WN: Hereditary hemolysis anemias associated with specific erythrocyte enzymopathies. California Med 108:280, 1968.

Valentine WN (editor): Hereditary deficiencies of erythrocytes. Seminars Hemat 8:307, 1971.

7. GLUCOSE-6-PHOSPHATE DEHYDROGENASE (G6PD) DEFICIENCY

This is a drug-induced acute hemolytic anemia which occurs in persons of particular racial groups who have genetically transmitted errors of metabolism. The defect is a deficiency of G6PD in the erythrocytes and, to a variable degree, in other tissues. The trait is X-linked and of intermediate dominance; it finds its full expression in males and homozygous females and intermediate expression in heterozygous females. Ten to 15% of American black males and 1–2% of American black females have the African variant of this disorder. The Mediterranean variant, which is found especially in Sardinians, Sicilians, Greeks, Sephardic Jews, Iranians, and Arabs, may produce more severe disease than the African variant; some of these individuals have chronic hemolytic anemia. Upon exposure to drugs or (in some cases) fava beans, a profound hemolytic anemia may develop. Other variants of the enzyme defect have been observed in northern Europeans and Chinese.

When not challenged by a drug, the red blood count, red cell indices, and red cell morphology are normal although the red cell survival time is slightly shortened. More than 40 drugs and other substances are capable of inducing hemolysis, including antimalarials, sulfonamides, eg, salicylazosulfapyridine, sulfamethoxypyridazine, sulfisoxazole; nitrofurans, antipyretics, analgesics, sulfones, water-soluble vitamin K, and uncooked fava beans. Favism occurs principally in the Mediterranean area and is most common in Sardinia. Hemolytic episodes in the absence of drug administration may be produced by hepatitis, other viral or bacterial infections, and diabetic acidosis. These drugs accelerate the oxygen consumption of red cells, thereby activating the pentose phosphate pathway. An enzyme defect in this pathway leads to oxidation of NADPH, which permits oxidation of protein sulfhydryl groups in the cell membrane and eventually causes oxidation of hemoglobin with irreversible changes and Heinz body formation.

Several laboratory methods have been devised for identifying susceptible individuals. There is a glutathione stability test, a dye reduction test using cresyl blue, a methemoglobin reduction test, and a commercially available dye reduction spot test.

Management consists of discontinuation of exposure to the offending drug or toxic substance. Recovery is the rule.

Beutler E: Drug induced hemolytic anemia. Pharmacol Rev 21:73, 1969.

Burka ER, Weaver Z, Marks PA: Clinical spectrum of hemolytic anemia associated with glucose-6-phosphate dehydrogenase deficiency. Ann Int Med 64:817, 1966.

Carson PE, Fisher H: G6PD deficiency and related disorders of the pentose phosphate pathway. Am J Med 41:744, 1966.

Grimes AJ: Laboratory diagnosis of enzyme defects in the red cell. Brit J Haemat 17:129, 1969.

8. MICROANGIOPATHIC HEMOLYTIC ANEMIA

This term describes a group of acquired hemolytic anemias due to various causes that are characterized by fragmented or helmet-shaped red cells, burr cells, or microspherocytes. Associated thrombocytopenia is common; normal donor cells are destroyed rapidly. This form of red cell distortion may be seen in association with the following conditions: thrombotic thrombocytopenic purpura, metastatic cancer, post-cardiotomy, drug toxicity (perhaps in association with glucose-6-phosphate dehydrogenase deficiency), the hemolytic-uremic syndrome of infancy and pregnancy, in postpartum malignant nephrosclerosis, malignant hypertension (rare), acute nephritis (rare), and uremia.

In some of these, small thrombi in arterioles and capillaries, especially in the kidney, may be found. Some degree of disseminated intravascular coagulation may be present.

Except for those that are drug-induced, these anemias carry a very poor prognosis.

Brain MC & others: Microangiopathic hemolytic anemia. New England J Med 281:833, 1969.

Finkelstein FO & others: Clinical spectrum of postpartum renal failure. Am J Med 57:649, 1974.

Hammond D & others: Hemolytic-uremic syndrome. Am J Dis Child 114:440, 1967.

ANEMIAS WITH INTRAMEDULLARY HEMOLYSIS*
(Ineffective Erythropoiesis)

An important pathologic process in several anemias is the destruction of immature, nucleated red cells while still in the marrow. The erythroblasts apparently are defective in some way and are sequestered by reticuloendothelial cells. Some of these disorders (eg, pernicious anemia) may be associated with frank megaloblastosis; others (eg, refractory normoblastic anemias) show erythroblasts that resemble megaloblasts. These disorders are characterized by marked

---

*Pernicious anemia, folic acid deficiency, and thalassemia are discussed elsewhere in this chapter.

erythroid hyperplasia in the marrow without elevation of reticulocyte counts. Radio-iron studies show greatly increased iron turnover and uptake by the marrow; delayed release from the marrow; and poor incorporation into circulating red cells with secondary accumulation in the liver. Red cell survival as measured with ^{51}Cr is usually only moderately shortened; the peripheral erythrocytes apparently represent the best cells made by the disordered marrow.

Examples of anemia with intramedullary hemolysis are the following:

Refractory Normoblastic Anemia

This is a heterogeneous group of chronic, moderate to severe anemias. Patients may have symptoms of anemia and perhaps slight splenic enlargement, but no other abnormal physical findings are present. Red cells are mostly normocytic and normochromic, but a few hypochromic microcytic cells may be seen. White cells and platelets may be slightly decreased. The bone marrow shows considerable erythroid hyperplasia and some erythrophagocytosis. Marrow hemosiderin is greatly increased and tends to aggregate in granules in normoblasts and histiocytes. Some of these patients respond to pyridoxine (see below).

Sideroachrestic Anemias

In this often familial group, most of the red cells are hypochromic and microcytic, serum iron is high, and iron deposits in the marrow, liver, and spleen are excessive. Many erythrocytes and erythroblasts contain nonhemoglobin iron ("ringed sideroblasts") in their mitochondria. The spleen is usually enlarged. Some of these patients respond to pyridoxine (see below).

Pyridoxine Responsive Anemias

In some of the above groups of anemias, hemoglobin may be restored to normal by large doses (50–200 mg IM daily) of pyridoxine; the microcytosis and hypochromia may persist. The patients have no other signs of pyridoxine deficiency such as CNS and skin involvement. A few patients have macrocytic anemia and megaloblastic bone marrow that do not respond to vitamin B_{12} or folic acid.

Dacie JV & others: Refractory normoblastic anemia. Brit J Haemat 5:56, 1959.

Horrigan DL, Harris JW: Pyridoxine responsive anemia. An analysis of 61 cases. Advances Int Med 12:103, 1964.

Kushner JP & others: Idiopathic refractory sideroblastic anemia. Medicine 50:139, 1971.

Symposium on sideroblastic anemia. Brit J Haemat 11:41, 1965.

ABNORMAL HEMOGLOBINS

The human red cell contains 200–300 million molecules of hemoglobin. Each molecule contains 4 heme groups and one globin molecule. The globin molecule is composed of 2 dissimilar pairs of polypeptide chains. The globin chains are designated a through δ, each chain being unique in amino acid composition. The members of each pair are identical. Each chain is made up of 141–146 amino acids. The production of the different globin chains is under the control of independent genetic loci.

Three different types of hemoglobin are normally present in adults; 97% is hemoglobin A, with 2 a and 2 β. The other 2 normal hemoglobins are present in trace amounts (1–3%). Hemoglobin A_2 possesses alpha chains, but in place of the beta chain has a pair of delta chains which differ from the beta chain probably in less than 10 amino acids. Fetal hemoglobin (hemoglobin F) also contains 2 a chains and contains 2 gamma chains instead of beta chains, and differs from the latter in numerous amino acid substitutions.

Hemoglobinopathies involve abnormalities in the hemoglobin chains. These are due to changes in the DNA template—a different order of bases in the one locus resulting in the production of different amino acids, and therefore a structurally and functionally altered protein. Differences between normal and abnormal hemoglobins are relatively minute. For example, sickle (S) hemoglobin differs from normal hemoglobin in the single amino acid substitution in the beta chains (composed of 146 amino acids). Valine instead of glutamic acid is the 6th amino acid from the terminal position. Yet this small difference has far-reaching clinical effects which produce sickle cell disease. Most of the well known hemoglobinopathies involve abnormalities of the beta chains. A few alpha chain abnormalities are known, eg, hemoglobin H disease.

Conley CL, Charache S: Inherited hemoglobinopathies. Hosp Practice 4:35, 1969.
Heller P: Hemoglobinopathic dysfunction of the red cell. Am J Med 41:799, 1966.
Ranney H: Clinically important variants of human hemoglobin. New England J Med 282:144, 1970.

1. HEREDITARY HEMOGLOBINOPATHIES

Certain hereditary hemolytic anemias seen almost exclusively in blacks are characterized by the genetically determined presence of an abnormal type of hemoglobin in the red cells.

The heterozygous hemoglobin trait syndromes usually represent asymptomatic carriers, eg, in sickle cell trait, which occurs in about 9% of American blacks, there is no anemia. With hemoglobin C trait, which occurs in about 3% of American blacks, there is no anemia but target cells are common. The relative frequency of some hemoglobinopathies (per 1000 blacks) is as follows: A/S, 90; S/S, 2; A/F, 10; S/C, 0.66; A/C, 30; C/C, 0.166.

The homozygous hemoglobin disorders usually cause some anemia. The most common and the most serious is sickle cell anemia, which occurs in 1 in 500 American blacks. Homozygous hemoglobin C disease occurs only in 1 in 6000 and is a relatively mild disease. Double heterozygous diseases, eg, combinations of hemoglobin S and C, occur with an incidence of 1 in 1500. In addition, S-thalassemia or C-thalassemia may occur, but they are much less severe than sickle cell anemia. Target cells are prominent in all, especially when the C trait is present.

In general, all of the homozygous disorders with the exception of sickle cell anemia and all of the double heterozygous disorders are characterized by splenomegaly. Fetal hemoglobin is increased in double heterozygous disorders when one of the genes is a thalassemia gene. Some fetal hemoglobin is also present in sickle cell anemia.

2. SICKLE CELL ANEMIA

Essentials of Diagnosis

- Recurrent attacks of fever, and pain in the arms, legs, or abdomen since early childhood in a black patient.
- Anemia, jaundice, reticulocytosis, positive sickle cell test, and demonstration of abnormal (S) hemoglobin.

General Considerations

Sickling of the chemically abnormal hemoglobin occurs at low oxygen tension, especially at a low pH. The S (sickle) hemoglobin is less soluble in deoxygenated (reduced) form, the viscosity of the whole blood consequently increases, and the result is stasis and obstruction of blood flow in the capillaries, terminal arterioles, and veins. Localized sickling, vascular occlusion, and perivascular edema cause pain and swelling in the involved organs.

Sickle cell anemia is a recessive hereditary disorder, essentially confined to blacks; the abnormal hemoglobin is transmitted as a dominant trait. Heterozygous carriers have mixtures of normal and sickle hemoglobin in all of their red blood cells.

Clinical Findings

A. Symptoms and Signs: Most patients with sickle cell anemia have moderately severe anemia. The anemia usually is not a major problem because a good oxygen supply to tissues is preserved by a shift of the oxygen dissociation curve to the right and an increased cardiac output. The disease is disabling because of the recurrent painful crises.

The diagnosis is usually made in childhood, but occasionally a patient will reach adult life before a well documented crisis develops. Patients with sickle cell anemia tend to be of asthenic build with long spindly legs. Constant scleral icterus of moderate degree is common. The crisis consists of attacks of bone and

Table 9—3. Hematologic findings in the hemoglobinopathies.*

Hemoglobin Disorder	Erythrocytes (mill/cu mm)	Hemoglobin (gm/100 ml)	RBC		Reticulocytes (%)	Target Cells (%)	Hemoglobins (%)		Fetal Hemoglobins (%)
			Size	Hgb Content					
Normal (adult men and women A/A)	4.2–6.2	12–18	82–92 cu μ	32–36 %	0.5–1.5	0	A A$_2$	97 2–3	0–2
A/S	N	N	N	N	N	0	A$_2$ S	3–4 22–48	0–2
S/S	1.5–4.0	2–11	N	N	5–30	Some	A$_2$ S	3–4 80–100	0–20
S-Thalassemia	2.0–5.0	6–14	Small	Decr	4–20	Many	A$_2$ S A	3–8 50–90 2–3	1–26
S/C	2.5–5.5	8.1–15.1	N	N	0.2–10	5–85	C S	37–67 30–60	0–8
S/D	2.5–4.0	7–12	N	N	7–13	2– Some	D S	23–75 25–77	Trace
S-Persistent F	3.5–5.0	11–15	N	N	N	0	S A$_2$	75 0–1	25
A/C	N	N	N	N	N	0–40	A C	50–70 30–50	0–2
C/C	3.1–5.0	7–14.5	N	Incr	1–12	20–100	C	97–100	0–3
A/D	N	N	N	N	N	0	D	<50	0–2
D/D	5.5–7.1	12–13	Small	N	1–1.5	50–80	D	100	0–2
H-Thalassemia	1.6–6.4	8–11	Small	Decr	2–22	1–30	A H A$_2$	60–85 15–40 0–1	Trace–4
Thalassemia minor	4.0–7.5	8.3–13.2	Small	Decr	0.5–9.0	0–10	A A$_2$	90+ 2–9	0–10
Thalassemia major	1.0–4.0	2–8	Small	Decr	1.5–38	0–50	A A$_2$	10–30 2–3	70–90
Hereditary persistence of fetal hemoglobin (A/F)	N	N	N	N	N	0	A A$_2$	70–90 0–1	10–30

*Modified from Dacie: *The Hemolytic Anemias, Congenital and Acquired,* 2nd ed. Part I. Grune & Stratton, 1960.

joint pain or abdominal pain, sometimes with fever, lasting hours or days. The tender, rigid abdomen may resemble surgical illness and may last for hours or days. Cerebral thrombosis may occur, producing headaches, paralysis, and convulsions.

B. Laboratory Findings: Hemoglobin values average about 8 gm/100 ml, with a range of 6–10 gm, and change only slightly during painful crises. The red cell indices are usually normal. In addition to the sickled cells, some target cells are commonly seen on the blood film. The reticulocyte count may be 15–20%. Serum iron is normal or slightly elevated. Serum LDH is often greatly elevated, and haptoglobin is usually absent. Serum bilirubin values usually vary between 2 and 4 mg/100 ml. Plasma hemoglobin is slightly elevated, and ^{51}Cr red cell survival is approximately 10 days.

Two screening tests are in common use: (1) The sodium metabisulfite test uses a drop of fresh 2% reagent mixed on a slide with 1 drop of patient's blood; sickling of most red cells will occur in a few minutes. Sodium metabisulfite is a strong reducing agent, and the deoxygenated red cells become distorted as their hemoglobin becomes insoluble. (2) "Sickledex" is a simple solubility test that does not require a microscope; sodium dithionite is used as a reducing agent, and saponin and phosphate buffer make up the precipitating agents. When 0.02 ml of blood are mixed with 2 ml of the reagent, normal blood will give a clear tube and S hemoglobin will produce a cloudy tube.

Differential Diagnosis

Sickle cell anemia is differentiated from other hemoglobinopathies by hemoglobin electrophoresis, the sickle cell test, and fetal hemoglobin determination. Hematuria may simulate genitourinary tumor, tuberculosis, or vascular disease. Bone and joint pain may resemble rheumatic fever. The abdominal pain may simulate surgical abdominal conditions; persistence of normal bowel sounds in sickle cell crisis may be a helpful differential diagnostic finding.

The spleen is not enlarged in adult sickle cell anemia. An anemic black patient with an enlarged spleen and a positive sickle cell preparation probably has a double heterozygous disorder instead (eg, "sickle thalassemia" rather than sickle cell anemia). The sickle cell test does not differentiate between sickle cell anemia (the homozygous disorder) and sickle cell trait (the heterozygous carrier state). In sickle cell anemia the red count is always low; the finding of a low hemoglobin with a normal red count in a black patient with a positive sickle cell preparation is not compatible with sickle cell anemia but suggests iron deficiency anemia plus sickle cell trait.

An electrophoretic pattern indistinguishable from that of sickle cell anemia may be found in the following: (1) Sickle cell-hemoglobin D disease: Hemoglobin D has the same electrophoretic mobility as hemoglobin S, but electrophoresis on agar gel at pH 6.0 differentiates these 2 hemoglobins. Hemoglobins A and D migrate together and ahead of hemoglobin S. (2) Some instances of sickle thalassemia: Hemoglobin A is sometimes absent in sickle thalassemia because the formation of normal beta chains is prevented by the sickle cell gene and is suppressed by the thalassemia gene. Family studies may distinguish sickle thalassemia from sickle cell anemia. Hemoglobin A_2 is usually elevated in S-thalassemia but normal in S/S. (3) Sickle cell-persistent fetal hemoglobin syndrome.

Complications

Complications include leg ulcers, bone infarction, aseptic necrosis of the femoral head, osteomyelitis (especially due to salmonella), cardiac enlargement with auscultatory findings similar to those of mitral stenosis, recurrent gross hematuria, and cholelithiasis. Following infection, there may be an aplastic crisis.

Treatment

Treatment is symptomatic. There is considerable variation in the frequency and severity of clinical manifestations.

A. Treatment of Clinical Crisis: Adequate hydration and analgesics should be provided. Oxygen therapy, local measures, alkalinizing measures, vasodilators, and urea have all been tried but have failed to give beneficial results.

B. Treatment of Hemolytic and Aplastic Crisis: Transfusions are mandatory. The hemoglobin level should be raised to 12–14 gm/100 ml. Adequate hydration is necessary. A careful search for infections should be made and appropriate antibiotic therapy instituted.

C. Treatment of Complications:

1. Leg ulcers—The legs are immobilized and elevated under a heat cradle. The ulcer area is cleansed and debrided. The patient is given sufficient blood to raise the hemoglobin level to 12–14 gm/100 ml.

2. Cholelithiasis or orthopedic disorders requiring surgery—Give sufficient preoperative blood to raise the

hemoglobin level to 12–14 gm/100 ml.

3. Sickle cell anemia appearing during pregnancy—Transfuse to 10–12 gm/100 ml in the third trimester.

4. Pulmonary thrombosis, pneumonia, or osteomyelitis—Treat by standard methods.

Prognosis

Many patients die in childhood of cerebral hemorrhage or shock. Others live beyond the age of 50 years. There is a tendency to progressive renal damage, and death from uremia may occur.

Desforges JF: Treatment of sickle cell crisis. New England J Med 284:913, 1971.

Diggs LW: Sickle cell crisis. Am J Clin Path 44:1, 1965.

Finch CA: Pathophysiologic aspects of sickle cell anemia. Am J Med 53:1, 1972.

Messer MI: Sickle cell disease. California Med 118:48, April 1973.

3. SICKLE CELL TRAIT

Sickle cell trait rarely causes symptoms or signs. Blood counts, red cell morphology, and red cell life span are normal. Gross hematuria occurs in 3–4% of cases; renal concentrating capacity is usually impaired; and pregnant women with the trait have an increased susceptibility to pyelonephritis. Splenic infarcts on high altitude flying as well as pulmonary infarcts develop occasionally. Under the stress of anoxia, as in congestive heart failure, acute alcoholism, or shock due to any cause, massive, fatal infarct may occur.

Bristow LA: The myth of sickle cell trait. Western J Med 121:177, 1974.

McCormick WF: The pathology of sickle cell trait. Am J Med Sc 241:329, 1961.

4. S/C HEMOGLOBIN DISEASE

Essentials of Diagnosis

- Recurrent attacks of abdominal, joint, or bone pain.
- Enlarged spleen.
- Minimal anemia.
- Positive sickle cell test; many target cells.

General Considerations

The racial incidence and mode of inheritance of hemoglobin S/C disease are similar to those of sickle cell anemia. It represents a double heterozygous state, ie, the patient must receive the gene for S from one parent and the gene for C from the other. The incidence is 1 in 1500 in the American black population.

Clinical Findings

A. Symptoms and Signs: The average age at time of diagnosis is 11 years. In addition to abdominal, bone, joint, or chest pain, there may be painless hematuria, vitreous hemorrhages, and pulmonary thromboses. Jaundice is minimal. The liver is slightly enlarged and the spleen is large in two-thirds of patients. Heart murmurs are uncommon.

B. Laboratory Findings: Red blood count and hemoglobin values are nearly normal unless a complication is present. Target cells are very prominent, but red cell indices are normal; a few sickled cells may be seen. The sickle cell test is positive. Red cell survival is slightly shortened. White cell and platelet counts are normal. The marrow shows increased erythropoiesis. On electrophoresis the percentages of hemoglobin S and hemoglobin C are nearly equal. Hemoglobin F is normal.

Differential Diagnosis

S/C hemoglobin disease is differentiated from sickle cell anemia by its more benign clinical picture and splenic enlargement and by its characteristic migration on hemoglobin electrophoresis. Sickle thalassemia is also more severe than S/C hemoglobin disease and is identified by hemoglobin electrophoresis. Other conditions with target cell formation include hemoglobin C disease and C trait, thalassemia minor, and jaundice, especially when due to cirrhosis and in patients who have undergone splenectomy.

Complications

Eye manifestations (eg, vitreous hemorrhages, retinal detachment), splenic infarcts, gross hematuria, or pulmonary thromboses may occur.

Treatment

Management is similar to that given for sickle cell anemia. Most patients require no therapy.

Prognosis

The outlook for these patients is considerably better than in sickle cell anemia. Some patients live into their 70s.

River GL, Robbins AB, Schwartz SO: S-C hemoglobin: A clinical study. Blood 18:385, 1961.

Serjeant GR & others: The clinical features of hemoglobin S-C in Jamaica. Brit J Haemat 24:491, 1973.

5. S-THALASSEMIA

Some patients with this disease may have frequent episodes of jaundice, enlargement of the liver and spleen, recurrent bouts of fever, joint pain, and occasional abdominal pain. Others may have no symptoms and no splenic enlargement. The blood shows hypochromic, microcytic red cells varying in size and shape, with target and sickle forms. Different electrophoretic patterns are recognized. Patients may have relatively large amounts of hemoglobin S and increased amounts of hemoglobin A_2 (up to 6%) and F (up to 15%), and hemoglobin A varies from none to 40%; these probably represent hemoglobin S/beta thalassemia disease. Others have more hemoglobin A than S, and normal or low fractions of A_2 and F; they are classified as hemoglobin S/alpha thalassemia and are clinically much milder. The severity of anemia varies from patient to patient and even may fluctuate in a given patient; normal hemoglobin values may be found.

Aksoy M: Alpha S-thalassemia. Blood 22:757, 1963.

Monti A & others: The thalassemia syndrome. *In:* Problems of Cooley's anemia. Ann New York Acad Med 119:474, 1964.

Serjeant GR & others: The clinical features of sickle-cell/β thalassemia in Jamaica. Brit J Haemat 24:19, 1973.

6. HEREDITARY PERSISTENCE OF FETAL HEMOGLOBIN

Individuals with this condition have no clinical abnormalities and are not anemic. They are characterized by the presence, throughout life, of large amounts of fetal hemoglobin in the erythrocytes. The trait is transmitted as a single factor allelic with the gene for hemoglobins S and C. The heterozygous (hemoglobin A/F) form occurs in 1 in 1000 American blacks.

The red cells appear normal, and the reticulocytes and serum bilirubin are not elevated. Fetal hemoglobin is uniformly distributed among the erythrocytes. Hemoglobin A_2 is decreased.

Heterozygotes carry 10–30% hemoglobin F and have no hematologic abnormalities. In individuals heterozygous for hereditary persistence of fetal hemoglobin and hemoglobin S or C, the hemoglobin pattern consists of approximately 20–35% hemoglobin F and the remainder is hemoglobin S or C; no hemoglobin A is present. Individuals heterozygous for hereditary persistence of fetal hemoglobin and hemoglobin S are healthy.

Conditions with lesser elevation of hemoglobin F include occasional cases of thalassemia minor and rare cases of aplastic anemia. Fetal hemoglobin values in this group may reach 20%.

Conley CL & others: Hereditary persistence of fetal hemoglobin. Blood 21:261, 1963.

Weatherall DJ, Clegg JB: Annotation. Brit J Haemat 29:191, 1975.

7. THALASSEMIA MINOR

Essentials of Diagnosis
- Mild but persistent anemia.
- Red blood count normal or elevated.
- Similar blood findings in one of the parents.
- Patient usually has a Mediterranean or southern Chinese racial background.

General Considerations
In thalassemia, an insufficient amount of hemoglobin is made to fill the red cells. The defect lies in reduced synthesis in one of the globin chains, apparently involving defective messenger RNA. In beta thalassemia, the beta chains are defective and the alpha chains are normal; in alpha chain thalassemia (see hemoglobin H disease), the reverse is true. Beta thalassemia is the more common type seen in the USA in individuals of southern Italian extraction, other Mediterraneans, southern Chinese, and some blacks. The greater the imbalance between beta chain production and alpha chain production, the more severe the disorder. The discrepancy is least in blacks, which is why the clinical disorder is milder in this racial group. The unbalanced synthesis leads to precipitation of the normal chains, which are in relative excess; the precipitated hemoglobin causes premature red cell death, either in the marrow (intramedullary hemolysis, ineffective erythropoiesis) or in the blood stream (shortened survival of red cells). In beta thalassemia, the other "nonalpha" chains, ie, the gamma chains and the delta chains, compensate to some extent for the lack of beta chains, producing increase in hemoglobin F or hemoglobin A_2, respectively. Thalassemia minor is the heterozygous form of the disorder; thalassemia major is the homozygous state.

Clinical Findings
A. Symptoms and Signs: There are usually no symptoms. The spleen may be slightly enlarged. Occasionally there is upper left quadrant pain.

B. Laboratory Findings: The red count may exceed 6 million/cu mm. The hemoglobin does not fall below 9 gm/100 ml in uncomplicated cases. The red cells are very small (MCV = 50–70 fl), and hemoglobin concentration often is only moderately reduced (MCHC = 29–31%). Target cells and stippled cells are common. Red cells vary considerably in size and shape—more than in iron deficiency anemia of a comparable hemoglobin level. Some hypochromic macrocytes may be seen. Red cell patterns vary from one family to another. One group may have many target cells; another group may have stippled cells. Reticulocytes vary from 1–9%; platelets and white cells are not remarkable.

The bone marrow shows increased numbers of nucleated red cells. White cells and megakaryocytes are normal. Hemosiderin is present. In patients of Mediterranean ancestry, hemoglobin A_2 (a slow-moving normal hemoglobin component demonstrated on starch or agar gel electrophoresis) is usually increased 2- to 3-fold. It represents a beta hemoglobin chain abnormality. Fetal hemoglobin may be increased up to 6% in about half of patients; it is unevenly distributed among the red blood cells. In a much less common form of beta thalassemia, hemoglobin F levels are increased to 10–20%, but A_2 levels are normal. Clinically these patients are similar to those with A_2 variant. When thalassemia minor is associated with normal A_2 and F components, it probably represents an alpha chain abnormality. (See Hemoglobin H Disease.)

Differential Diagnosis
Thalassemia minor must be differentiated principally from iron deficiency anemia. It is not a severe anemia; the hemoglobin level is almost always above 9 gm/100 ml, and serum iron, total iron-binding capacity, and marrow hemosiderin are normal.

Other hypochromic, microcytic anemias with normal or even increased serum iron and marrow hemosiderin are as follows:

A. Certain hemoglobinopathies, especially hemoglobin H and hemoglobin E disease and the so-called Lepore trait, are diagnosed by hemoglobin electrophoresis.

B. Sideroachrestic anemia, characterized by increased iron values, many sideroblasts, and biochemical evidence of disordered heme synthesis. Hemoglobin electrophoresis is normal.

Complications
Thalassemia does not respond to iron therapy, and unnecessary and prolonged treatment with parenteral iron could lead to excess iron storage.

Treatment & Prognosis
No treatment is required, and unnecessary iron therapy must be avoided. During pregnancy, transfusions may be necessary to maintain hemoglobin above 9 gm/100 ml. Patients with thalassemia minor have normal life spans.

Fink H (editor): Second conference on the problems of Cooley's anemia. Ann New York Acad Sc 165:1, 1969.

Marks PA: Thalassemia syndromes. New England J Med 275:1363, 1966.

Nathan DG, Gunn RB: Thalassemia. Am J Med 41:815, 1966.

Pearson HA & others: Screening for thalassemia trait by electronic measurement of mean corpuscular volume. New England J Med 288:351, 1973.

8. THALASSEMIA MAJOR

Essentials of Diagnosis
- Severe anemia starting in early infancy.
- Very large liver and spleen.
- Hypochromic, microcytic red cells with many erythroblasts.
- Greatly elevated fetal hemoglobin.

General Considerations

See discussion in previous section.

Clinical Findings

A. Symptoms and Signs: Severe anemia and a huge liver and spleen are usually recognized in early childhood. Jaundice is usually present.

B. Laboratory Findings: Severe microcytic, hypochromic anemia is present. Target cells and bizarre-shaped red cells are seen. Nucleated red cells are numerous. The reticulocyte count is moderately elevated. The platelet count and white count are normal or increased. Serum bilirubin is elevated. Haptoglobins are absent. Paper hemoglobin electrophoresis is normal. A_2 is not elevated, but fetal hemoglobin may be increased to 90%. The bone marrow shows tremendous erythroid hyperplasia and ample stainable iron.

C. X-Ray Findings: Skeletal lesions (evident on x-ray) are most prominent in the skull and long bones and consist of increase of the medullary portion and thinning of the cortex, the so-called hair on end appearance.

Differential Diagnosis

Other hemoglobinopathies involving varying mixtures of hemoglobin S, hemoglobin C, and others with thalassemia may give similar but less severe clinical pictures. Congenital nonspherocytic hemolytic anemia may resemble this disorder. Hemoglobin electrophoresis, determination of fetal hemoglobin, and family studies make the correct diagnosis. Family studies show that both parents have the thalassemia trait.

Treatment

Regularly spaced transfusions are often necessary to maintain life. Rarely, folic acid may be helpful for associated folic acid deficiency. When secondary hemolytic anemia develops with evidence of accelerated splenic sequestration of transfused red cells, splenectomy may be helpful.

Complications

There may be cardiorespiratory symptoms due to the chronic anemia. Leg ulcers and cholelithiasis may develop. Transfusion induced iron overload, with myocardial hemosiderosis, may lead to cardiac arrhythmia; intractable heart failure is a fairly common cause of death. Few patients survive into adult life.

Nathan D: Thalassemia. New England J Med 286:586, 1972.

Weatherall DJ: *The Thalassemia Syndromes,* 2nd ed. Blackwell, 1972.

9. ALPHA THALASSEMIA; HEMOGLOBIN H DISEASE

Hemoglobin H disease is an example of alpha thalassemia. Three other types of alpha thalassemia can be recognized: (1) The homozygous form is lethal; death occurs in utero or at birth as hydrops fetalis. (2) Alpha thalassemia trait resembles beta thalassemia minor. (3) The silent carrier is hematologically normal, but analysis of globin chain synthesis shows diminished alpha chain production.

These disorders are found in Filipinos, Chinese, Thais, and sometimes Greeks. The silent carrier state is often found in blacks. In hemoglobin H disease one of the parents usually has alpha thalassemia minor and the other is a silent carrier; it is thus a doubly heterozygous disorder. In the alpha thalassemias, hemoglobin F is not elevated; hemoglobin A_2 is lower than normal; and, at birth, hemoglobin Barts (4 gamma chains) is found in the cord blood.

Hemoglobin H disease is a hypochromic microcytic anemia that resembles thalassemia minor of the beta chain type. However, the morphologic abnormalities of the red cells are more striking, and at times the anemia becomes more severe, eg, with infections. Hemoglobin H has a very high affinity for oxygen, which means that it does not deliver oxygen well to the tissues. It is unstable, and acute hemolysis may follow the use of oxidant drugs.

The spleen is enlarged; a moderate degree of anemia is present, and the reticulocyte count is elevated. Hemoglobin H differs from normal hemoglobin by its more rapid electrophoretic mobility and by its instability. When blood from a patient with hemoglobin H disease is incubated for 30 minutes at room temperature with 1% brilliant cresyl blue, precipitates form in the red cells. Hemoglobin H, unlike hemoglobin I, the other "faster than normal" hemoglobin, migrates to the anode even at pH 6.5. Its iso-electric point is pH 5.6. Osmotic fragility is decreased; red cell life span is shortened to a half-life of 12–24 days; marrow erythropoiesis is effective; and glycolytic enzyme levels are normal. Hemoglobin H varies from a few percent up to 40% of the patient's hemoglobin. (It is composed of 4 beta chains.) A_2 hemoglobin is decreased.

Splenectomy may be helpful if anemia is severe.

Kan WY & others: Globin chain synthesis in the alpha thalassemia syndromes. J Clin Invest 47:2515, 1968.

Rigas DA & others: Hemoglobin H. J Lab Clin Med 47:51, 1956.

HYPERSPLENISM

Essentials of Diagnosis

- Large spleen.
- Pancytopenia.
- Active marrow.

General Considerations

The most common form of hypersplenism is congestive splenomegaly, often due to portal hypertension secondary to cirrhosis. Other causes are thrombosis, stenosis, atresia, or angiomatous deformity of the portal or splenic vein, external pressure due to cysts, and aneurysm of the splenic artery.

The spleen may be enlarged because of a specific infiltrate, as in Gaucher's disease, Niemann-Pick disease, Letterer-Siwe disease, tuberculosis, or Boeck's sarcoid. Nonspecific enlargement may occur, as in rheumatoid arthritis (Felty's syndrome).

In hypersplenism the platelet count, white count, and to some extent the red count are reduced because of pooling in or sequestration by the enlarged spleen.

Clinical Findings

A. **Symptoms and Signs:** Patients affected with hypersplenism due to congestive splenomegaly are usually under 35 years of age. Some have little difficulty; others may have sudden hematemesis due to esophageal varices. Gastrointestinal bleeding occurs in about half.

The large spleen may cause abdominal fullness. Sometimes the spleen is found accidentally during a routine examination. Some patients have purpura. In primary splenic neutropenia, fever and pain over the splenic region occur.

B. **Laboratory Findings:** The anemia is often mild, normocytic and normochromic; the reticulocyte count may be elevated. The ^{51}Cr red cell life span is decreased, with evidence of increased splenic sequestration. Platelets and white cells, particularly the granulocytes, are greatly decreased, with a shift to the left.

The bone marrow shows varying degrees of generalized hyperactivity.

Differential Diagnosis

Hypersplenism is characterized by "empty blood, full marrow," and a large spleen.

Leukemia and lymphoma are diagnosed by marrow or lymph node biopsy and examination of the peripheral blood (white count and differential). In hereditary spherocytosis there are spherocytes, osmotic fragility is increased, and platelets and white cells are normal. The hemoglobinopathies with splenomegaly are differentiated on the basis of hemoglobin electrophoresis. Thalassemia major becomes apparent in early childhood, and the blood smear morphology is characteristic. In myelofibrosis, marrow biopsy shows proliferation of fibroblasts and replacement of normal elements. In idiopathic thrombocytopenic purpura, the spleen is not enlarged. In aplastic anemia, the spleen is not enlarged and the marrow is fatty.

Complications

Gastrointestinal hemorrhage due to bleeding from esophageal varices may be fatal. Granulocytopenia may cause persistent leg ulcers or overwhelming infection.

Treatment

Therapy is usually that of the underlying condition. When the hematologic abnormalities are not severe, no treatment is required.

Splenectomy may be advisable for congestive splenomegaly due to a splenic vein abnormality alone and when leukopenia with recurrent infections or thrombocytopenic purpura are associated with the splenomegaly of tuberculosis, Gaucher's disease, Felty's syndrome, or sarcoidosis.

If congestive splenomegaly is due to liver or portal vein disease, splenectomy should be done only in conjunction with a splenorenal, splenocaval, or portacaval shunt.

Prognosis

The prognosis is that of the underlying disorder. The course in congestive splenomegaly due to portal hypertension depends upon the degree of venous obstruction and liver damage. Without hematemesis, the course may be relatively benign and splenectomy may not be necessary.

Baines CG & others: Felty's syndrome. Ann Rheumat Dis 30:359, 1971.
Bischel MD & others: Hypersplenism in the uremic hemodialyzed patient. Nephron 9:146, 1972.
Jandl JH, Aster RH: Increased splenic pooling and the pathogenesis of hypersplenism. Am J M Sc 253:383, 1967.

SECONDARY ANEMIAS

Under this heading are listed several diseases frequently accompanied by moderate to severe anemia. The anemia is usually caused by a combination of shortened red cell life span and inadequate bone marrow compensation, so-called relative bone marrow failure or sick cell syndrome. The red cells may be normal in appearance. The reticulocyte count may be slightly elevated. White cells are normal. Platelet counts may be elevated. No abnormal serum factors are demonstrable. The bone marrow is active and erythropoiesis may be increased. Some of these disorders have their own characteristics which are described below. It is important to recognize complicating iron deficiency or folic acid deficiency, which can be treated specifically.

Characteristically, these anemics have low transferrin, albumin, and erythropoietin.

Cartwright GE: Anemia of chronic disorders. Brit J Haemat 21:147, 1971.
Kernick JE: Mechanism of the anemia of chronic disorders. Arch Int Med 130:323, 1972.

1. ANEMIA OF CIRRHOSIS

Some degree of anemia is almost invariably seen in the patient with cirrhosis.

(1) Iron deficiency due to blood loss may occur with gastritis, esophageal varices, hemorrhoids, or associated peptic ulcer.

(2) Folic acid deficiency and the characteristic megaloblastic picture is seen in only 5% of cirrhotic patients with anemia, but some degree of folic acid deficiency can be demonstrated in most patients by serum folate levels.

(3) A moderately severe hemolytic anemia is seen most frequently. The red cells are thin, flat, macrocytic, and slightly hypochromic, and vary greatly in size but not in shape. Target cells are common, and the reticulocyte count is moderately elevated. The white count is normal or elevated, and the platelet count is usually increased. In some patients, particularly when the spleen is enlarged, white cell and platelet counts are decreased. ^{51}Cr red cell survival studies show a half-life of 15—25 days. The Coombs test is negative. The bone marrow is hyperplastic and contains many erythroblasts, frequent plasma cells, and increased numbers of megakaryocytes. With acute exacerbation of chronic hepatitis, histiocytes filled with fat may be seen. In the more severe cases, spur cells and acanthocytes may be seen; bile salts apparently inhibit serum transesterase; cholesterol is not esterified; and free cholesterol accumulates in the membrane and deforms it.

The hemolytic anemia of cirrhosis does not respond to any specific measures nor to corticosteroid therapy. The treatment is that of the underlying disorder.

(4) Acute hemolytic anemia develops occasionally after excessive alcohol intake. Jaundice, hyperlipemia, hypercholesterolemia, and spherocytosis are associated findings. Liver biopsy shows fatty infiltration and only minimal fibrosis. The syndrome improves rapidly with abstinence from alcohol.

Cooper RA, Shattil SJ: Mechanism of hemolysis. New England J Med 285:1514, 1971.

Eichner ER: The hematologic disorders of alcoholism. Am J Med 54:521, 1973.

Eichner ER, Hillman RS: The evolution of anemia in alcoholic patients. Am J Med 50:218, 1971.

Jandl JH: The anemia of liver disease: Observations on its mechanism. J Clin Invest 34:390, 1955.

Sherwood WC: The recognition of hemolytic disease in patients with portal cirrhosis. Am J Clin Path 57:618, 1972.

2. ANEMIA OF CANCER

Anemia of cancer may be due to any of the following:

(1) Chronic blood loss with subsequent development of iron deficiency anemia.

(2) Hemolysis, usually moderate and demonstrable only by ^{51}Cr red cell survival studies. Occasionally, hemolysis is severe and acute and features schistocytes.

(3) Replacement of functional marrow by the malignant tissue ("myelophthisic anemia").

Hyman GA, Harvey JL: The pathogenesis of anemia in patients with carcinoma. Am J Med 19:350, 1955.

3. ANEMIA OF INFECTION

Anemia usually develops only in chronic infections which are clinically obvious, eg, in patients with lung abscess, empyema, pelvic inflammatory disease, tuberculosis, or rheumatoid arthritis. The anemia in these cases is only moderately severe, and the hemoglobin rarely falls below 9 gm/100 ml. The cells are normocytic and may be slightly hypochromic. The reticulocyte count is normal, low, or slightly elevated. Platelets and white cells are not remarkable, although there may be toxic granulation of polymorphonuclear cells. The serum iron is low, but (in contrast to iron deficiency anemia) the total iron-binding capacity is also low. The red cell life span is moderately shortened and there is an insufficient increase in erythropoiesis. Red cell protoporphyrin levels are high. Erythropoietin activity is decreased. Iron reutilization is decreased. The bone marrow contains decreased, normal, or increased numbers of cells. Hemosiderin appears fuzzy and diffuse. No sideroblasts are seen. Severe anemia with a marked degree of hemolysis may develop during the course of subacute bacterial endocarditis, *Escherichia coli* infection, hemolytic streptococcus infection, or *Clostridium welchii* infection.

Cartwright GE, Wintrobe MM: The anemia of infection. XVII. A review. Advances Int Med 5:165, 1952.

4. ANEMIA OF AZOTEMIA

Anemia commonly develops during the course of renal insufficiency from any cause. The red cells are normocytic and normochromic, and there is little variation from normal in size and shape. "Acanthocytes" (cells with thorny outpocketings) and schistocytes (contracted cells) are occasionally seen. The reticulocyte count is normal, low, or slightly elevated. The bone marrow usually shows a striking decrease in the number of nucleated red cells. Erythropoietin levels are very low. Ferrokinetic measurements show decreased red cell life span and an inadequate increase in bone marrow erythropoiesis. Hemolysis is occasionally severe, with greatly shortened red cell survival time. Renal failure may be considered responsible for anemia if the NPN is above 75 mg/100 ml, the BUN above 50 mg/100 ml, or the serum creatinine above 2 mg/100 ml.

Adamson JW, Eschbach J, Finch CA: The kidney and erythropoiesis. Am J Med 44:725, 1968.

Desforges JF: Anemia in uremia. Arch Int Med 126:808, 1970.

Eisler A: Anemia of chronic renal disease. Arch Int Med
  126:774, 1970.
Nieman RS & others: Hypersplenism in the uremic hemodialyzed patient. Am J Clin Path 60:502, 1973.

•   •   •

LEUKEMIAS

1. ACUTE LEUKEMIA

Essentials of Diagnosis

- Weakness, malaise, anorexia, bone and joint pain.
- Pallor, fever, petechiae, lymph node swelling, splenomegaly.
- Leukocytosis; immature, abnormal white cells in peripheral blood and bone marrow.
- Anemia, thrombocytopenia.

General Considerations

Acute leukemia is a disorder of the blood-forming tissue characterized by proliferation of abnormal white cells. It is generally considered to be neoplastic, occurs in all races, and may develop at any age. The peak incidence of acute lymphatic leukemia is in the first 5 years of life.

Clinical Findings

A. Symptoms and Signs: Presenting complaints are often general, consisting of weakness, malaise, anorexia, fever, and purpura. Pain in the joints, lymph node swelling, or excessive bleeding after dental extraction may also be initial complaints. Petechiae are frequently seen early in the course of the disease. Spleen, liver, and lymph nodes are usually enlarged in acute lymphatic leukemia but in less than half of patients with acute myeloblastic leukemia. Sternal tenderness is common. Any organ may be involved.

B. Laboratory Findings: Normochromic, normocytic anemia occurs early. The platelet count is usually below 100,000/cu mm, while the white count varies from less than 10,000 to over 100,000/cu mm. One-third are leukopenic. On the blood smear immature and abnormal cells may be seen; on a thick or over-stained smear they may be mistaken for lymphocytes.

Auer bodies, red-staining rods in the cytoplasm of myeloblasts or monoblasts, occur in 10–20% and are pathognomonic of acute leukemia. Acute myelocytic leukemia may be differentiated from acute lymphocytic leukemia by the presence of peroxidase-staining cytoplasmic granules in the former.

There is massive proliferation of primitive malignant cells in the bone marrow even when leukopenia exists.

Skeletal involvement can be seen radiologically in almost all of the children and in half of the adults. Diffuse osteoporosis, periosteal elevation, osteolytic lesions, and radiolucent metaphyseal bands are the most common lesions.

Complications

Fatal gastrointestinal tract hemorrhage, pressure symptoms on the brain stem, brain hemorrhage, and overwhelming infection are the chief causes of death. Intracerebral hemorrhage occurs more frequently in patients with very high white cell counts (over 300,000/cu mm).

Differential Diagnosis

The combination of anemia, thrombocytopenia, and bone marrow proliferation of primitive white cells is found only in leukemia. Leukocytosis may or may not be present. Among the other features, petechiae may be seen in idiopathic thrombocytopenic purpura or in aplastic anemia, but there is no enlargement of lymph nodes, liver, or spleen. Enlarged lymph nodes and splenomegaly may be found in infectious mononucleosis, Hodgkin's disease, or in lymphosarcoma, but the bone marrow and peripheral red cells and platelets are usually normal. Marked lymphocytosis is often seen in whooping cough and infectious lymphocytosis, but the white cells are mature and red cell and platelet counts are normal. Malignant tumors, eg, neuroblastoma, osteosarcoma, and metastatic cancer, may cause bone pain, anemia, and leukocytosis; if there is marrow invasion, these conditions may resemble leukemia.

Treatment

A. Acute Lymphatic Leukemia: Because it is generally believed that unless every leukemic cell in the body is destroyed the residual cells will multiply and cause a relapse, attempts are now being made to cure this disease by using multiple agents in an effort to kill all leukemic cells. It is estimated that the total burden of malignant cells when leukemia first presents clinically is in the neighborhood of 10^{12}–10^{13} cells. Initial therapy will reduce that to 10^9 cells, which results in an apparent clinical and hematologic remission, ie, the marrow will appear normal. Consolidation therapy will reduce the total number of leukemic cells to 10^6 or fewer. As the total burden of cells decreases, it becomes more difficult to treat the leukemic cells without damaging normal cells. It is not clear whether the body's own immunologic defenses can cope with this residue or whether additional aggressive chemotherapy is required. Multiple drug therapy attacks the leukemic cells in different phases of the mitotic cycle—eg, vincristine arrests cells in mitosis, prednisone lyses lymphoblasts in their resting phases or prevents their entry into DNA synthesis, mercaptopurine inhibits DNA synthesis, and methotrexate inhibits DNA, RNA, and protein synthesis. Use of these drugs sequentially or in combination also avoids drug resistance to a large extent and improves the chances of destroying the leukemic cells that are in a "resting phase" (ie, nondividing) and are usually relatively insensitive to chemotherapy. Finally, prophylactic therapy to the CNS eradicates foci of malignant cells in "sanctuaries" not reached by systemic therapy.

The current schemes of multiple drug therapy and prophylactic CNS treatment as compared to single drug treatment have a considerably higher morbidity, are more costly, and often remove patients from their home environment for longer periods of time. In deciding which approach to use, the physician must weigh these problems against the chance of prolonging survival.

The following regimen incorporates most of the above considerations:

1. For rapid initial remission—

a. Vincristine, 0.05 mg/kg (2 mg/sq m) IV once a week for 4 weeks, plus—

b. Prednisone, 1 mg/kg (40 mg/sq m) orally daily.

2. For consolidation and further distribution of drug—Methotrexate, 15 mg/sq m orally twice a week.

3. To destroy residual leukemic blood in CNS—Radiation to cerebrospinal axis, 2400 R.

4. Prolonged maintenance—Mercaptopurine, 2.5 mg/kg daily orally, or methotrexate, 15 mg/sq m twice a week orally, or cyclophosphamide, 200 mg/sq m weekly orally.

5. Management of relapses—Acute relapses may be treated with vincristine and prednisone, as above, or cytarabine, 50—100 mg daily IV for 4 days, or daunomycin, 1 mg/kg IV daily for 4 days.

B. Acute Myeloblastic Leukemia: This is usually a disease of adults. The objective of therapy is prolonged remission since cure is not possible at present. The reasons for multiple drug therapy are similar to those that justify similar treatment of acute lymphatic leukemia, but the effective agents are different. Many schemes have been used. Intermittent therapy is in favor at present because it appears to minimize toxic suppression of normal cells. The following 2 regimens are most widely used in current practice:

1. Cytarabine and thioguanine—

a. Cytarabine, 2—3 mg/kg IV daily in 2 divided doses 12 hours apart for 4 days, plus—

b. Thioguanine, 2.5 mg/kg orally daily in 2 divided doses 12 hours apart for 4 days; repeat every 2 weeks.

2. "COAP"*—Cyclophosphamide, 100 mg/sq m orally daily for 4 days; vincristine, 2 mg IV once only; cytarabine, 100 mg/sq m IV daily for 4 days; and prednisone, 200 mg orally daily. Cycles are repeated every 2 weeks until the marrow is clear.

3. Other agents—Other agents that have been used in the treatment of acute myeloblastic leukemia include mercaptopurine (Purinethol), 2.5 mg orally daily; vincristine, 0.05 mg IV once a week; daunomycin, 1—2 mg/kg orally daily for 4 days; and cyclophosphamide, 100—150 mg/sq m IV daily for 4 days. For maintenance, one may use mercaptopurine, 2.5 mg/kg orally daily.

*Acronym for Cytoxan (cyclophosphamide), Oncovin (vincristine), Ara-C (cytarabine), and prednisone.

C. Treatment of Complications:

1. Local manifestations—Severe bone pain, massive lymph node enlargement interfering with respirations and swallowing, and CNS involvement with signs of increased intracranial pressure may be treated successfully with local irradiation. Intrathecal methotrexate, 5 mg dissolved in 10 ml of spinal fluid administered every 3 days until the spinal fluid is clear, may be a valuable adjunct to oral or intramuscular methotrexate.

2. Fever—In adult patients with leukemia, bacterial infection is ultimately proved in 75% of cases to be the cause of febrile episodes. Septicemia and infections of the throat, lungs, skin, urinary tract, and anorectal area are the usual causes. Gram-negative organisms—especially pseudomonas, but also *Escherichia coli,* klebsiella, proteus, and bacteroides—are frequently identified. In a febrile patient the following antibiotics should be started pending results of blood cultures and continued for 1 week: In a patient with adequate circulating granulocyte levels, one may use gentamicin, 1 mg/kg IV over 1 hour every 8 hours, plus cephalothin, 4 gm IV over one-half hour every 6 hours. In patients with significant granulocytopenia, also give carbenicillin, 5 gm IV over one-half hour every 4 hours. These drugs can be mixed in the intravenous infusion bottle and should be given over periods of one-half to 1 hour. Fungal infections, virus hepatitis, herpes zoster, cytomegalovirus, and infections with *Pneumocystis carinii* may also occur in the compromised host and call for specific management.

3. Hemorrhage—For patients with severe thrombocytopenia and bleeding, platelet concentrates should be given to raise the platelet count to at least 60,000/cu mm. To estimate dosage, assume that 1 unit will raise the count of a 70 kg subject by 10,000/cu mm.

4. Hyperuricemia—Allopurinol, which inhibits the formation of uric acid, should be administered to patients with high uric acid or high white count along with chemotherapy. A high fluid intake is also important. The usual dose of allopurinol is 100 mg 3—4 times daily. The dose of mercaptopurine must be reduced to 25—35% of the usual dose when allopurinol is being given.

Prognosis

A. Acute Lymphatic Leukemia: Over 90% of patients under 20 years of age treated as above can be brought into a state of remission. The mean duration of remissions is 1—3 years. Using the above approach or some variation of it, survival for several years can now be achieved in 15—25% of all patients.

B. Acute Myeloblastic Leukemia: Up to 50% of patients with acute myeloblastic leukemia will achieve remissions on the above 2 regimens. The median duration of remissions is 1 year or less, but survivals of several years occur occasionally.

Boggs DR, Wintrobe MM, Cartwright G: The acute leukemias. Medicine 41:163, 1962.

Clarkson B & others: Changing concepts of treatment in acute leukemia. M Clin North America 55:561, 1971.

Levi JA, Vincent PC, Gunz FW: Combination chemotherapy of adult acute nonlymphatic leukemia. Ann Int Med 76:397, 1972.

Levine AS & others: Hematologic malignancies and other marrow failure states: Progress in the management of complicating infections. Seminars Hemat 11:141, 1974.

Pinkel D: Five-year follow-up of total therapy of childhood lymphocytic leukemia. JAMA 216:648, 1971.

2. CHRONIC MYELOCYTIC LEUKEMIA

Essentials of Diagnosis

- Weakness, lassitude, fever, abdominal discomfort.
- Painless enlargement of spleen.
- Unexplained leukocytosis, immature white cells in peripheral blood and bone marrow.
- Anemia.

General Considerations

Chronic leukemia is characterized by proliferation of abnormal white cells, which invade the blood stream and may infiltrate any part of the body to cause local symptoms. It is inevitably fatal.

In addition to their immaturity, leukemic cells have certain distinguishing biochemical characteristics. Leukemic neutrophilic cells have less glycogen and alkaline phosphatase than normal or polycythemia white cells, whereas their histamine content is higher. Many of the immature myeloid cells in blood and marrow characteristically show the so-called Philadelphia chromosome, an abnormally small autosome.

Chronic myelocytic leukemia is primarily a disease of young adults, but it may be found at any age.

Clinical Findings

A. Symptoms and Signs: Pallor, weakness, sternal tenderness, fever, purpura, skin nodules, and retinal hemorrhages or exudate may be seen. There may be abdominal discomfort secondary to splenomegaly. Gum bleeding after dental extraction, or large ecchymoses or muscle bleeding after trauma—presumably manifestations of thrombasthenia—may be the presenting sign.

Some patients are diagnosed accidentally before the onset of symptoms when a high white count is found during a routine examination.

B. Laboratory Findings: The white count may exceed 500,000/cu mm, but fewer than 5% of the cells are "blasts." Nonfilamented neutrophils, metamyelocytes, and myelocytes predominate; the neutrophils are alkaline phosphatase negative; basophils, eosinophils, and platelets are increased; and a few normoblasts may be seen. Some degree of anemia is common. The marrow shows complete replacement of fat by cellular elements, mostly granulocytes, but few blasts.

Differential Diagnosis

In leukemoid reactions due to infection or metastatic cancer, eosinophils and basophils are decreased rather than increased, the leukocyte alkaline phosphatase is strongly positive, and the marrow is only moderately hyperplastic. In myelofibrosis, the spleen may be quite large but leukocytosis only moderate; the marrow is fibrotic, the granulocytes are usually alkaline phosphatase positive; and the Philadelphia chromosome is not seen.

Complications

Probably no part of the body is exempt from leukemic infiltration. Complications will depend upon the area infiltrated, eg, pressure symptoms or hemorrhage if the CNS is infiltrated. The spleen may become very large and painful. Half of the patients die in a "blastic" crisis.

Treatment

A. General Measures: The aim of therapy is palliation of symptoms and correction of anemia. Initial manifestations and each exacerbation should be treated promptly. Specific treatment of the anemia is unnecessary, as it is usually corrected by treatment directed at the leukemic process. Blood counts are checked weekly at first and then once or twice a month until a satisfactory remission is obtained. During remission patients are encouraged to resume normal activity, but follow-up visits are necessary every 1–3 months. The nature of the disease should be explained to the patient and the necessity for periodic observation and lifelong treatment should be impressed upon him.

B. Irradiation: X-ray therapy consists of total body irradiation or local therapy to the spleen, liver, or local infiltrates. (X-ray therapy localized to the spleen has a beneficial general effect on the hematopoietic system by mechanisms which are still unknown. Localized high-voltage x-ray over the spleen in doses of 50–100 R daily until a total of 600 R has been given is usually sufficient for clinical hematologic remission.) X-ray therapy (by a radiologist) is given over a period of a few weeks. X-ray is most effective in the treatment of local manifestations.

The results of treatment with radiophosphorus (^{32}P) are comparable to those of total body irradiation; it is less effective in the treatment of local manifestations. There is no radiation sickness. The dosage of ^{32}P depends upon the degree of leukocytosis. One mCi (millicurie) is equivalent to 15 R. If the white count is above 50,000/cu mm, the initial dosage of ^{32}P is 1–2.5 mCi IV; 2 weeks later, 1–1.5 mCi are given. Similar doses are given every 2 weeks until the white count is less than 20,000. During remission patients are seen every 1–3 months. When the white count rises above 25,000, an additional 1–1.5 mCi are given.

C. Chemotherapy: Busulfan (Myleran), an alkylating agent, is the drug of choice. Initial dosage is 2 mg 2–4 times daily, continued until the white count is less than 10,000/cu mm. As a rule, the white count begins to drop within a week and normal values are reached in 4–6 weeks. When the white count reaches about 10,000/cu mm, the drug may be discontinued or administered intermittently. Remissions may last for several months to more than a year. When relapse occurs, a course of busulfan may be repeated. Overtreatment results in general depression of myelopoiesis; irreversible thrombocytopenia may develop. Since thrombocytopenia may occur before any significant drop in hemoglobin, platelet counts should always be done as part of the routine count. The drug should be withheld if platelet values are below normal.

Melphalan (Alkeran) is quite effective. Mercaptopurine, vincristine, and prednisone are used for blastic crises.

Prognosis

The average life expectancy in chronic myelocytic leukemia is about 3–4 years. With appropriate therapy the course is frequently remittent, with periods of months during which the patient is free of symptoms.

Haut A & others: Busulfan in the treatment of chronic myelocytic leukemia. The effect of long term intermittent therapy. Blood 17:1, 1961.
Haut A, Wintrobe MM, Cartwright GE: The clinical management of leukemia. Am J Med 28:777, 1960.

3. CHRONIC LYMPHATIC LEUKEMIA

Essentials of Diagnosis

- Pallor.
- Superficial lymph node enlargement.
- Absolute lymphocytosis in adults.

General Considerations

This disorder involves progressive accumulation of small lymphocytes which have lost the capacity to divide. The life span of these metabolically abnormal cells may be lengthened to several years; the total body lymphocyte mass expands considerably, and may reach enormous proportions. The cells, which originate in lymph nodes, aggregate chiefly in the lymph nodes, spleen, blood, and marrow. The decline in levels of immunoglobulins commonly observed during the course of the disease may represent the replacement of normal, immunologically competent cells by cells that are functionally inert and have lost the ability to react to antigenic stimuli. These lymphocytes have a strikingly low mitotic rate.

The disorder may remain relatively quiescent for several years, free of symptoms and signs and with relatively stable lymphocyte counts; or it may become progressive, with various clinical manifestations and a rising blood count.

Chronic lymphatic leukemia is rare under the age of 30 and extremely rare in Orientals.

Clinical Findings

A. Symptoms and Signs: The onset is insidious, and the diagnosis is usually made accidentally during routine examination. Weakness and symptoms of hypermetabolism may be present. Enlarged lymph nodes may cause pressure symptoms (eg, tracheal compression with respiratory difficulty). The spleen, liver, and lymph nodes are not tender.

B. Laboratory Findings: At the time of diagnosis, the hemoglobin may be normal. Anemia develops as the disease progresses. Lymphocytosis usually precedes the rise in total white count. Eventually, the white count rises and may reach 100–500 thousand/cu mm. Over 90% of the cells are mature lymphocytes; "smudge" cells are common. The platelet count tends to be below normal. Early in the disease, the marrow architecture may be normal; lymphocytes make up more than 30% of cells.

Differential Diagnosis

Similar lymph node enlargement may be seen in lymphosarcoma and infectious mononucleosis. Differentiation is usually readily made on the basis of the blood smear.

Lymphocyte counts of 50–100 thousand/cu mm may be seen in children with whooping cough or infectious lymphocytosis. Lymphatic leukemoid reactions of moderate degree (with white counts of 20–30 thousand/cu mm) are occasionally seen with tuberculosis. Diffuse lymph gland enlargement may be found in lymphosarcoma and infectious mononucleosis, and rarely in tuberculosis, syphilis, carcinomatosis, hyperthyroidism, brucellosis, lupus erythematosus, and toxoplasmosis. In Hodgkin's disease, lymph node enlargement is usually asymmetric or only in a single site.

Complications

Severe hemolytic anemia, frequently with a positive Coombs test, develops in one-third of the patients. Thirty percent of patients have hypogammaglobulinemia and may be susceptible to infection.

Treatment

A. General Measures: It may be desirable to withhold therapy until clinical manifestations appear or until hematologic complications develop. Many older patients with this disorder remain relatively asymptomatic despite high leukocyte levels. All symptomatic patients and all patients with anemia or thrombocytopenia must be treated.

B. Irradiation: As for chronic myelocytic leukemia, but systemic control with splenic radiation is less frequent.

C. Chemotherapy:

1. Chlorambucil is widely used. The dosage is 0.1–0.2 mg/kg daily or 0.4–0.6 mg/kg as a single dose once every 4 weeks or, if necessary, every 2 weeks. Clinical and hematologic improvement may not be evident for 3–4 weeks and maximum improvement may not be achieved for 2–4 months. The drug should be discontinued when the white count falls to

5000–10,000/cu mm. Side-effects are relatively uncommon, although gastrointestinal irritation occurs. Pancytopenia may develop, but recovery usually occurs when the drug is discontinued.

2. Cyclophosphamide, 50–100 mg orally 1–3 times daily may be used.

D. Corticosteroids: Some patients respond well to relatively small doses of corticosteroids. Initially one may give prednisone (or equivalent), 40 mg daily until a response occurs; maintenance may be as little as 10–20 mg every 48 hours.

E. Treatment of Complications:

1. **Anemia**—Anemia is caused by a combination of 2 factors: increased rate of red cell destruction and inadequate bone marrow compensation. It often fails to respond to antileukemic therapy and transfusions have to be given. Prednisolone (or equivalent), 10–20 mg 4 times daily, is usually required. With remission of the anemia, corticosteroids may be gradually withdrawn. With severe hemolytic anemia and splenic sequestration of the red cells, splenectomy may have to be considered. Intercurrent anemia due to blood loss and iron deficiency is treated with iron.

2. **Hemorrhage**—Abnormal bleeding in leukemia is usually due to thrombocytopenia, which may be secondary to either the leukemic process or to therapy. If due to the leukemia, it may be improved by appropriate chemotherapy; if due to chemotherapy, the marrow-depressing drugs must be discontinued and corticosteroid therapy instituted until the marrow has had a chance to recover.

3. **Infections**—Infections are treated with specific antibiotics. Prophylactic use of antibiotics is not recommended. Some patients develop low levels of gamma globulin. With gamma globulin levels of 0.7 gm/100 ml or less, prophylactic gamma globulin is needed. Initially, 0.3 ml/lb is given in divided doses of 5 ml each; a maintenance dose of half this amount is administered once or twice a month.

Prognosis

The average life expectancy in chronic lymphatic leukemia is about 3–4 years. Most patients respond well to chemotherapy or x-ray therapy, and long periods of remission are the rule. In elderly patients the disease may remain inactive, even without treatment, for several years. A more aggressive variant is chronic lymphosarcoma cell leukemia, which may run a course of only 1–2 years.

Boggs DR & others: Factors influencing the duration of survival of patients with chronic lymphocytic leukemia. Am J Med 40:243, 1966.

Galton DAG: The pathogenesis of chronic lymphocytic leukemia. Canad MAJ 94:1005, 1966.

Silver RT: Treatment of chronic lymphatic leukemia. Seminars Hemat 6:344, 1969.

Zacharski LR, Linman JW: Chronic lymphocytic leukemia versus chronic lymphosarcoma cell leukemia. Am J Med 47:75, 1969.

MULTIPLE MYELOMA

Essentials of Diagnosis

- Weakness, weight loss, recurrent pneumonia.
- Constant, severe bone pain aggravated by motion, often associated with pathologic fractures.
- Anemia, rapid sedimentation rate, and elevated serum globulin.
- Immature, atypical plasma cells in bone marrow.

General Considerations

Malignant plasma cells synthesize one of the immunoglobulins to excess, usually IgG or IgA. This accounts for the spike on electrophoresis. Synthesis of normal immunoglobulins is usually decreased. The immunoglobulin consists of 2 pairs of polypeptide chains: a pair of "heavy" chains (molecular weight approximately 55,000 each) whose subunits determine whether the whole molecule belongs to the IgG, IgA, or IgM class; and a pair of "light" chains (molecular weight 20,000 each) which is the same for all 3 molecules. Dimers of light chains form Bence Jones protein, which has no heavy chains. Synthesis of heavy and light chains may be unbalanced, eg, an excess of light chain production leads to Bence Jones proteinuria. The malignant cells may also synthesize only part of an immunoglobulin molecule, eg, in Bence Jones myeloma, which is characterized by generalized hypogammaglobulinemia in the serum and excretion of large amounts of Bence Jones proteins in the urine, giving a paraprotein spike on electrophoresis. Much less commonly, only heavy chains—or portions of heavy chains—are synthesized. These "heavy chain diseases," which may involve excessive production of part of the IgG, IgA, or IgM molecule, clinically resemble lymphosarcoma more than they do multiple myeloma.

Myeloma usually appears in later life. It is seen in all races, and is twice as common in males as in females.

Amyloidosis, whether primary or secondary, is probably always associated with plasma cell neoplasia; abnormal gamma globulin products, particularly those of the Bence Jones type, are directly involved in these tissue ("amyloid") infiltrates.

Clinical Findings

A. Symptoms and Signs: Symptoms of anemia may be the only complaint, or there may be constant bone pain, especially on motion, and tenderness (especially of the back) and spontaneous fractures. Spleen and liver are usually not enlarged. Extramedullary plasma cell tumors are occasionally found in the oropharynx, on the skin, or near the spinal cord. Marked weight loss is common.

B. Laboratory Findings: Anemia is moderate and of the normocytic, normochromic type. Rouleau formation is marked and interferes with the technic of the red count, blood smear, typing, and cross-matching.

The sedimentation rate is greatly elevated; white count, platelet count, and morphology are usually normal. The bone marrow may show sheets of plasma cells with large nuclei and nucleoli.

Serum globulin may exceed 10 gm/100 ml. The electrophoretic pattern is characterized by a tall, sharp peak in contrast to the broad gamma peaks seen in other illnesses with hyperglobulinemia. The abnormal globulin peak may be in the alpha$_2$, beta, or gamma range for immunoglobulin gamma G, and in the gamma to beta range for gamma A. Exact identification of the immunoglobulin is made by immunoelectrophoresis. Cryoglobulin, a serum protein which precipitates in the cold, may be found. Serum calcium levels are often elevated, but phosphorus and alkaline phosphatase values remain normal. Nitrogen retention, proteinuria, and renal casts also occur. Bence Jones proteinuria is found in about 40% of myeloma patients.

The bony lesions appear on x-rays as rounded, punched-out, or mottled areas. New bone formation is lacking. Sometimes there is merely diffuse osteoporosis. In about 10% of cases x-rays are normal early in the disease. Bone scans are usually normal.

Differential Diagnosis

Pathologic fractures and osteolytic lesions are also found in reticulum cell sarcoma, lymphosarcoma, and in metastatic cancer, particularly if the origin is the breast, kidney, prostate, or thyroid. In most of these lesions some attempt at new bone formation is evident. Lymphosarcoma is particularly difficult to differentiate from multiple meyloma when there are bony tumors, oral cavity tumors, cord compression with paraplegia, or invasion of the bone marrow by atypical cells. Electrophoresis usually provides the answer.

Hyperparathyroidism is differentiated by low serum phosphorus and high alkaline phosphatase values. In primary macroglobulinemia (Waldenström), the electrophoretic pattern is similar to that of multiple myeloma, but hemorrhagic phenomena are prominent, bone lesions are, rare, and the pathologic cells resemble lymphocytes rather than plasma cells. The diagnosis is made by demonstration of "specific" macroglobulin paraprotein by immunoelectrophoresis. In the gamma heavy chain diseases, no light chains are demonstrable by immunoelectrophoresis.

In cirrhosis of the liver, cancer, infections, and hypersensitivity reactions, up to 25% of plasma cells may be seen in the bone marrow, but they tend to aggregate near histiocytes and blood vessels and do not form sheets of cells. Hyperglobulinemia may be seen in sarcoidosis, lupus erythematosus, cirrhosis, lymphogranuloma venereum, and kala-azar infections. In most of these disorders, however, the basic disorder is obvious, the plasma cells are adult, and the electrophoretic pattern shows a broad gamma elevation rather than a sharp peak.

A monoclonal "spike" on serum electrophoresis may be observed occasionally in patients who have no other clinical or laboratory stigmas of myeloma or macroglobulinemia. Lymphoma, leukemia, and cancer may be associated disorders; in some cases, no disease is found.

Complications

Complications include paraplegia due to cord tumor, hemorrhage due to thrombocytopenia or interference with the normal coagulation mechanism, recurrent infections due to disturbance of antibody formation, renal failure, and liver disease.

Treatment

A. General Measures: Treatment is supportive only, with the principal aims being control of pain and reduction of tumor masses. Antimetabolites are ineffective. Good urine output must be maintained to prevent protein precipitation in the renal tubules. Ambulation is encouraged to combat negative calcium balance, but patients must avoid exposure to trauma because of their susceptibility to fractures. Frequent blood transfusions may be necessary to combat the anemia. Analgesics may be necessary for control of pain.

B. Irradiation: X-ray therapy is valuable in controlling pain and decreasing tumor mass.

C. Alkylating Agents: Melphalan is probably the most effective agent available now. It is structurally similar to mechlorethamine but is administered orally. The usual dose is 6 mg daily for 2–3 weeks; the maintenance dose is 1–4 mg daily–or one may give 0.25 mg/kg 4 times daily every 4 weeks along with prednisone, 2 mg/kg.

D. Cyclophosphamide: This is another alkylating agent effective at times in the therapy of multiple myeloma. Give 50–100 mg orally 1–3 times daily for maintenance. Side-effects are nausea, alopecia (20%), and leukopenia.

E. Treatment of Complications:

1. Hypercalcemia–Mithramycin, 25 μg/kg IV daily for 4 days, or prednisone, 10 mg orally 4 times daily.

2. **Recurrent infections**–Gamma globulin, 10 ml IM every 2 weeks.

3. **Cord compression**–Laminectomy.

Prognosis

The average survival time after diagnosis is 1½–2 years. Occasionally a patient may live for many years in apparent remission.

Combined Staff Clinics: Plasma cell dyscrasias. Am J Med 44:256, 1968.

Hobbs JR: Paraproteins: Benign or malignant. Brit MJ 3:699, 1967.

Osserman EF, Takatsuki K: Plasma cell myeloma: Gamma globulin synthesis and structure. Medicine 42:357, 1963.

Stone MJ, Frenkel EP: The clinical spectrum of light chain myeloma. Am J Med 58:601, 1975.

MACROGLOBULINEMIA

Macroglobulinemia is a chronic neoplastic disease of the bone marrow which bears some clinical resemblance to both multiple myeloma and chronic lymphocytic leukemia. It is characterized by excessive production of gamma M (IgM) globulin. The disorder usually develops after the age of 50. Symptoms of anemia (weakness, easy fatigability), hemorrhagic phenomena (petechiae and ecchymoses, mucous membrane bleeding), signs of hypermetabolism (fever and weight loss), or peripheral neuropathy may be the presenting findings. Some patients have a moderately enlarged spleen or diffuse lymphadenopathy. The blood may show some degree of pancytopenia; rarely, abnormal white cells, and often some rouleau formation. The marrow may be difficult to aspirate, and biopsy may be necessary to demonstrate a diffuse infiltrate with lymphoid elements and some plasma cells. Precipitated protein may be seen on the marrow smear. Total serum globulin may exceed 7 gm/100 ml. Most sera with a concentration of macroglobulins greater than 2 gm/100 ml and with an electrophoretic mobility in the gamma region will give a positive Sia water (euglobulin) test. Serum protein electrophoresis shows a sharp peak and is indistinguishable from multiple myeloma. Differentiation from multiple myeloma is made by (1) ultracentrifugation, which shows the globulin to be of the S (Svedberg) 19 type or greater, implying a molecular weight in excess of 1 million; (2) immunoelectrophoresis; or (3) demonstration that the IgM is composed of a single light chain type, ie, kappa or lambda. About 10% of patients have Bence Jones protein in their urine. Renal tubule and osteolytic lesions are rare. Many patients have greatly increased blood volumes, and an increase in serum viscosity is common. Smaller amounts of macroglobulin, usually less than 15% of the total globulin, may be seen in malignant lymphomas, collagen diseases, sarcoidosis, cirrhosis, and nephrosis.

In some patients the course is benign over several years. The average survival is about 4 years.

Treatment is with chlorambucil, 0.1–0.2 mg/kg daily, as described on p 297; or melphalan as described above.

Block KJ & others: Gamma heavy chain disease. Am J Med 55:61, 1973.
Cohen R, Bohannon RA, Wallerstein RO: Waldenström's macroglobulinemia. Am J Med 41:278, 1966.
MacKenzie MR, Fudenberg HH: Macroglobulinemia: An analysis of forty patients. Blood 39:874, 1972.
McCallister BD & others: Primary macroglobulinemia: Review with a report on thirty-one cases and notes on the value of continuous chlorambucil therapy. Am J Med 43:394, 1967.

CRYOGLOBULINEMIA

Serum globulins that precipitate on cooling and redissolve on warming may occur in a variety of disorders (eg, myeloma, macroglobulinemia, malignant lymphoma, collagen diseases, glomerulonephritis, infectious mononucleosis, syphilis, and cytomegalovirus disease). They may represent homogeneous proteins that have become physically altered (myeloma), mixtures of immunoglobulins, or immune complexes (eg, IgG and IgM)—ie, antigen and antibody, possibly with complement (eg, lupus erythematosus). The finding of cryoglobulinemia is often without any apparent significance. It is assumed that when symptoms do occur as a result of cryoglobulinemia, the abnormal protein, on cooling, precipitates in smaller vessels and causes increased viscosity, stasis, thrombosis, or hemorrhage.

Clinical manifestations may include a Raynaud-like phenomenon on exposure to cold, oronasal bleeding, purpura, petechiae, retinal vascular constriction and hemorrhage, urticaria, and mottling, ulcerations, necrosis, and gangrene, especially in dependent areas. Cryoglobulins in significant concentrations (30 mg/100 ml) may be demonstrated in the blood.

Treatment consists of preventing exposure to cold and, when possible, treatment of the underlying disease. Penicillamine and immunosuppressive agents have been tried. In general, treatment is unsatisfactory.

Barnett EV & others: Cryoglobulinemia and disease. Ann Int Med 73:95, 1970.
Spalluto LO & others: Cryoglobulinemia based upon interaction between a gamma macroglobulin and 7S gamma globulin. Am J Med 32:142, 1962.

MYELOFIBROSIS
(Myelosclerosis, Agnogenic Myeloid Metaplasia)

Essentials of Diagnosis
- Weakness and fatigue.
- Large spleen.
- "Leukoerythroblastic" blood picture with poikilocytosis.
- "Dry tap" on bone marrow aspiration.

General Considerations
Myelofibrosis is a proliferative neoplastic disorder of the mesenchymal tissue and is probably related to other myeloproliferative disorders such as chronic myelocytic leukemia and polycythemia vera. There is progressive fibrosis of the marrow and myeloid metaplasia in the liver and spleen. The disease is usually seen in adults beyond middle age. In about 10% of cases it is preceded by polycythemia vera. Fibrosis of the marrow is occasionally associated with tuberculosis, metastatic cancer, or Hodgkin's disease.

Clinical Findings

A. Symptoms and Signs: Patients may complain of fatigue, weakness, weight loss, occasionally bone pain, abdominal discomfort, and symptoms of anemia. The spleen is almost always enlarged, usually markedly so. The liver may be enlarged. The lymph nodes are not affected.

B. Laboratory Findings: Anemia may be severe. The red cells vary greatly in size and shape; teardrop-shaped, distorted red cells, nucleated and stippled cells may be seen. The reticulocyte count is often slightly elevated. The white count may be high (20–50 thousand/cu mm), with a marked shift to the left and many basophils. The white cell alkaline phosphatase reaction is usually strongly positive, but may be negative in 10% of patients. The platelet count may be greatly increased initially, and giant platelets and megakaryocyte fragments may be seen. Bone marrow aspiration is usually unsuccessful, yielding only sheets of platelet and megakaryocyte fragments and a few erythroblasts and granulocytes. Bone marrow biopsy shows fibrous tissue replacing normal marrow spaces. Splenic puncture may show erythroblasts, megakaryocytes, and young granulocytes.

Complications

Rapid splenic enlargement may be painful. The patient may develop symptoms of hypermetabolism with fever, sweating, and weight loss.

Secondary hypersplenism may lead to thrombocytopenia and bleeding and to hemolytic anemia with splenic sequestration of red cells. Some patients die in an acute "blastic" crisis.

Differential Diagnosis

In chronic myelocytic leukemia the white cell alkaline phosphatase reaction is negative. Hemolytic anemias are readily differentiated by the great number of reticulocytes, hypercellularity, and red cell hyperplasia of the bone marrow. Lymphoma and metastatic cancer with "dry tap" are differentiated by marrow biopsy.

Treatment

If the spleen is not painful and the anemia only moderate, no treatment may be required. For severe anemia, an androgenic steroid may be used (see p 277). Many patients have to be maintained on multiple transfusions. For painful enlargement of the spleen give busulfan, 2 mg 1–3 times daily, or x-ray radiation. For hemolytic anemia with splenic sequestration give prednisolone (or equivalent), 10–20 mg 4 times daily orally, or consider splenectomy. For "blastic crisis," mercaptopurine, 2.5 mg/kg/day, may be tried.

Prognosis

The average survival from the time of diagnosis is 2–3 years. In some patients the disease remains quiescent for several years even without transfusions. Death is due to hemorrhage, secondary infection, or acute blastic crisis.

Bergsman KL, Van Slyck EJ: Acute myelofibrosis. Ann Int Med 74:232, 1971.

Bouroncle BA, Doan CA: Myelofibrosis: Clinical, hematologic, and pathologic study of 110 patients. Am J Med Sc 243:697, 1962.

Nakai GS & others: Agnogenic myeloid metaplasia. Ann Int Med 57:419, 1962.

Ward HP, Block MH: The natural history of agnogenic myeloid metaplasia. Medicine 50:397, 1971.

HODGKIN'S DISEASE

Essentials of Diagnosis

- Regional lymph nodes enlarged, firm, nontender, painless.
- Fever, weight loss, excessive sweating, pruritus, fatigue.
- Exacerbations and remissions.

General Considerations

Hodgkin's disease is seen in all races and occurs most commonly in young adults. It is characterized by abnormal proliferation, in one or several lymph nodes, of lymphocytes, histiocytes, eosinophils, and Reed-Sternberg giant cells. It starts most likely as a regionally localized process which tends to spread to contiguous lymphatic structures. Accurate measurement of the extent, or "staging," of the disease when first diagnosed is essential for proper management and prognosis. The "stage" of the disease (Table 9–4) is important in determining its course, and the histologic pattern also has prognostic value.

Clinical Findings

A. Symptoms and Signs: Regional unilateral lymphadenopathy (especially swelling of cervical nodes) is usually the presenting sign. The nodes are firm, nontender, and of various sizes. They may adhere to the deeper tissues, but the skin remains freely movable. If the mediastinum is involved early, respiratory difficulty may be the initial complaint. Hepatosplenomegaly and constitutional complaints—fever, excessive sweating, fatigue, and pruritus—usually appear late.

B. Laboratory and X-Ray Findings: The blood count may show an absolute lymphocytopenia, especially in the histologic types showing lymphocytic depletion. Occasionally some eosinophilia is seen. Anemia is a late finding. Diagnosis is made by lymph node biopsy, but the extent of the disease must be well established prior to therapy. This is done by chest x-ray, lower extremity lymphangiogram or inferior venacavagram, scintiscan of the liver and spleen, bone marrow biopsy, and liver function tests. With clinical evidence of disease in the upper abdomen—ie, a large spleen or radiographically demonstrable involvement of upper lumbar lymph nodes—exploratory laparotomy and splenectomy are indicated. The extensive pretherapy diagnostic work-up is important because

Table 9—4. Staging of Hodgkin's disease.

Stage*	Definition
0	No detectable disease due to prior excisional biopsy
I	Single abnormal lymph node
II	Two or more discrete abnormal nodes, limited to one side of diaphragm
III	Disease on both sides of diaphragm but limited to the lymph nodes, spleen, or Waldeyer's ring
IV	Involvement of bone, bone marrow, lung parenchyma, pleura, liver, skin, gastrointestinal tract, CNS, renal or sites other than lymph nodes, spleen, or Waldeyer's ring

*All stages are subclassified to describe the absence (A) or presence (B) of systemic symptoms.

many patients with apparent stage I or II disease actually have more extensive involvement, and this greatly influences the plan of therapy. Histopathologic classification of the tumor also is of prognostic value. In general, patients with lymphocytic predominance and nodular sclerosis do better than patients with a mixed pattern (histiocytes and lymphocytes) or lymphocytic depletion.

Differential Diagnosis

Hodgkin's disease must be distinguished from other diseases which involve lymph tissue. Anticonvulsive agents may produce lymph node changes similar to those seen in Hodgkin's disease. Differential diagnosis is made by biopsy, blood smear, or serologic tests.

Complications

Hemolytic anemia, intractable itching, superior vena cava obstruction, and pleural effusion occur. Painful and tender Hodgkin's sarcoma may develop. Paraplegia from extradural cord compression may occur.

Treatment

Radiation is used for stages I, II, and III in an effort to eradicate the disease. Chemotherapy is palliative for patients with advanced disease, especially if they have constitutional symptoms. Occasionally, the 2 methods are combined.

A. Irradiation: The treatment of choice for regionally localized disease is wide-field megavoltage radiotherapy to 3500—4000 R in 4 weeks. Some radiotherapists give similar doses to the involved areas in stage III disease. Depending on the site and extent of the disease, one ("extended field") or both ("total nodal") of the following fields will have to be irradiated: The "mantle" field covers the cervical, supraclavicular, infraclavicular, axillary, hilar, and mediastinal nodes to the level of the diaphragm; the "inverted Y" covers the splenic pedicle, celiac, para-aortic, iliac, inguinal, and femoral nodes.

B. Antitumor Chemotherapy (Stage III or IV):

1. Combination chemotherapy—This is the treatment of choice. To obtain maximal antitumor effect with minimal damage to healthy tissue, combinations of drugs with different mechanisms of action and various dose-limiting toxicities have been employed in preference to a large dose of a single drug. The following scheme ("MOPP")* has been used: mechlorethamine, 6 mg/sq m IV on days 1 and 8; vincristine, 1.4 mg/sq m IV on days 1 and 8; procarbazine, 100 mg/sq m orally daily for 14 days in each cycle; and prednisone, 40 mg/sq m orally daily for 14 days during cycles 1 and 4 only. A complete cycle consists of these 2 weeks of intensive therapy followed by a rest period of 2 weeks without any treatment. Cyclophosphamide, 650 mg/sq m IV, may be substituted for mechlorethamine. Three to 6 cycles are normally given.

2. Mechlorethamine (nitrogen mustard)—0.4 mg/kg of the powder is dissolved in sterile water and given within 5 minutes into an infusion of physiologic saline. Patients are best treated in the evening after a light lunch and no supper. The unpleasant immediate side-effects of nausea and vomiting should be controlled by premedication with sedatives and antiemetic agents. Improvement of symptoms and reduction in size of lymph node masses may begin in 1—3 days. Medication may be repeated every 2 months as long as there is no marrow depression.

3. Chlorambucil—Used for maintenance for 3—6 weeks after mechlorethamine therapy in severe cases or instead of mechlorethamine in less severe cases. Give 0.2 mg/kg orally in divided doses after meals. Improvement may not begin for 3—4 weeks, and maximum improvement may not be achieved for 2—4 months. Side-effects are rare, but medication must be discontinued if bone marrow depression occurs. Patients should be followed with weekly blood counts at first and less frequently thereafter (but at least once a month).

4. Cyclophosphamide, 2—3 mg/kg IV daily for 6 days followed by 50—100 mg orally 1—3 times daily for maintenance. The principal disadvantage of this drug is the high incidence (20%) of alopecia and chemical hemorrhagic cystitis.

5. Vinblastine sulfate (Velban) may be tried in resistant cases. Give 0.1—0.15 mg/kg IV once a week, depending upon the white count. Untoward reactions include nausea, peripheral neuropathy, and alopecia.

6. Procarbazine, 50—200 mg daily orally.

7. Bleomycin, 15—30 mg IV once a week.

C. Treatment of Complications:

1. Autoimmune hemolytic anemia—See p 279.

2. Fever—(See p 1.) For fever that does not respond to antibiotics, one may try indomethacin, 25 mg orally 4 times daily, or colchicine, 3 mg in 20 ml of saline solution given slowly IV.

3. Mediastinal or spinal cord compression is treated with mechlorethamine, 0.4 mg/kg IV, followed 24 hours later by x-ray therapy.

*Acronym for mechlorethamine, Oncovin (vincristine), procarbazine, and prednisone.

Prognosis

Patients with true stage I or II disease who receive intensive radiotherapy and who have no new manifestations for 5 years (about 50% of patients so treated) have at least a 95% chance of being cured. New manifestations, usually by extension of disease from the original site, occur in the other 50%, but usually within 2 years after initial therapy. Attempts are now being made to reduce the incidence of extension by prophylactically radiating apparently uninvolved contiguous areas. The overall 5-year survival in Hodgkin's disease appears to be about 30% at the present time.

DeVita VT & others: Combination chemotherapy in the treatment of advanced Hodgkin's disease. Ann Int Med 73:881, 1970.

Hellman S: Current status of Hodgkin's disease. New England J Med 290:894, 1974.

Kaplan HS, Rosenberg SA: The management of Hodgkin's disease. Cancer 36 (Suppl):796, Aug 1975.

Lukes RJ & others: Natural history of Hodgkin's disease as related to its pathologic picture. Cancer 19:317, 1966.

Rosenberg S: Splenectomy in the management of Hodgkin's disease. Brit J Haemat 23:271, 1972.

Rubin P: Updated Hodgkin's disease. JAMA 222:1292, 1972; 223:49, 1973.

MALIGNANT LYMPHOMA

The malignant lymphomas can be divided into the following categories, each of which may occur in a diffuse form or in a nodular form: (1) Lymphocytic, well differentiated. (The diffuse form may be hard to distinguish from chronic lymphatic leukemia or macroglobulinemia.) (2) Lymphocytic, poorly differentiated. (This corresponds to what was formerly called lymphosarcoma.) (3) Histiocytic (formerly reticulum cell sarcoma). (4) Mixed lymphocytic and histiocytic. (5) Undifferentiated or stem cell malignant lymphoma (occurs only in the diffuse form). (Burkitt's lymphoma is an example of this category.)

The nodular forms correspond to the former "giant follicular lymphoma." A complete histopathologic diagnosis may be as follows: "lymphocytic lymphoma, well differentiated, nodular type." In general, the nodular lymphomas do better than the diffuse ones and the well differentiated forms have a better prognosis than the poorly differentiated ones.

Diffuse enlargement of lymph nodes may be seen in rheumatoid arthritis, secondary syphilis, mononucleosis, toxoplasmosis, herpes simplex infection, or in association with anticonvulsant therapy with phenytoin (Dilantin). Often it is better to rule out these disorders by appropriate serologic tests before doing a lymph node biopsy.

The malignant lymphomas may arise in any lymphoid aggregate. Lymphadenopathy, usually painless, is the initial abnormality in most patients, occurring most frequently in the neck and usually unilaterally at first. Initial nasopharyngeal, mediastinal, or intra-abdominal involvement is not infrequent. The skin, gastrointestinal tract, nervous system, and bones are involved occasionally. Malaise, fever, weight loss, and sweating are the presenting findings. The liver or spleen is enlarged during the course of the illness in about a third of patients. The diagnosis is made by. lymph node biopsy, which shows destruction of node architecture and replacement with tightly packed lymphocytes, lymphoblasts, or histiocytes.

This is a disease of middle age, but it may also occur in children. The median survival is 2 years in adults, but less than a year in patients under age 16.

Unlike Hodgkin's disease, which is often unifocal initially and may be cured by intensive local or "mantle" irradiation, the malignant lymphomas are usually multifocal from the beginning, and therapy is merely palliative; local irradiation should rarely exceed 2500 R (in air). However, if careful staging indicates localized disease, intensive radiotherapy, as described in the section on Hodgkin's disease, is worthwhile to attempt a cure. Corticosteroids are often helpful in generalized disease. Chemotherapy is used as in Hodgkin's disease. Since lymphoid tissue may be destroyed rapidly, all patients should be on allopurinol, 100 mg 3 times daily, for the acute phase of therapy. Combination chemotherapy may be more effective than single agents, eg, "CVP" (cyclophosphamide, vincristine, prednisone). Give cyclophosphamide, 15 mg/kg IV on day 1, vincristine, 0.025 mg/kg IV on day 1, and prednisone, 0.6 mg/kg orally daily for 5 days. Give no therapy from day 6 to day 21. On day 22, repeat cyclophosphamide and vincristine. On day 42 start a new cycle. One usually gives 4–6 cycles.

Bagley CM & others: Advanced lymphosarcoma: Intensive cyclical combination chemotherapy with cyclophosphamide, vincristine, and prednisone. Ann Int Med 76:227, 1972.

DeVita VT Jr & others: Advanced histocytic lymphoma: A potentially curable disease. Lancet 1:248, 1975.

Jones SE & others: Non-Hodgkin's lymphomas. 4. Clinicopathologic correlation in 405 cases. Cancer 31:806, 1973.

Kaplan HS: Clinical evaluation and radiotherapeutic management of Hodgkin's disease and the malignant lymphomas. New England J Med 278:892, 1968.

Rappaport H, Winter WJ, Hicks EB: Follicular lymphoma: A reevaluation of its position in the scheme of malignant lymphoma, based on a survey of 253 cases. Cancer 9:792, 1956.

Schein PS & others: Potential for prolonged disease-free survival following combination chemotherapy of non-Hodgkin's lymphoma. Blood 43:181, 1974.

WHO Memorandum: Histopathological definition of Burkitt's tumor. Bull WHO 40:601, 1969.

HAIRY CELL LEUKEMIA
(Leukemic Reticuloendotheliosis)

This variant of malignant lymphoma is characterized by splenomegaly without lymphadenopathy, pancytopenia, and the typical "hairy" cells, ie, lymphoid cells with cytoplasmic projection on a freshly made peripheral blood film; these cells contain tartrate-resistant acid phosphatase. On biopsy, the marrow shows mononuclear cells with striking fibrosis. The clinical course is relatively benign. Splenectomy may be helpful. Chemotherapy is contraindicated.

Burke JS, Byrne GE Jr, Rapaport H: Hairy cell leukemia. Cancer 33:1399, 1974.

IMMUNOBLASTIC LYMPHADENOPATHY

This recently described entity resembles Hodgkin's disease but differs from it pathologically in several important ways. Patients have fever, sweats, weight loss, in some cases a rash, and diffuse, striking lymphadenopathy. Polyclonal hyperglobulinemia and hemolytic anemia are frequent findings. Lymph nodes show proliferation of arborizing blood vessels, interstitial amorphous acidophilic material, but no Reed-Sternberg cells. It is thought to represent a nonneoplastic hyperimmune proliferation of B lymphocytes, although occasional cases have been reported in association with combination treatment with cyclophosphamide, vincristine, and prednisone. The disorder is frequently fatal in a year or so.

Lukes RJ, Tindle BJ: Immunoblastic lymphadenopathy: A hyperimmune entity resembling Hodgkin's disease. New England J Med 292:1, 1975.

MYCOSIS FUNGOIDES

Mycosis fungoides is a malignant, progressive, proliferative disease, primarily of the skin. Initially, the lesions may resemble eczema, seborrheic dermatitis, psoriasis, or erythroderma; eventually they may become elevated and form tumors. Lymph nodes, liver, and spleen may become involved. Pathologically, the disease probably belongs to the lymphoma group; the malignant growth arises in the lymphoid-reticular system. The early histopathologic features are usually nonspecific. In the later stages of the disease, the characteristic findings are pleomorphic cellular infiltrates in the skin, with focal collections of mononuclear cells in the epidermis. When the cellular aggregates form tumors, they may break through the epidermis and ulcerate. At this stage, histologic distinction from reticulum cell sarcoma and Hodgkin's disease may be impossible. Generalized itching and lymph node enlargement are frequent systemic manifestations. The disorder resembles Sézary's syndrome (erythroderma with atypical lymphocytes).

The interval between the first appearance of a

seemingly benign chronic skin eruption and the definite diagnosis of mycosis fungoides may be several years. Most patients die within 3–4 years after the tissue diagnosis is made.

Treatment is palliative, but good results may be obtained with electron beam radiation to give very little skin penetration and permit total body irradiation without visceral damage. Chemotherapy with mechlorethamine, cyclophosphamide, or methotrexate is the alternative. Weekly topical application of mechlorethamine (10 mg in 50 ml of water) may be helpful in the early stages.

Block JB & others: Mycosis fungoides. Am J Med 34:228, 1963.
Epstein EH & others: Mycosis fungoides. Medicine 51:61, 1972.
Winkelmann RK, Linman JW: Erythroderma with atypical lymphoma. Am J Med 55:192, 1973.

SÉZARY'S SYNDROME

This syndrome is characterized by chronic skin lesions, chiefly intensely pruritic erythroderma with mononuclear infiltration of the dermis and many abnormal lymphoid cells in the blood; they are thought to be of thymic origin (T cells). The cells may contain PAS-positive, cytoplasmic granules that are resistant to diastase. The disorder resembles mycosis fungoides in several ways and is treated similarly.

Crossen P & others: The Sézary syndrome. Am J Med 50:24, 1971.

HISTIOCYTOSIS

The histiocytic cell series includes monoblasts, monocytes, and immature and mature tissue macrophages. Each of these cells may undergo malignant transformation.

Acute monocytic leukemia results from malignant transformation of the monoblast. Malignant lymphoma, histiocytic type (reticulum cell sarcoma), arises from poorly differentiated macrophages.

Histiocytic medullary reticulosis, which clinically resembles acute leukemia and is characterized by striking phagocytosis of red cells, white cells, and platelets, also arises from immature macrophages.

Histiocytosis X is a term that has been applied to a group of disorders including eosinophilic granuloma of bone, Hand-Schüller-Christian disease, and Letterer-Siwe disease. These conditions are of unknown cause. They are characterized by proliferation of well-differentiated histiocytes and reticulum cells, and they may be closely related, perhaps differing only in individual host resistance.

Eosinophilic granuloma of bone is a relatively

benign, usually solitary osteolytic lesion. It is frequently asymptomatic and is discovered only on x-ray. It may cause pain, tenderness, swelling, and pathologic fracture. Biopsy shows histiocytic proliferation with eosinophilic infiltration. It can be treated successfully by curettage, excision, or radiation; it may also recur at another site. It is most frequently seen in children and adolescents; the commonest sites are the pelvis, head, ribs, and vertebrae. The blood is usually not involved. It is not familial and is not restricted to any particular race.

Hand-Schüller-Christian disease is a disseminated disorder involving many bones, especially the flat bones, with multiple osteolytic lesions. It is a disease of childhood, not familial, and not restricted to any race. Clinically, it frequently causes diabetes insipidus. Other manifestations may be exophthalmos, eczema or eczematoid dermatitis, otitis media, and upper respiratory infections. The lymph nodes, liver, and spleen may be enlarged. The diagnosis is established by biopsy. The blood is usually not involved. Treatment may include radiation or chemotherapy with prednisone or vincristine.

Letterer-Siwe disease is characterized by proliferation of histiocytes in the skin, liver, spleen, lymph nodes, and sometimes the bones and lungs. It is not familial and may be seen in all races. Patients are often wasted; they have marked enlargement of the spleen and liver, maculopapular skin lesions, and recurrent infections. Pancytopenia is common, and the marrow may be replaced by histiocytes. It is most commonly seen in children under 3 years of age but it occurs also in older children, usually with a better prognosis. Prednisone and several antimetabolites may be used in therapy.

Abele DC & others: Histiocytic medullary reticulosis. Arch Dermat 106:319, 1972.

Cline MJ, Golde DW: A review and reevaluation of the histiocytic disorders. Am J Med 55:49, 1973.

Lahey ME: Prognosis in reticuloendotheliosis in children. J Pediat 60:664, 1962.

Lichtenstein L: Histiocytosis X (eosinophilic granuloma of bone, Letterer-Siwe disease, and Schüller-Christian disease). J Bone Joint Surg 46A:76, 1964.

Lieberman PH & others: A reappraisal of eosinophilic granuloma of bone, Hand-Schüller-Christian syndrome, and Letterer-Siwe syndrome. Medicine 48:375, 1969.

Vogel JM, Vogel P: Idiopathic histiocytosis. Seminars Hemat 9:349, 1972.

POLYCYTHEMIA VERA

Essentials of Diagnosis

- Malaise, fatigue, weakness.
- Florid facies, dusky redness of mucosa.
- Greatly increased red cell values and increase in total red cell mass.

General Considerations

Polycythemia vera is a myeloproliferative disorder which often involves one or several formed elements, such as red cells, white cells, or platelets in varying degrees. Symptoms are probably due to increased blood viscosity and hypermetabolism. Although the disease may occur at any age, it is usually a disorder of middle age. It is more common in men than in women. Erythropoietin production is greatly depressed.

Clinical Findings

A. Symptoms and Signs: Patients may complain of headache, inability to concentrate, some hearing loss, itching (especially after bathing), pain in the fingers and toes, and redness of the conjunctivas. They may have a decreased feeling of well-being and a loss of efficiency and energy. A dusky redness is particularly noticeable on the lips, fingernails, and mucous membranes. The retinal veins are frequently tortuous and black. There is no clubbing of the fingers. The spleen is palpable in about half of cases at initial examination.

B. Laboratory Findings: The red cell count is 6–10 million/cu mm; the hemoglobin is above 18 gm/100 ml in men and above 16 gm/100 ml in women; and the hematocrit is over 55%. The white count may be normal or as high as 20,000/cu mm, and there may be an increase in basophils. The leukocyte alkaline phosphatase content is increased; platelets often are elevated and may be above 1 million/cu mm, but may be normal. Some patients with greatly elevated platelet counts (over 1 million/cu mm) but hemoglobin concentrations in the normal range may have masked polycythemia vera. In these cases the increased red cell volume may be obscured by a simultaneous rise in plasma volume. In others, chronic gastrointestinal bleeding may keep the red cell volume within the normal range.

The bone marrow shows hyperactivity of all elements with a corresponding decrease in marrow fat; the increase in megakaryocytes may be striking.

The arterial oxygen saturation is normal or slightly low, but always above 91%. The uric acid is frequently elevated to 5–10 mg/100 ml. The red cell volume is increased above the upper normal of 33 ml/kg.

Differential Diagnosis

Polycythemia vera must be differentiated especially from high normal values (see below), which remain relatively stable and do not increase; and from stress erythrocytosis, a state of decreased plasma volume, normal red cell volume, and rapid fluctuations in blood values seen occasionally in tense individuals.

The upper limits of normal for males are as follows: Hemoglobin, 18 gm/100 ml; red blood cell count, 6.2 million; hematocrit, 54%. For women: Hemoglobin, 16 gm/100 ml; red blood cell count, 5.4 million; hematocrit, 47%.

In secondary polycythemia the basic pulmonary or cardiac disorder is usually obvious, as in cyanotic heart disease and pulmonary fibrosis. In marked obesity (Pickwickian syndrome), which may also result in hypoventilation, the arterial oxygen saturation is distinctly decreased, leukocytosis and thrombocytosis are absent, and bone marrow hyperplasia is limited to the erythroid series. (Emphysema rarely raises the hemoglobin more than 1–2 gm/100 ml above normal.)

Occasionally a structural hemoglobin abnormality is responsible for tight oxygen binding; only partial pressure of blood oxygen is decreased, and dissociation at the tissue level is below normal.

Polycythemia may occur in association with renal tumors or cysts, pyelonephritis, renal obstructive disease, cerebellar hemangioblastoma, uterine fibroids, and hepatoma. Some of these disorders may be responsible for excessive erythropoietin production. The spleen usually is not enlarged, and the white cells and platelets are not affected.

Complications

Hemorrhage (particularly gastrointestinal bleeding) and thrombosis (cerebral, pulmonary, or deep vein) may occur in uncontrolled polycythemia vera. Excessive bleeding at surgery is common. Secondary gout occurs in about 10% of patients.

Treatment

A. Radiophosphorus (^{32}P): The initial dosage varies from 3–5 mCi IV. If ^{32}P is given orally, the dose is increased by 25%.

After therapy the patient should be seen at intervals of 3–4 weeks until a remission has occurred. Platelets begin to fall at 2 weeks and reach a low point in 3–5 weeks. Red cells begin to decrease at 1 month and reach a low point at 3–4 months. At 2 months, if there has been no effect on platelets or red cells, patients are re-treated with an additional 2–3 mCi or with ^{32}P. If necessary, another 2–3 mCi dose is given at 6 months. When blood counts have returned to normal, patients are reexamined every 3 months.

Remissions may last 6 months to 2 years, and occasionally longer. Relapse is treated by the total initial effective dose but should not exceed 5 mCi.

B. Venesection (Phlebotomy): Remove 500–2000 ml of blood per week until the hematocrit reaches 45%, and repeat phlebotomy whenever the hematocrit rises 4–5%. The average maintenance is 500 ml every 2–3 months. When phlebotomy is the only therapy, medicinal iron must not be given. A low-iron diet is not practical, but certain foods of very high iron content should be avoided (clams, oysters, liver, legumes).

C. Chemotherapy: As an alternative to radiation, myelosuppressive agents may be used. Dosages for initial therapy until response occurs (which may require 3–5 months) are about twice as large as maintenance dosages. Some patients stay in remission without maintenance therapy.

1. Chlorambucil, 10–12 mg/day initially and then 3–4 mg/day.

2. Cyclophosphamide, 100–150 mg/day initially and then 50–75 mg/day.

3. Melphalan, 4–6 mg/day initially and then 2 mg/day or less for maintenance.

D. Treatment of Complications: Surgery in patients with polycythemia vera is frequently complicated by hemorrhage. Patients should be in hematologic remission before operation. Blood loss at surgery is replaced by whole blood transfusions. Fibrinogen (human), 4–6 gm, is given if the bleeding is due to fibrinogen deficiency. Gout is treated the same as primary gout.

Prognosis

In properly treated patients, survival averages approximately 13 years. Three stages of the disease can be recognized: (1) the "florid" stage, with a high red count and hemoglobin, may last many years; (2) compensated myelofibrosis, not requiring treatment, may continue for several more years; (3) the anemic phase, with severe myelofibrosis, megakaryocytic hyperplasia, and a very large spleen lasts for a few months up to 2 years. About 5% of patients die of acute leukemia.

Gardner F (editor): Polycythemia. Seminars Hemat 3:175, 1966.

Pollycove M & others: Classification and evaluation of patterns of erythropoiesis in polycythemia vera studied by iron kinetics. Blood 28:807, 1966.

Treatment of polycythemia: A panel discussion. Blood 32:483, 1968.

Wasserman LR: The management of polycythemia vera. Brit J Haemat 21:371, 1971.

Wasserman LR, Gilbert HS: The treatment of polycythemia vera. M Clin North America 50:1501, 1966.

AGRANULOCYTOSIS

Essentials of Diagnosis

- Chills, fever, sore throat, prostration.
- Ulceration of oral mucosa and throat.
- Granulocytopenia with relative lymphocytosis.
- Increased sedimentation rate.

General Considerations

Agranulocytosis may be secondary to the use of certain drugs and chemicals, eg, antithyroid drugs, sulfonamides, phenothiazines, phenylbutazone, and aminopyrine. Some of these agents lead to the production of circulating agglutinins against granulocytes; in other cases the cause of agranulocytosis is not known. Some drugs, eg, aminopyrine, cause an explosive onset of symptoms and leukopenia; others, eg, the antithyroid drugs and the phenothiazines, produce leukopenia only gradually after several days or weeks, even on readministration.

Clinical Findings

A. Symptoms and Signs: Onset is often sudden, with chills, fever, and extreme weakness. There may be a brownish-gray exudate of the throat and greenish-black membranous ulcers of the oral mucosa, respiratory tract, vagina, and rectum. Regional adenopathy is common. Macules and papules developing into bullae may develop on the skin. The spleen and liver are not enlarged, and there is no bone tenderness.

B. Laboratory Findings: Granulocytes disappear from the blood, and monocytes and lymphocytes may also be reduced in absolute numbers. Red cells and platelets are not affected. The bone marrow appears hypoplastic; only a few early myeloid cells are seen, but red cell series and megakaryocytes are normal. After the offending drug is removed, recovery takes place in 8–10 days; lymphocytes and monocytes reappear before the granulocytes. During recovery, a transient excess of lymphocytes followed by a phase of primitive granulocyte proliferation may be observed in the marrow.

Differential Diagnosis

Differentiate from aplastic anemia (thrombocytopenia and anemia) and from acute aleukemic leukemia (hyperplastic marrow, predominance of malignant cells).

Complications

Complications include sepsis, bronchial pneumonia, hemorrhagic necrosis of mucous membrane lesions, and parenchymal liver damage with jaundice.

Treatment

A. General Measures: Discontinue suspected chemical agents or drugs. Obtain a blood sample for bacterial culture and antibiotic sensitivity testing. Supportive measures include good oral hygiene, adequate fluid intake, and reduction of fever. Patients should be isolated if possible to reduce exposure to infection.

B. Antibiotics: The patient should receive carbenicillin, 20 gm/sq m/day given every 4 hours IV, plus cephalothin, 20–80 mg/kg/day given every 6 hours IV. Penicillin or other antibiotics should not be used "prophylactically." Broad-spectrum antibiotics are used only when specifically indicated on the basis of culture and sensitivity tests.

C. Corticosteroids: If the patient appears toxic, corticosteroids may have to be considered.

Prognosis

The mortality rate may approach 80% in untreated cases. With antibiotic therapy, the mortality rate is much lower, and when recovery occurs it is complete. Patients must be cautioned against reexposure to offending agents.

Pisciotta AV: Studies in agranulocytosis: Patterns of recovery. J Lab Clin Med 63:445, 1964.

Pisciotta AV & others: Agranulocytosis following administration of phenothiazine derivatives. Am J Med 25:210, 1958.

Pretty HM & others: Agranulocytosis: A report of 30 cases. Canad MAJ 93:1058, 1965.

HEMORRHAGIC DISORDERS

Coagulation Mechanisms (Fig 9–1.)

Blood clots when its fibrinogen is converted to fibrin by the action of thrombin. Prothrombin can be converted to thrombin either by a series of reactions involving factors VIII and IX and is generally referred to as the intrinsic clotting reaction, or it can be converted by tissue damage and the action of factor VII (extrinsic clotting reaction). One should note that in both reactions a complex of activated factors X and V, phospholipid ("platelet factor III"), and calcium acts on prothrombin to yield thrombin. Both intrinsic and extrinsic clotting reactions must be intact for normal hemostasis.

One can visualize the clotting factors as falling into 3 groups:

(1) Factors XII and XI concern surface control.

Coagulation Factor Synonyms	
Factor I:	Fibrinogen.
Factor II:	Prothrombin.
Factor III:	Thromboplastin.
Factor IV:	Calcium.
Factor V:	Proaccelerin, labile factor, AC globulin.
Factor VI:	(Originally felt to be the active form of V.)
Factor VII:	Proconvertin, stable factor, serum prothrombin conversion accelerator (SPCA).
Factor VIII:	Antihemophilic factor (AHF), antihemophilic globulin (AHG), antihemophilic factor A (AHF-A).
Factor IX:	Plasma thromboplastin component (PTC), antihemophilic factor B (AHF-B), Christmas factor.
Factor X:	Stuart factor, Stuart-Prower factor.
Factor XI:	Plasma thromboplastic antecedent (PTA).
Factor XII:	Hageman factor.
Factor XIII:	Fibrin stabilizing factor.

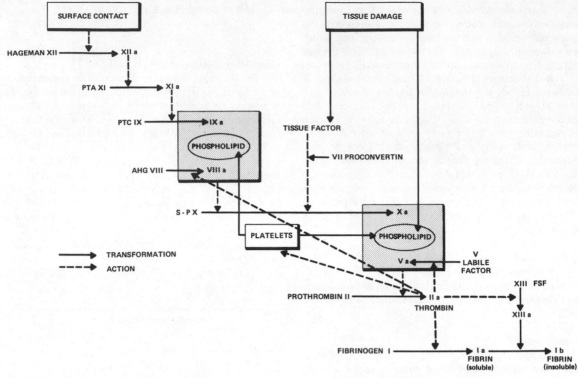

Figure 9—1. Current concept of the intrinsic and extrinsic systems of blood coagulation. (Reproduced with permission and adapted by JG Pool from schemes proposed by RG Macfarlane [Nature 202:498, 1964] and OD Ratnoff [Disease-A-Month for Nov 1965].)

(2) Factors II, VII, IX, and X all depend on vitamin K for their synthesis. They are relatively small, are stable in bank blood, can be adsorbed by barium sulfate, and require calcium for their activation.

(3) Factors V, VIII, and fibrinogen are consumed or altered by the action of thrombin. Factors V and VIII are relatively large and are unstable.

Diagnosis of Coagulation Problems

In the study of a coagulation problem the history is of utmost importance. The following questions must be answered:

(1) How long is the history of bleeding? Has bleeding been noted since early childhood, or is onset relatively recent? How many previous episodes have there been?

(2) What are the circumstances of the bleeding? Has it occurred after minor surgery, such as tonsillectomy or tooth extraction? Has it occurred after falls or participation in contact sports?

(3) What is the duration of the bleeding episode? (Prolonged oozing is more significant than massive hemorrhage.)

(4) Is there a family history of bleeding?

(5) What is the type or character of the bleeding? Purpuric spots suggest a capillary or platelet defect; they are not characteristic of hemophilia. Hematomas, hemarthroses, or large ecchymoses at the site of trauma suggest hemophilia. Sudden, severe bleeding from multiple sites after prolonged surgery or during obstet-

ric procedures suggests acquired fibrinogen deficiency. Massive bleeding from a single site without a history of purpura or previous bleeding suggests a surgical or anatomic defect rather than a coagulation defect.

Gaston LW: The blood clotting factors. (2 parts.) New England J Med 270:236, 290, 1964.

Ratnoff OD: The blood clotting mechanism and its disorders. Disease-A-Month, Nov 1965.

Ratnoff OD: The therapy of the hereditary disorders of blood coagulation. Arch Int Med 112:92, 1963.

HEMOPHILIA

Essentials of Diagnosis

- Lifelong history of bleeding in a male; usually congenital and familial.
- Slow, prolonged bleeding after minor injury.
- Recurrent hemarthroses and hematomas.
- Prolonged coagulation time.

General Considerations

Classical hemophilia is due to a deficiency of antihemophilic factor (AHF) activity, a constituent of normal plasma which is essential for thromboplastin formation. While the concentration of functional antihemophilic factor is reduced, the antigenic material

Table 9–5. Differential diagnosis of some bleeding disorders.

	Hemophilia (AHF, PTC)*		Idiopathic Thrombocytopenic Purpura	Vascular Hemophilia	Thrombasthenia (Glanzmann's)	Prothrombin Complex Deficiency	Defibrination Syndrome
	Severe	Mild					
Clinical Features:†							
Petechiae	–	–	++++	+	++	Ecchymoses	Ecchymoses
Hematoma, large	++++	++	–	–	–	–	–
Hemarthrosis	++++	±	–	±	–	–	–
Postsurgical bleeding	++++	++++	+	+++	+	++	++++
Onset in childhood	+	±	–	+	+	±	–
Hereditary	+	+	–	+	+	–	–
Laboratory:							
Bleeding time	N	N	Incr	Incr	N or incr	N	N
Clotting time	Incr	N	N	N	N	N or incr	No clot
Clot retraction time	N	N	Incr	N	Incr	N	No clot
Prothrombin time	N	N	N	N	N	Incr	Incr
Partial thromboplastin time (PTT)	Incr	Incr	Only platelets abnormal	Abnormal	Incr. Only platelets abnormal	N	Incr
Platelet count	N	N	Decr	N	Platelets look abnormal	N	Decr

*AHF = Antihemophilic factor. PTC = Plasma thromboplastin component.
†Frequency expressed on a scale of – to ++++.

related to antihemophilic factor is normal. The disorder is transmitted as an X-linked recessive gene by clinically unaffected female carriers to male offspring. AHF levels are decreased in one-third to one-half of female carriers. About 85% of congenital bleeders have classical hemophilia. One-third of these cases are sporadic, ie, they do not have a family history of bleeding.

Clinical Findings

A. Symptoms and Signs: Patients with hemophilia rarely have massive hemorrhages. Bleeding is characteristically a delayed and prolonged oozing or trickling, occurring after minor trauma or surgery, eg, tonsillectomy or tooth extraction. With extravasation of blood, painful hematomas form in the deep subcutaneous or intramuscular tissue. Joint deformity results from repeated hemorrhage into joint spaces. Gastrointestinal bleeding and hematuria are also prominent findings.

The frequency of bleeding episodes is variable. There may be periods of spontaneous bleeding from multiple sites followed by a phase during which there is neither spontaneous bleeding nor bleeding following minor trauma.

In mild cases a bleeding history may be lacking; the disease is suspected only after dental or surgical procedures.

B. Laboratory Findings: In patients with severe hemophilia, the coagulation time may range from 30 minutes to several hours. Partial thromboplastin time (PTT) is greatly prolonged. Antihemophilic factor (AHF) is virtually absent from the plasma. During clinically silent periods these laboratory tests remain abnormal. Capillary fragility, bleeding time (except after

ingestion of aspirin), prothrombin time, fibrinogen content, and platelet values are normal.

In mild cases the coagulation time is normal, but the PTT is prolonged. The plasma contains only 5–40% of antihemophilic factor (normal = 50–150%).

Differential Diagnosis

Plasma thromboplastin component deficiency (Christmas disease), which accounts for about 2–3% of congenital bleeders (15% of hemophiliacs), has the same clinical manifestations and hereditary transmission as classical hemophilia. Differentiation is by special coagulation studies and is essential if appropriate therapy is to specifically correct each of these deficiencies.

Plasma thromboplastin antecedent (PTA) deficiency accounts for 1% of hemophiliacs. It is an autosomal recessive trait, therefore affecting both males and females. It occurs almost exclusively in Jews. Patients have only mild bleeding tendencies. Spontaneous bleeding is unusual, though some patients bruise easily. Bleeding usually only occurs after injury and some surgical procedures; hemarthroses do not occur. The differentiation from factor VIII and IX deficiency is made by special coagulation studies. Treatment consists only of administering fresh frozen plasma; no therapeutic concentrate exists as yet.

Prothrombin complex disorders are characterized by a prolonged prothrombin time and a normal coagulation time.

In fibrinogen deficiency, the blood does not clot at all in the test tube, or a clot may form at a normal rate and then contract to a tiny residue.

Complications

Repeated hemarthroses may lead to ankylosis. Hematoma formation around the peripheral nerves may cause permanent damage with pain, anesthesia, or muscle atrophy. Retroperitoneal bleeding may be fatal. Autoimmune anticoagulants (anti-AHF) following repeated transfusions develop in approximately 5% of patients.

Treatment

A. General Measures: Aspirin-containing medication must not be given. Substitute acetaminophen, pentazocine, propoxyphene, or plain codeine to alleviate pain. Treatment is based on raising the level of AHF in the patient's blood and maintaining it at this level until hemostasis is obtained. The half-disappearance time of AHF in vivo is about 12 hours.

Treatment is evaluated by the clinical response. Correction of abnormal PTT is a useful indicator.

The management of factor IX deficiency is similar; however, since factor IX is stable at blood bank conditions for long periods, plasma need not be fresh.

B. AHF Concentrates: See Table 9–6.

C. Plasma: (Fresh frozen plasma, 140 units/200 ml.) Just prior to infusion the plasma is thawed at 37° C (98.6° F) until all solid material is liquefied. For maximum response it is administered as an initial dose of 15–20 ml/kg over a period of 1–2 hours.

For both concentrates and plasma, half the initial dose is repeated every 12 hours until bleeding stops.

D. Factor IX Complex: Proplex (Hyland) contains factors II, VII, IX, and X. The 30 ml bottle contains approximately 500 units of factor IX in a dried form. For common bleeding (eg, hemarthroses), give 1 bottle or approximately 10 units/kg. For severe bleeding and surgical procedures, give 20 units/kg.

Fresh frozen plasma—or any kind of plasma—may be used for factor IX deficiency. The dosage considerations are similar to those for factor VIII deficiency.

None of the concentrates listed in Table 9–6 are effective for factor IX deficiency.

E. Special Problems:

1. Bleeding—For the simpler bleeding episodes, give enough AHF concentrate to raise the plasma level to 50% (eg, cryoprecipitate, 1 bag/6 kg).

No further therapy is usually needed. In severe cases (eg, abdominal or retroperitoneal bleeding), one must raise the AHG level to 75% (1 bag/3 kg); this dose may have to be repeated in 24 and 48 hours. After dental work, one may give aminocaproic acid (Amicar) syrup, 1 tbsp (3.75 gm) 4 times daily for 8 days, starting 24 hours before surgery.

2. Surgical procedures—Patients are prepared by infusing, just prior to surgery, enough concentrate to reach 75% AHF levels (eg, one bag of cryoprecipitate/3 kg; one bag/6 kg at 6 hours and again at 12 hours; and then one bag/6 kg every 12 hours until the wound has healed, which may be 1–2 weeks after surgery). To assess efficacy of therapy, the AHF level must be determined; the PTT cannot be used for this.

Aminocaproic acid (Amicar, EACA) may be a valuable adjunct to therapy. Give 5 gm IV 24 hours before surgery and then 6 gm 4 times daily IV for 1 week. (Do not use with factor IX concentrate.)

3. Hemarthroses—During the bleeding phase the joint must be put at rest, in the position of comfort, and possibly packed with ice or put into a protective case. If pain is severe, aspiration may be necessary.

As soon as pain and bleeding have been controlled, usually within 3–5 days, muscle-setting exercises are begun. When swelling subsides, active motion of the joint is encouraged. Weight bearing is not permitted until the periarticular soft tissues have returned to nearly normal and motion and muscle power of the joint are normal.

4. Hematuria—Give oral prednisone (2 mg/kg/day) for 2 days; the dose is then tapered and stopped after 5 days.

5. Inhibitors of anticoagulants—Five to 10% of hemophiliacs develop inhibitors. Initial manifestations are uncontrolled bleeding and failure of PTT and factor VIII levels to normalize after appropriate therapy with concentrate. Addition of normal plasma to patient's plasma in vitro does not correct the PTT. (With low level inhibitor, an incubation period may be necessary to demonstrate binding of the antigen.)

Large amounts of concentrate are usually ineffective in overcoming the inhibitor. Immunosuppressive therapy with prednisone, 1–2 mg/kg/day, and cyclophosphamide, 2.5 mg/kg/day, occasionally is successful. Success has been reported with the use of factor IX concentrate (Proplex), 50–100 units/kg every 12 hours for 2 doses (approximately 2–3 bottles per 10 kg) in the treatment of patients with inhibitors to factor VIII.

Prognosis

Spontaneous hemorrhages into joints and bleeding from minor injuries or surgery are rarely dangerous. Major trauma and bleeding into loose tissues, eg, the

Table 9–6. AHF concentrates.

| | AHF Units | | | |
	Per Package	Per ml	Usual Dose to Reach 50% AHF	Storage Requirement
Cryoprecipitate*	100–150	4–6	1 bag/6 kg	Freeze
Hemofil (Hyland)	230	33	1 pg/12 kg	Refrigerate
AHG (Courtland)	200	8	1 vial/10 kg	Room temperature
Fibro-AHG (Merck)	75	0.75	1 vial/ 3–4 kg	Refrigerate
Factorate (Armour)	250	10	1 vial/12 kg	Refrigerate
Profilate (Abbott)	250	10	1 vial/12 kg	Refrigerate

*When a large number of units is required, as in some surgical cases, the cryoprecipitate should be type-specific.

retroperitoneal space, may be fatal despite therapy with plasma. Fatal, uncontrollable hemorrhage may also occur if inhibitors (anti-AHF factor) develop following multiple transfusions.

Aggeler PM & others: The mild hemophilias: Occult deficiencies of AHF, PTC, and PTA frequently responsible for unexpected surgical bleeding. Am J Med 30:89, 1961.

Biggs R, MacFarlane RG: Haemophilia and related conditions. A survey of 148 cases. Brit J Haemat 4:1, 1958.

Coleman RW: Immunologic heterogeneity of hemophilia. New England J Med 288:369, 1973.

Dallman PR, Pool JG: Treatment of hemophilia with factor VIII concentrates. New England J Med 278:199, 1968.

Perner JA, Kelly PE: Management of patients with factor VIII or IX inhibitors. Seminars Thromb Hemo 1:386, May 1975.

Ratnoff OD: The biology and pathology of the initial stages of blood coagulation (factors XII and XI deficiencies). Pages 220–245 in: *Progress in Hematology.* Vol 5. Grune & Stratton, 1966.

Walsh PN & others: Epsilon-aminocaproic acid therapy for dental extractions in hemophilia. Brit J Haemat 20:463, 1971.

PURPURA

Petechiae, ecchymoses, and easy bruisability may be caused by thrombocytopenia, qualitative platelet disorders, or vascular defects.

1. IDIOPATHIC (PRIMARY) THROMBOCYTOPENIC PURPURA

Essentials of Diagnosis

- Petechiae, ecchymoses, epistaxis, easy bruising.
- No splenomegaly.
- Decreased platelet count, prolonged bleeding time, poor clot retraction.

General Considerations

The thrombocytopenia is the result of increased platelet destruction; the platelet count is closely related to the rate of destruction. Normal platelet survival is 8–10 days. Survival is usually only 1–3 days in chronic idiopathic thrombocytopenic purpura, and even less in the acute form. An antiplatelet factor with the characteristics of antibody may be present in the plasma. Despite an apparent increase in the number of megakaryocytes in the marrow, platelet production is usually not increased; antibodies may disturb megakaryocytic development and lead to ineffective production. The disorder may be postinfectious, eg, following infectious mononucleosis or rubella; may be caused by isoimmunity, eg, following transfusions or in the neonatal period; may develop in diseases with auto-

immune manifestations, eg, lupus erythematosus or lymphoproliferative disorders; or may follow the use of certain drugs, eg, quinidine, quinine, thiazides, sulfonamides, phenylbutazone, acetazolamide, aminosalicylic acid, gold, and others.

The spleen, while not large, contributes to the thrombocytopenia in 2 ways: (1) It sequesters the subtly damaged platelets and (2) it manufactures some antibody.

Acute thrombocytopenic purpura is more common in children. Eighty-five percent of patients are less than 8 years old; it usually remits spontaneously in 2 weeks to a few months. Chronic thrombocytopenic purpura may start at any age and is more common in females. At onset it cannot be distinguished from the acute form by laboratory test. There may be clinical remissions and exacerbations, but the platelet count is always low.

Clinical Findings

A. Symptoms and Signs: The onset may be sudden, with petechiae, epistaxis, bleeding gums, vaginal bleeding, gastrointestinal bleeding, or hematuria. In the chronic form there may be a history of easy bruising and recurrent showers of petechiae, particularly in pressure areas. The spleen is not palpable.

B. Laboratory Findings: The platelet count is always below 100,000/cu mm and may be below 10,000/cu mm. Platelets may be absent on the peripheral blood smear. White cells are not affected; anemia, if present, is secondary to blood loss.

The bone marrow megakaryocytes are increased in number but not surrounded by platelets; they are abnormal, with single nuclei, scant cytoplasm, and often vacuoles. The chief value of the marrow examination is to rule out leukemia and aplastic anemia.

The bleeding time is prolonged, but PTT and PT are normal. Clot retraction is poor. Prothrombin consumption is decreased in severe cases. Capillary fragility (Rumpel-Leede test) is greatly increased. An antinuclear antibody (ANA) test and a prothrombin time should be done to look for lupus, which may present as purpura or with bleeding due to an anticoagulant.

Differential Diagnosis

Purpura may be the first sign of acute leukemia or macroglobulinemia. The diagnosis is made by finding the characteristic malignant cells in the blood or bone marrow. In thrombocytopenia accompanying aplastic anemia, the marrow fat is increased and megakaryocytes are decreased or absent. Thrombotic thrombocytopenic purpura is associated with hemolytic anemia, jaundice, CNS symptoms, fever, and schistocytes.

Thrombocytopenic purpura may also be seen in association with a variety of disorders causing splenomegaly and hypersplenism: congestive splenomegaly, Felty's syndrome, Gaucher's disease, tuberculosis, sarcoidosis, and myelofibrosis. Lupus erythematosus may be associated with thrombocytopenic purpura with or without splenomegaly. Other conditions that may have to be ruled out before making the diagnosis of idiopathic thrombocytopenic purpura include septicemia (especially with gram-negative organisms) and disseminated intravascular coagulation (often associated with schistocytes). Thrombocytopenia is relatively common in acute severe alcoholism.

In the newborn, thrombocytopenic purpura may also be caused by septicemia, congenital syphilis, cytomegalic inclusion disease, hemolytic disease of the newborn, a congenital lack of megakaryocytes, or a congenital giant hemangioma. In the Wiskott-Aldrich syndrome, thrombocytopenic purpura is associated with eczema, increased susceptibility to infection, and deficiency of isoagglutinins, immunoglobulins, and lymphocytes; it is an X-linked recessive disorder.

Scurvy may cause purpura and massive skin and muscle hemorrhage, especially into hair follicles of the legs and extensor surfaces of the arms. Coagulation tests are normal.

Complications

Fatal cerebral hemorrhage occurs in 1–5% of cases; hemorrhage from the nose and gastrointestinal and urinary tracts may be dangerously severe. Pressure of a hematoma on nerve tissue may cause pain, anesthesia, or paralysis. Children born to mothers with idiopathic thrombocytopenic purpura may have transient neonatal purpura.

Treatment

A. General Measures: Patients should avoid trauma, contact sports, elective surgery, and tooth extraction. All unnecessary medications and exposure to potential toxins must be discontinued.

Children with mild purpura following viral infections do not require any therapy. They should be observed until petechiae disappear and the platelet count returns to normal.

B. Corticosteroids: Corticosteroids are warranted in patients with moderately severe purpura of short duration, especially when there is bleeding from the gastrointestinal or genitourinary tract. Corticosteroids are also given to patients with purpura who have complications contraindicating surgery. Prednisolone (or equivalent), 10–20 mg 4 times daily, is usually required to control bleeding. The dosage is continued until the platelet count returns to normal, and then is gradually decreased.

C. Splenectomy: Splenectomy is indicated for all patients with well documented thrombocytopenic purpura of more than 1 year's duration; for all patients with moderately severe purpura who have relapsed 2–3 times after corticosteroid therapy; and for all patients with severe idiopathic thrombocytopenic purpura who do not respond to corticosteroids.

Corticosteroids should not be used immediately before surgery unless bleeding is severe. If splenectomy must be performed on a patient who has been on corticosteroids, full doses of corticosteroids should be maintained for 3 days after surgery and then decreased gradually.

The platelet count rises promptly following splenectomy, and often doubles within the first 24 hours. Maximum values are reached 1–2 weeks postoperatively. Sometimes the platelet count will exceed 1 million/cu mm before leveling off. Anticoagulant therapy is not necessary with even higher platelet counts. Splenectomy may be considered successful only when counts stay normal for at least 2 months.

Prognosis

Spontaneous and permanent recovery occurs in 75% of all childhood idiopathic thrombocytopenic purpura and in 25% of all adult cases. Splenectomy is curative in 70–90% of all patients.

In thrombocytopenia caused by drugs, the platelet count may rise promptly (within a few days) when the drug is discontinued and return to normal within a few weeks. Occasionally, this return to normal is delayed, and the initial rise may not take place for several weeks.

Baldini M: Idiopathic thrombocytopenic purpura. (3 parts.) New England J Med 274:1245, 1301, 1360, 1966.

Finch SC & others: Immunosuppressive therapy of chronic idiopathic thrombocytopenic purpura. Am J Med 56:4, 1974.

Karpatkin S: Drug induced thrombocytopenia. Am J Med Sc 262:69, 1971.

Sahud MA: Platelet disorders: A review of disturbances in adhesion, aggregation, and release reaction. California Med 116:21, Jan 1972.

2. DISORDERS WITH QUALITATIVE PLATELET DEFECTS

Skin purpura after minor trauma, dependent petechiae, and mucocutaneous bleeding may be seen. Some patients have abnormal bleeding after surgery. Platelet counts are usually normal but may be slightly low. Platelets may look abnormal on the blood smear; depending on the disorders, they may be small (Wiskott-Aldrich syndrome), large (May-Hegglin anomaly), or they may fail to aggregate (Glanzmann's disease). The Ivy bleeding time is prolonged in all of these disorders, especially after a test dose of 0.6 gm of aspirin. All of these patients should avoid the therapeutic use of aspirin. Other tests helpful in classifying the various entities in this group are clot retraction; platelet aggregation in response to collagen, adenosine diphosphate (ADP), epinephrine, and thrombin; and platelet factor 3 availability.

Thrombasthenia (Glanzmann's Disease)

This is an autosomal recessive disorder. The platelet count is normal, but the platelets appear isolated on the blood smear. Bleeding time is prolonged, clot retraction is absent or decreased, and platelets do not aggregate with ADP as measured on the aggregometer. Platelet fibrinogen content is low. Platelet factor 3 availability is impaired.

Primary Familial Platelet-ADP Release Dysfunction

This is a milder disorder than thrombasthenia, but the symptoms are similar. Easy bruising is a common finding. The bleeding time is less prolonged than in thrombasthenia, and the clot retraction is normal. The platelets look normal on the blood smear. Platelet aggregation is impaired or absent following exposure to collagen and epinephrine, and abnormal aggregation is seen following exposure to ADP.

Von Willebrand's Disease

This disorder (see below) may present with purpura.

Acquired Platelet Defects

In uremia, bleeding is caused largely by defective function of platelets. Adhesiveness and aggregation by ADP and epinephrine are impaired, and the bleeding time is prolonged.

Platelet function may be impaired in the myeloproliferative disorders, ie, polycythemia vera, myelofibrosis, and chronic myelocytic leukemia.

In macroglobulinemia and some cases of multiple myeloma, the abnormal globulin may coat the platelets and cause impaired aggregation and platelet factor III availability.

Sahud MA: Differential diagnosis of platelet dysfunction. California Med 112:66, March 1970.

3. HENOCH-SCHÖNLEIN SYNDROME
(Anaphylactoid Purpura)

This is an acquired hemorrhagic disorder characterized by general vasculitis involving multiple organ systems. It is much more common in children than in adults. Purpura may be associated with abdominal pain, intussusception, gastrointestinal bleeding, hematuria, proteinuria, glomerulonephritis, and arthralgia. The disorder is thought to be of immunologic origin. The purpura may be urticarial at first, followed by red macular lesions, often involving the palms and soles. All tests of coagulation, including bleeding tissue, are normal.

Cream JJ & others: Henoch-Schönlein purpura in the adult. Quart J Med 39:461, 1970.

HEREDITARY HEMORRHAGIC TELANGIECTASIA
(Rendu-Osler-Weber Disease)

Essentials of Diagnosis

- Telangiectatic lesions on face, mouth, nose, hands.
- Epistaxis or gastrointestinal bleeding.
- Familial involvement.

General Considerations

This is a vascular abnormality involving primarily the veins; vessels are dilated and their walls are thin. The disorder is inherited as a dominant trait. Males and females are involved equally. A positive family history can be obtained in 80% of cases.

Skin and mucous membrane lesions may be asymptomatic for many years; the diagnosis is established by inference when telangiectases and angiomas are noted in patients with a history of otherwise inexplicable attacks of epistaxis or gastrointestinal bleeding.

Clinical Findings

A. Symptoms and Signs: Multiple bright red lesions 1–4 mm in diameter that blanch on pressure are seen on the face, oral or nasopharyngeal membranes, and upper extremities in over 90% of patients. The lesions are often first noticed in childhood, but severe bleeding is unusual before the age of 30; the peak incidence of severity is in the 6th decade of life. Approximately 5% of patients have pulmonary arteriovenous fistulas.

Epistaxis is the most common form of bleeding; gastrointestinal bleeding occurs in about 15% of cases; it may be severe enough to require surgery, but the actual gastrointestinal lesions may be difficult to demonstrate at operation.

B. Laboratory Findings: The usual laboratory tests are helpful only in ruling out other causes of bleeding; bleeding and clotting times, prothrombin time, platelet count, clot retraction, and tourniquet tests are normal. Secondary iron deficiency anemia is common.

Differential Diagnosis

Petechiae do not blanch on pressure, are more purple, and are not particularly common on the lips and tongue. Spider angiomas are arteriolar, can be shown to pulsate on pressure, and have several fine channels extending from their centers.

Complications

Severe bleeding may cause chronic iron deficiency anemia. Bleeding may exceed 1000 ml per week from the gastrointestinal tract.

Treatment

There is no cure.

Asymptomatic lesions require no therapy. Local pressure and topical hemostatic agents may be tried in accessible bleeding areas. Cauterization of the nasal mucous membranes may be necessary.

For uncontrollable gastrointestinal bleeding, unsuitable for surgery, iron therapy is indicated. If bleeding is severe (50–100 ml/day), give iron dextran injection, 5–10 ml IV once weekly. For more severe bleeding, transfusions are necessary.

Halpern M & others: Hereditary hemorrhagic telangiectasia. Radiology 90:1143, 1968.

Smith CR & others: Hereditary hemorrhagic telangiectasia and gastrointestinal hemorrhage. Gastroenterology 44:1, 1963.

THROMBOTIC THROMBOCYTOPENIC PURPURA

This is a severe, acute illness with a poor prognosis. The major clinical manifestations are fever, jaundice, purpura, drowsiness with fluctuating neurologic signs, thrombocytopenia, hemolytic anemia with characteristically fragmented red blood cells, and renal abnormalities. Any one of these features may be absent, especially initially. The Coombs test is negative, red cell enzymes are not decreased, and Heinz bodies are absent.

The pathologic diagnosis depends upon vascular lesions located at arteriolocapillary junctions, with widespread distribution in many organs. The lesions consist of subintimal deposition of PAS-positive material, hyaline thrombi, and vessel wall weakening, leading to aneurysmal dilatations. The thrombotic phenomena are thought to be secondary reactions to the damaged vascular walls.

Treatment is usually of no avail. Occasional successes have been reported with large doses of corticosteroids, heparin, or splenectomy.

Amorosi EL, Ultman JE: Thrombotic thrombocytopenic purpura: Report of 16 cases and review of the literature. Medicine 45:139, 1966.

Lerner RC, Rapaport SI, Melitzer J: Thrombotic thrombocytopenic purpura: Serial clotting studies, relation to the generalized Shwartzman reaction, and remission after adrenal steroid and dextran therapy. Ann Int Med 66:1180, 1967.

VON WILLEBRAND'S DISEASE
(Vascular Hemophilia, Pseudohemophilia)

Essentials of Diagnosis

- History of excessive bruising and frequent nosebleeds since childhood.
- Prolonged bleeding time, normal platelet count.

General Considerations

This relatively common disorder resembles hemophilia in that it causes prolonged bleeding, particularly after oropharyngeal surgery or trauma; however, it occurs in both sexes, the bleeding time is prolonged, and the coagulation time is usually normal.

Von Willebrand's disease is characterized by low values of Willebrand factor activity, factor VIII antigen, and factor VIII activity. In contrast, in hemophilia, Willebrand factor and factor VIII antigen levels are normal. The lack of Willebrand factor is responsible for poor adherence of platelets, in vivo to cut vessels and to each other and in vitro to glass. It also is responsible for the prolonged bleeding time that occurs in this condition.

Clinical Findings

A. Symptoms and Signs: There is a history of frequent nosebleeds in childhood, prolonged bleeding from small cuts (eg, kitchen knife, razor cuts while shaving), excessive menstrual flow, prolonged oozing following oropharyngeal or minor gynecologic surgery, and easy bruisability. Other family members are usually affected also. Childbirth is usually uncomplicated by bleeding, and these patients can often undergo major abdominal surgery without hemorrhagic complications. Skin bleeding is ecchymotic rather than petechial.

B. Laboratory Findings: A prolonged bleeding time (Ivy) is essential for diagnosis; it is greatly prolonged following the ingestion of as little as 0.6 gm of aspirin. PTT is usually slightly prolonged, reflecting low factor VIII, which is usually in the range of 15–50%. If factor VIII levels are very low (less than 5%), even the coagulation time may be prolonged. Platelet adhesiveness, as measured by the Salzman test, in which blood is passed through a tube with fine glass beads, is characteristically decreased (ie, more platelets than normal pass through the tube without adhering). Platelet count, platelet aggregation, prothrombin time, and clot retraction are all normal.

Differential Diagnosis

Vascular hemophilia must be differentiated from conditions with qualitative platelet defects. Glanzmann's syndrome is also characterized by a prolonged bleeding time and a normal platelet count; platelet morphology is abnormal; bleeding is often severe and may even be fatal. In macroglobulinemic purpura, ecchymoses and prolonged bleeding time may occur. In the recently described platelet-collagen interaction defect, platelet aggregation is faulty. In all of these conditions, factor VIII levels are normal.

Treatment

For serious bleeding episodes, the low factor VIII level should be corrected by concentrates as described for AHF deficiency on p 310. If the bleeding site is accessible, bleeding is controlled by local pressure with thrombin-soaked gelfoam. Whole blood replacement may be necessary.

Prognosis

Bleeding is usually self-limited, although it may be prolonged. Fatal bleeding may occur, especially after minor surgical procedures. Childbirth and major abdominal procedures are less likely to be complicated by excessive bleeding. Bleeding tends to become less severe with increasing age.

Barrow EM, Graham JB: Von Willebrand's disease. Progr Hemat 4:203, 1964.

Caen JP: Congenital bleeding disorders with long bleeding time and normal platelet count. I. Glanzmann's thrombasthenia. Am J Med 41:4, 1966.

Larrieu MJ & others: Congenital bleeding disorders with long bleeding time and normal platelet count. II. Von Willebrand's disease. Am J Med 45:354, 1968.

Ratnoff OD: Hemophilia and von Willebrand's disease. Western J Med 120:226, 1974.

DISSEMINATED INTRAVASCULAR COAGULATION
(Defibrination Syndrome, Coagulopathy, DIC)

Essentials of Diagnosis
- Diffuse bleeding from the skin and mucous membranes.
- Poor, small clot.
- Reduced platelets or on smear.
- Prolonged prothrombin time.

General Considerations

This is a pathologic form of coagulation which differs from normal clotting in 3 principal ways: (1) it is diffuse rather than localized; (2) it damages the site of clotting instead of protecting it; and (3) it consumes several clotting factors to such a degree that their concentration in the plasma becomes so low that diffuse bleeding may occur. It is seen in certain obstetric catastrophes and following some types of surgery, particularly involving the lung, brain, or prostate. In some of these conditions and in malignancies (especially of the prostate), septicemia, hemolytic transfusion reaction, and hemolytic uremic syndrome in infancy, deposition of fibrin in small blood vessels may lead to serious and even fatal tissue necrosis. Examples are (1) glomerular capillary thrombosis leading to cortical necrosis or a pattern similar to that of acute tubular necrosis, (2) adrenal sinusoidal thrombosis with resultant hemorrhagic necrosis of the adrenals (Waterhouse-Friderichsen syndrome); and (3) hemorrhagic skin necrosis in purpura fulminans. These conditions are caused in part by a failure to clear fibrin. Some relationship may exist between irreversible endotoxin shock and disseminated intravascular clotting.

Unexpected, profuse, or uncontrollable bleeding in certain surgical or obstetric situations suggests acute defibrination. Multiple coagulation factors are involved. The syndrome is acquired and results from intravascular coagulation.

Clinical Findings

A. Symptoms and Signs: The most common manifestation is diffuse bleeding from many sites at surgery and from needle puncture. Minimal trauma may cause severe bleeding, or there may be spontaneous ecchymoses, epistaxis, or gastrointestinal hemorrhage. Uncontrollable postpartum hemorrhage may be a manifestation of intravascular coagulation.

B. Laboratory Findings: The combination of a poor, small clot, reduced platelets on the blood smear, and a prolonged prothrombin time is very suggestive of this disorder. Clotting time is usually normal. With marked fibrinogen depletion (fibrinogen < 75 mg/ml), the clot that forms in a test tube may be quite flimsy and friable. It may be so small and retracted that it may not even be visible, thus simulating fibrinolysis. The contents of the test tube should be poured into a Petri dish or onto a piece of filter paper for closer examination. If a clot can be demonstrated, it suggests that fibrinogen depletion, and not fibrinolysis, is the primary process.

A form of hemolytic anemia associated with fragmentation of the red blood cells (microangiopathic hemolytic anemia) may accompany some of these conditions.

Platelet counts usually vary from 30–120 thousand/cu mm. Prothrombin time is usually less than 40% and may be less than 10%. Screening tests for fibrinogen (Hyland Laboratories Fi test) usually indicate values of less than 100 mg/100 ml. The activated PTT (normal: < 47 seconds) is prolonged to as much as 100 seconds. The thrombin time is prolonged. The bleeding time is usually prolonged when platelet levels are below 70,000. Factors V and VIII fall markedly.

It is usually quite helpful to obtain laboratory evidence of fibrinolysis when investigating a case of suspected intravascular coagulation. Acute fibrinolysis, while occasionally a primary process, is most commonly seen in association with intravascular coagulation. The 2 most commonly used tests are demonstration of fibrin degradation products in plasma or serum and the determination of euglobulin clot lysis.

Fibrin degradation products result from the digestion of fibrinogen or fibrin by plasmin or other enzymes. These products cannot be coagulated by thrombin; they actually inhibit the thrombin-fibrinogen reaction and cause a prolonged thrombin time, and also inhibit platelet aggregation, thromboplastin formation, and fibrin polymerization. They make the Fi test for fibrinogen difficult to interpret. Fibrin degradation products are usually demonstrated by immunologic methods and can be quantitated by a tanned red cell hemagglutination inhibition test. A simple latex test (Thrombo-Wellco) has recently become available which is quite sensitive to fibrin monomer and all 4 fragments, X, Y, D, and E—especially the latter two. Soluble fibrin monomer complexed with fibrinogen or fibrin split products also gives rise to a positive protamine test. If thrombin has been formed intravascularly, the blood will contain fibrin monomer (ie, fibrinogen from which peptides A and B have been cleaved). In the protamine test, the monomer is precipitated, making the test useful in detecting DIC.

The time necessary for a euglobulin clot to lyse is a measure of fibrinolytic activity. In normal individuals more than 2 hours is required for the clot to lyse. Significant fibrinolysis is evident when a euglobulin clot liquefies in less than 60 minutes.

Plasminogen levels are low; plasminogen is the inactive precursor of fibrinolysin (plasmin). Since it is activated to plasmin in acute fibrinolysis, its activity is characteristically low in this disorder.

Demonstration of the characteristic clotting factor pattern by individual factor assay is of great help in differential diagnosis. In primary fibrinolysis, in fibrinogen deficiency from underproduction rather than excessive utilization, in hepatic necrosis, and following heparin administration (eg, excessive dose by error), clot formation or retraction may be grossly abnormal, but factor VII levels are not decreased.

Differential Diagnosis

Disseminated intravascular coagulation—which, like all clotting, is associated with secondary fibrinolysis—must be distinguished from primary fibrinolysis, a much rarer clinical phenomenon requiring very different management. This latter syndrome may occur with disseminated carcinoma (especially of the prostate), with septicemia, and with very severe liver disease. Diffuse bleeding similar to that encountered in intravascular coagulation does not occur, and platelets, factor V, and factor VIII are less strikingly decreased; a clot may form initially but dissolves completely in less than 2 hours. As in secondary fibrinolysis, fibrinogen is low or absent; consequently, prothrombin and thrombin times are prolonged, plasminogen is low, and plasmin levels are increased.

Other conditions where clots fail to form in vitro are circulating anticoagulant and heparin administration. In vitro clotting may be greatly prolonged to 1 hour or more in the hemophilias and in factor XII deficiency.

Treatment

If possible, treat the underlying disorder, eg, shock or sepsis. Heparin may be effective to stop pathologic clotting, and it may also control bleeding. In adults, the usual dose of heparin is 100 USP units/kg every 4–6 hours IV; in children, 50 units/kg every 4 hours after an initial dose of 100 units. If the diagnosis of intravascular coagulation was correct and therapy is effective, fibrin degradation products should fall and fibrinogen levels, PTT, and PT should rise within 24 hours and platelet count within a few days. Whole blood may be necessary to combat shock. With severe fibrinogen deficiency, human fibrinogen in doses of 4–6 gm may be given IV, but the risk of hepatitis is considerable. Platelet concentrates may be used in severe platelet deficiency.

Prognosis

In fibrinogen deficiency due to liver disease or cancer, the prognosis is usually that of the underlying disorder. Excessive bleeding during brain or lung surgery or at delivery may be completely and permanently corrected by intravenous administration of fibrinogen if fibrinolysins have not been activated.

Abildgaard CF: Recognition and treatment of intravascular coagulation. J Pediat 74:163, 1969.

Deykin D: The clinical challenge of disseminated intravascular coagulation. New England J Med 283:636, 1970.
Kwaan HC: Disseminated intravascular coagulation. M Clin North America 56:177, 1972.
Marcus A: Heparin therapy for disseminated intravascular coagulation. Am J Med Sc 264:365, 1972.
Verstraete M & others: Excessive consumption of blood coagulation components as cause of hemorrhagic diathesis. Am J Med 38:899, 1965.

ACQUIRED PROTHROMBIN COMPLEX DISORDERS
(Factors V, VII, X, & Prothrombin)

Essentials of Diagnosis

- Ecchymoses and epistaxis, spontaneously or after minimal trauma.
- Postoperative wound hemorrhage.
- Bleeding from venipuncture.

General Considerations

In all of these disorders an underlying process is usually evident, eg, liver disease or anticoagulant therapy. Regardless of which member of the prothrombin complex is deficient (prothrombin, factors V, VII, or X), the Quick prothrombin time is prolonged.

There are 3 forms of prothrombin complex deficiency.

A. Vitamin K Deficiency: This may be seen in obstructive jaundice, in the malabsorption syndrome, after prolonged antibiotic therapy, in hemorrhagic diseases of the newborn, and following continued ingestion, therapeutic or surreptitious, of coumarin anticoagulants. The pattern of vitamin K deficiency is characterized by reduction of factors II, VII, and X but not of factor V. Administration of warfarin (Coumadin) results in the synthesis of physiologically inactive prothrombin protein, which cannot bind calcium and does not adsorb onto barium sulfate; it is defective in carboxyglutamic acid.

B. Severe Liver Disease: There is primarily a deficiency of factor V, but factors II, VII, IX, and X may also be low.

C. Excessive Utilization: See Intravascular Coagulation.

Clinical Findings

A. Symptoms and Signs: There is no previous history of hemorrhagic manifestations. Ecchymoses and epistaxis may occur spontaneously or after minimal trauma. Gastrointestinal bleeding and postoperative wound hemorrhage are common. Bleeding into joints does not occur.

B. Laboratory Findings: The Quick prothrombin time measures deficiencies in any member of the prothrombin complex, ie, if there is a deficiency in prothrombin, factor V, factor VII, or factor X, or if the fibrinogen levels are less than 125 mg/100 ml, the prothrombin time will be prolonged. Conversely, if the prothrombin time is normal one can assume that all prothrombin complex components are adequate. Specific tests for these factors are of value when a congenital defect is suspected or when the underlying cause of the prolonged prothrombin time is not evident.

In these acquired prothrombin complex disorders the prothrombin time is usually below 40–50%; surgical bleeding may occur below 50%; spontaneous bleeding at 10–15%. Prothrombin consumption, coagulation time, bleeding time, capillary fragility, and clot retraction are normal unless there is associated thromboplastin deficiency.

Treatment

A. General Measures: Deficiency due to vitamin K lack or coumarin compound excess is successfully treated by cessation of coumarin therapy and administration of appropriate medication. The deficiency of liver disease, however, does not respond to vitamin K. Replacement therapy with whole blood or plasma is generally unsatisfactory because of the lability of factor V in vitro and the very rapid disappearance rate of factor VII in vivo.

B. Vitamin K:

1. Phytonadione (fat-soluble vitamin K_1; Mephyton) for the treatment of warfarin excess—To restore prolonged prothrombin time to normal, give 5 mg orally. For major bleeding, 10–15 mg of Aqua-Mephyton given slowly IV at a rate not exceeding 10 mg/minute will shorten the prothrombin time in 2 hours and produce safe therapeutic levels in 4–6 hours.

2. Synthetic, water-soluble vitamin K (menadione sodium bisulfite [Hykinone], menadiol [Synkayvite]) is used for the treatment of vitamin K deficiency due to malabsorption. The dosage is 5 mg daily.

Prognosis

Vitamin K deficiency and the effect of coumarin excess can be corrected by parenteral or oral administration of vitamin K. The prognosis in other conditions depends upon the underlying disorder.

Deykin D: Heparin therapy. New England J Med 283:691, 801, 1970.

Koch-Weser J, Sellers EM: Drug interaction with coumarin anticoagulants. New England J Med 285:487, 547, 1971.

O'Reilly RA, Aggeler PM: Surreptitious ingestion of coumarin anticoagulant drugs. Ann Int Med 64:1034, 1966.

Woolf IL, Babior BM: Vitamin K and warfarin. Am J Med 53:261, 1972.

CIRCULATING ANTICOAGULANTS

Essentials of Diagnosis

- Ecchymoses.
- Gastrointestinal bleeding.
- Hemarthroses.
- Prolonged coagulation time.

General Considerations

A circulating anticoagulant is an abnormal blood component which inhibits the coagulation of normal blood. Most circulatory anticoagulants interfere with thromboplastin formation, probably by immune antibody production; the majority are directed against AHF and occur either in patients with hemophilia after many transfusions or spontaneously and transiently 8–10 weeks after obstetric delivery. Other circulatory anticoagulants interfere with the action of thromboplastin and may be associated with lupus erythematosus and similar disorders. Circulating anticoagulants may appear at any age and in either sex.

Clinical Findings

A. Symptoms and Signs: Patients develop sudden spontaneous hemorrhages characterized by ecchymoses, subcutaneous and intramuscular hematomas, hematuria, hemarthroses, gastrointestinal bleeding, and bleeding into the tongue and pharynx. Abnormal uterine bleeding may occur in women.

B. Laboratory Findings: In all patients the coagulation time is prolonged (30 minutes to several hours), but once a clot forms it is of good quality and contracts normally. PTT is prolonged. Prothrombin time is normal in the hemophilia-like group but may be prolonged in the type of circulating anticoagulants seen in lupus erythematosus. Bleeding time and platelet counts are normal. The existence of circulatory anticoagulants can be proved if relatively small amounts (20–40%) of patient's blood or plasma inhibit coagulation of normal blood or plasma. If circulating anticoagulants are present only in small amounts, more refined methods of demonstrating the inhibitory effect are necessary.

Differential Diagnosis

Coagulation time is prolonged also in hemophilia, fibrinogen deficiency, in the presence of fibrinolysins, and in patients receiving heparin. However, in fibrinogen deficiency or in the presence of fibrinolysins, either no clot forms at all or it forms at a normal rate and then lyses or contracts to a small nubbin. Another group of inhibitors of coagulation causing hemorrhagic phenomena (chiefly petechiae, epistaxis, and abnormal uterine bleeding) are the abnormal proteins, macroglobulins, myelomas, and cryoglobulins.

Treatment

The therapy of a bleeding hemophiliac with a circulating anticoagulant to AHF may require massive doses of AHF concentrate (Hyland Antihemophilic Factor-Method Four) to overload the inhibitor.

Prednisolone orally in relatively large doses (15–20 mg 4 times daily) with cyclophosphamide (Cytoxan), 2.5 mg/kg/day, may be tried.

Occasionally, success has been reported by giving factor IX concentrate (eg, Proplex).

Prognosis

The presence of circulating anticoagulants in the blood is a severe and dangerous disorder. If anticoagulants develop in the course of hemophilia, the outcome is often fatal. Circulating anticoagulants which develop after pregnancy disappear spontaneously after several months.

Margolius A & others: Circulating anticoagulants. Medicine 40:145, 1961.
Shapiro SS: Characterization of factor VIII antibodies. Ann New York Acad Sc 240:350, 1975.

BLOOD TRANSFUSIONS

Blood transfusions are used to restore blood volume after hemorrhage; to improve the oxygen-carrying capacity of the blood in severe chronic anemia; and to combat shock in acute hemolytic anemia. Blood volume or red cell mass should be restored to approximately 70% of normal after hemorrhage. Adequate oxygen-carrying capacity can usually be maintained in chronic anemia by raising the hemoglobin value to 50–70% of normal. Shock in acute hemolytic or acute aplastic anemia can be prevented by maintaining hemoglobin values at 50–70% of normal.

Amount of Blood for Transfusion
A. Adults: Two units of whole blood or red cell mass will raise the hemoglobin by 2–3 gm in the average adult (70 kg) (red blood count 0.8–1 million/cu mm, hematocrit 8–9%). (Ten ml/kg of whole blood or 5 ml/kg of cells will produce a 10% hemoglobin rise.)
B. Children:
1. Over 25 kg–Give 500 ml of whole blood or 400 ml of red cells.
2. Under 25 kg–Give 20 ml/kg of whole blood or 15 ml/kg of red cells.
3. Premature infants–Give 10 ml/kg of whole blood or red cells.

Rate of Transfusion
Except in the case of emergencies, blood should be given at a rate of 80–100 drops/minute, or 500 ml in 1½–2 hours. For rapid transfusions, it is best to use a 15 gauge needle and allow the blood to run freely. The use of pressure is dangerous unless it can be applied by gentle compression of collapsible plastic blood containers.

Serologic Considerations
The antigens for which routine testing should always be performed in donors and recipients are A, B, and D (Rh$_0$). Pretransfusion compatibility tests use the serum of the recipient and the cells of the donor (major cross-match). To ensure a maximal margin of safety, each transfusion should be preceded by a 3-part compatibility procedure: (1) at room temperature in saline; (2) at 37° C fortified by the addition of albumin; and (3) at 37° C followed by an antiglobulin test.

Miscellaneous Considerations
The age of the blood (within the expiration period) is relatively unimportant in restoring volume deficits or repairing oxygen-carrying capacity defects. Fresh blood is required only if functioning platelets are needed; relatively fresh blood (less than 4 days old) is used in exchange transfusions. Red cell mass (hematocrit about 70%), infused through 17–18 gauge needles, is the treatment of choice in chronic anemias. Precipitates of platelets, leukocytes, and fibrinogen or fibrin in some bank bloods may clog the filters in administration sets and cause the infusion rate to slow down; when this happens, the filters should be replaced.

General principles of blood transfusion. Transfusion 3:301, 1963.
Hinkes E, Steffen RO: Current transfusion therapy. California Med 118:38, May 1973.
Uses of blood and blood components. Med Lett Drugs Ther 14:89, 1972.

FRESH BLOOD

Concern about the freshness of blood has to do with 4 considerations: (1) **Platelets:** Platelets are in adequate supply in whole blood up to about 24 hours after collection. (2) **Factors V and VIII:** All coagulation factors except V and VIII are stable in banked blood for at least 21 days; factors V and VIII decline fairly rapidly within a few days after collection. (3) **Levels of 2,3-diphosphoglycerate (2,3-DPG):** As red cells age–usually after a week or so–levels of 2,3-DPG decline, which causes increased affinity of hemoglobin for oxygen and results in less supply to the tissues. While normal affinity is restored in a few hours after transfusion, massive infusions of older blood to a critically ill patient may make him worse. The problem of declining 2,3-DPG levels may be largely solved when citrate-phosphate-dextrose (CPD) replaces acid-citrate-dextrose (ACD) as the standard anticoagulant in blood banking. (4) **Levels of plasma potassium, lactic acid, and ammonia:** Plasma levels rise very little above baseline for the first 4–5 days and become potentially important only after 2 weeks. Most transfusions are given for acute blood loss–either post-traumatic, during surgery where blood loss is inevitable, or in patients with acute hemorrhage from the gastrointestinal tract. In none of these 3 categories is the age of blood particularly important, and fresh blood should not be ordered.

The recognized occasions when the age of the blood may be specified are the following:
(1) Open heart surgery, where heparinized blood is needed. Heparinized blood cannot be used later than 24 hours after procurement.
(2) Exchange transfusions for hemolytic disease of the newborn. Blood should not be more than 2–3 days old to avoid immediate hemolysis of older cells,

which would put an undue burden on the immature liver of the newborn; and to avoid decline in red cell 2,3-DPG content.

(3) Massive transfusions, ie, more than 10 units in a few hours. Platelets may become a problem (see next section).

Fresh blood is an imprecise term; to most blood bank personnel, it means "same day's procurement," ie, blood no more than 24 hours old. It is needed where platelet problems exist. Relatively fresh blood (1–3 days old) is used for exchange transfusions. It is also used in critically ill, usually injured patients who require several units of blood. In renal dialysis and in patients with liver failure, blood can be given within a week after procurement. Some surgeons experienced in major trauma believe that "warm" blood, ie, used without refrigeration within 1–3 hours after collection, provides severely injured patients hemostasis not provided by "same day's procurement" blood. Until objective data on this become available, the use of "warm" blood must be considered experimental and its use restricted to those who can collect meaningful data.

TRANSFUSIONS IN BLEEDING PROBLEMS

Fresh frozen plasma, which contains all the clotting factors except platelets, may be used in a patient who continues to ooze postoperatively for several days if the suspicion of some type of hemophilia is strong and diagnostic results are not immediately available. Plasma is not a clinically useful source of fibrinogen because its fibrinogen concentration is too low.

When over 10 units of bank blood have to be given in a few hours, the levels of factors V and VIII may decrease sufficiently to cause prolongation of the PTT, but they usually do not fall below hemostatically adequate levels. Thrombocytopenic bleeding may become a problem and may have to be treated. Platelet concentrates are available in 30 ml volumes and contain three-fourths of the platelets formed in a unit of fresh blood. Two units of platelet concentrate will raise the platelet count by approximately 15,000/cu mm 1 hour after infusion in an average sized adult; 8 units are the minimum effective dose. Compatibility tests are not necessary for platelet concentrates; either type-specific or type O blood should be given.

Aggeler PM: Physiologic basis for transfusion therapy in hemorrhagic disorders. Transfusion 1:71, 1961.

HEMOLYTIC TRANSFUSION REACTIONS

Essentials of Diagnosis
- Chills and fever during blood transfusion.
- Pain in the back, chest, or abdomen.
- Hemoglobinemia and hemoglobinuria.

General Considerations
In all significant hemolytic transfusion reactions there is immediate, grossly visible hemoglobinemia. A normal serum color during or immediately after a transfusion rules out hemolysis as the cause of even severe symptoms.

In transfusion reaction due to ABO incompatibility the donor cells are hemolyzed instantaneously in the general circulation. In reactions due to incompatibility in some of the other blood groups (such as Rh), hemolysis is more gradual and may last hours, most of the destruction occurring in the reticuloendothelial tissues.

Serious transfusion reactions are often caused by clerical errors such as improper labeling of specimens or improper identification of patients.

Incompatibility due to uncommon blood group antibodies may be detected only by a Coombs test.

Clinical Findings
A. Symptoms and Signs: There may be chills and fever, and pain in the vein at the local injection site or in the back, chest, or abdomen. Anxiety, apprehension, and headache are common. In the anesthetized patient, spontaneous bleeding from different areas may be the only sign of a transfusion reaction.

B. Laboratory Findings: Post-transfusion blood counts fail to show the anticipated rise in hemoglobin; spherocytes may be present on the blood smear; and initial leukopenia at 1–2 hours is followed by a slight leukocytosis. Free hemoglobin can be detected within a few minutes. Methemalbumin, an acid hematin-albumin complex giving a brown color to the serum, may appear after a few hours and persist for several days. Elevated bilirubin levels, when present, are usually greatest 3–6 hours after the transfusion. Haptoglobin disappears from the serum. Hemoglobinuria and oliguria may occur.

After the reaction occurs it is essential to draw a fresh specimen from the patient, perform a direct Coombs test, and check it against the blood in the transfusion bottle (not the pilot tube) by the indirect Coombs test. If the indirect Coombs test is positive, exact identification of the offending antibody may be made by matching the patient's serum against a panel of known test cells. Unusual antibodies found in transfusion reactions are anti-c, anti-K (Kell), anti-E, anti-Fy[a] (Duffy), anti-Le[a] (Lewis), anti-Jk[a] (Kidd), anti-C, and anti-P.

Differential Diagnosis
Transfusion in the presence of leukoagglutinins,

which usually develop after 5 or more transfusions or after previous pregnancy, may cause severe chills and high fever. There is no fall in hematocrit, a cross-match is compatible, there are no pigmentary changes in the serum, and leukoagglutinins can be demonstrated in vitro when the patient's serum is matched against several white cell donors. In allergic transfusion reactions, the above tests also are negative and no leukoagglutinins are present.

Complications

Acute tubular necrosis and azotemia may follow a severe transfusion reaction.

Treatment

Hives, chills, and fever following the transfusion of blood are not necessarily due to hemolysis; if the patient's serum remains clear, the transfusion may be continued. However, once the diagnosis of hemolysis is well established by appropriate tests the main problems are to combat shock and treat possible renal damage.

A. Treatment of Shock: After antibody screening of the patient's serum, transfusions with properly matched blood may be advisable. If no satisfactory answer can be found to the reason for the transfusion reaction, plasma expanders, such as dextran, and plasma may have to be used instead of whole blood. Pressor agents may be necessary.

B. Treatment of Renal Failure: Some studies suggest that osmotic diuretics such as mannitol can prevent renal failure following a hemolytic transfusion reaction. After an apparent reaction and in oliguric patients, a test dose of 12.5 gm of mannitol (supplied as 25% solution in 50 ml ampules) is administered IV over a period of 3–5 minutes; this dose may be repeated if no signs of circulatory overload develop. A satisfactory urinary output following the use of mannitol is 60 ml/hour or more. Mannitol can be safely administered as a continuous intravenous infusion; each liter of 5–10% mannitol should be alternated with 1 liter of normal saline to which 40 mEq of KCl have been added to prevent serious salt depletion. If oliguria develops despite these efforts, treat as for acute renal failure.

Prognosis

The hemolysis is self-limited. Renal involvement is comparatively infrequent. The death rate from hemolytic transfusion reactions is about 10%.

Davidsohn I, Stern K: Blood transfusion reactions: Their causes and identification. M Clin North America 44:281, 1960.

POST-TRANSFUSION HEPATITIS

The risk of contracting hepatitis from a unit of whole blood is approximately 0.3%. It is only one-third as high when blood from donors negative for hepatitis B antigen (HB Ag) is used. Approximately 0.1–1% of potential donors are positive; it is thought that only one-third of hepatitis-transmitting donors can be detected by current methods, but severe cases may be entirely eliminated by screening for positive donors. Many cases of hepatitis following transfusion are not due to HB Ag.

The incidence of hepatitis with blood from positive donors is 50–75%. The risk of hepatitis from fibrinogen may approach 25%; the risk from pooled plasma is about 10%.

Blumberg BS & others: Australia antigen and hepatitis. New England J Med 283:349, 1970.

Feinstone SM & others: Transfusion-associated hepatitis not due to viral hepatitis A or B. New England J Med 292:767, 1975.

Gitnick GL: Australia antigen and the revolution in hepatology. California Med 116:28, April 1972.

10 . . .
Gastrointestinal Tract & Liver

John V. Carbone, Lloyd L. Brandborg, & Sol Silverman, Jr.

NONSPECIFIC MANIFESTATIONS

HALITOSIS
("Bad Breath")

Halitosis can result from many causes, including improper oral hygiene; chronic nasal and sinus disease; dental caries, gum infections, tonsillar infections; systemic diseases, fevers, and toxemias; chronic pulmonary disease (eg, lung abscess); gastrointestinal disease at almost any level of the gastrointestinal tract; and neuropsychiatric disorders where only the subjective complaint of "bad breath" is present.

In the absence of disease, oral malodor results from the production of odorous metabolic end products by some bacteria of the oral flora. Factors favoring odor production are stagnation of saliva in local areas within the oral cavity, a slightly alkaline pH, and the depletion of available carbohydrate.

Treatment is directed at the underlying cause. Thorough brushing of the teeth after each meal and the use of antiseptic rinses to reduce the number of microorganisms effectively decrease intrinsic odor formation.

McNamara TF & others: The role of microorganisms in the production of oral malodor. Oral Surg 34:41, 1972.

PYROSIS
("Heartburn")

Pyrosis, a disagreeable substernal burning pain, may result from any irritating stimulus of the distal esophagus. Its most important association is with reflux of acid-peptic gastric contents, ie, peptic esophagitis. The incidence of heartburn in pregnancy is very high (42–48%). Heartburn tends to improve in the final weeks of pregnancy and to disappear shortly after delivery.

Antacids are often effective in relieving symptoms, although it is not clear that they act by neutral-izing gastric hydrochloric acid. Reduction of acidity has the effect of reducing gastric secretion and increasing the pressure in the lower esophageal sphincter, thereby reducing reflux. The treatment is usually small dry meals, elevation of the head of the bed, maintaining an erect position after eating, weight reduction, and avoidance of tight clothing (eg, girdles and belts).

Briggs DW: Heartburn of pregnancy. Practitioner 200:824, 1968.
Castell DO, Levine SM: Lower esophageal sphincter response to gastric alkalinization: A new mechanism for treatment of heartburn with antacids. Ann Int Med 74:223, 1971.

NAUSEA & VOMITING

These symptoms may occur singly or concurrently, and may be due to a wide variety of causes. The vomiting center of the medulla may be stimulated by afferent impulses from gastrointestinal structures and other viscera. Correction is therefore dependent upon treatment of the underlying cause: irritation, inflammation, or mechanical disturbance at any level of the gastrointestinal tract (from pharynx to rectum); irritating impulses arising in any diseased viscera, eg, cholecystitis; disturbances of semicircular canals, eg, seasickness; and toxic action of cardiac drugs, eg, digitalis. Central (vomiting center) causes also include central emetics (emetine, apomorphine, morphine); exogenous and endogenous toxins, increased intracranial pressure, and cerebral hypoxia due to cerebral anemia or hemorrhage and psychologic factors.

Severe or prolonged nausea may reflect severe underlying gastrointestinal or systemic disease, eg, gastric outlet obstruction, small bowel obstruction, uremia, congestive failure, or pancreatitis.

Complications of vomiting include pulmonary aspiration of vomitus, post-emetic rupture of the esophagus (Boerhaave's syndrome), and gastroesophageal mucosal tear (Mallory-Weiss syndrome).

Treatment

Simple acute vomiting such as occurs following dietary or alcoholic indiscretion or in the morning sickness of early pregnancy may require little or no treatment. Severe or prolonged nausea and vomiting require careful medical management. Specific causes must be corrected. The following general measures may be utilized as adjuncts to specific medical or surgical measures:

1. Fluids and nutrition—Maintain adequate hydration and nutrition. Withhold foods temporarily and give 5—10% glucose in saline solution intravenously. When oral feedings are resumed, begin with dry foods in small quantities, eg, salted crackers, graham crackers. With "morning sickness" these foods may best be taken before arising. Later, change to frequent small feedings of simple, palatable foods. Hot beverages (tea and clear broths) and cold beverages (iced tea and carbonated liquids, especially ginger ale) are tolerated quite early. Avoid lukewarm beverages. Always consider the patient's food preferences.

2. Medical measures—*Note:* All unnecessary medication should be withheld from pregnant women during the critical early phase of fetal development. Unless nausea and vomiting of pregnancy are severe or progressive, caution should be observed in using medication for this purpose. The possible teratogenic effects of many classes of drugs are now being investigated.

(1) Sedative-antispasmodic drugs may be of value.

(2) Chlorpromazine hydrochloride may be administered deeply IM in doses of 25—50 mg every 4—6 hours as necessary, or orally in doses of 10—50 mg every 4—6 hours as necessary.

(3) Prochlorperazine, 5 mg 3—4 times daily orally when feasible; 25 mg by rectal suppository twice daily.

3. Psychotherapy—Attempt to determine the psychic basis of the nausea and vomiting, but avoid aggressive psychotherapy during the acute phase of the illness. Hospitalization may be necessary. Visiting should be restricted. Avoid unpleasant psychic stimuli such as strange odors, foul-smelling or foul-tasting medication, emesis basins or other unattractive objects, and foods which are improperly prepared or served.

Hill OW: Psychogenic vomiting. Gut 9:348, 1968.

Lumsden K, Holden WS: The act of vomiting in man. Gut 10:173, 1969.

Midwinter A: Vomiting in pregnancy. Practitioner 206:743, 1971.

HICCUP
(Singultus)

Hiccup, usually a benign, transient phenomenon, may occur as a manifestation of many diseases. It is important to rule out specific causes such as neuroses, CNS disorders, phrenic nerve irritation, cardiorespiratory disorders, gastrointestinal disorders, renal failure, infectious diseases, and other diseases. It may be the only symptom of peptic esophagitis.

Treatment

Countless measures have been suggested for interrupting the rhythmic reflex that produces hiccup. None of these may be successful, however, and the symptom may be so prolonged and severe as to jeopardize the patient's life.

A. Simple Home Remedies: These measures probably act by diverting the patient's attention; they consist of distracting conversation, fright, painful or unpleasant stimuli, or of having the patient perform such apparently purposeless procedures as holding his breath, sipping ice water, or inhaling strong fumes.

B. Medical Measures:

1. Sedation—Any of the common sedative drugs may be effective, eg, pentobarbital sodium, 0.1 gm orally or 0.13 gm by rectal suppository.

2. Stimulation of nasopharynx—A soft catheter can be introduced nasally to stimulate the nasopharynx and pharynx with frequent success.

3. Local anesthetics—Viscous lidocaine may be of some use. General anesthesia may be tried in intractable cases.

4. Antispasmodics—Atropine sulfate, 0.3—0.6 mg, may be given subcut.

5. Amyl nitrite inhalations may be effective.

6. CO_2 inhalations—Have the patient rebreathe into a paper bag for 3—5 minutes, or give 10—15% CO_2 mixture by face mask for 3—5 minutes.

7. Tranquilizers—Chlorpromazine hydrochloride and promazine hydrochloride have been used successfully for prolonged or intractable hiccup.

8. Antacids.

C. Surgical Measures: Various phrenic nerve operations, including bilateral phrenicotomy, may be indicated in extreme cases which fail to respond to all other measures and which are considered to be a threat to life.

Davis JN: An experimental study of hiccup. Brain 93:851, 1970.

Salem MR & others: Treatment of hiccoughs by pharyngeal stimulation in anesthetized and conscious subjects. JAMA 202:32, 1967.

Souadjian JV, Cain JC: Intractable hiccup: Etiologic factors in 220 cases. Postgrad MJ 43:72, 1968.

CONSTIPATION

The frequency of defecation and the consistency of stools vary greatly in normal individuals. The complaint of constipation often reflects the attitude of the patient with respect to the pattern of bowel movements. The patient should be considered to be constipated only if defecation is unexplainably delayed for a matter of days or if the stools are unusually hard, dry, and difficult to express. Specific causes of constipation include colonic or rectal lesions, hypometabolism, and neuroses. Be especially suspicious of organic causes when there are sudden unexplained changes in bowel habits. Inadequate fluids and highly refined low-residue foods may have a constipating effect. Constipation is a frequent complication of physical inactivity or prolonged bed rest. Many commonly used drugs may cause constipation: belladonna and derivatives, narcotics, diuretics, salts of bismuth, calcium, and iron, and aluminum hydroxide or aluminum phosphate gels.

Treatment

The patient should be told that (1) a daily bowel movement is not essential to health or well-being, (2) so-called "auto-intoxication" theories are unfounded, and (3) many symptoms (eg, lack of "pep") attributed to constipation have no such relationship.

A. Reestablishment of Regular Evacuation: Set aside a regular period after a meal for a bowel movement, even when the urge to defecate is not present. Cathartics and enemas should not be used for simple constipation since they interfere with the normal bowel reflexes. If it seems inadvisable to withdraw such measures suddenly from a patient who has employed them for a long time, bland laxatives and mild enemas (see below) can be used temporarily. Cathartic and enema "addicts" often defy all medical measures, and treatment is especially difficult when there is a serious underlying psychiatric disturbance.

B. Diet: The diet may be modified to satisfy the following requirements:

1. Adequate volume—Often "constipation" is merely due to inadequate food intake.

2. Adequate bulk or residue—Foods containing high fiber content such as bran and raw fruits and vegetables may be helpful unless specifically contraindicated (eg, intolerance).

3. Vegetable irritants—Unless there is a specific contraindication (eg, intolerance), stewed or raw fruits or vegetables may be of value, especially in the "atonic" type of constipation.

4. Adequate fluids—The patient should be encouraged to drink adequate quantities of fluids so that sufficient water will be available in the intestinal tract for passage of intestinal contents. Six to 8 glasses of fluid per day, in addition to the fluid content of foods, are ordinarily sufficient. A glass of hot water taken one-half hour before breakfast seems to exert a mild laxative effect.

C. Exercise: Moderate physical exercise is essential. Bed patients may require active and passive exercises. Good tone of the external abdominal muscles is important. Corrective physical therapy may be employed in patients with protuberant abdomens.

D. Medications: Bland laxatives may be employed temporarily. They should be withdrawn as soon as the constipation improves. The bulk-producing laxatives must be administered with an adequate or high fluid intake.

1. Liquid petrolatum (mineral oil) (a lubricant laxative), 15—30 ml 1—2 times daily as needed. Do not use mineral oil over prolonged periods, since it may interfere with intestinal absorption, particularly fat-soluble vitamins. There is also a slight risk of lipoid pneumonia, even from its oral use.

2. Agar with mineral oil, 15—30 ml 1—2 times daily as needed.

3. Olive oil, 15—30 ml 1—2 times daily as needed.

4. Vegetable mucilages (bulk-forming laxatives), eg, psyllium hydrophilic mucilloid (Metamucil), 4—12 ml 2—3 times daily after meals in a full glass of water.

5. Cascara sagrada aromatic fluidextract, a mild stimulant laxative, 4—8 ml at bedtime.

6. Magnesia magma (milk of magnesia), 15—30 ml at bedtime, is a common saline laxative. It should not be used in patients with impaired renal function.

7. Sodium phosphate, 4—8 gm in hot water before breakfast.

8. Dioctyl sodium sulfosuccinate (Colace, Doxinate), a surface wetting agent, in recommended doses varying from 50—480 mg/day.

9. Bisacodyl (Dulcolax), a mild colonic stimulant laxative, 10—15 mg at bedtime.

E. Enemas: Because they interfere with restoration of a normal bowel reflex, enemas should ordinarily be used only as a temporary expedient in chronic constipation or fecal impaction. In some instances it may be necessary to administer enemas, as required, for a prolonged period.

1. Saline enema (nonirritating)—Warm physiologic saline solution, 500—2000 ml as necessary.

2. Warm tap water (irritating)—500—1000 ml as necessary.

3. Soapsuds (SS) enema (irritating)—75 ml of soap solution per liter of water.

4. Oil retention enema—180 ml of mineral oil or vegetable oil instilled in the rectum in the evening and retained overnight. The oil is evacuated the following morning. This is continued until a "bowel rhythm" is reestablished.

Hinton JM, Lennard-Jones JE: Constipation: Definition and classification. Postgrad MJ 44:720, 1968.

FECAL IMPACTION

Hardened or putty-like stools in the rectum or colon may interfere with the normal passage of feces; if the impaction is not removed manually, by enemas, or by surgery, it can cause partial or complete intestinal obstruction. The impaction may be due to organic causes (painful anorectal disease, tumor, or neurogenic disease of the colon) or to functional causes (bulk laxatives, antacids, residual barium from x-ray study, low-residue diet, starvation, drug-induced colonic stasis, or prolonged bed rest and debility). The patient may give a history of obstipation, but more frequently there is a history of watery diarrhea. There may be blood or mucus in the stool. Physical examination may reveal a distended abdomen, palpable "tumors" in the abdomen, and a firm stool in the rectum. The impaction may be broken up digitally or dislodged with a sigmoidoscope. Cleansing enemas (preferably in the knee-chest position) or, in the case of impaction higher in the colon, colonic irrigations may be of value. Daily oil retention enemas followed by digital fragmentation of the impaction and saline enemas may be necessary.

FLATULENCE
(Tympanites)

The amount of intestinal gas varies normally from individual to individual. Intestinal gas comes from air swallowed unavoidably during eating and drinking (aerophagia), from gases in foods, and from the action of colonic bacteria. Flatulence may be due to functional and organic disease of the digestive system. Some of the gas is normally absorbed from the intestine, and the remainder is expelled as flatus.

Treatment

A. Specific Treatment: Eliminate specific causes if known.

B. Correction of Aerophagia: Anxiety states are often associated with deep breathing and sighing and the consequent swallowing of considerable quantities of air. When possible, treat underlying anxiety features.

C. Correction of Physical Defects: These sometimes interfere with normal swallowing or breathing. (1) Structural deformities of the nose and nasopharynx, eg, nasal obstruction and adenoids. (2) Spatial defects of the teeth or ill-fitting dentures.

D. Good Hygiene and Eating Habits: Instruct the patient to avoid dietary indiscretions, eating too rapidly and too much, eating while under emotional strain, drinking large quantities of liquids with meals, taking laxatives, and chewing gum.

E. Diet: The diet should be nutritious as tolerated and enjoyed by the patient. Milk and milk products and certain other foods (eg, beans, aromatic vegetables, carbonated beverages) may lead to excessive flatulence in susceptible individuals.

F. Medications: Drugs are generally unsatisfactory and at times are only of placebo value.

1. Anticholinergic-sedative drugs—These agents serve to diminish the flow of saliva (which is often excessive in these patients), thereby reducing the aerophagia which accompanies swallowing.

2. Spirit of peppermint, 0.5 ml 3 times daily in a small glass of water after meals.

3. Sedatives.

Berk JE (editor): Gastrointestinal gas. Ann New York Acad Sc 150:1, 1968.

Levitt MD: Intestinal gas production. J Am Dietet A 60:487, 1972.

Thompson WG: Burbulence (indigestion due to gas). Canad MAJ 106:1220, 1972.

DIARRHEA

Etiology

The causes of diarrhea, with examples, may be classified as follows:

(1) Psychogenic disorders: "nervous" diarrhea.

(2) Intestinal: Viral enteritis, bacterial infection due to salmonella, shigella, pathogenic *Escherichia coli* and yersinia, coccidiosis, giardiasis, amebiasis, heavy metal poisoning, catharsis habituation, antibiotic therapy, fecal impaction, gastrocolic fistula, inflammatory bowel disease, carcinoma.

(3) Malabsorption: Celiac sprue, vagotomy, short bowel syndrome.

(4) Pancreatic disease: Pancreatic insufficiency, pancreatic endocrine tumors.

(5) Cholestatic syndromes: Biliary atresia.

(6) Reflex from other viscera: Pelvic disease (extrinsic to gastrointestinal tract).

(7) Neurologic disease: Tabes dorsalis, diabetic neuropathy.

(8) Metabolic disease: Hyperthyroidism.

(9) Immunodeficiency disease: IgA deficiency.

(10) Malnutrition: Marasmus, kwashiorkor.

(11) Food allergy.

(12) Dietary factors: Excessive fresh fruit intake.

(13) Factitious: Surreptitious laxative ingestion.

(14) Unknown.

Treatment

Eliminate the specific cause whenever possible.

A. Correct Physiologic Changes Induced by Diarrhea: In addition to the necessity for control of hyperperistalsis, it is essential that the following secondary or complicating features be treated.

1. Fluid imbalance (dehydration).

2. Mineral imbalance (eg, hypocalcemia, hypokalemia, hyponatremia, hypomagnesemia).

3. Nutritional disturbances (eg, hypoproteinemia and other deficiencies).

4. Psychogenic disturbances (eg, fixation on gastrointestinal tract or anxiety regarding sphincter mishaps in cases of long-standing diarrhea).

B. Diet:

1. Acute—If diarrhea is severe, food should be withheld for the first 24 hours or restricted to clear liquids. Frequent small soft feedings are added as tolerated.

2. Convalescent—Food should be incorporated into the diets of patients convalescing from acute diarrhea as tolerated. Nutritious food, preferably all cooked, in small frequent meals, is usually well tolerated. *Avoid* raw vegetables and fruits, fried foods, bran, whole grain cereals, preserves, syrups, candies, pickles, relishes, spices, coffee, and alcoholic beverages.

A diet free of milk and milk products and all foods cooked is a restricted diet. These patients may require vitamin supplements if this diet is prolonged.

C. Antidiarrheal Agents:

1. Bismuth preparations—Any of the following

may be used for acute or chronic diarrheas:

a. Bismuth subcarbonate, 1–2 gm, after liquid bowel movements or 4 times daily.

b. Bismuth magma (bismuth hydroxide and subcarbonate), 4 ml after liquid bowel movements or 4 times daily.

c. Bismuth and paregoric—

R Bismuth subcarbonate   15–30.0
Paregoric, qs ad   120.0

> Sig: Shake well. One tsp after liquid bowel movements or 4 times daily.

2. Pectin-kaolin compounds—Useful proprietary mixtures are available (eg, Kaopectate). Give 15–30 ml 3 times daily, before meals and at bedtime, or after liquid bowel movements as needed.

3. Diphenoxylate with atropine (Lomotil), 2.5 mg 3–4 times daily as needed, is an effective antidiarrheal agent, but it must be used cautiously in patients with advanced liver disease and in those who are addiction-prone or who are taking barbiturates and other addicting drugs.

4. Opiates must be avoided in chronic diarrheas and are preferably avoided in acute diarrheas unless there is intractable diarrhea, vomiting, and colic. Always exclude the possibility of acute surgical abdominal disease before administering opiates. Give either of the following:

a. Paregoric, 4–8 ml after liquid movements as needed or with bismuth (see above).

b. Codeine phosphate, 15–65 mg subcut, if patient is vomiting, after liquid bowel movements as needed.

5. Strong opiates—Morphine and hydromorphone should be reserved for selected patients with severe acute diarrhea who fail to respond to more conservative measures.

6. Antispasmodic-sedative drugs are frequently useful. The antispasmodic drugs, particularly when used in combination with the barbiturates, exert a mild antiperistaltic action in acute and chronic diarrheas associated with anxiety tension states. It may be necessary to administer the various belladonna or belladonna-like alkaloids to a point near toxicity in order to achieve the desired effect.

D. Psychotherapy: Many cases of chronic diarrhea are of psychogenic origin. A survey of anxiety-producing mechanisms should be made in all patients with this complaint. Antidepressant therapy may be useful.

Barrett-Connor E: Travellers' diarrhea. California Med 118:1, March 1973.

Donovan EJ: A diagnostic approach to chronic diarrhea. Dis Colon Rectum 12:364, 1969.

Fordtran JS: Speculations on the pathogenesis of diarrhea. Fed Proc 26:1405, 1967.

Kraft AR, Tompkins RK, Zollinger RM: Recognition and management of the diarrheal syndrome caused by nonbeta islet cell tumors of the pancreas. Am J Surg 119:163, 1970.

Low-Beer TS, Read AE: Diarrhea: Mechanisms and treatment. Gut 12:1021, 1971.

Phillips SF: Diarrhea: A current view of the pathophysiology. Gastroenterology 63:495, 1972.

Read AE: Anti-diarrheal agents. Practitioner 206:69, 1971.

PSYCHOLOGIC GASTROINTESTINAL DISORDERS

This common group of disorders has many names, eg, nervous indigestion, functional dyspepsia, pylorospasm, irritable colon, spastic "colitis," functional "colitis," mucous "colitis," intestinal neurosis, and laxative or cathartic "colitis." All or a portion of the gastrointestinal tract may be involved. These disorders are characterized by hyperirritability and altered motility and secretion of the gastrointestinal tract, and they have a common origin in psychic factors or abnormal living habits (or both).

It is essential to eliminate the possibility of organic gastrointestinal disease. A history of "nervousness," neuropathic traits, and emotional disturbances can usually be obtained. The patient's living habits are irregular and unhygienic, eg, improper diet and irregular meals. Bowel consciousness and cathartic and enema habits are a prominent feature. There is a highly variable complex of gastrointestinal symptoms: nausea and vomiting, anorexia, foul breath, sour stomach, flatulence, cramps, and constipation or diarrhea, and a definite relationship can usually be established between symptoms and emotional stress or strain.

Nocturnal diarrhea, awakening the patient from a sound sleep, almost invariably is due to organic disease of the bowel.

Examination discloses generalized abdominal tenderness (variable), particularly along the course of the colon. X-ray shows sphincter spasm and altered gastrointestinal motility without other evidence of abnormalities.

Treatment

A. Diet: No single diet is applicable to all of these patients. Exclusion of milk and milk products may prove helpful. All foods should be cooked.

B. Personal Habits and Hygiene: Regular hours and meals and adequate sleep, exercise, and recreation are important. Restriction of alcohol and tobacco may be indicated.

C. Symptomatic Treatment: Sedative-antispasmodic medication is of particular value in these disorders.

D. Vegetable Mucilages: Eg, psyllium hydrophilic mucilloid (Metamucil).

E. Psychotherapy: This may consist of simple reassurance or more intensive technics. Reassurance as to the absence of organic disease, after careful examination, is most important.

Connell AM: The irritable colon syndrome. Postgrad MJ 44:668, 1968.

Esler MD, Goulston KJ: Levels of anxiety in colonic disorders. New England J Med 288:16, 1973.

Goulston K: Clinical diagnosis of the irritable colon syndrome. MJ Australia 1:1122, 1972.

Hislop IG: Psychological significance of the irritable colon syndrome. Gut 12:452, 1971.

MASSIVE UPPER GASTROINTESTINAL HEMORRHAGE

Massive upper gastrointestinal hemorrhage is a common emergency. It may be defined as rapid loss of sufficient blood to cause hypovolemic shock. The actual volume of blood loss required to produce shock varies with the size, age, and general condition of the patient and with the rapidity of bleeding. Sudden loss of 20% or more of blood volume (blood volume is approximately 75 ml/kg of body weight) produces hypotension, tachycardia, and other signs of shock. For example, a previously well 70 kg man who develops shock as a result of gastrointestinal hemorrhage will have lost at least 1000–1500 ml of blood. The immediate objectives of management are (1) to restore an effective blood volume and (2) to establish a diagnosis on which definitive treatment can be based.

The major causes of gastrointestinal bleeding are peptic ulceration of the duodenum, stomach, or esophagus, esophageal varices, and gastritis. In addition, bleeding may be due to Mallory-Weiss syndrome or hemorrhagic gastritis due to an ulcerogenic drug such as aspirin.

Clinical Findings

A. Symptoms and Signs: There is usually a history of sudden weakness or fainting associated with or followed by tarry stools or vomiting of blood. Melena occurs in all patients, and hematemesis in over 50%. Hematemesis is especially common in esophageal varices (90%), gastritis, and gastric ulcer. The patient may or may not be in shock when first seen, but he will at least be pale and weak if major blood loss has occurred. If the patient is not vomiting, a stomach tube will often help determine if the bleeding is in the upper gastrointestinal tract. There may be a history of peptic ulcer, chronic liver disease, other predisposing disease, alcoholic excess, or severe vomiting.

There is usually no pain, and the pain of peptic ulcer disease often stops with the onset of bleeding. Abdominal findings are not remarkable except when hepatomegaly, splenomegaly, or a mass (neoplasm) is present.

The etiology of bleeding should be established promptly, if possible, since the decision whether to operate or to continue with medical measures will often depend upon the diagnosis. The most critical differentiation is between peptic ulcer and esophageal varices, since emergency surgery may be indicated and successful in peptic ulcer but less often indicated or successful in varices. Specific diagnosis is of value also because of the difficulties of entering the abdomen in search of the unknown bleeding point.

A history of peptic ulcer or ingestion of antacids favors a diagnosis of peptic ulcer. A history of alcoholism or jaundice favors liver disease. Jaundice, hepatosplenomegaly, spider angiomas, liver palms, fetor hepaticus, ascites, and hepatic encephalopathy are suggestive of liver disease.

The principal diagnostic procedures in the investigation of gastrointestinal bleeding, to be carried out after instituting necessary emergency treatment, are outlined below.

B. Laboratory Findings: When the cause of the massive gastrointestinal hemorrhage cannot be established, certain laboratory studies should be conducted:

1. Liver function studies—Bilirubin, transaminases, serum protein electrophoresis, alkaline phosphatase, prothrombin time, and BSP retention determinations on the blood are useful in diagnosis of liver disease (portal hypertension and varices) as a possible cause of bleeding.

2. Coagulation studies—Studies of the clotting mechanism, bleeding time, prothrombin concentration, partial thromboplastin time, and platelet count may prove useful.

C. Endoscopy: Fiberoptic esophagogastroduodenoscopy should be done as the first definitive diagnostic examination if an experienced endoscopist is available. This procedure identifies bleeding sites and lesions more precisely than does x-ray. It is the only means of diagnosing hemorrhagic gastritis and is sensitive in detecting esophageal varices. Sigmoidoscopy should be done in all patients with gastrointestinal bleeding, particularly if they have not had hematemesis. Fiberoptic colonoscopy has not proved useful because of the difficulty in cleansing the colon.

D. X-Ray Findings: The cause of upper gastrointestinal bleeding can be demonstrated on x-ray in up to 75% of cases. If upper gastrointestinal endoscopy does not reveal the bleeding site, elective arteriography is indicated if the bleeding persists. Arteriography may not be successful if the bleeding is less than 1 ml/minute.

If the arteriogram fails to demonstrate the site of bleeding, then the upper gastrointestinal small bowel series is done. The patient's vital signs should be monitored during the procedure (tachycardia, postural syncope, hypotension).

Treatment

A. General Measures: The patient should be under the observation of both an internist and a surgeon from the outset. Bed rest and charting of fluid intake, urine output, and temperature are ordered. Insert a large-bore nasogastric tube, a Foley catheter, and a central venous pressure line. Blood pressure, pulse, and respiration are recorded every 15–60 minutes. Blood is obtained immediately for complete blood count and hematocrit, as well as grouping and cross-matching of at least 3 or 4 units of blood. In interpreting the red blood count and hematocrit it should be kept in mind that, after acute blood loss, a period of 24–36 hours may be required for reequilibration of body fluids. Meanwhile, the hematocrit poorly reflects extent of blood loss. Frequent determination of vital signs, especially those associated with postural changes, is helpful in estimating acute blood loss. Replacement therapy through a large intravenous needle (18 gauge minimum) or catheter is started immediately with lactated Ringer's injection or 5% dextrose in normal saline. If shock is severe, plasma is given while blood transfusion is being prepared. Aqueous vasopressin (Pitressin), 20 units in 200–250 ml of 5% glucose in water IV over a 30- to 40-minute period, causes temporary arteriolar vasoconstriction and lowering of the portal venous pressure. Although used primarily for variceal bleeding, it has been used for slowing arterial bleeding anywhere in the gastrointestinal tract.

Infusions of vasopressin may be repeated every 2–3 hours as necessary, but the clinician must be alert to the possibility of myocardial ischemia. Selective arterial perfusion of posterior pituitary extract has been reported to successfully control angiographically localized acute gastric hemorrhage. Water-soluble vitamin K (menadiol sodium diphosphate [Synkayvite], 5–10 mg orally or IM daily) is given empirically if hepatobiliary disease is suspected. Restlessness may be due to continued hemorrhage, shock, or hypoxia.

B. Blood Replacement: Treatment of shock by blood transfusion is begun without delay. Hematocrit or hemoglobin determinations are done every few hours until stabilized. The objective of blood replacement is to relieve shock and restore effective blood volume. The volume of blood required to accomplish this must be estimated empirically. Assume that blood volume is 75 ml/kg of body weight and calculate the patient's normal blood volume. If moderate shock is present (eg, blood pressure is 70–90, pulse rate 110–130, and there are clinical signs of hypovolemia such as faintness, pallor, cold and moist skin), transfusion equivalent to 25% of the normal blood volume will probably be required for resuscitation. If shock is severe, with blood pressure below 70, the initial volume of blood transfusion required may be 40–50% of normal blood volume. Shock should be controlled promptly and completely by rapid administration of blood. When blood pressure and pulse have been restored to relatively normal levels and clinical signs of hypovolemia have been relieved, blood transfusion may be slowed and the total volume of blood to be given is then determined by the course of the disease. A poor response usually means continued bleeding (see below) or inadequate replacement. A central venous pressure catheter is useful in gauging blood replacement and detection of over-transfusions and congestive heart failure.

C. Medical Measures: Acid peptic digestion is a causative or aggravating factor in many cases of massive upper gastrointestinal hemorrhage, perhaps including varices. Feedings and oral medications for ulcer are begun as soon as shock and nausea have subsided. Continued slight bleeding is no contraindication to the following regimen:

1. **Diet**—Liquid diet for the first 24 hours, followed by mechanically soft diet.

2. **Antacids**—Aluminum hydroxide-magnesium hydroxide mixture, 30 ml every hour. The clinician must be aware of the possibility of severe constipation and fecal impaction.

3. **Mild sedation.**

4. **A nasogastric tube** may be useful to permit evacuation of blood by lavage with ice water or an ice water-antacid mixture until returns are clear. Antacids may then be administered hourly through the tube, which is aspirated periodically to determine the presence of fresh blood.

D. Management of Bleeding Esophageal Varices: When varices are the cause of bleeding, special measures are indicated (see p 383).

E. Indications for Emergency Operation: Except when esophageal varices are the cause of bleeding, emergency surgery to stop active bleeding should be considered under any of the following circumstances: (1) When the patient has received 2 liters or more of blood but shock is not controlled or recurs promptly. (2) When acceptable blood pressure and hematocrit cannot be maintained with a maximum of 500 ml of blood every 8 hours. (3) When bleeding is slow but persists more than 2–3 days. (4) When bleeding stops initially but recurs massively while the patient is receiving adequate medical treatment. (5) When the patient is over 50. It has been shown that the death rate from exsanguination in spite of conservative measures is greater in the older age group. Massive bleeding is less well tolerated and is less likely to stop in older patients or small children, who will therefore require operative intervention more frequently.

Prognosis

The overall mortality of about 14% indicates the seriousness of massive upper gastrointestinal hemorrhage. Fatality rates vary greatly, depending upon the etiology of the bleeding and the presence of other serious systemic disease. Overall operative mortality for emergency surgery to stop bleeding is high, and best results are obtained when bleeding can be controlled medically and surgery deferred until the patient has recovered from the effects of the bleeding. Hemorrhage from duodenal ulcer causes death in about 3% of treated cases, whereas in bleeding varices the mortality rate may be as high as 50%.

Baum S, Nusbaum M: The control of gastrointestinal hemorrhage by selective mesenteric arterial infusion of vasopressin. Radiology 98:497, 1971.

Cooke AR: Intra-arterial vasopressin infusion: A therapeutic advance? New England J Med 290:624, 1974.

Frey CF, Reuter SR, Bookstein JJ: Localization of gastrointestinal hemorrhage by selective angiography. Surgery 67:548, 1970.

Halmagyi AF: A critical review of 425 patients with upper gastrointestinal hemorrhage. Surg Gynec Obst 130:419, 1970.

Lord JW & others: Portasystemic shunts in the management of massive hemorrhage from esophageal varices due to cirrhosis of the liver. Am J Surg 121:241, 1971.

Malt RA: Control of massive upper gastrointestinal hemorrhage. New England J Med 286:1043, 1972.

McGuire HH, Haynes BW: Massive hemorrhage from diverticulosis of the colon: Guidelines for therapy based on bleeding patterns observed in fifty cases. Ann Surg 175:847, 1972.

Menguy R: Acute gastric mucosal bleeding. Ann Rev Med 23:297, 1972.

Pitcher JL: Safety and effectiveness of the modified Sengstaken-Blakemore tube: A prospective study. Gastroenterology 61:291, 1971.

Renert WA & others: Mesenteric venous thrombosis and small bowel infarction following infusion of vasopressin into the superior mesenteric artery. Radiology 102:299, 1972.

Walls WD & others: Early investigations of haematemesis and melaena. Lancet 2:387, 1971.

Zollinger RM, Nick WV: Upper gastrointestinal tract hemorrhage. JAMA 212:2251, 1970.

DISEASES OF THE MOUTH

CARIES
(Dental Decay)

It is well established that 3 essentials are required to produce the carious lesion: bacteria, a substrate, and a susceptible tooth. Although animal studies indicate a relationship between caries and certain metabolic disorders, this association has not been confirmed in humans. Conditions that predispose to xerostomia (eg, tranquilizers and belladonna type drugs, Sjögren's syndrome, head and neck irradiation) may promote caries.

The diagnosis is based on x-ray examination (radiolucencies of the enamel and dentin) and clinical observation of an area of tooth structure that is soft, necrotic, discolored, and often sensitive. Both types of examination are necessary to a complete evaluation of the presence and extent of dental caries. There is no absolute correlation between extent of caries and symptoms. Absence of dental pain does not imply absence of caries.

Prevention & Treatment

The following empiric approach is suggested:

(1) Restorative dentistry to remove decay is the single most important measure. Do not neglect caries in deciduous teeth, since bone infection or premature loss of these teeth affects the health and eventual positions of the permanent dentition.

(2) Proper mouth hygiene will reduce bacterial flora and substrate. Frequent brushing with dentifrices and the use of mouth rinses are both helpful. Electric toothbrushes increase efficiency in cleansing tooth surfaces, but a relationship to reduced caries incidence has not been proved. Therapeutic ingredients other than fluoride added to dentifrices have no recognized beneficial effects.

(3) Reduction of carbohydrate (mainly sucrose) and sticky foods (eg, jams, cookies, foods that tend to adhere to tooth surfaces for prolonged periods) will reduce available substrate and acid production and decalcification.

(4) Topical applications (by a dentist) of fluoride will form a more acid-resistant tooth structure (fluoroapatite instead of hydroxyapatite). This procedure should be considered if a clinical problem of caries control exists even if the patient has been exposed to a fluoridated water supply during dental development. If water supplies are not fluoridated, daily oral fluoride supplements are recommended for the child up to age 12 (during tooth development). (The amount of supplementation depends upon the concentration of fluoride occurring naturally in the water supply and should not exceed a total daily intake of 1 mg.)

The evidence available does not give clear support to the use of fluoride as a prenatal supplement for caries prevention in children.

Carlos JP & others: Caries research: The current status. J Am Dent A 87:998, 1973.

DISCOLORED TEETH

The most common causes of discolored teeth are food stains, bacteria, habits (such as tobacco use), and drugs. These can be managed by altering habits and by dental prophylaxis. There may be pulpal hemorrhage induced by trauma, resulting in a deposition of hemosiderin on the internal crown surface. This causes a darkening of the tooth, which usually remains sterile and asymptomatic but nonvital. These teeth can be effectively bleached for aesthetic reasons. Occasionally, however, discoloration is due to changes in tooth structure caused by tetracyclines, congenital defects of enamel or dentin, fluorosis, and erythroblastosis fetalis.

Tetracycline discoloration occurs in some patients when these antibiotics (tetracycline, oxytetracycline, chlortetracycline, and demethylchlortetracycline) are given by mouth during the period of tooth development (infancy and childhood). Since an entire layer of dentin may be calcified in a few days, a small dosage over a short period may be incorporated into and appear to involve an entire tooth. The discoloration is gray-brown or yellow-brown. A typical yellow fluorescence is seen under ultraviolet light in undecalcified sections.

The teeth are not harmed. Treatment (by a

crown) is indicated only for aesthetic reasons. Preliminary reports indicate that bleaching technics utilizing 30% hydrogen peroxide (Superoxol) may be effective.

Dental fluorosis occurs most frequently when the fluoride in the water supply exceeds 2 ppm (1 ppm is the recommended concentration). Fluorosis can also be caused when the daily ingestion of fluoride-vitamin combinations exceeds the recommended levels (maximum of 1 mg of fluoride). The frequency and intensity of the discoloration are proportionate to the concentration in the water and the amount consumed during tooth development. The discoloration can vary from chalky-white to yellow-brown stains, often irregular in appearance. Deciduous teeth are not affected, possibly because the amount of fluorine available in utero is very low. These teeth can be effectively bleached as required with 30% hydrogen peroxide (Superoxol).

Rare hereditary congenital defects may cause brownish discoloration of the teeth. Treatment is primarily for aesthetic reasons.

Moffitt JM & others: Prediction of tetracycline-induced tooth discoloration. J Am Dent A 88:547, 1974.

ABSCESSES OF THE TEETH
(Periapical Abscess)

Dental decay is not self-limiting; unless it is removed it will lead to infection of the pulp and subsequent periapical abscess. Death of the pulp and periapical infection may also result from physical and chemical trauma. The only treatment is root canal therapy (cleansing and filling of the entire canal) or extraction.

In the early stage of pulp infection the symptoms may not be localized to the infected tooth. Intermittent throbbing pain is usually present, and is intensified by local temperature change. In the later putrescent stage the pain is extreme and continuous, and may be accentuated by heat but is often relieved by cold. After the infection reaches the bone, the typical syndrome is localization, pain upon pressure, and looseness of the tooth. Symptoms may then disappear completely, and, if drainage occurs, a parulis (gumboil) may be the only finding. When drainage is inadequate, swelling, pain, lymphadenopathy, and fever are often present. At this stage, antibiotics are advisable before local therapy is undertaken. Diagnosis depends upon symptoms, pulp testing (hot, cold, electricity), percussion, x-rays (may not show the diagnostic periapical radiolucency), looseness, deep decay or fillings, parulis, and swelling. Rule out sinusitis, neuralgia, and diseases affecting the cervical lymph nodes.

Incision and drainage are indicated whenever possible. Antibiotics and analgesics may be given as necessary. Unless contraindicated from a history of hypersensitivity, penicillin is the antibiotic of choice. Do not use antibiotic troches.

If not eventually treated by root canal therapy or extraction, the abscess may develop into a more extensive osteomyelitis or cellulitis (or both), or may eventually become cystic, expand, and slowly destroy bone without causing pain.

Johnson RH, Dachi SF, Haley JV: Pulpal hyperemia: A correlation of clinical and histologic data from 706 teeth. J Am Dent A 81:108, 1970.

VINCENT'S INFECTION
(Necrotizing Ulcerating Gingivitis, Trench Mouth)

Vincent's infection is an acute inflammatory disease of the gums which may be accompanied by pain, bleeding, fever, and lymphadenopathy. The etiology is not known, and it is doubtful if the disease is communicable. It may occur as a response to many factors, such as poor mouth hygiene, inadequate diet and sleep, alcoholism, and various other diseases such as infectious mononucleosis, nonspecific viral infections, bacterial infections, thrush of mouth, blood dyscrasias, and diabetes mellitus. The presence of fusiform and spiral organisms is of no importance since they occur in about one-third of clinically normal mouths and are absent in some cases of Vincent's infection.

Management depends upon ruling out underlying systemic factors and treating the signs and symptoms as indicated with systemic antibiotics, oxygenating mouth rinses (3% hydrogen peroxide in an equal volume of warm water), analgesics, rest, and appropriate dietary measures. Refer the patient to a dentist for further treatment (eg, curettage).

PERIODONTAL DISEASE

Periodontal disease is related to accumulations of microorganisms and substrate (plaque) on tooth surfaces. These may calcify and be recognized as calculus. Food, bacteria, and calculi which are present between the gums and teeth in areas called "dental pockets" may cause an inflammatory process and the formation of pus (pyorrhea) with or without discomfort or other symptoms. If this continues unchecked, the involved teeth will become loose and eventually will be lost as a result of resorption of supporting alveolar bone. If there is no drainage, accumulation of pus will lead to acute swelling and pain (lateral abscess).

The diagnosis depends upon a combination of findings, including localized pain, loose teeth, demonstration of dental pockets, erythema, and swelling or suppuration. X-ray may reveal destruction of alveolar bone.

As in periapical abscess, the severity of signs and symptoms will determine the advisability of antibiotics. Local drainage and oxygenating mouth rinses (3% hydrogen peroxide in an equal volume of warm water) will usually reverse the acute symptoms and allow for routine follow-up procedures. Curettage or gingivectomy (or both) to reduce excess gum tissue help prevent formation of the "dental pockets" which predispose to acute periodontal infections. In some cases, because of the advanced nature of the lesion (bone loss) or the position of the tooth (third molars in particular), extraction is indicated.

In some cases, periodontal disease occurs even in the presence of good hygiene and without obvious cause. Programs of regular dental care (periodic curettage and gingival or bone procedures) and home care (brushing, flossing, and rinsing) to remove dental plaque will at least slow the process of alveolar bone destruction.

•

Glickman I: Periodontal disease. New England J Med 284:1071, 1971.

Rizzo AA & others: Periodontal disease research. J Am Dent A 87:1019, 1973.

APHTHOUS ULCER
(Canker Sore, Ulcerative Stomatitis)

An aphthous ulcer is a shallow mucosal ulcer with flat, fairly even borders surrounded by erythema. The ulcer is often covered with a pseudomembrane. It has never been adequately demonstrated that this lesion is due to a virus or any other specific chemical, physical, or microbial agent. One or more ulcers may be present, and they tend to be recurrent. They are often painful. Nuts, chocolates, and irritants such as citrus fruits often cause flare-ups of aphthous ulceration, but abstinence will not prevent recurrence. Stresses of various types have also been shown to be contributory. Aphthous ulcers may be associated with inflammatory bowel disease, Behçet's syndrome, infectious mononucleosis, and prolonged fever. The diagnosis depends mainly upon ruling out similar but more readily identifiable disease, a history of recurrence, and inspection of the ulcer.

Bland mouth rinses and hydrocortisone-antibiotic ointments reduce pain and encourage healing. Hydrocortisone in an adhesive base (Orabase) has been particularly useful. Sedatives, analgesics, and vitamins may help indirectly. Vaccines and gamma globulins have not proved significantly beneficial. Although caustics relieve pain by cauterizing the fine nerve endings, they also cause necrosis and scar tissue. Systemic antibiotics are contraindicated. Systemic corticosteroids in high doses for a short period of time may be very helpful for severe debilitating recurrent attacks.

Healing, which usually occurs in 1–3 weeks, may be only slightly accelerated with treatment. Occasionally, aphthous ulcers take the form of periadenitis, in which they are larger, persist sometimes for months, and may leave a residual scar. This form can be confused with carcinoma.

Ulcerative stomatitis is a general term for multiple ulcerations on an inflamed oral mucosa. It may be secondary to blood dyscrasias, erythema multiforme (allergies), bullous lichen planus, acute herpes simplex infection, pemphigoid, pemphigus, and drug reactions. If the lesions cannot be classified, they are referred to as aphthae.

Brody HA, Silverman S Jr: Studies on recurrent aphthae. 1. Clinical and laboratory comparisons. Oral Surg 27:27, 1969.

Francis TC: Recurrent aphthous stomatitis and Behçet's disease. Oral Surg 30:476, 1970.

HERPETIC STOMATITIS

Herpetic infections of the mouth can be primary (one episode) or secondary (recurrent attacks).

Primary gingivostomatitis due to herpesvirus I (HSV I) occurs in about 90% of the population before age 10. The disease has diverse manifestations, ranging from mild, almost unrecognizable signs and symptoms to multiple intraoral and lip ulcerations, erythema, edema, fever, cervical lymphadenopathy, and malaise. The course of the illness usually entails an increase in signs and symptoms for 1 week and then 1 week of progressive improvement as antibodies are produced (serum antibody titers will increase at least 4-fold). Adults who never have been infected or who have not developed adequate immunity may develop similar disease. Increasing susceptibility is seen in patients on immunosuppressive drugs. Once afflicted with HSV, a patient develops permanent immunity.

Herpetic gingivostomatitis must be differentiated from aphthous stomatitis, which is not due to a virus. The diagnosis is established by the history (no prior attack and short duration), characteristic signs and symptoms, and a confirmatory cytologic smear (pathognomonic pseudo-giant cells). Direct cultures for HSV are positive but impractical.

There is no evidence that the disease is contagious; however, this might be explained by existing immunologic resistance among the contacts.

Treatment is palliative (analgesics, bland mouth rinses, fluids, soft diet, and rest). In the differential diagnosis, erythema multiforme, infectious mononucleosis, and pemphigus must be considered.

Recurrent intraoral herpetic infections are extremely rare and only occur on the mucosa covering bone (gingiva and palate). The ulcers are small, shallow, and irregular in size and shape. They can be mistaken for traumatic abrasions. There is no effective therapy, and the infection is self-limiting within 2 weeks.

Herpes labialis (cold sore) is due to recurrent HSV infections. These lesions usually have a burning premonitory stage and are first manifested by small vesicles that soon rupture and scab. Factors that trigger HSV migration by nerve pathways to the lip range from unidentifiable stimuli to temperature changes, chemical and physical irritants, or "stress."

The diagnosis is based on the history and the appearance of the lesions. The differential diagnosis includes carcinoma, syphilitic chancre, and erythema multiforme. No treatment has been uniformly successful. Improvement has been claimed by the use of idoxuridine ointment, chloroform, or ether applications, and, for recurrent lesions on the lips, topical 0.1% neutral red or 0.1% proflavine (dyes that alter viral DNA by photodynamic inactivation utilizing a cool light source).

There is no firm evidence that HSV I is associated either primarily or secondarily with oral carcinoma.

Silverman S Jr, Beumer J: Adult onset primary herpetic gingivostomatitis. Oral Surg 36:496, 1973.

CANDIDIASIS
(Moniliasis, Thrush)

Thrush of the mouth is due to overgrowth of *Candida albicans*. It is characterized by creamy-white, curd-like patches anywhere in the mouth. The adjacent mucosa is usually erythematous, and scraping the lesions usually uncovers a raw bleeding surface. Pain is commonly present, and fever and lymphadenopathy are sometimes present also. Although this fungus occurs in about one-third of normal-appearing mouths, overgrowth does not occur unless the "balance" of the oral flora is disturbed, eg, by debilitating or acute illnesses or by anti-infective therapy. Concomitant candidiasis of the gastrointestinal tract may occur.

The diagnosis is based upon the rather typical clinical picture, and may be confirmed by cultures.

Treatment is not uniformly successful; the infection usually persists in spite of treatment as long as the causative factors are present. The patient should have a nutritious diet with vitamin supplementation, and should receive sufficient rest. Saline solution mouth rinses every 2 hours give local relief and promote healing. Specific antifungal therapy consists of nystatin mouth rinses, 500,000 units 3 times daily (100,000 units/ml in a flavored vehicle), held in the mouth and then swallowed; vaginal troches (100,000 units) to be dissolved orally 4 times daily; and 1% aqueous gentian violet solution painted on affected areas 3 times daily.

In some instances, primarily under dentures, a candidal lesion may appear as a slightly granular or irregularly eroded erythematous patch. In these cases,

a diagnosis can be established by a heavy overgrowth of *Candida albicans* in culture or a biopsy revealing hyphae of candida invading epithelium (PAS stain). Nystatin powder, 100,000 units/gm, applied 4 times daily for several weeks, is frequently effective in reversing signs and symptoms.

Chronic angular cheilitis is often a manifestation of candidiasis. It is best treated with nystatin powder or Mycolog (nystatin-neomycin-gramicidin-triamcinolone) cream.

Cawson RA, Lehner T: Chronic hyperplastic candidiasis: Candidal leukoplakia. Brit J Dermat 80:9, 1968.

LEUKOPLAKIA

Leukoplakia (a white patch) of the oral mucous membranes is occasionally a sign of carcinoma; it is important to rule out malignancy.

The most common cause of leukoplakia is epithelial hyperplasia and hyperkeratosis, usually in response to an irritant. In many cases the cause cannot be determined.

Leukoplakia is usually asymptomatic. It is often discovered upon routine examination or by patients feeling roughness in their mouths. Because there is no reliable correlation between clinical features and microscopic findings, a definitive diagnosis may be established only by histopathology. However, because of the extensiveness of some intraoral leukoplakias, cytologic smears from the surface are helpful in supplementing both clinical and biopsy information.

Treatment consists of removing all irritants (eg, tobacco, ill-fitting dentures). If the leukoplakia is not reversible, excision should be performed when feasible. However, since some leukoplakias occur so diffusely that complete excision is often impractical, careful clinical examination and follow-up are essential. It must be remembered that the diagnosis must be reaffirmed periodically, since a leukoplakia may unpredictably be transformed into a malignancy. Electrodesiccation, cryosurgery, vitamin A, and proteolytic enzymes have not given predictably favorable results.

Silverman S Jr, Rozen RD: Observations on the clinical characteristics and natural history of oral leukoplakia. J Am Dent A 76:772, 1968.

SIALADENITIS

Acute inflammation of a parotid or submandibular salivary gland is usually due to viral or bacterial infection or, less commonly, blockage of the duct. The gland is swollen and tender. Observation of Wharton's and Stensen's ducts may show absent or scanty secretion with fluctuation of swelling, especially during meals, which indicates blockage; or a turbid secretion, which suggests infection. Clinical examination and x-ray may disclose ductal or glandular calcific deposits. Sialograms are of help in differentiating normal and diseased glands. Probing the ducts may reveal an inorganic plug or organic stenosis.

Inflammation of the salivary glands due to bacterial, chemical, or other unidentified factors may also cause xerostomia. When the dryness is not responsive to therapy and acute signs are not apparent, systemic sialagogues or local troches may stimulate salivation. Sjögren's syndrome must be considered.

Tumors may be confused with nonneoplastic inflammation. In these situations biopsy (usually excisional) should be performed, but only after other diagnostic and therapeutic procedures have failed to yield a diagnosis. Neoplasms are usually not associated with an acute onset and, at least in the early phases, are not painful. The lymph nodes are intimately associated with the salivary glands, and consideration must be given to diseases in which lymphadenopathy is a prominent finding, eg, lymphomas and metastatic malignancy.

In the acute stage, antibiotics, heat, and analgesics are indicated. Ductal stones which are too large for removal by massage and manipulation must be removed surgically (when the acute phase has subsided). If calcification or infection of the gland recurs often, extirpation of the gland must be considered. Radiation therapy may be effective in curing acute or recurrent sialadenitis which does not respond to other types of therapy.

Daniels TE & others: The oral component of Sjögren's syndrome. Oral Surg 39:875, 1975.

Epker BN: Obstructive and inflammatory diseases of the major salivary glands. Oral Surg 33:2, 1972.

GLOSSITIS

Inflammation of the tongue (usually associated with partial or complete loss of the filiform papillae, which creates a red, smooth appearance) may be secondary to a variety of diseases such as anemia, nutritional deficiency, drug reactions, systemic infection, and physical or chemical irritations. Treatment is based on identifying and correcting the primary cause if possible and palliating the tongue symptoms as required. Many obscure cases are due to such conditions as geographic tongue and median rhomboid glossitis.

The diagnosis is usually based on the history and laboratory studies, including cultures as indicated. Empiric therapy may be of diagnostic value in obscure cases.

When the cause cannot be determined and there are no symptoms, therapy is not indicated.

Dreizen S: Oral indications of the deficiency states. Postgrad Med 49:97, 1971.

GLOSSODYNIA, GLOSSOPYROSIS
(Chronic Lingual Papillitis)

Burning and pain, which may involve the entire tongue or isolated areas and may occur with or without glossitis, may be associated findings in hypochromic or pernicious anemia, nutritional disturbances, diabetes mellitus, or other disorders, and may be the presenting symptoms. In those cases due to diabetes the 2-hour glucose tolerance test is often positive when the screening urinalysis is negative. Allergens (eg, in dentifrices) are rare causes of tongue pain. Certain foods may cause flare-ups but are not the primary causes. Dentures, poor oral hygiene, and dental infections are usually of no etiologic significance.

Although most cases occur in postmenopausal women, these disorders are neither restricted to this group nor indicative of hypoestrogenemia.

In most cases a primary cause cannot be identified. Cultures are of no value since the offending organisms are usually present also in normal mouths. Many clinicians believe that these symptoms occur on a primarily functional basis.

Treatment is mainly empiric. Antihistamines, sedatives and tranquilizers, and vitamins are occasionally of value. Placebos are of value in differentiating functional and organic disease. Ointments and mouth rinses are of no value.

Partial xerostomia occasionally contributes to the symptoms. This may be remedied by sucking on nonmedicated troches or the administration of pilocarpine, 10–20 mg daily in divided doses.

Brody HA, Prendergast JJ, Silverman S Jr: The relationship between oral symptoms, insulin release, and glucose intolerance. Oral Surg 31:777, 1971.

Silverman S Jr: Oral changes in metabolic diseases. Postgrad Med 49:106, 1971.

PIGMENTATION OF GINGIVAS

Abnormal pigmentation of the gingiva is most commonly a racially controlled melanin deposition in the epithelial cytoplasm. It is most prevalent in nonwhite peoples. The color varies from brown to black, and the involvement may be in isolated patches or a diffuse speckling. Nongenetic causes include epithelial or dermal nevi (rare), drugs (eg, bismuth, arsenic, mercury, or lead), and amalgam fragments which become embedded in the gums during dental work. (Mercury from this source has not been determined to be a health hazard.) Similar lesions may also appear during the menopause or in Addison's disease, intestinal polyposis, neurofibromatosis, and several other disorders associated with generalized pigmentations.

The most important consideration is to rule out malignant melanoma (extremely rare in the mouth), which is suggested by rapid growth and slight elevation.

Hansen LS, Silverman S Jr, Beumer J: Primary malignant melanoma of the oral cavity. Oral Surg 26:352, 1968.
Rupp NW, Paffenbarger GC: Significance to health of mercury used in dental practice: A review. J Am Dent A 82:1401, 1971.

ORAL CANCER

Cancers of the lips, tongue, floor of the mouth, buccal mucosa, palate, gingivas, and oropharynx account for about 5% of all malignancies. Estimates from various surveys indicate that the average 5-year survival rate for all patients with oral cancer is less than 30%. However, with early detection, the 5-year survival rates are almost doubled. (By definition, detection is "early" when lesions are less than 2 cm in diameter without evidence of metastases.) Therefore, early diagnosis followed by adequate treatment appears to be the most effective means of controlling oral cancer.

The lips and tongue are the most frequent sites of involvement. Squamous cell carcinoma is the most common type, accounting for over 90% of all oral cancers. Oral cancer is a disease of older people; over 90% occur in persons over 45, and the average age is about 60. The male/female ratio is about 2:1.

The etiology of oral cancer is not known. A genetic factor is not apparent. There is a definite increased risk with the use of tobacco and alcohol. Oral leukoplakia is an important precancerous lesion.

There are no reliable signs or symptoms in early oral carcinoma, although pain is the most frequent first complaint. An early cancer may appear as a small white patch (leukoplakia), an aphthous-like or traumatic ulcer, an erythematous plaque, or a small swelling. Biopsy is the only method of definitely diagnosing a carcinoma. However, immediate biopsy of every ill-defined or innocuous-appearing lesion is impractical and not indicated. Exfoliative cytology is a simple, reliable, and acceptable means of differentiating benign and early malignant neoplasms. In the case of small lesions whose gross appearance would be altered by a biopsy, the clinician who will give the treatment should see the lesion before the biopsy is taken so he can judge the extent of resection or radiation required. Lymph nodes should not be incised for biopsy for fear of causing dissemination of tumor cells.

Curative treatment consists of surgery and radiation, alone or in combination. An attempt should be made to save the teeth necessary to support prostheses. Many teeth exposed to irradiation remain relatively free of disease and functional for long periods. The periodontium is maintained in optimal condition by periodic routine dental procedures. When areas that have been directly in the beam of irradiation are treated, extreme care is exercised and antibiotics may be selectively administered. Frequent fluoride applications appear to aid in minimizing tooth decalcification and caries. Daily mouth rinses containing 1 mg fluoride per 5 ml are a practical source. Alterations of taste and saliva are usually reversible; if not, there is no effective remedy. In many cases, pilocarpine solution, 5 mg 2–4 times daily, will selectively increase salivation and add to the patient's comfort.

Rubin P & others: Cancer of the head and neck. JAMA 215:1, 1971.

DISEASES OF THE ESOPHAGUS

ACHALASIA OF THE ESOPHAGUS

Achalasia is a disease of unknown cause in which there is dysergia, dysphagia, and dilatation of the esophagus. It is the result not of organic obstruction but impaired integration of parasympathetic stimulation. Peristalsis in the body of the esophagus is nonpropulsive and uncoordinated, and the lower sphincter remains closed because the impulses which should induce relaxation are disrupted. Difficult swallowing is variable at first in frequency and degree; later, it tends to become more persistent and severe. Although achalasia may appear in infancy or old age, it more commonly afflicts men in the fourth to sixth decades. It may predispose to esophageal carcinoma.

Two types of achalasia of the esophagus can be defined on the basis of differences in pathologic anatomy, symptoms, and radiographic findings. The first type (about 75% of cases) is characterized by narrowing of the distal 5 cm of the esophagus. The more proximal portion is markedly dilated and tortuous, with the ultimate appearance of an elongated sigmoid configuration. Stasis of intraluminal contents is responsible for varying degrees of esophagitis. Patients with this form of achalasia characteristically experience dysphagia without chest pain. However, regurgitation frequently causes soilage of the tracheobronchial tree with resultant pneumonitis, bronchiectasis, lung abscess, or pulmonary fibrosis.

In the second form of achalasia, the circular muscle fibers of the distal segment of the esophagus are hypertrophied and the proximal dilatation is not marked. Retrosternal or subxiphoid pain may appear early and is caused by esophageal spasm.

Dysphagia may initially be intermittent, with

food apparently sticking at the level of the xiphoid cartilage, and is associated with variable discomfort in the retrosternal or subxiphoid areas. Precipitation or accentuation of difficult swallowing may inconstantly follow the ingestion of solids or large quantities of cold beverages and may be related to emotionally stressful situations. Continued esophageal dilatation with retention of food and liquids results in a sensation of fullness behind the sternum. Pain (when present) may also radiate to the back and neck and may occur independently of swallowing. Because increased hydrostatic pressure facilitates swallowing, patients soon learn to drink extra water, followed by performance of the Valsalva maneuver, enabling more ready entry of esophageal contents into the stomach. However, prolonged impairment of alimentation may cause varying degrees of malnutrition.

Radiographic diagnosis is based on the characteristic tapering of the distal esophagus in a conical fashion to a markedly narrowed distal segment, 1–3 cm long, which usually lies above the diaphragm. Fluoroscopy, cinefluorography, and films of the proximal esophagus reveal purposeless and ineffectual peristalsis as well as varying degrees of dilatation. The subcutaneous administration of 5–10 mg of methacholine (Mecholyl) to a patient with achalasia can also be seen to cause violent peristalsis and mass contractions of the esophagus with retrograde propulsion of barium toward the mouth. Severe chest pain will usually occur at the same time, making it mandatory that atropine be available to terminate this response.

After a clear liquid diet for 24–36 hours and pre-endoscopic aspiration and lavage, esophagoscopy should be performed at least once in every case of achalasia to ascertain the severity of esophagitis and to eliminate the possibility of occult carcinoma.

Brusque dilatation, using a pneumatic bag under fluoroscopic guidance—designed to split muscle fibers of the esophagogastric vestibule—is the definitive form of nonsurgical treatment. Passage of mercury-filled bougies is, at best, only palliative, but may be employed in a preparatory way to enable easier emptying of esophageal contents prior to pneumatic dilatation. Esophagocardiomyotomy is required in approximately 20–25% of patients.

Benedict EG: Forceful dilatation and surgery in treatment of achalasia. JAMA 188:105, 1965.

Bennett NR: Achalasia of the cardia: Reflections upon a clinical study of over 100 cases. Brit MJ 1:1135, 1964.

Cohen BR & others: The clinical value of esophageal motility study. JAMA 187:819, 1964.

Ellis FH & others: Esophagomyotomy for esophageal achalasia: Experimental, clinical, and manometric aspects. Ann Surg 166:640, 1967.

Fleshler B: Diffuse esophageal spasm. Gastroenterology 52:559, 1967.

Gillies M & others: Clinical, manometric, and pathological studies in diffuse esophageal spasm. Brit MJ 1:527, 1967.

Hendrix TR, Bennett JR: Diffuse esophageal spasm: A disorder with more than one cause. Gastroenterology 59:272, 1970.

Just-Viera JO, Haight C: Achalasia and carcinoma of the esophagus. Surg Gynec Obst 128:1081, 1969.

Palmer ED: Hiatus hernia associated with achalasia of the esophagus. Gastrointest Endosc 17:177, 1971.

ESOPHAGEAL WEBS

Esophageal webs are thin membranous structures which include in their substance only mucosal and submucosal coats. They are occasionally congenital but more commonly appear to be the sequelae of ulceration, local infection, hemorrhage, or mechanical trauma. Cervical vertebral exostoses are believed to be the most common cause. Most webs are found in the proximal portion of the esophagus and produce significant dysphagia with occasional laryngospasm. Difficult swallowing secondary to a web—when combined with iron deficiency anemia, splenomegaly, glossitis, and spooning of the nails and occurring almost invariably in premenopausal women—is called Plummer-Vinson syndrome. In this condition, a diaphanous web is usually located immediately below the cricopharyngeus and is associated with an atrophic pharyngoesophagitis. Esophagoscopy, which is essential to rule out carcinoma effectively, ameliorates dysphagia by disrupting the web. However, bougienage with Mahoney or Hurst dilators may occasionally be necessary.

Postlethwait RW, Sealy WC: Experiences with the treatment of 59 patients with lower esophageal web. Ann Surg 165:786, 1967.

Seaman WB: The significance of webs in the hypopharynx and upper esophagus. Radiology 89:32, 1967.

Smiley TB & others: Sideropenic dysphagia and hiatus hernia. Lancet 2:7, 1963.

LOWER ESOPHAGEAL RING
(Schatzki's Ring)

The finding of a static but distensible lower esophageal ring usually signifies the presence of a sliding hiatus hernia which may or may not be symptomatic. Most rings histologically represent the esophagogastric junction. Manometric studies have also confirmed that the lower esophageal ring physiologically represents the point at which the esophagus and stomach meet. However, biopsies from both sides of the ring have rarely revealed esophageal mucosa, thus indicating that some rings can be purely esophageal in origin.

The classical ring is 4 mm or less in thickness, is composed of a connective tissue core with muscularis mucosae, and is covered on the upper side by squamous (esophageal) epithelium and on the lower side by columnar (gastric) epithelium. Submucosal fibrosis is present, but esophagitis is usually absent. This correlates well with the clinical absence of "heartburn," suggesting that significant gastroesophageal reflux is not present.

Not all lower esophageal rings are mucosal in nature. Some are due to muscular contractions of the esophagus. Distention of the lower esophagus with barium does not obliterate a mucosal ring but rather accentuates it. Dysphagia is likely to be present when the ring reduces the internal esophageal lumen to a diameter of 13 mm or less.

Most rings can be seen at endoscopy with fiberoptic instruments and can frequently be successfully treated simply by passing an esophagoscope through the ring, thereby dilating it. In the event of a tight ring, multiple biopsies can be taken around its circumference. If this does not relieve difficult swallowing, it will at least facilitate peroral dilatation.

Goyal RK, Glancy JJ, Spiro HM: Lower esophageal ring. (2 parts.) New England J Med 282:1298, 1355, 1970.

Rinaldo JA & others: The narrow lower esophageal ring. Am J Digest Dis 11:257, 1966.

Sanowski RA, Riegel N: Pneumatic dilatation of lower esophageal ring. Am J Digest Dis 15:407, 1970.

ESOPHAGEAL CYSTS

Esophageal cysts probably result from buds of the primitive foregut or tracheobronchial branches. They may be asymptomatic but can cause dysphagia, dyspnea, cough, cyanosis, or chest pain, either because of their location or because they tend to contain acid-secreting epithelium which may produce peptic ulceration. The cysts are in the lower half of the esophagus between the muscle layers of the esophageal wall. Diagnosis is made by demonstration of a mediastinal mass on x-ray or at surgery. Surgical excision may be necessary.

Desforges G, Strieder JW: Esophageal cysts. New England J Med 262:60, 1960.

ESOPHAGEAL DIVERTICULOSIS

Essentials of Diagnosis

- Dysphagia progressing as more is eaten; bad breath, foul taste in mouth.
- Regurgitation of undigested or partially digested food representing first portion of a meal.
- X-ray (barium) confirms diagnosis.

General Considerations

Although it has been customary for almost a cen-tury to divide diverticula of the esophagus into traction and pulsion types, the clinical picture and pathologic effects of esophageal diverticulosis are to a large extent dictated by the location of the lesion. Additionally, it is therefore convenient to distinguish pharyngoesophageal (pulsion or Zenker's), midesophageal (traction), and epiphrenic (traction-pulsion) diverticula by their locations. The first (pharyngoesophageal) develops through the space of Lannier-Hackerman in the posterior line at the junction of the hypopharynx and esophagus; occurs chiefly in middle-aged men; and may attain large size. The second (midesophageal) type rarely is larger than 2 cm; may be multiple; frequently arises opposite the pulmonary hilar region; occurs with equal frequency in men and women; and usually causes no symptoms. The third and least common (epiphrenic) type occurs primarily in men in the esophageal segment immediately proximal to the hiatus; may be congenital in origin; and progressively enlarges so that afflicted individuals become symptomatic in middle age. Pharyngoesophageal and epiphrenic diverticula frequently produce nocturnal regurgitation and aspiration with resultant bronchitis, bronchiectasis, and lung abscess.

Clinical Findings

A. Symptoms and Signs: The main symptoms of pharyngoesophageal (Zenker's) diverticula are dysphagia, regurgitation, gurgling sounds in the neck, nocturnal coughing, halitosis, and weight loss. Enlargement of the pouch results in its downward dissection between the postesophageal septum of the deep cervical fascia and the prevertebral fascia. When filled with food, the pouch may appear as a swelling at the side of the neck, and internally is able to compress from behind to produce obstruction of the proximal esophagus. There is frequently so much compression of the esophagus that its entrance becomes slitlike, making it difficult to find endoscopically, and readily explaining the difficulty in swallowing and impaired nutrition.

Epiphrenic diverticula, which are occasionally associated with achalasia, usually cause no symptoms at first but ultimately may produce dysphagia, pain, and pulmonary complications.

Although midesophageal diverticula may rarely be responsible for mediastinal abscess or esophagobronchial fistulas and inconstantly may cause dysphagia, these lesions generally produce no symptoms.

B. X-Ray Diagnosis: Barium swallow will usually demonstrate the 3 types of diverticula without difficulty.

Differential Diagnosis

Regurgitation and difficult swallowing associated with diverticula must be distinguished from that caused by neoplasm, vascular anomalies, hiatus hernia, stenoses, or motility dysfunctions of the esophagus. Epiphrenic diverticula must also be differentiated from esophageal ulcer. Physical examination, radiography, and endoscopy totally clarify the situation.

Treatment & Prognosis

Large and symptom-producing pharyngoesophageal and epiphrenic diverticula should be treated surgically by amputation. Although recurrence or postoperative dysphagia is occasionally seen following operation for the former, long-term results are usually excellent. Cricopharyngeal sphincter myotomy has been advocated for pharyngoesophageal diverticula secondary to an abnormal sphincter. Since midesophageal pouches rarely produce complications or significant symptoms, therapy is usually not required.

Allen T, Clagett OT: Changing concepts in the surgical treatment of pulsion diverticula of the lower esophagus. J Thoracic Cardiovas Surg 50:455, 1965.

Cross FS: Esophageal diverticula and related neuromuscular problems. Ann Otol Rhin Laryng 77:914, 1968.

Ellis FH Jr: Cricopharyngeal myotomy for pharyngoesophageal diverticulum. Ann Surg 170:340, 1969.

Welsh GF, Payne WS: The present status of one-stage pharyngeo-esophageal diverticulectomy. S Clin North America 53:953, 1973.

REFLUX ESOPHAGITIS

Peptic esophagitis is probably secondary only to duodenal ulcer as a discernible cause of upper gastrointestinal symptoms. The esophagus is damaged whenever it is exposed to the contents of either the stomach or the small intestine. Since the condition occurs in situations in which there is achlorhydria—and since bile is known to be irritating—the "acid-pepsin theory" as the primary cause is apparently not adequate. The common denominator in the genesis of reflux esophagitis, therefore, is reflux of either acid or alkaline gastric juice. The lower esophageal sphincter functions as a high pressure zone between the stomach and esophagus and is an important protective mechanism against reflux. That portion of the esophagus which is normally infradiaphragmatic is responsive to increases in intragastric pressure induced by elevation of intra-abdominal pressure and maintains the barrier between the stomach and the thoracic esophagus. Among conditions which contribute to reflux are (1) hiatus hernia, (2) short esophagus, (3) pregnancy, (4) pernicious vomiting, and (5) nasogastric intubation.

Symptoms include pyrosis, which is often worsened by recumbency and ameliorated by antacids, waterbrash (the combination of regurgitation and increased salivation), dysphagia, and odynophagia. Blood tinging of regurgitated material or (occasionally) frank hematemesis, anemia, and stricture formation are later manifestations.

The diagnosis is based primarily on the history, radiography, and esophagoscopy. Cinefluorography, acid perfusion (Bernstein) test, esophageal manometry, and biopsy are complementary modalities.

Successful treatment depends on preventing reflux or ameliorating its effects. Therefore, conditions which predispose to increased intra-abdominal pressure, eg, tight belts or corsets, should be avoided. Elevation of the head of the bed and frequent administration of antacids are important concomitants of effective therapy. Keeping patients in a sitting position during the course of nasogastric intubation is prophylactically important to avoid reflux and potential stenosis. Dysphagia secondary to stricture formation is effectively managed by esophageal dilatation, using either Puestow "stringless" dilators or mercury-filled bougies.

If medical management is not successful, surgical treatment is indicated, and it is ultimately designed to modify anatomically those conditions which produce reflux or correct its sequelae. Accordingly, repair of reflux due to hiatus hernia and relief of esophageal stricture give highly satisfactory results in carefully selected patients.

Benz LJ & others: A comparison of clinical measurements of gastroesophageal reflux. Gastroenterology 62:1, 1972.

Bombeck CT, Aoki T, Nyhus LM: Anatomic etiology and operative treatment of peptic esophagitis: An experimental study. Ann Surg 165:752, 1967.

Cocco AE, Brantigan OL: Esophagitis: Diagnosis and surgical treatment. Ann Surg 169:857, 1969.

Crozier RE & others: Obscure chest pain as a symptom of reflux esophagitis. M Clin North America 56:771, 1972.

Windsor CWO: Gastroesophageal reflux after partial gastrectomy. Brit MJ 2:1233, 1964.

BARRETT'S ESOPHAGUS

Barrett's esophagus is an acquired disorder of unknown cause in which the lower one-third to one-half of the esophagus is lined by columnar rather than by squamous epithelium. While nests of columnar cells may occur at any level of the esophagus, that organ is normally lined by squamous epithelium. However, there is histologic proof that transition of this normal lining to columnar epithelium may follow the chronic inflammation associated with peptic esophagitis. The theorized sequence of events would seem to be (1) gastroesophageal reflux, (2) esophagitis, (3) regeneration of columnar rather than squamous epithelium, and (4) cephalad or circumferential extension of the abnormal lining, with progressive involvement of the distal esophagus. The previously described phenomena may well represent a protective adaptation of the esophagus to gastric reflux.

The principal symptoms are pyrosis or dysphagia. The entity should be thought of when there is radiographic evidence of a high, seemingly benign stricture followed by a normal-appearing esophagus with or without accompanying hiatus hernia or a discrete "peptic ulcer" of the lower gullet. Esophagoscopy and biopsy are required to establish the histologic characteristics of the mucosal lining and to differentiate esophageal ulcer from epiphrenic diverticulum.

Treatment is basically the same as for esophagitis, ie, neutralization of the effects of gastric reflux by gravity or antacids, early consideration of surgical repair of hiatus hernia, and dilatation of esophageal strictures.

Adler RH: The lower esophagus lined by columnar epithelium: Its association with hiatal hernia, ulcer, stricture, and tumor. J Thoracic Cardiovas Surg 45:13, 1963.

Cohen BR & others: Correlation of manometric, esophagoscopic and radiologic findings in the columnar lined gullet (Barrett syndrome). Gut 4:406, 1963.

De La Pava S & others: Ectopic gastric mucosa of the esophagus: A study on histogenesis. New York J Med 64:1831, 1964.

Trier JS: Morphology of the epithelium of the distal esophagus in patients with midesophageal peptic strictures. Gastroenterology 58:444, 1970.

BENIGN STRICTURE OF THE ESOPHAGUS

Healing of any inflammatory lesion of the esophagus may result in stricture formation. Common causes are peptic esophagitis secondary to gastroesophageal reflux; Barrett's epithelium and ulcer formation; ingestion of corrosive substances; acute viral or bacterial infectious diseases; and, rarely, injuries caused by endoscopes.

The principal symptom is dysphagia, which may not appear for years after the initial insult. In patients who have swallowed caustics, the initial difficulty with swallowing caused by edema may be short-lived. However, it may be followed weeks or months later by stricture formation. Ability to swallow liquids is maintained the longest.

Odynophagia (painful swallowing) occurs not infrequently in association with difficult swallowing. The patient's description of the point at which he senses "hang-up" of food conforms with amazing accuracy to the level of the obstruction.

X-ray demonstration of smooth narrowing with no evidence of mucosal irregularity is usually diagnostic. However, esophagoscopy, biopsy, and cytologic examination are mandatory in all cases to rule out the possibility of malignancy.

Dilatation is the definitive form of treatment, using Puestow dilators or mercury-filled (Mahoney or Hurst) bougies to attain a lumen size of 45—60F. However, both the patient and the physician must be prepared for a continuing program of bougienage, since recurrence of stenosis will invariably ensue if dilatation is terminated once swallowing again becomes normal. Monthly passage of the largest bougie which the patient can tolerate usually prevents regression. If dilatation is unsuccessful, resection of the stricture with esophagogastrostomy or jejunal or colonic interposition will be indicated.

Adler RH: The lower esophagus lined by columnar epithelium: Its association with hiatal hernia, ulcer, stricture, and tumor. J Thoracic Cardiovas Surg 45:13, 1963.

Hill LD & others: Simplified management of reflux esophagitis with stricture. Ann Surg 172:638, 1970.

Jordon PH Jr, Longhi EH: Diagnosis and treatment of an esophageal stricture (ring) in a patient with Barrett's epithelium. Ann Surg 169:355, 1969.

Law SW, Sheehan EE: Benign esophageal stricture and the lower esophagus lined by columnar epithelium: Report of two cases. Dis Chest 48:214, 1965.

HIATUS HERNIA
(Diaphragmatic Hernia)

Essentials of Diagnosis

- Pressure sensation, severe pain, burning behind lower sternum (any one or all 3).
- Pain aggravated by recumbency or increase of abdominal pressure, relieved by upright position.
- Cough, dyspnea, palpitation, and tachycardia may be present.
- X-ray and esophagoscopy demonstrate the herniation.

General Considerations

The esophageal hiatus is a "teardrop"-shaped opening in the right crus of the diaphragm, lying anteriorly and to the left of the upper part of the abdominal aorta. The only anatomic attachment between the esophagus and diaphragm at the hiatus is the diaphragmatico-esophageal ligament, an insubstantial structure which offers little support to this area. Therefore, it is not surprising that conditions which greatly increase intra-abdominal pressure such as obesity, pregnancy, or crush injuries and poor musculature promote herniation of part of the stomach through the hiatus.

There are essentially 2 types of hiatus hernia: (1) The most common (75—80%) is the sliding hiatus hernia in which a portion of the stomach slides up through the hiatus, carrying a peritoneal sac with it. The esophagus is of normal length, but the esophagogastric junction lies above the diaphragm. In the short esophageal type (12%), the esophagogastric junction is above the hiatus and the stomach is converted into a funnel-like structure that is drawn up through the hiatus into the mediastinum. (2) In the relatively rare para-esophageal type (7%), the fundus of the stomach herniates either through the hiatus or through a separate opening in the diaphragm lateral to the hiatus but the esophagogastric junction maintains its normal relation to the hiatus.

Clinical Findings

A. Symptoms and Signs: Pyrosis ("heartburn") is the most common symptom and is inconstantly indicative of the degree of esophagitis which is secondary to reflux. It is frequently severe, occurring 30—60 minutes after eating, and is initiated or accentuated by recumbency and relieved by sitting upright. Pain at the lower sternal level or xiphoid frequently radiates into the interscapular area, neck, jaw, or down the arms. Dysphagia may occur if there is ulceration or esophagitis with secondary stenosis. Regurgitation may result in soilage of the tracheobronchial tree with resultant cough and dyspnea.

B. X-Ray Findings: There is usually no problem in the radiographic identification of hernias of the para-esophageal type or those which are associated with a shortened esophagus. However, the radiologist not infrequently has difficulty in demonstrating hernias of the sliding type, despite placement of the patient in the Trendelenburg position. Diagnosis hinges on showing both gastric mucosa and the esophagogastric junction above the diaphragm. Demonstration of an esophageal ring almost always indicates a hiatus hernia. Reflux of barium from the stomach into the esophagus occurs frequently in individuals with sliding type hernias but may also occur in the absence of that abnormality. There is usually complete reduction of the hernia on the upright films.

C. Special Examinations: Esophagoscopic visualization of the junction of esophageal and gastric mucosa in relationship to the diaphragm enables accurate diagnosis of hernias of the sliding type but is not helpful in evaluation of the para-esophageal variety. Accurate assessment of esophagitis can only be accomplished by esophagoscopy, the severity of the process being related to the presence or degree of **hyperemia, friability, erosion,** and **exudation.** Endoscopy is mandatory in patients in whom symptoms persist despite adherence to a good treatment program and in those who have dysphagia. The acid perfusion (Bernstein) test and esophageal manometry are confirmatory studies for establishing the presence or absence of reflux.

Differential Diagnosis

The differentiation of the retrosternal chest pain of hiatus hernia from that of angina pectoris or myocardial infarction requires sequential ECGs, enzyme determinations, and close clinical observation. Gastroduodenal ulcer disease, presenting with similar symptoms, can usually be distinguished by radiographic study.

Complications

Esophagitis, stenosis, and esophageal ulcer are the most common complications. However, significant gastritis in the herniated portion of the stomach is often a cause of occult blood and anemia.

Treatment

Since obesity is an associated or precipitating factor in sliding hiatus hernia, weight reduction is essential. Conditions which predispose to increased intra-abdominal pressure, eg, tight belts or corsets, should be avoided. The patient should also be advised to avoid lying down immediately after meals and to sleep with the head of the bed elevated 20–25 cm

(8–10 inches) with wooden blocks. Despite the well-documented association of occasionally low or absent gastric acidity with pyrosis, frequent administration of antacids is nevertheless helpful in markedly symptomatic individuals or in those with endoscopic documentation of severe esophagitis.

Large hiatus hernias or those of the para-esophageal type will frequently require surgical repair because of failure to respond to medical treatment or significant complications such as hemorrhage, persistent anemia, or pulmonary fibrosis secondary to regurgitation and aspiration. Paradoxically, small sliding hiatus hernias frequently produce pain which is not ameliorated by conservative measures and may necessitate operation to allay varying incapacity.

Prognosis

Most patients (85–90%) with hiatus hernias respond to weight reduction and other conservative measures. Surgical repair of hiatus hernia is unsuccessful either in relieving symptoms not due to reflux or in restoring and maintaining normal anatomic relationships. However, the prognosis is usually good in patients with esophageal reflux who have been carefully selected prior to operation.

Berman JK: The balanced procedure for the treatment of hiatal hernia complex: A reaffirmation. S Clin North America 53:529, 1973.

Cohen S, Harris LD: Does hiatus hernia affect competence of the gastroesophageal sphincter? New England J Med 284:1053, 1971.

Ellis FH Jr: Esophageal hiatus hernia. New England J Med 287:646, 1972.

Forstner GG, Bogoch A: Gastritis of the herniated stomach in patients with esophageal hiatus hernia. Canad MAJ 88:16, 1963.

Fraser K & others: Hiatus hernia: Follow-up after surgery. Brit J Surg 53:691, 1966.

Palmer ED: The hiatus hernia-esophagitis-esophageal stricture complex: Twenty-year prospective study. Am J Med 44:566, 1968.

Pearson JEG, Wilson RSE: Diffuse pulmonary fibrosis and hiatus hernia. Thorax 26:300, 1971.

Texter EC & others: Criteria for the diagnosis of hiatal hernia. Arch Int Med 110:827, 1962.

BENIGN NEOPLASMS OF THE ESOPHAGUS

Benign tumors of the esophagus are quite rare and are generally found accidentally by either the radiologist or prosector in the lower half of the esophagus. The most common of the benign neoplasms is the leiomyoma, which arises from one of the smooth muscle coats of the esophagus. This lesion may be circumferential or multiple, gradually increases in size (up to 2–2.5 cm or ¾–1 inch), and may ultimately compromise the esophageal lumen or normal peristalsis, producing dysphagia. Other uncommon benign tumors are fibromas, lipomas, lymphangiomas, hemangiomas, and schwannomas. The diagnosis is made by barium swallow and esophagoscopy. Cytologic examination is not definitive, and biopsy may be inadequate or technically not feasible.

Surgical removal is curative.

Barrett N: Benign smooth muscle tumor of the esophagus. Thorax 19:185, 1964.
Schmidt A, Lockwood K: Benign neoplasms of the esophagus. Acta chir scandinav 133:640, 1967.

CARCINOMA OF THE ESOPHAGUS

In the USA, carcinoma of the esophagus is predominantly a disease of men in the 5th–8th decades. It usually arises from squamous epithelium. Stasis-induced inflammation such as is seen in achalasia or esophageal stricture and chronic irritation induced by excessive use of alcohol seemingly are etiologically important in the development of this neoplasm. Malignant tumors of the distal esophagus are frequently adenocarcinomas, which originate in the stomach and spread cephalad to the gullet. Conversely, squamous cell carcinoma of the esophagus rarely invades the stomach. Primary adenocarcinoma of the esophagus is rare and probably arises in Barrett's epithelium. An even more unusual lesion is esophageal carcinosarcoma. Regardless of cell type, the prognosis for malignancy of the esophagus is usually poor.

Clinical Findings

A. Symptoms and Signs: Dysphagia, which is progressive and ultimately prevents swallowing of even liquids, is the principal symptom. Anterior or posterior chest pain which is unrelated to eating implies local extension of the tumor, whereas significant weight loss over a short period is an ominous sign. Swallowing times are abnormally prolonged or absent.

B. X-Ray Findings: Barium swallow is positive for an irregular, frequently annular, space-occupying lesion, usually localized to the midesophagus.

C. Special Examinations: Esophagoscopy, biopsy, and cytologic examination confirm the diagnosis.

Differential Diagnosis

Achalasia can be differentiated by endoscopy, esophageal manometry (with or without methacholine), and cinefluorography. Since there is a significant association of stricture with malignancy, any compromise of the esophageal lumen should be evaluated by esophagoscopy and biopsy.

Treatment & Prognosis

Although once considered a hopeless disease, dramatic improvements during the last 2 decades in anesthesia, surgical technics, and radiation therapy have substantially improved survival of patients with esophageal carcinoma. Irradiation generally is the best form of therapy, particularly for lesions in the proximal half of the gullet. When there is no evidence of metastases, tumors of the lower half of the esophagus may be treated by resection and esophagogastrostomy or jejunal or colonic interpositions. After dilatation of tumor-bearing portions of the esophagus, effective palliation can often be accomplished by the use of prosthetic tubes which are inserted through the mouth to facilitate swallowing.

Gastrostomy is supposed to improve nutrition but does not prolong survival, and the inability of completely obstructed patients to swallow even saliva makes the operation of questionable value for palliation.

Anticancer drugs have not proved to be of value.

Mercer JL, MacArthur AM: Use of Gourevitch tube in unresectable lesions of esophagus. Thorax 24:39, 1969.
Nakayama K & others: Surgical treatment combined with preoperative concentrated irradiation for esophageal cancer. Cancer 20:778, 1967.
Palmer ED: Peroral prosthesis for the management of incurable esophageal carcinoma. Am J Gastroenterol 59:487, 1973.
Pearson JG: The value of radiotherapy in the management of esophageal cancer. Am J Roentgenol 105:500, 1969.
Takita H: Endoesophageal intubation for advanced esophageal carcinoma. New York J Med 71:2526, 1971.

DISEASES OF THE STOMACH

ACUTE SIMPLE GASTRITIS

Acute gastritis, probably the most common disturbance of the stomach, is frequently accompanied by generalized enteritis. It occurs in all age groups. The causes are as follows: (1) chemical irritants, eg, alcohol, salicylates; (2) bacterial infections or toxins, eg, staphylococcal food poisoning, scarlet fever, pneumonia; (3) viral infections, eg, "viral gastroenteritis," measles, hepatitis, influenza; and (4) allergy, eg, to shellfish.

Clinical Findings

A. Symptoms and Signs: Anorexia is always present and may be the only symptom. More commonly there is epigastric fullness and pressure and nausea and vomiting. Hemorrhage is frequent with chemical irritants (eg, salicylates). Diarrhea, colic, malaise, fever, chills, headache, and muscle cramps are common with toxins or infections. The patient may be prostrated and dehydrated. Examination shows mild epigastric tenderness.

B. Laboratory Findings: Mild leukocytosis may be present. Leukopenia may be present with viral infections.

C. Special Examinations: Upper gastrointestinal endoscopy for hemorrhage may differentiate acute simple gastritis from erosive gastritis, peptic ulcer, or a mucosal laceration (Mallory-Weiss syndrome).

Treatment & Prognosis

Treat specific infections. Correct water and electrolyte disturbances. Give nothing by mouth until acute symptoms of pain and nausea have subsided. Then give clear liquid and progress to a soft diet as tolerated. Sedatives, phenothiazine tranquilizers, or opiates may be used as indicated. Symptoms last 1–7 days.

ACUTE CORROSIVE ESOPHAGITIS & GASTRITIS

Ingestion of corrosive substances is most common in children but may occur in cases of attempted suicide. The substances most commonly swallowed are strong acids (sulfuric, nitric), alkalies (lye, potash), oxalic acid, iodine, bichloride of mercury, arsenic, silver nitrate, and carbolic acid. The esophagus is most severely injured. Gastric changes vary from superficial edema and hyperemia, deep necrosis and sloughing, to perforation.

Corrosion of the lips, tongue, mouth, and pharynx and pain and dysphagia due to esophageal lesions are usually present. Nitric acid causes brown discoloration; oxalic acid causes white discoloration of mucous membranes. There is severe epigastric burning and cramping pain, nausea and vomiting, and diarrhea. The vomitus is often blood-tinged. Severe prostration with a shock-like picture and thirst may occur. Palpation of the abdomen may show epigastric tenderness or extreme rigidity. Leukocytosis and proteinuria are present.

Immediate treatment is supportive, including nasogastric suction, analgesics, intravenous fluids and electrolytes, sedatives, and antacids. Although the specific antidote (see Chapter 30) should be administered immediately, supportive measures must not be neglected. The benefit to be expected from the antidote appears minuscule if a large amount of corrosive has been ingested and of doubtful benefit considering that tissue damage occurs almost immediately. Avoid emetics and lavage if corrosion is severe because of the danger of perforation.

The outcome depends upon the extent of tissue damage. Careful fiberoptic endoscopy may serve to determine tissue necrosis. Emergency laparotomy may be indicated to resect the area of gangrene and potential perforation. If alkali has been ingested, prednisone, 20 mg orally every 8 hours started immediately, may prevent esophageal stricture. This dose should be tapered slowly over several weeks.

After the acute phase has passed, place the patient on a peptic ulcer regimen. If perforation has not occurred, recovery is the rule. However, pyloric stenosis may occur early or late, requiring gastric aspiration, parenteral fluid therapy, and surgical repair.

The amount of the corrosive substance, its local and general effects, and the speed with which it is removed or neutralized determine the outcome. If the patient survives the acute phase, gastric effects are usually overshadowed by esophageal strictures, although chronic gastritis or stricture formation at the pylorus may follow.

Allen R & others: Corrosive injuries of the stomach. Arch Surg 100:409, 1970.
Arena JN: Treatment of caustic alkali poisoning. Mod Treat 4:729, 1967.
Thompson CE, Ashurst PM, Butler TJ: Survey of haemorrhagic erosive gastritis. Brit MJ 3:283, 1968.

CHRONIC GASTRITIS

Essentials of Diagnosis

- Symptoms, if present, consist of vague, nondescript upper abdominal distress.
- Mild epigastric tenderness or no physical findings whatever.
- Gastric biopsy is the definitive diagnostic technic.

General Considerations

At best, a very poor correlation exists between the gastroscopic appearance considered to be gastritis and the histopathology.

Chronic gastritis is a wastebasket diagnosis to which symptoms should never be attributed until all other causes of abdominal distress have been excluded. Although the disorder is seen in association with gastric ulcer and gastric carcinoma, a cause and effect relationship has not been established.

Clinical Findings

A. Symptoms and Signs: The vast majority of persons with chronic gastritis do not have symptoms. Gastrointestinal symptoms, if they occur, may include anorexia, epigastric pressure and fullness, heartburn, nausea, vomiting, specific food intolerance, peptic ulcer-like syndrome, and anemia or gross hemorrhage.

Physical findings are often absent or consist only of mild epigastric tenderness.

B. Laboratory Findings: The laboratory findings may be entirely normal. Hematologic studies may reveal evidence of macrocytic anemia. The Schilling test may be abnormal. Gastric analysis, although not diagnostic, frequently shows achlorhydria.

C. X-Ray Findings: Although the x-ray in chronic hypertrophic gastritis may show heavy folds, these findings are not diagnostic and not specific to the lesion.

Differential Diagnosis

Since clinical and pathologic findings correlate so poorly, the diagnosis of chronic gastritis should be made only on the basis of anatomic findings obtained via gastric biopsy, surgery, or autopsy.

Treatment & Prognosis

The treatment of chronic gastritis, except in those cases associated with pernicious anemia or iron deficiency anemia, is not very successful. A peptic ulcer regimen, elimination of possible aggravating factors such as alcohol, salicylates, and caffeine, anticholinergic drugs, and mild tranquilizers may give symptomatic relief.

MacDonald WC, Rubin CE: Gastric biopsy: A critical evaluation. Gastroenterology 53:143, 1967.

Morrissey JF: Gastrointestinal endoscopy. Gastroenterology 62:1241, 1972.

Siurala M & others: Prevalence of gastritis in a rural population: Bioptic study of subjects selected at random. Scandinav J Gastroent 3:211, 1968.

PEPTIC ULCER

A peptic ulcer is an acute or chronic benign ulceration occurring in a portion of the digestive tract which is accessible to gastric secretions. An active peptic ulcer does not occur in the absence of acid-peptic gastric secretions.

Other factors in peptic ulceration (besides the presence of gastric acidity) include hypersecretion of hydrochloric acid and decreased tissue resistance.

Peptic ulcer may occur during the course of drug therapy (adrenocortical hormones, phenylbutazone, salicylates, reserpine, and indomethacin). It may occur as a result of severe tissue injury such as extensive burns or intracranial surgery, and may be associated with endocrine tumors producing gastrin, which stimulates hypersecretion of hydrochloric acid and a very refractory peptic ulcer diathesis (Zollinger-Ellison syndrome).

Kirsner JB: Peptic ulcer: A review of the recent literature on various clinical aspects. (2 parts.) Gastroenterology 54:611, 945, 1968.

1. DUODENAL ULCER

Essentials of Diagnosis

- Epigastric distress 45–60 minutes after meals, or nocturnal pain, both relieved by food, antacids, or vomiting.
- Epigastric tenderness and guarding.
- Chronic and periodic symptoms.
- Gastric analysis shows acid in all cases and hypersecretion in some.

- Ulcer crater or deformity of duodenal bulb on x-ray.
- Visualization of a crater during fiberoptic duodenoscopy.

General Considerations

Duodenal ulcer occurs in about 10% of people at some time. Although the average age at onset is 33 years, duodenal ulcer may occur at any time from infancy to the later years. It is 4 times as common in males as in females. Occurrence during pregnancy is unusual.

Duodenal ulcer is 4 or 5 times as common as benign gastric ulcer. Morbidity due to peptic ulcer is a major public health problem.

About 95% of duodenal ulcers occur in the duodenal bulb or cap, ie, the first 5 cm (2 inches) of the duodenum. The remainder are between this area and the ampulla. Ulcers below the ampulla are rare. The majority are near the lesser curvature. The ulceration varies from a few mm to 1–2 cm in diameter and extends at least through the muscularis mucosae, often through to the serosa and into the pancreas. The margins are sharp, but the surrounding mucosa is often inflamed and edematous. The base consists of granulation tissue and fibrous tissue, representing healing and continuing digestion.

Clinical Findings

A. Symptoms and Signs: Symptoms may be absent or vague and atypical. In the typical case pain is described as gnawing, burning, cramp-like, or aching, or as "heartburn"; it is usually mild to moderate, located over a small area near the midline in the epigastrium near the xiphoid. The pain may radiate below the costal margins, into the back, or, rarely, to the right shoulder. Nausea may be present, and vomiting of small quantities of highly acid gastric juice with little or no retained food may occur. The distress usually occurs 45–60 minutes after a meal; is usually absent before breakfast; worsens as the day progresses; and may be most severe between 12 midnight and 2:00 a.m. It is relieved by food, milk, alkalies, and vomiting, generally within 5–30 minutes.

Spontaneous remissions and exacerbations are common. Precipitating factors are often unknown but may include trauma, infections, or physical or emotional distress.

Signs include superficial and deep epigastric tenderness, voluntary muscle guarding, and unilateral (rectus) spasm over the duodenal bulb.

B. Laboratory Findings: Bleeding, hypochromic anemia, and occult blood in the stools occur in chronic ulcers. Gastric analysis shows acid in all cases and gastric hypersecretion of hydrochloric acid (> 5 mEq/hour) in some.

C. X-Ray Findings: An ulcer crater is demonstrable by x-ray in 50–70% of cases but may be obscured by deformity of the duodenal bulb. When no ulcer is demonstrated, the following are suggestive of ulceration: (1) irritability of the bulb with difficulty in retaining barium there; (2) point tenderness over the bulb; (3) pylorospasm; (4) gastric hyperperistalsis; and (5) hypersecretion or retained secretions.

D. Special Examinations: Duodenoscopy has proved to be a valuable adjunct in the diagnosis of the duodenal ulcer which has not been demonstrated radiographically. Duodenoscopy may also demonstrate duodenitis, a disorder which may have a pathogenetic mechanism in common with duodenal ulcer.

Differential Diagnosis

When symptoms are typical, the diagnosis of peptic ulceration can be made with assurance; when symptoms are atypical, duodenal ulcer may be confused clinically with functional gastrointestinal disease, gastritis, gastric carcinoma, and irritable colon syndrome. Final diagnosis often depends upon x-ray or endoscopic visualization.

Complications

A. Intractability to Treatment: Most cases of apparently intractable ulcer are probably due to an inadequate medical regimen or failure of cooperation on the part of the patient. The designation "intractable" should be reserved only for those patients who have received an adequate supervised trial of therapy. The possibility of occult etiologic and aggravating factors as well as complications of the ulcer must always be considered.

B. Hemorrhage Due to Peptic Ulcer: Hemorrhage is caused either by erosion of an ulcer into an artery or vein or, more commonly, by bleeding from granulation tissue. The majority of bleeding ulcers are on the posterior wall. The sudden onset of weakness, faintness, dizziness, chilliness, thirst, cold moist skin, desire to defecate, and the passage of loose tarry or even red stools with or without coffee-ground vomitus is characteristic of acute gastrointestinal hemorrhage.

The blood findings (hemoglobin, red cell count, and hematocrit) lag behind the blood loss by several hours and may give a false impression of the quantity of blood lost. Postural hypotension and tachycardia and central venous pressure are more reliable indicators of hypovolemia than the hematocrit (see p 326).

C. Perforation: Perforation occurs almost exclusively in males 25–40 years of age. The symptoms and signs are those of peritoneal irritation and peritonitis; ulcers which perforate into the lesser peritoneal cavity cause less dramatic symptoms and signs. A typical description of perforated peptic ulcer is an acute onset of epigastric pain, often radiating to the shoulder or right lower quadrant and sometimes associated with nausea and vomiting, followed by a lessening of pain for a few hours, and then by board-like rigidity of the abdomen, fever, rebound tenderness, absent bowel sounds, leukocytosis, tachycardia, and even signs of marked prostration. X-ray demonstration of free air in the peritoneal cavity confirms the diagnosis.

D. Penetration: Extension of the crater beyond the duodenal wall into contiguous structures without extension into the free peritoneal space occurs fairly frequently with duodenal ulcer and is one of the important causes of failure of medical treatment. Penetration generally occurs in ulcers on the posterior wall, and extension is usually into the pancreas; but the liver, biliary tract, or gastrohepatic omentum may be involved.

Radiation of pain into the back, night distress, inadequate or no relief from eating food or taking alkalies, and, in occasional cases, relief upon spinal flexion and aggravation upon hyperextension—any or all of these findings in a patient with a long history of duodenal ulcer usually signify penetration.

E. Obstruction: Minor degrees of pyloric obstruction are present in about 20–25% of patients with duodenal ulcer, but clinically significant obstruction is much less common. The obstruction is generally caused by edema and spasm associated with an active ulcer, but it may occur as a result of scar tissue contraction even in the presence of a healed ulcer.

The occurrence of epigastric fullness or heaviness and, finally, copious vomiting after meals—with the vomitus containing undigested food from a previous meal—suggests obstruction. The diagnosis is confirmed by the presence of an overnight gastric residual of greater than 50 ml containing undigested food, and x-ray evidence of obstruction, gastric dilatation, and hyperperistalsis. A succussion splash on pressure in the left upper quadrant may be present, and gastric peristalsis may be visible.

Treatment

The rationale and efficacy of the various dietary and pharmacologic measures for the treatment of peptic ulcer have been seriously challenged. Despite the difficulty of documenting the influence of the different traditional treatment measures in inducing remissions or preventing recurrences of peptic ulcer, the clinician usually finds it necessary to provide symptomatic treatment by such measures. The limiting factor in therapy, in the light of present knowledge, is the fact that although ulcers heal, the ulcer diathesis remains.

A. Acute Phase:

1. General measures—The patient should have 2 or 3 weeks' rest from work if possible. If the home situation is unsatisfactory or if the patient is unable to cooperate, hospitalization is recommended. If the patient must continue to work, he should be given careful instructions about the medical program. Arrangements should be made for rest periods and sufficient sleep. Anxiety should be relieved whenever possible, but active psychotherapy during the acute phase is usually not indicated.

Alcohol should be strictly forbidden. If the patient can quit smoking without too much distress, he should do so.

The following drugs may aggravate peptic ulcer or may even cause perforation and hemorrhage: corticotropin, the adrenal corticosteroids, rauwolfia, phenylbutazone, and large doses of salicylates. They should be discontinued.

2. Diet—Numerous dietary regimens have been designed for the treatment of peptic ulcer. There is considerable doubt regarding the value or advisability of the strict smooth, bland diets so widely used in the past. All of the controlled clinical studies have documented that the kind, content, and consistency of the diet have no relationship to ulcer healing. Diets which include large amounts of milk and cream are associated with a striking increase in the incidence of death due to myocardial infarction in ulcer patients.

The important principles of dietary management of peptic ulcer are as follows: (1) nutritious diet; (2) regularity of meals; (3) restriction of substances which stimulate gastric secretion, especially coffee, tea, cola beverages, and alcohol; and (4) avoidance of foods known to produce symptoms in a given individual.

In the acute phase with partial gastric outlet obstruction, it is often useful to begin with a full liquid diet and hourly antacids. The diet may be liberalized rapidly to a regular diet in unobstructed patients. Some patients may require a "bland diet" for the placebo effect. Do not give milk as "therapy."

Interval feedings should be avoided. Food, regardless of content, kind, or consistency, has been shown to markedly stimulate gastric acid secretion and to be ineffective as a buffer of acid in the stomach.

It is doubtful that dietary measures, other than for the elimination of known aggravating factors, play a significant role in preventing ulcer recurrence.

3. Antacids—Antacids usually relieve ulcer pain promptly. Antacid dosage should be selected on the basis of neutralizing capacity. The response to antacids varies widely according to the preparation, the dosage, and the individual patient. Most tablet aluminum hydroxide preparations are considerably less effective than the liquid preparations and should not be given. *Caution:* All patients on antacid therapy should be watched for diarrhea, constipation, fecal impaction, phosphate depletion, hypercalcemia, or "milk-alkali syndrome."

In order to be effective, antacids must be taken frequently. During the acute phase they must be taken every hour during the day and at night if necessary. They should be continued on an hourly basis during the day to complete healing if possible. A patient who does not achieve pain relief on this regimen is either emptying his stomach rapidly or secreting more acid than the antacid can neutralize. (Suspect Zollinger-Ellison syndrome.)

a. Aluminum hydroxide gel—These agents have enjoyed popularity because they are convenient to administer and have less tendency to cause alkalosis. However, they are constipating. Prolonged ingestion may lead to phosphate depletion. The preparations that contain magnesium compounds are generally more effective than aluminum hydroxide gel alone but may cause diarrhea in some individuals. Among the effective preparations are Mylanta II, Maalox, and Aludrox. The usual dosage is 15–30 ml taken hourly. Dosage and frequency of use may have to be altered according to the patient's response.

b. Magnesium oxide-calcium carbonate mixtures—

R Magnesium oxide   15.0–60.0
  Calcium carbonate, qs ad   120.0

Sig: Take ½–1 tsp in ½ glass of water as directed.

Magnesium oxide is a laxative drug and calcium carbonate tends to produce constipation. By varying the amount of magnesium oxide in this prescription, the laxative or constipating effects of the 2 ingredients may be effectively balanced. The powder may be given in alternating doses with aluminum hydroxide gels. Effective calcium carbonate-containing tablets include Dicarbosil, Tums, Alkets, and Titralac. The usual dosage is 2 tablets hourly.

Calcium carbonate has an excellent neutralizing action. A paradoxic calcium-induced gastric hypersecretion has been reported but probably has no clinical significance. Patients must be checked for hypercalcemia 2–3 weeks after beginning treatment or sooner if symptoms develop (polydipsia, polyuria, anorexia, nausea, constipation).

c. Aluminum hydroxide, calcium carbonate, magnesium hydroxide mixtures—These (Ducon, Camalox) are among the more effective antacids. The usual dosage is 10–15 ml hourly.

4. Sedatives—Tense and apprehensive patients will usually profit greatly from sedation. The barbiturates or other sedatives may be used, alone or in combination with antispasmodic drugs. Hypnotic doses of the barbiturates may be necessary to ensure sleep.

5. Parasympatholytic (anticholinergic, antispasmodic) drugs—Although the parasympatholytic drugs have enjoyed a wide and long-standing therapeutic popularity for the treatment of peptic ulcer, their effectiveness is questionable. The usefulness of the compounds is limited largely to the relief of refractory pain. The dosage necessary to produce significant gastric antisecretory effect may cause blurring of vision, constipation, urinary retention, and tachycardia. If patients have gastric retention, the danger of drug-induced pyloric obstruction must be considered. Belladonna preparations in proper dosage are as effective as the synthetic parasympatholytic agents and have the advantage of being less expensive.

Note: Belladonna and other anticholinergic drugs should be avoided in patients with glaucoma, hiatal hernia, gastric ulcer, pyloric obstruction, cardiospasm, gastrointestinal hemorrhage, bladder neck obstruction, or serious myocardial disease.

a. Belladonna tincture, 10–20 drops in one-half glass of water 20–30 minutes before meals and at bedtime.

b. Belladonna extract, 8–24 mg (with or without sedatives) 20–30 minutes before meals and at bedtime.

c. Atropine, 0.25–0.5 mg orally 20–30 minutes before meals and at bedtime.

d. Synthetic parasympatholytics—Numerous proprietary tertiary and quaternary amines are available as belladonna or atropine substitutes. Although they do not have CNS side-effects, it is difficult to substantiate other therapeutic advantages.

B. Convalescent Phase:

1. Reexamination—Once the diagnosis is established, it is unnecessary to repeat the gastrointestinal series unless complications develop. Anticholinergic therapy, if used, should be discontinued 72 hours prior to x-ray examination for duodenal ulcer.

2. Education of patient regarding recurrences—The chronic and recurrent nature of the illness should be explained to the patient, and he should be warned about the complications of careless or improper treatment. Although the cause of ulcer recurrence is not known, it may be associated with irregular eating habits, irregular living habits (long or irregular hours), use of alcohol or tobacco, emotional stress, and infections, particularly of the upper respiratory tract. The patient should be instructed to return to the ulcer regimen if symptoms recur or if he recognizes that he is exposing himself to conditions known to aggravate the ulcer. Antacids and other medications should be readily available.

3. Rest and recreation—Provisions should be made for rest and recreation to promote physical and mental relaxation.

C. Treatment of Complications:

1. Hemorrhage—Institute immediate emergency measures for treatment of hemorrhage and shock (see p 326).

2. Perforation—Acute perforation constitutes a medical emergency. Immediate surgical repair, preferably by simple surgical closure, is indicated. More extensive operations may be unwise at the time of the acute episode because of the increased operative hazard due to the patient's poor physical condition. If the patient has had no previous therapy or if previous therapy has been inadequate, he should be treated by means of a conservative medical regimen.

The morbidity and mortality depend upon the amount of spillage and especially the time lapse between perforation and surgery. Surgical closure of the perforation is indicated as soon as possible. If surgery is delayed beyond 24 hours, gastric suction, antibiotics, and intravenous fluids are the treatment of choice.

3. Obstruction—Obstruction due to spasm and edema can usually be treated adequately by gastric decompression and ulcer therapy; obstruction due to scar formation requires surgery. It must be remembered that the obstruction may not represent a complication of an ulcer but may be due to a primary neoplastic disease, especially in those patients with no history or only a short history of peptic ulcer.

a. Medical measures (for obstruction due to spasm or edema) consist of bed rest, preferably in a hospital, continuous gastric suction for 48 hours, and parenteral administration of electrolytes and fluids. After 48 hours, begin liquid feedings. Aspirate gastric juice every 12 hours to measure gastric residual. Do not use anticholinergic drugs since they delay gastric emptying. Give sedative or sedative-tranquilizer drugs, and a pro-

gressive diet as tolerated. Hourly antacids should be employed as for treatment of uncomplicated ulcer.

b. Surgical measures (for obstruction due to scarring) are indicated only after a thorough trial of conservative measures. (See Moore reference, below.)

Prognosis

Duodenal ulcer tends to have a chronic course with remissions and exacerbations. Many patients can be adequately controlled by medical management. About 25% develop complications, and 5–10% ultimately require surgery.

Babb RR: Diagnosis of Zollinger-Ellison syndrome: Ulcerogenic tumor of the pancreas. California Med 113:1, July, 1970.

Belber J: Endoscopic examination of the duodenal bulb. Gastroenterology 61:55, 1971.

Briggs RI & others: Myocardial infarction in patients treated with Sippy and other high-milk diets: An autopsy study of fifteen hospitals in the USA and Great Britain. Circulation 21:538, 1960.

Buchman E & others: Unrestricted diet in the treatment of duodenal ulcer. Gastroenterology 56:1016, 1969.

Burdette WJ, Rasmussen B: Perforated peptic ulcer. Surgery 63:576, 1968.

Clarke JS & others: Gastroduodenal stress ulcer. California Med 116:32, Jan 1972.

Clayman C & others: Gastric irradiation in the treatment of peptic ulcer. Gastroenterology 55:403, 1968.

Conn JH & others: Massive hemorrhage from peptic ulcer: Evaluation of methods of surgical control. Ann Surg 169:784, 1969.

Dragstedt LR: Peptic ulcer: An abnormality in gastric secretion. Am J Surg 117:143, 1969.

Fisher RD, Ebert PA, Zuidema GD: Obstructing peptic ulcer: Results of treatment. Arch Surg 94:724, 1967.

Fordtran JS & others: In vivo and in vitro evaluations of liquid antacids. New England J Med 288:923, 1973.

Hinshaw DB & others: Vagotomy and pyloroplasty for perforated duodenal ulcer: Observations in 180 cases. Am J Surg 115:173, 1968.

Lennard-Jones JE, Barbouris N: A comparison between two "therapeutic" diets and freely-chosen meals. Gut 6:113, 1965.

Levant JA, Walsh JH, Isenberg JI: Stimulation of gastric secretion and gastrin release by single oral doses of calcium carbonate in man. New England J Med 289:555, 1973. [See also editorial on p 587, same issue.]

Moore FD: Operative treatment of duodenal ulcer: Transatlantic data and opinion. New England J Med 290:906, 1974.

Morrissey JF, Barreras RF: Antacid therapy. New England J Med 290:550, 1974.

Schiff ER: Treatment of uncomplicated peptic ulcer disease. M Clin North America 55:305, 1971.

2. ZOLLINGER-ELLISON SYNDROME

Essentials of Diagnosis

- Severe peptic ulcer disease.
- Gastric hypersecretion.
- Elevated serum gastrin.
- Nonbeta islet cell tumor of pancreas.

General Considerations

Zollinger-Ellison peptic ulceration syndrome, although uncommon, is not rare. Sixty percent of patients are males. Onset may be at any age from early childhood on but is most common in persons 20–50 years old. Most patients have the gastrin-secreting tumor in the pancreas; a few have tumors in the submucosa of the duodenum and stomach, hilus of the spleen, and regional lymph nodes. They may be either single or multiple. Approximately two-thirds of Zollinger-Ellison tumors are malignant with respect either to their biologic behavior or to their histologic appearance.

Clinical Findings

A. Symptoms and Signs: Pain is of the typical peptic ulcer variety but is more difficult to control by medical means. Diarrhea may occur as a result of excessively low proximal small bowel pH with impaired fat absorption. Hemorrhage, perforation, and obstruction occur commonly.

B. Laboratory Findings: The most reliable means of establishing the diagnosis of Zollinger-Ellison syndrome is measurement of serum gastrin by radioimmunoassay. Patients with Zollinger-Ellison syndrome usually have serum gastrin levels > 300 pg/ml. Serum calcium levels are useful in revealing hypercalcemia to evaluate the possibility of hyperparathyroidism and multiple endocrine adenomatosis. Gastric analysis reveals gastric hypersecretion (> 15 mEq/hour). Maximal acid output (MAO) following stimulation with histamine or betazole (Histalog) does not show the increased rate of gastric acid secretion as much as in normals or patients with peptic ulcer disease not of the Zollinger-Ellison type. In the Zollinger-Ellison patient, the basal acid output (BAO) is greater than 60% of the MAO, while in ordinary peptic ulcer disease the BAO is usually substantially less than 60% of the MAO.

C. X-Ray Findings: Gastrointestinal series reveal that 75% of the ulcers are in the first part of the duodenum and stomach and that the ulcers are usually not multiple. Ulcers occurring in the second, third, or fourth portion of the duodenum or in the jejunum are strongly suggestive of Zollinger-Ellison syndrome. Coarseness of the proximal jejunal folds and radiographic evidence of gastric hypersecretion also suggest Zollinger-Ellison syndrome.

Treatment

Medical treatment is unsatisfactory for long-term management. Surgical treatment consisting of total gastrectomy is the procedure of choice. Occasionally, excision of a solitary adenoma will result in cure. Following surgery, vitamin B_{12} supplementation and iron replacement are indicated.

Amberg JR & others: Roentgenographic observations in the Zollinger-Ellison syndrome. JAMA 190:185, 1964.
Way LW, Goldman L, Dunphy JE: Zollinger-Ellison syndrome. Am J Surg 116:293, 1968.
Zollinger RM, Ellison EH: Primary peptic ulcerations of the jejunum associated with islet cell tumors of the pancreas. Ann Surg 142:709, 1955.

3. GASTRIC ULCER

Essentials of Diagnosis

- Epigastric distress on an empty stomach, relieved by food, alkalies, or vomiting.
- Epigastric tenderness and voluntary muscle guarding.
- Anemia, occult blood in stool, gastric acid.
- Ulcer demonstrated by x-ray or gastroscope.

General Considerations

Benign gastric ulcer is in many respects similar to duodenal ulcer. Acid gastric juice is necessary for its production, but decreased tissue resistance appears to play a more important role than hypersecretion.

About 60% of benign gastric ulcers are found within 6 cm of the pylorus. The ulcers are generally located at or near the lesser curvature and most frequently on the posterior wall. Another 25% of the ulcers are located higher on the lesser curvature.

If the radiographic appearance of the ulcer is benign, the occurrence of carcinoma is about 3.3%. If it is indeterminate (features of both benignancy and malignancy), it is approximately 9.5%. With evidence of associated duodenal ulcer, it is about 1%.

Clinical Findings

A. Symptoms and Signs: There may be no symptoms or only vague and atypical symptoms. The epigastric distress is typically described as gnawing, burning, aching, or "hunger pangs," referred at times to the left subcostal area. Episodes occur usually 45–60 minutes after a meal and are relieved by food, alkalies, or vomiting. Nausea and vomiting are frequent complaints. There may be a history of remissions, with exacerbations occurring in the winter months. Weight loss, constipation, and fatigue are common.

Epigastric tenderness or voluntary muscle guarding is usually the only finding.

B. Laboratory Findings: If bleeding has occurred, there may be hypochromic anemia or occult blood in the stool. The gastric analysis always shows an acid pH after betazole (Histalog) and the presence of low normal to normal secretion.

C. Other Examinations: Upper gastrointestinal series, gastroscopy with multiple biopsies (6–10), and a direct vision brush biopsy of the ulcer serves to confirm the benignancy of the lesion. If these studies do not demonstrate malignancy in a clinically suspicious lesion, cytologic examination of a specimen obtained by lavage is indicated.

Differential Diagnosis

The symptoms of gastric ulcer, especially if atypical, need differentiation from those of irritable colon, gastritis, and functional gastrointestinal distress.

Most important is the differentiation of benign gastric ulcer from malignant gastric ulcer. A favorable response to hospital management is presumptive evidence that the lesion is benign and not malignant. Malignant ulcers may respond initially, but residual changes at the site usually demonstrate the true nature of the process.

Complications

Hemorrhage, perforation, and obstruction may occur (see Complications of Duodenal Ulcer, above).

Treatment

Ulcer treatment (as for duodenal ulcer) should be intensive, and failure to respond in 3—4 weeks with significant healing should be regarded as an indication for surgical resection. However, even a carcinoma may show improvement on an ulcer regimen, and clinical relief does not necessarily mean that the ulcer is benign. Follow-up at 6 weeks, 3 months, and 6 months after apparently complete healing is therefore indicated. In the event of recurrence under intensive medical management, perforation, obstruction, or massive uncontrollable hemorrhage, surgery is mandatory.

Prognosis

Gastric ulcers tend to be recurrent. There is no evidence that malignant degeneration of gastric peptic ulceration ever occurs. Recurrent uncomplicated ulcer is not a serious event and in fact may heal more readily than the previous ulcer.

Brandborg LL, Wenger J: Cytological examination in gastrointestinal tract disease. M Clin North America 52:1315, 1968.

Kukral JC: Gastric ulcer: An appraisal. Surgery 63:1024, 1968.

Nelson SW: The discovery of gastric ulcers and the differential diagnosis between benignancy and malignancy. Radiol Clin North America 7:5, 1969.

Rhodes J: Etiology of gastric ulcer. Gastroenterology 63:171, 1972.

VA Cooperative Study on Gastric Ulcer. Gastroenterology 61 (Suppl 2):567, 1971.

preoperative ulcer pain, and is located lower in the epigastrium, even below the umbilicus and often to the left. The pain often covers a wider area and may radiate to the back.

The "food-pain rhythm" of peptic ulcer distress frequently occurs earlier (within an hour) in marginal ulcer as a result of more rapid emptying time; and relief with antacids, food, and milk may be incomplete and of short duration. Nausea, vomiting, and weight loss are common. Hematemesis occurs frequently. Low epigastric tenderness with voluntary muscle guarding is usually present. An inflammatory mass may be palpated. Anemia and occult blood in the stool are common. On gastric analysis, acid can be demonstrated, although rapid emptying and reflux of intestinal contents make the procedure difficult. On x-ray the ulcer niche at the stoma is often difficult to demonstrate, although compression films are helpful. Gastroscopy is the most effective means of diagnosing stomal ulcer.

Stomal ulcer must be differentiated from functional gastrointestinal distress, especially in a patient concerned about the possibility of recurrence of an ulcer after surgery. Atypical symptoms must be differentiated from "bile" gastritis and from biliary tract or pancreatic disease. Consider the possibility of Zollinger-Ellison syndrome.

Complications include gross hemorrhage, perforation, stenosis of the stoma, and gastrojejunocolic fistula.

Stomal ulcers are often resistant to medical therapy; vagotomy or a more extensive gastrectomy is usually necessary to decrease the acid secretion of the stomach.

X-ray therapy to the stomach (1800—2000 R) will substantially reduce the gastric secretion of hydrochloric acid and in some instances may induce achlorhydria for varying periods of time. The use of x-ray therapy to the stomach should be restricted to those instances of complicating disease leading to increased surgical risk and to elderly patients. The procedure is also of value in similar patients with duodenal and benign gastric ulcer.

Andros G & others: Anastomotic ulcers. Ann Surg 165:955, 1967.

4. STOMAL (MARGINAL) ULCER
(Jejunal Ulcer)

Marginal ulcer should be suspected when there is a history of operation for an ulcer followed by recurrence of abdominal symptoms after a symptom-free interval of months to years. The marginal ulcer incidence after simple gastroenterostomy is 35—75%; after subtotal gastrectomy or vagotomy, about 5%. Nearly all of the ulcers are jejunal, and the others are located on the gastric side of the anastomosis. The abdominal pain is burning or gnawing, often more severe than the

POSTGASTRECTOMY SYNDROMES

Dumping Syndrome

Postgastrectomy (dumping) syndrome probably occurs in about 10% of patients after partial gastrectomy. The pathogenesis is complex and incompletely understood. The disorder is provoked mainly by soluble, hypertonic carbohydrates. The following phenomena occur: a rapid flow of fluid into the small intestine, an increase in free plasma kinins, increase in peripheral blood flow, and a modest drop in plasma volume with a corresponding increase in hematocrit and a mild decrease in serum potassium. Whether sympathetic vasomotor responses contribute to the syndrome is uncertain.

One or more of the following symptoms occurs within 20 minutes after meals: sweating, tachycardia, pallor, epigastric fullness and grumbling, warmth, nausea, abdominal cramps, weakness, and, in severe cases, syncope, vomiting, or diarrhea. Nonspecific ECG changes may be noted. Blood sugar is not low during an attack.

It is important to distinguish this syndrome from reactive hypoglycemia which occurs in some postgastrectomy patients and is associated with a low blood sugar. This latter syndrome occurs much later after the meal (1–3 hours) and is relieved by the ingestion of food.

Changing the diet to frequent, small, equal feedings high in protein, moderately high in fat, and low in carbohydrate usually reduces the severity of symptoms. Fluids should be taken between meals and not with meals. Sedative and anticholinergic drugs may be of value.

Buchwald H: The dumping syndrome and its treatment. Am J Surg 116:81, 1968.
Moore HG Jr: Complications of gastric surgery. Pages 665–734 in: *Surgery of the Stomach and Duodenum*, 2nd ed. Harkins HN, Nyhus LM (editors). Little, Brown, 1969.
Wong PY & others: Kallikrein-kinin system in postgastrectomy dumping syndrome. Ann Int Med 80:577, 1974.

Afferent Loop Syndrome

The afferent loop syndrome occurs after either Billroth II gastrectomy or gastrojejunostomy. The symptoms are due to distention of and stasis within the afferent loop of the gastrojejunostomy. Typically, abdominal pain occurs 15–30 minutes after eating and is relieved by vomiting of bile fluid which does not contain food. Stasis and afferent loop contents may lead to bacterial overgrowth with malabsorption. Overgrowth of bacteroides leads to deconjugation of bile salts with subsequent impairment of micellar function in the gut. Steatorrhea with malabsorption of the fat-soluble vitamins may occur. In addition, vitamin B_{12} absorption may be impaired as a consequence of binding of this vitamin by the organisms in the intestinal lumen.

Surgical reconstruction of the afferent loop is the procedure of choice. However, if stasis of the afferent loop with bacterial overgrowth and malabsorption is the major manifestation of the syndrome, satisfactory results can be obtained by the use of broad-spectrum antibiotics such as tetracycline, 250 mg 2–4 times daily, or lincomycin, 500 mg twice daily. Bacterial resistance may develop. This can be avoided by changing antibiotics or intermittent antibiotic therapy.

Mitty WF Jr, Grossi G, Nealon TF Jr: Chronic afferent loop syndrome. Ann Surg 172:996, 1970.

Wardward ER: The pathophysiology of the afferent loop syndrome. S Clin North America 46:411, 1963.

Bile Reflux

Bile reflux following gastric surgery is one of the most debilitating complications of this surgical procedure. Typically, the patient experiences nausea, substernal distress, and anorexia. Vomiting or reflux of clear bile-stained fluid may occur.

Medical management is unsatisfactory. The surgical approach is a diversion of bile from the stomach. The Roux-en-Y procedure serves this end.

Torrance HB, Watson A: Bilious vomiting after gastric surgery. J Roy Coll Surg Edinb 14:161, 1969.

CARCINOMA OF THE STOMACH

Essentials of Diagnosis

- Upper gastrointestinal symptoms with weight loss in patients over age 40.
- Palpable abdominal mass.
- Anemia, occult blood in stools, positive cytologic examination.
- Gastroscopic and x-ray abnormality.

General Considerations

Carcinoma of the stomach is a common cancer of the digestive tract. It occurs predominantly in males over 40 years of age. Delay of diagnosis is caused by absence of definite early symptoms and by the fact that patients treat themselves instead of seeking early medical advice. Further delays are due to the equivocal nature of early findings and to temporary improvement with symptomatic therapy.

A history of the following possibly precancerous conditions should alert the physician to the danger of stomach cancer:

(1) **Atrophic gastritis of pernicious anemia:** The incidence of adenomas and carcinomas is significantly increased.

(2) **Chronic gastritis, particularly atrophic gastritis:** There is a wide variation in the reported incidence of gastritis with cancer, and a definite relationship has not been proved.

(3) **Gastric ulcer:** The major problem is in the differentiation between benign and malignant ulcer.

(4) **Achlorhydria:** The incidence of lowered secretory potential in early life is higher in those patients who later develop carcinoma.

Carcinoma may originate anywhere in the stomach. Grossly, lesions tend to be of 4 types (Borrmann):

Type I: Polypoid, intraluminal mass.
Type II: Noninfiltrating ulcer.
Type III: Infiltrating ulcer.
Type IV: Diffuse infiltrating process (to linitis plastica).

Gross typing generally correlates better with prognosis than the histologic grading of malignancy, ie, type I has a better prognosis than type II, etc.

Clinical Findings

A. Symptoms and Signs: Early gastric carcinoma, such as is detected in the mass surveys in Japan, causes no symptoms. The appearance of symptoms implies relatively advanced disease. The patient may complain of vague fullness, nausea, sensations of pressure, belching, and heartburn after meals, with or without anorexia, especially for meat. These symptoms in association with weight loss and decline in general health and strength in a man over 40 years of age should suggest the possibility of stomach cancer. Diarrhea, hematemesis, and melena may be present.

Specific symptoms may be determined in part by the location of the tumor. A peptic ulcer-like syndrome generally occurs with ulcerated lesions (types II and III) and in the presence of acid secretion, but may occur with complete achlorhydria. Unfortunately, symptomatic relief with antacids tends to delay diagnosis. Symptoms of pyloric obstruction are progressive postprandial fullness to retention type vomiting of almost all foods. Lower esophageal obstruction causes progressive dysphagia and regurgitation. Early satiety usually occurs with linitis plastica but may be seen with other cancers.

Physical findings are usually limited to weight loss and, if anemia is present, pallor. In about 20% of cases, a palpable abdominal mass is present; this does not necessarily mean that the lesion is inoperable. Liver or peripheral metastases may also be present.

B. Laboratory Findings: Achlorhydria (gastric pH > 6.0) after stimulation with betazole (Histalog), 1.5 mg/kg subcut, in the presence of a gastric ulcer is pathognomonic of malignancy. The presence of acid does not exclude malignancy. If bleeding occurs, there will be occult blood in the stool and mild to severe anemia. With bone marrow invasion, the anemia may be normochromic and normocytic.

C. Other Examinations: Endoscopic biopsy and directed cytology and expert lavage cytology with chymotrypsin will provide the correct diagnosis in almost every patient. These methods will also establish the important differential diagnosis between adenocarcinoma and the malignant lymphomas.

Differential Diagnosis

The symptoms of carcinoma of the stomach are often mistaken for those of benign gastric ulcer, chronic gastritis, irritable colon syndrome, or functional gastrointestinal disturbance; x-ray and gastroscopic findings must be differentiated from those of benign gastric ulcer or tumor. Nonhealing ulcers or ulcers which are enlarging with a strict ulcer regimen require surgery. Most of these will still be benign.

The clinical history of gastric leiomyosarcoma may be indistinguishable from that of carcinoma. Bleeding, particularly massive, is more common. These tumors account for approximately 1.5% of gastric cancers. A palpable mass is more frequent than in gastric carcinoma, and the x-ray picture is characteristically that of a well-circumscribed intramural mass with, frequently, a central crater.

With the decreasing incidence of carcinoma of the stomach in the USA, gastric lymphoma now accounts for about 10% of gastric cancers. Treatment consists of resection, if possible, followed by irradiation therapy. The prognosis is much more favorable than in patients with carcinoma, and cure may be anticipated in over half of patients if the tumor is confined to the stomach.

Treatment

Surgical resection is the only curative treatment. Signs of metastatic disease include a hard, nodular liver, enlarged left supraclavicular (Virchow's) nodes, skin nodules, ascites, rectal shelf, and x-ray evidence of osseous or pulmonary metastasis. If none of these are present and there is no other contraindication to operation, exploration is indicated. The presence of an abdominal mass is not a contraindication to laparotomy, since bulky lesions can often be totally excised. Palliative resection or gastroenterostomy is occasionally helpful. High-voltage x-ray therapy may be of some value. Combined therapy with fluorouracil and the newer nitrosoureas may provide palliation and prolong life. These agents should be given by specialists in oncology because of their toxicity.

Prognosis

There is wide variation in the biologic malignancy of gastric carcinomas. In many the disease is widespread before symptoms are apparent; in a fortunate few, slow growth may progress over years and be resectable even at a late date. Approximately 10% of all patients with gastric carcinoma will be cured by surgical resection.

Brandborg LL, Tankersley CB, Uyeda F: "Low" vs "high" concentration chymotrypsin in gastric exfoliative cytology. Gastroenterology 57:500, 1969.

Kelsey JR: *Cancer of the Stomach.* Thomas, 1967.

Kovach JS & others: A controlled study of 1,3-bis-(2-chlorethyl)-1-nitrosourea and 5-fluorouracil therapy for advanced gastric and pancreatic cancer. Cancer 33:563, 1974.

McNeer G, Pack GT: *Neoplasms of the Stomach.* Lippincott, 1967.

Prolla JC, Kobayashi S, Kirsner JB: Gastric cancer. Arch Int Med 124:238, 1969.

Ringerta N: The pathology of gastric carcinoma. Nat Cancer Inst Monogr 25:275, 1967.

Silverberg E, Holleb AI: Cancer statistics, 1972. CA 22:2, 1972.

BENIGN TUMORS OF THE STOMACH

Most benign tumors do not cause symptoms and often are so small that they are overlooked on x-ray examination. Their importance lies in the problem of differentiation from malignant lesions, their precancerous possibilities, and the fact that they occasionally cause symptoms.

These tumors may be of epithelial origin (eg, adenomas, papillomas) or mesenchymal origin (eg, leiomyomas, fibromas, hemofibromas, lipomas, hemangiomas). The mesenchymal tumors, which are intramural, rarely undergo malignant change.

Clinical Findings

A. Symptoms and Signs: Large tumors may cause a vague feeling of epigastric fullness or heaviness; tumors located near the cardia or pylorus may produce symptoms of obstruction. If bleeding occurs it will cause symptoms and signs of acute gastrointestinal hemorrhage (eg, tarry stools, syncope, sweating, vomiting of blood). Chronic blood loss will cause symptoms of anemia (fatigue, dyspnea). If the tumor is large, a movable epigastric mass may be palpable.

B. Laboratory Findings: The usual laboratory findings may be present.

C. X-Ray Findings: The x-ray is characterized by a smooth filling defect, clearly circumscribed, which does not interfere with normal pliability or peristalsis. Larger tumors may show a small central crater.

Treatment & Prognosis

If symptoms occur (particularly hemorrhage), surgical resection is necessary. Adenomas rarely, if ever, become malignant. If there are no symptoms, the patient does not require surgery. These tumors may even regress spontaneously.

Beard EJ & others: Non-carcinomatous tumours of the stomach. Brit J Surg 55:535, 1968.
Elsborg L & others: Gastrocamera screening in pernicious anemia with special reference to the occurrence of gastric polyps and cancer. Scandinav J Gastroenterol 8:5, 1973.

DISEASES OF THE INTESTINES

REGIONAL ENTERITIS
(Regional Ileitis, Regional Enterocolitis, Granulomatous Ileocolitis, Crohn's Disease)

Essentials of Diagnosis

- Insidious onset.
- Intermittent bouts of diarrhea, low-grade fever, and right lower quadrant pain in a young adult.
- Fistula formation or right lower quadrant mass and tenderness.
- X-ray evidence of abnormality of the terminal ileum.

General Considerations

Regional enteritis is a chronic inflammatory disease of the small intestine causing fever, weight loss, and disturbed bowel function. It generally occurs in young adults and runs an intermittent clinical course with mild to severe disability and frequent complications.

The etiology is not known. The terminal ileum is the typical primary site, but involvement may extend up to the duodenum and into the colon, at times as "skip lesions" with normal intestine intervening. There is marked thickening of the submucosa with lymphedema, lymphoid hyperplasia, and nonspecific granulomas, and often ulceration of the overlying mucosa. A marked lymphadenitis occurs in the mesenteric nodes.

Clinical Findings

A. Symptoms and Signs: The disease is characterized by exacerbations and remissions. Abdominal pain, colicky or steady, in the right lower quadrant or periumbilical area, is present at some time during the course of the disease and varies from mild to severe. Diarrhea may occur, usually with intervening periods of normal bowel function or constipation. Fever may be low-grade or, rarely, spiking with chills. Anorexia, flatulence, malaise, and weight loss are present. Milk products and chemically or mechanically irritating foods may aggravate symptoms.

Abdominal tenderness, especially in the right lower quadrant, with signs of peritoneal irritation and an abdominal or pelvic mass in the same area, is usually present. The mass is tender and varies from a sausage-like thickened intestine to matted loops of intestine. The patient usually appears chronically ill.

Regional enteritis may pursue various clinical patterns. In certain instances, the course is indolent and symptomatology mild. In other instances, the course is toxic, with fever, toxic erythemas, arthralgias, anemia, etc. Still other patients pursue courses complicated by stricture of the bowel, perforation of the bowel, and suppurative complications of intra-abdominal perforation.

B. Laboratory Findings: There is usually a hypochromic (occasionally macrocytic) anemia and occult blood in the stool. The x-ray shows mucosal irregularity, ulceration, stiffening of the bowel wall, and luminal narrowing in the terminal ileum. Sigmoidoscopic examination may show an edematous hyperemic mucosa or a discrete ulcer when the colon is involved.

Differential Diagnosis

Acute regional enteritis may simulate acute appendicitis. Location in the terminal ileum requires differentiation from intestinal tuberculosis and lymphomas. Regional enteritis involving the colon must be distinguished from idiopathic ulcerative colitis, amebic colitis, and infectious disease of the colon. The sigmoidoscopic and x-ray criteria distinguishing these various entities may not be absolute, and definitive diagnosis may require cultures, examinations of the stool for parasites, and biopsy in selected instances.

Complications

Ischiorectal and perianal fistulas occur frequently. Fistulas may occur to the bladder or vagina and even to the skin in the area of a previous scar. Mechanical intestinal obstruction may occur. Nutritional deficiency due to malabsorption may produce a sprue-like syndrome. Generalized peritonitis is rare because perforation occurs slowly. The incidence of colon or rectal cancer in regional enteritis patients is greater than in a controlled population.

Treatment & Prognosis

A. General Measures: The diet should be generous, high-calorie, high-vitamin, and adequate in proteins, excluding raw fruits and vegetables. Treat anemia, dehydration, diarrhea, and avitaminosis as indicated.

B. Antimicrobial Agents: In our present state of knowledge about this disease, it appears that the beneficial effect of sulfonamides and antimicrobials can only be achieved by prolonged administration, perhaps even for life.

1. Sulfonamides—The sulfonamides may exert a beneficial effect; give sulfisoxazole, 2—4 gm/day orally, or salicylazosulfapyridine (Azulfidine), 2—8 gm/day orally.

2. Ampicillin—In cases of acute suppuration (manifested by tender mass, fever, leukocytosis), ampicillin, 4—8 gm/day IV or 2—4 gm/day orally, may be extremely useful.

3. Tetracycline—In cases where internal fistulization has led to a defunctionalized loop with bacterial overgrowth or where stricture formation has led to small bowel stasis with malabsorption, tetracycline, 1—2 gm/day orally, may be valuable in combating the bacterial overgrowth in the bowel and in correcting absorptive malfunction.

C. Adrenocortical Hormones: These agents are often of use in the diffuse form of the disease and are particularly helpful in the toxic forms (arthritis, anemia, toxic erythemas). The complications of long-term therapy can be minimized by administering the drug on an alternate-day schedule (eg, prednisone, 15—40 mg every other day).

D. Surgical Measures: Surgical treatment of this disease is best limited to the management of its complications. Resection of the small bowel, particularly the extensive resection often necessary in regional enteritis, leads to a "short bowel" syndrome (diminished absorptive surface), ie, malabsorption of vitmain B_{12} to varying degrees (loss of terminal ileum), hyperoxaluria, steatorrhea, osteomalacia, and macrocytic anemia (due to folic acid and vitamin B_{12} deficiency). Short-circuiting operations may lead to blind loops (intestinal defunctionalization with bacterial overgrowth) with similar difficulties in absorption. When surgery is necessary in this disease, study of postsurgical bowel function is indicated to detect the possibility of impaired bowel function. If defects in absorption are present, appropriate therapy may prevent serious complications.

Alexander-Williams J & others: A comparison of results of excision and bypass for ileal Crohn's disease. Gut 13:973, 1972.

Brooke BN: The pathogenesis of ulcerative and granulomatous colitis. S Clin North America 52:971, 1972.

Chadwich VS & others: Mechanism of hyperoxaluria in patients with ileal dysfunction. New England J Med 289:172, 1973.

Crohn's disease of the large bowel. (Leading article.) Brit MJ 1:125, 1972.

Fischer JE & others: Hyperalimentation as primary therapy for inflammatory bowel disease. Am J Surg 125:165, 1973.

Goldstein MJ & others: Ulcerative and "granulomatous" colitis: Validity of differential diagnostic criteria. Ann Int Med 72:841, 1970.

Kraft SC, Kirsner JB: Immunological apparatus of the gut and inflammatory bowel disease. Gastroenterology 60:922, 1971.

Lennard-Jones JE, Williams CB: Azathioprine in the treatment of Crohn's disease. Proc Roy Soc Med 65:291, 1972.

LiVolsi VA, Jaretski A: Granulomatous esophagitis. Gastroenterology 64:313, 1973.

Schachter H, Kirsner JB: Ulcerative and Crohn's (granulomatous) colitis. Postgrad Med 51:175, 1972.

Stankler L & others: Crohn's disease of the mouth. Brit J Dermat 87:501, 1972.

Weedon DD & others: Crohn's disease and cancer. New England J Med 289:1009, 1973.

Williams JA: The place of surgery in Crohn's disease. Gut 12:739, 1971.

TUMORS OF THE SMALL INTESTINE

Benign and malignant tumors of the small intestine are rare. There may be no symptoms or signs, but bleeding or obstruction (or both) may occur. The obstruction consists either of an intussusception with the tumor in the lead or a partial or complete occlusion in the lumen by growth of the tumor. Bleeding may cause weakness, fatigability, lightheadedness, syncope, pallor, sweating, tachycardia, and tarry stools. Obstruction causes nausea, vomiting, and abdominal pains. The abdomen is tender and distended, and bowel sounds are high-pitched and active. Malignant lesions produce weight loss and extra-intestinal manifestations (eg, pain due to stretching of the liver capsule, flushing due to carcinoid). In the case of a duodenal carcinoma, a peptic ulcer syndrome may be present. A palpable mass is rarely found.

If there is bleeding, melena and hypochromic anemia occur. X-ray (small bowel series) may show the tumor mass or dilatation of the small bowel if obstruction is present; in the absence of obstruction, it is extremely difficult to demonstrate the mass.

Benign Tumors

Benign tumors may be symptomatic or may be incidental findings at operation or autopsy. Treatment consists of surgical removal.

Benign **adenomas** constitute 25% of all benign

bowel tumors. **Lipomas** occur most frequently in the ileum; the presenting symptom is usually obstruction due to intussusception. **Leiomyomas** are usually associated with bleeding and may also cause intussusception. **Angiomas** behave like other small bowel tumors but have a greater tendency to bleed.

Multiple intestinal polyposis of the gastrointestinal tract (any level) associated with mucocutaneous pigmentation (Peutz-Jeghers syndrome) is a benign condition. Malignant change has been reported but is rare, and the entity becomes a problem only with complications such as obstruction or bleeding. The polyps are hamartomas and the pigment is melanin. The pigment is most prominent over the lips and buccal mucosa.

Colonic polyposis associated with osteomas and soft tissue tumors (Gardner's syndrome) is a condition with malignant potential. The colonic polyps are adenomatous. The soft tissue tumors are diffuse and may be sebaceous cysts, lipomas, fibromas, or leiomyomas. The bone tumors occur primarily in the mandible, sphenoid, and maxilla. This is a premalignant lesion. Consideration must be given to total colectomy or colectomy with ileorectal anastomosis. Careful follow-up is essential.

Malignant Tumors

The treatment of malignant tumors and their complications is usually surgical.

Adenocarcinoma is the most common malignancy of the small bowel, occurring most frequently in the duodenum and jejunum. Symptoms are due to obstructions or hemorrhage. The prognosis is very poor. **Lymphomas** are also first manifested by obstruction or bleeding. Perforation or malabsorption may also occur. Postoperative radiation therapy may occasionally be of value. **Sarcomas** occur most commonly in the mid small bowel and may first be manifested by mass, obstruction, or bleeding. The prognosis is guarded.

Carcinoid tumors arise from the argentaffin cells of the gastrointestinal tract. Ninety percent of these tumors occur in the appendix and 75% of the remainder occur in the small intestine (usually the distal ileum). Carcinoids may arise in other sites, including the stomach, colon, bronchus, pancreas, and ovary. Most small bowel carcinoids do not produce carcinoid syndrome. The main problem is metastases. Carcinoid syndrome occurs only in the instance of hepatic metastases. The tumor may secrete serotonin, and the systemic manifestations may consist of (1) paroxysmal flushing and other vasomotor symptoms, (2) dyspnea and wheezing, (3) recurrent episodes of abdominal pain and diarrhea, and (4) symptoms and signs of right-sided valvular disease of the heart. The diagnosis is confirmed by finding elevated levels of 5-hydroxyindoleacetic acid in the urine. The primary tumor is usually small, and obstruction is unusual. The metastases are usually voluminous and surprisingly benign. Treatment is symptomatic and supportive; surgical excision may be indicated if the condition is recognized before widespread metastases have occurred. Response to treatment with serotonin antagonists has been irregular. Repeated administration of corticotropin or the corticosteroids may occasionally be of value. The prognosis for cure is poor, but long-term survival is not unusual.

Calabro JJ: Hereditable multiple polyposis syndromes of the gastrointestinal tract. Am J Med 33:276, 1962.

Cohen A & others: Neoplasms of the small intestine. Am J Digest Dis 16:815, 1971.

Kenwright S: Coeliac disease and small bowel carcinoma. Postgrad MJ 48:673, 1972.

MECKEL'S DIVERTICULITIS

Meckel's diverticulum, a remnant of the omphalomesenteric duct, is found in about 2% of persons, more frequently in males. It arises from the ileum 2 or 3 feet from the ileocecal valve and may or may not have an umbilical attachment. Most are silent, but various abdominal symptoms may occur. The blind pouch may be involved by an inflammatory process similar to appendicitis; its congenital bands or inflammatory adhesions may cause acute intestinal obstruction; it may induce intussusception; or, in the 16% which contain heterotopic islands of gastric mucosa, it may form a peptic ulcer.

The symptoms and signs of the acute appendicitis-like disease and the acute intestinal obstruction caused by Meckel's diverticulitis cannot be differentiated from other primary processes except by exploration. Ulcer-type distress, if present, is localized near the umbilicus or lower and, more important, is not relieved by alkalies or food. If ulceration has occurred, blood will be present in the stool. Other laboratory findings often cannot be differentiated from those of appendicitis or other causes of obstruction. Massive gastrointestinal bleeding and perforation may occur.

Meckel's diverticulitis should be resected, either for relief or for differentiation from acute appendicitis. Surgery is curative.

Berquist TH & others: Diagnosis of Meckel's diverticulum by radioisotope scanning. Mayo Clin Proc 48:98, 1973.

Dalinka MK, Wunder JF: Meckel's diverticulum and its complications with emphasis on roentgenologic demonstration. Radiology 106:295, 1973.

MESENTERIC VASCULAR INSUFFICIENCY

1. CHRONIC MESENTERIC VASCULAR ISCHEMIA
(Abdominal Angina)

The syndrome of intestinal angina has received increasing attention of late. Progress in angiographic technics and vascular surgery has led to effective diagnostic and therapeutic approaches. The entity may be secondary to atherosclerosis and may precede vascular occlusion (see below). In some instances it is secondary to compression of the vessels either by the crura of the diaphragm or by anomalous bands.

Localized or generalized postprandial pain is the classical picture. The intensity of pain may be related to the size of the meal; the relationship to eating leads to a diminution in food intake and eventually weight loss. An epigastric bruit may be heard. Laboratory evidence of malabsorption may be present. The small bowel series may reveal a motility disorder. Visceral angiograms are necessary to confirm the narrowing of the celiac or mesenteric arteries.

Surgical revascularization of the bowel is the treatment of choice if the patient's condition permits. In certain instances, small, frequent feedings prove helpful.

2. ACUTE MESENTERIC VASCULAR OCCLUSION

Essentials of Diagnosis

- Severe abdominal pain with nausea, fecal vomiting, and bloody diarrhea.
- Severe prostration and shock.
- Abdominal distention, tenderness, rigidity.
- Leukocytosis, hemoconcentration.

General Considerations

Mesenteric arterial or venous occlusion is a catastrophic abdominal disorder. Arterial occlusion is occasionally embolic but is more frequently thrombotic. Both occur more frequently in men and in the older age groups.

The superior mesenteric artery or its branches are often involved. The affected bowel becomes congested, hemorrhagic, and edematous, and may cease to function, producing intestinal obstruction. True ischemic necrosis then develops.

Intestinal infarction may occur in the absence of mesenteric vascular thrombosis. Most patients have been in severe congestive heart failure or shock or in a state of hypoxia. Although many patients with this syndrome have been receiving digitalis glycosides, the relationship of this agent to the bowel problem is unclear. Occlusive vascular disease may also play a role in reducing perfusion of the bowel in these patients.

Clinical Findings

A. Symptoms and Signs: Generalized abdominal pain often comes on abruptly and is usually steady and severe, but it may begin gradually and may be intermittent with colicky exacerbations. Nausea and vomiting occur; the vomitus is rarely bloody. Bloody diarrhea and marked prostration, sweating, and anxiety may occur. For a period following the occlusion, the symptoms are severe but the physical findings are meager.

Shock may be evident. Abdominal distention occurs early, and audible peristalsis (evident early) may later disappear. As peritoneal irritation develops, diffuse tenderness, rigidity, and rebound tenderness appear.

B. Laboratory Findings: Hemoconcentration, leukocytosis (over 15,000/cu mm with a shift to the left), and often blood in the stool may occur.

C. X-Ray Findings: A plain film of the abdomen shows moderate gaseous distention of the small and large intestines and evidence of peritoneal fluid.

Differential Diagnosis

Differentiate from acute pancreatitis and a perforated viscus. The elevated amylase in pancreatitis and free peritoneal air in perforation may help to differentiate these conditions.

Treatment & Prognosis

The treatment of acute mesenteric arterial thrombosis consists of the measures necessary to (1) restore fluid, colloid, and electrolyte balance; (2) decompress the bowel; and (3) prevent sepsis by administration of antimicrobial drugs. Unless there are absolute contraindications to surgery, laparotomy should be done as soon as possible and gangrenous bowel resected. If the infarction is due to an isolated thrombus or embolus of the superior mesenteric artery, embolectomy or thrombectomy may be possible. Anticoagulants are not indicated. The mortality rate is extremely high in the acute disease. The treatment of nonthrombotic intestinal infarction poses a therapeutic dilemma. Basically, the principles are the same, namely, maintenance of fluid, electrolyte, and colloid balance. However, in the face of congestive failure, this can be most difficult. Careful monitoring by a central venous catheter provides useful information but is not the solution to this problem. Surgical resection of gangrenous bowel in a patient with congestive failure is a formidable undertaking but should be tried if at all possible. The prognosis in either event is grave; survival is unusual.

Friedman G, Sloan WC: Ischemic enteropathy. S Clin North America 52:1001, 1972.

Marston A: Diagnosis and management of intestinal ischemia. Ann Roy Coll Surg England 50:29, 1972.

Mathews JE, White RR: Primary mesenteric venous occlusive disease. Am J Surg 122:579, 1971.

Stemmer EA, Connolly JE: Mesenteric vascular insufficiency: Identification and management. California Med 118:18, March 1973.

ACUTE ORGANIC SMALL INTESTINAL OBSTRUCTION

Essentials of Diagnosis

- Colicky abdominal pain, vomiting, constipation, borborygmus.
- Tender distended abdomen without peritoneal irritation.
- Audible high-pitched tinkling peristalsis or peristaltic rushes.
- X-ray evidence of gas or gas and fluid levels without movement of gas.
- Little or no leukocytosis.

General Considerations

Acute organic intestinal obstruction usually involves the small intestine, particularly the ileum. Major inciting causes are external hernia and postoperative adhesions. Less common causes are gallstones, neoplasms, granulomatous processes, intussusception, volvulus, internal hernia, and foreign bodies.

Clinical Findings

A. Symptoms and Signs: Colicky abdominal pain in the periumbilical area becomes more constant and diffuse as distention develops. Vomiting, at first of a reflex nature associated with the waves of pain, later becomes fecal. Borborygmus and consciousness of intestinal movement, obstipation, weakness, perspiration, and anxiety are often present. The patient is restless, changing position frequently with pain, and is often in a shock-like state with sweating, tachycardia, and dehydration. Abdominal distention may be localized, with an isolated loop, but usually is generalized. The higher the obstruction, the less the distention; the longer the time of obstruction, the greater the distention. Audible peristalsis, peristaltic rushes with pain paroxysms, high-pitched tinkles, and visible peristalsis may be present. Abdominal tenderness is absent to moderate, and generalized, and there are no signs of peritoneal irritation. Fever is absent or low-grade. A tender hernia may be present.

B. Laboratory Findings: Hemoconcentration may occur with dehydration. Leukocytosis is absent or mild. Vomiting may cause electrolyte disturbances.

C. X-Ray Findings: Abdominal x-ray reveals gas-filled loops of bowel, and the gas does not progress downward on serial x-rays. Fluid levels may be visible.

Differential Diagnosis

Differentiate from other acute abdominal conditions such as inflammation and perforation of a viscus or renal or gallbladder colic. The absence of both rigidity and leukocytosis helps distinguish the obstruction from inflammation and perforation; the location, radiation, and the absence of distention or fecal vomiting distinguish the colic. Differentiate also from mesenteric vascular disease and torsion of an organ (eg, ovarian cyst). In the late stages of obstruction it may be impossible to distinguish acute organic intestinal obstruction from the late stage of peritonitis.

Complications

Strangulation (necrosis of the bowel wall) occurs with impairment of the blood supply to the gut. Strangulation is difficult to determine clinically, but fever, marked leukocytosis, and signs of peritoneal irritation should alert the clinician to this possibility. Strangulation may lead to perforation, peritonitis, and sepsis. Strangulation increases the mortality rate of intestinal obstruction to about 25%.

Treatment

A. Supportive Measures:

1. Decompression of the intestinal tract by nasogastric suction should relieve vomiting, reduce intestinal distention, and prevent aspiration. Tube decompression may be successful in relieving partial small bowel obstruction.

2. Correct fluid, electrolyte, and colloid deficits.

3. Give broad spectrum antibiotic therapy (gentamicin, ampicillin, or kanamycin) if strangulation is suspected.

B. Surgical Measures: Complete obstruction of the intestine is treated surgically after appropriate supportive therapy. The danger of strangulation is always present as long as obstruction is present, and the presence of fever, leukocytosis, peritoneal signs, or blood in the feces are indications that strangulation may have occurred and immediate surgery is indicated.

If the bowel is successfully decompressed during the preoperative preparation period, with cessation of pain and passage of flatus and feces, surgery may be delayed. Otherwise, surgical relief of the obstruction is indicated. Surgery consists of relieving the obstruction and removing gangrenous bowel with reanastomosis.

Prognosis

Prognosis varies with the causative factor and the presence of strangulation.

Giuffre JC: Intestinal obstruction: Ten-year experience. Dis Colon Rectum 15:426, 1972.

Greene WW: Bowel obstruction in the aged: A review of 300 cases. Am J Surg 118:541, 1969.

Rickham PP: Intraluminal intestinal obstruction. Progr Pediat Surg 2:73, 1971.

Silen W, Hein MF, Goldman L: Strangulation obstruction of the small intestine. Arch Surg 85:121, 1962.

Zachary RB: Intestinal obstruction. Progr Pediat Surg 2:57, 1971.

FUNCTIONAL OBSTRUCTION
(Adynamic Ileus, Paralytic Ileus)

Essentials of Diagnosis

- Continuous abdominal pain, distention, vomiting, and obstipation.
- History of a precipitating factor (surgery, peritonitis, pain).
- Minimal abdominal tenderness; decreased to absent bowel sounds.
- X-ray evidence of gas and fluid in bowel.

General Considerations

Adynamic ileus is a neurogenic impairment of peristalsis which may lead to intestinal obstruction. It is a common disorder due to a variety of intra-abdominal causes, eg, direct gastrointestinal tract irritation (surgery), peritoneal irritation (hemorrhage, ruptured viscus, pancreatitis, peritonitis), and anoxic organic obstruction. Renal colic, vertebral fractures, spinal cord injuries, pneumonia and other severe infections, uremia, and diabetic coma also may cause adynamic ileus.

Clinical Findings

A. Symptoms and Signs: There is mild to moderate abdominal pain, continuous rather than colicky, associated with vomiting (which may later become fecal) and obstipation. Borborygmus is absent. The symptoms of the initiating condition may also be present, eg, fever and prostration due to a ruptured viscus.

Abdominal distention is generalized and may be massive, with nonlocalized minimal abdominal tenderness and no signs of peritoneal irritation unless due to the primary disease. Bowel sounds are decreased to absent. Dehydration may occur after prolonged vomiting. Other signs of the initiating disorder may be present.

B. Laboratory Findings: With prolonged vomiting hemoconcentration and electrolyte imbalance may occur. Leukocytosis, anemia, and elevated serum amylase may be present depending upon the initiating condition.

C. X-Ray Findings: X-ray of the abdomen shows distended gas-filled loops of bowel in the small and large intestines and even in the rectum. There may be evidence of air-fluid levels in the distended bowel.

Differential Diagnosis

The symptoms and signs of obstruction with absent bowel sounds and a history of a precipitating condition leave little doubt as to the diagnosis. It is important to make certain that the adynamic ileus is not secondary to an organic obstruction, especially anoxic, where conservative management is harmful and immediate surgery may be lifesaving.

Treatment

Most cases of adynamic ileus are postoperative and respond to restriction of oral intake with gradual liberalization of the diet as the bowel function returns. Severe and prolonged ileus may require gastrointestinal suction and complete restriction of oral intake. Parenteral restoration of fluids and electrolytes is essential in such instances. When conservative therapy fails it may be necessary to operate for the purpose of decompressing the bowel by enterostomy or cecostomy and to rule out mechanical obstruction.

Those cases of adynamic ileus secondary to other diseases (eg, electrolyte imbalance, severe infection, intra-abdominal or back injury, pneumonitis) are managed as above plus treatment of the primary disease.

Prognosis

The prognosis varies with that of the initiating disorder. Adynamic ileus may resolve without specific therapy when the cause is removed. Intubation with decompression is usually successful in causing return of function.

Neely J, Catchpole B: Ileus: The restoration of alimentary-tract motility by pharmacological means. Brit J Surg 58:21, 1971.

INTESTINAL PSEUDO-OBSTRUCTION

Small Bowel Pseudo-obstruction

Apparent obstruction of the small bowel for which no mechanical cause can be found is termed pseudo-obstruction. It can occur transiently secondary to renal failure, pancreatitis, pneumonia, congestive heart failure, spinal injury, or electrolyte imbalance. Chronic pseudo-obstruction can occur secondary to myxedema, scleroderma, hypo- or hyperparathyroidism, sprue, mesenteritis, amyloidosis, Chagas' disease, myotonia dystrophica, Hirschsprung's disease, drug toxicity, or autonomic nervous system disorders. It may be idiopathic.

The presenting symptoms are cramping abdominal pain, abdominal distention, vomiting, and diarrhea. Weight loss and exacerbations and remissions characterize the course of the chronic disease.

Plain abdominal films show large distended loops of small bowel. Esophagograms may demonstrate motility disorders in the lower two-thirds of the esophagus. Barium meal and follow-through show hypomotility of the small bowel and a decreased rate of transit.

Treatment of secondary pseudo-obstruction consists of treatment of the primary disorder. No consistently effective treatment for idiopathic psuedo-obstruction is known. Antibiotic therapy for bacterial overgrowth has been transiently effective.

Idiopathic pseudo-obstruction leads to disability due to repeated episodes of obstruction with a possible progression to advanced malnutrition, electrolyte derangement, and death.

Large Bowel Pseudo-obstruction

Pseudo-obstruction of the colon may occur secondary to intra-abdominal inflammation, retroperitoneal disease or manipulation, hypoxia, congestive heart failure, myocardial infarction, or systemic infections. It may be idiopathic.

The presenting symptoms are cramping abdominal pain, abdominal distention, and vomiting. Plain films of the abdomen show a distended, gas-filled colon and rectum. Barium enema demonstrates the absence of a mechanical obstruction.

Treatment is surgical, with cecostomy the apparent procedure of choice. Secondary pseudo-obstruction of the colon does not recur following recovery from the primary disease. Idiopathic pseudo-obstruction of the colon tends to recur.

Caves PK, Crockard HA: Pseudo-obstruction of the large bowel. Brit MJ 2:583, 1970.

Maldonado JE & others: Chronic idiopathic intestinal pseudo-obstruction. Am J Med 49:203, 1970.

Moss AA & others: Idiopathic intestinal pseudo-obstruction. Am J Roentgenol 115:312, 1972.

Wanebo H, Connolly B: Pseudo-obstruction of the colon. Surg Gynec Obst 133:44, 1971.

SPRUE SYNDROME
(Malabsorption Syndrome, Tropical Sprue, Celiac Sprue, Idiopathic Steatorrhea)

Essentials of Diagnosis

- Bulky, pale, frothy, foul-smelling, greasy stools with increased fecal fat on chemical analysis of the stool.
- Weight loss and signs of multiple vitamin deficiencies.
- Impaired intestinal absorption of glucose, vitamins, fat; large amounts of fat in the stool.
- Hypochromic or megaloblastic anemia; "deficiency" pattern on small bowel x-ray.

General Considerations

Sprue syndromes are diseases of disturbed small intestine function characterized by impaired absorption, particularly of fats, and motor abnormalities. Celiac sprue responds to a gluten-free diet, whereas tropical sprue does not. The polypeptide gliadin is the offending substance in gluten. Although an infectious cause has not been conclusively demonstrated, tropical sprue behaves clinically like an infectious disease. It responds to folic acid and broad-spectrum antibiotics.

The clinical severity of sprue syndrome varies depending upon the extent of the lesion in the small intestine and the duration of the disease. Severe wasting, gastrointestinal protein loss, multiple vitamin deficiencies, and adrenal and pituitary deficiency may be associated with the severe forms of the disease. A flat intestinal mucosa without villi in the small intestine is noted, and some observers have described degenerative changes in the myenteric nerve plexuses.

Rare secondary varieties of sprue syndrome in which the cause of the small intestine dysfunction is known include gastrocolic fistulas, obstruction of intestinal lacteals by lymphoma, Whipple's disease, extensive regional enteritis, and parasitic infections such as giardiasis, strongyloidiasis, and coccidiosis.

Clinical Findings

A. Tropical Sprue: The main symptom is diarrhea; at first it is explosive and watery; later, stools are fewer and more solid and characteristically pale, frothy, foul-smelling, and greasy, with exacerbations on high-fat diet or under stress. Indigestion, flatulence, abdominal cramps, weight loss (often marked), pallor, asthenia, irritability, paresthesias, and muscle cramps may occur. Quiescent periods with or without mild symptoms often occur, especially on leaving the tropics.

Vitamin deficiencies cause glossitis, cheilosis, angular stomatitis, cutaneous hyperpigmentation, and dry rough skin. Abdominal distention and mild tenderness are present. Edema occurs late.

Anemia is usually megaloblastic, and, with blood loss or malabsorption of iron, may be hypochromic, microcytic, or mixed. The fecal fat is increased. Absorption of other substances is decreased, giving flat oral vitamin A tolerance and glucose tolerance curves. The intravenous glucose tolerance, however, is normal. Plasma carotene and proteins and serum calcium, phosphorus, cholesterol, and prothrombin are low. Gastric hypochlorhydria is present. The pancreatic enzymes are normal.

X-rays using nonflocculating barium show dilatation of the intestine and occasionally excess fluid and gas.

B. Celiac Sprue: This disorder is characterized by defective absorption of fat, protein, vitamin B_{12}, carbohydrate, and water. Absorption of fat-soluble vitamins A, D, and K is impaired. Osteomalacia may ensue. Protein loss from the intestine may occur. Elimination of gluten from the diet causes dramatic improvement.

In one-third of patients with celiac sprue, symptoms begin in early childhood. Symptoms may persist into adult life, but there is usually a latent phase of apparent good health. The anemia is usually hypochromic and microcytic. The complications of impaired absorption are more severe: infantilism, dwarfism, tetany, vitamin deficiency signs, and even rickets may be seen. The definitive diagnosis of steatorrhea requires quantitation measurement of fecal fat, preferably on a known fat intake.

Differential Diagnosis

It is necessary to differentiate between the various causes of malabsorption to permit selection of specific therapy, if any. Anatomic abnormalities such as fistulas, blind loops, and jejunal diverticulosis may be found on x-ray. Regional enteritis usually has a characteristic appearance but must be distinguished from intestinal tuberculosis. The small bowel x-ray appearance in Whipple's disease, intestinal lymphoma, and amyloidosis is abnormal but not specific or diagnostic. In primary diseases of the small intestine, mucosal suction biopsy is the most effective way of making the diagnosis. In some diseases, the pathologic response is patchy and multiple specimens may be required. Pancreatic insufficiency may be diagnosed by a low water and bicarbonate secretion in response to intravenous secretin.

Treatment

A. Celiac Sprue: Strict elimination of gluten from the diet will lead to clinical recovery. If there is no response, another diagnosis must be sought. The diet should be high in calories and protein, low in fat, and gluten-free. Prothrombin deficiency is treated by means of water-soluble vitamin K orally or, if urgent, parenterally. Treat hypocalcemia or tetany with calcium phosphate or gluconate, 2 gm orally 3 times daily, and vitamin D, 5−20 thousand units. Multiple vitamin supplements may also be advisable. Macrocytic anemia usually responds to vitamin B_{12}, 100 μg IM every month. When the steatorrhea disappears, vitamin B_{12} may be discontinued.

B. Tropical Sprue: Folic acid, 10−20 mg daily orally or IM for a few weeks, corrects diarrhea, anorexia, weight loss, glossitis, and anemia. Tetracycline, 250 mg orally 4 times daily, is given at the outset of treatment. When complete remission occurs, the patient may be maintained on 5 mg of folic acid daily. If the patient has achlorhydria, vitamin B_{12} should also be considered. Hypochromic anemia is treated with oral iron. A high-calorie, high-protein, low-fat diet is given.

C. Corticosteroids: The corticosteroids may be advantageous in certain patients with malabsorption since they increase the absorption of nitrogen, fats, and other nutrients from the gastrointestinal tract.

Prognosis

With proper treatment, the response is good.

Brandborg LL: Structure and function of the small intestine in some parasite diseases. Am J Clin Nutr 24:124, 1971.

Finkelstein JD: Malabsorption. M Clin North America 52:1339, 1968.

Greenberger NJ, Skillman TG: Medium-chain triglycerides: Physiologic considerations and clinical implications. New England J Med 280:1045, 1969.

Isselbacher KJ: Biochemical aspects of fat absorption. Gastroenterology 50:78, 1966.

Jeffries GH, Weser E, Sleisinger MH: Malabsorption. Gastroenterology 56:777, 1969.

Klipstein FA: Tropical sprue. Gastroenterology 54:275, 1968.

Kowlessar OD, Phillips LD: Celiac disease. M Clin North America 54:647, 1970.

Krone CL & others: Studies on the pathogenesis of malabsorption. Medicine 47: 89, 1968.

Mann JG, Brown WR, Kern F Jr: The subtle and variable clinical expression of gluten-induced enteropathy (adult celiac disease, non-tropical sprue). Am J Med 48:357, 1970.

Roggin GM: Malabsorption in the chronic alcoholic. Johns Hopkins Med J 125:321, 1969.

Rubin CE, Dobbins WO III: Peroral biopsy of the small intestine: A review of its diagnostic usefulness. Gastroenterology 49:676, 1965.

Rubin CE, Eidelman S, Weinstein WM: Sprue by any other name. Gastroenterology 58:409, 1970.

Trier JS: Diagnostic value of peroral biopsy of the proximal small intestine. New England J Med 285:1470, 1971.

DISACCHARIDASE DEFICIENCY

The specific disaccharidase deficiencies in the intestinal mucosa have become increasingly important in our understanding of malabsorption. The congenital absence of these enzymes leads to an acidic diarrhea (fecal pH 4.5−6.0). There are large amounts of lactic acid in the stool. The infant fails to thrive. The onset of the clinical picture in the adult may follow intestinal surgery, regional enteritis, ulcerative colitis, or the sprue syndromes. The diagnosis is confirmed by a flat oral tolerance to the specific disaccharide and the onset of an acidic diarrhea with ingestion of the offending sugar.

Thus far lactose, sucrose-isomaltose, and glucose-galactose intolerances have been described as congenital defects. Secondary disaccharidase deficiencies have been described in both children and adults with giardiasis, celiac disease, ulcerative colitis, short bowel syndrome, cystic fibrosis, and after gastrectomy. Removal of the offending sugar from the diet will result in remission.

Herber R: Dissaccharidase deficiency in health and disease. California Med 116:23, June 1972.

Kretchmer N: Lactose and lactase: A historical perspective. Gastroenterology 61:805, 1971.

Peternel WW: Disaccharidase deficiency. M Clin North America 52:1355, 1968.

Welsh TD & others: Human intestinal disaccharidase activity. Arch Int Med 117:488, 1966.

INTESTINAL LIPODYSTROPHY
(Whipple's Disease)

Whipple's disease is an uncommon malabsorption disorder of unknown cause with widespread systemic manifestations. Histologic examination of a small bowel mucosal biopsy specimen reveals characteristic large, foamy mononuclear cells filled with cytoplasmic material which gives a positive periodic acid-Schiff (PAS) staining reaction. Electron microscopic studies reveal bacterial bodies in the epithelium and lamina propria. The disease occurs primarily in middle-aged men and is of insidious onset; the course, without treatment, is usually downhill. The clinical manifestations include abdominal pain, diarrhea, steatorrhea, gastrointestinal bleeding, fever, lymphadenopathy, polyarthritis, edema, and gray to brown skin pigmentation. Anemia and hypoproteinemia are common.

Treatment consists of tetracycline, 250 mg 4 times daily, or oral penicillin G, 600,000 units twice daily. The duration of treatment should be at least 6 months. Reappearance of symptoms after therapy or while on therapy suggests emergence of resistant organisms, and the antibiotic should be changed.

Clemett AR, Marshak RH: Whipple's disease: Roentgen features and differential diagnosis. Radiol Clin North America 7:105, 1969.

Fearrington EL, Monroe EW: Whipple's disease. Postgrad Med 44:103, 1968.

Trier JS & others: Whipple's disease: Light and electron microscope correlation of jejunal mucosal histology with antibiotic treatment and clinical status. Gastroenterology 48:684, 1965.

PROTEIN-LOSING ENTEROPATHY

Leakage of plasma proteins into the intestinal lumen is an integral phase of the metabolism of plasma proteins. In certain intestinal disease states, excessive protein loss into the intestinal lumen may be responsible for hypoproteinemia noted in these entities. Excessive loss of plasma protein may be due to increased mucosal permeability to protein, inflammatory exudation, excessive cell desquamation, or direct leakage of lymph from obstructed lacteals. Gastrointestinal diseases associated with protein-losing enteropathy include gastric carcinoma, lymphoma, gastric rugal hypertrophy, sprue, allergic gastroenteropathy, regional enteritis, diffuse jejuno-ileitis, and others.

Treatment consists of management of the primary disorder.

Jeffries GH, Holman HR, Sleisenger MH: Plasma proteins and the gastrointestinal tract. New England J Med 266:652, 1962.

Sleinfeld JL & others: Mechanism of hypoproteinemia in patients with regional enteritis and ulcerative colitis. Am J Med 29:405, 1960.

PSEUDOMEMBRANOUS ENTEROCOLITIS

Pseudomembranous enterocolitis is a necrotizing lesion of the gut which may extend from the stomach to the rectum. Grossly it is characterized by a friable, grayish-yellow membrane loosely adherent to the underlying mucosa or submucosa. Microscopically, mucosal necrosis, leukocytes, and necrotic debris are enmeshed in the fibrin membrane. Gram-positive cocci and other bacteria may be present in the membrane.

The etiology is not completely understood, but the evidence points to the enterotoxin of the hemolytic *Staphylococcus aureus* as the precipitating factor. Suppression of other intestinal bacteria by antibiotics leads to the overgrowth of staphylococci. In clindamycin-associated colitis, staphylococci and other pathogens have not been found.

The disease usually becomes manifest from the 2nd—12th day after surgery or after antibiotic therapy. The patient usually has had or is taking antibiotics. The initial symptoms are usually diarrhea and fever. Diarrhea is profuse and watery and the stools may resemble serum and have a peculiar necrotic odor. Some patients may show abdominal distention or vomiting. The patient's condition rapidly deteriorates, with tachycardia, hypotension, shock, dehydration, oliguria, and electrolyte and protein loss. Liquid stools may exceed 10 liters/day. Leukocyte counts are normal or elevated. Hemoconcentration frequently occurs. Stools may contain membrane, leukocytes, and gram-positive cocci.

Pseudomembranous enterocolitis must be distinguished from other postoperative complications such as peritonitis, mesenteric thrombosis, and hypovolemia due to blood loss. The history of antibiotic therapy and major surgery (especially gastrointestinal) are important in the differential diagnosis.

All antibiotics the patient is receiving at the outset of the disease must be discontinued. Combat the marked dehydration and electrolyte depletion which occurs with electrolyte solutions containing sodium and potassium according to the patient's needs. Administer plasma, whole blood, and corticosteroids to combat shock. Vancomycin, 250—500 mg IV, is the treatment of choice if staphylococci are present; otherwise, give cephalothin, 1 gm IV, every 6 hours until toxicity subsides and staphylococci disappear from the stools. In noninfective pseudomembranous colitis failing to respond to treatment, colectomy has been suggested when the disease is confined to the colon.

Pseudomembranous enterocolitis is an extremely grave condition. Mortality statistics vary from 30—90% if the condition is not recognized. In clindamycin-associated colitis, stopping the antibiotic results in cure in most cases.

Ecker JA & others: Pseudomembranous enterocolitis: An unwelcome gastrointestinal complication of antibiotic therapy. Am J Gastroenterol 54:214, 1970.

Groll A & others: Fulminating noninfective pseudomembranous colitis. Gastroenterology 58:88, 1970.

Tedesco FJ, Barton RW, Alpers DH: Clindamycin-associated colitis: A prospective study. Ann Int Med 81:429, 1974.

APPENDICITIS

Essentials of Diagnosis

- Right lower quadrant abdominal pain and tenderness with signs of peritoneal irritation.

- Anorexia, nausea, vomiting, constipation.
- Low-grade fever and mild polymorpho-nuclear leukocytosis.

General Considerations

Appendicitis is initiated by obstruction of the appendiceal lumen by a fecalith, inflammation, foreign body, or neoplasm. Obstruction is followed by infection, edema, and frequently infarction of the appendiceal wall. Intraluminal tension develops rapidly and tends to cause early mural necrosis and perforation. All ages and both sexes are affected, but appendicitis is more common in males between 10 and 30 years of age.

Appendicitis is one of the most frequent causes of acute surgical abdomen. The symptoms and signs usually follow a fairly stereotyped pattern, but appendicitis is capable of such protean manifestations that it should be considered in the differential diagnosis of every obscure case of intra-abdominal sepsis and pain.

Clinical Findings

A. Symptoms and Signs: An attack of appendicitis usually begins with epigastric or periumbilical pain associated with 1−2 episodes of vomiting. Within 2−12 hours the pain shifts to the right lower quadrant, where it persists as a steady soreness which is aggravated by walking or coughing. There is anorexia, moderate malaise, and slight fever. Constipation is usual, but diarrhea occurs occasionally.

At onset there are no localized abdominal findings. Within a few hours, however, progressive right lower quadrant tenderness can be demonstrated; careful examination will usually identify a single point of maximal tenderness. The patient can often place his finger precisely on this area, especially if asked to accentuate the soreness by coughing. Light percussion over the right lower quadrant is helpful in localizing tenderness. Rebound tenderness and spasm of the overlying abdominal muscles are usually present. Psoas and obturator signs, when positive, are strongly suggestive of appendicitis. Rectal tenderness is common and, in pelvic appendicitis, may be more definite than abdominal tenderness. Peristalsis is diminished or absent. Slight to moderate fever is present.

B. Laboratory Findings: Moderate leukocytosis (10,000−20,000/cu mm) with an increase in neutrophils is usually present. It is not uncommon to find a few red cells on microscopic examination of the urine, but otherwise the urinalysis is not remarkable.

C. X-Ray Findings: There are no characteristic changes on plain films of the abdomen. However, visualization in the right lower quadrant of a radiopaque shadow consistent with fecalith in the appendix may heighten suspicion of appendicitis.

Factors Which Cause Variations From the "Classical" Clinical Picture

A. Anatomic Location of Appendix: Abdominal findings are most definite when the appendix is in the iliac fossa or superficially located. When the appendix extends over the pelvic brim, the abdominal signs may be minimal, greatest tenderness being elicited on rectal examination. Right lower quadrant tenderness may be poorly localized and slow to develop in retrocecal or retroileal appendicitis. Inflammation of a high-lying lateral appendix may produce maximal tenderness in the flank. Bizarre locations of the appendix may rarely occur in association with a mobile or undescended cecum; in such cases symptoms and signs may be localized in the right upper or the left lower quadrant.

B. Age:

1. Infancy and childhood—In infancy appendicitis is relatively rare, but when it occurs the diagnosis is difficult because of the problem of interpretation of history and physical findings. The disease tends to progress rapidly and, when rupture occurs, to result in generalized peritonitis because of poor localizing mechanisms.

2. Old age—Elderly patients frequently have few or no prodromal symptoms. Abdominal findings may be unimpressive, with slight tenderness and neglible muscle guarding until perforation occurs. Fever and leukocytosis may also be minimal or absent. When the white count is not elevated, a shift to the left is significant evidence of inflammation.

3. Obesity—Obesity frequently increases the difficulty of evaluation by delaying the appearance of abdominal signs and by preventing their sharp localization.

4. Pregnancy—See discussion in Chapter 12.

Differential Diagnosis

Acute gastroenteritis is the disorder most commonly confused with appendicitis. In rare cases it either precedes or is coincident with appendicitis. Vomiting and diarrhea are more common. Fever and white blood count may rise sharply and may be out of proportion to abdominal findings. Localization of pain and tenderness is usually indefinite and shifting. Hyperactive peristalsis is characteristic. Gastroenteritis frequently runs an acute course. A period of observation usually serves to clarify the diagnosis.

Mesenteric adenitis may cause signs and symptoms identical with appendicitis. Usually, however, there are some clues to the true diagnosis. Mesenteric adenitis is more likely to occur in children or adolescents; respiratory infection is a common antecedent; localization of right lower quadrant tenderness is less precise and constant; and true muscle guarding is infrequent. In spite of a strong suspicion of mesenteric adenitis, it is often safer to advise appendectomy than to risk a complication of appendicitis by procrastination.

Meckel's diverticulitis may mimic appendicitis. The localization of tenderness may be more medial, but this is not a reliable diagnostic criterion. Because operation is required in both diseases, the differentiation is not critical. When a preoperative diagnosis of appendicitis proves on exploration to be erroneous, it is essential to examine the terminal 5 feet of the ileum for Meckel's diverticulitis and mesenteric adenitis.

Regional enteritis, perforated duodenal ulcer, ureteral colic, acute salpingitis, mittelschmerz, ruptured ectopic pregnancy, and twisted ovarian cyst may at times also be confused with appendicitis.

Complications

A. Perforation: Appendicitis may rarely subside spontaneously, but it is an unpredictable disease with a marked tendency (about 95%) to progression and perforation. Because perforation rarely occurs within the first 8 hours, diagnostic observation during this period is relatively safe. Signs of perforation include increasing severity of pain, tenderness, and spasm in the right lower quadrant followed by evidence of generalized peritonitis or of a localized abscess. Ileus, fever, malaise, and leukocytosis become more marked. If perforation with abscess formation or generalized peritonitis has already occurred when the patient is first seen, the diagnosis may be quite obscure.

Treatment of perforated appendicitis is appendectomy unless a well-localized right lower quadrant or pelvic abscess has already walled off the appendix. Supportive measures are as for acute peritonitis.

1. Generalized peritonitis—This is a common sequel to perforation. Clinical findings and treatment are discussed elsewhere in this chapter.

2. Appendiceal abscess—This is one of the possible complications of untreated appendicitis. Malaise, toxicity, fever, and leukocytosis vary from minimal to marked. Examination discloses a tender mass in the right lower quadrant or pelvis. Pelvic abscesses tend to bulge into the rectum or vagina.

Abscesses usually become noticeable 2–6 days after onset, but antibiotic therapy may delay their appearance. Appendiceal abscess is occasionally the first and only sign of appendicitis and may be confused with neoplasm of the cecum, particularly in the older age group in whom systemic reaction to the infection may be minimal or absent.

Treatment of early abscess is by intensive combined antibiotic therapy (eg, penicillin and streptomycin or tetracycline, or both). On this regimen, the abscess will frequently resolve. Appendectomy should be performed 6–12 weeks later. A well-established, progressive abscess in the right lower quadrant should be drained without delay. Pelvic abscess requires drainage when it bulges into the rectum or vagina and has become fluctuant.

B. Pylephlebitis: Suppurative thrombophlebitis of the portal system with liver abscesses is a rare but highly lethal complication. It should be suspected when septic fever, chills, hepatomegaly, and jaundice develop after appendiceal perforation. Intensive combined antibiotic therapy is indicated.

C. Other Complications: These include subphrenic abscess and other foci of intra-abdominal sepsis. Intestinal obstruction may be caused by adhesions.

Treatment

A. Preoperative Care:

1. Observation for diagnosis—Within the first 8–12 hours after onset the symptoms and signs of appendicitis are frequently indefinite. Under these circumstances a period of close observation is essential. The patient is placed at bed rest and given nothing by mouth. *Note:* Laxatives should not be prescribed when appendicitis or any form of peritonitis is suspected. Parenteral fluid therapy is begun as indicated. Narcotic medications are avoided if possible, but sedation with barbiturates or tranquilizing agents is not contraindicated. Abdominal and rectal examinations, white blood count, and differential count are repeated periodically. Abdominal films and an upright chest film must be obtained as part of the investigation of all difficult diagnostic problems. In most cases of appendicitis, the diagnosis is clarified by localization of signs to the right lower quadrant within 12 hours after onset of symptoms.

2. Intubation—Preoperatively, a nasogastric tube is inserted if there is sufficient peritonitis or toxicity to indicate that postoperative ileus may be troublesome. In such patients the stomach is aspirated and lavaged if necessary, and the patient is sent to the operating room with the tube in place.

3. Antibiotics—In the presence of marked systemic reaction with severe toxicity and high fever, preoperative administration of antibiotics (eg, penicillin and streptomycin) is advisable.

B. Surgical Treatment: In uncomplicated appendicitis, appendectomy is performed as soon as fluid imbalance and other significant systemic disturbances are controlled. Little preparation is usually required. Early, properly conducted surgery has a mortality of a fraction of 1%. The morbidity and mortality that occur as a result of this disease are due primarily to the complications of gangrene and perforation which occur when operation is delayed.

C. Postoperative Care: In uncomplicated appendicitis, postoperative gastric suction is usually not necessary. Ambulation is begun on the first postoperative day. The diet is advanced from clear liquids to soft solids during the 2nd–5th postoperative days, depending upon the rapidity with which peristalsis and gastrointestinal function return. Parenteral fluid supplements are administered as required. Enemas are contraindicated. Mineral oil, milk of magnesia, or a similar milk laxative may be given orally at bedtime daily from about the third day onward if necessary. Antibiotic therapy (eg, penicillin with streptomycin or tetracycline, or both) is advisable for 5–7 days or longer if abdominal fluid at operation was purulent or malodorous, if culture was positive, or if the appendix was gangrenous. Primary wound healing is the rule, and the period of hospitalization is usually 1 week or less. Normal activity can be resumed in 2–3 weeks after surgery in uncomplicated cases, especially if a McBurney type incision was used.

D. Emergency Nonsurgical Treatment: When surgical facilities are not available, treat as for acute peritonitis. On such a regimen acute appendicitis will frequently subside and complications will be minimized.

Prognosis

With accurate diagnosis and early surgical removal of the appendix mortality and morbidity are minimal. Delay of diagnosis still produces significant mortality and morbidity if complications occur.

Recurrent acute attacks may occur if the appendix is not removed. "Chronic appendicitis" does not exist.

Burgos WF, Johnson DG: Appendicitis: A computer study. Postgrad Med 44:110, 1968.
Burkitt DP: The aetiology of appendicitis. Brit J Surg 58:695, 1971.
Jones FC, Martin JD: Present problems of acute appendicitis. Am Surgeon 38:247, 1972.
Kazarian K, Roeder WJ, Mersheimer WL: Decreasing mortality and increasing morbidity from acute appendicitis. Am J Surg 119:681, 1970.

ACUTE MESENTERIC LYMPHADENITIS

Essentials of Diagnosis

- Acute right lower quadrant or periumbilical pain in a child.
- Anorexia, nausea, vomiting, fever up to 39.5° C (103.1° F).
- Right lower quadrant tenderness with minimal or no peritoneal irritation.
- Leukocytosis generally over 15,000/cu mm.
- History of recent or current upper respiratory infection.

General Considerations

Mesenteric lymphadenitis is an acute benign inflammation of the mesenteric lymph nodes causing fever and abdominal pain. It is usually a disease of children, may be recurrent, and presents a major problem in differentiation from acute appendicitis, Meckel's diverticulitis, renal infection or colic, and right lower lobe pulmonary infections in children with pain referred to the right lower quadrant. Episodes are frequently preceded by or accompanied by upper respiratory infections. Various bacteria (staphylococci, streptococci, yersiniae) and viruses have been implicated.

Clinical Findings

A. Symptoms and Signs: There is an acute onset of abdominal pain in the right lower quadrant of periumbilical area, generally steady from the onset rather than colicky, and associated with nausea, vomiting, and anorexia. Diarrhea often occurs. Abdominal tenderness is mild to severe and usually greatest in the right lower quadrant; point localization of pain is unusual. Peritoneal irritation and right vault rectal tenderness are mild or absent. Fever to 37.8–39.5° C (100–103.1° F) is usually present.

B. Laboratory Findings: There is a polymorphonuclear leukocytosis with a shift to the left, generally over 15,000/cu mm and higher than would be expected from the findings.

Treatment & Prognosis

Exploration may be warranted to be certain that the patient does not have appendicitis. Complete resolution is the rule.

Blattner RL: Acute mesenteric lymphadenitis. J Pediat 74:479, 1969.
Donhauser JL: Primary acute mesenteric lymphadenitis. Arch Surg 74:528, 1957.

INTESTINAL TUBERCULOSIS
(Tuberculous Enterocolitis)

In the USA tuberculosis of the intestinal tract is almost always secondary to pulmonary tuberculosis. The incidence rises sharply in far-advanced lung disease.

The mode of infection is by ingestion of tubercle bacilli with the formation of ulcerating lesions in the intestine, particularly the ileocecal region, and involvement of the mesenteric lymph nodes.

Symptoms may be absent or minimal even with extensive disease. When present they usually consist of fever, anorexia, nausea, flatulence, distention after eating, and food intolerance. There may be abdominal pain and mild to severe cramps, usually in the right lower quadrant and often after meals. Constipation may be present, but mild to severe diarrhea is more characteristic.

Abdominal examination is not characteristic, although there may be mild right lower quadrant tenderness. Fistula-in-ano may be evident. Weight loss occurs.

There are no characteristic laboratory findings. The presence of tubercle bacilli in the feces does not correlate with intestinal involvement.

X-ray examination reveals irritability and spasm, particularly in the cecal region, irregular hypermotility of the intestinal tract; ulcerated lesions and irregular filling defects, particularly in the right colon and ileocecal region; and pulmonary tuberculosis.

The prognosis varies with that of the pulmonary disease. The intestinal lesions usually respond to chemotherapy and rest when reexposure to infecting material is prevented. Operation may be required for intestinal obstruction.

Lewis EA: Tuberculous ileocolitis in Ibadan: A clinicoradiological review. Gut 13:646, 1972.
Tandon HD, Prakash A: Pathology of intestinal tuberculosis and its distinction from Crohn's disease. Gut 13:260, 1972.

DISEASES OF THE COLON & RECTUM

NONSPECIFIC ULCERATIVE COLITIS

Essentials of Diagnosis

- Bloody diarrhea with lower abdominal cramps.
- Mild abdominal tenderness, weight loss, fever.
- Anemia; no stool pathogens.
- Specific x-ray and sigmoidoscopic abnormalities.

General Considerations

Ulcerative colitis is an inflammatory disease of the colon of unknown etiology characterized by bloody diarrhea, a tendency to remissions and exacerbations, and involvement mainly of the left colon. It is primarily a disease of adolescents and young adults but may have its onset in any age group.

The pathologic process is that of acute nonspecific inflammation in the colon, particularly the rectosigmoid area, with multiple, irregular superficial ulcerations. Repeated episodes lead to thickening of the wall with scar tissue, and the proliferative changes in the epithelium may lead to polypoid structures. Pseudopolyps are usually indicative of severe ulceration. The etiology is not known; it may be multiple.

Clinical Findings

A. Symptoms and Signs: This disease may vary from mild cases with relatively minimal symptoms to acute and fulminating, with severe diarrhea and prostration. Diarrhea is characteristic; there may be up to 30 or 40 discharges daily, with blood and mucus in the stools, or blood and mucus may occur without feces. Blood in the stool is the cardinal manifestation of ulcerative colitis. Constipation may occur instead of diarrhea.

Nocturnal diarrhea is usually present when daytime diarrhea is severe. Rectal tenesmus may be severe, and anal incontinence may be present. Cramping lower abdominal pain often occurs but is generally mild. Anorexia, malaise, weakness, and fatigability may also be present. A history of intolerance to dairy products can often be obtained, and there is a tendency toward remissions and exacerbations.

Fever, weight loss, and evidence of toxemia vary with the severity of the disease. Abdominal tenderness is generally mild and occurs without signs of peritoneal irritation. Abdominal distention may be present in the fulminating form and is a poor prognostic sign. Rectal examination may show perianal irritation, fissures, hemorrhoids, fistulas, and abscesses.

B. Laboratory Findings: Hypochromic microcytic anemia due to blood loss is usually present. In acute disease a polymorphonuclear leukocytosis may also be present. The sedimentation rate is elevated. Stools contain blood, pus, and mucus but no pathogenic organisms. Hypoproteinemia may occur. In the fulminating disease electrolyte disturbances may be evident.

C. X-Ray Findings: On x-ray the involvement may be regional to generalized and may vary from irritability and fuzzy margins to pseudopolyps, decreased size of colon, shortening and narrowing of the lumen, and loss of haustral markings. When the disease is limited to the rectosigmoid area, the barium enema may even be normal.

D. Special Examinations: Sigmoidoscopic changes are present in over 90% of cases and vary from mucosal hyperemia, petechiae, and minimal granularity in mild cases to ulceration and polypoid changes in severe cases. The mucosa, even when it appears grossly normal, is almost invariably friable when wiped with a cotton sponge.

Differential Diagnosis

Differentiate from bacillary dysentery and amebic dysentery on the basis of specific stool pathogens. When rectal strictures have developed, differentiate from lymphogranuloma venereum by history and Frei test. Other points in the differential diagnosis are functional diarrhea, Crohn's colitis, intestinal neoplasm, and diverticulitis. It is imperative that cultures and parasitology specimens be taken prior to barium examinations or initiation of therapy.

Complications

A. Local Complications: Local complications in and around the large bowel include ischiorectal abscess, fistula-in-ano, rectovaginal fistula, rectal prolapse, fibrous stricture of the rectum or colon, colonic perforation, toxic dilatation of the colon, carcinoma, and massive colonic hemorrhage.

B. Systemic Complications: Systemic complications include pyoderma gangrenosum, erythema nodosum, polyarthritis, ankylosing spondylitis, ocular lesions (including iritis, uveitis, and conjunctivitis), liver disease (including fatty liver and pericholangitis), anemia, thrombophlebitis, and impaired growth and sexual development in children.

The incidence of carcinoma is significantly greater in patients with ulcerative colitis. It appears to be related to 2 factors. The first is the extent of involvement. Involvement of the entire colon carries a greater risk than minimal disease. The second factor is duration of the disease. The risk rises from approximately 2% at 10 years to 10–15% at 20 years.

Treatment

Ulcerative colitis is a chronic disease. Symptomatic remission is not the only index of response. Treatment should be prolonged until the sigmoidoscopic and x-ray appearance of the colon have returned to normal.

A. General Measures: Bed rest is necessary during the acute phase of the disease, and may substantially reduce intestinal cramping and diarrhea. The diet should be nutritious and supplemented liberally with vitamins. All foods should be cooked to reduce intestinal cramping and diarrhea, and milk and milk products should be eliminated from the diet. The diet may be liberalized when the disease process has improved.

These patients need understanding and reassurance. Mild sedation is often necessary for nervousness.

Care should be used in the administration of antiperistaltic agents so that excessive amounts are not used; dilation of the colon may occur. Narcotics should be avoided except for severe diarrhea.

B. Medical Measures: The pathogenesis of ulcerative colitis is unknown. The role of autoimmunity or bacteria and the nature of precipitating events have not yet been discerned. Whatever the pathogenesis, corticotropin, adrenocorticosteroids, and the sulfonamides have provided the best means of control.

1. Adrenocorticosteroid hormones—Corticotropin and hydrocortisone are the most effective drugs for inducing remissions, and are definitely indicated in the severe toxic form of the disease. The hospitalized patient may be given corticotropin as IV drip (20–40 units over a period of 8 hours) or 80–100 units of gel subcut, or hydrocortisone (100–300 mg/day). Prednisone or prednisolone, 20–80 mg/day or equivalent, may be preferred. These drugs may be given parenterally if oral therapy seems ineffective. If the response to corticotropin is satisfactory, the dosage may be reduced or oral therapy with prednisone (20–40 mg/day) may be substituted and gradually reduced at weekly intervals over a period of 1–3 months. General measures include diet, rest, and sulfonamide drugs. These are essential during this phase of the illness.

The choice of adrenocortical hormone therapy should be in large part dictated by the severity of the disease. If the course is fulminant and rapid action is essential to the patient's welfare, the use of intravenous hydrocortisone becomes essential. In less fulminant forms of the disease, parenteral corticotropin or oral adrenocortical hormones are the agents of choice. If the disease is effectively managed by topical corticosteroids (by enema), these agents are the method of choice because of reduced side-effects.

Long-term suppression of ulcerative colitis with these agents leads to hyperadrenocorticism, osteoporosis, toxic psychosis, peptic ulcer, hypokalemia, and hyperglycemia. Local therapy of the colon by enema makes possible the long-term treatment with steroids with a negligible risk of hyperadrenocorticism and other complications. Give hydrocortisone hemisuccinate (100 mg) or prednisolone-21-phosphate (20 mg) in 100 ml of saline once or twice daily by slow rectal drip or retention enema; or hydrocortisone in oil (100 mg/2 oz) every night as a retention enema. The patient should preferably lie on his left side with the buttocks elevated. Hydrocortisone is the least expensive and can be prepared for home use by mixing 1.6 gm of hydrocortisone powder in 1 quart of vegetable oil.

2. Anti-infective agents—Sulfonamides are not curative but may be useful in management. In one carefully controlled study, sulfonamide (salicylazosulfapyridine) therapy reduced the incidence of recurrence and severity of individual attacks. Although the poorly absorbable sulfonamides are preferred by many clinicians, there are no critical data confirming the superiority of the nonabsorbable over the absorbable drugs or of one drug over another. Sulfisoxazole, 2–4 gm/day orally, or salicylazosulfapyridine, 2–8 gm/day orally, is useful in the mild to moderate forms of the disease. Adverse effects of salicylazosulfapyridine (gastrointestinal, hematologic, generalized) necessitate periodic follow-up examinations, and the side-effects can often be overcome if the drug is stopped temporarily or reduced in dosage or if the enteric-coated drug is employed. In case of sulfonamide hypersensitivity, ampicillin, 2–4 gm/day orally, or cephalexin monohydrate, 2–4 gm/day orally, may be useful. The observation that long-term sulfonamide (salicylazosulfapyridine) therapy reduces the rate of recurrence of acute attacks of ulcerative colitis suggests that prolonged therapy with sulfonamides may be indicated in many of these patients.

Penicillin, streptomycin, chloramphenicol, or other antibiotics may be indicated in certain instances (eg, localized perforation or systemic infection).

C. Surgical Measures: Surgical excision of the colon is required for patients with refractory disease, severe extracolonic complications (growth suppression), prolonged widespread colon disease, massive hemorrhage, or extensive perirectal disease. The usual procedure is total colectomy with a permanent ileostomy. In some instances, the rectum may be preserved and a primary reanastomosis or subsequent reanastomosis carried out if the rectum appears normal or minimally involved.

Prognosis

The disease may have many remissions and exacerbations over many years. At times the course is fulminant. Permanent and complete cure on medical therapy is unusual, and life expectancy is shortened. The incidence of bowel cancer in patients with active disease rises with each decade after the diagnosis. Medical measures control the majority of cases, but colectomy is often necessary for fulminant, refractory disease and for complications.

Das KM & others: Adverse reactions during salicylazosulfapyridine therapy and the relation with drug metabolism and acetylator phenotype. New England J Med 289:491, 1973.

Devroede GJ & others: Cancer risk and life expectancy of children with ulcerative colitis. New England J Med 285:17, 1971.

Eade MN: Liver disease in ulcerative colitis. 1. Analysis of operative liver biopsy in 138 consecutive patients having colectomy. Ann Int Med 72:475, 1970.

Eade MN, Cooke WT: Hepatobiliary disease associated with ulcerative colitis. Postgrad Med 53:112, 1973.

Edwards FC, Truelove SC: The course and prognosis of ulcerative colitis. 1. Short-term prognosis. 2. Long-term prognosis. 3. Complications. 4. Carcinoma of the colon. Gut 4:299, 1963; 5:1, 1964.

Friedland GW & others: Inflammatory bowel disease: A symposium. California Med 119:14, Nov 1973.

Glotzer DJ & others: Comparative features and course of ulcerative and granulomatous colitis. New England J Med 282:582, 1970.

Jalan KN & others: Influence of corticosteroid on the results of surgical treatment for ulcerative colitis. New England J Med 282:588, 1970.

Jewell DP, Truelove SC: Azathioprine in ulcerative colitis: An interim report on a controlled therapeutic trial. Brit MJ 1:709, 1972.

Margulis AR: Radiology of ulcerating colitis. Radiology 105:251, 1972.

Margulis AR & others: The overlapping spectrum of ulcerative and granulomatous colitis: A roentgenographic-pathologic study. Am J Roentgenol 113:325, 1971.

Misiewicz JJ & others: Controlled trial of sulphasalazine [salicylazosulfapyridine; Azulfidine®] in maintenance therapy for ulcerative colitis. Lancet 1:185, 1965.

Nugent FW, Bulan MB: Extracolonic manifestations of ulcerative colitis. Am Family Physician-GP 5:68, Jan 1972.

Schachter H & others: Ulcerative and "granulomatous" colitis: Validity of differential diagnostic criteria. Ann Int Med 72:841, 1970.

Wall AJ, Kirsner JB: The management of ulcerative and granulomatous colitis. Mod Treat 8:944, 1971.

Warwick RRG & others: Colonoscopy and double contrast barium enema examination in chronic ulcerative colitis. Am J Roentgenol 117:292, 1973.

TOXIC DILATATION OF THE COLON
(Toxic Megacolon)

Toxic megacolon is a life-threatening complication of idiopathic ulcerative colitis or Crohn's disease of the colon. It results from extensive damage to the mucosa with areas of mucosal denudation and inflammation of the submucosal layers. It is manifested clinically by evidence of systemic toxicity, fever, leukocytosis, tachycardia, and abdominal distention. Radiographically, the colon is dilated. Colonic dilatation per se without signs of systemic toxicity may be the result of potassium deficiency or anticholinergic or opiate therapy. The mortality rate of this fulminant complication is high, and treatment, both medical and surgical, should be instituted as soon as possible.

Treatment consists of the following urgent measures: (1) Decompress the bowel and pass an intestinal tube to prevent swallowed air from further distending the colon. (2) Restore fluid, electrolyte, colloid, and blood volume. Remember that diarrhea and adrenal steroid therapy significantly reduce total body potassium with an effect on colonic function. (3) Suppress the inflammatory reaction with hydrocortisone, 100 mg IV every 8 hours. (4) Prevent sepsis with broad-spectrum antibiotics (gentamicin, kanamycin, chloramphenicol).

Careful observation with frequent abdominal films during the period of 6–8 hours while the above therapy is being given determines whether or not the patient will require surgical treatment. If the colon decompresses, medical therapy is continued; if not, colectomy should be considered. These patients are desperately ill, and if surgery is necessary the procedure of choice is subtotal colectomy. This reduces operating time and the extent of operative trauma.

Norland CC, Kirsner JB: Toxic dilatation of colon (toxic megacolon): Etiology, treatment and prognosis in 42 patients. Medicine 48:229, 1969.

GRANULOMATOUS COLITIS

Transmural colitis (Crohn's granulomatosis) may be difficult or impossible to distinguish from the mucosal form of colitis (idiopathic ulcerative colitis) by clinical criteria alone. The most distinguishing feature is transmural involvement in Crohn's colitis. Table 10–1 briefly summarizes the features of these 2 entities. However, the differential diagnostic criteria, when tested against the pathologic findings following colectomy, show a substantial overlap in clinical, radiographic, and histologic criteria.

The most common clinical manifestations are abdominal cramping, diarrhea, and weight loss. Extracolonic manifestations such as erythema nodosum, spondylitis, polyarthritis, and perirectal disease may antedate the colonic manifestations of the disease.

The treatment of granulomatous colitis is essentially the same as for idiopathic ulcerative colitis. The response to treatment, however, is usually not so dramatic.

Table 10–1. Differential features of ulcerative colitis and granulomatous colitis.*

	Ulcerative Colitis	Granulomatous Colitis
Clinical		
Toxicity	Common	Rare
Bleeding	Common	Rare
Perianal disease	Rare	Common
Fistula	Rare	Common
Perforation	Rare	Common
Sigmoidoscopy	Diffuse, friable superficial ulceration	Discrete, occasionally diffuse
X-ray		
Distribution	Continuous	Segmental
Mucosa	Serrated	Fissures to deep ulcers
Stricture	Rare	Common
Pathology	Mucosal microabscesses	Transmural involvement, granulomas

*Reference: Margulis AR & others: The overlapping spectrum of ulcerative and granulomatous colitis: A roentgenographic-pathologic study. Am J Roentgenol 113:325, 1971.

ISCHEMIC PROCTOCOLITIS

Infarction of the colon or rectum due to deprivation of arterial blood causes ischemic proctocolitis. Most patients are in their 6th or 7th decades. Younger women taking oral contraceptives are also at risk.

Presenting symptoms are lower abdominal pain of sudden onset, fever, vomiting, and the passage of bright red blood and clots per rectum. A neutrophil leukocytosis is usual. The sigmoidoscopic examination is nonspecific. The appearance may vary from that of nonspecific proctocolitis to multiple ulcers, polypoid or nodular lesions, and, in some instances, hemorrhagic or necrotic membrane formation.

Plain films of the abdomen may show generalized dilatation of the colon. Barium enema shows a single lesion, usually localized near the splenic flexure or in the rectum. It is characterized by a variable combination of thumbprinting (edematous mucosal folds), saw-toothed mucosal irregularity, tubular narrowing, and sacculation. The rectum and colon are not involved simultaneously. Angiograms may show vascular occlusion, but absence of such evidence does not exclude the diagnosis. Inflammatory bowel involvement by Crohn's disease, idiopathic ulcerative colitis, and infection and stricture due to carcinoma must be ruled out.

Severe ischemia leading to gangrene is treated by replacement of blood volume, antibiotics (chloramphenicol, kanamycin, gentamicin), and excision of the necrotic bowel. Less severe ischemia leading to stricture formation is treated by resection of the stricture. Transient ischemia requires no specific treatment.

The prognosis is good in transient proctocolitis. The mortality rate is high when gangrene occurs.

Kilpatrick ZM & others: Ischemic proctitis. JAMA 205:74, 1968.

Marston A & others: Ischemic colitis. Gut 7:1, 1966.

CONGENITAL MEGACOLON
(Hirschsprung's Disease)

Hirschsprung's disease is a congenital disorder characterized by massive dilatation of the proximal colon due to loss of propulsive function in the distal sigmoid and rectum. The basic pathophysiologic abnormality is absent or reduced ganglion cells in the rectum and lower sigmoid with loss of propulsive activity in this segment. Dilatation and muscular hypertrophy above this level are compensatory.

Symptoms include recurrent fecal impactions that are relatively refractory to cathartics and more responsive to enemas, infrequent bowel movements, and an enlarging abdomen. The periods between defecations may be 3–4 weeks or longer. Stools are large and have an offensive odor. Secondary symptoms include displacement of the thoracic contents, causing dyspnea, edema of the extremities, and audible borborygmus.

Abdominal distention is often massive and associated with costal flaring. Fecal masses and gas-filled loops of bowel are palpable in the abdomen, and sluggish visible peristalsis may be evident. Signs of poor nutrition may be present, such as multiple vitamin deficiencies, emaciation, and retarded growth. Secondary signs such as abdominal hernia, thinning of the abdominal wall, and diastasis recti abdominis are frequently present.

X-ray shows a normal or narrowed segment in the lower sigmoid or rectum and a dilated proximal colon.

In mild forms treatment may consist only of dietary supervision (avoiding high-residue foods) and giving stool softeners and lubricating agents. Frequent enemas are necessary. Parasympathomimetic drugs are useful on occasion.

If surgery is necessary the colon must be completely emptied and the gastrointestinal tract sterilized preoperatively. Cecostomy or colostomy is not definitive, but is a useful preliminary step until definitive surgery is feasible or as a lifesaving procedure in a critically ill child.

The surgical procedure of choice is abdominoperineal removal of the rectosigmoid, the so-called "pull-through" operation (Swenson).

Abdominoperineal resection and anastomosis will yield excellent results in 80% of cases.

Davis PW, Foster DBE: Hirschsprung's disease: A clinical review. Brit J Surg 59:19, 1972.

Ehrenpreis T: Progress report: Hirschsprung's disease. Am J Digest Dis 16:1032, 1971.

Howard ER: Hirschsprung's disease: A review of the morphology and physiology. Postgrad MJ 48:471, 1972.

Soper RT, Miller FE: Congenital aganglionic megacolon (Hirschsprung's disease). Arch Surg 96:554, 1968.

Tobon F & others: Nonsurgical test for diagnosis of Hirschsprung's disease. New England J Med 278:188, 1968.

DIVERTICULAR DISEASE OF THE COLON

Essentials of Diagnosis

- Intermittent, cramping left lower abdominal pain.
- Constipation or alternating constipation and diarrhea.
- Tenderness in the left lower quadrant.
- X-ray evidence of diverticula, thickened interhaustral folds, narrowed lumen.

General Considerations

Diverticula of the colon become more frequent with advancing age and may be entirely asymptomatic. The inflammatory complication, diverticulitis, probably affects 20–25% of the patients with diverticulosis at some time.

Colonic diverticula occur primarily in the pressure areas of the colon. They tend to dissect along the course of the nutrient vessels, and they consist of a mucosal coat and a serosa. Although diverticula may occur throughout the gut, excluding the rectum, they are most common in the sigmoid colon and occur with increasing frequency after age 40.

Inflammatory changes in diverticulitis vary from mild infiltration in the wall of the sac to extensive inflammatory change in the surrounding area (peridiverticulitis) with perforation or abscess formation. The changes are comparable to those that occur in appendicitis.

Clinical Findings

A. Symptoms and Signs: Left lower quadrant pain may be steady and severe and last for days or may be cramping and intermittent and relieved by a bowel movement. Constipation is usual, but diarrhea may occur. Occult blood is found in the stool in about 20% of cases. Massive hemorrhage may occur and is the most common cause of colonic hemorrhage.

B. Laboratory Findings: Noncontributory in uncomplicated diverticular disease.

C. X-Ray Findings: X-ray examination reveals diverticula and in some cases spasm, interhaustral thickening, or narrowing of the colonic lumen.

Complications

Diverticulitis is a complication of diverticular disease in which micro- or macroperforation of the diverticulum has occurred. The clinical manifestations vary with the extent of the inflammatory process and may include pain, signs of peritoneal irritation, chills, fever, sepsis, ileus, and partial or complete colonic obstruction. Peritonitis and abscess formation may also occur. Urinary frequency and dysuria are associated with bladder involvement in the inflammatory process. Fistula formation usually involves the bladder (usually vesicosigmoid) but may also be to the skin, perianal area, or small bowel. Laboratory examination reveals polymorphonuclear leukocytosis. Red and white blood cells may be seen in the urine. Blood cultures may be positive.

Differential Diagnosis

The constrictive lesion of the colon seen on x-ray or visualized at sigmoidoscopy must be differentiated from carcinoma of the colon. The appearance of a short lesion with abrupt transition to normal bowel suggests carcinoma. Colonoscopy with biopsy can be very useful in these instances.

Treatment

The treatment of uncomplicated diverticular disease consists of (1) a diet high in residue; (2) bulk additives (with appropriate caution about possible bowel obstruction), eg, psyllium hydrophilic mucilloid (Metamucil); (3) a stool softener such as dioctyl sodium sulfosuccinate (Colace, etc), 240 mg/day; and (4) anticholinergic drugs such as Donnatal, Librax, and propantheline (Pro-Banthine). Vegetable oils (olive oil), mineral oil (for short periods), and vegetable gum laxatives may be used.

The treatment of acute diverticulitis requires antibiotic therapy. The antibiotic of choice is ampicillin. Other useful antibiotic drugs include cephalothin and combined treatment with penicillin and streptomycin.

Recurrent attacks of diverticulitis or the presence of perforation, fistulization, or abscess formation require surgical resection of the involved portion of the colon.

Massive diverticular hemorrhage usually stops spontaneously. Adequate blood replacement and careful endoscopic and barium studies to rule out other causes of bleeding are indicated. In certain instances, selective arteriography may localize the site of the bleeding and make it possible to control the bleeding with vasopressin.

Prognosis

The usual case is mild and responds well to dietary measures and antibiotics.

Berman PM, Kirsner JB: Current knowledge of diverticular disease of the colon. Am J Digest Dis 17:741, 1972.

Botsford TW, Zollinger RM Jr: Diverticulitis of the colon. Surg Gynec Obst 128:1209, 1969.

Fleischner G: Diverticular disease of the colon: New observations and revised concepts. Gastroenterology 60:316, 1971.

Judd ES: Massive bleeding of colonic origin. S Clin North America 49:977, 1969.

Lewis EE, Schnug GE: Importance of angiography in the management of massive hemorrhage from colonic diverticula. Am J Surg 124:573, 1972.

Shulman AG: High bulk diet for diverticular disease of the colon. Western J Med 120:278, 1974.

Tagart RE: Diverticular disease of the colon: Clinical aspects. Brit J Surg 56:417, 1969.

Zollinger RW, Zollinger RM: Diverticular disease of the colon. Advances Surg 5:255, 1971.

POLYPS OF THE COLON & RECTUM
(Intestinal Polyps)

Adenomatous polyps of the colon and rectum are common benign neoplasms which are usually asymptomatic but may cause painless rectal bleeding. They may be single or multiple, occur most frequently in the sigmoid and rectum, and are found incidentally in about 9% of autopsies. The incidence of polyps increases with age. The diagnosis is established by sigmoidoscopy and double contrast barium enema. When a polyp is found in the rectum, the colon should be studied by x-ray.

Whether polyps are precancerous is an important question. Pedunculated, adenomatous polyps probably have negligible malignant potential and may usually be treated by simple polypectomy through the sigmoidoscope or colonoscope. In most patients, more aggressive operation is not indicated unless the polyp grows on repeated observation or causes symptoms such as bleeding. Papillary (villous) adenomas are sessile lesions which are known to become metastasizing carcinoma and should be removed. The overwhelming majority of cancers of the colon and rectum arise de novo.

Familial intestinal polyposis is a rare hereditary disease characterized by innumerable adenomatous polyps of the colon and rectum. Cancer frequently develops in the large bowel, sometimes at a very early age. Colectomy with ileoproctostomy is the treatment of choice and may be followed by spontaneous regression of the rectal polyps. The rectum should be examined regularly and residual polyps removed through the sigmoidoscope. If this is not possible, the rectum should also be excised.

Buntain WL & others: Premalignancy of polyps of the colon. Surg Gynec Obst 134:499, 1972.
Bussey HJR: Progress report: Gastrointestinal polyposis. Gut 11:970, 1970.
Drexler J: Asymptomatic polyps of the rectum and colon. Arch Int Med 121:62, 1968.
Haenszel W, Correa P: Cancer of the colon and rectum and adenomatous polyps: A review of epidemiological findings. Cancer 28:14, 1971.
Thomas KE & others: Natural history of Gardner's syndrome. Am J Surg 115:218, 1968.

COLONIC OBSTRUCTION

Colonic obstruction may be acute or chronic. It may be simple, strangulating, paralytic, or closed loop. The most common cause of subacute and chronic obstruction of the colon is carcinoma. Other conditions include fecal impaction, scleroderma, strictures caused by granulomatous colitis, and diverticular disease of the colon. Acute obstruction is usually due to volvulus, intussusception, or inguinal herniation of the colon.

Clinical Findings

A. Symptoms and Signs: Simple obstruction with constipation or obstipation may lead to the insidious development of pain. Severe continuous pain suggests strangulation. Borborygmus may be prominent. Nausea and vomiting are late signs. Physical examination discloses abdominal distention and tympany. High-pitched tinkles may be heard on auscultation. Localized mass suggests carcinoma, intussusception, or strangulated closed loop. Peritoneal signs suggest perforation. Blood in the rectum suggests intussusception or carcinoma.

B. Laboratory Findings: Noncontributory unless strangulation has occurred.

C. X-Ray Findings: Colonic distention can be demonstrated by plain abdominal films. The barium enema will demonstrate the site of obstruction, but this procedure is contraindicated if there is ischemia with necrosis of the bowel wall. Barium by upper gastrointestinal series should never be given if there is any possibility of colonic obstruction.

Differential Diagnosis

In paralytic ileus the abdomen is silent and cramping does not occur. Signs of peritonitis are present, or there is a history of drug ingestion or trauma to the back or pelvis.

In small bowel obstruction, vomiting is more common and occurs earlier. The abdominal pain is usually more severe, and x-ray may reveal the ladder configuration of distended small bowel with little or no colonic distention.

Complications

Delay in treatment may lead to strangulation with perforation, peritonitis, and sepsis.

Treatment

The treatment of colonic obstruction is surgical. Although an occasional sigmoid volvulus or intussusception may be reduced by barium enema, the usual medical treatment is to prepare the patient for surgery with attention to fluid, electrolyte, cardiac, and pulmonary status.

Morton JH, Schwartz SI, Gramiak R: Ileus of the colon. Arch Surg 81:425, 1960.
Shepherd JJ: Treatment of volvulus of the sigmoid colon: A review of 425 cases. Brit MJ 1:280, 1968.

CANCER OF THE COLON & RECTUM

Essentials of Diagnosis

- Altered bowel function (constipation or diarrhea).
- Blood in the feces, unexplained anemia, weight loss.
- Palpable mass involving colon or rectum.
- Sigmoidoscopic or x-ray evidence of neoplasm.

General Considerations

Carcinoma is the only common malignancy of the colon and rectum. Lymphoma, carcinoid, melanoma, fibrosarcoma, and other types of sarcoma occur rarely. The treatment of all is essentially the same.

Carcinoma of the colon and rectum causes more deaths than any other form of cancer. The only known predisposing causes are familial multiple polyposis, chronic ulcerative colitis, chronic lymphogranuloma venereum, chronic granuloma inguinale, and perhaps adenoma. Males are affected more commonly than females in a ratio of 3:2. The highest incidence is in patients about 50 years of age, but occasional cases have been reported in younger persons and even in children. The anatomic distribution of cancer of the large bowel is approximately 16% in the cecum and ascending colon, 5% in the transverse colon, 9% in the descending colon, 20% in the sigmoid, and 50% in the rectum.

Of all lesions of the colon and rectum, half to two-thirds lie within reach of the examining finger or sigmoidoscope and therefore can be biopsied on the first visit.

Clinical Findings

Symptoms vary depending upon whether the lesion is in the right or the left side of the colon. In either case, a persistent change in the customary bowel habits almost always occurs and should invariably alert the physician to investigate the colon. Bleeding is a cardinal diagnostic point. An acute abdominal emergency may be precipitated by perforation or colonic obstruction (due to circumferential narrowing, not intussusception). The definitive diagnostic procedures in all cases of colon and rectal cancer are sigmoidoscopy and barium enema.

A. Carcinoma of the Right Colon: Because the fecal stream is fluid and the bowel lumen large in the right half of the colon, symptoms of obstruction occur less frequently than in left-sided tumors. Vague abdominal discomfort is often the only initial complaint. This may progress to cramp-like pain, occasionally simulating cholecystitis or appendicitis. Secondary anemia with associated weakness and weight loss is found in half of patients with right colon lesions. The stools are usually positive for occult blood but rarely show gross blood. The patient is likely to have diarrhea. The first indication of cancer may be the discovery of a palpable mass in the right lower quadrant.

B. Carcinoma of the Left Colon: Obstructive symptoms predominate, particularly increasing constipation. There may be short bouts of diarrhea. Occasionally the first sign is acute colonic obstruction. A small amount of bright red blood with bowel movements is common, and anemia is found in about 20% of cases. At times a mass is palpable. About half of patients give a history of weight loss.

Differential Diagnosis

Cancer of the colon may need to be differentiated from diverticulitis, which is usually associated with fever and has a different x-ray appearance. Functional bowel distress may also simulate cancer of the colon symptomatically.

Treatment

The only curative treatment in cancer of the large bowel is wide surgical resection of the lesion and its regional lymphatics after adequate bowel preparation and appropriate supportive measures. When a significant degree of mechanical obstruction is present, a preliminary transverse colostomy or cecostomy is necessary. Even in the presence of metastatic disease, palliative resection may be of value to relieve obstruction, bleeding, or the symptoms of local invasion. Preoperative irradiation, 2000–2500 rads in 10 fractions given over 12 days, has been shown to increase resectability and improve survival in patients undergoing abdominoperineal resection.

Care of the Colostomy

The commonest permanent colostomy is the sigmoid colostomy made at the time of combined abdominoperineal resection.

Colostomy irrigation is begun about 1 week after operation. Each day, a well-lubricated catheter or rectal tube is gently inserted about 15 cm (6 inches) into the colostomy and 500–1000 ml of water are instilled from an enema can or bag held 30–60 cm (12–24 inches) above the colostomy. After the bowel has become accustomed to regular enemas, evacuation will occur within about one-half hour after the irrigation. Some individuals have regular movements without irrigation. A small gauze or disposable tissue pad worn over the colostomy, held in place by a wide elastic belt or ordinary girdle, is usually all the protection required during the day. If the stoma is tight, it is advisable for the patient to dilate it daily for several months by insertion of the index finger. Commercial colostomy kits make care simple and convenient.

Three important principles of colostomy management are routine time for bowel evacuation; complete emptying after irrigation; and regulation of diet to avoid diarrhea. The patient with a colostomy can live a normal life.

Stricture, prolapse, and wound hernia are late colostomy complications requiring surgical correction. Skin irritation is less likely to occur than with ileostomy.

Prognosis

Over 90% of patients with carcinoma of the colon and rectum are suitable for either curative or palliative resection, with an operative mortality of 3–6%. The overall 5-year survival rate after resection is about 50%. If the lesion is confined to the bowel and there is no evidence of lymphatic or blood vessel invasion, the 5-year survival rate is 60–70%. Local recurrence of carcinoma in the anastomotic suture line or wound area occurs in 10–15% of cases. The incidence of local recurrence can be decreased if special precautions are taken at operation to avoid implantation of malignant cells. About 5% of patients develop multiple primary colon cancers. Early identification of resectable local recurrence or a new neoplasm depends upon careful follow-up with sigmoidoscopy and barium enema every 6 months for 2 years and yearly thereafter.

Bartholomew LG, Schutt AJ: Systemic syndromes associated with neoplastic disease including cancer of the colon. Cancer 28:170, 1971.

Beahrs OH, Sanfelippo PM: Factors in prognosis of colon and rectal cancer. Cancer 28:213, 1971.

Cole WH: Cancer of the colon and rectum. S Clin North America 52:871, 1972.

Dykes PW, King J: Progress report: Carcinoembryonic antigen (CEA). Gut 13:1000, 1972.

First National Conference on Cancer of the Colon and Rectum. Cancer 28:1, 1971.

Gallagher EG, Zeigler MG: Rectal carcinoma in patients in the second and third decades of life. Am J Surg 124:655, 1972.

Hardin WJ: Unusual manifestations of malignant disease of the large intestine. S Clin North America 52:287, 1972.

Roswit B, Higgins GA Jr, Keehn RJ: Preoperative irradiation for carcinoma of the rectum and rectosigmoid colon: Report of a national Veterans Administration randomized study. Cancer 35:1597, 1975.

DISEASES OF THE ANUS

HEMORRHOIDS

Essentials of Diagnosis

- Rectal bleeding, protrusion, and vague discomfort.
- Mucoid discharge from rectum.
- Characteristic findings on external anal inspection or anoscopic examination.

General Considerations

Internal hemorrhoids are varices of that portion of the venous hemorrhoidal plexus which lies submucosally just proximal to the dentate margin. External hemorrhoids arise from the same plexus but are located subcutaneously immediately distal to the dentate margin. There are 3 primary internal hemorrhoidal masses: right anterior, right posterior, and left lateral. Three to 5 secondary hemorrhoids may be present between the 3 primaries. Straining at stool, constipation, prolonged sitting, and anal infection are contributing factors and may precipitate complications such as thrombosis. Diagnosis is suspected on the history of protrusion, anal pain, or bleeding, and confirmed by proctologic examination.

Carcinoma of the colon or rectum not infrequently aggravates hemorrhoids or produces similar complaints. Polyps may be present as a cause of bleeding which is wrongly attributed to hemorrhoids. For these reasons, the treatment of hemorrhoids is always preceded by sigmoidoscopy and barium enema. When portal hypertension is suspected as an etiologic factor, investigations for liver disease should be carried out. Hemorrhoids which develop during pregnancy or parturition tend to subside thereafter and should be treated conservatively unless persistent after delivery.

Clinical Findings

The symptoms of hemorrhoids are usually mild and remittent, but a number of disturbing complications may develop and call for active medical or surgical treatment. These complications include pruritus, incontinence, recurrent protrusion requiring manual replacement by the patient, fissure, infection, or ulceration, prolapse and strangulation, and secondary anemia due to chronic blood loss. Carcinoma has been reported to develop very rarely in hemorrhoids.

Treatment

Conservative treatment suffices in most instances of mild hemorrhoids, which may improve spontaneously or in response to low-roughage diet and regulation of the bowel habits with mineral oil or other nonirritating laxatives to produce soft stools. Local pain and infection are managed with warm sitz baths and insertion of a soothing anal suppository 2 or 3 times daily. Benzocaine and similar types of anal ointments should be avoided so as not to sensitize the patient to these agents. Prolapsed or strangulated hemorrhoids may be treated conservatively by gentle reduction with the lubricated gloved fingers, the buttocks strapped, and the prone position maintained for a few days; or by immediate surgical resection.

For severe symptoms or complications, complete internal and external hemorrhoidectomy is advisable and is a highly satisfactory procedure when properly done. Excision of a single external hemorrhoid, evacuation of a thrombosed pile, and the injection treatment of internal hemorrhoids fall within the scope of office practice. Injection therapy is effective, but there is a recurrence rate of more than 50%.

Evacuation of Thrombosed External Hemorrhoid

This condition is caused by the rupture of a vein at the anal margin, forming a clot in the subcutaneous tissue. The patient complains of a painful lump, and examination shows a tense, tender, bluish mass covered with skin. If seen after 24–48 hours when the pain is subsiding–or if symptoms are minimal–hot sitz baths are prescribed. If discomfort is marked, removal of the clot is indicated. With the patient in the lateral position, the area is prepared with antiseptic and 1% procaine or lidocaine is injected intracutaneously around and over the lump. A radial ellipse of skin is then excised and the clot evacuated. A dry gauze dressing is held in place for 12–24 hours by taping the buttocks together, and daily sitz baths are then begun.

Parks AG: Hemorrhoidectomy. Advances Surg 5:1, 1971.

Rowe RJ: Symposium: Management of hemorrhoidal disease. Dis Colon Rectum 11:127, 1968.

CRYPTITIS & PAPILLITIS

Anal pain and burning of brief duration with defecation is suggestive of cryptitis and papillitis. Digital and anoscopic examination reveals hypertrophied papillae and indurated or inflamed crypts. Treatment consists of mineral oil by mouth, sitz baths, anal suppository after each bowel movement, and local application of 5% phenol in oil or carbolfuchsin compound to the crypts. If these measures fail, surgical excision of involved crypts and papillae should be considered.

Hirschman LJ, Nigro ND, Burke RM: The scope of office proctology: Cryptitis and papillitis. S Clin North America 35:1506, 1955.

FISSURE-IN-ANO
(Anal Fissure)

Acute fissures represent linear disruption of the anal epithelium due to various causes. They usually clear if bowel movements are kept regular and soft (eg, with mineral oil). The local application of a mild styptic such as 1–2% silver nitrate or 1% gentian violet solution may be of value.

Chronic fissure is characterized by (1) acute pain during and after defecation; (2) spotting of bright red blood at stool with occasional more abundant bleeding; (3) tendency to constipation through fear of pain; and (4) the late occurrence of a sentinel pile, a hypertrophied papilla, and spasm of the anal canal (usually very painful on digital examination). Regulation of bowel habits with mineral oil or other stool softeners, sitz baths, and anal suppositories (eg, Anusol), twice daily, should be tried. If these measures fail, the fissure, sentinel pile, or papilla and the adjacent crypt must be excised surgically. Postoperative care is along the lines of the preoperative treatment.

Alexander RM, Manheim SD: Anal fissures in infants and children. Am J Dis Child 96:29, 1958.
Hayden EP: Proctology. New England J Med 260:420, 1959.

ANAL ABSCESS

Perianal abscess should be considered the acute stage of an anal fistula until proved otherwise. The abscess should be adequately drained as soon as localized. Hot sitz baths may hasten the process of localization. The patient should be warned that after drainage of the abscess he may have a persistent fistula. It is painful and fruitless to search for the internal opening of a fistula in the presence of acute infection. The presence of an anal abscess should alert the clinician to the possibility of inflammatory bowel disease.

FISTULA-IN-ANO

About 95% of all anal fistulas arise in an anal crypt, and they are often preceded by an anal abscess. If an anal fistula enters the rectum above the pectinate line and there is no associated disease in the crypts, ulcerative colitis, regional ileitis, rectal tuberculosis, lymphogranuloma venereum, cancer, or foreign body should be considered in the differential diagnosis.

Acute fistula is associated with a purulent discharge from the fistulous opening. There is usually local itching, tenderness, or pain aggravated by bowel movements. Recurrent anal abscess may develop. The involved crypt can occasionally be located anoscopi-

cally with a crypt hook. Probing the fistula should be gentle because false passages can be made with ease, and in any case demonstration of the internal opening by probing is not essential to the diagnosis.

Treatment is by surgical incision or excision of the fistula under general anesthesia. If a fistula passes deep to the entire anorectal ring so that all the muscles must be divided in order to extirpate the tract, a 2-stage operation must be done to prevent incontinence.

Jackman RJ: Anorectal fistulas: Current concepts. Dis Colon Rectum 11:247, 1968.

ANAL CONDYLOMAS

These wart-like papillomas of the perianal skin and anal canal flourish on moist, macerated surfaces, particularly in the presence of purulent discharge. They are not true tumors but are infectious and autoinoculable, probably due to a virus. They must be distinguished from condyloma lata caused by syphilis. The diagnosis of the latter rests on the positive serologic test for syphilis or the discovery of *Treponema pallidum* on dark-field examination.

Treatment consists of accurate application of 25% podophyllin in tincture of benzoin to the lesion (with bare wooden or cotton-tipped applicator sticks to avoid contact with uninvolved skin). Condylomas in the anal canal are treated through the anoscope and the painted site dusted with powder to localize the application and minimize discomfort. Electrofulguration under local anesthesia is useful if there are numerous lesions. Local cleanliness and the frequent use of a talc dusting powder are essential.

Condylomas tend to recur. The patient should be observed for several months and advised to report promptly if new lesions appear.

Shah IC, Hertz RE: Giant condylomata of the anorectum: Report of two cases. Dis Colon Rectum 15:207, 1972.
Swerdlow DB, Salvati EP: Condyloma acuminatum. Dis Colon Rectum 14:226, 1971.

BENIGN ANORECTAL STRICTURES

Congenital

Anal contracture or stenosis in infancy may result from failure of disintegration of the anal plate in fetal life. The narrowing is treated by careful repeated dilatation, inserting progressively larger Hegar dilators until the anus admits first the little and then the index finger.

Traumatic

Acquired stenosis is usually the result of surgery

or trauma which denudes the epithelium of the anal canal. Hemorrhoid operations in which too much skin is removed or which are followed by infection are the commonest cause. Constipation, ribbon stools, and pain on defecation are the most frequent complaints. Stenosis predisposes to fissure, low-grade infection, and occasionally fistula.

Prevention of stenosis after radical anal surgery is best accomplished by local cleanliness, hot sitz baths, and gentle insertion of the well-lubricated finger twice weekly for 2–3 weeks beginning 2 weeks after surgery. When stenosis is chronic but mild, graduated anal dilators of increasing size may be inserted daily by the patient. For marked stenosis a plastic operation on the anal canal is advisable.

Inflammatory

A. Lymphogranuloma Venereum: This infectious disease is the commonest cause of inflammatory stricture of the anorectal region. Acute proctitis due to lymphatic spread of the organism occurs early, and may be followed by perirectal infections, sinuses, and formation of scar tissue (resulting in stricture). Frei and complement fixation tests are positive.

The tetracycline drugs are curative in the initial phase of the disease. When extensive chronic secondary infection is present or when a stricture has formed, repeated biopsies are essential because epidermoid carcinoma develops in about 4% of strictures. Local operation on a stricture may be feasible, but a colostomy or an abdominoperineal resection is often required.

B. Granuloma Inguinale: This disease may cause anorectal fistulas, infections, and strictures. The Donovan body is best identified in tissue biopsy when there is rectal involvement. Epidermoid carcinoma develops in about 4% of cases with chronic anorectal granuloma.

The early lesions respond to tetracyclines. Destructive or constricting processes may require colostomy or resection.

Holder WR, Duncan WC: Lymphogranuloma venereum. Clin Obst Gynec 15:1004, 1972.
Samenius B, Hansson HPJ: Venereal diseases of the anorectum. Mod Treat 8:875, 1971.
Santulli TV, Schulinger LN, Amoury RA: Malformations of the anus and rectum. S Clin North America 45:1253, 1965.

ANAL INCONTINENCE

Obstetric tears, anorectal operations (particularly fistulotomy), and neurologic disturbances are the most frequent causes of anal incontinence. When incontinence is due to surgery or trauma, surgical repair of the divided or torn sphincter is indicated. Repair of anterior laceration due to childbirth should be delayed for 6 months or more after parturition.

Duthie HL: Progress report: Anal continence. Gut 12:844, 1971.

SQUAMOUS CELL CARCINOMA OF THE ANUS

These tumors are relatively rare, comprising only 1–2% of all malignancies of the anus and large intestine. Bleeding, pain, and local tumor are the commonest symptoms. Because the lesion is often confused with hemorrhoids or other common anal disorders, immediate biopsy of any suspicious lesion or mass in the anal area is essential. These tumors tend to become annular, invade the sphincter, and spread upward into the rectum.

Except for very small lesions (which can be adequately excised locally), treatment is by combined abdominoperineal resection. Radiation therapy is reserved for palliation and for patients who refuse or cannot withstand operation. Metastases to the inguinal nodes are treated by radical groin dissection when clinically evident. The 5-year survival rate after resection is about 50%.

Hickey RC & others: Anal cancer with special reference to the cloacogenic variety. S Clin North America 52:943, 1972.
Khier S & others: Cloacogenic carcinoma of the anal canal. Arch Surg 104:407, 1972.
Sawyers JL: Squamous cell cancer of the perianus and anus. S Clin North America 52:935, 1972.

DISEASES OF THE LIVER & BILIARY TRACT

JAUNDICE

Classification

A. **Prehepatic (Hemolytic):**

1. **Intramedullary**—"Shunt" hyperbilirubinemia.

2. **Extramedullary**—Hemolysis due to drugs, infections, etc.

B. **Hepatic:**

1. **Congenital**—

a. **Indirect (unconjugated) hyperbilirubinemia**—Constitutional hepatic dysfunction (Gilbert's disease), glucuronyl transferase deficiency.

b. **Direct (conjugated) hyperbilirubinemia**—Dubin-Johnson-Sprinz-Nelson syndrome, benign intermittent cholestasis, intermittent jaundice of pregnancy.

2. **Acquired**—

a. **Cholestatic**—

(1) Due to drugs, eg, chlorpromazine, methyltestosterone.

(2) Due to infection—Viral hepatitis, infectious mononucleosis.

b. Noncholestatic—

(1) Due to drugs—Halothane (Fluothane), isoniazid.

(2) Due to infection—Viral, spirochetal.

C. Posthepatic: Extrahepatic obstruction.

1. Intermittent, eg, choledocholithiasis, carcinoma of ampulla of Vater.

2. Complete, eg, carcinoma of head of pancreas.

Manifestations of Diseases Associated With Jaundice

A. Prehepatic: Hemolysis, weakness. Abdominal or back pain may occur with acute hemolytic crises. Normal stool and urine color. Jaundice. Splenomegaly, except in sickle cell anemia. Hepatomegaly is variable.

B. Hepatic:

1. **Acquired—**Malaise, anorexia, low-grade fever, right upper quadrant discomfort. Dark urine, jaundice, amenorrhea. Enlarged, tender liver, vascular spiders, palmar erythema, ascites, gynecomastia, sparse body hair, fetor hepaticus, asterixis.

2. **Congenital—**May be asymptomatic; the intermittent cholestasis is often accompanied by pruritus, light-colored stools, and occasionally malaise.

C. Posthepatic: Colicky right upper quadrant pain, weight loss (carcinoma), jaundice, dark urine, light-colored stools. Fluctuating jaundice and intermittently colored stools indicate intermittent obstruction due to stone or to carcinoma of the ampulla or junction of the intrahepatic ducts. Blood in stools suggests malignancy. Hepatomegaly, visible and palpable gallbladder (Courvoisier's sign), ascites, rectal (Blumer's) shelf, and weight loss indicate malignancy. Chills and fever suggest stone with cholangitis.

SGOT and SGPT are invaluable in the assessment of liver disease. However, their diagnostic usefulness is enhanced when combined with complementary studies such as alkaline phosphatase, lactate dehydrogenase, and their isoenzymes and serum immunoglobulins.

Percutaneous liver biopsy is a safe and accurate way of diagnosing diffuse hepatic disease. It is of less value in differentiating intrahepatic from extrahepatic cholestasis, and is only occasionally successful in defining liver metastases.

Liver scans using ^{99m}Tc sulfur colloid may be of value in detecting space-occupying lesions of the liver (tumors, abscesses, or cysts) and for demonstrating the extent of hepatic enlargement.

Clermont RJ, Chalmers TC: The transaminase tests in liver disease. Medicine 46:197, 1967.

Harris RC: Current thoughts on bilirubin problems. Present Concepts Int Med 2:37, 1969.

Lester R, Troxler RF: Recent advances in bile pigment metabolism. Gastroenterology 56:143, 1969.

Lorenzo GA, Beal JM: Recent diagnostic advances in obstructive jaundice. S Clin North America 51:211, 1971.

Lucey J & others: Prevention of hyperbilirubinemia of prematurity by phototherapy. Pediatrics 41:1047, 1968.

Schimmel EM: Diagnostic procedures in liver disease. M Clin North America 52:1407, 1968.

Table 10–2. Liver function tests: Normal values and changes in 2 types of jaundice.

Tests	Normal Values	Hepatocellular Jaundice	Uncomplicated Obstructive Jaundice
Bilirubin			
Direct	0.1–0.4 mg/100 ml	Increased	Increased
Indirect	0.2–0.7 mg/100 ml	Increased	Increased
Urine bilirubin	None	Increased	Increased
Urine urobilinogen	0–4 mg/24 hours	Increased	Markedly decreased in complete obstruction
Stool urobilinogen	40–280 mg/24 hours	Unchanged or lowered	Decreased
Protein electrophoresis (gm/100 ml)	Albumin, 3.3–6.5 Alpha$_1$ globulin, 0.04–0.41 Alpha$_2$ globulin, 0.3–0.9 Beta globulin, 0.7–1.5 Gamma globulin, 0.3–1.4 Total protein, 6.5–8.4	Albumin decreased	Unchanged
Alkaline phosphatase	2–4.5 Bodansky units	Increased (++)	Increased (++++)
Cholesterol			
Total	100–250 mg/100 ml	Decreased if damage severe	Increased
Esters	60–70% of total	Decreased if damage severe	Normal
Prothrombin time	40–100%. After vitamin K, 15% increase in 24 hours.	Prolonged if damage severe	Prolonged if obstruction marked
SGPT, SGOT	SGPT, 5–35 units SGOT, 5–40 units	Increased in hepatocellular damage, viral hepatitis	Usually unchanged, may be increased

Trujillo NP: The isoenzymes of LDH in pulmonary embolism, hepatic disease, postoperative state and other conditions. Arch Int Med 119:333, 1967.

Wieme RJ: Lactic dehydrogenase in hepatic injury. Ann New York Acad Sc 94:898, 1961.

Zimmerman HJ: The differential diagnosis of jaundice. M Clin North America 52:1417, 1968.

VIRAL HEPATITIS
("Infectious," Short Incubation Period, Hepatitis A; "Serum," Long Incubation Period, Hepatitis B)

Essentials of Diagnosis

- Anorexia, nausea, vomiting, malaise, symptoms of upper respiratory throat infection or "flu"-like syndrome, aversion to smoking.
- Fever; enlarged, tender liver; jaundice.
- Normal to low white cell count; abnormal hepatocellular liver function tests.
- Liver biopsy shows characteristic hepatocellular necrosis and mononuclear infiltrate.

General Considerations

"Infectious" hepatitis (hepatitis A, short incubation period hepatitis) is a viral infection of the liver which may occur sporadically or in epidemics. The liver involvement is part of a generalized infection but dominates the clinical picture. Transmission of the virus is usually by the fecal-oral route. Stools from patients with type A hepatitis have been shown to contain particles 27 nm in diameter. Marmoset monkeys and chimpanzees appear to be the only susceptible animals, and livers of infected marmoset monkeys have been shown to contain the 27 nm particles. In infected volunteers, virus particles appear in the stools 5 days prior to elevation of the serum transaminase. The viral particles disappear from the stools when the serum transaminase levels are at their highest. This is consistent with the clinical impression that the disease becomes noninfective as it becomes overt.

Antibodies to type A hepatitis appear early in the course of the illness and tend to persist in the serum. Volunteers infected with type A hepatitis could not be reinfected.

The viral agent of hepatitis A has been characterized as an RNA virus inactivated by ultraviolet light, by heating to 100° C (212° F) for 5 minutes, and by exposure to formalin solution 1:4000.

"Serum" hepatitis (hepatitis B, long incubation period hepatitis) is a viral infection of the liver usually transmitted by inoculation of infected blood or blood products. However, since it has been estimated that 5–10% of infected individuals become carriers, a substantial reservoir of infection exists, and transmission by shared objects such as razors or toothbrushes is possible. Sexual transmission is increasingly being recognized, and type B hepatitis is an important venereal

disease. Forty to 70% of infants born to $HB_s Ag$-positive mothers will develop antigens to hepatitis B in the blood stream. Fecal-oral transmission of virus B has also been documented.

The large Dane particle probably represents the complete virion. This particle consists of a core in the nucleus of the liver cell and double-shelled surface particles formed in the cytoplasm. The surface antigen is the antigen routinely measured in blood ($HB_s Ag$). In acute infection, the core antibody ($HB_c Ab$) rises shortly after the $HB_s Ag$ is detected and tends to persist. $HB_s Ab$ appears later in the course of the disease. $HB_c Ab$ is unusual in a blood donor population but is usually constant in carriers of $HB_s Ag$. When more readily available, $HB_c Ab$ may prove useful in screening donors when the $HB_s Ag$ is negative.

The incubation period of type B viral hepatitis is 6 weeks to 6 months. The histologic findings are identical to those of type A viral hepatitis. The clinical features are also similar; however, the onset in type B hepatitis tends to be more insidious. (See Table 10–3.)

The histologic findings in both diseases are those of varying degrees of necrosis of the liver parenchymal cells and variable numbers of lymphocytes and plasma cells in the portal areas and in areas of necrosis. The reticulum framework is well preserved, although there may be varying degrees of collapse if the insult is too severe. Healing occurs by regeneration from surviving cells—usually without distortion of the normal architecture.

Clinical Findings

The clinical picture is extremely variable, ranging from asymptomatic infection without jaundice to a fulminating disease and death in a few days.

A. Symptoms:

1. Prodromal phase—The speed of onset varies from abrupt to insidious with general malaise, myalgia, arthralgia, easy fatigability, upper respiratory symptoms (nasal discharge, pharyngitis), and severe anorexia out of proportion to the degree of illness. Nausea and vomiting are frequent, and diarrhea or constipation may occur. Fever is generally present but is rarely over

Table 10–3. Differentiating features of infectious hepatitis and serum hepatitis.

	Hepatitis A ("Infectious")	Hepatitis B ("Serum")
Incubation period	Relatively short (30–40 days)	Relatively long (41–180 days)
Onset	Acute	Insidious
Urticarial rash, arthralgias	Usually absent	Often present
Abnormal transaminase activity	Brief (30 days)	Prolonged (35–200 days)
Hepatitis-associated antigen ($HB_s Ag$)	Not present*	Present ($HB_s Ag$)

*Absence of $HB_s Ag$ does not imply that the diagnosis is hepatitis A.

39.5° C (103.1° F). Defervescence often coincides with the onset of jaundice. Chills or chilliness may mark an acute onset.

Abdominal pain is usually mild and constant in the upper right quadrant or right epigastrium and is often aggravated by jarring or exertion. (On rare occasions, upper abdominal pain may be severe enough to simulate cholecystitis or cholelithiasis.) A distaste for smoking, paralleling anorexia, may occur early.

2. Icteric phase—Clinical jaundice occurs after 5–10 days but may appear at the same time as the initial symptomatology. Some patients never develop clinical icterus. With the onset of jaundice, there is often an intensification of the prodromal symptoms, followed by progressive clinical improvement.

3. Convalescent phase—There is an increasing sense of well-being, return of appetite, and disappearance of jaundice, abdominal pain and tenderness, and fatigability.

B. Signs: Hepatomegaly—rarely marked—is present in over half of cases. Liver tenderness is usually present. Splenomegaly is reported in 15% of patients, and soft, enlarged lymph nodes—especially in the cervical or epitrochlear areas—may occur. Signs of general toxemia vary from minimal to severe.

C. Laboratory Findings: The white cell count is normal to low. (Abnormal or "atypical" lymphocytes may suggest the presence of infectious mononucleosis. A positive "mono spot" test lends additional support to that diagnosis.) Mild proteinuria is common, and bilirubinuria often precedes the appearance of jaundice. Acholic stools are often present during the initial icteric phase. Liver function tests tend to reflect hepatocellular damage, with abnormal SGOT, SGPT, and LDH values, increased gamma globulin, and urobilinogenuria. In the cholangiolitic variety, the alkaline phosphatase is significantly elevated. HB_sAg may be positive in hepatitis B.

Liver biopsy usually shows the characteristic pathologic picture.

Differential Diagnosis

It is necessary to differentiate viral hepatitis from other diseases that cause hepatitis or involve the liver such as leptospirosis (Weil's disease), amebiasis, cirrhosis, infectious mononucleosis, and toxic hepatitis. The prodromal phase or the nonicteric form of the disease must be distinguished from other infectious diseases such as influenza, upper respiratory infections, and the prodromal stages of the exanthematous diseases. In the obstructive phase of viral hepatitis, it is necessary to rule out other obstructive lesions such as choledocholithiasis, chlorpromazine toxicity, and carcinoma of the head of the pancreas. Determination of HB_sAg may help in differentiating the 2 types of viral hepatitis since they are clinically indistinguishable.

Prevention

Strict isolation of patients is not necessary, but thorough handwashing by medical attendants who come into contact with contaminated utensils, bedding, or clothing is essential. Disinfection of feces is not necessary when water-borne sewage is available. Hepatitis B is for the most part transmitted by the parenteral route, but the possibility of fecal-oral infection as well as venereal dissemination must be considered. Screening by means of HB_sAg and SGOT determinations can remove potentially infectious individuals from blood donor lists. Unfortunately, there is increasing evidence that other viruses are responsible for similar clinical states. In blood donors, routine screening for HB_sAg has reduced the incidence of posttransfusion hepatitis by 25%. In the USA the avoidance of unnecessary transfusions and the exclusion of commercially obtained blood along with clinical studies of the donor as well as the HB_sAg and serum transaminase determinations may be helpful in excluding potential sources of infectious blood. It may enable the detection of one-third of infected donors. The use of disposable needles and syringes protects medical attendants as well as other patients. Gamma globulin should be routinely given to all persons who have been exposed to patients with infectious hepatitis. An arbitrary dose of 5 ml for an adult has been found to be protective for hepatitis A if administered during the incubation period. It is also desirable that individuals traveling or residing in endemic regions receive gamma globulin

Table 10–4. Comparison of various features in different forms of liver injury.

	Poison	Alcohol	Drug Idiosyncrasy	Virus A	Virus B
Incubation	1–3 days	Years	2–4 weeks	4 ± 1 week	10 ± 4 weeks
Onset	Abrupt	Often complications	Abrupt	Abrupt	May be less abrupt
Early symptoms	Coma	Fever, ascites	Fever, pain	Gastroenteritis, flu-like	Rash, arthralgias, fever
Laboratory	SGOT > SGPT BUN elevated	SGOT > SGPT Cholesterol elevated	SGPT > SGOT Delayed hypersensitivity	SGPT > SGOT	SGPT > SGOT HB_sAg-positive
Pathology	Central necrosis	Fat and Mallory bodies	Spotty or massive necrosis	Spotty necrosis	Spotty or massive necrosis
Chronicity	No	Yes	Some drugs	Usually no	Yes

within 2 weeks after having arrived in those areas. In the event of prolonged residence, a second dose should be given 5–6 months after the first.

Treatment

A. General Measures: Bed rest should be at the patient's option during the acute initial phase of the disease when he is most symptomatic. Bed rest beyond the most acute phase is not warranted. However, return to normal activity during the convalescent period should be gradual. If nausea and vomiting are significant problems or when oral intake is substantially decreased, the intravenous administration of 10% glucose solution is indicated. If the patient shows signs of impending coma, protein should be temporarily interdicted and gradually reintroduced and increased as clinical improvement takes place. In general, dietary management consists of giving palatable meals as tolerated without overfeeding. Patients with infectious hepatitis should avoid strenuous physical exertion, alcohol, and hepatotoxic agents. While the administration of small doses of barbiturates is safe, it is traditionally recommended that morphine sulfate be avoided.

B. Corticotropin and Corticosteroids: These agents are recommended only in the presence of fulminant hepatitis. They should not be given in the routine and uncomplicated case of viral hepatitis.

Prognosis

In most cases of infectious hepatitis, clinical recovery is complete in 3–16 weeks. Laboratory evidence of disturbed liver function may persist for a longer period, but the bulk of such patients usually go on to complete recovery. Overall mortality is less than 1%, but is reportedly higher in older individuals (particularly in postmenopausal women). Cirrhosis of the postnecrotic or macronodular type and chronic active (aggressive) hepatitis are infrequent.

Hepatitis tends to be more severe and potentially has a poorer prognosis in the elderly or in those with other complicating illnesses. Posttransfusion hepatitis occurs as a complication in 0.25–3% of blood transfusions and as many as 12% of pooled plasma transfusions. The asymptomatic carrier state and persistent viremia after acute disease make control of contamination in donor blood extremely difficult.

Del Prete S & others: Detection of a new serum antigen in three epidemics of short incubation hepatitis. Lancet 2:579, 1970.

Feinman SV & others: Clinical and epidemiological significance of the HB$_S$Ag (Australia antigen) carrier state. Gastroenterology 68:113, 1975.

Feinstone SM & others: Transfusion associated hepatitis not due to viral hepatitis type A or B. New England J Med 292:767, 1975.

Krugman S, Giles JP: Viral hepatitis: New light on an old disease. JAMA 212:1019, 1970.

Lewis TL & others: Hepatitis-B antigen and antibody in hospital personnel. New England J Med 289:647, 1973.

McCollum RW: The natural history of hepatitis. Bull New York Acad Med 45:127, 1969.

Sabesin SM, Koff RS: Pathogenesis of experimental viral hepatitis. (2 parts.) New England J Med 290:944, 996, 1974.

Shulman NR & others: Viral hepatitis. Ann Int Med 72:257, 1970.

Sutnick AI: Australia antigen: Progress report. M Clin North America 57:1029, 1973.

Virus hepatitis updated. (Editorial.) Lancet 1:1365, 1975.

VARIANTS OF INFECTIOUS HEPATITIS

Cholangiolitic Hepatitis

There is usually a cholestatic phase in the initial icteric phase of infectious hepatitis, but in occasional cases this is the dominant manifestation of the disease. The course tends to be more prolonged than that of ordinary hepatitis. The symptoms are often extremely mild, but jaundice is deeper and pruritus is often present. Laboratory tests of liver function indicate cholestasis with hyperbilirubinemia, biliuria, and elevated alkaline phosphatase and cholesterol.

Differentiation from extrahepatic obstruction may be difficult even with liver biopsy. Liver biopsy itself should be undertaken with considerable caution in the presence of extrahepatic biliary obstruction.

Gall EA, Braunstein H: Hepatitis with manifestations simulating bile duct obstruction (so-called "cholangiolitic hepatitis"). Am J Clin Path 25:1113, 1955.

Fulminant Hepatitis

Hepatitis may take a rapidly progressive course terminating in less than 10 days. Extensive necrosis of large areas of the liver gives the typical pathologic picture of acute liver atrophy. Toxemia and gastrointestinal symptoms are more severe, and hemorrhagic phenomena are common. Neurologic symptoms of hepatic coma develop (see Nodular Cirrhosis, p 381). Jaundice may be absent or minimal, but laboratory tests show extreme hepatocellular damage.

The use of corticosteroids is inconstantly effective in management. Exchange transfusions have also been advocated in fulminant hepatitis. Although the hepatic coma may be transiently improved, the prognosis in this form of the disease is apparently unaffected. Since patients die in and not from hepatic coma, the procedure is not generally recommended.

Davis M & others: Appraisal of the mortality in acute fulminant viral hepatitis. New England J Med 278:1248, 1968.

Katz R & others: Corticosteroids in the treatment of acute hepatitis in coma. Gastroenterology 42:250, 1962.

Trey C & others: Treatment of hepatic coma by exchange blood transfusion. New England J Med 274:473, 1966.

Turcotte JA & others: Experimental hepatic coma: Effect of exchange transfusion on metabolism and survival. Surgery 62:189, 1967.

CHRONIC HEPATITIS

Chronic hepatitis is defined as a chronic inflammatory reaction in the liver as demonstrated by (1) abnormal liver function tests, (2) abnormal liver histology, and (3) persistent illness without improvement for at least 6 months. From the point of view of patient care, the crucial factor to be determined is whether the chronic hepatitis will resolve, remain static, or progress to cirrhosis. The cause of chronic hepatitis is only partially defined. Chronic hepatitis may be associated with HB_sAg in the serum and may be considered a sequela of this infection. Type A virus may also be responsible. Additionally, identical clinical entities may be associated with drug reactions, including oxyphenisatin, methyldopa, and isoniazid. Wilson's disease can also present as chronic liver disease, and a_1 antitrypsin deficiency is also associated with chronic liver disease.

1. CHRONIC PERSISTENT HEPATITIS

This form of chronic hepatitis represents an essentially benign condition with a good prognosis. The diagnosis is confirmed by liver biopsy. The biopsy may show either mild hepatitis or portal zone infiltration with primarily mononuclear and plasma cells. The borderline between portal tracts and parenchyma remains sharp, and there is little or no "piecemeal necrosis" (a process in which the liver cells are gradually destroyed and replaced by fibrous tissue septa). In essence, the architecture of the hepatic lobule remains intact. The symptomatology varies from the asymptomatic state to various vague manifestations including fatigability, anorexia, malaise, and lassitude. The diagnosis may also be suspected when liver function studies remain abnormal or if HB_sAg persists. Physical examination is usually normal.

After careful study—including liver biopsy—establishes the diagnosis of persistent hepatitis, the treatment is principally that of reassurance. Corticosteroids and immunosuppressive drugs should not be given. Dietary restrictions, excessive vitamin supplementation, and prolonged bed rest are not necessary. The prognosis is excellent. Rarely does the disease progress to chronic active hepatitis.

2. CHRONIC ACTIVE HEPATITIS

This form of chronic hepatitis is usually characterized by progression to cirrhosis, although milder cases may resolve spontaneously. The histologic changes include chronic inflammatory infiltration involving portal zones and extending into the parenchyma, with piecemeal necrosis and the formation of intralobular septa. The piecemeal necrosis transcends zonal boundaries extending from one lobule to another and from portal zone to central zone. The process is known as bridging. In severe cases, the piecemeal necrosis is severe enough to obscure the hepatic architecture completely, making it difficult if not impossible to exclude cirrhosis. In milder cases, it may be difficult to distinguish this entity from persistent hepatitis. Liver biopsies repeated at varying intervals may be necessary to make this distinction between persistent and active chronic hepatitis.

Clinical Findings

A. Symptoms and Signs:

1. Chronic active hepatitis (lupoid type)—This is generally a disease of young people, particularly young women. However, the disease can occur at any age. The onset is usually insidious, but about 25% of cases present as an acute attack of hepatitis. Although the serum bilirubin is usually increased, 20% of these patients have anicteric disease. Examination often reveals a healthy-appearing young woman, with multiple spider nevi, cutaneous striae, acne, and hirsutism. Amenorrhea may be a feature of this disease. Multisystem involvement, including kidneys, joints, lungs, bowel, and Coombs-positive hemolytic anemia are associated with this clinical entity.

2. Chronic active hepatitis (HB_sAg-positive type)—This type of hepatitis clinically resembles the lupoid type of disease. The histologic pictures of these 2 types of chronic active hepatitis are indistinguishable. The HB_sAg form of chronic active hepatitis appears to affect males predominantly. It may be noted as a continuum of acute hepatitis or be detected only by biochemical abnormalities of liver function. Serum smooth muscle antibody, if present, occurs in low titer; serum mitochondrial antibodies are absent; and lupus erythematosus cells are rarely found in this form of the disease.

B. Laboratory Findings: The serum bilirubin is usually only modestly increased (4.5–7 mg/100 ml); SGOT, SGPT, IgG, IgM, and gamma globulin are elevated. Serum albumin levels are usually decreased late in the course of the disease. Significant prolongation of the prothrombin time, with a tendency to bleed, may occur early in the course of the disease. Antinuclear and smooth muscle antibodies are positive 15–50% of the time. Latex fixation tests for rheumatoid arthritis and anticytoplasmic and immunofluorescent antimitochondrial antibodies are positive in 28–50% of patients. Hepatitis B antigen is not found in the blood of patients with classical "lupoid" hepatitis.

The activity of chronic active hepatitis can be defined practically and accurately in terms of objective criteria. Thus, the magnitudes of transaminase and gamma globulin elevations and the degree of hepatocellular necrosis are suitable means of defining activity and judging the response to treatment. Activity in chronic liver disease can be defined quantitatively quite readily by establishing arbitrary biochemical standards. For example, either a 10-fold increase in serum transaminase level or a 5-fold elevation of SGOT with a 2-fold increase in gamma globulin concentration constitutes "high-grade" activity.

A definite diagnosis of chronic active hepatitis may be difficult while the lobular changes of acute viral hepatitis are still present, since in the latter the edges of the portal tracts are usually not sharply defined. The terminal phase is that of stable postnecrotic cirrhosis arising from any cause. The intermediate phase is usually quite characteristic and consists of piecemeal necrosis, aggressive early fibrosis with isolation of cell groups, rosette formation, and marked mononuclear and plasma cell infiltration.

Differential Diagnosis

Chronic active hepatitis can be confused with 4 other chronic liver conditions: cholestatic viral hepatitis, persistent viral hepatitis, subacute hepatic necrosis, and postnecrotic cirrhosis of unknown cause. The differentiation is made on the basis of the clinical course, sequential laboratory testing, and liver biopsy. It may occasionally be difficult to distinguish persistent from active hepatitis, but repeated examination of the patient, persistence of normal albumin and gamma globulin levels, and absence of piecemeal necrosis and fibrosis in liver biopsy specimens make differentiation possible.

Treatment

Prolonged or enforced bed rest has not been shown to be beneficial. Activity should be modified according to the patient's symptoms. The diet should be well balanced, without specific limitations other than sodium or protein restrictions as dictated by water retention or encephalopathy.

Controlled trials of corticosteroids and immunosuppressive agents showed a decided reduction in the frequency of early deaths due to chronic active hepatitis. Prednisone has been shown to decrease the serum bilirubin, SGOT, and gamma globulin levels and to reduce the piecemeal necrosis in the liver biopsy. Prednisone or an equivalent drug is given initially in doses of 30 mg orally daily, with gradual reduction to the lowest maintenance level (usually 15–20 mg/day) that will control the symptomatology and reduce the abnormal liver function. If symptoms are not controlled, azathioprine (Imuran), 50–150 mg/day orally, is added. Azathioprine imposes a significant hazard of hyperbilirubinemia, thrombocytopenia, and leukopenia, and complete blood counts should be obtained at least weekly or more frequently as dictated by the hematologic picture. In general, the combination of prednisone, 10–15 mg/day, and azathioprine, 25–50 mg/day, enables therapeutic efficacy with a paucity of significant side-effects of both drugs. Corticosteroids alone or combined with immunosuppressive agents are not only helpful in ameliorating symptoms but also decrease short-term mortality and may perhaps even prolong life.

Prognosis

If chronic active hepatitis is divided into hepatic and cirrhotic phases, the total life expectancy without treatment is 3–5 years. The hepatic phase has few symptoms or signs, and is characterized primarily by variable biochemical aberrations. Fatigue, hepatomegaly, jaundice, splenomegaly, and marked derangement of laboratory tests occur in the intermediary phase. The cirrhotic stage (macronodular cirrhosis) is attended by the recognized complications of liver failure and portal hypertension. Finally, it is important to realize that chronic active hepatitis can progress within a few weeks or months from acute viral hepatitis to end-stage of cirrhosis.

Mistilis SP, Blackburn CRB: Active chronic hepatitis. Am J Med 48:484, 1970.

Sherlock S: *Chronic Hepatitis in Diseases of the Liver and Biliary System,* 5th ed. Blackwell, 1974.

Sherlock S: Progress report: Chronic hepatitis. Gut 15:581, 1974.

Soloway RD & others: Clinical, biochemical, and histological remission of severe chronic, active liver disease: A controlled study of treatments and early prognosis. Gastroenterology 63:820, 1972.

Summerskill WHJ: Chronic active liver disease reexamined: Prognosis hopeful. Gastroenterology 66:450, 1974.

ALCOHOLIC HEPATITIS

Alcoholic hepatitis is an acute or chronic inflammation of the liver that occurs as a result of parenchymal necrosis induced by alcohol abuse. Although a variety of terms were used in the past to describe this type of hepatitis in chronic alcoholics, the term alcoholic hepatitis is now regarded as the most appropriate one to describe this injury, which is currently accepted as the precursor of alcoholic cirrhosis.

While alcoholic hepatitis is often a reversible disease, it is the most common cause of cirrhosis in the USA. This is especially significant since cirrhosis ranks among the most common causes of death of adults in this country. Alcoholic hepatitis does not develop in all chronic heavy drinkers; the exact prevalence and incidence are not known but have been estimated to be about one-third. Women appear to be more susceptible than men.

Alcoholic hepatitis usually occurs after years of excessive drinking. Although it may not develop in many patients even after several decades of alcohol abuse, it can appear in a few individuals within a year. Over 80% of patients with alcoholic hepatitis were drinking 5 years or more before developing any symptoms that could be attributed to liver disease. In general, the longer the duration of drinking (10–15 or more years) and the larger the alcoholic consumption (more than 160 gm/day), the greater the probability of developing alcoholic hepatitis and cirrhosis. It is also important to realize that while drinking of large amounts of alcoholic beverages is essential for the development of alcoholic hepatitis, drunkenness is not. In drinking individuals, the rate of ethanol metabolism can be sufficiently high to permit the consumption of large quantities of spirits without raising their blood alcohol level over 80 mg/100 ml, the concentration at which the conventional breath analyzer begins to detect ethanol.

The roles of proteins, vitamins, and calories in the development of alcoholic hepatitis or in the progression of this lesion to cirrhosis are not understood.

Only liver biopsy can establish the diagnosis with certainty, since any of the manifestations of alcoholic hepatitis can be seen in other types of alcoholic liver disease such as fatty liver or cirrhosis.

Clinical Findings

A. Symptoms and Signs: Alcoholic hepatitis is usually seen after a recent period of heavy drinking. That history in addition to complaints of anorexia and nausea and the objective demonstration of hepatomegaly and jaundice strongly suggest the diagnosis. Abdominal pain and tenderness, splenomegaly, ascites, fever, and encephalopathy support the diagnosis. The clinical presentation of alcoholic hepatitis can vary from an essentially asymptomatic patient with an enlarged liver to a critically ill individual who dies quickly.

B. Laboratory Findings: Anemia is variable, to a large extent reflecting the socioeconomic status of the patient. Leukocytosis is common and is seen more frequently in patients with severe disease. Leukopenia is occasionally seen and disappears after cessation of drinking. About 10% of patients have thrombocytopenia.

SGOT is normal in 15–25% of patients; when increased, it is usually under 300 mU/ml. Values over 300 mU/ml imply increasing severity of the disease and correlate well with biopsy findings. Serum alkaline phosphatase is generally elevated, but rarely more than 3 times the normal value. Serum bilirubin is increased in 60–90% of patients, and when levels greater than 5 mg/100 ml are demonstrated it can be assumed that the process is severe. The serum albumin is depressed, and the gamma globulin is elevated in 50–75% of individuals with alcoholic hepatitis even in the absence of cirrhosis.

Liver biopsy is diagnostic.

C. Special Procedures: Scintiphotographic evaluation (liver scanning) using ^{99m}Tc sulfur colloid is nonspecific and nondiagnostic, revealing "patchy" hepatic uptake of the isotope and inferential evidence of splenomegaly.

Differential Diagnosis

Nausea, vomiting, abdominal pain, jaundice, fever, right upper abdominal tenderness, leukocytosis, and elevated serum alkaline phosphatase with concomitantly minimal to moderate elevation of the SGOT occur in both alcoholic hepatitis and diseases of the hepatobiliary tree such as cholecystitis and choleli-

thiasis. A history of chronic insobriety and recent debauch is helpful but far from conclusive. Percutaneous liver biopsy, if there is no contraindication, is the only reliable means of differentiation.

Complications

Clinical deterioration and worsening abdominal pain and tenderness may result in the unfortunate decision to perform celiotomy. The postoperative mortality rate of acutely ill patients with alcoholic hepatitis is far greater than that of those who are operated on for intra- or extrahepatic cholestasis.

Treatment

A. General Measures: During periods of anorexia, every effort should be made to provide sufficient amounts of carbohydrate and calories to reduce endogenous protein catabolism and gluconeogenesis. Although the clinical value of intravenous hyperalimentation has not been established, the judicious administration of parenteral fluids is most important. Caloric intake is gratifyingly improved by the use of palatable liquid formulas during the transitional period between totally intravenous alimentation and normal feeding. The administration of vitamins, particularly folic acid, is an important part of treatment, and is frequently associated with dramatic clinical improvement in patients with alcoholic liver disease.

B. Steroids: The use of corticosteroids in this disorder has been evaluated over a period of more than 20 years, with reports of sporadic success. However, recent carefully controlled studies have shown that these drugs exert no beneficial effect on the course of alcoholic hepatitis. Similar conclusions have been drawn after evaluation of the therapeutic effects of anabolic steroids.

Prognosis

A. Short-Term: The severity of liver injury, which can be ascertained clinically, biochemically, and histologically, enables valid speculation about prognosis. The presence of asterixis seems to be associated with an increased likelihood of death. Biochemically, it has been shown that when the prothrombin time is short enough to permit performance of liver biopsy without risk, the mortality rate is 7.1%, rising to 18% if there is progressive prolongation of that parameter during hospitalization. Individuals in whom the prothrombin time is so prolonged that liver biopsy cannot be attempted have a 42% mortality rate.

B. Long-Term: In the USA, the mortality rate over a 3-year period of persons who recover from acute alcoholic hepatitis is 10 times greater than that of average individuals of comparable age. The histologically severe form of the disease is associated with continued excessive mortality after 3 years, whereas the death rate is not increased after the same period in those whose liver biopsies show only mild alcoholic hepatitis.

The most important prognostic consideration is the indisputable fact that continued excessive drinking is associated with reduction of life expectancy in these individuals. The prognosis is indeed poor if the patient is unwilling to abstain from drinking or markedly decrease his use of alcohol.

Fung W & others: Differentiation between acute alcoholic hepatitis and acute infectious (viral) hepatitis. Am J Gastroenterol 59:221, 1973.

Gregory DH, Levi DF: The clinical-pathologic spectrum of alcoholic hepatitis. Am J Digest Dis 17:479, 1972.

Hardison WG & others: Prognosis in acute liver disease of the alcoholic patient. New England J Med 275:61, 1966.

Harinasuta U, Zimmerman HJ: Alcoholic steatonecrosis. Gastroenterology 60:1036, 1971.

Kramer K & others: Increasing mortality attributed to cirrhosis and fatty liver in Baltimore (1957–1966). Ann Int Med 69:273, 1968.

Rubin E, Lieber CS: Fatty liver, alcoholic hepatitis, and cirrhosis produced by alcohol in primates. New England J Med 290:128, 1974.

Tischner MW & others: Natural history of alcoholic hepatitis. 1. The acute disease. Am J Digest Dis 16:481, 1971.

UNCOMMON HYPERBILIRUBINEMIA STATES

1. CONSTITUTIONAL HEPATIC DYSFUNCTION (Gilbert's Syndrome)

This is a benign form of jaundice which must be distinguished from hemolytic disease and chronic hepatitis. The serum bilirubin is primarily in the unconjugated form, and the defect may be due to a deficiency of the bilirubin-conjugating liver enzyme, glucuronyl transferase. Increase in the degree of hyperbilirubinemia follows a 24- to 36-hour fast. Occasional demonstration of compensated hemolysis is possible with radioisotope technics. The remainder of the laboratory examination is normal. Physical examination and liver biopsy are unremarkable. The symptoms are usually of iatrogenic or psychoneurotic origin.

The prognosis is excellent.

Arias M & others: Chronic non-hemolytic unconjugated hyperbilirubinemia in Gilbert's syndrome. Am J Med 47:395, 1969.

Redeker A & others: The reciprocal relation between caloric intake and the degree of hyperbilirubinemia in Gilbert's syndrome. New England J Med 283:170, 1970.

2. CRIGLER-NAJJAR SYNDROME

This is a rare form of severe hereditary nonhemolytic jaundice, appearing shortly after birth. Total absence of the bilirubin-conjugating liver enzyme, glu-

curonyl transferase, results in the type I form of the syndrome, which always leads to kernicterus. A severe deficiency of glucuronyl transferase produces the type II form, which is a milder disease and may persist into adult life. Crigler-Najjar syndrome is the only one of the hyperbilirubinemic states that is due to absence of a specific enzyme. The administration of phenobarbital to patients with type II Crigler-Najjar syndrome is beneficial. There is no satisfactory treatment for the type I form of the disease.

Crigler JF, Najjar VA: Congenital familial nonhemolytic jaundice with kernicterus. Pediatrics 10:169, 1952.

Lars W: Congenital non-hemolytic jaundice. Acta paediat scandinav 56:552, 1967.

3. FAMILIAL CHRONIC IDIOPATHIC JAUNDICE (Dubin-Johnson-Sprinz-Nelson Syndrome)

This form of jaundice is believed to be due to a faulty excretory function of liver cells and is characterized by elevated serum bilirubin (conjugated form), elevated BSP (conjugated form), and normal alkaline phosphatase. The gallbladder does not visualize on oral cholecystograms, and the liver biopsy shows a coarsely granular pigment which is localized to the centrizonal areas. Grossly, the liver appears dark brown to black.

The prognosis is excellent.

Blanck C & others: Chronic idiopathic jaundice (Dubin-Johnson syndrome) in three sisters. Acta paediat scandinav 55:329, 1966.

Butt HR & others: Studies of chronic idiopathic jaundice (Dubin-Johnson syndrome). Gastroenterology 51:619, 1966.

4. ROTOR'S SYNDROME

This condition is similar to Dubin-Johnson-Sprinz-Nelson syndrome and, in fact, may be a variant of it. Pigmentation of the liver, however, does not occur in Rotor's syndrome, and the gallbladder is visualized on oral cholecystography.

Dubin IN: Rotor's syndrome and chronic idiopathic jaundice. Arch Int Med 110:823, 1962.

Peck OC & others: Familial jaundice with free and conjugated bilirubin in the serum and without liver pigmentation. Gastroenterology 39:625, 1960.

5. BENIGN INTERMITTENT CHOLESTASIS

The patient with intermittent cholestasis characteristically has prolonged periods of pruritus, jaun-

Table 10–5. Uncommon hyperbilirubinemic disorders.

	Nature of Defect	Type of Hyper-bilirubinemia	Clinical and Pathologic Characteristics
Constitutional hepatic dysfunction (Gilbert's syndrome)	Glucuronyl transferase deficiency	Unconjugated (indirect) bilirubin	Benign, asymptomatic hereditary jaundice. Hyperbilirubinemia increased by 24–36 hour fast. No treatment required. Prognosis excellent.
Crigler-Najjar syndrome			Severe, nonhemolytic hereditary jaundice of neonates of type I sustain CNS damage (kernictcrus). Milder cases (type II) may persist into adult life and may benefit from treatment with phenobarbital.
Familial chronic idiopathic jaundice (Dubin-Johnson syndrome)	Faulty excretory function of liver cells (hepatocytes)	Conjugated (direct) bilirubin	Benign, asymptomatic hereditary jaundice. BSP excretion impaired. Gallbladder does not visualize on oral cholecystography. Liver darkly pigmented on gross examination. Biopsy shows centrilobular brown pigment. Prognosis excellent.
Rotor's syndrome			Similar to Dubin-Johnson syndrome but liver is not pigmented and the gallbladder is visualized on oral cholecystography. Prognosis excellent.
Benign intermittent cholestasis	Cholestatic liver dysfunction	Unconjugated plus conjugated (total) bilirubin	Benign intermittent idiopathic jaundice, itching, and malaise. Onset in early life and may persist for lifetime. Alkaline phosphatase and BSP retention are increased. Cholestasis found on liver biopsy. (Biopsy is normal during remission.)
Recurrent jaundice of pregnancy			Benign cholestatic jaundice of unknown cause, usually occurring in the third trimester of pregnancy. Itching, gastrointestinal symptoms, and abnormal liver excretory function tests. Cholestasis noted on liver biopsy. Prognosis excellent, but recurrence with subsequent pregnancies is characteristic.

dice, and malaise. The cause is unknown. Typically, the serum bilirubin, alkaline phosphatase, and BSP retention are increased. The condition appears early in life and may persist throughout the patient's lifetime. Liver biopsy is positive for cholestasis. However, during remissions, there is no significant histologic abnormality.

Tygstrup N: Intermittent possibly familial intrahepatic cholestatic jaundice. Lancet 1:1171, 1960.

6. RECURRENT JAUNDICE OF PREGNANCY

This form of cholestatic liver dysfunction is manifested by the onset of pruritus and jaundice in the third trimester of pregnancy. In the milder forms, patients may experience only itching. Hepatic dysfunction clears rapidly after delivery, and the jaundice and pruritus usually abate within 2 weeks after confinement. The condition is benign but characteristically recurs with subsequent pregnancies. Liver biopsy reveals cholestasis. These women may have an increased tendency to cholestasis with hormonal agents employed to regulate ovulation.

Kreek MJ & others: Recurrent cholestatic jaundice of pregnancy with demonstrated estrogen sensitivity. Am J Med 43:795, 1967.

DRUG- & TOXIN-INDUCED LIVER DISEASE

The continuing synthesis, testing, and introduction of new drugs into clinical practice has resulted in an increase in toxic reactions of many types. Not infrequently, the site of the toxic reaction is the liver.

The diagnosis of drug-induced liver disease is not always easy, and in many instances the diagnosis is not made until long-term observation or repeated administration of an agent defines the relationship. Drug-induced liver disease can mimic infectious hepatitis or obstructive jaundice. The clinician must be aware of these reactions and carefully question the patient with respect to the use of various drugs before he can dismiss drug-induced liver disease as a possibility.

One percent of persons taking chlorpromazine for at least 1 week develop jaundice. In half of all people who take this drug for 1 month, BSP retention and elevation of the serum alkaline phosphatase occur. These statistics illustrate the extent of cholestatic drug jaundice as a problem in clinical practice. The phenothiazine tranquilizers are the most common offenders, but numerous drugs are implicated, including the arsenicals, thiazide diuretics, sulfonylureas, sulfonamides, testosterone, methimazole, chlortetracycline, nitrofurantoin, and nicotinic acid. Jaundice usually occurs within the first 4 weeks of therapy with the offending agent.

Illness begins with an acute prodrome similar to that of infectious hepatitis. Malaise, low-grade fever, nausea, and mild abdominal pain last for 4–5 days. Pruritus often precedes the jaundice. Anorexia is milder than in viral hepatitis. Jaundice with acholic stools and dark urine occur within 1 week of systemic symptoms. Pruritus becomes severe. Besides the jaundice, physical findings are sparse. There may be low-grade temperature elevation. The liver is only slightly enlarged and is usually not tender.

Laboratory results are those of obstructive jaundice. The bilirubin is mostly conjugated. The alkaline phosphatase is markedly elevated. SGOT and SGPT are seldom greater than 200 IU/ml. Peripheral eosinophilia is a differentiating feature but is only seen early, diminishing as jaundice deepens.

Liver biopsy reveals bile stasis in the Kupffer cells and canaliculi. Bile lakes are not seen, these being virtually diagnostic of extrahepatic obstruction. Focal necrosis may be seen. Portal zones show an increased cellular infiltrate with round cells predominating. Eosinophils may be seen early, decreasing in number as jaundice progresses, correlating with the peripheral eosinophilia.

Acute cholestatic drug jaundice appears to be an allergic or hypersensitivity phenomenon. The timing of the illness following initial exposure and the eosinophilia strongly support this concept. Since some individuals do not develop jaundice on reexposure and others have recovered without withdrawal of the offending drug, some doubt exists about the true mechanism. Icterus usually lasts 1–4 weeks, and complete recovery is the rule. However, on rare occasions, jaundice or liver function test abnormalities have persisted for as long as 18 months. A few patients have died, following initial use of the offending agent or when hepatotoxic drugs were reinstituted in susceptible patients.

No specific therapy, including corticosteroids, is effective. Cholestyramine is occasionally useful in controlling pruritus.

Hepatotoxic Group

A. Substances Which May Act Like Poisons: Some substances that lead to fatty metamorphosis and centrolobular necrosis are listed below.

Alcohol	Tetracyclines
Carbon tetrachloride	Stilbamidine and related
Chloroform	stilbenes
Heavy metals	Phosphorus

B. Drugs Producing a Picture Similar to That of Viral Hepatitis:

Cinchophen	Phenylacetylurea
Chloramphenicol	Phenylbutazone
Chlortetracycline	Pyrazinamide
Halothane	Streptomycin
Iproniazid	Sulfamethoxypyridazine
Isoniazid	Zoxazolamine

Cholestatic-Cholangiolitic Groups

The substances in this group, although unrelated structurally, cause a reaction resembling extrahepatic obstruction clinically, functionally, and occasionally histologically:

Arsenicals (organic)	Norethandrolone
Aminosalicylic acid	Para-aminobenzyl
Chlorpromazine	caffeine
Chlorpropamide	Phenindione
Chlorothiazide	Prochlorperazine
Ectylurea	Promazine
Erythromycin estolate	Sulfadiazine
Mepazine	Thiouracil
Methimazole	Toluenediamine
Methyltestosterone	

Liver Dysfunction Due to Oral Contraceptives (Cholestatic)

Abnormalities of liver function, including elevated transaminases, serum bilirubin, and BSP retention, have been reported with the use of oral contraceptive agents. Histologic changes have been demonstrated. Serum transaminase abnormalities may revert to normal with continuing therapy. Studies suggest that the hepatotoxic effect of oral contraceptives is due primarily to their progesterone content.

Bailey WC & others: Fatal hepatic necrosis in a woman receiving chemoprophylaxis with isoniazid. Am J Gastroenterol 59:512, 1973.

Conney AH: Drug metabolism and therapeutics. New England J Med 280:653, 1969.

Dujovne CA, Shoeman DW: Hepatotoxicity of laxatives. Clin Pharmacol Therap 13:602, 1972.

Kappas A: Studies in endocrine pharmacology. New England J Med 278:378, 1968.

Lewis M & others: Studies on the pathogenesis of tetracycline-induced fatty liver. Am J Digest Dis 12:429, 1967.

Ockner RK, Davidson CS: Hepatic effects of oral contraceptives. New England J Med 276:331, 1967.

Peters RL & others: Hepatic necrosis associated with halothane anesthesia. Am J Med 47:748, 1969.

Read AE & others: Effects of chlorpromazine in patients with hepatic disease. Brit MJ 3:497, 1969.

Recknagel RO: Carbon tetrachloride hepatotoxicity. Pharmacol Rev 19:145, 1967.

Zimmerman HJ: The spectrum of hepatotoxicity. Perspectives Biol Med 12:135, 1968.

FATTY LIVER

It was formerly believed that malnutrition rather than ethanol was responsible for steatosis (fatty metamorphosis) of the liver in the alcoholic. More recently, it has come to be agreed that the role of deficient nutrition in such individuals has been overemphasized. However, it cannot be ignored that inadequate diets—specifically, those deficient in choline, methionine, and dietary protein—can produce fatty liver (kwashiorkor) in children.

Other nonalcoholic causes of steatosis are starvation, obesity, diabetes mellitus, poisons (carbon tetrachloride and yellow phosphorus), endocrinopathies such as Cushing's syndrome, tetracycline toxicity, and, rarely, pregnancy.

Regardless of the cause, there are apparently at least 5 factors, acting in varying combinations, which are responsible for the accumulation of fat in the liver: (1) Increased mobilization of fatty acids from peripheral adipose depots; (2) decreased utilization or oxidation of fatty acids by the liver; (3) increased hepatic fatty acid synthesis; (4) increased esterification of fatty acids into triglycerides; and (5) decreased secretion or liberation of fat from the liver.

Percutaneous liver biopsy is diagnostic.

Treatment consists of removing or modifying the offending factor.

Kramer K & others: Increasing mortality attributed to cirrhosis and fatty liver in Baltimore (1957–1966). Ann Int Med 69:273, 1968.

Lieber CS, Spritz N: Effects of prolonged ethanol intake in man: Role of dietary, adipose and endogenously synthesized fatty acids in pathogenesis of alcoholic fatty liver. J Clin Invest 45:1400, 1966.

NODULAR CIRRHOSIS

The concept of cirrhosis that evolved during the past few decades includes only those cases in which hepatocellular injury leads to both fibrosis and nodular regeneration throughout the liver. These features delineate cirrhosis as a serious and irreversible disease which is characterized not only by variable degrees of hepatic cell dysfunction but also by portosystemic shunting and portal hypertension. Fibrosis alone, regardless of its severity, is excluded by the previous definition. Also excluded by definition are the earlier stages of chronic biliary obstruction and hemochromatosis, neither of which forms regenerating nodules until late.

An important part of this concept is the realization that the type of cirrhosis changes with the passage of time in any one patient. Terms such as "portal" and "postnecrotic" refer not so much to separate disease states with different causes as to stages in the evolution of cirrhosis.

Attempts to classify cirrhosis on the basis of cause or pathogenesis are usually unsuccessful when applied to individual patients. Such persons often represent end-stage cirrhosis, enabling only speculation about the evolutionary process. The use of a purely anatomic and descriptive categorization facilitates easier and more practical classification. One such classification which is currently employed divides cirrhosis into micronodular, mixed, and macronodular forms. It is important, however, to remember that these are stages of development rather than separate diseases.

(1) Micronodular cirrhosis is the form in which the regenerating nodules are no larger than the original lobules, ie, approximately 1 mm in diameter or less. This feature has been suggested as due to the persistence of the offending agent (alcohol), a substance that prevents regenerative growth.

(2) Macronodular cirrhosis is characterized by larger nodules, which can measure several centimeters in diameter. This form corresponds more or less to postnecrotic cirrhosis but does not necessarily follow episodes of massive necrosis and stromal collapse.

(3) Mixed macro- and micronodular cirrhosis points up the fact that the features of cirrhosis are highly variable and not always easy to classify. In any case, the configuration of the liver is determined by the mixture of liver cell death and regeneration as well as the deposition of fat, iron, and fibrosis.

Finally, it should be emphasized that there does exist a limited relationship between anatomic types and etiology as well as between anatomic types and prognosis. For example, alcoholics who continue to drink tend to have that form of cirrhosis which remains micronodular for long periods. The presence of fatty micronodular cirrhosis, although not an infallible criterion, is strongly suggestive of chronic alcoholism. On the other hand, liver cell carcinoma not uncommonly arises in macronodular rather than micronodular cirrhosis. Although speculative and subject to dispute, it is possible that this propensity to malignancy is related either to the increased regeneration in macronodular cirrhosis or to the longer period required for the process to develop.

Clinical Findings

A. Symptoms and Signs: Micronodular (Laennec's) cirrhosis may cause no symptoms for long periods, both at the onset and later in the course (compensated phase). The onset of symptoms may be insidious or, less often, abrupt. Weakness, fatigability, and weight loss are common. In advanced cirrhosis, anorexia is usually present and may be extreme, with associated nausea and occasional vomiting. Abdominal pain may be present and is related either to hepatic enlargement and stretching of Glisson's capsule or to the presence of ascites. Diarrhea is frequently present, but some patients are constipated. Menstrual abnormalities (usually amenorrhea), impotence, loss of libido, sterility, and painfully enlarged breasts in men (rare) may occur. Hematemesis is the presenting symptom in 15–25%.

In 70% of cases the liver is palpable, firm if not hard, and has a blunt edge. Skin manifestations consist of spider nevi (usually only on the upper half of the body), palmar erythema (mottled redness of the thenar and hypothenar eminences), telangiectases of exposed areas, and evidence of vitamin deficiencies (glossitis and cheilosis). Weight loss, wasting, and the appearance of chronic illness are present. Jaundice—usually not an initial sign—is mild at first, increasing in severity during the later stages of the disease. Ascites, pleural effusion, peripheral edema, and purpuric lesions are late findings. The precoma state (asterixis, tremor, dysarthrias, delirium, and drowsiness) and encephalopathy or coma also occur very late. Gynecomastia, pectoral and axillary alopecia, and testicular atrophy may be present. Fever is present in 35% of cases and may reflect the presence of alcoholic hepatitis. (Peritonitis, secondary to tuberculosis, pneumococci or *E coli* infection should also be considered in any cirrhotic patient who is febrile for a prolonged period without a readily demonstrable cause.) Splenomegaly is present in 35–50% of cases. The superficial veins of the abdomen and thorax are dilated and represent the intrahepatic obstruction to portal blood flow.

B. Laboratory Findings: Excluding increased BSP retention, laboratory abnormalities are either absent or minimal in latent or quiescent cirrhosis. Anemia is a frequent finding and represents, in the heavy drinker, direct suppression of erythropoiesis by alcohol as well as folate deficiency and insidious or overt blood loss from the gastrointestinal tract. The white count may be low, elevated, or normal, reflecting hypersplenism or infection. The sedimentation rate is nonspecifically increased. Coagulation abnormalities may be present as a result of failure of synthesis of clotting constituents in the liver. Proteinuria may be present, and oliguria is frequent in active or decompensated disease with ascites.

Liver function tests show primarily hepatocellular dysfunction, reflected by elevations of SGOT, LDH, alkaline phosphatase, and bilirubin. Serum albumin is low, whereas gamma globulin is increased.

Liver biopsy shows cirrhosis.

C. X-Ray Findings: Radiographic examinations may reveal the presence of esophageal or gastric varices if these vessels are sufficiently large.

D. Special Examinations: Esophagogastroscopy demonstrates or confirms the presence of varices and detects specific causes of bleeding in the esophagus, stomach, and proximal duodenum. Splenoportography and arteriography are complementary modalities. Hepatic scanning, using ^{99m}Tc sulfur colloid, is helpful in documentation of splenomegaly or intrahepatic lesions such as hepatoma. Peritoneoscopy is especially helpful in judging the type of cirrhosis present.

Differential Diagnosis

As previously noted, differentiation of one type of cirrhosis from another can be difficult. Actual visualization of the liver by peritoneoscopy, when correlated with biopsy results and the history, facilitates classification. Hemochromatosis may be associated with "bronzing" of the skin and diabetes mellitus. Special staining of liver biopsies will be positive for increased iron deposition in the hepatic parenchyma. Biliary cirrhosis tends to occur more frequently in women and is associated with significant elevation of the alkaline phosphatase as well as positive antimitochondrial antibodies.

Complications

Upper gastrointestinal tract bleeding may occur from varices, hemorrhagic gastritis, or gastroduodenal ulcers. Hemorrhage may be massive, resulting in fatal exsanguination or in portosystemic encephalopathy. Liver failure may also be precipitated by alcoholism, surgery, and infection. Carcinoma of the liver and portal vein thrombosis occur more frequently in patients with cirrhosis. Lowered resistance often leads to serious infections, particularly of the lungs.

Treatment

A. General Measures: The principles of treatment include abstinence from alcohol and adequate rest, especially during the acute phase. The diet should be palatable, with adequate calories and protein (75–100 gm/day) and, in the stage of fluid retention, sodium restriction. In the presence of hepatic precoma or coma, protein intake should be low or drastically reduced. Vitamin supplementation is desirable.

B. Special Problems:

1. Ascites and edema due to sodium retention, hypoproteinemia, and portal hypertension—Removal of ascites by paracentesis is usually not indicated unless it is critically important to relieve respiratory distress or patient discomfort becomes intolerable.

In many patients, there is a rapid diminution in ascites on dietary sodium restriction alone. In individuals who pose more significant problems of fluid retention and who are considered to have "intractable" ascites, the urinary excretion of sodium is less than 5 mEq/liter. Mechanisms which have been postulated to explain sodium retention in cirrhosis include impaired liver inactivation of aldosterone or hepatic production of a humoral stimulator of aldosterone secretion. If such persons are permitted unrestricted fluids, serum sodium progressively falls, representing dilution. By imposing a 200 mg sodium diet and 500 ml allowance of oral fluids per day, ascites production ceases and the patient's abdominal discomfort abates.

a. Restoration of plasma proteins—This is dependent upon improving liver function and serves as a practical index of recovery. The use of salt-poor albumin intravenously is expensive, and the benefits are negligible.

b. Diuretics—Spironolactone should be used after documentation of secondary aldosteronism, as evidenced by markedly low urinary sodium. Starting with spironolactone, 25 mg 4 times daily, and monitoring the aldosterone-antagonist effect, reflected by the urinary sodium-potassium ratio and the fact that sodium excretion exceeds sodium intake, the dose of spironolactone is increased 100 mg every 2—4 days (up to a daily dosage of 1000 mg) until the urinary sodium-potassium ratio is greater than 1. Diuresis commonly occurs at this point and may be augmented by the addition of a potent agent such as furosemide, a potent diuretic which poses the risk of maintaining its effect even in the face of falling glomerular filtration rate (GFR) with resultant severe renal damage. The dose of furosemide ranges from 80—120 mg/day, and the drug should be administered with careful monitoring of serum electrolytes.

Ethacrynic acid, 50 mg orally every 2—3 days and increasing to a maximum daily dose of 150—200 mg (if necessary), may be employed if sodium restriction and thiazides have proved ineffective.

Both furosemide and ethacrynic acid should be used only in the hospitalized patient. They are potentially hazardous because of their potency.

2. Hepatic encephalopathy—Ammonia produced by bacterial decomposition of protein in the large bowel is either ineffectively removed by damaged liver cells or, because of portal obstruction, bypassed directly into the systemic circulation. The amount of ammonia produced is dependent upon the protein content, the bacterial flora, and the motility of the colon. Hepatic encephalopathy may also be further aggravated by the invasion of colonic organisms through the blood stream. Bleeding into the intestinal tract from varices or ulcerations may significantly increase the amount of protein in the bowel and may precipitate rapid development of liver coma. Other factors which may precipitate hepatic encephalopathy include potassium deficiency induced by most diuretics, narcotics, hypnotics, and sedatives; medications containing ammonium or amino compounds, paracentesis with attendant hypovolemia; and hepatic or systemic infection.

Dietary protein may be drastically curtailed or completely withheld for short periods during acute episodes. Parenteral nutrition is usually indicated.

Gastrointestinal bleeding should be treated by all necessary medical and surgical means to prevent further bleeding and to remove blood. Give milk of magnesia, 30 ml 4 times daily, or magnesium sulfate, 10—15 gm by indwelling nasogastric tube.

Control the intestinal flora with neomycin sulfate, 0.5—1 gm orally every 6 hours for 5—7 days.

Treat shock as outlined in Chapter 1.

Treat infection with antibiotic agents chosen on the basis of culture and sensitivity studies. In some cases, broad-spectrum antimicrobials are indicated if the patient's condition is deteriorating.

If agitation is marked, give sodium phenobarbital, 15—30 mg IM, cautiously as indicated. Avoid narcotics, tranquilizers, and sedatives excreted by the liver.

3. Anemia—For hypochromic anemia, give ferrous sulfate, 0.3 gm enteric-coated tablets, one tablet 3 times daily after meals. Folic acid, 5 mg/day orally is indicated in the treatment of macrocytic anemia.

4. Hemorrhagic tendency—A bleeding tendency due to hypoprothrombinemia may be treated with vitamin K preparations. This treatment is ineffective in the presence of severe hepatic disease when other coagulation factors are deficient. Blood transfusions (fresh) may be necessary to control bleeding tendencies. Give menadione, 1—3 mg orally 3 times daily after meals; or menadione sodium bisulfite, 2 mg IV or IM every other day for a few days.

5. Hemorrhage from esophageal varices—Posterior pituitary extract for surgical use (Pituitrin S), 20 units in 50 ml 5% dextrose in water by IV infusion over a 20- to 30-minute period, may be tried and repeated in an effort to control hemorrhage due to esophageal or gastric varices. If this is not successful, bleeding can usually be controlled by the use of the triple-lumen (Sengstaken-Blakemore) tube. Emergency surgical decompression of portal hypertension may be considered in selected patients. However, morbidity and mortality rates will be substantially decreased if the various shunting procedures can be performed electively.

6. Hemochromatosis—A program of phlebotomy (intermittent bleeding) over a period of months and years results in removal of intrahepatic iron and concomitant improvement of liver disease. The use of deferoxamine (Desferal) as a chelating agent has resulted in a high degree of iron mobilization and increased urinary iron excretion. Although more iron can be eliminated by phlebotomy in the treatment of hemochromatosis, deferoxamine can be reserved for anemic patients or combined with venesection in the management of advanced cases of abnormal iron storage.

Prognosis

The prognosis in advanced cirrhosis has shown little change over the years. A major factor determining the duration of the patient's life is his ability to discontinue the use of alcohol. In established cases with severe hepatic dysfunction, only 50% survive 2 years and only about 35% survive 5 years. Hematemesis, jaundice, and ascites are unfavorable signs.

Many latent cases go unrecognized, and are discovered only at autopsy.

Anderson RP, Wolfman EF Jr: Portal hypertension: Current status. California Med 111:25, 1969.

Chalmers TC: The management of hepatic coma: A continuing problem. M Clin North America 52:1475, 1968.

Close JH: Use of amino acid precursors in nitrogen accumulation disorders. New England J Med 290:663, 1974.

Epstein FH: Ascites and its delivery. New England J Med 282:713, 1970.

Epstein M & others: Renal failure in patients with cirrhosis: The role of active vasoconstriction. Am J Med 49:175, 1970.

Gall EA, Dobrogorski O: Hepatic alterations in obstructive jaundice. Am J Clin Path 42:126, 1964.

Joseph RR: A rational approach to the treatment of ascites in Laennec's cirrhosis. M Clin North America 53:1359, 1969.

Leevy CM, Baker H: Nutritional deficiencies in liver disease. M Clin North America 54:467, 1970.

Liebowitz HR: Pathogenesis of ascites in cirrhosis of the liver. New York J Med 69:1895, 1969.

MacDonald RA, Mallory GK: The natural history of post-necrotic cirrhosis: A study of 221 autopsy cases. Am J Med 24:334, 1958.

Schaffner F (editor): Symposium on the treatment of liver disease. Mod Treat 6:121, 1969.

Sherlock S & others: Complications of diuretic therapy in hepatic cirrhosis. Lancet 1:1049, 1966.

Steignmann Mejicano R: The impact of diuretics on chronic liver disease. Am J Gastroenterol 52:37, 1969.

Stone WD & others: The natural history of cirrhosis. Quart J Med 37:119, 1968.

Webster LT Jr: Hepatic coma: A biochemical disorder of the brain. Gastroenterology 49:698, 1965.

Zieve L: Pathogenesis of hepatic coma. Arch Int Med 118:211, 1966.

BILIARY CIRRHOSIS
(Primary & Secondary)

Biliary cirrhosis is a chronic disease of the liver clinically manifested by cholestasis. Bile flow is most commonly obstructed in an extrahepatic site by calculus, neoplasm, scarring, or congenital atresia. Stasis alone may produce cirrhosis, but the frequently superimposed infection hastens the process. The less common intrahepatic obstructions may have no identifiable cause but have been noted to follow viral hepatitis—particularly the cholangiolitic type—and intrahepatic cholangitis. Some cases may be due to hepatotoxins. The disease is far more common in women (particularly the intrahepatic type).

The pathologic findings vary with the cause and the stage of the process, but the following are characteristic: bile stasis with bile thrombi, pigmentation, extensive multiplication of bile ducts, nodular loss of normal architecture, marked cellular infiltration in the fibrous septa, little evidence of hepatic necrosis or regeneration, and absence of fatty metamorphosis. Bile lakes and bile infarcts are characteristic of extrahepatic obstruction.

Clinical Findings

A. Symptoms and Signs: In extrahepatic obstruction, symptoms of the primary lesion may predominate (eg, carcinoma of the pancreas, choledocholithiasis). Jaundice and pruritus are initial symptoms. Jaundice is of varying intensity but is often marked. Cholangitis may cause chills and fever. Mild right upper quadrant aching pain may be present. Anorexia, weight loss, and weakness may occur late in the illness.

The liver is enlarged and firm but is usually not tender. Splenomegaly is a late finding when it occurs. The usual signs of cirrhosis—ascites, peripheral edema, hematemesis, hemorrhagic manifestations in the skin and mucous membranes, bleeding gums, and epistaxis—are usually late manifestations. Spider nevi and palmar erythema are not usually present. Xanthomatous lesions may occur in the skin of the eyelids, around the joints, and within the tendons. Nutrition may remain good until the terminal phase.

B. Laboratory Findings: Hemograms are normal except insofar as they reflect the inciting lesion, eg, choledocholithiasis with cholangitis. The stools are acholic, and frequently diarrheal and steatorrheic. Stool urobilinogen is reduced. The urine is dark and contains bile. Liver function tests initially show the pattern of obstruction (elevated alkaline phosphatase, leucine aminopeptidase, serum cholesterol, and bilirubin, primarily in the conjugated fraction). Prothrombin time is prolonged. As obstruction persists—often complicated by infection—evidence of hepatocellular dysfunction appears. Hyperlipidemia, with a predominant increase in cholesterol and phospholipids, may reach extreme levels of over 3 gm/100 ml. The serum, however, remains clear in appearance.

Liver biopsy, obtained percutaneously or at surgery, usually demonstrates the typical pathologic findings, although in late stages differentiation from other forms of cirrhosis may be difficult. Antimitochondrial antibodies may be helpful in diagnosis.

C. X-Ray Findings: X-ray may show the inciting lesion on intravenous cholangiography or may demonstrate varices on upper gastrointestinal series.

Treatment

Exploration is indicated to establish the diagnosis of primary or secondary biliary cirrhosis. If no obstruction can be found with operative cholangiography, therapy is supportive, incorporating adequate nutrition and control of pruritus with cholestyramine. In the primary form of the disease corticosteroids and immunosuppressant agents may occasionally offer palliation. Extrahepatic obstruction, if present, should be relieved to ameliorate the secondary form of the disease. Infections should be treated with antimicrobial agents.

Prognosis

The intrahepatic form is generally progressive. Occasional clinical improvement and prolongation of life have followed the use of continuous immunosuppression. Death due to liver failure, infections, or hemorrhage usually occurs in about 5 years.

The course and prognosis of biliary cirrhosis secondary to extrahepatic obstruction depends upon the nature of the causative lesion. If the obstruction can be relieved and associated infection controlled, the early stage fibrosis will not progress.

Goudie RB & others: Serological and histological diagnosis of primary biliary cirrhosis. J Clin Path 19:527, 1966.

Sherlock S, Scheuer PJ: The presentation and diagnosis of 100 patients with biliary cirrhosis. New England J Med 289:674, 1973.

HEMOCHROMATOSIS

Primary or idiopathic hemochromatosis is considered to be a genetically determined disorder of iron metabolism characterized by increased accumulation of dietary iron. This iron is deposited as hemosiderin in the liver, pancreas, heart, adrenals, testes, and kidneys. Eventually the patient may develop hepatic, pancreatic, and cardiac insufficiency. The disease usually occurs in males and is rarely recognized before the 5th decade. Clinical manifestations include hepatomegaly and evidence of hepatic insufficiency, occasional skin pigmentation (slate gray due to iron and brown due to melanin), cardiac enlargement and insufficiency, and diabetes mellitus with its complications. Bleeding from esophageal varices and hepatic carcinoma may occur.

Laboratory findings include elevated plasma iron, saturated iron-binding protein in plasma, and the characteristic liver biopsy which stains positive for iron.

Treatment consists initially of weekly phlebotomies (500 ml of blood for months—occasionally up to 2 or 3 years) until plasma iron and hematocrit determinations indicate depletion of iron stores. During the past few years there has been increasing confirmation of the efficacy of a chelating agent, deferoxamine, which, when administered intramuscularly to patients with hemochromatosis, has been shown to produce urinary excretion of up to 5–18 gm of iron per year. This rate of urinary excretion compares very favorably with the rate of 10–20 gm of iron removed annually by weekly or biweekly phlebotomies. Symptomatic and supportive treatment of diabetic, hepatic, and cardiac complications may be necessary.

Although the long-term benefits of iron depletion therapy have not been completely established, available data indicate that the course of the disease may be favorably altered by chelation or bleeding.

Crosby WH: Intestinal response to the body's requirement for iron: Control of iron absorption. JAMA 208:347, 1969.

Hallberg L, Hedenberg L: The effect of desferrioxamine on iron metabolism in man. Scandinav J Haemat 2:67, 1965.

Hallberg L & others: Liver iron and desferrioxamine-induced urinary iron excretion. Scandinav J Haemat 3:85, 1966.

Heilmeyer L: Pathogenesis of hemochromatosis. Medicine 46:209, 1967.

Johnson BF: Hemochromatosis resulting from prolonged oral iron therapy. New England J Med 278:1100, 1968.

WILSON'S DISEASE

Wilson's disease (hepatolenticular degeneration) is a rare familial disorder which is inherited in an autosomally recessive manner and occurs in both males and females between the first and third decades. The condition is characterized by excessive deposition of copper in the liver and brain.

Awareness of the entity is important since it may masquerade as chronic hepatic or neurologic disease. It is potentially reversible, and appropriate therapy will prevent neurologic and hepatic damage.

The major physiologic aberration in Wilson's disease is excessive absorption of copper from the small intestine. Ceruloplasmin, the plasma copper protein, is low, whereas large quantities of copper are excreted in the urine and deposited in the tissues.

Wilson's disease can present primarily as a neurologic abnormality, with liver involvement appearing later; or the reverse may be true, with hepatic disease being the initial manifestation. It may first be clinically recognized when jaundice appears in the first few years of life. The diagnosis should always be considered in any child with manifestations of atypical hepatitis, splenomegaly with hypersplenism, hemolytic anemia, and portal hypertension. The appearance of neurologic or psychiatric abnormalities in childhood should also excite suspicion.

The neurologic manifestations are related to basal ganglia dysfunction and are characterized by rigidity or parkinsonian tremor. Hepatic involvement is evidenced by signs of cirrhosis, portal hypertension, and biochemical confirmation of hepatocellular insufficiency. The pathognomonic sign of the condition is the Kayser-Fleischer ring, which represents fine pigmented granular deposits in Descemet's membrane in the cornea close to the endothelial surface. Scattering and reflection of light by these deposits give rise to the typically brownish or gray-green appearance of the ring. The ring itself is not always complete and is usually most marked at the superior and inferior poles of the cornea. It can frequently be seen with the naked eye and almost invariably by slitlamp examination.

The diagnosis is based on demonstration of increased urinary copper excretion (> 100 mg/24 hours) or low serum ceruloplasmin levels (< 20 mg/100 ml), elevated hepatic copper concentration (> 100 μg/gm of dry liver) and increased urinary copper excretion (> 100 μg/24 hours). Histologically, liver biopsy reveals only cirrhosis, which is indistinguishable from the usual varieties.

Treatment involves removal of copper before it can produce neurologic or hepatic damage. Oral penicillamine ($1-1.5$ gm/day in divided doses) is the drug of choice, making possible urinary excretion of chelated copper. A recent report has suggested that triethylenetetramine may have an important place in the treatment of patients with Wilson's disease who have developed intolerance to penicillamine. The use of copper-restricted diets has not been beneficial and is superfluous when penicillamine is employed. The prognosis is excellent in patients who are effectively treated before liver or brain damage has occurred.

Sternlieb I, Scheinberg IH: Prevention of Wilson's disease in asymptomatic patients. New England J Med 278:352, 1968.

Walshe JM: Copper chelation in patients with Wilson's disease: A comparison of penicillamine and triethylene tetramine dihydrochloride. Quart J Med 42:441, 1973.

Walshe JM: Wilson's disease: The presenting symptoms. Arch Dis Childhood 37:253, 1962.

Walshe JM, Briggs J: Ceruloplasmin in liver disease: A diagnostic pitfall. Lancet 2:263, 1963.

PYOGENIC HEPATIC ABSCESS

Single or multiple local collections of pus in the liver which are large enough to be seen with the naked eye are presently quite rare, principally because of the use of antibiotics and improved methods of diagnosis of appendicitis, which was formerly the most common precursor of liver abscess. Although the actual clinical incidence cannot be determined because the condition is aborted or modified by antimicrobial treatment, hepatic abscess is still reported in 0.5–1.5% of autopsy specimens. It is equally distributed between men and women, usually in the sixth or seventh decade.

There are apparently 5 ways in which the liver can be invaded by bacteria: (1) by way of the portal vein; (2) by way of ascending cholangitis in the common duct; (3) by way of the hepatic artery, secondary to bacteremia; (4) by direct extension from an infectious process; and (5) by traumatic implantation of bacteria through the abdominal wall.

Although mitigated by antimicrobial drugs, liver abscess secondary to appendicitis still occurs in 10% of cases. Another 10% have no demonstrable cause and are classified as idiopathic. At present, ascending cholangitis is the most common cause of hepatic abscess in the USA. Bacterial infection of the hepatobiliary tree is more likely to accompany obstruction by stone than by carcinoma of the head of the pancreas and is probably attributable to dissemination of bacteria from an acutely inflamed gallbladder. The most frequently encountered organisms are *Escherichia coli, Proteus vulgaris,* and *Enterobacter aerogenes.*

Clinically, fever is almost always present and may antedate other symptoms or signs. Pain is prominent and is localized to the right hypochondrium or epigastric area. Jaundice, tenderness in the right upper abdomen, and either steady or swinging fever are the primary physical findings.

Laboratory examination reveals leukocytosis with a shift to the left. Chest roentgenograms will usually reveal elevation of the diaphragm if the abscess is on the right side. Left-sided abscess does not produce significant diaphragmatic elevation. Liver scanning, using ^{99m}Tc sulfur colloid, may reveal the presence of intrahepatic defects.

Treatment should consist of antimicrobial agents which are effective against coliform organisms. If adequate response to therapy is not rapidly evident, surgical drainage should be undertaken. Failure to recognize and treat the condition is attended by mortality rates of about 60% in patients with multiple abscesses.

Joseph WL, Kahn AM, Longmire WP Jr: Pyogenic liver abscess: Changing patterns in approach. Am J Surg 115:63, 1968.

Pyrtek LJ, Barters SA: Hepatic pyemia. New England J Med 272:551, 1965.

Stokes JF: Cryptogenic liver abscess. Lancet 1:355, 1960.

NEOPLASMS OF THE LIVER

Neoplasms of the liver arise either in the hepatic parenchymal cells or in the biliary ductules. A tumor that arises from parenchymal cells is called a hepatoma; one that originates in the ductular cells is called a cholangioma.

Although hepatoma was formerly thought to occur only in underdeveloped parts of the world where malnutrition and parasitism are prevalent, it has now become apparent that its incidence is increasing in the USA. This neoplasm occurs in up to 20% of cases of macronodular cirrhosis. In the Orient, *Clonorchis sinensis,* the liver fluke, is etiologically significant.

Histologically, the tumor may be made up of cords or sheets of cells that roughly resemble the hepatic parenchyma. In the case of a cholangioma, a fibrous stroma or tissue containing structures which simulate bile ducts will be seen. Blood vessels such as portal or hepatic veins are commonly involved by tumor.

The presence of a hepatoma may be unsuspected until there is deterioration in the condition of a cirrhotic patient who was formerly stable. Cachexia, weakness, and weight loss are associated symptoms. The sudden appearance of ascites, which may be bloody, suggests portal or hepatic vein thrombosis by tumor.

Physical examination is positive for tender enlargement of the liver with an occasionally palpable mass. Auscultation may reveal a bruit over the tumor, or a friction rub may be heard when the process has extended to the surface of the liver.

Laboratory tests may reveal leukocytosis, as opposed to the leukopenia that is frequently encountered in cirrhotic patients. Sudden and sustained elevation of the serum alkaline phosphatase in a patient who was formerly stable is a common finding. Alpha$_1$-fetoglobulin—not usually found in adults—is demonstrable in 30–50% of patients with hepatoma. Cytologic study of ascitic fluid may reveal malignant cells.

Arteriography is frequently diagnostic, revealing a tumor "blush" which reflects the highly vascular nature of the tumor. Liver scanning with ^{99m}Tc sulfur colloid is occasionally helpful. Liver biopsy is diagnostic.

No therapy, including hepatic perfusion with cytotoxic agents, has proved effective. Attempts at surgical resection are usually fruitless because of the presence of cirrhosis and the wide dissemination of the tumor.

Alpert M & others: Hepatoma in Uganda. Lancet 1:1265, 1968.

Lee FI: Cirrhosis and hepatoma in alcoholics. Gut 7:77, 1966.

Manderson W & others: Incidence of primary carcinoma of the liver in the west of Scotland between 1949 and 1965. Gut 9:480, 1968.

ACUTE CHOLECYSTITIS

Essentials of Diagnosis

- Steady, severe pain and tenderness in the right hypochondrium or epigastrium.
- Nausea and vomiting.
- Jaundice.
- Fever and leukocytosis.

General Considerations

Cholecystitis is associated with gallstones in over 90% of cases. It occurs when a calculus becomes impacted in the cystic duct and inflammation develops behind the obstruction. Vascular abnormalities of the bile duct or pancreatitis may rarely produce cholecystitis in the absence of gallstones. If the obstruction is not relieved, pressure builds up within the gallbladder as a result of continued secretion. Primarily as a result of ischemic changes secondary to distention, gangrene may develop, with resulting perforation. Although generalized peritonitis is possible, the leak usually remains localized and forms a chronic, well-circumscribed abscess cavity.

Clinical Findings

A. Symptoms and Signs: The acute attack is often precipitated by a large or fatty meal and is characterized by the relatively sudden appearance of severe, minimally fluctuating pain which is localized to the epigastrium or right hypochondrium and which in the uncomplicated case may gradually subside over a period of 12−18 hours. Vomiting occurs in about 75% of patients, and in half of instances affords variable relief. Tenderness in the right upper quadrant of the abdomen is almost always present and is usually associated with muscle guarding and rebound pain. A palpable gallbladder is present in about 15% of cases. Jaundice is present in approximately 25% of cases, and when persistent or severe suggests the possibility of choledocholithiasis. Fever is usually present.

B. Laboratory Findings: The white count is usually high (12−15 thousand/cu mm). Total serum bilirubin values of 1−4 mg/100 ml may be reported even in the absence of common duct obstruction. Serum transaminase and alkaline phosphatase are often elevated—the former as high as 300 mU/ml. Serum amylase may be as high as 1000 units/100 ml.

C. X-Ray Findings: Films of the abdomen may show gallstones (15%). Intravenous cholangiography is helpful since visualization of the gallbladder usually rules out the possibility of acute cholecystitis.

Differential Diagnosis

The disorders most likely to be confused with acute cholecystitis are perforated peptic ulcer, acute pancreatitis, appendicitis in a high-lying appendix, perforated carcinoma or diverticulum of the hepatic flexure, liver abscess, hepatitis, and pneumonia with pleurisy on the right side. The definite localization of pain and tenderness in the right hypochondrium with fre-quent radiation to the infrascapular area strongly favors the diagnosis of acute cholecystitis.

Complications

A. Gangrene of the Gallbladder: Continuation or progression of right upper quadrant abdominal pain, tenderness, muscle guarding, fever, and leukocytosis after 24−48 hours suggest severe inflammation and possible gangrene of the gallbladder. Necrosis may occasionally develop without definite signs in either the obese or the elderly.

B. Cholangitis: Intermittently high fever and chills strongly suggest choledocholithiasis.

Treatment

Acute cholecystitis will usually subside on a conservative regimen (interdiction of oral feedings, intravenous alimentation, analgesics and antibiotics if indicated). Cholecystectomy can be performed a few days after institution of hospitalization or can be scheduled for 2−3 months later, depending on the surgeon's preference and the clinical aspects of the individual case. If, as occasionally happens, recurrent acute symptoms develop during this waiting period, cholecystectomy is indicated without delay. If conservative treatment has been elected, the patient (especially if diabetic or elderly), should be watched carefully for evidence of gangrene of the gallbladder or cholangitis.

Operation is mandatory when there is evidence of gangrene or perforation. Operation during the first 24 hours can be justified as a means of reducing overall morbidity in good-risk patients in whom the diagnosis is unequivocal. It is usually best to defer surgery, if possible, in the presence of acute pancreatitis.

A. Conservative Treatment: During the acute period, the patient should be observed frequently, with careful abdominal examination and sequential determination of the white count several times a day. Anticholinergic agents such as parenteral atropine or propantheline should be used with an analgesic such as pentazocine, or, if that fails to control pain, meperidine. (Morphine sulfate is known to produce spasm of the sphincter of Oddi and may also produce spurious elevations of the serum amylase.) Appropriate antimicrobial agents should be employed in all but the most mild and rapidly subsiding cases.

B. Surgical Treatment: When surgery is elected for acute cholecystitis, cholecystectomy is the procedure of choice. Cholangiography should be performed at the time of operation to ascertain the need for common duct exploration. In the poor-risk patient or when technical difficulties preclude cholecystectomy, cholecystostomy can be performed under local anesthesia.

Prognosis

Mild acute cholecystitis usually subsides, but recurrences are common. Symptomatic cholecystitis is a definite indication for surgery. Persistence of symptoms after removal of the gallbladder implies either mistaken diagnosis or technical error, since cholecystectomy is curative.

Gunn A, Keddie N: Some clinical observations on patients with gallstones. Lancet 2:239, 1972.

Munster AM, Brown JR: Acalculous cholecystitis. Am J Surg 113:730, 1967.

Valberg LS & others: Biliary pain in young women in the absence of gallstones. Gastroenterology 60:1020, 1971.

CHOLELITHIASIS

Gallstones are more common in women than in men and increase in incidence in both sexes and all races with aging. Data are available which indicate that in the USA 10% of men and 20% of women between the ages of 55 and 65 years have gallstones, and that the overall total exceeds 15 million people. Although it is less common in black people, cholelithiasis attributable to hemolysis has been encountered in over a third of individuals with sickle cell disease. As many as 70% of Pima Indian women over age 25 have cholelithiasis. The incidence of gallstones is also high in individuals with certain diseases such as regional enteritis. Approximately one-third of individuals with inflammatory involvement of the terminal ileum have cholesterol gallstones. Cholelithiasis is also increased in incidence in patients with diabetes mellitus. Pregnancy as a significant cause of gallstones has been overemphasized.

The simplest classification of gallstones is according to chemical composition: stones containing predominantly cholesterol and stones containing predominantly calcium bilirubinate. The latter comprise less than 5% of the stones found in Europe or the USA but 30–40% of stones found in Japan.

Three compounds comprise 80–95% of the total solids dissolved in bile: conjugated bile salts, lecithin, and cholesterol. Cholesterol is a neutral sterol; lecithin is a phospholipid; and both are almost completely insoluble in water. However, bile salts are able to form multimolecular aggregates (micelles) which solubilize lecithin and cholesterol in an aqueous solution. Bile salts alone are relatively inefficient in solubilizing cholesterol (approximately 50 molecules of bile salt are necessary to solubilize 1 molecule of cholesterol), but the solubilization of lecithin in bile salt solutions results in a mixed micelle which is 7 times more efficient in the solubilization of cholesterol. Precipitation of cholesterol microcrystals may come about through a simultaneous change in all 3 major components.

Cholelithiasis is frequently asymptomatic and is discovered fortuitously in the course of routine radiographic study, operation, or autopsy. Although there is disagreement about the desirability of cholecystectomy in patients with "silent" gallstones, it is generally agreed that diabetic patients should undergo gallbladder removal to avoid complications. Operation is mandatory for symptomatic cholelithiasis.

Chemical dissolution of gallstones in vivo with chenodeoxycholic acid may be useful in certain cases, but experience has been limited, and recurrence of cholelithiasis has followed cessation of the agent.

Danzinger RG & others: Dissolution of cholesterol gallstones by chenodeoxycholic acid. New England J Med 286:1, 1972.

Gunn A, Keddie N: Some clinical observations on patients with gallstones. Lancet 2:239, 1972.

Javitt NB & others: Conference on gallstone prophylaxis and therapy. Am J Digest Dis 19:81, 1974.

Javitt NB, McSherry CK: Pathogenesis of cholesterol gallstones. Hosp Practice 8:39, 1973.

Redinger RN, Small DM: Bile composition, bile salt metabolism and gallstones. Arch Int Med 130:618, 1972.

Schkar E & others: The fate of the nonvisualized gallbladder. Am J Digest Dis 14:80, 1969.

Soloway RD & others: Hepatic lipid secretion and cholelithiasis. Am J Digest Dis 16:437, 1971.

Thistle JL, Hoffman AF: Efficiency and specificity of chenodeoxycholic acid therapy for dissolving gallstones. New England J Med 289:655, 1973.

Thistle JL, Schoenfield LJ: Induced alterations in composition of bile of persons having cholelithiasis. Gastroenterology 61:488, 1971.

Thistle JL, Schoenfield LJ: Lithogenic bile among young Indian women. New England J Med 284:177, 1971.

CHOLESTEROLOSIS
(Strawberry Gallbladder)

"Strawberry gallbladder" is characterized by abnormal deposits of cholesterol esters in fat-laden macrophages situated in the lamina propria of the gallbladder. The lesion may be diffuse or localized. Diffuse involvement is generally associated with good function of the gallbladder, and, since it presents no specific radiologic features, is rarely diagnosed by cholecystography. The localized form consists of single or multiple polypoid lesions which may be either sessile or pedunculated. Radiographically, these appear as fixed filling defects. These gallbladders usually visualize well on oral cholecystography. When gallstones are not present, the gallbladder often has soft walls, and on microscopic examination there is no evidence of inflammation. A fine to coarse yellowish speckled marking, often diffuse but at times circumscribed, appears at the level of the mucous membrane folds. This gives the characteristic strawberry appearance. However, inflammation, cholesterol concretions, and polyps may also occur. Microscopically, the cholesterol is seen to be in the form of esters in the foam-like cells of the submucous connective tissue. The cause of the deposits is not known, although the disease has been attributed to excessive cholesterol absorption across the gallbladder mucosa. Strawberry gallbladders are frequently found in stone-free organs that have been removed because of severe intractable pain. It would therefore appear that cholesterolosis and adenomyomatosis are associated with or are capable of producing symptoms which are indistinguishable from those of cholelithiasis.

Lubera RJ & others: Cholecystitis and the hyperplastic cholecystoses: A clinical, radiologic and pathologic study. Am J Digest Dis 12:696, 1967.

ADENOMYOMATOSIS OF THE GALLBLADDER

Adenomyomatosis—hyperplasia of the gallbladder wall—is characterized by excessive proliferation of the surface epithelium and thickening of the muscle layer. When the process is well established, the mucosal folds are increased in number as well as height and project into or through the muscularis as tubules, crypts, and saccules. These outpouchings are called intramural diverticula or Rokitansky-Aschoff sinuses. The hyperplasia of the muscularis may be so pronounced as to present the appearance of a myoma. Epithelial and muscular hyperplasia may involve the entire viscus or only part of it. Consequently, 3 main forms may be recognized: generalized, segmental, and localized. The name adenomyoma is a misnomer.

Adenomyomatosis is more common in women than in men, and the incidence increases with age, particularly after the fourth decade. It is generally agreed that the risks of malignant degeneration are low, although one such case has been reported.

The clinical significance and management of this condition continue to be controversial. However, it would appear that in the majority of instances the lesion does not produce symptoms. In a few patients with acalculous adenomyomatosis, biliary type pain had been present for periods of almost 20 years. Following cholecystectomy in these individuals, pain disappeared or decreased. None of these gallbladders had stones or inflammatory changes. It would therefore appear that pain is produced by excessive neuromuscular activity of the hyperplastic gallbladder.

Juytsd JA, Levesque H: Adenomyoma and adenomyomatosis of the gallbladder. Radiol Clin North America 4:483, 1966.

CYSTIC DUCT SYNDROMES

Precholecystectomy

A small group of patients (mostly women) has been reported in whom right upper quadrant abdominal pain occurred frequently following meals. Conventional radiographic study of the upper gastrointestinal tract and gallbladder—including intravenous cholangiography—was unremarkable. Using cholecystokinin (CCK) as a gallbladder stimulant, contraction and evacuation of the viscus did not take place, as usually occurs in the 3- to 5-minute period after injection of the hormone. However, the gallbladder assumed a "golf ball" configuration, and biliary type pain was reproduced. At the time of cholecystectomy, the gallbladders were found to be enlarged and could not be emptied by manual compression. Anatomic and histologic examination of the operative specimens revealed obstruction of the cystic ducts either because of fibrotic stenosis at their proximal ends or because of adhesions and kinking.

Postcholecystectomy

If the cystic duct is not removed as close to the common duct as possible, the remaining portion undergoes dilatation. This seems to predispose to the formation or retention of calculi with attendant abdominal pain. Although cystic duct remnants are frequently associated with choledocholithiasis, the relationship may be due more to failure to perform common duct exploration at the time of cholecystectomy than to new stone formation.

Pain secondary to cystic duct remnant may also be due to neuroma formation in the ductal wall. Traction on the common duct may result from a long stump with resultant kinking.

Symptoms tend to appear about 3 years after removal of the gallbladder, although in a few cases recurrent abdominal pain has first appeared 20 years after operation.

Treatment consists of surgical removal of the stump after the diagnosis of cystic duct remnant has been established.

Cozzolino HJ & others: The cystic duct syndrome. JAMA 85:100, 1963.

Hayes MA: Retained cystic duct stump. Connecticut Med 26:390, 1962.

CHRONIC CHOLECYSTITIS

The most common disability that results from cholelithiasis is chronic cholecystitis. It is characterized pathologically by varying degrees of chronic inflammation on macro- or microscopic examination of the gallbladder. Calculi are usually present, but the gallbladder may or may not visualize on cholecystography. The diagnosis is often erroneously applied to collections of symptoms that are only vaguely or indirectly related to gallbladder dysfunction.

Clinical Findings

Chronic cholecystitis is associated with discrete bouts of right hypochondriac and epigastric pain which is either steady or intermittent. Discomfort is usually persistent, but, if intermittent, the height of pain may be separated by 15- to 60-minute intervals.

The onset of pain is usually abrupt, with maximum intensity and plateau reached within 15 minutes to 1 hour. Attacks of biliary colic may persist for as long as several hours or be as brief as 15—20 minutes, the average duration being about 1 hour. Pain referral to the interscapular area is occasionally noted.

Chronic indigestion is considered by many to be frequently caused by gallbladder disease. Fatty food intolerance, belching, flatulence, a sense of epigastric heaviness, upper abdominal pain of varying intensity, and pyrosis are some of the symptoms that have been erroneously considered to be suggestive of cholelithiasis and cholecystitis. Efforts have therefore been made to evaluate "dyspeptic" symptomatology in relationship to objective evidence of gallbladder disease. In one prospective study of 142 women who experienced "chronic indigestion," only 24 had either gallstones or nonvisualization of the gallbladder on oral cholecystograms. Sixty-three (53%) of the 118 who had normal cholecystograms complained of "dyspepsia." Accordingly, it can be assumed that the association of chronic indigestion and gallstones is purely fortuitous. If cholecystectomy is performed in patients with calculi who have complained of a constellation of "dyspeptic" symptoms, the results of operation may be unpredictable and frequently unsatisfactory.

Physical examination is nonspecific, revealing abdominal tenderness which may be localized to the right hypochondrium and epigastric area but which may also be diffuse. Hydrops of the gallbladder results when subsidence of acute cholecystitis occurs but cystic duct obstruction persists, producing distention of the gallbladder with a clear mucoid fluid. The gallbladder in that circumstance is palpable in the right upper abdomen. The presence of jaundice obviously supports the diagnosis of cholecystitis with choledocholithiasis.

Laboratory studies are usually not diagnostic.

Films of the abdomen taken prior to oral cholecystography may reveal opacification of the gallbladder caused by high concentrations of calcium carbonate (limy bile) or radiopaque stones. Nonvisualization of the gallbladder implies cholecystitis, but it is important to remember the following technical reasons for nonvisualization: failure to ingest the dye, vomiting or diarrhea, gastric outlet obstruction or esophageal stricture, intestinal malabsorption, abnormal location of the gallbladder, liver disease (including preicteric hepatitis), Dubin-Johnson-Sprinz-Nelson syndrome, fat-free diet prior to cholecystography, and previous cholecystectomy.

Iophendylate is quickly absorbed from an inflamed gallbladder but not from the normal organ. Conversely, meglumine iodipamide, which is used for intravenous cholangiography, is water-soluble and poorly absorbed from the gastrointestinal tract and is not conjugated prior to biliary excretion.

Accordingly, if a gallbladder fails to visualize with iophendylate but shows normal opacification with meglumine iodipamide, it is likely that gallbladder absorption of iophendylate, implying cholecystitis, produced nonvisualization. If the gallbladder is not shown on either the oral or intravenous study, it can be assumed that the cystic duct is obstructed. Finally, the main value of intravenous cholangiography after nonvisualization on oral cholecystography is the possibility of demonstrating calculi in either the gallbladder or the common duct.

Differential Diagnosis

When nonspecific symptoms are present, it is necessary to consider the possibilities of gastroduodenal ulcer disease, chronic relapsing pancreatitis, irritable colon syndrome, and malignant neoplasms of the stomach, pancreas, hepatic flexure, or gallbladder. Barium enema and upper gastrointestinal series complement cholecystography and cholangiography. Microscopic examination of bile, obtained by biliary drainage, is occasionally helpful in demonstrating calculous disease of the gallbladder. (The test is valid only in the absence of hepatic and pancreatic disease.)

Complications

The presence of cholelithiasis with chronic cholecystitis can result in acute exacerbation of gallbladder inflammation, common duct stone, cholecystenteric fistulization, pancreatitis, and, rarely, carcinoma of the gallbladder.

Treatment

Although proved cholelithiasis and cholecystitis ideally should be managed surgically, significant metabolic and cardiovascular disease or other factors may preclude operation. Nonspecific and "dyspeptic" symptoms such as heartburn, belching, abdominal pain, bloating, flatulence, and constipation will frequently be ameliorated by the judicious use of low-fat diets, weight reduction, and anticholinergic and sedative medication in conjunction with antacids and hydrophilic agents.

Surgical treatment is the same as for acute cholecystitis, with transhepatic and operative cholangiography employed if there is a possibility of choledocholithiasis.

Prognosis

The overall mortality after cholecystectomy is less than 1%, but hepatobiliary tract surgery is a more formidable procedure in the elderly and has a mortality rate of 5–10%. A technically successful surgical procedure in an appropriately selected patient is generally followed by complete cessation of symptoms.

Achkar E & others: The fate of the nonvisualized gallbladder. Am J Digest Dis 14:81, 1969.

Doyle JL, Zanca P: Infusion "drip" cholangiography. Clin Med 75:46, 1968.

French EB: Gallstones and flatulent dyspepsia. Lancet 1:681, 1967.

Gunn A, Keddie N: Some clinical observations on patients with gallstones. Lancet 2:239, 1972.

Lasser EC: Pharmacodynamics of biliary contrast media. Radiol Clin North America 4:511, 1966.

Meyer KA & others: Personal experiences with 1261 cases of acute and chronic cholecystitis and cholelithiasis. Surgery 61:661, 1967.

CHOLEDOCHOLITHIASIS

Essentials of Diagnosis

- Often a history of biliary colic or jaundice.
- Sudden onset of severe right upper quadrant or epigastric pain, which may radiate to the right scapula or shoulder.

- Nausea and vomiting.
- Fever, often followed by hypothermia and gram-negative shock.
- Jaundice.
- Leukocytosis.
- Abdominal films may reveal gallstones.

General Considerations

About 15% of patients with gallstones have choledocholithiasis. The percentage rises with age, and the incidence in elderly people may be as high as 50%. Common duct stones usually originate in the gallbladder but may also form spontaneously in the common duct. The stones are frequently "silent," as no symptoms result unless there is obstruction.

Clinical Findings

A. Symptoms and Signs: A history suggestive of biliary colic or prior jaundice can usually be obtained. The additional features that suggest the presence of a common duct stone are (1) frequently recurring attacks of right upper abdominal pain which is severe and persists for hours; (2) chills and fever associated with severe colic; and (3) a history of jaundice which was chronologically associated with abdominal pain. The combination of pain, fever (and chills), and jaundice represents Charcot's triad and denotes the classical picture of cholangitis. The presence of altered sensorium, lethargy, and septic shock connotes acute suppurative cholangitis accompanied by pus in the obstructed duct and represents a surgical emergency.

Biliary colic in choledocholithiasis is apparently caused by rapidly increasing biliary pressure which is secondary to sudden obstruction to the flow of bile. Radiation of pain into the interscapular area may be helpful in differentiating choledocholithiasis from cholecystolithiasis. Hepatomegaly may be present in calculous biliary obstruction, and tenderness is usually present in the right hypochondrium and epigastrium. Generally, however, there are no specific physical findings.

B. Laboratory Findings: Bilirubinuria and elevation of serum bilirubin are present if the common duct is obstructed. Serum alkaline phosphatase and leucine aminopeptidase elevation is especially suggestive of obstructive jaundice. Because prolongation of obstruction of the common duct results in hepatocellular dysfunction, SGOT, SGPT, and serum immunoglobulins will be abnormal. Prolongation of the prothrombin time will occur when there is disturbance of the normal enterohepatic circulation of bile with its exclusion from the intestinal tract. When extrahepatic obstruction persists for more than a few weeks, liver damage occurs and differentiation of obstruction from primarily inflammatory disease becomes progressively more difficult.

C. X-Ray Findings: If the serum bilirubin level is below 3 mg/100 ml, intravenous cholangiography may visualize the common duct.

Differential Diagnosis

The most common cause of obstructive jaundice is common duct stone. Next in frequency is carcinoma of the pancreas, ampulla of Vater, or common duct. Metastatic carcinoma (usually from the gastrointestinal tract) and direct extension of gallbladder cancer are other important causes of obstructive jaundice. Hepatocellular jaundice can usually be differentiated by the history, clinical findings, and liver function tests.

Complications

A. Biliary Cirrhosis: Prolonged common duct obstruction results in severe liver damage. Hepatic failure with portal hypertension commonly occurs in untreated cases.

B. Cholangitis: If bacteria enter the duct proximal to the obstruction and inoculation of these organisms into the blood stream occurs as the result of elevated biliary pressure in the ductal system, fever (and chills), jaundice, and pain will appear (Charcot's triad). Cholangitis may be nonsuppurative or suppurative. The former usually responds well to antimicrobial therapy while the latter is a surgical emergency. Untreated cholangitis is the most common cause of multiple pyogenic hepatic abscesses, resulting in a progressively downhill course and septic death.

C. Hypoprothrombinemia: Patients with obstructive jaundice or liver disease may bleed excessively as a result of prolonged prothrombin times. If the hypoprothrombinemia is due to faulty vitamin K absorption, the following preparations are of value. The comparison of prothrombin response to parenteral versus oral administration additionally corroborates the nature of the underlying lesion—hepatocellular versus obstructive.

1. Intravenously or subcutaneously—Phytonadione (AquaMephyton, Konakion), 10 mg daily, is the preparation of choice. Menadione sodium bisulfite (Hykinone), 10 mg daily, may be used if phytonadione is not available.

2. Orally—Menadiol sodium diphosphate (Synkayvite), 5 mg twice daily, is the preferred oral agent. It is water-soluble and is absorbed from the intestinal tract in the absence of bile. Menadione, 5 mg twice daily after meals, may also be used.

Treatment

Common duct stone is treated by cholecystectomy and choledochostomy.

A. Preoperative Preparation: Emergency operation is rarely necessary; a few days devoted to careful evaluation and preparation will be well spent.

Liver function should be evaluated thoroughly. Prothrombin time should be restored to normal by parenteral administration of vitamin K preparations (see above). Nutrition should be restored by a high-carbohydrate, high-protein diet and vitamin supplementation. Cholangitis, if present, should be controlled with antimicrobials.

B. Indications for Common Duct Exploration: At every operation for cholelithiasis, the advisability of exploring the common duct must be considered. Operative cholangiography via the cystic duct is a very useful procedure for demonstrating common duct stone. Evidence of common duct stone may be an indication for choledochostomy.

1. Preoperative findings suggestive of choledocholithiasis include a history (or the presence) of obstructive jaundice; frequent attacks of biliary colic; cholangitis; a history of pancreatitis; and an intravenous cholangiogram, showing stone, obstruction, or dilatation of the duct.

2. Operative findings of choledocholithiasis are palpable stones in the common duct; dilatation or thickening of the wall of the common duct; gallbladder stones small enough to pass through the cystic duct; and pancreatitis.

C. Postoperative Care:

1. **Antibiotics**—Postoperative antibiotics are not administered routinely after biliary tract surgery. Cultures of the bile are always taken at operation. If biliary tract infection was present preoperatively or is apparent at operation, penicillin and streptomycin or a tetracycline is administered postoperatively until sensitivity tests on culture specimens are available.

2. **Management of the T tube**—Following choledochostomy, a simple catheter or T tube is placed in the common duct for decompression. It must be attached securely to the skin or dressing because accidental removal of the tube may be disastrous. A properly placed tube should drain bile at the operating table and continuously thereafter; otherwise, it should be considered blocked or dislocated. The volume of bile drainage varies from 100–1000 ml daily (average, 200–400 ml). Above-average drainage may be due to obstruction at the ampulla (usually by edema), increased bile output, low resistance or siphonage effect in the drainage system, or a combination of these factors.

3. **Cholangiography**—A cholangiogram should be taken through the T tube on about the 7th or 8th postoperative day. Under fluoroscopic control, a radiopaque medium is aseptically and gently injected until the duct system is outlined and the medium begins to enter the duodenum. The injection of air bubbles must be avoided since on x-ray they resemble stones in the duct system. Spot films are always taken. If the cholangiogram shows no stones in the common duct and the opaque medium flows freely into the duodenum, the tube is clamped overnight and removed by simple traction on the following day. A small amount of bile frequently leaks from the tube site for a few days. A rubber tissue drain is usually placed alongside the T tube at operation. This drain is partially withdrawn on the 5th day and shortened daily until it is removed completely on about the 7th day.

Custer MD Jr, Clore JN Jr: Source of error in operative cholangiography. Arch Surg 100:664, 1970.

Kune GA: Gall stones in diverticula of the lower common bile duct. Gut 6:95, 1965.

Larson RE & others: The early and long-term results of 500 consecutive explorations of the common duct. Surg Gynec Obst 122:744, 1966.

Mackay C & others: The composition of hepatic and gallbladder bile in patients with gallstones. Gut 13:759, 1972.

Mullen JL & others: The diagnosis of choledocholithiasis. Surg Gynec Obst 133:774, 1971.

Way LW & others: Management of choledocholithiasis. Ann Surg 176:347, 1972.

BILIARY STRICTURE

Benign biliary strictures are the result of surgical trauma in about 95% of cases. The remainder are caused by blunt external injury to the abdomen or, infrequently, by erosion of the duct by a gallstone.

Signs of injury to the duct may or may not be recognized in the immediate postoperative period. If complete occlusion has occurred, jaundice will develop rapidly; but more often a tear has been accidentally made in the duct, and the earliest manifestation of injury may be excessive or prolonged loss of bile from the surgical drains. Bile leakage contributes to the production of localized infection, which in turn accentuates scar formation and the ultimate development of a fibrous stricture.

Cholangitis is the most common syndrome produced by stricture. Typically, the patient notices episodes of pain, fever, chills, and jaundice within a few weeks to months after cholecystectomy. With the exception of jaundice during an attack of cholangitis and right upper quadrant abdominal tenderness, physical findings are usually not significant.

Serum alkaline phosphatase and leucine aminopeptidase are usually elevated. Hyperbilirubinemia is variable, fluctuating during exacerbations and usually remaining in the range of 5–10 mg/100 ml. Blood cultures may be positive during an episode of cholangitis. If total serum bilirubin is below 3 mg/100 ml, intravenous cholangiography may define the lesion. In the presence of clinical icterus, percutaneous transhepatic cholangiography can be valuable in demonstrating the stricture.

Differentiation from choledocholithiasis may require surgical exploration. Operative treatment of a stricture frequently necessitates performance of choledochojejunostomy or hepaticojejunostomy to reestablish bile flow into the intestine.

Biliary stricture is not a benign condition, since significant hepatocellular disease will inevitably occur if it is allowed to continue uncorrected. The death rate for untreated stricture ranges from 10–15%.

Warren KW & others: Management of strictures of the biliary tract. S Clin North America 51:711, 1971.

Way LW, Dunphy JE: Biliary stricture. Am J Surg 124:387, 1972.

PRIMARY SCLEROSING CHOLANGITIS

Primary sclerosing cholangitis is a rare disease of unknown cause that on occasion has seemingly had more than a fortuitous association with ulcerative colitis. It may occur at any period of life and may initially simulate a slowly growing bile duct carcinoma. However, the chronicity of the process militates against neoplasm. The criteria for making the diagnosis of primary sclerosing cholangitis are as follows: (1) progressive obstructive jaundice; (2) absence of calculi in the gallbladder or biliary ducts; (3) absence of prior surgical injury to the biliary tract; (4) absence of diseases causing cholangitis; (5) absence of congenital biliary anomalies; (6) thickening and narrowing of the biliary ductal system, demonstrated by palpation at surgery, biopsy, or x-ray technics; (7) absence of biliary cirrhosis; and (8) exclusion of cholangiocarcinoma by long-term follow-up and multiple liver biopsies.

The disease is characterized by diffuse inflammation of the biliary tract, ultimately leading to fibrosis and stenosis of the common duct. Clinically, the disease presents as progressively obstructive jaundice. Treatment consists of surgical bypass such as cholecystoduodenostomy. Corticosteroids and broad-spectrum antimicrobial agents have been employed with rare success, but generally the results have been inconstant and unpredictable. The prognosis is regarded as poor, with few individuals living more than a few years after the appearance of symptoms.

Grua OE, McMurrin JA: Sclerosing cholangitis: Review and presentation of an unusual pathologic variant. Am J Surg 116:659, 1968.

Warren KW & others: Primary sclerosing cholangitis: A study of 42 cases. Am J Surg 111:23, 1966.

CARCINOMA OF THE BILIARY TRACT

Carcinoma of the gallbladder occurs in approximately 2% of all people operated on for biliary tract disease. It is notoriously insidious, and the diagnosis is usually made unexpectedly at surgery. Spread of the cancer—by direct extension into the liver or to the peritoneal surface—may be the initial manifestation.

Carcinoma of the extrahepatic bile ducts accounts for 3% of all cancer deaths in the USA. It affects both sexes equally but is more prevalent in individuals age 50–70. There is a questionable increased incidence in patients with chronic nonspecific ulcerative colitis.

Progressive jaundice is the most common and is usually the first sign of obstruction of the extrahepatic biliary system. Pain is usually present in the right upper abdomen and radiates into the back. Anorexia and weight loss are common and are frequently associated with fever and chills. Rarely, hematemesis may be a confusing presentation which results from erosion of tumor into a blood vessel. Fistulization between the biliary system and adjacent organs may also occur. The course is usually one of rapid deterioration, with death occurring within a few months.

Physical examination will reveal profound jaundice. A palpable gallbladder with obstructive jaundice usually signifies malignant disease. Courvoisier's law states that the most frequent cause of obstructive jaundice distal to the cystic duct with a normal gallbladder wall is neoplasm. This clinical generalization has been proved to be accurate about 90% of the time. Hepatomegaly is usually present and is associated with liver tenderness. Ascites may occur with peritoneal implants. Pruritus and skin excoriations are common.

Laboratory examinations reveal hyperbilirubinemia, predominantly of the conjugated variety. Total serum bilirubin values range from 5–30 mg/100 ml. There is usually concomitant elevation of the alkaline phosphatase and its hepatic isoenzyme, leucine aminopeptidase, and serum cholesterol. SGOT and SGPT are normal or minimally elevated.

The most helpful radiographic study prior to surgery is the percutaneous transhepatic cholangiogram. This procedure should be done to define the pathologic anatomy (ductal obstruction). Differentiation of benign strictures of the ductal system from progressive sclerosing cholangitis is suggested by the history of prior exploration of the hepatobiliary tree with resultant injury that was unrecognized at the time of the initial celiotomy.

Unless there are overwhelming contraindications, palliative surgery is indicated to decompress the hepatobiliary system and relieve jaundice. This can be accomplished by cholecystoduodenostomy or by T tube drainage of the common duct. The prognosis is poor, few patients surviving for more than 6 months after surgery.

DenBesten L, Liechty RD: Cancer of the biliary tree. Am J Surg 109:587, 1965.

ElDomeiri AA, Brasfield RD, O'Quinn JL: Carcinoma of the extrahepatic bile ducts. Ann Surg 169:525, 1969.

Litwin MS: Primary carcinoma of the gallbladder. Arch Surg 95:236, 1967.

Pemberton LB & others: The surgical significance of carcinoma of the gallbladder. Am J Surg 122:381, 1971.

DISEASES OF THE PANCREAS

ACUTE PANCREATITIS
(Acute Hemorrhagic Pancreatitis, Acute Interstitial Pancreatitis)

Essentials of Diagnosis

- Abrupt onset acute epigastric pain, often with back radiation.

- Nausea, vomiting, prostration, sweating.
- Abdominal tenderness and distention, fever.
- Leukocytosis, elevated serum and urinary amylase and lipase.
- History of previous episodes or alcoholic or dietary excess.

General Considerations

Acute pancreatitis is a severe abdominal disease produced by acute inflammation in the pancreas and associated "escape" of pancreatic enzymes from the acinar cells into the surrounding tissue. The pathogenesis is not known. Although more than 80 clinical causes have been related to acute pancreatitis, a large percentage of cases occur with biliary tract disease and alcoholism. Another large group is called idiopathic. Vascular and allergic causes have also been postulated. Pancreatitis may occur in association with hyperparathyroidism, hyperlipidemias, vasculitis, abdominal trauma, and during therapy with prednisone or thiazides. Pancreatitis associated with severe type IV hyperlipidemia has been reported in women who are taking oral contraceptives. Surgical manipulation in the upper abdomen may also be followed by acute pancreatitis.

Pathologic changes vary from acute edema and cellular infiltration to necrosis of the acinar cells, hemorrhage from necrotic blood vessels, and intra- and extrapancreatic fat necrosis. A portion of the gland or the entire pancreas may be involved.

Clinical Findings

A. Symptoms and Signs: Epigastric abdominal pain, generally abrupt in onset, is steady and severe, and is often made worse by lying supine and better by sitting and leaning forward. The pain usually radiates into the back but may radiate to the right or left. Nausea, vomiting, and constipation are present; and severe prostration, sweating, and anxiety are often present. There may be a history of alcoholic intake or a heavy meal immediately preceding the attack, or a history of similar, milder episodes in the past.

The abdomen is tender mainly in the upper abdomen, most often without guarding, rigidity, or rebound. The abdomen may be distended, and bowel sounds may be absent in associated paralytic ileus. Fever of 38.4–39° C (101.1–102.2° F), tachycardia, hypotension (even true shock), pallor, and a cool clammy skin are often present. Mild jaundice is common in acute pancreatitis. An upper abdominal mass may be present but is not characteristic.

B. Laboratory Findings: Leukocytosis (10,000–30,000/cu mm), proteinuria, casts (25% of cases), glycosuria (10–20% of cases), hyperglycemia and abnormal glucose tolerance curves (50% of cases), and elevated serum bilirubin may be present. BUN and serum alkaline phosphatase may be elevated and coagulation tests abnormal. Decrease in serum calcium correlates well with severity of disease; it is lowest on about the 6th day; levels < 7 mg/100 ml are associated with tetany and an unfavorable prognosis.

The serum enzymes are elevated. Serum amylase is elevated within 24 hours (in 90% of cases) and returns to normal by the third day; serum lipase rises more slowly and persists a few days longer. Urine amylase and amylase activity in the peritoneal fluid (may be very high) remain elevated longer than serum amylase.

Peritoneal fluid is yellow to reddish brown, with microscopic fat globules, and its pancreatic enzyme content is very high.

C. X-Ray Findings: X-rays may show gallstones, a "sentinel loop" of gas-distended small intestine in the left upper quadrant, or linear focal atelectasis or pleural fluid in the left pleural cavity. These findings suggest acute pancreatitis but are not diagnostic.

D. ECG Findings: ST–T wave changes may occur, but they usually differ from those of myocardial infarction. Abnormal Q waves do not occur as a result of pancreatitis.

Differential Diagnosis

Acute pancreatitis may be almost impossible to differentiate from common duct stone or perforated peptic ulcer with elevated serum amylase. It must be differentiated also from acute mesenteric thrombosis, renal colic, dissecting aortic aneurysm, acute cholecystitis, and acute intestinal obstruction. The serum amylase may also be elevated in high intestinal obstruction, mumps, and after abdominal surgery or administration of narcotics.

Complications

Pancreatic abscess is a suppurative process in necrotic tissue with rising fever, leukocytosis, and localized tenderness and epigastric mass.

Pseudocyst (a cystic structure formed from necrotic areas) develops outside the pancreas and may become very large.

Chronic pancreatitis develops in about 10% of cases.

Permanent diabetes mellitus and exocrine pancreatic insufficiency occur uncommonly.

Prevention

All associated etiologic factors should be corrected, eg, biliary tract disease, duodenal ulcers. The patient should be warned not to eat large meals or foods which are high in fat content and not to drink alcohol. The most common precipitating factor in acute pancreatitis is alcoholic indulgence.

Treatment

A. Emergency Measures for Impending Shock: Withhold food and fluids by mouth and initiate continuous nasogastric suction. The patient should be placed at bed rest and given meperidine (Demerol), 100–150 mg subcut, or pentazocine (Talwin), 30–60 mg IM, as necessary for relief of pain. Morphine may be used in cases of severe pain that cannot be controlled with other drugs. Atropine sulfate, 0.4–0.6 mg subcut, should be given as an antispasmodic.

Give 250–500 ml of plasma IV immediately and follow with subsequent infusions as necessary to correct disturbed fluid balance and maintain normal hematocrit. Two to 3 liters of 5% glucose in normal saline may be used initially if plasma is not available to correct plasma volume depletion. If shock persists after adequate volume replacement, levarterenol may be required. Central venous pressure should be monitored during parenteral fluid treatment.

Calcium gluconate must be given intravenously if there is evidence of hypocalcemia with tetany. The use of prophylactic antibiotics is controversial. If the fever exceeds 39° C (102.2° F) and blood, urine, sputum, and effusions (if present) have been cultured, it is reasonable to begin antibiotic therapy. Ampicillin, chloramphenicol, gentamicin, kanamycin, and other antibiotics have been used.

The patient should be constantly attended, and vital signs should be checked every 15–30 minutes, as indicated, during the acute phase. Blood count, hematocrit, serum amylase, and serum lipase should be observed closely.

B. Follow-Up Care: After the patient has recovered from shock (or if shock does not develop) it is necessary to choose between conservative or expectant medical management and exploratory surgery. Conservative therapy is preferred. Observe the patient closely for evidence of continued inflammation of the pancreas or related structures. A surgeon should be consulted in all cases of suspected acute pancreatitis. If the diagnosis is in doubt and there is a possibility of a serious and surgically correctable lesion (eg, perforated peptic ulcer), exploration is indicated.

In general, conservative measures are indicated when the diagnosis of pancreatitis has been established. However, in patients with severe hemorrhagic pancreatitis not responding to conservative treatment, it may be advisable to perform a laparotomy in order to remove the fluid collection or drain an abscess.

When acute pancreatitis is unexpectedly found on exploratory laparotomy, it is usually wise to close without intervention of any kind. If the pancreatitis appears mild and cholelithiasis is present, cholecystostomy or cholecystectomy may be justified. Patients with unsuspected pancreatitis who receive the least intra-abdominal manipulation have the least morbidity and mortality after laparotomy except that sump suction drainage as noted above may be indicated in severe hemorrhagic pancreatitis.

The development of a pancreatic abscess is an indication for prompt drainage, usually through the flank. If a pseudocyst develops and persists, surgical treatment may be required.

The patient should be examined frequently. Periodic blood counts, blood glucose determinations, and serum and urine enzyme determinations should be carried out as indicated. Antibiotic therapy should be reserved for patients with septic complications.

No fluid or foods should be given by mouth for at least 48 hours, and continuous nasogastric suction should be maintained for that period. After 48–72 hours, small quantities of liquid foods may be introduced gradually by mouth as tolerated. Gastric suction may be temporarily discontinued several times during the day for small oral feedings and then gradually discontinued, depending upon clinical progress. Give parenteral fluids as necessary to replace lost fluid, electrolytes, albumin, and whole blood.

Atropine sulfate, 0.4–0.6 mg subcut, may be administered 3 times daily.

C. Convalescent Care: When clinical evidence of pancreatic inflammation has cleared, place the patient on a low-fat diet and give belladonna extract, 15 mg 3 times daily, or atropine sulfate, 0.4–0.6 mg 3 times daily. Antacids should be given at hourly intervals until the acute attack subsides.

Prognosis

Recurrences are common. The mortality rate for acute hemorrhagic pancreatitis is high, especially when hepatic, cardiovascular, or renal impairment is present. Surgery is indicated only when the diagnosis is in doubt, when the patient is desperately ill despite conservative therapy, or in the presence of an associated disorder such as stones in the biliary tract.

Acosta JM, Ledesma CL: Gallstone migration as a cause of acute pancreatitis. New England J Med 290:484, 1974.

Davidoff F, Tishler S, Rosoff C: Marked hyperlipidemia and pancreatitis associated with oral contraceptive therapy. New England J Med 289:552, 1973.

Geokas MC: Acute pancreatitis. California Med 117:25, Aug 1972.

Lawson DW & others: Surgical treatment of acute necrotizing pancreatitis. Ann Surg 172:605, 1970.

Roth JA: Patients with hyperbilirubinemia and hyperamylasemia: Is the diagnosis pancreatitis or biliary lithiasis? Am J Surg 40:321, 1974.

Wyatt AP: Diagnosis and management of acute pancreatitis. Ann Roy Coll Surg England 54:229, 1974.

CHRONIC PANCREATITIS
(Chronic Relapsing Pancreatitis)

Chronic pancreatitis occurs most often in patients with alcoholism, hereditary pancreatitis, hypercalcemia, and hyperlipoproteinemias (types I, IV, and V). Progressive fibrosis and destruction of functioning glandular tissue occur as a result. Pancreaticolithiasis and obstruction of the duodenal end of the pancreatic duct are often present. Pancreatitis associated with cholelithiasis rarely recurs after cholecystectomy.

Clinical Findings

A. Symptoms and Signs: Persistent or recurrent episodes of epigastric and left upper quadrant pain with referral to the upper left lumbar region are typical. Anorexia, nausea, vomiting, constipation, and flatulence are common. Abdominal signs during attacks consist chiefly of tenderness over the pancreas, mild muscle guarding, and paralytic ileus. Attacks may last only a few hours or as long as 2 weeks; pain may eventually be almost continuous. Steatorrhea (as indicated by bulky, foul, fatty stools) and other types of intestinal malabsorption may occur.

B. Laboratory Findings: Serum amylase and bilirubin may be elevated during acute attacks. Glycosuria may be present. Excess fecal fat may be demonstrated on chemical analysis of the stool.

C. X-Ray Findings: Plain films often show pancreaticolithiasis and mild ileus. A cholecystogram may reveal biliary tract disease, and upper gastrointestinal series may demonstrate a widened duodenal loop.

Complications

Narcotic addiction is common. Other frequent complications include diabetes mellitus, pancreatic pseudocyst or abscess, cholestatic liver disease with or without jaundice, steatorrhea, malnutrition, and peptic ulcer.

Treatment

Correctable coexistent biliary tract disease should be treated surgically.

A. Medical Measures: A low-fat diet and anticholinergic drugs should be prescribed. Alcohol is forbidden because it frequently precipitates attacks. Mild sedatives may be helpful. Narcotics should be avoided if possible. Steatorrhea is treated with pancreatic supplements (Viokase, Cotazym), 3–4 gm orally during and following meals. Treat associated diabetes as for any other diabetic patient. Every effort is made to manage the disease medically.

B. Surgical Treatment: The only indication for surgery in chronic pancreatitis, other than internal drainage of persistent pseudocysts or to treat other complications, is to attempt to relieve pain. The objectives of surgical intervention are to eradicate biliary tract disease, ensure a free flow of bile into the duodenum, and eliminate obstruction of the pancreatic duct. When obstruction of the duodenal end of the duct can be demonstrated by operative pancreatography, dilatation of the duct or resection of the tail of the pancreas with implantation of the distal end of the duct by pancreaticojejunostomy may be successful. Anastomosis between the longitudinally split duct and a defunctionalized limb of jejunum without pancreatectomy may be in order. In advanced cases it may be necessary, as a last resort, to do subtotal or total pancreatectomy.

Prognosis

This is a serious disease and often leads to chronic invalidism. The prognosis is best when patients with acute pancreatitis are carefully investigated with their first attack and are found to have some remediable condition such as chronic cholecystitis and cholelithiasis, choledocholithiasis, stenosis of the sphincter of Oddi, or hyperparathyroidism. Surgical relief of these aggravating conditions may prevent recurrent pancreatic disease.

Berk JE, Guth PH: Chronic pancreatitis. M Clin North America 54:479, 1970.

Warren KW: Surgical management of chronic relapsing pancreatitis. Am J Surg 117:24, 1969.

CARCINOMA OF THE HEAD OF THE PANCREAS & THE PERIAMPULLARY AREA

Essentials of Diagnosis

- Obstructive jaundice, which may be painless.
- Enlarged gallbladder may be painful.
- Upper abdominal pain with radiation to back, weight loss, and thrombophlebitis are usually late manifestations.

General Considerations

Carcinoma is the commonest neoplasm of the pancreas. About 75% are in the head and 25% in the body and tail of the organ. Carcinomas involving the head of the pancreas, the ampulla of Vater, the common bile duct, and the duodenum are considered together because they are usually indistinguishable clinically.

Clinical Findings

A. Symptoms and Signs: Abdominal pain, jaundice, weight loss, and a palpable gallbladder are the most frequent findings in these tumors. Pain, which is present in over 70%, is often vague and diffuse in the epigastrium and is rarely comparable to biliary colic. Later, more persistent, severe pain develops and often radiates to the back. This usually indicates that the lesion has spread beyond the pancreas and is inoperable. The jaundice is obstructive and must be differentiated from the hepatocellular type. Unfortunately, it is rarely possible to make the diagnosis before jaundice occurs. Diarrhea is seen occasionally. Migratory thrombophlebitis is a rare sign. It is a useful clinical rule (Courvoisier's law) that jaundice associated with a palpable gallbladder is indicative of obstruction by neoplasm. The gallbladder is usually not palpable. A hard, fixed, occasionally tender mass may be present.

B. Laboratory Findings: There may be mild anemia. Glycosuria, hyperglycemia, and impaired glucose tolerance or true diabetes mellitus are found in 10–20% of cases. The serum amylase or lipase is occasionally elevated. Liver function responses are those of obstructive jaundice. Steatorrhea is rare. The secretin test of exocrine secretion usually has a low volume with normal bicarbonate concentration. In a few cases, duodenal cytology has shown malignant cells. Occult blood in the stool is suggestive of carcinoma of the ampulla of Vater.

C. X-Ray Findings: Hypotonic duodenography and selective celiac and superior mesenteric arteriography may be most helpful by demonstrating either the encroachment of the duodenum or abnormal vessels in the region of the pancreas. X-ray examination is usually noncontributory in involvement of the body and tail. With carcinoma of the head of the pancreas, the gastrointestinal series may show a widening of the duodenal loop, mucosal abnormalities in the duodenum ranging from edema to invasion or ulceration, or spasm or compression.

Treatment

Abdominal exploration is usually necessary to confirm the diagnosis and determine resectability, which is about 30%. Radical pancreaticoduodenal resection is indicated for lesions which are strictly limited to the head of the pancreas, periampullary zone, and duodenum. When resection is not feasible, cholecystojejunostomy is performed to relieve the jaundice. A gastrojejunostomy is also done if duodenal obstruction is expected to develop later.

Prognosis

Carcinoma of the head of the pancreas has a very poor prognosis. Five-year survival rate ranges from 2.3–5.2%. Lesions of the ampulla, common duct, and duodenum are more favorable, with a 5-year survival rate of 20–40% after resection. The operative mortality rate of radical pancreaticoduodenectomy is 10–15%.

Bowden L: Cancer of the pancreas. CA 22:275, 1972.
Dreiling DA: The early diagnosis of pancreatic cancer. Scandinav J Gastroenterol 5 (Suppl 6):115, 1970.
Kalberer JT Jr: Cancer of the pancreas. J Surg Oncol 6:1, 1974.

CARCINOMA OF THE BODY & TAIL OF THE PANCREAS

About 25% of pancreatic cancers arise in the body or tail. Islet cell tumors arise in the pancreas, as do the non-β-cell gastrin-secreting tumors associated with the Zollinger-Ellison syndrome. There are no characteristic findings in the early stages. The initial symptoms are vague epigastric or left upper quadrant distress. Anorexia and weight loss usually occur. Later, pain becomes more severe and frequently radiates through to the left lumbar region. A mass in the mid or left epigastrium may be palpable. The spontaneous development of thrombophlebitis is suggestive. The diagnosis is usually made only by abdominal exploration. Resection is rarely feasible, and cure is rarer still.

Arlen M, Brockunier A Jr: Clinical manifestations of carcinoma of the tail of the pancreas. Cancer 20:1920, 1967.
Mani JR, Zboralske FF, Margulis AR: Carcinoma of the body and tail of the pancreas. Am J Roentgenol 96:429, 1966.

ACUTE PERITONITIS

Essentials of Diagnosis

- History of abdominal illness.
- Abdominal pain, vomiting, fever, and prostration.
- Abdominal rigidity and diffuse or local tenderness (often rebound).
- Later, abdominal distention and paralytic ileus.
- Leukocytosis.

General Considerations

Localized or generalized peritonitis is the most important complication of a wide variety of acute abdominal disorders. Peritonitis may be caused by infection or chemical irritation. Perforation or necrosis of the gastrointestinal tract is the usual source of infection. Chemical peritonitis occurs in acute pancreatitis and in the early stages of gastroduodenal perforation. Regardless of the etiology, certain typical features are usually present.

Clinical Findings

A. Systemic Reaction: Malaise, prostration, nausea, vomiting, septic fever, leukocytosis, and electrolyte imbalance are usually seen in proportion to the severity of the process. If infection is not controlled, toxemia is progressive and toxic shock may develop terminally.

B. Abdominal Signs:

1. Pain and tenderness—Depending upon the extent of involvement, pain and tenderness may be localized or generalized. Abdominal pain on coughing, rebound tenderness referred to the area of peritonitis, and tenderness to light percussion over the inflamed peritoneum are characteristic. Pelvic peritonitis is associated with rectal and vaginal tenderness.

2. Muscle rigidity—The muscles overlying the area of inflammation usually become spastic. When peritonitis is generalized (eg, after perforation of a peptic ulcer), marked rigidity of the entire abdominal wall may develop immediately. Rigidity is frequently diminished or absent in the late stages of peritonitis, in severe toxemia, and when the abdominal wall is weak, flabby, or obese.

3. Paralytic ileus—Intestinal motility is markedly inhibited by peritoneal inflammation. Diminished to absent peristalsis and progressive abdominal distention are the cardinal signs. Vomiting occurs as a result of pooling of gastrointestinal secretions and gas, 70% of which is swallowed air.

C. X-Ray Findings: Abdominal films show gas and fluid collections in both large and small bowel, usually with generalized rather than localized dilatation. The bowel walls, when thrown into relief by the gas patterns, may appear to be thickened, indicating the presence of edema or peritoneal fluid. A gentle barium enema will resolve whether large bowel obstruction is present.

D. Diagnostic Abdominal Tap: Occasionally useful.

Differential Diagnosis

Peritonitis, which may present a highly variable clinical picture, must be differentiated from acute intestinal obstruction, acute cholecystitis with or without choledocholithiasis, renal colic, gastrointestinal hemorrhage, lower lobe pneumonias, porphyria, periodic fever, hysteria, and CNS disorders (eg, tabes).

Treatment

The measures employed in peritonitis as outlined below are generally applicable as supportive therapy in most acute abdominal disorders. The objectives are (1) to control infection, (2) to minimize the effects of paralytic ileus, and (3) to correct fluid, electrolyte, and nutritional disorders.

A. Specific Measures: Operative procedures to close perforations, to remove sources of infection such as gangrenous bowel or an inflamed appendix, or to drain abscesses are frequently required. The cause of the peritonitis should always be identified and treated promptly.

B. General Measures: No matter what specific operative procedures are employed, their ultimate success will often depend upon the care with which the following general measures are performed:

1. Bed rest in the medium Fowler (semi-sitting) position is preferred.

2. Nasogastric suction is started as soon as peritonitis is suspected to prevent gastrointestinal distention. Suction is continued until peristaltic activity returns and the patient begins passing flatus. A self-tending sump tube should be used, but it must be checked frequently for patency. In persistent paralytic ileus, the intestinal tract may be more adequately decompressed by means of a long intestinal tube (eg, Miller-Abbott), although passage of such a tube into the small bowel is frequently difficult because of poor intestinal motility. In rare cases, combined gastric and long intestinal tube suction may be necessary to relieve or prevent distention.

3. Give nothing by mouth. Oral intake can be resumed slowly after nasogastric suction is discontinued.

4. Fluid and electrolyte therapy and parenteral feeding are required.

5. Narcotics and sedatives should be used liberally to ensure comfort and rest.

6. Antibiotic therapy—If infection with mixed intestinal flora is probably present, combined therapy with penicillin and streptomycin is begun empirically. When cultures are available, antibiotics are chosen according to sensitivity studies.

7. Blood transfusions are used as needed to control anemia.

8. Toxic shock, if it develops, requires intensive treatment.

Complications & Prognosis

The most frequent sequel of peritonitis is abscess formation in the pelvis, in the subphrenic space, between the leaves of the mesentery, or elsewhere in the abdomen. Antibiotic therapy may mask or delay the appearance of localizing signs of abscess. When fever, leukocytosis, toxemia, or ileus fails to respond to the general measures for peritonitis, a collection of pus should be suspected. This will usually require surgical drainage. Liver abscess and pylephlebitis are rare complications. Adhesions may cause early or, more frequently, late intestinal obstruction.

If the cause of peritonitis can be corrected, the infection, accompanying ileus, and metabolic derangement can usually be managed successfully.

Bose B & others: Primary pneumococcal peritonitis. Canad MAJ 110:305, 1974.
Long WB & others: Peritonitis. J Roy Coll Surg Edinb 15:158, 1970.

. . .

PERIODIC DISEASE
(Benign Paroxysmal Peritonitis, Familial Mediterranean Fever, Periodic Fever, Recurrent Polyserositis)

Periodic disease is a heredofamilial disorder of unknown pathogenesis, probably metabolic, characterized by recurrent episodes of abdominal or chest pain, fever, and leukocytosis. It is usually restricted to people of Mediterranean ancestry, primarily Armenians, Sephardic Jews, Turks, Arabs, Greeks, and Italians. The disease suggests surgical peritonitis, but the acute attacks are recurrent, self-limited, and not fatal. Amyloidosis of the primary type occurs in some cases, and death may result from renal or cardiac failure. Acute episodes may be precipitated by emotional upsets, alcohol, or dietary indiscretion. Treatment is symptomatic and supportive. It has been suggested that a low-fat diet will reduce the number and severity of attacks.

Özer FL, Kaplaman E, Zileli S: Familial Mediterranean fever in Turkey: A report of twenty cases. Am J Med 50:336, 1971.
Sohar E & others: Familial Mediterranean fever: A survey and review of the literature. Am J Med 43:227, 1967.

11...
Diseases of the Breast

John L. Wilson

CARCINOMA OF THE FEMALE BREAST

Essentials of Diagnosis

- Be alert to the diagnosis in women who have never married or borne children; those with a family history of breast cancer; and those with a history of previous breast disease.
- Early findings: Single, nontender, firm to hard breast mass with ill-defined margins.
- Later findings: Skin or nipple retraction, axillary lymphadenopathy, breast enlargement, hardness, redness, pain, fixation of mass to skin or chest wall.
- Nipple erosion may be the only indication of early Paget's carcinoma.

General Considerations

Carcinoma of the breast is among the most common malignant tumors and is a major cause of death in women. It is the leading cause of death from cancer among women in the USA. The peak incidence is between the ages of 40 and 50, but breast cancer occurs frequently at all ages past 30. The annual incidence of breast carcinoma is about 72 per 100,000 women, and the age-adjusted death rate is about 23 per 100,000 women in the USA. In 1974, there were about 89,000 new cases and 33,000 deaths from breast cancer in American women. It is estimated that one out of every 15 American women will develop the disease at some time during her lifetime, and that 20% of deaths from cancer among women are attributable to breast cancer. There has been no great reduction in the mortality rate of this disease in the past 35 years.

Breast cancer occurs 100 times more frequently in women than in men.

Although the mean duration of life in untreated carcinoma of the breast is about 3 years, the biologic behavior of the disease is highly variable; some untreated patients succumb within a few months after the diagnosis is made, whereas others survive for 5–30 years. In general, the course of mammary cancer is related to histologic type and grade: well-differentiated tumors tend to progress more slowly. However, the choice of treatment is based primarily upon the extent of the disease and not upon the microscopic pattern of the lesion.

The relative frequency of carcinoma in various anatomic sites in the breast is as follows: upper outer quadrant, 45%; lower outer quadrant, 10%; upper inner quadrant, 15%; lower inner quadrant, 5%; central (subareolar or diffuse), 25% (Fig 11–1). Metastasis to regional lymph nodes is the principal initial mode of spread. Axillary metastases are found on microscopic study in 50–60% of patients undergoing radical mastectomy. The internal mammary nodes are invaded in about one-third of patients who have clinically advanced disease of borderline operability. When the tumor is in the center or inner half of the breast and when the axillary nodes have already been invaded, the internal mammary chain is involved in up to two-thirds of patients.

Hematogenous spread of breast cancer is common; the bones (especially the pelvis, spine, femur, ribs, skull, and humerus), lungs, and liver are most frequently affected.

The high mortality rate of breast cancer can be most effectively reduced by early detection and adequate surgical treatment. The patient herself is able to discover the early lesions when they are palpable. Regular monthly self-examination of the breasts after

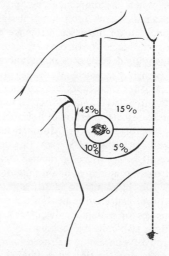

Figure 11–1. Frequency of breast carcinoma at various anatomic sites. (Reproduced, with permission, from Dunphy JE, Way LW [editors]: *Current Surgical Diagnosis & Treatment,* 2nd ed. Lange, 1975.)

each menstrual period should be practiced by all women over 30. Periodic screening examination, including mammography, is effective in detecting early breast cancer, and the mammogram may be positive before the cancer is palpable. The general availability of screening service would significantly reduce the mortality rate from carcinoma of the breast.

Etiology

The cause of breast cancer is not known, but certain conditions are associated with a higher incidence of the disease. A predisposition to breast cancer can be inherited, but the mechanism of inheritance is not clear. Numerous investigations have shown that female relatives of women with mammary carcinoma have a higher rate of disease than the general population. There is evidence that a woman has as much as twice the risk of breast cancer (as compared to the general population) if her family history includes breast cancer in her mother, aunts, or sisters. Reports of symmetric mammary cancer in monozygotic twins support the conclusion that inheritance plays a role in some cases.

Marital status and parity also influence the incidence of breast cancer. Single and nulliparous women have a slightly higher death rate from breast cancer than married and parous women. Women with 3 or more children have a lower risk than women with fewer children. Menarche after age 15 and artificial menopause are associated with a slightly lower incidence of breast cancer. These observations regarding fertility and ovarian function suggest that hormonal factors have some influence on the incidence of breast cancer. Lactation probably does not protect from breast cancer, as formerly thought. Breast cancer patients do not differ from unaffected women with respect to a history of lactation if account is taken of the fact that breast cancer patients tend to be of low parity.

Mammary dysplasia (cystic disease of the breast), particularly when accompanied by proliferative changes, papillomatosis, or solid hyperplasia, is possibly associated with an increased incidence of malignancy. This association is controversial because of the occurrence of varying degrees of mammary dysplasia in over 50% of breasts examined at autopsy in women dying of causes other than breast carcinoma. The suspected relationship between malignancy and mammary dysplasia again raises the question of hormonal factors in the etiology of breast cancer. Although the pathogenesis of cystic disease is not known, this disorder is believed to result either from a relative or absolute increase in estrogen or a relative or absolute decrease in progesterone. The inference is inescapable that the variations in hormonal environment which cause the pathologic changes of mammary dysplasia may under certain conditions also induce neoplasia.

Contraceptives containing estrogens and progestins may produce proliferation of epithelial elements within the breast and stimulation of the intralobular and interlobar connective tissues. The reaction in the ductal epithelium is particularly noticeable. Tenderness of the breasts, nodularity, galactorrhea, and fibroadenomas are among the gross breast changes which may rarely occur. While there is no definite evidence that oral contraceptives are related to human breast cancer, breast changes caused by these agents may be important to consider in differential diagnosis macroscopically and microscopically. Further information on the long-term effects of these hormonal preparations is needed. Administration of estrogens to postmenopausal women has not been found to increase the incidence of breast cancer, although fibrocystic and other benign changes in the breast are occasionally seen.

Many studies have been done in an attempt to determine whether women with breast cancer or with a predisposition to the disease show an abnormal pattern of excretion of estrogens, androgens, or hydroxycorticosteroids. These studies have proved very difficult to conduct, control, and interpret. As a result, evidence based on hormonal assays is conflicting, and it is not now possible to identify by these means those women with a high risk of developing malignancy of the breast. It does appear, however, that a significant percentage of women with carcinoma of the breast may have an abnormal hormonal environment which will be of diagnostic importance when better understood.

There is no evidence that trauma to the breast causes cancer. Both breast trauma and cancer are common. When trauma precedes the discovery of cancer, it can be taken as coincidence rather than a cause and effect relationship.

Age-adjusted female cancer death rates show that, in general, rates reported from developing countries are low, whereas rates are high in developed countries, with the notable exception of Japan. Some of the variability may be due to underdiagnosis and underreporting in the developing countries or to differences in reporting practices, but undoubtedly there are environmental, dietary, hormonal, fertility, genetic, or other factors yet to be determined. There has been great interest in the low breast cancer rate in Japanese women, which is well illustrated by statistics from California. Although their breast cancer rates remain relatively low, Japanese women who have migrated to the USA and their daughters born in the USA show some increase in rates over those who stay in Japan.

Routine scanning of data from a multipurpose survey of inpatients in hospitals in the Boston area revealed an association between reserpine use and breast cancer (Boston Collaborative Drug Surveillance Program; Lancet 2:669, 1974). Similar findings were reported from England and Finland (Lancet 2:672, 1974; Lancet 2:675, 1974). More recent surveys by O'Fallon WM & others (Lancet 2:292, 1975), Laska EM & others (Lancet 2:296, 1975), and Mack TM & others (New England J Med 292:1366, 1975) have failed to confirm the relationship between chronic reserpine administration and breast cancer. An editorial by Jick H (JAMA 233:896, 1975) points out the difficulty of disproving the hypothesis that there is an association between reserpine and breast cancer. Pending further study of this question, individual physicians, together with their patients, must exercise their own judgment regarding the use of reserpine.

Clinical Findings

A. Symptoms and Signs: The primary complaint in about 80% of patients is a lump (usually painless) in the breast. Less frequent symptoms are breast pain; erosion, retraction, enlargement, discharge, or itching of the nipple; and redness, generalized hardness, enlargement, or shrinkage of the breast. Rarely, an axillary mass, swelling of the arm, or bone pain (from metastases) may be the first symptom.

A lesion smaller than 1 cm in diameter may be difficult or impossible for the examiner to feel and yet may be discovered by the patient. She should always be asked to demonstrate the location of the mass; if the physician fails to confirm her suspicions, he should repeat the examination in 1 month. During the premenstrual phase of the cycle, increased innocuous nodularity may suggest neoplasm or may obscure an underlying lesion. If there is any question regarding the nature of an abnormality under these circumstances, the patient should be asked to return after her period.

Examination of the breast should be meticulous, methodical, and gentle. Careful inspection, with the patient sitting, arms at her sides and overhead, and palpation, with the patient supine, arms abducted, are essential; unless this procedure is followed at all physical examinations, early lesions may be missed. In some series, 5–10% of cases of breast carcinoma have been discovered during physical examinations performed for other purposes.

The axillary and cervical regions must be examined carefully for lymphadenopathy. The location, size, consistency, and other physical features of all lesions should be recorded on a drawing of the breast for future reference.

Breast cancer usually consists of a nontender firm or hard lump with poorly delimited margins (caused by local infiltration). Slight skin or nipple retraction is an important sign. Minimal asymmetry of the breast may be noted. Very small (1–2 mm) erosions of the nipple epithelium may be the only manifestation of carcinoma of the Paget type. Watery, serous, or bloody nipple discharge is an infrequent early sign. The following are characteristic of advanced carcinoma: edema, redness, nodularity, or ulceration of the skin; the presence of a large breast mass; fixation to the chest wall; enlargement, shrinkage, or retraction of the breast; marked axillary lymphadenopathy; ipsilateral supraclavicular lymphadenopathy; and distant metastases.

B. Special Clinical Forms of Breast Carcinoma:

1. Paget's carcinoma—The basic lesion is intraductal carcinoma, usually well differentiated and multicentric in the nipple and breast ducts. The nipple epithelium is infiltrated, but gross nipple changes are often minimal and a tumor mass may not be palpable. The first symptom is often itching or burning of the nipple accompanied by a superficial erosion or ulceration. The diagnosis is readily established by biopsy of the erosion.

Paget's carcinoma is not common (about 3% of all breast cancers), but it is important because it appears innocuous. It is frequently diagnosed and treated as dermatitis or bacterial infection, leading to unfortunate delay in diagnosis. When the lesion consists of nipple changes only, the incidence of axillary metastases is about 5%. When a breast tumor is also present, the incidence of axillary metastases rises to about 67% with an associated marked decrease in prospects for cure by surgical or other treatment.

2. Inflammatory carcinoma—This is the most malignant form of breast cancer and comprises about 3% of all cases. The clinical findings consist of a rapidly growing, sometimes painful mass which enlarges the breast. The overlying skin becomes erythematous, edematous, and warm. The diagnosis should be made clinically only when the redness involves more than one-third of the skin over the breast. The inflammatory changes, often mistaken for an infectious process, are caused by carcinomatous invasion of the dermal lymphatics with resulting edema and hyperemia (Ellis DL, Teitelbaum SL: Cancer 33:1045, 1974; Saltzstein SL: Cancer 34:82, 1974). These tumors may be caused by a variety of histologic types. Metastases occur early and widely in all cases, and for this reason inflammatory carcinoma is virtually incurable. Radical mastectomy is rarely indicated. Radiation and hormone therapy are usually of little value but may be tried.

C. Laboratory Findings: Carcinoma localized to the breast and axillary nodes causes no abnormalities detectable by clinical laboratory examinations. Certain tests may be useful as clues to the presence of more widespread disease. A consistently elevated sedimentation rate may be the result of disseminated cancer. Liver metastases may be associated with elevation of alkaline phosphatase. Hypercalcemia is an occasional important finding in advanced malignancy of the breast.

D. X-Ray Findings: Because of the frequency of metastases to the bones and lungs, preparation for a radical mastectomy should include posteroanterior and lateral chest films. Anteroposterior and lateral views of the lumbar spine and pelvis and lateral skull x-ray should also be taken preoperatively in all except early lesions. Mammography of the unaffected breast, either preoperatively or after the diagnosis has been established in a potentially curable lesion of the opposite breast, is advisable as an aid in identifying occult carcinoma. A baseline mammogram of the unaffected breast is also of value for comparison with future examinations.

E. Radionuclide Scanning: Bone scans utilizing a bone-seeking nuclide such as ^{85}Sr, ^{87m}Sr, or ^{18}F with a rectilinear scanner or gamma camera are more sensitive than skeletal x-rays in detecting metastatic breast cancer. Therefore, the use of bone scan in the diagnostic evaluation of patients with breast cancer prior to radical surgery has been advocated even in the absence of symptoms or of findings on roentgenograms (Hoffman HC, Marty R: Am J Surg 124:194, 1972). Unexpected bony metastases, even in early breast cancer, have been discovered on bone scans with sufficient frequency to warrant giving serious consideration to this relatively simple procedure before performing mastectomy for cancer. On the other hand, experience at the Memorial Hospital for Cancer and Allied Diseases in New York suggests that routine bone scan or skeletal x-rays (or both) prior to definitive therapy are not warranted "unless the patient has a borderline operable situation or has bone pain" (Robbins GF & others: Cancer 29:1702, 1972).

Radionuclide scanning of liver and brain is of value when metastases are suspected in these areas.

F. Mammography: A mammogram is a special soft tissue x-ray of the breast which is of great diagnostic value. Mammography is the only reliable means of detecting breast cancer prior to the appearance of signs and symptoms. Many breast cancers can be diagnosed by mammography as long as 2 years prior to their clinical recognition, and recent reports indicate that certain premalignant conditions of the breast may be identifiable.

The 2 methods in common use for obtaining mammograms are ordinary film radiography and xeroradiography. In the latter method, in lieu of a roentgen film, an aluminum plate with an electrically charged selenium layer is exposed to x-rays and the electrostatic image is transferred to paper by a special process.

Xeroradiography is the superior technic for mammography because xeroradiographs require less radiation, afford more soft tissue detail, are more accurate, and are easier and faster to interpret (Wolfe JN & others: Cancer 28:1569, 1971).

Various other technics of earlier detection such as thermography, ultrasonography, isotope scanning, and angiography are still experimental. There has now been considerable experience with thermography, which has not yet proved to be a reliable screening method because of the high incidence of false-negative and false-positive examinations (Lewis JD & others: Arch Surg 110:903, 1975).

1. Indications—Indications for mammography include the following:

a. To supplement the annual physical examination of women, particularly those with a family history of breast cancer; and to accompany physical examination in mass screening for breast cancer.

b. To survey the opposite breast at the time a diagnosis of breast cancer is made and annually thereafter as a means of ensuring early diagnosis of a second primary.

c. As an aid in evaluating breasts with ill-defined or questionable masses; multiple masses; nipple discharge, erosion, or retraction; skin change; or pain.

d. As an aid to prebiopsy evaluation to determine the most useful biopsy site.

e. As an aid in the search for occult primary cancer in the presence of metastatic disease from an unknown primary.

f. To serve as follow-up for inoperable cases treated by chemotherapy.

g. To serve as reassurance for women with can-

cerophobia.

Both false-positive and false-negative results are obtained with mammography, but if mammography is employed proficiently and extensively the percentage of malignant lesions reported on biopsy remains around 35%—and this in spite of the fact that more biopsies are done. Screening programs which include mammography result in earlier diagnosis and reduced mortality from breast cancer.

2. Usefulness and limitations—The advantages of mammography are as follows: (1) It may demonstrate early and operable breast neoplasms when clinical findings are minimal or absent; (2) a negative result helps to confirm the surgeon's impression of the benign nature of a lesion; and (3) in proved carcinoma of the breast, mammography can at times demonstrate unsuspected carcinoma of the opposite breast.

Although false-negative and false-positive readings occur, the experienced radiologist can interpret mammograms correctly in about 90% of cases.

G. Biopsy: The ultimate diagnosis of breast tumors depends upon examination of tissue removed by surgical biopsy. The safest course is to biopsy all suspicious masses found on physical examination and, in the absence of a mass, suspicious lesions demonstrated by mammography.

Treatment of breast cancer should never be undertaken without an unequivocal histologic diagnosis. It is often appropriate to accomplish this by biopsy performed under local or general anesthesia in the operating room without admitting the patient to the hospital. Needle biopsy, which is an office procedure, may be adequate in some cases. If the tumor is malignant and suitable for surgical treatment, the patient is then scheduled for early hospital admission and definitive operation. As an alternative, the patient may be admitted to the hospital where the diagnosis is established by open biopsy with frozen section, usually under general anesthesia. If the frozen section is positive, the surgeon proceeds immediately with mastectomy. This latter approach subjects many patients to unnecessary hospitalization since cancer is found in only about 35% of patients who require biopsy for a breast lump.

H. Cytology: Cytologic examination of nipple discharge or cyst fluid may rarely be helpful. Breast biopsy is generally required for bloody or questionable secretions.

Differential Diagnosis

The diagnosis of a breast lump should be established without delay, either by biopsy or by careful observation of the clinical course. The following lesions are most likely to be confused with carcinoma: mammary dysplasia (cystic disease of the breast), fibroadenoma, intraductal papilloma, and fat necrosis.

Differential diagnosis usually depends upon biopsy. Indications for biopsy of the breast include the following: (1) persistent mass, (2) bloody nipple discharge, (3) eczematoid nipple, and (4) positive mammography. Unexplained axillary adenopathy calls for biopsy of the enlarged node. Random or mirror image biopsy of the contralateral breast is practiced in some centers when the diagnosis of operable breast cancer is established. This procedure is most clearly justified in lobular carcinoma, which is frequently bilateral. In patients at high risk of developing breast cancer, biopsy for minimal or equivocal change is justified.

In experienced hands, needle aspiration of discrete, spherical lesions of the breast is a useful means of distinguishing the benign cysts of mammary dysplasia from a solid tumor which may be cancer. Turbid greenish or amber fluid is characteristic of a benign cyst which should disappear completely without residual mass when aspirated. Cytologic examination of the fluid should be considered. Blood-tinged fluid or a persistent mass after aspiration is an indication for biopsy. In any case, patients who develop cysts possibly have an increased risk of breast cancer and should be followed regularly. A baseline mammogram should be obtained. When in doubt regarding the diagnosis of a mass in the breast, biopsy should be performed.

Clinical Staging

Patients with breast cancer can be grouped into stages according to the characteristics of the primary tumor (T), regional lymph nodes (N), and distant metastases (M). Physical, radiologic, and other clinical examinations, usually including biopsy of the primary lesion, are used in determining the stage, which is based on all information available before therapy. Staging is useful in estimating the prognosis and deciding on the type of treatment to be advised. The International Union Against Cancer and the American Joint Committee on Cancer Staging and End Results Reporting have each formulated a standard TNM system to be used by physicians in breast cancer staging.

From the practical point of view, it is useful to remember that the International and American systems of staging differ only in detail from the following brief definition of stages:

Stage I: The tumor is confined to the breast. There may be early signs of skin involvement such as dimpling or nipple retraction, but there are no signs of axillary or distant metastases.

Stage II: The primary tumor is as in stage I, but there are movable, suspicious nodes in the ipsilateral axilla.

Stage III: The primary tumor is infiltrating the skin or chest wall, or the axillary nodes are matted or fixed.

Stage IV: Distant metastases are present.

The clinician must decide treatment and prognosis in breast cancer patients whose extent of disease ranges from minimal to advanced. Judgment on management and outlook is improved if patients are systematically classified or "staged" in a manner which allows comparison with similar cases treated by others. Both the International and the American staging systems provide sound criteria for the clinical classification of patients with breast cancer (Table 11-1).

Table 11-1. Five-year survival after radical mastectomy according to stage of breast cancer.

Stage	International System	American System
I	80%	75%
II	70%	65%
III	50%	45%
IV	0	0

Pathologic Types

The behavior of breast cancer can be correlated with the histologic appearance of the lesion. Information on the microscopic characteristics of the neoplasm is therefore helpful in determining treatment and prognosis. Kouchoukos NT & others (Cancer 20:948, 1967) have distinguished 4 types of mammary carcinoma on the basis of cellular differentiation and invasiveness. Type I lesions, as exemplified by noninvasive intraductal, papillary, or lobular carcinoma, rarely metastasize (about 13% of cases have positive axillary nodes). Type II cancers, as exemplified by invasive but relatively well differentiated tumors, metastasize somewhat more frequently (about 34% positive axillary nodes). Type III and type IV lesions are generally less well differentiated cancers which have a greater tendency to metastasize (55–60% positive nodes).

In most statistical studies of survival after treatment for carcinoma of the breast, the various pathologic types are not separately identified. More attention is now being given to histologic appearance, which clearly influences the frequency of metastases and curability.

Curative Treatment

Treatment may be curative or palliative. Curative treatment is advised for clinical stage I and stage II disease and for selected patients in stage III. Palliative treatment by radiation, hormones, endocrine ablation, or chemotherapy is recommended for patients in stage IV (distant metastases), for stage III patients unsuitable for curative efforts, and for previously treated patients who develop distant metastases or ineradicable local recurrence.

A. Types of Curative Treatment:

1. Standard radical mastectomy—This operation involves en bloc removal of breast, pectoral muscles, and axillary nodes and has been the standard curative procedure for breast cancer since the turn of the century, when W. S. Halsted and Willy Meyer independently described their versions of the technic. Experience with radical mastectomy is extensive, and no other form of therapy has produced better results in properly selected patients. Radical mastectomy removes the local lesion and the axillary nodes with a wide safety margin of surrounding tissue. If the disease has already spread to the internal mammary or supraclavicular nodes or to more distant sites, radical mastectomy alone will not cure the patient.

2. Extended radical mastectomy—This procedure involves, in addition to standard radical mastectomy, the removal of the internal mammary nodes. It does not appear that extended radical mastectomy is significantly more effective than irradiation in preventing recurrence from internal mammary metastases. For that reason, extended radical mastectomy has few advocates at this time.

3. Modified radical mastectomy—This procedure involves complete removal of all breast and subcutaneous tissue (as in standard radical mastectomy) and dissection in continuity of the axillary lymphatic bed up to the level of the coracoid process. The difference between the modified and the standard radical mastectomy is that the standard operation also removes the pectoralis major and minor muscles and the highest group of axillary nodes just inferior to the clavicle. There is now considerable evidence that morbidity, mortality, survival, and local recurrence rates for standard and modified radical mastectomy are essentially the same for stage I and stage II breast cancer. Prospective controlled clinical studies will be needed to settle the issue in a definitive manner, but there is already a notable shift in major centers to the use of modified radical mastectomy in patients who, a few years ago, would have been treated by standard radical mastectomy.

4. Simple mastectomy—If the malignancy is confined to the breast without spread to the adjacent muscles or to the regional nodes or beyond (true clinical stage I disease), simple mastectomy (or even wide local excision) should be effective in eradicating the cancer. Clinical experience bears this out in certain cases. The problem is the inability to determine with certainty, prior to their resection and pathologic examination, that the axillary nodes are not involved. Physical examination is highly unreliable in detecting axillary metastases. Simple mastectomy must, therefore, be considered an inadequate operation for breast cancer until more is known about the risk associated with leaving axillary metastases until they become clinically evident.

5. Local excision—Limited procedures such as local excision ("lumpectomy"), quadrant excision, partial mastectomy, and subcutaneous mastectomy have been suggested as definitive treatment for early breast cancer such as small stage I lesions in the periphery of the breast laterally, particularly if the tumor is of histologic type I. Crile (Crile G Jr, Hoerr SO: Surg Gynec Obst 132:780, 1971; Crile G Jr: Lancet 1:549, 1972) has been the most prominent recent advocate of limited resection. Although patients with strictly localized disease adequately excised will be cured by local excision, the hazards of local recurrence and of leaving unsuspected metastases in axillary nodes are as yet undetermined and are possibly serious (Anglem JJ, Leber RE: Ann Surg 176:625, 1972; CA 23:330, 1973). Limited surgical procedures which remove less than the entire breast have not been scientifically proved to be as effective as mastectomy and are therefore not recommended for operable breast cancer except under carefully controlled conditions such as a prospective clinical trial.

6. Supervoltage irradiation—The efficacy of supervoltage irradiation in sterilizing the primary lesion and the axillary and internal mammary nodes has made radiation therapy with or without simple mastectomy (or wedge resection) an important option for primary treatment of certain breast cancers, particularly those that are locally advanced or when the patient refuses mastectomy.

B. Choice of Primary Treatment for Breast Cancer: There is evidence that control of mammary cancer confined to the breast and axillary nodes can be achieved by a number of different approaches as outlined above. Variability in tumor-host relationships from patient to patient and the unpredictability of occult metastases make it difficult to determine with precision the relative merits of current competing forms of treatment without controlled prospective clinical trials. Relying on the evidence now at hand, modified radical mastectomy is recommended as the primary treatment of choice in stage I and stage II lesions.

In considering the overall program of treatment for patients with stage II disease (positive axillary nodes), it is essential to keep in mind that most of these patients already have occult metastases elsewhere in the body. This is shown by the treatment failure and survival information which has recently been obtained from a 10-year follow-up of patients in the National Surgical Adjuvant Breast Project clinical trial begun in 1958. This study showed that, following radical mastectomy, 76% of all patients with positive axillary nodes (65% with 1–3 and 86% of those with 4 or more positive) were treatment failures by 10 years. The survival of those with 1–3 positive nodes was 37.5%; it was only 13.4% when more than 4 nodes contained tumor. Especially disturbing was the observation that 25% of patients with negative nodes were treatment failures by 10 years (Fisher B, Wolmark N: Cancer [Suppl] 36:627, 1975). This underscores the significance of recent clinical trials which indicate the effectiveness of adjuvant chemotherapy after mastectomy in increasing the tumor-free period in patients with positive axillary nodes (see p 981).

Stage III lesions are a borderline group and may or may not be suitable for surgical treatment by standard or modified radical mastectomy. Radical surgical treatment is usually contraindicated in stage III lesions with the following characteristics: (1) Extensive edema involving more than one-third of the skin of the breast. (2) Satellite nodules on the skin. (3) Carcinoma of the inflammatory type. (4) Parasternal tumor nodules. (5) Edema of the ipsilateral arm. (6) Palpable ipsilateral infraclavicular lymph nodes (metastases suspected or proved by biopsy). (7) Two or more of the following grave signs of locally advanced carcinoma: (a) ulceration of the skin; (b) limited edema involving less than one-third of the skin of the breast; (c) fixation of axillary lymph nodes to the skin or the deep structures of the axilla; (d) axillary lymph nodes measuring 2.5

cm or more in transverse diameter; (e) pectoral muscle or chest wall attachment.

The features listed above are signs of advanced disease and are almost invariably associated with spread to the internal mammary or supraclavicular nodes or other distant sites outside the scope of either standard or modified radical mastectomy. Under these circumstances, operation is not curative and may actually encourage dissemination of the disease locally or systemically. Radiotherapy with or without simple mastectomy (or wedge resection) is a more effective approach in these advanced stage III cases.

There remain those stage III lesions which do not exhibit the advanced signs listed above. A modified radical mastectomy may be performed if the primary tumor and the enlarged axillary nodes can clearly be excised with an adequate margin by this procedure. Attachment to the pectoral muscles, high axillary nodes, large primary tumor or nodes, or other technically unfavorable conditions would make standard radical mastectomy the preferred operation. Adjunctive chemotherapy should be considered in all stage III lesions.

C. Radiotherapy as Adjunct to Radical Mastectomy: The purposes of preoperative or postoperative radiotherapy in association with modified or standard radical mastectomy are (1) to reduce the incidence of local recurrence from residual cancer in the operative field and (2) to sterilize metastatic cancer in the internal mammary and supraclavicular lymph nodes. Patients are, therefore, selected for radiotherapy on the basis of the likelihood of local recurrence or of the existence of disease in unresected regional nodes. According to these criteria, completely resectable lesions confined to the breast (stage I) do not call for radiotherapy. On the other hand, stage II and stage III patients may be considered for radiotherapy before or after modified or standard radical mastectomy. Only supervoltage irradiation should be advised as adjunctive therapy. Orthovoltage irradiation for this purpose is outmoded.

1. Preoperative radiotherapy—The beneficial results of preoperative radiotherapy are more definite than those of postoperative radiotherapy. Preoperative irradiation reduces the incidence of local recurrence and may improve the 10-year survival rate. One investigator (Fletcher GH: JAMA 200:140, 1967; Cancer 29:545, 1972) demonstrated a 5% local recurrence rate after preoperative radiotherapy—compared to a 16% local recurrence rate following postoperative radiotherapy. Preoperative radiotherapy is possibly also of value in making inoperable patients curable by radical mastectomy, although in such patients the results may not be superior to those obtainable by radiotherapy alone.

Indications for preoperative irradiation include the following: (1) Primary tumor larger than 5 cm. (2) Limited skin edema or direct skin involvement over tumor. (3) Multiple low or midaxillary nodes. (4) A prior surgical intervention which may have disseminated the tumor locally. A 4000–6000 rad tumor dose is delivered to the axillary, supraclavicular, and internal mammary nodes, and the chest wall and breast are treated tangentially. Radical mastectomy is performed 5–6 weeks after completion of radiotherapy.

2. Postoperative radiotherapy—The efficacy of postoperative irradiation in improving survival or recurrence rates has not been demonstrated. However, in view of the proved ability of supervoltage radiotherapy to destroy cancer cells in the breast and regional nodes, postoperative radiotherapy is commonly recommended under the following conditions: (1) The tumor is cut through or there is a high likelihood that residual tumor has been left in the operative field. (2) The tumor is larger than 5 cm or is located in the central or medial portion of the breast. (3) There are metastases to the axillary nodes. Radiotherapy is begun as soon after operation as the patient's general condition and state of the wound permit. A tumor dose in the range of 4000–6000 rads is delivered in 4–5 weeks, primarily to the internal mammary and supra- and infraclavicular nodal areas. The chest wall may also be irradiated.

When irradiation is properly managed, delayed wound healing, pulmonary damage, and lymphedema of the arm are infrequent problems.

D. Chemotherapy as Adjunct to Radical Mastectomy: Chemotherapy is now recognized as an important adjunct to primary therapy of breast cancer in patients with stage II and III disease who are selected for curative treatment by surgery or irradiation (see Chapter 32).

Palliative Treatment

A. Radiotherapy: Palliative radiotherapy may be advised for locally advanced cancers with distant metastases in order to control ulceration, pain, and other manifestations in the breast and regional nodes. Radical irradiation of the breast and chest wall and the axillary, internal mammary, and supraclavicular nodes should be undertaken in an attempt to cure locally advanced and inoperable lesions when there is no evidence of distant metastases. A small number of patients in this group are cured in spite of extensive breast and regional node involvement. Adjuvant chemotherapy should be considered for such patients.

Palliative irradiation is also of value in the treatment of certain bone or soft tissue metastases to control pain or avoid fracture, particularly when hormonal therapy, endocrine ablation, and chemotherapy are either inappropriate or ineffective. Radiotherapy is especially useful in the treatment of the isolated bony metastasis.

B. Hormone Therapy: When distant metastases have occurred in breast cancer, the patient is incurable, but disseminated disease may be kept under control or made to regress for sustained periods by various forms of endocrine therapy including administration of hormones or ablation of ovaries, adrenals, or hypophysis. About one-third of breast cancer patients will respond to one or more of these endocrine measures. The incidence of hormonal responsiveness is approximately the same in premenopausal women as in older postmenopausal women, although the methods of treatment used may be quite different.

Ablation of ovarian secretion by oophorectomy or irradiation of the ovaries is, in the premenopausal patient, the simplest and most reliable method of obtaining tumor regression in advanced breast cancer. Administration of estrogen to premenopausal patients—or to patients whose tumor has responded favorably to castration—may stimulate tumor growth. These observations have led to the hypothesis of estrogen dependence to explain the tumor regression seen in some breast cancers after castration, bilateral adrenalectomy, or hypophysectomy. According to this hypothesis, reactivation of tumor growth after control by castration is due to increasing estrogen secretion from the adrenal cortex. Bilateral adrenalectomy at this stage is known to cause further tumor regression in some cases. Subsequently, when the tumor reactivates after control by adrenalectomy, hypophyseal ablation may have an effect by eliminating secretion of both FSH and ACTH, which are capable of activating ectopic adrenal sources of estrogen. The assumption of estrogen dependence thus appears to explain the clinical remission of tumor growth seen after endocrine ablation therapy in some patients with late breast cancer. However, biochemical methods of estrogen determination have failed to show a correlation between clinical response and quantitative change in estrogen secretion. Furthermore, the estrogen dependence hypothesis cannot explain regression of some tumors after estrogen, androgen, or progestin therapy. Therefore, a combination of direct effect by metabolic products of the steroid on the tumor and of indirect effect via the pituitary (eg, alteration in prolactin or other pituitary secretion) is a postulated cause of tumor regression in steroid therapy of breast cancer. Since different tumors probably vary in their response to hormonal therapy (depending on the hormonal environment in which they have developed), the choice of a suitable steroid for therapy in each patient may be difficult. Nevertheless, certain general principles can be followed as guides to endocrine therapy.

Endocrine therapy is employed when surgery and irradiation have failed or when widespread metastases have rendered them useless. Many patients are candidates for a trial of hormone treatment because about half of all patients with breast cancer and 60–80% of those having positive axillary nodes at the time of mastectomy will develop metastatic lesions. The major forms of hormone treatment are (1) estrogen, (2) androgen, and (3) corticosteroid therapy.

Methods for the identification of those patients most likely to benefit from the administration of hormones or ablation of endocrine glands are now available. Normal mammary cells contain cytoplasmic or membrane receptor sites for estrogen. When malignant transformation occurs, those breast cancers which retain all or part of the estrogen receptor sites are most susceptible to endocrine control, and their growth may be reduced by altering the hormonal environment. Those breast cancers which do not retain estrogen receptor sites are unlikely to respond to endocrine abla-

tion or hormonal therapy. It is now possible to assay breast cancer tissue from either the primary tumor or metastases for the presence of estrogen receptors. In view of the importance of this information as a guide to future treatment, it is advisable to obtain an estrogen receptor analysis on every breast cancer at the time of initial diagnosis if possible (McGuire WL: Cancer [Suppl] 36:638, 1975).

1. Estrogen therapy—Estrogens should be reserved for postmenopausal women. The best results of estrogen administration are obtained in women more than 5 years past the menopause. Estrogen is capable of causing exacerbation of tumor growth in 50% of premenopausal women and should not be given to them or to recently postmenopausal women until the vaginal smear ceases to show evidence of estrogenic activity. Tumor remission rates from estrogen (and androgen as well) tend to increase with increasing number of years past the menopause.

Estrogen administered as primary therapy will induce tumor regression in over 30% of postmenopausal patients with advanced breast cancer. Objective evidence of tumor regression is seen most commonly in soft tissue metastases in older patients, and over 40% of this group show remission of tumor growth. Both local soft tissue and visceral lesions show a higher remission rate from estrogen than from androgen therapy. The reverse is true for bone metastases. When estrogen receptor assay of the cancer is positive, the response rate to estrogen therapy is about 65%. When the assay is negative for estrogen receptors, the response rate is only about 9% (McGuire WL: Cancer [Suppl] 36:638, 1975).

Treatment usually consists of giving diethylstilbestrol, 5 mg 3 times daily orally (or equivalent) and should be continued as long as it is beneficial.

Initial evidence of regression of metastatic cancer is usually not seen until about 4 weeks after beginning estrogen therapy, but the trial of estrogen should not be abandoned in less than 2 months except in case of obvious exacerbation or serious side-effects. The average duration of remission is about 16 months, but remissions of soft tissue lesions of over 5 years are occasionally seen. The survival time of those who respond to estrogen therapy is about twice that of nonresponders.

The commonest side-effects are anorexia, nausea, and vomiting. These usually disappear within a few weeks, but when symptoms of toxicity are severe the dosage should be reduced temporarily until tolerance is acquired. Pigmentation of nipples, areolas, and axillary skin; enlargement of the breasts; and sodium and water retention are other side-effects of estrogen therapy. Uterine bleeding occurs in the majority of postmenopausal patients when estrogen therapy is stopped, and patients should be told of this possibility to avoid anxiety. Severe bleeding can usually be controlled by administration of testosterone proprionate, 100 mg IM daily for 3 or 4 doses.

There is evidence that various synthetic progestins with antiestrogenic action such as megestrol acetate

(Megace) are also moderately effective in the treatment of disseminated breast cancer (Ansfield FJ & others: Cancer 33:607, 1974).

2. Androgen therapy—Androgen administration causes temporary amenorrhea in premenopausal women. Tumor regression is noted in 20% of such patients with advanced breast cancer. However, because of the more frequent and prolonged remission from castration, this procedure is preferred as initial treatment in the premenopausal group. Androgen therapy may be usefully added to castration in patients under 35 years of age, or in the presence of bone metastases, because of the poor results from castration alone in such patients. Failure of response to castration may be considered an indication for a trial of androgen therapy because of the low likelihood of a favorable response by these patients to adrenalectomy or hypophysectomy.

Estrogen therapy is not advisable in recently postmenopausal women until the vaginal smear ceases to show evidence of estrogenic activity because of the danger of exacerbating the disease. A trial of androgen therapy is warranted in this group, but the expectation of favorable response is only about 15% of patients.

Since bone metastases are commonly more responsive to androgen than to estrogen therapy, a trial of androgen may be advantageous when osseous lesions are present, particularly before adrenalectomy or hypophysectomy is undertaken. About 25% of patients more than 5 years past the menopause with bone metastases will respond to androgen therapy. Patients failing to respond can still be subjected to operation if indicated, and surgery will usually have been delayed only about 6 weeks.

Postmenopausal patients who have shown a favorable response to castration or estrogen therapy and have then relapsed may be given a trial of androgen therapy with a 20–30% chance of favorable response. In patients more than 5 years past the menopause, bony metastases which have failed to respond to estrogens are more likely to regress on secondary androgen therapy than are soft tissue metastases. Occasionally, androgen administration will cause tumor regression in the completely hypophysectomized patient.

When estrogen receptor assay of the cancer is positive, the response rate to androgen therapy is about 45%. When the assay is negative, the response rate is only about 8% (McGuire WL: Cancer [Suppl] 36:638, 1975).

Androgen may be given continuously as long as tumor regression persists. It is probably preferable, however, to administer androgen until the tumor has regressed maximally and then discontinue administration until reactivation occurs, at which time resumption of androgen therapy will often lead to another regression. Intermittent therapy of this kind has the advantage of reducing the tendency to virilization while varying the hormonal environment of the tumor, thereby possibly postponing the development of autonomy in the tumor.

The androgen preparation frequently employed is testosterone propionate, 100 mg IM 3 times a week. However, it is simpler and equally effective to give fluoxymesterone (Halotestin), 20–40 mg daily orally. An orally administered nonvirilizing androgen, testolactone (Teslac), in a dosage of 1000–2000 mg daily, is reported to be slightly less effective than testosterone propionate in causing tumor regression. The major interest in this compound is that, since it appears to be relatively inert hormonally, it may have a direct effect on the breast cancer.

About 3 months of androgen therapy are usually required for maximal response. Pain relief may be achieved in up to 80% of patients with osseous metastases. In addition, androgen therapy usually results in a sense of well-being and an increase in energy and weight, particularly in postmenopausal patients. The principal adverse side-reactions are increased libido and masculinizing effects, eg, hirsutism, hoarseness, loss of scalp hair, acne, and ruddy complexion. Virilization occurs in practically all women taking testosterone propionate for longer than 6 months but in only about one-third of patients on fluoxymesterone. Fluid retention, anorexia, vomiting, and hepatotoxicity are among the rarer side-effects of androgen therapy.

Estrogen and androgen therapy is generally of limited value in patients with metastases to the liver or lungs.

3. Corticosteroids—Corticosteroids are especially valuable in the management of the serious acute symptoms which may result from such conditions as hypercalcemia, brain and lung metastases, and hepatic metastases with jaundice. Corticosteroid therapy is also indicated for patients who are too ill for major endocrine ablation therapy and for those whose tumors do not respond to other endocrine therapy. The combination of systemic corticosteroid and the intracavitary injection of an alkylating agent (see Chapter 32) may be effective in controlling pleural effusion due to metastatic breast cancer.

The patient's age and previous response to sex hormone therapy are not correlated with response to corticosteroid therapy, which probably acts through a local effect upon the tumor or the tumor bed. Previous response to corticosteroids does not predict a similar response to adrenalectomy. Objective evidence of tumor regression following corticosteroid administration is less than that following adrenalectomy. Remission on corticosteroid therapy averages about 6 months, whereas that following adrenalectomy is over 12 months.

The subjective response of the seriously ill patient to corticosteroid administration is often striking. Appetite, sense of well-being, and pain from bone or visceral metastases may be markedly improved. However, objective regression of soft tissue lesions occurs in only about 15% of patients. The relief of coma from brain metastases and dyspnea from lung metastases is often encouraging but transient. Hypercalcemia is probably improved by specific action on calcium metabolism.

Cortisone, 150 mg, or prednisone or prednisolone, 30 mg, is an average daily oral dose. Twice or 3 times this dosage may be required temporarily for control of severe, acute symptoms. A variety of other corticosteroids have been employed in equivalent dosage with similar results. The dosage of corticosteroids must be reduced slowly if they have been used for prolonged periods because of the adrenocortical atrophy that is induced.

Adrenocortical hormones may cause numerous undesirable systemic effects and serious complications such as uncontrollable infection, bleeding peptic ulcer, muscle weakness, hypertension, diabetes, edema, and features of Cushing's syndrome.

The best overall tumor remission rate from hormonal therapy in postmenopausal patients can probably be obtained when treatment is individualized. In general, those patients with soft tissue and intrathoracic metastases will respond best to estrogen therapy. Androgen therapy is usually more effective in patients with bone metastases. Corticosteroid therapy should be particularly considered for those with brain and liver metastases.

C. Therapeutic Endocrine Ablation:

1. Castration—Oophorectomy in premenopausal women with advanced, metastatic, or recurrent breast cancer results in temporary regression in about 35% of cases, with objective improvement lasting an average of about 10 months. Life is definitely prolonged in those who respond favorably. Patients not responding to castration usually fail to respond favorably to adrenalectomy, hypophysectomy, or specific hormones. Authorities differ on whether castration should be given a trial in all premenopausal women before advising bilateral adrenalectomy or hypophysectomy. Of those patients responding favorably to castration, 40–50% will respond to bilateral adrenalectomy or hypophysectomy. Of those not responding to oophorectomy, only 10–15% show tumor regression after one of those major procedures. According to some authorities, simultaneous oophorectomy and adrenalectomy is the palliative treatment of choice in premenopausal women with disseminated breast cancer. However, prophylactic castration of all premenopausal women with breast cancer is not of proved value and is not recommended.

Castration can be performed by bilateral oophorectomy or irradiation. Surgical removal of the ovaries is preferable because it rules out the possibility of residual ovarian function. Therapeutic castration is essentially confined to premenopausal women and is of no value in truly postmenopausal women. Ovarian function may persist for a few years after cessation of menses, and this can be determined by means of the vaginal smear; if evidence of persistent estrogenic activity is found, castration may be beneficial.

2. Adrenalectomy or hypophysectomy—Regression of advanced breast cancer occurs in about 30% of patients after either of these procedures. Patients who respond to castration or to hormone administration are most likely to benefit from removal of the adrenals or pituitary. This information is helpful in the selection of patients for one of these major ablation procedures.

Adrenalectomy is preferred over hypophysectomy because of its wider availability and greater ease of postoperative endocrine management. The mortality rate of both procedures is in the range of 5%.

Corticosteroid replacement therapy is required after bilateral adrenalectomy. The following regimen is suggested:

Day before operation, 6 p.m.: Hydrocortisone sodium succinate (Solu-Cortef), 100 mg IM

Day of operation:
Preoperatively: Solu-Cortef, 100 mg IM
During operation: Solu-Cortef, 100 mg IV
Postoperatively: Solu-Cortef, 50 mg IV every 4 hours

Postoperative day:
First day: Solu-Cortef, 100 mg IV or IM every 8 hours
Second day: Solu-Cortef, 50 mg IV or IM every 6 hours
Third day: Solu-Cortef, 50 mg IV or IM every 12 hours
Fourth day: Solu-Cortef, 25 mg IV or IM every 8 hours, or cortisone acetate, 25 mg orally every 8 hours
Fifth day and thereafter as maintenance dose: Cortisone acetate, 25 mg orally twice daily

Maintenance dose of cortisone must be supplemented in some patients by fludrocortisone, 0.1–0.25 mg orally daily or every other day, for its sodium-retaining effect. Diet following adrenalectomy should include at least 3 gm of salt daily, which may be achieved by liberal salting of food. Adrenal insufficiency will occur if the cortisone maintenance regimen is inadequate or is neglected. Resulting symptoms may include extreme weakness, nausea and vomiting, rapid weight loss, or hypotension. Increased stress calls for increased cortisone dosage. Acute crises of adrenal insufficiency require immediate hospitalization and intensive treatment.

In premenopausal women, when oophorectomy alone is followed by a remission and adrenalectomy is withheld until progression of the tumor resumes, the overall palliation and length of survival are better than when adrenals and ovaries are removed at the same operation. Menopausal and postmenopausal women should be treated by simultaneous oophorectomy and adrenalectomy.

The response of metastatic breast carcinoma to administration of hormones or to ablation of endocrine glands is most likely to be favorable under the following circumstances: (1) slowly growing tumor (eg, free interval between diagnosis and development of metastases exceeds 24 months); (2) hormone therapy is begun promptly when metastases appear; (3) metastases localized to soft tissues, bones, and pleuropulmonary region (as opposed to visceral areas such as liver and brain); (4) advanced age; and (5) previous response to hormone therapy or castration. However, favorable responses may occur occasionally when none of these conditions exist.

Adrenalectomy or hypophysectomy will be of no benefit to two-thirds of patients on whom the operation is performed. Obviously, it is of great importance to develop methods of selection which will identify the patients who will respond and thus avoid unnecessary major surgery in the remainder. Jensen EV & others (Nat Cancer Inst Monogr 34:55, Dec 1971), using incubated tissue slices or homogenates of patient's tumor, demonstrated that certain tumors contain estrogen receptor protein capable of binding estrogen. In a limited series of patients treated by oophorectomy, hypophysectomy, or adrenalectomy, they found that tumors lacking estrogen receptors rarely responded to endocrine ablation but that the presence of estrogen receptors was correlated with over 90% response to endocrine ablation.

More recent studies (McGuire WL: Cancer [Suppl] 36:638, 1975) confirm the significance of estrogen receptors in breast cancer tissue as an indicator of responsiveness to endocrine therapy by either hormone administration or endocrine ablation. In 94 patients with negative tumor estrogen receptor values, only 8 (8%) responded to endocrine ablation (adrenalectomy, hypophysectomy, or castration), whereas, in 107 patients with positive tumor estrogen receptor values, 59 (55%) responded to endocrine ablation. About 30% of patients with borderline tumor estrogen receptor values also responded. The prognostic significance of endocrine receptor assay does not appear to depend upon the type of tissue examined. Estrogen receptor values from primary tumors or metastatic lesions predict equally well. The percentage of primary tumors reported to contain estrogen receptors has risen in recent years from 50% to 70–85%, probably because of increased sensitivity of assay methods. Most investigators have found that tumors from postmenopausal patients contain higher estrogen receptor values than those from premenopausal patients. Although there is no definite correlation between the histologic type of tumor and the presence of estrogen receptors, available data suggest that morphologically undifferentiated tumors are less likely to contain estrogen receptors. In view of these findings, it is advisable to obtain an estrogen receptor assay on the tumor of every patient with primary or metastatic breast cancer as a guide to future treatment, particularly when adrenalectomy or hypophysectomy is under consideration.

As noted above, the success rate for endocrine therapy in breast cancer can be improved to 55–60% by selecting for therapy only those patients whose tumors contain estrogen receptors. It is important to develop a method for identifying the 40% of estrogen receptor positive but endocrine resistant tumors whose growth cannot be inhibited either by administration of hormones or by endocrine ablation. In an effort to achieve this goal, the significance of progesterone receptors in breast cancer tissue is currently being studied (Horwitz KB & others: Science 189:726, 1975).

Progesterone receptors were found in 56% of a small series of breast cancers all of which contained estrogen receptors, but progesterone receptors were absent from cancers which did not contain estrogen receptors. Preliminary clinical trials showed that only those cancers with progesterone receptors regressed after endocrine therapy. If these results are confirmed, the presence of progesterone receptors in breast cancer may prove to be a sensitive predictor of responsiveness to endocrine therapy.

D. Chemotherapy:* Anticancer chemotherapy should be considered for palliation of advanced breast cancer when visceral metastases are present or when hormone treatment is unsuccessful or the patient becomes unresponsive to it. Chemotherapy is most likely to be effective in patients who previously responded to hormonal therapy. The most useful single chemotherapeutic agent to date is doxorubicin (Adriamycin), an anthracycline antibiotic administered intravenously, with a response rate of 40–50%. The remissions tend to be brief, and, in general, experience with single agent chemotherapy in patients with disseminated disease has not been too encouraging.

Combination chemotherapy using multiple agents has proved to be more effective, with objectively observed favorable responses achieved in 60–80% of patients with stage IV disease. Various combinations of drugs have been used, and clinical trials are continuing in an effort to improve results and to reduce undesirable side-effects of treatment. Doxorubicin and cyclophosphamide produced an objective response in 87% of 46 patients who had an adequate trial of therapy (Jones SE & others: Cancer 36:90, 1975). Other chemotherapeutic regimens have used various combinations of drugs including cyclophosphamide, vincristine, methotrexate, and fluorouracil with response rates ranging up to 60–70% (Otis PT, Armentrout SA: Cancer 36:311, 1975). The value of chemotherapy has been underestimated in the past because it has typically been reserved for use after hormone administration and endocrine ablation have failed.

Of special interest is the use of chemotherapy as an adjunct to the surgical treatment of patients who are found at radical mastectomy to have positive axillary nodes. The poor prognosis of this group of patients has already been noted (see p 404). In 1958, a clinical trial was begun by the National Surgical Adjuvant Breast Project to determine whether thiotepa, when administered on the day of and for 2 successive days following radical mastectomy, would reduce treatment failure and increase patient survival. Follow-up studies at 5 years and 10 years showed a significant decrease in recurrence rate for premenopausal women with 4 or more positive nodes who received thiotepa. There was a 20% improvement in survival in this group (Fisher B, Wolmark N: Cancer [Suppl] 36:627, 1975; Carbone PP: Cancer [Suppl] 36:633, 1975). Another more recent multi-institutional, randomized, prospective cooperative clinical trial was undertaken to eval-

*A more detailed discussion is presented in Chapter 32.

uate the efficacy of prolonged oral administration of melphalan (Alkeran) as an adjuvant to radical mastectomy (conventional or modified) in lengthening the disease-free interval of women with potentially curable breast cancer having one or more axillary nodes involved with cancer (Fisher B & others: New England J Med 292:117, 1975). In premenopausal women, the difference with respect to disease-free interval between treated and control groups was highly significant. A treatment failure occurred in 30% of premenopausal patients receiving placebo and in only 3% of those treated with melphalan. A similar trend was observed in postmenopausal patients, but the difference was not statistically significant at the time of publication. This demonstration of the effectiveness of melphalan as an adjuvant to radical mastectomy, and preliminary reports of similar results with the use of combination chemotherapy, indicate that adjuvant chemotherapy should be given serious consideration in the management of patients who are found after radical mastectomy to have positive axillary nodes. Studies are continuing in order to develop improved treatment programs and to determine the possible long-range adverse effects of the chemotherapeutic agents themselves.

Malignant pleural effusion develops at some time in almost half of patients with breast cancer. When severe and persistent, the effusion is best controlled by closed tube drainage of the chest and intrapleural chemotherapy. Fracchia AA & others (Cancer 26:626, 1970) achieved an objective response rate in about half of their patients by the combined use of a weighted pleural catheter and suction with chemotherapeutic agents. An intercostal tube (if available, use a tube weighted at the tip so that it sinks to the lowest portion of the pleural space) is inserted and placed on suction and water-seal drainage until as much fluid as possible has been removed. Then mechlorethamine (0.4 mg/kg, up to 20 mg) or thiotepa (30–45 mg, or 0.8 mg/kg) in 40 ml of saline is injected through the tube, which is clamped for 6 hours. Suction drainage is then reinstituted for 4–6 days–or until no further fluid is obtained–before removing the catheter. The procedure may be repeated in 3–4 weeks if necessary. Toxicity due to intrapleural mechlorethamine or thiotepa is usually mild and consists of occasional nausea or vomiting and infrequent bone marrow depression.

E. Hypercalcemia in Advanced Breast Cancer:* Breast cancer is the most common single cause of hypercalcemia that occurs transiently or terminally in about 10% of women with advanced disease. The hypercalcemia of breast cancer is usually but not always associated with osteolytic metastases. Increased blood calcium may be related in some cases to the regular occurrence in the blood of breast cancer patients of phytosteryl esters which have calcium-mobilizing properties similar to that of vitamin D. Immobilization exaggerates the tendency of direct bony invasion or humoral processes to produce hypercalcemia. Breast cancers do not produce parathyroid

*A more detailed discussion is presented in Chapter 32.

hormone, and the hypercalcemia is therefore not associated with low serum phosphate or low tubular reabsorption of phosphate (TRP) (unless artifactually produced by glucose or corticosteroid administration). Thus, the presence of hypercalcemia, hypophosphatemia, and low TRP in a patient with breast cancer indicates an additional diagnosis such as parathyroid adenoma. Although estrogens and androgens were once erroneously thought to cause hypercalcemia in breast cancer, it now appears that they are actually beneficial in the condition. It is possible, however, that acute hypercalcemia may be precipitated by the nausea, vomiting, and dehydration which may occur with hormone therapy—particularly estrogens—and radiotherapy.

The symptoms of hypercalcemia are protean, and its course is treacherous. Initial symptoms usually include diffuse CNS changes, alterations of renal function, vomiting, and dehydration. Rapid deterioration, anuria, coma, and death may occur.

Prevention is important and consists of (1) adequate hydration (at least 2 liters of fluid per day), (2) maintenance of as much physical activity as possible, and (3) a low-calcium diet (avoidance of milk, cheese, ice cream, and vitamin.D).

Treatment for mild hypercalcemia in patients with only moderate elevation of serum calcium (eg, 11–12 mg/100 ml) consists of hydration to induce diuresis, preferably with sodium-containing fluids to facilitate tubular rejection of calcium. In severe hypercalcemia with calcium levels above 12 mg/100 ml, corticosteroid is administered orally or intravenously in the form of prednisone, 30–100 mg/day (or equivalent), in order to decrease calcium mobilization from bone. Corticosteroid treatment is usually required only until restoration of a normal serum calcium level, which is subsequently maintained by 3 liters per day of oral fluids and avoidance of milk, cheese, and immobilization.

When the above measures prove inadequate to control high levels of serum calcium, the administration of isotonic solution of sodium sulfate intravenously is valuable. Sodium sulfate forms a calcium complex which is readily excreted by the kidney. There is current interest in mithramycin as an antitumor agent which regularly lowers both normal and elevated serum calcium levels at dosages which are relatively nontoxic. Major endocrine ablation may be advisable after hypercalcemia is controlled or may rarely be necessary as a control measure.

After subsidence of an episode of hypercalcemia, many patients survive for months or years with essentially the same relationship to their disease.

Complications of Radical Mastectomy

Except for local recurrence, usually due to implantation of tumor cells in the wound at operation, the only important late complication of radical mastectomy is edema and pain in the arm on the involved side. Significant edema occurs in 10–30% of cases. When it appears in the early postoperative period, it is usually caused by lymphatic obstruction due to infection in the axilla. Late or secondary edema of the arm may develop years after radical mastectomy as a result of infection in the hand or arm with obliteration of lymphatic channels. After radical mastectomy, the lymphatic drainage of the arm is always compromised and the extremity is more susceptible to infection from minor injuries than formerly. The patient should be warned of this and treatment instituted promptly if infection occurs. Specific instruction should be given to the patient who has had radical mastectomy to avoid breaks in the skin of the hand and arm on the operated side and to refrain from tasks likely to cause superficial wounds and infections. Well-established chronic edema is treated by elevation and the wearing of an elastic sleeve tailored to fit the arm snugly. Periodic use of an intermittent positive pressure sleeve may be helpful in severe cases. These measures will not cure the condition but will reduce the edema and minimize its reaccumulation.

Prognosis

In the USA, the annual mortality rate for breast cancer is about 28 per 100,000 females. Death rates are slightly higher among the nonwhite population (92% black) than among whites through ages 45–49, but lower thereafter. Age-adjusted death rates for female breast cancer differ throughout the world. In general, reported rates are higher in developed countries (with the notable exception of Japan) and are low in underdeveloped countries. Reported differences may be due in part to underdiagnosis, underreporting, and variable certification practices.

When cancer is confined to the breast, the 5-year clinical cure rate by radical mastectomy is 75–90%. When axillary nodes are involved, the rate drops to 40–60% at 5 years and, by the end of 10 years after radical mastectomy, the clinical cure rate is only about 25% in this group of patients. Operative mortality is about 1%. The most unfavorable anatomic site for breast carcinoma is the medial portion of the inner lower quadrant. Breast cancer is probably more malignant in young than in old women, but the difference is not great. The prognosis of carcinoma of the breast occurring during lactation or pregnancy is generally poor since over one-fourth are inoperable; but when radical mastectomy is feasible and the axillary nodes are not involved, the overall 5-year clinical cure rate in this group of patients is 60–70%. The presence of axillary metastases in patients who are pregnant or lactating is an extremely poor prognostic sign, and the 5-year clinical cure rate after radical mastectomy under these conditions is only 5–10%.

Most of the local and distant metastases occur during the first 3 years after radical mastectomy. During this period the patient should be examined every 3–4 months. Thereafter, a follow-up examination is done every 6–12 months for the life of the patient with special attention to the opposite breast because of the increased risk in such patients of developing a second primary lesion. In some cases, metasta-

ses are dormant for long periods and may appear up to 10–15 years or longer after removal of the primary tumor.

Anderson CB, Philpott GW, Ferguson TB: The treatment of malignant pleural effusion. Cancer 33:916, 1974.
Cady B: Total mastectomy and partial axillary dissection. S Clin North America 53:313, 1973.
Egan RL: *Mammography,* 2nd ed. Thomas, 1972.
Farrow JH: Current concepts in the detection and treatment of the earliest of the early breast cancers. Cancer 25:468, 1970.
Fisher ER & others: The pathology of invasive breast cancer. Cancer 36:1, 1975.
Goldenberg IS & others: Androgenic therapy for advanced breast cancer in women: A report of the Cooperative Breast Cancer Group. JAMA 223:1267, 1973.
Haagensen CD, Lane N, Lattes R: Neoplastic proliferation of the epithelium of the mammary lobules: Adenosis, lobular neoplasia and small cell carcinoma. S Clin North America 52:497, 1972.
Haagensen CD & others: Treatment of early mammary carcinoma: A cooperative international study. Ann Surg 170:875, 1969.
Kennedy BJ: Hormone therapy in inoperable breast cancer. Cancer 24:1345, 1969.
Kline TS, Hunter SN: Needle biopsy: A pilot study. JAMA 224:1143, 1973.
Lee JM & others: An evaluation of five drug combination chemotherapy in the management of recurrent carcinoma of the breast. Surg Gynec Obst 138:77, 1974.
Lynch HT & others: Tumor variation in families with breast cancer. JAMA 222:1631, 1972.
Marty R, Hoffman HC: Bone scan helps detect breast cancer metastases. JAMA 221:1215, 1972.
McGuire WL: *Estrogen Receptors in Human Breast Cancer.* Raven Press, 1975.
M.D. Anderson Hospital: *Breast Cancer: Early and Late.* Year Book, 1970.
Oberfield RA & others: A multidisciplined approach for the management of breast cancer. M Clin North America 56:651, 1972.
O'Brien PH: Preoperative irradiation in cancer therapy [breast]. S Clin North America 51:66, 1971.
Papaioannou AN: Etiologic factors in cancer of the breast in humans. Surg Gynec Obst 138:257, 1974.
Robbins GF & others: Metastatic bone disease developing in patients with potentially curable breast cancer. Cancer 29:1702, 1972.
Welbourne RB, Burn JI: Treatment of advanced mammary cancer. New England J Med 287:398, 1972.
Wolfe JN: *Xeroradiography of the Breast.* Thomas, 1972.

CARCINOMA OF THE MALE BREAST

Male breast cancer, since it is rare and usually asymptomatic, is often ignored by the patient and overlooked by the physician. It may occur at any time after age 20, but the peak incidence is in the 50s. The chief local finding is a painless mass not infrequently associated with nipple retraction, encrustation, or discharge.

Treatment consists of radical mastectomy in operable patients, who should be chosen by the same criteria as for female breast carcinoma. Radiation therapy is also advised according to similar indications as in female patients. Irradiation is the first step in the treatment of localized metastases in the skin, lymph nodes, or skeleton which are causing symptoms. Since male breast cancer is so frequently a disseminated disease, endocrine therapy is of considerable importance in its management. Castration in advanced breast cancer is the most successful palliative measure and is more beneficial than the same procedure in the female. Objective evidence of regression may be seen in 60–70% of male patients who are castrated—approximately twice the proportion seen in the female. Bilateral adrenalectomy (or hypophysectomy) has been proposed as the procedure of choice when a tumor has reactivated after castration. Corticosteroid therapy is considered by some to be more efficacious than major endocrine ablation. Male breast cancer is too rare to enable this issue to be decided in a definitive manner at this time. Either approach may be temporarily beneficial. Estrogen therapy (5 mg of diethylstilbestrol 3 times daily orally) may rarely be effective, and androgen therapy may exacerbate bone pain. Castration, bilateral adrenalectomy, and corticosteroids are the main lines of therapy for advanced male breast cancer. Nonhormonal combination chemotherapy will probably be used with increasing frequency in the future as an alternative mode of treatment.

The absolute 5-year survival of men with breast cancer is about 30%. Following radical mastectomy, the 5-year survival is about 40%. Huggins and Taylor reported a 5-year survival in only 35% of 14 stage I cases of male breast cancer. Palliative therapy is frequently required in this disease because of the frequency of occult metastases and the tendency to present in an advanced stage.

Crichlow RW, Kaplan EL, Kearney WH: Male mammary cancer: Analysis of 32 cases. Ann Surg 175:489, 1972.

MAMMARY DYSPLASIA

Essentials of Diagnosis

- Painful, often multiple, frequently bilateral masses in the breast.
- Rapid fluctuation in the size of the masses is common.
- Frequently, pain occurs or increases and size increases during premenstrual phase of cycle.
- Most common age is 30–50. Rare in postmenopausal women.

General Considerations

This disorder, also known as chronic cystic mastitis of the breast, is the most frequent lesion of the breast. It is common in women 30–50 years of age but rare in postmenopausal women, which suggests that it is related to ovarian activity. Estrogen hormone is considered an etiologic factor. The typical pathologic change in the breast is the formation of gross and microscopic cysts from the terminal ducts and acini. Large cysts are clinically palpable and may be several cm or more in diameter.

Clinical Findings

Mammary dysplasia may produce an asymptomatic lump in the breast which is discovered by accident, but pain or tenderness often calls attention to the mass. There may be discharge from the nipple. In many cases discomfort occurs or is increased during the premenstrual phase of the cycle, at which time the cysts tend to enlarge rapidly. Fluctuation in size and rapid appearance or disappearance of a breast tumor are common in cystic disease. Multiple or bilateral masses are not unusual, and many patients will give a past history of transient lump in the breast or cyclic breast pain. Pain, fluctuation in size, and multiplicity of lesions are the features most helpful in differentiation from carcinoma. However, if skin retraction is present, the diagnosis of cancer should be assumed until disproved by biopsy.

Differential Diagnosis

Pain, fluctuation in size, and multiplicity of lesions help to differentiate these lesions from carcinoma and adenofibroma. Final diagnosis often depends on biopsy. Mammography may be helpful.

Treatment

Because mammary dysplasia is frequently indistinguishable from carcinoma on the basis of clinical findings, it is advisable to biopsy suspicious lesions in the operating room. General anesthesia is usually required, but small lesions may be suitable for excision under local anesthesia. Provision is made for immediate diagnosis by frozen section. If cancer is present, definitive surgery such as mastectomy may be deferred for a few days without risk pending further discussion with the patient and additional studies as needed. When it is planned to proceed at once with mastectomy, the patient must be prepared preoperatively. Discrete cysts or small localized areas of cystic disease should be excised when cancer has been ruled out by microscopic examination. Surgery in mammary dysplasia should be conservative, since the primary objective of surgery is to exclude malignancy. Simple mastectomy or extensive removal of breast tissue is rarely, if ever, indicated.

When the diagnosis of mammary dysplasia has been established by previous biopsy or is practically certain because the history is classical, aspiration of a discrete mass suggestive of a cyst is indicated. The skin and overlying tissues are anesthetized by infiltration with 1% procaine, and a No. 20 gauge needle is introduced. If a cyst is present, typical watery fluid (straw-colored, gray, greenish, brown, or black) is easily evacuated and the mass disappears. Cytologic examination of the fluid should be considered. The patient is reexamined at intervals of 2—4 weeks for 3 months and every 6—12 months thereafter throughout life. If no fluid is obtained, if a mass persists after aspiration, or if at any time during follow-up an atypical persistent lump is noted, biopsy should be performed without delay.

Breast pain associated with generalized mammary dysplasia is best treated by avoidance of trauma and by wearing (night and day) a brassiere which gives good support and protection. Hormone therapy is not advisable because it does not cure the condition and has undesirable side-effects.

Prognosis

Exacerbations of pain, tenderness, and cyst formation may occur at any time until the menopause, when the symptoms of mammary dysplasia subside. The patient should be taught to examine her own breasts each month just after menstruation and to inform her physician if a mass appears. Although there is lack of agreement on whether mammary dysplasia predisposes to breast cancer, Davis HB & others (Cancer 17:957, 1964) concluded from a thorough review of the world literature that the risk of breast cancer in women with mammary dysplasia is about twice that of women in general.

Fechner RE: Fibrocystic disease in women receiving oral contraceptive hormones. Cancer 25.1332, 1970.

Sartwell PE, Arthes FG, Tonascia JA: Epidemiology of benign breast lesions: Lack of association with oral contraceptive use. New England J Med 288:551, 1973.

Steinhoff NG, Black WC: Florid cystic disease preceding mammary cancer. Ann Surg 171:501, 1970.

FIBROADENOMA OF THE BREAST

This common benign neoplasm occurs most frequently in young women, usually within 20 years after puberty. It is somewhat more frequent and tends to occur at an earlier age in black than in white women. Multiple tumors in one or both breasts are found in 10—15% of patients.

The typical fibroadenoma is a round, firm, relatively movable, nontender mass 1—5 cm in diameter. The tumor is usually discovered accidentally. Clinical diagnosis in young patients is generally not difficult. In women over 30, cystic disease of the breast and carcinoma of the breast must be considered. Fibroadenoma does not normally occur after the menopause, but postmenopausal women may occasionally develop fibroadenoma after administration of estrogenic hormone.

Treatment in all cases is excision and pathologic examination to determine if the lesion is cancerous.

Cystosarcoma phyllodes is a type of fibroadenoma with cellular stroma which tends to grow rapidly. This tumor may reach a large size, and if inadequately excised will recur locally. The lesion is rarely malignant. Treatment is usually by local excision of the mass with a margin of surrounding breast tissue.

DIFFERENTIAL DIAGNOSIS OF NIPPLE DISCHARGE

In order of frequency, the following lesions cause nipple discharge: intraductal papilloma, carcinoma, mammary dysplasia, and ectasia of the ducts. The discharge is usually serous or bloody. It should be checked for occult blood with the benzidine or guaiac test. When papilloma or cancer is the cause, a tumor can frequently (but not always) be palpated beneath or close to the areola.

The site of the duct orifice from which the fluid exudes is a guide to the location of the involved duct. Gentle pressure on the breast is made with the fingertip at successive points around the circumference of the areola. A point will often be found at which pressure produces discharge. The dilated duct or a small tumor may be palpable here. The involved area should be excised by a meticulous technic which ensures removal of the affected duct and breast tissues immediately adjacent to it. If a tumor is present it should be biopsied and a frozen section done to determine whether cancer is present.

When localization is not possible and no mass is palpable, the patient should be reexamined every week for one month. When unilateral discharge persists, even without definite localization or tumor, exploration must be considered. The alternative is careful follow-up at intervals of 1—3 months. Mammography should be done. Cytologic examination of nipple discharge for exfoliated cancer cells occasionally may be helpful in differential diagnosis.

Although none of the benign lesions causing nipple discharge are precancerous, they may coexist with cancer and it is not possible to distinguish them definitely from malignancy on clinical grounds. Patients with carcinoma almost always have a palpable mass, but in rare instances a nipple discharge may be the only sign. For these reasons chronic nipple discharge, especially if bloody, is usually an indication for resection of the ducts.

Funderburk WW, Syphax B: Evaluation of nipple discharge in benign and malignant breast diseases. Cancer 24:1290, 1969.

Leis HP Jr, Dursi J, Mersheimer WL: Nipple discharge: Significance and treatment. New York J Med 67:3105, 1967.

FAT NECROSIS

Fat necrosis is a rare lesion of the breast but is of clinical importance because it produces a mass, often accompanied by skin or nipple retraction, which is indistinguishable from carcinoma. Trauma is presumed to be the cause, although only about half of patients give a history of injury to the breast. Ecchymosis is occasionally seen near the tumor. Tenderness may or may not be present. If untreated, the mass associated with fat necrosis gradually disappears. As a rule the safest course is to obtain a biopsy. When carcinoma has been ruled out, the mass should be excised.

BREAST ABSCESS

During nursing, an area of redness, tenderness, and induration not infrequently develops in the breast. In the early stages the infection can often be reversed by discontinuing nursing with that breast and administering an antibiotic. If the lesion progresses to form a localized mass with local and systemic signs of infection, an abscess is present and should be drained.

A subareolar abscess may develop in young or middle-aged women who are not lactating. These infections tend to recur after incision and drainage unless the area is explored in a quiescent interval with excision of the involved collecting ducts at the base of the nipple.

Except for the subareolar type of abscess, infection in the breast is very rare unless the patient is lactating. Therefore, findings suggestive of abscess in the nonlactating breast require incision and biopsy of any indurated tissue.

Benson EA, Goodman MA: An evaluation of the use of stilbestrol and antibiotics in the early management of acute puerperal breast abscess. Brit J Surg 57:255, 1970.

Benson EA, Goodman MA: Incision with primary suture in the treatment of acute puerperal breast abscess. Brit J Surg 57:55, 1970.

Habif DV & others: Subareolar abscess associated with squamous metaplasia of lactiferous ducts. Am J Surg 119:523, 1970.

GYNECOMASTIA

Hypertrophy of the male breast may result from a variety of causes. Pubertal hypertrophy is very common during adolescence and is characterized by a tender discoid enlargement 2–3 cm in diameter beneath the areola with hypertrophy of the breast. The changes are usually bilateral and subside spontaneously within a year in the majority of cases.

Men between 50 and 70 occasionally develop hypertrophy (often unilateral) similar to that occurring at puberty.

Certain organic diseases may be associated with gynecomastia: cirrhosis of the liver, hyperthyroidism, Addison's disease, testicular tumors (especially chorioepithelioma), and adrenocortical tumors. Antihypertensive treatment (reserpine, methyldopa) and estrogen therapy for carcinoma of the prostate may cause gynecomastia.

If there is uncertainty about the diagnosis of the breast lesion, a biopsy should be done to rule out cancer. Otherwise, the treatment of gynecomastia is nonsurgical unless the patient insists on excision for cosmetic reasons. In this case, at least 2 years should be allowed before operation for possible subsidence.

Levy DM & others: Gynecomastia. Postgrad Med 36:234, 1964.

12 ...
Gynecology & Obstetrics

Ralph C. Benson

GYNECOLOGY

PRECOCIOUS ISOSEXUAL PUBERTY

Precocious puberty or unusually early sexual maturation—arbitrarily defined as < 8 years for girls and < 10 years for boys—is an uncommon abnormality which affects females more often than males. Two types of precocious puberty are recognized: (1) The primary, constitutional, cryptogenic or idiopathic variety occurs sporadically without known cause and is associated with actual advanced pituitary and ovarian function, including the production of mature ova and the development of all sex characteristics. (2) A slightly smaller group known as secondary or pseudo-precocious puberty in which only secondary sex characteristics develop early, usually as the result of intracranial, adrenal, or ovarian disease. In rare cases, idiopathic precocious puberty may be familial, but no race or culture seems predisposed. At least 60% of all cases of early sexual development in females are of the constitutional type; about 15% are due to intracranial disease; most of the remainder have hyperadreno-corticism; and a few have a gonadal tumor.

Pubertal development in girls varies with respect to environment, age at onset, and the rate of development. The sequence of development also varies: Pubic hair appears before the breasts enlarge in about 20% of girls, and breast development usually precedes menses.

Genetic, nutritional, and general health factors also influence pubertal development, especially the age at onset. In countries with advanced social and medical standards, the age of menarche has dropped from about age 16 to 13 during the past century.

Clinical Findings

A. Symptoms and Signs: The diagnosis of constitutional sexual precocity must be made by exclusion. Enlargement of the breasts and pigmentation of the nipples; the appearance of pubic hair; enlargement of the external genitalia (especially the labia majora) and the ovaries; and uterine bleeding are manifestations of pubescence. Secretory endometrium occurs periodically with ovulation, but observation and repeated evaluations over months or years may be necessary to prove or disprove this point.

In pseudoprecocious puberty, there may be no uniformity of somatic and sexual development. Nevertheless, consistently abnormal physical, laboratory, and x-ray findings will in time direct attention to the basic disorder. Uterine bleeding is from a nonsecretory endometrium. Early sexual maturation may precede CNS symptomatology, or the reverse may occur in pseudoprecocious puberty.

B. X-Ray and Laboratory Findings: X-ray studies of bone age and laboratory findings in cases of idiopathic sexual precocity approach but never exceed normal values for children of about the same somatic age. Measurable amounts of pituitary gonadotropins are not always present, but estrogenic vaginal smears are noted and estrogen excretion is much increased for patients of that chronologic age.

C. Special Examinations: Electroencephalography, cerebral angiography, or pneumoencephalography may identify cerebral disease. Intravenous urography, reproperitoneal pneumography, and assays of urinary 17-ketosteroids and 17-hydroxycorticosteroids help to diagnose an adrenal problem. Peritoneoscopy, culdoscopy, and x-ray studies may reveal an ovarian tumor.

Note: Surgical exploration is unwarranted in the absence of convincing preliminary evidence of neoplasm.

D. Diagnostic Procedures: The following diagnostic procedures (after Huffman) are recommended for the evaluation of the sexually precocious girl:

1. **History**—Family and childhood.
2. **General physical examination.**
3. **Gynecologic examination**—Clinical, vaginal cytology smear, pneumoperitoneography.
4. **Neurologic examination**—Clinical, ophthalmologic, EEG, skull x-rays, pneumoencephalography (rare), brain scan.
5. **Laboratory**—Estrogen titer (often not necessary), pituitary gonadotropin titer, pregnanediol titer, 17-ketosteroid titer, chorionic gonadotropin titer (rarely), thyroid function tests.
6. **Roentgenography**—Bone age, long bones.
7. **Surgery**—Exploratory laparotomy (rarely), curettage (very rarely).

Differential Diagnosis

In precocious puberty, the differential diagnosis is based on the history, physical findings, x-ray studies, and hormone assays. Obesity, hirsutism, and early virilization (adrenogenital syndrome) are consistent with a diagnosis of posterior pituitary tumor (Cushing's disease) or primary hyperadrenocorticism (Cushing's syndrome). A pelvic mass and hyperestrogenism suggest a functional ovarian neoplasm. In the CNS form of the disease, there may be neurologic malfunction and often mental deficiency.

Treatment

Precocious puberty is not a gynecologic problem alone; special problems of education, psychology, marriage, and pregnancy must be considered. Children with precocious puberty due to any cause—and especially those with mental retardation—must be protected against sexual exploitation.

A. Idiopathic Precocious Puberty: The child must receive sex education and menstrual and feminine hygiene information early. Precocious puberty may invite precocious pregnancy. No acceptable therapy will alter accelerated growth. Nevertheless, periodic progestogen therapy will suppress uterine bleeding and sometimes decreases breast size in girls with precocious puberty. Medroxyprogesterone acetate (Depo-Provera), 50 mg IM every 10 days, may be helpful for this purpose.

B. Secondary Precocious Puberty: Therapy depends upon the underlying disorder. CNS, adrenal, and ovarian tumors should be removed if possible.

Prognosis

When abnormally early breast development and the appearance of pubic hair coincide, uterine bleeding probably will occur soon thereafter.

In constitutional sexual precocity, somatic growth usually ceases prematurely at about 10 years of age. The patient's ultimate height will be related directly to her age at onset of puberty. Reproductive ability develops earlier, and menopause may be advanced slightly. Most patients enjoy good health and an average life span.

Bilateral ovariectomy will arrest abnormal growth and development, but partial resection will not benefit the patient. On the other hand, removal of the ovaries will not prevent adult dwarfism.

Abnormal maturation and uterine bleeding can be checked only if the cause of secondary precocious puberty can be eliminated or controlled. Patients with nonsurgical CNS disorders such as postinfectious encephalopathy or diffuse fibrous dysplasia are usually not helped by any therapy.

Brainstein GD & others: In vivo and in vitro production of human chorionic gonadotrophin and alpha fetoprotein by a virilizing hepato-blastoma (precocious puberty). J Clin Endocrinol 35:857, 1972.

Cognat M & others: Laparoscopy in infants and adolescents. Obst Gynec 42:515, 1975.

Sadeghi-Nejad A: Sexual precocity: An unusual complication of propylthiouracil therapy. J Pediat 79:833, 1971.

NORMAL UTERINE BLEEDING

Menstruation is uterine bleeding which occurs at intervals of 24–32 days in the normal woman during the reproductive years. The pituitary gonadotropins and estrogen are responsible, although progesterone, thyroid hormones, and the adrenocorticosteroids also influence menstruation.

Ovulation and the resulting production of estrogen and progesterone result in bleeding (**ovulatory menstruation**) from a secretory endometrium when pregnancy does not occur. In the absence of ovulation, bleeding (**anovulatory menstruation**) is from a nonsecretory endometrium.

Menarche, which generally occurs between ages 11–14, marks the onset of menstrual periods. Menstruation ceases with the **menopause** at 45–55 years of age.

The average duration of menstrual bleeding is 3–7 days, and a blood loss of 50–100 ml is usual. Characteristically, menstrual blood will not clot because it has already clotted within the uterine cavity and has reliquefied. Uterine cramping often occurs with ovulatory cycles, but anovulatory bleeding is usually painless.

Menstrual aberrations are often indications of disease or deficiency states, emotional tension, and pregnancy.

Beller FK: Observation on the clotting of menstrual blood and clot formation. Am J Obst Gynec 111:535, 1971.

Dann TC, Roberts DF: End of a trend? A 12-year study of age at menarche. Brit MJ 3:265, 1973.

Doolittle TL, Engebretsen J: Performance variations during the menstrual cycle. J Sports Med Phys Fitness 12:54, 1972.

Ferdman J: Survey of recent literature on the menstrual cycle and behavior. J Asthma Res 11:27, 1973.

Keye WR Jr & others: New concepts on the physiology of the menstrual cycle. Clin Endocrinol 2:451, 1975.

Moghissi KS & others: A composite picture of the menstrual cycle. Am J Obst Gynec 114:405, 1972.

Nearing MP & others: The effect of the menstrual cycle in tests of physical fitness. J Sports Med Phys Fitness 12:38, 1972.

Shaw ST Jr & others: Quantitation of menstrual blood loss: Further evaluation of the alkaline hematin method. Contraception 5:497, 1972.

Sommer B: The effect of menstruation on cognitive and perceptual motor behaviour: A review. Psychosom Med 35:515, 1975.

Staymore ML & others: Hormonal factors in human ovulation. Am J Obst Gynec 114:445, 1972.

Weir J & others: Race and age at menarche. Am J Obst Gynec 111:594, 1971.

ABNORMAL PREMENOPAUSAL UTERINE BLEEDING

Abnormal uterine bleeding means either (1) excessive or prolonged bleeding during the normal time of flow (hypermenorrhea, menorrhagia) or (2) any bleeding during the intermenstrual interval (metrorrhagia). Abnormal uterine bleeding is a matter of concern to almost every woman at some time between the menarche and the menopause. The bleeding is always disturbing, often debilitating, and occasionally critical.

The causes of abnormal bleeding may be classified according to whether bleeding occurs during or between periods. Common causes of **hypermenorrhea** (menorrhagia) are myoma, endometrial polyposis, irregular shedding of the endometrium, functional hypertrophy of the uterus, blood dyscrasias, and psychologic syndromes. **Polymenorrhea** (uterine bleeding which occurs more often than once every 24 days) may be due to a short cycle (proliferative phase less than 10 days, or secretory phase less than 14 days), or to premature interruption of the cycle due to physical or emotional stress. **Metrorrhagia** (irregular flow at times other than the normal menstrual period) may be due to hormonal imbalance or miscellaneous pelvic abnormalities. Hormonal causes include endometrial cystic glandular hyperplasia, ovulation bleeding (mittelschmerz), administration of estrogens, anovulatory bleeding, and hypothyroidism. Pelvic abnormalities which cause metrorrhagia include cervical or endometrial polyposis, submucous myoma; carcinoma or sarcoma of the cervix, corpus uteri, or fallopian tubes; and endometritis (postabortion, or due to tuberculosis or cervical stenosis).

Clinical Findings

A. Symptoms and Signs: The diagnosis of the disorders underlying the bleeding usually depends upon a careful description of the extent and amount of flow, related pain, if any, relationship to LMP and PMP, and a past history or family history of pertinent illnesses. All medications the patient has taken during the previous month must be accounted for to rule out estrogenic stimulation or androgenic inhibition of flow. The following signs are significant: fullness of the abdomen, cutaneous lesions, edema, exaggerated vascular patterns, abdominal or pelvic floor herniation, tenderness or guarding of the abdomen, adenopathy, dullness or shifting dullness, and swelling, tenderness, or discharge in the vicinity of Skene's or Bartholin's glands. The rectovaginal examination may reveal tenderness, induration, nodulation, mass formation, and the presence of intraperitoneal fluid.

B. Laboratory Findings: Vaginal smears should be obtained (before digital examination) for cytologic and bacteriologic study. Vaginal smears taken during active bleeding and fixed in alcohol-ether can be laked of red cells (after fixation) with 1% HCl; the epithelial detritus which remains may reveal tumor or trophoblastic cells from a uterine abortion. "Jet washings" with saline may enhance the value of simple vaginal smear technics. In addition to urinalysis and routine hematocrit, STS, white and differential count, and sedimentation rate, blood studies (when necessary) should include bleeding time, clotting time, clot retraction time, platelet count, and a tourniquet test for capillary fragility. T_4 and T_3 tests are indicated to rule out abnormal thyroid function (see Chapter 18).

C. X-Ray Findings: X-rays should be ordered only if tumors, fluid collections, or anatomic deformities are suspected, in which case a plain film of the abdomen, hysterosalpingography, cystography, and barium enema studies are indicated.

D. Special Examination: Cervical biopsy and curettage are usually necessary to establish a definitive diagnosis of the cause of bleeding. Polyps, tumors, and submucous fibroids are commonly identified in this way. Cancer of the cervix or endometrium may require cone or multiple-quadrant biopsy of the cervix and differential curettage of the cervix and uterine cavity.

Complications

Continued or excessive blood loss leads to anemia, which favors local or systemic infection. Tumors may cause infertility. Cervical, uterine, or tubal neoplasm must be found and removed before metastasis occurs.

Treatment

A. Emergency Measures: If bleeding has been massive, place the patient in the Trendelenburg position and give sedation, intravenous fluids, and blood transfusions as required. Hemostasis is best achieved with surgical dilatation and curettage because this procedure has both therapeutic and diagnostic advantages. Temporary hemostasis (for 1–2 days) with diethylstilbestrol, 25 mg orally every 15 minutes for 8 doses or 100 mg twice daily for 2 days, is often effective. Intravenous Premarin has been recommended by some.

B. Curettage: Surgical curettage is the treatment of choice. After biopsy and curettage, hormonal therapy may be used for several months for the further control of bleeding.

C. Corrective Hormone Therapy After Proper Diagnosis:

1. **Estrogens and progestogens—**

a. To control **hypermenorrhea** (not metrorrhagia)—Progesterone aqueous suspension, 35 mg IM on the 24th day after the onset of LMP; hydroxyprogesterone caproate (Delalutin), 125 mg IM on the 21st day; norethindrone (Norlutin), 10 mg orally daily for 7 days beginning on the 21st day; norethynodrel with mestranol (Enovid), 10 mg orally daily for 7 days beginning on the 21st day; medroxyprogesterone acetate (Provera), 5 mg orally daily for 4 days beginning on the 21st day.

b. In **metrorrhagia** the following may be used—Estradiol valerate (Delestrogen), 5 mg IM on the 14th day and hydroxyprogesterone caproate (Delalutin), 250 mg IM on the 21st day; norethynodrel with mestranol (Enovid), 10 mg orally daily from the 5th through the 20th days.

2. Androgens—Androgens should be administered cautiously to adolescent girls or young adult women because even minimal doses may cause permanent voice change and irreversible hirsutism. The following regimen should be used only in patients over 45 years of age: Testosterone enanthate (Delatestryl), 200 mg IM on the 5th day of the cycle; after 7 days, methyltestosterone, 10 mg sublingually daily for 2 weeks; after 7 days, methyltestosterone, 10 mg sublingually every other day for 3 weeks of each month for 2 months.

3. Thyroid hormone is indicated if it is certain that hypothyroidism is present and is the only cause of abnormal bleeding.

4. Chorionic gonadotropin, 1000–2000 units IM daily for 12 days following ovulation, will extend the postovulatory (luteal) phase and may thus enhance fertility.

5. Clomiphene citrate (Clomid), 50 mg orally daily for 5 days, is of value in proved anovulatory bleeding states and in the Stein-Leventhal syndrome but is not effective for hypermenorrhea or metrorrhagia due to other causes.

D. Irradiation Therapy: X-ray or radium therapy to terminate menses is indicated only for poor-risk or menopausal patients and is of doubtful value.

E. Surgical Therapy: Intractable bleeding, particularly in women over age 40, may occasionally require hysterectomy. Prior to the menopause, the ovaries should be preserved if they appear to be normal, particularly in younger women.

Prognosis

In the absence of cancer, large tumors, and salpingitis, about 50% of patients with hypermenorrhea and almost 60% of patients with metrorrhagia will resume normal menstrual periods after curettage alone. Giving thyroid hormone or progesterone when indicated will increase the recoveries by another 10–15%.

Aksel S, Jones GS: Etiology and treatment of dysfunctional uterine bleeding. Obst Gynec 44:1, 1974.

Chamberlain G: Excessive menstruation. Practitioner 208:465, 1972.

Cole SK & others: Hematological characteristics and menstrual blood losses. J Obstet Gynaec Brit Common 79:994, 1972.

Cope E: Physiology of abnormal bleeding. Brit MJ 2:573, 1971.

Smith RA: Investigation and classification of oligomenorrhea and amenorrhea. M Clin North America 56:931, 1972.

Smith RA, Litwak O: Endocrine aspects of menstrual irregularity. M Clin North America 58:869, 1974.

POSTMENOPAUSAL VAGINAL BLEEDING

Vaginal bleeding which occurs 6 months or more following cessation of menstrual function may be due to local or systemic causes. Carcinoma of the cervix or endometrium accounts for 35–50% of cases. Administration of estrogens in excessive amounts or in noncyclic manner is the second most important cause. Other causes include atrophic vaginitis, trauma, polyps, hypertensive cardiovascular disease, submucous myomas, trophic ulcers of the cervix associated with prolapse of the uterus, blood dyscrasias, and endogenous estrogen production by a feminizing ovarian tumor. Uterine bleeding is usually painless, but pain will be present if the cervix is stenotic, if bleeding is severe and rapid, or in the presence of infection or torsion or extrusion of a tumor.

Bleeding varies from a bright ooze or brown discharge to frank hemorrhage. The patient may report a single episode of spotting or profuse bleeding for days or months. Laboratory examination of vaginal fluid may disclose exfoliated neoplastic cells, infection, or free basal epithelial cells and white cells (but no cornified epithelial cells in the absence of exogenous or endogenous estrogen). Passage of a sound into the uterus will demonstrate cervical stenosis and hematocolpos; will cause an intracervical or endometrial neoplasm to bleed (Clark test); or may outline a cervical or uterine tumor. Aspiration biopsy or suction curettage often provides sufficient endometrial tissue for the purpose of examining for cancer, endometrial hyperplasia, endometritis, and other local disorders.

Treatment

The patient should be hospitalized for thorough evaluation and definitive care. Dilatation and curettage (with polypectomy if indicated) will cure about half of all patients with postmenopausal bleeding. Withdraw all sex steroid drugs and do not reinstitute therapy until the cause of bleeding has been identified and bleeding has been controlled for at least 3 months. If bleeding recurs after a second curettage in a patient who is not taking estrogens, total hysterectomy and bilateral salpingo-oophorectomy may be indicated.

Prognosis

Curettage will cure many cases. The prognosis for women whose bleeding is due to neoplastic disease depends upon the extent of invasion and the success of antitumor therapy.

Balger JT: When the postmenopausal woman bleeds. Patient Care 7:70, 1973.

Coyle MG: Gynaecological disorders of old age. Practitioner 208:480, 1972.

Gambrell RD Jr: Postmenopausal bleeding. J Am Geriatrics Soc 22:337, 1974.

Lin TJ & others: Clinical and cytologic responses of postmenopausal women to estrogen. Obst Gynec 41:97, 1973.

The menopause and estrogen therapy. (Symposium.) J Reprod Med 11:233, 1973.

Notelovitz M: Beware the weeping womb. South African MJ 47:1653, 1973.

Schaefer G & others: Postmenopausal endometrial tuberculosis. Am J Obst Gynec 112:681, 1972.

PREMENSTRUAL TENSION SYNDROME

Essentials of Diagnosis
- Recurrent, marked, periodic weight gain, agitation, or depression prior to menstruation of ovulatory cycles.
- Emotional, unmarried, or nulliparous women between 30–40 years of age are most commonly affected.

General Considerations
The premenstrual tension syndrome is a recurrent (monthly) disorder characterized by fluid retention, autonomic over-response, and hyper- or hypoactivity. It involves about 50% of women to some degree, especially during the 3rd and 4th decades of life. The disorder appears to be an exaggerated physiologic and psychologic reaction to the onset of menstruation, and is often accompanied by antisocial behavior (even crimes of violence).

Although slight hypoglycemia has been reported on occasion, no gross endocrine or other physical dysfunction distinguishes the patient with premenstrual tension syndrome. This disorder aggravates mental illness, hypermetabolism, chronic cystic mastitis, and obesity.

Dread of an impending period and concern regarding pregnancy, elimination, and femininity are basic problems. The woman experiences ego depreciation and often blames her mother for her menstrual difficulties. Atypical pelvic pain and primary dysmenorrhea may be associated problems.

Clinical Findings
A. **Symptoms and Signs**: Anxiety, agitation, insomnia, inability to concentrate, and a feeling of inadequacy are reported. Patients complain of mastalgia, nausea and vomiting, and diarrhea or constipation. Depression and self-pity may color the woman's affect, or she may be contentious and aggressive. Peculiar drives or unusual appetites are commonplace.

The emotional build-up parallels weight gain (edema) of up to 6–8 lb. The general and pelvic examinations are not otherwise specific. A prompt weight loss by diuresis follows the onset of the period.

B. **Laboratory Findings**: Blood counts and urinalysis are not diagnostic. Slight functional hypoglycemia may occasionally be noted during the period of tension. Estrogen and progestogen production and excretion studies generally relate to an ovulatory cycle.

C. **Special Examinations**: Psychologic testing and consultation may be required.

Differential Diagnosis
Rule out hyperthyroidism, hyperaldosteronism, hyperinsulinism, extreme psychoneurosis, and psychosis.

Treatment
Prescribe diuretics together with tranquilizers for agitated patients, or diuretics and stimulant drugs for depressed patients. Reassurance, positive suggestion, and specific psychotherapy are most helpful. A medium caloric, low-sodium, high-protein diet with frequent small feedings is helpful. Encourage an active life and discourage invalidism. An attempt should be made to redirect the patient's attitudes, with emphasis on pride in her feminine role. Suppress ovulation by small doses of a progestin-dominant, combination type oral contraceptive when acceptable.

Prognosis
Considerable symptomatic relief and improvement in behavior can be achieved in responsive, cooperative patients.

Cullberg J: Mood changes and menstrual symptoms with different gestagen/estrogen combinations: A double-blind comparison with a placebo. Acta psychiat scandinav Suppl 236:1, 1972.
Jordheim O: The premenstrual syndrome: Clinical trials of treatment with a progestogen combined with a diuretic compared with both a progestogen alone and with a placebo. Acta obst gynec scandinav 51:77, 1972.
Liskey NE: Accidents: Rhythmic threat to females during premenstrual and menstrual phases of the cycle. Accident Anal Prev 4:1, 1972.
Wong WH & others: Changes in the capillary filtration coefficient of cutaneous vessels in women with premenstrual tension. Am J Obst Gynec 114:950, 1972.

PRIMARY DYSMENORRHEA
(Essential or Functional Dysmenorrhea)

Essentials of Diagnosis
- Prodromal signs of breast engorgement, agitation, abdominal bloating, pelvic heaviness.
- Intermittent aching or cramping in lower midline of abdomen at onset of bleeding.
- Tenderness upon pelvic and abdominal examination.

General Considerations
Pain with menstrual periods for which no organic cause can be found (primary or essential dysmenorrhea) accounts for about 80% of cases of painful menses. The pain is always secondary to an emotional problem. Although primary dysmenorrhea is particularly common during adolescence, it may occur at any time from the menarche to the menopause. Dysmenorrhea and general menstrual discomfort are often described together as "menorrhalgia."

Clinical Findings
Agitation, abdominal bloating, breast engorgement, and pelvic heaviness often precede the flow. Intermittent aching to cramp-like discomfort in the lower midline usually accompanies the onset of bleed-

ing. Circulatory engorgement of the vagina and cervix, slight patulousness of the os, and bogginess of the uterus (all evidence of the pelvic congestion syndrome) are frequently recorded before and during bleeding. Uterine, parametrial, and adnexal tenderness are often described as well.

Dysmenorrhea equivalents—periodic headache, nausea, diarrhea, urinary frequency and urgency—indicate monthly dysfunction of other organ systems.

Differential Diagnosis

Menstrual cramps which develop more than 5 years after the menarche are usually due to organic causes. Generalized abdominal pain or particularly well-localized right- or left-sided pelvic pain are indicative of organic disease. Typical patterns of referred pain also suggest secondary dysmenorrhea.

Treatment

A. Specific Measures: The definitive management of primary dysmenorrhea must be directed at the underlying psychodynamics. The gynecologist who is interested in these problems must be prepared to spend considerable time with the patient at each visit and to pursue a cure over a long period of time. Patients with severe emotional disorders should be treated by a psychiatrist.

B. General Measures: Analgesics may be warranted until the diagnosis is established. Narcotics should be avoided. Ovulation can be suppressed and dysmenorrhea usually prevented by any of the oral contraceptives. Minimal dosage is recommended to reduce side-effects. Administration of diethylstilbestrol, 0.5 mg orally daily for 14 days beginning with the first day of the period, or methyltestosterone, 5 mg orally 3 times daily from the 5th through the 10th days after the onset of menstruation (for 2 or 3 months), is a valuable temporary expedient. Methyltestosterone does not interfere with ovulation in this dosage.

C. Surgical Measures: Primary presacral neurectomy is rarely justified, and hysterectomy is never indicated.

Prognosis

In women with insight who are cooperative and want to be cured, the prognosis is good. Very little can be done for the patient who prefers to use menstrual symptoms as a monthly refuge from responsibility and participation.

Berry C, McGuire TL: Menstrual distress and acceptance of sexual role. Am J Obst Gynec 114:83, 1972.

Nakano R, Takemura H: Treatment of functional dysmenorrhea: A double blind study. Acta obstet gynaecol jap 18:41, 1971.

LEUKORRHEA
("White Vaginal Discharge")

Leukorrhea may occur at any age and affects almost all women at some time. It is not a disease but the manifestation of ovulation or of a local or systemic disorder. The most common cause is infection of the lower reproductive tract; other causes are inflammation, estrogenic or psychic stimulation, tumors, and estrogen depletion.

Leukorrheic discharge is usually white because of the presence of exfoliated or inflammatory cells. The persistence of some vaginal mucus is normal. Nevertheless, when soiling of the clothing or distressing local symptoms occur, the discharge must be considered abnormal.

Any moisture may add to normal body odor and may be a source of self-consciousness. Frequent bathing and drying of the parts will suffice. In contrast, a seriously objectionable odor may be an indication of vaginal (or vulvar) infection.

Clinical Findings

A. Symptoms and Signs: Vaginal discharge, with or without discomfort, may be associated with itching when urine contaminates the inflamed introitus. The patient may complain of pudendal irritation, proctitis, vaginismus, and dyspareunia. There may be no symptoms in other cases.

Inflammation or ulceration of the vulvovaginal surfaces or cervix and a copious, white or colored, usually odorous discharge are usually present.

B. Laboratory Findings: Blood findings may suggest low-grade infection. Cytologic study of a smear of vaginal secretion is indicated for all parous patients and others over 25 years of age or whenever malignancy is suspected. The same preparation can be stained to show trichomonads, candida, or other organisms. Trichomonads are often seen in freshly voided urine contaminated with leukorrheic discharge. If these organisms are noted in a catheterized specimen, urethral and bladder involvement by the flagellate is likely. Culture of the trichomonad is difficult but may be successful when Trichosel medium is used.

Leukorrhea associated with a positive serology may be due to syphilis; a positive Frei test suggests lymphogranuloma venereum; the dmelcos skin test is positive in chancroid.

Inspect a fresh wet preparation of the vaginal fluid first for motile *Trichomonas vaginalis*. Look for heavy clouding of the spread and especially the covering of epithelial cells ("clue cells") by myriads of small, darker bacteria; these will probably be *Haemophilus vaginalis*. Then add 10% potassium hydroxide to lake blood cells as an aid in visualization of candida hyphae and spores. Examination of a gram-stained smear will identify intracellular gram-negative diplococci (*Neisseria gonorrhoeae*), other predominant bacteria, and helminths. If possible, culture the vaginal fluid anaerobically and aerobically to identify bacterial

Table 12–1. Differential diagnosis of the causes of leukorrhea.

Color	Consistency	Amount	Odor	Probable Causes
Clear	Mucoid	+ to ++	None	Normal ovulation, excessive estrogen stimulation, emotional tension.
Milky	Viscid	+ to +++	None to acrid	Cervicitis, *Haemophilus vaginalis* vaginitis.
White	Thin with curd-like flecks	+ to ++	Fusty	Vaginal mycosis.
Pink	Serous	+ to ++	None	Hypoestrinism, nonspecific infection.
Yellow-green	Frothy	+ to +++	Fetid	*Trichomonas vaginalis* vaginitis.
Brown	Watery	+ to ++	Musty	Vaginitis, cervicitis. Cervical stenosis, endometritis; neoplasm of the cervix, endometrium, or tube. Post-irradiational.
Gray, blood-streaked	Thin	+ to ++++	Foul	Vaginal ulcer. Pyogenic vaginitis-cervicitis (trauma, long-retained pessary, forgotten tampon). Vaginal, cervical, endometrial, tubal neoplasm.

pathogens. Thioglycollate bacterial medium is most useful in the culture of haemophilus microorganisms.

Inoculate Nickerson's, Sabouraud's, Pagano-Levin, or a similar medium to demonstrate candida.

Secure a vaginal smear for acid-fast staining and an inoculum for culture (or guinea pig inoculation) for *Mycobacterium tuberculosis* when tuberculosis is suspected.

Prevention

The husband should use a condom if infection or reinfection is likely. Sexual promiscuity and borrowing of douche tips, underclothing, or other possibly contaminated articles should be avoided.

Antibiotic therapy over long periods of time may cause candida vaginitis due to the overgrowth of these yeasts.

Treatment

A. Specific Measures: Treat infection with the specific drugs listed below. If sensitivity develops, discontinue medication and substitute another drug as soon as practicable. Continue treating the patient during menstrual flow. Choose a mode of therapy (eg, suppositories, oral therapy) which need not be discontinued because of bleeding.

1. *Trichomonas vaginalis* **vaginitis**—It may be necessary to treat the patient for several months; change the medication after 2–3 months in resistant cases: (1) Metronidazole (Flagyl), 250 mg orally 3 times daily for 10 days. The physician should treat the husband similarly during the same interval. Insist upon condom protection against reinfection during coitus until both partners are free of *Trichomonas vaginalis* organisms. *(Caution:* This drug may encourage the growth of candida organisms or mask gonorrhea. See p 852 for other remarks on the toxicity of metronidazole.) (2) Diiodohydroxyquin (Diodoquin), dextrose, lactose, and boric acid (Floraquin), carbarsone, or

Devegan suppositories, 1 vaginally twice daily for 8 weeks. Additional vaginal insufflation with the same preparation in powder form twice weekly for the first month is also helpful. (3) Furazolidone-nifuroxime (Tricofuron) vaginal suppositories, 1 twice daily for 8 weeks.

2. *Candida albicans*—Discontinue oral contraception; substitute condom protection temporarily. (1) Nystatin (Mycostatin) vaginal suppositories, each containing 100,000 units, 1 daily for 2 weeks, are most effective. (2) Propionic acid gel (Propion Gel), 1 application vaginally daily for 3 weeks. (3) Gentian violet, 2% aqueous solution applied topically to the vulva, vagina, and cervical area twice weekly for 3 weeks. (4) Gentian violet, lactic acid, and acetic acid (Gentia Jel), 1 application vaginally daily for 3 weeks.

3. *Haemophilus vaginalis* **vaginitis**—(1) Sulfathiazole, sulfacetamide, and benzylsulfanilamide in cream form (Sultrin), 1 application daily for 2 weeks. (2) Acidified 0.1% hexetidine gel (Sterisil), 1 application daily for 2 weeks.

4. Atrophic (senile) vaginitis—(1) Diethylstilbestrol, 0.5 mg vaginal suppository, 1 every third day for 3 weeks. Omit medication for 1 week (to avoid uterine bleeding); then resume cyclic therapy indefinitely unless contraindicated. (2) Dienestrol or Premarin vaginal cream, one-third of an applicator every third day for 3 weeks. Omit medication for 1 week, then resume cyclic therapy. (3) Diethylstilbestrol, 0.2–0.5 mg (or equivalent), orally daily for 3 weeks each month.

5. Gonorrheal vaginitis—Treat as directed in Chapter 23. *Caution:* Treatment will be inadequate unless 3 sets of slides or, preferably, cultures of discharge from Skene's ducts and the cervical canal reveal no gonococci. Perform a serologic test for syphilis prior to treatment and repeat 2 months later.

B. General Measures: Utilize internal menstrual tampons to reduce vulvar soiling, pruritus, and odor. Coitus should be avoided until a cure has been achieved. Trichomonal and candidal infections require treatment of the husband also. Relapses are often reinfections. Re-treat both parties.

Antipruritic medications are disappointing unless an allergy is present. Specific and local therapy will usually control itching promptly.

C. Local Measures: Occasional warm saline or acetic acid douches (2 tbsp of distilled [white] vinegar per liter of water) may be beneficial in the treatment of leukorrhea. *Caution:* Never prescribe alkaline (soda) douches. They are unphysiologic and often harmful because they discourage the normal vaginal flora by raising vaginal pH.

Douches are not essential to cleanliness or marital hygiene. Too frequent douches of any kind tend to increase mucus secretion. Irritating medications cause further mucus production.

In severe, resistant, or recurrent trichomonal or candidal vaginitis, treat the cervix (even when it is apparently normal) by chemical or light thermal cauterization. Investigate the urinary tract and Skene's and Bartholin's ducts and treat these areas if they appear to be reservoirs of reinfection.

D. Surgical Measures: Cauterization, cryosurgery, conization of the cervix, incision of Skene's glands, or bartholinectomy may be required. Cervical, uterine, or tubal disease (tumors, infection) may necessitate laparotomy, irradiation, or other appropriate measures.

Prognosis

Leukorrhea in pregnant, debilitated, or diabetic women is difficult to cure, especially when due to *Trichomonas vaginalis, Candida albicans,* or *Haemophilus vaginalis.* Repeated or even continuous treatment over 3–4 months may be required until the patient is delivered or the diabetes is controlled.

The prognosis is good if the exact diagnosis is made promptly and intensive therapy instituted. Treatment of only one of several causes may be the reason for failure of therapy.

Aimakhu VE: Treatment of trichomonal vaginitis with a single oral dose of tinidazole. Internat J Gynaec Obstet 12:84, 1974.

Akerlund M, Mardh PA: Isolation and identification of *Corynebacterium vaginale (Haemophilus vaginalis)* in women with infections of the lower genital tract. Acta obst gynec scandinav 53:85, 1973.

Banner EA: Vaginitis. M Clin North America 58:759, 1974.

Davidson F: Short-term high dose metronidazole for vaginal trichomoniasis. J Obstet Gynaec Brit Common 80:368, 1973.

Hesseltine HC: Identifying the organism in vulvovaginal infections. Am Family Physician 9:151, 1974.

Hilton AL & others: Chlamydia A in the female genital tract. Brit J Ven Dis 50:1, 1974.

Hirsch HA, Dedes M: Local and systemic treatment of vaginal candidiasis. Postgrad MJ 50:83, 1974.

Josey WE & others: The epidemiology of type 2 (genital) herpes simplex infection. Obst Gynec Surv 27:295, 1972.

Lee L, Schmale JD: Ampicillin for *Corynebacterium vaginale (Haemophilus vaginalis)* vaginitis. Am J Obst Gynec 115:786, 1973.

Legal HP: The treatment of trichomonas and candida vaginitis with clotrimazole vaginal tablets. Postgrad MJ 50:81, 1974.

Nelson WB: Accurate office diagnosis of vaginitis. Am Family Physician 10:105, 1974.

Paredes FR, Hawkins SF: Sensitivity of *Trichomonas vaginalis* to chemotherapeutic agents. J Obstet Gynaec Brit Common 80:86, 1973.

Swate TE, Weed JC: Boric acid treatment of vulvovaginal candidiasis. Obst Gynec 43:893, 1974.

CERVICITIS

Cervicitis is the most common of all gynecologic disorders. Over 60% of parous women have cervicitis, usually as a result of pre- or postpartum infections. Gonorrhea and mixed infections frequently cause acute and chronic cervicitis in nonpregnant women. Chronic cervical infection is the most common cause of leukorrhea and a major etiologic factor in infertility, dyspareunia, abortion, and intrapartum infection. Chronic cervicitis may even predispose to cervical cancer. At least three-fourths of all women have cervicitis at some time during their adult lives.

Vaginitis or cervical instrumentation and lacerations may initiate cervicitis.

Cervicitis is characterized by erosion (a transient ulceration of the endo- and ectocervix) and eversion (ectropion), which is due to outward growth of endocervical cells.

The characteristics of cervical mucus vary with the menstrual cycle. In the absence of infection, the cervical mucus is thin, clear, and acellular at the time of ovulation or after moderate estrogen stimulation. In cervicitis the mucus is mucopurulent, even bloodstreaked, and may be tenacious and viscid at midcycle. Microscopic examination of a smear of cervical mucus from a patient with clinical cervicitis or bleeding never shows the normal "fern" formation. The acidity of the mucus and the presence of bacteria are noxious to sperm.

The symptoms include leukorrhea, low back pain, hypogastric pain, dyspareunia, dysmenorrhea, dysuria, urinary frequency and urgency, metrorrhagia, and cervical dystocia.

Cervical cancer, venereal infections, and cervical tuberculosis must be ruled out.

Treatment

A. Acute Cervicitis: Treat acute infections with appropriate antibiotics. Avoid instrumentation and vigorous topical therapy during the acute phase and before the menses, when an upward spread of the infection may occur.

B. Chronic Cervicitis: Replace and retain a free retroverted uterus (which both aggravates and predisposes to cervicitis) with a vaginal pessary to reduce chronic passive congestion of the cervix and corpus.

1. For mild cervicitis, cauterize the ecto- and

endocervix during the midcycle with 5% silver nitrate solution or 2% sodium hydroxide solution.

2. In more severe or resistant cases, give diethylstilbestrol, 0.1 mg orally, and sulfisoxazole (Gantrisin), 0.5 gm orally twice daily for 15 days, beginning with the first day of menstruation.

3. In deep hypertrophic chronic cervicitis, cauterize the cervix with the galvanocautery ("hot" or nasal tip cautery) or by means of cryosurgery or diathermy (high frequency or "cold" cautery), coagulating lightly with radial strokes of the instrument. Treat only portions of the canal and portio at any one visit, preferably during the first half of the cycle. Treatment may be repeated monthly if necessary. Immediately after cauterization, prescribe warm saline douches or furazolidone-nifuroxime (Tricofuron) or sulfonamide cream or suppositories locally for 3–4 days to suppress infection. Sound and dilate the cervical canal periodically to prevent stenosis.

4. Trachelorrhaphy (cervical repair), conization, and hysterectomy are justified only occasionally for intractable cervicitis.

Prognosis

Mild chronic cervicitis usually responds to local therapy in 4–8 weeks; more severe chronic cervicitis may require 2–3 months of treatment. The prognosis for acute cervicitis is excellent if an accurate diagnosis by means of smears and cultures is made and appropriate antibiotic treatment given.

Acosta AA, Kaufman RH: Cryosurgical treatment of chronic cervicitis. J Reprod Med 9:17, 1972.

Dooley RR & others: Polypoid cervicitis in cystic fibrosis patients receiving oral contraceptives. Am J Obst Gynec 118:971, 1974.

Haswell JN: Cryosurgery and practical gynecology. J Indiana MA 64:1123, 1971.

Miller JF, Elstein M: A comparison of electrocautery and cryocautery for treatment of cervical erosions and chronic cervicitis. J Obstet Gynaec Brit Common 80:658, 1973.

Nunez-Montiel TJ & others: Colposcopic aspects of endocervicitis. J Reprod Med 12:197, 1974.

Oriel JD & others: Chlamydial infections of the cervix. Brit J Ven Dis 50:11, 1974.

Peck JE: Cryosurgery for benign cervical lesions. Brit MJ 2:198, 1974.

Stepto RC: Treatment of the Nabothian cyst. Am Family Physician 4:82, 1971.

CYST & ABSCESS OF BARTHOLIN'S DUCT & GLAND

Gonorrhea and other infections often involve Bartholin's duct and, to a lesser degree, the gland itself. Obstruction prevents drainage of secretions and exudations, which leads to pain and swelling. The infection resolves and pain disappears, but stenosis of the distal portion of the duct and distention of the proximal duct persist. Reinfection causes recurrent tenderness and further enlargement of the duct.

The principal symptoms are periodic painful swelling on either side of the introitus and dyspareunia. Fullness in one or both of the labia and soft distortion of the introitus are apparent. A fluctuant swelling 1–4 cm in diameter in the inferior portion of either labium minus is a sign of occlusion of Bartholin's duct. Tenderness is evidence of active infection.

Differentiate from inclusion cysts (after laceration or episiotomy), large sebaceous cysts, hydradenoma, congenital anomalies, and cancer of Bartholin's gland or duct (rare).

Treat infection with broad-spectrum antibiotics and local heat. If an abscess develops, incise and drain. After the acute process has subsided, marsupialize the affected duct or excise the duct and gland.

The prognosis is excellent.

Roberts DB, Hester LL: Progressive synergistic bacterial gangrene arising from abscesses of the vulva and Bartholin's gland duct. Am J Obst Gynec 114:285, 1972.

Swenson RM & others: Anaerobic bacterial infections of the female genital tract. Obst Gynec 42:538, 1973.

Tchang F & others: Adenocarcinoma of Bartholin's gland associated with Paget's disease of vulvar area. Cancer 31:221, 1973.

URETHRAL CARUNCLE

Urethral caruncles may occur at any age, but postmenopausal women are most commonly affected. Caruncle may be due to infection, ectropion, papilloma, angioma, or benign or malignant neoplasms. Most caruncles represent eversions of the urethral mucosa or bacterial infections at the meatus (or both). Consider cancer when the lesion is ulcerative or progressive.

Dysuria, frequency, tenderness, vaginal bleeding, leukorrhea, and dyspareunia are the usual complaints, but a few caruncles are asymptomatic. A small, bright red tumor or sessile mass protruding from the urethral meatus may bleed, exude, or cause pain depending upon its etiology and size.

Complications include local ulceration, urethritis, and vaginitis. Bleeding is rarely excessive. An occasional caruncle may represent malignant change in a granuloma or a primary urethral or vulvar cancer.

Treatment

Obtain tissue for biopsy and exudate for smear and culture. If the growth is benign and infection is minimal, fulgurate lightly under topical anesthesia and apply nitrofurazone (Furacin) cream or other chemotherapeutic agent. Repeated light fulguration is preferred to extensive coagulation initially. A bladder sedative compound will usually relieve urinary distress. Surgical excision may also be a valuable procedure, but care must be taken to avoid causing stenosis of the urethra. Local or systemic cyclic estrogen therapy is helpful before and after treatment in the postmenopausal patient. The prognosis in benign cases is excellent.

If the growth is malignant, the patient should receive radical surgery or irradiation therapy.

Blath RG, Boehm FH: Carcinoma of the female urethra. Surg Gynec Obst 136:574, 1973.

Desai S & others: Primary carcinoma of the female urethra. J Urol 110:693, 1973.

URETHRAL DIVERTICULUM

One or more diverticula occasionally develop in the urethra, generally in the mid or distal portion, as the result of inflammation, trauma, or a wolffian duct cyst. Most patients with a diverticulum are parous females 40–50 years of age. Urethritis, venereal disease, or trauma due to obstetric, surgical, or urologic procedures or the passage of a stone may be the immediate cause of the diverticulum.

Clinical Findings

A. Symptoms and Signs: Recurrent exacerbations of urinary distress, postvoiding dribbling, painful coitus, and fullness in the anterior or mid urethra, perhaps dating from urethritis or trauma, are described. There may be a doughy or cystic anterior vaginal mass. Stones are found in 10% of diverticula, and carcinoma may develop in the sacculations also.

Panendoscopy with catheterization of the diverticula generally will identify the problem.

B. Laboratory Findings: Expression and examination of the purulent, sanguineous, or uriniferous discharge from the urethra will reveal local inflammation.

C. X-Ray Findings: Fill the bladder with 60 ml of radiopaque material and 100 ml of sterile water. Require the patient to void but suddenly stop the stream by occluding the urethral meatus with the finger. Lateral and anteroposterior x-rays generally reveal the contrast medium in diverticula.

Differential Diagnosis

Urethrocele—not a herniation but a sagging urethra—usually is associated with cystocele and is not a separate or discrete fullness. Gartner's duct and inclusion cysts are always lateral to and never communicate with the urethra. Firm, nontender masses may be urethral or para-urethral stones or benign or malignant tumors.

Treatment

A. General Measures: Prescribe broad-spectrum antibiotic therapy, warm vinegar douches, and analgesics. Aspiration of the fluid from an occluded, acutely inflamed diverticulum may give marked relief.

B. Surgical Measures: Transvaginal diverticulectomy generally is required. The bladder should be drained by means of an inlying catheter for 7–10 days postoperatively.

Prognosis

Excision of a diverticulum generally is successful, but fistula or stricture formation may occur, and the diverticulum may recur.

Busch FM, Carter FH: Vaginal flap incision for urethral diverticulectomy. J Urol 111:773, 1974.

Pathak UN & others: Diverticulum of the female urethra. Obst Gynec 36:789, 1970.

CARCINOMA OF THE UTERINE CERVIX

Essentials of Diagnosis

- Abnormal uterine bleeding and vaginal discharge.
- Cervical lesion may be visible on inspection as a tumor or ulceration.
- Vaginal cytology usually positive; must be confirmed by biopsy.

General Considerations

Cancer of the cervix is the third most common malignancy in women (exceeded only by breast and colon cancer). Squamous cell cancer accounts for about 95% of cases; adenocarcinoma is responsible for almost 5%.

Cancer appears first in the intra-epithelial layers (the preinvasive stage, or carcinoma in situ). Preinvasive cancer is a common diagnosis in women 30–40 years of age, but most patients with invasive carcinoma are 40–50 years old. Five to 10 years probably are required for carcinoma to penetrate the basement membrane and invade the tissues in most instances. After invasion, death usually occurs in 3–5 years in the untreated or unresponsive patient.

Invasion is associated with ulceration and spotting. Sanguineous vaginal discharge or abnormal bleeding does not occur until the cancer has penetrated into the substance of the cervix.

Clinical Findings

A. Symptoms and Signs: The most common findings are metrorrhagia and cervical ulceration. Hypermenorrhea occurs later. Leukorrhea (sanguineous or purulent, odorous, and nonpruritic) appears after the invasion. Vesical and rectal dysfunction or fistulas and pain are late symptoms. Anemia, anorexia, and weight loss are signs of advanced disease.

Cervical carcinoma in situ is not visible unless one employs the colposcope. Occasionally a small patch of leukoplakia may represent preinvasive carcinoma, or a thickened area in an everted cervix may show malig-

Table 12-2. Clinical staging and lymph node metastases of cancer of the cervix.*

Stage	Direct Extension	Lymph Node Metastases
0	Preinvasive carcinoma (carcinoma in situ).	None
I	Carcinoma strictly confined to the cervix (extension to the corpus disregarded).	About 10%
Ia	Minimal stromal invasion (preclinical invasive carcinoma, ie, cases which cannot be diagnosed by routine clinical examination).	
Ib	All other cases of stage I.	
II	Carcinoma extends beyond the cervix but has not extended to pelvic wall; vagina (but not the lower third) is involved.	Slightly over 20%
IIa	Carcinoma has not infiltrated parametrium.	
III	Carcinoma has extended to pelvic wall. Rectal examination shows no cancer-free space between tumor and pelvic wall. Lower third of vagina is involved.	30–35%
IV	Carcinoma has extended beyond true pelvis or has involved the mucosa of the bladder or rectum. However, the presence of bullous edema is not sufficient evidence to classify a case as stage IV.	At least 75%

*Approved by the International Federation of Obstetricians and Gynecologists.

nant changes. Punch biopsy or cold conization of the cervix is required for diagnosis.

Schiller test: Aqueous solutions of iodine stain the surface of the normal cervix mahogany-brown because normal cervical epithelial cells contain glycogen. Zones of cancer within the epithelium over the cervix do not contain glycogen and so fail to stain with Lugol's or Schiller's iodine reagent. Scars, areas of erosion or eversion, cystic mucous glands, and zones of nonmalignant leukoplakia also fail to take the stain, however, and so this test is useful only in identifying abnormal areas.

B. "Staging" or Estimate of Gross Spread of Cancer of the Cervix: The depth of penetration of the malignant cells beyond the basement membrane is a reliable clinical guide to the extent of primary cancer within the cervix and the likelihood of secondary or metastatic cancer. It is customary to stage cancers of the cervix as shown in Table 12-2. (Percentages given are approximations.)

C. Cytologic Examination (Papanicolaou): Vaginal cytology is usually suggestive or positive. If the smear is negative but cancer is still suspected, biopsy is required. Biopsy confirmation of a positive cytologic examination is always required before definitive treatment is given. Vaginal smears for cytologic examina-

tion should be prepared as requested by the pathologist who will examine the slides. A frequently used technic is as follows:

Material from the vagina can be obtained by aspiration or with a spatula or cut tongue depressor. After vaginal fluid is obtained, a vaginal speculum (moistened in warm water) is inserted and the cervix is visualized. No lubricant should be used. The second specimen is taken from the region of the squamocolumnar junction by scraping with a cut tongue depressor or plastic spatula. Because this is the focus from which most cancers of the cervix develop, these scrapings provide the most reliable specimen for finding carcinoma in situ. Specimens should be taken from any clinically abnormal area of the cervix.

While the scrapings taken directly from the cervix provide material for highly accurate interpretation, the vaginal smear gives reliable results as well, ranging from 80–95%. The advantage of the vaginal smear is that it may reveal malignant cells not only from the cervix but also from the endometrium, the ovaries, and even other abdominal viscera.

Smears to be mailed to a laboratory for staining and interpretation should remain in the alcohol fixative for at least 1 hour. After fixation fit the slides into the mailing container. Wrap the history form around the container and secure with a rubber band for further protection of the slides against breakage in mailing.

If a serial study is desired, most patients can learn to aspirate, smear, and fix their own slides.

The cytologic report from the pathology laboratory (Table 12-3) usually describes the cell specimens as (1) "normal," repeat in 1 year; (2) "suspicious," repeat stage II smears in 6 months and stage III smears immediately; or (3) "positive," take biopsy. Any additional information of value is added—eg, degree of inflammation, the presence of pathogens, and hormonal evaluation.

Perhaps the most important caution relates to the "suspicious" smear. Repeat smears should be done to pinpoint the source of danger since trichomonas infec-

Table 12-3. American Cancer Society terminology of Papanicolaou smears.

American Cancer Society	Papanicolaou Stage	Characteristics
Normal	I	Negative for malignant cells.
Suspicious	II	Negative for malignant cells but containing atypical benign elements (including evidences of infection or radiation changes).
	III	Markedly atypical cells suspicious of malignancy.
Positive	IV	Probably malignant cells.
	V	Cells cytologically conclusive of malignancy.

tion, atrophic changes, or other clinical conditions unreleated to cancer may be the reason for the abnormal or atypical cells.

Note: In no case, including that of the positive smear, is treatment justified until definitive diagnosis has been established through biopsy studies.

An excess of exudate can be dropped into Bouin's or Zenker's fixative (10% formalin causes too much shrinkage) and subsequently treated as a "button" for sectioning. The following information should be included with the request for cytologic examination: patient's name, date, record of previous vaginal smear (Yes or No; Positive or Negative), age, marital status, gynecologic complaints, menstrual history, LMP, surgical procedures, endocrine administration, x-ray or radium irradiation, provisional diagnosis, and the purpose of the study.

D. Cold Conization and Differential Curettage: These procedures may be necessary to determine invasion and extent of the cancer.

E. Colposcopic Examination and Biopsy: May be required for diagnosis.

F. X-Ray Findings: Chest and skeletal x-rays may reveal metastases in advanced disease.

Differential Diagnosis

Abnormal bleeding and vaginal discharge are also found in cervicitis, venereal cervical lesions, and cervical polyps. A visible suspicious cervical lesion may be found in benign cervical polyps, cervical ulceration, nabothian cyst, cervical endometriosis, and cervical pregnancy or tuberculosis.

Complications

Metastases to regional lymph nodes occur with increasing frequency from stage I to stage IV. Paracervical extension occurs in all directions from the cervix. The ureters are often obstructed lateral to the cervix, causing hydroureter and hydronephrosis and consequently impaired kidney function. Almost two-thirds of patients with carcinoma of the cervix die of uremia when ureteral obstruction is bilateral. Pain in the back and in the distribution of the lumbosacral plexus is often indicative of neurologic involvement. Gross edema of the legs may be indicative of vascular and lymphatic stasis due to tumor.

Pelvic infections which complicate cervical carcinoma are most often due to streptococci and staphylococci.

Vaginal fistulas to the gastrointestinal and urinary tracts are severe late complications. Incontinence of urine and feces is a major complication, particularly in debilitated individuals.

Hemorrhage is the cause of death in 10–20% of patients with extensive invasive carcinoma.

Prevention

The causes of cervical cancer are still unknown. Nevertheless, complete chastity is associated with almost total freedom from this malignancy. Theoretically, carcinoma of the cervix (and penis) before middle age may be considered to be a carcinogen-induced neoplasm. The incidence of cervical cancer should therefore be reduced by the following health measures: (1) Improved personal hygiene. Prevention and prompt treatment of vaginitis and cervicitis, male circumcision in infancy, and precoital washing of the penis or habitual use of condoms. (2) Avoidance of intercourse at an early age; limitation of the number of consorts. (3) Frequent cancer cytoscreening of all women, especially parous individuals in lower socioeconomic groups and those who are sexually promiscuous. (4) Prompt removal of suspicious cervical lesions such as epithelial anaplasia, dysplasia, and atypical or equivocal foci.

Treatment

A. Emergency Measures: Vaginal hemorrhage originates from gross ulceration and cavitation in stage II–IV cervical carcinoma. Ligation and suturing are usually not feasible, but ligation of the uterine or hypogastric arteries may be lifesaving when other measures fail. Styptics such as Negatan, 10% silver nitrate solution, and acetone are effective, although delayed sloughing may result in further bleeding. Vaginal packing is helpful. Irradiation therapy usually controls bleeding.

B. Specific Measures:

1. Noninvasive carcinoma (stage 0)–In a woman over 40 with in situ carcinoma of the cervix, total hysterectomy with removal of a wide vaginal cuff is the surgical treatment of choice; irradiation therapy may be used alternatively in women who are poor operative risks. In a younger woman who wishes to have another baby, deep conization of the cervix may be acceptable. This is a calculated risk and imposes the absolute necessity of vaginal smears every 6 months for an indefinite time.

2. Invasive carcinoma–Irradiation (by a specialist) is generally the best treatment for invasive carcinoma of the cervix. The objectives of irradiation treatment are (1) the destruction of primary and secondary carcinoma within the pelvis and (2) the preservation of tissues not invaded. Gamma emissions derived from x-rays, ^{60}Co, radium, the cyclotron, the linear accelerator, and comparable sources are employed. All stages of cancer may be treated by this method, and there are fewer medical contraindications to irradiation than to radical surgery. Optimal results have been achieved with externally applied roentgen therapy combined with intracavitary and paracervical vaginal radium therapy. Selected cases can be treated satisfactorily with radical surgical procedures by appropriately trained pelvic surgeons.

Prognosis

The overall 5-year arrest rate for squamous cell carcinoma or adenocarcinoma originating in the cervix is about 45% in the major clinics. Percentage arrest rates are inversely proportionate to the stage of the cancer: stage 0, 99%; stage I, 77%; stage II, 65%; stage III, 25%; stage IV, about 5%.

Antibol MM & others: Management of the abnormal cervical smear and carcinoma of the cervix during pregnancy. Am J Obst Gynec 117:904, 1973.

Beral V: Cancer of the cervix: A sexually transmitted infection? Lancet 1:1037, 1974.

Brown GD & others: Leukoplakia of the cervix. Am J Obst Gynec 116:214, 1973.

Cunningham JJ & others: Radiographic manifestations of carcinoma of the cervix and complications of its treatment. Radiol Clin North America 12:93, 1974.

Curches CK & others: Treatment of carcinoma of the cervix by a combination of irradiation and operation. Am J Obst Gynec 118:1033, 1974.

Halpin TF & others: Critical points of failure in the therapy of cancer of the cervix: A reappraisal. Am J Obst Gynec 114:755, 1972.

Kelso JW, Funnell JD: Combined surgical and radiation treatment of invasive carcinoma of the cervix. Am J Obst Gynec 116:205, 1973.

May D: Error rates in cervical cytological screening tests. Brit J Cancer 29:106, 1974.

Sall S & others: Surgical management of invasive carcinoma of the cervix in pregnancy. Am J Obst Gynec 118:1, 1974.

Savage EW: Microinvasive carcinoma of the cervix. Am J Obst Gynec 113:708, 1972.

Tasker JT, Collins JA: Adenocarcinoma of the uterine cervix. Am J Obst Gynec 118:344, 1974.

Terris M & others: Relation of circumcision to cancer of the cervix. Am J Obst Gynec 117:1056, 1973.

Thomas DB: An epidemiologic study of carcinoma in situ and squamous dysplasia of the uterine cervix. Am J Epidem 98:10, 1973.

Van Nagell JR Jr & others: Small bowel injury following radiation therapy for cervical cancer. Am J Obst Gynec 118:163, 1974.

CARCINOMA OF THE ENDOMETRIUM
(Corpus or Fundal Cancer)

Adenocarcinoma of the endometrium is the second most common malignancy of the female genital tract. It occurs with greatest frequency in women 60–70 years of age. Abnormal uterine bleeding is the presenting sign in 80% of cases. A watery, serous or sanguineous, malodorous vaginal discharge is occasionally present. Pyometra or hematometra may be due to carcinoma of the endometrium. Pain occurs late in the disease, with stasis, or when the uterus becomes infected.

Surgical dilatation and differential curettage and pathologic examination of curretings are the most reliable means of diagnosis. Cytologic examination of aspirated material from the upper endocervical canal is diagnostic in only 80–85% of cases. Uterine lavage of the endometrial cavity with 3–5 ml of normal saline (eg, using the Gravlee Jet Washer) may yield cells identifiable as malignant elements in suspected endometrial cancer. However, curettage is essential for confirmation before definitive therapy is initiated.

The **Clark test** is performed by gently passing a blunt curved uterine sound through the endocervical os and into the uterine cavity, and then removing it without further manipulation. Bleeding constitutes a positive test, and is presumptive evidence of fundal cancer. However, benign polyps, submucous myomas, and even an early pregnancy may also cause bleeding. Tissue is therefore required to make the diagnosis of cancer. Hysterography shows hypertrophic folds of endometrium, an irregular bulky tumor tending to fill the cavity, or gross papillary growths within the cavity.

Prevention

Routine screening of all women by periodic vaginal smears and prompt dilatation and curettage of patients who report abnormal menstrual bleeding or postmenopausal uterine bleeding will uncover many incipient as well as clinical cases of endometrial cancer.

Treatment

A. General Measures: Patients with carcinoma of the uterus are often weak, anemic, obese, diabetic, or hypertensive; they should be restored to maximum health before surgery.

B. Specific Measures: Treatment usually consists of total hysterectomy and bilateral salpingo-oophorectomy. Preliminary external irradiation or intracavitary radium therapy is probably indicated if the cancer is poorly differentiated, if the uterus is definitely enlarged in the absence of myomas, or if invasion deep into the myometrium has occurred.

Prognosis

With early diagnosis and treatment, the 5-year cure rate is 80–85%.

Boyd IE & others: Preoperative intramuscular progestogen in the treatment of endometrial carcinoma. J Obstet Gynaec Brit Common 80:360, 1973.

Burk JR & others: Inadequacy of Papanicolaou smears in detection of endometrial cancer. New England J Med 291:191, 1974.

De Müelenaere GFGO: Vaginal metastases in endometrial carcinoma. Am J Obst Gynec 118:168, 1974.

Hofmeister FJ: Endometrial biopsy: Another look. Am J Obst Gynec 118:773, 1974.

Kay S: Squamous cell carcinoma of the endometrium. Am J Clin Path 61:264, 1974.

Keller D & others: Management of the patient with early endometrial carcinoma. Cancer 33:1108, 1974.

Maudsley RF, Johnson FL: An appraisal of office endometrial suction curettage. Am J Obst Gynec 118:349, 1974.

Mouson RR & others: Postoperative irradiation in carcinoma of the endometrium. Cancer 31:630, 1973.

Muenzer RW & others: An acceptable yearly screening device for endometrial carcinoma. Am J Obst Gynec 119:31, 1974.

Reagan J: Cellular pathology and uterine cancer. Am J Clin Path 62:150, 1974.

Rodriguez MA & others: Evaluation of endometrial jet wash technique (Gravlee) in 303 patients in a community hospital. Obst Gynec 43:392, 1974.

Rozier JC Jr, Underwood PB Jr: Use of progestational agents in endometrial adenocarcinoma. Obst Gynec 44:60, 1974.

CERVICAL POLYPS

Cervical polyposis is a common disorder which may occur at any time after the menarche but which is only occasionally noted in postmenopausal women. The cause is not known, but inflammation may play a role in etiology. The principal symptoms are leukorrhea and abnormal vaginal bleeding. A cervical polyp is visible on pelvic examination unless it is high in the canal, in which case hysterosalpingography or sounding of the cervix may be required. Vaginal cytologic examination demonstrates infection and metaplasia.

Cervical polyp must be differentiated from neoplastic disease of the endometrium, small submucous pedunculated myoma, endometrial polyp, and the products of an aborted conception.

Treatment

A. Medical Measures: Cervical discharge should be submitted for culture and sensitivity tests and antibiotic therapy instituted as indicated.

B. Surgical Measures: All cervical polyps should be removed surgically. They can often be removed in the office by avulsion, scalpel excision, or high-frequency electrosurgery. All tissue recovered should be examined by a pathologist to rule out malignant change. If the cervix is soft, patulous, or definitely dilated and the polyp is large, surgical dilatation and curettage in a hospital is required (especially if the pedicle is not readily visible). Exploration of the cervical and uterine cavities with the polyp forceps and curet may reveal multiple polyps or other important lesions. Daily warm saline douches may be indicated for 3–7 days after removal.

Prognosis

Simple removal is almost always curative.

Overstreet EW: Clinical aspects of endometrial polyps. S Clin North America 42:1013, 1962.

MYOMA OF THE UTERUS
(Fibroid Tumor, Fibromyoma)

Essentials of Diagnosis

- Irregular enlargement of the uterus (may be asymptomatic).
- Hypermenorrhea, metrorrhagia, dysmenorrhea, and leukorrhea (variable).
- Acute and recurrent pelvic pain if the tumor becomes twisted on its pedicle.
- Symptoms due to pressure on neighboring organs (large tumors).
- X-ray evidence of calcification of some degenerative myomas.

General Considerations

Myoma is the most common neoplasm of the female genital tract. It is a discrete, round, firm, benign uterine tumor composed of smooth muscle and connective tissue. At least 10% of all gynecologic disorders of women are related to myoma. Only 2% are solitary, and several hundred have been found in one uterus. Some myomas become quite large; the largest on record weighed over 100 lb. The most convenient classification is by anatomic location: (1) intramural, (2) submucous, (3) subserous, (4) intraligamentous, (5) parasitic, ie, deriving its blood supply from an organ to which it becomes attached, and (6) cervical.

Clinical Findings

A. Symptoms and Signs: Intramural, subserous, and intraligamentary tumors may distort or obstruct neighboring viscera, causing pain and bleeding. Submucous myomas large enough to displace adjacent organs cause dysmenorrhea, leukorrhea, hypermenorrhea, and metrorrhagia. Cervical myomas cause vaginal discharge, bleeding, dyspareunia, and infertility. Parasitic myomas cause intestinal obstruction if they are large enough to involve the omentum or bowel.

In nonpregnant women the manifestations of myoma are often minimal, eg, pelvic pressure or distention, urinary frequency, menometrorrhagia, constipation, dysmenorrhea. Infertility may be due to a myoma which obstructs or distorts the genital tract.

In pregnant women myomas cause additional hazards: abortion, malpresentation, failure of engagement, premature labor, pain, dystocia, ineffectual labor, and postpartum hemorrhage.

B. Laboratory Findings: The red blood cell count may reveal polycythemia due (curiously) to the tumor or anemia as a result of blood loss.

C. X-Ray Findings: A flat film of the pelvis may demonstrate opacities if calcific degeneration has occurred. Hysterography (contraindicated during pregnancy) may reveal a cervical or submucous tumor.

D. Special Examination: In the nonpregnant woman, vaginal examination under general anesthesia and surgical dilatation and curettage can be used in doubtful cases to establish the diagnosis.

Differential Diagnosis

The irregular enlargement of the uterus observed with myomas must be differentiated from the similar but regular enlargement that may occur with uterine pregnancy, adenomyosis, benign uterine hypertrophy, sarcoma, and adherent adnexa or viscera. Uterine bleeding, dysmenorrhea, and leukorrhea may also occur with other types of neoplastic disease, cervicitis, cervical stenosis, and other gynecologic disorders. These possibilities must be considered even when the diagnosis of myoma has been established.

Treatment

A. Emergency Measures: Give blood transfusions if necessary. Emergency surgery is required for acute torsion of a pedunculated myoma or intestinal obstruction. The only emergency indication for myomectomy during pregnancy is torsion. Abortion is not inevitable.

B. Specific Measures:

1. Nonpregnant women—In nonpregnant women, small asymptomatic myomas should be left undisturbed and observed at intervals of 6 months. Intramural and subserous myomas do not require surgery unless they are larger than a 14 week pregnancy, multiple, or distorting. Cervical myomas larger than 3–4 cm in diameter should be removed.

2. Pregnant patients—If the uterus is no larger than a 6 month pregnancy by the 4th month of gestation, an uncomplicated course can be anticipated. If the mass (especially a cervical tumor) is the size of a 5 or 6 month pregnancy by the second month of gestation, abortion will probably occur. Wherever possible, defer surgery until 6 months after delivery, at which time involution of the uterus and regression of the tumor will be complete.

C. Surgical Measures: Surgery is indicated for the removal of large, rapidly growing or seriously symptomatic myomas in the nonpregnant patient. The measures available for the treatment of myoma are myomectomy, total or subtotal abdominal or vaginal hysterectomy, and, if surgery is contraindicated, irradiation. Myomectomy is the treatment of choice during the childbearing years. The ovaries should be preserved if possible in women under age 45. Subtotal hysterectomy has been virtually abandoned because it is a difficult procedure and there is no advantage to leaving the cervix. Radium should not be used for submucous tumors.

Prognosis

Surgical therapy is curative. Future pregnancies are not endangered by myomectomy, although cesarean delivery may be necessary after wide dissection. Careful hysterectomy with retention of normal ovaries does not hasten menopause.

Ogunbode O & others: Uterine fibroids and obstructed labor. Obst Gynec 42:71, 1973.
Pietila K, Kauppila A: Modified phlebography and hysterography in diagnosis of uterine myomas. Acta obst gynec scandinav 51:375, 1972.
Scharfenberg JC, Geary WL: Intravenous leiomyomatosis. Obst Gynec 43:909, 1974.
Solomon S & others: Fibromyomata of the uterus with hemothorax: Meigs' syndrome? Arch Int Med 127:307, 1971.
Spellacy WN & others: Plasma growth hormone and estradiol levels in women with uterine myomas. Obst Gynec 40:829, 1972.
Spurlin GW & others: Uterine myomas and erythrocytosis. Obst Gynec 40:646, 1972.
Stearns HC: Uterine myomas: Clinical and pathologic aspects. Postgrad Med 51:165, 1972.

ENDOMETRIOSIS & ADENOMYOSIS

Aberrant growth of endometrium outside the uterine cavity (endometriosis) and benign invasion of endometrium into the uterine musculature (adenomyosis) are common causes of abnormal uterine bleeding and dysmenorrhea. Endometriosis frequently causes dyspareunia, painful defecation, or rectal bleeding. The pain tends to be constant, beginning 2–7 days before the onset of menses and becoming increasingly severe until flow slackens. Pelvic examination may disclose tender indurated nodules in the cul-de-sac, especially if the examination is done at the onset of menstruation.

Endometriosis and adenomyosis must be distinguished from pelvic inflammatory disease (differentiated by the presence of fever and leukocytosis), from tuberculosis, and from myomas and other neoplasia of the reproductive organs. Only in pelvic inflammatory disease and endometriosis are the symptoms usually aggravated by menstruation. Dilatation and curettage will generally distinguish adenomyosis from submucous myoma and cancer of the endometrium. Bowel invasion by endometrial tissue may produce clinical findings which may be almost indistinguishable from bowel neoplasm; differentiation in these rare instances depends upon biopsy.

Laboratory findings are of no value in the diagnosis of these disorders. X-ray contrast studies are helpful in the delineation of colonic involvement in endometriosis; and contrast hysterography is diagnostic in adenomyosis if the medium penetrates the glands. Laparoscopy is very useful.

Endometriosis is a significant cause of infertility.

Treatment

A. Endometriosis:

1. Medical treatment—Young married women with mild but advancing endometriosis should be advised to become pregnant without delay to secure a family and retard the progress of the disease. If the patient does not want a child or cannot become pregnant, exogenous hormone therapy is indicated with one of the following regimens:

(1) Enovid (or Enovid-E), 2.5 mg daily for 1 week; 5 mg daily for 2 weeks; increase by 2.5 mg for breakthrough bleeding.

(2) Norlestrin (2.5 mg), 1 tablet daily; increase by 1 tablet for breakthrough bleeding.

(3) Deluteval 2X, 1 ml IM weekly; increase by 0.5 ml for breakthrough bleeding.

(4) Depo-Provera, 2 ml (100 mg) IM every 2 weeks for 4 doses; then 2 ml every 4 weeks; add oral estrogen or Delestrogen, 30 mg IM, for breakthrough bleeding.

Give analgesics with codeine as necessary.

2. Surgical measures—The surgical treatment of moderately extensive endometriosis depends upon the patient's age and her desire to preserve reproductive function. If the patient is under 35, resect the lesions, free adhesions, and suspend the uterus. At least 20% of patients so treated will become pregnant, although half must undergo surgery again when the disease progresses. If the patient is over 35 years old and both ovaries are involved, both ovaries, the tubes, and the uterus must be excised.

Extensive endometriosis almost invariably necessitates ablation of both ovaries and tubes and the uterus regardless of the patient's age, unless it is possible to improve the patient's condition by inducing pseudopregnancy with progestins (see above) so that a less radical procedure will suffice.

3. **X-ray therapy**—If surgery is contraindicated or refused, castration doses of x-ray will relieve the symptoms and cause almost complete regression of the lesions. X-ray therapy cannot be condoned unless the diagnosis of advanced endometriosis is unequivocal.

B. Adenomyosis: The only treatment is surgical. A distinct zone of involvement is rarely found at operation. Hysterectomy is the treatment of choice because adenomyosis is such a widespread process. Prior to the menopause, normal ovaries should be retained. Irradiation therapy is effective but should be avoided in young women because it induces menopause.

Prognosis

The prognosis for reproductive function in early or moderately advanced endometriosis is good with conservative therapy. Castration is curative in severe and extensive endometriosis; if it is refused, hormone therapy may be beneficial.

Complete relief of symptoms is the rule following corrective surgery for adenomyosis.

Andrews WC, Larsen GD: Endometriosis: Treatment with hormonal pseudopregnancy and/or operation. Am J Obst Gynec 118:643, 1974.

Baggish MS, Woodruff JD: Uterine stromatosis: Clinicopathologic features and hormone dependency. Obst Gynec 40:487, 1972.

Bird CC & others: Elusive adenomyosis of the uterus: Revisited. Am J Obst Gynec 112:583, 1973.

Bullock JL & others: Symptomatic endometriosis in teenagers: A reappraisal. Obst Gynec 43:896, 1974.

Fagan CJ: Endometriosis: Clinical and roentgenographic manifestations. Radiol Clin North America 12:109, 1974.

Gray LA: Endometriosis of the bowel: Role of bowel resection, superficial excision and oophorectomy in treatment. Ann Surg 177:580, 1973.

Lamm DL & others: Ectopic endometrial glands in lymph nodes masquerading as metastatic adenocarcinoma. J Urol 111:770, 1974.

Pauli T, Tedeschi LG: Perineal endometriosis at the site of episiotomy scar. Obst Gynec 40:28, 1972.

Schifrin BS & others: Teenage endometriosis. Am J Obst Gynec 116:973, 1973.

Venable JH: Endometriosis of the ileum: Four cases with obstruction. Am J Obst Gynec 113:1054, 1972.

Voight JC: Carcinomatous change in ovarian endometriosis. Internat Surg 57:563, 1972.

CYSTOCELE

Essentials of Diagnosis

- Feeling of vaginal fullness and looseness, and incomplete emptying of the bladder.
- Soft, reducible mass, bulging into the anterior vagina, increased by straining.
- Residual urine collection.
- Urinary frequency, dysuria, stress or urgency incontinence (frequently).

General Considerations

Herniation of the posterior bladder wall and trigone into the vagina almost always are the result of laceration, during parturition, of the subvesical fibroareolar pseudofascia. Birth of a large baby and multiple or operative delivery increase the likelihood and degree of cystocele. Cystocele may be accompanied by urethrocele, a sagging of the urethra stripped from its attachments beneath the symphysis during childbirth. Prolapse of the uterus and rectocele and enterocele may be associated with cystocele. Concomitant with involution, which is marked after the menopause, the pelvic floor supports become attenuated, so that cystocele often becomes symptomatic after middle life.

Residual urine (60 ml or more) commonly complicates cystocele. Chronic, recurrent cystitis may follow, and problems of voiding usually result. When the normal posterior urethrovesical angle becomes considerably reduced with enlarging cystocele, stress incontinence develops.

Clinical Findings

A. Symptoms and Signs: Patients with cystocele describe vaginal looseness and a sense of the presence of urine even after voiding. A thin, reducible, nontender bulge into the vagina is noted forward of the cervix when cystocele is present. The woman may learn to manually reduce the sagging bladder to void completely. Residual urine usually is contaminated by bacteria. Hence, urgency, frequency, and dysuria, symptomatic of chronic urinary infection, may persist or recur. Stress incontinence is likely when the bladder herniation is extensive.

B. Laboratory Findings: Catheter drainage of the bladder after voiding will reveal more than 60 ml of residual urine in moderate or marked cystocele. Urinalysis of a catheterized or "clean-catch" specimen may reveal evidence of urinary tract infection.

C. X-Ray Findings: Anteroposterior and, especially, lateral films following introduction of x-ray contrast medium or a metal bead chain into the bladder will demonstrate bladder herniation.

Differential Diagnosis

Large bladder stones and tumors are firm and easily outlined. The bulge of a prolapsed cervix is readily seen with a speculum. An anterior cul-de-sac hernia is rare, but the small bowel within the sac may be felt to crepitate. This intestinal hernia may be visualized during gastrointestinal x-ray studies.

Treatment

A. Emergency Measures: Acute urinary retention secondary to overfilling of the bladder or marked uterine prolapse requires bladder catheterization.

B. Surgical Measures: Anterior vaginal colporrhaphy is most effective for cystocele repair. Transabdominal cystocele correction or obliterative vaginal operations (Le Fort's operation or colpectomy) may be chosen for correction of cystocele in special instances.

C. Supportive Measures: Pessaries (Menge, Gellhorn, Gehrung, ball) may reduce and support cystocele in patients who refuse or cannot withstand surgery. In postmenopausal women, estrogen therapy, eg, conjugated estrogenic substances (Premarin), 1.25 mg every other day (or equivalent) for an indefinite period, and the Kegel isometric exercises may improve urinary control.

D. Medical Measures: Treat urinary infections vigorously and adequately with antibiotics selected by culture and sensitivity tests.

Prognosis

The prognosis following surgery is excellent in the absence of pregnancy or stress due to increased intra-abdominal pressure (chronic ascites, bronchitis, asthma, bronchiectasis) or degenerative neurologic disorders affecting the pelvic floor structures.

Beecham CT, Beecham JB: Correction of prolapsed vagina or enterocele with fascia lata. Obst Gynec 42:542, 1973.
Cantor EB: Limited vaginal surgery for urinary stress incontinence. J Urol 105:867, 1971.
Wiser WL & others: Management of bladder drainage following vaginal plastic repairs. Obst Gynec 44:65, 1974.

RECTOCELE

Essentials of Diagnosis

- Chronic constipation or painful evacuation of feces.
- Soft posterior vaginal fullness.

General Considerations

Rectocele is a rectovaginal hernia caused by rupture, during childbirth, of the fibrous connective tissue layer separating these 2 structures. It may be due to the trauma of rapid delivery or forceps or breech extraction, particularly of a large fetus. Multiparous women are commonly affected. The quality of the tissues, the degree of damage, and the elimination habits of the patient are important factors in the development of rectocele and in its symptomatology. Constipation is aggravated by feces collection in the rectocele pouch. Straining at stool increases the defect, and hemorrhoids, anal fissures, uterine prolapse, enterocele, and cystocele may develop also. Although rectocele occasionally is diagnosed soon after a particularly difficult delivery, the abnormality usually becomes apparent after age 35–40 years. Digital rectocele compression, enemas, or frequent laxatives may be required to facilitate regular, easy bowel movements.

Clinical Findings

A. Symptoms and Signs: A sense of vaginal and rectal fullness and the constant urge for a bowel movement are typical complaints. A soft, thin-walled, reducible, nontender fullness involving the lower two-thirds of the posterior vagina may be seen (even without a speculum) and felt, often while the patient is straining, by depression of the perineum. A rectal examination easily confirms sacculation of the rectum into the vagina.

B. X-Ray Findings: Lateral films during a barium enema will delineate the rectocele.

Differential Diagnosis

Enterocele may develop above a rectocele. The apex of the rectocele should be identified by digital examination. Rectovaginal examination with the patient standing is helpful for confirmation of the diagnosis of enterocele because this hernia may protrude only when the patient is erect. A vaginal speculum will usually expose a prolapsed cervix or soft cervical or pedunculated uterine tumor, which are rarely confused with rectocele.

Treatment

A. Surgical Measures: Posterior colpoperineorrhaphy (often with correction of a true or potential enterocele) usually is curative of rectocele.

B. Supportive Measures: Avoidance of straining, coughing, and heavy lifting, improved diet and bowel habits, laxatives, and rectal suppositories are helpful. Good muscular relaxation during the second stage of labor, episiotomy, and prophylactic forceps delivery will often avoid or limit rectocele occurrence.

Prognosis

The prospects for cure after surgery are good provided subsequent vaginal delivery and straining at stool are avoided.

Marek CB: Transverse repair for rectocele. South MJ 62:749, 1969.
Nichols DH & others: Surgical significance of the rectovaginal septum. Am J Obst Gynec 108:215, 1970.

ENTEROCELE

Essentials of Diagnosis

- Uncomfortable heaviness in the vagina.
- Abdominal cramping several hours after eating (occasionally); constipation.
- Fullness or bulge in the vaginal vault, usually in menopausal or older parous women.

General Considerations

Cul-de-sac hernias may involve the pouch of Douglas (common) or may be anterior to the uterus (rare). Either type may be congenital or, by far most commonly, acquired. The congenital form may be noted in nulliparous patients. Enterocele frequently appears after severe coughing or straining. Birth trauma (usually forceps or breech extraction) develops or extends a sacculation between the uterosacral ligaments involving especially the posterior wall of the cul-de-sac. The thin enterocele sac, lined by peritoneum, generally contains small bowel which rarely is adherent. Uterine prolapse often is associated with enterocele, and, if procidentia is progressive, the hernial pouch also becomes larger. A sense of weight in the pelvis and fullness in the vagina may be associated with gastrointestinal discomfort several hours after meals, or constipation may be troublesome. Spontaneous obstruction almost never occurs in an enterocele. The differential diagnosis involves rectocele (posterior hernia) or cystocele (anterior hernia) and uterine descensus.

Clinical Findings

A. Symptoms and Signs: The pelvic and abdominal symptoms are vague and nonspecific. A sense of weight and distention of the upper vagina rarely is severe. Vaginal palpation will reveal a fullness in the upper vagina with enterocele. To distinguish a posterior cul-de-sac hernia, the examiner should place one finger in the rectum and one in the vagina; when the patient strains, the enterocele may be felt between the fingers in the rectovaginal septum. The hernia ia always more marked when the patient is standing or is in the high Fowler position.

B. X-Ray Findings: Lateral (erect) pelvic x-rays taken during small bowel study may reveal an enterocele.

Differential Diagnosis

Distinguish enterocele from cystocele when an anterior enterocele is suspected, or from rectocele when a posterior cul-de-sac hernia is possible. Prolapse of the vaginal vault (colpocele) following hysterectomy is almost always an enterocele. Uterine descensus may be confusing until the cervix is visualized, palpated, and identified.

Treatment

A. Emergency Measures: If bowel obstruction occurs, immediate laparotomy and release will be required.

B. Surgical Measures: Enterocele excision may be done transvaginally or transabdominally after dissection of the sac, high ligation, and fixation of the point of closure and reinforcement of the zone of weakness. Rectocele and cystocele repair and correction of uterine prolapse (or hysterectomy) should be done concomitantly.

C. Supportive Measures: Treat cough and constipation and limit straining and heavy lifting. Help the obese patient reduce.

Prognosis

The prognosis following proper (complete) surgery is good. Hysterectomy without closure of a true

or potential pelvic hernia will be followed by enterocele.

Fox PF, Kowalczyk AS: Ruptured enterocele. Am J Obst Gynec 111:592, 1971.
Nichols DH: Types of enterocele and principles underlying choice of operation for repair. Obst Gynec 40:257, 1972.
Zacharia RF, Hamilton NT: The problem of the large enterocele. Australian New Zealand J Obstet Gynaec 12:105, 1972.

MALPOSITION OF THE UTERUS
("Tipped Uterus")

Various types of uterine malposition have been said to cause pelvic pain, backache, abnormal uterine bleeding, and infertility. However, current opinion holds that a relationship between malposition of the uterus and definite symptomatology can be established only after specific, careful evaluation. Back pain, for example, is usually due to an orthopedic disorder. Anteflexion of the uterus almost never causes symptoms and requires no treatment. Lateral displacements of the uterus are frequently due to far more serious pelvic disease (usually neoplasms). Retrodisplacements may cause symptoms and require treatment.

The diagnosis of any type of uterine malposition depends upon abdominal and rectovaginal examination, and can be confirmed and documented by hysterography. If a woman complaining of pain, bleeding, or infertility is found to have a retroverted or retroflexed uterus, and if other more common causes of these complaints have been ruled out, a trial of pessary support is warranted. If the vaginal pessary consistently relieves symptoms and the symptoms return when the pessary is removed, it may be advisable to suspend the uterus surgically. If surgery is contraindicated or refused, the pessary may be worn intermittently until the menopause, at which time regression of uterine tissue will probably relieve symptoms altogether.

Knee-chest exercises are of doubtful value.

Soderberg G: Influence of abdominal and vaginal pessaries on the position of the uterus, especially during pregnancy and the puerperium. Acta obst gynec scandinav 50 (Suppl 13):1, 1971.

UTERINE PROLAPSE

Essentials of Diagnosis

- Firm mass in the lower vagina or protrusion of the cervix beyond the introitus.
- Sense of heaviness in the pelvis.
- Low backache or dragging sensation in the groins.

General Considerations

Uterine prolapse most commonly occurs as a delayed result of childbirth injury to the pelvic floor (particularly the transverse cervical and uterosacral ligaments). Unrepaired lacerations of the levator musculature and perineal body aggravate the weakness. Attenuation of the pelvic structures with aging, congenital weakness, neurologic injury to the sacral nerves, ascites, and internal genital tumors accelerate the development of prolapse.

Retroposition of the uterus usually develops with prolapse, whereupon the corpus, now in the axis of the vagina, exerts a piston-like action with each episode of increased intra-abdominal pressure. The cervix often becomes elongated for unknown reasons.

In slight prolapse the uterus descends only part way down the vagina. In moderate prolapse the corpus descends to the introitus and the cervix protrudes slightly beyond. In marked prolapse (procidentia) the entire cervix and uterus protrude beyond the introitus and the vagina is inverted.

Clinical Findings

A firm mass is palpable in the lower vagina. In moderate prolapse the cervix protrudes just beyond the introitus. The patient complains of a sense of heaviness in the pelvis, low backache, and a "dragging" sensation in the inguinal regions.

Pelvic examination with the patient bearing down or straining in the supine or standing position will demonstrate downward displacement of a prolapsing cervix and uterus. Herniation of the bladder, rectum, or cul-de-sac is diagnosed in a similar way. Consider uterine or adnexal neoplasms and ascites as possible causes of prolapse.

Rectovaginal examination may reveal rectal fullness (rectocele) or hernia of the pouch of Douglas behind and below the cervix. A metal sound or firm catheter within the bladder may be used to determine the extent of cystocele.

Differential Diagnosis

Uterine prolapse, a reducible sacropubic hernia, is the descensus of the cervix and uterus down the vagina to or beyond the introitus. If the uterus protrudes outside the introitus, the condition is known as uterine procidentia. Prolapse is generally associated with a compressible vaginal herniation of the bladder (cystocele), rectum (rectocele), and of the small bowel (enterocele). These defects may occur singly or in combination. Tumors of the cervix or uterus and fecal impaction in a rectocele must be differentiated from a sagging cervix and uterus.

Complications

Abnormal uterine bleeding and abortion may result from disordered uterine circulation. Ulceration in procidentia predisposes to cancer.

Prevention

Avoidance of obstetric trauma, and postpartum exercises to strengthen the levator musculature (Kegel), will prevent or minimize subsequent prolapse. Prolonged cyclic estrogen therapy for the postmenopausal woman will often conserve the strength and tone of the pelvic floor.

Treatment

Selection of the surgical approach depends upon the patient's age, the extent of prolapse, and her desire for menstruation, pregnancy, and coitus. Uterine suspension or ventrofixation is not effective in the treatment of prolapse.

Palliative therapy with a well-fitted vaginal pessary (eg, inflatable doughnut type, Gellhorn pessary) may give relief if surgery is refused or contraindicated.

Estrogen supplements improve tissue tone and correct atrophic vaginitis in postmenopausal patients.

Prognosis

Prolapse may remain constant for months or years, but it never regresses and will ultimately become more extreme unless corrected surgically.

Ekerling B, Goldman JA: Conservative treatment of utero-vaginal prolapse and stress incontinence. Internat Surg 57:221, 1972.

Elkin M & others: Ureteral obstruction in patients with uterine prolapse. Radiology 110:289, 1974.

Lavery JP, Boey CS: Uterine prolapse with pregnancy. Obst Gynec 42:681, 1973.

Mahran U: Vesical calculi complicating uterovaginal prolapse. Obstet Gynaec Brit Common 79:1146, 1972.

Ogunbode O, Aimakhu VE: Uterine prolapse during pregnancy in Ibadan. Am J Obst Gynec 116:622, 1973.

Myerscough PR: Genital prolapse. Practitioner 208:470, 1972.

Ubachs JMH & others: Partial colpocleisis by a modification of Le Fort's operation. Obst Gynec 42:415, 1973.

SALPINGITIS

Essentials of Diagnosis

- Severe cramp-like, nonradiating, lower abdominal pain; adnexal tenderness.
- Chills, moderately high intermittent fever.
- Venereal contact, leukorrhea.
- Abnormal menstruation or abortion.
- White count 20,000/cu mm with marked leukocytic preponderance; rapid sedimentation rate.
- Intracellular gram-negative diplococci are present in cervical, urethral, or Bartholin duct discharge with initial *Neisseria gonorrhoeae* infection.

General Considerations

Salpingitis, or inflammation of the fallopian tubes (also called pelvic inflammatory disease, PID), is directly or indirectly involved in almost one-fifth of all gynecologic problems. It may be acute or chronic and unilateral or bilateral. It is almost always due to bacterial infection, usually with gonococci, streptococci, tubercle bacilli, or a mixed bacterial flora. Tuberculous salpingitis usually occurs in prepuberal girls or in infertile or postmenopausal women. Women in the child-bearing years are most susceptible to pyogenic infection. Predisposing factors include venereal contact, infected abortions (including therapeutic abortion), hysterosalpingography with excess of oily contrast medium, degenerative cervical or uterine neoplasms, operative delivery, and peritonitis of bowel origin.

Clinical Findings

A. Symptoms and Signs: The manifestations of acute salpingitis include severe, cramp-like lower abdominal (usually bilateral) nonradiating pain, chills and fever, menstrual disturbances, leukorrhea, and adnexal tenderness. In the chronic stage, dysmenorrhea, dyspareunia, infertility, recurrent low-grade fever, and tender pelvic masses are described.

B. Laboratory Findings: The white count is elevated and the sedimentation rate is increased. The causative organisms may be demonstrated by appropriate smears and cultures of the vaginal discharge.

Differential Diagnosis

Acute appendicitis is typified by generalized lower abdominal pain, nausea, vomiting, and altered bowel function, with localization of pain in the right lower quadrant. Ectopic pregnancy is the preferred diagnosis when persistent lower quadrant pain of sudden onset is associated with a tender, soft adnexal mass, uterine bleeding, and a history of recent menstrual irregularity. In infected intrauterine abortion with adnexitis, the cervix is patulous, the lochia bloody and foul-smelling, and one or both ovaries are enlarged and tender.

Treatment

A. Specific Measures: For nontuberculous salpingitis give ampicillin, 500 mg orally 4 times daily for 5–7 days, or the equivalent in other antibacterial drugs. Tuberculous salpingitis is treated with streptomycin, 1 gm IM twice weekly; isoniazid, 150–300 mg orally daily; and aminosalicylic acid, 12–20 gm orally daily for at least 6 months.

B. General Measures: Control pain with hypnotics and analgesics. Delay or prevent menstruation for 1–2 months by oral sequential contraceptive hormone therapy such as Enovid, 10–15 mg/day.

C. Surgical Measures: Defer surgery during the acute phase. Consider surgery for pelvic abscess, large pelvic inflammatory masses, demonstrable pelvic disease causing persistent pain which cannot be controlled by medication, repeated episodes of abnormal uterine bleeding unresponsive to therapy, and whenever tuberculous masses do not resolve or fistulas develop in spite of massive prolonged antibiotic therapy. Adnexectomy and perhaps hysterectomy may be required for the treatment of extensive chronic incapacitating bilateral salpingitis.

Prognosis

Inflammation confined to one or both fallopian tubes, treated early and adequately, usually resolves rapidly, although obstruction may occur. If an abscess develops within or near the tube, recurrent salpingitis is the rule, and infertility is almost an unavoidable result.

Fraser AC: Surgical treatment of acute pelvic sepsis. J Obstet Gynaec Brit Common 79:560, 1972.

Josey WE, Staggers SR: Heparin therapy in septic pelvic thrombophlebitis: Study of 46 cases. Am J Obst Gynec 120:228, 1974.

Marshall BR, Jinguiji MS: Fatal *Streptococcus pyogenes* septicemia associated with intrauterine device (Dalkon Shield). Obst Gynec 41:83, 1973.

Phillips JC: A spectrum of radiologic abnormalities due to tubo-ovarian abscess. Radiology 110:307, 1974.

Swenson RM & others: Anaerobic bacterial infections of the female genital tract. Obst Gynec 42:538, 1973.

OVARIAN TUMORS

Follicle (Retention) Cysts

Follicle cysts are common, frequently bilateral and multiple cysts which appear on the surface of the ovaries as pale blebs filled with a clear fluid. They vary in size from microscopic to 4 cm in diameter (rarely larger). These cysts represent the failure of an incompletely developed follicle to reabsorb. They are commonly found in prolapsed adherent ovaries or when a thickened previously inflamed ovarian capsule prevents extrusion of the ovum. Symptoms are usually not present unless torsion or rupture with hemorrhage occurs, in which case the symptoms and signs of an abdominal emergency are often present. Large or numerous cysts may cause aching pelvic pain, dyspareunia, and occasionally abnormal uterine bleeding. The ovary may be slightly enlarged and tender to palpation, and the vaginal smear will often show a high estrogen level and a lack of progesterone stimulation.

Pelvic inflammatory disease and endometriosis must be considered in the differential diagnosis.

Most follicle cysts disappear spontaneously within 60 days without any treatment; when symptoms are disturbing, pelvic diathermy and attempt at reestablishment of ovulation with progesterone medication may be helpful. Malignant change does not occur.

Any cyst which becomes larger than 5 cm in diameter or which persists longer than 60 days probably is not a follicle cyst.

Smeaton TC, Robertson HA: Studies on the growth and atresia of the Graafian follicle in the ovary. J Reprod Fertil 25:243, 1971.

Spenos WJ: Preoperative hormone therapy of cystic ovarian masses. Am J Obst Gynec 116:551, 1973.

Van Campenhout J & others: Gonadotropin-resistant ovaries in primary amenorrhea. Obst Gynec 40:6, 1972.

Corpus Luteum Cysts

Corpus luteum cysts are functional, nonneoplastic enlargements of the ovary caused by the unexplained increase in secretion of fluid by the corpus luteum which occurs after ovulation or during early pregnancy. They are 4–6 cm in diameter, raised, and brown; and are filled with tawny serous fluid. An organizing blood clot is often found within the cavity.

Corpus luteum cysts may cause local pain and tenderness and either amenorrhea or delayed menstruation followed by brisk bleeding after resolution of the cyst. They are usually readily palpable. Corpus luteum cyst may encourage torsion of the ovary, causing severe pain, or it may rupture and bleed, in which case laparotomy is usually required to control hemorrhage into the peritoneum. Unless these acute complications develop, symptomatic therapy is all that is required. The cyst will disappear within 2 months in nonpregnant women and will gradually become smaller during the last trimester in pregnant women.

Theca Lutein Cysts

Theca lutein cysts range in size from minute to 4 cm in diameter. They are usually bilateral, are filled with clear straw-colored and occasionally bloody serous fluid, and are found only in association with hydatidiform mole and chorio-epithelioma or after excessive chorionic gonadotropin therapy. The cysts may rupture and bleed. The primary disease is suggested when an extremely high titer of chorionic gonadotropin is found in association with ovarian cysts. The remote possibility of bilateral papillary cystadenoma should be considered in the differential diagnosis.

These cysts disappear spontaneously following elimination of the molar pregnancy or destruction of the chorio-epithelioma.

Dick JS: Bilaterial theca lutein cysts associated with apparently normal pregnancy. J Obstet Gynaec Brit Common 79:852, 1972.
Judd HL & others: Maternal virilization developing during a twin pregnancy: Demonstration of excess ovarian androgen production associated with theca lutein cysts. New England J Med 288:118, 1973.

Endometrial Ovarian Cysts

Ectopic endometrium which develops on the ovary causes periodic (nonhormonally induced) bleeding. Attempts at "healing" follow each period, but invasion of the endometrial tissue eventually results in cyst formation. These cysts vary from microscopic in size up to 10–12 cm in diameter. They are filled with thick, chocolate-colored (old) blood and are often adherent to neighboring viscera. The symptoms are infertility, hypermenorrhea, dyspareunia, and secondary or acquired dysmenorrhea. Not all "chocolate cysts" are of endometrial origin, since bleeding into any cystic cavity will result in the accumulation of decomposed blood.

The treatment of large endometrial ovarian cysts is surgical removal, leaving as much functioning ovarian tissue as possible. Small cysts may be destroyed by electrocautery.

Aure JC & others: Carcinoma of the ovary and endometriosis. Acta obst gynec scandinav 50:63, 1971.
Voight JC: Carcinomatous change in ovarian endometriosis. Internat Surg 57:563, 1972.

Fibromas of the Ovary

About 5% of ovarian tumors are fibromas. They are unilateral, firm, nonfunctional (no hormone production), and benign, being composed principally of fibrous connective tissue. Fibromas are smooth, round, lobulated, nonadherent, and generally small, although a few have been reported which weighed as much as 5 lb. Fibromatous tumors are the principal cause of **Demons-Meigs syndrome.** The ascitic fluid is thought to be ovarian tumor transudate which is transferred in an undetermined manner to the thoracic cavity. The abdomen enlarges and the patient complains of orthopnea, tachycardia, and chest oppression. Torsion often occurs, causing agonizing pain in the affected lower quadrant and nausea and vomiting. Larger tumors cause a sense of pelvic heaviness. The tumor is usually palpable on pelvic examination.

Demons-Meigs syndrome must be distinguished from primary pulmonary and abdominal disease causing hydrothorax and ascites.

Treatment consists of surgical removal. Hydrothorax and ascites disappear promptly after removal of the tumor. Unless sarcoma is found on pathologic examination, the prognosis is excellent.

Chalvardjian A, Scully RE: Sclerosing stromal tumors of the ovary. Cancer 31:664, 1973.
Imin HK & others: Classification of fibroma and thecoma of the ovary: An ultrastructural study. Cancer 27:438, 1971.

Brenner Tumor

A Brenner tumor is a unilateral, firm, nonencapsulated, nonfunctioning neoplasm which consists of nests of epithelioid cells surrounded by whorls of dense connective tissue. It is often mistaken for fibroma. These tumors comprise 1% of all ovarian neoplasms. They are believed to arise from Walthard cell rests but are occasionally found in the wall of a pseudomucinous cystadenoma. Brenner tumors may grow to 30 cm in diameter, although most are less than 2–3 cm. They are most common in women over 40 years of age and are occasionally associated with Demons-Meigs syndrome. They are almost never malignant.

Brenner tumors produce symptoms only by virtue of their size and situation, ie, unilateral pelvic discomfort and a sense of fullness and heaviness in the lower abdomen. If torsion occurs it causes acute abdominal pain with nausea and vomiting.

Treatment consists of ovariectomy.

Bransilver BR & others: Brenner tumors and Walthard cell nests. Arch Path 98:76, 1974.

Fox H & others: The Brenner tumor of the ovary: A clinico-pathological study of 54 cases. J Obstet Gynaec Brit Common 79:661, 1972.

Hameed K: Brenner tumor of the ovary with Leydig cell hyperplasia: A histologic and ultrastructural study. Cancer 30:945, 1972.

Hull MGR, Campbell GR: The malignant Brenner tumor. Obst Gynec 42:527, 1973.

Nissen ED, Goldstein AJ: Ovarian tumors with functioning stromal cells: Case report of a feminizing Brenner tumor. Internat J Gynaec Obstet 11:213, 1973.

Teratoid Tumors

Teratoid tumors are of unknown origin. They are composed of one, 2, or 3 germinal layers which may grow into any possible combination of imperfectly formed structures. If one type of tissue predominates, the appearance will be that of a single-tissue tumor; such is the case in struma ovarii, the thyroid (iodine-containing) tumor of the ovary. Dermoid cysts, the most common type of teratoid tumor, contain ectodermal (and often mesodermal) tissue in the form of macerated skin, hair, bone and teeth; the cyst is filled with a heavy, greasy sebaceous material and integumental structures. Teratoid tumors occur primarily in women 18–40 years of age. Orientals are prone to develop dermoids. Dermoids account for 10% and solid teratomas 0.1% of all ovarian tumors. About 15% are bilateral.

The clinical manifestations of teratoid tumor are produced when the freely shifting mass distorts and displaces neighboring viscera. A teratoid is relatively light and rarely adherent. It tends to "float" upward in the abdomen, which encourages the development of a long pedicle; when torsion occurs, sudden, excruciating, persistent pain results. Rupture of a dermoid due to trauma or during pregnancy results in chemical peritonitis. If the neoplasm is large, the patient may complain of constipation and urinary frequency. Calcification may be observed on x-ray in the form of teeth or bone.

Teratoid tumor must be differentiated from pedunculated uterine myomas.

The treatment of teratoma is surgical removal and examination and aspiration of the other ovary to make certain that another dermoid is not present. Care should be taken not to spill the contents into the pelvic cavity, and teratomas should never be needled through the cul-de-sac for therapeutic or diagnostic reasons since leakage into the abdomen causes irritation and peritonitis.

The prognosis is excellent. Malignant change, though uncommon, implies a guarded prognosis.

Cox CT, Kitay DZ: Spontaneous rupture of an ovarian cystic teratoma in pregnancy. J Reprod Med 7:179, 1971.

Garden AS, Best PV: Ovarian teratoma with intraabdominal dissemination. J Obstet Gynaec Brit Common 79:1139, 1972.

Philippe E & others: Benign cystic teratoma of the ovaries: An anatomic and clinical study of 481 cases. Gynec Obst 70:513, 1971.

Sinniah R, O'Brien FV: Pigmented progonoma in a dermoid cyst of the ovary. J Path 109:357, 1973.

Cystadenomas (Pseudomucinous & Serous Cystadenomas)

Cystadenomas are the most common of ovarian neoplasms, representing 70% of all ovarian tumors. These tumors produce no hormone and are most common in women between the ages of 45 and 65. Serous and pseudomucinous cystadenomas occur with about equal frequency.

Pseudomucinous cystadenoma grows more sluggishly and becomes larger than the serous type; some have been reported to weigh over 100 lb. These tumors are in a sense teratomas composed entirely of entoderm. They are usually multilocular; contain a thick, viscid, brownish liquid; are lined by tall columnar epithelial and goblet cells; and are contained in a tough membranous capsule. About 5% are found to be malignant at surgery.

Serous cystadenomas do not become as large as pseudomucinous cystadenomas; most weigh 10–20 lb. They are multilocular, filled with a thin yellowish fluid, are lined by cuboidal or short columnar cells, and tend to develop papillary excrescences on both their inner and outer surfaces. Serous cystadenomas, like the pseudomucinous type, are also contained in a parchment-like capsule. Small sand-like, sharp, calcareous concretions (psammoma bodies) are often present within the tumor. Serous cystadenomas are believed to arise from invagination of the germinal epithelium of the surface of the ovary.

Cystadenomas are silent tumors because they do not produce hormones, pedicles form rarely, and the capsule does not rupture easily. Symptoms are produced only when the tumor becomes large enough to cause increased abdominal girth and weight gain, pelvic heaviness, constipation, and urinary frequency. The tumor is easily palpable on abdominal examination, and x-rays may show psammoma bodies. About 50% eventually become malignant.

Treatment consists of surgical removal of benign tumors by oophorocystectomy and, if malignant change has occurred, panhysterectomy and bilateral salpingo-oophorectomy. Radiation or systemic chlorambucil or another cancer chemotherapeutic drug is indicated if peritoneal or visceral metastases are found.

All ovarian cysts over 7 cm in diameter and those which persist for over 90 days should be removed.

Fazekas JT, Maier JG: Irradiation of ovarian carcinoma: A prospective comparison of the open-field and moving strip techniques. Am J Roentgenol 120:118, 1974.

Jensen RD, Morris HJ: Epithelial tumors of the ovary: Occurrence in children and adolescents less than 20 years of age. Arch Path 94:29, 1972.

Julian C, Woodruff JD: Biologic behavior of low-grade papillary serous carcinoma of the ovary. Obst Gynec 40:860, 1972.

Malkasian GD Jr: Chemotherapy for ovarian cancer. M Clin North America 58:779, 1974.

Mesonephroma

Mesonephroma is an uncommon nonfunctioning ovarian tumor which clinically and grossly resembles papillary serous cystadenoma. Most cases occur in patients over 35 and are probably of teratogenous origin. The tumor is often 10–20 cm in diameter when first discovered. Thirty percent are malignant. Salpingo-oophorectomy is necessary for cure. If it is likely that malignant change has occurred, panhysterectomy is required. Radiation therapy should be considered also.

Fine G & others: Mesonephroma of the ovary: A clinical, morphological and histogenetic appraisal. Cancer 31:398, 1973.
Hayes D: Mesonephroid tumors of the ovary. J Obstet Gynaec Brit Common 79:728, 1972.
Parmley TH, Woodruff JD: The ovarian mesothelioma. Am J Obst Gynec 120:234, 1974.

Arrhenoblastoma

Arrhenoblastoma is a rare ovarian tumor (fewer than 175 cases have been reported). It occurs most frequently during the reproductive years and is assumed either to arise from sexually ambivalent cells noted in the ovary of the 6- to 7-week embryo or to be of teratoid origin. The tumor is unilateral (slightly more often on the right side) and may be minute or may fill the entire pelvis. Twenty-five percent become malignant, but metastases are usually late.

Arrhenoblastomas are often hormonally active, producing androgenic substances which cause both defeminization and virilization, manifested by varying degrees of amenorrhea, acne, hirsutism, recession of the hairline at the forehead, slight alopecia, loss of feminine contour, breast and genital atrophy, clitoral hypertrophy, and deepening of the voice. Urinary excretion of 17-ketosteroids is slightly to moderately increased; urinary dehydroepiandrosterone levels are strikingly high. Urinary hydroxysteroids are not elevated. The FSH titer is normal or minimally reduced.

Arrhenoblastoma must be distinguished from the adrenocortical disorders, a much more frequent cause of virilization, which usually cause less virilization and a much more pronounced elevation of the urinary 17-ketosteroids.

Arrhenoblastoma should be removed surgically together with other pelvic reproductive organs unless the patient desires children and the tumor is clinically and histologically benign, in which case unilateral oophorectomy and salpingectomy are sufficient. Hormonal evaluation should be repeated after several months to determine recurrence.

Cruikshank DP & others: Arrhenoblastomas and associated pathology. Obst Gynec 43:539, 1974.
Greenblatt RB & others: Arrhenoblastoma: Three case reports. Obst Gynec 39:567, 1972.
Gupta PK: Cytohormonal studies in arrhenoblastoma. Acta cytol 16:1, 1972.
Younglai EV & others: Arrhenoblastoma: In vivo and in vitro studies. Am J Obst Gynec 116:401, 1973.

Virilizing Lipoid Cell Tumors

Virilizing lipoid cell tumors of the ovary are a group of rare small neoplasms occurring in women over 50 years of age and causing symptoms and signs of virilization, such as hirsutism, masculine hair distribution, odorous perspiration, acne, and clitoral hypertrophy. Obesity is common. Hypertension, polycythemia, and diabetes mellitus are sometimes associated. The tumor may be too small to be palpated. The excretion of 17-oxysteroids and 17-ketosteroids is elevated, and the urinary pregnanetriol level may be high.

These tumors must be differentiated from arrhenoblastoma and primary adrenal abnormalities. About 20% are malignant.

Treatment consists of surgical removal.

Verhoeven AT & others: Virilization in pregnancy coexisting with an (ovarian) mucinous cystadenoma: A case report and review of virilizing ovarian tumors in pregnancy. Obst Gynec Surv 28:597, 1973.

Stein-Leventhal Syndrome

Bilateral polycystic ovaries, secondary amenorrhea or oligomenorrhea, and infertility in females 15–30 years of age typify the classical Stein-Leventhal or polycystic ovarian syndrome. Hirsutism and obesity often are associated problems. Defective intermediate metabolism of sex steroids, perhaps familial, is postulated as the cause, and a deficiency of the enzymes 3β-ol-dehydrogenase and 10-hydroxylase in the ovary probably is responsible. Anovulation accounts for the menstrual aberration and infertility. Hirsutism probably is due to overstimulation by intrinsic androgen. The slightly enlarged gonads, often described as "oyster ovaries," are pearly-white, smooth, and firm. A condensation of tissue in the peripheral cortex forming a pseudocapsule with many small, persistent follicle cysts beneath luteinization of the theca interna (but rarely of the ovarian stroma) may be noted.

The history and palpably enlarged ovaries (in about half of cases) permit a presumptive diagnosis. Pelvic pneumography, culdoscopy, peritoneoscopy, or culdotomy adds confirmatory evidence. Laboratory studies reveal slight elevation of the urinary 17-ketosteroids and plasma testosterone. The urinary estrogen, FSH, and adrenocorticosterone excretion remain normal. An increased output of Δ4-androstenedione, 17α-hydroxyprogesterone, or dehydroepiandrosterone has been described.

Adrenocortical hyperplasia or tumor is ruled out by the normal hydroxycorticosteroid excretion. A masculinizing neoplasm is unlikely because of bilateral ovarian enlargement.

Initial treatment (still empiric) should be medical. Courses of clomiphene citrate (Clomid), 50 mg orally daily for 5 days each month, or 50 mg daily for 3–4 months, may induce ovulation and correct the menstrual problem. Larger doses may cause macrocystic ovaries, rupture, and hematoperitoneum and should not be given. If the patient is unresponsive to clomiphene, wedge resection of one-third to one-half of each ovary may be beneficial. The hirsutism and obesity do not respond to the above therapy, but these side-effects can be overcome by epilation and diet.

Judd HL & others: Familial hyperthecosis: Comparison of endocrinologic and histologic findings with polycystic ovarian disease. Am J Obst Gynec 117:976, 1973.

Nebel L & others: Coelomic mesothelium-like cells in the ovarian stroma of patients with polycystic ovarian syndrome (Stein-Leventhal syndrome). Am J Obst Gynec 111:766, 1971.

Stahl NL & others: Ovarian adrenal and peripheral testosterone levels in the polycystic ovarian syndrome. Am J Obst Gynec 117:194, 1973.

Stahl NL & others: Serum testosterone levels in hirsute women: A comparison of adrenal, ovarian and peripheral vein values. Obst Gynec 41:650, 1973.

Theca Cell Tumors*

Theca cell tumors are rare functional, feminizing ovarian neoplasms derived from ovarian stromal anlagen. They occur most frequently in young girls and postmenopausal women, and vary in size from minute nodules to masses 30 cm in diameter. The ratio of theca cell tumors to granulosa cell tumors is 1:8, and pure theca cell tumors are rare. About 1% become malignant. The tumor is almost invariably unilateral.

Clinical and laboratory findings are identical with those of granulosa cell tumors. As is true of granulosa cell tumors also, theca cell tumors may rarely virilize rather than feminize for obscure reasons.

As the cause of abnormal uterine bleeding, theca cell tumors must be differentiated from idiopathic precocious puberty, granulosa cell tumors, and uterine neoplasms.

Treatment for benign theca cell tumors is unilateral ovariectomy. Malignant tumors require total hysterectomy and bilateral salpingo-oophorectomy.

Granulosa Cell Tumor*

Granulosa cell tumors, the most common ovarian neoplasms of sex gland derivation, represent 3–4% of all ovarian tumors. They are solid tumors which vary in size from microscopic to 9 kg (20 lb) and often produce estrogens. A rare tumor may be virilizing, however. Granulosa cell tumors are most often seen in women 50–70 years of age. Ten percent are bilateral. Both granulosa and theca cells are always found together. About 15–20% are malignant, but metastasis is almost always confined to neighboring genital organs.

The clinical manifestations of granulosa cell tumors are secondary to the production of large amounts of estrogen. In children, this causes early development of pubic hair, hypertrophy of the breasts, and enlargement of the labia, cervix, and uterus (pseu-

*Pure granulosa cell tumors of the ovary are rare; theca cells are almost always present also. It would be more appropriate to speak of granulosa-theca cell tumors or theca-granulosa cell tumors, depending upon which type of cell predominates. The 2 types are dealt with separately here in order to simplify discussion.

doprecocious puberty). Advanced bone age and early epiphyseal closure (dwarfism) will occur if hormonal stimulation is continued for a long period. In the functional years menometrorrhagia is usually the only symptom. In postmenopausal women refeminization and reinstitution of uterine bleeding occur. Very large tumors may cause symptoms secondary to abdominal distention, displacement of the pelvic structures, or torsion of the pedicle. Ascites often occurs when the neoplasm is malignant. On pelvic examination a mobile, often soft and cystic mass is palpable in the adnexa. Laboratory findings consist of elevated urinary estrogens and a high degree of cornification as demonstrated in the vaginal smear.

Granulosa cell tumors must be differentiated from other causes of postmenopausal bleeding or abnormal menstruation, and other functional tumors (eg, lipoid cell tumors and theca cell tumors of the ovary).

Treatment consists of surgical removal. In patients in the functional or prepuberal years, benign tumors are removed by ovariectomy; in postmenopausal women, total hysterectomy and bilateral salpingo-oophorectomy are indicated.

Anderson WR & others: Granulosa-theca cell tumors: Clinical and pathologic study. Am J Obst Gynec 110:32, 1971.

Gough HM, Walther GL: Thecoma in pregnancy. Canad MAJ 108:595, 1973.

Mecca JT & others: Thecoma with extensive calcification. Brit J Radiol 47:492, 1974.

Dysgerminoma

Dysgerminoma is a nonfunctioning, potentially malignant ovarian tumor. About 4% of all primary malignant ovarian tumors are dysgerminomas and about one-third of dysgerminomas are cancerous. Dysgerminoma is bilateral in one-third of cases and is most common in females 10–30 years of age. It is thought to be of teratoid origin. Although usually small when found (4–7 cm in diameter), dysgerminomas may grow rapidly to fill the entire pelvis. The tumor is often discovered in patients with underdeveloped secondary sex characteristics such as occur in female pseudohermaphrodites. The same tumor found in a male is called a seminoma.

Symptoms are usually due to abdominal enlargement caused by rapid tumor growth and ascites. Severe abdominal distress and acute pain may result if the thin capsule ruptures. Weakly false-positive pregnancy tests have been reported in some cases.

Other nonfunctioning ovarian tumors (eg, teratoma, cystadenoma) must be considered in the differential diagnosis.

Treatment usually consists of surgical removal of the tumor and all pelvic reproductive organs, but if the tumor is small, unilateral, and histologically benign, and if the patient desires to maintain reproductive function, partial oophorectomy may be feasible.

Underdeveloped secondary sex characteristics do not improve after removal of the tumor.

Fun KM, Poddar DL: Dysgerminoma of the ovary: Malignancy prognosis and treatment. J Obstet Gynaec India 24:183, 1974.

Talerman A & others: Dysgerminoma: Clinicopathological study of 22 cases. Obst Gynec 41:137, 1973.

Williamson HO, Pratt-Thomas HR: Bilateral gonadoblastoma with dysgerminoma: A case report. Obst Gynec 39:263, 1972.

Secondary Ovarian Cancer

In 10% of cases of fatal malignant disease in women, the ovary is found to be secondarily involved by metastasis or extension of malignancy, usually from the uterus or the ovary. One-third represent metastasis from stomach cancer. The intestine, breast, thyroid, kidney, and adrenals may also be primary foci. One of the most important carcinomas which metastasizes to the ovaries is the Krukenberg tumor, which usually originates in the stomach, involves both ovaries, and presents as a large mucin-producing, buff-colored, solid, lobulated, often kidney-shaped, nonadherent tumor with a heavy capsule. At laparotomy it is important to distinguish these secondary ovarian cancers from primary ovarian tumors clinically and by frozen section.

Hudson CV, Dendy PP: Aspects of treatment of more advanced cases of ovarian cancer. Proc Roy Soc Med 67:798, 1974.

Percival R: Cancer and the ovary. Proc Roy Soc Med 67:381, 1974.

Ramachandran G & others: Ovarian neoplasms: A study of 903 cases. J Obstet Gynaec India 22:309, 1972.

Timm J: Ovarian carcinoma: A 10-year series from a provincial hospital. Acta obst gynec scandinav 52:103, 1973.

URINARY STRESS INCONTINENCE

Involuntary leakage of urine during moments of increased intra-abdominal pressure is one of the most common gynecologic complaints. It may occur as a result of congenital or acquired disorders of the urinary tract, pelvic musculature, or nervous system. Compression of the bladder by the pregnant uterus, pelvic tumors, or ascites may also reduce the ability to retain urine. Leakage usually occurs upon coughing, sneezing, laughing, or sudden lifting of objects. Most women with urinary stress incontinence have suffered childbirth injuries or have developed weakness of the pelvic floor structures following menopause. Relaxation of the supports to the bladder and urethra is noted, often with cystocele, rectocele, and uterine prolapse. Lateral cystourethrograms generally reveal loss of the normal posterior urethrovesical angle.

Urinary stress incontinence must be differentiated from neurogenic bladder and bladder irritability. Paradoxic incontinence or overflow voiding may be due to neurologic disorders or to partial urethrovesical obstruction.

Treatment

A trial of medical treatment is always indicated before surgery is considered. Medical disorders such as myasthenia gravis, diabetes mellitus, extreme obesity, and asthma, which aggravates stress incontinence, should be controlled if possible. Postmenopausal women should receive cyclic estrogen therapy, eg, with diethylstilbestrol, 0.25 mg orally daily for 3 weeks each month. Patients who do not have serious neurologic disorders and have not sustained severe physical injury can be taught to contract the pubococcygeus and sphincter ani muscles repeatedly to reestablish urinary control (Kegel exercises).

Patients who fail to respond to exercises may be candidates for surgery, particularly when cystocele or prolapse of the bladder and uterus is present. A useful surgical prognostic test is to fill the bladder and elevate the anterior vaginal wall lateral to the urethra at the urethrovesical junction with the fingers or an instrument. If loss of urine does not occur with stress, the prognosis is good.

Medical therapy alone is curative in about half of cases. The overall surgical cure rate in patients who require operation is about 85%.

Arnoed EP: Urodynamics of female incontinence: Factors in fluencing the results of surgery. Am J Obst Gynec 117:805, 1973.

Beck RP & others: Recurrent urinary stress incontinence treated by fascia lata sling procedure. Am J Obst Gynec 120:613, 1974.

Brocklehurst JC: Treatment of urinary incontinence in the elderly. Postgrad Med 51:184, 1972.

Cantor EB: The management of female urinary stress incontinence. Internat J Gynaec Obstet 11:153, 1973.

Crist T & others: Stress incontinence and the nulliparous patient. Obst Gynec 40:13, 1972.

Edwards EL: The investigation and management of incontinence of urine in women. Ann Roy Coll Surg England 52:69, 1973.

Furlow WL: Evaluation of the Kaufman anti-incontinence procedure with 14 patients. J Urol 108:770, 1972.

Kursch ED & others: The Pereyra procedure and urinary stress incontinence. J Urol 108:591, 1972.

Moolaoker AS & others: The diagnosis and management of urinary incontinence in the female. J Obstet Gynaec Brit Common 79:481, 1972.

Morgan JE: The suprapubic approach to primary stress urinary incontinence. Am J Obst Gynec 115:316, 1973.

Nichols DH, Milley PS: Identification of pubourethral ligaments and their role in transvaginal surgical correction of stress incontinence. Am J Obst Gynec 115:123, 1973.

Nielsen E, Lundwall T: Urethrovaginal fixation to Cooper's ligament (Burch) in the treatment of incontinence. Acta chir scandinav 443(Suppl):118, 1973.

Roman-Lopez JJ, Barclay DL: Bladder dysfunction following Schauta hysterectomy. Am J Obst Gynec 115:81, 1973.

Williams TJ: Urinary incontinence in the female. M Clin North America 58:729, 1974.

DYSPAREUNIA

Dyspareunia (painful coitus) may be functional or organic; may be due to decreased vaginal secretion, particularly in the region of the vulva; or may be due to a combination of causes. It may occur early (primary) or late (secondary) in marriage. The location of discomfort may be external (at the introitus) or internal (deep within the genital canal or beyond), and some women describe both types of pain.

External dyspareunia may be due to occlusive or rigid hymen, vaginal contracture due to any cause, or traumatic or inflammatory disorders of the vulva, vagina, urethra, or anus.

Organic causes of internal dyspareunia include hourglass contracture of the vagina, septate vagina, severe cervicitis or retroposition of the uterus, prolapse or neoplastic disease of the uterus, tubo-ovarian disease, and pelvic endometriosis.

Pelvic examination often reveals marked contraction of the perineal and levator musculature, with adduction of the thighs. Genital hypoplasia and other congenital disorders, urethral caruncle, scarring or contracture of the vagina, vulvovaginitis, kraurosis vulvae, and rectal or bladder abnormalities may be present.

Treatment

A. Specific Measures: Functional dyspareunia can only be treated by counseling and psychotherapy. The importance of preplay before sexual intercourse must be emphasized. An appropriate vaginal lubricant may be useful. Adequate estrogen treatment is often required for older women. Patients should be cautioned against the unwarranted use of douches, especially prolonged or employing detergent solution. Both partners should be interviewed. The treatment of organic dyspareunia depends upon the underlying cause.

B. General Measures: Mild sedation, eg, phenobarbital, 15 mg orally 3 times daily, or prochlorperazine, 15 mg orally daily, is of value for the relief of extreme emotional tension.

C. Local Measures: For functional dyspareunia, hymeneal-vaginal dilatations with a conical (Kelly) dilator or test tubes of graduated sizes may give relief. Anesthetic ointment applied to the introitus gives some relief but is of no permanent value. Organic dyspareunia due to vaginal dryness may be treated with a water-soluble lubricant. Estrogen therapy is indicated for senile vulvovaginitis.

D. Surgical Measures: Hymenectomy, perineotomy, and similar procedures should be performed only on clear indications. Significant obstructive lesions should be corrected. Treat chronic symptomatic cervicitis by cauterization or shallow conization.

Prognosis

Few patients with functional dyspareunia are quickly and easily cured. Organic dyspareunia subsides promptly after elimination of the cause.

Rankin PR Jr: The use of Z-plasty in gynecologic operations: Case report. Am J Obst Gynec 117:231, 1973.
Serreyn R, Vande Kerckhove D: Lacerations of the broad ligament: A critical approach to the Allen-Masters syndrome. Europ J Obstet Gynaec 2:133, 1972.

PSYCHOGENIC PELVIC PAIN

Functional pelvic pain is variously reported to occur in 5–25% of gynecologic patients. The diagnosis is established by ruling out organic causes and, wherever possible, by eliciting a consonant history. A fairly characteristic "profile" of the typical woman with psychogenic pain is as follows: she is egotistical and vain, demanding and self-indulgent, shallow, dramatic, emotionally labile and inconsistent, and coquettish but relatively frigid.

Treatment

Any woman who complains of pelvic pain must have a thorough diagnostic evaluation, in a hospital if necessary. Reassurance and symptomatic therapy are always indicated, and may be all that the physician can provide. Since the basic disorder is a psychic one, the physician must be prepared to spend a great deal of time with these women. Do not give narcotics and do not operate except upon definite surgical indications. Be wary of prescribing sedatives as these patients may commit suicide when depressed.

Prognosis

Since these women often refuse therapy, withdraw from a treatment program soon after it is well

Table 12–4. Differential diagnosis of organic psychogenic pain.

	Organic Pain	Psychogenic Pain
Type	Sharp, cramping, intermittent.	Dull, continuous.
Time of onset	Any time. May awaken patient.	Usually begins well after waking, when social obligations are pressing.
Radiation	Follows definite neural pathways.	Bizarre pattern or does not radiate.
Localization	Localizes with typical point tenderness.	Variable, shifting, generalized.
Progress	Soon becomes either better or worse.	Remains the same for weeks, months, years.
Provocation	Often reproduced or augmented by manipulation, not by mood.	Not triggered or accentuated by examination but by interpersonal relationships.

under way, and change physicians frequently, their medical future is bleak. In general, they are unwilling to abandon invalidism as a way of life.

Of those patients who can be persuaded to seek psychiatric treatment, over half will show marked improvement and many will be cured. Reassurance and symptomatic therapy result in temporary improvement in about three-fourths of cases.

DeSousa-Alan PC & others: Psychological aspects in gynaecological disorders. Clinician 37:443, 1973.

Frangenheim H, Kleindienst W: Chronic pelvic pain of unknown origin. J Reprod Med 13:23, 1974.

Hartnett LJ: Venography of the female pelvis. Obst Gynec 41:507, 1973.

Sloan D: Pelvic pain and dysmenorrhea. P Clin North America 19:669, 1972.

GYNECOLOGIC CAUSES OF BACKACHE

Gynecologic causes of backache are uncommon. Backache occurs most frequently as a gynecologic complaint during the childbearing years, and is more common among women who have had several children. Multiple causes are the rule (gynecologic combined with orthopedic, urologic, or neurologic disease). Gynecologic causes include the following: (1) Traction or pulsion on the peritoneum, the supportive structures of the generative organs, or the pelvic floor (tumors, ascites, uterine prolapse). (2) Inflammation of the pelvic contents: bacterial infection (peritonitis, salpingitis) or chemical irritation (due to iodides used in salpingography, fluid from a ruptured dermoid cyst). (3) Invasion of pelvic tissues or bone by tumor or endometriosis. (4) Obstruction of the genital tract (cervical stenosis). (5) Torsion or constriction of pelvic viscera (ovary enmeshed in adhesions, twisted ovarian cyst). (6) Congestion of internal genitalia (turgescence of the retroposed uterus, backache during menstruation). (7) Psychologic tension (anxiety, apprehension). (8) Masters-Allen syndrome (avulsion of uterus from parauterine supports), also called the "universal joint syndrome."

Clinical Findings

A. Symptoms and Signs: Constant lumbosacral or sacral backache is often due to salpingitis, pelvic abscess, or a twisted ovarian cyst. Back pain due to endometriosis of the cul-de-sac is referred to the coccygeal region or rectum. Ovarian, renal, and ureteral backache commonly radiates down the back into the buttocks or along the distribution of the sciatic nerves.

The major symptoms and signs of the underlying pelvic disease are almost always present.

B. Laboratory Findings: Infection will be reflected in the routine blood studies. Cytologic study of vaginal exudate may reveal neoplastic cells or bacteria.

C. X-Ray Findings: Anteroposterior and lateral films of the spine often disclose a postural, degenerative, neoplastic, or other orthopedic cause of backache. Myelograms may be required to demonstrate a herniated intervertebral disk.

Treatment

Successful treatment of the underlying disease is the only curative procedure. Supportive measures include the following: (1) Bed rest on a firm mattress, permitting the patient to seek the most comfortable position. (2) Local heat as necessary. (3) Aspirin or aspirin with codeine as needed. (4) Sedatives, eg, phenobarbital, 15 mg 3 times daily to reduce emotional tension.

Prognosis

Gynecologic backache almost always subsides with treatment of the underlying pelvic disorder.

INFERTILITY

A couple is said to be infertile (1) if pregnancy does not result after 1 year of normal marital relations without contraceptives; (2) if the woman conceives but aborts repeatedly; or (3) if the woman bears one child but aborts repeatedly or fails to conceive thereafter. About 10% of marriages are infertile. Female infertility may be due to nutritional deficiencies, hormonal imbalance, developmental anomalies of the reproductive organs, infections, or tumors. Male infertility is usually due to sperm deficiencies (low sperm count, morphologic abnormalities, or impaired motility). The male partner is accountable for about 40% of cases of infertility.

Diagnostic Survey

Successful treatment of infertility is possible only if an early and accurate diagnosis can be established. Over a period of at least 3 months, with 4 office visits for the wife and 2–3 for the husband, both partners usually can be evaluated and the cause of infertility determined.

A. First Visit: (Wife and husband.) In a joint interview, the physician explains the problem of infertility and its causes to the husband and wife. Separate private consultations are then conducted, allowing appraisal of marital adjustments without embarrassment or criticism. Pertinent details (eg, venereal disease or prior illegitimate pregnancies) must be obtained concerning marital, premarital, and extramarital sexual activities. A complete medical, surgical, and obstetrical history must be taken. The gynecologic history should include queries regarding the menstrual pattern (eg, pain, metrorrhagia, and leukorrhea) and the type of menstrual protection worn, either internal or external. The present history includes marital adjustment, difficulties, use of contraceptives and types, douches, libido, sex technics, orgasm, frequency and success of coitus, and correlation of intercourse with ovulation. Family history includes familial traits, liabilities, illnesses, repeated abortions, and abnormal children.

The husband is instructed to bring a complete ejaculate for spermatozoal analysis at the next visit. Sexual abstinence for at least 4 days before the semen is obtained is emphasized. Semen may be collected either by coitus or masturbation. A clean, dry, wide-mouthed bottle for collection is preferred, but a vaginal (Doyle) spoon can be used. Condoms should not be employed. The stoppered bottle should be transported to the laboratory in a paper bag held away from the body. Chilling of the bottle should also be avoided.

Semen should be examined (by the physician himself) within 1–2 hours after collection.

B. Second Visit: (Wife and husband; 2–4 weeks after first visit.) The woman receives a complete physical and pelvic examination. Do not overlook irritations, discharges, tenderness, maldevelopments, and masses. The husband's general physical examination, with emphasis on the genital and rectal examination, is done next. Penile, urethral, testicular, epididymal, and prostatic abnormalities are sought. The results of the spermatozoal analysis are explained to the couple without undue optimism or pessimism. Laboratory studies for both husband and wife include urinalysis, complete blood count (including hematocrit determination), and STS. Thyroid function should be determined.

C. Third Visit: (Wife; 1 month after second visit. The husband is not required to return for a third visit if his physical examination and initial semen analysis are normal. Spermatozoal analysis is repeated on the third visit if the previous study was abnormal.)

1. Tubal insufflation (Rubin test)—Uterotubal insufflation in infertile patients has both diagnostic and therapeutic value. It is best done during the early preovulatory period. The test is a safe office procedure in properly selected patients if CO_2 is employed and if the pressure is kept below 200 mm Hg. Tubal insufflation at or about the time of ovulation is most likely to be revealing and successful. Pneumoperitoneum (and shoulder pain) is proof of tubal patency. Auscultation over the lower abdomen during insufflation may disclose the whistle of gas passing through one tubal ostium or the other. It is most helpful to secure a kymographic record of insufflation; tubal peristalsis, patency, leakage in the system, tubal spasm, partial obstruction, or release of tubal obstruction may be revealed in this way.

2. Hysterosalpingography is preferred by many but may not be required if gas insufflation is unimpeded.

D. Fourth Visit: (Wife; 1 month following the third visit.) The patient returns just prior to ovulation within 6 hours after coitus. The cervical mucus should be thin, clear, and alkaline. Spinnbarkheit or elasticity is an expression of the viscosity of mucus. When a drop of cervical fluid is placed between 2 fingers, for example, the mucus will stretch into a thin strand when the fingers are separated slowly. The mucus is more viscid

before and after ovulation. At the time of ovulation, the mucus can often be stretched 10 cm or more. Infection and bleeding also reduce spinnbarkheit. A good spinnbarkheit (stretching to a fine thread 4 cm or more in length) is desirable. A small drop of cervical mucus should be obtained for the fern test and the Sims-Huhner test. The presence or absence of active sperms is noted. The presence in the cervical mucus of 10–15 active sperms per high power field constitutes a satisfactory Sims-Huhner test. The fern test should show clear arborizations: frond-like crystal patterns in the dried mucus. If no motile spermatozoa are found, the Sims-Huhner test should be repeated (assuming that active spermatozoa were present in the semen analysis).

E. Later Tests: (As indicated.) Testicular biopsy is indicated if azoospermia or oligospermia is present. A vaginal smear and an endometrial biopsy may be required to determine if ovulation is occurring. This is best taken from the side wall in the fundus to avoid a pregnancy which usually implants high in the uterus anteriorly or posteriorly. If tests of tubal patency were unsatisfactory, hysterosalpingography is done. Peritoneoscopy or culdoscopy may be required if tubal adhesions or endometriosis are suspected. Laparotomy will be necessary for salpingostomy, lysis of adhesions, and removal of ovarian abnormalities. Sterility on the basis of disorders of the sex chromosomes should be ruled out by examination for Barr bodies and sex chromatin analysis of desquamated buccal or vaginal cells.

Cystoscopy and catheterization of ejaculatory duct orifices, using a fluid x-ray contrast medium, may be required to demonstrate duct stenosis. Vasography by direct injection of the vas near its origin may demonstrate an occlusion. Needle aspiration of the upper pole of the epididymis (globus major) suggests inflammatory closure of the tract if no spermatozoa are recovered.

Treatment

Treatment in all cases depends upon correction of the underlying disorder or disorders suspected of causing infertility.

A. Infertility in the Female:

1. Medical measures—Fertility may be restored by proper treatment in many patients with endocrine imbalance, particularly those with hypo- or hyperthyroidism. The alleviation of cervicitis is of value in the return of fertility.

2. Surgical measures—Surgical correction of congenital or acquired abnormalities (including tumors) of the lower genital tract or uterus may frequently renew fertility. Surgical excision of ovarian tumors or ovarian foci of endometriosis frequently restores fertility. Surgical relief of tubal obstruction due to salpingitis will reestablish fertility in fewer than 20% of cases. In special instances of cornual or fimbrial block, the prognosis after surgery is much better.

3. Induction of ovulation—An attempt should be made to induce ovulation in cases of infertility due to anovulation which has persisted longer than 6 months (includes brief secondary amenorrhea, oligomenorrhea), galactorrhea, recurrent dysfunctional uterine bleeding, and polycystic ovarian disease (Stein-Leventhal syndrome).

a. Clomiphene citrate (Clomid)—The mechanism of action of this drug is not clearly understood.

Give 50 mg orally daily for 5 days. If ovulation does not occur, increase the dosage to 100 mg orally daily for 5 days. If ovulation still does not occur, repeat the course of 100 mg daily for 5 days and add chorionic gonadotropin, 2000 units IM daily.

Ovulation is likely to occur in women with polycystic ovarian disease and those who are amenorrheic after having used oral contraceptive agents. In other types of patients, the results are unpredictable. Multiple pregnancies occur with a frequency of 1:16; abortion occurs in 20–25% of pregnancies. The long-range effectiveness of this treatment is poor.

b. Corticosteroids (glucocorticoids)—In patients with hyperadrenocorticism (hyperplasia) and polycystic ovarian disease, give prednisone (minimal sodium retention), 7.5–15 mg orally in 3–4 divided doses daily (or equivalent). Treatment must be continued indefinitely for women with adrenal hyperplasia; for others, a therapeutic trial of 6–8 months is indicated.

About 30% of patients with polycystic ovarian disease will ovulate as a result of corticosteroid therapy. Discontinue treatment if ovulation does not occur after 6–8 months. Polycystic ovarian disease patients are generally improved for months after cessation of therapy.

c. Ovarian wedge resection—Wedge resection is indicated when medical measures are not effective.

d. Human menopausal gonadotropins (HMG) (Pergonal)—HMG is indicated in cases of hypogonadotropism and most other types of anovulation (exclusive of ovarian failure) after previous treatment failure. Begin with 75 IU of FSH plus 75 IU of LH (1 ampule) IM daily for 9–12 days. Determine 24-hour urinary estrogen. If < 100 μg, give 10,000 IU chorionic gonadotropin (HCG) IM when a good estrogen effect (clear, thin cervical mucus) indicates advanced follicle development. Arrange daily coitus following the last injection of HMG for 3 days. If pregnancy does not occur, repeat the cycle of treatment twice more. If pregnancy still does not result, increase the dosage to 2 ampules of HMG daily for 9–12 days, plus HCG (if not contraindicated by elevated estrogen). The cost is considerable.

Ovulation is likely to occur, and multiple pregnancies (mostly twins) occur in 20% of pregnancies.

B. Infertility in the Male: Surgical correction of congenital or acquired abnormalities of the penis and urethra may permit successful vaginal penetration and normal insemination. Testicular hypofunction secondary to hypothyroidism or diabetes mellitus is often corrected by appropriate treatment. Surgical correction of varicocele and hydrocele may restore fertility.

Mumps orchitis requires prompt testicular decompression by surgical excision of the tunica albuginea to preserve fertility.

Artificial insemination using the husband's specimen (AIH), as in oligospermia, has been most disappointing. Artificial insemination with a donor's specimen (AID) is very successful—assuming normal female function and acceptability of AID by the couple.

Prognosis

The prognosis for conception and normal pregnancy is good if minor (even multiple) disorders can be identified and treated early; poor if the causes of infertility are severe, untreatable, or of prolonged duration.

No treatment is effective for infertility due to marked uterine hypoplasia. Congenital deficiency or absence of the ovaries is a hopeless sterility problem. Perioophoritis defies medical and surgical treatment. Agenesis or dysgenesis of the testes resists all treatment. Infertility due to prostatitis, seminal vesiculitis, and obstruction in the sperm conduit system rarely responds to treatment.

If treatment is not successful within 1 year, the physician must consider whether he should recommend adoption.

Brandl E, Mettler L: Timing of ovulation in sterility patients. Internat J Fertil 19:13, 1974.

Conaughton JF Jr & others: Induction of ovulation with cisclomiphene and a placebo. Obst Gynec 43:697, 1974.

Cox LW: Infertility, practice, and practicability. Australian New Zealand J Obstet Gynaec 12:126, 1972.

DeGeorge FV, Nesbitt REL Jr: The relationship of certain variables to conception in treated infertility patients. Am J Obst Gynec 114:175, 1972.

Ferriman D: The significance of the polycystic ovary. Postgrad MJ 48:20, 1972.

Gnarpe H, Friberg J: Mycoplasma and human reproductive failure. 1. The occurrence of different mycoplasmas in couples with reproductive failure. Am J Obst Gynec 114:727, 1972.

Haub EJ: Prognosis for the infertile couple. Fertil Steril 23:320, 1972.

Isojima S & others: Further studies on sperm immobilizing antibody found in the sera of unexplained cases of sterility in women. Am J Obst Gynec 112:199, 1972.

Jette NT, Glass RH: Prognostic value of the postcoital test. Fertil Steril 23:29, 1972.

MacNaughton MC: Treatment of female infertility. Clin Endocrinol 2:545, 1973.

Mettler L & others: Sperm antibody production in female sterility. Internat J Fertil 19:7, 1974.

Parekh MC, Arronet GH: Diagnostic procedures and methods in the assessment of the female organs, with specific reference to infertility. Clin Obst Gynec 15:1, 1972.

Pontifex G & others: Hysterosalpingography in the diagnosis of infertility (statistical analysis of 3437 cases). Fertil Steril 23:829, 1972.

Roland M, Leisten D: Tuboplasty in 130 patients: Improved results due to stents and preoperative endoscopy. Obst Gynec 39:57, 1972.

Rowley MJ, Heller CG: The testosterone rebound phenomenon in the treatment of male infertility. Fertil Steril 23:498, 1972.

Ulstein M: Evaluation of a capillary tube sperm penetration

method for fertility investigations. Acta obst gynec scandinav 51:287, 1972.

Umezaki C & others: Pregnancy rates after reconstructive surgery on the fallopian tubes. Obst Gynec 43:418, 1974.

Vande Wiele RL: Treatment of infertility due to ovulatory failure. Hosp Practice 7:119, Oct 1972.

Vaucer-Vleit WL, Hafez ESE: Survival and aging of spermatozoa: A review. Am J Obst Gynec 118:1006, 1974.

Zauartu J & others: Induction of ovulation with synthetic gonadotropin-releasing hormone in women with constant anovulation. Brit MJ 1:605, 1974.

CONTRACEPTION

Contraception is the voluntary prevention of pregnancy either for medical or personal reasons. In the USA, the prescription, demonstration, and sale of contraceptives is now legal in all states. All faiths accept the principle of family planning; the Roman Catholic Church alone requires that this be accomplished by total or periodic abstinence.

The "perfect" contraceptive should be simple, acceptable, effective, safe, economical, and reversible. No contraceptive method yet devised satisfies all of these criteria. The following is a selection based upon efficacy and general patient acceptance:

"Rhythm" Method

The "rhythm" method, using the basal body temperature to identify the period of ovulation ("unsafe period"), requires the cooperation of both parties and may be effective depending upon the care with which it is used and the regularity of the woman's menstrual cycle. It is useless postpartum until regular cycles are established.

A. Method of Ogino: After the length of the menstrual cycle has been observed for at least 8 months (preferably for 1 year), the following calculations are made: (1) The first fertile day is determined by subtracting 18 days from the shortest cycle. (2) The last fertile day is determined by subtracting 11 days from the longest cycle. For example, if the observed cycles run from 24–28 days, the fertile period would extend from the 6th day of the cycle (24 minus 18) through the 17th day (28 minus 11). It is essential to base the calculations upon a written record of the woman's menstrual periods—not on her memory or testimony alone. Other variations of this method are also used.

B. Basal Body Temperature Method: A great deal of effort and interest is required on the part of the patient to make sure that a truly basal temperature chart is being recorded. (The temperature must be taken immediately upon awakening, before any activity.) A drop in temperature usually occurs 1–1½ days before ovulation, and a rise of about 0.7° F occurs 1–2 days after ovulation. The high temperature continues throughout the remainder of the cycle. The third day after the rise marks the end of the fertile period.

1. HORMONAL SUPPRESSION OF OVULATION
(See Table 18–21.)

Inhibition of ovulation by means of estrogens or progestogens, alone or in combination, has been possible for many years, but only recently has the availability of potent synthetic progestational agents (mainly 19-nortestosterone and 17-hydroxyprogesterone compounds, now called "gestagens") made effective oral contraception generally practical and widely acceptable.

Methods of Suppression

A. Single Hormone Therapy: Moderate to large daily doses of estrogen for 3 weeks per month will prevent ovulation because the estrogen suppresses LTH, LH, and FSH. However, unpleasant side-effects, particularly nausea and menometrorrhagia, invariably develop. For this reason, this hormone alone is impractical for long-term use. The possibility of vaginal adenocarcinoma in offspring, should pregnancy occur, must also be considered.

Combined daily small dosage gestagens (Micronor, Nor-QD) are now considered to be a useful method of contraception. Although they have a lower rate of adverse reactions, there is a higher pregnancy rate and a greater frequency of menstrual cycle disturbances. Ovulation usually continues with this "minipill" therapy, but pregnancy does not occur mainly because the cervical mucus becomes hostile to sperm penetration. This promising new approach may soon be available to more patients.

B. Combined Hormone Therapy:

1. The "classic pill" is a synthetic progestin or gestagen plus estrogen (Enovid, Ortho-Novum, etc). One tablet per day is prescribed, beginning on the 5th day from the start of the period and continuing for 20 days. Bleeding usually begins 1–4 days after cessation of the medication. The patient then resumes the same dosage on the 5th day of the cycle.

This type of hormonal contraception is effective because it (1) interferes with pituitary function by blocking LH release, (2) alters tubal motility to discourage fertilization, (3) modifies endometrial maturation, and (4) renders cervical mucus impervious to sperm migration.

2. The "sequential pill" (Oracon) contains a higher daily dosage of estrogen than the "classic pill" alone. The estrogen is given alone for 15 days, and estrogen and gestagen are given each day for the last 5 days. The dosage program is similar to that outlined for (1) above. Estrogen inhibits ovulation, and progestogen is added at the end of the cycle to produce a more physiologic endometrium, normalize menstruation, and thicken the cervical mucus, adding to the contraceptive effect of the medication.

The sequential pill inhibits ovulation by suppressing release of FSH. It probably also affects the physiology of the tubes, endometrium, and cervix.

3. Continuous nonestrogen pill (Micronor, Nor-

QD)—This preparation is less effective but may be necessary in patients who cannot take estrogens.

Caution: Maximal protection against pregnancy with combined therapy may not be assured until the second cycle because ovulation occasionally occurs early during the first month of medication.

In general, a dose of $\leqslant 50$ μg of estrogen per pill is preferred as a means of avoiding serious side-effects.

Effects of Oral Contraceptives (Table 12–5.)

In general, most patients "feel better" on this medication, although libido remains about the same. Most women with dysmenorrhea and many with premenstrual tension are relieved by oral contraception. A few of the latter become worse.

Some undesirable side-effects relating to dosage and tolerance develop in at least 25% of patients on oral contraceptives. Approximately 20% of women placed on this routine discontinue it, largely because of one or more of the following problems: Nausea (rarely emesis) affects 10–15% of all patients but is most marked during the first few cycles and usually subsides thereafter. Headache and mastalgia occur initially in 3–5% of patients but are less troublesome after 2–3 months of therapy. Initial weight gain (edema) of 2–5 lb or more is reported by about 50% of women. This weight is lost during menstruation but recurs each month despite fair control by diet and diuretics. Breakthrough bleeding develops in 5–8% of patients. This complication usually is controlled by the administration of an extra one-half tablet daily for the remainder of that cycle only. The next month, the patient may resume a 1 tablet per day regimen.

Some patients describe depression, abdominal cramps, lethargy, chloasma, or acne.

A. Effect on Menstrual Cycle: Oral contraceptive therapy helps to regulate and maintain normal menstrual bleeding. Many patients develop scanty periods, and a few cease to menstruate. However, an occasional patient will experience breakthrough bleeding. *Caution:* Cancer may cause abnormal uterine bleeding also, and vaginal cytology alone may not detect cancer. Women over 35 years of age who experience repeated breakthrough bleeding should cease taking oral contraceptive therapy and submit to multiple cervical biopsy or conization and dilatation and curettage to rule out malignancy.

B. Thromboembolic Disorders: There may be a slight increase in the incidence of thromboembolic disorders in women over 35 who are on oral contraceptives. The mechanism of this process is uncertain, but prethrombotic plasma changes, including an increase in prothrombin, proconvertin, fibrinogen, and Stuart factor levels, have been blamed. The incidence of lipid anomalies of genotypic origin (ie, familial hyperlipidemia) is about 3% of the general population. It is possible that in such women anovulatory steroids may facilitate the occurrence of intravascular coagulation due to interference by anomalous lipids. Women with a history of varices or thrombophlebitis—especially those over 35 years of age—should use another contraceptive method.

C. Liver Dysfunction: Increase in serum transaminase levels and interference with bile secretion by

Table 12–5. Hormone-related side-effects of oral contraceptives.*

Common side-effects	
Estrogen excess	**Estrogen deficiency**
Gastric disturbances	Nervousness, irritability
Fluid retention	Early and midcycle bleeding
Mucorrhea	Decreased menstrual flow
Premenstrual tension	
Increased size of fibroids	
Progestogen excess	**Progestogen deficiency**
Depression, lassitude, reduced libido	Delayed onset of menses
Decreased menstrual flow	Late breakthrough spotting and bleeding
Acne, hirsutism	Irregular cycles
Increased appetite; anabolic weight gain	Hypermenorrhea
Candidal vaginitis	
Melasma	
Mastodynia; leg cramps	
Uncommon side-effects	
Alopecia	Galactorrhea
Gingivitis (epulis)	Coronary or hypertensive disease
Visual disturbances	Jaundice (hypercholestasis)
Cerebral arterial insufficiency (stroke, severe headache)	Ureteral dilatation
Cystic mastitis; fibroadenoma	Venous thromboembolism
	Rheumatic symptomatology

*After R.M. Nelson.

hepatic cells—even cholestatic jaundice—are reported occasionally. Oral contraception should not be used by women with liver disorders or cholelithiasis.

D. Carbohydrate Intolerance: Reduced glucose tolerance may develop after several months of medication. Women with diabetes mellitus on oral contraceptives require especially close supervision of their metabolism.

E. Lactation: The amount of milk produced is decreased in about one-third of patients who are given oral contraceptives in the late puerperium. A rare non-pregnant woman may for unexplained reasons develop slight lactation when on oral contraceptives.

F. Effect on Endocrine System: (See also Table 12–5.) Even with long-term therapy, most normal women have not been found to be adversely affected by oral contraceptive drugs. Nevertheless, it has been recommended by some clinicians that patients discontinue oral contraceptive therapy every year for approximately 2 months and that pituitary, thyroid, and adrenal performance be checked if normal function does not resume.

High-dosage or continuous administration of progestin-estrogen combinations finally results in gonadotropin repression to undetectable levels. Low-dosage combined oral contraceptives prevent the LH and FSH midcycle peaks. Sequential anovulants depress FSH.

G. Subsequent Fertility: Approximately three-fourths of women desirous of pregnancy will conceive within 2 months following discontinuation of oral contraceptive therapy. This indicates prompt resumption of endocrine function, even after prolonged use of the pill. Unfortunately, a few develop amenorrhea for unexplained reasons.

H. Miscellaneous Effects: Oral contraceptives may cause plasma triglyceride levels to rise almost as high as those of men of comparable age, suggesting that these drugs may have atherogenic potential.

Increased plasma triglyceride levels in normal young women taking oral contraceptives may result from a decrease in postheparin lipolytic activity and impaired triglyceride removal. Concomitant elevation of serum insulin suggests the stimulation of endogenous hepatic triglyceride synthesis and its secretion into the plasma.

Oncology and "The Pill"

There is no convincing evidence that oral contraceptives are cancerogenic. Patients who have had an estrogen-dependent breast tumor or endometrial cancer, however, should not be given an oral estrogen-containing contraceptive. On the other hand, progestogens encourage endometrial slough at the time of the period and may actually have an anti-cancer effect. Patients with uterine myomas should not receive continued gestagen-estrogen medications because these tumors often enlarge considerably after 2–3 months.

Contraceptive Effectiveness

Unless medically contraindicated, oral contraceptives are by far the most effective method of contraception now in use as long as women remember to take the daily pill. The effectiveness of the various types of oral contraception has been reported to be 0.2–1.5 pregnancies per 100 woman years.

Selection of the Proper Oral Contraceptive

The initial choice of oral contraceptives should be based on (1) a thorough knowledge of the differences in composition of the various pills, (2) an estimate of the woman's natural hormone status and requirements, and (3) a consideration of her age and desire for future pregnancies.

For younger patients (16–20 years of age), endocrine maturity may lag behind social sophistication. These girls often have anovulatory, irregular menses. In young women and in older women (over 40 years of age) who do not have estrogen sensitivity, sequential regimens with an estrogen dominance are best. The patient should be asked about nausea and vomiting in previous pregnancies, fluid retention, weight gain, acne, etc. Keep the dosage low in both patient groups to avoid oversuppression of the pituitary in the young and thromboembolism in older women. Sequentials can be prescribed for most patients because intermenstrual spotting is not often associated with their use. Moreover, the duration of flow can be reduced by sequentials with 6 rather than 5 days of progestogen. Nevertheless, if oligomenorrhea occurs in the young patient, oral contraception is contraindicated.

If the patient has estrogen sensitivity, give a combination pill; the length of the cycle will determine the potency of the progestogen. A good index of the woman's progestogen requirement is the amount and duration of the menstrual flow. When bleeding is heavy and long, potent progestins are needed and a larger dose combination pill (eg, Norlestrin, 2.5 mg; Norinyl, 2 mg) is useful. This avoids breakthrough bleeding. Patients with a short flow do best with a weaker progestogen, estrogen dominant product. Intermediate progestogen products are Norlestrin, 1 mg; Ovulen; Ortho-Novum, 1 mg; and Enovid.

Side-effects are not inevitable but are due to too much or not enough estrogen or progestogen. Selection of the proper oral contraceptive is possible in most cases without impractical biochemical or cytologic studies. If the first choice is poor and the patient has unpleasant side-effects, select another pill in an attempt to avoid the problems described.

If the patient has progestogen sensitivity, give a sequential with low progestogen content (eg, Oracon).

The "minipill" (norethindrone acetate, 0.2 mg daily) can be given to most women with reasonably regular, average periods because side-effects, save for intermenstrual spotting, are virtually absent.

Contraindications to Oral Contraceptives

Oral contraceptives are contraindicated in the presence of (or if the patient has a history of) any of the following: Strong family history of stroke, severe migraine, cerebral arterial insufficiency, cardiovascular disease, liver disease, severe diabetes mellitus, nephritis, genital or breast cancer, thrombophlebitis or thromboembolism, large uterine myomas.

Astedt B & others: Thrombosis and oral contraceptives: Possible predisposition. Brit MJ 4:631, 1973.

Badaracco MA, Vessey MP: Recurrence of venous thromboembolic disease and use of oral contraceptives. Brit MJ 1:215, 1974.

Barsivala V & others: Thyroid functions of women taking oral contraceptives. Contraception 9:305, 1974.

Beaconsfield P & others: Amenorrhea and infertility after the use of oral contraceptives. Surg Gynec Obst 138:571, 1974.

Buttram VC Jr & others: Post "pill" amenorrhea. Internat J Fertil 19:37, 1974.

Corfman PA: Coordinated studies of the effects of oral contraceptives. Contraception 9:109, 1974.

Darlington LG: Erythema nodosum and oral contraceptives. Brit J Dermat 90:209, 1974.

Doar JWH: Metabolic side-effects of oral contraceptives. Clin Endocrinol 2:503, 1973.

Drill VA: Benign cholestatic jaundice of pregnancies and benign cholestatic jaundice from oral contraceptives. Am J Obst Gynec 119:165, 1974.

Drill VA: Oral contraceptives and thromboembolic disease. 1. Prospective and retrospective studies. JAMA 219:583, 1972.

Fisch IR & others: Oral contraceptives, pregnancy and blood pressure. JAMA 222:1507, 1972.

Klopper A: Endocrinological effects of oral contraceptives. Clin Endocrinol 2:489, 1973.

Kuchera LK: Postcoital contraception with diethylstilbestrol: Updated. Contraception 10:47, 1974.

Nelson JH: The use of the mini-pill in private practice. J Reprod Med 10:139, 1973.

Shearman RP, Smith ID: Statistical analysis of the relationship between oral contraceptives, secondary amenorrhea and galactorrhea. J Obstet Gynaec Brit Common 79:654, 1972.

Worth AV, Boyes DA: Case control study into possible effects of birth control pills on preclinical carcinoma of the cervix. J Obstet Gynaec Brit Common 79:673, 1972.

Zuck TF, Bergin JJ: Thrombotic predisposition associated with oral contraceptives. Obst Gynec 41:427, 1973.

2. DIAPHRAGM & JELLY

The cervical diaphragm used in combination with spermatocidal vaginal jelly or cream is fairly acceptable and effective. The cost is not insignificant.

Wiggins P: Use effectiveness of the diaphragm in selected family planning population in the United Kingdom. Contraception 9:15, 1974.

3. FOAMS & JELLIES

Spermatocidal foam (Delfen, Emko) transferred from an aerosol container to the vagina by an applicator is a good, aesthetic contraceptive of moderate cost and effectiveness. Koromex, a water-soluble jelly, is a comparable alternative.

4. CONDOM

The male sheath of rubber or animal membrane affords good protection against pregnancy—equivalent to that of a diaphragm and spermatocidal jelly; it is also to a degree a venereal disease prophylactic. The disadvantages are expense, psychologic dulling of sensation, and sperm loss due to tearing, slipping, or leakage with detumescence of the penis.

5. INTRAUTERINE CONTRACEPTIVE DEVICE (IUCD)

Plastic or metal coils, spirals, or rings, when retained in the uterus for the prevention of pregnancy, are as effective as other methods excepting hormone suppression of ovulation. Fertilization may occur, but nidation is prevented because tubal mobility is so increased by IUCD that the endometrium is unprepared for implantation. The IUCD is particularly useful and popular among couples in the lower socioeconomic classes because it offers semipermanent, reversible protection at minimal cost and no personal effort or reference to the calendar. The most successful IUCD's are the Lippes loop and the double coil (Saf-T-Coil). Insertion 6 weeks postpartum or immediately after a menstrual period is recommended; removal can be accomplished at any time. Difficulty in insertion and removal of the IUCD (especially in nulliparas), initial cramping, and extrusion of the IUCD (particularly within the first 2–3 months) are disadvantages. Excessive bleeding, cramping, extrusion, perforation, and infection may occur.

Allen J & others: Removal of intrauterine contraceptive devices after uterine perforation. Obst Gynec 40:225, 1972.

Davis HL: Intrauterine contraceptive devices: Present status and future prospects. Am J Obst Gynec 114:134, 1972.

Goldman JA: Infected ovarian cysts and the IUD. Contraception 8:521, 1973.

Goldsmith A & others: Immediate postabortal intrauterine contraceptive device insertion: Double-blind study. Am J Obst Gynec 112:957, 1972.

Hagenfeldt K & others: Intrauterine contraception with the copper T device. 3. Effect on endometrial morphology. Contraception 6:207, 1972.

Israel R & others: Comparative quantitation of menstrual blood loss with Lippes Loop, Dalkon Shield, and Copper T intrauterine devices. Contraception 10:63, 1974.

Mishell DR Jr: Assessing the intrauterine device. Fam Plann Perspect 7:103, 1975.

Mishell DR Jr, Israel R, Freid N: A study of the copper T intrauterine contraceptive device (TCu 200) in nulliparous women. Am J Obst Gynec 116:1092, 1973.

Newton J & others: Intrauterine contraception with the Copper 7: Evaluation after two years. Brit MJ 3:447, 1974.

Ostergard DR, Broen EM: The insertion of intrauterine devices by physicians and paramedical personnel. Obst Gynec 41:257, 1973.

Piiroinew O: Ultrasonic localization of intrauterine contraceptive devices. Acta obst gynec scandinav 51:203, 1972.

Sobrero AJ: Intrauterine devices in clinical practice. Fam Plann Perspect 3:10, 1972.

COMMON SURGICAL PROCEDURES IN OBSTETRICS & GYNECOLOGY

SURGICAL DILATATION & CURETTAGE (D&C)

Curettage is the instrumental exploration of the cervical canal and endometrial cavity and the removal of tissue for diagnostic and therapeutic purposes. Curettage requires the use of dilators for the introduction of instruments beyond the internal os.

Surgical curettage is the most frequently performed of all gynecologic operations. In contrast to aspiration curettage, surgical curettage requires general anesthesia. The relaxation that occurs with anesthesia provides an excellent opportunity for examination and yields far more information and tissue than suction collection or biopsy of the endometrial cavity.

Curettage should not be done if there is any reason to suspect that an intrauterine pregnancy is present nor in the absence of definite indications. Hysterosalpingography can sometimes give the desired information. In septic shock due to late abortion, control of shock and hysterectomy with D&C may be lifesaving.

Indications for Surgical Dilatation & Curettage

A. Childhood:

1. Diagnostic indications—Suspected genital tract anomalies (hypoplastic uterus, bicornuate uterus); uterine bleeding (eg, due to endometrial tuberculosis, cancer).

2. Therapeutic indications—Control of bleeding.

B. Adolescence and Adulthood:

1. Diagnostic indications—Suspected neoplasms of the cervix and uterus; abnormal uterine bleeding; investigation of possible malformations, including position of fundus; endometritis; confirmation of ovulation and determination of consistency of endometrial maturation relative to time in cycle (in study of infertility).

2. Therapeutic indications—Removal of polyps and excessive tissue overgrowth (endometrial hyperplasia) in the management of abnormal uterine bleeding. Early therapeutic abortion.

C. Postmenopausal Age Group:

1. Diagnostic indications—Bleeding or discharge due to possible cancer, polyps, or infection.

2. Therapeutic indications—Drainage of hematometra or pyometra. (Drain first and perform curettage when infection subsides and the uterus is smaller.)

Edelman DA & others: Effectiveness and complications of abortion by dilatation and vacuum operation versus dilatation and rigid metal curettage. Am J Obst Gynec 119:473, 1974.

Fraser IS, Baird DS: Endometrial cystic glandular hyperplasia in adolescent girls. J Obstet Gynaec Brit Common 79:1009, 1972.

Jensen PA, Stomme WB: Amenorrhea secondary to puerperal curettage (Asherman's syndrome). Am J Obst Gynec 113:150, 1972.

Newton BW: Laminaria tent: Relic of the past or modern medical device? Am J Obst Gynec 113:442, 1972.

Richards MT: Uterine curettage as an office procedure. Canad MAJ 107:133, 1972.

Saudmire HF, Austin SD: Curettage as an office procedure. Am J Obst Gynec 119:82, 1974.

Saunders P, Rowland R: Vacuum curettage of the uterus without anesthesia: A comparison with conventional curettage. J Obstet Gynaec Brit Common 79:168, 1972.

Smith RK, Gibson JL: Low cost outpatient curettage. Obst Gynec 39:329, 1972.

OVARIECTOMY

The ovary performs numerous functions. It is a repository for primordial sex cells, the woman's chromosomal endowment for procreation. During the functional years, it is the organ for the production, "ripening," and monthly release of mature ova. The ovary produces steroid sex hormones. Estrogens are produced from childhood until about age 65; after puberty until the menopause, ovulation is associated with the production of progestogens; and from maturity and into the climacteric, small amounts of androgens are produced. Estrogens, most of all, have specific effects on virtually every gland and tissue in the body.

In benign ovarian disease before the menopause, inspection, bisection, and, perhaps, frozen section of the other ovary at laparotomy are necessary in order not to miss serious abnormalities. If an ovary appears normal, it should not be removed until after the menopause. Ovarian hormones "cushion" the patient into the climacteric and help to prevent atherosclerosis, osteoporosis, and vaginitis.

Unless the ovaries are seriously diseased or obviously inactive, they should be protected and retained. Even though synthetic ovarian hormones can be given exogenously, they are expensive and troublesome and less satisfactory than natural estrogens.

Ovariectomy is not warranted in the case of small, unilateral, nontender ovarian enlargements in premenopausal women, nor for the management of asymptomatic postinflammatory tubo-ovarian cysts. There is no justification for ovariectomy for cancer prevention during the functional years. Unilateral ovariectomy for benign cystoma is followed by reoperation involving the other ovary in 5–10% of cases; nevertheless, the chance of the remaining ovary developing cancer is only about 6%. After age 50, the occurrence of ovarian cancer falls to about 1%.

Indications for Ovariectomy

(1) A persistent or enlarging ovarian tumor > 6–7 cm diameter in premenopausal women or > 4 cm in postmenopausal patients. The enlargement should be substantiated by 2 or more examinations over a 3-month period.

(2) Sudden acute and then persistent adnexal pain and tenderness associated with ovarian enlargement—all indicative of an ovarian tumor on a twisted pedicle.

(3) Unresectable ovarian dermoid, endometriosis, or obviously benign tumor.

(4) Ovarian inflammatory destruction or abscess.

(5) Serous cystadenoma containing numerous solid areas or exteriorization of papillary projections. Remove the other ovary and uterus if malignancy seems likely.

(6) Both ovaries should be removed when carcinoma of the ovary, fallopian tube, or endometrium is being treated by hysterectomy.

(7) An ovary that contains a functional ovarian tumor larger than 3–4 cm should be removed.

(8) Remove both ovaries for cancer prevention in women who undergo hysterectomy after the menopause or those over age 65 who are subjected to laparotomy for other reasons.

(9) Bilateral ovariectomy is justified premenopausally for palliation of estrogen-dependent mammary cancer.

Aitken JM & others: Osteoporosis after oophorectomy for nonmalignant disease in premenopausal women. Brit MJ 2:325, 1973.

Lee RA: Sigmoid complications of left ovarian enlargement. Minnesota Med 55:565, 1972.

Utian WH: True clinical features of postmenopause and oophorectomy and their response to estrogen therapy. South African MJ 46:732, 1972.

Williams TJ & others: Management of unilateral and encapsulated ovarian cancer in young women. Gynecol Oncol 1:143, 1973.

HYSTERECTOMY

The menstrual and procreative functions of the uterus have great psychologic significance for women, and the physician should attempt to preserve the uterus in premenopausal women if at all possible. There are absolute indications for hysterectomy such as uterine sarcoma and uncontrollable hemorrhage, but most hysterectomies are performed for less compelling

reasons. The patient's age, marital status, and parity must be considered in the decision whether or not to remove the uterus.

Hysterectomy is not warranted for control of pain or bleeding or for contraception or sterilization when other less extreme measures will suffice. It should be avoided if possible in those women who have a psychologic need for menstruation; in those who are inordinately apprehensive of major surgery; and in any case where the uterus is needed as a repository for radium in the management of residual pelvic cancer.

Indications for Hysterectomy

(1) **Gynecologic indications:** Chronic, disabling pelvic inflammatory disease or rupture of pelvic abscess; extensive endometriosis not amenable to hormone therapy or conservative surgery; generative tract anomalies of uncorrectable dysfunctional type causing habitual abortion (eg, hypoplastic uterus); uterine perforation at curettage, causing intraperitoneal or retroperitoneal hemorrhage, hematoperitoneum, pelvic floor lacerations, uterine prolapse, abnormal uterine bleeding that cannot be controlled by curettage or hormonal therapy, menometrorrhagia complicating sex steroid therapy for osteoporosis.

Bilateral adnexectomy for tubo-ovarian disease should include hysterectomy unless the uterus is required as a receptacle for radium therapy of pelvic malignancy.

(2) **Neoplastic diseases:** Symptomatic myoma or adenomyosis of the uterus; bilateral serous adnexal cystadenoma; sarcoma or carcinoma of the uterus; hemorrhagic chorio-epithelioma of the uterus unresponsive to chemotherapy; stage I epidermoid carcinoma of the cervix; in conjunction with bilateral oophorectomy for control of residual estrogen-dependent mammary carcinoma; as part of exenteration for pelvic recurrence of rectal carcinoma.

(3) **Obstetric indications:** Ruptured interstitial pregnancy, placenta accreta, advanced hydatidiform mole, sterilization, septic shock due to clostridia (correct shock first).

(4) **Medical indications:** Hypertensive cardiovascular disease causing abnormal bleeding due to "uterine apoplexy"; hypermenorrhea due to pseudohemophilia.

Types of Hysterectomy

A. Subtotal Hysterectomy: Subtotal (incomplete) hysterectomy is rarely justified because the cervix, a potentially serious focus of disease, is left behind.

B. Total Hysterectomy:

1. Abdominal hysterectomy is advisable for the treatment of inflammatory problems; large, multiple uterine tumors; adnexal neoplasms; obstetric complications; for wide exploration or dissection; or whenever previous surgery or scarring has restricted the uterus.

2. Vaginal hysterectomy usually is preferred for removal of a prolapsed uterus, especially when pelvic floor weakness and associated vaginal hernias require correction.

C. Extended hysterectomy (Wertheim, Schauta, Okabiachi) is warranted only for the elimination of invasive cancer by one fully qualified in this highly specialized area of surgery.

Coulam CB, Pratt JH: Vaginal hysterectomy: Is previous pelvic operation a contraindication? Am J Obst Gynec 116:252, 1973.

Hampton PT, Tarnasky WG: Hysterectomy and tubal ligation: A comparison of the psychological aftermath. Am J Obst Gynec 119:949, 1974.

Ledger WJ, Child MA: Hospital care of patients undergoing hysterectomy: Analysis of 12,026 patients from the Professional Activity Study. Am J Obst Gynec 117:423, 1973.

Nissen EJ, Goldstein AI: A prospective investigation of the etiology of febrile morbidity following abdominal hysterectomy. Am J Obst Gynec 113:111, 1972.

Parrott MH: Elective hysterectomy. Am J Obst Gynec 113:531, 1972.

Sprague AD, van Nagell JR Jr: The relationship of age and endometrial histology to blood loss and morbidity following vaginal hysterectomy. Am J Obst Gynec 118:805, 1974.

Van Nagell JR Jr & others: Vaginal hysterectomy following conization in the treatment of carcinoma in situ of the cervix. Am J Obst Gynec 113:948, 1972.

OBSTETRICS

DIAGNOSIS & DIFFERENTIAL DIAGNOSIS OF PREGNANCY

In about one-third of cases it is difficult to make a definitive diagnosis of pregnancy before the second missed period because of the variability of the physical changes induced by pregnancy, the possibility of tumors, and because obesity and poor patient relaxation often interfere with the examination. Even experienced physicians sometimes make "false-positive" and "false-negative" diagnoses of pregnancy. The potentially grave emotional and legal consequences of an incorrect diagnosis of pregnancy should make the physician cautious; if he is in any doubt, he should schedule a reexamination in 3—4 weeks. If the patient demands earlier confirmation, a pregnancy test can be ordered (Tables 12—6 and 12—7).

Manifestations of Pregnancy
A. Presumptive Manifestations: The following symptoms and signs are usually due to pregnancy, but even 2 or more are not diagnostic. A record or history of time and frequency of coitus may be of considerable value.

Table 12—6. Immunodiagnostic tests for pregnancy.*

Name	Procedure	Interpretation and Remarks
Hemagglutination inhibition test (Pregnosticon)	Red cells sensitized to human chorionic gonadotropin (HCG) + urine (?HCG) + anti-HCG serum.	Immunodiagnostic test depends upon: (1) HCG injected into a rabbit which develops anti-HCG serum. (2) Sheep red cells are tanned, formalinized, and sensitized to HCG. (3) When antibodies are bound or "coated" to red cells, hemagglutination results, but addition of urine from a pregnant woman blocks the reaction between antibody and red cells. Therefore, clumping (ring formation in bottom of test tube) indicates that the patient is not pregnant; no clumping, patient is pregnant.
Agglutination inhibition test (Gravindex)	Anti-HCG serum + urine + HCG antigen (latex particles). Interpret in 3 minutes.	Similar to above but latex particles with adsorbed HCG used instead of red cells.

*Accuracy is satisfactory, with increasing reliability from the 40th day after the first day of LMP.

Table 12—7. Clinical pregnancy tests.*

Name	Procedure	Interpretation and Remarks
Estrogen-progesterone	Progesterone, 20 mg, and estradiol benzoate, 2 mg IM	If bleeding does not occur within 10 days after administration of estrogen-progesterone or 7 days after administration of progesterone, norethindrone, or norethynodrel, and if other causes of amenorrhea have been ruled out, pregnancy is probable. *Note:* If bleeding occurs, the test is negative for pregnancy.
Progesterone	Delalutin, 250 mg (2 ml) IM	
Norethindrone	Norethindrone (Norlutin), 20 mg orally	
Norethynodrel	Norethynodrel (Enovid), 20 mg orally	

*Accuracy is high.

1. Symptoms—Amenorrhea, nausea and vomiting (first trimester), breast tenderness and tingling (after 1–2 weeks), urinary frequency and urgency (first trimester), "quickening" (may appear at about the 16th week), weight gain.

2. Signs—Skin pigmentation (after 16th week), epulis (after first trimester), breast changes (enlargement, vascular engorgement, colostrum), abdominal enlargement, cyanosis of vagina and cervical portio (about the 6th week), softening of the cervix (4th or 5th week), softening of the cervicouterine junction (5th or 6th week), irregular softening and slight enlargement of the fundus (about the 5th week), generalized enlargement and diffuse softening of the corpus (after 8th week).

B. Probable Manifestations (After 28th Week): Uterine enlargement, uterine souffle (bruit), uterine contractions.

C. Positive Manifestations: Any of the following, none of which is usually present until the 4th month, is undeniable medical and legal proof of pregnancy: auscultation of the fetal heart, palpation of the fetal outline, recognition of fetal movements by the physician, demonstration of fetal skeleton by x-ray. (Radiation exposure should be kept to a minimum.)

Differential Diagnosis of Pregnancy

All of the presumptive and probable symptoms and signs of pregnancy can be caused by other conditions, and all the clinical and laboratory tests indicative of pregnancy may be positive in the absence of conception. Clinical experience and often the passage of time with reexamination are required to establish the correct diagnosis. The most common disorders which may be confused with pregnancy are uterine and adnexal tumors.

Arkin C, Uoto TA: A false positive immunologic pregnancy test with tubo-ovarian abscess. Am J Clin Path 58:314, 1972.

Cochrane WJ: Early obstetric diagnosis by diagnostic ultrasound. Med Ann DC 41:148, 1972.

Edelman DA & others: An evaluation of the Pregnosticon Dri-Dot test in early pregnancy. Am J Obst Gynec 119:521, 1974.

Gal I: Risks and benefits of the use of hormonal pregnancy test tablets. Nature 240:241, 1972.

Horwitz CA & others: Evaluation of a latex tube agglutination inhibition pregnancy test: An analysis of 1776 specimens. Am J Obst Gynec 116:626, 1973.

Killip M: Experience with gonavislide: A new slide test for pregnancy. Australia New Zealand J Obst Gynec 12:250, 1972.

Laudesman R & others: Menstrual extraction: Review of 400 procedures at the Somen's Services, N.Y. (including Pregnosticon Dri Dot pregnancy test). Contraception 8:527, 1973.

MINOR DISCOMFORTS OF NORMAL PREGNANCY*

Backache

Virtually all pregnant women suffer from at least minor degrees of lumbar backache during gestation. Postural and other back strain, especially during the last trimester, and relaxation of the pelvic joints due to the steroid sex hormones and perhaps relaxin are also responsible for backache.

The following measures are valuable both as prevention and treatment.

(1) Stress correct ("tall") posture, with abdomen flattened as much as possible, the pelvis tilted forward, and the buttocks "tucked under" to straighten the back.

(2) Daily body exercises to maintain normal muscle strength and tone.

(3) Heels for general wear should be of medium height to further strengthen the back, particularly when flat footwear has been worn extensively.

(4) A firm mattress. Avoid sag which may cause painful, prolonged flexion of the back (after exaggerated extension while erect). Bedboards between the springs and mattress often provide welcome support.

(5) Local heat and light massage to relax tense, taut back muscles.

(6) A maternity girdle may be indicated for patients with backache due to extreme lordosis or kyphoscoliosis or associated with obesity or multiple pregnancy.

(7) Analgesics will be adequate for mild distress. Carisoprodol, 350 mg orally 4 times daily (or a comparable sedative or muscle relaxant drug), gives temporary relief.

(8) Orthopedic evaluation is necessary when disability results from backache. Note neurologic signs and symptoms indicative of intervertebral disk syndrome or other nerve compression problems, radiculitis, and similar disorders.

Pomerance JJ & others: Physical fitness in pregnancy: Its effect on pregnancy outcome. Am J Obst Gynec 119:867, 1974.

Syncope & Faintness

Syncope and faintness are most common in early pregnancy. Vasomotor instability, often associated with postural hypotension, results in transient cerebral hypoxia and pooling of blood in the legs and in the splanchnic and pelvic areas, especially after prolonged sitting or standing in a warm room. Hypoglycemia before or between meals, more common during pregnancy, may result in "lightheadedness" or even fainting.

These attacks can be prevented by avoiding inactivity and utilizing deep breathing, vigorous leg motions, and slow change of position. Encourage the patient to take 6 small meals a day rather than 3 large

*Morning sickness is discussed with Vomiting of Pregnancy.

ones. Stimulants (spirits of ammonia, coffee, tea, or amphetamines) are indicated for attacks due to hypotension; food for hypoglycemia.

Urinary Symptoms

Urinary frequency, urgency, and stress incontinence are quite common, especially in advanced pregnancy. They are due to reduced bladder capacity and the pressure of the presenting part upon the bladder.

Suspect urinary tract disease, especially infection, if dysuria or hematuria is reported.

When urgency is particularly troublesome, the patient should avoid tea, coffee, spices, and alcoholic beverages. Bladder sedatives are available in various forms. Levamine (Repetabs), one orally twice daily, may be beneficial.

Heartburn

Heartburn (pyrosis or "acid indigestion") results from gastroesophageal regurgitation. In late pregnancy, this may be aggravated by displacement of the stomach and duodenum by the uterine fundus.

About 15% of all pregnant patients experience severe pyrosis (as well as nausea and vomiting) during the latter portion of pregnancy because of diaphragmatic hiatus hernia. This develops with "tenting" of the diaphragm and flaring of the lower ribs after the 7th or 8th month of pregnancy. The hernia is reduced spontaneously by parturition. Symptomatic relief, not surgery, is recommended.

A. Neostigmine Bromide (Prostigmin): Give 15 mg orally 3 times daily as necessary to stimulate gastrointestinal secretion and motility.

B. Acidifying Agents: Glutamic acid hydrochloride, 0.3 gm 3 times daily before meals. (Hydrochloric acid solutions damage the teeth.) Avoid antacids during early pregnancy because gastric acidity is already low at this time.

C. Other Measures: Hard candy, hot tea, and change of posture are helpful. In late pregnancy, antacids containing aluminum hydroxide gel to reduce gastric irritation are beneficial.

Atlay RD & others: A fresh look at pregnancy heartburn. J Obstet Gynaec Brit Common 80:63, 1973.

Constipation

Bowel sluggishness is common in pregnancy. It is due to suppression of smooth muscle motility by increased steroid sex hormones and pressure upon and displacement of the intestines by the enlarging uterus. Constipation frequently causes hemorrhoids and aggravates diverticulosis and diverticulitis.

A. General Measures: Stress good bowel habits. The patient should attempt to have an evacuation at the same time every day. The diet should consist of bulk foods, including roughage (unless contraindicated by gastrointestinal intolerance), laxative foods (citrus fruits, apples, prunes, dates, and figs), and a liberal fluid intake. Encourage exercise (walking, swimming, calisthenics).

B. Medical Treatment:

1. To soften the stool, give bulk laxatives and "smoothage" agents which are neither absorbed by nor irritating to the bowel. By accumulating fluid volume, they increase peristalsis. Dioctyl sodium sulfosuccinate (Colace, Doxinate) is detergent. Psyllium hydrophilic mucilloid (Metamucil) is hydrophilic.

2. Prescribe mild laxatives in more severe cases. These include cascara and phenolphthalein. Milk of magnesia and Epsom salts are also useful.

3. Avoid purges for fear of inducing labor. Do not prescribe mineral oil since it prevents absorption of fat-soluble vitamins when administered in large amounts.

Greenhalf JO, Leonard HSD: Laxatives in the treatment of constipation in pregnant and breast feeding mothers. Practitioner 210:259, 1973.

Hemorrhoids

Straining at stool and bearing down at delivery often cause hemorrhoids, especially in women prone to varicosities. For these reasons it is best to prevent or treat constipation early and to spare the patient's having to strain during the second stage of labor by elective low forceps delivery with episiotomy when feasible.

For treatment, see discussion in Chapter 10.

Injection treatments to obliterate hemorrhoids during pregnancy are contraindicated. They may cause infection and extensive thrombosis of the pelvic veins, and are rarely successful because of the great dilatation of many vessels.

Breast Soreness

Physiologic breast engorgement may cause discomfort, especially during early and late pregnancy. A well-fitting brassiere worn 24 hours a day affords relief. Ice caps are temporarily effective. Hormone therapy is of no value.

Headache

Headache is most disturbing during the first and third trimesters. Emotional tension is the most common cause; consider anxiety, uncertainty, and similar psychic causes when headache is migrainous, band-type, occipital, or more or less constant. Refractive errors and ocular imbalance are not caused by normal pregnancy, but the pregnant woman tends to be sedentary and may read or sew more despite "eyestrain." Hormonal stimulation causes vascular engorgement of the nasal turbinates, and the resultant congestion contributes to sinusitis and headache. The belief that pituitary swelling during normal pregnancy causes headache is without foundation.

Callaghan N: The migraine syndrome in pregnancy. Neurology 18:197, 1968.

Ankle Swelling

Edema of the lower extremities not associated

with toxemia develops in two-thirds of women in late pregnancy. Edema is due to sodium and water retention as a result of ovarian, placental, and adrenal steroid hormones and the normally increased venous pressure in the legs. Varicose veins develop from venous congestion, prolonged sitting or standing, and elastic garters and panty girdles.

Treatment is largely preventive and symptomatic, since nothing can be done about the level of the pregnancy hormones. The patient should elevate her legs frequently and sleep in a slight Trendelenburg position. Circular garters and clothing which interfere with venous return should not be worn.

Restrict salt intake and provide elastic support for varicose veins (see below).

Hytten FE: Water storage in normal pregnancy. Int J Gynaec Obstet 8:343, 1970.

Robertson EG: The natural history of oedema during pregnancy. J Obstet Gynaec Brit Common 78:520, 1971.

Varicose Veins

Varicosities are usually a problem of the multipara, and may cause severe complications. They are due to weakness of the vascular walls, increased venous stasis in the legs due to the hemodynamics of pregnancy, inactivity and poor muscle tone, and obesity, since the excessive tissue mass requires increased circulation, and fatty infiltration of connective tissue impairs vascular support.

Serious phlebothrombosis and thrombophlebitis often complicate the puerperium but are uncommon during pregnancy. Pulmonary emboli are rare.

The vulvar, vaginal, and even the inguinal veins may be markedly enlarged during pregnancy. Damaged vulvovaginal vessels give rise to hemorrhage at delivery.

Large vulvar varices cause pudendal discomfort. A vulvar pad wrapped in plastic film, snugly held by a menstrual pad belt or T-binder and elastic leotards gives relief.

Anticoagulants may be required in acute thrombophlebitis. Heparin is preferred to dicumarol since it does not cause fetal damage, is more easily controlled, and is not excreted in the milk. Fortunately, whether administered before or during labor, increased bleeding from the uterus is not common since efficient mechanical compression of the myometrial vessels prevents excessive blood loss despite increased blood coagulation time. Cervical, vaginal, and perineal lacerations may bleed more briskly if the patient has received heparin or dicumarol.

Injection treatment of varicose veins during pregnancy is futile and hazardous.

Vascular surgery can be performed during the first 2 trimesters, but vein stripping is best delayed until after the puerperium. In all other respects, management is the same as in nonpregnant women (see Chapter 8).

Fanfera FJ, Palmer LH: Pregnancy and varicose veins. Arch Surg 96:33, 1968.

Mabatoff RA, Pincus JA: Management of varicose veins during pregnancy. Obst Gynec 36:928, 1970.

Leg Cramps

Cramping or "knotting" of the muscles of the calves, thighs, or buttocks may occur suddenly after sleep or recumbency after the first trimester of pregnancy. For unknown reasons it is less common during the month prior to term. Sudden shortening of the leg muscles by "stretching" with the toes pointed precipitate the cramp. It is believed that cramps are due to reduction in the level of diffusible serum calcium or increase in the serum phosphorus level (or both). This follows excessive dietary intake of phosphorus in milk, cheese, meat, or dicalcium phosphate, diminished calcium intake, or impaired calcium absorption. Fatigue and sluggish circulation in the extremities are contributory factors.

A. Immediate Treatment: Require the patient to stand barefooted on a cold surface (eg, a tiled bathroom floor). Rub and "knead" the contracted, painful muscle. Passively flex the foot to lengthen the calf muscles. Apply local heat.

B. Preventive and Definitive Treatment:

1. Reduce dietary phosphorus intake temporarily by limiting meat to one serving daily and milk to 1 pint daily. Discontinue dicalcium phosphate and other medications containing large amounts of phosphorus.

2. Eliminate excess phosphorus by absorption with aluminum hydroxide gel, 0.5−1 gm orally in liquid or tablet form with each meal.

3. Increase the calcium intake by giving calcium lactate, 0.6 gm (or equivalent) orally 3 times daily before meals. Even larger doses may be required if the absorption of calcium from the intestinal tract is impaired.

4. Walk with the toes pointed forward, but lead with the heel.

Abdominal Pain

Intra-abdominal alterations causing pain during pregnancy include the following:

A. Pressure: Pelvic heaviness, a sense of "sagging" or "dragging," relate to the weight of the uterus on the pelvic supports and the abdominal wall. Frequent rest periods in the supine or lateral recumbent position and a maternity girdle are recommended.

B. Round Ligament Tension: Tenderness along the course of the round ligament (usually the left) during late pregnancy is due to traction on this structure by the uterus with rotation of the uterus and change of the patient's position. Local heat and treatment as for pressure pain are effective.

C. Flatulence, Distention, and Bowel Cramping: Large meals, fats, gas-forming foods, and chilled beverages are poorly tolerated by pregnant women. Mechanical displacement and compression of the bowel by the enlarged uterus, hypotonia of the intestines, and constipation predispose to gastrointestinal distress. Correct and simplify the diet, and reduce food intake at any one meal. Maintain regular bowel functions and prescribe mild laxatives when indicated. Recommend regular exercise and frequent change of body position.

D. Uterine Contractions: Braxton Hicks contractions of the uterus are a normal phenomenon which may be startling to hyperreactive women. The onset of premature labor must always be considered when forceful contractions develop, but if contractions remain infrequent and brief, the danger of early delivery is not significant. Analgesics and sedatives (including alcohol) may be of value. Codeine is rarely required.

E. Intra-abdominal Disorders: Pain due to obstruction or inflammation involving the gastrointestinal, urinary, nervous, or vascular system must be diagnosed and treated specifically.

F. Uterine or Adnexal Disease: Consider and treat pathologic pregnancy and tubal or ovarian disease appropriately.

VOMITING OF PREGNANCY
(Morning Sickness) &
HYPEREMESIS GRAVIDARUM
(Pernicious Vomiting of Pregnancy)

Essentials of Diagnosis

- Morning or evening nausea and vomiting usually begins soon after the first missed period and ceases after the 4th–5th month of gestation.
- Dehydration, acidosis, and nutritional deficiencies develop.

General Considerations

About three-fourths of women, most of them primiparas, complain of nausea and vomiting during pregnancy ("morning sickness"). Persistent severe vomiting during pregnancy—hyperemesis gravidarum—can be fatal if it is not controlled. About one woman in 500 develops hyperemesis gravidarum and requires hospitalization.

The cause of vomiting during pregnancy is not known, although various physiologic mechanisms have been postulated to account for it. Psychogenic factors are prominent in most cases.

Clinical Findings

A. Symptoms and Signs: The onset is most commonly during the 5th or 6th week of pregnancy, and the disorder usually persists only until the 14th to 16th week. Symptoms are most severe in the morning upon arising. Nutritional deficiencies are almost never noted. Hyperemesis gravidarum which continues unchecked is characterized clinically by dehydration, weight loss, avitaminosis, and jaundice.

B. Laboratory Findings: Severe vomiting causes hemoconcentration, decreased serum proteins and alkali reserves, and elevation of BUN, serum sodium

chloride, and serum potassium. Ketone bodies are present in the concentrated urine specimen. Slight proteinuria is a common finding.

C. Ophthalmoscopic Examination: Retinal hemorrhages and retinal detachment are unfavorable prognostic signs.

Differential Diagnosis

Vomiting during pregnancy may be due to any of the diseases with which vomiting is usually associated, eg, infections, poisoning, neoplastic diseases, hyperthyroidism, gastric disorders, gallbladder disease, intestinal obstruction, hiatus hernia, diabetic acidosis, uremia due to any cause, and hydatidiform mole.

Complications

The most serious complication of hyperemesis gravidarum is jaundice due to so-called "toxic hepatitis." Intraocular hemorrhage and retinal detachment may cause permanent blindness.

Treatment

A. Mild Nausea and Vomiting of Pregnancy: Reassurance and dietary restrictions are all that is required in many instances. In general, dry foods at frequent intervals are indicated. Restrict fats, odorous foods, spiced dishes, and items which do not appeal to the patient.

Sedatives and antiemetics may be required. Vitamins are of no value unless deficiencies have developed. Antihistamines are useful for their sedative effect. Amphetamines may be given for their mood-elevating effect. Narcotics have no place in the treatment of digestive disorders of pregnancy.

Note: The possibility of teratogenicity of many drugs, including some antiemetics, cannot be overlooked in selecting patients for medical treatment of nausea of pregnancy and in deciding which drugs to use and in what dosages (Table 12–8). In general, it is probably best to give medication only when urgently required; to avoid new and experimental drugs and all drugs which have been suggested as potential teratogens; and to give the lowest dosage which is consistent with clinical efficacy. Sedative-antispasmodic medication may be used with discretion.

B. Hyperemesis Gravidarum: Hospitalize the patient in a private room at complete bed rest without bathroom privileges. Allow no visitors (not even the husband) until vomiting ceases and the patient is eating. Give nothing by mouth for 48 hours, and maintain normal electrolyte balance by giving appropriate parenteral fluids and vitamin and protein supplements as indicated. If there is no response after 48 hours, institute nasogastric tube feeding of a well-balanced liquid baby formula by slow drip. As soon as possible, place the patient on a dry diet consisting of 6 small feedings daily with clear liquids 1 hour after eating. Chlorpromazine suppositories may be useful, and psychiatric consultation is often advisable.

If the clinical situation continues to deteriorate in spite of therapy, therapeutic abortion may be required.

Table 12—8. Teratogenic and fetotoxic drugs.

Maternal Medication	Fetal or Neonatal Effect
Established teratogenic agents	
Antineoplastic agents	Multiple anomalies, abortion
Antimetabolites (amethopterin, fluorouracil, DON, 6-azauridine, etc)	
Alkylating agents (cyclophosphamide, etc)	
Antibiotics (amphotericin B, mitomycin, etc)	
Estrogens	Vaginal adenocarcinoma in daughter in later years *
Other sex hormones (androgens, progestogens, estrogens)	Masculinization, advanced bone age
Thalidomide	Fetal death or phocomelia; deafness; cardiovascular, gastrointestinal, or genitourinary anomalies
Organic mercury	Cerebral palsy
Polychlorinated biphenyls (PCBs) (contaminants in manufacture of rice cooking oil)	"Cola"-colored neonates with other developmental defects
Possible teratogens	
Antihistamines	Anomalies
Antithyroid drugs (thioureas, potassium iodide)	Goiter, mental retardation
Corticosteroids	Cleft palate, harelip
Insulin (shock or hypoglycemia)	Anomalies
LSD	"Fractured chromosomes," anomalies
Sulfonylurea derivatives	Anomalies
Vitamin D	Cardiopathies
Fetotoxic drugs	
Analgesics, narcotics	
Heroin, morphine	Neonatal death or convulsions, tremors
Salicylates (excessive)	Neonatal bleeding
Cardiovascular drugs	
Ammonium chloride	Acidosis
Hexamethonium	Neonatal ileus
Reserpine	Nasal congestion, drowsiness
Coumarin anticoagulants	Fetal death or hemorrhage
Poliomyelitis immunization (Sabin)	Death or neurologic damage
Sedatives, hypnotics, tranquilizers	
Meprobamate	Retarded development
Phenobarbital (excessive)	Neonatal bleeding
Phenothiazines	Hyperbilirubinemia
Smallpox vaccination	Death or fetal vaccinia
Tetracyclines	Dental discoloration and abnormalities
Thiazides	Thrombocytopenia
Tobacco smoking	Undersized babies
Vitamin K (excessive)	Hyperbilirubinemia

*FDA Drug Bulletin, Nov 1971: Diethylstilbestrol contraindicated in pregnancy.

The urgent indications are delirium, blindness, tachycardia at rest, jaundice, anuria, and hemorrhage.

Prognosis

Vomiting of pregnancy is self-limited, and the prognosis is good. Intractable hyperemesis gravidarum is a threat to the life of the mother and the fetus.

Caselnova DA: Hyperemesis gravidarum with retinal hemorrhage. Internat J Gynaec Obstet 12:19, 1974.

Weston PV, Lindheimer MD: Intermittent intestinal obstruction simulating hyperemesis gravidarum. Obst Gynec 37:106, 1971.

ECTOPIC PREGNANCY

Essentials of Diagnosis

- Abnormal menstrual bleeding with symptoms suggestive of pregnancy.
- Cramping pains in the lower abdomen.
- Vaginal bleeding, frequently with passage of decidual tissue.
- A tender mass palpable outside the uterus.

General Considerations

Any pregnancy arising from implantation of the

ovum outside the cavity of the uterus is ectopic. Ectopic implantation occurs in about one out of 200
pregnancies. About 98% of ectopic pregnancies are
tubal. Other sites of ectopic implantation are the abdomen, the ovary, and the cervix. Peritonitis, salpingitis, abdominal surgery, and pelvic tumors may predispose to abnormally situated pregnancy. Combined
extrauterine and intrauterine pregnancy may occur.
Only tubal ectopic pregnancy will be discussed in the
following paragraphs.

Clinical Findings

A. Symptoms and Signs: The cardinal symptoms
and signs of tubal pregnancy are (1) amenorrhea or a
disordered menstrual pattern, followed by (2) uterine
bleeding, (3) pelvic pain, and (4) pelvic (adnexal) mass
formation. It may be acute or chronic.

**1. Acute (about 40% of tubal ectopic pregnan-
cies)**—Severe lower quadrant pain occurs in almost
every case. It is sudden in onset, lancinating, intermittent, and does not radiate. Backache is present during
attacks. Abnormal uterine bleeding is present in 80%
and a pelvic mass is palpable in 70%. Collapse and
shock occur in about 10%, often after pelvic examination. Two-thirds of patients give a history of abnormal
menstruation; most have been infertile.

**2. Chronic (about 60% of tubal ectopic pregnan-
cies)**—Blood leaks from the tube over a period of days,
and considerable blood may accumulate in the peritoneum. Slight but persistent vaginal spotting is reported,
and a pelvic mass can be palpated. Discoloration of the
umbilicus by blood pigment (Cullen-Hofstätter sign),
although it is not commonly seen, is diagnostic of
hematoperitoneum.

B. Laboratory Findings: Blood studies show anemia, increased icteric index, slight leukocytosis, elevated serum amylase (variable), and reticulocytosis.
Urine urobilinogen is elevated in ectopic pregnancy
with internal hemorrhage. Pregnancy tests are of little
value in diagnosis.

C. X-Ray Findings: A plain posteroanterior film
of the abdomen may reveal a pelvic mass or other evidence of ectopic pregnancy. Percutaneous retrograde
femoral arteriography and hysterosalpingography are
believed by most American obstetricians to be dangerous procedures which are not essential to the diagnosis
of ectopic pregnancy.

D. Special Examinations: Culdocentesis and similar procedures are of value principally for demonstrating hematoperitoneum.

Differential Diagnosis

The presence of clinical and laboratory findings
suggestive or diagnostic of pregnancy will distinguish
ectopic pregnancy from many acute abdominal illnesses, such as acute appendicitis, a ruptured corpus
luteum cyst or ovarian follicle, a twisted ovarian cyst,
and urinary calculi. Uterine enlargement with clinical
findings similar to those found in ectopic pregnancy is
also characteristic of an aborting uterine pregnancy or
hydatidiform mole.

Complications

The principal complications are hemorrhage and
shock from acute ectopic tubal pregnancy. The most
serious sequelae are chronic pelvic inflammatory disease, infertility, and urinary tract infection.

Treatment

Surgical treatment is imperative, since the patient
may bleed to death if internal hemorrhage is not
promptly brought under control. Devitalized tissue and
blood must be removed to prevent complications.

An ectopic pregnancy is "neglected" if surgery is
delayed more than a few hours after the first physician
has examined the patient. Transfusion should be
started before surgery is begun.

A. Emergency Treatment: Hospitalize the patient
at once if there is a reasonable likelihood of ectopic
pregnancy. Ideally, 6 pints of blood for transfusion
should be available if the patient is in shock or if internal bleeding is suspected. Give blood under pressure
into 2 large veins or intra-arterially. External heat,
morphine, oxygen, slight Trendelenburg position, and
moderately snug tourniquets around the upper legs
may be lifesaving while preparations for surgery are
being made.

B. Surgical Treatment: *Stop the bleeding!* The
products of conception must be removed. Gross blood
in the abdomen should be evacuated. If it is fresh and
unclotted, autotransfusion is feasible, especially if
adequate bank blood is not available. Blood for autotransfusion must be filtered through several layers of
gauze into a flask containing a solution of 3.8% sodium
citrate (1 part citrate solution to 5 parts blood).

Utilize an anesthetic agent which will stimulate
respiration and ensure adequate oxygen, eg, ether or
cyclopropane. Thiopental may cause depression of
vital centers, and spinal or caudal anesthesia is often
accompanied by severe, uncontrollable hypotension in
patients verging upon shock. Most women with a
ruptured ectopic pregnancy require only a light anesthetic for the brief procedure necessary to control
hemorrhage.

1. Salpingectomy (not excision of a portion of
the tube) is indicated if gross tubal damage has occurred. Cornual excision must be done to prevent subsequent tubal or cornual pregnancy and endosalpingo-
sis in the tubal stump.

2. Salpingostomy—Enucleation of the products of
conception, with ligation of bleeding points (but without closure of the tube), has many advocates. The tube
heals readily without stenosis. This procedure is especially appropriate when the other tube is absent or
diseased. Although pregnancy may occasionally recur
in such a tube, the majority of these patients become
normally pregnant.

Salpingostomy for the purpose of eliminating the
pregnancy is not condoned by the Roman Catholic
Church.

C. Postoperative Care: Transfusions and iron therapy are indicated postoperatively, together with a high-
vitamin, high-protein diet.

Prognosis

Maternal mortality in the USA from ectopic pregnancy is 1–2%. The mortality is lowest where adequate surgical facilities are available for immediate intervention.

Repeat tubal gestation occurs in about 10% of cases, but this should not be regarded as a contraindication to future pregnancy.

Campbell JS & others: Acute hemoperitoneum, IUD, and occult ovarian pregnancy. Obst Gynec 43:438, 1974.

Esposito JM: The laparoscope: An aid in the diagnosis of the intact ectopic gestation. J Reprod Med 9:158, 1972.

Franklin EW III, Zeiderman AM: Tubal ectopic pregnancy: Etiology and obstetric and gynecologic sequelae. Am J Obst Gynec 117:220, 1973.

Glover JS Jr: Interstitial pregnancy. North Carolina Med J 34:365, 1973.

Harralson JD & others: Operative management of ruptured tubal pregnancy. Am J Obst Gynec 115:995, 1973.

Kosana TS & others: Use of radioimmunoassay specific for human chorionic gonadotropin in diagnosis of early ectopic pregnancy. Obst Gynec 42:868, 1973.

Leir S: Diagnostic use of ultrasonics in abortion (including extrauterine): A study of 250 patients. Internat J Gynaec Obstet 11:195, 1973.

Rothe DJ, Birnbaum SJ: Cervical pregnancy: Diagnosis and management. Obst Gynec 42:675, 1973.

Scheuker JG & others: Fertility after tubal surgery. Surg Gynec Obst 135:74, 1972.

Stromme WB: Conservative surgery for ectopic pregnancy: A 20-year review. Obst Gynec 41:215, 1973.

Swolen K, Fall M: Ectopic pregnancy: Recurrence, postoperative fertility and aspects of treatment based on 182 patients. Acta europ fertil 3:147, 1972.

Van Iddekinge B: Ectopic pregnancy: A review. South African MJ 46:1844, 1972.

PREECLAMPSIA-ECLAMPSIA
(Toxemia of Pregnancy)*

Essentials of Diagnosis

- Headache, vertigo, irritability, convulsions, coma.
- Scintillating scotomas, partial or complete blindness, retinal hemorrhages.
- Nausea, vomiting, epigastric pain, hepatic enlargement and tenderness.
- Elevated blood pressure, edema, proteinuria, oliguria, anuria.

General Considerations

Preeclampsia-eclampsia usually occurs in the last trimester of pregnancy or early in the puerperium. The term **preeclampsia** denotes the nonconvulsive form; with the development of convulsions and coma, the disorder is termed **eclampsia.** Ten to 20% of pregnant

*The term toxemia is a misnomer and is being abandoned in the literature of obstetrics.

women in the USA develop preeclampsia-eclampsia. Primigravidas are most commonly affected. Uncontrolled toxemia causes permanent disability and may be fatal. Five percent of cases of preeclampsia-eclampsia progress to eclampsia; 10–15% of women with eclampsia die.

The cause is not known. Malnutrition—especially reduced protein ingestion—may play a role. Predisposing factors include vascular and renal disease and sodium retention, which seems to "sensitize" an otherwise healthy pregnant woman.

Clinical Findings

A. Preeclampsia: Headache, vertigo, malaise, and nervous irritability are due in part to cerebral edema; scintillating scotomas and visual impairment are due to edema of the retina, retinal hemorrhage, and retinal detachment; epigastric pain, nausea, and liver tenderness are due to congestion, thrombosis of the periportal system, and subcapsular hepatic hemorrhages.

Preeclampsia-eclampsia is diagnosed by observing both of the following: (1) persistent hypertension or a sudden rise of blood pressure and (2) generalized edema and proteinuria during the last 4 months of pregnancy. Urine protein determinations are the only laboratory tests of positive value in the diagnosis. Ophthalmoscopic examination in severe preeclampsia and eclampsia reveals variable arteriolar spasm, edema of the optic disks, and, with increasing severity, cotton-wool exudates and even retinal detachment.

B. Eclampsia: The symptoms of eclampsia are those of severe preeclampsia. The signs are as follows: (1) generalized tonic-clonic convulsions; (2) coma followed by amnesia and confusion; (3) 3–4+ proteinuria; (4) marked hypertension preceding a convulsion, and hypotension thereafter (during coma or vascular collapse); (5) stertorous breathing, rhonchi, frothing at the mouth; (6) twitching of muscle groups (eg, face, arms); (7) nystagmus; and (8) oliguria or anuria.

Laboratory findings in eclampsia are hemoconcentration, greatly reduced blood CO_2 combining power and content, and increased serum uric acid, nonprotein nitrogen, and urea nitrogen.

Ophthalmoscopic examination generally reveals one or more of the following: papilledema, retinal edema, retinal detachment, vascular spasm, arteriovenous "nicking," and hemorrhages. Repeated ophthalmoscopic examination is helpful in judging the success of treatment.

Differential Diagnosis

The combination of renal, neurologic, and hypertensive findings in a previously normal pregnant woman distinguishes preeclampsia-eclampsia from primary hypertensive, renal, or neurologic disease.

Treatment

Treatment must be prompt and vigorous. In most cases, the best form of treatment is termination of pregnancy by the most expeditious means available which is least harmful to the patient and her baby.

Cesarean section after the 36th week of pregnancy may be indicated for patients who are not good candidates for induction of labor. Avoid delaying more than 3 weeks in severe preeclampsia because fetal death in utero and permanent maternal vascular damage may result.

A. Preeclampsia: The objectives of treatment are (1) to prevent eclampsia, permanent cardiovascular and renal damage, and vascular accidents; and (2) to deliver a normal baby that will survive. Place the patient at bed rest and give sedatives. Give antihypertensive drugs as indicated. Delivery should be delayed, if possible, until the disease is under control or until improvement is marked.

1. Home management—Most patients can be managed at home (at bed rest with sedation) under alert supervision, including frequent blood pressure readings, daily urine protein determinations, and careful recording of fluid intake and output. Sodium restriction (less than 3 gm of salt per day) must be rigidly enforced. If improvement does not occur in 48 hours, transfer the patient to a hospital.

2. Hospital care—Any patient who does not respond to home management (as above) after 48 hours must be hospitalized at absolute bed rest in a single room with no visitors (not even the husband). Determine blood pressure, serum electrolytes, and urine protein at frequent intervals. Examine the ocular fundi every day, noting particularly arteriolar spasm, edema, hemorrhages, and exudates. The diet should be salt-poor (less than 1 gm salt per day), low-fat, high-carbohydrate, and with a moderate protein content. If the urine output exceeds 500 ml/day, a zero water balance is essential; limit fluid intake to 500 ml/day from all sources, plus salt-free fluids to compensate visible losses. Sedatives, diuretics, and antihypertensive drugs should be given as indicated.

B. Eclampsia:

1. Emergency care—If the patient is convulsing, turn her on her side to prevent aspiration of vomitus and mucus and to prevent the caval syndrome. Insert a padded tongue blade or plastic airway between the teeth to prevent biting the tongue and to maintain respiratory exchange. Aspirate fluid and food from the glottis or trachea. Give oxygen by face cone or tent. (Masks and nasal catheters produce excessive stimulation.) Give magnesium sulfate, 10 ml of 25% aqueous solution IV or IM; repeat half of this dose 4 times daily to prevent or control convulsions, lower blood pressure, and encourage diuresis. (Do not repeat magnesium sulfate if the urinary output is less than 100 ml/hour, the respirations are less than 16/minute, or the knee jerk reflex is absent.) In cases of overdosage, give calcium gluconate (or equivalent), 20 ml of a 10% aqueous solution IV slowly, and repeat every hour until urinary, respiratory, and neurologic depression have cleared. (Do not give more than 8 injections of a calcium salt within 24 hours.)

2. General care—Hospitalize the patient in a single, darkened, quiet room at absolute bed rest, lying on her side, with side rails for protection during convulsions. Allow no visitors. Do not disturb the patient for unnecessary procedures (eg, baths, enemas, douches), and leave the blood pressure cuff on her arm. Typed and cross-matched whole blood must be available for immediate use because patients in eclampsia often develop premature separation of the placenta with hemorrhage and are susceptible to shock.

3. Laboratory evaluation—Insert a retention catheter for accurate measurement of the quantity of urine passed. Determine the protein content of each 24-hour specimen until the 4th or 5th postpartum day. Serum BUN, CO_2 combining power and content, serum electrolytes, and serum protein should be determined as often as the severity and progression of the disease indicate. If serum protein is below 5 gm/100 ml, give 250—500 ml of serum albumin. If salt-poor serum albumin is not available, give plasma or serum.

4. Physical examination—Check blood pressure frequently during the acute phase and every 2—4 hours thereafter. Observe fetal heart tones every time the blood pressure is obtained. Perform ophthalmoscopic examination once a day. Examine the face, extremities, and especially the sacrum (which becomes dependent when the patient is in bed) for signs of edema.

5. Diet and fluids—If the patient is convulsing, give nothing by mouth. Record fluid intake and output for each 24-hour period. If she can eat and drink, give a salt-poor (less than 1 gm salt per day), high-carbohydrate, moderate-protein, low-fat diet. Provide potassium chloride as a salt substitute. If the urine output exceeds 700 ml/day, replace the output plus visible fluid loss with salt-free fluid (including parenteral fluid) each day. If the output is less than 700 ml/day, allow no more than 2000 ml of fluid per day (including parenteral fluid). Give 200—300 ml of a 20% solution of dextrose in water 2—3 times a day during the acute phase to protect the liver, to replace fluids, and to aid nutrition. (Do not give 50% glucose; it will sclerose the veins.) Use no sodium-containing fluids (eg, Ringer's injection). Give 25—50 ml salt-poor albumin or 250—500 ml of plasma or serum if the patient is oliguric or if the serum protein is low.

6. Diuretics—Hydrochlorothiazide, 25—50 mg orally or IV, may be given to promote diuresis in patients who are not anuric or severely oliguric.

7. Sedatives—Give phenobarbital on admission and maintain sedation until improvement is established. Give parenteral magnesium sulfate as necessary.

8. Delivery—Because severe hypertensive disease, renal disease, and toxemia of pregnancy are usually aggravated by continuing pregnancy, the most direct method of treatment of any of these disorders is termination of pregnancy. Control eclampsia before attempting induction of labor or delivery. Induce labor, preferably by amniotomy alone, when the patient's condition permits. Use oxytocin (Pitocin) to stimulate labor if necessary. Regional anesthesia (preferably pudendal block) is the technic of choice. Nitrous oxide (70%) and oxygen (30%) may be given with contractions, but 100% oxygen should be administered between contractions.

Vaginal delivery is preferred. If the patient is not at term, if labor is not inducible, if she is bleeding, or if there is a question of disproportion, cesarean section may be necessary. If so, use procaine (or equivalent) for local infiltration of the abdominal wall. After the baby is delivered, give thiopental anesthesia for abdominal closure.

Prognosis

The maternal mortality rate in eclampsia is 10–15%. Most patients improve strikingly in 24–48 hours with appropriate therapy, but early termination of pregnancy is usually required.

Although babies of mothers with preeclampsia-eclampsia are small for their gestational age (probably because of placental malfunction), they fare better than premature babies of the same weight born of women who do not develop preeclampsia-eclampsia.

Baskett TF, Bradford CR: Active management of severe preeclampsia. Canad MAJ 109:1209, 1975.

Beecham JB, Watson WJ, Clapp JF III: Eclampsia, preeclampsia, and disseminated intravascular coagulation. Obst Gynec 43:576, 1974.

Craig CJT: Eclampsia and the anesthetist. South African MJ 46:248, 1972.

Del Greco F, Krumlovsky FH: The renal pressor system in human pregnancy. J Reprod Med 8:98, 1972.

Ehrlich EN, Lindheimer MD: Sodium metabolism, aldosterone and the hypertensive disorders of pregnancy. J Reprod Med 8:106, 1972.

Joyce VG: The use of diazepam and hydralazine in the treatment of severe preeclampsia. J Obstet Gynaec Brit Common 79:250, 1972.

Kitzmiller JL & others: Hematologic assays in preeclampsia. Am J Obst Gynec 118:363, 1974.

Lopez-Leera M, Hernandez-Horta JL: Pregnancy after eclampsia. Am J Obst Gynec 119:193, 1974.

McAllister CJ & others: Amniotic fluid levels of uric acid and creatinine in toxemia patients: Possible relation to diuretic use. Am J Obst Gynec 115:560, 1973.

Pahe EW: On the pathogenesis of preeclampsia and eclampsia. J Obstet Gynaec Brit Common 79:883, 1972.

Perel ID & others: Thrombotic thrombocytopenic purpura presenting as eclampsia. Australian New Zealand J Obstet Gynaec 12:257, 1972.

Roach CJ: Renovascular hypertension in pregnancy. Obst Gynec 42:856, 1973.

Sprague AD & others: Pheochromocytoma associated with pregnancy. Obst Gynec 39:887, 1972.

Sullivan M: Blood pressure elevation in pregnancy. Progr Cardiovas Dis 16:375, 1974.

Vardi J, Fields GA: Microangiopathic hemolytic anemia in severe preeclampsia: A review of the literature and pathophysiology. Am J Obst Gynec 119:617, 1974.

Vardi J, Halbrecht J: Toxemia of pregnancy. 1. Antigens associated with toxemia of pregnancy in placental connective tissue. Am J Obst Gynec 118:552, 1974.

Wiser WL & others: Laboratory characteristics in toxemia. Obst Gynec 39:866, 1972.

Yogman MW & others: Child development after pregnancies complicated by low urinary estriol excretion and preeclampsia. Am J Obst Gynec 114:1069, 1972.

ANEMIA DURING PREGNANCY

Physiologic and pathologic changes in the maternal organism during pregnancy make the determination of anemia difficult. Not only do blood values during pregnancy differ from those in the nonpregnant patient, but these factors also vary with the course of pregnancy. If deficiencies of a significant degree are noted, the patient is anemic and specific therapy is indicated.

In every evaluation of clinical and laboratory data, the following questions must be answered: (1) Is anemia present? (2) Is there evidence of iron deficiency? (3) Are megaloblasts present in the blood smear? (4) Are there signs of hemolysis? (5) Is there bone marrow deficiency?

Iron Deficiency Anemia

Iron deficiency anemia in pregnancy is usually due to iron deprivation from previous pregnancies. It occurs in at least 20% of pregnancies in the USA. About 95% of pregnant women with anemia have the iron deficiency type. Pregnancy increases the woman's iron requirements because an increase of about 30% in total blood volume is necessary to meet the needs of the enlarged uterus and augmented vascular system.

Because so many women are iron deficient, oral iron should be administered to all patients during pregnancy and for at least 1 month following delivery. If iron is given prophylactically, the great majority of patients will maintain an acceptable hemoglobin concentration.

Folic Acid Deficiency Anemia
("Pernicious" or Megaloblastic Anemia of Pregnancy)

"Pernicious" anemia of pregnancy is caused by folic acid—not vitamin B_{12}—deficiency. This disorder is most common in multiparas over age 30. The reported incidence varies from 1:40–1:200 deliveries. Folic acid deprivation is most common where dietary resources are inadequate, although some women on apparently adequate diets may be deficient. Curiously, only a small percentage of women with low serum folic acid levels have megaloblastic anemia. Folic acid deficiency anemia follows malnutrition, and is often associated with alcoholism or protracted vomiting. It may be associated with multiple pregnancy or toxemia and may accompany sprue or sickle cell disease. It often occurs in epileptic patients who have received prolonged primidone, phenytoin, or barbiturate medication.

Lassitude, progressive anorexia, mental depression, and nausea are the principal complaints. Pallor is often not marked. Glossitis, gingivitis, vomiting, and diarrhea occur frequently. There are no abnormal neurologic findings.

Folic acid deficiency results in hematologic findings similar to those of true pernicious anemia (vitamin B_{12} deficiency), which is very rare in the pregnancy age group. With folic acid lack, blood changes appear sooner. The hemoglobin may be as low as 4—6 gm/100 ml. The red blood cell count may be < 2 million/cu mm in severe cases. Extreme anemia often is associated with leukopenia and thrombocytopenia. The MCV is normal or increased. The peripheral white blood cells are hypersegmented. The bone marrow is hyperplastic and megaloblastic. Free gastric hydrochloric acid is present in normal amounts. Serum iron values are high, and serum vitamin B_{12} levels are normal.

Treatment consists of giving folic acid, 5—10 mg/day orally or parenterally, until a hematologic remission is achieved. Megaloblastic anemia of pregnancy does not usually respond to vitamin B_{12} even in large doses. Administer iron orally or parenterally (or both) as indicated. Prescribe a high-vitamin, high-protein diet. Transfusions are rarely necessary except when anemia is extreme, especially if the patient is near term.

Megaloblastic anemia during pregnancy is not apt to be severe unless it is associated with systemic infection or toxemia. If the diagnosis is made at least 4 weeks before term, treatment can often raise the hemoglobin to normal or nearly normal levels. The outlook for mother and baby is good if there is adequate time for treatment. Spontaneous remissions usually occur after delivery. Anemia usually recurs only when the patient becomes pregnant again.

Aplastic Anemia

Aplastic anemia is rare, but it may be devastating during pregnancy. The anemia may be a toxic sequel to drugs such as chloramphenicol, phenylbutazone, mephenytoin, or alkylating chemotherapeutic agents. Hair dyes, insecticides, and cleaning fluids may be implicated also. In about half of cases, the cause cannot be identified.

Fetal death or premature labor may ensue. Infection or hemorrhage may be the terminal event for the mother. Severe bone marrow depression carries a 50% threat of death due to hemorrhage or infection within weeks or months. Partial or complete remissions do occur, however.

Sickle Cell Anemia (Sickle Cell Disease)

Pregnancy is very deleterious to patients with sickle cell disease. Almost 50% of these pregnancies are complicated by anemia (often with folic acid and iron deficiency overlay), pyelonephritis, thrombosis, and bone and joint pain. (Iron and folic acid should be given to all pregnant patients with sickle cell disease.)

Symptomatic therapy is required. For sickle cell anemia which occurs during pregnancy, consider exchange transfusion and bring the hemoglobin to 10—12 gm/100 ml in the third trimester. Bed rest and analgesics are helpful. Sodium bicarbonate (3.5 mEq/kg/hour IV) or 5% glucose with 0.45% sodium chloride IV may relieve pain. Elimination of infection and transfusion are required for an aplastic crisis.

The risk to the fetus is increased considerably because of the complications, although the offspring will suffer no specific adverse effects.

The maternal mortality rate may be as high as 5—10%. Cesarean section should be done on obstetric indications. Limitation of pregnancy—often by sterilization—is indicated.

Beydoun SN & others: Maternal nutrition. 1. The urinary urea nitrogen/total nitrogen ratio as an index of protein nutrition. Am J Obst Gynec 114:190, 1972.

Carr MC: The diagnosis of iron deficiency in pregnancy. Obst Gynec 43:15, 1974.

Cohenour SH, Calloway DH: Blood, urine and dietary pantothenic acid levels of pregnant teenagers. Am J Clin Nutr 25:512, 1972.

Desforges J: Anemia complicating pregnancy. J Reprod Med 10:111, 1973.

Fleming AF: Maternal anemia and fetal outcome in pregnancies complicated by thalassemia minor and stomatocytosis. Am J Obst Gynec 116:309, 1973.

Fleming AF: Urinary excretion of folate in pregnancy. J Obstet Gynaec Brit Common 79:916, 1972.

Hall MH: Blood and neoplastic diseases: Pregnancy anemia. Brit MJ 2:661, 1974.

Hashmi JA, Afroze N: Plasma fibrinogen and serum lipids in anemia of pregnancy. Am J Obst Gynec 112:821, 1972.

Hendrickse JPDV & others: Pregnancy in homozygous sickle cell anemia. J Obstet Gynaec Brit Common 79:396, 1972.

Hibbard BM: Prophylaxis in pregnancy anaemia. Prevention 1:35, 1972.

Hibbard BM, Hibbard ED: Anemia and folate status in late pregnancy in a mixed Asiatic population. J Obstet Gynaec Brit Common 79:584, 1972.

Kaminetzky HA & others: The effect of nutrition in teenage gravidas on pregnancy and the status of the neonate. 1. A nutritional profile. Am J Obst Gynec 115:639, 1973.

Kazazian HH Jr: Antenatal detection of sickle cell anemia. New England J Med 287:41, 1972.

Kuah KB: Total dose of Imferon® in obstetrics. Med J Malaya 26:186, 1972.

McFee JG: Anemia in pregnancy: A reappraisal. Obst Gynec Surv 28:769, 1973.

Molina RA & others: Nutritional anemia during pregnancy: A comparative study of 2 socio-economic classes. J Obstet Gynaec Brit Common 81:544, 1974.

Nunnelley PP Jr & others: Pregnancy and hemoglobin SD disease. Am J Obst Gynec 113:844, 1972.

Rao KPR: The role of triple therapy in severe iron deficiency anemias of pregnancy. J Obstet Gynaec India 22:164, 1972.

Tan PM: Megaloblastic anemia in pregnancy and the puerperium. Ann Acad Med Singapore 1:79, 1972.

ABORTION

Essentials of Diagnosis

- Vaginal bleeding in a pregnant woman.
- Uterine cramping.
- Disappearance of symptoms and signs of pregnancy.
- Negative or equivocal pregnancy tests.
- The products of conception may or may not be expelled.

General Considerations

Abortion is defined as termination of gestation before the fetus becomes viable. Viability is usually reached at 28 weeks, when the infant weighs slightly more than 1 kg (2.2 lb). About three-fourths of abortions occur before the 16th week of gestation; of these, three-fourths occur before the 8th week. At least 12% of all pregnancies terminate in spontaneous abortion. Criminally induced abortions are less frequent in areas where legal termination of pregnancy exists.

About 50–60% of spontaneous abortions result from ovular defects; 15% are caused by maternal factors (trauma, infections, dietary deficiencies, diabetes mellitus, hypothyroidism, poisoning, anatomic malformations). There is no good evidence that abortion may be induced by psychic stimuli such as severe fright, grief, anger, or anxiety. In about one-fourth of cases, the cause of abortion cannot be determined.

Clinical Findings

A. Symptoms and Signs: Abortion is classified clinically as (1) inevitable, (2) complete, (3) incomplete, and (4) missed. In threatened abortion the previable gestation is in jeopardy but the pregnancy often continues.

1. Inevitable abortion—In inevitable abortion the passage of some or all of the products of conception is momentarily impending. Bleeding and cramps do not subside.

2. Complete abortion—In complete abortion all of the conceptus is expelled. When complete abortion is impending the symptoms of pregnancy often disappear; sudden bleeding then begins, followed by cramping. The fetus and the rest of the conceptus may be expelled separately. When the entire conceptus has been expelled, pain ceases but slight spotting persists.

3. Incomplete abortion—In incomplete abortion a significant portion of the pregnancy (usually a placental fragment) remains in the uterus. Only mild cramps are reported, but bleeding is persistent and often excessive.

4. Missed abortion—In missed abortion the pregnancy has been terminated for at least 1 month but the conceptus has not been expelled. Symptoms of pregnancy disappear and the BBT is not elevated. There is a brownish vaginal discharge but no free bleeding. Pain is not present. The cervix is semi-firm and slightly patulous; the uterus becomes smaller and irregularly softened; the adnexa are normal.

B. Laboratory Findings: Pregnancy tests are negative or equivocally positive. Blood and urine findings are those usually observed in infection and anemia if these complications have occurred.

C. X-Ray Findings: In late abortion a plain film of the abdomen may demonstrate a distorted angulated fetal skeleton and often intrauterine gas.

Differential Diagnosis

The bleeding which occurs in abortion of a uterine pregnancy must be differentiated from the abnormal bleeding of an aborting ectopic pregnancy, hyperestrinism in a nonpregnant woman, and membranous dysmenorrhea. The passage of hydropic villi in the bloody discharge is diagnostic of the abortion of a hydatidiform mole.

Complications

Hemorrhage in abortion is a major cause of maternal death. Infection is most common after criminally induced abortion; death results from salpingitis, peritonitis, septicemia, and septic emboli. Less common complications are perforation of the uterus, chorioepithelioma, and infertility.

Treatment

A. Emergency Measures: If abortion has occurred after the first trimester, the patient should be hospitalized. In all cases induce uterine contraction with oxytocics, eg, oxytocin (Pitocin), IM or IV (not ergot preparations), to limit blood loss and aid in the expulsion of clots and tissues. Ergonovine maleate (Ergotrate) should be given only if the diagnosis of complete abortion is certain. Give antishock therapy, including blood replacement, to prevent collapse after hemorrhage.

B. General Measures: Place the patient at bed rest and give sedatives to allay uterine irritability and limit bleeding. Coitus and douches are contraindicated. Stilbestrol and its analogues and derivatives should not be given because of the possible induction of clear cell carcinoma of the vagina or cervix in female offspring. These drugs are useless in any case in the prevention of abortion. Antibiotics are indicated if criminal abortion is likely or if signs of infection are present.

C. Surgical Measures:

1. Cerclage (Shirodkar) during the second trimester for closure of an incompetent internal cervical os.

2. Dilatation and curettage for possible retained tissue. Start an intravenous drip of oxytocin (Pitocin) before surgery to avoid uterine penetration.

Bland BJ, Lowry RB: Use of spontaneous abortions and stillbirths in genetic counseling. Am J Obst Gynec 118:322, 1974.

Boyce J, Hales J: Problems in the management of patients who have abortions. Drug Therapy 4:59, Feb 1974.

Brotherton J, Craft IL: A clinical and pathologic survey of 91 cases of spontaneous abortion. Fertil Steril 23:289, 1972.

Connally WJ, Breen JL: Aggressive management of septic abortion: Report of 262 cases. South MJ 65:1480, 1972.

Corbett TH: Anesthetics as a cause of abortion. Fertil Steril 23:866, 1972.

Hill EC: Clear cell carcinoma of the cervix and vagina in young women: A report of six cases with association of maternal stilbestrol therapy and adenosis of the vagina. Am J Obst Gynec 116:470, 1973.

Little HM Jr: Managing incomplete abortion. Am Family Physician 9:136, 1974.

McLennan MT, McLennan CE: Use of vaginal wall cytologic smears to predict abortion in high risk pregnancies. Am J Obst Gynec 114:857, 1972.

Papaevangelou G & others: The effect of spontaneous and induced abortion on prematurity and birthweight. J Obstet Gynaec Brit Common 80:418, 1973.

Poole RM & others: A case of abortion consequent upon infection with *Brucella abortus* biotype 2. J Clin Path 25:882, 1972.

Ratten GJ: Resumption of ovulation after incomplete abortion. Australian New Zealand J Obstet Gynaec 12:217, 1972.

Wallner HJ: The fate of the child after threatened abortion. J Perinatal Med 2:54, 1974.

HABITUAL ABORTION

Habitual abortion implies loss of 3 or more previable (< 1000 gm) pregnancies in succession. Emotionally immature women are prone to habitual abortion.

Habitual abortion is a clinical, not a pathologic diagnosis. Hormonal aberrations often seem to be responsible for habitual abortion. Habitual abortion occurs in about 0.4% of all pregnancies or 4% of all spontaneous abortions and is usually the result of recurrent (persistent) rather than random (accidental) factors. Many habitual abortions result from abnormal genetic disorders. About 15% are due to maternal organic disease.

The clinical findings are similar to those observed in other types of abortion (see above).

Treatment

The entire program of therapy rather than any single aspect of it will be responsible for success or failure. Most regimens of therapy include psychotherapy. A special clinic or individualized therapy, preferably by one therapist who has established good rapport with the patient, is most desirable.

A. General Measures:

1. Preconception therapy is aimed at detection of maternal or paternal defects which may contribute to abortion. A thorough general and gynecologic examination is essential. Psychic factors, including emotional conflicts in marriage and during previous pregnancies, must be evaluated. The competence of the cervical os must be determined. Hysterography (for tumor or congenital anomalies), PBI, vaginal smears, and other tests should be performed as indicated. Endometrial tissue should be examined in the postovulation stage of the cycle to determine the adequacy of the response of the endometrium to hormones. Every attempt should be made to restore good physical and emotional health.

2. Postconception therapy—Provide early prenatal care and schedule frequent office visits. Repeated gentle abdominopelvic examinations are indicated so that abnormal uterine development can be noted early. Permit unrestricted telephone calls. Give adequate sedatives. Insert a vaginal pessary if retroposition of the uterus is a possible cause of symptoms. Be prepared to hospitalize the patient promptly at the first sign of impending abortion.

Prescribe an adequate diet high in vitamins (especially vitamins C and K). The patient should strive to achieve and maintain an appropriate pregnancy weight for her height and build. Give thyroid hormone only as indicated. Vitamin E is of no value.

Insist that the patient avoid intercourse during the entire pregnancy. Hot baths and douches are likewise contraindicated. Complete bed rest is justified, however, only for bleeding or pain. Empiric steroid sex hormone therapy is not warranted. Excessive smoking should be curbed.

If arborization of the cervical mucus occurs, with or without therapy, the pregnancy is lost.

B. Surgical Measures: Incompetency of the cervical os should be corrected by means of the Lash, MacDonald, or Shirodkar type of operation. Trachelorrhaphy may be required for severe cervical lacerations. Uterine suspension, myomectomy, and a unification operation (for double uterus) may be justified for treatment of habitual abortion.

Prognosis

The prognosis is good if the cause of abortion can be corrected. If a woman has lost 3 previous pregnancies, she has a 70–80% chance of carrying a fetus to viability. If she has aborted 4 or 5 times, her likelihood of a successful pregnancy is 65–70%.

Holman MR: An aid for cervical cerclage. Obst Gynec 42:468, 1973.

Kuptsow P: Cerclage in the treatment of the incompetent cervix. J Am Osteopath A 72:1094, 1973.

Lanersen WH, Fuchs F: Experience with Shirodkar's operation and postoperative alcohol treatment. Acta obst gynec scandinav 52:77, 1973.

McLaren HC: Management of recurring abortion. Practitioner 209:661, 1972.

Southern PM Jr: Habitual abortion and toxoplasmosis: Is there a relationship? Obst Gynec 39:45, 1972.

THERAPEUTIC ABORTION

The indications for and legal restraints on therapeutic abortion have been greatly liberalized in recent years, and all physicians should become familiar with the professional practices and standards in their communities. This discussion will be limited to a description of the methods employed and the complications that may arise.

Methods

A. Dilatation and Curettage: Almost two-thirds of therapeutic abortions are performed transvaginally by dilatation of the cervix and evacuation of the uterus. Before the 12th week of pregnancy, the vaginal route is usually chosen for therapeutic abortions unless sterilization is to be performed also, in which case laparotomy and abdominal hysterotomy are required. After the 12th week, abdominal hysterotomy is safer than dilatation of the cervix and evacuation of the uterus from below.

The preoperative preparation is similar to that employed for dilatation and curettage or cesarean section if hysterotomy is chosen. Postoperative management is comparable to postpartal care, although the patient can usually resume full activity in 2–3 weeks.

B. Suction Therapeutic Abortion: Suction curettage has supplanted mechanical curettage in many hospitals for the interruption of early pregnancy. The following advantages and disadvantages are recognized.

1. Advantages—Suction evacuation of the products of early conception has the following advantages:

a. Less dilatation of the cervix is necessary than for surgical dilatation and curettage (lessens likelihood of cervical tears and incompetent cervix).

b. The negative pressure is powerful enough so that the tip of the instrument need not come into contact with the entire uterine cavity surface (even the uterine "dead space" is denuded).

c. Separation of the placenta occurs at its surface contact, thus protecting the basalis and muscularis. Therefore, traumatic amenorrhea and intrauterine adhesion (Asherman's syndrome) are less likely.

d. Suction aspiration is much more rapid and expeditious than surgical dilatation and curettage (3 minutes average).

e. Less anesthesia and analgesia are required (basal analgesia and paracervical block may suffice).

f. When the uterine cavity is quickly evacuated, rapid contraction of the uterus occurs, minimizing blood loss. Measurement of blood lost is possible.

g. The short operating time and the minimal use of instruments reduce the danger of infection.

h. Blunt suction tubes are less traumatic than curets.

2. Disadvantages—

a. The suction tube is not delicate enough to distinguish minor changes in architecture of the uterus (small polyps, partial septa).

b. In pregnancy of more than 10 weeks' duration, the instrument can be blocked by fetal-placental fragments.

c. The negative pressure is produced by an electric motor, and mechanical or current failure may occur.

d. More distortion and fragmentation of the tissues occur with suction.

e. If there is a tight fit at the cervix and prolonged suction is applied, excessive blood loss may occur.

C. Intra-amniotic Injection of Hypertonic Solutions: Therapeutic abortion after the 14th week and evacuation of the uterus following fetal death can be accomplished medically within 12–14 hours, almost without exception, by aseptic transabdominal aspiration of amniotic fluid and immediate very slow replacement by a similar amount of sterile aqueous 20% sodium chloride or 50% glucose solution. Saline should not be used for patients with eclamptogenic toxemia or other disorders in which sodium restriction is desirable. Labor generally requires only 2–3 hours; its cause is uncertain. Whether labor is the result of

progestogen block or reduced progestogen production by the placenta is debated.

After voiding (to prevent injury to the bowel or bladder), the patient is placed in the slight Trendelenburg position. A site half-way between the symphysis and umbilicus and slightly lateral to the midline is chosen for amniocentesis. Under aseptic operating room conditions, after preparation with antiseptic, the skin is anesthetized with procaine or comparable solution. A No. 14 or 16, 4–6 inch needle with obturator is inserted slowly into the uterine cavity. Ideally, 100–200 ml of fluid are withdrawn. In second trimester pregnancy and missed abortion, only small amounts of amniotic fluid may be available. In such instances, at least 60–90 ml of solution should be injected if possible.

The recovered placenta reveals extensive edema and submembranous degeneration. Signs of hypoxia are noted when fetal death follows injection of hypertonic solutions.

D. Prostaglandins are under investigation.

Complications

Therapeutic abortion is a potentially dangerous operation even in healthy women. Perforation of the uterus, pelvic infection, hemorrhage, and embolism are the most common complications. The primary mortality in elective first trimester abortion is 0.05–0.1% (Scandinavia). A 5% morbidity (fever, pelvic infection) is recorded in the first trimester and over 15–20% in such second-trimester, state-authorized interruptions of pregnancy.

The mortality is 1–2% in the seriously ill pregnant patient whose physical or emotional disease may justify abortion. The postoperative morbidity is proportionate.

Protracted feelings of guilt commonly result from interruption of pregnancy, particularly when religious conflicts complicate the decision and the patient feels responsible for the loss of the baby.

Baudry F, Wiener A: The pregnant patient in conflict about abortion: A challenge for the obstetrician. Am J Obst Gynec 119:705, 1974.

Berger GS & others: Maternal mortality associated with legal abortions in New York State: July 1, 1970–June 30, 1972. Obst Gynec 43:315, 1974.

Bradley-Watson PJ & others: Injuries to the cervix after induced mid trimester abortion. J Obstet Gynaec Brit Common 80:284, 1973.

Brenner WE & others: Coagulation changes during abortion induced by prostaglandin F_{2a}. Am J Obst Gynec 117:1080, 1973.

Craft I: Intra-amniotic prostaglandin E_2 and F_2 for induction of abortion: A dose response study. J Obstet Gynaec Brit Common 80:46, 1973.

Dillon TF & others: The efficacy of prostaglandin F_{2a} in a second-trimester abortion. Am J Obst Gynec 118:688, 1974.

Embrey MP & others: Induction of abortion by extra-amniotic administration of prostaglandins E_2 and F_{2a}. Brit MJ 3:146, 1972.

Golditch IM, Glasses MH: The use of laminaria tents for cervical dilatation prior to vacuum aspiration abortion. Am J Obst Gynec 119:481, 1974.

Gullattee AC: Psychiatric aspects of abortion. J Nat Med A 64:308, 1972.

Hodgson JE, Portmann KC: Complications of 10,543 consecutive 1st trimester abortions: Prospective study. Am J Obst Gynec 120:802, 1974.

Kerenyi TD & others: Five thousand consecutive saline inductions. Am J Obst Gynec 116:593, 1973.

Lee J, Wessler S, Avioli LV: Prostaglandins as therapeutic agents. Arch Int Med 131:294, 1973.

Nanthanson BM: The postabortal pain syndrome: A new entity. Obst Gynec 41:739, 1973.

Ng AYH, Ratuam SS: Outpatient termination of pregnancy by vacuum aspiration. Singapore MJ 14:23, 1973.

Paine JM & others: Use of hypertonic urea solution as the method of choice for mid-trimester abortion. Obst Gynec 43:295, 1974.

Roht LH, Aoyama H: Induced abortion and its sequelae: Prevalence and associations with the outcome of pregnancy. Internat J Epidem 2:103, 1973.

Rovinsky JJ: Abortion recidivism: A problem in preventive medicine. Obst Gynec 39:649, 1972.

Sedaghat A, Ayromlooi J: Disseminated intravascular coagulation resulting in severe hemorrhage, following the intra-amniotic injection of hypertonic saline to induce abortion. Am J Obst Gynec 114:841, 1972.

Tietze C: The effect of legalization of abortion on population growth and public health. Fam Plann Perspect 7:123, 1975.

Walton LA: Immediate morbidity on a large abortion service. New York State J Med 72:919, 1972.

Weinberg PC, Shepard MK: Intra-amniotic urea for induction of mid-trimester abortion. Obst Gynec 41:451, 1973.

STERILIZATION

Sterilization is any procedure which renders the individual, man or woman, incapable of reproduction. Sterilization may be done electively in all states but Utah (where a medical indication is required), to limit the number of children; or may be compulsory, if the individual or couple are considered unfit to bear children because of hereditary diseases or mental incapacity.

The indications for sterilization are usually grouped as neuropsychiatric, medical, surgical, obstetric, and socioeconomic. In general, when irremediable conditions constitute a bona fide indication for therapeutic abortion, prevention of subsequent pregnancy by sterilization is warranted. The Roman Catholic Church forbids sterilization without exception.

Surgical sterilization of women may be accomplished by the abdominal, vaginal, transuterine, or inguinal approach. The most commonly used technic is to occlude the tubes by ligation. However, part or all of the tubes may be excised or closed by coagulation. Hysterectomy may be the best means of sterilization if tumors, bleeding problems, or relaxation of the pelvic floor justifies the major procedure required.

The safety of tubal ligation, the sterilization operation most commonly employed, varies with the procedure, whether the woman has just been delivered, and by what route. If done at cesarean section, a 1—2% failure rate must be expected with the Pomeroy method. In the nonpregnant patient (or 24 hours following vaginal delivery), failures (Pomeroy) are about 1:300.

The effectiveness of sterilization depends upon the method employed. The only certain and safe methods are bilateral oophorectomy and hysterectomy.

Ballard CA: Therapeutic abortion and sterilization by vaginal hysterectomy. Am J Obst Gynec 118:891, 1974.

Bazley WS, Crisp WE: Postpartum hysterectomy for sterilization. Am J Obst Gynec 119:139, 1974.

DiMusto JC & others: A follow-up study of 100 sterilized women. J Reprod Med 12:112, 1974.

Hulka JF & others: Complications Committee of the American Association of Gynecological Laparoscopists: First annual report. J Reprod Med 10:301, 1973.

Poulson AM Jr: Analysis of female sterilization techniques. Obst Gynec 42:131, 1973.

Stoot JEGM, Ubachs JMH: Sterilization by salpingectomy through posterior colpotomy. Contraception 8:577, 1973.

Thompson BH, Wheeless CR Jr: Gastrointestinal complications of laparoscopy sterilization. Obst Gynec 41:669, 1973.

Wheeless CR Jr, Thompson BH: Laparoscopic sterilization: Review of 3,600 cases. Obst Gynec 42:751, 1973.

HYDATIDIFORM MOLE & CHORIO-EPITHELIOMA

Essentials of Diagnosis

- Uterine bleeding at 6—8 weeks.
- Excessive nausea and vomiting.
- Uterus larger than expected for duration of pregnancy.
- Presence of vesicles passed from vagina.
- Urinary chorionic gonadotropins high.

General Considerations

Hydatidiform mole is a degenerative disorder of the chorion which occurs as a complication of about one in 1500 pregnancies in the USA, usually during the first 18 weeks. It is characterized by prominent, pale yellow, grape-like vesicular enlargements of the villi and vascular incompetence of the villous tree. Although it is assumed to be of placental (fetal) origin, the precise cause is not known. Hydatidiform mole is more common among women over 40, and is over 5 times more prevalent in the Orient than in the Occident. Malignant change (chorio-epithelioma) occurs in about 4% of cases in the USA and is often fatal when it does occur.

Clinical Findings

A. Symptoms and Signs: Excessive nausea and vomiting occur in over one-third of patients with hydatidiform mole. Uterine bleeding, beginning at 6—8 weeks, is observed in virtually all instances and is indicative of threatened or incomplete abortion. In about one-fifth of cases, the uterus is larger than would be expected in a normal pregnancy of the same duration. Intact or collapsed vesicles may be passed through the vagina.

Eclamptogenic toxemia, frequently of the fulminating type, may develop during the second trimester of pregnancy.

Chorio-epithelioma may be manifested by continued or recurrent uterine bleeding after evacuation of a mole or by the presence of an ulcerative vaginal tumor, pelvic mass, or evidence of distant metastatic tumor. The diagnosis is established by pathologic examination of curettings or by biopsy.

B. **Laboratory Findings**: Hydatidiform mole or chorio-epithelioma is probably present when the FSH exceeds 0.5 million rat units/liter of urine and the LH titer is above 0.2 million rat units/liter. The urinary 17-ketosteroid level is often twice the normal pregnancy level (10—15 μg/100 ml). The vaginal smear reveals distinct, heavy cell groupings, a predominance of superficial cells, acidophilia, and pyknosis in about half of the exfoliate cells.

C. **X-Ray Findings**: Amniography after the third month, either by the transcervical or transcutaneous route, utilizing intravenous urographic media, may demonstrate a honeycomb appearance of the uterine contents.

D. **Special Examinations**: Preserve any tissue passed spontaneously. Identification of placental hydatids will establish the diagnosis.

Differential Diagnosis

The excessive nausea and vomiting which occurs in hydatidiform mole must be distinguished from hyperemesis gravidarum; the excessively large uterus from multiple pregnancy, hydramnios, and uterine tumors; and the vaginal bleeding from threatening or complete abortion. The presence of a large uterus and laboratory findings of pregnancy with the absence of a fetal skeleton by x-ray makes the diagnosis of a mole very probable.

Treatment

A. **Emergency Measures**: Hemorrhage indicative of abortion requires immediate hospitalization. Type and cross-match the patient's blood, and have at least 2 units of blood available for transfusion. Free bleeding will cease as soon as the uterine contents are evacuated and firm uterine contraction with oxytocin is established. Curettage will probably be required for removal of adherent tissue.

B. **Specific (Surgical) Measures**:

1. **Empty the uterus** as soon as possible after the diagnosis of hydatidiform mole is established. Suction evacuation followed by careful dilatation and curettage is the preferred method of treatment. If the uterus is larger than a 3-month pregnancy, pack the cavity for 6—12 hours after curettage to reduce bleeding and aid in the removal of tissue missed by the curet. Give ergonovine maleate (Ergotrate), 0.2 mg orally every 4 hours after curettage for 4 doses. A second D&C in 3—4 weeks may be required if bleeding persists or fever develops.

2. **Hysterotomy**—If the uterus is larger than a 5-month pregnancy and the cervix is resistant to wide dilatation, hysterotomy may be indicated (vaginal if infection is clinically evident; otherwise, anterior abdominal). Do not resect ovarian cysts or remove the ovaries; spontaneous regression will occur with elimination of the mole.

3. **Hysterectomy** rarely is curative. If malignant tissue is found at surgery or follow-up, chemotherapy is indicated. Methotrexate is the most promising chemotherapeutic agent.

C. **Antitumor Chemotherapy**: Methotrexate, 3 mg/kg IM in divided doses over a 5-day period, is recommended. The side-effects—anorexia, nausea and vomiting, stomatitis, rash, diarrhea, and bone marrow depression—usually are reversible in about 3 weeks. They can be ameliorated by the administration of folic acid or folinic acid. Death occurs occasionally from agranulocytosis or toxic hepatitis. Repeated courses of methotrexate 1 month apart generally are required to destroy the trophoblast and maintain a zero chorionic gonadotropin titer. If liver disease complicates the problem or if the tumor is resistant, give dactinomycin (Cosmegen), 10 μg/kg IV (well diluted), over a period of 5 days in monthly courses.

D. **Supportive Measures**: Replace blood and give iron and vitamins. If infection is suspected, give broad-spectrum antibiotics for 24 hours before and 3—4 days after surgery.

Prognosis

A 5-year arrest after courses of chemotherapy, even when metastases have been demonstrated, can be expected in about 75% of cases of chorio-epithelioma. The risk of chronic abortion is not great in women who have had hydatidiform mole.

Bagshawe KD & others: Follow-up after hydatidiform mole: Studies using radioimmunoassay for urinary human chorionic gonadotrophin (HGC). J Obstet Gynaec Brit Common 80:461, 1973.

Dawood MY & others: Serum estradiol-17β and serum human chorionic gonadotropin in patients with hydatidiform moles. Am J Obst Gynec 119:904, 1974.

Goldstein DP: Prevention of gestational trophoblastic disease by use of actinomycin D in molar pregnancies. Obst Gynec 43:475, 1974.

Jones WB, Lewis JL Jr: Treatment of gestational trophoblastic disease. Am J Obst Gynec 120:14, 1974.

Pastorfidi GB, Goldstein DP: Pregnancy after hydatidiform mole. Obst Gynec 42:67, 1973.

Rao S & others: Hydatidiform mole. Clinician 38:129, 1974.

Scheer KI, Goldstein DP: An alternative in trophoblastic disease follow-up. Am J Obst Gynec 114:838, 1972.

Teoh ES & others: The source of circulating progesterone and 17α-hydroxyprogesterone in hydatidiform mole. Acta endocrinol 71:773, 1972.

THIRD TRIMESTER BLEEDING

Five to 10% of women have vaginal bleeding in late pregnancy. Multiparas are more commonly affected. Obstetric bleeding is the major cause of maternal mortality and morbidity. The physician must distinguish between placental causes of obstetric bleeding (placenta previa, premature separation of the placenta) and nonplacental causes (systemic disease or disorders of the lower genital tract).

The approach to the problem of bleeding in late pregnancy should be conservative and expectant.

The patient should be hospitalized at once, preferably by ambulance, at complete bed rest. Perform a complete, gentle abdominal examination but no rectal or vaginal examination. Obtain placentography, type and match. Have blood ready for possible need at examination. Over 90% of patients with third trimester bleeding will cease to bleed in 24 hours on bed rest alone. If bleeding is profuse and persistent, however, vaginal examination is indicated after preparation and blood replacement. The operating room should be ready for cesarean section before this examination is done.

If the patient is less than 36 weeks pregnant and the fetus is too small for survival, it may be necessary to keep her in the hospital or at home at bed rest until the chances of delivering a viable infant improve. If bleeding stops, it is likely that it will start again.

Baum SE: Coagulation disorders in pregnancy: Pathophysiology and treatment. J Am Osteopath A 71:1055, 1972.

Cohen WN & others: Correlation of ultrasound and radioisotope placentography. Am J Roentgenol 116:843, 1972.

Czapek EE: Coagulation problems. Internat Anesth Clin 11:175, 1973.

Kawathekar P & others: Etiology and trends in the management of transverse lie. Am J Obst Gynec 117:39, 1973.

Lunan CB: The management of abruptio placentae. J Obstet Gynaec Brit Common 80:120, 1973.

Moss ML, Freeman LM: Scintiphotographic diagnosis of abruptio placentae. J Nuclear Med 14:297, 1973.

Naftolin F & others: The syndrome of chronic abruptio placentae, hydrorrhea, and circumvallate placenta. Am J Obst Gynec 116:347, 1973.

Scheer K: Ultrasonic diagnosis of placenta previa. Obst Gynec 42:707, 1973.

Schlesinger ER & others: The impact of placenta previa on survivorship of offspring to four years of age. Am J Obst Gynec 116:657, 1973.

Varma TR: Fetal growth and placental function in patients with placenta previa. J Obstet Gynaec Brit Common 80:311, 1973.

POSTPARTUM HEMORRHAGE

Postpartum hemorrhage has been defined arbitrarily as the loss of at least 500 ml of blood following delivery. However, since a small woman can lose blood less safely than a large one, it is felt that the loss of 1% or more of body weight (expressed in terms of ml of blood) would be a more proper definition. Postpartum hemorrhage is the major cause of maternal mortality in the USA.

The most common causes are uterine atony, lacerations during delivery, and blood dyscrasias or coagulation defects.

Prevention

The following types of patients are especially prone to develop postpartum bleeding: women with multiple pregnancies, polyhydramnios, a history of postpartum hemorrhage, primary or secondary uterine inertia, desultory or prolonged labor, uterine infections, placenta previa, abruptio placentae, after heavy analgesia or anesthesia, and those who are delivered by cesarean section. Measures to prevent postpartum bleeding in these patients are as follows:

(1) Start 500 ml of 5% glucose in water slowly IV through a No. 18 needle near the end of the first stage of labor.

(2) Immediately after delivery, add 0.5 ml oxytocin (Pitocin) to the infusion (not into the tubing).

(3) On completion of the third stage of labor, give ergonovine maleate (Ergotrate), 0.2 mg IM. Avoid giving excessive amounts of analgesics and anesthesia.

(4) Maneuver the uterus up and out of the pelvis and, by raising it with a large sponge on a forceps in the vagina, massage it gently until it becomes firm and remains so.

(5) Keep the patient in the delivery room or recovery room for 1 hour after delivery.

Treatment

A. Emergency Measures: Control bleeding promptly by suture, manual recovery or expression of the placenta, or intravenous oxytocin (Pitocin) as indicated. Packing of the uterus (and vagina) controls bleeding by the pressure applied to bleeding points and because packing stimulates uterine contractions. However, packing must be used with discretion for the following reasons: (1) The uterus relaxes slowly and bleeding often recurs, even when packing is very tight. (2) Tight packing may actually prevent uterine contractions. (3) If packing fails to check bleeding, further blood loss may make a necessary hysterectomy even more hazardous. (4) The risk of infection is greater with packing than when other methods of hemostasis are used.

B. General Measures: Reinspect the placenta for missing fragments. Examine for lacerations of the birth canal. Note the quality of contractions of the elevated uterus, determine bleeding and clotting time, and obtain typed and cross-matched blood for transfusion.

Prognosis

The mortality rate in postpartum hemorrhage depends upon the amount and rapidity of blood loss, the patient's general health, and the speed and adequacy of treatment.

Fox H: Placenta accreta 1945—1969. Obst Gynec Surv 27:475, 1972.

Hammond H: Death from obstetrical hemorrhage. California Med 117:16, Aug 1972.

Loring TW: Pregnancy and uterine malformations: A report of 2 unusual cases (including retained placenta). Am J Obst Gynec 116:505, 1973.

O'Leary JL, O'Leary JA: Uterine artery ligation for control of postcesarean section hemorrhage. Obst Gynec 43:849, 1974.

Paydar M, Ostooarzadeh M: Late postpartum hemorrhage. Internat J Gynaec Obstet 12:141, 1974.

Volenson DA, Beard RJ: A lost placenta: An unusual presentation of uterine rupture in labor. J Obstet Gynaec Brit Common 79:860, 1972.

HIGH-RISK PREGNANCY

A high-risk pregnancy is one in which the mother or fetus has a significantly increased chance of death—either before, during, or after birth—or of later disability. The infant may be jeopardized by maternal dysfunction or disease and by fetal problems, including genetic, traumatic, infectious, toxic, or respiratory disorders. Hazard may also develop from the treatment of maternal or perinatal complications.

The scope of the problem of high-risk pregnancy is enormous. The mother may die during pregnancy, labor, delivery, or the puerperium from hemorrhage, toxemia, infection, heart disease, or respiratory problems. In other cases, the woman may sustain serious sequelae (eg, cerebrovascular accident during eclampsia; bacteremic shock from puerperal sepsis). Most newborns who die during the first 4 weeks of life are of low birth weight. The death rate for these individuals is 40 times that of the full-sized term newborn. The incidence of cerebral palsy associated with prematurity is 10 times, mental deficiency 5 times, and serious malformations 7 times that of the average term infant. Visual and hearing defects, emotional disorders, and social problems are far greater for the person who was undergrown at birth.

Diagnostic Evaluation

At least 20% of all women fall into the groupings shown in the box opposite. These women account for over 50% of all perinatal deaths. Most perinatal deaths are associated with 6 obstetric complications: breech presentation, premature separation of the placenta, toxemia of pregnancy, multiple pregnancy, pyelonephritis, and hydramnios. Exposure to teratogens (drugs, viral diseases, irradiation, etc) may also complicate pregnancy. Ignorance, poverty, unwanted pregnancy, and irresponsible parenthood add a considerable additional burden to the pregnancy outcome.

A. Initial Screening: Initial screening of the gravida must include the following:

1. A complete general physical examination (including height, weight, development, etc) and diagnosis of systemic disease, dysfunction, or abnormality.

High-Risk Obstetric Categories
(Modified after Wigglesworth, 1968)

History of Any of the Following:

Hereditary abnormality (osteogenesis imperfecta, Down's syndrome, etc).

Premature or small-for-dates neonate (most recent delivery).

Congenital anomaly, anemia, blood dyscrasia, toxemia, etc.

Severe social problem (teen-age pregnancy, drug addiction, alcoholism, etc).

Long-delayed or absent prenatal care.

Age < 18 or > 35 years.

Teratogenic viral illness or dangerous drug administration in the first trimester.

A 5th or subsequent pregnancy, especially when the gravida is > 35 years of age.

Prolonged infertility or essential drug or hormone treatment.

Significant stressful or dangerous events in the present pregnancy (critical accident, excessive exposure to irradiation, etc).

Heavy cigarette smoking.

Pregnancy within 2 months of a previous delivery.

Diagnosis of Any of the Following:

Height under 60 inches or a prepregnant weight of 20% less than or over the standard for height and age.

Minimal or no weight gain.

Obstetric complications (toxemia, multiple pregnancy, hydramnios, etc).

Abnormal presentation (breech, presenting part unengaged at term, etc).

A fetus that fails to grow normally or is disparate in size from that expected.

A fetus > 42 weeks gestation.

---

2. Careful abdominopelvic evaluation with special reference to the following:

a. Uterus—Configuration, size, fundal height, patient girth, fetal size (estimate), fetal presentation, position, engagement, amount of amniotic fluid.

b. Cervix—Position, epithelialization, effacement, dilatation.

c. Spine, pelvis, and extremities—Abnormalities, measurement of pelvic diameters.

3. Laboratory tests—Hematocrit, urinalysis, urine culture, STS, rubella and antibody screening, blood type, Rh determination, vaginal cytology for infection, hormone status, and malignant elements. Special studies may be required for particular problems (eg, glucose tolerance test in diabetes mellitus).

B. Antenatal Visits: Antenatal visits should be more frequent for high-risk than for normal obstetric patients. This allows for more accurate appraisal of the course of the pregnancy and identification and correction of problems (eg, anemia, urinary tract infection). Obstetric disorders which may require special treatment or decision (eg, toxemia of pregnancy, uterine bleeding) must be identified early. Visits also provide the opportunity for education about hygiene, nutrition, use of drugs, and care of the newborn and for psychiatric counseling.

C. Assessment of Fetal Growth, Maturity, and Well-Being:

1. Indirect (noninvasive) methods—

a. Recalculation of gestational age of the fetus (LMP, BBT, date of quickening, first FHT).

b. Growth of uterus (fundal height, patient's girth).

c. Engagement.

d. Roentgenography (ossification centers, anomalies).

e. Sonography (fetal biparietal diameter), amnioscopy.

2. Direct (invasive) methods—

a. Amniocentesis (amniotic fluid volume, enzyme studies, osmolality, optical density, creatinine content, bilirubin concentration, lecithin-sphingomyelin ratio, percentage of fat-laden cells), urinary estriol or total estrogen.

b. Amniography (anomaly, placental situation).

c. Cytology of amniotic fluid cells (culture, cytochemistry, chromosome studies, etc to determine heritable disorders in the fetus).

Differential Diagnosis

A "large" uterus for dates may indicate multiple pregnancy, hydramnios, or uterine tumors. A uterus that is smaller than expected from the LMP may signify dysmaturity of the fetus (placental insufficiency), oligohydramnios, incorrect estimation of the duration of pregnancy, or fetal disease (eg, rubella, cytomegalic inclusion disease) or anomaly.

Treatment

Maternal disease must be treated cautiously to avoid harm to the fetus. Fetal perinatal mortality and morbidity can sometimes be reduced by extension of gestation—eg, in the case of premature labor, multiple pregnancy, placenta previa, cervical incompetence, slight premature separation of the placenta, or thyroid dysfunction. Judicious early delivery may be necessary to rescue the fetus if the membranes rupture before 34 weeks or in the case of toxemia of pregnancy, severe isoimmunization, clinical diabetes mellitus, persistent urinary tract infection, considerable hydramnios, or placental insufficiency.

The reader should consult the references listed below for the diagnosis and treatment of obstetric problems, the course and conduct of labor, and perinatal complications and their therapy.

Prognosis

Although improved obstetric care has reduced the maternal mortality rate in the USA from 660 per 100,000 births in 1930 to 27 per 100,000 in 1970, two-thirds to three-fourths of the latter were still probably preventable. Some investigators feel that less rigid dietary restriction for weight control in pregnancy could further reduce the infant mortality rate. Moreover, the present perinatal mortality rate in this country is about 30 per 100,000 births, and at least one-third to one-half of these losses could have been avoided. Socioeconomic factors undoubtedly play a role. The vast majority of maternal and perinatal deaths are in the high-risk category.

Barham K: Amnioscopy, amniotomy: A look at surgical induction of labor. Am J Obst Gynec 117:35, 1973.

Brackbill Y & others: Obstetric premedication and infant outcome. Am J Obst Gynec 118:377, 1974.

Burton BK & others: Present status of intrauterine diagnosis of genetic defects. Am J Obst Gynec 118:718, 1974.

Dawes G: The distribution and action of drugs on foetus in utero. Brit J Anaesth 45:766, 1973.

Gabert HA, Stenchever MA: Electronic fetal monitoring in association with paracervical block. Am J Obst Gynec 116:1143, 1973.

Gabert HA, Stenchever MA: Electronic fetal monitoring as a routine practive in an obstetric service: A progress report. Am J Obst Gynec 118:534, 1974.

Goldstein AS & others: A comparison of the lecithin/sphingomyelin ratio and shake test for estimating fetal pulmonary maturity. Am J Obst Gynec 118:1132, 1974.

Hobel CJ & others: Prenatal and intrapartum high-risk screening. 1. Prediction of high-risk neonate. Am J Obst Gynec 117:1, 1973.

Hon EH: The present status of electronic monitoring of the human fetal heart. Internat J Gynec Obst 10:191, 1972.

Lipshaw LA & others: A rapid method of measuring the lecithin-sphingomyelin ratio in amniotic fluid. Obst Gynec 42:93, 1973.

Low JA, Galbraith RS: Pregnancy characteristics of intrauterine growth retardation. Obst Gynec 44:122, 1974.

Lubs MLE: Racial differences in maternal smoking effects on the newborn infant. Am J Obst Gynec 115:66, 1973.

Mandelbaum B: Gestational meconium in the high-risk pregnancy. Obst Gynec 42:87, 1973.

Masson GM: Plasma estriol in retarded intrauterine fetal growth. J Obstet Gynaec Brit Common 80:423, 1973.

Paul RH: Intrapartum fetal monitoring: Current status and future. Obst Gynec 28:453, 1973.

Persianinov LS: The effect of normal and abnormal labor of the fetus: A survey. Acta obst gynec scandinav 52:29, 1973.

Prenatal care: Which drugs for the pregnant patient? (Editorial.) Patient Care 8:54, March 1, 1974.

Rothbard M & others: The foam test as a prognosticator of fetal pulmonary maturity. Am J Obst Gynec 119:924, 1974.

Walker PA: Drugs used in labour: An obstetrician's view. Brit J Anaesth 45:787, 1973.

Ward H & others: Hormone and enzyme levels in normal and complicated pregnancy. Am J Obst Gynec 116:1105, 1973.

MEDICAL CONDITIONS
COMPLICATING PREGNANCY

Diabetes Mellitus

Changes in carbohydrate and fat metabolism and increased clearance of glucose complicate the management of diabetes in the pregnant woman. The prevention of common hazards of diabetes, such as hypoglycemia, ketosis, and diabetic coma, requires greater effort and attention to detail on the part of both the physician and the patient. Although pregnancy does not appear to alter the ultimate severity of diabetes, retinopathy and nephropathy may appear or become worse during pregnancy.

Even in carefully managed diabetics, the incidence of obstetric complications such as hydramnios, toxemia, infections, and prematurity are increased. The infants are larger than those of nondiabetic women. There is a marked increase in unexplained fetal mortality in the last few weeks of pregnancy as well as a high rate of neonatal deaths.

Optimal care requires cooperative management of the patient and offspring (by internist, obstetrician, and pediatrician) and delivery 2—4 weeks before term. Under these circumstances, maternal mortality is not significantly higher than in the nondiabetic. However, the fetal and neonatal mortality remains about 10—20%.

Bates GW: Management of gestational diabetes. Postgrad Med 55:55, 1974.

Fisher PM & others: The effect of pregnancy on intravenous glucose tolerance. J Obstet Gynaec Brit Common 81:285, 1974.

Gaither D, Clark JFJ: Pregnancy and latent diabetes. J Nat Med A 65:139, 1973.

Khojandi M & others: Gestational diabetes: The dilemma of delivery. Obst Gynec 43:1, 1974.

O'Sullivan JG & others: Medical treatment of the gestational diabetic. Obst Gynec 43:817, 1974.

Pedersen J, Molsted-Pedersen L, Andersen B: Assessors of fetal perinatal mortality in diabetic pregnancy: Analysis of 1332 pregnancies in the Copenhagen series, 1946—1972. Diabetes 23:302, 1974.

Pedersen J & others: Perinatal fetal mortality in 1245 diabetic pregnancies: Secular trends 1946—1971 and variations according to the White and PBSP classifications. Acta chir scandinav (Suppl) 433:191, 1973.

Spellacy WN & others: Usefulness of rapid blood glucose measurements in obstetrics: Dextrostix/reflectance meter system. Obst Gynec 41:299, 1973.

Ursell W & others: Placental lactogen levels in diabetic pregnancy. Brit MJ 2:80, 1973.

Glomerulonephritis Complicating Pregnancy

The initial attack of acute glomerulonephritis rarely occurs during pregnancy; most obstetric problems relating to glomerulonephritis involve transitional chronic forms of the disease.

Pregnancy does not aggravate glomerulonephritis, although infertility, abortion, premature delivery, fetal death in utero, premature separation of the normally implanted placenta, and placental dysmaturity occur with greater frequency in women with glomerulonephritis than in normal women. Nephritis causes hypertension, predisposes to eclamptogenic toxemia, and is associated with a high incidence of perinatal mortality and morbidity.

The medical treatment of glomerulonephritis is discussed in Chapter 15. Therapeutic abortion may be justified for acute, severe exacerbation of glomerulonephritis with renal insufficiency. Glomerulonephritis may be an indication for cesarean section when placental dysmaturity or eclamptogenic toxemia occurs.

Fairbanks WL, Loomis GW: Nephrotic syndrome in pregnancy. Nebraska MJ 57:432, 1972.

Weisman SA & others: Nephrotic syndrome in pregnancy. Am J Obst Gynec 117:867, 1973.

Tuberculosis

Tuberculosis of the bronchi, lungs, and pleura is not directly affected by pregnancy, but urologic tuberculosis may be. A pregnant patient with tuberculosis is slightly more prone to spontaneous abortion and premature delivery than other women. Tuberculous endometritis and placentitis occur in advanced cases, but congenital tuberculosis is rare. Interruption of pregnancy because of pulmonary tuberculosis is almost never justified on medical grounds since the advent of antituberculosis drugs. Babies born of tuberculous mothers are no more likely to develop the disease than others provided they are separated from the infected mother and unfavorable environment at birth.

Elwood JH: Infant mortality in Belfast and Dublin: 1900—1969 (including tuberculosis). Irish J Med Sc 142:166, 1973.

Maheswaran C, Nenwirth RS: An unusual case of postpartum fever: Acute hematogenous tuberculosis. Obst Gynec 41:765, 1973.

Wilson EA & others: Tuberculosis complicating pregnancy. Am J Obst Gynec 115:526, 1973.

Heart Disease Complicating Pregnancy

About 5% of maternal deaths are due to heart disease. Pregnancy causes a significant increase in pulse rate, an increase of cardiac output of more than 30%, a rise in plasma and blood volume, and expansion of the red cell mass. Both vital capacity and oxygen consumption rise only slightly during pregnancy.

Over 90% of cases of heart disease complicating pregnancy in the USA are of rheumatic origin, and three-fourths of these patients have mitral stenosis. Congenital heart disease constitutes an obstetric problem in fewer than 5% of cardiac patients.

The physical stress of labor, delivery, and the puerperium imposes moderate to extreme burdens on the maternal heart. These increase to a peak at about 28—32 weeks, when maximal cardiac strain must be anticipated.

In general, patients with class I or class II functional disability (80% of pregnant women with heart disease) do well obstetrically. Over 80% of maternal deaths due to heart disease occur in women with class III or IV cardiac disability. Congestive failure is the usual cause of death. Three-fourths of these deaths occur in the early puerperium. The perinatal fetal death rate is greatly increased when the mother is a class III–IV cardiac.

Therapeutic abortion may be justified in certain cases of pregnancy associated with class III–IV cardiac disease. Cesarean section should be performed only upon obstetric indications. The indications for sterilization should be liberalized for women with class III–IV heart disease not amenable to surgery.

Cabaniss CD: Management of heart disease in pregnancy. J Reprod Med 8:51, 1972.

Hillstad L: Aortic coarctation and pregnancy. Acta obst gynec scandinav 51:95, 1972.

Ibarra-Perez C, Del Bosque-Ruiz M: Pregnancy in 6 patients with Starr-Edwards heart prostheses. Am J Cardiol 30:565, 1972.

Kitchen DH: Dissecting aneurysm of the aorta in pregnancy. J Obstet Gynaec Brit Common 81:410, 1974.

Lee YK: Complete heart block in pregnancy. Ann Acad Med Singapore 2:14, 1973.

Lewis JP: Myocardial infarction during pregnancy, with associated myocardial bacteroides abscess. South MJ 66:379, 1973.

Messer JV: Heart disease in pregnancy. J Reprod Med 10:102, 1973.

Szekely P & others: Pregnancy and the changing pattern of rheumatic heart disease. Brit Heart J 35:1293, 1973.

Ueland K & others: Hemodynamic response of patients with heart disease to pregnancy and exercise. Am J Obst Gynec 113:47, 1972.

Wilber JA: The management of hypertension during pregnancy. J Reprod Med 8:53, 1972.

Urinary Tract Infection During Pregnancy

The urinary tract is especially vulnerable to infections during pregnancy because the altered secretions of steroid sex hormones and the pressure exerted by the gravid uterus upon the ureters and bladder cause hypotonia and congestion and predispose to urinary stasis. Cervicitis and vaginitis also predispose to urinary infection. The trauma of labor and delivery and urinary retention postpartum may initiate or aggravate infection in the urinary system. *Escherichia coli* is an offending organism in over two-thirds of cases.

Almost 10% of pregnant women suffer from urinary tract infection. Chronic pyelonephritis, a major cause of death in older women, often follows recurrent acute urinary tract infections during successive pregnancies. Urinary tract infection increases the likelihood of premature delivery and the incidence of perinatal mortality.

The diagnosis should be based on stained smear and culture of a catheterized or clean-catch specimen of urine. Bacillary infection should be treated initially with sulfisoxazole, 2 gm orally and then 1 gm 4 times daily, or nitrofurantoin (Furadantin), 75 mg orally 4 times daily. If cocci are present, give penicillin G, 1 million units IM and then 600,000 units IM twice daily. Mixed infections should be treated with strepto-

mycin, 1 gm IM, and penicillin G, 600,000 units IM, and then 0.5 gm of streptomycin and 600,000 units of penicillin twice daily. Change to other drugs as dictated by the results of laboratory studies.

In late pregnancy, the treatment of urinary tract infections with certain drugs (eg, sulfonamides, tetracyclines, streptomycin) may be harmful, and unless the infection is critical, treatment may be best deferred in the last few weeks of pregnancy.

Force fluids and alkalinize the urine. Give analgesics, laxatives, and antipyretic drugs as indicated.

Bobeck S, Schasten B: Detection and diagnosis of bacteriuria in pregnancy: A study from general practice. Practitioner 212:257, 1974.

Harkins JL & others: Acute renal failure in obstetrics. Am J Obst Gynec 118:331, 1974.

McFadyen IR & others: Bacteriuria in pregnancy. 1. Prevalence and natural history. J Obstet Gynaec Brit Common 80:385, 1973.

Simpson JW & others: Transvaginal aspiration of bladder in screening for bacteriuria. Obst Gynec 43:215, 1974.

Syphilis & Gonorrhea

Untreated syphilis acquired shortly before conception usually causes midtrimester abortion or fetal death in utero, and the fetus almost invariably bears the stigmas of syphilis. Syphilis contracted at conception often results in the premature delivery of an infant with congenital syphilis. If syphilis is acquired late in pregnancy, the infant may or may not have the disease at birth. Syphilis contracted in early pregnancy responds in a manner similar to syphilis contracted in late pregnancy but untreated; premature delivery of an infant with congenital syphilis is to be expected. Syphilis contracted during mid pregnancy often results in congenital syphilis in the infant. (See Chapter 24.)

Gonorrhea now is one of the most common infectious diseases in the USA. It must be diagnosed and treated successfully before delivery because gonococcal ophthalmia in neonates may occur even in babies who supposedly received silver nitrate drops in the conjunctival sacs immediately after birth.

False-positive (and false-negative) serologic tests for syphilis are not uncommon. Intensive treatment with penicillin or, in the case of penicillin sensitivity, other antisyphilitic drugs is indicated whenever syphilis is proved or presumed to be present. The possibility that other venereal diseases may be present also must always be considered in any patient with syphilis.

Asoba AO, Onifade A: Venereal disease among pregnant women in Nigeria. West African MJ 22:23, 1973.

Bellingham FR: Syphilis in pregnancy: Transplacental infection. MJ Australia 2:647, 1973.

Brown D: Gonococcal arthritis in pregnancy. South MJ 66:693, 1973.

Caldwell JG: Masking of syphilis. [Leading article.] Brit MJ 3:206, 1971.

Hare MJ: Serological tests for treponemal disease in pregnancy. J Obstet Gynaec Brit Common 80:515, 1973.

Monif GRG: The problem of maternal syphilis after serologic surveillance during pregnancy. Am J Obst Gynec 117:268, 1973.

Notelovitz M: The antenatal detection of asymptomatic disease. South African MJ 48:178, 1974.

Schofield CBS: Serological tests for syphilis in pregnancy: False and missed positive reactions. Brit J Ven Dis 49:420, 1973.

Herpes Genitalis*

Infection of the lower genital tract by herpesvirus type II is a venereal disease of increasing frequency and seriousness. The incidence varies greatly but may be 1:750 in gynecologic clinic patients and twice this frequency in obstetric patients of comparable lower socioeconomic status. This is many times the frequency of occurrence in private patients, whose hygiene is far better. This incidence probably exceeds that of syphilis and is approaching that of gonorrhea in some social groups.

Herpesvirus type II is associated with later cervical dysplasia and may be a carcinogenic agent. Necrotizing cervicitis due to herpesvirus may even resemble a stage 2 squamous cell carcinoma. The infection during pregnancy is responsible for higher incidence of spontaneous abortion, stillbirth, and neonatal death.

Patients with this infection complain of fever, malaise, anorexia, local genital pain, leukorrhea, dysuria, and even vaginal bleeding. Typical genital lesions are multiple, shallow ulcerations, vesicles, and erythematous papules. Painful bilateral inguinal adenopathy is usually present. Scrapings and biopsies may reveal a characteristic homogenous "ground glass" appearance of cellular nuclei with numerous small intranuclear vacuoles, small scattered basophilic particles, and acidophilic inclusion bodies. Cultures may reveal type II; serum antibodies to this virus may be expected in well-established cases.

Local analgesic ointments, eg, 2% lidocaine, may limit severe pain, especially during vesiculation and ulceration. One must avoid sensitization. Hence, treatment for less than 2 weeks is suggested. Topical or systemic corticosteroids are not helpful in vulvovaginal herpes. Douching is not recommended because this may induce spread of the lesions.

Genital herpes is especially susceptible to secondary infection by *Candida albicans.* Nystatin vaginal suppositories may be used prophylactically or therapeutically for this associated problem. Gonorrhea and syphilis must be excluded.

Genital herpes during pregnancy is especially devastating to the fetus. The overall risk to the offspring after 32 weeks is about 10%. When herpes genitalis is present at delivery, the neonate will be affected in over 40% of cases unless elective cesarean section can be undertaken less than 4 hours after rupture of the membranes. Even then, cesarean section is no guarantee that fetal infection will not occur. If the mature fetus contracts the disorder, his serum IgM

*See also discussion on p 51 for recent advances in treatment.

generally will be elevated. The fetus or neonate who contracts the disease probably will die of viremia. Only supportive therapy is available. Strict isolation of the mother and fetus is mandatory. Contraception and long-term follow-up studies for possible cervical neoplasia should be arranged.

Anderson FD & others: Recurrent herpes genitalis: Treatment with *Mycobacterium bovis* (BCG). Obst Gynec 43:797, 1974.

Friedrich EG Jr: Relief of herpes vulvitis. Obst Gynec 41:74, 1973.

Hurley R: Contemporary obstetrics and gynecology: Viral diseases in pregnancy. Brit J Hosp Med 12:86, 1974.

Roberts JK: A case of genital herpesvirus infection in pregnancy. J Obstet Gynaec Brit Common 80:188, 1973.

Shevach A: Concomitant herpetic vulvovaginitis in mother and child due to *Herpesvirus hominis* type T. J Florida MA 60:26, 1973.

Smith RN, Hanna L: Herpesvirus infections in pregnancy: A comparison of neutralizing antibody titers in mothers and their infants. Am J Obst Gynec 119:314, 1974.

Thyrotoxicosis

Toxic goiter is not common during pregnancy, but it often develops soon after delivery and may have serious consequences. Thyrotoxicosis during pregnancy may result in fetal maldevelopment and goiter.

Radioactive isotope therapy may cause athyreosis in the fetus and therefore must never be given during pregnancy. Antithyroid drugs may be given cautiously, but hypothyroidism must be avoided at all costs to ensure normal fetal development. Elective thyroidectomy following preparation with iodine is recommended by some clinicians in preference to medical management during and after pregnancy.

Ayromlovi J & others: Thyrotoxicosis in pregnancy. Am J Obst Gynec 117:818, 1973.

Chew PCT & others: Hyperthyroidism in pregnancy: A study of 37 pregnancies in 34 patients. Singapore MJ 14:95, 1973.

Emslander RF & others: Hyperthyroidism and pregnancy. M Clin North America 58:835, 1974.

Goluboff LG & others: Hyperthyroidism associated with pregnancy. Obst Gynec 44:107, 1974.

Worley RJ, Crosby WM: Hyperthyroidism during pregnancy. Am J Obst Gynec 119:150, 1974.

Parathyroid Dysfunction & Tetany

Pregnancy normally causes a slight (secondary) hyperparathyroidism. Severe, chronic hyperparathyroidism causing osteitis fibrosa cystica is rare during pregnancy except in patients with long-standing renal disease. The most serious problems relating to parathyroid dysfunction during pregnancy are hypoparathyroid tetany and muscle cramps. Tetany is usually associated with a deficiency of calcium or excess of phosphate (eg, due to intake of calcium phosphate prenatal capsules), or lack of vitamin D and parathormone. It may follow infection or the hypocalcemia which sometimes occurs during lactation, or may be seen during the latter months of pregnancy if calcium supplements are inadequate. Hyperventilation during labor may precipitate tetany. Tetany of the newborn is unusual in breast-fed infants, but it may occur transiently if phosphate intake is excessive (eg, if too much cow's milk is given or as a result of relative hypoparathyroidism in the neonatal period).

Cushard WG Jr & others: Physiologic hyperparathyroidism in pregnancy. J Clin Endocrinol 34:767, 1972.
Johnstone RE & others: Hyperparathyroidism during pregnancy. Obst Gynec 40:580, 1972.

The Exanthematous Diseases

Maternal mortality is increased in smallpox and severe epidemic chickenpox. The effects of these viral diseases on the pregnant woman and on the fetus depend upon the virulence of the strain and the degree of the mother's immunity to the disease. High fever, toxicosis, and fetal viremia may result in death of the fetus.

Infants born of women with smallpox, measles, or chickenpox may have the disease at birth, but congenital malformations are rarely present. Congenital anomalies occur in up to 50% of infants born to women who contract sporadic rubella during the first trimester. Gamma globulin will not prevent deformity even if it is given to exposed women before the rash appears. Congenital disorders may result, however, even if the disease never becomes clinically apparent and gamma globulin is given.

Bolognese RJ & others: Evaluation of possible transplacental infection with vaccination during pregnancy. Am J Obst Gynec 117:939, 1973.
Fleet WF Jr & others: Fetal consequences of maternal rubella immunization. JAMA 227:621, 1974.
Giles PFH: Rubella and the obstetrician: A review of recent advances. Australian New Zealand J Obstet Gynaec 13:77, 1973.
Mair HJ, Buchan AR: Rubella vaccination and termination of pregnancy. Brit MJ 4:271, 1972.
Northrop RL & others: Rubella reinfection during early pregnancy. Obst Gynec 39:524, 1972.
Rekant SI: Eczema herpeticum and pregnancy. Obst Gynec 41:387, 1972.
Siegal M: Congenital malformations following chicken pox, measles, mumps and hepatitis. JAMA 226:1521, 1973.

SURGICAL COMPLICATIONS DURING PREGNANCY

Elective major surgery should be avoided during pregnancy. However, normal, uncomplicated pregnancy has no debilitating effect and does not alter operative risk except as it may interfere with the diagnosis of abdominal disorders and increase the technical problems of intra-abdominal surgery. Abortion is not a serious hazard after operation unless peritoneal sepsis or other significant complication occurs.

During the first trimester, congenital anomalies may be induced in the developing fetus by hypoxia. It is preferable to avoid surgical intervention during this period; if surgery does become necessary, the greatest precautions must be taken to prevent hypoxia and hypotension.

The second trimester is usually the optimum time for operative procedures.

Wilson F, Schwartz DP: Gunshot and war projectile wounds of the gravid uterus: Case report and review of the literature. J Nat Med A 64:8, 1972.

Ovarian Tumors in Pregnancy

Ovarian tumors in pregnancy are important because of (1) delay in diagnosis and palliation of possible malignant neoplasm; (2) obstruction of the birth canal by the tumor; and (3) the possibility of rupture and chemical peritonitis or intraperitoneal spread of tumor. Tumors with a high malignancy potential include the serous and pseudomucinous cystadenomas, which often are bilateral and large. Teratoid tumors may involve both ovaries, and when they rupture they may cause serious irritation and obstruction. Pelvic examination done early and repeated later in pregnancy may reveal discrete adnexal masses. If these are persistent, greater than 6 cm in diameter, and increasing in size or bilateral, laparotomy is indicated despite an advancing pregnancy.

White KC: Ovarian tumors in pregnancy: A private hospital 10-year survey. Am J Obst Gynec 116:544, 1973.

Colon & Rectal Carcinoma

Pregnancy increases the likelihood of spread of carcinoma of the colon or rectum. Malignant tumors of the lower bowel are often neglected or palliated during pregnancy with tragic results. The prognosis is extremely poor for the pregnant carcinoma patient unless prompt radical surgery is possible.

The symptoms of rectal and colon carcinoma include constipation of increasing severity, often alternating with transient diarrhea, and rectal bleeding or blood-streaked stools. Anemia and weight loss are late signs.

In almost two-thirds of cases of carcinoma of the colon and rectum, the lesion can be reached by the examining finger and biopsied through the sigmoidoscope even during pregnancy. Barium x-ray studies may reveal the site and extent of the lesion.

The treatment of apparently curable carcinoma of the rectum and colon during pregnancy depends upon the duration of the pregnancy at the time of the diagnosis as well as the extent of the malignancy.

(1) **Four to 20 weeks:** Radical resection and colostomy via the abdominoperineal approach is indicated, avoiding the pregnant uterus. In the absence of obstetric contraindications, vaginal delivery at term should be permitted.

(2) **Twenty-one to 28 weeks:** Sacrifice the pregnancy by hysterectomy and then do an abdominoperineal resection and colostomy.

(3) After the 28th week: Cesarean section should be done as soon as fetal viability seems likely. Resect the cancerous bowel and construct a colostomy 3—4 weeks after delivery.

For the incurable patient, cesarean section is indicated as soon as the fetus is viable. Palliative resection should be done at delivery or afterward to prevent intestinal obstruction.

Lea AW: Pregnancy following rectal operation for rectal carcinoma. Am J Obst Gynec 113:504, 1972.

Carcinoma of the Breast

Cancer of the breast is diagnosed approximately once in 3500 pregnancies and accounts for about 2.5% of breast cancers in women. Pregnancy accelerates the growth of cancer of the breast. Inflammatory carcinoma is an extremely serious type of breast cancer which occurs most commonly during lactation in young, obese women with pendulous breasts.

If breast biopsy confirms the diagnosis of cancer, radical mastectomy should be done regardless of the stage of the pregnancy. (An exception is inflammatory carcinoma, which invariably is far-advanced when correctly diagnosed. Surgery or irradiation will not benefit such a patient, for whom the prospect is hopeless.) If spread to the regional glands has occurred, x-ray therapy should be given also. Therapeutic abortion or interruption of pregnancy is usually of no value. Cesarean section should be performed only upon obstetric indications. After delivery, oophorectomy, adrenalectomy, and hypophysectomy may be considered for palliation of advanced breast cancer.

The 5-year survival rate in patients with stage I cancer of the breast diagnosed during pregnancy and treated by radical surgery is 60—70%; with stage II breast cancer, the survival rate drops to less than 10% even with radical surgery and x-ray therapy.

Birks DM & others: Carcinoma of the breast in women 30 years of age or less. Surg Gynec Obst 137:21, 1973.
Helman P & others: Interim report on trial of treatment of operable breast cancer. South African MJ 46:1374, 1972.
Lynch GA: Breast cancer associated with pregnancy. Ulster MJ 38:34, 1969.
Zeigerman JH & others: Inflammatory mammary cancer during pregnancy and lactation. Obst Gynec 32:373, 1968.

Choledocholithiasis & Cholecystitis

Severe choledocholithiasis and cholecystitis are not common during pregnancy despite the fact that women tend to form gallstones (one-third of all women over 40 have gallstones). When they do occur, it is usually in late pregnancy or in the puerperium. About 90% of patients with cholecystitis have gallstones.

Symptomatic relief may be all that is required. Meperidine and atropine are effective in alleviating pain and ductal spasm. Morphine is contraindicated in cholelithiasis or cholecystitis because it may induce spasm of the sphincter of Oddi.

Gallbladder surgery in pregnant women should be attempted only in extreme cases (eg, obstruction) because it greatly increases the fetal mortality rate (up to about 15%). Cholecystostomy and lithotomy may be all that is feasible during advanced pregnancy, deferring cholecystectomy until after delivery. On the other hand, withholding surgery when it is definitely needed may result in necrosis and perforation of the gallbladder and peritonitis. Intermittent high fever, jaundice, and right upper quadrant pain may indicate cholangitis due to impacted common duct stone. Surgical removal of gallstones and establishment of biliary drainage are essential in such cases.

Therapeutic abortion or early delivery (by induction or cesarean section) is not warranted.

Friley MD, Douglas G: Acute cholecystitis in pregnancy and the puerperium. Am Surg 38:314, 1972.

Ileus

Adynamic (paralytic) ileus is the result of diminished or absent contractility of the bowel and causes intestinal obstruction. Ileus is rare before delivery, but moderate ileus is common in the postpartum period, especially after cesarean section. Obstetric complications such as peritonitis, renal or ureteral stone, or torsion of the adnexa and bladder atony may be associated with adynamic ileus.

A "silent" bowel is indicative of reduced or absent peristalsis. Abdominal tenderness and pain are present. A "laddering" effect of gas in the bowel segments in the small and large intestine on x-ray films supports the diagnosis of adynamic ileus.

It is essential to differentiate paralytic ileus from ileus due to mechanical obstruction. In the latter form, the bowel is hyperactive and x-rays reveal distention of the intestine proximal to the obstruction.

The treatment of paralytic ileus is discussed in Chapter 10. Ileus due to mechanical obstruction usually requires surgery.

Hudson CN: Ileostomy in pregnancy. Proc Roy Soc Med 65:281, 1972.
McCorriston CC: Non-obstetrical abdominal surgery required during pregnancy. J Abdom Surg 15:85, 1973.
See also reference under Hernia, below.

Hernia

Pregnancy gives temporary protection from umbilical, incisional, and often inguinal hernias even though it widens the hernial rings. The enlarging uterus displaces the intestines, so that the bowel will usually not enter a defect in the body wall. Many abdominal hernias are reduced spontaneously during pregnancy; a few irreducible ones may result in obstruction of the involved intestine. After delivery, hernia again becomes a hazard, but the chance of incarceration is not increased.

Incarcerated hernias must be reduced surgically during pregnancy if severe pain or obstruction develops. Elective herniorrhaphy should be deferred until after delivery. The necessity for repair of hernias is not an indication for cesarean section. Women with abdominal hernias should be delivered by the low forceps technic to prevent straining before and during labor.

Goldstein AI & others: Strangulated diaphragmatic hernia in pregnancy presenting as empyema. J Reprod Med 9:135, 1972.

Ureteral Stone

Ureteral stone is more common during pregnancy than otherwise because of the dilatation of the renal pelvis and ureter which occurs in response to high titers of steroid sex hormones and the minor (physiologic) obstructive uropathy characteristic of pregnancy. Small stones, previously retained, are thus permitted to enter the proximal ureter. Most ureteral stones are passed in the urine, albeit painfully; others become impacted. Sudden, agonizing pain in the costovertebral angle and flank with radiation to the lower quadrant and vulva, urinary urgency, and hematuria without—initially—pyuria or fever are characteristic of ureteral stone. X-ray films rarely reveal a stone, but intravenous urography may demonstrate partial obstruction.

Symptomatic therapy with hypnotics and antispasmodics is always indicated. Paravertebral or caudal block may sometimes be used for relief of pain and to relax the spastic ureter. Retrograde catheter manipulation may dislodge the stone and permit it to pass, or the stone may be extracted transureterally. If such efforts are unsuccessful and if severe pain persists and progressive hydronephrosis develops, remove the stone by extraperitoneal ureterolithotomy irrespective of the patient's obstetric status. In the absence of dystocia, normal delivery at term is the rule.

Harris RE, Dunnihoo DR: Incidence and significance of urinary calculi in pregnancy. Am J Obst Gynec 99:237, 1967.

Appendicitis During Pregnancy

Appendicitis occurs in about one of 1200 pregnancies. Management is more difficult than when the disease occurs in nonpregnant persons since the appendix is carried high and to the right, away from McBurney's point, and localization of infection does not usually occur. The distended uterus displaces the colon and small bowel; uterine contractions prevent abscess formation and walling-off; and the intestinal relationships are disturbed. In at least 20% of obstetric patients, the correct diagnosis is not made until the appendix has ruptured and peritonitis has become established. Delay may lead to premature labor or abortion.

Early appendectomy is indicated. If the diagnosis is made during labor at or near term, do an extraperitoneal cesarean section and appendectomy to minimize peritonitis. Therapeutic abortion is never indicated with appendicitis. If drains are necessary, they should be transabdominal, not transvaginal.

With early diagnosis and appendectomy, the prognosis is good for the mother and her baby.

Todd DW & others: Chronic appendicitis: Report of a case coexistent with pregnancy. Am J Obst Gynec 107:650, 1970.
Wilson EA & others: Appendectomy incidental to postpartum sterilization procedures. Am J Obst Gynec 116:76, 1973.

PREVENTION OF HEMOLYTIC DISEASE OF THE NEWBORN
(Erythroblastosis Fetalis)

The antibody anti-Rh_O(D) is responsible for most severe instances of hemolytic disease of the newborn (erythroblastosis fetalis). The Rh_O(D) antigen, also called the Rh factor, is inherited by approximately 85% of Caucasians. The remaining 15% are Rh-negative or, more properly, Rh_O(D)-negative. An Rh_O(D)-negative woman who carried an Rh_O(D)-positive fetus often develops the antibody anti-Rh_O(D). This antibody, once produced, remains in the woman's circulation during subsequent pregnancies. It poses a serious threat of hemolytic disease for subsequent fetuses whose red cells carry the antigen.

Immunization against hemolytic disease of the newborn now is possible with human Rh_O(D) immune globulin (RhoGAM). This purified concentrate of antibodies against Rh_O(D) antigen is obtained from Rh-negative women immune to the D-antigen. A passive immunity is conferred when such a preparation is injected into another individual. Unfortunately, passive immunity is brief. Nevertheless, passive antibodies can prevent active immunity from occurring, as in a mother who is producing anti-Rh_O(D).

When fetal Rh-positive red cells enter the mother's blood stream, she does not begin to produce anti-Rh_O(D) immediately. If passive anti-Rh_O(D) is injected soon after delivery (< 72 hours), therapeutically administered anti-Rh_O(D) will attack and destroy fetal Rh-positive cells so that Rh_O(D) antigen is removed from her circulation. Once the antigen is eliminated, the mother will not produce anti-RH_O(D), and she does not become actively immune to Rh_O(D). Hence, during her next Rh-positive gestation, there will be no anti-Rh_O(D) antibodies in her blood stream to react to fetal red cells, and erythroblastosis will be prevented during that pregnancy.

The immunizing dose of human Rh_O(D) immune globulin is 2 ml IM.

Aickin DR & others: Urinary estriol excretion in pregnancies complicated by Rhesus immunization. Australian New Zealand J Obstet Gynaec 12:86, 1972.
Douglas R, Staveley SM: Quantitative measurement of anti-D during pregnancy using a low ionic strength antoanalyzer system. New Zealand MJ 76:184, 1972.
Goplerud CP & others: The first Rh-isoimmunized pregnancy. Am J Obst Gynec 115:632, 1973.

Jonasson LE: Clinical value of amniotic fluid analysis in pregnancies complicated by Rh isoimmunization or hepatitis. Acta obstet gynec scandinav 52:113, 1973.

Ladipo OA: Management of the third stage of labor, with particular reference to reduction of feto-maternal transfusion. Brit MJ 1:721, 1972.

Mackay EV & others: Levels of fetal erythrocytes in the puerperal patient with particular reference to mode of delivery and ABO status. MJ Australia 1:1281, 1972.

Massi GB & others: Low dosage anti-immunoglobulin in the prevention of rhesus isoimmunization. J Obstet Gynaec Brit Common 81:87, 1974.

PREVENTION OF PREMATURE LABOR

The successful prevention of premature labor and delivery should reduce perinatal mortality and morbidity enormously. Nevertheless, the onset of labor is a complex biologic phenomenon controlled by multiple regulatory mechanisms most of which are only partially understood. CNS control appears to be exerted through the release of oxytocin, secreted in the hypothalamus, and stored in the posterior pituitary gland. Ethyl alcohol administered intravenously to the point of inebriation will inhibit the pituitary release of oxytocin, an impetus for labor. Alcohol can be given as 10% solution in 500 ml of 5% dextrose in water. The first 100–200 ml must be allowed to run in rapidly and the drip then slowed to 10–20 ml/hour for maintained sedation. This dosage is safe for both mother and fetus.

The administration of certain beta-adrenergic drugs inhibits myometrial contractions. Isoxsuprine (Vasodilan), 10 mg IV in 50 ml of 5% dextrose in water over a period of 1–2 hours, may be effective. This can be repeated over a 24-hour span, after which 10 mg orally every 3 hours may be substituted. Isoxsuprine may cause maternal hypotension, syncope, or fetal bradycardia, and its administration requires careful control. Ritodrine hydrochloride, an analogue of isoxsuprine, has recently been reported to be effective in obliterating uterine contractions.

Treatment measures to prolong pregnancy should be avoided for women with complications of pregnancy if those complications create hazards for the mother or fetus that are greater than the hazards of premature delivery. Ideally, the patient should be 32–36 weeks pregnant.

Although premature labor is associated with increased perinatal mortality and morbidity rates, it does not follow that the administration of a drug which will arrest premature labor will eliminate all reproductive wastage. In many instances, prematurity and perinatal death are related to some serious pathologic processes, but this may be impossible to determine clinically antepartum.

For this reason, one must identify those cases in which untimely delivery is the sole threat to the life or health of the infant. This requires that an effort be made to eliminate the following: (1) maternal conditions which compromise the intrauterine environment and make premature birth the lesser risk, eg, eclampsia; (2) fetal conditions which either are helped by early delivery or make attempts to stop premature labor meaningless, eg, severe erythroblastosis fetalis; and (3) clinical situations in which it is likely that attempts to stop labor will be futile, eg, ruptured membranes, cervix fully effaced and dilated > 3 cm, strong labor in progress.

Other drugs mentioned as of possible value in prevention of premature labor include pregneninolone sulfate, an adrenal steroid hormone and precursor of placental progesterone; and prostaglandin antagonists such as indomethacin and aspirin. Other drugs such as the opiates and anesthetics, possibly harmful to the fetus, may slow uterine contractions but will not always stop established labor and are therefore contraindicated.

Barden TP & others: Premature labor: Its management and therapy. J Reprod Med 9:93, 1972.

Bieniarz J & others: Uterine and cardiovascular effects of ritodrine in premature labor. Obst Gynec 40:65, 1972.

Mosler KH & others: Tocolytic therapy in obstetrics. J Perinatal Med 2:3, 1974.

Renand R & others: Use of ritodrine in treatment of premature labor. J Obstet Gynaec Brit Common 81:182, 1974.

Unbehaun V: Effects of sympathomimetic tocolytic agents on the fetus. J Perinatal Med 2:17, 1974.

Zuspan FP (coordinator): Premature labor—its management and therapy: A symposium. J Reprod Med 9:93, 1972.

SUPPRESSION OF LACTATION

If the patient does not wish to suckle her infant and wishes to "dry up" her breasts, this can be done by estrogen or androgen (or combination estrogen-androgen) administration or by mechanical inhibition of lactation. Hormones presumably suppress lactation by inhibiting the secretion of pituitary hormone. Hormonal suppression is effective only if started immediately after delivery. Postpartum bleeding may be increased.

Suppression With Estrogens
    A. Oral Estrogens: Eg, ethinyl estradiol, 1.3 mg (26 tablets containing 0.05 mg each), administered as follows: (Comparable doses for diethylstilbestrol.)
    1. Four tablets (0.2 mg) twice daily, first postpartum day.
    2. Three tablets (0.15 mg) twice daily, second day.
    3. Two tablets (0.1 mg) twice daily, third day.
    4. One tablet (0.05 mg) twice daily, 4th–7th days.
    B. Depot Estrogens: Estradiol valerate (Delestrogen), 3 ml of a solution containing 10 mg/ml immediately after delivery.

Suppression With Estrogen & Progestin

High-dosage estrogen-progestogen combinations with estrogen dominance (eg, Enovid, 5 mg) are moderately effective in suppressing lactation. Inhibition is principally due to the suppressive effect of estrogen on hypothalamic-pituitary function.

Suppression With Androgens

Methyltestosterone, 10 mg buccal tablets dissolved in the cheek pouch 5 times daily on the second and third postpartum days.

Suppression With Estrogens & Androgens

Testosterone enanthate, 180 mg/ml, and estradiol valerate, 8 mg/ml (Deladumone), 2 ml injected IM immediately after delivery, are very effective.

Mechanical Suppression of Lactation

If the patient begins to nurse and then for any reason wishes to transfer her baby to formula feedings and dry up her breasts (eg, if mastitis develops or the baby is to be weaned), hormones will not be effective and mechanical suppression is indicated. The patient should cease attempting to nurse and should not express milk or pump her breasts. Apply a tight compression "uplift" binder for 72 hours and a snug brassiere thereafter. Ice packs and analgesics, eg, aspirin and codeine, can be used as necessary. Fluid restriction and laxatives are of no value.

The breasts will become distended, firm, and tender. After 48–72 hours, lactation will cease and pain will subside. Involution will be complete in about 1 month.

The uncommon but impressive occurrence of thromboembolic phenomena in parturients on high-dosage estrogen or estrogen-progestogen medication is reminiscent of similar problems ascribed to the oral contraceptives. When the likelihood of vascular occlusion is increased, as in postcesarean section patients, those who have had a difficult vaginal delivery, a fe-brile course, etc, mechanical suppression of lactation is the logical choice when nursing is not elected.

Schwartz DJ & others: A clinical study of lactation suppression. Obst Gynec 42:599, 1973.
Zuckerman H, Carmel S: The suppression of lactation by clomiphene. J Obstet Gynaec Brit Common 80:822, 1973.

PUERPERAL MASTITIS

Postpartum inflammation of the breast occurs most often in clinic patients after several weeks or more of nursing. Infection is via the ducts following contamination of the nipple, and is often related to fissures in the nipple or obstructed milk flow. The hemolytic *Staphylococcus aureus* is the causative agent in most cases. Inflammation is unilateral in three-fourths of patients; primiparas are most often affected.

The onset is with chills, fever, malaise, and regional pain, tenderness, and induration. Localization, mass formation, fluctuation, and axillary adenopathy occur later. In most cases, once infection is well established, abscess formation is unavoidable.

Treatment consists of suppression of lactation, constant support of the breasts, antipyretics and analgesics, and intensive broad-spectrum antibiotic therapy. Incision and drainage are required if abscess formation occurs.

Prevention consists of proper initial nursing procedure and breast hygiene.

Hemingway L: Breast feeding and the family doctor. 2. Lactation problems. Australian Fam Physician 2:90, 1973.
Ramadan MA: The effect of breast infection on the composition of human milk. J Reprod Med 9:84, 1972.
Sweet RL, Ledger WJ: Puerperal infectious morbidity: A two-year review. Am J Obst Gynec 117:1093, 1973.

13 ...
Arthritis & Allied Rheumatic Disorders

Ephraim P. Engleman & Milton J. Chatton

Examination of the Patient

The specific diagnosis of a rheumatic disease can often be made at the bedside or in the office.

The examination depends upon a careful history and physical examination, with special attention to signs of articular inflammation (eg, heat, soft tissue swelling, effusion) and the functional status of the joints (eg, range of motion, ankylosis, deformity, atrophy). Certain laboratory procedures, depending upon the suspected diagnosis, complete the study. These most commonly include a complete blood count, urinalysis, ESR, tests for rheumatoid factor and antinuclear antibodies, serum uric acid determination, synovianalysis, and x-rays of key joints. These studies are not only important for diagnosis but may also serve as a baseline for judging the results of therapy.

Examination of Joint Fluid (See Table 13—1.)

Synovial fluid examination may provide valuable diagnostic and prognostic information in the management of joint disease. It also demonstrates the severity of synovial tissue inflammation. The skin overlying the joint to be aspirated is cleansed with soap and water and then prepared with an antiseptic solution. With sterile technic, the puncture site is infiltrated with a local anesthetic. The knee, by far the easiest joint to tap, is entered with an 18 gauge needle slightly superior and 2 cm (¾ inch) lateral (or medial) to the patella with the joint fully extended. From this position, the suprapatellar space is entered. After as much fluid has been removed as possible, the needle is withdrawn and the puncture site is covered with a sterile bandage or adhesive dressing.

The following studies should then be performed:

(1) Gross examination: Carefully note consistency and appearance. If fluid is green or purulent, examination with Gram's stain may be indicated. If grossly bloody, consider a bleeding disorder, trauma, or "traumatic tap." Note if the fluid is xanthochromic.

(2) Microscopic examination:

(a) Cytology: Collect 2—5 ml in a heparinized bottle (to prevent clotting). The red and white cells are counted, using the same equipment and technic as for a standard white count. The diluent, however, should be normal saline since the usual acidified diluent causes the fluid to clot in the pipet (see below). One drop of methylene blue added to the saline makes the cells distinguishable. Differential counts are performed on thin smears with Wright's stain.

(b) Crystals: Compensated polarized light microscopy identifies the existence and type of crystals: uric acid, calcium pyrophosphate, or cholesterol.

(3) Mucin clot tests for hyaluronate: Several drops of fluid are placed in a test tube containing 10 ml of 5% acetic acid. The resulting clot is graded from good to very poor according to its integrity.

Table 13—1. Examination of joint fluid.

Measure	Normal	Group I (Noninflammatory)	Group II (Inflammatory)	Group III (Septic)
Volume (ml) (knee)	< 3.5	Often > 3.5	Often > 3.5	Often > 3.5
Clarity	Transparent	Transparent	Translucent-opaque	Opaque
Color	Clear	Yellow	Yellow to opalescent	Yellow to green
Viscosity	High	High	Low	Variable
WBC (per cu mm)	< 200	200—2000	2000—100,000	> 100,000*
Polymorphonuclear leukocytes (%)	< 25%	< 25%	50% or more	75% or more*
Culture	Negative	Negative	Negative	Often positive
Mucin clot	Firm	Firm	Friable	Friable
Glucose (mg/100 ml)	Nearly equal to blood	Nearly equal to blood	> 25, lower than blood	< 25, much lower than blood

*Counts are lower with infections caused by organisms of low virulence or if antibiotic therapy has been started.

477

Table 13—2. Differential diagnosis by joint fluid groups.*

Group I (Noninflammatory)	Group II (Inflammatory)	Group III (Septic)	Hemorrhagic
Degenerative joint disease Trauma† Osteochondritis dissecans Osteochondromatosis Neuropathic arthropathy† Subsiding or early inflammation Hypertrophic osteoarthropathy‡ Pigmented villonodular synovitis†	Rheumatoid arthritis Acute crystal-induced synovitis (gout and pseudogout) Reiter's syndrome Ankylosing spondylitis Psoriatic arthritis Arthritis accompanying ulcerative colitis and regional enteritis Rheumatic fever‡ Systemic lupus erythematosus‡ Progressive systemic sclerosis (scleroderma)‡	Bacterial infections	Hemophilia or other hemorrhagic diathesis Trauma with or without fracture Neuropathic arthropathy Pigmented villonodular synovitis Synovioma Hemangioma and other benign neoplasm

*Reproduced from Rodman GP (editor): Primer on the rheumatic diseases, 7th ed. JAMA 224 (Suppl):662, 1973.
†May be hemorrhagic.
‡Groups I or II.

(4) **Culture:** Collect 1 ml of fluid in a sterile culture tube and perform routine cultures as well as special studies for gonococci, tubercle bacilli, or fungi as indicated.

(5) **Sugar:** Collect 2—3 ml of fluid in a fluoride tube. The patient must be in a fasting state, and the blood sugar must be determined at the time of joint aspiration.

Interpretation: Synovial fluid studies are not diagnostic unless a specific organism is identified in the culture or unless the urate crystals of gouty synovitis or the calcium pyrophosphate crystals of pseudogout are demonstrated. There is considerable overlap in the cytologic and biochemical values obtained in different diseases. These studies do, however, make possible a differentiation according to severity of inflammation. Thus, joint fluids in inflammatory diseases such as infections and rheumatoid arthritis are often turbid, with an elevated white count (usually well above 3000 cells/cu mm, with over 50% polynucleated forms), a poor mucin clot, and a synovial fluid sugar content which is considerably lower than the blood sugar. In diseases characterized by relatively mild articular inflammation, such as degenerative joint disease or traumatic arthritis, the synovial fluid is usually clear with a low white cell count (usually below 3000/cu mm) and a good mucin clot; and the synovial fluid and blood sugar levels are within 10 mg/100 ml of each other.

Meyers MH: Practical aspects of synovial fluid aspiration: The approaches to major extremity joints and examination of the aspirate. Western J Med 121:100, 1974.

CONNECTIVE TISSUE (COLLAGEN) DISEASES

The connective tissue disorders are a protean group of acquired diseases which appear to have in common widespread immunologic and inflammatory alterations of connective tissue. A variety of other names has been given to the group (eg, collagen diseases, collagenoses, diffuse vascular diseases, collagen vascular diseases, visceral angiitides), but no completely satisfactory term has been found. This group of acquired diseases must be distinguished from rare heritable disorders of connective tissue (see Chapter 20).

The acquired connective tissue diseases generally include the following clinical entities: rheumatoid arthritis, systemic lupus erythematosus, dermatomyositis, scleroderma, necrotizing vasculitis, rheumatic fever, glomerulonephritis, relapsing polychondritis, and Sjögren's syndrome.

These entities have certain features in common, and differentiation among them is often difficult because of overlapping features. Common findings include synovitis, pleuritis, myocarditis, endocarditis, pericarditis, peritonitis, vasculitis with or without fibrinoid necrosis, myositis, subcutaneous nodules, characteristic and nonspecific skin lesions, iritis and episcleritis, changes in skin and appendages, nephritis, and alterations of many connective tissues with scarring, hyperplasia, or distortions. Laboratory tests may reveal combinations of nonspecific findings, such as Coombs-positive hemolytic anemia, thrombocytopenia, leukopenia, B and T cell alterations, immunoglobulin excesses or deficiencies, impaired or accentuated delayed hypersensitivity, antinuclear antibodies, rheumatoid factors, cryoglobulins and other globulins, false-positive STS, elevated muscle enzymes, antithyroid antibodies, alterations in serum complement, and changes in acute phase reactants.

Although the connective tissue disorders are regarded as acquired diseases, the underlying causes cannot be determined in most instances, and it is unlikely that the established clinical entities have similar causes. Heredity, infection or other environmental antigen, immunoglobulin deficiency or hyperactivity (T cells), drug allergy, antigen-antibody-complement immune complexes, anaphylaxis, cytolysis, or some combination of all of these factors appear to play varying roles, but exactly what roles they have are unknown.

Some of the laboratory alterations that occur in this group of diseases (eg, false-positive STS) may occur in asymptomatic individuals and should suggest the possibility of the presence or future development of one of the connective tissue diseases. It is interesting to note also that these alterations in laboratory values may be demonstrated in certain asymptomatic relatives of patients with connective tissue diseases.

RHEUMATOID ARTHRITIS

Essentials of Diagnosis

- A systemic disease.
- Prodromal symptoms: malaise, fever, weight loss, sweating or paresthesias (or both) of the hands or feet, morning stiffness (prolonged).
- Onset usually insidious and in small joints; progression is centripetal and symmetric; deformities common.
- X-ray findings: changes characteristic of juxta-articular osteoporosis and (particularly) joint erosions.
- Serologic test for rheumatoid factor usually positive.
- Extra-articular manifestations: vasculitis, atrophy of skin and muscle, subcutaneous nodules, lymphadenopathy, splenomegaly, and leukopenia.

General Considerations

Rheumatoid arthritis is a chronic systemic inflammatory disease of unknown cause. Its incidence in the general population is 1–3%; female patients outnumber males almost 3:1. The usual age at onset is 20–40 years; however, rheumatoid arthritis may begin at any age.

The pathologic findings in the joint include chronic synovitis with pannus formation. The pannus erodes cartilage, bone, ligaments, and tendons. In the acute phase, effusion and other manifestations of inflammation are common. In the late stage, organization may result in fibrous ankylosis; true bony ankylosis is rare. In both acute and chronic phases, inflammation of soft tissues around the joints may be prominent.

The histologic findings most characteristic of rheumatoid arthritis are those in the subcutaneous nodule. This is a granuloma with a central zone of necrosis, a surrounding palisade of radially arranged elongated connective tissue cells, and a periphery of chronic granulation tissue. Pathologic alterations indistinguishable from those of the subcutaneous nodule are occasionally seen in the myocardium, pericardium, endocardium, heart valves, visceral pleura, lungs, sclera, dura mater, spleen, and larynx as well as in the synovial membrane, periarticular tissues, and tendons. Nonspecific pericarditis and pleuritis are found in 25–40% of patients at autopsy. Additional nonspecific lesions associated with rheumatoid arthritis include inflammation of small arteries, pulmonary fibrosis, round cell infiltration of skeletal muscle and perineurium, and hyperplasia of lymph nodes. Secondary amyloidosis may also be present.

Clinical Findings

A. Symptoms and Signs: The onset of articular signs of inflammation is usually insidious, with prodromal symptoms of malaise, weight loss, vasomotor disturbances (eg, paresthesias, Raynaud's phenomenon), and vague periarticular pain or stiffness. Less often, the onset is acute, apparently triggered by a stressful situation such as infection, surgery, trauma, emotional strain, or the postpartum period. In any case there is characteristically symmetric joint swelling with associated stiffness, warmth, tenderness, and pain. Pain and stiffness are prominent in the morning and subside during the day with moderate use. Stiffness may recur after daytime inactivity and may be much more severe after strenuous activity. Stiffness is a useful indication of active disease. Although any joint may be affected, the proximal interphalangeal and metacarpophalangeal joints of the fingers, wrists, knees, ankles, and toes are most often involved. Monarticular disease is occasionally seen early, especially in children. Synovial cysts and rupture of joint capsules may occur. Entrapment syndromes are not unusual—particularly entrapment of the median nerve at the carpal tunnel of the wrist. Palmar eyrthema is seen occasionally, as are tiny hemorrhagic infarcts in the nail folds or finger pulps and other signs of vasculitis. An evanescent morbilliform rash is commonly observed in children. Twenty percent of adult patients have subcutaneous nodules. These are most commonly situated over bony prominences but are also observed in the bursas and tendon sheaths. Five to 10% of patients have an enlarged spleen, and about 30% have lymph node enlargement. Low-grade fever, anorexia, weight loss, fatigue, and weakness are often present; chills do not occur except in children with severe disease. After months or years, thickening of the periarticular tissue, flexion deformities, subluxation, and ankylosis, usually fibrous, may occur. Atrophy of skin or muscle is common. Dryness of the eyes (also of the mouth and other mucous membranes), with corneal and conjunctival staining characteristic of keratoconjunctivitis sicca, is found especially in advanced disease (see Sjögren's Syndrome). Other ocular manifestations worthy of note include episcleritis, scleromalacia, scleral nodules, and nongranulomatous iritis. Pericarditis and pleuropulmonary diseases, when present, are frequently unsuspected clinically; these are found commonly at autopsy.

B. Laboratory Findings: Serum protein abnormalities are often present. Various serologic technics are used to detect certain macroglobulins which constitute the so-called rheumatoid factor. One of these, the F2 latex fixation test, is positive in 60–75% of cases. More sensitive tests will yield even higher percentages of positivity. False-positive reactions are not unusual, especially with old age, liver disease, subacute bacterial endocarditis, chronic lung disease, and syphilis and in symptom-free relatives of patients with rheumatoid arthritis. Antinuclear antibodies are often demonstrable, although their titers are usually lower in rheumatoid arthritis than in active systemic lupus erythematosus.

During both the acute and chronic phases the ESR and the gamma globulins are usually elevated. A moderate hypochromic normocytic anemia is common. The white cell count is normal or slightly elevated, but leukopenia may occur, especially in the presence of splenomegaly. Joint fluid examination is valuable, reflecting abnormalities which are associated with varying degrees of inflammation. (See Table 13–1.)

C. X-Ray Findings: Early signs are osteoporosis around the involved joint and erosion of the peripheral "bare space" of bone surface which is not covered by cartilage. Later, extensive erosion of cartilage causes joint space narrowing. Bony cysts result from invasion by granulation tissue. Rheumatoid synovium may invade the joint capsule, ligaments, and tendons, and it may add to joint instability induced by destruction of cartilage and bone. After some years, the degenerative changes of secondary osteoarthritis may be superimposed.

Special attention should be directed to the upper cervical spine and especially to C1–2, where subluxation may result in serious neurologic complications.

Differential Diagnosis

The differentiation of rheumatoid arthritis from other diseases of connective tissue can be exceedingly difficult, even impossible. However, certain clinical features are often helpful. Rheumatic fever is characterized by the migratory nature of the arthritis, the dramatic and objective response to salicylates in adequate doses, the more common occurrence of carditis, skin rashes, and chorea, and the elevated antistreptolysin titer. Butterfly rash, discoid lupus erythematosus, photosensitivity, alopecia, positive LE preparations, and renal disease point to the diagnosis of systemic lupus erythematosus. Degenerative joint disease (osteoarthritis) is not associated with constitutional manifestations, and the joint pain is characteristically relieved by rest, frequently in contrast to the morning stiffness of rheumatoid arthritis. Signs of articular inflammation, prominent in rheumatoid arthritis, are usually minimal in degenerative joint disease. Gouty arthritis may be confused with rheumatoid arthritis, but acute onset in one joint, hyperuricemia, the identification of urate crystals in the joint fluid, the presence of tophi, and the dramatic response to colchicine indicate gout. Pyogenic arthritis can be distinguished by chills as well as fever, the demonstration of the causative organism in the joint fluid, and the frequent presence of a primary focus elsewhere, eg, gonococcal urethritis.

Treatment

A. Basic Program (Conservative Management): All evidence indicates that conservative management offers a long-term prognosis that is often as good as or better than that of more spectacular methods. Since none of the latter measures are curative, and because their administration is often accompanied by undesirable side-effects, a conservative approach is preferable.

The primary objectives of treatment of rheumatoid arthritis are reduction of inflammation and pain, preservation of function, and prevention of deformity. A simple regimen consisting of rest, physical therapy, and salicylates is the best means of rehabilitating the patient without trading existing problems for others which may be even more devastating. In any event, these measures are so basically necessary as to warrant their continuation even when more heroic steps must be taken. They constitute the basic program of treatment to which other treatment may be added.

1. Systemic rest—There is a great deal of empirical evidence for the benefits of systemic rest. That rheumatoid arthritis is a systemic disease and not a disease limited to the joints has been shown above. Rest may be considered a common therapeutic denominator, treating as it does the person as a whole. Although the investigators in a recent clinical study questioned the beneficial effects of prolonged bed rest, the preponderance of evidence supports the view that intermittent rest has definite value. Rest, in some measure, should be prescribed when the diagnosis of active disease is made. It is assumed that bed rest is supervised and that other aspects of care are not neglected.

The amount of rest required depends upon the severity of the disease. Complete bed rest may be desirable and even imperative, particularly in patients with profound systemic and articular involvement. In mild disease, 2–4 hours of rest each day may suffice, allowing the patient to continue his work by restricting only his avocational activities. The duration of the rest program depends upon the course. In general, rest should be continued until significant improvement is sustained for at least 2 weeks; thereafter, the program may be liberalized. However, the increase of physical activity must proceed gradually and with appropriate support for any involved weight-bearing joints. Recrudescence of the disease is an indication for retarding the rate of physical restoration.

2. Emotional rest—The importance of emotional factors in rheumatoid arthritis and the need for psychologic support cannot be overemphasized. This support depends upon rapport between the patient and his doctor and is especially necessary during the early phase of the illness as well as during periods of increased disease activity.

3. Articular rest—Decrease of articular inflammation may be expedited by articular rest. Relaxation and stretching of the hip and knee muscles, to prevent flexion contractures, can be accomplished by having the patient lie in the prone position for 15 minutes (or preferably 1–2 hours) several times daily in addition to nighttime rest. Sitting in a flexed position for prolonged periods is a poor form of joint rest. Appropriate adjustable supports or splints provide rest for inflamed weight-bearing joints, relieve spasm and thus pain, and prevent or reduce deformities due to muscle spasm, soft tissue contracture, or ligamentous instability. The supports must be removable to permit daily range of motion and exercise of the affected extremities (see below). When ambulation is started, care must be taken to avoid weight-bearing, which will aggravate flexion deformities. This is accomplished with the aid of supports such as crutches and braces until the tendency to contracture has subsided.

4. Exercise—This is the most important measure in the physical therapy of rheumatoid arthritis. The management of rheumatoid arthritis is based on the concomitant administration of rest and therapeutic exercise, always in proper balance. Therapeutic exercises are designed to preserve joint motion and muscular strength and endurance. Most effective are exercises of the active-assistive type. These should be performed, within the limits of pain tolerance, from the outset of management. As tolerance for exercise increases and the activity of the disease subsides, progressive resistance exercises may be introduced. (Specific instructions for exercises are contained in *Home Care Programs in Arthritis,* a booklet published by the Arthritis Foundation, 475 Riverside Dr., Room 240, New York NY 10027.

5. Heat and cold—These are used primarily for their muscle relaxing and analgesic effect. Radiant or moist heat is generally most satisfactory. The ambulatory patient will find warm tub baths most convenient. Exercise may be better performed after exposure to heat. Some patients derive more relief of joint pain from local application of cold.

6. Salicylates—Aspirin and sodium salicylate are the analgesic drugs of choice. There is evidence that salicylates also exert an anti-inflammatory effect. The proper dose is that amount that provides optimal relief of symptoms without causing toxic reactions. Most adults can tolerate daily doses of 4–6 gm. Tinnitus and gastric irritation are early manifestations of toxicity. If tinnitus occurs, the daily dose should be decreased by decrements of 0.6 or 0.9 gm until this symptom disappears. The addition of antacids, especially at bedtime, may lessen symptoms of gastric irritation. This may also be accomplished by the ingestion of salicylates with meals and at bedtime with antacid. The use of enteric-coated tablets may also reduce gastric irritation, but enteric coating may interfere with the absorption of salicylates.

7. Other analgesic drugs—Anti-inflammatory analgesic drugs (see below) may be required for pain relief in progressive and severe disease. Codeine, in a bedtime dose of 30 mg, should be reserved for patients with severe nocturnal pain. Use of other narcotics should be discouraged. (See Chapter 1.)

8. Diet—The diet should be well balanced and adjusted to each individual's requirements. There is no specific food contraindication. If dietary intake is normal, there is usually no need to use supplemental vitamins.

9. Hematinic agents—These are not beneficial in the treatment of the anemia of rheumatoid arthritis. If iron deficiency coexists, however, iron salts are useful—eg, ferrous sulfate, 0.2 gm orally 3 times daily. Significant iron deficiency is not unusual following long-term loss of microscopic amounts of blood per rectum associated with the prolonged use of salicylates.

B. Anti-inflammatory Drugs: One or another of the drugs discussed below may be considered for use in patients with progressive disease following a reasonable trial (3–6 months) of conservative management. Their use must be regarded as a supplement to and not a substitute for the comprehensive approach outlined above.

1. Gold salts (chrysotherapy)—Although the value of gold salts in the treatment of rheumatoid arthritis remains controversial, this form of therapy has regained some of its former popularity in recent years. The exact mode of action is not known, but these agents are known to be lysosomal stabilizers.

a. Indications—Active disease responding unfavorably to conservative management; contraindications to corticosteroids; and erosive disease.

b. Contraindications—Previous gold toxicity; other drug allergy; systemic lupus erythematosus (misdiagnosed as rheumatoid arthritis); significant renal, hepatic, or hematopoietic dysfunction; general debility.

c. Preparations of choice—Gold thiomalate or gold thioglucose.

d. Weekly intramuscular dose—10 mg the first week; 25 mg the second week; and 50 mg weekly thereafter until toxic reactions appear, response is adequate, or a total dose of 1–1.2 gm has been given without improvement. If the response is good, continue to give 50 mg every 2 weeks and, as improvement continues, every 3 and then every 4 weeks for an indefinite period.

e. Toxic reactions—About 32% of patients (range in various series: 4–55%) experience toxic reactions to gold therapy; the mortality rate is less than 0.4%. The manifestations of toxicity are similar to those of poisoning by other heavy metals (notably arsenic) and include dermatitis (mild to exfoliative), stomatitis, agranulocytosis and other signs of bone marrow impairment, nephritis, and nitritoid reactions (especially to gold thiomalate and presumably due to its vehicle). In order to prevent or reduce the severity of toxic reactions, do not give gold salts to patients with any of the contraindicating disorders listed above and observe all patients carefully during the course of gold therapy. Before each injection, ask the patient how he has felt since the previous injection; examine the skin and mucous membranes for dermatitis or purpura; examine the urine for protein and microscopic hematuria; determine the hemoglobin and white cell count; and inspect a blood smear for differential white cell count values and for platelets. Platelet counts or liver function tests should be performed periodically. Warn the patient against exposure to strong light.

If signs of toxicity appear, withdraw the drug immediately. Severe toxicity may require corticosteroids for control, but failure to respond might then be an indication for the cautious use of penicillamine or dimercaprol (BAL).

2. Corticosteroids (cortisone, hydrocortisone, prednisone, prednisolone, triamcinolone, methylprednisolone, dexamethasone, betamethasone)—These agents represent an important advance in the management of rheumatoid arthritis. However, they must be considered as a nonspecific supplement to and not a substitute for the comprehensive approach outlined above. Some clinicians feel that the corticosteroids should not be employed unless the patient is also receiving maximal doses of salicylates. Perhaps the greatest disadvantage which might stem from their use, aside from the serious problem of untoward reactions, lies in the tendency of patient and physician to neglect the less spectacular but proved benefits which may be derived from general supportive treatment, physical therapy, and orthopedic measures. While corticosteroids usually produce immediate and dramatic symptomatic relief, they do not alter the natural progression of the disease; furthermore, clinical manifestations of active disease commonly reappear when the drug is discontinued.

a. Indications—Active and progressive disease which does not respond favorably to conservative management; contraindications to gold salts.

b. Contraindications and precautions—See p 718.

c. Daily oral dose—Give the least amount that will permit functional improvement but not more than 10–15 mg of prednisone or equivalent. Short- or intermediate-acting steroids, in a single daily dose, produce fewer undesirable side-effects. Many patients do reasonably well on 5–7.5 mg daily. (The use of 1 mg or 2.5 mg tablets is to be encouraged.) Efforts should be made to lower the daily dose by decrements of 0.5–1 mg every 2–4 weeks.

d. Intra-articular corticosteroids (hydrocortisone or newer analogues of hydrocortisone esters) may be helpful if one or 2 joints are the chief source of difficulty. Intra-articular hydrocortisone esters, 25–50 mg, may be given for symptomatic relief but no oftener than 4 times a year.

3. Chloroquines (antimalarials)—It appears probable that chloroquine phosphate and hydroxychloroquine sulfate have slight antirheumatic properties in selected patients with mild rheumatoid arthritis. Giving a daily dose of only 250 mg (1 tablet) of chloroquine or hydroxychloroquine (200 mg) minimizes the likeli-

hood of major toxic reactions (eg, retinitis, keratitis). Nevertheless, use of dark glasses and periodic ophthalmologic examination are required if these drugs are used.

4. Phenylbutazone—This analgesic drug is of limited usefulness in peripheral rheumatoid arthritis (see Ankylosing Spondylitis, below).

5. Indomethacin—This drug is probably no more effective in rheumatoid arthritis than the salicylates, but its untoward effects are far greater.

6. Ibuprofen (Motrin)—Ibuprofen is a propionic acid derivative which is probably no more effective in rheumatoid arthritis than the salicylates. However, it may cause fewer gastrointestinal side-effects.

7. Drug interreaction—Corticosteroids, the butazones, and indomethacin often cause sodium retention and gastrointestinal irritation; they should be used with caution in combination with sodium-containing antacids or sodium salicylate.

C. Cytotoxic Drugs: Cyclophosphamide, azathioprine, and chlorambucil have been used in patients with severe rheumatoid arthritis. Response to treatment is not invariably correlated with laboratory parameters of rheumatoid activity. The toxicity of these drugs and their potential teratogenic and oncogenic capacities are such that they should not be used until further experimental studies have been carried out.

D. Physical Therapy: See p 500 for additional measures.

Prognosis

The course of rheumatoid arthritis is totally unpredictable, although spontaneous remissions and relapses are common early in the disease. Occasionally, in well-established cases, permanent spontaneous remission occurs, with either return to normal function of the involved joints (if involvement is early and minimal) or some decrease in the degree of disability (if of longer duration). Although the disease is commonly progressive—and although some degree of permanent deformity may result—it must be emphasized that after 10 years half of patients are still capable of self-care and fully employable.

Bland JH (editor): Symposium on rheumatoid arthritis. M Clin North America 52:477, 1968.
Brewer EJ Jr: *Juvenile Rheumatoid Arthritis.* Saunders, 1970.
Bunch TW & others: Synovial fluid complement: Usefulness in diagnosis and classification of rheumatoid arthritis. Ann Int Med 81:32, 1974.
Cooperating Clinics Committee of the American Rheumatism Association: A controlled trial of cyclophosphamide in rheumatoid arthritis. New England J Med 283:883, 1970.
Duff IF, Carpenter JO, Neukom JE: Comprehensive management of patients with rheumatoid arthritis: Some results of the regional Arthritis Control Program in Michigan. Arthritis Rheum 17:635, 1974.
Duthie JJR & others: Course and prognosis in rheumatoid arthritis: A further report. Ann Rheumat Dis 23:193, 1964.
Engleman EP: Conservative management of rheumatoid arthritis. M Clin North America 52:699, 1968.

Ganda OP, Caplan HI: Rheumatoid disease without involvement. JAMA 228:338, 1974.

Goldman JA, Hesse EV: Treatment of rheumatoid arthritis—1970. Bull Rheumat Dis 21:609, 1971.

MacKenzie AH: An appraisal of chloroquine. Arthritis Rheum 13:280, 1970.

McCarty DJ: Treatment of rheumatoid joint inflammation with triamcinolone hexacetonide. Arthritis Rheum 15:157, 1972.

Mills JA & others: Value of bed rest in patients with rheumatoid arthritis. New England J Med 284:453, 1971.

Nomeir A & others: Cardiac involvement in rheumatoid arthritis. Ann Int Med 79:800, 1973.

Paulus HE, Whitehouse MW: Nonsteroid anti-inflammatory agents. Ann Rev Pharmacol 13:107, 1973.

Ruddy S, Colten HR: Rheumatoid arthritis: Biosynthesis of complement proteins by synovial tissue. New England J Med 290:1284, 1974.

Sharp JT & others: Observations on the clinical, chemical and serological manifestations of rheumatoid arthritis, based on the course of 154 cases. Medicine 43:41, 1964.

Sigler JW & Others: Gold salts in the treatment of rheumatoid arthritis: A double-blind study. Ann Int Med 80:21, 1974.

Smith PH & others: Natural history of rheumatoid cervical luxations. Ann Rheumat Dis 31:431, 1972.

Tibin WE, Jeffreys DE: Detection of the carpal tunnel syndrome. Arch Phys Med 54:373, 1973.

Urowitz M & others: Azathioprine in rheumatoid arthritis: A double-blind study comparing full dose to half dose. J Rheum 1:274, 1974.

Williams RC: *Rheumatoid Arthritis as a Systemic Disease.* Saunders, 1974.

SYSTEMIC (DISSEMINATED) LUPUS ERYTHEMATOSUS

Essentials of Diagnosis

- Occurs predominantly (85%) in young women.
- Multiple organ system manifestations (eg, arthritis, nephritis, pleuritis).
- Weakness, malaise, fever, and weight loss.
- Erythematous rash on face or other areas exposed to sunlight.
- Anemia, leukopenia, thrombocytopenia, hyperglobulinemia, and increased ESR.
- LE cells may be demonstrated in blood and other tissues.
- Antinuclear antibodies usually found.
- Raynaud's phenomenon.
- Chronic false-positive STS.

General Considerations

Systemic lupus erythematosus (SLE) is an inflammatory syndrome of unknown cause which primarily involves the vascular and connective tissues of many organs with a resultant multiplicity of local and systemic manifestations.

Virus-like structures—or "defective" or "altered" viruses—have been suggested as possible causes. Virus-like inclusions have been demonstrated in the capillary endothelial cells from a variety of sites (eg, glomerular, synovial) in patients with SLE, but the presence of these structures does not correlate well with the activity or extent of the disease, and they have also been demonstrated in such related disorders as scleroderma and dermatomyositis. Increased antibody titers to the Epstein-Barr (EB) virus, certain myxoviruses (measles and parainfluenza type 1), and Australia antigen have been reported. Antibodies have also been found to other antigens, including platelets, erythrocytes, leukocytes, thrombin, cytoplasm, lysozyme, and muscle.

The disease (or at least an SLE-like syndrome) may be initiated by the use of certain drugs: diphenylhydantoin and other anticonvulsants, hydralazine, isoniazid, phenothiazines, procainamide, quinidine, sulfonamides, and thiouracils.

Heredity probably plays a role in SLE; antinuclear antibodies have been found with increased frequency in families of patients. SLE has been reported in several sets of identical twins.

Although the pathogenesis of SLE has been studied extensively, the underlying mechanisms remain unclear. The pathologic changes in SLE apparently involve an alteration of the immune mechanism. Antibody to DNA is found in most patients with severe, active SLE. Antinuclear antibody, although a frequent serologic finding in SLE, can also be demonstrated in normal older individuals, particularly women, as well as in clinical disorders other than SLE. Absence of antinuclear antibody in active untreated SLE is unusual. Free DNA is a frequent finding in the serum of patients with SLE. It is felt that the anticomplementary activity of SLE serum is due to complement (C') consumption by circulating DNA antigen-antibody complexes. Fluorescent antibody studies of renal glomeruli of SLE patients demonstrate antigen, antibody, and complement, pointing to immune complex deposition in the pathogenesis of renal lesions. Serum complement is normal in drug-induced SLE, which may account for decreased renal involvement in the drug-induced disease. It has been reported that serious renal disease is less frequent in patients with precipitating antibodies to RNA-protein antigen than in those who have complement fixation antibodies to double-stranded DNA.

The type, severity, time of onset, and duration of the pathologic involvement may result in a highly variable clinical pattern and prognosis. Pathologic changes are nonspecific but include widespread fibrinoid vascular changes and disseminated arteritis.

Pathologic changes as demonstrated by ordinary postmortem and light microscope studies do not necessarily reflect the clinical severity of the condition. Patients who die of fulminant disease may show subtle nonspecific changes, whereas biopsies of living patients with moderate clinical disease may show necrotizing vasculitis. "Hematoxylin bodies"—homogeneous masses of nuclear material staining purple with hematoxylin—are histochemically identical with LE cell inclusions in polymorphonuclear cells. Vasculitis may vary from cellular infiltrates to fibrinoid necrosis in almost any organ, including onion-skinning of the vessels of the spleen. Renal lesions may be focal proliferative, diffuse proliferative, or membranous; and immunofluorescence studies usually show DNA-IgG-complement immune complex deposits; these appear as electron-dense deposits under the electron microscope.

Clinical Findings

In 1971, the American Rheumatism Association selected 14 clinical manifestations as being the most characteristic of SLE: "butterfly rash," discoid lupus, Raynaud's phenomenon, alopecia, photosensitivity, oral ulcers, nondeforming arthritis, LE cells, false-positive STS, profuse proteinuria, cellular casts, serositis, CNS symptoms, and hematologic changes. It was recommended that a diagnosis of SLE could be made with reasonable certainty if 4 or more of these criteria were present serially or simultaneously. This approach has usefulness, but false-positives and false-negatives occur.

A. Symptoms and Signs:

1. Systemic reaction—Weakness, fatigue, malaise, fever, sweating, and weight loss may occur.

2. Skin—Discoid lupus erythematosus may occasionally precede the systemic disease. Conversely, discoid lesions may develop during the course of the systemic disease. Erythema of exposed surfaces due to sensitivity to sunlight—especially the classical symmetric malar erythema (so-called butterfly rash)—and erythematous rashes of the neck, elbows, and hands are the most common dermatologic manifestations. Purpura, angioneurotic edema, alopecia, vitiligo, mucosal ulceration, or hyperpigmentation occurs less frequently.

3. Lymph nodes and spleen—Half of patients have generalized lymphadenopathy. One-fourth have splenomegaly.

4. Eyes—Corneal involvement and retinopathy, including cotton wool retinal exudates, have been reported in about 20–25% of patients.

5. Hematopoietic system—Hematologic involvement occurs in all patients. There may be severe hemolytic anemia or thrombocytopenic purpura. Hypersplenism has been described. Splenomegaly occurs in about 20–25% of cases.

6. Lungs—Pulmonary dysfunction with basilar atelectatic pneumonitis, and pleurisy with or without effusion, are common.

7. Cardiovascular system—Pericarditis, with or without effusion, occurs in about half of cases. Myocarditis with tachycardia, gallop rhythm, and disturbances of rhythm may result in heart failure. Verrucous endocarditis may occur. Coronary arteritis is a rare but serious complication. Arterial hypertension may be a manifestation of renal disease. Raynaud's phenomenon is common, and vasculitis of nearly any blood vessel may occur.

8. Gastrointestinal system—Ulcerative lesions of the mucous membranes, especially the mouth, are very common. There may be anorexia, nausea and vomiting, dysphagia, diarrhea, abdominal pains, ileus, peritonitis, and bloody stools. The intestinal involvement may be the result of extensive vasculitis, of ulceration or perforation, or of coexisting ulcerative colitis or ileocolitis.

9. Liver—Hepatomegaly, often accompanied by evidence of hepatic dysfunction, occurs in about one-third of cases. Chronic, active hepatitis—with LE cells, hyperglobulinemia, and other immunologic phenomena—has been mistakenly termed "lupoid hepatitis" but is not true SLE.

10. Kidneys—Renal complications are a serious feature of SLE. Three different types of lupus nephritis have been described. Focal proliferative lupus nephritis is characterized by proteinuria and microscopic hematuria, but nephrotic syndrome and renal failure are rare. Response to corticosteroids is favorable. Diffuse proliferative lupus nephritis and membranous lupus nephritis are usually characterized by the nephrotic syndrome and renal insufficiency. Although remissions can be induced in some of the latter group, the prognosis is generally unfavorable, and most patients die of the complications of renal failure within 3 years.

11. Musculoskeletal system—Myalgia and arthralgia occur in over 90% of patients. Myositis, with elevation of muscle enzymes, is common. About a third of patients develop polyarthritis which is difficult to distinguish from rheumatoid arthritis. However, advanced destruction of articular cartilage, ankylosis, contractures, spinal involvement, and pannus formation are uncommon. "Rheumatoid" nodules and cysts of synovial surfaces may cause pain and deformity of the involved joints.

12. Nervous system—Involvement of the CNS is common and may vary from mild neurotic traits to psychosis, mild to severe convulsions, hemiplegia, and coma. Peripheral neuritis is not uncommon.

B. Laboratory Findings: A mild to moderate normochromic, normocytic anemia is found in the majority of patients. Hemolytic anemia occurs infrequently but may be severe. The Coombs test is frequently positive. Mild leukopenia with lymphopenia is common. The sedimentation rate is high in almost all cases, often even during periods of remission. Serum globulin is increased in about half of cases, usually in the alpha$_2$ and gamma (especially IgG) fractions. Cryoglobulins and many other serum protein abnormalities of unknown significance have been described. Antinuclear antibodies are found in over 97% of cases. The antibody to native DNA (double-stranded), although found less frequently than anti-DNA, is considered to be more specific. Serum complement levels are usually low during periods of active SLE. Tests for rheumatoid factor may be positive, but less often than in rheumatoid arthritis. Liver function tests and muscle enzymes are frequently abnormal. Biologic false-positive STS (sometimes including FTA and TPI) are found in 20% of cases. Protein, white cells, red cells, and casts in the urine reflect the type and degree of renal involvement. Finding the characteristic LE cell in venous blood or in other tissues is of great value in diagnosis, although the LE cell is not pathognomonic. An absence of LE cells does not rule out the diagnosis of systemic lupus erythematosus. The LE cell, which is apparently due to a specific antibody (anti-IgG), is typically a polymorphonuclear leukocyte containing a globular mass of homogeneous material, reddish purple when stained with Wright's stain, which fills a large portion of the cell. This material may also occur extracellularly. The LE cell may be found in many other disease states.

Fluorescent antibody technics may detect characteristic antibody fluorescence in skin and kidney biopsy specimens.

Differential Diagnosis

Since SLE involves many organ systems, it may be confused with a variety of diseases, especially other collagen diseases and musculoskeletal, dermatologic, and hematologic disorders. It must also be differentiated from many acute and chronic infectious diseases, particularly syphilis because of the positive STS.

Treatment

It is extremely difficult to evaluate the results of presently available treatment in a disease with such variable dominant features, severity, and course. Patients with CNS involvement or diffuse proliferative or membranous nephritis generally do not respond to treatment as well as those without involvement of these systems, and they have a poorer prognosis. Although treatment may be followed by subjective improvement, reduction in anti-DNA titers, increase in complement, and decrease in proteinuria, controlled studies now in progress have not been continued long enough to determine the effect on longevity or the course of the disease. Use of cytotoxic immunosuppressive agents should be reserved for symptomatic patients or those with life-threatening disease which fails to respond to more conservative therapy.

A. Corticosteroids and Corticotropin: These drugs may exert a favorable effect in some patients, but the results are variable. Treatment with 7–15 mg of prednisone daily orally is usually more effective in the early phases of the illness. Many patients obtain marked temporary benefit during acute episodes or when there is involvement of vital organs. Large doses (1 mg/kg prednisone daily) may be necessary for patients with hemolytic anemia, thrombocytopenia, pericarditis, diffuse renal disease, or CNS involvement.

When improvement has occurred, cautious reduction in the total daily dose is begun, with the goal of controlling the disease with the least possible amount of drug. In patients requiring large doses for long periods of time, gradual change to alternate-day therapy may control the disease and reduce the cushingoid side-effects. All possible clinical parameters should be assessed in treatment and may include serum complement studies and search for anti-DNA antibodies. Caution should be used in trying to follow activity with tests such as the erythrocyte sedimentation rate or urinary protein studies without relating them to the total disease activity. Renal lesions, previously considered to be irreversible, may respond favorably to large doses of corticosteroids over a prolonged period.

B. Other Measures: A high-caloric, high-vitamin diet is advised. Iron salts or blood transfusions may be necessary to correct anemia. Patients should be cautioned against undue exposure to sunlight or to other ultraviolet radiation. If Raynaud's phenomenon occurs, protect against exposure to cold. All drugs previously mentioned as causative should be avoided. Appropriate anti-infective treatment should be instituted for pneumonia or other infections. Salicylates and other analgesics and physical therapy may be indicated for musculoskeletal aches and pains.

In patients who fail to respond to adequate corticosteroid therapy, a trial of immunosuppressive agents such as the purine antagonists (eg, mercaptopurine or azathioprine) or alkylating agents (eg, mechlorethamine, cyclophosphamide) is indicated although their value has not been proved. Severe side-effects and an increased incidence of neoplastic disease may occur with their use.

Many clinicians feel that chloroquine and other antimalarial drugs are not justified because of the risk of toxic retinopathy. However, these drugs may be useful in selected patients who can be examined frequently by an ophthalmologist.

Course & Prognosis

SLE may be relatively mild or it may be fulminant, with severe symptoms leading to death in a few weeks despite treatment. More frequently, the disease follows an episodic pattern with recurrent involvement of one or more organ systems over many years. The mortality rate decreases after the 4th year. Patients with the chronic illness can perhaps be helped to live longer by proper corticosteroid therapy. (A 5-year survival rate of 75% has been reported.)

Ackerman GL: Alternate-day steroid therapy in lupus nephritis. Ann Int Med 72:511, 1970.

Atkins CJ, Kondon JJ: The choroid plexus in systemic lupus erythematosus. Ann Int Med 76:65, 1972.

Baldwin DS & others: The clinical course of the proliferative and membranous forms of lupus nephritis. Ann Int Med 73:929, 1970.

Decker JL & others: Cyclophosphamide in lupus nephritis: A controlled test. Ann Int Med 75:165, 1971.

Dubois EL (editor): *Lupus Erythematosus,* 2nd ed. Univ of Southern California Press, 1974.

Eisenberg H & others: Diffuse interstitial lung disease in systemic lupus erythematosus. Ann Int Med 79:37, 1973.

Epstein WV: Immunologic events preceding clinical exacerbation of systemic lupus erythematosus. Am J Med 54:631, 1973.

Epstein WV, Grausz H: Favorable outcome in diffuse proliferative glomerulonephritis of systemic lupus erythematosus. Arthritis Rheum 17:129, 1974.

Estes D, Christian CL: The natural history of systemic lupus erythematosus by prospective analysis. Medicine 50:85, 1971.

Gibson TP: Use of the American Rheumatism Association's preliminary criteria for the classification of systemic lupus erythematosus. Ann Int Med 77:754, 1972.

Hahn BH, Bagby MK, Osterland CK: Abnormalities of delayed hypersensitivity in systemic lupus erythematosus. Am J Med 55:25, 1973.

Hardin JG Jr: Steroid-induced morbidity mimicking active systemic lupus erythematosus. Ann Int Med 78:558, 1973.

Holman HR: The nephritis of systemic lupus erythematosus. California Med 117:49, Nov 1972.

Perry HM: Late toxicity to hydralazine resembling systemic lupus erythematosus or rheumatoid arthritis. Am J Med 54:58, 1973.

Sharon E, Kaplan D, Diamond HS: Exacerbations of systemic lupus erythematosus after withdrawal of azathioprine therapy. New England J Med 288:122, 1973.

Soloway RD & others: "Lupoid" hepatitis, a non-entity in the spectrum of chronic active liver disease. Gastroenterology 63:458, 1972.

Whittingham S & others: Antinuclear antibody response to procainamide in man and laboratory animals. Am Heart J 84:228, 1972.

POLYARTERITIS (PERIARTERITIS) NODOSA

Essentials of Diagnosis

- Symptoms and signs referable to multiple organ systems.
- Weakness, malaise, fever, weight loss.
- Renal involvement, hypertension, asthma, heart failure, cutaneous eruptions, abdominal pain, musculoskeletal aches and pains, peripheral neuritis.
- Proteinuria and hematuria, leukocytosis, eosinophilia, elevated erythrocyte sedimentation rate, hyperglobulinemia.
- Biopsy of painful areas may show necrotizing arteritis.

General Considerations

Polyarteritis nodosa is one of a group of several overlapping syndromes of systemic vasculitis of unknown cause. The highly variable clinical manifestations are similar to those of other forms of vasculitis and are due to multiple organ system involvement. Polyarteritis nodosa is characterized by sequential inflammation and necrosis of medium-sized arteries with resultant fibrosis of vessel walls (granulomas), aneurysms, and infarction. Although any organ may be involved, the arterial lesions occur most frequently in the kidneys, muscles, peripheral nerves, heart, lungs, gastrointestinal tract, and liver. A wide variety of antigens, including Australia antigen, may be responsible for the immunologic reactions and vascular damage associated with polyarteritis. A history of drug sensitization occurs in some cases. Drug sensitivity reactions resembling polyarteritis nodosa have been described in drug abusers and in a small number of patients receiving allopurinol and guanethidine.

Clinical Findings

A. Symptoms and Signs: The mode of onset, the clinical findings, and the course of the disease may be highly variable. The most common manifestations are hypertension, renal disease, musculoskeletal aches and pains, and peripheral neuritis. Acute oliguric renal failure may develop early, without significant evidence of other organ involvement. Other manifestations include fever, malaise, weakness, weight loss, bronchial asthma, bronchial pneumonia, angina, congestive failure, nausea, abdominal pain, hematemesis, and melena. Skin lesions may include papular eruptions, purpura, vesicles, bullae, or subcutaneous periarterial nodules.

B. Laboratory Findings: Leukocytosis and mild normocytic anemia are common. Eosinophilia may occur. The erythrocyte sedimentation rate and the serum globulin level are frequently elevated. Proteinuria, hematuria, pyuria, and casts are common urinary findings.

Renal biopsy or biopsy of multiple sections of muscle or of subcutaneous nodules from painful areas may establish the diagnosis, although negative pathologic findings do not necessarily rule out the possibility of the disease. Histologic evidence of vasculitis may also appear in the other connective tissue diseases.

C. X-Ray Findings: Arteriographic studies may reveal rather characteristic aneurysms in the renal, celiac, mesenteric, hypogastric, and hepatic arteries.

Differential Diagnosis

The diagnosis of polyarteritis is suggested by the very multiplicity of clinical involvement and the rapid progression of the illness. Polyarteritis must be differentiated from the other angiitides such as those of systemic lupus erythematosus, scleroderma, and Wegener's granulomatosis as well as from rheumatic fever, rheumatoid arthritis, glomerulonephritis, and pyelonephritis. It may at times be confused with acute and chronic infections, the lymphomas, and other granulomatous diseases.

Treatment

Treatment is symptomatic and supportive. Corticosteroids may occasionally be beneficial, especially if vital organs are involved. The healing of arteritis may be accompanied by thrombosis. In so-called "paradoxic" adverse reactions, the corticosteroid dosage should be reduced. Intercurrent infections may be treated with antibiotics.

Prognosis

The disease usually runs a fulminating course, death often occurring within a few months after diagnosis. In occasional instances the patient may live comfortably for several years, especially with corticosteroid therapy. Recovery is unpredictable.

Dornfeld L, Lecky JW, Peter JB: Polyarteritis and intrarenal artery aneurysms. JAMA 215:1950, 1971.

Fronhert PP, Sheps SG: Long-term follow-up study of periarteritis nodosa. Am J Med 43:8, 1967.

Gocke DJ & others: Association between polyarteritis and Australia antigen. Lancet 2:1149, 1970.

Mills RM: Severe hypersensitivity reactions to allopurinol. JAMA 216:799, 1971.

Yust I, Schwartz J, Dreyfuss F: A cytotoxic serum factor in polyarteritis nodosa and related conditions. Am J Med 48:472, 1970.

DIFFUSE SCLERODERMA
(Progressive Systemic Sclerosis)

Scleroderma is a chronic disease of undetermined cause characterized by insidious onset of connective tissue proliferation in the dermis and in multiple internal organs. There is early and progressive small arterial involvement disproportionate to the fibrosis. The disease occurs most frequently in middle-aged women.

The localized forms of scleroderma are usually benign; 50% of the nodular localized forms, however, progress to systemic forms. The overlapping syndromes of scleroderma (mixed connective tissue syndrome, sclerodermatomyositis) are distinguished by definite skin changes of scleroderma, definite myositis that is usually responsive to small doses of corticosteroids, and a high incidence of positive findings on search for antinuclear antibodies. The systemic syndromes (progressive systemic sclerosis) are of 2 types: the rare diffuse progressive form (5% of cases) that shows rapid systemic progression with little or no incidence of Raynaud's phenomenon, and the common form of progressive systemic sclerosis (95% of cases), which is often dominated in early stages by Raynaud's phenomenon and acrosclerosis.

Stiffness of the hands, sweating of the hands and feet, and Raynaud's phenomenon may at times be present for years before the condition becomes recognized. The skin eventually becomes hard, thick, parchment-like, and glossy without evidence of pitting edema, and the fingers and toes become fixed in position. Gradually, the entire integument becomes involved; and telangiectasia, pigmentation and depigmentation, widespread or local calcification of the skin (especially around the joints), and paronychia and ulceration of the fingers and toes may occur. Esophageal involvement with cardioesophageal sphincter incompetence and dysphagia may occur early. Disturbance of gastrointestinal motility may occur. Sclerodermatous constriction of the thorax, pulmonary fibrosis, and recurrent bronchial pneumonia may lead to decreased vital capacity, decreased compliance, and low diffusing capacity even in patients whose chest x-rays show no abnormality. Pericardial disease is usually subtle. Myocardial disease may result in arrhythmias or congestive heart failure; the latter is a bad prognostic sign. Arthritis may occur, but the findings are not conspicuous. Neurologic manifestations may occur but are uncommon. Laboratory findings are not diagnostic. The erythrocyte sedimentation rate and serum globulin may be elevated. The LE phenomenon or a rise in numbers of antinuclear antibodies may occur in 50% of cases. Concomitant autoimmune hematologic disorders (eg, thrombocytopenia and hemolytic anemia) are rare. Proteinuria and casts are found frequently. In rare cases, renal involvement is extensive, with a progressive course ending in death within months. X-rays show subcutaneous calcification, osteoporosis of bone, and destruction of the distal phalanges. Gastrointestinal x-rays may show loss of normal peristalsis.

Scleroderma-like lesions have been described in patients with carcinoid syndrome.

Treatment is symptomatic and supportive. Orally administered doses of reserpine may improve the capillary blood flow in patients with Raynaud's phenomenon. Corticosteroids should be used only if definite polymyositis is a component.

The condition is usually slowly progressive for several years. The prognosis for long survival is best in young white women. Only about a third of all patients with scleroderma survive beyond 7 years. Death is usually due to renal or cardiac failure or to sepsis.

Cannon PJ & others: The relationship of hypertension and renal failure in scleroderma (progressive systemic sclerosis) to structural and functional abnormalities of the renal circulation. Medicine 53:1, 1974.

D'Angelo WA & others: Pathologic observations in systemic sclerosis (scleroderma): A study of 58 autopsy cases and 58 matched controls. Am J Med 46:428, 1969.

Medsger TA Jr & others: Survival with systemic sclerosis (scleroderma): A life-table analysis of clinical and demographic factors in 309 patients. Ann Int Med 75:369, 1971.

Sharp GC & others: Mixed connective tissue disease: An apparently distinct rheumatic disease associated with a specific antibody to an extractable nuclear antigen (ENA). Am J Med 52:148, 1972.

Siegel RC: Progressive systemic sclerosis. California Med 119:35, Aug 1973.

DERMATOMYOSITIS
(Polymyositis)

Dermatomyositis is a chronic, nonsuppurative inflammatory disease of undetermined origin which involves primarily the skin and striated muscles. The inflammatory process may be limited largely to the muscles—hence the term polymyositis. Recent studies suggest that the lymphocytes of patients with dermatomyositis are sensitized to muscle antigen. There is an unexplained high incidence (10–20%) of associated neoplastic disease. Some workers have speculated that the dermatomyositis is a metabolic or immunologic manifestation of the primary neoplastic disease.

The onset, although usually insidious, may at times be acute. Weakness, fatigue, mild fever, weight loss, and muscular aching are early symptoms. Diffuse erythema of the face and neck may occur, and a purplish periorbital edema is often noted. Erythema, with or without edema, may occur in other skin areas, especially the extensor surfaces of the arms and legs. Desquamation, pigmentary changes, and subcutaneous induration and calcification may occur. Aching, tenderness, and weakness of muscles is characteristic. Muscular involvement may be generalized, but it is most marked in the flexor muscles of the upper and lower extremities and the neck flexors. Slowly progressive muscle weakness, with or without muscle aching and tenderness, occurs in nearly all patients. Involvement of special muscle groups may result in ocular palsies, dysphagia, or respiratory embarrassment. Raynaud's phenomenon and arthritic manifestations occur in about one-third of patients. Multiple gastrointestinal ulcers may occur. There may be a mild normocytic anemia, increased erythrocyte sedimentation rate, and increased serum globulin. Serum enzyme (eg, SGOT, CPK, aldolase) levels are elevated and are useful not only in diagnosis but in following the effectiveness of therapy. Creatinuria parallels muscle destruction. Biopsies show variable dermatitis and chronic inflammatory, degenerative, and necrotic changes in muscles. The electromyogram is useful for the early detection and differentiation of dermatomyositis from the neuromuscular disorders.

Appropriate investigations to rule out malignant neoplastic disease are indicated for all patients who develop dermatomyositis in adult life.

Treatment is symptomatic and supportive. Large doses of salicylates may be of value. Corticosteroids generally lead to marked improvement. Doses of prednisone as large as 60 mg/day may be required to bring enzyme levels toward normal, at which time the dosage should be gradually reduced. Methotrexate may help in cases resistant to corticosteroids, or it may be steroid-sparing when large doses are required. Emergency measures to provide an adequate airway may be necessary. Removal of an associated neoplastic lesion may result in regression of the disease.

Dermatomyositis is usually moderately progressive, undulating in severity, and crippling over a period of years, but it may at times be fulminating.

Dawkins RL, Mastaglia FL: Cell-mediated cytotoxicity to muscle in polymyositis. New England J Med 288:434, 1973.

Medager TA & others: Factors affecting survivorship in polymyositis: A life-table study of 124 patients. Arthritis Rheum 14:249, 1971.

Rose AL, Watson JN: Polymyositis: A survey of 89 cases with particular reference to treatment and prognosis. Brain 89:747, 1966.

Sokoloff MC, Pearson CM, Goldberg LS: Treatment of corticosteroid-resistant polymyositis with methotrexate. Lancet 1:14, 1971.

SJÖGREN'S SYNDROME
(Sicca Syndrome)

Sjögren's syndrome is a generalized connective tissue disorder of undetermined cause which occurs most frequently in women over 50 years of age. Dryness of the eyes, mouth, nose, trachea, bronchi, vagina, and skin, with hypofunction of the lacrimal and parotid glands, is characteristic. Bilateral parotid swelling may occur.

The "sicca complex" is due to defective secretion by the lacrimal and salivary glands, giving rise to keratoconjunctivitis sicca and xerostomia (mouth dryness), which may become so severe as to cause corneal ulceration and inability to swallow and chew foods without sipping liquids. The salivary glands are often swollen, either chronically or recurrently. Secretory insufficiency may also involve the nasopharynx, laryngotracheobronchial tree, or vagina. Ophthalmologic examination and biopsy of the small salivary glands in the lower lip usually confirm the diagnosis. About half of patients have rheumatoid arthritis or some other connective tissue disorder. Even when there is no clear evidence of associated specific connective tissue syndromes, patients often have such manifestations as splenomegaly, vasculitis, peripheral neuropathy, Raynaud's phenomenon, hypergammaglobulinemic purpura, renal tubular acidosis, Hashimoto's thyroiditis, hepatomegaly, achlorhydria, pancreatitis, polymyositis, anemia, rheumatoid factor, antinuclear antibodies, LE cells, and antibodies to salivary duct tissue.

Many treatment methods have been proposed, but results have not been uniformly good. Local treatment of eye dryness with irrigating solution or artificial tears (methylcellulose, 0.12% in saline) instilled into the eyes every 3 hours is simple and effective in minimizing keratoconjunctivitis and corneal ulceration. Treatment with corticotropin or the corticosteroids is warranted, especially in the systemic disease, but should be used with caution if corneal infection or ulceration is present. There is no known treatment for the mouth dryness.

The disease is subject to remissions and exacerbations but is usually not progressive. The overall prognosis depends upon the associated systemic involvement or connective tissue disease. There is an increased incidence of reticulum cell sarcoma and other lymphomas after several years.

Cummings NA & others: Sjögren's syndrome: Newer aspects of research, diagnosis and therapy. Ann Int Med 75:937, 1971.

Shearn MA: *Sjögren's Syndrome.* Saunders, 1971.

Steinberg AD, Talal N: The coexistence of Sjögren's syndrome and systemic lupus erythematosus. Ann Int Med 74:55, 1971.

Talal N & others: Extrasalivary lymphoid abnormalities in Sjögren's syndrome: Reticulum cell sarcoma, "pseudolymphoma," macroglobulinemia. Am J Med 43:50, 1967.

POLYMYALGIA RHEUMATICA
& TEMPORAL ARTERITIS

These disorders, seen most often in elderly women, often begin abruptly with severe pain and stiffness in the shoulders, hips, pectoral and pelvic girdles, and proximal limb muscles. Unlike those in polymyositis, all muscle enzymes and muscle biopsy findings are normal. There may be fever, malaise, weight loss, and some degree of anemia, but an elevated erythrocyte sedimentation rate is the most important and most common laboratory finding. Giant cell arteritis, now recognized as a form of systemic vasculitis, can often be demonstrated by biopsy of the temporal artery. There appears to be a relationship between polymyalgia rheumatica and temporal or cranial arteritis. Blindness is a serious threat if arteritis coexists; thus, temporal artery biopsy is almost mandatory whenever the diagnosis of polymyalgia rheumatica is suspected.

In most patients, the disease responds well to small doses of corticosteroids, eg, 10 mg or less of prednisone daily. The erythrocyte sedimentation rate is a helpful guide to treatment. Large doses of corticosteroids are required if there is giant cell arteritis. In some cases the drug may be gradually discontinued over a period of several months, but prolonged treatment is commonly required.

Fauchald P, Rygvold O, Oystese B: Temporal arteritis and polymyalgia rheumatica. Ann Int Med 77:845, 1972.
Fessel WJ, Pearson CM: Polymyalgia rheumatica and blindness. New England J Med 276:1403, 1967.
Healy L & others: Polymyalgia rheumatica and giant cell arteritis. Arthritis Rheum 14:138, 1971.
Mowat AG, Hazleman BL: Polymyalgia rheumatica: A clinical study with particular reference to arterial disease. J Rheum 1:190, 1974.

WEGENER'S SYNDROME
(Wegener's Granulomatosis)

Wegener's syndrome is a rare generalized progressive disorder of undetermined cause characterized by severe necrotizing granulomatous involvement of the upper and lower respiratory tracts, multiplicity of symptoms resulting from generalized focal necrotizing vasculitis of arteries and veins, and terminal renal insufficiency caused by focal necrotizing glomerulitis. Limited forms of the disease have been described. The onset is usually marked by nasal, paranasal sinus, or pulmonary symptoms, including chronic productive cough or hemoptysis. Fever, malaise, weakness, or weight loss may be severe. Progressive destruction of the cartilage of the nose and the bony structures around the paranasal sinuses occurs later. Chemosis, papillitis, and exophthalmos may occur. There may be parotitis, carditis, musculoskeletal aches and pains, prostatitis, or polyneuritis. Microangiopathic hemolytic anemia may occur in association with rapidly progressive renal failure. Proteinuria, hematuria, and white cells and casts in the urine are evidence of marked renal involvement.

Corticosteroids may give temporary relief or induce temporary remissions early in the course of the disease. Bacterial infections are treated with appropriate antibiotics.

Immunosuppressive treatment with methotrexate and other cytotoxic agents has been reported to induce remissions lasting over 2 years. Combined treatment with corticosteroids and cytotoxic agents has resulted in remission for as long as 8 years.

Gullion DS: Wegener's granulomatosis. Western J Med 121:123, 1974.
Raitt JW: Wegener's granulomatosis: Treatment with cytotoxic agents and adrenocorticoids. Ann Int Med 74:344, 1971.

ANKYLOSING SPONDYLITIS
(Rheumatoid Spondylitis, Marie-Strümpell Disease)

Essentials of Diagnosis
- Chronic backache in a young man.
- Progressive limitation of back motion and of chest expansion.
- Transient (50%) or permanent (25%) peripheral joint involvement indistinguishable from peripheral rheumatoid arthritis.
- Diagnostic x-ray changes in sacroiliac joints.
- Uveitis in 20–25%.
- Accelerated erythrocyte sedimentation rate and negative serologic tests for rheumatoid factor.
- A positive test for the histocompatibility antigen HL-A 27 (80–90% of cases).

General Considerations
Ankylosing spondylitis, frequently familial, is a chronic inflammatory disease of the joints of the axial skeleton, manifested clinically by pain and progressive stiffening of the spine. While the synovitis of ankylosing spondylitis is histologically identical with that of peripheral rheumatoid arthritis, certain features tend to distinguish this disease from rheumatoid arthritis: its preponderance among males (approximately 10:1); age at onset (usually in late teens or early 20s); the relatively high incidence of uveitis; a pathologically distinctive lesion of the aorta; and absence of "rheumatoid factor." In addition to the synovitis, a second pathologic feature of ankylosing spondylitis involves the intervertebral fibrocartilages: the annulus fibrosis may gradually ossify, with fusion of vertebral bodies.

Clinical Findings
A. Symptoms and Signs: The onset is usually gradual, with intermittent bouts of back pain which may radiate down the thighs. As the disease advances, symptoms progress in a cephalad direction and back motion becomes limited, with the normal lumbar curve flattened and the thoracic curvature exaggerated. Atrophy of the trunk muscles is common. Chest expansion is often limited as a consequence of costovertebral joint involvement. Radicular symptoms may occur.

Sciatica or the cauda equina syndrome may occur and is frequently progressive. In advanced cases the entire spine becomes fused, allowing no motion in any direction. Transient, acute arthritis of the peripheral joints occurs in about 50% of cases, and permanent changes in the peripheral joints—most commonly the hips, shoulders, and knees—are seen in about 25%. Spondylitic heart disease, characterized chiefly by atrioventricular conduction defects, aortic insufficiency, and cardiac enlargement, occurs in 3–10% of patients. Nongranulomatous uveitis may occur in as many as 25% of cases and may be a presenting feature. About 8% of patients develop evidence of amyloidosis. Constitutional symptoms similar to those of rheumatoid arthritis may occasionally be present.

B. Laboratory Findings: The erythrocyte sedimentation rate is accelerated in 85% of cases, but serologic tests for rheumatoid factor are usually negative. There may be leukocytosis and anemia. The CSF protein is frequently elevated.

The remarkable frequency in patients with ankylosing spondylitis of the histocompatibility (transplantation) antigen HL-A 27 (80–90%, as opposed to 4–8% among normal individuals) makes this an important diagnostic test. While the cellular membrane antigens determined by the major histocompatibility locus in man (HL-A system) are found with greater than normal frequency in some other diseases, the most striking association is that between HL-A 27 and certain rheumatic diseases—notably ankylosing spondylitis, Reiter's syndrome, and the sacroiliitis and spondylitis associated with psoriasis and inflammatory bowel disease (see below). Family studies support the notion that HL-A 27 is a genetic marker which predisposes the individual to one of these disorders; thus, its presence may portend the diagnosis. Indeed, the diagnosis of one of these disorders is only suspect in the absence of HL-A 27.

Persons with other rheumatic diseases such as rheumatoid arthritis, degenerative joint disease (osteoarthritis), and gout do not show a higher than normal incidence of HL-A 27.

C. X-Ray Findings: Early in the course of ankylosing spondylitis, x-ray shows early erosion and sclerosis of the sacroiliac joints; later, one sees involvement of the apophyseal joints of the spine, ossification of the annulus fibrosis, calcification of the anterior and lateral spinal ligaments, and squaring and generalized demineralization of the vertebral bodies. The term "bamboo spine" has been used to describe the late radiographic changes.

Additional x-ray findings include periosteal new bone formation on the iliac crest, ischial tuberosities, and calcanei and alterations of the symphysis pubis and sternomanubrial joint similar to those of the sacroiliacs. Radiologic changes in peripheral joints, when present, resemble those of rheumatoid arthritis.

Differential Diagnosis

Although peripheral rheumatoid arthritis may ultimately involve the spine, it does so characteristi-

cally in the cervical region, usually sparing the sacroiliac joints. Other features which differentiate ankylosing spondylitis from peripheral rheumatoid arthritis are the rare involvement of the small joints of the hands and feet, the absence of subcutaneous nodules, and the negative serologic tests for rheumatoid factor in spondylitis. The history and physical findings of ankylosing spondylitis serve to distinguish this disorder from other causes of low back pain such as degenerative disk disease, degenerative joint disease, osteoporosis, soft tissue trauma, and tumors. The single most valuable distinguishing radiologic sign of ankylosing spondylitis is the appearance of the sacroiliac joints, although a similar pattern may be seen in juvenile rheumatoid arthritis; in arthritis associated with psoriasis, ulcerative colitis, regional enteritis, and Whipple's disease; and as a sequel to Reiter's syndrome, especially after frequent recurrences. The x-ray appearance of the sacroiliac joints in spondylitis should be distinguished from that in osteitis condensans ilii. In some geographic areas and in persons with appropriate occupations, brucellosis and fluoride poisoning may be important in the differential diagnosis.

Treatment

A. Basic Program: In general, treatment is as for rheumatoid arthritis. The importance of postural and breathing exercises should be stressed. When spondylitis is associated with chronic ulcerative colitis, regional enteritis, or psoriasis, appropriate treatment of these disorders sometimes (but not often) improves the spondylitis.

B. Drug Therapy: Phenylbutazone and oxyphenbutazone are potent analgesic and anti-inflammatory agents which in small doses are often remarkably effective against ankylosing spondylitis and may be used cautiously if response to salicylates is inadequate. They are contraindicated by peptic ulcer, cardiac decompensation, or significant renal, hepatic, or hematopoietic dysfunction. Give the least amount that will provide symptomatic improvement. Start with 100 mg daily and increase if necessary to 100 mg every 12 hours or every 8 hours, but do not give more than 300 mg daily except for very short periods during flare-ups. The drug may be continued cautiously as long as required for symptomatic relief unless toxic reactions occur. Special precautions include blood counts twice weekly for 4 weeks, once weekly for the next 4 weeks, and once every 2 or 3 weeks thereafter. Toxic reactions include salt and water retention, rash, agranulocytosis and other hematologic abnormalities, and peptic ulcer. If toxicity occurs, withdraw the drug immediately. Corticosteroids or corticotropin may be helpful in the treatment of agranulocytosis.

Indomethacin is also an effective anti-inflammatory analgesic drug which would seem at present to be less toxic than the butazones. The initial dosage is 25 mg twice daily, increasing weekly to the lowest effective dose (but not to exceed 50 mg 3 times daily). Indomethacin may produce a variety of untoward reactions, including headache, giddiness, nausea and vomiting, peptic ulcer, depression, and psychosis.

C. X-ray radiation to painful areas of the spine often provides symptomatic relief but has lost favor because of the high incidence of leukemia in patients so treated.

D. Corticosteroids may be given as for rheumatoid arthritis.

E. Physical Therapy: See p 500.

Prognosis

Spontaneous remissions and relapses are common and may occur at any stage. Occasionally, the disease progresses to ankylosis of the entire spine. In general, the functional prognosis is good unless the hips are seriously and permanently involved.

Brewerton D & others: Perspective: The histocompatibility antigen (HL-A27) and its relation to disease. J Rheum 1:249, 1974.

Calabro JJ, Maltz BA: Ankylosing spondylitis. New England J Med 282:606, 1970.

Espinoza L & others: Ankylosing spondylitis: Family studies and HL-A27 antigen distribution. J Rheum 1:254, 1974.

Godfrey RG & others: A double-blind crossover trial of aspirin, indomethacin, and phenylbutazone in ankylosing spondylitis. Arthritis Rheum 15:110, 1972.

Polley HF: Ankylosing spondylitis. Postgrad Med 51:53, 1972.

Schlosstein L & others: High association of an HL-A antigen, W27, with ankylosing spondylitis. New England J Med 288:704, 1973.

ARTHRITIS & INFLAMMATORY INTESTINAL DISEASES

Arthritis is a common complication of ulcerative colitis, regional enteritis, and Whipple's disease. Occasionally, such joint disease is indistinguishable from rheumatoid arthritis and may represent a coincidence of the 2 disorders. More commonly, however, the so-called "intestinal arthritis" is asymmetric, affects large joints, parallels the course of the bowel disease, and rarely results in residual deformity. Ankylosing spondylitis affects 2–5% of patients, is indistinguishable from true ankylosing spondylitis, and usually runs a course separate from bowel disease activity.

The synovitis is pathologically nonspecific. Rheumatoid factor is usually absent from the serum. The test for HL-A 27 antigen is positive in the presence of sacroiliitis or spondylitis. Treatment of the joint disorder that resembles rheumatoid arthritis is the same as for rheumatoid arthritis; that of intestinal arthritis involves control of intestinal inflammation and use of supportive anti-inflammatory drugs; that of ankylosing spondylitis is the same as for idiopathic ankylosing spondylitis.

Haslock I, Wright V: Arthritis associated with intestinal disease. Bull Rheumat Dis 24:973, 1974.

Reynolds MD, Rankin TJ: Diagnosis of "rheumatoid variants": Ankylosing spondylitis, the arthritides of gastrointestinal disease and psoriasis, and Reiter's syndrome. Western J Med 120:441, 1974.

Russell A & others: HL-A (transplantation) antigens in ankylosing spondylitis and Crohn's disease. J Rheum 1:203, 1974.

ARTHRITIS & PSORIASIS

In many patients with coexisting joint disease and psoriasis, the arthritic component is indistinguishable from rheumatoid arthritis. There is, however, a group of persons with psoriasis whose articular findings are sufficiently distinct to warrant classification as a separate category: psoriatic arthritis. In them, the psoriasis usually, but not invariably, precedes the onset of arthritis; the articular and cutaneous lesions may recur together and relapse simultaneously. The joint manifestations occur more frequently with generalized than with local psoriatic involvement. In contrast with that of rheumatoid arthritis, the onset of psoriatic arthritis is often in the distal rather than the proximal interphalangeal joints of the fingers or toes. The distal interphalangeal joint disease of psoriasis is almost always associated with psoriasis of the nails. Any peripheral joint may be affected, but—again in contrast with rheumatoid arthritis—the distribution of joint involvement is often asymmetric, fewer joints are usually involved, subluxation is uncommon, and there is little tendency to ulnar drift of the digits. Low back pain and spondylitis, when they occur, are usually late manifestations. Rheumatoid nodules are absent, and serologic tests for rheumatoid factor are negative. Serum uric acid may be elevated, especially in generalized psoriasis, as a consequence of rapid turnover of nucleoproteins in psoriatic skin. The test for the histocompatibility antigen HL-A 27 is positive in at least 25% of patients with psoriatic arthritis and in nearly all of those who have sacroiliitis or spondylitis.

Radiologic findings in psoriatic arthritis are often distinctive. These include multiple articular erosions in the distal interphalangeal and other peripheral joints, little or no osteoporosis, frequent synostosis, and fluffy periosteal new bone formation adjacent to capsules and tendons, notably those of the calcaneus, with resulting painful heel. Severe osteolysis and wide gaps between bones may be observed. These are especially common in affected digits, where bony proliferation at the base of the distal phalanx may be seen. X-ray evidence of sacroiliac involvement and spondylitis is seen in 25–35% of patients with psoriatic arthritis.

The treatment of arthritis with psoriasis is similar to that of rheumatoid arthritis or ankylosing spondylitis, depending on whether peripheral or spinal arthritis is present. However, drugs causing skin reactions should be avoided when possible. Serious adverse effects (eg, cirrhosis) have tempered the early enthusiasm for cytotoxic agents such as methotrexate.

Engleman EP: Psoriatic arthritis and Reiter's syndrome. Postgrad Med 51:37, 1972.
Metzgar A & others: HL-AW 27 in psoriatic arthropathy. Arthritis Rheum 18:111, 1975.
Muller SA, Farrow GM, Martalock DL: Cirrhosis caused by
methotrexate in the treatment of psoriasis. Arch Dermat
100:523, 1969.
Wright V, Moll J: Psoriatic arthritis. Bull Rheumat Dis 21:627,
1971.

REITER'S SYNDROME

Reiter's syndrome is a clinical tetrad of unknown
cause consisting of nonspecific urethritis, conjunctivitis
(or, less commonly, uveitis), mucocutaneous manifestations, and arthritis. It occurs most commonly in
young men. It may follow (within a few days to 4
weeks) sexual intercourse or diarrhea, and is usually
accompanied by a systemic reaction, including fever
(without chills). The arthritis is most commonly asymmetric, and frequently involves the large weight-bearing joints (chiefly the knee and ankle); sacroiliitis or
ankylosing spondylitis may occur. The mucocutaneous
lesions may include balanitis, stomatitis, and kerato-
derma blennorrhagica, resembling pustular psoriasis
with involvement of the skin and nails. Carditis and
aortic regurgitation may occur. While most signs of the
disease disappear within days or weeks, the arthritis
may persist for several months or even years. The test
for HL-A 27 antigen is positive in 80–90% of patients
and may thus be diagnostic. (See p 487 for further
discussion of HL-A 27.) Characteristically, the initial
attack is self-limited and terminates spontaneously.

Recurrences involving any combination of the
clinical manifestations are common and are sometimes
followed by permanent sequelae, especially in the
joints. X-ray signs of permanent or progressive joint
disease may be seen in the sacroiliac as well as the
peripheral joints.

Reiter's syndrome must be distinguished from
gonococcal arthritis, postgonococcal rheumatoid arthritis, rheumatoid arthritis, or ankylosing spondylitis
that follow nonspecific urethritis incidentally and from
psoriatic arthritis.

Treatment is symptomatic. The most effective
analgesic and anti-inflammatory drugs are usually
phenylbutazone, oxyphenbutazone, and indomethacin.
(See p 490 for drug therapy of ankylosing spondylitis.)

Engleman EP, Weber HM: Reiter's syndrome: Rheumatic mani-
festations of systemic disease. Clin Orthop 57:19, 1968.
McClusky OE & others: HL-A27 in Reiter's syndrome and
psoriatic arthritis: A genetic factor in disease susceptibil-
ity and expression. J Rheum 1:263, 1974.
Morris R & others: HL-A W27: A clue to the diagnosis and
pathogenesis of Reiter's syndrome. New England J Med
290:554, 1974.
Paulus HE, Pearson CM, Pitts W Jr: Aortic insufficiency in
Reiter's syndrome. Am J Med 53:464, 1972.
Sholkoff SD, Glickman MG, Steinbach HL: Roentgenology of
Reiter's syndrome. Radiology 97:497, 1970.

• • •

DEGENERATIVE JOINT DISEASE
(Osteoarthritis)

Essentials of Diagnosis

- A degenerative disorder without systemic
  manifestations.
- Pain relieved by rest.
- Articular inflammation minimal.
- X-ray findings: Narrowed joint space, osteophytes, increased density of subchondral
  bone, bony cysts.
- Commonly secondary to other articular disease.

General Considerations

Degenerative joint disease is a chronic, progressive
arthropathy characterized by degeneration of cartilage
and by hypertrophy of bone at the articular margins.
Inflammation is usually minimal, and thus the popular
term osteoarthritis is inappropriate. Hereditary and
mechanical factors may be variably involved in the
pathogenesis.

Degenerative joint disease is traditionally divided
into 2 types: (1) primary, which most commonly affects the terminal interphalangeal joints (Heberden's
nodes) and less commonly the proximal interphalangeal joints (so-called Bouchard's nodes), the metacarpophalangeal and carpometacarpal joints of the thumb,
the hip (malum coxae senilis), the knee, the metatarsophalangeal joint of the big toe, and the cervical and
lumbar spine; and (2) secondary, which may occur in
any joint as a sequel to articular injury resulting from
either intra-articular (including rheumatoid arthritis) or
extra-articular causes. The injury may be acute, as in a
fracture; or chronic, as that due to overweight, bad
posture, occupational overuse of a joint, or metabolic
diseases (eg, hyperparathyroidism, hemochromatosis,
ochronosis). The articular cartilage is first roughened
and finally worn away, and spur formation and lipping
occur at the edge of the joint surface. The synovial
membrane becomes thickened, with hypertrophy of
the villous processes; the joint cavity, however, never
becomes totally obliterated, and the synovial membrane does not form adhesions. As indicated above,
inflammation is characteristically minimal except for
that observed in acute interphalangeal joint involvement (Heberden's node) and in "primary generalized
osteoarthritis," in which many small joints may be
affected, especially those of the fingers (exclusive of
the metacarpophalangeal joints).

Clinical Findings

A. Symptoms and Signs: The onset is insidious.
Initially, there is articular stiffness; this develops later
into pain on motion of the affected joint and is made
worse by prolonged activity and relieved by rest. Deformity may be absent or minimal; however, bony

enlargement is occasionally prominent, and flexion contracture or valgus or varus deformity of the knee is not unusual. There is no ankylosis, but limitation of motion of the affected joint or joints is common. Coarse crepitus may often be felt in the joint. Joint effusion and other articular signs of inflammation are mild. There are no systemic manifestations.

B. Laboratory Findings: Elevated sedimentation rate and other laboratory signs of inflammation or dysproteinemia are not present.

C. X-Ray Findings: X-rays may reveal narrowing of the joint space, sharpened articular margins, osteophyte formation and lipping of marginal bone, and damaged and thickened, dense subchondral bone. Bone cysts may also be present.

Differential Diagnosis

Because articular inflammation is minimal and systemic manifestations are absent, degenerative joint disease should seldom be confused with other arthritides. The appearance of the hands in degenerative joint disease may mimic that in rheumatoid arthritis. Bony rather than soft tissue swelling and lack of involvement of the metacarpophalangeal joints are helpful indications in diagnosis. The neurogenic arthropathy of Charcot is easily distinguished by x-ray and neurologic examination. Degenerative joint disease may coexist with any other type of joint disease. Furthermore, one must be cautious in attributing all skeletal symptoms to degenerative changes in joints, especially in the spine, where metastatic neoplasia, osteoporosis, multiple myeloma, or other bone disease may coexist.

Treatment

A. General Measures:

1. Rest—Physical activity that induces physiologic or traumatic strain should be avoided. Occupational or recreational overuse of an affected joint must be prevented. If weight-bearing joints are involved, such weight-bearing activities as climbing stairs, walking, or prolonged standing should be minimized. Postural strain should be corrected. Supports which relieve strain due to pendulous abdomen or breasts should be supplied.

2. Diet should be adjusted to meet the patient's needs. In obese patients, weight reduction helps to diminish stress on the joints.

3. Local heat in any form and other forms of physical therapy are often of symptomatic value.

B. Analgesic Drugs: Salicylates (as for rheumatoid arthritis) are indicated for the relief of pain. Indomethacin, 50—75 mg/day in divided doses, may be effective temporarily, especially in joint disease of the hip.

C. Intra-articular corticosteroids (as for rheumatoid arthritis) may give transient relief.

D. Orthopedic Measures: * Orthopedic measures

*See General Measures in the Management of Arthritic Joints, p 500. For cervical traction, see p 512.

to correct developmental anomalies, deformities, disparity in leg length, and severely damaged joint surfaces may be required.

Prognosis

Although marked disability is less common than in rheumatoid arthritis, symptoms may be quite severe and limit activity markedly. This is especially true of involvement of the hips, knees, and cervical spine. Although there is no cure, proper treatment may greatly relieve symptoms and thereby improve function.

Bollet AJ: An essay on the biology of osteoarthritis. Arthritis Rheum 12:152, 1969.

Howell DS & others: A comprehensive regimen for osteoarthritis. M Clin North America 55:457, 1971.

Kellgren JH & others: Genetic factors in generalized osteoarthritis. Ann Rheumat Dis 22:237, 1969.

Radin EL & others: Pattern of degenerative arthritis: Preferential involvement of distal finger-joints. Lancet 1:377, 1971.

NEUROGENIC ARTHROPATHY
(Charcot Joint)

Neurogenic arthropathy is joint destruction resulting from loss or diminution of proprioception, pain, and temperature perception. Although traditionally associated with tabes dorsalis, it is more frequently seen in diabetic neuropathy, syringomyelia, spinal cord injury, subacute combined degeneration of pernicious anemia, and peripheral nerve injury. Prolonged administration of hydrocortisone by the intra-articular route may also cause Charcot joint. As normal muscle tone and protective reflexes are lost, a marked traumatic (secondary) degenerative joint disease ensues; this results in an enlarged, boggy, painless joint with extensive erosion of cartilage, osteophyte formation, and multiple loose joint bodies. X-ray changes, although sometimes "classical," may be degenerative or hypertrophic in the same patient.

Treatment is directed against the primary disease; mechanical devices are used to assist in weight-bearing and prevention of further trauma. In some instances, amputation becomes unavoidable.

Sinha S, Munichoodappa CS, Kozak GP: Neuro-arthropathy (Charcot joints) in diabetes mellitus: Clinical study of 101 cases. Medicine 51:191, 1972.

ACUTE INFECTIOUS (SEPTIC) ARTHRITIS

Essentials of Diagnosis

- Sudden onset of acute arthritis, usually monarticular, most often in large weight-bearing joints and wrists, frequently preceded by migratory arthralgia.

- Frank chills and fever.
- Joint fluid findings often diagnostic.
- Dramatic therapeutic response to appropriate antibiotic.
- Similar infection commonly found elsewhere in body.

General Considerations

The pyogenic cocci (gonococcus, meningococcus, staphylococcus, pneumococcus, and streptococcus), *Haemophilus influenzae,* and gram-negative bacilli are the usual causes of this form of arthritis. The organisms may enter the joints directly, as in local trauma or needling or by extension from adjacent bone; or indirectly, by hematogenous spread. In recent years this type of disease has been seen more commonly as a result of the development of resistant strains of organisms, the increasing therapeutic use of intra-articular injections, and the decreasing mortality of premature infants, in whom the incidence of septic arthritis is relatively high. The worldwide increase of gonococcal infections, particularly antibiotic-resistant, has posed a special problem. Pathologic changes include varying degrees of acute inflammation with synovitis, effusion, abscess formation in synovial or subchondral tissues, and, if treatment is not adequate, articular destruction.

Clinical Findings

A. Symptoms and Signs: The onset is usually sudden; the joint becomes acutely painful, hot, and swollen; and chills and fever are often present. In gonococcal infections, disseminated infections may be seen in individuals whose primary infection may be asymptomatic. The large weight-bearing joints and the wrists are most frequently affected. Although only one or 2 joints are affected, there may be a prodromal period of migratory arthralgia which may last for several days; this is especially true during the period of bacteremia.

Special attention is called to the systemic manifestations of gonococcal infection. Disseminated infection is seen not uncommonly in individuals whose anogenital or throat infection may be asymptomatic. Dissemination in females usually occurs during pregnancy or menstruation. The initial bacteremic stage may persist for weeks and may be characterized not only by migratory arthralgia but also by chills and fever or normal temperature and by typical skin lesions. The latter are commonly tiny red papules or petechiae which may disappear or progress through transient vesicular, pustular, and bullous stages. The organism may be recovered from these lesions. Tenosynovitis is commonly observed. Less common systemic complications are liver function abnormalities, myocarditis or pericarditis, meningitis, and endocarditis.

B. Laboratory Findings: The leukocyte count of the synovial fluid may be as high as 100,000/cu mm, with 90% or more polymorphonuclear cells. Synovial fluid sugar is usually low. The organisms are often demonstrated by smear or culture. However, there is increasing evidence that articular infection starts in the periarticular tissues and that organisms do not appear in synovial fluid unless the infective focus ulcerates into the joint cavity. In gonococcal arthritis, for example, the gonococcus is recovered from joint fluid in only half of cases. Throat and anorectal cultures for gonococci as well as blood and genital cultures are required whenever infection with this organism is suspected.

C. X-Ray Findings: X-rays are usually normal early in the disease, but radiologic evidence of demineralization may be present within days of onset. Bony erosions and narrowing of the joint space followed by osteomyelitis and periostitis may be seen within 2 weeks.

Differential Diagnosis

The septic course with chills and fever, the acute systemic reaction, the joint fluid findings, evidence of similar infection elsewhere in the body, and the dramatic response to appropriate antibiotics are diagnostic of pyogenic arthritis. Gout and pseudogout are excluded by the absence of hyperuricemia and the failure to find crystals on synovial fluid analysis. Acute rheumatic fever and rheumatoid arthritis commonly involve many joints and are not associated with chills. Pyogenic arthritis may be superimposed on other types of joint disease, notably rheumatoid arthritis, and must be excluded (by joint fluid examination) in any apparent acute relapse of the primary disease, particularly when a joint has been needled or one is more strikingly inflamed than the others.

Treatment

Prompt systemic antibiotic therapy should be based on the best clinical judgement of the causative organism and the results of smear and culture of joint fluid, blood, urine, or other specific sites of potential infection. If the organism cannot be determined clinically, treatment should be started with bactericidal antibiotics effective against staphylococci, pneumococci, gonococci, and gram-negative organisms. Cultures for gonococci require immediate inoculation of Thayer-Martin medium.

Frequent (even daily) local aspiration is sometimes indicated. Incision and drainage are required rarely. Relieve pain with local hot compresses and by immobilizing the joint with a splint or traction (or both). Rest, immobilization, and elevation are used at the onset of treatment. Early active motion exercises within the limits of tolerance will hasten recovery.

Prognosis

With prompt antibiotic therapy (within 7–10 days of onset), functional recovery is usually complete. Bony ankylosis and articular destruction commonly occur if treatment is inadequate.

Brandt KD, Cathcart ES, Cohen AS: Gonococcal arthritis: Clinical features correlated with blood, synovial fluid and genitourinary cultures. Arthritis Rheum 17:503, 1974.

Goldenberg DL & others: Treatment of septic arthritis: Comparison of needle aspiration and surgery as initial modes of joint drainage. Arthritis Rheum 18:83, 1975.

Holmes KK & others: Disseminated gonococcal infection. Ann Int Med 74:979, 1971.

Medical Staff Conference, University of California, San Francisco: Gonococcal sepsis and arthritis. California Med 114:18, Jan 1971.

Nelson JD: Antibiotic concentrations in septic joint effusions. New England J Med 284:349, 1971.

Russell AS, Ansel BM: Septic arthritis. Ann Rheumat Dis 31:40, 1972.

Schmid FR, Parker RH: Ongoing assessment of therapy in septic arthritis. Arthritis Rheum 12:529, 1969.

The goal of treatment is eradication of infection and restoration of maximum joint function. Bacterial sensitivity tests provide a basis for selection of antimicrobial drugs to be used as an adjunct to surgical operations. Operative destruction of the joint by arthrodesis, debridement, saucerization of bone, or resection is often necessary.

Jergesen F, Jawetz E: Pyogenic infections in orthopaedic surgery: Combined antibiotic and closed wound treatment. Am J Surg 106:152, 1963.

Warren CPW: Arthritis associated with salmonella infection. Ann Rheumat Dis 29:483, 1970.

CHRONIC PYOGENIC ARTHRITIS

Chronic pyogenic arthritis follows untreated or unsuccessfully treated acute primary or secondary pyogenic arthritis. Inadequacy of treatment may be manifested by persistence of infection, but the course of the chronic disease is either intermittent or continuous at a slow rate. One or more pathogens may induce a purulent inflammatory response within a joint; pyogenic cocci and enteric gram-negative rods are more common. Although a previously identified pathogen is likely to persist, superinfection may occur, especially after open surgical treatment and antibiotics. The original bacterial strain may be eliminated by antimicrobial treatment only to be supplanted by another, or it may persist with the new invader to cause a mixed infection.

Chronic pyogenic arthritis is likely to produce variable but characteristic clinical pictures. An overt or manifest infection may be continuously or recurrently active. Uninterrupted progress from the acute stage is characterized by continued local pain and swelling, restriction of joint motion, sinus formation, and increasing deformity. X-rays show progressive destruction of cartilage, manifested by narrowing of the joint cleft, erosion of bone, and even infraction or cavitation. Even though the course is indolent, it is that of continued deterioration. In the recurrent type, apparent abatement may follow intermittent treatment, notably with antibiotics; but these episodes of comparative clinical quiescence reflect only temporary dormancy. Occult or covert infections are characterized by insidiousness and indolence. They may be unrecognized for long periods since they do not produce striking clinical findings. They may occur concomitantly with other joint lesions or complicate surgical operations on joints, especially after surgical implants or antibiotic prophylaxis of postoperative infection. Culture of synovial tissue taken for biopsy examination may be necessary.

Chronic pyogenic arthritis must be differentiated from all chronic nonpyogenic microbial infections of joints, gout, rheumatoid arthritis, and symptomatic degenerative arthritis.

INTERMITTENT HYDRARTHROSIS

Intermittent hydrarthrosis is a rare clinical entity of unknown cause which is characterized by episodes of often painless joint effusions, particularly in the knee, usually recurring at regular intervals and lasting several hours to several days. The attacks characteristically begin in adolescent females; the joints appear normal between attacks, and attacks frequently terminate or lessen with pregnancy or advancing age. A significant number of patients will later develop rheumatoid arthritis. Other causes of joint effusion must be carefully excluded before the diagnosis is considered.

Treatment is symptomatic and may include removal of joint fluid.

Ehrlich GE: Intermittent and periodic rheumatic syndromes. Bull Rheumat Dis 24:746, 1974.

PALINDROMIC RHEUMATISM

Palindromic rheumatism is a disease of unknown cause characterized by frequent recurring attacks (at irregular intervals) of acutely inflamed joints. Periarticular pain and swelling and transient subcutaneous nodules may also occur. The attacks cease within several hours to several days. The knee and finger joints are most commonly affected, but any peripheral joint may be involved. Systemic manifestations do not occur. Although hundreds of attacks may take place over a period of years, there is no permanent articular damage. Laboratory findings are usually normal. Palindromic rheumatism must be distinguished from acute gouty arthritis and an atypical, acute onset of rheumatoid arthritis.

Symptomatic treatment is usually all that is required during the attacks. Chrysotherapy may be of value in preventing recurrences.

Williams MH & others: Palindromic rheumatism: Clinical and immunologic studies. Ann Rheumat Dis 30:375, 1971.

GOUTY ARTHRITIS

Essentials of Diagnosis

- Acute onset, usually monarticular, involving the metatarsophalangeal joint of the big toe in about 50% of cases.
- Dramatic therapeutic response to colchicine.
- Postinflammatory desquamation and pruritus are almost pathognomonic.
- Hyperuricemia.
- Identification of urate crystals in joint fluid or tophi.
- Asymptomatic periods between acute attacks.
- Urate deposits in subcutaneous tissue, bone, cartilage, joints, and other tissues.
- Familial disease; 95% males.

General Considerations

Gout is a metabolic disease of heterogeneous nature, often familial, associated with abnormal amounts of urates in the body and characterized early by a recurring acute arthritis, usually monoarticular, and later by chronic deforming arthritis.

Primary gout is a heritable metabolic disease in which hyperuricemia is usually due to overproduction or underexcretion of uric acid—sometimes both. It is rarely due to a specifically determined genetic aberration (eg, Lesch-Nyhan syndrome). Secondary gout, which may have some latent heritable component, is related to acquired causes of hyperuricemia, eg, myeloproliferative disorders, multiple myeloma, hemoglobinopathies, chronic renal disease, thiazide drugs, and lead poisoning.

About 90% of patients with gout are men, usually over 30 years of age. In women the onset is usually postmenopausal. The characteristic histologic lesion is the tophus, a nodular deposit of monosodium urate monohydrate crystals, and an associated foreign body reaction. These may be found in cartilage, subcutaneous and periarticular tissues, tendon, bone, the kidneys, and elsewhere. Urates have been demonstrated in the synovial tissues (and fluid) during acute arthritis; indeed, the acute inflammation of gout is believed to be activated by the phagocytosis by polymorphonuclear cells of urate crystals with the ensuing release from the PMNs of chemotactic and other substances capable of mediating inflammation. The precise relationship of hyperuricemia to acute gouty arthritis is still obscure, since hyperuricemia may occur in patients who never have gouty arthritis. Recent studies suggest that rapid fluctuations in serum urate levels, either increasing or decreasing, are important factors in precipitating acute gout. The mechanism of the late, chronic stage of gouty arthritis is better understood. This is characterized pathologically by tophaceous invasion of the articular and periarticular tissues, with structural derangement and secondary degeneration (osteoarthritis).

Uric acid kidney stones are present in 10–20% of patients with gouty arthritis. Nephrosclerosis with renal dysfunction is common. The term gouty nephropathy (or "gouty nephritis"), which is much less common, refers to kidney disease due to tophaceous deposition in the renal parenchyma, chiefly the pyramids and the renal vasculature. It is often associated with pyelonephritis.

Hyperuricemia often occurs in patients without arthritis, urinary stones, or tophaceous deposits. Unless the serum uric acid levels are consistently higher than 11 mg/100 ml or are associated with rapid breakdown of cellular nucleic acid following aggressive treatment of leukemia or lymphoma, drug treatment need not be instituted until arthritis, renal calculi, or tophi become apparent. Psoriasis, sarcoidosis, and diuretic drugs are commonly overlooked causes of hyperuricemia. An adequate fluid intake and urinary output may suffice as treatment for uncomplicated hyperuricemia.

Clinical Findings

A. Symptoms and Signs: The acute arthritis is characterized by its sudden onset, frequently nocturnal, either without apparent precipitating cause or following rapid fluctuations in serum urate levels from food and alcohol excess, surgery, infection, diuretics, chemicals (eg, meglumine diatrizoate, Urografin), or uricosuric drugs. The metatarsophalangeal joint of the great toe is the most susceptible joint, although others, especially those of the feet, ankles, and knees, are commonly affected. More than one joint may occasionally be affected during the same attack; in such cases, the distribution of the arthritis is usually asymmetric. As the attack progresses, the pain becomes intense. The involved joints are swollen and exquisitely tender and the overlying skin tense, warm, and dusky red. Fever, headache, malaise, anorexia, and tachycardia are common. Local desquamation and pruritus during recovery from the acute arthritis are almost pathognomonic of gout but are not always present. Tophi may be found in the external ears, hands, feet, olecranon, and prepatellar bursas. They are usually seen only after several attacks of acute arthritis.

Asymptomatic periods of months or years commonly follow the initial acute attack. Later, gouty arthritis may become chronic, with symptoms of progressive functional loss and disability. Gross deformities, due usually to tophaceous invasion, are seen. Signs of inflammation may be absent or superimposed.

Hypertension, renal stones, and renal failure may be associated with gouty arthritis.

B. Laboratory Findings: The serum uric acid is practically always elevated (> 7.5 mg/100 ml) unless uricopenic drugs are being given (see p 1019). During an acute attack, the erythrocyte sedimentation rate white cell count are usually elevated. Examination of the material aspirated from a tophus shows the typical crystals of sodium urate and confirms the diagnosis. Further confirmation is obtained by identification of sodium urate crystals by compensated polariscopic examination of wet smears prepared from joint fluid aspirates. Such crystals are negatively birefringent and needle-like and may be found free or in cells.

C. X-Ray Findings: Early in the disease, x-rays show no changes. Later, punched-out areas in the bone (radiolucent urate tophi) are seen. Although bony punched-out areas may also be seen in rheumatoid arthritis, a punched-out area is diagnostic of gout if it is adjacent to a soft tissue tophus.

Differential Diagnosis

Once the diagnosis of acute gouty arthritis is suspected, it is easily confirmed by the presence of hyperuricemia, dramatic response to full doses of colchicine, local desquamation and pruritus as the edema subsides, positive identification of tophi, a positive family history, and polariscopic examination of joint fluid. Acute gout is often confused with cellulitis. Appropriate bacteriologic studies should exclude acute pyogenic arthritis. Acute chondrocalcinosis (pseudogout) may be distinguished by the identification of calcium pyrophosphate crystals in the joint fluid, usually normal serum uric acid, the x-ray appearance of chondrocalcinosis, and the relative therapeutic ineffectiveness of colchicine.

Chronic tophaceous arthritis may rarely mimic chronic rheumatoid arthritis. In such cases, the diagnosis of gout is established conclusively by the demonstration of urate crystals in the contents of a suspected tophus. Biopsy may be necessary to distinguish tophi from rheumatoid nodules. An x-ray appearance similar to that of gout may be found in rheumatoid arthritis, sarcoid, multiple myeloma, hyperparathyroidism, or Hand-Schüller-Christian disease.

Treatment

A. Acute Attack:

1. Colchicine, which may inhibit the chemotactic property of leukocytosis and thus interfere with the inflammatory response to urate crystals, is the traditional drug; it is used diagnostically as well as therapeutically. It should be given as early as possible in the acute attack or during the prodrome to obtain maximum benefit, since 75% of patients with acute gouty arthritis respond to colchicine, and failure of relief in the remainder may be related to a delay in the initiation of treatment. Trial with colchicine should not replace joint aspiration for diagnosis when an aspirable joint is readily accessible, since 80% of patients receiving colchicine have significant abdominal cramping, diarrhea, nausea, or vomiting. Give 0.5 or 0.6 mg every hour or 1 mg every 2 hours until pain is relieved or until nausea or diarrhea appears, and then stop the drug. The usual total dose required is 4—8 mg. The pain and swelling will subside in 24—72 hours. Once the patient knows how much will produce toxic symptoms, the drug should be given in a dose of about 1 mg less than the toxic dose. Colchicine-induced diarrhea is controlled with paregoric, 4 ml after each bowel movement. The incidence of gastrointestinal side-effects of colchicine can be reduced by intravenous administration in an initial dose of 1—3 mg in 10—20 ml of saline solution. This may be repeated in a few hours, but no more than 4—6 mg should be given IV within a period of 24 hours for a single attack. Colchicine occasionally causes local pain and tissue damage from occasional extravasation during injection. This route of administration of colchicine is rarely necessary and is inadvisable if the oral route can be used. Administration of usual doses of colchicine to patients with significant renal or hepatic disease may result in serious toxicity.

2. Phenylbutazone and oxyphenbutazone are remarkably effective anti-inflammatory agents in acute gout and are the drugs of choice when the diagnosis is well established. The initial dose is 400 mg, followed by 200 mg every 6 hours until the attack subsides; do not continue for more than 3 days. Toxicity is rarely a problem in such short-term use of phenylbutazone, except in the presence of active ulcer.

3. Indomethacin is said to be as effective as phenylbutazone in acute gout. Give 50 mg every 6 hours for 3—4 doses. When a response occurs, reduce dosage to 25 mg 3—4 times daily for 4—5 days. Active peptic ulcer is a contraindication.

4. Corticotropin (ACTH) and the corticosteroids often give dramatic symptomatic relief in acute episodes of gout, and if given for a sufficient length of time will control most acute attacks. However, when corticotropin and corticosteroids are discontinued shortly after termination of attacks, many patients promptly undergo relapse unless colchicine is given. Since colchicine, phenylbutazone, and indomethacin are equally or more effective and provide a more lasting effect, these agents are preferred.

5. Analgesics—At times the pain of an acute attack may be so severe that analgesia is necessary before a more specific drug becomes effective. In these cases, codeine or meperidine may be given. Cinchophen and neocinchophen should not be used because they cause severe liver damage.

6. Bed rest is very important in the management of the acute attack and should be continued for about 24 hours after the acute attack has subsided. Early ambulation may precipitate a recurrence. Physical therapy is of little value during the acute attack, although hot or cold compresses to or elevation of the affected joints may make some patients more comfortable.

B. Management Between Attacks: Treatment during symptom-free periods is intended to minimize urate deposition in tissues, which causes chronic tophaceous arthritis, and to reduce the frequency and severity of recurrences. There is evidence that these objectives are in fact attainable.

1. Diet—From a dietary standpoint, it would appear that it is most important simply to avoid obesity, fasting, dehydration, and acidosis. Rigid diets are nutritionally inadequate and often fail to influence the hyperuricemia or the course of gouty arthritis. Since dietary sources of purines contribute very little to the causation of the disease, restriction of foods high in purine (eg, kidney, liver, sweetbreads, sardines, anchovies, meat extracts) cannot be expected to contribute significantly to the management of the disease. Spe-

cific foods or alcoholic beverages that precipitate attacks should be avoided. However, there is little evidence that alcohol in moderation will precipitate attacks or is otherwise harmful in patients with gout. A high liquid intake and, more important, a daily urinary output of 2 liters or more will aid urate excretion and minimize urate precipitation in the urinary tract.

2. Colchicine—The daily administration of colchicine in a dose of 0.5 mg 3 times daily should be started simultaneously with uricosuric drugs or allopurinol in order to suppress the acute attack that may be precipitated by these drugs. After several weeks of such treatment, it is usually possible to lower the daily dose of colchicine to 0.5 mg. There is some suggestion that colchicine, even in this small dosage, has preventive value and should be continued indefinitely.

3. Reduction of serum uric acid—Indications include persistent serum uric acid levels greater than 9 mg/100 ml (colorimetric), frequent acute arthritis not controlled by colchicine prophylaxis, tophaceous deposits, or renal damage. It is emphasized that mild hyperuricemia which is either asymptomatic or associated only with infrequent attacks of arthritis may not require treatment.

Two classes of agents may be used to lower the serum uric acid—the uricosuric drugs and allopurinol (neither is of value in the treatment of acute gout).

a. Uricosuric drugs—These drugs, by blocking tubular reabsorption of filtered urate and reducing the metabolic pool of urates, prevent the formation of new tophi and reduce the size of those already present. Furthermore, when administered concomitantly with colchicine, they may lessen the frequency of recurrences of acute gout. The indications for uricosuric treatment are either the appearance of tophi on physical or x-ray examination, or increasing frequency or severity of the acute attacks.

The following uricosuric drugs may be employed:

(1) Probenecid (Benemid), starting with 0.5 gm daily and gradually increasing to 1–2 gm daily.

(2) Sulfinpyrazone (Anturane), starting with 100 mg daily and gradually increasing to 200–400 mg daily. In any case, the maintenance dose is determined by observation of the serum uric acid response and the urinary uric acid response. Ideally, one attempts to maintain a normal serum urate level.

Hypersensitivity to either uricosuric drug in the form of fever and rash occurs in 5% of cases; gastrointestinal complaints occur in 10%.

Precautions with uricosuric drugs: It is important to maintain a daily urinary output of 2000 ml or more in order to minimize the precipitation of uric acid in the urinary tract. This can be further prevented by giving alkalinizing agents to maintain a urine pH of above 6.0. If a significant uricosuric effect is not obtained in the presence of overt renal dysfunction, do not increase the dose of the drug beyond the limits stated above. Uricosuric drugs are probably contraindicated in patients with a history of uric acid lithiasis. Avoid using salicylates since they antagonize the action of uricosuric agents.

b. Allopurinol—The xanthine oxidase inhibitor allopurinol (Zyloprim) promptly lowers plasma urate and urinary uric acid concentrations and facilitates tophus mobilization. The drug is of special value in uric acid overproducers (as defined by urinary excretion of uric acid in excess of 800 mg per day while on a purine-free diet); in patients unresponsive to the uricosuric regimen; and in gouty patients with renal insufficiency or uric acid renal stones. It should be used cautiously in patients with renal insufficiency. The most frequent adverse effect is the precipitation of an acute gouty attack. However, the commonest sign of hypersensitivity to allopurinol (occurring in 5% of cases) is a pruritic rash which may progress to toxic epidermal necrolysis. Diffuse angiitis, renal failure, and death may also ensue if the drug is not discontinued as soon as signs of sensitivity appear.

The daily dose is determined by the serum uric acid response. A normal serum uric acid level is often obtained with a daily dose of 200–400 mg. Occasionally (and in selected cases) it may be helpful to continue the use of allopurinol with a uricosuric drug. Neither of these drugs is of help in acute gout.

Severe and potentially fatal hypersensitivity reactions associated with allopurinol have been reported.

C. Chronic Tophaceous Arthritis: There is good evidence that in the presence of adequate renal function tophaceous deposits can be made to shrink in size and occasionally to disappear altogether. The treatment is essentially the same as that outlined for the intervals between acute attacks. Surgical excision of large tophi offers immediate mechanical improvement in selected deformities and may lessen the load on renal function.

Prognosis

Without treatment, the acute attack may last from a few days to several weeks, but proper treatment quickly terminates the attack. The intervals between acute attacks vary up to years, but the asymptomatic periods often become shorter if the disease progresses. Chronic tophaceous arthritis occurs after repeated attacks of acute gout, but only after inadequate treatment. Although the deformities may be marked, only a small percentage of patients become bedridden. The younger the patient at the onset of disease, the greater the tendency to a progressive course. Destructive arthropathy is rarely seen in patients whose first attack is after age 50.

Patients with gout have an increased incidence of hypertension, renal disease (eg, nephrosclerosis, tophi, pyelonephritis), diabetes mellitus, hypertriglyceridemia, and atherosclerosis, although these relationships are not well understood.

Casagrande PA: Surgery of tophaceous gout. Seminars Arthritis Rheum 15:317, 1972.

Grahame R, Scott JT: Clinical survey of 354 patients with gout. Ann Rheumat Dis 29:461, 1970.

Gutman AB: Medical management of gout. Postgrad Med 51:47, 1972.

Hadler N: Acute polyarticular gout. Am J Med 56:715, 1974.

McCarty DJ Jr: Mechanisms of the crystal deposition diseases: Gout and pseudogout. Ann Int Med 78:767, 1973.

Rieselbach RE, Steele T: Influence of kidney upon urate homeostasis in health and disease. Am J Med 56:665, 1974.

Seegmiller JE & others: Purine overproduction in man associated with increased phosphoribosylpyrophosphate synthetase activity. Science 179:1123, 1973.

Spilberg I: Current concepts of the mechanism of acute inflammation in gouty arthritis. Arthritis Rheum 18:129, 1975.

Wallace SL: The treatment of gout. Arthritis Rheum 15:317, 1972.

Wyngaarden JB: Metabolic defects of primary hyperuricemia of gout. Am J Med 56:651, 1974.

CHONDROCALCINOSIS & PSEUDOGOUT

The term chondrocalcinosis refers to the presence of calcium-containing salts in articular cartilage. It is most often first diagnosed radiologically. It may be familial and is commonly associated with a wide variety of metabolic disorders, eg, hemochromatosis, hyperparathyroidism, ochronosis, diabetes mellitus, and true gout. Pseudogout, most often seen in persons age 60 or older, is characterized by acute recurrent arthritis which usually involves large joints (principally the knees) and is almost always accompanied by chondrocalcinosis of the affected joints. Identification of calcium pyrophosphate crystals in joint aspirates is diagnostic of pseudogout. Like the intra-articular urate crystals of gouty synovitis, calcium pyrophosphate crystals are believed to induce the synovitis of pseudogout. They may be seen with the ordinary light microscope but are best visualized under polarized light, in which they exhibit a weakly positive birefringence; like gouty crystals, they may be intracellular or extracellular. X-ray examination shows not only calcification (usually symmetric) of cartilaginous structures but also signs of advanced degenerative joint disease (osteoarthritis). Unlike gout, pseudogout is usually associated with normal serum urate levels and is not ordinarily benefited by colchicine.

Treatment of chondrocalcinosis is directed at the primary disease, if present. Some of the anti-inflammatory agents (eg, salicylates, indomethacin, phenylbutazone, corticosteroids) are helpful in the treatment of acute episodes of pseudogout. Aspiration of the inflamed joint and intra-articular injection of a hydrocortisone ester is also of benefit in resistant cases.

McCarty DJ & others: Disease associated with calcium pyrophosphate dihydrate crystal deposition. Am J Med 56:704, 1974.

Moskowitz RW, Garcia F: Chondrocalcinosis articularis (pseudogout syndrome). Arch Int Med 132:87, 1973.

ARTHRITIS IN SARCOIDOSIS

The frequency of arthritis among patients with sarcoidosis is variously reported between 10% and 37%. It is usually acute in onset, but articular symptoms may appear insidiously and often antedate other manifestations of the disease. Knees and ankles are most commonly involved, but any joint may be affected. Distribution of joint involvement is usually, but not always, polyarticular and symmetric. The arthritis is commonly self-limiting after several weeks or months; infrequently, the arthritis is recurrent or chronic. Despite its occasional chronicity, the arthritis is rarely associated with joint destruction or significant deformity. Although sarcoid arthritis is often associated with erythema nodosum, the diagnosis is contingent upon the demonstration of other extra-articular manifestations of sarcoidosis and, notably, biopsy evidence of epithelioid tubercles. In chronic arthritis, x-ray shows rather typical changes in the bones of the extremities with intact cortex and cystic changes. Typical sarcoid granulomas may be demonstrated by a biopsy of a chronically involved synovial membrane. Rheumatoid factor is sometimes present in low titers in the serum of patients with sarcoidosis, but this is a nonspecific finding and is unrelated to the joint disease.

Treatment of arthritis in sarcoidosis is usually symptomatic and supportive. Colchicine may be of value. A short course of corticosteroids may be effective in patients with severe and progressive joint disease.

The occurrence of joint disease is usually a favorable prognostic sign with respect to the course of sarcoidosis.

Spilberg I, Siltzbach LE, McEwen C: The arthritis of sarcoidosis. Arthritis Rheum 12:126, 1969.

BURSITIS

Bursae are closed sacs lined with a cellular membrane resembling synovium. They facilitate motion of tendons and muscles over bony prominences. Local pain and nonspecific inflammation may be provoked by friction or trauma or may occur without obvious cause. Bursitis may also be secondary to such other rheumatic diseases as rheumatoid arthritis or gout. Common sites of bursitis are the subdeltoid, olecranon, trochanteric, ischial ("weaver's bottom"), and prepatellar ("housemaid's knee") areas.

Tendinitis and bursitis are occasionally associated with periarticular calcific deposits, which may be present before the onset of pain and disappear weeks after the cessation of pain. Such attacks often simulate acute arthritis. They may occur in only one site but may involve multiple sites. They are referred to as calcific tendinitis or periarthritis, but there is usually no evidence of systemic or metabolic disorder in these cases.

Treatment of bursitis includes rest, immobilization, analgesia, local heat or other forms of physical therapy, and local injection of corticosteroids or systemic treatment with anti-inflammatory drugs.

Swannell AJ, Underwood FA, Dixon AS: Periarticular calcific deposits mimicking acute arthritis. Ann Rheumat Dis 29:380, 1970.

•   •   •

GENERAL PRINCIPLES IN THE PHYSICAL MANAGEMENT OF ARTHRITIC JOINTS

Proper physical management of arthritic joints can improve patient comfort and help preserve joint and muscle function and total well-being. In order to obtain optimal results, as well as to conserve financial resources and time, it is important for the physician to be as specific as possible in his instructions to the patient or to the occupational and physical therapists conducting treatment.

Exercise

A. Passive Range of Motion: Since someone other than the patient puts the joints through the range of motion once or twice daily, the patient is not directly involved and maintenance of muscle tone is not assisted. Passive exercises should be ordered infrequently and only for specific purposes.

B. Active Range of Motion: This type of exercise requires the patient to contract his own muscles in order to put joints through the range of motion. The prescribed motions should be repeated 3–10 times once or twice daily. Such active exercise should be encouraged since it involves the patient, costs no money, protects joint motion, and assists in maintaining muscle tone.

C. Isometric Exercise: With this type of exercise the muscle is contracted but not shortened, while the joint is minimally moved, for 3–10 repetitions several times daily. This maintains or even increases muscle strength and tone; the patient is involved, joint use is minimal, and the cost is nil. Isometric exercise should be used to supplement passive or active range of motion exercises.

D. Isotonic Exercise: In isotonic exercise, the muscle is contracted and shortened and the joint is maximally moved and stressed. This type of exercise should seldom be used (see below).

E. Hydrotherapy: The buoyancy of water permits maximum isotonic and isometric exercise with no more stress on joints than active range-of-motion exer-

cises. Though ideal for arthritic patients, its cost often precludes use and it is generally prescribed only for specific short-term goals.

F. Active-Assistive Exercise: The therapist provides direct supervision, physical support, and exercise guidance. Although this is ideal for arthritic patients, cost again often precludes its use except for specific short-term goals. A member of the family may be taught to assist the patient in his exercises on a long-term basis.

Note: Any exercise in the arthritic patient may be associated with some pain, but pain lasting for hours after exercise is an indication for a change in the duration or type of exercise.

Heat, Cold, & Massage

A. Heat: Most patients with chronic arthritis find that some form of heat gives temporary muscle relaxation and relief of pain. Generally, moist heat is more effective than electric pads or heat lamps. Tub baths may require some bar supports for ease of entry and exit. Paraffin dips may spare the patient the "dishpan hands" caused by water.

B. Cold: Some patients with particularly acute arthritis or acutely injured arthritic joints find that cold (ice pack or bag) relieves pain more effectively than does heat.

C. Massage: While massage is helpful in relaxing muscles and giving psychologic support, it provides only temporary relief, and its cost is usually high.

Splints

Splints may provide joint rest, reduce pain, and prevent contracture, but certain principles should be adhered to.

(1) Night splints of the hands or wrists (or both) should maintain the extremity in the position of optimum function. The elbow and shoulder lose motion so rapidly that other local measures and corticosteroid injections are usually preferable to splints.

(2) The best "splint" for the hip is prone-lying for several hours a day on a firm bed. For the knee, prone-lying may suffice, but splints in maximum tolerated extension are frequently needed. Ankle splints are of the simple right-angle type.

(3) Splints should be applied for the shortest period needed, should be made of light-weight materials for comfort, and should be easily removable for range-of-motion exercises once or twice daily to prevent loss of motion.

(4) Corrective splints, such as those for overcoming knee flexion contractures, should be used under the guidance of a physician familiar with their proper use.

Note: Avoidance of prolonged sitting or knee pillows may decrease the need for splints.

Braces

Unstable joints—particularly the knee and wrist—can be supported, and the pain of weight-bearing may be relieved, by appropriately prescribed braces.

Assistive Devices

Patient-oriented publications (see references at end of section), physical therapists, occupational therapists, and home health nurses can be of help to the patient in securing appropriate bars, raised toilet seats, long-handled reachers, and other assistive devices that are available to help arthritic patients deal with the activities of daily living.

Referral of the Patient for Surgical Opinion by an Orthopedist

A. Synovectomy: This procedure has been used for over 50 years to attempt to retard joint destruction by invasive synovial pannus of rheumatoid arthritis. It remains a controversial procedure because (1) it is chiefly of value if done early and debridement is feasible, but this is a time when both the doctor and the patient find it difficult to determine the future course of the disease; and (2) recurrences are not uncommon. In selected cases, the areas where synovectomy is most likely to be successful are the metacarpophalangeal joints, the wrists and overlying tendons, and the knees. The major indication for synovectomy is intractable pain in an isolated joint, most commonly the knee.

B. Joint Replacement: Total hip replacement by methylmethacrylate has a high degree of success. Infection, the major complication of this procedure, is uncommon. The long-term effects of replacement of the knee—and more recently the ankle, shoulder, and metacarpophalangeal joints—have not been fully determined.

C. Arthroplasty: Realignment and reconstruction of the knee, wrist, and small joints of the hand are feasible in a small number of selected patients.

D. Tendon Rupture: This is a fairly common complication in rheumatoid arthritis and requires immediate orthopedic referral. The most common sites are the finger flexors and extensors, the patellar tendon, and the Achilles tendon.

E. Arthrodesis: Arthrodesis (fusion) is being used less now than formerly, but a chronically infected, painful joint may be an indication for this surgical procedure.

Joint Protection Program

Physical and occupational therapists can instruct patients in changing their daily habits and their occupational and recreational activities to lessen damage to joints, maintain range of motion, and lessen pain and muscle atrophy.

Harris WH: Surgical management of arthritis of the hip. Seminars Arthritis Rheum 1:35, 1971.

Home Care Programs in Arthritis: A Manual for Patients. Arthritis Foundation, 1969.

Katz S & others: Outpatient care in rheumatoid arthritis. JAMA 206:1249, 1968.

Kenright J, Duthie RB: Surgical management of arthritis of the knee. Seminars Arthritis Rheum 1:35, 1971.

Lowman EW: Clinical management of disability due to rheumatoid arthritis. Arch Phys Med Rehabil 48:136, 1967.

Swezey RL: Dynamic factors in deformity of the rheumatoid arthritic hand. Bull Rheumat Dis 22:649, 1971.

14 . . .
Bone & Joint Diseases

Floyd H. Jergesen

INFECTIONS OF BONES & JOINTS

OSTEOMYELITIS

Osteomyelitis is acute or chronic inflammation of bone due to infection. It may be classified according to the mechanism of introduction of the causative agent (ie, as primary or secondary) or on the basis of microbial etiology.

Primary osteomyelitis is caused by direct implantation of microorganisms into bone and is likely to be localized to the site of inoculation. Open (compound) fractures, penetrating wounds (especially those due to firearms), and surgical operations on bone commonly provide access for microbial contamination. Diagnostic intramedullary aspiration or injection of drugs accounts for an occasional infection. Operative treatment is usually necessary; the principal adjunctive treatment is with antimicrobial drugs. Because the selection of a particular operative technic depends in part upon the type of associated bone lesion, primary osteomyelitis is usually discussed in conjunction with open fractures, penetrating wounds, and postoperative wound complications.

The route of infection of **secondary osteomyelitis** is usually through the arteries. Exceptions are spread through veins to the bones of the pelvis or spine and direct extension from neighboring articular or soft tissue infections. Infected soft tissue wounds caused by small-diameter objects (eg, nail puncture wound of the foot) and animal or human bites may obscure early manifestations of complicating osteomyelitis. Episodes of osteomyelitis secondary to prolonged or repetitive therapeutic cannulation or self-administration among drug addicts are encountered with increasing frequency.

1. ACUTE PYOGENIC OSTEOMYELITIS

Essentials of Diagnosis
- Fever, chills, malaise, sweating.
- Pain, tenderness, swelling, limitation of joint motion.
- Culture of the blood or lesion is essential for precise etiologic diagnosis.

General Considerations

About 95% of cases of acute secondary osteomyelitis are caused by pyogenic organisms, usually a single strain. Further contamination during open surgical treatment or "superinfection" during antibiotic treatment with a different organism may produce a mixed infection.

Acute hematogenous osteomyelitis occurs predominantly during the period of skeletal growth, with the peak incidence during childhood rather than during infancy or adolescence. Staphylococci account for about 75% of infections, and group A beta-hemolytic streptococci are the next most common pathogens. The remainder of cases are caused by a wide variety of organisms. Preexisting infection of other organ systems—most commonly the skin, respiratory tract, and genitourinary tract—can be identified in about one-half of cases. A history of trauma is frequently present.

Clinical Findings

A. Symptoms and Signs: In infants the onset is often precipitate, with alarming systemic symptoms of toxicity; an insidious onset may be characterized by subtle generalized symptoms. Voluntary movement of the extremity is likely to be inhibited. Tenderness in the region of the involved bone usually occurs before swelling or redness, which are later manifestations frequently associated with extra-osseous abscess formation.

In children, the onset may be accompanied by high fever, chills, and prostration; it may be less dramatic, especially when drug therapy for a predisposing infection has been given. Local pain may indicate an area of tenderness and even soft tissue swelling. Passive joint motion of the extremity may be inhibited because of muscle guarding.

The onset in adults is likely to be less striking than in infants and children. Generalized toxic symptoms of bacteremia may be absent, and vague, shifting, or evanescent local pain may be the earliest manifestation. Depending upon the duration and extent of bone involvement, tenderness may be present or absent.

Limitation of joint motion may be marked, especially in patients with spine involvement or when lesions are near joints.

B. Laboratory Findings: The precise diagnosis at any age depends upon the recovery and identification of the causative organism. Early in the course—especially during the stage of invasion—blood cultures are likely to be positive; repeated cultures may be necessary. Acceleration of the ESR and leukocytosis occur commonly, but their absence does not rule out osteomyelitis.

When the infection is severe, secondary anemia is likely to occur early.

C. X-Ray Findings: Significant changes in bone cannot be identified by x-ray examination until 7–10 days after the onset in infants and 2–4 weeks after onset in adults. Therefore, treatment should not be delayed until these findings appear. Extra-osseous soft tissue swelling (caused by exudates) adjacent to the osseous focus may be the earliest significant finding, appearing within 3–5 days after the onset of symptoms. Xeroradiography may demonstrate subtle changes in extracortical soft tissues that are not apparent on routine x-ray films. Later, architectural alteration of cancellous bone and destruction of compact bone are indicative of processes that have been active for days or weeks. Subperiosteal new bone formation is a late manifestation of a healing reaction.

D. Special Examinations: Early diagnosis is facilitated by recovery of material from the local lesion for culture studies. Exudates may be recovered by aspiration of extra-osseous tissues in areas of tenderness. Otherwise, when localizing symptoms are clearly manifest—especially in the region of a metaphysis, where the cortex is comparatively thin—the medulla can be aspirated with a small bore trocar to obtain material for culture. Joint effusion may complicate metaphyseal infection. It may be irritative (nonmicrobial) or a manifestation of complicating suppurative arthritis. To avoid possible intra-articular contamination, arthrocentesis should precede metaphyseal puncture. If symptoms are severe and the process has been active for more than 48 hours, specimens for culture may be obtained during open surgical treatment. In addition to microbial culture of the specimen recovered by aspiration or open operation, careful microscopic examination of appropriately stained preparations may be helpful in the initial diagnosis, noting the character and incidence of the cell population (eg, polymorphonuclear leukocytosis) and the morphology of identifiable bacteria.

Radionuclide imaging may help to localize an occult focus of infection before routine x-ray studies become diagnostic.

Differential Diagnosis

Acute hematogenous osteomyelitis must be differentiated from suppurative arthritis, rheumatic fever, and cellulitis. The pseudoparalysis associated with acute osteomyelitis of infancy may simulate poliomyelitis at the onset. With mild symptoms, it may initially mimic transient synovitis of the hip joint or Legg-Perthes disease. Acute forms with mixed symptoms and subacute forms must be differentiated from tuberculosis and mycotic infections of bone and Ewing's sarcoma.

Complications

The most common complication of acute secondary osteomyelitis is chronic osteomyelitis, which can be due to delayed diagnosis or inadequate early treatment. Waiting for manifest x-ray evidence, treatment by nonspecific measures, or ineffective antimicrobial drug therapy may abet progressive destruction of bone and soft tissues.

Other complications include soft tissue abscess formation, septic arthritis from extension into joints, and metastatic infections from the initial osteomyelitic focus.

Pathologic fracture may occur at the site of extensive bone destruction.

Treatment

A. General Measures: The severity of systemic symptoms partly determines the general management. Attention must be given to fluid balance of the acutely toxic patient. Immobilization of the affected extremity by splinting, plaster encasement, or suspension in an orthopedic apparatus is advisable for relief of pain and protection against pathologic fracture. During the acute stage, secondary anemia is best corrected by whole blood replacement. Pain should not be completely abolished by uninterrupted use of drugs since its intensity can be an important clue to the effectiveness of treatment.

B. Specific Measures: Although the antibiotics have provided new concepts of treatment, rational therapy continues to rest upon surgical principles and drug therapy is mainly adjunctive. The selection of specific measures depends in part upon the type of infecting organism, the stage of progress of the lesion, and the general response of the patient. Treatment must be individualized, and only broad guides will be outlined here.

1. Operative treatment—During the first 2–3 days after the onset of acute infection, open surgical treatment can be avoided in some cases, especially in infants and children. If vigorous general care and appropriate antibiotic therapy are instituted promptly, the progress of the local lesion may be controlled and spread of the infection halted before suppuration and significant tissue destruction have occurred.

If an abscess has formed beneath the periosteum or has extended into soft tissues of infants and children, it should be drained at least once daily by aspiration. Pain and fever that persist longer than 2–3 days after initiating aspiration and antimicrobial therapy suggest spread of the infection. Surgical decompression of the medullary cavity by drilling or fenestration should be done promptly with the hope of minimizing progression of bone necrosis. Subsequent treatment of the local lesion may be by open or closed technics.

2. Antibiotics—Rational antibiotic treatment is based upon an understanding of the disease and laboratory isolation of the pathogen followed by antibiotic sensitivity studies. In the seriously ill patient, antibiotic therapy should be instituted as soon as culture material has been collected; treatment should not be withheld until laboratory studies have been completed. If the initial clinical findings are compatible with the understanding that the most common causes of acute osteomyelitis in infants and children are staphylococci or group A beta-hemolytic streptococci, drug treatment can be started promptly. If no contraindication (such as a history of drug sensitivity) exists, begin treatment immediately intravenously with a β-lactamase-resistant semisynthetic penicillin such as methicillin, oxacilllin, or nafcillin in dosages sufficient to produce a bactericidal serum level. The dosage of the appropriate antibiotic may be guided in part by the serum assay, which determines in vitro the comparative efficacy of the drug against the etiologic microbial strain. Broad-spectrum antibiotics alone, with the exception of semisynthetic penicillins or cephalosporins, should be avoided because prolonged treatment is required and resistant strains are likely to emerge rapidly.

In the seriously ill adult patient, it is often necessary to begin treatment before the causative organism has been isolated. The initial selection of drugs requires a critical clinical appraisal. The most common microbial causes of acute hematogenous osteomyelitis are gram-positive cocci and gram-negative enteric bacilli. A likely primary focus such as a skin, respiratory tract, or genitourinary tract infection may offer a clue. If a gram-positive coccal infection is suspected, a semisynthetic penicillin resistant to penicillinase (β-lactamase) is the drug of first choice. Cephalosporin and vancomycin are alternatives. Gram-negative bacilli have widely different drug sensitivities, and combinations of drugs must be given until the causative microorganism has been isolated and its precise drug sensitivities determined. Various combinations have been advocated, eg, kanamycin plus polymyxin B given intravenously. Recent studies have indicated that the combination of carbenicillin and cephalothin is as effective in the control of severe gram-negative infections in patients with disseminated cancer as the triple combination of carbenicillin, cephalothin, and gentamicin. Gentamicin, with or without cephaloridine, may also be effective for acute severe infections presumably caused by gram-negative bacteria. When endotoxic shock is present, specific measures for its treatment must be used in addition to chemotherapy.

Chemotherapy should be continued for about 2–3 weeks after the patient is afebrile or repeated wound cultures fail to show growth.

Rational drug therapy is based upon drug sensitivity tests. Properly executed disk sensitivity studies will give early guidance concerning the probable efficacy of drugs that might be selected for the treatment of infections due to staphylococci or group A streptococci. However, the disk sensitivity technic does not indicate the likely effective dosage, which should be in the bactericidal range. A more reliable laboratory guide is assay of the drug concentration in the patient's serum against the isolated strain. Adjustment of dosage or selection of alternative drugs may then be indicated. Although disk sensitivity studies may provide reliable guidance for treatment of infections caused by the microorganisms mentioned above (and others), these tests cannot be relied upon for optimal help when enteric bacilli or enteric cocci are involved. Tube dilution sensitivity studies are more reliable under these circumstances. Other advantages of the tube dilution methods include a more realistic indication of drug dosage, determination of drug combinations that may have additive or synergistic effects, and indications of effective drug selections when the flora are mixed.

C. Treatment of Complications: Treatment of the common complications of acute hematogenous osteomyelitis is essentially as for acute suppurative arthritis and chronic osteomyelitis, which are discussed elsewhere. "Superinfection" in the form of bacteremia due to a different microbial strain requires, in addition, the same treatment as primary infection.

Course & Prognosis

The mortality rate in treated acute osteomyelitis is probably no more than 1%. Morbidity, however, continues to be high. If effective treatment can be instituted within 48 hours after onset, prompt recovery can be expected in about two-thirds of cases. Chronicity and recurrence of infection are likely when treatment is delayed.

Brand RA, Black H: Pseudomonas osteomyelitis following puncture wounds in children. J Bone Joint Surg 56A:1637, 1974.

Capitanio MA, Kirkpatrick JA: Early roentgen observations in acute osteomyelitis. Am J Roentgenol 108:488, 1970.

Klastersky J & others: Gram-negative infections in cancer: Study of empiric therapy comparing carbenicillin-cephalothin with and without gentamicin. JAMA 227:45, 1974.

Letts RM & others: Technetium bone scanning as an aid in the diagnosis of atypical osteomyelitis in children. Surg Gynec Obst 140:899, 1975.

Waldvogel FA & others: Osteomyelitis: A review of clinical features, therapeutic considerations and unusual aspects. (3 parts.) New England J Med 282:198, 260, 316, 1970.

2. SALMONELLA OSTEOMYELITIS & ARTHRITIS

Infection of bones and joints occurs as a complication in less than 1% of cases of typhoid fever. The symptoms and the local lesions of hematogenous osteoarticular infections due to *Salmonella typhi* are not characteristic and may simulate the clinical manifestations of infection caused by other Salmonella species. The precise diagnosis depends upon recovery of *S typhi* from the osteoarticular focus, and treatment is essentially the same as that for other salmonella infections. The incidence of infection with *S typhi* has decreased in the USA during the past 25 years, but the incidence of infection by other species has increased.

More than 1000 serotypes of salmonella have been identified, and all can be assumed to be pathogenic. The actual rate of clinically apparent infection of bones and joints following epidemic salmonellosis has been estimated to be less than 1% in the USA. Salmonellae cause most bacteremias of sickle cell disease and account for almost 10 times as many cases of osteomyelitis among patients with hemoglobinopathies as other pyogenic bacteria (see Waldvogel reference, below). The species that most frequently cause bone and joint infections are *S choleraesuis, S typhimurium,* and *S paratyphi* B.

Patients without predisposing systemic disease are likely to show a somewhat different pattern of distribution, frequency, and anatomic location of osteomyelitic lesions than is seen in infants and children with sickle cell disease. In otherwise healthy patients, the bone lesion of salmonellosis is more likely to be solitary and may exhibit any of the protean gross pathologic manifestations of acute or chronic pyogenic osteomyelitis. In infants and children, the focus is commonly in the metaphysis of a major long bone, especially the lower femur, proximal humerus, or distal tibia. In the adult, in addition to the shafts of long bones, the lesion may be found in the metaphyses or epiphyses; other locations include the ribs and spine.

Infants and children with sickle cell disease complicated by antecedent episodes of marrow thrombosis and bone infarction can present a somewhat different pathologic picture of salmonella osteomyelitis from that seen in otherwise healthy patients. Engh & others (see reference) have noted the tendency toward diaphyseal involvement, the multiplicity of foci, and the propensity toward symmetric localization.

The onset of osteoarticular infection is likely to occur during the subacute phase of salmonellosis, but it may be delayed until convalescence or even for months or many years. Attention is called to the site of active osteoarticular infection by pain, tenderness, restriction of joint motion, and swelling; fever may be intensified or may recur. Painful swelling of the hands or feet or both (hand-foot syndrome of sickle cell disease) in a black infant or child may represent thrombotic marrow crisis, osteomyelitis, or a combination of both because of simultaneous involvement of different bones (see Constant reference, below).

Positive culture of material recovered from the osteoarticular focus is necessary for precise diagnosis. Positive cultures from blood, feces, or iliac marrow (see Robertson reference) during the febrile phase of enteritis or significant serologic agglutination titers (Widal) give support to a tentative diagnosis.

The x-ray findings of bone or joint infection caused by salmonellae are not characteristic and are essentially those of pyogenic osteomyelitis or arthritis in the acute or chronic stage.

The chief complication is chronicity with persistence of infection and recurrence of clinical findings.

The lesions of bones or joints caused by salmonellae are not characteristic and must be differentiated from those due to other pyogenic bacteria, *Mycobacterium tuberculosis,* and certain fungi. Thrombotic marrow crises of sickle cell disease may mimic osteomyelitis.

Dogmatic recommendations are not offered for open operative treatment during the early stages of osteoarticular infection. Open drainage of major joint infections to relieve tension during the purulent stage may be obviated by periodic aspiration or closed catheter drainage. If systemic drug administration is rational and adequate, open drainage of acute bone infections is not usually necessary, although periodic aspiration or closed catheter drainage of an enlarging abscess may be indicated. Previous episodes of thrombotic marrow crises in infants and children with sickle cell disease can cause bone infarction which may negate or limit the benefits of operative treatment for infection (see Engh & others reference). Recurrent or chronic infections may require open operation in addition to antimicrobial therapy.

The drug sensitivity of the causative strain should be promptly determined. Chloramphenicol is generally effective, but some strains may be resistant to it as well as to other antimicrobials (see Gill & Hook reference). Ampicillin is also likely to be effective. The adequacy of drug dosage may be estimated by serum assay.

Constant E & others: Salmonella osteomyelitis of both hands and the hand-foot syndrome. Arch Surg 102:148, 1971.
Engh CA & others: Osteomyelitis in the patient with sickle-cell disease. J Bone Joint Surg 53A:1, 1971.
Gill FA, Hook EW: Salmonella strains with transferable antimicrobial resistance. JAMA 198:1267, 1966.
Robertson RP & others: Evaluation of chloramphenicol and ampicillin in salmonella enteric fever. New England J Med 278:171, 1968.
Waldvogel FA & others: Osteomyelitis: A review of clinical features, therapeutic considerations and unusual aspects. (3 parts.) New England J Med 282:198, 260, 316, 1970.

3. BRUCELLA OSTEOMYELITIS

Brucella infection as a complication or sequel of brucellosis is not common but may involve the skeletal system or bursae around joints, especially the shoulder or elbow. Infections both by *Brucella melitensis* and *Br abortus* have been reported. Bone lesions are likely to be found in the lumbar spine or sacroiliac joints. The lesion is usually granulomatous, although abscess formation may occur. Osteophytes may form early in the course of the disease and subsequently, by coalescence, cause spontaneous fusion of the spine.

It may not be possible to recover organisms from the blood or from specimens taken from the local lesion. Presumptive diagnosis of active infections will depend upon a rising titer of serologic agglutination tests during the acute stage or brucellergen skin tests which, when positive, do not indicate relative activity of the disease.

Bradstreet CMP & others: Intradermal tests and serological tests in suspected brucella infection in man. Lancet 2:653, 1970.

Kelly PJ & others: Brucellosis of the bones and joints. JAMA 174:347, 1960.

Seal PV, Morris CA: Brucellosis of the carpus: Report of a case. J Bone Joint Surg 56B:327, 1974.

Serre H & others: Sacro-iliitis due to brucellosis. Sem Hôp Paris 46:3311, 1970.

4. CHRONIC PYOGENIC OSTEOMYELITIS

Essentials of Diagnosis

- Pain, tenderness, swelling, edema, and redness of overlying skin.
- Sinus tract formation.

General Considerations

Chronic pyogenic osteomyelitis may occur as a consequence of missed diagnosis or ineffective treatment of acute infection, or it may appear without preceding acute infection as an indolent, slowly progressive process with no striking symptoms. Recurrent infection is manifested by exacerbation of symptoms with or without drainage after a quiescent period of days, weeks, or years. Chronic osteomyelitis at the site of an unhealed fracture is generally discussed under the treatment of fractures.

Clinical Findings

A. Symptoms and Signs: Symptoms may be so mild and the onset so insidious that there is little or no disability. There may be a history of injury. Local manifestations are variable, ranging from no symptoms at all to unremitting pain and persistent discharge. A nidus of infection of bone or soft tissue may communicate through a sinus to the skin surface. Periodic or constant discharge of pus in small quantities may cause no great disability, and the patient may care for it himself by frequent dressing changes. Other manifestations of chronicity are recurrent fever, swelling, pain, and increased drainage.

B. Laboratory Findings: Leukocytosis, anemia, and acceleration of the ESR are inconstant and cannot be relied upon as diagnostic criteria.

C. X-Ray Findings: Architectural alterations of bone depend upon the stage, extent, and rate of progress of the disease. Destruction of bone may be diffuse or focal and may appear as areas of radiolucency. Bone necrosis, apparent as areas of increased density, is due to differentially increased absorption of calcium from surrounding vascularized bone. Involucrum and new bone formation are healing responses which may be identified beneath the periosteum or within bone.

Subperiosteal new bone may be seen as a lamellar pattern. Resorption of sclerotic bone and re-formation of the normal trabecular pattern also suggest healing in cancellous bone.

Tomography may be helpful in identifying deep areas of bone destruction. Sinograms made with aqueous radiographic media (hypaque, 25%; Renografin, 30%) frequently aid in localization of sequestra and points of persistent infection. They also demonstrate the anatomic course and configuration of sinus tracts. Occasionally, radionuclide imaging may aid in the localization of occult infection when x-ray examination by usual technics is inconclusive.

D. Special Examinations: The causative organisms should be determined by culture, and drug sensitivity studies performed. Culture of exudates from sinus orifices may be misleading because skin contaminants are likely to be present. More reliable specimens for culture can be recovered by taking multiple samples of suspected tissue at operation or by deep aspiration at a distance from points of external drainage.

Differential Diagnosis

Chronic pyogenic osteomyelitis should be differentiated from benign and malignant tumors; from certain forms of osseous dysplasia; from fatigue fracture; and from specific infections discussed in this section.

Complications

The most common complication is persistence of infection and acute recurrences. Chronic infection may cause deterioration of health evidenced by anemia, weight loss, weakness, and amyloidosis. Chronic osteomyelitis may act as a focus of infection for seeding other areas.

Acute exacerbations can be complicated by sympathetic effusions into adjacent joints or frank purulent arthritis.

Constant erosion and progressive destruction of bone occasionally lead to pathologic fracture.

Prior to epiphyseal closure, overgrowth of a long bone may occur as a result of chronic hyperemia.

Rarely, and only after many years of drainage, squamous cell carcinoma or a fibrosarcoma arises in persistently and actively infected tissues.

Treatment

A. General Measures: Rigid rules of treatment cannot be laid down because of the varied clinical and pathologic manifestations of this disease. During the quiescent phase, no treatment is necessary and the patient lives an essentially normal life. Minor exacerbations accompanied by drainage may be managed adequately with changes of dressings. More acute episodes may require immobilization of the part, bed rest, local heat, and mild analgesics. Anemia and malnutrition should be treated as indicated.

B. Specific Measures: Occasionally, when the drug sensitivities of the causative organism are known, systemic antibiotic therapy alone and without surgical interference is advantageous in conjunction with general measures. This is especially true during the early phase of a recurrence without external drainage or abscess formation.

Evidence is lacking at this time of the efficacy of hyperbaric oxygen therapy in the treatment of chronic osteomyelitis caused by aerobic microorganisms.

Copious drainage and clinical and x-ray evidence of progressive bone destruction and sequestration require more aggressive treatment.

1. Operative treatment—Soft tissue abscesses occasionally form without certain evidence of reactivated infection of bone; they can be treated adequately after diagnostic operative exploration by open or closed drainage. In addition to curettement, similar treatment may also suffice for **Brodie's abscess,** a unique and rare localized infection of bone.

When localized chronic or recurrent infection of superficial bones (especially the tibia or the ulna) is treated by simple sequestrectomy, saucerization, or craterization, lack of skin and subcutaneous tissue may prevent primary wound closure and closed treatment of the infection. Under such circumstances, modified closed treatment can be used with intermittent local antibiotic instillation and suction drainage during the first 1 or 2 weeks after operation while vascularization of exposed bone surface occurs. The soft tissue defect is treated subsequently by split thickness skin grafting. Concomitant systemic antibiotic treatment is frequently unnecessary. The transfer of pedicle flaps of skin and subcutaneous fat from distant sites for more adequate coverage of defects in superficial bones should be deferred until there is reasonable assurance that the infection has been suppressed. In some cases, it may be months or years before minor but frequent recurrences of infection can be eliminated.

More extensive and long-standing infections require more extensive surgery to remove sinus tracts, abscess walls, thick soft tissue scars, and infected bone which is either sequestered or attached. In very serious cases, destructive operations such as diaphysectomy or amputation are required.

Before antibiotic drugs became available, primary wound closure was generally followed by persistent drainage, and most surgeons preferred open wound treatment. With local and systemic antibiotic therapy, it is now possible to close the wound and drain it intermittently by tube suction. Obliteration of cavities is essential for successful early wound closure. Some deep cavities can be obliterated by transferring an adjacent muscle into the cavity.

2. Antibiotics—Rational antibiotic therapy is based upon careful sensitivity studies of material cultured from the wound. Antimicrobial drugs in high concentrations can be introduced intermittently into the wound for topical therapy. Although the systemic use of a single antibiotic is often successful for the treatment of staphylococcal and beta-hemolytic streptococcal infections, optimal treatment of gram-negative infections often necessitates combinations of drugs. The principle of combined antibiotic action can also be applied by using poorly absorbed, more toxic

agents such as kanamycin, neomycin, vancomycin, or polymyxin B locally and well absorbed, less toxic drugs systemically. Periodic cultures of wound secretions are necessary to determine the effectiveness of treatment. Serum concentrations of systemically administered drugs should be determined periodically as a guide for drug selection and dosage.

Course & Prognosis

Even after vigorous treatment, recurrence of infection is likely. The most frequent technical cause of recurrence is failure to remove all areas of infected soft tissue scar or necrotic and unseparated bone no matter how small. It is assumed that these abnormal tissues harbor bacterial "persisters." The altered metabolic activity or (perhaps) the altered morphology of "persisters" probably permits them to remain in relatively unaggressive states in the tissues for prolonged periods. The mechanisms of survival of microorganisms are not well understood, but their causative roles in recurrence of infection are well recognized.

Cabanela ME & others: Osteomyelitis appearing as neoplasms: A diagnostic problem. Arch Surg 109:68, 1974.

Deysine M & others: Diagnosis of chronic and postoperative osteomyelitis with gallium 67 citrate scans. Am J Surg 129:632, 1975.

Gordon SL & others: Recurrent osteomyelitis: Report of four cases culturing L-form variants of staphylococci. J Bone Joint Surg 53A:1150, 1971.

Johnson LL, Kempson RL: Epidermoid carcinoma in osteomyelitis. J Bone Joint Surg 47A: 133, 1965.

West WF & others: Chronic osteomyelitis. 1. Factors affecting the results of treatment in 186 patients. JAMA 213:1837, 1970.

SPECIFIC INFECTIONS OF BONES & JOINTS*

MYCOTIC INFECTIONS

Fungus infections of the skeletal system are usually secondary to a primary infection in another organ system, frequently the lower pulmonary tract. Although skeletal lesions have a predilection for the cancellous extremities of long bones and the bodies of vertebrae, the predominant lesion—a granuloma with varying degrees of necrosis and abscess formation—does not produce a characteristic clinical picture.

Differentiation from other chronic focal infections depends upon culture studies of synovial fluid or tissue obtained from the local lesion. Serologic and skin tests and histologic studies provide presumptive support of the diagnosis.

*Acute and chronic pyogenic arthritis is discussed in Chapter 13.

Baum GL, Schwarz J: Diagnosis and treatment of systemic mycoses. M Clin North America 58:661, 1974.

Bennett JE: Chemotherapy of systemic mycoses. (2 parts.) New England J Med 290:30, 320, 1974.

1. COCCIDIOIDOMYCOSIS

Coccidioidomycosis of bones and joints is usually secondary to primary pulmonary infection. The focus in the lungs may not be visible by x-ray examination when the skeletal lesion appears. During the initial phase of pulmonary infection, arthralgia with periarticular swelling, especially in the regions of the knees and ankles, should be differentiated from organic bone and joint involvement. Osseous lesions commonly occur in cancellous bone of the vertebrae or near the ends of long bones. Because of the predilection for the latter sites, redness and swelling of the skin over bony prominences may be the first to call attention to the local process; abscess and sinus formation follow. Joint infection may be due to direct spread via the blood stream, or it may be caused by extension from a nearby osseous focus. The granulomatous lesions of bone or the villonodular synovitis of the joints cannot be differentiated microscopically from other mycotic infections. Histologic demonstration of spherules containing endospores supports the diagnosis but is not pathognomonic. Changes in bone seen in x-rays simulate those of tuberculosis. Local atrophy of bone progresses to focal destruction, which may appear cystic, indicating coalescence of granulomas or abscess formation. Subperiosteal new bone formation and sclerosis characterize the healing response. Sequestration is uncommon.

The precise diagnosis depends upon recovery of *Coccidioides immitis* from the lesion by mycotic culture, which is hazardous except in a specially equipped laboratory. A safer technic is microscopic examination of the inoculated testis of a guinea pig. Significant complement fixation or agar gel precipitin inhibition titers are indicative of disseminated coccidioidomycosis and offer presumptive identification of a concomitant osteoarticular lesion. The organism may not be recovered from synovial fluid, especially after systemic treatment with amphotericin B. Histologic examination of grossly suspicious synovium obtained by open biopsy may demonstrate the presence of the organism when the synovial fluid is negative.

Systemic treatment with amphotericin B should be tried for bone and joint infections. It may also be of value for instillation into joints during the early stages of infection or after synovectomy. Immobilization of joints by plaster casts and avoidance of weight bearing provide beneficial rest. Chronic infection of bone may respond to operative treatment by curettage or saucerization. Amputation may be the only solution for stubbornly progressive infections which do not respond to less drastic measures. Synovectomy and joint debridement are reserved for more advanced joint infections. Contaminated dressings and plaster casts should be carefully handled to prevent spread of infection to others.

Dalinka MK & others: Roentgenographic features of osseous coccidioidomycosis and differential diagnosis. J Bone Joint Surg 53A:1157, 1971.

Pankovich AM, Jevtic MM: Coccidioidal infection of the hip: A case report. J Bone Joint Surg 55A:1525, 1973.

Wallraff EB, Wachs EE: Recent developments in serologic methods for diagnosis of coccidioidomycosis: Soluble antigen fluorescent antibody test. Am J Clin Path 55:418, 1971.

2. HISTOPLASMOSIS

Focal skeletal or joint involvement in histoplasmosis is rare and generally represents dissemination from a primary focus in the lungs. Skeletal lesions may be single or multiple. The granulomatous lesions are not characteristic, and the diagnosis depends upon the recovery of *Histoplasma capsulatum* by culture studies of biopsy material from skeletal foci. Complement fixation tests may provide presumptive support of a diagnosis.

Surgical debridement of the focal lesion has been recommended. Amphotericin B has been useful for treatment of some patients, and recovery is more likely to occur in patients treated with amphotericin B than in untreated patients.

Perlman R & others: Histoplasmosis of the common palmar tendon sheath. J Bone Joint Surg 54A:676, 1972.

Sarosi GA & others: Disseminated histoplasmosis: Results of long-term follow-up. Ann Int Med 75:511, 1971.

3. CRYPTOCOCCOSIS
(Torulosis)

Cryptococcosis (torulosis or European blastomycosis) is an uncommon but worldwide chronic granulomatous pulmonary disease which may be disseminated to the nervous system and rarely to the skeletal system. The granulomatous lesions of bone are not characteristic. Diagnosis depends upon culture of the yeast-like fungus, *Cryptococcus neoformans,* from the osseous lesion; agglutination tests for the specific antigen and antibody, when positive, give presumptive support to the diagnosis. Surgical removal of diseased bone is believed to enhance healing and minimize further dissemination.

Systemic treatment with amphotericin B, alone or in combination with flucytosine, should supplement any operative procedure.

Cowen NJ: Cryptococcosis of bone. Case report and review of the literature. Clin Orthop 66:174, 1969.

Gordon MA, Vedder DK: Serologic tests in diagnosis and prognosis of cryptococcosis. JAMA 197:961, 1966.

4. NORTH AMERICAN BLASTOMYCOSIS
(Gilchrist's Disease)

Osteoarticular blastomycosis represents dissemination from a focus more likely primary in the lungs but occasionally from a cutaneous lesion. The granulomatous and suppurative lesions, which are predominantly osteolytic, may localize in any part of the skeleton but appear most frequently in the cancellous extremities of major long bones, the vertebrae, and the carpal and tarsal bones. The clinical picture is essentially that of chronic osteomyelitis. The x-ray patterns are not characteristic; the destructive process may be focal or diffuse in cancellous bone. Lesions may involve any part of the vertebrae and are likely to mimic tuberculosis.

Suppurative arthritis as a complication of systemic blastomycosis tends to appear in a single major appendicular joint, especially the knee. Unless the precise diagnosis is established early in the course and effective treatment instituted, progressive destruction of the joint follows.

Diagnosis depends upon identification by culture of *Blastomyces dermatitidis* from the osteoarticular focus. The budding spherules may be demonstrated in histologic preparations, tissue exudates, or joint fluid.

Conservative surgical treatment of the local lesion is advocated. Although not specific for the disease, systemically administered amphotericin B is likely to be more beneficial than hydroxystilbamidine.

Cushard WG & others: Blastomycosis of bone: Treatment with intramedullary amphotericin-B. J Bone Joint Surg 51A:704, 1969.

Gehweiler JA & others: Observations on the roentgen patterns in blastomycosis of bone. Am J Roentgenol 108:497, 1970.

Liggett AS, Silberman Z: Blastomycosis of the knee joint. J Bone Joint Surg 52A:1445, 1970.

Riegler HF & others: Blastomycosis osteomyelitis. Clin Orthop 100:225, 1974.

SYPHILIS OF BONES & JOINTS

Syphilitic arthritis or osteitis may occur during any stage of the congenital or acquired systemic disease. Neurotrophic arthropathy (Charcot's joints) can be caused indirectly by syphilitic disease of the spinal cord; thus, the joint lesion is not a local response to *Treponema pallidum*. Although the incidence contin-ually decreases in the USA, syphilis and its skeletal manifestations continue to be significant problems in some parts of Africa and southeast Asia.

In **infancy**, a typical manifestation of congenital syphilis is epiphysitis and metaphysitis. Radiologically, a zone of sclerosis appears adjacent to the growth plate but is separated from another similar zone by one of rarefaction. Partial replacement of the rarefied bone by inflammatory tissue precedes suppuration and abscess formation, which may in turn cause epiphyseal displacement because of structural weakening. Focal periosteal thickening about the anterior fontanel causes Parrot's nodes.

Periostitis and osteoperiostitis are manifestations of congenital syphilis in **childhood** and **adolescence**. Bone involvement is frequently symmetric, and periosteal proliferation along the tibial crest causes the classical "saber shin." A painless bilateral effusion of the knees (Clutton's joints) is a rare manifestation of the congenital disease.

In **adulthood**, a tertiary manifestation of either congenital or acquired syphilis is gumma formation. This granulomatous process is characterized by localized destruction of bone accompanied by surrounding areas of sclerosis of varying extent. Extensive destruction with accompanying rarefaction may cause pathologic fracture because of structural weakening. Periostitis in the adult is likely to occur in the bones of the thorax and in the shafts of long bones. The x-ray picture of syphilitic osteitis in the adult is not diagnostic, but bone production is generally more pronounced than bone destruction.

Clinical suspicion is diagnostically useful because syphilis can mimic so many diseases. Osteoarticular lesions due to other causes that simulate those of *T pallidum* must be differentiated in patients who have received either adequate or inadequate treatment of the systemic disease. When localized clinical symptoms with compatible x-ray studies are supported by a history of congenital or acquired infection, thorough serologic studies will probably provide confirmatory evidence. Biopsy is not necessary to establish a direct diagnosis, but it may differentiate a gumma from other lesions. A favorable response of the lesion to specific drug treatment supports the diagnosis and can be a useful method of differentiation from other lesions which would be refractory to the specific agent.

The only local treatment that is necessary for the skeletal lesion is immobilization to provide comfort or protection from fracture if extensive weakening of bone is judged to be present. Lesions of bones and joints respond favorably and promptly to adequate chemotherapy of the systemic disease.

Fleming TC, Bardenstein MB: Congenital syphilis. J Bone Joint Surg 53A:1648, 1971.

Johns D: Syphilitic disorders of the spine. J Bone Joint Surg 52B:724, 1970.

McGladdery H: Osteolytic bone syphilis. J Bone Joint Surg 32B:226, 1950.

TUBERCULOSIS OF BONES & JOINTS

Essentials of Diagnosis

- Pain, tenderness, swelling, limitation of joint motion.
- Known primary infection in another organ system.

General Considerations

Practically all tuberculous infections in the USA are caused by the human strain of *Mycobacterium tuberculosis*. Infection of the musculoskeletal system is commonly caused by hematogenous spread from a primary lesion of the respiratory or gastrointestinal tract. Tuberculosis of the thoracic or lumbar spine may be associated with an active lesion of the genitourinary tract. It is a disease of childhood, occurring most commonly before puberty. Adult infection is uncommon except in the debilitated geriatric patient.

Clinical Findings

A. Symptoms and Signs: The onset of symptoms is generally insidious and not accompanied by alarming general manifestations of fever, sweating, toxicity, or prostration. Pain in the region of an involved joint may be mild at onset and accompanied by a sensation of stiffness. It is commonly accentuated at night. Limping is a mechanism to protect a weight-bearing joint. Restriction of joint motion due to muscle guarding during the early phase of the infection is another protective mechanism. As the disease process progresses, limitation of joint motion becomes fixed because of muscle contractures, organic destruction of the joint, and the progressive healing response in soft tissue and bone.

Local findings during the early stages may be limited to tenderness, soft tissue swelling, joint effusion, and increase in skin temperature about the involved area. As the disease progresses without treatment, muscle atrophy and deformity become apparent. Abscess formation with spontaneous drainage externally leads to sinus formation. Progressive destruction of bone in the spine may cause a gibbus, especially in the thoracolumbar region.

B. Laboratory Findings: The precise diagnosis rests upon the recovery of the causative acid-fast pathogen from joint fluid, tissue exudates, or tissue specimens by artificial culture methods or animal inoculation. Biopsy of the lesion or of a regional lymph node may demonstrate the characteristic histologic picture of acid-fast bacillary infection but does not differentiate tuberculosis from other nontuberculous mycobacterial lesions.

C. X-Ray Findings: X-ray manifestations are not characteristic. There is a latent period between the onset of symptoms and the initial positive x-ray finding. The earliest changes of tuberculous arthritis are those of soft tissue swelling and distention of the capsule of effusion. Subsequently, bone atrophy causes thinning of the trabecular pattern, narrowing of the cortex, and enlargement of the medullary canal. As

joint disease progresses, destruction of cartilage is manifested by narrowing of the joint cleft and focal erosion of the articular surface, especially at the margins. Extensive destruction of joint surfaces causes deformity. As healing takes place, osteosclerosis becomes apparent around areas of necrosis and sequestration. Where the lesion is limited to bone, especially in the cancellous portion of the metaphysis, the x-ray picture may be that of single or multilocular cysts surrounded by sclerotic bone. As intra-osseous foci expand toward the limiting cortex and erode it, subperiosteal new bone formation takes place.

D. Special Examinations: An important step toward establishment of a precise diagnosis is to obtain material from the focal lesion for animal inoculation or microbial culture studies. Exudates may be collected by aspiration or representative tissues removed by either percutaneous or open biopsy. Cutaneous reaction to protein derivatives of various mycobacteria are of presumptive diagnostic value insofar as the local lesion is concerned.

Differential Diagnosis

Tuberculosis of the musculoskeletal system must be differentiated from all subacute and chronic infections, rheumatoid arthritis, gout, and occasionally from osseous dysplasia. Infections caused by nontuberculous mycobacteria can be differentiated only by laboratory procedures which require expert knowledge.

Complications

Clinical infection probably occurs only in persons with inadequate immunologic defense following massive exposure to this ubiquitous pathogen. In people with inadequate defense mechanisms, children, and elderly people with other systemic disease, tuberculosis is likely to have an accelerated rate of progress. Destruction of bones or joints may occur in a few weeks or months if adequate treatment is not provided. Deformity due to joint destruction, abscess formation with spread into adjacent soft tissues, and sinus formation are common. Paraplegia is the most serious complication of spinal tuberculosis. As healing of severe joint lesions takes place, spontaneous fibrous or bony ankylosis follows.

Treatment

The modern treatment of tuberculosis of the skeletal system consists of 3 phases: general care, surgery, and chemotherapy.

A. General Measures: This is especially important when prolonged recumbency is necessary and includes skillful nursing care, adequate diet, and appropriate treatment of associated lesions (pulmonary, genitourinary, etc).

B. Surgical Treatment: No rigid recommendations can be made for the operative treatment of tuberculosis because the stage of the infection and the character of the lesion are the determinants. In acute infections where synovitis is the predominant feature, treatment can be conservative, at least initially: Immobilization by splint or plaster, aspiration, and chemotherapy may suffice to control the infection. This treatment is desirable for the management of infections of large joints of the lower extremities in children during the early stage of the infection. Immobilization may also be used in adults either as definitive treatment of early and mild infections or preliminary to operative management. Synovectomy may be valuable for less acute hypertrophic lesions which involve tendon sheaths, bursae, or joints.

Various types of operative treatment are necessary for chronic or advanced tuberculosis of bones and joints depending upon the location of the lesion and the age and general condition of the patient. The availability of effective drugs for systemic use has broadened the indications for synovectomy and debridement. Conversely, the need for more radical surgical procedures such as arthrodesis and amputation has diminished. Even though the infection is active and all involved tissue cannot be removed, supplementary chemotherapy permits healing to proceed. In general, arthrodesis of weight-bearing joints is preferred when useful function cannot be salvaged.

C. Chemotherapy: Modern chemotherapy of tuberculosis is based essentially on the systemic administration of drugs to which the strain of pathogen is likely to be susceptible as indicated by in vitro testing. Resistant strains are likely to emerge during administration of single drugs. Therefore, combinations of antituberculosis agents are recommended. Although isoniazid (INH) plus aminosalicylic acid (PAS) with or without streptomycin have been used widely in the past, combinations of isoniazid and ethambutol or rifampin and ethambutol are now employed more frequently. Other useful but more toxic drugs include viomycin, capreomycin, pyrazinamide, cycloserine, and ethionamide.

Ellis W: Multiple bone lesions caused by Avian-Battey mycobacteria. J Bone Joint Surg 56B:323, 1974.

Friedman B, Kapur V: Management of tuberculosis of the knee joint. Am Rev Resp Dis 101:265, 1970.

Popescu E & others: Local diffusibility of rifampicin in tuberculous lesions of bone and joint. Respiration (Suppl) 28:44, 1971.

Tuli SM: Results of treatment of spinal tuberculosis by "middle-path" regime. J Bone Joint Surg 57B:13, 1975.

Wilkinson MC: Tuberculosis of the hip and knee treated by chemotherapy, synovectomy, and debridement. J Bone Joint Surg 51A:1343, 1969.

Wolinsky E: New antituberculosis drugs and concepts of prophylaxis. M Clin North America 58:697, 1974.

GONORRHEAL ARTHRITIS

Gonorrheal arthritis (gonococcal arthritis, gonorrheal rheumatism) is an acute inflammatory disease caused by *Neisseria gonorrhoeae* which is almost always secondary to infection of the genitourinary tract. At one time, joint involvement occurred in 2–5% of all gonococcal infections. Currently, gonorrheal arthritis is encountered more frequently in women who have occult genitourinary infections and occasionally in children. Symptoms related to the musculoskeletal system are likely to appear during the third week of inadequately treated infection.

Joint infection is via the blood stream. Clinical evidence of involvement of multiple joints is often present at onset, but symptoms are likely to be transient in all joints except one. Large weight-bearing joints are affected most frequently. Systemic symptoms may accompany the essential clinical features of the local lesion, which are those of acute arthritis. Initially, the process may only consist of synovitis with effusion, but as it progresses the exudate becomes purulent and destruction of cartilage follows which may lead to fibrous or bony ankylosis. Tenosynovitis about the wrist and maculopapular eruptions on the palms and forearms may accompany the acute articular infection.

The precise diagnosis is established by recovery of the causative microorganism from the involved joint by culture. This may be successful in only a minority of acute cases. A positive complement fixation test of joint exudate is said to be more significant than a positive reaction in the blood. Identification of gonococcal antibody in serum by the fluorescent technic is more reliable than the complement fixation test. Other presumptive evidence is obtained from positive cultures from the lower genitourinary tract.

Gonorrheal arthritis must be differentiated from rheumatoid arthritis, although there may be a concomitant gonococcal infection of the genitourinary system; from pyogenic arthritis caused by other organisms; from acute synovitis; from Reiter's disease; and from gout.

Nonspecific treatment includes immobilization of the joint, bed rest, and analgesics as necessary for pain. Systemic treatment of gonorrhea by antimicrobial drugs is discussed in Chapter 23. If the joint fluid is purulent, contains parent organisms, and recurs rapidly in large quantities, systemic treatment can be supplemented by instillation into large joints of 25–50 thousand units of penicillin G in 5 ml of saline, and repeated once or twice at daily intervals.

The prognosis for preservation of joint function is good if the diagnosis is established promptly and treatment is vigorous.

Cooke CL & others: Gonococcal arthritis. JAMA 217:204, 1971.

Hess EV, Hunter DK, Ziff M: Gonococcal antibodies in acute arthritis. JAMA 191:531, 1965.

Holmes KK & others: Recovery of *Neisseria gonorrhoeae* from "sterile" synovial fluid in gonococcal arthritis. New England J Med 284:318, 1971.

CERVICOBRACHIAL PAIN SYNDROMES

A large group of articular and extra-articular disorders is characterized by pain that may involve simultaneously the neck, shoulder girdle, and upper extremity. Diagnostic differentiation is often difficult. Some of these entities and clinical syndromes represent primary disorders of the cervicobrachial region; others are local manifestations of systemic diseases. The clinical picture is further complicated when 2 or more of these conditions occur coincidentally.

Some of the more common disorders in this category are discussed below.

OSTEOARTHRITIS OF THE CERVICAL SPINE
(Cervical Spondylosis, Degenerative Arthritis, Hypertrophic Arthritis)

This entity consists of degenerative disease of the apophyseal joints and intervertebral disk joints with or without neurologic manifestations. Osteoarthritis of the articular facets is characterized by progressive thinning of articular cartilage, subchondral osteosclerosis, and osteophytic proliferation around the joint margins.

Although degeneration of cervical disks does occur in adolescence, it increases in frequency after age 40 and is marked by gradual narrowing as demonstrated by x-ray examination. The nucleus pulposus may extrude through a tear in the annulus fibrosus, or a portion of the annulus may protrude; either can cause nerve root or spinal cord compression. Osteocartilaginous proliferation occurs around the margins of the vertebral body and gives rise to osteophytic ridges which may encroach upon the intervertebral foramens and the spinal canal, causing compression of the neurovascular contents. A large anterior osteophyte may occasionally cause dysphagia. Pain may be limited to the posterior neck region or, depending upon the level of the symptomatic joint, may radiate segmentally (sclerotomally) to the occiput, anterior chest, shoulder girdle region, arm, forearm, and hand. It may be intensified by active or passive neck motions. The general distribution of pain and paresthesias, when they are a feature, corresponds roughly to the involved dermatome in the upper extremity. Radiating pain in the upper extremity is often intensified by hyperextension of the neck and deviation of the head to the involved side. Limitation of cervical movements is the most common objective finding. Neurologic signs depend upon the extent of compression of nerve roots or the spinal cord. Severe compression of the spinal cord may cause long tract involvement resulting in paraparesis or paraplegia.

An early x-ray finding is loss of the normal anterior convexity of the cervical curve. Comparative reduc-

tion in height of the involved disk space is a frequent finding in adults, and characteristic changes around the apophyseal joint clefts are late changes observed predominantly in the lower cervical spine. The most common late x-ray finding is osteophyte formation anteriorly adjacent to the disk, which should be differentiated from vertebral osteophytosis. Other sites of proliferative changes are frequently about the "joints" of Luschka. Myelography is the single most valuable x-ray means of demonstrating nerve root or spinal cord compression. The diagnostic value of cervical discography remains moot.

This entity should be differentiated from other cervicobrachial pain syndromes, rheumatoid arthritis, ankylosing spondylitis, chronic cervical sprains ("whiplash" injuries), primary and metastatic tumors of bone, and other causes of cervical myelopathy intrinsic to the cord.

Acute symptoms usually respond to rest of the cervical spine, which may be provided by a thick, firm pillow at night and external cervical support with a nonrigid surgical collar or a neck brace. Cervical traction, either continuously in recumbency or periodic, may be necessary for severe pain. Analgesics may be given for temporary relief, but prolonged use of narcotics may only obscure and delay the recognition of a more serious associated disorder. Chronic pain, especially when it radiates into the upper extremity, usually requires more positive methods of providing cervical rest such as bracing.

Surgical fusion of the cervical spine alone is rarely necessary for control of pain. When compression of nerve roots or the spinal cord causes significant neurologic deficit, laminectomy (with or without spine fusion) or anterior disk removal with spine fusion is necessary to prevent further damage.

Osteoarthritis is progressive, and symptoms are likely to recur. The cervical segment that first caused symptoms may become asymptomatic, but symptoms may arise from a previously uninvolved segment.

Carlson MJ & others: Ankylosing vertebral hyperostosis causing dysphagia. Arch Surg 109:197, 1974.

DePalma AF & others: Anterior interbody fusion for severe cervical disc degeneration. Surg Gynec. Obst 134:755, 1972.

Holt EP Jr: Further reflections on cervical discography. JAMA 231:613, 1975.

Murphey F & others: Surgical treatment of laterally ruptured cervical disc: Review of 648 cases, 1939 to 1972. J Neurosurg 38:679, 1973.

THORACIC OUTLET SYNDROMES

Thoracic outlet syndromes include certain disorders with varied manifestations which are caused by compression of the neurovascular structures supplying the upper extremity: cervical rib syndrome, costoclavicular syndrome, scalenus anticus and scalenus medius syndromes, pectoralis minor syndrome, Wright's syndrome, "effort thrombosis" of the axillary and subclavian veins, and the subclavian steal syndrome. (Cervical rib syndrome is discussed in Chapter 16.)

Symptoms and signs may arise from intermittent or continuous pressure on elements of the brachial plexus and the subclavian or axillary vessels by a variety of anatomic structures of the shoulder girdle region. The neurovascular bundle can be compressed between the anterior or middle scalene muscles and a normal first thoracic rib or a cervical rib. Descent of the shoulder girdle may continue in adulthood and cause compression. Faulty posture, chronic illness, occupation, and advancing age are other predisposing factors. The components of the median nerve that encircle the axillary artery may cause compression and vascular symptoms. Sudden or repetitive strenuous physical activity may initiate "effort thrombosis" of the axillary or subclavian vein.

Pain may radiate from the point of compression to the base of the neck, the axilla, the shoulder girdle region, arm, forearm, and hand. Paresthesias are frequently present and are commonly distributed to the volar aspect of the 4th and 5th digits. Sensory symptoms may be aggravated at night or by prolonged use of the extremities for daily tasks. Weakness and muscle atrophy are the principal motor symptoms. Vascular symptoms consist of arterial ischemia characterized by pallor of the fingers on elevation of the extremity, sensitivity to cold, and, rarely, gangrene of the digits or venous obstruction marked by edema, cyanosis, and engorgement.

Deep reflexes are usually not altered. When the site of compression is between the upper rib and clavicle, partial obliteration of subclavian artery pulsation may be demonstrated by abduction of the arm to a right angle with the elbow simultaneously flexed and rotated externally at the shoulder so that the entire extremity lies in the coronal plane. The position of the neck or arm has no effect on the diminished pulse, which remains constant in the subclavian steal syndrome (see Heath reference, below).

X-ray examination is most helpful in differential diagnosis. The value of clinical plethysmography as an objective method of recording brachial arterial pulsations has been emphasized by Winsor and Brow. When venous or arterial obstruction is thought to be intravascular, venography or arteriography is likely to demonstrate the location of the occlusion. Determinations of the conduction velocities of the ulnar and other peripheral nerves of the upper extremity may help to localize the site of their compression.

Thoracic outlet syndrome must be differentiated from symptomatic osteoarthritis of the cervical spine, tumors of the cervical spinal cord or nerve roots, periarthritis of the shoulder, and other cervicobrachial pain syndromes.

Conservative treatment is directed toward relief of compression of the neurovascular bundle. The patient is instructed to avoid any physical activity that is likely to precipitate or aggravate symptoms. Overhead pulley exercises are useful to improve posture. Shoulder bracing, although uncomfortable to many patients, provides a constant stimulus to improve posture. When lying down, the shoulder girdle should be bolstered by arranging pillows in an inverted "V" position.

Operative treatment may be necessary when conservative measures are not successful.

Symptoms may disappear spontaneously or may be relieved by carefully directed conservative treatment. Operative treatment is more likely to relieve the neurologic rather than the vascular component that causes symptoms.

Benzian SR, Mainzer F: Erect arteriography: Its use in the thoracic outlet syndrome. Radiology 111:275, 1974.
Heath RD: The subclavian steal syndrome: Cause of symptoms in the arm. J Bone Joint Surg 54A:1033, 1972.
Lord JW: Thoracic outlet syndromes: Current management. Ann Surg 173:700, 1971.
Urschel HC Jr & others: Objective diagnosis (ulnar nerve conduction velocity) and current therapy of thoracic outlet syndrome. Ann Thoracic Surg 12:608, 1971.

SCAPULOHUMERAL PERIARTHRITIS
(Adhesive Capsulitis, Frozen Shoulder)

Periarthritis of the shoulder joint is an inflammatory disorder of multiple etiology involving primarily the soft tissues. The condition may be divided into a primary type, in which no obvious etiologic disease can be identified, and a secondary type associated with an organic articular lesion (eg, rheumatoid arthritis, osteoarthritis, fracture or dislocation). The primary type is most common in the minor shoulder among women after the 4th decade. It may be manifest as inflammation of the articular synovia, the tendons around the joint, the intrinsic ligamentous capsular bands, the paratendinous bursae (especially the subacromial), and the bicipital tendon sheath. Calcareous tendinitis and attritional disease of the rotator cuff, with or without tears, are incidental lesions.

The onset of pain, which is aggravated by extremes of shoulder joint motion, may be acute or insidious. Pain may be most annoying at night and may be intensified by pressure on the involved extremity when sleeping in the lateral decubitus position. Tenderness upon palpation is often noted near the tendinous insertions into the greater tuberosity or over the bicipital groove. Although a sensation of stiffness may be noted only at onset, restriction of shoulder joint motion soon becomes apparent and is likely to progress unless effective treatment is instituted.

Opinion differs on how best to treat this disorder. Pain can usually be controlled with mild analgesics. Passive exercise of the shoulder by an overhead pulley mechanism should be repeated slowly for about 2 minutes 4 times daily. Forceful manipulation of the shoulder joint during this exercise should be avoided. Injection of tender areas with local anesthetics or corticosteroids gives at best only transitory relief. Some surgeons prefer closed manipulation of the shoulder under anesthesia, but this is likely to aggravate rather than relieve pain and restriction of motion. Operative treatment has been advocated by some but should be reserved for the occasional refractory case.

Hammond GJ: Complete acromionectomy in the treatment of chronic tendinitis of the shoulder: A follow-up of ninety operations on eighty-seven patients. J Bone Joint Surg 53A:173, 1971.

Lundberg BJ: The frozen shoulder. Acta orthop scandinav 119 (Suppl):1, 1969.

Steinbrocker O, Argyros TG: Frozen shoulder: Treatment by local injections of depot corticosteroids. Arch Phys Med 55:209, 1974.

SCAPULOHUMERAL CALCAREOUS TENDINITIS

Calcareous tendinitis of the shoulder joint is an acute or chronic inflammatory disorder of the capsulotendinous cuff (especially the supraspinatous portion) characterized by deposits of calcium salts among tendon fibers. It is the most common cause of acute pain near the lateral aspect of the shoulder joint in men over age 30. The calcium deposit may be restricted to the tendon substance or may rupture into the overlying subacromial bursa.

Symptoms consist of pain (at times quite severe), tenderness to pressure over the deposit, and restriction of shoulder joint motion. Chronic symptoms may be intermittent and similar to those of scapulohumeral periarthritis.

X-ray examination confirms the diagnosis and demonstrates the site of the lesion.

Calcareous tendinitis must be differentiated from other cervicobrachial pain syndromes, pyogenic arthritis, osteoarthritis, gout, and tears of the rotator cuff.

The aim of treatment is to relieve pain and restore shoulder joint function. Pain is best treated by multiple needling of the lesion under local anesthesia. In the occasional refractive case, operative evacuation of the calcium deposit is necessary to relieve pain. After either type of treatment, early recovery of shoulder joint function should be fostered by judiciously supervised exercises. Acute symptoms occasionally subside after spontaneous rupture of the calcium deposit into the subacromial bursa. Chronic symptoms may be treated by analgesics, exercises, injection of local anesthetics or corticosteroids with or without needling of the deposit, and x-ray therapy. Large deposits that appear dense on x-ray may require surgical evacuation.

When x-ray examination shows that a deposit has disappeared, recurrence of that deposit is rare. Symptoms of periarthritis may persist if shoulder joint motion is not completely regained.

Quigley TB: Injection therapy of calcium deposits. S Clin North America 43:1495, 1963.

SCAPULOCOSTAL SYNDROME

The scapulocostal syndrome has been attributed to fatigue associated with habitually faulty posture which exerts tension on the deep cervical fascia and adjacent muscles, causing dull, aching pain in the posterior cervical region. Pain may radiate to the occiput, the medial border of the scapula, and down the arm and forearm to the ulnar side of the hand, or along the vertebral border of the scapula to the region of the 4th and 5th ribs posteriorly. Tenderness is commonly present near the insertion of the levator muscle into the vertebral border of the scapula. A sensation of stiffness around the shoulder girdle and diffuse tenderness in the region of the trapezius muscle may also be present.

This disorder must be differentiated from other cervicobrachial pain syndromes—especially osteoarthritis, which is manifested predominantly by degenerative disk disease in the lower cervical spine—and from generalized disorders such as polymyositis and fibrositis.

Treatment consists of correction of faulty posture by exercise, periodic rest to relieve fatigue, local applications of heat or cold (whichever provides greater comfort) to the posterior cervical region, and infiltration with local anesthetics or spraying the skin overlying "trigger points" with ethyl chloride. If symptoms do not subside in response to these measures, the diagnosis should be reconsidered.

Michele AA, Eisenberg J: Scapulocostal syndrome. Arch Phys Med 49:383, 1968.

CAUSALGIA
(Reflex Sympathetic Dystrophy)

The term causalgia will be restricted here to denote an uncommon pain syndrome that affects either the lower or upper extremity. (A more complete discussion is offered in Chapter 8.) The precise cause is unknown, but upper extremity causalgia is most often due to complete or incomplete laceration of the median nerve or the brachial plexus. The cardinal symptom, which appears immediately or within a few weeks after injury, is severe, burning pain, often paroxysmally precipitated by friction or even drafts of air and commonly restricted to the area of sensory supply of the affected nerve. Intolerance to dryness and relief by cold, wet applications are characteristic. Vasomotor or trophic changes of skin appear and are evidenced by coolness, color changes (redness or cyanosis), glossiness, edema, and dryness. The small joints of the hand become stiff, and bone atrophy is demonstrable by x-ray. Relief of pain by stellate ganglion block is a useful confirmatory test.

In its major form, causalgia must be differentiated from pseudocausalgia (minor causalgia), Sudeck's atrophy (see Chapter 8), and other reflex dystrophies of the upper extremity.

Symptomatic treatment consists of wet dressings, analgesics, repeated sympathetic blocks, and protection of the part from irritation, all of which are temporizing measures. Operative sympathetic denervation gives permanent relief of intractable pain of true causalgia in the majority of critically selected patients (see Buker reference).

Buker RH & others: Causalgia and transthoracic sympathectomy. Am J Surg 124:724, 1972.
Wirth FP Jr, Rutherford RB: A civilian experience with causalgia. Arch Surg 100:633, 1970.

EPICONDYLITIS
(Tennis Elbow, Epicondylalgia) ✓

Epicondylitis is a pain syndrome affecting the midportion of the upper extremity; no single causative lesion has been identified. It has been postulated that chronic strain of the forearm muscles due to repetitive grasping or rotatory motions of the forearm causes microscopic tears and subsequent chronic inflammation of the common extensor or common flexor tendon at or near their respective osseous origins from the epicondyles. Inflamed and redundant, synovium-covered fibrofatty projections in the posterior radiohumeral joint may also play an etiologic role.

Epicondylitis occurs most frequently during middle life in the major extremity. Pain is predominantly on the medial or lateral aspect of the elbow region; may be aggravated by grasping; and may radiate proximally into the arm or distally into the forearm. The point of maximal tenderness to pressure is 1–2 cm distal to the epicondyle but may also be present in the muscle bellies more distally. Resisted dorsiflexion or volar flexion of the wrist may accentuate the pain. X-ray examination generally reveals no significant change, but occasionally a discrete, amorphous deposit of calcium salts adjacent to the epicondyle in the tendinous fibers is demonstrated.

Epicondylitis must be differentiated from other cervicobrachial pain syndromes as well as from gout and rheumatoid arthritis.

Treatment is directed toward relief of pain and tenderness. Most acute or subacute symptoms can be relieved by avoidance of repetitive grasping. An elastic bandage applied firmly about the proximal forearm may temporarily ameliorate discomfort when the patient is grasping forcefully. Chronic symptoms may require restrictive immobilization such as that provided by an Ilfeld elbow brace or a volar plaster splint. Physi-

cal therapy is ineffective except for relief of mild symptoms. Infiltration of "trigger points" by local anesthetic solutions with or without corticosteroids may be helpful. If 3–4 injections do not provide lasting relief of pain, other treatment should be given. Operative treatment is reserved for chronic, refractory cases.

Symptoms usually respond to rest and conservative measures.

Boyd HB, McLeod AC Jr: Tennis elbow. J Bone Joint Surg 55A:1183, 1973.
Coonrad RW, Hooper WR: Tennis elbow: Its course, natural history, conservative and surgical management. J Bone Joint Surg 55A:1177, 1973.

CARPAL TUNNEL SYNDROME ✓

Carpal tunnel syndrome is a painful disorder caused by compression of the median nerve between the essentially inelastic carpal ligament and other structures within the carpal tunnel. The volume of the contents of the tunnel can be increased by organic lesions such as synovitis of the tendon sheaths or carpal joints, recent or malhealed fractures, tumors, and occasionally congenital anomalies. Even though no anatomic lesion is apparent, flattening or even circumferential constriction of the median nerve may be observed during operative section of the ligament. Carpal tunnel syndrome can be a feature of systemic diseases such as rheumatoid arthritis, amyloidosis, acromegaly, myxedema, and diabetes. The occurrence of this syndrome during pregnancy or after menopause has been attributed to changes in tissue turgor. Extremes of volar flexion or dorsiflexion of the wrist may intensify existing symptoms or precipitate acute complaints. This syndrome is most frequently encountered in postmenopausal women and is not a feature of occupations that require strenuous and repetitive use of the hands.

Pain in the distribution of the median nerve, which may be burning and tingling (acroparesthesia), is the initial symptom. Aching pain may radiate proximally into the forearm and even to the shoulder joint. Pain may be episodic or constant, and is exacerbated by manual activity. It may be only nocturnal. Impairment of sensation in the median nerve distribution may not be apparent when symptoms are recent, and subtle disparity between the affected and opposite sides can be demonstrated by requiring the patient to identify different textures of cloth by rubbing them between the tips of the thumb and the index finger. Tinel's and Phalen's tests may be positive. Muscle weakness or atrophy, especially of the abductor pollicis brevis, appears later than sensory disturbances. Useful special examinations include electromyography and determinations of sensory and motor conduction delay. Distal median sensory conduction delay may be evident before motor delay.

This syndrome should be differentiated from other cervicobrachial pain syndromes and from compression syndromes of the median nerve in the forearm or arm.

Treatment is directed toward relief of pressure on the median nerve. Conservative treatment usually relieves mild symptoms of recent onset. When a primary lesion is discovered, specific treatment should be given. When soft tissue swelling is a cause, elevation of the extremity may relieve symptoms. Splinting of the hand and forearm at night may be beneficial. When nonspecific inflammation of the ulnar bursa is thought to be a cause, some authors recommend injection of corticosteroids into the carpal tunnel.

Conservative treatment, especially splinting of the wrist, may be helpful in relieving pain of recent duration but should not be prolonged when median nerve motor or sensory impairment is present.

Operative division of the volar carpal ligament gives lasting relief from pain which usually subsides within a few days. Muscle strength returns gradually, but complete recovery cannot be expected when atrophy is pronounced.

Frymoyer JW, Bland J: Carpal-tunnel tyndrome in patients with myxedematous arthropathy. J Bone Joint Surg 55A:78, 1973.

Hoffman DE: Carpal tunnel syndrome: Importance of sensory nerve conduction studies in diagnosis. JAMA 233:983, 1975.

SHOULDER-HAND SYNDROME

Shoulder-hand syndrome (accepted by some as a clinical entity) is a variable complex of symptoms and signs arising from various painful disorders of the shoulder joint and hand of the same extremity. According to the current view, it is a manifestation of reflex neurovascular dystrophy. The syndrome is essentially a combination of scapulohumeral periarthritis and Sudeck's atrophy of the hand and wrist.

Shoulder-hand syndrome occurs with increasing frequency during the middle years of life. Shoulder symptoms may precede or follow hand involvement, or both may begin at the same time. The elbow joint is usually spared; when the elbow is involved, painful restriction of motion is the principal manifestation.

This syndrome should be differentiated from other cervicobrachial pain syndromes and from rheumatoid arthritis, polymyositis, scleroderma, and gout.

In addition to specific treatment of the underlying disorder, treatment is directed toward restoration of function. Therapy described for scapulohumeral periarthritis (see above) and Sudeck's atrophy (see Chapter 8) is given simultaneously. The prognosis depends in part upon the stage in which the lesions of the shoulder joint and hand are encountered and the extent and severity of associated organic disease. Early treatment offers the best prognosis for recovery.

Steinbrocker O: The shoulder-hand syndrome: Present perspective. Arch Phys Med 49:388, 1968.

Woolf D: Shoulder-hand syndrome. Practitioner 213:176, 1974.

CERVICOBRACHIAL PAIN OF INTRATHORACIC ORIGIN

Pain in the shoulder girdle region and upper extremity due to myocardial ischemia of arteriosclerotic heart disease is discussed in Chapter 8. This is a frequent cause of shoulder-hand syndrome.

Bronchogenic carcinoma (see Chapter 6) in the region of the pulmonary apex is an uncommon cause of cervicobrachial pain. Because of the frequency of bronchogenic carcinoma among older people, it is likely to coexist with other organic lesions which cause pain in the anatomic regions under discussion here. X-ray examination of the upper thorax by lordotic projections or tomography may reveal lesions that are not demonstrated by routine x-ray technics employed for the diagnosis of lung, shoulder girdle, and cervical spine disorders.

Spengler DM & others: Orthopaedic aspects and early diagnosis of superior sulcus tumor of lung (Pancoast). J Bone Joint Surg 55A:1645, 1973.

TUMORS & TUMOR-LIKE LESIONS OF BONE

Essentials of Diagnosis

- Persistent pain, swelling, or tenderness of a skeletal part.
- Limitation of motion of an affected part.
- Pathologic ("spontaneous") fractures.
- Suspicious areas of bony enlargement, deformity, radiodensity, or radiolucency on x-ray.
- Histologic evidence of bone neoplasm on biopsy specimen.

General Considerations

Primary tumors of bone are relatively uncommon in comparison with secondary or metastatic neoplasms. They are, however, of great clinical significance because of the possibility of malignancy and because some of them grow rapidly and metastasize widely.

Although tumors of bone have been categorized classically as primary or secondary, there is some disagreement about which tumors are primary to the skeleton. Tumors of mesenchymal origin that reflect skeletal tissues (eg, bone, cartilage, and connective tissue) and tumors developing in bones that are of hematopoietic, nerve, vascular, fat cell, and notochordal origin should be differentiated from secondary malignant tumors that involve bone by direct extension or hematogenous spread.

Because of the great variety of bone tumors, it is difficult to establish a satisfactory simple classification of bone neoplasms. Lichtenstein's classification of benign and malignant primary bone tumors serves as a useful framework.

Persistent skeletal pain and swelling, with or without limitation of motion of adjacent joints or spontaneous fracture, are indications for prompt clinical, x-ray, laboratory, and possibly biopsy examination. X-rays may reveal the location and extent of the lesion and certain characteristics which may suggest the specific diagnosis. The so-called classical x-ray findings of certain tumors (eg, punched-out areas of the skull in multiple myeloma, "sun ray" appearance of osteogenic sarcoma, and "onion peel" effect of Ewing's sarcoma), although suggestive, are not pathognomonic. Even histologic characteristics of the tumor, when taken alone, cannot provide infallible information about the nature of the process. The age of the patient, the duration of complaints, the site of involvement and the number of bones involved, and the presence or absence of associated systemic disease—as well as the histologic characteristics—must be considered collectively for proper diagnosis and treatment.

The possibility of benign developmental skeletal abnormalities, metastatic neoplastic disease, or infections (eg, osteomyelitis), collagenoses, or metabolic disease of bone must always be kept in mind. If bone tumors occur in or near the joints, they may be confused with the various types of arthritis, especially monarticular arthritis.

The diagnosis of bone tumors is most precise when it is made in close consultation between the clinician, radiologist, and pathologist.

Although prompt action is essential for optimal treatment of certain bone tumors, accurate diagnosis is required because of the great potential for harm which may result either from temporization or from radical or ablative operations or unnecessary irradiation. If conservative treatment is elected, careful clinical and x-ray follow-up and expert consultation are necessary.

The clinical features, treatment, and prognosis of a few primary bone tumors are summarized in Table 14–1.

Aegerter E, Kirkpatrick JA Jr: *Orthopedic Diseases,* 4th ed. Saunders, 1975.

Campbell CJ & others: New therapies for osteogenic sarcoma. J Bone Joint Surg 57A: 143, 1975.

Cortes EP & others: Amputation and adriamycin in primary osteosarcoma. New England J Med 291:998, 1974.

Douglass HO Jr & others: Improvement in the results of treatment of osteogenic sarcoma. Surg Gynec Obst 140:693, 1975.

Jaffee N & others: Adjuvant methotrexate and citrovorum-factor treatment of osteogenic sarcoma. New England J Med 291:994, 1974.

Lichtenstein L: *Bone Tumors,* 4th ed. Mosby, 1972.

Rosen G & others: High-dose methotrexate with citrovorum factor rescue and adriamycin in childhood osteogenic sarcoma. Cancer 33:1151, 1974.

Tachdjian MO: *Pediatric Orthopedics.* 2 vols. Saunders, 1972.

. . .

OSTEOGENESIS IMPERFECTA
(Fragilitas Ossium, Brittle Bones, Osteopsathyrosis)

Essentials of Diagnosis

- Clinical triad: (1) Fragility of bone manifest by pathologic fracture. (2) Clearness or blue coloration of ocular scleras. (3) Deafness.
- Family history.
- Ligamentous laxity.
- Proneness to bruising.
- Dentinogenesis imperfecta.

General Considerations

Osteogenesis imperfecta is a heritable disorder of mesenchymal tissue usually transmitted as an autosomal dominant, though some cases may be autosomal recessive. A positive family history of this disorder may be lacking, especially among those afflicted by the congenita type. It has been debated whether this is a single disorder or a conglomeration of unsorted entities. Two recognized clinical types may occur: **osteogenesis imperfecta congenita** (fetal type), in which fractures occur in utero and skeletal deformities are apparent at birth; and **osteogenesis imperfecta tarda,** in which fractures and deformities occur after birth. Although subdivision of the latter type into 2 categories has been proposed, general agreement is lacking on the criteria of diagnosis with the exception of bowing deformity of the long bones (especially of the lower extremity).

Epiphyseal cartilaginous proliferation and maturation appear normal, but enchondral ossification lags as a result of inadequate osteoid formation by osteoblasts. Disturbance of intramembranous bone formation is identified in the congenita type by softness of the calvarium to palpation (caput membranaceum), temporal and occipital bulges, flattening of the vertex, and secondary centers of ossification (Wormian bones). A defect of collagen formation has been repeatedly proposed, but its nature has not been identified with certainty. Immaturity and deficiency of cardiovascular connective tissue have been observed in the congenita type.

Clinical Findings

A. Symptoms and Signs: Fragility of bones is the single most obvious diagnostic criterion. A nodular or "lumpy" appearance, with angular or bow-like deformities of the extremities, directs attention at birth to other clinical manifestations. Repeated fractures in childhood should suggest the underlying disorder.

Table 14—1. "Primary" bone tumors.

Name and Source	Age and Sex Incidence	Clinical Features*	X-Ray Findings	Treatment	Prognosis
Osteoid osteoma Osteoblastic connective tissue origin	Older children and adolescents. M 2:1	Small, painful (especially nocturnal), tender tumor of almost any bone, but more often in the femur and tibia.	Dense sclerotic lesion with radiolucent center.	Surgical removal.	Good. Removal is curative.
Osteogenic sarcoma Osteoblastic connective tissue derivation	Peak incidence 20 years. Rare over 40 years. Slight male preponderance.	Gradually progressive pain with variable swelling, local heat, venous engorgement, and tenderness, commonly at metaphyses of major long bones; about 50% involve the knee region. Other sites include pelvis, slender long bones, and flat bones. Weight loss, anemia, and elevation of serum alkaline phosphatase occur later. Histologic examination of biopsy specimen is the most useful laboratory procedure.	Variable, depending upon the osteolytic or sclerosing nature of the tumor. Penetration of cortical bone usually occurs with periosteal elevation and extension into soft tissues. Bone spicules perpendicular to the normal cortical surface—"sunburst" effect—may appear in sclerosing lesions. Chest x-ray may reveal pulmonary metastases.	Local control by amputation or resection of accessible lesions and adjuvant chemotherapy with multiple drugs. Chemotherapy with or without radiation for palliation if tumor is inoperable.	Poor. Smallest and most distal lesions offer best prognosis. Prognosis less favorable for large tumors and trunk tumors. Five-year overall survival is 5—20%. Death due to metastases or toxic effects of drug therapy.
Fibrosarcoma Nonosteoblastic connective tissue derivation	Adults 30—70 years, but also seen in second decade. M = F	Similar to above. Differentiation from osteogenic sarcoma depends upon histologic findings. May be a history (very rare) of irradiation exposure of bone many years previously.	Similar to above.	Amputation if accessible, with or without preliminary irradiation.	Poor, but perhaps slightly better than for osteogenic sarcoma.
Enchondroma Cartilaginous derivation	Adults. Rare before 10 years. M = F	Mild pain, tenderness, or swelling or spontaneous fracture of bones of hands or feet or of metaphyses of major long bones or flat bones. Lesions may be multiple. Histologic examination confirms diagnosis.	Discrete foci of radiolucency with mottling and compartmentalization. Cortical expansion occurs without extensive erosion.	Curettement of solitary nodules.	Usually good. Pelvic lesions may become malignant.
Chondromyxoid fibroma Cartilaginous derivation	Young adults 10—30 years. Rare before 10 years. M = F	Pain, swelling, tenderness at metaphyses of major long bones, bones of hands or feet, and flat bones. Histologic examination confirms the diagnosis.	Not characteristic. Ovoid or elongated focus of rarefaction and cortical expansion with erosion. May be multiple foci of osteolysis.	Thorough curettement or excision.	Good.
Chondrosarcoma Cartilaginous derivation	Adults 30—60 years, but also found in childhood and adolescence. M = F	Slow development of pain and swelling of almost any bone, especially long bones, with delayed tendency to metastasis (compare with osteogenic sarcoma).	Irregularly mottled and calcified interior of long bones with fuzzy localized destruction of cortex. Peripheral lesions present a dense, blotchy peripheral outline.	Radical surgical excision or amputation.	If excision is complete, prognosis is excellent. If incomplete, recurrence and progression.

	Age/Sex	Clinical Findings	X-Ray Findings	Treatment	Prognosis
Giant cell tumor (osteoclastoma) Nonosteoblastic connective tissue derivation	10–50 years. M = F	Pain and swelling at ends of major long bones, especially near knee and lower radius. Also found in other bones of extremities and spine.	Eccentrically located osteolytic focus with expansion and cortical erosion. Roughly spherical foamlike areas in cancellous ends of femur and tibia or in distal radial metaphyses.	Excision preferred to curettement when feasible.	About half are biologically benign and have a favorable outcome regardless of treatment. About a third are aggressive, recur, and require further treatment. The rest are frankly malignant.
Chondroblastoma (Epiphyseal giant cell tumor) Cartilaginous derivation	Almost always under 20 years. Predominantly male.	Pain and swelling in epiphyseal areas of major tubular bones and in flat bones.	Ovoid areas of mottled translucency in epiphyses or adjacent metaphyses with demarcating wall of sclerotic bone.	Thorough curettement usually adequate.	Almost always benign. Instances of malignancy reported.
Ewing's sarcoma Mesenchymal connective tissue derivation	Adolescents and young adults, but may occur in children. Slight male preponderance.	Pain, swelling, and tenderness of single or multiple lesions of shafts of major tubular bones, vertebrae, or flat bones of trunk. Later findings include fever, anemia, leukocytosis, and increased sedimentation rate. Biopsy essential for diagnosis. Course may be slow, with remissions and exacerbations to progression with metastases.	Diffuse osteosclerosis of cortex with fusiform configuration, subperiosteal lamination ("onion peel") and occasionally "sunburst" periosteal reaction and medullary destruction evidenced by diffuse rarefaction or mottling.	Supervoltage radiation and adjuvant multi-drug chemotherapy.	Very poor. Mortality rate about 85% with local radiation alone.
Plasma cell myeloma (Multiple myeloma) Hematopoietic origin	Adults over 40 years. M 2:1	Multifocal skeletal involvement. Local pain, swelling, and tendency to pathologic fractures. Spine involvement can cause kyphosis and decreased stature. Late findings include anemia, hypercalcemia, hypercalciuria, hyperglobulinemia, Bence Jones proteinuria, and hyperuricemia. Marrow aspiration or bone biopsy essential for diagnosis. Course may be slow, with remissions and exacerbations.	Variable. Diffuse osteoporosis. Focal lesions appear as diffuse or circumscribed (punched-out) areas of rarefaction without surrounding sclerosis and sometimes with cortical expansion.	X-ray therapy for relief of pain. Chemotherapy (alkylating agents).	Chemotherapy may relieve symptoms and sometimes prolongs life. Average survival is about 1–2 years but may be much longer.

*Local pain, swelling, and tenderness—and occasionally pathologic fractures—are common features of all bone tumors.

Clearness or blue coloration of the scleras is not pathognomonic of this syndrome. Deafness (consistent with otosclerosis) occurs in about half of cases. Spinal deformities (scoliosis and kyphosis) emphasize the clinical pattern of dwarfism.

No obvious hematologic defect has been identified to explain the proneness to bruising in these patients. Defective dentin formation (dentinogenesis imperfecta) of both deciduous and permanent teeth is characterized by a translucent or opalescent appearance after eruption and subsequent pink, gray, or even amber discoloration of the teeth. Ligamentous laxity causes joint hypermobility. Other manifestations of connective tissue dysplasia include hernias and hyperelasticity of the skin. Neurologic symptoms may be caused by hydrocephalus or compression of the spinal cord at the foramen magnum or in the kyphotic cervical spine.

B. X-Ray Findings: A wide variety of structural abnormalities may be identified in the skull, vertebral bodies, and pelvis. The major long bones in the congenita type may exhibit the "thick form," in which the cortices are thin and the marrow cavities are broad. In the late type, the bones may be "slender," with narrow shafts, reduced marrow cavities, and bell-shaped widening of the epiphyses. The trabecular markings of the spongiosa are absent or faint. Callus formation after fracture may be meager or luxuriant. Hyperplastic callus formation may occur with or without apparent fracture.

At birth, the congenita form should be differentiated from achondroplasia, hydrocephalus, and hypophosphatasia. The milder cases of the late form may simulate idiopathic juvenile or menopausal osteoporosis. Joint hypermobility and spinal deformities occur in Marfan's syndrome. Articular laxity, with dislocations and proneness to bruising, may simulate some manifestations of Ehlers-Danlos syndrome. Hyperplastic callus formation, especially when it occurs without evidence of fracture, may simulate osteogenic sarcoma.

Treatment

No successful treatment has been developed for the apparent defect in formation of adequate osteoid.

Most severe orthopedic lesions require specific treatment. Most fractures require immobilization for the relief of pain and prevention of malhealing. They can generally be treated by closed technics, but prolonged and extensive external immobilization is to be avoided because of the threat of further bone weakening as a result of atrophy. A simple osteotomy or osteoclasis occasionally can correct a minor deformity of a long bone. Extensive deformities of the diaphysis of a major long bone require more elaborate surgical treatment. Surgical treatment of kyphoscoliosis may have to be delayed until late adolescence, when skeletal structures are stronger.

X-ray therapy in small doses has been advocated for amelioration of hyperplastic callus formation.

Prognosis

Because of the protean manifestations of this disease, the course and prognosis are variable. Severe manifestations of the congenita form, especially multiple fractures, may be associated with death of the fetus or premature birth and neonatal death. Transmission of the more severe traits is probably prevented by death before puberty or by prevention of reproduction of invalids. The incidence of fracture and the extent of ligamentous laxity are likely to decrease after puberty, and this favorable turn tends to continue through adolescence into later life. Severe deformities of major long bones that require extensive operative procedures for correction have a tendency to recur as growth continues.

A considerable number of patients with milder expressions of the disease will survive and be capable of productive lives in sedentary occupations.

Albright JA, Grunt JA: Studies of patients with osteogenesis imperfecta. J Bone Joint Surg 53A:1415, 1971.

Bauze RJ & others: A new look at osteogenesis imperfecta: A clinical, radiological and biochemical study of forty-two patients. J Bone Joint Surg 57B:2, 1975.

Falvo KA, Bullough PG: Osteogenesis imperfecta: A histometric analysis. J Bone Joint Surg 55A:275, 1973.

Falvo KA & others: Osteogenesis imperfecta: Clinical evaluation and management. J Bone Joint Surg 56A:783, 1974.

King JD, Bobechko WP: Osteogenesis imperfecta: An orthopaedic description and surgical review. J Bone Joint Surg 53B:72, 1971.

Tiley F, Albright JA: Osteogenesis imperfecta: Treatment by multiple osteotomy and intramedullary rod insertion. J Bone Joint Surg 55A:701, 1973.

15 . . .
Genitourinary Tract

Marcus A. Krupp

NONSPECIFIC MANIFESTATIONS

Pain

The localization, pattern of referral, and type of pain are important clues to the diagnosis of genitourinary tract disease.

(1) Pain caused by **renal disease** is usually felt as a dull ache in the "flanks" or costovertebral angle, often extending along the rib margin toward the umbilicus. Because many renal diseases do not produce sudden distention of the capsules of the kidney, absence of pain is common.

(2) **Ureteral pain** is related to obstruction and is usually acute in onset, severe, and colicky, and radiates from the costovertebral angle down the course of the ureter into the scrotum or vulva and the inner thigh. The site of the obstruction may be determined by the location of the radiation of the pain: high ureteral pain is usually referred to the testicle or vulva; mid-ureteral pain to the right lower quadrant of the abdomen; and low ureteral pain to the bladder.

(3) **Bladder pain** accompanies overdistention of the bladder in acute urinary retention and distention of a bladder wall altered by tuberculosis or interstitial cystitis. Relief comes with emptying the bladder. Pain due to bladder infection is usually referred to the distal urethra and accompanies micturition.

(4) Pain caused by **chronic prostatic disease** is uncommon.

(5) Pain caused by **testicular inflammation or trauma** is acute and severe and is occasionally referred to the costovertebral angle. Pain associated with infection of the epididymis is similar to that associated with testicular inflammation.

Urinary Symptoms

Infection, inflammation, and obstruction produce symptoms associated with urination.

(1) **Frequency, urgency, and nocturia** are commonly experienced when inflammation of the urinary tract is present. Severe infection produces a constant desire to urinate even though the bladder contains only a few ml of urine. Frequency and nocturia occur when bladder capacity is diminished by disease or when the bladder cannot be emptied completely, leaving a large volume of residual urine. Nocturia associated with a large urine volume may occur with heart failure, renal insufficiency, mobilization of edema due to any cause, diabetes insipidus, hyperaldosteronism, and ingestion of large amounts of fluid late in the evening.

(2) **Dysuria and burning pain in the urethra on urination** are associated with infection of the bladder and prostate.

(3) **Enuresis** may be due to urinary tract disease but is most often caused by neural or psychogenic disorders.

(4) **Urinary incontinence** may be due to anatomic abnormality, physical stress, the urgency associated with infection or nervous system disease, and the dribbling associated with an overdistended flaccid bladder.

Characteristics of Urine

(1) **Urinalysis**, an essential part of the examination of all patients, is critical in the study of patients who may have renal disease. Organic and inorganic materials in solution in the urine are diagnostic of metabolic disease (inherited or acquired) and of renal disease. The urinary sediment provides evidence of renal disease that is not available from other sources, and some elements are characteristic of the type and extent of renal disease. Whenever possible, the physician himself should review the sediment, particularly if renal disease may be present. The significance of elements appearing in the urine will be explained below in the discussion of each disease.

(2) **Cloudy urine** is most frequently the result of the urates or phosphates which precipitate out as urine collects in the bladder, and is usually of no significance.

(3) **Hematuria** is always of grave significance. It may be due to glomerular disease, neoplasms, vascular accidents, infections, anomalies, stones, or trauma to the urinary tract. When blood appears only during the initial period of voiding, the likely source is the anterior urethra or prostate. When blood appears during the terminal period of voiding, the likely source is the posterior urethra, vesical neck, or trigone. Blood mixed in with the total urine volume is from the kidney, ureters, or bladder.

Renal Function Tests

Recognition of renal diseases and evaluation of renal function are dependent on laboratory determinations. As renal function becomes impaired, laboratory observations provide reliable indices of the capacity of the kidney to meet the demands of excretion, reabsorption, and secretion and to fulfill its role in maintaining homeostasis.

Useful tests may be categorized according to the physiologic function measured, as follows:

A. Glomerular Filtration Rate (GFR): Inulin clearance is the reference method for measuring GFR. After a single intravenous injection of ^{51}Cr edetate or of ^{131}I iothalamate, the slope of decreasing concentration in plasma can be determined to give a precise measure of GFR. For routine clinical use, the less precise endogenous creatinine clearance is adequate. Plasma creatinine or urea levels reflect GFR, rising as the filtration rate diminishes.

B. Renal Plasma Flow (RPF): There is no simple clinical test of RPF. Measurement of clearance of para-aminohippurate or of radioiodine-tagged compounds utilized in urography may be used.

C. Tubular Function: Clinical means of assessing tubular function include the ability to produce urine that is more concentrated or less concentrated than the osmolality of plasma; the ability to acidify the urine; and, of lesser value, the ability to excrete phenolsulphonphthalein (PSP).

Renal Biopsy

Renal biopsy is a valuable diagnostic procedure which also serves as a guide to rational treatment. The technic has become well established, frequently providing sufficient tissue for light and electron microscopy and for immunofluorescent examination. Absolute contraindications include anatomic presence of only one kidney, severe malfunction of one kidney even though function is adequate in the other, bleeding diathesis, the presence of hemangioma, tumor, or large cysts, abscess or infection, hydronephrosis, and an uncooperative patient. Relative contraindications are the presence of serious hypertension, uremia, severe arteriosclerosis, and unusual difficulty in doing a biopsy due to obesity, anasarca, or inability of the patient to lie flat.

Clinical indications for renal biopsy, in addition to the necessity for establishing a diagnosis, include the need to determine prognosis, to follow progression of a lesion and response to treatment, to confirm the presence of a generalized disease (collagen disorder, amyloidosis, sarcoidosis), and to follow rejection response in a transplanted kidney.

ROENTGENOGRAPHIC EXAMINATION

Renal Radiography

Radiography is an essential resource for the diagnosis and evaluation of renal disease amenable to medical as well as surgical treatment. Kidney size, shape, and position may be critical elements of infor-

mation. Routine films, tomography, urography, and angiography are sources of anatomic and physiologic data that often are definitive, revealing details of circulation, structure, and calcification available by no other means. Collaboration with the radiologist provides the greatest opportunity for properly performed and interpreted radiographic examinations.

Ultrasound (Sonography)

Ultrasound is a noninvasive technic that involves no hazard to the patient. Radar-like devices utilizing high-frequency sound waves are capable of delineating solid or fluid-filled organs or masses. Kidney size and shape can often be distinguished clearly enough to identify tumors or cysts and anomalies such as horseshoe kidney. Calcification within the kidney and urinary tract can sometimes be demonstrated better in this way than by any other means.

DISORDERS OF THE KIDNEYS

GLOMERULONEPHRITIS

Information obtained from experimentally induced glomerular disease in animals and from correlations with evidence derived by modern methods of examination of tissue obtained by biopsy and at necropsy have provided a new concept of glomerulonephritis.

The clinical manifestations of renal disease are apt to consist only of varying degrees of hematuria, excretion of characteristic formed elements in the urine, proteinuria, and renal insufficiency and its complications. Alterations in glomerular architecture as observed in tissue examined by light microscopy are also apt to be minimal and difficult to interpret. For these reasons, attempts to correlate clinical syndromes with histologic features of renal tissue have failed to provide a satisfactory basis for precise diagnosis, treatment, and prognosis.

More recently, however, immunologic technics for demonstrating a variety of antigens, antibodies, and complement fractions have led to new concepts of the origins and pathogenesis of glomerular disease. Electron microscopy has complemented the immunologic methods.

Briefly, then, glomerular disease resulting from immunologic reactions may be divided into 2 groups:

(1) **Immune complex disease**, in which soluble antigen-antibody complexes in the circulation are trapped in the glomeruli. The antigens are not derived from glomerular components; they may be exogenous (bacterial, viral, chemical, including antibiotics and other drugs) or endogenous (circulating native DNA, thyroglobulin). Factors in the pathogenic potential of

the antigen include its origin, quantity, and route of entry and the host's duration of exposure to it. The immune response to the antigen depends in part upon the severity of inflammation or infection and in part on the host's capacity to respond (immunocompetency).

In the presence of antigen excess and, in some cases, antibody excess, antigen-antibody complexes form in the circulation and are trapped in the glomeruli as they are filtered through capillaries rendered permeable by the action of vasoactive amines. The antigen-antibody complexes bind components of complement, particularly C3. Activated complement provides chemoactive factors which attract leukocytes whose lysosomal enzymes incite the injury to the glomerulus.

By immunofluorescent methods and by electron microscopy, these complexes appear as lumpy deposits between the epithelial cells and the glomerular basement membrane. IgG, IgM, occasionally IgA, β1C, and C3 are demonstrable.

(2) Anti-GBM (glomerular basement membrane) disease, in which antibodies are generated against the glomerular basement membrane of the kidney and often against lung basement membrane, which appears to be antigenically similar to GBM. The autoantibodies may be stimulated by autologous GBM altered in some way or combined with an exogenous agent. The reaction of antibody with GBM is accompanied by activation of complement, the attraction of leukocytes, and the release of lysosomal enzymes. The presence of thrombi in glomerular capillaries is often accompanied by leakage of fibrinogen and precipitation of fibrin in Bowman's space with subsequent development of epithelial "crescents" in the space.

Immunofluorescent technics and electron microscopy show the anti-GBM complexes as linear deposits outlining the GBM. IgG and C3 are usually demonstrable.

The current classification of glomerulonephritis is based on the immunologic concepts described above. However, the discussions in the following pages will be organized according to the traditional clinical categories.

I. Immunologic Mechanisms Likely

A. Immune Complex Disease:

Glomerulonephritis clearly poststreptococcal

Glomerulonephritis associated with infectious agents, including staphylococci, pneumococci, bacterial endocarditis, secondary syphilis, malaria, viruses of hepatitis (HB-Ag) and measles

Lupus erythematosus

Glomerulonephritis associated with other systemic (? autoimmune) disease such as polyarteritis nodosa, scleroderma, anaphylactoid purpura, and idiopathic cryoglobulinemia

Membranous glomerulonephritis, cause unknown

Membranoproliferative glomerulonephritis, cause unknown

Focal glomerulonephritis

Rapidly progressive glomerulonephritis (some cases)

B. Anti-GBM Disease:

Goodpasture's syndrome

Rapidly progressive glomerulonephritis (some cases)

II. Immunologic Mechanisms Not Clearly Shown

Lipoid nephrosis

Focal glomerulonephritis (some cases)

Chronic sclerosing glomerulonephritis

Diabetic glomerulosclerosis

Amyloidosis

Hemolytic-uremic syndrome and thrombohemolytic thrombocytopenic purpura

Wegener's granulomatosis

Alport's syndrome

Sickle cell disease

1. POSTSTREPTOCOCCAL GLOMERULONEPHRITIS

Essentials of Diagnosis

- History of preceding streptococcal infection.
- Malaise, headache, anorexia, low-grade fever.
- Mild generalized edema, mild hypertension, retinal hemorrhages.
- Gross hematuria; protein, red cell casts, granular and hyaline casts, white cells, and renal epithelial cells in urine.
- Elevated antistreptolysin O titer, variable nitrogen retention.

General Considerations

Glomerulonephritis is a disease affecting both kidneys. In most cases recovery from the acute stage is complete, but progressive involvement may destroy renal tissue and renal insufficiency results. Acute glomerulonephritis is most common in children 3–10 years of age, although 5% or more of initial attacks occur in adults over the age of 50. By far the most common cause is an antecedent infection of the pharynx and tonsils or of the skin with group A β-hemolytic streptococci, certain strains of which are nephritogenic. Nephritis occurs in 10–15% of children and young adults who have clinically evident infection with a nephritogenic strain. In children under age 6, pyoderma (impetigo) is the most common antecedent; in older children and young adults, pharyngitis is a common and skin infection a rare antecedent. Nephritogenic strains commonly encountered include, for the skin, M types 49 (Red Lake), 2, and provisional 55; for pharyngitis, types 12, 1, and 4. Rarely, nephritis may follow infections due to pneumococci, staphylococci, some bacilli and viruses, or *Plasmodium malariae,* and exposure to some drugs. Rhus dermatitis and reactions to venom or chemical agents may be associated with renal disease clinically indistinguishable from glomerulonephritis.

The pathogenesis of the glomerular lesion has been further elucidated by the use of new immunologic technics (immunofluorescence) and electron microscopy. A likely sequel to infection by nephritogenic strains of β-hemolytic streptococci is injury to the mesangial cells in the intercapillary space. The glomerulus may then become more easily damaged by antigen-antibody complexes developing from the immune response to the streptococcal infection. The C3 component of complement is deposited in association with IgG or alone in a granular pattern on the epithelial side of the basement membrane and occasionally in subendothelial sites as well.

Gross examination of the involved kidney shows only punctate hemorrhages throughout the cortex. Microscopically, the primary alteration is in the glomeruli, which show proliferation and swelling of the mesangial and endothelial cells of the capillary tuft. The proliferation of capsular epithelium produces a thickened crescent about the tuft, and in the space between the capsule and the tuft there are collections of leukocytes, red cells, and exudate. Edema of the interstitial tissue and cloudy swelling of the tubule epithelium are common. As the disease progresses, the kidneys may enlarge. The typical histologic findings in glomerulitis are enlarging crescents which become hyalinized and converted into scar tissue and obstruct the circulation through the glomerulus. Degenerative changes occur in the tubules, with fatty degeneration and necrosis and ultimate scarring of the nephron. Arteriolar thickening and obliteration become prominent.

Clinical Findings

A. Symptoms and Signs: Often the disease is very mild, and there may be no reason to suspect renal involvement unless the urine is examined. In severe cases, about 2 weeks following the acute streptococcal infection, the patient develops headache, malaise, mild fever, puffiness around the eyes and face, flank pain, and oliguria. Hematuria is usually noted as "bloody" or, if the urine is acid, as "brown" or "coffee-colored." Respiratory difficulty with shortness of breath may occur as a result of salt and water retention and circulatory congestion. There may be moderate tachycardia and moderate to marked elevation of blood pressure. Tenderness in the costovertebral angle is common.

B. Laboratory Findings: The diagnosis is confirmed by examination of the urine, which may be grossly bloody or coffee-colored (acid hematin) or may show only microscopic hematuria. In addition, the urine contains protein (1–3+) and casts. Hyaline and granular casts are commonly found in large numbers, but the classical sign of glomerulitis, the erythrocyte cast (blood cast), may be found only occasionally in the urinary sediment. The erythrocyte cast resembles a blood clot formed in the lumen of a renal tubule; it is usually of small caliber, intensely orange or red, and

under high power with proper lighting may show the mosaic pattern of the packed red cells held together by the clot of fibrin and plasma protein.

With the impairment of renal function (decrease in GFR and blood flow) and with oliguria, plasma or serum urea nitrogen and creatinine become elevated, the levels varying with the severity of the renal lesion. The sedimentation rate is rapid. A mild normochromic anemia may result from fluid retention and dilution. Infection of the throat with nephritogenic streptococci is frequently followed by increasing antistreptolysin O (ASO) titers in the serum, whereas high titers are usually not demonstrable following skin infections. Production of antibody against streptococcal deoxyribonuclease B (anti-DNase B) is more regularly observed following both throat and skin infections. Serum complement levels are usually low.

Confirmation of diagnosis is made by examination of the urine, although the history and clinical findings in typical cases leave little doubt. The finding of erythrocytes in a cast is proof that erythrocytes were present in the renal tubules and did not arise from elsewhere in the genitourinary tract.

Differential Diagnosis

Although considered to be the hallmark of glomerulonephritis, erythrocyte casts also occur along with other abnormal elements in any disease in which glomerular inflammation and tubule damage are present, ie, polyarteritis nodosa, disseminated lupus erythematosus, dermatomyositis, sarcoidosis, subacute bacterial endocarditis, "focal" nephritis, Goodpasture's syndrome, Henoch's purpura, or poisoning with chemicals toxic to the kidney.

Complications

In severe cases, signs compatible with cardiac failure appear as a result of salt and water retention rather than of myocardial failure per se: cardiac enlargement, tachycardia, gallop rhythm, pulmonary passive congestion, pleural fluid, and peripheral edema.

With severe hypertension, signs of left ventricular failure often develop and the symptoms and signs of hypertensive encephalopathy may predominate: severe headache, drowsiness, muscle twitchings and convulsions, vomiting, and at times papilledema and retinal hemorrhage.

Any infection occurring in a patient with glomerulonephritis must be regarded as a serious complication.

Treatment

A. Specific Measures: There is no specific treatment. Eradication of beta-hemolytic streptococci with penicillin or other antibiotic is desirable. Adrenocorticosteroids and corticotropin are of no value and may be contraindicated because they increase protein catabolism, sodium retention, and hypertension. Immunosuppressive and cytotoxic drugs have been ineffective in this form of nephritis. (See Nephrotic Syndrome.)

B. General Measures: In uncomplicated cases, treatment is symptomatic and designed to prevent overhydration and hypertension. Hospitalization is indicated if oliguria, nitrogen retention, and hypertension are present. Bed rest is of great importance and should be continued until clinical signs abate. Blood pressure and BUN should be normal for more than 1–2 weeks before activity is resumed. A guide to duration of bed rest is the urine: When protein excretion has diminished to near normal and when white and epithelial cell excretion has decreased and stabilized, activity may be resumed on a graded basis. Excretion of protein and formed elements in the urine will increase with resumption of activity, but such increases should not be great. Erythrocytes may be excreted in large numbers for months, and the rate of excretion is not a good criterion for evaluating convalescence. If the sedimentation rate increases or if urinary findings become more pronounced with activity, return to bed rest and restricted activity are indicated for 10 days to 2 weeks before trial of activity is repeated.

In the presence of elevated BUN and oliguria, severe dietary protein restriction is indicated. If severe oliguria is present, no protein should be given. If no nitrogen retention is apparent, the diet may contain 0.5 gm of protein/kg ideal weight. Carbohydrates should be given liberally to provide calories and to reduce the catabolism of protein and prevent starvation ketosis. With severe oliguria, potassium intoxication may occur.

Sodium restriction varies with the degree of oliguria; in severe cases no sodium should be allowed. As recovery progresses, sodium intake can be increased.

Fluids should be restricted in keeping with the ability of the kidney to excrete urine. If restriction is not indicated, fluids can be consumed as desired. Occasionally, when nausea and vomiting preclude oral consumption, fluids must be given intravenously in amounts depending upon the severity of the oliguria. Glucose must be given in sufficient quantities to spare protein and prevent ketosis.

If edema becomes severe, a trial of an oral diuretic such as furosemide is in order. Treatment of extreme fluid overload and oliguria may require dialysis.

If anemia becomes severe (hematocrit less than 30%), blood transfusions in the form of packed red cells may be given.

C. Treatment of Complications:

1. Hypertensive encephalopathy should be treated vigorously as a medical emergency. Drowsiness and confusion accompanied by severe headache, nausea, blurred vision, and twitching progress to stupor and coma. A greatly elevated blood pressure (often > 250/150 mm Hg) and evidence of retinal arteriolar spasm with or without papilledema and hemorrhages are characteristic. The goal of therapy is to reduce blood pressure to near normal levels without further impairing renal function. The first-line drugs include diazoxide, hydralazine, methyldopa, reserpine, and nitroprusside. Diuretics employed concurrently are furosemide and ethacrynic acid. Sympathetic ganglionic blocking agents should be avoided if at all possible. Therapy may be initiated with diazoxide, 300 mg bolus rapidly IV (*caution:* the solution has a high pH; avoid extravasation). Maximal response occurs within 10–30 minutes and may last for as long as 18 hours. The dose may be repeated every 4–6 hours to maintain blood pressure at a desirable level. Furosemide, 40–80 mg IV, or ethacrynic acid, 50–100 mg IV, should be given simultaneously and repeated as required. Hydralazine, 10–50 mg, is administered IV or IM every 4–6 hours to titrate the dose required to hold blood pressure in the 150–170/100–90 mm Hg range. Methyldopa or reserpine may be employed but often produces an undesirable degree of drowsiness. Patients must be closely monitored during aggressive treatment with these potent drugs.

Diphenylhydantoin may be of value in controlling seizures.

2. Heart failure should be treated as any case of left ventricular failure, ie, with severe restriction of fluid and sodium intake and the use of digitalis and oxygen. To reduce fluid overload, an oral diuretic such as furosemide may be helpful.

3. Infection should be promptly eradicated with appropriate antibiotics. Prophylactic penicillin for several months after the acute phase has been advocated, but its value is not proved.

Prognosis

The progression of glomerulonephritis to healing or advancing disease is depicted in Fig 15–1. Most patients with the acute disease recover completely within 1–2 years; 5–20% show progressive renal damage. If oliguria, heart failure, or hypertensive encephalopathy is severe, death may occur during the acute attack. Even with severe acute disease, however, recovery is the rule, particularly in children.

See references under Latent Glomerulonephritis, below.

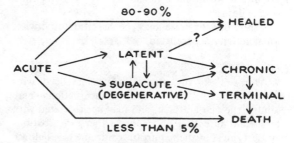

Figure 15–1. Prognosis in glomerulonephritis.

2. CHRONIC GLOMERULONEPHRITIS

Progressive destruction of the kidney may continue for many years in a clinically latent or subacute form. The subacute form is similar to the latent form (see below) except that symptoms occur, ie, malaise, mild fever, and sometimes flank pain and oliguria. Treatment is as for the acute attack. Exacerbations may appear from time to time, reflecting the stage of evolution of the disease.

3. LATENT GLOMERULONEPHRITIS

If acute glomerulonephritis does not heal within 1–2 years, the vascular and glomerular lesions continue to progress and tubular changes occur. In the presence of smoldering, active nephritis, the patient is usually asymptomatic and the evidence of disease consists only of the excretion of abnormal urinary elements.

The urinary excretion of protein, red cells, white cells, epithelial cells, and casts (including erythrocyte casts, granular casts, and hyaline and waxy casts) continues at levels above normal. As renal impairment progresses, signs of renal insufficiency appear (see below).

The differential diagnosis is the same as that given for acute glomerulonephritis. Recent studies of tissue obtained by renal biopsy in cases of recurrent or persistent hematuria indicate a high incidence of mesangial deposition of immune complexes made up of IgM or IgA (rarely IgG) and fractions of complement.

Prevention

Treat intercurrent infections promptly and vigorously as indicated. Avoid unnecessary vaccinations.

Treatment

Treat exacerbations as for the acute attack, nephrotic state, or incipient renal insufficiency as indicated. A normal diet, adequate for growth in childhood and adolescence, is desirable. A protein intake of 0.5–1 gm/kg is permissible as long as renal function is adequate to maintain a normal BUN. A liberal fluid intake is desirable.

Strenuous exercise may be harmful; otherwise, normal activity is permitted.

Prognosis

Worsening of the urinary findings may occur with infection, trauma, or fatigue. Exacerbations may resemble the acute attack, and may be associated with intercurrent infection or trauma. Other exacerbations may be typical of the nephrotic syndrome (see below). Death in uremia is the usual outcome, but the course is variable and the patient may live a reasonably normal life for 20–30 years.

Baldwin DS & others: The long-term course of poststreptococcal glomerulonephritis. Ann Int Med 80:342, 1974.

Ballard HS & others: Renal manifestations of the Henoch-Schönlein syndrome in adults. Am J Med 49:328, 1970.

Bricker NS: Renal function in chronic renal disease. Medicine 44:263, 1965.

Carpenter CB: Immunologic aspects of renal disease. Ann Rev Med 21:1, 1970.

Cream JJ & others: Schönlein-Henoch purpura in the adult: A study of 77 adults with anaphylactoid or Schönlein-Henoch purpura. Quart J Med 39:461, 1970.

Dixon FJ: The pathogenesis of glomerulonephritis. Am J Med 44:493, 1968.

Fish AJ & others: Epidemic acute glomerulonephritis associated with type 49 streptococcal pyoderma. 2. Correlative study of light, immunofluorescent and electron microscopic findings. Am J Med 48:28, 1970.

Gutman RA & others: The immune complex glomerulonephritis of subacute bacterial endocarditis. Medicine 51:1, 1972.

Kaplan EL & others: Epidemic acute glomerulonephritis associated with type 49 streptococcal pyoderma. 1. Clinical and laboratory findings. Am J Med 48:9, 1970.

Lewis EJ: Rapidly progressive glomerulonephritis. The Kidney 6:1, Jan 1973.

McCluskey RT, Leber PD: An evaluation of immunologic mechanisms. Page 694 in: *Controversy in Internal Medicine.* Vol 2. Ingelfinger FJ & others (editors). Saunders, 1974.

Merrill JP: Glomerulonephritis. (3 parts.) New England J Med 290:257, 313, 374, 1974.

Morel-Maroger L, Leathem A, Richet G: Glomerular abnormalities in nonsystemic diseases. Am J Med 53:170, 1972.

Rapoport A & others: Idiopathic focal proliferative glomerulonephritis associated with persistent hematuria and normal renal function. Ann Int Med 73:921, 1970.

Sagel I & others: Occurrence and nature of glomerular lesions after group A streptococci infections in children. Ann Int Med 79:492, 1973.

Wilson CB: Immunological mechanisms of glomerulonephritis. California Med 116:47, Jan 1972.

Wilson CB, Dixon FJ: The importance of immunologic mechanisms. Page 685 in: *Controversy in Internal Medicine.* Vol 2. Ingelfinger FJ & others (editors). Saunders, 1974.

4. ANTI-GLOMERULAR BASEMENT MEMBRANE NEPHRITIS (Goodpasture's Syndrome)

The patient usually gives a history of recent hemoptysis and often of malaise, anorexia, and headache. The clinical syndrome is that of a severe acute glomerulonephritis accompanied by diffuse hemorrhagic inflammation of the lungs. The urine shows gross or microscopic hematuria, and laboratory findings of severely suppressed renal function are usually evident. Biopsy shows glomerular crescents, glomerular adhesions, and inflammatory infiltration interstitially. Electron microscopic examination shows an increase in basement membrane material and deposition of fibrin beneath the capillary endothelium. In some cases, circulating antibody against glomerular basement membrane can be identified. IgG and C3 complement can be demonstrated as linear deposits on the basement membranes of the glomeruli and the lung. Antiglomerular basement membrane antibody also reacts with lung basement membrane.

Only rare cases of survival have been documented.

Adrenal corticosteroid therapy in combination with immunosuppressive therapy may be useful. Hemodialysis and nephrectomy with renal transplantation may offer the only hope for rescue. Transplantation should be delayed until circulating antiglomerular antibodies have disappeared.

Occasionally, acute renal disease with a similar clinical and immunologic pattern may occur without associated lung disease. Termed **idiopathic rapidly progressive glomerulonephritis**, it characteristically progresses to severe renal insufficiency in a few weeks.

Benoit FL & others: Goodpasture's syndrome: A clinicopathologic entity. Am J Med 37:424, 1964.

Proskey AJ & others: Goodpasture's syndrome: A report of five cases and a review of the literature. Am J Med 48:162, 1970.

CHRONIC RENAL INSUFFICIENCY

Essentials of Diagnosis

- Weakness and easy fatigability, headaches, anorexia, nausea and vomiting, pruritus, polyuria, nocturia.
- Hypertension with secondary encephalopathy, retinal damage, heart failure.
- Anemia, azotemia, and acidosis, with elevated serum potassium, phosphate, and sulfate; and decreased serum calcium and protein.
- Urine specific gravity low and fixed; mild to moderate proteinuria; few red cells, white cells, and broad renal failure casts.

General Considerations

The pathologic picture varies with the cause of the damage to the kidney. Extensive scarring with decrease in kidney size, hyalinization of glomeruli, and obliteration of some tubules and hypertrophy and dilatation of others produce great distortion of renal architecture. The vascular changes are due to the effects of scar formation and of prolonged hypertension, with thickening of the media, fragmentation of elastic fibers, intimal thickening, and obliteration of the lumens in some areas. In diabetic nephropathy the typical glomerular lesions of intercapillary sclerosis are often distinct. The vascular lesions of periarteritis or of systemic lupus erythematosus often serve to establish these diagnoses. Obstructive uropathy presents the classical picture of hydronephrosis with compression and destruction of the renal parenchyma. Polycystic disease, multiple myeloma, persistent hypercalcemia, amyloid disease, and other rarer causes of renal failure usually can be identified by characteristic pathologic lesions.

Clinical Findings

The clinical symptoms and signs of metabolic and

hypertensive components of renal failure appear insidiously and may not be noted until the effects are severe.

A. Symptoms and Signs: Metabolic and vascular abnormalities incident to renal insufficiency produce typical symptoms and signs. The metabolic defect is due to failure of the kidney to excrete the daily load of nitrogenous waste and to excrete or conserve water and electrolytes as required to maintain balance. The result is the clinical picture of uremia with its 3 cardinal signs: anemia, azotemia, and acidosis. The uremic patient often is weak and tired, complains of anorexia and nausea and vomiting, and may have diarrhea. He is often short of breath. Pruritus is common and the excoriations may be purpuric. Pallor and a waxy appearance of the skin are often observed. Polyuria reflects the inability of the kidney tubules to absorb water; as glomerular filtration becomes greatly reduced, oliguria appears. Terminal manifestations are severe nausea, diarrhea, muscle twitching, hyperpnea, pruritus, bleeding from mucous membranes, and somnolence. Urea frost on the skin and fibrinous pericarditis and pleurisy are associated with marked elevations of BUN.

Hypertension may become severe and may produce headache, convulsions, and left heart failure. Retinopathy with papilledema, hemorrhages, exudates, and severe changes of the arterioles often produce impairment of vision. Encephalopathy produces convulsions. Left heart failure is often accompanied by overt pulmonary edema.

Bone disease (osteitis fibrosa and osteomalacia) and peripheral neuropathy may be disabling.

B. Laboratory Findings: Laboratory studies reveal the functional and chemical defects. The urine usually is dilute, contains small amounts of protein, few red cells, white cells, and epithelial cells, and a few granular and waxy casts some of which are broad in caliber (broad renal failure casts). The anemia is usually normochromic, and the hemoglobin often in the range of 6–9 gm/100 ml. BUN and serum creatinine and (often) uric acid are greatly elevated. Serum sodium concentration may be slightly lower than normal, serum potassium slightly to markedly elevated, and serum calcium concentration decreased. With retention of phosphate, sulfate, and (frequently) chloride, plasma bicarbonate concentration is decreased. Retention of organic acids and loss of sodium and of bicarbonate buffer are accompanied by a decrease of plasma pH. Deficient hydrogen ion secretion by damaged tubules contributes to acidosis.

Differential Diagnosis

Chronic renal insufficiency presents symptoms and signs related to the functional disability resulting from a reduction in the number of functioning nephrons rather than to the cause of the renal damage. It is often impossible to distinguish between renal insufficiency due to chronic glomerulonephritis, pyelonephritis, malignant hypertension, diabetic nephropathy, and collagen disease. The presence of large kidneys characteristic of polycystic disease should serve to identify this cause of renal failure.

The physician must identify remediable causes of renal insufficiency such as obstruction, infection, persistent hypercalcemia, gout, myeloma, and drug toxicity.

Treatment

Hypertension or heart failure should be treated as indicated with agents that sustain renal function and coronary artery blood flow.

A. Diet and Fluids: Limitation of protein of high biologic value to 0.5 gm/kg/day helps to reduce azotemia, acidosis, and hyperkalemia. Trials of mixtures of essential amino acids or of amino acid precursors such as a-keto and a-hydroxy acid analogues are promising approaches to protein replacement.

The diet should include adequate calories and a multivitamin product plus folic acid, 5 mg, particularly when protein is severely restricted. Sodium should not be restricted. Fluid intake should be sufficient to maintain an adequate urine volume, but no attempt should be made to force diuresis. Obligatory water loss may be quite high because of the large solute load (eg, sodium and urea) which must be excreted by a reduced number of nephrons. Intake of up to 2–3 liters may be required when creatinine clearance is reduced to 10–20 ml/minute. With decreasing clearance, urine volume decreases. Intake must be sufficient to maintain renal function without causing excessive diuresis or water retention. If edema is present, a cautious trial of furosemide or ethacrynic acid is indicated with careful monitoring of serum electrolytes. *Caution:* Water restriction for laboratory examination or tests of renal function is hazardous.

B. Electrolyte Replacement:

1. Sodium supplements may be required to restore sodium losses resulting from failure of the kidney to provide NH_4^+ and H^+ for sodium conservation. A mixture of NaCl and $NaHCO_3$ in equal parts, 1–2 gm 2–3 times daily with meals, may be required in addition to dietary sources. Weight loss and a decreasing urine volume indicate a need for additional sodium; hypertension and edema are signs that a trial of sodium restriction is in order.

2. Potassium intake may have to be restricted or supplemented. In severe hyperkalemia, active measures to remove potassium may be required (see discussion in Chapter 2). Measurement of the serum potassium concentration will provide indications.

3. Serum phosphate levels may be lowered and secondary hyperparathyroidism ameliorated by reducing absorption of phosphate in the gastrointestinal tract with administration of aluminum hydroxide gel, 30 ml, or (as tablets) 4–5 gm 3–4 times daily.

4. Calcium lactate, 4 gm 2–3 times daily, may be given to relieve hypocalcemic tetany. Intravenous administration of calcium gluconate may be required at times.

C. Transfusions: Transfusion should be avoided unless the hematocrit falls below 20% or the anemia produces symptoms of angina or shortness of breath. If renal transplantation is contemplated, transfusion should be avoided if at all possible in order to protect against sensitization that will increase the possibility of rejection. Packed red cells that are leukocyte poor or frozen blood are preferred for transfusion when needed. Iron therapy is usually ineffective.

D. General Measures: Nausea and vomiting may be alleviated with chlorpromazine, 15–25 mg orally or 10–20 mg IM (or equivalent amounts of related compounds). The barbiturate drugs may be used for sedation as required.

Hypertension is a common manifestation of uremia. Most often an expanded extracellular fluid volume is responsible for hypertension, and the circumstances can be ameliorated by reduction of extracellular fluid volume by hemodialysis. Some cases of hypertension are due to elevated concentrations of renin in peripheral blood. Combinations of hydralazine and propranolol may be effective; methyldopa is useful in patients on hemodialysis; diazoxide is also a promising drug. Bilateral nephrectomy may be necessary to rescue the patient from persistent hypertension. (See references for details of management of hypertension in the presence of renal failure.)

E. Approach to Drug Therapy: Because the half-life of many drugs is prolonged in patients with renal failure, the physician must monitor the effects of drugs closely. The dosage of drugs often must be reduced and guided by blood levels.

F. Extracorporeal Dialysis and Kidney Transplants: These approaches to the treatment of renal insufficiency due to any cause have been under investigation for many years, and encouraging experience has prompted expansion of facilities for scheduled repeated extracorporeal dialysis. The growing success that has been achieved with renal transplantation holds promise for extending the life of the patient with chronic renal disease.

Amelioration of complications such as neuropathy, hyperparathyroidism, and anemia can be frequently achieved by dialysis or transplantation.

1. Simplified mechanisms for dialysis with the artificial kidney and ingenious cannulas and arteriovenous fistulas permit periodic dialysis with a minimum of professional supervision in hospital centers and in the patient's home. Patients with creatinine clearances of 0–2 ml/minute have been kept alive for 6–10 years in reasonable health and activity by dialysis once or twice a week. The criteria for selection of patients are now clear. Centers are being established for the treatment of chronic renal insufficiency and home units are generally available, although considerable skill is demanded of those who operate the devices. A recent survey indicates a 1-year survival rate on dialysis of 87%, a 2-year survival rate of 73%, and, in the 20- to 45-year age group, a 6-year survival rate of 60%.

2. Transplantation of kidneys from one human to another has been technically feasible for many years. Survival of such grafts has been limited by rejection of

the foreign organ by the recipient except when donor and recipient were identical twins. Blood typing and leukocyte typing for multiple antigens have improved the matching of donor and recipient, with an encouraging decrease in the rejection rate. Further experience with immunosuppressive drugs (azathioprine or cyclophosphamide) and adrenal corticosteroids has improved protection of the homologous transplant from rejection for extended periods. The use of antilymphocytic globulin (ALG) to suppress immunity has been impressively effective, but evaluation requires more experience. Survival data since January 1970 are much improved over prior experience. When the donor is a parent or sibling, recipient survival with the first transplant still functional at 1 year is 74% or greater and at 3 years 70%. When the transplant is a cadaver kidney, recipient survival with the first transplant still functional at 1 year is about 50% and at 3 years 42%. A national collaborative effort to select cadaver kidneys compatible by HL-A type and other criteria should improve the experience with cadaver kidneys.

Prognosis

The prognosis depends upon the degree of renal failure. Intercurrent infections will hasten the downhill course.

Anderson CF & others: Nutritional therapy for adults with renal disease. JAMA 223:68, 1973.

Armbruster KF & others: Nondialytic treatment of chronic renal insufficiency. Ration Drug Ther 7:1, May 1973.

Bennett WM, Singer I, Coggins CH: A guide to drug therapy in renal failure. JAMA 230:1544, 1974.

Berlyne GM: *Nutrition in Renal Disease.* Livingstone, 1968.

Burton BT & others: National registry of long-term dialysis patients. JAMA 218:718, 1971.

Busch GJ, Galvanek EG, Reynolds ES Jr: Human renal allografts: Analysis of lesions in long term survivors. Human Pathol 2:253, 1971.

Dempster WJ: Functional aspects of the rejection of transplanted kidneys. California Med 115:17, Dec 1971.

Ginn HE, Walker PJ: Intermittent hemodialysis. The Kidney, Vol 7, No. 4, July 1974.

Grossman RA, Goldberg M: The use of diuretics in renal disease. The Kidney, Vol 7, No. 5, September 1974.

Kolff WJ: Hemodialysis in the management of renal disease. Ann Rev Med 23:321, 1972.

Lazarus JM & others: Hypertension in chronic renal failure. Arch Int Med 133:1059, 1974.

Lowrie EG & others: Cardiovascular disease in dialysis patients. New England J Med 290:737, 1974.

Merrill JP, Hampers CL: Uremia. (2 parts.) New England J Med 282:953, 1014, 1970.

Milne MD (editor): Management of renal failure. Brit M Bull 27:95, 1971.

The 12th Report of the Human Renal Transplant Registry. JAMA 233:787, 1975.

RENAL OSTEODYSTROPHY

Essentials of Diagnosis

- Chronic renal insufficiency with uremia and hyperphosphatemia.
- Clinical or radiologic evidence of bone disease (osteitis fibrosa or osteomalacia).
- Evidence of secondary hyperparathyroidism (usually occult but may be overt with symptoms due to hypercalcemia).

General Considerations

In patients with chronic renal failure, skeletal abnormalities occur as a result of derangements of metabolism of calcium, phosphate, and vitamin D and of secretion of parathyroid hormone. Osteitis fibrosa reflects parathyroid hyperplasia; osteomalacia reflects resistance to vitamin D secondary to impairment of renal function.

The pathogenesis of resistance to vitamin D may be the loss of ability of the kidney to convert 25-hydroxycholecalciferol to the active compound 1,25-dihydroxycholecalciferol. Osteomalacia occurs more commonly in areas where there is less sunshine and lower intake of vitamin D.

Secondary hyperparathyroidism with resultant osteitis fibrosa appears to be the result of inability to excrete phosphate with consequent hyperphosphatemia. With increase of concentration of phosphate in extracellular fluids, ionized calcium is decreased, and this stimulates secretion of parathyroid hormone.

Clinical Findings

A. Symptoms and Signs: Clinical manifestations are not often present. Patients may complain of bone pain and may suffer pathologic fractures. Itching (common in uremia) may also occur as a result of increased calcium content of the skin. Soft tissue calcifications may occur in periarticular tissues, in the media of large arteries, in the bulbar conjunctiva, and around the edges of the cornea (band keratopathy) as well as in the skin.

The syndrome of secondary hyperparathyroidism may be exacerbated in the course of hemodialysis. Hypercalcemia and its associated symptoms may be persistent and may require subtotal parathyroidectomy for control of symptoms. Renal transplantation may be followed by regression of bone disease.

B. Laboratory Findings: Serum phosphorus is elevated and serum calcium is usually lower than normal, although it often becomes elevated when hyperparathyroidism becomes overt. Alkaline phosphatase of bone origin is often increased in the serum. Parathyroid hormone levels in the plasma are elevated.

C. X-Ray Findings: Radiologic evidence of bone disease is commonly present long before overt symptoms and clinical signs appear.

Treatment

Treatment is directed primarily at reduction of

serum phosphate by reducing phosphate intake and by interfering with phosphate absorption with aluminum hydroxide (30 ml of gel or 4–5 gm as tablets 4 times a day). Oral supplements of calcium to provide 1500 mg of calcium (15 gm of calcium gluconate) per day and vitamin D in the range of 50,000 units or more per day are indicated. Serum phosphorus and calcium should be monitored frequently. Levels of calcium and magnesium in the dialysis bath must be regulated accurately. If control cannot be achieved with conservative therapy, subtotal parathyroidectomy is indicated.

Bricker NS & others: Calcium, phosphorus and bone in renal disease and transplantation. Arch Int Med 123:543, 1969.

Massry SG, Coburn JW: Renal osteodystrophy: Pathogenesis, clinical features and treatment. The Kidney 5:1, Jan 1972.

Massry SG & others: Secondary hyperparathyroidism in chronic renal failure: The clinical spectrum in uremia, during hemodialysis and after renal transplantation. Arch Int Med 124:431, 1969.

Wilson RE & others: Subtotal parathyroidectomy in chronic renal failure: A seven-year experience in a dialysis and transplant program. Ann Surg 174:640, 1971.

NEPHROTIC SYNDROME

Essentials of Diagnosis

- Massive edema.
- Proteinuria > 3.5 gm/day.
- Hypoalbuminemia < 3 gm/100 ml.
- Hyperlipidemia: Cholesterol > 300 mg/100 ml.
- Lipiduria: Free fat, oval fat bodies, fatty casts.

General Considerations

Because treatment and prognosis vary with the cause of nephrotic syndrome (nephrosis), renal biopsy and appropriate examination of an adequate tissue specimen are important. Light microscopy, electron microscopy, and immunofluorescent identification of immune mechanisms provide critical information for identification of most of the causes of nephrosis.

Glomerular diseases associated with nephrosis include the following:

(1) **Minimal glomerular lesions:** Lipoid nephrosis accounts for about 20% of cases of nephrosis in adults. No abnormality is visible by examination of biopsy material with the light microscope. With the electron microscope, alterations of the glomerular basement membrane with swelling and vacuolization and loss of organization of foot processes of the epithelial cells (foot process disease) are evident. There is no evidence of immune disease by immunofluorescent studies. The response to treatment with adrenocortical steroids is satisfactory. Renal function remains good.

(2) **Membranous glomerulonephritis:** (About 25–27% of cases.) Examination of biopsy material

with the light microscope shows thickening of the glomerular capillary walls and some swelling of mesangial cells but no cellular proliferation. With the electron microscope, irregular lumpy deposits appear between the basement membrane and the epithelial cells and new basement membrane material protrudes from the glomerular basement membrane as spikes or domes. Immunofluorescent studies show diffuse granular deposits of immunoglobulins (especially IgG) and complement (C3 component). As the membrane thickens, glomeruli become sclerosed and hyalinized. This disease does not respond to any therapy. It usually progresses to renal failure within 10 years.

(3) **Membranoproliferative (hypocomplementemic) glomerulonephritis:** (About 5% of cases.) Light microscopy shows thickening of glomerular capillaries accompanied by mesangial proliferation and obliteration of glomeruli. With the electron microscope, subendothelial deposits and growth of mesangium into capillary walls are demonstrable. Immunofluorescent studies show the presence of the C3 component of complement and, rarely, the presence of immunoglobulins. There is no known treatment.

(4) **Proliferative glomerulonephritis:** (About 5% of cases.) This is considered to be a stage in the course of poststreptococcal nephritis.

Clinical Findings

A. Symptoms and Signs: Edema may appear insidiously and increase slowly; often it appears suddenly and accumulates rapidly. As fluid collects in the serous cavities, the abdomen becomes protuberant and the patient may complain of anorexia and become short of breath. Symptoms other than those related to the mechanical effects of edema and serous sac fluid accumulation are not remarkable.

On physical examination massive edema is apparent. Signs of hydrothorax and ascites are common. Pallor is often accentuated by the edema, and striae commonly appear in the stretched skin of the extremities. Hypertension, changes in the retina and retinal vessels, and cardiac and cerebral manifestations of hypertension may be demonstrated more often when collagen disease, diabetes mellitus, or renal insufficiency is present.

B. Laboratory Findings: The urine contains large amounts of protein, 4–10 gm/24 hours or more. The sediment contains casts, including the characteristic fatty and waxy varieties; renal tubule cells, some of which contain fatty droplets (oval fat bodies); and variable numbers of erythrocytes. A mild normochromic anemia is common, but anemia may be more severe if renal damage is great. Nitrogen retention varies with the severity of impairment of renal function. The plasma is often lipemic, and the blood cholesterol is usually greatly elevated. Plasma protein is greatly reduced. The albumin fraction may fall to less than 2 gm or even below 1 gm/100 ml. Some reduction of gamma globulin occurs in pure nephrosis, whereas in systemic lupus erythematosus the protein of the gamma fraction may be greatly elevated. Serum complement is usually low in active disease. The serum electrolyte concentrations are often normal, although the serum sodium may be slightly low; total serum calcium may be low, in keeping with the degree of hypoalbuminemia and decrease in the protein-bound calcium moiety. During edema-forming periods, urinary sodium excretion is very low and urinary aldosterone excretion elevated. If renal insufficiency (see above) is present, the blood and urine findings are usually altered accordingly.

Renal biopsy is essential to confirm the diagnosis and to indicate prognosis.

Differential Diagnosis

The nephrotic syndrome (nephrosis) may be associated with a variety of renal diseases, including glomerulonephritis (membranous and proliferative), collagen diseases (disseminated lupus erythematosus, polyarteritis, etc), amyloid disease, thrombosis of the renal vein, diabetic nephropathy, myxedema, multiple myeloma, malaria, syphilis, reaction to toxins such as bee venom, Rhus antigen, drugs such as trimethadione, and heavy metals, and with constrictive pericarditis. In small children, nephrosis may occur without clear evidence of any cause.

Treatment

There is no specific treatment except for syphilis or for heavy metal poisoning. Bed rest is indicated for patients with severe edema or those who have infections. Infections should be treated vigorously and promptly with appropriate antibiotics. Hospitalization is desirable if corticosteroid therapy is given. The diet should provide a normal protein ration (0.75−1 gm/kg/day), with adequate calories. Sodium intake should be restricted to 0.5−1 gm/day. Potassium need not be restricted.

Experience over the last decade has proved the value of adrenocorticosteroids in treating the nephrotic syndrome in children and in adults when the underlying disease is the minimal glomerular lesion (lipoid nephrosis), systemic lupus erythematosus, proliferative glomerulonephritis, or idiosyncrasy to toxin or venom. Corticosteroid therapy is less often efficacious in the presence of membranous disease and membranoproliferative lesions of the glomerulus. It is of little or no value in amyloidosis or renal vein thrombosis, and is contraindicated in diabetic nephropathy.

The goals of therapy are (1) to induce diuresis, (2) to produce a protein-free urine, (3) to elevate the serum albumin to normal levels, and (4) to reduce lipidemia toward normal. With increasing experience, the trend has been toward longer courses of therapy extending well into periods of clinical remission.

Although prednisone is widely used, other corticosteroids may be employed in equivalent doses. Give prednisone (1−2 mg/kg/day for children or 80−120 mg daily for adults) in divided doses orally for 10 days to 3 or 4 weeks. If diuresis begins early in the course of treatment, the dosage of corticosteroid may be reduced slowly over a period of 3−4 weeks, seeking the smallest dose that will fulfill the goals of therapy and maintain the remission. When there is no response to corticosteroid therapy, rapid reduction of intake of corticosteroid may be followed by diuresis and improvement. If there is no response upon withdrawal of the corticosteroid, additional courses using high doses daily should be tried before concluding that the patient's disease is refractory to corticosteroids.

When diuresis is well established and proteinuria and edema are diminishing, therapy can be altered from daily to intermittent administration of corticosteroid. Alternate day therapy appears to maintain remission satisfactorily. The total dose administered for 48 hours on the daily schedule is administered orally as one dose at breakfast every other day. On this regimen there is usually no evidence of adrenal suppression; normal growth may be expected in children; and cushingoid changes and hypertension are very rare. In some instances, initiation of therapy on the 48-hour schedule has been successful.

Another form of intermittent therapy consisting of prednisone, 60 mg orally daily in divided doses on 3 consecutive days of the week, with no corticosteroid on the succeeding 4 days, has been employed extensively. Disadvantages include the high incidence of the customary side-effects of high doses of corticosteroid with signs of adrenal suppression manifest during the 4 days of rest.

At present it is considered justifiable to continue intermittent therapy for a year if the patient remains edema-free and if proteinuria is reduced to negligible amounts. If exacerbations occur, therapy can be intensified. Potassium supplements may be desirable during corticosteroid therapy, although none may be required on the alternate day schedule.

Diuretics are often ineffective. The most useful are the thiazide derivatives, eg, hydrochlorothiazide, 50−100 mg every 12 hours; other thiazide derivatives, chlorthalidone, and other diuretics may be employed in comparable effective dose levels. Spironolactone may be helpful when employed concurrently with thiazides. Salt-free albumin, dextran, and other oncotic agents are of little help and their effects are transient.

Caution: Elevation of serum potassium, development of hypertension, and sudden severe increase in edema contraindicate continuation of corticosteroid therapy. Such complications usually arise during the first 2 weeks of continuous therapy.

Immunosuppressive drugs, including alkylating agents, cyclophosphamide, mercaptopurine, azathioprine, and others, are under trial in the treatment of the nephrotic syndrome. The use of corticosteroids plus immunosuppressive agents is similar to that employed in reversing rejection of homotransplants in man. Experience is still meager, but increasingly encouraging results have been reported in children and adults with proliferative or membranous lesions and with systemic lupus erythematosus. Those with minimal lesions refractory to corticosteroid therapy did no better when immunosuppressive agents were added. Improvement was shown in the glomerular changes and renal function in many responding well to treatment.

The incidence of improvement has not been established.

Serious side-effects related both to corticosteroids and to the cytotoxic agents are common. At present this form of therapy should be employed only by those experienced in treating the nephrotic syndrome in patients who have proved refractory to well-established treatment regimens.

For renal vein thrombosis, the treatment is directed against progress of thrombus formation with heparin and long-term use of coumarin drugs.

Prognosis

The course and prognosis depend upon the basic disease responsible for the nephrotic syndrome. In about 50% of cases of childhood nephrosis, the disease appears to run a rather benign course when properly treated, and to leave insignificant sequelae. Of the others, most go inexorably into the terminal state with renal insufficiency. Adults with nephrosis fare less well, particularly when the fundamental disease is glomerulonephritis, systemic lupus erythematosus, amyloidosis, renal vein thrombosis, or diabetic nephropathy. In those with minimal lesions, remissions, either spontaneous or following corticosteroid therapy, are common. Treatment is more often unsuccessful or only ameliorative when the other glomerular lesions are present. Hypertension and nitrogen retention are serious signs.

Bhorade MS & others: Nephropathy of secondary syphilis: A clinical and pathological spectrum. JAMA 216:1159, 1971.

Cameron JS & others: Long term stability of remission in nephrotic syndrome after treatment with cyclophosphamide. Brit MJ 4:7, 1974.

Hamilton CR Jr & others: Renal vein thrombosis and pulmonary embolism. Johns Hopkins Med J 124:331, 1969.

Hayslett JP & others: Clinicopathological correlation in the nephrotic syndrome due to primary renal disease. Medicine 52:93, 1973.

Hopper J Jr & others: Lipoid nephrosis in 31 adult patients: Renal biopsy study by light, electron and fluorescence microscopy with experience in treatment. Medicine 49:321, 1970.

Medical Research Council Working Party: Controlled trial of azathioprine and prednisone in chronic renal disease. Brit MJ 2:239, 1971.

Miller RB & others: Long term results of steroid therapy in adults with idiopathic nephrotic syndrome. Am J Med 46:919, 1969.

Moncrieff MW & others: Cyclophosphamide therapy in the nephrotic syndrome in childhood. Brit MJ 1:666, 1969.

Rosen S: Membranous glomerulonephritis: Current status. Human Path 2:209, 1972.

Rosenmann E, Pollak VE, Pirani CL: Renal vein thrombosis in the adult: A clinical and pathological study based on renal biopsies. Medicine 47:269, 1968.

Skinner MD, Schwartz RS: Immunosuppressive therapy. (2 parts.) New England J Med 287:221, 281, 1972.

Steinberg AD & others: Cyclophosphamide in lupus nephritis: A controlled trial. Ann Int Med 75:165, 1973.

HEMOLYTIC-UREMIC SYNDROME

This rare syndrome—characterized by severe hemolytic anemia, thrombocytopenia, and renal failure—occurs more commonly in young children than in adults. The cause is unknown, but the syndrome has features relating it to disseminated intravascular coagulation and to thrombotic thrombocytopenic purpura. After an attack of gastroenteritis or respiratory infection, there is an abrupt onset of weakness, jaundice, purpura, and severe oliguria. Glomeruli show platelet aggregations and fibrin thrombi obstructing the capillaries and terminal arterioles. Only about half of the patients survive, and of those who do about 10% have hypertension. Hemodialysis may be useful; anticoagulant therapy appears to be ineffectual.

ARTERIOLAR NEPHROSCLEROSIS

Intimal thickening of the afferent arteriole of the glomerulus is the characteristic finding. Obliteration of the arteriole or severe narrowing of the lumen deprives the nephron of its blood supply and produces areas of infarction and scar formation. Obliteration of glomeruli is common. If the disease is "malignant" and rapidly progressive, points of hemorrhage are found and vascular changes, resembling an endarteritis with severe intimal thickening associated with malignant hypertension, become marked. Renal insufficiency occurs when the kidney is scarred and contracted.

The symptoms and signs are those of hypertension and renal insufficiency and, occasionally, heart failure and hypertensive encephalopathy.

Treatment is directed against hypertension and chronic renal insufficiency.

The course is progressively downhill. The patient usually succumbs to renal failure, and death is sometimes hastened by intercurrent infection.

DISEASES OF THE RENAL TUBULES & INTERSTITIUM

1. ACUTE RENAL FAILURE

Essentials of Diagnosis

- Sudden onset of oliguria; urine volume 20–200 ml/day.
- Proteinuria and hematuria; isosthenuria with a specific gravity of 1.010–1.016.
- Anorexia, nausea and vomiting, lethargy, elevation of blood pressure. Signs of uremia.
- Progressive increase in serum BUN, creati-

nine, potassium, phosphate, sulfate; decrease in sodium, calcium, CO_2.

- Spontaneous recovery in a few days to 6 weeks.

General Considerations

Acute renal failure is a term applied to a state of sudden cessation of renal function following a variety of insults to normal kidneys. Among the causes of acute renal failure are the following: (1) Toxic agents, eg, carbon tetrachloride, methoxyflurane, sulfonamides, aminoglycoside antibiotics, amphotericin B, mercury bichloride, arsenic, diethylene glycol, and mushroom poisoning. (2) Traumatic shock due to severe injury, surgical shock, or myocardial infarction, and ischemia associated with surgery on the abdominal aorta. (3) Tissue destruction due to crushing injury, burns, intravascular hemolysis (transurethral resection of the prostate, incompatible blood transfusion). (4) Infectious diseases, eg, leptospirosis, hemorrhagic fever, septicemia due to gram-negative bacteria with shock. (5) Severe water and electrolyte depletion. (6) Complications of pregnancy, eg, bilateral cortical necrosis.

Return of renal function can be expected, but even with the best treatment the mortality rate is high.

Renal tubular necrosis is the characteristic finding. In some instances, after exposure to a specific toxin, the proximal tubule may be primarily damaged; and renal tubule cell disintegration and desquamation with collection of debris in the lumens of the tubules are found uniformly throughout both kidneys. In other cases, tubule cell destruction and basement membrane disruption are scattered throughout both kidneys. In cases due to hemolysis or crushing injury, heme or myoglobin casts may be present, but it is unlikely that such casts produce tubule cell destruction. The spotty distribution of the damage caused by ischemic necrosis is consistent with a great reduction in cortical blood flow in addition to a moderate to marked decrease in total renal blood flow. In bilateral cortical necrosis, ischemic infarcts are distributed throughout both kidneys.

Clinical Findings

The cardinal sign of acute renal failure is acute reduction of urine output following injury, surgery, a transfusion reaction, or other causes listed above. The daily volume of urine may be reduced to 20–30 ml/day or may be as high as 400–500 ml/day. After a few days to 6 weeks the daily urine volume slowly increases. Anorexia, nausea, and lethargy are common symptoms. Other symptoms and signs are related to the causative agent or event.

The course of the disease may be divided into the oliguric and diuretic phases.

A. Oliguric Phase: During the oliguric phase, the urine excretion is greatly reduced. The urine contains protein, red cells, and granular casts, and the specific gravity of the urine is usually 1.010–1.016. The rate of catabolism of protein determines the rate of increase of metabolic end products in body fluids. In the presence of injury or fever, the serum BUN, creatinine, potassium, phosphate, sulfate, and organic acids increase rapidly. Typically, because of dilution and intracellular shifts, the serum sodium concentration drops to 120–130 mEq/liter with a corresponding fall in serum chloride. As organic acids and phosphate accumulate, serum bicarbonate concentration decreases. Normochromic anemia is common. With prolonged oliguria, signs of uremia appear with nausea, vomiting, diarrhea, neuromuscular irritability, convulsions, somnolence, and coma. Hypertension frequently develops and may be associated with retinopathy, left heart failure, and encephalopathy. During this phase of the disease, therapy modifies the clinical picture significantly. Overhydration produces signs of water intoxication with convulsions, edema, and the serious complication of pulmonary edema. Excess saline administration may produce edema and congestive failure. Failure to restrict potassium intake or to employ agents to remove potassium at the proper time may result in potassium intoxication. High extracellular potassium levels produce neuromuscular depression which progresses to paralysis and interference with the cardiac conduction system, resulting in arrhythmias; death may follow respiratory muscle paralysis or cardiac arrest. The ECG changes as the potassium level rises, first showing peaked T waves, then broadening of the QRS complex and lack of P waves; later, a biphasic ventricular complex; and, finally, cardiac arrest or ventricular fibrillation. With proper treatment, potassium intoxication is almost always reversible, and death should seldom occur because of it.

B. Diuretic Phase: After a few days to 6 weeks of oliguria, the diuretic phase begins, signifying that the nephrons have recovered to the point that urine excretion is possible. The urine volume usually increases in increments of a few ml to 100 ml/day until 300–500 ml/day are excreted, after which the rate of increase in flow is usually more rapid. Rarely, the urine volume increases rapidly during the first day or so of diuresis. Diuresis may be the result of impaired nephron function, with loss of water and electrolytes; but this is uncommon and true deficits of water, sodium, and potassium seldom occur. More often, diuresis represents an unloading of excess extracellular fluid which has accumulated during the oliguric phase, either as a result of overhydration during therapy or unusual metabolic production of water. Diuresis usually occurs when the total nephron function is still insufficient to excrete nitrogenous metabolic products, potassium, and phosphate, and the concentration of these constituents in the serum may continue to rise for several days after urine volumes exceed 1 liter/day. Renal function returns slowly to normal, and blood chemical findings become normal.

Differential Diagnosis

Because acute glomerulonephritis, ureteral obstruction due to edema at the ureterovesical junction following ureteral catheterization, ureteral obstruction by neoplasm, bilateral renal artery occlusion due to embolism or dissecting aneurysm, and, rarely, a ruptured bladder may present with symptoms and signs indistinguishable from those of tubular necrosis, appropriate diagnostic procedures should be employed as suggested by the history and by physical examination. Occasionally a profound state of dehydration may produce severe oliguria; rapid infusion of 500–1000 ml of 0.45% saline will restore blood volume temporarily to the point that glomerular filtration will increase and urine will be excreted.

Treatment

A. Specific Treatment: Immediate treatment of the cause of oliguria is essential.

1. Shock—Vigorous measures to restore normal blood pressure levels are mandatory in order to overcome renal ischemia. Early in the course of renal ischemia, tubular necrosis may be prevented by rapid administration of mannitol, 25 gm, as a 20% solution given IV. *Caution:* When it becomes apparent that tubular necrosis has occurred, the volume of fluids administered must be sharply curtailed; if vasopressor drugs are required, they must be given in the limited amount of fluid permitted.

2. Transfusion reaction—See Chapter 9.

3. Obstruction of ureters—Cystoscopy and catheterization of ureters may be necessary.

4. Heavy metal poisoning—Dimercaprol (BAL) may be of use in mercury or arsenic poisoning, although by the time the renal lesion is apparent it may be too late.

B. General Measures: The following discussion of conservative medical management often serves adequately for the uncomplicated case. If oliguria persists beyond a week or if the patient has sustained severe trauma or is in a severe "catabolic state," from infection or toxic materials, dialysis is indicated. Hemodialysis is more effective, but peritoneal dialysis may be adequate. Dialysis is useful prophylactically to prevent the uremic state. Indications for dialysis include threatening hyperkalemia, serious electrolyte or water excess, inability to maintain a relatively stable state with continuing oliguria, or severe oliguria that persists for more than 4 or 5 days.

1. Oliguric phase—The objectives of therapy are to maintain normal body fluid volume and electrolyte concentration, reduce tissue catabolism to a minimum, and prevent infection until healing occurs.

a. Bed rest—"Reverse isolation" to protect the patient from exposure to hospital infections.

b. Fluids—Restrict fluids to a basic ration of 400 ml/day for the average adult. Additional fluid may be given to replace unusual losses due to vomiting, diarrhea, sweating, etc. The metabolism of fat, carbohydrate, and protein provides water of combustion; and catabolism of tissues provides intracellular water. These sources must be included in calculations of water balance, thus leaving only a small ration to be provided as "intake" (see ¶ e, below).

c. Diet—In order to limit sources of nitrogen,

potassium, phosphate, and sulfate, no protein should be given. Glucose, 100–200 gm/day, should be given to prevent ketosis and to reduce protein catabolism. Although fat may be given as butter or as an emulsion for oral or intravenous use, it is usually better to permit the patient to fulfill caloric needs from his own fat deposits.

The fluid and glucose may be given orally or intravenously. When administered intravenously as a 20–50% glucose solution, the 400 ml of fluid should be given continuously through the 24-hour period through an intravenous catheter threaded into a large vein to reduce the likelihood of thrombosis. Vitamin B complex and vitamin C should be provided.

d. Electrolyte replacement—Replace preexisting deficits. Otherwise, electrolyte therapy is not necessary unless clear-cut losses are demonstrable, as in vomiting, diarrhea, etc. *Note:* Potassium must not be administered unless proved deficits exist, and then only with caution.

e. Observations—Daily records of fluid intake and output are essential; an indwelling catheter is usually required to permit accurate measurement of urine output. Weight should be recorded daily whenever possible. Because the patient is consuming his own tissues, he should lose about 0.5 kg/day. If he fails to lose weight, he is receiving too much fluid. Frequent (often daily) measurements of serum electrolytes (especially potassium) and creatinine are essential. The ECG may be helpful in evaluating potassium levels.

f. Infection—Treat vigorously with appropriate antibiotics, bearing in mind that the drug may not be excreted. "Reverse isolation" is a useful protective measure.

g. Congestive heart failure—See discussion in Chapter 7.

h. Anemia—A hematocrit of less than 30% is an indication for cautious transfusion with a small volume of packed fresh red blood cells.

i. Potassium intoxication—See discussion in Chapter 2.

j. Uremia—Hemodialysis and peritoneal dialysis are effective, but they require expert management in a well-equipped hospital. With appropriate facilities, dialysis has proved to be of great value if employed "prophylactically" when it is evident that conservative therapy is inadequate to prevent acidosis, advance of azotemia, and clinical deterioration.

k. Convulsions and encephalopathy—Give paraldehyde rectally. Barbiturates should be restricted to pentobarbital sodium or amobarbital sodium, which are metabolized by the liver. Chlorpromazine and promazine are also useful. Dialysis is useful.

2. Diuretic phase—Unless water and electrolyte deficits clearly exist, no attempt should be made to "keep up" with the diuresis; collections of excess water and electrolyte are usually being excreted. Fluid and diet intake can be liberalized as diuresis progresses until a normal daily intake is reached. Protein restriction should be continued until serum BUN and creatinine levels are declining. Infection is still a hazard.

Occasionally diuresis will be accompanied by sodium retention, hypernatremia, and hyperchloremia associated with confusion, neuromuscular irritability, and coma. When this happens, water and glucose must be given in sufficient quantities to correct hypernatremia. Serum electrolytes and BUN or creatinine should be measured frequently.

Prognosis

If severe complications of trauma and infection are not present, skillful treatment often will tide the patient over the period of oliguria until spontaneous healing occurs. Death may occur as a result of water intoxication, congestive heart failure, acute pulmonary edema, potassium intoxication, and encephalopathy. With recovery there is little residual impairment of renal function.

Flamenbaum W: Pathophysiology of acute renal failure. Arch Int Med 131:911, 1973.

Harrington JT, Cohen JJ: Current concepts: Acute oliguria. New England J Med 292:89, 1975.

Hollenberg NH & others: Acute oliguric renal failure in man: Evidence for preferential renal cortical ischemia. Medicine 47:455, 1968.

Lewers DT & others: Long-term follow-up of renal function and histology after acute tubular necrosis. Ann Int Med 73:515, 1970.

Maher JF, Schreiner GE: Cause of death in acute renal failure. Arch Int Med 110:493, 1962.

Merrill JP: Kidney disease: Acute renal failure. Advances Int Med 10:127, 1960.

Muehrcke RC: *Acute Renal Failure: Diagnosis and Management.* Mosby, 1969.

Nienhuis LI: Clinical peritoneal dialysis. Arch Surg 93:643, 1966.

Papper S: Renal failure. M Clin North America 55:335, 1971.

2. INTERSTITIAL NEPHRITIS

Acute interstitial disease may be due to systemic infections such as syphilis and sensitivity to drugs, including antibiotics (penicillins, colistin, sulfonamides), phenindione, and diphenylhydantoin. Recovery may be complete.

Chronic interstitial nephritis is characterized by focal or diffuse interstitial fibrosis accompanied by infiltration with inflammatory cells ultimately associated with extensive atrophy of renal tubules. It represents a nonspecific reaction to a variety of causes: analgesic abuse, lead and cadmium toxicity, nephrocalcinosis, urate nephropathy, radiation nephritis, sarcoidosis, Balkan nephritis, and some instances of obstructive uropathy. There are a few cases in which antitubule basement membrane antibodies have been identified by means of immunofluorescent linear staining of IgG and C3.

3. ANALGESIC NEPHROPATHY

Renal papillary necrosis has usually been associated with fulminating urinary tract infection in the presence of diabetes mellitus. Since 1953, however, increasing numbers of cases have been associated with long-term ingestion of phenacetin alone or in analgesic mixtures. The typical patient is a middle-aged woman with chronic and recurrent headaches or a patient with chronic arthritis who habitually consumes large amounts of analgesic mixtures containing phenacetin. The ensuing damage to the kidneys usually is detected late, after renal insufficiency has developed.

The kidney lesion is pathologically nonspecific, consisting of peritubular and perivascular inflammation with degenerative changes of the tubule cells (chronic interstitial nephritis). There are no glomerular changes. Renal papillary necrosis extending into the medulla may involve many papillae.

Hematuria is a common presenting complaint. Renal colic occurs when necrotic renal papillae slough away. Polyuria may be prominent. Signs of acidosis (hyperpnea), dehydration, and pallor of anemia are common. Infection is a frequent complication. The history of phenacetin ingestion may be concealed by the patient.

The urine usually is remarkable only for the presence of blood and small amounts of protein. Hemolytic anemia is usually evident. Elevated BUN and creatinine and the electrolyte changes characteristic of renal failure are typically present.

Urograms show typical cavities and ring shadows of areas of destruction of papillae.

Treatment consists of withholding analgesics containing phenacetin and aspirin. Renal failure and infection are treated as outlined elsewhere in this chapter.

Abel JA: Analgesic nephropathy: A review of the literature, 1967–1970. Clin Pharmacol Therap 12:583, 1971.

4. URIC ACID NEPHROPATHY

See section on gout, p 496.

Crystals of urate produce an interstitial inflammatory reaction. Urate may precipitate out in acid urine in the calyces distally in the ureters to form uric acid stones. Patients with myeloproliferative disease under treatment may develop hyperuricemia and are subject to occlusion of the upper urinary tract by uric acid crystals. Alkalinization of the urine and a liberal fluid intake will help prevent crystal formation. Allopurinol is a useful drug to prevent hyperuricemia and hyperuricosuria.

5. OBSTRUCTIVE UROPATHY

Interstitial nephritis due to obstruction may not be associated with infection. Tubular conservation of salt and water is impaired. Following relief of obstruction, diuresis may be massive and may require vigorous but judicious replacement of water and electrolyte.

6. MYELOMATOSIS

Features of myelomatosis which contribute to renal disease include proteinuria (including filtrable Bence Jones protein and κ and λ chains) with precipitation in the tubules leading to accumulation of abnormal proteins in the tubule cells, hypercalcemia, and occasionally increase in viscosity of the blood associated with macroglobulinemia. A Fanconi-like syndrome may develop.

Plugging of tubules, giant cell reaction around tubules, tubular atrophy, and, occasionally, the accumulation of amyloid are evident on examination of renal tissue.

Renal failure may occur acutely or may develop slowly. Hemodialysis may rescue the patient during efforts to control the myeloma with chemical agents.

HEREDITARY RENAL DISEASES

The importance of inheritance and the familial incidence of disease warrants inclusion of the classification of hereditary renal diseases suggested by Perkoff (see reference below). Although relatively uncommon in the population at large, hereditary disease must be recognized to permit early diagnosis and treatment in other family members and to prepare the way for genetic counseling.

Many of the renal diseases that can occur as heritable abnormalities are listed in Chapter 31 (Some Diseases With Known Modes of Inheritance). Selected diseases are discussed briefly below.

1. HEREDITARY CHRONIC NEPHRITIS

Evidence of the disease usually appears in childhood, with episodes of hematuria often following an upper respiratory infection. Renal insufficiency commonly develops in males but only rarely in females. Survival beyond the age of 40 is rare.

In many families, deafness and abnormalities of the eyes accompany the renal disease. Another form of the disease is accompanied by polyneuropathy. Infec-

tion of the urinary tract is a common complication.

The anatomic features in some cases resemble proliferative glomerulonephritis; in others, there is thickening of the glomerular basement membrane or podocyte proliferation and thickening of Bowman's capsule. In a few cases there are fat-filled cells (foam cells) in the interstitial tissue or in the glomeruli.

Laboratory findings are commensurate with existing renal function.

Treatment is symptomatic.

2. CYSTIC DISEASES OF THE KIDNEY

Congenital structural anomalies of the kidney must always be considered in any patient with hypertension, pyelonephritis, or renal insufficiency. The manifestations of structural renal abnormalities are related to the superimposed disease, but management and prognosis are modified by the structural anomaly.

Polycystic Kidneys

Polycystic kidney disease is familial and often involves not only the kidney but the liver and pancreas as well.

The formation of cysts in the cortex of the kidney is thought to result from failure of union of the collecting tubules and convoluted tubules of some nephrons. New cysts do not form, but those present enlarge and, by pressure, cause destruction of adjacent tissue. Cysts may be found in the liver and pancreas. The incidence of cerebral vessel aneurysms is higher than normal.

Cases of polycystic disease are discovered during the investigation of hypertension, by diagnostic study in patients presenting with pyelonephritis or hematuria, or by investigating the families of patients with polycystic disease. At times, flank pain due to hemorrhage into a cyst will call attention to a kidney disorder. Otherwise the symptoms and signs are those commonly seen in hypertension or renal insufficiency. On physical examination the enlarged, irregular kidneys are easily palpable.

The urine may contain leukocytes and red cells. With bleeding into the cysts there may also be bleeding into the urinary tract. The blood chemical findings reflect the degree of renal insufficiency. X-ray examination shows the enlarged kidneys, and urography demonstrates the classical elongated calyces and renal pelves stretched over the surface of the cysts.

No specific therapy is available, and surgical interference is contraindicated unless ureteral obstruction is produced by an adjacent cyst. Hypertension, infection, and uremia are treated in the conventional manner.

Because persons with polycystic kidneys may live in reasonable comfort with slowly advancing uremia, it is difficult to determine when renal transplantation is in order. Hemodialysis can extend the life of the patient, but recurrent bleeding and continuous pain indicate the need for a transplant.

Although the disease may become symptomatic in childhood or early in early adult life, it usually is discovered in the 4th or 5th decades. Unless fatal complications of hypertension or urinary tract infection are present, uremia develops very slowly and patients live longer than with other causes of renal insufficiency.

Cystic Disease of the Renal Medulla

Two syndromes have been recognized with increasing frequency as their diagnostic features have become better known.

Medullary cystic disease is a familial disease which may become symptomatic during adolescence. Anemia is usually the initial manifestation, but azotemia, acidosis, and hyperphosphatemia soon become evident. Hypertension may develop. The urine is not remarkable, although there is often an inability to produce a concentrated urine. Many small cysts are scattered through the renal medulla. Renal transplantation is indicated by the usual criteria for the operation.

Sponge kidney is asymptomatic and is discovered by the characteristic appearance of the urogram. Enlargement of the papillae and calyces and small cavities within the pyramids are demonstrated by the contrast media in the excretory urogram. Many small calculi often occupy the cysts, and infection may be troublesome. Life expectancy is not affected, and only symptomatic therapy for ureteral impaction of a stone or for infection is required.

Gardner KD Jr: Evolution of clinical signs in adult-onset cystic disease of the renal medulla. Ann Int Med 74:47, 1971.

Hatfield PM, Pfister RC: Adult polycystic disease of the kidneys (Potter type 3). JAMA 222:1527, 1972.

MacDougall JA, Prout WG: Medullary sponge kidney: Clinical appraisal and report of 12 cases. Brit J Surg 55:130, 1968.

Medical Staff Conference: Renal cystic disease. California Med 119:36, Nov 1973.

Osathanondh V, Potter EL: Pathogenesis of polycystic kidneys. Arch Path 77:459, 1964.

Perkoff GT: Hereditary renal diseases. New England J Med 277:79, 1967.

Strauss MB: Clinical and pathological aspects of cystic disease of the renal medulla. Ann Int Med 57:373, 1962.

Wahlqvist L: Cystic disorders of kidney: Review of pathogenesis and classification. J Urol 97:1, 1967.

3. ANOMALIES OF THE PROXIMAL TUBULE

Defects of Amino Acid Reabsorption

A. Congenital Cystinuria: Increased excretion of cystine results in the formation of cystine calculi in the urinary tract. Ornithine, arginine, and lysine are also excreted in abnormally large quantities. There is also a defect in absorption of these amino acids in the jejunum. Nonopaque stones should be examined chemically to provide a specific diagnosis.

Maintain a high urine volume by giving a large fluid intake. Maintain the urine pH above 7.0 by giving sodium bicarbonate and sodium citrate plus acetazolamide (Diamox) at bedtime to ensure an alkaline night urine. In refractory cases a low-methionine (cystine precursor) diet may be necessary. Penicillamine has proved useful in some cases.

B. Aminoaciduria: Many amino acids may be poorly absorbed, resulting in unusual losses. Failure to thrive and the presence of other tubular deficits suggests the diagnosis.

There is no treatment.

C. Hepatolenticular Degeneration: In this congenital familial disease, aminoaciduria is associated with cirrhosis of the liver and neurologic manifestations. Hepatomegaly, evidence of impaired liver function, spasticity, athetosis, emotional disturbances, and Kayser-Fleischer rings around the cornea constitute a unique syndrome. There is a decrease in synthesis of ceruloplasmin with a deficit of plasma ceruloplasmin and an increase in free copper which may be etiologically specific.

Give penicillamine to chelate and remove excess copper. Edathamil (Versenate, EDTA) may also be used to remove copper.

Multiple Defects of Tubular Function (De Toni-Fanconi-Debré Syndrome)

Aminoaciduria, phosphaturia, glycosuria, and a variable degree of renal tubular acidosis characterize this syndrome. Osteomalacia is a prominent clinical feature; other clinical and laboratory manifestations are associated with specific tubular defects described separately above.

The proximal segment of the renal tubule is replaced by a thin tubular structure constituting the "swan neck" deformity. The proximal segment also is shortened to less than half the normal length.

Treatment consists of replacing cation deficits (especially potassium), correcting acidosis with bicarbonate or citrate, replacing phosphate loss with isotonic neutral phosphate (mono- and disodium salts) solution, and a liberal calcium intake. Vitamin D is usually useful, but the dose used must be controlled by monitoring serum calcium and phosphate.

Defects of Phosphorus & Calcium Absorption

A. Vitamin D-Resistant Rickets: Excessive loss of phosphorus and calcium result in rickets or osteomalacia which respond poorly to vitamin D therapy. Treatment consists of giving large doses of vitamin D and calcium supplementation of the diet.

B. Pseudohypoparathyroidism: As a result of excessive reabsorption of phosphorus, hyperphosphatemia and hypocalcemia occur. Symptoms include muscle cramps, fatigue, weakness, tetany, and mental retardation. The signs are those of hypocalcemia; in addition, the patients are short, round-faced, and characteristically have short 4th and 5th metacarpal and metatarsal bones. The serum phosphorus is high, serum calcium low, and serum alkaline phosphatase normal. There is no response to parathyroid hormone.

Vitamin D therapy and calcium supplementation may prevent tetany.

Defects of Glucose Absorption (Renal Glycosuria)

This results from an abnormally low ability to reabsorb glucose, so that glycosuria is present when blood glucose levels are normal. Ketosis is not present. The glucose tolerance response is usually normal. In some instances, renal glycosuria may precede the onset of true diabetes mellitus.

There is no treatment for renal glycosuria.

Defects of Glucose & Phosphate Absorption (Glycosuric Rickets)

The symptoms and signs are those of rickets or osteomalacia, with weakness, pain, or discomfort of the legs and spine, and tetany. The bones become deformed, with bowing of the weight-bearing long bones, kyphoscoliosis, and, in children, signs of rickets. X-ray shows markedly decreased density of the bone, with pseudofracture lines and other deformities. Nephrocalcinosis may occur with excessive phosphaturia, and renal insufficiency may follow. Urinary calcium and phosphorus are increased and glycosuria is present. Serum glucose is normal, serum calcium is normal or low, serum phosphorus is low, and serum alkaline phosphatase is elevated.

Treatment consists of giving large doses of vitamin D and calcium supplementation of the diet.

Defects of Bicarbonate Reabsorption

A form of renal tubular acidosis in which proximal tubular wasting of bicarbonate is the characteristic defect may be associated with multiple dysfunctions of the proximal tubule, often genetically transmitted. Excretion of excessive amounts of bicarbonate occurs even in the presence of low plasma bicarbonate.

For a complete discussion, see Morris RC Jr: New England J Med 281:1405, 1969.

4. ANOMALIES OF THE DISTAL TUBULE

Defects of Hydrogen Ion Secretion & Bicarbonate Reabsorption (Classical Renal Tubular Acidosis)

Failure to secrete hydrogen ion and to form ammonium ion results in loss of "fixed base": sodium, potassium, and calcium. There is also a high rate of excretion of phosphate. Vomiting, poor growth, and symptoms and signs of chronic metabolic acidosis are accompanied by weakness due to potassium deficit and the bone discomfort due to osteomalacia. Nephrocalcinosis, with calcification in the medullary portions of the kidney, occurs in about half of cases. The urine is alkaline and contains larger than normal quantities of sodium, potassium, calcium, and phosphate. The blood chemical findings are those of metabolic acidosis (low HCO_3^- or CO_2) with hyperchloremia, low serum calcium and phosphorus, low serum potassium, and, occasionally, low serum sodium.

Treatment consists of replacing deficits and increasing the intake of sodium potassium, calcium, and phosphorus. Sodium and potassium should be given as bicarbonate or citrate. Additional vitamin D may be required.

Excess Potassium Secretion (Potassium "Wastage" Syndrome)

Excessive renal secretion or loss of potassium may occur in 4 situations: (1) Chronic renal insufficiency with diminished H^+ secretion. (2) Renal tubular acidosis and the De Toni-Fanconi syndrome, with cation loss resulting from diminished H^+ and NH_4^+ secretion. (3) Aldosteronism and hyperadrenocorticism. (4) Tubular secretion of potassium, the cause of which is yet unknown. Hypokalemia indicates that the deficit is severe. Muscle weakness, metabolic alkalosis, and polyuria with dilute urine are signs attributable to hypokalemia.

Treatment consists of correcting the primary disease and giving supplementary potassium.

Defects of Water Absorption (Renal Diabetes Insipidus)

Nephrogenic diabetes insipidus occurs more frequently in males. Unresponsiveness to antidiuretic hormone is the key to differentiation from pituitary diabetes insipidus.

In addition to congenital refractoriness to antidiuretic hormone, obstructive uropathy, lithium, methoxyflurane, and demeclocycline may also render the tubule refractory.

Symptoms are related to an inability to reabsorb water with resultant polyuria and polydipsia. The urine volume approaches 12 liters/day, and osmolality and specific gravity are low. Mental retardation, atonic bladder, and hydronephrosis occur frequently.

Treatment consists primarily of an adequate water intake. Chlorothiazide may ameliorate the diabetes; the mechanism of action is unknown, but the drug may act by increasing isosmotic reabsorption in the proximal segment of the tubule.

5. UNSPECIFIED RENAL TUBULAR ABNORMALITIES

In **idiopathic hypercalciuria**, decreased reabsorption of calcium predisposes to the formation of renal calculi. Serum calcium and phosphorus are normal. Urine calcium excretion is high; urine phosphorus excretion is low.

Treatment is discussed on p 545.

Courey WR, Pfister RC: The radiographic findings in renal tubular acidosis. Radiology 105:497, 1972.

Frimpter GW: Aminoacidurias due to inherited disorders of metabolism. (2 parts.) New England J Med 289:835, 895, 1974.

Lee DBN & others: The adult Fanconi syndrome. Medicine 51:107, 1972.

Morris RC Jr: Renal tubular acidosis: Mechanisms, classification and implications. New England J Med 281:1405, 1969.

Perkoff GT: Hereditary renal diseases. (2 parts.) New England J Med 277:79, 129, 1967.

Stanbury JB, Wyngaarden JB, Frederickson DS (editors): *The Metabolic Basis of Inherited Disease,* 3rd ed. McGraw-Hill, 1972.

6. CONGENITAL ANOMALIES

Renal Agenesis

Occasionally one kidney, usually the left, is congenitally absent. The remaining kidney is hypertrophied. Before performing a nephrectomy for any reason, it is mandatory to prove the patient has a second kidney.

Horseshoe Kidney

A band of renal tissue or of fibrous tissue may join the 2 kidneys. Associated abnormalities of the ureterocalyceal system, or hydronephrosis resulting from ureteral obstruction by aberrant vessels, predispose to pyelonephritis.

Ectopic Kidney

The kidney may occupy a site in the pelvis and the ureter may be shorter than normal. Infection is common in ectopic kidneys compromised by ureteral obstruction or urinary reflux.

Nephroptosis

Unusual mobility of the kidney permits it to move from its normal position to a lower one. The incidence of ureteral occlusion due to movement of a kidney is extremely low.

Megaloureter & Hydronephrosis

These anatomic abnormalities may occur congenitally but are more commonly the result of vesicoureteral urinary reflux.

Glenn JF: Analysis of 51 patients with horseshoe kidney. New England J Med 216:684, 1959.

Kissane JM: Congenital malformations. In: *Pathology of the Kidney,* 2nd ed. Heptinstall RH. Little, Brown, 1974.

INFECTIONS OF THE URINARY TRACT*

The term urinary tract infection (UTI) denotes a wide variety of clinical entities in which the common denominator is the presence of a significantly large number of microorganisms in any portion of the urinary tract. Microorganisms may be evident only in the urine (bacteriuria), or there may be evidence of infection of an organ, eg, urethritis, prostatitis, cystitis, pyelonephritis. At any given time, any one of these organs may be asymptomatic or symptomatic. Infection in any part of the urinary tract may spread to any other part of the tract.

Symptomatic urinary tract infection may be acute or chronic. The term relapse implies recurrence of infection with the same organism; the term reinfection implies infection with another organism.

Pathogenesis

Urine secreted by normal kidneys is sterile until it reaches the distal urethra. Bacteria can reach the urinary tract by the ascending route or by hematogenous spread. The latter occurs during bacteremia (eg, with staphylococci) and results in abscess formation in the cortex or the perirenal fat. Far commoner is ascending infection, where bacteria are introduced into the distal urethra (from fecal flora on the perineum or the vaginal vestibule, or by instrumentation) and travel up the urinary tract to reach the bladder, ureters, or renal pelvis. The most important factor in aiding or perpetuating ascending infection is anatomic or functional obstruction to free urine flow. Free flow, large urine volume, and acid pH are important antibacterial defenses.

Age & Sex Distribution of Urinary Tract Infection

In infants, urinary tract infection occurs more frequently in boys than in girls, in keeping with a higher incidence of obstructive anomalies of the urinary tract. After the first year of life, urinary tract infection is more frequent in girls because of the contamination of the vaginal vestibule with fecal flora and the short urethra. In surveys of school children, only 0.05% of boys have been found to have bacteriuria, whereas at least 2% of girls have bacteria in their urine specimens. In later life, urinary tract infection is rare among men until the age of prostatic hypertrophy (over 40), but there is a regular increase in incidence among women until age 70, when about 10% of women have urinary tract infection. There is some correlation of the incidence of urinary tract infection with sexual activity in women, as well as with parity.

Infecting Microorganisms

Virtually any microorganism which is introduced into the urinary tract may cause urinary tract infec-

*By Ernest Jawetz, PhD, MD.

tion. However, the vast majority of cases of urinary tract infection are caused by aerobic members of the fecal flora, especially escherichia, enterobacter, klebsiella, enterococci, pseudomonas, and proteus. Other organisms are occasionally found in spontaneous urinary tract infection, but their significance must be assessed as described below.

Significant Bacteriuria

The concept of significant bacteriuria is basic to the accurate interpretation of urine cultures. Urine secreted by the normal kidney is sterile and remains so while it travels to the bladder. However, the normal urethra has a microbial flora, and any voided urine in normal persons may therefore contain thousands of bacteria per milliliter derived from this normal flora. To differentiate this smaller number of microorganisms from the larger number commonly found in urinary tract infection, it is essential to count the number of bacteria in fresh, properly collected urine specimens by appropriate methods (quantitative culture). In general, active urinary tract infections are characterized by more than 100,000 bacteria per ml. If such numbers are found in 2 consecutive specimens of urine, and if they are of a single type, there is more than a 90–95% chance that an active urinary tract infection is present.

Pathology

Acute urinary tract infection shows inflammation of any part of the tract and sometimes intense hyperemia or even bleeding of the mucous membranes. The prominent lesion in the kidney is acute inflammation of the interstitial tissue, which may progress to frank suppuration and patchy necrosis. Chronic urinary tract infection may cause only minimal changes or progressively more severe scarring in any part of the tract. Chronic pyelonephritis may lead to widespread fibrosis and scarring of functional cortical and medullary tissue, resulting in renal insufficiency. Chronic interstitial nephritis may result from bacterial infection or from other causes.

Collection of Urine for Culture*

A. Voided Midstream Specimen: This is the optimal method, involving no risk to the patient. The urethral meatus or vaginal vestibule is cleansed, the labia are spread, and the first part of the stream is discarded. The mid part of the stream is aseptically collected in a sterile container.

B. Specimen Obtained by Catheterization: Each urethral catheter insertion carries a 1–2% risk of introducing microorganisms into the bladder and thus initiating urinary tract infection. Results of quantitative culture from a single catheterized urine specimen yielding more than 100,000 bacteria of a single species per ml indicate—with 95% reliability—that an active urinary tract infection is present.

*Details of the methods of urine collection are given in Kunin CM: *Detection, Prevention and Management of Urinary Tract Infections*, 2nd ed. Lea & Febiger, 1974.

C. Specimen Obtained by Suprapubic Aspiration: While the bladder is distended, the suprapubic skin is aseptically prepared and a sterile needle is then thrust into the bladder. This permits aspiration of bladder urine, free from urethral contamination. It is especially useful in infants (from whom a satisfactory specimen for culture may be difficult to obtain) and in patients with equivocal counts on several occasions.

Examination of Urine

Urine must be cultured or examined microscopically within 1 hour of collection or after no more than 18 hours of refrigeration. Urine is a good culture medium for many microorganisms, and growth can occur at room temperature.

A. Microscopic Examination: A drop of fresh urine or a drop of resuspended sediment from centrifuged fresh urine is placed on a microscope slide, covered with a cover glass, and examined with the high-dry objective under reduced illumination. More than 10 bacteria (often motile) per field in the unstained specimen suggest the presence of more than 100,000 bacteria per ml of urine. Smears may also be made from fresh urine, stained with Gram's stain, and examined under the oil immersion objective. The interpretation is similar. By immunofluorescence, bacteria in urine are coated with immunoglobulin if they are derived from tissue infection (especially chronic pyelonephritis, prostatitis) but are not so coated if the infection is limited to the outflow system (cystitis, urethritis).

B. Urine Culture: Only quantitative cultures are used. For most accurate determinations, 0.1 ml of undiluted urine, 0.1 ml of urine diluted 1:100, and 0.1 ml of urine diluted 1:10,000 are spread over an agar plate containing suitable medium. After incubation, colonies are counted and multiplied by the dilution factor to yield the bacterial count per ml. A number of simplified semiquantitative culture methods are available which are readily performed in the physician's office at nominal cost. The dip-slide method and its several variations involve dipping an agar-coated slide or spoon into fresh urine, incubating it, and then comparing the resultant growth with optical density standards. Alternatively, measured amounts of urine (or dilutions) may be aspirated into agar-coated pipettes which are then drained and incubated and the resultant growth optically compared with standards.

C. Chemical Tests of Urine: The presence and number of bacteria can also be estimated by various chemical tests which rely on the enzymatic activity of viable bacteria, eg, the reduction of nitrate. These indirect tests are much less reliable than tests employing quantitative estimates of bacterial growth.

D. Identification of Microorganisms: In a majority of cases of acute urinary tract infection, detailed identification of the etiologic organism may not be required. However, in chronic or recurrent urinary tract infection, identification of the organism by standard microbiologic methods is desirable. Antimicrobial drug susceptibility tests are often not done in the first attack of urinary tract infection (a vast majority of which are caused by coliform organisms), which is often treated with sulfonamides. In chronic or recurrent urinary tract infection, antimicrobial drug susceptibility tests by standard methods are required.

ACUTE URINARY TRACT INFECTION

Clinical Findings

A. Lower Tract Involvement:

1. Symptoms and signs—Sudden or more gradual onset of burning pain on urination, often with turbid, foul-smelling, or dark urine, and lower abdominal discomfort. There are usually no positive physical findings unless the upper tract is involved also.

2. Laboratory findings—Microscopic examination of a properly collected urine specimen usually shows significant bacteriuria and pyuria and occasionally hematuria. The bacteriuria is confirmed by culture. Leukocytosis is rare unless the upper tract is also involved.

B. Upper Tract Involvement:

1. Symptoms and signs—Headache, malaise, vomiting, chills and fever, costovertebral angle pain and tenderness, and abdominal pain. The absence of upper tract involvement does not exclude bacterial invasion of the upper tract.

2. Laboratory findings—Significant bacteriuria is often accompanied by proteinuria and pyuria. The bacteria in the urine are often coated with immunoglobulin, as revealed by immunofluorescence. Leukocytosis is common, with a marked shift to the left. Blood culture is occasionally positive.

Differential Diagnosis

Acute urinary tract infection may occasionally present as an "acute abdomen," acute pancreatitis, or basal pneumonia. In all of these circumstances, the presence of significant bacteriuria usually establishes the diagnosis.

Treatment

A. Specific Treatment:

1. First attack of urinary tract infection—Give sulfisoxazole or trisulfapyrimidines USP, 4 gm daily in divided doses by mouth, for 10 days. Co-trimoxazole (sulfamethoxazole, 400 mg, plus trimethoprim, 80 mg), 1 tablet 6 times daily, is an alternative drug. Tetracycline, 1–2 gm daily, or ampicillin, 1–2 gm daily, may also be used. Maintain an alkaline urine pH. If symptoms have not subsided by day 4 of treatment, reexamine the urine for possible resistant microorganisms. Follow-up at 2 and 6 weeks after treatment is stopped should demonstrate absence of bacteriuria; otherwise, continued management is indicated.

2. Recurrence of urinary tract infection—Select an antimicrobial drug on the basis of antimicrobial susceptibility tests of cultured organisms. Give the drug for 10–14 days in doses sufficient to maintain high urine levels. Reexamine the urine 2 and 6 weeks after treatment is stopped.

3. Second recurrence, or failure of bacteriuria to be suppressed—Perform tests of renal function and excretory urograms and consider referral to a urologist for a work-up for possible obstruction, reflux, and localization of infection in the upper or lower tract. (For details, see Kunin reference, p 543.)

B. General Measures: Forcing fluids may relieve signs and symptoms but should be limited to amounts which will avoid undue dilution of antimicrobials in the urine. Analgesics may be required briefly for pain. Metabolic abnormalities such as diabetes mellitus must be identified and treated.

Prevention

Certain women have a high rate of urinary reinfection, sometimes related to sexual activity. In the latter situation, 1 or 2 doses of an effective antimicrobial (eg, trimethoprim/sulfamethoxazole [co-trimoxazole], ampicillin) taken after intercourse tend to prevent establishment of infection. In other women, recurrences can be greatly reduced if the patient takes daily one-half tablet of co-trimoxazole (ie, 40 mg trimethoprim and 200 mg sulfamethoxazole) for many months.

In patients who must have an indwelling catheter postoperatively and in whom closed sterile drainage is established, the acquisition of bacteriuria is delayed if antimicrobial drugs (eg, cephalosporins) are given during the first 3 days after insertion. Thereafter, there is no benefit.

Prognosis

Initial attacks of acute urinary tract infection, in the absence of obstruction, tend to heal with treatment or spontaneously. The symptoms subside and bacteriuria often disappears. This is not true in recurrent or chronic urinary tract infection. About 20% of pregnant women with asymptomatic bacteriuria develop symptomatic urinary tract infection—often upper tract infection—later in pregnancy.

CHRONIC URINARY TRACT INFECTION

Essentials of Diagnosis

- Recurrent episodes of lower or upper tract involvement.
- Absence of symptoms or signs referable to the urinary tract but persistent asymptomatic bacteriuria.
- Impairment of renal function with nitrogen retention, anemia, acidosis, uremia, or hypertension.

General Considerations

Chronic or recurrent episodes of urinary tract

infection may produce no permanent harm or may lead to dysfunction or scarring of the lower or upper tract. Chronic bacterial pyelonephritis may progress to inflammation of interstitial tissue, scarring, atrophy, and, rarely, progressive renal failure or hypertension. In any patient with hypertension, a search for bacterial pyelonephritis should be made. If unilateral pyelonephritis should be found, nephrectomy may be curative. With bilateral pyelonephritis, chronic suppression of infection may permit improved renal function. The end stage of renal failure resulting from chronic bacterial pyelonephritis may be indistinguishable from that resulting from chronic glomerulonephritis or nephrosclerosis. Over a significant extent of its natural history, chronic urinary tract infection is asymptomatic, manifested mainly by bacteriuria or by recurrent episodes of acute urinary tract infection.

Clinical Findings

A. Symptoms and Signs: There are often no positive clinical findings in chronic urinary tract infection except chronic significant bacteriuria. There may be episodes of recurrent acute or subacute urinary tract infection with symptoms referable to the lower or to the upper urinary tract. Hypertension, anemia, or uremia may appear in the late stages of chronic pyelonephritis.

Whenever chronic bacteriuria is discovered, it is mandatory to perform a complete urologic study, including excretory urograms, cystograms, and voiding cystourethrograms, followed by procedures to localize the source of bacteriuria to one or both sides and to the lower or upper tract. Surgical correction of any abnormality (reflux, obstruction, etc) found in these studies must be considered while chronic suppression of bacteriuria is undertaken.

B. Laboratory Findings: The white blood count is usually normal, but significant anemia may be present in early renal failure. Blood urea, serum creatinine, and other measures of nitrogen retention may be elevated; creatinine clearance and other measures of excretory function may be reduced. The crucial laboratory procedure as a guide to medical treatment is repeated and meticulous urine culture. If significant bacteriuria is discovered, an attempt may be made to eradicate or suppress it (see below). If no significant bacteriuria is found, infection by tubercle bacilli, anaerobic bacteria, or fungi must be considered.

Bacteria derived from tissue infection are usually found coated with immunoglobulin by immunofluorescence, eg, in pyelonephritis and prostatitis. No such staining occurs if bacteria are coming from the ureter or bladder.

The concentrating ability of the kidney is one of the earliest functions to be impaired in chronic pyelonephritis. Determination of urine osmolality under controlled fluid intake is a good guide to changes in kidney status under antimicrobial treatment.

Treatment

A. Specific Treatment: Specific treatment may

consist of surgical correction of functional or anatomic abnormalities by the urologist or antimicrobial treatment. The latter usually involves attempts to eradicate the infectious agent by short-term treatment and, if bacteriuria recurs, long-term suppression of the bacteria by administration of urinary antiseptics.

1. If the same organism is isolated from at least 2 sequential urine cultures, antimicrobial drug sensitivity tests should be performed. From the group of drugs to which the organism is susceptible in vitro, the least toxic is selected (for choice of drugs, see Chapter 28) and administered daily in full systemic doses orally for 4 weeks. Urine pH must be adjusted to be optimal for the selected drug. The urine must be checked after 3 days of treatment and then at weekly intervals to make certain that bacteriuria is suppressed and that reinfection with another organism has not occurred. At the end of the treatment period, all drug administration is stopped and, 2 and 6 weeks later, the urine is checked again. If bacteriuria is not found, it may be assumed that the particular organism has been eradicated. Repeated follow-up examinations for bacteriuria are necessary to confirm absence of infection.

2. If the foregoing measures fail to eradicate the infection, chronic suppression of bacteriuria is attempted by daily dosage with a urinary antiseptic, eg, nitrofurantoin, methenamine mandelate or hippurate, nalidixic acid, or acidifying agents (see Chapter 28). Urinary pH must be adjusted to the optimum for the drug selected and usually should be held below pH 6.0. The patient is instructed to check his urine pH with indicator paper daily. At the end of the first week of treatment, and at monthly intervals thereafter, urine must be examined to ascertain the absence of bacteriuria. Chronic suppression is continued for at least 6 months or even longer provided the patient can tolerate the drug and superinfection does not occur. If the latter should occur, a specific antimicrobial drug may be selected, by laboratory test, for a 14-day course of treatment, and suppression with another urinary antiseptic may then be continued. At the end of 1 year of suppressive treatment, renal function and bacteriuria are reevaluated. During suppressive long-term treatment, instrumentation of the urinary tract should be strenuously avoided.

B. General Measures: Water diuresis may often provide relief from minor discomfort of lower urinary tract symptoms. Water and electrolyte balance must be maintained and renal failure managed as described on p 534. For management of hypertension, see Chapter 7. Prevention of infection is all-important, particularly by the avoidance of catheterization and instrumentation and by adherence to the principles of good hygiene. In selected cases, the prophylactic administration of penicillin G or ampicillin immediately after sexual intercourse can prevent recurrences of urinary tract infection. Similar claims have been made for trimethoprim/sulfamethoxazole (co-trimoxazole).

Prognosis

Probably 10% or less of asymptomatic bacteriuria

patients develop renal failure attributable to the infection; hypertension can be attributed to urinary tract infection even more rarely. Chronic urinary tract infection is eradicated by short-term therapy (2–6 weeks) in about one-fourth to one-third of patients. Some of the others have relapses caused by the same organism; some have reinfection caused by other organisms.

Long-term suppression (more than 6 months) with urinary antiseptics eradicates bacteriuria in about two-thirds of patients, but some may become reinfected later. Many elderly patients tolerate recurrent urinary tract infection well, and treatment should be directed mainly at symptomatic relief by the best tolerated measures.

Freeman RB & others: Prevention of recurrent bacteriuria with continuous chemotherapy. Ann Int Med 69:655, 1968.

Garibaldi RA & others: Factors predisposing to bacteriuria during indwelling urethral catheterization. New England J Med 291:215, 1974.

Harding GKH, Ronald AR: A controlled study of antimicrobial prophylaxis of recurrent urinary infection in women. New England J Med 291:597, 1974.

Kunin CM: *Detection, Prevention and Management of Urinary Tract Infections,* 2nd ed. Lea & Febiger, 1974.

Norden WW & others: Predictive effect of urinary concentrating ability upon response to antimicrobial therapy in bacteriuria of pregnancy. J Infect Dis 121:588, 1970.

Stamey TA & others: The localization and treatment of urinary tract infections. Medicine 44:1, 1965.

Straffon RA: Urinary tract infection. M Clin North America 58:545, 1974.

Turck M & others: Relapse and reinfection in chronic bacteriuria. (2 parts.) New England J Med 275:70, 1966; 278:422, 1968.

TUBERCULOSIS OF THE URINARY TRACT

Essentials of Diagnosis

- Fever, easy fatigability, night sweats, or other signs of systemic infection.
- Symptoms or signs of upper or lower urinary tract infection.
- Urine may contain leukocytes and erythrocytes but no visible bacteria. Urine culture is negative.
- Special culture of urine for mycobacteria reveals *M tuberculosis.*
- Excretory urogram may show deformed or "moth-eaten" calcyes and varying types of kidney tissue destruction.
- Cystoscopy may reveal ulcers or granulomas of bladder wall.

General Considerations

Hematogenous dissemination of tubercle bacilli from foci in the lung or lymph nodes is the usual source of tuberculosis of the kidney; rarely does the infection originate in the genital tract. The genital organs may become infected by hematogenous spread or secondary to kidney infection. The prostate, seminal vesicles, epididymides, and, rarely, the testes may be infected. The fallopian tubes are more frequently involved than the ovaries and uterus.

The kidney and ureter may show little gross change. Caseous nodules in the renal parenchyma and abscess formation with destruction of tissue and fibrosis often produce extensive damage. Calcification in the lesions is common. The ureter and calyces are thickened, and stenosis may occur with total destruction of functioning renal tissue above. The bladder shows mucosal inflammation and submucosal tubercles which become necrotic and form ulcers. Fibrosis of the bladder wall occurs late or upon healing. Tubercles with caseous necrosis and calcification are found in the genital organs. Microscopically, typical tubercles are found, and demonstration of the tubercle bacilli in the lesions is usually easily accomplished.

Note: The search for tuberculosis elsewhere in the body must be complete whenever urinary tract tuberculosis is found.

Clinical Findings

A. Symptoms and Signs: Symptoms are not characteristic or specific. Manifestations of chronic infection with malaise, fever, fatigability, and night sweats may be present. Kidney and ureter infection is usually silent. Bladder infection produces frequency, burning on urination, nocturia, and, occasionally, tenesmus. If bleeding occurs with clot formation, ureteral or vesical colic may occur. Gross hematuria is fairly common. There may be nodular induration of the testes, epididymis, or prostate and thickened seminal vesicles. Occasionally there is pain and tenderness in the costovertebral angle. A draining sinus may form from any of these sites.

B. Laboratory Findings: The urine contains "pus without bacteria," red cells, and usually protein. Culture for tubercle bacilli confirms the diagnosis. If renal damage is extensive, signs of renal insufficiency can be demonstrated: elevated BUN and serum electrolyte abnormalities characteristic of uremia. A mild anemia usually is present, and the sedimentation rate is rapid.

C. X-Ray and Cystoscopic Findings: Excretory urograms will reveal the moth-eaten appearance of the involved calyces or the obliteration of calyces, stenosis of calyces, abscess cavities, ureteral thickening and stenosis, and the nonfunctioning kidney (autonephrectomy). Calcification of involved tissues is common. Thorough cystoscopic examination is required to determine the extent of bladder wall infection and to provide biopsy material if needed. Culture of urine obtained from ureteral catheters will help establish whether one or both kidneys are affected.

Differential Diagnosis

The "sterile" pyuria of chronic pyelonephritis and chronic nonspecific urethritis and cystitis may mimic tuberculous infection. Culture should serve to distinguish tuberculosis from these.

Treatment

Intensive and prolonged antituberculosis therapy is indicated, employing 2 or 3 drugs simultaneously for at least 18 months (see Chapter 28). In 1975–1976 the drugs of choice (and dosages) appear to be isoniazid, 5–8 mg/kg/day (usually 300 mg daily orally); ethambutol, 15 mg/kg/day in a single oral dose; and rifampin, 10–20 mg/kg/day (usually 600 mg as a single oral dose). Alternative antituberculosis drugs are listed in Chapter 28.

Pyridoxine, 100 mg/day orally, is usually given simultaneously to prevent neurotoxic reactions to isoniazid. Surgical procedures are generally limited to situations where extensive destruction of one kidney makes it unlikely that infection can be eradicated and meaningful function restored, or where obstruction in the tract interferes with proper function, or when erosion of a vessel leads to severe bleeding.

Prognosis

The outlook depends largely on the degree of destruction of renal tissue and impairment of renal function. If urinary tract tuberculosis is detected early, prolonged drug treatment can suppress and arrest the infectious process successfully. Structural defects resulting from infection or fibrosis require surgical correction.

Christensen WI: Genitourinary tuberculosis. Medicine 53:377, 1974.
Lattimer JK & others: Current treatment for renal tuberculosis. J Urol 102:2, 1969.

PROSTATITIS

Bacteria may reach the prostate from the blood stream (eg, tuberculosis) or from the urethra. Prostatitis is thus commonly associated with urethritis (eg, gonococcal, chlamydial, mycoplasmal) or with active infection of the lower urinary tract. Perineal pain, lumbosacral backache, fever, and dysuria and frequency may be symptoms of prostatic bacterial infection ("prostatosis").

Prostatitis may be acute or chronic. However, acute prostatitis commonly develops into a chronic state, and overmanipulation of chronic prostatitis gives rise to acute stage symptoms.

Clinical Findings

A. Symptoms and Signs: Symptoms of acute prostatitis usually are perineal pain, fever, dysuria, frequency, and urethral discharge. To the palpating finger, the prostate feels enlarged, boggy, and very tender; fluctuation occurs only if an abscess has formed. Even gentle palpation of the prostate results in expression of copious purulent discharge.

Symptoms of chronic prostatitis may include lumbosacral backache, perineal pain, mild dysuria and frequency, and scanty urethral discharge. Palpation reveals an irregularly enlarged, firm, and slightly tender prostate.

B. Laboratory Findings: With acute febrile prostatitis, there is often leukocytosis. The expressed prostatic fluid shows pus cells and bacteria on microscopy and culture. During the acute phase, prostatic palpation may express frank pus. The first glass of urine contains a far larger number of pus cells and bacteria than subsequent urine specimens.

Differential Diagnosis

Prostatitis should be differentiated from lower urinary tract infection, although it may form part of it. In the latter case, the infected prostate may serve as a source of recurrent lower urinary tract infections. Other perirectal infections may be considered, as well as epididymitis, gonococcal infection, and tuberculosis.

Complications

Epididymitis and cystitis as well as urethritis commonly accompany acute prostatitis. Chronic prostatitis commonly predisposes to recurrent urinary tract infection and occasionally to urethral obstruction and acute urinary retention.

Treatment

A. Specific Treatment: For acute prostatitis, initial treatment may consist of co-trimoxazole (sulfamethoxazole, 400 mg, plus trimethoprim, 80 mg), 6–8 tablets daily, or tetracycline, 2 gm daily by mouth, until culture of prostatic fluid and susceptibility tests indicate the drug of choice. Treatment for 2 weeks usually results in subsidence of the acute inflammation, but chronic prostatitis may continue.

Eradication of bacteria in chronically infected prostatic tissue is exceedingly difficult. Antimicrobial drugs diffusing best into prostatic acini must be lipid-soluble and basic (eg, trimethoprim/sulfamethoxazole [co-trimoxazole]). Erythromycins are quite active in the prostate but effective mainly against gram-positive organisms, which are rare in urinary tract infections and prostatitis. Conversely, most drugs which are active against gram-negative coliform bacteria (the commonest cause of prostatitis) fail to reach the prostatic acini.

B. General Measures: During the acute phase the patient must be kept at bed rest with adequate hydration and given analgesics, stool softeners, and sitz baths. Urethral instrumentation and prostatic massage must be avoided.

Chronic prostatitis should be treated by prolonged antimicrobial therapy accompanied by vigorous prostatic massage once weekly to promote drainage. Total prostatectomy is curative but has a high morbidity and a significant mortality rate. Transurethral prostatectomy offers only uncertain benefits. Surgical drainage of an abscess is mandatory.

Prognosis

While the symptoms of acute prostatitis usually

subside with treatment, the prospects for the elimination of chronic prostatitis are discouraging.

Gibder MJ: Prostatitis. S Clin North America 45:1449, 1965.

Meares EM: Bacterial prostatitis vs "prostatosis." JAMA 224, 1372, 1973.

Meares EM: Observations on activity of trimethoprim-sulfamethoxazole in the prostate. J Infect Dis 128 (Suppl):S679, 1973.

Stamey TA & others: Chronic bacterial prostatitis and the diffusion of drugs into prostatic fluid. J Urol 104:559, 1970.

URINARY STONES

Urinary stones and calcification in the kidney may be associated with metabolic disease, may be secondary to infection in the urinary tract, may occur in sponge kidney, tuberculosis of the kidney, or papillary necrosis, or may be idiopathic. The incidence of urinary tract calculus is higher in men.

NEPHROCALCINOSIS

Essentials of Diagnosis
- Asymptomatic, or symptoms of primary disease producing hypercalciuria.
- Physical signs of the primary disease.
- Anemia is common.
- Blood chemical findings of primary disease plus variable degrees of renal insufficiency.

General Considerations

Chronic hypercalciuria and hyperphosphaturia may result in precipitation of calcium salts in the renal parenchyma. The commonest causes are hyperparathyroidism, hypervitaminosis D (particularly with associated high-calcium intake), and excess calcium and alkali intake. Chronic pyelonephritis predisposes to nephrocalcinosis. Other causes include acute osteoporosis following immobilization, sarcoidosis, renal tubular acidosis, the De Toni-Fanconi syndrome, and destruction of bone by metastatic carcinoma.

Clinical Findings

The symptoms, signs, and laboratory findings are those of the primary disease. The diagnosis is usually established by x-ray demonstration of calcium deposits in the kidney, which appear as minute calcific densities with linear streaks in the region of the renal papillae. True renal stones may be present as well.

Differential Diagnosis

Differentiate from renal calculi, renal tuberculosis, and medullary sponge kidney.

Treatment

Specific treatment is directed at the primary disorder. Particular attention is directed to treatment of urinary tract infection and renal insufficiency. When renal tubular acidosis or the De Toni-Fanconi defect is present, it is essential to maintain a high fluid intake, to replace cation deficit, and to alkalinize the urine with sodium bicarbonate, 1–1.5 mEq/kg/day in 3 divided doses, or with Shohl's solution (hydrated crystalline sodium citrate, 98 gm, and citric acid, 140 gm, in 1000 ml water). One ml of Shohl's solution equals 1 mEq of bicarbonate. Give 50–150 ml/day in 3 divided doses. Potassium supplements may be required and can be given as 50% potassium citrate solution (4 ml 3 times daily provides approximately 50 mEq/day). Even with adequate treatment, the prognosis is poor.

McMillan DE, Freeman RB: The milk-alkali syndrome: A study of the acute disorder with comments on the development of the chronic condition. Medicine 44:485, 1965.

Morris RC Jr: Renal tubular acidosis: Mechanisms, classification and implications. New England J Med 281:1405, 1969.

Mortensen JD, Baggenstoss AH: Nephrocalcinosis: A review. Am J Clin Path 24:45, 1954.

Rodriquez-Soriano J, Edelman CM Jr: Renal tubular acidosis. Ann Rev Med 20:363, 1969.

Seldin DW, Wilson IO: Renal tubular acidosis. In: *The Metabolic Basis of Inherited Disease*, 3rd ed. Stanbury JB, Wyngaarden JB, Fredrickson DS (editors). McGraw-Hill, 1972.

RENAL STONE

Essentials of Diagnosis
- Often asymptomatic.
- Symptoms of obstruction of calyx or ureteropelvic junction, with flank pain and colic.
- Nausea, vomiting, abdominal distention.
- Hematuria.
- Chills and fever and bladder irritability if infection is present.

Etiology

A. Excessive Excretion of Relatively Insoluble Urinary Constituents:

   1. Calcium–

      a. With hypercalcemia and hypercalciuria–

        (1) Primary hyperparathyroidism (see p 675) produces increased excretion of calcium and phosphate in the urine. Serum calcium is high and serum phosphorus low.

        (2) High vitamin D intake increases dietary calcium absorption, which increases the load of calcium excreted by the kidney.

        (3) Excessive intake of milk and alkali.

        (4) Prolonged immobilization (due to spi-

nal cord injury, poliomyelitis, fractures).

(5) Destructive bone disease due to neoplasm or of metabolic origin (Cushing's syndrome, hyperthyroidism).

b. With hypercalciuria but normal or low serum calcium—

(1) Idiopathic hypercalciuria.

(2) Distal renal tubular acidosis.

2. **Oxalate**—Over half of urinary stones are composed of calcium oxalate or calcium oxalate mixed with calcium phosphate.

a. Congenital or familial oxaluria.

b. High oxalate intake (cabbage, spinach, tomatoes, rhubarb, chocolate).

c. Ileal disease, including ileal bypass or resection.

d. Methoxyflurane anesthesia.

3. **Cystine**—Hereditary cystinuria.

4. **Uric acid**—

a. Gout—Stone may form spontaneously or due to treatment with uricosuric agents.

b. Therapy of neoplastic disease with agents which cause rapid tissue breakdown, resulting in increased excretion of uric acid.

c. Myeloproliferative disease such as leukemia, myeloid metaplasia, polycythemia vera.

B. **Physical Changes in the Urine:**

1. Increased concentration of urinary constituents when fluid intake is low.

2. Urinary pH—Inorganic salts are ordinarily less soluble at high pH. Organic substances are least soluble at low pH.

C. **Nucleus (Nidus) for Stone Formation:**

1. Organic material, particularly bits of necrotic tissue or blood clot, may serve as a nucleus for stone formation.

2. Clumps of bacteria, particularly when infection is accompanied by stasis or obstruction.

D. **Congenital or Acquired Deformities of the Kidneys:**

1. Sponge kidney.

2. Horseshoe kidney.

3. Local obstruction of calyceal system.

General Considerations

The location and size of the stone and the presence or absence of obstruction determine the changes which occur in the kidney and calyceal system. The pathologic changes may be modified by ischemia due to pressure or by infection.

Clinical Findings

A. **Symptoms and Signs:** Often a stone trapped in a calyx or in the renal pelvis is asymptomatic. If a stone produces obstruction in a calyx or at the ureteropelvic junction, dull flank pain or even colic may occur. Hematuria and symptoms of accompanying infection may be present. Nausea and vomiting may suggest enteric disease. Flank tenderness and abdominal disten-

tion may be the only physical findings.

B. **Laboratory Findings:** Leukocytosis may be present if there is an infection. The urine may contain red cells, white cells, and protein; pus and bacteria occur with infection. Crystals in the urine may provide a clue to the type of stone, eg, uric acid or cystine. Chemical abnormalities in the blood and urine will confirm the diagnosis of the primary metabolic disease (eg, hyperparathyroidism, gout, cystinuria, renal tubular acidosis).

C. **X-Ray Findings:** The x-ray examination will reveal radiopaque stones, delineate kidney size, demonstrate bone lesions of parathyroid disease, gout, and metastatic neoplasm. Excretory and retrograde urograms help to delineate the site and degree of obstruction and to confirm the presence of nonopaque stones (uric acid, cystine).

Differential Diagnosis

Differentiate from acute pyelonephritis, renal tumor, renal tuberculosis, and infarction of the kidney.

Complications

Infection and hydronephrosis are complications which may destroy renal tissue.

Prevention of Further Stone Formation

Obtain a stone for analysis whenever possible.

Treat predisposing disease, eg, surgical removal of parathyroid tumor or hyperplastic parathyroid glands; treat gout, cystinuria, and renal tubular acidosis as indicated.

Thiazide diuretics plus modest restriction of salt intake reduce calcium excretion and may also increase excretion of magnesium, which has the effect of inhibiting stone formation.

Recently, cellulose phosphate has been shown to be an apparently safe agent for the purpose of binding calcium in the gut and preventing its absorption, thus reducing the hypercalciuria secondary to increased absorption of dietary calcium.

For calcium phosphate and calcium oxalate stones (excluding those associated with renal tubular acidosis), inorganic orthophosphate has proved useful. Give potassium acid phosphate (K-Phos), 6 gm daily divided into 3–4 doses before meals and at bedtime. If gastrointestinal irritability results from the acid phosphate, give a mixture of monobasic and dibasic phosphate (Neutra-Phos), available as a powder 2¼ oz of which is added to 1 gallon of warm water. The usual dose is 12–15 oz of solution per day, divided into 3–4 doses.

A high fluid intake throughout the 24 hours to produce 3–4 liters of urine a day is important. This program is aimed at prevention of new stone formation and must be maintained indefinitely. It may be used in hyperparathyroidism while awaiting surgical attack on the parathyroid. A low calcium diet may be helpful.

Prevention of uric acid stones by inhibiting the formation of uric acid is now possible by blocking the conversion of xanthine to uric acid with the xanthine oxidase inhibitor allopurinol. The usual adult dose of allopurinol is 600 mg/day (300 mg every 12 hours). This will reduce elevated serum uric acid to normal levels and markedly reduce the excretion of uric acid. It is even effective in the presence of renal failure associated with gouty nephropathy. The drug is well tolerated and apparently produces no alteration of renal function. Treatment should be continued indefinitely in patients with gout (see Chapter 13) or myeloproliferative disorders. Allopurinol may be used in association with antileukemia and anticancer agents. While the allopurinol effect is developing, treatment should include a high fluid intake and alkalinization of the urine with sodium bicarbonate, 10–12 gm/day in divided doses.

Cystine stone formation can be reduced by forcing fluids to produce a urine output of 3–4 liters/day and alkalinizing the urine with sodium bicarbonate, 10 12 gm daily, or sodium citrate, 50% solution, 4–8 ml 4 times daily or oftener. Urine pH should be maintained at 7.5 or higher, at which levels cystine solubility is greatly increased. A low-methionine diet may help, but protein deprivation must be avoided. Patients with severe cystinuria may require penicillamine, which complexes cysteine and reduces the total excretion of cystine. There are many side-effects which appear to be dose-related.

Treatment

Small stones may be passed. They do no harm if infection is not present. Larger stones may require surgical removal if obstruction is present or renal function threatened. Nephrectomy may be necessary.

Force fluids to maintain a dilute urine and restrict calcium intake.

Combat infection with appropriate antibiotics.

Prognosis

If obstruction can be prevented and infection eradicated, the prognosis is good.

URETERAL STONE

Essentials of Diagnosis

- Obstruction of ureter produces severe colic with radiation of pain to regions determined by position of the stone in the ureter.
- Gastrointestinal symptoms common.
- Urine usually contains fresh red cells.
- May be asymptomatic.
- Exacerbations of infection when obstruction occurs.

General Considerations

Ureteral stones are formed in the kidney but produce symptoms as they pass down the ureter.

Clinical Findings

A. **Symptoms and Signs:** The pain of ureteral

colic is intense. The patient may be in mild shock, with cold, moist skin. There is marked tenderness in the costovertebral angle. Abdominal and back muscle spasm may be present. Referred areas of hyperesthesia may be demonstrated.

B. **Laboratory Findings:** As for renal stone.

C. **X-Ray and Instrumental Examination:** X-rays may show the stone lodged in the ureter or at the ureterovesical junction. Nonopaque stones can be demonstrated by excretory urograms, which reveal the site of obstruction and the dilated ureteropelvic system above it. Because of the danger of infection, cystoscopy and ureteral catheterization should be avoided unless retrograde urography is essential.

Differential Diagnosis

Differentiate from clots due to hemorrhage, from tumor, acute pyelonephritis, and acute cholecystitis.

Prevention

As for renal stone. Every effort should be made to obtain a stone for analysis.

Treatment

A. **Specific Measures:** Most stones will pass spontaneously if spasm of the ureter is relieved and fluids are forced. Surgical removal by cystoscopy or cystotomy may be necessary if the stone is large or if infection is present which does not respond readily to treatment.

B. **General Measures:** Morphine or other opiates should be given in doses adequate to control pain. Morphine sulfate, 8 mg (or equivalent dosage of other drugs), may be given IV and repeated in 5–10 minutes if necessary. Thereafter, subcutaneous administration is usually adequate. Atropine sulfate, 0.8 mg subcut, or methantheline bromide, 0.1 gm IV, may be used as antispasmodics.

Prognosis

If obstruction and infection can be treated successfully, the outlook is excellent.

VESICAL STONE

Essentials of Diagnosis

- Bladder irritability with dysuria, urgency, and frequency.
- Interruption of urinary stream as stone occludes urethra.
- Hematuria.
- Pyuria.

General Considerations

Vesical stones occur most commonly when there is residual urine infected with urea-splitting organisms (eg, proteus, staphylococci). Thus, bladder stones are associated with urinary stasis due to bladder neck or urethral obstruction, diverticula, neurogenic bladder, and cystocele. Foreign bodies in the bladder act as foci for stone formation. Ulceration and bladder inflammation predispose to stone formation.

Most vesical stones are composed of calcium phosphate, calcium oxalate, or ammonium magnesium phosphate. Uric acid stones are common in the presence of an enlarged prostate and uninfected urine.

Clinical Findings

A. Symptoms and Signs: Symptoms of chronic urinary obstruction or stasis and infection are usually present. Dysuria, frequency and urgency, and interruption of the urinary stream (causing pain in the penis) when the stone occludes the urethra are common complaints. Physical findings include prostatic enlargement, evidence of distended (neurogenic) bladder, a cystocele. Occasionally the stone may be palpable.

B. Laboratory Findings: The urine usually shows signs of infection and contains red cells.

C. X-Ray and Cystoscopic Examination: X-ray examination shows the calcified stone, and urograms show the bladder abnormalities and upper urinary tract dilatation due to long-standing back pressure. Direct cystoscopic examination may be necessary for final diagnosis.

Differential Diagnosis

Differentiate from pedunculated vesical tumor.

Treatment

A. Specific Measures: Surgical removal of the stone is indicated, either by transurethral manipulation or cystotomy. Any prostatic or urethral obstruction must be eliminated.

B. General Measures: Give analgesics as required and treat infection with appropriate antibiotics. Anti-infective measures are usually of little value until stone is removed and obstruction is relieved.

Prognosis

If obstruction and infection can be prevented, the prognosis is excellent.

Earll JM, Kolb FO: Treatment of cystinuria and cystine stone disease. Mod Treat 4:539, 1967.

Ettinger B, Kolb FO: Inorganic phosphate treatment of nephrolithiasis. Am J Med 55:32, 1973.

Maurice PF, Henneman PH: Medical aspects of renal stones. Medicine 40:315, 1961.

Pak CYC & others: Successful treatment of recurrent nephrolithiasis (calcium stones) with cellulose phosphate. New England J Med 290:175, 1974.

Smith LH: The diagnosis and treatment of metabolic stone disease. M Clin North America 56:977, 1972.

Williams HE: Nephrolithiasis. New England J Med 290:33, 1974.

TUMORS OF THE GENITOURINARY TRACT

ADENOCARCINOMA OF KIDNEY
(Hypernephroma)

Essentials of Diagnosis

- Painless gross hematuria.
- Fever.
- Enlarged kidney may be palpable.
- Evidence of metastases.

General Considerations

The commonest malignant tumor of the kidney is adenocarcinoma, which occurs more frequently in males. This tumor metastasizes early to the lungs, liver, and long bones.

Adenocarcinoma of the kidney apparently arises from renal tubule cells or adenomas. It invades blood vessels early. Microscopically the cells resemble renal tubule cells arranged in cords and varying patterns.

Clinical Findings

A. Symptoms and Signs: Gross hematuria is the most frequent sign. Fever is often the only symptom. A flank mass may be palpable. Vena cava occlusion may produce characteristic patterns of collateral circulation and edema of the legs.

A hypernephroma may not produce classical symptoms of renal tumor. It may produce symptoms and signs suggesting a wide variety of diseases: fever of obscure origin, leukemoid reaction, refractory anemia, polycythemia, liver or biliary disease, hypercalcemia, peripheral neuropathy, and an abdominal mass of indeterminate origin.

B. Laboratory Findings: Polycythemia occasionally develops as a result of increased secretion of erythropoietin by the tumor. Anemia is more commonly found. Hematuria is almost always present. The erythrocyte sedimentation rate is rapid. Carcinoembryonic antigen (CEA) levels may be elevated in plasma or urine.

C. X-Ray Findings: X-ray examination may show an enlarged kidney. Metastatic lesions of bone and lung may be revealed. Excretory or retrograde urography (or both) must be employed to establish the presence of a renal tumor.

Differential Diagnosis

Differentiate from focal nephritis, hydronephrosis, polycystic kidneys, renal cyst, and renal tuberculosis.

Treatment

Nephrectomy is indicated if no metastases are present. Even when metastases are present, nephrectomy may be indicated if bleeding or pain is intractable.

X-ray irradiation of metastases may be of value, although the lesions are usually fairly radioresistant. Isolated single pulmonary metastases can occasionally be removed surigcally. At present, chemotherapy is ineffective. Palliation may be achieved with medroxyprogesterone.

Prognosis

The course is variable. Some patients may not develop metastases for 10–15 years after removal of the primary tumor. About 25% of patients live more than 5 years.

Rubin P (editor): Cancer of the urogenital tract: Kidney. (3 parts.) JAMA 204:219, 603, 981, 1968.

Skinner DG & others: Diagnosis and management of renal cell carcinoma. Cancer 28:1165, 1971.

Utz DC, Kelalis PP: Hypernephroma: The new image. Minnesota Med 54:503, 1971.

Weigensberg LJ: The many faces of metastatic renal carcinoma. Radiology 98:353, 1971.

EMBRYOMA OF THE KIDNEY
(Wilms's Tumor)

Embryoma is a highly malignant mixed tumor which occurs almost exclusively in children under 6 years of age. It metastasizes early to the lungs, liver, and brain.

Weight loss and anorexia are the most common signs. Pain occurs rarely. The enlarged kidney is usually easily palpable. Metastases produce an enlarged liver. Hypertension is common. Anemia may be present. The urine is not remarkable. X-ray examination demonstrates the tumor and metastases in the lung. Excretory urograms and gastrointestinal examination help to determine the size of the tumor.

Wilms's tumor must be differentiated from hydronephrosis, polycystic kidney disease, and neuroblastoma of the adrenal medulla.

Treatment consists of nephrectomy followed by local irradiation and irradiation of metastases. Antitumor chemotherapy with dactinomycin (actinomycin D) increases the cure rate and is usually effective in controlling local recurrences and metastases. Vincristine and doxorubicin (Adriamycin) have also been effective.

Cure can be achieved if metastases have not occurred before nephrectomy.

Aron BS: Wilms' tumor: A clinical study of eighty-one patients. Cancer 33:637, 1974.

Perez CA & others: Treatment of Wilms' tumor and factors affecting prognosis. Cancer 32:609, 1973.

TUMORS OF THE RENAL PELVIS & URETER

Epithelial tumors of the renal pelvis and ureter are relatively rare. They are usually papillary and tend to metastasize along the urinary tract. Epidermoid tumors are highly malignant and metastasize early. Transitional cell tumors have occurred in cases of interstitial nephritis and papillary necrosis due to phenacetin abuse.

Painless hematuria is the most common complaint. Colic occurs with obstruction due to blood clot or tumor. Tenderness in the flank may be found. Anemia due to blood loss occurs. The urine contains red cells and clots; white cells and bacteria are present when infection is superimposed. Urography should reveal the filling defect in the pelvis or show obstruction and dilatation of the ureter. At cystoscopy, the bleeding from the involved ureter may be seen and satellite tumors identified. Exfoliative cytologic studies should be done.

Radical removal of the kidney, the involved ureter, and the periureteral portion of the bladder should be done unless metastases are extensive.

Irradiation of metastases is usually of little value.

The prognosis depends upon the type of tumor. With anaplastic neoplasms, death usually occurs within 2 years.

TUMORS OF THE BLADDER

Essentials of Diagnosis

- Hematuria.
- Suprapubic pain and bladder symptoms associated with infection.
- Visualization of tumor at cystoscopy.

General Considerations

Bladder tumors are second to prostatic tumors in frequency. At least 75% of bladder tumors occur in males over the age of 50. Tumors usually arise at the base of the bladder and involve ureteral orifices and the bladder neck. The common tumor is transitional in type; epidermoid tumors, adenocarcinomas, and sarcomas are rare. Metastases involve regional lymph nodes, bone, liver, and lungs.

Clinical Findings

A. Symptoms and Signs: Hematuria is the commonest symptom. Cystitis with frequency, urgency, and dysuria is a frequent complication. With encroachment on the bladder neck, the urinary stream is diminished. Suprapubic pain occurs as the tumor extends beyond the bladder. Obstruction of the ureters produces hydronephrosis, frequently accompanied by renal infection and in which case the signs of urinary tract infection may be present. Physical examination is not remarkable. The bladder tumor may be palpable on bimanual (abdominorectal or abdominovaginal) examination. Exfoliative cytology is often diagnostic.

B. Laboratory Findings: Anemia is common. The urine contains red cells, white cells, and bacteria. Exfoliative cytology is usually confirmatory.

C. X-Ray and Instrumental Examination: Excretory urography may reveal ureteral obstruction. Cystograms usually show the tumor. Cystoscopy and biopsy confirm the diagnosis.

Differential Diagnosis

Hematuria and pain can be produced by other tumors of the urinary tract, urinary calculi, renal tuberculosis, acute cystitis, or acute nephritis.

Treatment

A. Specific Measures: Transurethral resection may be adequate to remove local and superficial tumors. Cystectomy with ureterosigmoidostomy or another urinary diversion procedure is required for invasive tumors. Radiation therapy may be useful for more anaplastic tumors. Chemotherapy has not been effective. Thiotepa instillations may be effective in eradicating superficial and papillary bladder epithelial tumors.

B. General Measures: Urinary tract infection should be controlled with appropriate antibiotics. Anastomosis of ureters to an isolated loop of ileum or sigmoid colon, one end of which is brought to the skin to act as a conduit, is relatively free of renal complications and of alteration of body fluid electrolytes. An isolated loop of ileum or sigmoid colon can be used as a urinary conduit when anastomosed to the ureters.

Prognosis

There is a tendency toward recurrence and increasing malignancy. With infiltrating carcinomas the outlook is poor even with radical resection.

Cummings KB & others: Renal pelvic tumors. J Urol 113:158, 1975.

Grabstald H, Whitmore WF, Melamed MR: Renal pelvic tumors. JAMA 218:845, 1971.

Rubin P (editor): Cancer of the urogenital tract: Bladder cancer. (4 parts.) JAMA 206:1761, 2719, 1968; 207:341, 1131, 1969.

Veenema RJ & others: Chemotherapy for bladder cancer. Urology 3:135, 1974.

BENIGN PROSTATIC HYPERPLASIA

Essentials of Diagnosis

- Prostatism: hesitancy and straining to initiate micturition, reduced force and caliber of the urinary stream, nocturia.
- Acute urinary retention.
- Enlarged prostate.
- Uremia follows prolonged obstruction.

General Considerations

Hyperplasia of the prostatic lateral and subcervical lobes which are invaded by periurethral glands results in enlargement of the prostate and urethral obstruction.

Clinical Findings

A. Symptoms and Signs: The symptoms of prostatism increase in severity as the degree of urethral obstruction increases. Symptoms may be overlooked or not reported when the progress of obstruction is slow. On rectal examination, the prostate is usually found to be enlarged. Infection commonly occurs with stasis and retention of "residual urine." Hematuria may occur. Uremia may result from prolonged back pressure and severe bilateral hydronephrosis. Determination of BUN may provide the only clue to slowly advancing and relatively asymptomatic obstructive disease. Residual urine can be measured by postvoiding catheterization. In the presence of prostatism, ganglionic blocking agents and parasympatholytic drugs used in the treatment of hypertension, as well as tranquilizers, weaken the power of detrusor contraction, thus causing symptoms simulating vesical neck obstruction and in some cases urinary retention.

B. X-Ray and Cystoscopic Examination: Excretory urograms reveal the complications of back pressure: ureteral dilatation and hydronephrosis and postvoiding urinary retention. Cystoscopy will reveal the enlargement of the prostate and the secondary bladder wall changes such as trabeculation, diverticula, inflammation due to infection, and vesical stone.

Differential Diagnosis

Other causes of urethral obstruction include urethral stricture, vesical stone, bladder tumor, neurogenic bladder, or carcinoma of the prostate.

Treatment

A. Specific Measures: Conservative (nonsurgical) management should be undertaken only in collaboration with a urologist. Relieve acute urinary retention by catheterization. Maintain catheter drainage if the degree of obstruction is severe. Surgery is usually necessary. There are various indications for each of the 4 approaches: transurethral resection or prostatectomy by suprapubic, retropubic, and perineal procedures.

B. General Measures: Treat infection of the urinary tract with appropriate antibiotics. The patient who develops postobstructive diuresis must be sustained with appropriate water and electrolyte replacement.

Prognosis

Surgical resection will relieve symptoms. The surgical mortality rate is low.

Finestone AJ, Rosenthal RS: Silent prostatism. Geriatrics 26:89, 1971.

Mad P & others: Human prostatic hyperplasia. Arch Path 79:270, 1965.

Vaughan ED Jr, Gillenwater JY: Diagnosis, characterization and management of postobstructive diuresis. J Urol 109:286, 1973.

CARCINOMA OF THE PROSTATE

Essentials of Diagnosis
- Prostatism.
- Hard consistency of the prostate.
- Metastases to bone produce pain, particularly in the low back.
- Anemia. Elevated serum acid phosphatase with extension of the cancer beyond the prostatic capsule.

General Considerations
Cancer of the prostate is rare before the age of 60. It metastasizes early to the bones of the pelvis and locally may produce urethral obstruction with subsequent renal damage. The growth of the tumor is increased by androgens and inhibited by estrogens. The prostatic tissue is rich in acid phosphatase, and when cancer has extended beyond the prostate to the periprostatic tissue, or to bone, the serum acid phosphatase is increased; when bone metastases occur, the serum alkaline phosphatase is increased. The serum acid phosphatase concentration thus provides a good index of the extent and growth of the tumor, and serum alkaline phosphatase its extension to bone.

Clinical Findings
A. Symptoms and Signs: Obstructive symptoms similar to those of benign prostatic hyperplasia are common. Rectal examination reveals a stone-hard prostate which is often nodular and fixed. Low back pain occurs with metastases to the bones of the pelvis and spine. Pathologic fractures may occur at the sites of metastases. Obstruction may produce renal damage and the symptoms and signs of renal insufficiency.

B. Laboratory Findings: Anemia may be extreme if bone marrow is replaced by tumor. The urine may show evidence of infection. Serum acid phosphatase is increased when metastases have occurred, and serum alkaline phosphatase may be elevated as new bone is formed at the site of metastases. Biopsy by transurethral resection or by needle aspiration through the perineum establishes the diagnosis.

C. X-Ray Findings: X-ray examination of the bones of the pelvis, spine, ribs, and skull will reveal the typical osteoblastic metastases. Excretory urograms delineate changes secondary to urethral obstruction and the back pressure of urine retention. Lymphangiography may demonstrate metastases to pelvic nodes.

Differential Diagnosis
Differentiate from benign prostatic hyperplasia, urethral stricture, vesical stone, bladder tumor, and neurogenic bladder.

Treatment
Cure may be obtained before metastasis has occurred by radical resection of the prostate, including the seminal vesicles and a portion of the bladder neck with or without lymph node dissection. Palliative therapy includes transurethral resection to relieve obstruction. Antiandrogen therapy slows the rate of growth and extension of the cancer. Orchiectomy and diethylstilbestrol, 5 mg daily (or equivalent of another estrogen), or estrogen therapy alone, are often effective. Radiotherapy with the linear accelerator or radioactive cobalt has provided good remission. Irradiation of bone metastases may afford relief.

The effectiveness of therapy can be judged by clinical response and by periodic measurements of the serum acid and alkaline phosphatase.

Prognosis
Palliative therapy is often not effective for long. Most patients die within 3 years; a few survive for 5–10 years.

Boyd HL: Combined hormone control therapy and radical prostatectomy in the treatment of selected cases of advanced carcinoma of the prostate: A retrospective study based on 25 years of experience. J Urol 101:86, 1969.

Gilbertsen VA: Cancer of the prostate gland: Results of early diagnosis and therapy undertaken for cure of the disease. JAMA 215:81, 1971.

Jewitt HJ & others: Radical prostatectomy in the management of carcinoma of the prostate: Probable causes of some therapeutic failures. J Urol 107:1034, 1972.

Rubin P: Cancer of the urogenital tract: Prostatic cancer. JAMA 209:1695, 1969.

Rubin P: Cancer of the urogenital tract: Prostatic cancer, advanced and metastatic. JAMA 210:1072, 1969.

TUMORS OF THE TESTIS
(See also Chapter 18.)

Essentials of Diagnosis
- Painless enlargement of the testes.
- Mass does not transilluminate.
- Evidence of metastases.

General Considerations
The incidence of testicular tumors is about 0.5% of all types of cancer in males. Tumors occur most frequently between the ages of 20 and 35 and are often malignant. Classification of tumors of the testes is based upon their origin from germinal components or from nongerminal cells. The most common are the germinal tumors: seminomas; embryonal tumors, including embryoma, choriocarcinoma, embryonal carcinoma, teratocarcinoma, and adult teratoma; and the gonadoblastomas of intersexes. Nongerminal tumors include those of interstitial cell, Sertoli cell, and stromal origin. Rarely, lymphomas, leukemias, plasmacytomas, and metastatic carcinoma may involve the testis.

Seminomas, the most common testicular tumors, tend to spread slowly via the lymphatics to the iliac and periaortic nodes and disseminate late. Embryonal tumors invade the spermatic cord and metastasize early, particularly to the lungs. Seminomas are usually radiosensitive; embryonal tumors are usually radioresistant. Chemotherapy may be helpful in choriocarcinoma.

Secretion of gonadotropic hormones occurs with only about 10% of tumors. The literature on tumor-hormonal relationships is limited and confusing, but gonadotropin secretion is usually indicative of a carcinomatous tumor.

Gynecomastia may be associated with testicular tumors. Interstitial cell tumors, which occur at any age and are rarely malignant, are occasionally associated with gynecomastia and with sexual precocity and virilization.

Clinical Findings

A. Symptoms and Signs: Painless enlargement of the testes is typical. The enlarged testis may produce a dragging inguinal pain. The tumor is usually symmetrical and firm, and pressure does not produce the typical testicular pain. The tumors do not transilluminate. Attachment to the scrotal skin is rare. Gynecomastia may be present. Virilization may occur in preadolescent boys with Leydig cell tumors.

Metastases to regional lymph nodes and to the lungs and liver may be evident. Hydrocele may develop.

B. Laboratory Findings: Gonadotropins may be present in high concentrations in urine and plasma in cases of choriocarcinoma, and pregnancy tests are positive. 17-Ketosteroids are normal or low in Leydig cell tumors. Estrogens may be elaborated in both Sertoli cell and Leydig cell tumors.

C. X-Ray Findings: Pulmonary metastases are demonstrated by chest films. Lymphangiography will reveal enlarged iliac and periaortic nodes. Displacement of ureters by enlarged lymph nodes can be demonstrated by urography or venacavograms.

Differential Diagnosis

Tuberculosis, syphilitic orchitis (gumma of the testicle), hydrocele, spermatocele, and tumors or granulomas of the epididymis may produce similar local manifestations.

Treatment

The testicle should be removed and the lumbar and inguinal nodes examined. Radical resection of iliac and lumbar nodes is usually indicated except for seminoma, which is radiosensitive. Radiation is the treatment of choice following removal of the testis bearing a seminoma. Radiation is employed following radical surgery for other malignant tumors. Chemotherapy (Table 32–2) is effective against chorionic tumors (choriocarcinoma). Mithramycin and doxorubicin (Adriamycin) have been effective in a variety of testicular tumors that have metastasized.

Prognosis

The presence of metastases or high gonadotropin secretion indicates a poor prognosis. Seminomas are least malignant, with 90% 5-year cures. Almost all patients with choriocarcinoma are dead within 2 years. Less than half of those with other tumors will live 5 years.

Collins DH, Pugh RCB: The pathology of testicular tumors. Brit J Urol 36 (Suppl):1, 1966.

Jacobs EM: Combination chemotherapy of metastatic testicular germinal cell tumors and soft part sarcomas. Cancer 25:324, 1970.

Keough B & others: Urinary gonadotropins in management and prognosis of testicular tumor. Urology 5:496, 1975.

Nefzger MD, Mostofi FK: Survival after surgery for germinal malignancies of the testis: 1. Rates of survival in tumor groups. 2. Effects of surgery and radiation therapy (2 parts). Cancer 30:1225, 1233, 1972.

Rubin P & others: Cancer of the urogenital tract: Testicular tumors. JAMA 213:89, 1970.

16...
Nervous System

Joseph G. Chusid

DISORDERS OF CONSCIOUSNESS

Disturbances of the sensorium may be associated with decreased motor activity (eg, stupor or coma) or increased motor activity (eg, excitement, delirium, mania). Sensorial disturbances may range from partial clouding to complete obliteration of consciousness. The pattern of reaction of these disorders depends upon the nature and intensity of the stimulus and the physical, mental, and emotional status of the patient. Causative factors include trauma, cerebrovascular accidents, drug and other poisonings, fever, metabolic disorders, meningitis, overwhelming infection, brain tumors, convulsive disorders, and cardiac decompensation.

STUPOR & COMA

Stupor ranges from partial to almost complete loss of consciousness. Coma is complete unconsciousness from which the patient cannot be aroused even by the most painful stimuli.

Etiology of Coma

Coma may be of intracranial or extracranial origin. Examples are given below.

A. Intracranial: Head injuries, cerebrovascular accidents, CNS infections, tumors, convulsive disorders, degenerative diseases, increased intracranial pressure.

B. Extracranial: Vascular (shock or hypotension, as with severe hemorrhage, myocardial infarction, arterial hypertension); metabolic (diabetic acidosis, hypoglycemia, uremia, hepatic coma, addisonian crisis, electrolyte imbalance); intoxications (alcohol, barbiturates, narcotics, bromides, analgesics, tranquilizers, carbon monoxide, heavy metals); miscellaneous (hyperthermia, hypothermia, electric shock, anaphylaxis, severe systemic infections).

Clinical Findings

A. History: Interrogate the patient during lucid intervals. Valuable information may also be obtained from the patient's friends, relatives, and attendants. Inquire specifically about the patient's occupation; previous physical, mental, or emotional illness; trauma, the use of alcohol and drugs, epilepsy, and hypertension.

B. Physical Examination: Place particular emphasis on vital signs, evidence of injury or intoxication, and neurologic abnormalities. Do not assume that sensorial disturbances are due to alcoholic intoxication merely because an alcoholic breath is detected. Inspect the head and body carefully for evidence of injury. Discoloration of the skin behind the ear often is associated with skull fractures (Battle's sign).

Observe respiration, which may be deep and labored (suggesting diabetic acidosis) or of the Cheyne-Stokes type. Puffing out of one cheek with each expiration indicates paralysis of that side of the face.

Spontaneous movements may indicate which areas are normal parts or may represent the onset of focal motor convulsions.

Paralysis of extremities may be determined by lifting each extremity and allowing it to fall. In light coma the paralyzed limb will fall heavily, whereas a normal limb will gradually sink to the bed. Vigorous stimulation of the feet may cause a normal leg to react, where a paralyzed leg will not. Passive motion may disclose diminished tone of affected limbs in acute or recent flaccid hemiplegia.

Decerebrate rigidity or the presence of tonic neck reflexes suggests dysfunction at a brain stem level.

Check the eyes carefully. Hemianopsia may be demonstrable in stupor by failure of flinching on threatening hand gestures initiated from the hemianopsic side. Pupillary differences may be of vital diagnostic importance; an enlarged pupil is often present with ipsilateral subdural hematoma. Papilledema indicates elevated intracranial pressure and is a grave prognostic sign.

Oculomotor paralysis of one eye is often associated with a ruptured aneurysm of the anterior portion of the circle of Willis.

Pronounced nuchal rigidity usually signifies meningeal irritation (meningitis, subarachnoid bleeding) or herniation of the cerebellar tonsils due to intracranial tumor or vascular accident.

C. Laboratory Findings: Catheterize the patient if

necessary and examine the urine especially for protein, blood, glucose, and acetone. Take hemoglobin, white blood count, differential count, and hematocrit. Draw blood for electrolytes, blood gases, pH, NPN, glucose, and blood ammonia when indicated (for diagnosis of uremia, diabetic coma, or hepatic coma). Lumbar puncture should be considered when meningitis, encephalitis, or subarachnoid hemorrhage is suspected. CSF examination and culture may be helpful. Special studies may be indicated, eg, blood cultures and analysis of body fluids for evidence of toxins. Skull x-rays, EEG, echoencephalography, brain scan, cerebral angiography, and pneumography are valuable aids in brain tumor and subdural hematoma suspects. Order chest x-ray and other x-rays as indicated.

Treatment

A. Emergency Measures: The immediate objective is to maintain life until a specific diagnosis has been made and appropriate treatment can be started.

1. Maintain adequate ventilation—First determine the cause of any respiratory difficulty (eg, obstruction, pulmonary disease, depression of respiratory center, vascular collapse).

Keep airways open. Place the patient on his side or abdomen with his face to the side and his head well extended (*never* on his back or with the head flexed). If necessary, pull the tongue forward with fingers or forceps and maintain in an extended position (eg, by pharyngeal airways). Aspirate mucus, blood, and saliva from the mouth and nose with a lubricated soft rubber catheter. If no suction apparatus is available, use a 25–50 ml syringe. Endotracheal catheterization or tracheostomy may be necessary. (*Caution:* If the endotracheal tube remains in place for more than 2 hours, there is danger of laryngeal edema and further obstruction upon its removal.) The services of a trained anesthetist or otolaryngologist are desirable.

Artificial respiration may be administered if respirations have ceased or are failing. Closed chest cardiac massage may be necessary. (See Appendix.)

Oxygen may be administered by mask, catheter, or tent as indicated (see Chapter 6).

2. Shock—Institute immediate treatment if the patient is in shock or if shock is threatened (see Chapter 1).

B. General Measures: The patient must be observed constantly. Change body positions every 30–60 minutes to prevent hypostatic pneumonia and skin ulcerations. Catheterize the patient if coma persists for longer than 8–12 hours and the patient fails to void. If necessary, insert an indwelling catheter (with appropriate aseptic technic).

Provide proper fluid and nutrition with intravenous glucose, amino acids, and saline solutions for the first few days until the patient is able to take fluids by mouth. If the patient is comatose for more than 2–3 days, tube feedings should be employed.

Whenever possible, avoid sedation or other depressant medications until a specific diagnosis has been made. Sedation with paraldehyde, barbiturates, or tranquilizers may be necessary for mild restlessness in coma which is not due to barbiturate or other drug toxicity.

Corticosteroids: Parenteral corticosteroids may be used to treat cerebral edema associated with brain tumor, head injury, subarachnoid hemorrhage, x-ray irradiation, and other causes. Give dexamethasone, 8–40 mg/day IV or IM.

Hypertonic solutions (such as 15% mannitol in water) may be used to reduce increased intracranial pressure quickly.

Increased intracranial pressure may be reduced for 3–10 hours by intravenous administration of urea. Give urea as 30% sterile solution (in 10% invert sugar) in a dosage of about 1 gm/kg at a rate of about 60 drops/minute. Poor renal function or active intracranial bleeding is a contraindication.

C. Specific Measures: Treat specific causes, such as fevers, infections, and poisonings. In the absence of hypothermia or sedation, irreversible brain damage or brain death may be suspected when there is areflexia, loss of spontaneous respirations, fixed dilated pupils, motor and sensory paralysis, and an iso-electric (flat) EEG for 24 hours.

Barrett R, Merritt HH, Wolf A: Depression of consciousness as a result of cerebral lesions. Res Publ A Nerv Ment Dis 65:241, 1967.

Ivan LP: Spinal reflexes in cerebral death. Neurology 23:650, 1973.

Locke S: The neurological aspects of coma. S Clin North America 48:251, 1968.

Mohandas A, Chou SN: Brain death: A clinical and pathological study. J Neurosurg 35:211, 1971.

Penn AS, Rowland LP, Fraser DW: Drugs, coma and myoglobinuria. Arch Neurol 26:336, 1972.

Plum F, Posner J: *The Diagnosis of Stupor and Coma,* 2nd ed. Davis, 1972.

Sabin TD: The differential diagnosis of coma. New England J Med 290:1062, 1974.

Silverman D & others: Irreversible coma associated with electrocerebral silence. Neurology 20:521, 1970.

NARCOLEPSY

Narcolepsy is a chronic clinical syndrome of unknown etiology characterized by recurrent episodes of uncontrollable desire to sleep. It is frequently associated with a transient loss of muscle tone (cataplexy), especially during emotional reactions (laughing, crying). Inability to move in the interval between sleep and arousal (sleep paralysis) and hallucinations at the onset of sleep (hypnagogic hallucinations) may also occur. The attacks of sleep may occur once or several times a day and may last minutes to hours. The sleep is similar to that of normal sleep, but is apt to occur at inappropriate times, such as during work or while walking or driving. Narcolepsy is about 4 times as frequent in males as in females.

Treatment

A. Amphetamine Sulfate (Benzedrine): The average dose is 10–20 mg 3 times daily, but more may be required for some patients. The optimal dosage may be determined by starting with 10 mg each morning and increasing the dosage as necessary to control symptoms.

B. Dextroamphetamine Sulfate (Dexedrine): Give 5 mg each morning initially and increase as necessary. Long-acting capsules (Dexedrine Spansules) are available in 5, 10, and 15 mg doses.

C. Methylphenidate Hydrochloride (Ritalin): Used in doses of 5–10 mg 3–4 times daily (or more if necessary).

D. Ephedrine Sulfate: Ephedrine is not as satisfactory as amphetamine but is helpful in many cases. The average dose is 25–50 mg 2–4 times daily.

Prognosis

Narcolepsy usually persists throughout life. Although the attacks of somnolence and sleep may be relieved by medical treatment, the cataplexy and attacks of muscular weakness which accompany emotional reactions (laughing, crying) are usually not affected by drug therapy. (See Sleep Disturbances, p 625.)

Guilleminault C, Carskadden M, Dement WC: On the treatment of rapid eye movement narcolepsy. Arch Neurol 30:90, 1974.
Guilleminault C, Wilson RA, Dement WC: A study on cataplexy. Arch Neurol 31:255, 1974.
Kales A, Kales JD: Sleep disorders. New England J Med 290:487, 1974.
Wyatt RG & others: Treatment of intractable narcolepsy with a monoamine oxidase inhibitor. New England J Med 285:987, 1971.
Zarcone V: Narcolepsy. New England J Med 288:1156, 1973.

SYNCOPE & VERTIGO

VASODEPRESSOR SYNCOPE
(Vasovagal Syncope, Simple Fainting, Benign Faint)

Vasodepressor syncope, the most common type, is usually characterized by a sudden fall in blood pressure and a slowing of the heart. The causative stimuli may be sensory (eg, sudden pain) or entirely emotional (eg, grief or bereavement). The patient is usually upright when the faint occurs; recumbency rapidly restores consciousness. In the early phase there may be motor weakness, epigastric distress, perspiration, restlessness, yawning, and sighing respirations. The patient may appear anxious, with a pale face and cold, moist extremities. After several minutes, lightheadedness, blurring of vision, and sudden loss of consciousness with decreased muscle tone may occur. If the patient remains erect, a brief but mild convulsion may follow. Syncope is believed to occur when the arterial pressure drops below 70 mm Hg systolic and is usually precipitated by fear, anxiety, or pain. Electroencephalographic changes occur after the onset of unconsciousness in a syncopal attack.

The patient should be placed in the recumbent position with his head lower than the rest of his body. Inhalation of aromatic spirits of ammonia may help revive the patient in a faint.

Ebert EV: Syncope. Circulation 27:1148, 1963.
Ruetz PP & others: Fainting: A review of its mechanism and a study in blood donors. Medicine 46:363, 1967.
Thomas JE, Rooke ED: Fainting. Proc Staff Meet Mayo Clin 38:397, 1963.
Wayne HH: Syncope: Physiological considerations and an analysis of the clinical characteristics in 570 patients. Am J Med 30:418, 1961.

ORTHOSTATIC HYPOTENSION
(Postural Hypotension)

Syncope may occur as the patient assumes an upright position. This type of syncope is characterized by repeated fainting attacks associated with a sudden drop in arterial blood pressure when the patient stands up. Recognized contributory factors are prolonged convalescence and recumbency, idiopathic disorders of postural reflexes, sympathectomy, peripheral venous stasis, chronic anxiety, and the use of antihypertensive drugs. Idiopathic orthostatic hypotension (Shy-Drager's syndrome) may be associated with dysarthria, rigidity, tremor, ataxia, monotonous speech, diplegia, vertigo, and incontinence; degenerative changes in the autonomic ganglia, basal ganglia, and cortex may be found.

Treatment is directed toward the underlying cause when possible. Withdraw or reduce the dosage of hypotensive drugs. Caution the patient against rising too rapidly from the sitting or lying position. If abdominal ptosis is present, an abdominal belt may help. Elastic stockings may be of value. Vasoconstrictor drugs may be tried but usually do not help.

Ephedrine sulfate, up to 75 mg daily, may be useful. Fludrocortisone acetate has also been reported to be effective in daily doses of 0.1 mg or more.

Hoehn MM: Levodopa-induced postural hypotension. Arch Neurol 31:255, 1974.
Meyer JS & others: Cerebral dysautoregulation in central neurogenic orthostatic hypotension (Shy-Drager syndrome). Neurology 23:262, 1973.
Roessman U, van den Noort S, McFarland DE: Idiopathic orthostatic hypotension. Arch Neurol 24:403, 1971.
Streeten DHP & others: Hyperbradykininism: A new orthostatic syndrome. Lancet 2:1048, 1972.
Thomas JE, Schirger A: Idiopathic orthostatic hypotension. Arch Neurol 22:289, 1970.

CAROTID SINUS SYNCOPE

Patients who suffer from attacks of carotid sinus syncope usually give a history of fainting associated with spells of dizziness between attacks. A definite relation between the attacks and sudden turning or raising of the head or the wearing of a tight collar may be elicited. The diagnosis is usually confirmed by reproducing an attack by firm pressure and massage over the carotid sinus for 10–20 seconds. *Caution:* Stimulate only one carotid sinus at a time. In stimulating the sinuses in elderly patients, care must be taken not to precipitate cerebrovascular accidents.

Three types of carotid sinus syncope are known to occur: (1) The vagal type (most common) is most often seen in older persons. Carotid sinus pressure slows the heart rate. This response can be abolished by the injection of atropine sulfate, 1 mg IV. (2) The vasomotor or depressor type occurs more frequently in younger individuals. Carotid sinus pressure causes a fall in blood pressure which can be abolished by injection of 0.5 ml of epinephrine, 1:1000 solution, but is unaffected by atropine sulfate. (3) In the cerebral type carotid sinus pressure affects neither heart rate nor blood pressure, and neither epinephrine nor atropine affects the reflex. A direct cerebral effect is postulated.

Treatment

Correct all abnormalities whenever possible. Eliminate emotional problems and forbid the use of tight collars. In severe cases, denervation of the sinuses may be necessary. Local anesthesia of the carotid sinuses abolishes all types of carotid sinus syncope.

A. Vagal Type: Atropine sulfate, 0.4–0.6 mg 3–4 times daily (or more, if needed), will usually abolish attacks. Ephedrine sulfate, 25 mg, with phenobarbital, 15 mg 3–4 times daily, or amphetamine sulfate, 5–10 mg, may be used.

B. Vasomotor Type: Ephedrine and phenobarbital as above will usually prevent attacks.

C. Cerebral Type: Drugs are of no value.

Brodie RE, Dow RS: Studies in carotid compression and carotid sinus sensitivity. Neurology 18:1047, 1968.
Hutchinson EC, Stock JPP: The carotid sinus syndrome. Lancet 2:445, 1960.
Ramirez A: Demand pacemaker for the treatment of carotid sinus syncope. J Thoracic Cardiovas Surg 66:287, 1973.
Smiddy J, Lewis HD, Dunn M: The effect of carotid massage in older men. J Gerontol 27:209, 1972.
Thomas JE: Hyperactive carotid sinus reflex and carotid sinus syncope. Mayo Clin Proc 44:127, 1969.

SYNCOPE DUE TO CARDIOVASCULAR DISORDERS

Syncope due to cerebral anoxia resulting from a temporary fall in cardiac output may occur in Stokes-Adams syndrome, myocardial infarction, pulmonary embolism, and the onset of paroxysmal tachycardia; and occurs in certain other types of heart disease (eg, aortic stenosis and tetralogy of Fallot). Syncope may occur with "cyanotic crisis" (low arterial oxygen saturation and low cardiac output). The use of a Holter monitor may assist in documenting cardiac arrhythmia as a cause of syncope.

Treatment consists of correcting the underlying abnormality.

Formel PF: Neurologic manifestations of cardiac disease. New York J Med 73:968, 1973.
Reed RL, Siekert RG, Merideth J: Rarity of transient focal cerebral ischemia in cardiac dysrhythmia. JAMA 223:893, 1973.
Stockard JJ, Bickford RG, Schauble JF: Pressure-dependent cerebral ischemia during cardiopulmonary bypass. Neurology 23:521, 1973.

SYNCOPE DUE TO METABOLIC DISTURBANCES

In some types of syncope, impaired cerebral metabolism may be the most significant factor. These varieties include (1) anoxemia, as in patients with congenital heart disease; (2) severe chronic debilitating anemias; (3) hypoglycemia, as in labile diabetics after overexertion, or failure to eat after taking insulin; (4) acidosis, as in some patients with uncontrolled diabetes mellitus; (5) drug intoxication, as with barbiturates; (6) acute alcoholism; and (7) hyperventilation with associated respiratory alkalosis and tetany.

Treat the specific cause whenever possible. Consciousness may be restored in hyperventilation by rebreathing into a paper bag, breath-holding, or administration of 5–10% CO_2 with oxygen by mask. Recurrent attacks of hyperventilation syndrome suggest that psychiatric consultation should be considered.

Bell WE, Samaan NA, Longnecker DS: Hypoglycemia due to organic hyperinsulinism in infancy. Arch Neurol 23:330, 1970.
Burton RA, Raskin NH: Alimentary (postgastrectomy) hypoglycemia. Arch Neurol 23:14, 1970.
Gabrilove JL: Neurologic and psychiatric manifestations in the classic endocrine syndromes. Res Publ Assoc Nerv Ment Dis 63:419, 1966.
Senior RM & others: The recognition and management of myxedema coma. JAMA 217:61, 1971.

SYNCOPE DUE TO IMPAIRED BRAIN CIRCULATION

Impairment of brain circulation may lead to syncopal attacks. Syncope associated with transient focal neurologic findings is encountered among elderly patients with arteriosclerotic cerebrovascular disease. Dizziness followed by syncope can occur following abrupt head movements in patients with recent head injuries. Lightheadedness, and occasionally syncope, may occur in migraine in association with diminished cranial arterial blood flow. A type of syncope associated with hypersensitivity of the carotid sinus may occur with profound fall in blood pressure and consequent impaired brain circulation. In some patients with brain tumors or vascular malformations, syncopal episodes sometimes occur which may be related to displacement, engorgement, or insufficiency of cranial circulation. (See Cerebrovascular Accidents, p 566.)

Gray FD, Horner GJ: Survival following extreme hypoxemia. JAMA 211:1815, 1970.

Koch-Weser J: Hypertensive emergencies. New England J Med 290:487, 1974.

Livingston S: Breath-holding spells in children. JAMA 212: 2231, 1970.

Slosberg P: Treatment and prevention of stroke. 2. Cerebrovascular insufficiencies. New York J Med 73:758, 1973.

VERTIGO
(Dizziness)

The terms "vertigo" and "dizziness" are generally used to denote the subjective sensation of rotatory movement, either of the individual or his environment, and imply an inability to orient the body in relation to surrounding objects. Vertigo is found mainly in disease processes involving the labyrinths, the vestibular portion of the 8th cranial nerve, and their nuclei or connections. True vertigo is usually manifested by nystagmus, falling to one side, and abnormal reaction to tests of vestibular function. Among the more common causes are Ménière's syndrome; acute labyrinthitis; organic brain damage involving the vestibular nerve, its end organs or connections, or the cerebellum; and drug and chemical toxicity.

Treatment is based upon accurate diagnosis of the underlying disorder. (See Diseases of the Ear, pp 88–95.)

Cappon D: Dizziness. Postgrad Med 48:317, 1970.

Drachman DA, Hart CW: An approach to the dizzy patient. Neurology 22:323, 1972.

Hicks JJ, Hicks JW, Cooley HN: Ménière's disease. Arch Otolaryng 86:610, 1967.

Koenigsberger MB & others: Benign paroxysmal vertigo of childhood. Neurology 20:1108, 1970.

Paparella MM: The dizzy patient. Postgrad Med 52:97, 1972.

MOTION SICKNESS

Motion sickness is an acute illness characterized by anorexia, nausea, dizziness, and vomiting. The principal factors in its etiology are visual, kinesthetic, and psychologic. Physiologically, the vestibular apparatus appears to be involved.

Prevention

Preventive measures are often effective. Attacks of motion sickness are difficult to treat successfully.

A. The antihistamines appear to be of benefit. Dimenhydrinate or diphenhydramine hydrochloride, 50–100 mg 4 times daily, may be effective.

B. Meclizine hydrochloride, 50 mg every 6–12 hours as needed, is a long-acting effective agent.

C. Cyclizine hydrochloride is effective in oral or IM doses of 50 mg every 4–6 hours as needed.

D. Parasympathetic depressants, alone or in combination with mild sedatives: scopolamine hydrobromide or atropine sulfate, 0.2–0.4 mg every 3–6 hours.

E. Mild Sedation: Phenobarbital, 15–30 mg every 3–6 hours, may help prevent attacks.

Chinn HI, Smith PK: Motion sickness. Pharmacol Rev 7:33, 1955.

Greenblatt DJ, Shader RI: Anticholinergics. New England J Med 288:1215, 1973.

Ley A & others: Chronic and subacute labyrinthine disorders: A major causative agent in some neurological syndromes. J Nerv Ment Dis 147:91, 1968.

Preston FS: Motion sickness. Practitioner 206:609, 1971.

HEADACHE

Headache is a common symptom which may be due to a wide variety of causes, including emotional disorders, head injuries, migraine, fever, intracranial vascular disorders, dental disease, diseases of the eyes, ears, or nose, or intracranial masses.

Certain types of headache are frequently observed to be associated with specific clinical entities. Throbbing, pulsating headache is more likely to be encountered in vascular diseases such as migraine, arterial hypertension, and intracranial vascular malformations. Pressure headache, a sensation of tightness with a constricting, band-like feeling about the head, is often due to emotional disorders. A steady, dull headache is often encountered in patients with intracranial masses or head injuries.

The most severe headaches are believed to be those associated with migraine, meningitis, high degrees of fever, and ruptured intracranial aneurysms. A relatively prolonged, minor grade of headache may

occur with such serious disorders as intracranial hematoma, brain tumor, or abscess. Whereas the skull, the
brain parenchyma, the choroid plexuses, and most of
the dura mater and pia-arachnoid are not sensitive to
pain, the tissues covering the cranium, especially the
arteries, are sensitive to pain.

Under some circumstances, the characteristics of
headaches may be modified by physical measures.
Abrupt increase in intracranial pressure, as is produced
by coughing, sneezing, or straining, will usually exaggerate most headaches associated with intracranial
masses or bleeding. Headache following lumbar puncture is usually made more severe by elevation of the
head and improved by lowering the position of the
head relative to the rest of the body. Manual compression of the common carotid artery in the neck or the
major cranial branches of the external carotid artery
may relieve the headache of migraine. Headaches following head injuries are frequently made worse by
abrupt alteration in position of the head. Pressure
headaches associated with emotional disorders may be
greatly relieved by local gentle massage of the affected
region. Nocturnal headaches of the migraine type
sometimes are exaggerated by the recumbent position
and relieved when the patient stands erect.

Since headache may occur as a symptom of many
clinical disorders, it may not always be possible to determine the cause in a given case despite elaborate diagnostic procedures. The choice of a particular study frequently reflects the tentative diagnosis and, indirectly,
the physician's clinical orientation. Thus the internist
may feel that no patient with headache has been adequately studied without allergy tests; the psychiatrist
may consider an elaborate psychometric assay essential; and the neurosurgeon may not feel satisfied until
pneumoencephalographic, angiographic, and cervical
myelographic studies have been exhausted. In some
clinics, routine skull x-rays and electroencephalograms
are made as initial "screening" tests in all patients with
headaches, and further specific test procedures are
then adapted to the particular diagnostic needs as
necessary. Among the clinical types are the following:

(1) **Traumatic headache:** Following head injury,
with or without obvious evidence of injury to the skull
and adjacent soft tissues; following injury to the upper
cervical spine or its associated soft parts (ligaments,
muscles, fascia, and intervertebral disks).

(2) **Inflammatory headache:** Associated with
paranasal sinusitis, mastoiditis, meningitis; febrile
systemic illnesses, especially those with acute onset of
high fever or fluctuations in temperature; myositis or
arthritis involving tissues of the head or neck; or angiitis, as in temporal arteritis.

(3) **Tumor headache:** Associated with primary or
metastatic tumors of the head and neck or intracranial
hematoma (eg, subdural, intracerebral).

(4) **Vascular headache:** Migraine, histaminic cephalalgia, intracranial aneurysms and vascular malformations, essential hypertension, and syncope (recovery
phase).

(5) **Metabolic headache:** Hypothyroidism, ovarian

dysfunction, anemias and blood dyscrasias, and drug
intoxications (eg, alcohol, carbon monoxide).

(6) **Emotional headache:** Anxiety or pain, conversion neuroses.

(7) **Miscellaneous:** Neuralgias (occipital, trigeminal), ocular disorders (refractive errors, glaucoma), or
following lumbar puncture.

Friedman AP: Reflections on the treatment of headache. Head-
ache 11:148, 1972.
Friedman AP, Merritt HH: *Headache: Diagnosis and Treatment.*
Davis, 1959.
Friedman AP & others: Classification of headache. JAMA
179:717, 1962.
Wolff HG: *Headache and Other Head Pain,* 2nd ed. Oxford Univ
Press, 1963.

HEADACHE DUE TO MENINGEAL INVOLVEMENT

This is the most severe type of headache. Salicylate analgesics are usually effective, but narcotics may
be necessary if pain is severe. Lumbar puncture performed very cautiously sometimes relieves headache
due to increased intracranial pressure (eg, subarachnoid
hemorrhage). It is contraindicated for relief of increased pressure in posterior fossa tumors.

Lumbar puncture headaches are believed to be
due to leakage of CSF from the puncture site, and are
more likely to occur when a large-bore needle is used.
If headache is mild upon arising, aspirin may suffice.
Intrathecal injection of small quantities of sterile normal saline may afford relief in severe cases.

Elkins AH, Friedman AP: Review of headache. (3 parts.) New
York J Med 67:255, 426, 552, 1967.
MacNeal PS: The patient with headache. Postgrad Med 42:249,
1967.
Petito F, Plum F: The lumbar puncture. New England J Med
290:225, 1974.
Symposium on headache: Its mechanism, diagnosis and manage-
ment. Neurology 13:1, 1963.

MIGRAINE

Migraine is characterized by paroxysmal attacks
of headache often preceded by psychologic or visual
disturbances and sometimes followed by drowsiness. It
is said to affect about 8% of the population. It is more
frequent among women than men and occurs more
commonly among persons with a background of inflex-
ibility and shyness in childhood and with perfectionis-
tic, rigid, resentful, and ambitious character traits in
adult life. There is commonly a history of similar headaches in blood relations.

The headache of migraine is believed to result from vascular changes. An initial episode of cerebral, meningeal, and extracranial arterial vasoconstriction is believed to occur (accounting for the visual and other prodromal phenomena), followed by dilatation and distention of cranial vessels, especially of the external carotid artery. Increased amplitude of pulsation is said to determine the throbbing nature of the headache. Rigid, pipe-like vessels result from persistent dilatation, and the headache becomes a steady ache. A phase of muscle contraction, with pain, is believed to follow.

Migraine often begins in childhood; about half of migraine patients report their initial attack before the age of 15 years. Characteristically, the headache occurs in episodes associated with gastrointestinal or visual symptoms (nausea, vomiting, scintillating scotomas, photophobia, hemianopsia, blurred vision).

Prevention

Methysergide maleate (Sansert) may be effective in preventing vascular headache. The average daily dose is 4–8 mg, preferably 2 mg with each meal. This drug is contraindicated in pregnancy, peripheral vascular disease, and arteriosclerosis. Retroperitoneal fibrosis may occur with this drug.

The use of sedatives, tranquilizers, antidepressants, and psychotherapy may help reduce the frequency of attacks.

Treatment

A. Treatment of Acute Attack:

1. Ergotamine tartrate (Gynergen), 0.25–0.5 mg IM, will relieve headache within an hour in most cases. Administer the drug as early in the attack as possible. Do not repeat more often than once weekly. Oral or sublingual administration is less effective, and if the patient vomits it is impossible to know how much of the drug he has absorbed. The dosage is 4–5 mg sublingually or orally; continue with 2 mg every hour until headache has disappeared or until a total of 11 mg has been administered.

Toxicity: Do not administer ergotamine to patients in septic or infectious states or who have peripheral vascular or arteriosclerotic heart disease, or to pregnant women. A few patients complain of numbness and tingling of extremities and some muscle pains and tension.

2. Dihydroergotamine (DHE 45), in doses of 1 mg IM or IV, may be substituted for ergotamine tartrate. Repeat in 1 hour if necessary.

3. Ergotamine with caffeine (Cafergot) or atropine is sometimes more effective by the oral route alone and requires a smaller total dose. It is available as suppositories for rectal use if vomiting prevents oral administration.

4. Pressure on the external carotid artery or one of its branches early in the attack may abolish pain. Oxygen, 100%, by nasal mask may relieve the acute attack.

B. General Measures: Until the drug begins to relieve headache, have the patient at rest in a chair. After headache has been relieved, he should rest in bed for at least 2 hours in a quiet, darkened room without food or drink. This will promote relaxation and is necessary to prevent another attack from occurring immediately.

C. Aborting an Attack: When the patient feels an attack of migraine coming on he should seek relaxation and rest in bed in a quiet, darkened room. The following drugs may help: Pentobarbital, 0.1 gm orally; ergotamine tartrate (Gynergen), 3–4 mg sublingually; or even aspirin, with or without codeine. An ergotamine inhaler may be effective.

Anthony M, Lance JW: Monoamine oxidase inhibition in the treatment of migraine. Arch Neurol 21:263, 1969.

Aring CD: The migrainous scintillating scotoma. JAMA 220:519, 1972.

Friedman AP: The migraine syndrome. Bull New York Acad Med 44:45, 1968.

Friedman AP & others: How should migraine be prevented and relieved? Hosp Med 9:92, 1973.

Hachinski VC, Porchawka J, Steele JC: Visual symptoms in the migraine symptom. Neurology 23:570, 1973.

Whitty CWM, Hockaday JM: Migraine: A follow-up study of 92 patients. Brit MJ 1:735, 1968.

CLUSTER HEADACHES
(Histaminic [Horton's] Cephalalgia)

"Histaminic cephalalgia" (or cluster headaches) is characterized by a sudden onset of severe unilateral pain. The pain is of short duration and subsides abruptly but may recur several times daily. Associated signs include redness of the eye, lacrimation, rhinorrhea or stuffiness of the nostril, swelling of the temporal vessels on the affected side, and dilatation of the vessels of the pain area. The headache involves the orbital area, frequently radiating to the temple, nose, upper jaw, and neck. Typical attacks can be induced by injection of small quantities of histamine diphosphate. Attacks occur most frequently during sleep.

Treatment

Methysergide maleate (UML-491, Sansert) may be effective in preventing vascular headache. The average daily dose is 4–8 mg, preferably 2 mg with each meal. This drug is contraindicated in pregnancy, peripheral vascular disease, and arteriosclerosis.

Although Horton initially recommended "desensitization" to histamine, these headaches are now treated as migraine variants. Because of the short duration of individual attacks and frequent spontaneous long remissions, evaluation of therapy is difficult.

Duvoisin R: The cluster headache. JAMA 222:1403, 1972.

Graham JR: Cluster headache. Headache 11:175, 1972.

Nelson RF: Cluster migraine: An unrecognized common entity. Canad MAJ 103:1026, 1970.

Robinson BW: Histaminic cephalgia. Medicine 37:161, 1958.

Stowell A: Physiologic mechanism and treatment of histaminic or petrosal neuralgia. Headache 9:187, 1970.

CONVULSIVE DISORDERS
(EPILEPSY)

HEADACHES DUE TO MUSCULOSKELETAL INVOLVEMENT

Muscle contraction or spasm may be caused by disease of the muscle or adjacent structures or may be associated with excessive fatigue or emotional tension. The muscles attached to the occiput are most frequently involved and cause the characteristic "occipital" headache. There may also be a feeling of pressure or tightness or a band-like constriction around the head associated with emotional tension.

Tension headaches are by far the most commonly encountered of all types. However, since emotionally disturbed patients may have headaches due to other causes, a complete and adequate history and examination is always necessary.

Tension headaches seem to have no precise localization and usually do not conform to the distribution of cranial or peripheral nerves or roots. The headache is described as being dull, drawing, pressing, burning, or vague in character, and is usually occipital and supraorbital. Medications, including potent analgesics, may not give complete relief. Exacerbation of complaints and association with anxiety, worry, or other emotional upsets is not always obvious to the patient.

Treatment

Muscle spasm due to organic disease and bone or joint pain may be relieved by appropriate physical therapeutic measures. Analgesics are usually also of value. Specific therapy should be directed at the underlying disease.

For muscle tension headache rest, relaxation, and freedom from emotional stress are of primary importance. Heat to the involved muscles by means of hot towels, a heating pad, or a warm bath will help relieve the discomfort. Gentle massage of the muscles will usually also be of benefit. Drugs may be of value in acute cases, but prolonged use should be avoided. Phenobarbital, 15–30 mg 4 times daily, will temporarily relieve many headaches due to "nervous tension." Aspirin or sedatives plus tranquilizers may also be of benefit.

Dutton CB, Riley LH: Cervical migraine. Am J Med 47:141, 1969.
Farbman AA: Neck sprain: Associated factors. JAMA 223: 1010, 1973.
Rooke ED: Benign exertional headache. M Clin North America 52:801, 1968.

Essentials of Diagnosis

- Abrupt onset of paroxysmal, transitory, recurrent alterations of brain function, usually accompanied by alterations in consciousness.
- Signs may vary from behavioral abnormalities to continuous prolonged motor convulsions.
- Primary brain disorder may be present.
- Family history of epilepsy may be present.

General Considerations

Convulsive disorders are characterized by abrupt transient symptoms of a motor, sensory, psychic, or autonomic nature, frequently associated with changes in consciousness. These changes are believed to be secondary to sudden transient alterations in brain function associated with excessive rapid electric discharges in the gray matter. Seizures are more apt to occur in a patient with organic brain disease than in one with a normal CNS. Symptomatic epilepsy may be produced by a variety of pathologic states and intoxications (eg, brain tumor, cerebrovascular accidents, head trauma, intracranial infections, uremia, hypoglycemia, hypocalcemia, and overhydration). In idiopathic epilepsy, morphologic changes may not be demonstrable. Individuals may inherit a convulsive tendency. The onset of idiopathic epilepsy is usually before the age of 30 years. Later age of onset suggests organic disease.

Some seizures tend to occur during sleep or following physical stimulation (eg, light or sound). In some patients emotional disturbances play a significant "trigger" role.

Clinical Findings

A. Classification of Seizures:

1. Grand mal (major epilepsy)—(Grand mal and petit mal may coexist.) A typical aura may herald a major seizure; it may be stereotyped for an individual, eg, an "odd" sensation in the epigastrium, memory phenomena, or a particular unpleasant taste or smell. The aura may consist of a motor phenomenon (eg, spasm of a limb, turning of the head and eyes) or a sensory aberration (eg, numbness). The patient may remember or actually "see" a scene or event from his past.

Consciousness is apt to be lost soon after the appearance of the aura; the subject may fall to the floor and emit a cry. The skeletal muscles then undergo strong tonic contractions; dyspnea and cyanosis may be present. Severe generalized clonic convulsive movements of the body begin a few seconds later, usually becoming less frequent as the attack persists. Frothing at the mouth, loss of bladder and bowel control, tongue biting, bruises, and contusions commonly occur at this time. A period of flaccid coma follows

Table 16—1. International classification of epileptic seizures.*

I. Partial seizures (seizures beginning locally):
  A. Partial seizures with elementary symptomatology (generally without impairment of consciousness):
    1. With motor symptoms (includes jacksonian seizures).
    2. With special sensory or somatosensory symptoms.
    3. With autonomic symptoms.
    4. Compound forms.
  B. Partial seizures with complex symptomatology (generally with impairment of consciousness) (temporal lobe or psychomotor seizures):
    1. With impairment of consciousness only.
    2. With cognitive symptomatology.
    3. With affective symptomatology.
    4. With "psychosensory" symptomatology.
    5. With "psychomotor" symptomatology (automatisms).
    6. Compound forms.
  C. Partial seizures secondarily generalized.
II. Generalized seizures (bilaterally symmetric and without local onset):
    1. Absences (petit mal).
    2. Bilateral massive epileptic myoclonus.
    3. Infantile spasms.
    4. Clonic seizures.
    5. Tonic seizures.
    6. Tonic-clonic seizures (grand mal).
    7. Atonic seizures.
    8. Akinetic seizures.
III. Unilateral seizures (or predominantly).
IV. Unclassified epileptic seizures (due to incomplete data).

*Abstracted from Gastaut H: Clinical and electroencephalographical classification of epileptic seizures. Epilepsia 11:102, 1970.

Table 16—2. International classification of the epilepsies.*

I. Generalized epilepsies:
  1. Primary generalized epilepsies (includes petit mal and grand mal seizures).
  2. Secondary generalized epilepsies.
  3. Undetermined generalized epilepsies.
II. Partial (focal, local) epilepsies (includes jacksonian, temporal lobe, and psychomotor seizures).
III. Unclassifiable epilepsies.

*Abstracted from Merlis JK: Proposal for an international classification of the epilepsies. Epilepsia 11:114, 1970.

during which the pupils may be dilated, corneal and deep reflexes absent, and the Babinski reflex positive. The patient may remain confused and disoriented during the initial stage of recovery. A period of deep sleep often follows. Upon awakening, the patient may complain of sore muscles.

2. Petit mal (minor epilepsy)—(Petit mal and grand mal may coexist.) The so-called "petit mal triad" includes myoclonic jerks, akinetic seizures, and brief absences (blank spells) without associated falling and body convulsions. A specific 3/second spike and wave EEG pattern is present.

Petit mal epilepsy is more often encountered in children. There may be momentary or transient loss of consciousness, so fleeting or hidden in ordinary activity that neither the patient nor his associates are aware of it. Classic petit mal is characterized by a sudden vacant expression, cessation of motor activity, and loss of muscle tone. Consciousness and mental and physical activity return abruptly. As many as 100 attacks may occur daily.

3. Jacksonian epilepsy—This type of epilepsy consists of a focal convulsion during which consciousness is often retained. The seizure may be motor, sensory, or autonomic in type. The seizure commonly starts in part of a limb (eg, thumb or great toe) or face (eg, at the angle of the mouth) as a localized clonic spasm, and spreads in a more or less orderly fashion. For example, a seizure may pass from the hand along the upper extremity to involve the shoulder, trunk, thigh, and leg muscles.

Loss of consciousness is apt to occur when the seizure spreads to the opposite side and becomes generalized.

The seizure may remain confined to the site of origin, waxing and waning in intensity ("epilepsia partialis continua").

4. Psychomotor seizures—In this category are included most types of attacks which do not conform to the classical criteria of grand mal, jacksonian seizures, or petit mal. Automatisms, patterned movements, apparently purposeful movements, incoherent speech, turning of head and eyes, smacking of the lips, twisting and writhing movements of the extremities, clouding of consciousness, and amnesia commonly occur. Temporal lobe foci (spikes, sharp waves, or combinations of these) are frequently noted in the EEG, and striking accentuation of these abnormalities is often seen during light phases of sleep.

5. Status epilepticus—Recurrent severe seizures with short or no intervals between seizures are frequently of serious import. Patients who remain comatose are apt to become exhausted and hyperthermic, and may die.

6. Febrile convulsions—In the very young, convulsions may be associated with or precipitated by a febrile illness. A febrile convulsion is sometimes the initial convulsion of an epileptic child, and many of these children subsequently develop psychomotor seizures. Febrile convulsions are more common in children with a family history of epilepsy. Nonfebrile con-

Table 16—3. Drugs used in epilepsy.*

Drug	Average Daily Dose	Indications	Toxicity and Precautions
Phenytoin sodium (Dilantin)	0.3—0.6 gm in divided doses	Safest drug for grand mal, some cases of psychomotor epilepsy. May accentuate petit mal.	Gum hypertrophy (dental hygiene); nervousness, rash, ataxia, drowsiness, nystagmus (reduce dosage).
Mephenytoin (Mesantoin)	0.3—0.5 gm in divided doses	Grand mal, some cases of psychomotor epilepsy. Effective when grand mal and petit mal coexist.	Nervousness, ataxia, nystagmus (reduce dosage); pancytopenia (frequent blood counts); exfoliative dermatitis (stop drug if severe skin eruption develops).
Ethotoin (Peganone)	2—3 gm in divided doses	Grand mal.	Dizziness, fatigue, skin rash (decrease dose or discontinue).
Trimethadione (Tridione)	0.3—2 gm in divided doses	Petit mal.	Bone marrow depression, pancytopenia, exfoliative dermatitis (as above); photophobia (usually disappears; dark glasses); nephrosis (frequent urinalysis; discontinue if renal lesion develops).
Paramethadione (Paradione)	0.3—2 gm in divided doses	Petit mal.	Toxic reactions said to be less than with trimethadione. Other remarks as for trimethadione.
Phenacemide (Phenurone)	0.5—5 gm in divided doses	Psychomotor epilepsy.	Hepatitis (liver function tests at onset; follow urinary urobilinogen at regular intervals); benign proteinuria (stop drug; may continue if patient is having marked relief); dermatitis (stop drug); headache and personality changes (stop drug if severe).
Carbamazepine (Tegretol)	0.3—1.2 gm in divided doses	Psychomotor epilepsy, grand mal epilepsy.	Diplopia, transient blurred vision, drowsiness, ataxia; bone marrow depression (frequent blood counts).
Phenobarbital	0.1—0.4 gm in divided doses	One of the safest drugs for all epilepsies, especially as adjunct. May aggravate psychomotor seizures.	Toxic reactions rare. Drowsiness (decrease dosage); dermatitis (stop drug and resume later; if dermatitis recurs, stop drug entirely).
Mephobarbital (Mebaral)	0.2—0.9 gm in divided doses	As for phenobarbital.	As for phenobarbital. Usually offers no advantage over phenobarbital and must be given in twice the dosage.
Metharbital (Gemonil)	0.1—0.8 gm in divided doses	Grand mal. Especially effective in seizures associated with organic brain damage and in infantile myoclonic epilepsy.	Drowsiness (decrease dosage).
Primidone (Mysoline)	0.5—2 gm in divided doses	Grand mal. Useful in conjunction with other drugs.	Drowsiness (decrease dosage); ataxia (decrease dosage or stop drug).
Bromides (potassium or sodium)	3—6 gm in divided doses	All epilepsies, especially as adjuncts. Rarely used now. Effective at times when all else fails.	Psychoses, mental dullness, acneiform rash (stop drug; may resume at lower dose).
Phensuximide (Milontin)	0.5—2.5 gm in divided doses	Petit mal.	Nausea, ataxia, dizziness (reduce dosage or discontinue); hematuria (discontinue).
Methsuximide (Celontin)	1.2 gm in divided doses	Petit mal, psychomotor epilepsy.	Ataxia, drowsiness (decrease dosage or discontinue).
Ethosuximide (Zarontin)	750—1500 mg in divided doses	Petit mal.	Drowsiness, nausea, vomiting (decrease dosage or discontinue).

*Modified and reproduced, with permission, from Chusid JG: *Correlative Neuroanatomy & Functional Neurology,* 15th ed. Lange, 1973.

Table 16–3 (cont'd). Drugs used in epilepsy.

Drug	Average Daily Dose	Indications	Toxicity and Precautions
Acetazolamide (Diamox)	1–3 gm in divided doses†	Grand mal, petit mal.	Drowsiness, paresthesias (reduce dosage).
Chlordiazepoxide (Librium)	15–60 mg in divided doses	Mixed epilepsies. Useful in patients with behavior disorders; also in status epilepticus (by intravenous infusion).	Drowsiness, ataxia (decrease dosage or discontinue).
Diazepam (Valium)	8–30 mg in divided doses		
Meprobamate (Equanil, Miltown)	1.2–2 gm in divided doses	Absence attacks, myoclonic seizures.	Drowsiness (decrease dosage or discontinue).
Dextroamphetamine sulfate (Dexedrine)	20–50 mg in divided doses	Absence and akinetic attacks. Counteracts sleepiness. Useful in narcolepsy.	Anorexia, irritability, insomnia (decrease dosage or discontinue).
Methamphetamine (Desoxyn)	2.5–10 mg in divided doses		

†Begin with 0.25 gm 3 times daily.

vulsions often occur in patients with a history of febrile convulsions.

7. Massive spasms—This type of seizure is most commonly encountered in the first 2 years of life, especially in children with evidence of motor and mental retardation. Sudden strong contraction of most of the body musculature occurs, often resulting in transient doubling up of the body and flexion-adduction of the limbs. A characteristic EEG pattern ("hypsarhythmia") is often present. A favorable response to treatment with corticotropin has been reported for some patients.

B. Laboratory Findings: EEG is the most important test in the study of epilepsy. In some cases provocative measures (eg, hyperventilation, sleep, drugs, photic stimulation) are of diagnostic value.

Skull x-rays, CSF studies, blood glucose and blood calcium determinations, pneumograms, brain scans, and cerebral angiograms may aid in determining the cause of convulsions.

Differential Diagnosis

In syncope there is an associated drop in blood pressure, the muscles are flaccid, there are no convulsive movements initially, and the attack subsides with increased brain blood flow in recumbency.

In hysteria there is usually no loss of consciousness, incontinence, tongue biting, or self-injury. The patient may be resistive, and the "convulsion" is erratic and atypical.

Narcolepsy is characterized by irreversible sleep attacks of brief duration, frequently associated with catalepsy (sudden loss of muscle tone with no loss of consciousness, precipitated by acute emotional disturbances such as fright or laughter).

Complications

Fractures and soft tissue injuries may occur during seizures. Mental and emotional changes, particularly in poorly controlled epileptics, sometimes occur. Behavioral or emotional components may mask an underlying convulsive disorder. Examples are disorientation, hallucinations, excitement, incoherent speech, erratic behavior, automatisms, mental dullness, and irritability.

Treatment

The objective of therapy is complete suppression of symptoms, though in many cases this is not possible. Epileptics may continue to receive anticonvulsant therapy throughout life. However, if seizures are entirely controlled for 3–5 years, the dosage may be slowly reduced (over a period of 1–2 years) and finally withdrawn to ascertain if seizures will recur.

The patient must be acquainted with his disease and encouraged to become a member of local branches of groups interested in the welfare of epileptics, such as the Epilepsy Association of America. Patients may receive information regarding research and treatment from these organizations.

Epileptic patients should avoid hazardous occupations and driving. It is important to maintain a regular program of activity to keep the patient in optimal physical condition but avoiding excessive fatigue. Forbid all alcohol. Treat emotional factors as indicated. Impress upon the patient the absolute necessity of faithful adherence to the drug regimen. An epilepsy identification card should be carried at all times.

Except in status epilepticus, no specific treatment is usually given during an attack except to protect the patient from injury. Anticonvulsant measures (see also

Table 16—3) in the 4 principal types of epilepsy are as follows:

A. Grand Mal: *Caution:* Never withdraw anticonvulsant drugs suddenly.

1. Phenytoin sodium (Dilantin) is the drug of choice. Give 0.1 gm after the evening meal for 3—7 days, increasing dosage by 0.1 gm daily every week until seizures are brought under control. If attacks are severe and frequent, it may be necessary to begin with 0.3 gm daily on the first visit. The average dose is 0.3—0.6 gm daily. After convulsive seizures are controlled, the dosage may be reduced if desired, but the dosage should immediately be raised again if symptoms return. A therapeutic level of serum phenytoin is believed to be 10—20 μg/ml (1—2 mg/100 ml).

2. Phenobarbital—If the patient is on maximum dosage of phenytoin and there is inadequate response, give phenobarbital in addition to phenytoin, increasing dosage as with phenytoin, while maintaining full dosage of phenytoin. Some clinicians prefer to begin with phenobarbital and maintain without phenytoin if possible. In many cases the 2 drugs used in combination are more effective than either drug used alone.

3. Mephenytoin (Mesantoin)—If excessive gum hypertrophy results from the use of phenytoin, mephenytoin may be tried in its place. The dosage is the same. This drug may be effective where grand mal and petit mal coexist. Do not change suddenly to mephenytoin, but gradually substitute for phenytoin. Combinations of both may prove more useful than the individual drugs.

4. Bromides, primidone (Mysoline), mephobarbital (Mebaral), or ethotoin (Peganone) may be tried (Table 16—3).

B. Petit Mal: In very mild petit mal, if attacks are rare, treat only with phenobarbital.

For moderate and severe petit mal, the succinimides (ethosuximide [Zarontin], methsuximide [Celontin], and phensuximide [Milontin]) and the diones (trimethadione [Tridione] and paramethadione [Paradione]) are highly effective. Unfortunately, trimethadione is not an entirely safe drug since it causes bone marrow depression in some patients. *Caution:* Whenever this drug is used, perform a complete blood count once or twice a week for the first month, then every 2 weeks for 2—3 months, and monthly thereafter. Begin with 0.3 gm daily and increase the daily dose by 0.3 gm every 7 days until attacks are controlled. Do not give more than 2 gm daily.

If grand mal seizures occur also, trimethadione may aggravate this tendency; it may therefore be necessary to administer medication for grand mal seizures simultaneously, and in some cases to stop the trimethadione. Paramethadione is said to be less toxic than trimethadione. It is almost as effective as trimethadione in petit mal attacks, and may be effective where other drugs fail. Observe precautions as for trimethadione.

Phenobarbital, acetazolamide (Diamox), or mephobarbital (Mebaral) may prove useful (Table 16—3). Ethosuximide (Zarontin) is very effective in petit mal and is the drug of choice.

C. Status Epilepticus: Amobarbital sodium (Amytal Sodium), 0.5—1 gm IV, may be given. Intravenous phenobarbital sodium, 0.4—0.8 gm, injected slowly, may be used. Paraldehyde, 1—2 ml diluted in a triple volume of saline IV slowly, is an effective alternative. If the convulsion continues, repeat the intravenous dose *very slowly and cautiously,* or give 8—12 ml IM. Phenytoin sodium (Dilantin Sodium) may be injected intravenously at a rate not exceeding 50 mg/minute. A total dosage of 150—500 mg may be required. General anesthesia may be used if all measures fail. Phenytoin sodium, 250—500 mg IM daily, or phenobarbital sodium, 30—60 mg IM 4 times daily (or both), may be required until the patient is able to take medication orally. Diazepam (Valium), 10 mg IV, is effective and may be repeated once or twice as necessary. Hypotension and respiratory depression may occur as side-effects.

D. Psychomotor Epilepsy: Patients must be watched and guarded to prevent injury to themselves or others. Phenytoin sodium (Dilantin), with or without phenobarbital, as for grand mal epilepsy, is the treatment of choice. Phenacemide (Phenurone) is also effective. Give initially 0.5 gm 3 times daily and increase (until symptoms are controlled) up to 5 gm daily in 3—5 equal doses. Mephenytoin (Mesantoin), mephobarbital (Mebaral), primidone (Mysoline), acetazolamide (Diamox), and methsuximide (Celontin), alone or in combination with other drugs, are frequently useful. Carbamazepine (Tegretol), 200 mg 3—4 times daily, is effective.

Prognosis

In symptomatic epilepsy due to identifiable lesions, the outcome varies with the underlying disease. In idiopathic epilepsy, skillful use of anticonvulsant drugs causes significant improvement in the great majority of cases.

Borofsky LG, Louis S, Kutt H: Diphenylhydantoin in children. Neurology 23:967, 1973.

Carter S, Gold A: Convulsions in children. New England J Med 278:315, 1968.

Cereghino JJ & others: Carbamazepine for epilepsy: A controlled prospective evaluation. Neurology 24:401, 1974.

Karnes WE: Medical treatment for convulsive disorders. M Clin North America 52:959, 1968.

Kutt H, Penry JK: Usefulness of blood levels of antiepileptic drugs. Arch Neurol 31:283, 1974.

Millichap GE: Drug treatment of convulsive disorders. New England J Med 286:464, 1972.

Nicol CF, Tutton JC, Smith BH: Parenteral diazepam in status epilepticus. Neurology 19:332, 1969.

Robb P: Epilepsy: A review of basic and clinical research. NINDB Monograph No. 1, 1965.

Symposium on post-traumatic epilepsy. Epilepsia 11:1, 1970.

Troupin AS, Green JR, Levy RH: Carbamazepine as an anticonvulsant: A pilot study. Neurology 24:863, 1974.

CONGENITAL CNS DEFECTS

SYRINGOMYELIA

Essentials of Diagnosis

- Loss of pain and temperature sense but preservation of other sensory function (painless burning or injury to hands).
- Weakness, hyporeflexia or areflexia, wasting of muscles at level of spinal cord involvement (usually upper limbs and hands).
- Hyperreflexia and spasticity at lower levels.

General Considerations

Syringomyelia is a disease of the spinal cord and brain stem of unknown cause, associated with gliosis and cavitation of the spinal cord and brain stem. The onset of symptoms is usually in the 3rd or 4th decade. Although the etiology is not known, a developmental defect has been inferred because other congenital defects are usually present also. A coincidence of syringomyelia and intramedullary tumors (gliomas, hemangiomas) has also been noted.

Clinical Findings

The characteristic clinical picture is that of muscular wasting and weakness, dissociation and loss of the pain-temperature sense, and signs of injury to the long tracts.

A. Symptoms and Signs: The most common form is cervical syringomyelia involving the cervical spinal cord. Loss of pain and temperature sensibility in the cervical and thoracic dermatomes in shawl-like distribution is characteristic. The following are variably present: painless burns of the fingers or forearms, atrophy of the small muscles of the hands (usually present), weakness and atrophy of the shoulder girdle muscles, Horner's syndrome, nystagmus, vasomotor and trophic changes of the upper extremities, absence of deep reflexes of the upper extremities, Charcot joints in affected limbs, spasticity and ataxia of the lower extremities, and neurogenic bladder.

Involvement of the lumbosacral spinal cord may also occur, with weakness and atrophy of the lower extremities and pelvic girdle, dissociated sensory loss in the lumbosacral area, bladder paralysis, and vasomotor and trophic disturbances of the lower extremities.

When the medulla oblongata of the brain stem is involved, the process may be referred to as syringobulbia. This is characterized by atrophy and fibrillation of the tongue, loss of pain and temperature sensibility in the face, and nystagmus. Dysphonia and respiratory stridor may occur.

B. Laboratory Findings: Myelography discloses the presence in many cases of partial or complete block in the zone of the syringomyelia. A characteristic deformity of the contrast column may be noted on the myelogram.

Differential Diagnosis

Spinal cord tumor gives a characteristic myelographic deformity, and is more apt to be associated with complete subarachnoid spinal block.

In multiple sclerosis the symptoms are intermittent and there are usually no associated trophic changes or scoliosis and no dissociation or loss of pain and temperature sensibility.

Amyotrophic lateral sclerosis is characterized by symmetric, widespread muscle wasting with no sensory loss, and fasciculations of muscle. In tabes dorsalis, serology is usually positive. Argyll Robertson pupils may be present, and the areas of cutaneous sensory deficit are smaller.

Platybasia and cervical spine anomalies show characteristic skull and cervical spine x-rays and characteristic myelograms.

Treatment

The treatment varies with the degree of clinical involvement and evidence of block on myelography. Laminectomy and decompression may be required, with needle aspiration or myelotomy through the posterior median fissure of the spinal cord in properly selected cases. Roentgen therapy of the affected area of the spinal cord has also been recommended, but the effects are poor.

Prognosis

Syringomyelia is slowly progressive over a period of many years. Severe incapacity may occur because of paralysis, muscular atrophies, and sensory defects. In spinal cases, intercurrent infections, especially of the bladder, commonly occur. In syringobulbia, death may occur in several months because of the destruction of vital medullary nuclei.

Ball MJ, Dayan AD: Pathogenesis of syringomyelia. Lancet 2:799, 1972.

Di Chiro G & others: Computerized axial tomography in syringomyelia. New England J Med 292:13, 1975.

McIlroy WJ, Richardson JC: Syringomyelia: A clinical review of 75 cases. Canad MAJ 93:731, 1965.

McLean DR & others: Post-traumatic syringomyelia. J Neurosurg 39:485, 1973.

CERVICAL RIB (NAFFZIGER'S) SYNDROME
(Scalenus Anticus Syndrome; Thoracic Outlet Syndrome)

The brachial plexus and subclavian artery may be compressed in the neck by a rudimentary cervical rib, fibrous band, first thoracic rib, or tight scalene muscle, giving rise to sensory, motor, or vascular symptoms in one or both upper extremities. The onset of symptoms has been related by some to the loss of tone in shoulder girdle muscles with age or excessive trauma to these parts incurred by lifting or straining.

Clinical Findings

Cervical ribs, rudimentary or fully developed, are relatively common although frequently asymptomatic. Although they are often bilateral, cervical ribs may give rise to unilateral complaints. Prominence of the lower neck above the clavicle on one or both sides may be obvious on inspection. Pressure in this region will give rise to local pain as well as pain referred to the hand and arm. Pain and paresthesia, particularly in the ulnar portion of the hand and forearm, most commonly occur. Impaired perception of pain and light touch in the hand or forearm, and muscular weakness of small hand muscles, may also be present. Coldness and blueness of the hand and diminished pulsation in the radial and ulnar arteries may be noted. Horner's syndrome, resulting from damage to cervical sympathetics, has occurred. Adson's test or maneuver is usually positive on the affected side. The patient, seated with hands resting on thighs, takes a rapid deep inspiration, holds his breath, hyperextends his neck, and turns his head as far as possible first to one side and then the other. Obliteration of the pulse on one side is considered a positive test.

Treatment & Prognosis

The clinical course is variable. Frequent remissions or slow progression occur. Temporary relief may be obtained by wearing a sling support on the affected extremity. Rest in bed, traction on the neck, and the use of pillows to support the shoulders are also helpful. Surgical removal of cervical ribs, division of fibrous bands, or section of the scalenus anticus muscles may give permanent relief.

Frankel SA, Hirata I Jr: The scalenus anticus syndrome and competitive swimming. JAMA 215:1796, 1971.

Moore M Jr: Scalenus anticus syndrome. South MJ 59:954, 1966.

Schlesinger EB: The thoracic outlet syndrome from a neurosurgical point of view. Clin Orthop 51:49, 1967.

Urschel HC, Razzuk MA: Management of the thoracic outlet syndrome. New England J Med 286:1140, 1972.

VASCULAR DISEASES OF THE CNS

CEREBROVASCULAR ACCIDENTS
(Strokes)

Essentials of Diagnosis

- Sudden onset of neurologic complaints varying from focal motor or hypesthesia and speech defects to profound coma.
- May be associated with vomiting, convulsions, or headaches.
- Nuchal rigidity frequently found.

General Considerations

Cerebrovascular accident or stroke is a focal neurologic disorder due to a pathologic process in a blood vessel. In most cases the onset is abrupt and evolution rapid, and symptoms reach a peak within seconds, minutes, or hours. Partial or complete recovery may occur over a period of hours to months.

Three basic processes account for most cerebrovascular accidents: thrombosis, embolism, and hemorrhage. Other infrequent causes include recurrent ischemic attacks, hypertensive encephalopathy, migrainous hemiplegia, and syncope.

Cerebrovascular accident is uncommon in persons under 40 years of age. The most frequent predisposing illnesses in cerebral thrombosis are cerebral arteriosclerosis, syphilis and other infections, dehydration, and trauma. Cerebral embolism may consist of small pieces of blood clot, tumor, or fat, or clumps of bacteria. Cerebral hemorrhage is usually caused by rupture of an arteriosclerotic cerebral vessel. Subarachnoid hemorrhage is usually due to rupture of a congenitally weak blood vessel or aneurysm.

Occlusion of a cerebral artery by thrombosis or embolism results in a cerebral infarction with its associated clinical effects. Other conditions may on occasion also produce cerebral infarction and thus may be confused with cerebral thrombosis or embolism. These include cerebral venous thrombosis, cerebral arteritis, systemic hypotension, reactions to cerebral angiography, and transient cerebral ischemia.

Transient cerebral ischemia may also occur without producing a cerebral infarction. Premonitory recurrent focal cerebral ischemic attacks may occur and are apt to be in a repetitive pattern in a given case. Attacks may last for 10 seconds to 1 hour, but the average duration is 2—10 minutes. As many as several hundred such attacks may occur.

Narrowing of the extracranial arteries (particularly the internal carotid artery at its origin in the neck and, in some cases, the intrathoracic arteries) by arteriosclerotic patches has been incriminated in a significant number of cases of transient cerebral ischemias and infarction.

Clinical Findings

A. **Early Symptoms and Signs:** Variable degrees and types occur. The onset may be violent, with the patient falling to the ground and lying inert like a person in deep sleep, with flushed face, stertorous or Cheyne-Stokes respirations, full and slow pulse, and one arm and leg usually flaccid. Death may occur in a few hours or days. Lesser grades of stroke may consist of slight derangement of speech, thought, motion, sensation, or vision. Consciousness need not be altered. Symptoms may last seconds to minutes or longer, and may persist indefinitely. Some degree of recovery is usual.

Premonitory symptoms may include headache, dizziness, drowsiness, and mental confusion. Focal premonitory symptoms are more likely to occur with thrombosis.

Generalized neurologic signs are most common with cerebral hemorrhage and include fever, headache, vomiting, convulsions, and coma. Nuchal rigidity is frequent with subarachnoid hemorrhage or intracerebral hemorrhage. Mental changes are commonly noted in the period following a stroke and may include confusion, disorientation, and memory defects. Specific focal signs and symptoms are apt to be associated with disorders of particular arteries:

1. Middle cerebral artery—Contralateral monoparesis or hemiparesis, numbness, tingling; dysphasia, homonymous hemianopsia, scintillating scotomas.

2. Anterior cerebral artery—Weakness or numbness of the opposite leg; reflex incontinence.

3. Posterior cerebral artery—Hemianopsia, scintillating scotomas, possibly blindness.

4. Internal carotid artery—Contralateral weakness, numbness, or dysphagia; mental confusion, poor memory, motor aphasia and personality changes; transient blindness or amblyopia, and decreased central retinal artery pressure (by ophthalmodynamometry) on the involved side.

5. Vertebral and basilar arteries—Dizziness; monoparesis, hemiparesis, or quadriparesis; bilateral numbness, staggering gait, ataxia, diplopia, dysphagia, dysarthria, blindness, deafness, confusion, or loss of memory and consciousness.

6. Great vessels of aortic arch—Diminished or absent pulsation in the common carotid, intermittent claudication, localized bruit and blood pressure differences in the 2 arms.

7. Subclavian and innominate artery—Occlusion of these vessels (subclavian steal syndrome) may cause collateral vertebral artery circulation on the involved side, resulting in retrograde flow and reduced blood supply to the brain, with dizzy spells and other cerebral symptoms.

B. Late Symptoms and Signs: usually resembling the acute manifestations and related to the location and degree of brain infarction or hemorrhage. Recovery is sometimes remarkably complete, so that altered brain function may be hardly demonstrable even with special tests (EEG, psychometrics, pneumoencephalography, etc). Generally, however, patients have lesser degrees of their initial defects (eg, hemiparesis, numbness, aphasia, hemianopsia, impaired mentation). Paralyzed limbs and parts in this later stage usually show signs of upper motor neuron disease: spastic weak muscles with little muscle atrophy, hyperactive deep reflexes, diminished or absent superficial reflexes, and pathologic reflexes such as a Babinski sign. The patient may remain disoriented or comatose for prolonged periods. Death is often due to pneumonia.

C. Laboratory Findings: Careful lumbar puncture will reveal bloody CSF, often under increased pressure, in cerebral or subarachnoid hemorrhage.

D. X-Ray Findings: Cerebral angiography is essential for the diagnosis of aneurysms and vascular malformations, and may show narrowing, occlusion, or other abnormality of extracranial as well as intracranial vessels. Skull x-rays may show a displaced pineal gland, or calcification within the vascular malformation or aneurysm. Arteriography should usually consist of a series of studies which include all 4 arteries to the brain. An aortic arch study may be done first, usually by means of a catheter inserted into the arch through the right axillary or brachial artery or through one of the femoral arteries, usually using the percutaneous method of catheterization.

E. Special Studies: The EEG is abnormal in most major cerebrovascular accidents and may be used serially to help follow the clinical course. ECG may establish the presence of "silent" recent myocardial infarct, which is a contributing factor in certain cerebral infarctions. Serial brain scans may show increased uptake in affected areas.

Differential Diagnosis

In brain tumor there is a progression of clinical findings, elevated CSF pressure and protein, and papilledema. Focal neurologic signs are common.

Patients with subdural hematoma may give a history of head trauma, and there may be visible evidence of head injury, a shift of the pineal gland on skull x-ray, and a characteristic angiogram.

Meningitis and encephalitis are differentiated on the basis of CSF changes (clouding; increased cells, protein, pressure; positive culture).

Hypertensive encephalopathy is associated with elevated blood pressure, and the episodes are frequently transient.

Multiple sclerosis shows diffuse neurologic findings, and the clinical course is characterized by remission and then progression.

Treatment

A. Acute Stage or Onset:

1. General measures—Place the patient at complete bed rest and handle him carefully to avoid injury. If he is agitated, give tranquilizers or sedatives as necessary. If he is unconscious or unable to swallow, maintain nutrition with tube feedings or by parenteral means; do not attempt to give feedings by mouth. Catheterization may be necessary if spontaneous voiding does not occur.

2. Lumbar puncture—If hemorrhage has occurred, lumbar puncture should be performed very cautiously.

3. Anticoagulant therapy—Maintenance on anticoagulant therapy (see Chapter 8) has been advocated for treatment and prevention of cerebral thrombosis or insufficiency of the carotid or vertebral-basilar system. However, recent studies by several groups suggest that anticoagulant therapy helps only a few individuals in any large series of patients with the clinical picture of stroke. The evidence is most promising for transient cerebral ischemia. The risk of hemorrhage, particularly in hypertensive patients, is great.

4. Surgery—Narrowing of the extracranial arteries (eg, internal carotid) as shown on angiography may be an indication for surgical correction. Surgery may restore a more normal blood flow to the brain, and improvement may result if the collateral flow has not

Table 16—4. Diagnosis of cerebrovascular disorders.*

	Intracerebral Hemorrhage	Cerebral Thrombosis	Cerebral Embolism	Subarachnoid Hemorrhage	Vascular Malformation and Intracranial Bleeding
Onset	Generally during activity. Severe headache (if patient is able to report findings).	Prodromal episode of dizziness, aphasia, etc, often with improvement between attacks. Unrelated to activity.	Onset usually within seconds or minutes. No headache. Usually no prodrome. Unrelated to activity.	Sudden onset of severe headache unrelated to activity.	Sudden "stroke" in young patient. No headache. Unrelated to activity.
Course	Rapid hemiplegia and other phenomena over minutes to 1 hour.	Gradual progression over minutes to hours. Rapid improvement at times.	Rapid improvement may occur.	Variable; apt to be at worst in initial few days after onset.	Most critical period is usually in early stages.
History and related disorders	Suspect diagnosis especially if other hemorrhagic manifestations are present and in acute leukemia, aplastic anemia, thrombocytopenic purpura, and cirrhosis of the liver.	Evidence of arteriosclerosis, especially coronary, peripheral vessels, aorta. Associated disorders: diabetes mellitus, xanthomatosis.	Evidence of recent emboli: (1) other organs (spleen, kidneys, lungs), extremities, intestines; (2) several regions of brain in different cerebrovascular areas.	History of recurrent stiff neck, headaches, subarachnoid bleeding.	History of repeated subarachnoid hemorrhages, epilepsy.
Sensorium	Rapid progression to coma.	Relative preservation of consciousness.	Relative preservation of consciousness.	Relatively brief disturbance of consciousness.	Relatively brief disturbance of consciousness.
Neurologic examination	Focal neurologic signs or special arterial syndromes; nuchal rigidity.	Focal neurologic signs or special arterial syndromes.	Focal neurologic signs or special arterial syndromes.	Focal neurologic signs frequently absent; nuchal rigidity, positive Kernig and Brudzinski signs.	Focal neurologic signs; cranial bruit.
Special findings	Hypertensive retinopathy, cardiac hypertrophy, and other evidences of hypertensive cerebrovascular disease may be present.	Evidence of arteriosclerotic cardiovascular disease frequently present.	Cardiac arrhythmias or infarction (source of emboli usually in the heart).	Subhyaloid (preretinal) hemorrhages.	Subhyaloid (preretinal) hemorrhages and retinal angioma.
Blood pressure	Arterial hypertension.	Arterial hypertension frequent.	Normotensive.	Arterial hypertension frequent.	Normotensive.
CSF	Grossly bloody.	Clear.	Clear.	Grossly bloody.	Grossly bloody.
Skull x-ray	Shift of pineal to opposite side.	Calcification of internal carotid artery siphon visible; shift of pineal to opposite side may occur.	Pineal apt to show little if any displacement.	Partial calcification of walls of aneurysm sometimes noted.	Characteristic calcifications in skull x-rays may be present.
Cerebral angiography	Hemorrhagic area seen as avascular zone surrounded by stretched and displaced arteries and veins.	Arterial obstruction or narrowing of circle of Willis (internal carotid, etc).	Arterial obstruction of circle of Willis branches (internal carotid, etc).	Typical aneurysmal pattern in circle of Willis arteries (internal carotid, middle cerebral, anterior cerebral, etc).	Characteristic pattern showing cerebral arteriovenous malformation.
Brain scan	May show increased uptake in affected cerebral area. Most marked in 2—3 weeks, with diminution or clearing thereafter.			Apt to be normal.	Increased uptake may be seen in area of arteriovenous malformation.
Echoencephalography	May show shift of midline toward opposite side in those patients with a cerebral lesion acting as a mass.				

*Reproduced, with permission, from Chusid JG: *Correlative Neuroanatomy & Functional Neurology,* 15th ed. Lange, 1973.

been adequate. Surgery may provide some future protection to the brain from damage due to a progression of the arterial disease with further reduction of total blood flow, or from emboli to the brain originating in the areas of stenosis. Stenoses that narrow the lumen less than 50% are not significant and should be left alone; "prophylactic" surgery on stenotic vessels in patients with no CNS symptoms is seldom indicated.

Emergency surgery for acute stroke has been disappointing, and fatal postoperative bleeding into an area of infarcted brain is not infrequent. In most cases, particularly if the patient is in coma or semi-coma, arterial studies and surgery should probably be deferred until the condition has stabilized and the collateral circulation has become better established. Patients with intermittent symptoms or constant mild neurologic defects—or those who have recovered well from a major vascular insult—should be evaluated for surgery. Patients with complete hemiplegia who show no signs of recovery will probably not be benefited by an operation to improve the blood supply to the damaged brain. If the occlusion of the internal carotid artery is complete and is more than a few hours old, the vessel will probably be thrombosed beyond the cervical segment of the internal carotid artery. Surgery to reestablish flow through this vessel is often unsuccessful.

Although the occlusive lesions of the larger intrathoracic vessels lend themselves best to surgical therapy, the results are also quite satisfactory in the surgical treatment of the stenotic lesions of the proximal internal carotid artery. Stenosis of the smaller vertebral artery may also be treated successfully, but if carotid disease also exists it should be treated in preference to the vertebral stenosis. Surgery for complete occlusion of the internal carotid or vertebral arteries or for significant and persistent CNS changes yields poor results in most cases.

B. Stage of Recovery and Convalescence: The rehabilitation of the patient with a stroke should be started early and should be intensive. The rehabilitation goals are: (1) achievement of mobility and ambulation, (2) achievement of self-care, (3) psychosocial adjustment to disability, and (4) prevention of secondary disability. Since stroke patients have various disabilities, the rehabilitation program has to be related to the functional loss. Rehabilitation of patients whose only disability is hemiplegia is relatively simple. The program can be divided into 4 phases: bed phase, standing phase, stair-climbing phase, and cane-walking phase.

1. Bed Phase—The bed phase starts on the second or third day after onset or as soon as the patient is conscious. The patient's bed should be of chair height and should have side rails and an overhead trapeze mechanism.

a. Exercises—Start with 10 minutes of exercise every 4 hours and increase gradually.

(1) With the uninvolved arm and leg, turn from back to side to abdomen and return.

(2) With the uninvolved hand on the trapeze, pull to a sitting position.

(3) Move sideways, upward, and downward in bed.

(4) Sit up on the edge of the bed, legs dangling; move along the edge of the bed with the aid of the good arm and leg.

b. Self-care—Done with the uninvolved hand.

(1) Toilet activities—Wash face and hands, comb hair, shave.

(2) Feeding activities—At first in bed with the back rolled up; later, sitting on the edge of the bed.

2. Standing phase—This phase starts 3–5 days after the beginning of the bed phase.

a. Exercise—The patient is placed in an armchair with his unaffected side next to the foot of the bed, the vertical bar of the overhead frame in reach of his uninvolved hand, and the paralyzed arm in a sling. Each of the following exercises is done 10 times every 4 hours, holding on with the uninvolved hand:

(1) Rise to a standing position using the uninvolved leg. Sit back.

(2) Stand up. Perform a slight knee bend and straighten up. Repeat with gradually deeper knee bends. Sit down.

(3) Stand up. Go up on toes, come back down. Sit down.

b. Self-care—Use the uninvolved hand.

(1) Toilet activities—Complete bath in bed.

(2) Dressing activities—Dress and undress except for shoes.

3. Stair-climbing phase—The stair-climbing phase starts 2–10 days after the beginning of the standing phase.

a. Exercise—The patient is placed in a chair facing the foot of a flight of stairs, his uninvolved arm next to the banister. The paralyzed arm is in a sling, and the paralyzed leg is braced if necessary.

(1) Pull to a standing position, holding to the banister; step up one step with the uninvolved leg, and then pull the paralyzed leg up to the same step. Continue for several steps.

(2) Step backward and down with the paralyzed leg and put the uninvolved leg down next to it.

b. Self-care—Complete toilet, feeding, and dressing activities should be possible by this time.

c. Bracing—

(1) If the patient has a foot drop during stair climbing, he should wear a short-leg brace with a 90° posterior stop at the ankle.

(2) If the patient shows evidence of inversion of the foot, he should have a short-leg brace with a T-strap.

(3) If the paralyzed leg remains completely flail, a long-leg brace is needed.

4. Cane-walking phase—This phase starts as soon as the patient is able to walk up and down a whole flight of stairs without tiring. A cane is held with the uninvolved hand.

a. Slow gait—(For fearful patients or patients with poor balance.) Move the cane forward, place the uninvolved foot next to the cane, and move the paralyzed foot next to it.

b. Fast gait—Standing on the uninvolved leg, move the cane and the paralyzed leg forward simultaneously and put weight on them. Swing the uninvolved leg through in front of the cane and the paralyzed leg and put weight on it. Continue in this fashion.

C. Special Problems in Hemiplegic Patients:

1. Care of the paralyzed upper extremity—In most cases no useful function returns to the paralyzed upper extremity. The sling may be discarded when the shoulder muscles become spastic. With his uninvolved hand, the patient should move the paralyzed fingers, wrist, and elbow through the full range of motion twice a day. In order to move the paralyzed shoulder through the full range of motion, the patient may use an overhead pulley by means of which the paralyzed arm, tied at the wrist, can be pulled up with the uninvolved arm. Ninety percent of hemiplegics develop a painful shoulder due to trauma during initial care. Careful positioning in bed and the arm sling may prevent injury. Treatment of painful shoulder consists of analgesics, immobilization, and gentle range of motion exercises.

If only partial function returns to the paralyzed extremity, the patient should use it only to the extent to which it is helpful or expedient.

2. Treatment of aphasia—If aphasia occurs, speech therapy (daily in half-hour periods) should be started as soon as possible. If sensory or receptive aphasia is present, the above program may be rendered extremely difficult since it is based on the ability of the patient to understand what is required of him.

3. Care of hemianopsia—(A minor problem.) If hemianopsia is present, the patient should be trained to turn his head to the hemianopsic side in order to bring his visual field in front of him.

4. Care of sphincters—Some hemiplegics are incontinent in the early phase. An indwelling catheter is rarely necessary. The patient should be reminded to empty his bladder voluntarily at hourly intervals. These intervals can be gradually increased.

5. Organic brain syndrome—Impaired mentation is an obstacle to the rehabilitation program. The confusion may be present at one time and absent at another, and advantage should be taken of the patient's lucid periods. The organic brain syndrome occurs more often in patients who have had several strokes. The patient's mental state improves considerably during an active rehabilitation program.

6. Medications—All CNS depressing drugs, even in small doses, may have a detrimental effect on the stroke patient. They may cause or aggravate confusion, aphasia, lack of balance, and incontinence. If used as hypotensive or anticonvulsive agents, they should be replaced if possible by nondepressive drugs (eg, chlorothiazide instead of reserpine). On the other hand, CNS stimulating drugs can help improve function in the confused and depressed patient. Dextroamphetamine (one long-acting dose daily, 10–15 mg) is particularly useful.

Prognosis

In cerebral thrombosis, the outcome is determined to a great extent by the location and extent of the infarct as well as the general condition of the patient. The greater the delay in improvement, the poorer the prognosis.

In cerebral embolism, the underlying condition and the presence of emboli in other organs are significant factors.

In intracerebral hemorrhage, the prognosis is poor, particularly in the presence of hypertension and arteriosclerosis.

If the patient survives the acute attack, the prognosis for life may be good. With active rehabilitation, many patients are able to walk and care for themselves. Return of useful function to the upper extremity occurs infrequently. The prognosis for functional recovery is poor in patients with severe residual organic mental syndrome or receptive aphasia.

Alter M & others: Cerebral infarction: Clinical and angiographic correlations. Neurology 22:590, 1972.

Bauer R & others: Oral contraceptives and increased risk of cerebral ischemia or thrombosis. New England J Med 288:871, 1973.

Brown M, Glassenberg M: Mortality factor in patients with acute stroke. JAMA 224:1493, 1973.

Browne TR, Poskanzer DC: Treatment of strokes. (2 parts.) New England J Med 281:594, 650, 1969.

Dyken ML & others: Complete occlusion of common or internal carotid arteries. Arch Neurol 30:343, 1974.

Hass WK: Occlusive cerebrovascular disease. M Clin North America 56:1281, 1972.

Hirschberg GG, Bard G, Robertson K: Technics of rehabilitation of hemiplegic patients. Am J Med 35:536, 1963.

Locksley HB: Hemorrhagic strokes: Principal causes, natural history, and treatment. M Clin North America 52:1193, 1968.

Mundall J & others: Transient monocular blindness and increased platelet aggregability treated with aspirin. Neurology 22:280, 1972.

Ott KH & others: Cerebellar hemorrhage: Diagnosis and treatment. Arch Neurol 31:160, 1974.

Patterson RH Jr: Risk of carotid surgery with occlusion of the contralateral carotid artery. Arch Neurol 30:188, 1974.

Reagan TJ, Okazaki H: The thrombotic syndrome associated with carcinoma. Arch Neurol 31:390, 1974.

Sedzimir CB, Robinson J: Intracranial hemorrhage in children and adolescents. J Neurosurg 38:269, 1973.

Toole JF & others: Transient ischemic attacks due to atherosclerosis. Arch Neurol 32:5, 1974.

Ziegler DK & others: Correlation of bruits over the carotid artery with angiographically demonstrated lesions. Neurology 21:860, 1971.

INTRACRANIAL ANEURYSM
(Subarachnoid Hemorrhage)

Essentials of Diagnosis

Before Rupture:

● Headache on effort.

- Disorder of cranial nerves II, III, and V.
- Cranial bruit.
- Often asymptomatic.

After Rupture:

- Sudden onset of severe headache without apparent cause.
- Only brief disturbance of consciousness.
- Nuchal rigidity.
- Bloody CSF.

General Considerations

Intracranial aneurysms vary in size from 5–6 mm to 10 cm in diameter, and individual aneurysms may vary in size from time to time. Larger aneurysms may erode the bones of the skull and sella turcica and compress adjacent cerebral tissue and cranial nerves. Most are located near the basilar surface of the skull, and almost half arise from the internal carotid or middle cerebral arteries. They usually occur singly. A coincidence of congenital intracranial aneurysms and polycystic kidneys and coarctation of the aorta has been noted. Saccular aneurysms are rare in childhood; their peak incidence is between 35 and 65 years of age.

Fusiform dilatation of the basilar arteries or the terminal portions of the internal carotids may occur as a consequence of diffuse arteriosclerotic changes. Miliary, saccular aneurysms frequently occur near the bifurcation of a vessel in the circle of Willis and are associated with congenital abnormalities of the muscularis. A mycotic aneurysm, the result of an arteritis produced by bacterial emboli, is relatively infrequent. Larger aneurysms may be partially or completely clot-filled; occasionally they are calcified.

Clinical Findings

A. **Symptoms and Signs:** Prior to rupture, aneurysms may be asymptomatic or may cause symptoms depending upon their location and size. Headache on effort and symptoms of involvement of cranial nerves II, III, and V may be present. A bruit is sometimes heard over the affected site.

Following rupture, the symptoms are those of acute subarachnoid hemorrhage. Recurrent unilateral headaches which clinically resemble those of migraine sometimes occur. Convulsions due to cortical irritation by blood may occur; blood pressure is often elevated.

B. **X-Ray Findings:** By use of carotid or vertebral arterial angiography, an aneurysm may be demonstrated on x-ray.

Differential Diagnosis

Differentiate from intracranial tumor or other causes of sudden intracranial hemorrhage.

Treatment & Prognosis

In most cases the patient survives the first attack of hemorrhage, but recurrence of bleeding is likely. Because of the high mortality rate associated with spontaneous subarachnoid bleeding and the probability of recurrence of subarachnoid hemorrhage, intracranial aneurysms are considered a serious pathologic entity.

Antifibrinolytic agents such as aminocaproic acid (Amicar) may be used during active bleeding to prevent recurrence. The choice of surgical as opposed to medical treatment rests upon many circumstances, including the size and location of the aneurysm, the clinical status of the patient, the skill and experience of the surgeon, and the current enthusiasm for a particular therapeutic regimen. Various surgical procedures, including "trapping" the aneurysm with clips on either side, clipping the neck of the sac, and packing muscle around the aneurysm, have been successful in some cases.

Alvord EC Jr & others: Subarachnoid hemorrhage due to ruptured aneurysm. Arch Neurol 27:273, 1972.

Bailey WL, Loeser JD: Intracranial aneurysms. JAMA 216: 1993, 1971.

Nijenson DE, Saez RJ, Reagan TJ: Clinical significance of basilar aneurysms. Neurology 24:301, 1974.

Okawara S: Warning signs prior to rupture of an intracranial aneurysm. J Neurosurg 38:575, 1973.

Richardson A: Subarachnoid hemorrhage. Brit MJ 4:89, 1969.

Sahs AL & others: *Intracranial Aneurysms and Subarachnoid Hemorrhage: A Cooperative Study.* Lippincott, 1969.

Sundt TM: Intracranial aneurysms and subarachnoid hemorrhage: A subject review for the clinician. Mayo Clin Proc 45:455, 1970.

Thomas JE, Reagan TJ: Nonhemorrhagic complications of intracranial aneurysms of the internal carotid artery. Neurology 20:1043, 1970.

Tovi D: The use of antifibrinolytic drugs to prevent early recurrent aneurysmal subarachnoid hemorrhage. Acta neurol scandinav 49:163, 1973.

CEREBRAL ANGIOMA

Subarachnoid hemorrhage from a cerebral angioma may bear a close clinical resemblance to a ruptured intracranial aneurysm. This type of angioma may vary from a small (2–3 mm) blemish in the cortex to large masses of tortuous channels (arteriovenous shunt), and may be designated as capillary, venous, or arterial (although the vessels are all abnormal). Clinically, cerebral angiomas are often associated with seizures which usually start in youth and are focal in nature. The patient may be aware of a pulsating noise in the head, and a bruit may be audible. Roentgenograms may show crescentic linear calcifications in the vessel walls.

The prognosis for ruptured angioma is generally believed to be better than for rupture of an aneurysm of the circle of Willis, and depends upon the size and site of the lesion. Surgical removal, when feasible, is performed at most centers; however, since a severe neurologic deficit may follow surgery, particularly if the dominant cerebral hemisphere is involved, the choice of operative versus nonoperative treatment often presents the clinician with a thereapeutic dilemma.

Berry RC, Alpers BJ, White JC: The site, structure and frequency of intracranial aneurysms, angiomas and arteriovenous malformations. Res Publ A Nerv Ment Dis 61:40, 1966.

Forster DMC, Steiner L, Håkanson S: Arteriovenous malformations of the brain: A long-term clinical study. J Neurosurg 37:562, 1972.

Henderson WR, Gomez RDL: Natural history of cerebral angiomas. Brit MJ 1:571, 1967.

McCormick WF, Hardman JM, Boulten TR: Vascular malformations ("angiomas") of the brain with special reference to those occurring in the posterior fossa. J Neurosurg 28:241, 1968.

Pool JL: Excision of cerebral arteriovenous malformations. J Neurosurg 29:312, 1968.

BRAIN ABSCESS ✓

Essentials of Diagnosis

- A history of preceding infection (eg, otitis media, mastoiditis, bronchiectasis, septicemia) is often present.
- Progressive or focal neurologic features.
- Evidence of increased intracranial pressure may be present.

General Considerations

Localized suppurations may occur within the brain as in other portions of the body. Following acute purulent infection, pus in brain tissue may be free or encapsulated. Abscesses vary in size from microscopic to an area covering most of a cerebral hemisphere.

Brain abscess is usually caused by staphylococci or pneumococci, although any of the common pyogenic bacteria may be found. The organism may gain access to the brain by direct extension from otitis media, mastoiditis, sinusitis, and infected head injuries, or, more rarely, via the blood stream from distant sources, such as lung infections and bacteremias.

Abscesses occurring by extension from infections of the middle ear or mastoid are usually located within the temporal lobe or cerebellum. Abscesses occurring by extension from the paranasal sinuses usually occur in the frontal lobe. Abscesses following bacteremia are apt to be multiple. Metastatic abscesses are commonly secondary to suppurative pulmonary infections.

Clinical Findings

A. Symptoms and Signs: A history or evidence of preceding infection is usually present. Otitis media, mastoiditis, sinusitis, bronchiectasis, or pneumonia is frequently present. Focalizing manifestations may occur, producing visual field defects, motor and other sensory changes, aphasia, and cranial nerve palsies similar to those caused by any other intracranial mass.

Signs of increased intracranial pressure may occur, such as papilledema, headache, and slowed pulse and respirations. Mild meningeal signs may be present, such as a mild rigidity of the neck and a positive Kernig sign. Somnolence and slowing of the mental processes are common. The temperature is mildly elevated and rarely exceeds 102° F (39° C) if complications such as meningitis do not occur.

B. Laboratory Findings: EEG, brain scan, air ventriculography, pneumoencephalography, or cerebral angiography is frequently necessary to determine the site of abscess.

C. Special Examinations: Brain abscesses may be located at operation with the use of needle aspiration.

Differential Diagnosis

Brain abscesses may be confused with other clinical entities such as brain tumors, leptomeningitis, or encephalitis. In brain tumor, a history or evidence of preceding infection is usually absent and the CSF cell count is usually normal. Leptomeningitis can usually be differentiated by means of a positive culture of the CSF. Acute fulminating leptomeningitis is easily distinguished clinically from brain abscess; mild leptomeningitis, such as tuberculous and syphilitic leptomeningitis, may be clinically indistinguishable. Encephalitis usually fails to exhibit the focalizing signs of brain abscess and usually provokes more profound and severe changes in the sensorium and personality.

Treatment & Prognosis

Treatment consists of operative drainage of pus. Surgery is usually delayed until the abscess is firmly encapsulated. If the abscess is well encapsulated and if it is practicable to do so, excision in toto is sometimes performed. Marsupialization of the cavity, packing of the cavity, and various types of incision and drainage are commonly employed. After surgical drainage has been instituted, irrigations of the abscess cavity with antibiotic solutions are helpful. Treatment of the original focus of infection, such as a chronic mastoiditis, is sometimes necessary before a brain abscess will heal completely.

The use of chemotherapy has improved the outlook for brain abscess. It has even been maintained that the formation of brain abscesses—eg, in debilitated patients with pyogenic infections elsewhere—can be aborted with the use of appropriate antibiotic drugs. Without treatment, brain abscess is usually fatal.

Brewer NS, MacCarty CS, Wellman WE: Brain abscess: A review of recent experiences. Ann Int Med 82:571, 1975.

Carey ME, Chou SN, French LA: Experience with brain abscesses. J Neurosurg 36:1, 1972.

Morgan H, Wood WW, Murphy F: Experience with 88 consecutive cases of brain abscess. J Neurosurg 38:698, 1973.

Sutherland JB & others: Brain scanning and brain abscesses. J Canad A Radiol 23:176, 1972.

Tarkkanen J, Kohonen A: Otogenic brain abscesses. Arch Otolaryng 91:91, 1970.

TRAUMATIC DISEASES
OF THE CNS

HEAD INJURY ✓

Emergency Evaluation

Any patient who gives a history of head injury followed by unconsciousness, and any unconscious patient who may have sustained a head injury, should receive careful neurologic evaluation. Particular effort should be made to detect focal or progressive neurologic changes. Skull x-rays should be taken as soon as possible.

The following are the most important features of the examination:

(1) **State of consciousness**—The depth and duration of unconsciousness usually reflect the degree of trauma. However, an initially alert and well-oriented patient may become drowsy, stuporous, and comatose as a result of progressive intracranial hemorrhage. During the first 24–48 hours it may be necessary to awaken the patient hourly to evaluate his degree of orientation, alertness, and general response to stimulation. *Caution:* Do not discharge the patient to home care unless it is certain that a responsible person will be on hand to awaken him from "sleep" every hour and to summon aid if he cannot be completely aroused.

(2) **Vital signs**—Temperature, pulse, respirations, and blood pressure should be observed at intervals of 30 minutes to 12 hours, depending upon the extent of injury.

(3) **Paralysis**—In the stuporous or unconscious patient, paralysis can be demonstrated only by careful examination. Loss of strength and motion, although of minimal grade, may indicate intracranial hemorrhage.

(4) **Ocular signs**—The pupils should be observed regularly along with the vital signs. A fixed dilated pupil often means an ipsilateral epidural or subdural hemorrhage or ipsilateral brain damage. Ophthalmoscopic examination may reveal evidence of papilledema (due to intracranial pressure) or retinal hemorrhage.

(5) **Convulsions**—Convulsions are apt to occur soon after a head injury; focal (jacksonian) convulsions suggest an irritative lesion of the contralateral cerebral hemisphere. Cerebral contusion and laceration, often in association with epidural, subdural, or intracranial hemorrhage causes focal convulsions.

(6) **Nuchal rigidity**—Although nuchal rigidity may result from the subarachnoid bleeding that is often associated with head injuries, cervical spine injury must be ruled out by appropriate x-ray and clinical examinations.

(7) **Bleeding from the ear**—Otorrhagia suggests basilar fracture through the petrous pyramid of the temporal bone, but it may also occur as a result of traumatic rupture of the tympanic membrane or laceration of the mucous membranes without perforation of the drum.

General Considerations

Craniocerebral injuries are frequently classified on the basis of the nature of the injury to the skull, although the prognosis for recovery depends primarily upon the nature and severity of the damage to the brain.

Closed head injuries are those in which there is no injury to the skull or in which the skull injury is limited to simple undisplaced fracture of the skull. They may be considered clinically as mild, moderate, or severe. Mild head injuries are characterized by brief loss of consciousness (seconds to minutes) without demonstrable neurologic changes (usually the same as cerebral concussion). CSF findings are usually normal. Retrograde amnesia may be present. Moderate head injuries are characterized by longer periods of unconsciousness, frequently with abnormal neurologic signs, and are often associated with cerebral edema and contusion. Severe head injuries cause prolonged unconsciousness and abnormal neurologic signs and are usually associated with cerebral contusion and laceration.

Open head injuries include scalp lacerations, compound fractures of the skull, and various degrees of cerebral destruction. If fragmentation of bone occurs, there will be extensive associated contusion and laceration of the brain. Consciousness may not be impaired at first, although depression of consciousness may occur later if progressive intracranial bleeding or edema occurs. Scalp lacerations should be sutured immediately unless they overlie a depressed fracture or penetrating wound of the skull, in which case the skin wound is treated in conjunction with the fracture in the operating room.

Fractures may be simple or compound, and linear (with no displacement of fragments), comminuted, or depressed.

Cerebral edema may follow head injury. Clinically, there is considerable variation in the severity of the findings. Localizing signs such as convulsions, hemiplegia, and aphasia are not uncommon. CSF pressure is usually slightly increased. At operation, the brain looks very pale and swollen.

Contusion or bruising of the brain at or directly contralateral to the zone of impact (contrecoup injury) may be limited to the superficial cortex, or associated hemorrhage into the underlying brain may also occur. Contusions frequently occur along the base of the posterior frontal lobes and the adjacent temporal lobe tips. Brain contusion is often clinically indistinguishable from concussion or laceration of the brain.

Brain laceration (a tear in the substance of the brain) usually occurs at the point of application of great force to the head or directly opposite (contrecoup effect). Lacerations involving the base of the brain usually cause death in a short time. Focal neurologic signs may persist after the acute episode has subsided. Associated subarachnoid or intracerebral hemorrhage is usually present, and the CSF is bloody. Brain laceration (or contusion) may occur with no injury (or minimal injury) to the skull. The frontal and temporal lobes are common sites. Minor injuries may cause tearing of the brain and meninges and extensive hemorrhagic necrosis of the cortex and subcortical white matter. Associated hemorrhage of the basal ganglia and brain stem may also occur. Laceration of arachnoidal vessels may result in subarachnoid bleeding or the formation of subdural hematoma. Tearing of the middle meningeal artery or the dural sinuses or veins may be followed by bleeding into the extradural spaces.

Clinical Findings

A. Symptoms and Signs: Transient loss of consciousness lasting seconds to minutes occurs classically with concussion of the brain. In coma which lasts for several hours or days there is a likelihood of edema or of contusion and laceration of the brain. The period of coma depends upon the extent and site of injury; in severe cases it may last for several hours, days, or weeks.

After the patient recovers consciousness, symptoms and signs are related to the severity and nature of associated brain injury. With mild concussion, the patient may be normal within a few minutes; with laceration or contusion of the brain, mental confusion is apt to be present. Hemiplegia, aphasia, cranial nerve paralysis, and other focal neurologic signs may also be noted depending upon the nature and extent of the brain injury. The ipsilateral pupil is often dilated in dural hemorrhage.

In the recovery phase and for months thereafter there may be complaints of headache, dizziness, and personality changes ("post-traumatic cerebral syndrome").

Loss of memory for the period immediately after recovery of consciousness (post-traumatic amnesia) and for the period immediately preceding the injury (pretraumatic or retrograde amnesia) may occur and is often related to the extent of brain damage.

If the patient remains unconscious, diagnosis of a progressive intracranial hemorrhagic lesion is difficult. Vital signs (pulse rate, respirations, blood pressure) may change, although these are not reliable. In case of deepening or unusually prolonged coma, exploratory trephination is indicated; cerebral angiography may show pathognomonic features of subdural, epidural, or intracerebral hemorrhage. Prolonged unconsciousness is believed to indicate severe damage to the brain stem, usually due to secondary hemorrhage or compression of the brain stem.

B. Laboratory Findings:

1. Lumbar puncture may establish the presence of subarachnoid hemorrhage and establish a baseline appearance and pressure of the CSF. CSF is frequently normal in all respects in brain concussion or cerebral edema. With contusion or laceration of the brain, bloody CSF under increased pressure may be found.

2. Skull x-rays should be taken as soon as the patient's physical condition permits. Cerebral angiography may help demonstrate subdural or intracerebral hematoma. A pneumogram often is useful in demonstrating ventricular distortion, shift, or dilatation following head injury.

3. EEG and brain scans may be of diagnostic and prognostic aid in selected cases.

Differential Diagnosis

The history of a blow to the head makes the etiology of the unconsciousness evident; however, especially where a history of trauma is lacking, it is necessary to differentiate head injury from other causes of unconsciousness such as diabetic, hepatic, or alcoholic coma, cerebrovascular accident, and epilepsy (where trauma to the head may actually occur during the attack).

Differentiate the neurologic findings following head injury from those caused by epidural hematoma, subdural hematoma, brain tumor, etc.

Complications & Sequelae

The complications of head injuries include vascular lesions (hemorrhage, thrombosis, aneurysm formation), infections (meningitis, abscess, osteomyelitis), rhinorrhea and otorrhea, pneumatocele, leptomeningeal cysts, cranial nerve injuries, and focal brain lesions. The sequelae include convulsive seizures, psychoses, mental disturbances, and the post-traumatic cerebral syndrome.

A. Subarachnoid Hemorrhage: Bleeding into the subarachnoid space is often associated with other types of brain injury and is relatively common in traumatized patients who have been unconscious for 1 hour or more. The clinical and diagnostic features of traumatic and spontaneous subarachnoid hemorrhage are similar. Painful stiffness of the neck and the presence of fresh blood in the CSF are the usual findings.

B. Subdural Hematoma: Acute subdural hematoma may occur after a head injury in association with contusion or laceration of the brain. In such cases, especially when the subdural hematoma is not massive, the patient's clinical course may be unaffected by evacuation of the subdural hematoma. In chronic subdural hematomas, particularly when a history of head injury is not obtained, the clinical course may be variable or suggestive of an intracranial mass.

In infants, the diagnosis may be readily established by direct needle aspiration of the subdural space at the lateral margin of the open anterior fontanelle (subdural tap). In others, the cerebral angiogram remains the single most reliable diagnostic test, since a highly specific angiographic pattern is usually found. However, changes suggestive of subdural hematoma may also be noted in skull x-ray (shift of pineal), pneumogram (shift and distortion of ventricle), and electroencephalogram (focal low amplitude or slow waves).

C. Extradural Hemorrhage: Extradural hemorrhage classically follows traumatic rupture of the middle meningeal artery or vein, and may be difficult to detect early. A blow on the temporal area, with dazing or transient loss of consciousness and apparent quick return to normal, usually occurs. A "lucid interval," lasting as long as a day or more in extreme cases, customarily follows; during this time the patient develops signs of increased intracranial pressure. This is caused by the continued steady accumulation of blood in the extradural space from the bleeding middle meningeal vessel.

Trephining of the skull is frequently necessary to make the diagnosis. Blood may then be evacuated through the trephine openings.

A fracture which by x-ray is found to cross the middle meningeal groove should raise the suspicion that this syndrome may be present.

D. Intracerebral Hemorrhage: A large subcortical hematoma may develop, but the most common findings are multiple small intracerebral hemorrhages near the contused area. The angiographic pattern is characteristic.

E. Rhinorrhea and Otorrhea: Rhinorrhea (leakage of CSF from the nose) may follow fracture of the frontal bone with associated tearing of the dura mater and arachnoid. Erect posture, straining, and coughing usually cause an increase in the flow of fluid. Replacement of lost fluid by air entering the cranial vault through the same (or a similar) pathway may give rise to an aerocele. Otorrhea (leakage of CSF from the ear) is usually of serious prognostic importance since it is caused by injuries to the more vital areas of the base of the brain.

Infection and meningitis are potential hazards in both instances and may be prevented by the early use of prophylactic antibiotic therapy. In the case of rhinorrhea, surgical repair of the dural tear may be necessary to stop the flow of CSF and to close off a potential route of infection.

F. Cranial Nerve Paralysis: Injury to the cranial nerves may occur. Commonly affected nerves are the olfactory (anosmia), facial (paralysis), auditory (tinnitus and deafness), and optic (atrophy).

G. Post-Traumatic Syndrome: The post-traumatic syndrome is more common after serious head injuries, but severe symptoms may be produced by relatively minor injuries. Headache, giddiness, easy fatigability, memory defects, and impaired ability to concentrate are common complaints. Personality changes are not uncommon. Changes of posture, exposure to sunlight or heat, exercise, and alcohol ingestion are apt to make the symptoms worse.

On pathologic examination the brain may appear normal or may show severe cortical atrophy and ventricular dilatation.

H. Post-Traumatic Epilepsy: The exact incidence of seizures following head injuries is not known. In general, the more severe the injury, the greater the possibility of seizures. EEG studies are important in establishing the diagnosis.

I. Other Complications of Head Injuries:

1. Increased intracranial pressure may be manifested by changes in the level of consciousness, headache, restlessness, unequal pupils, a slowly falling respiratory rate, a falling pulse rate, a slowly rising blood pressure, papilledema, hemiparesis, and elevated CSF pressure. Intracranial bleeding (subdural, epidural, or intracerebral) must be ruled out.

2. Wound infection or osteomyelitis may be pre-

vented by prophylactic antibiotic therapy in patients with compound or depressed fractures of the skull, rhinorrhea, otorrhea, or extensive scalp lacerations, and by meticulous aseptic technic for all dressings.

3. Pulmonary infections or atelectasis may be prevented or treated by the proper use of suction, positioning on the side, or, if necessary, intubation or tracheostomy.

4. Hyperthermia may result from injury to the hypothalamus or brain stem, local or general infection, or marked dehydration.

5. Shock may occur in patients with head injuries complicated by other severe injuries to the trunk and extremities, and must be treated at once.

Treatment

A. Emergency Measures:

1. Treat shock if present; parenterally administered fluids and blood may be required (see Chapter 1).

2. Maintenance of an adequate airway and pulmonary ventilation is vital. The patient should be placed prone, with head turned to one side to facilitate drainage of secretions from the mouth and keep the tongue from obstructing the pharynx. Endotracheal intubation or tracheostomy may be necessary to maintain an open airway. Give oxygen if necessary.

B. General Measures:

1. During the acute or initial phases, restlessness may be a disturbing factor. Special nursing care and sedatives may be required. Avoid morphine because of its medullary depressant effects. Catheterization of a full bladder may ameliorate restlessness.

2. Antibiotic treatment is always indicated if there is active bleeding or discharge from the nose or ears. Give procaine penicillin G, 600,000 units twice daily, or broad-spectrum antibiotics, until the danger of infection is past.

3. Continued careful observation is essential.

Course & Prognosis

Prognosis and course are related to the severity and site of cranial injury. With simple concussion recovery is usually rapid. With laceration of the brain, mortality may be 40–50%.

Subdural or epidural hematoma ordinarily requires prompt surgical evacuation in order to prevent death or serious neurologic complications.

In general, residual symptoms and signs in patients with head trauma are likely to be more extensive and incapacitating in those with the more severe types of brain injury. It is not uncommon, however, for patients to remain symptomatic (headache, dizziness, impaired memory, personality changes) even though neurologic diagnostic studies are negative.

Predictions regarding the clinical outcome are more accurate when made 6–12 months after the injury or when the clinical status of the patient has stabilized. Great variations occur in individual cases. A patient in whom subdural hematoma has been successfully removed may recover completely. On the other hand, many patients continue to have severe complaints after an apparently trivial head injury. A complicating factor in many cases is the role played by the "secondary gain" for the patient via lawsuits, insurance, and other types of compensation.

Bender MB, Christoff N: Nonsurgical treatment of subdural hematoma. Arch Neurol 31:73, 1974.

De Jesus PV Jr, Poser CM: Subdural hematomas: A clinicopathologic study of 100 cases. Postgrad Med 44:172, 1968.

Evans JP: Acute trauma to the head: Fundamentals of management. Postgrad Med 39:27, 1966.

Fell DA & others: Acute subdural hematoma: Review of 144 cases. J Neurosurg 42:37, 1975.

Gjerris F, Schmidt K: Chronic subdural hematoma: Surgery or mannitol treatment. J Neurosurg 40:639, 1974.

Javid M: Head injuries. New England J Med 291:890, 1974.

Mannarino E, McLaurin RL: Management of head injuries. S Clin North America 48:723, 1968.

Taylor AR: Post-concussional sequelae. Brit MJ 3:62, 1967.

LOW BACK PAIN*

Low back pain may be associated with a variety of causes, and careful examination of such a patient may yield important clues regarding the site and cause of the disorders. Such a patient may be subjected to a larger number of laboratory, x-ray, and diagnostic procedures with ambiguous or disappointing results. This may in turn often reflect the inadequate clinical evaluation of the patient and commonly results from failure to utilize the information which a properly conducted physical and neurologic examination may supply. The increasing overdependence of the clinician upon the laboratory is unnecessarily exaggerated when the physician fails to obtain vital information available at the bedside examination.

Inspection and palpation of the painful area are important. Since pain from nerve roots or nerves is commonly referred toward the periphery, the entire nerve lengths leading from the painful area should be explored, noting the presence of any masses or tenderness and, where possible, the size and consistency of nerves.

Rectal and vaginal examination should be part of the examination so that local lesions and involvement of accessible lumbodorsal plexuses can be ruled out if possible.

Muscle spasm and tenderness to percussion and deep pressure may give evidence suggesting radicular irritation, particularly when associated with local deformity or restriction of spinal motion.

The range of motion of joints and the effect of movement on the pain should be determined, since pain from areas such as the hip may be referred distally and severe distal peripheral pain may be referred to the entire limb.

The regional blood vessels and those of the extremity should be checked for adequacy of pulsation

*Gynecologic causes of backache are discussed in Chapter 12.

and aneurysmal dilatation.

The straight leg raising test (Lasègue's sign) should be elicited. The relaxed, extended lower extremity is gently lifted from the bed or table with the patient supine. The presence and amount of pain and the extent to which the straight leg may be raised are noted. Pain and limitation of motion often accompany radiculopathy, especially that which occurs with herniated lumbar or lumbosacral disks.

The "f-ab-er-e" sign (Patrick's sign) is tested for. The patient lies supine, and the heel of the lower extremity being tested is passively placed on the opposite knee. Then the knee on the side being tested is pressed laterally and downward by the examiner as far as it will go. The test is considered positive if motion is involuntarily restricted, and pain frequently accompanies this limitation of motion. The test is positive in hip joint disease and negative in sciatica. "F-ab-er-e" is a mnemonic formula: "f" for flexion, "ab" for abduction, "er" for external rotation, and "e" for extension motions of the hip.

Kernig's sign is elicited with the patient supine. The examiner flexes the hip and then extends the knee as far as possible without producing significant pain. A positive Kernig test consists of an involuntary spasm of the hamstring muscles which limits extension of the knee and often causes pain. Its clinical significance is similar to that of a positive straight leg raising test.

Lumbar paraspinal muscle spasm frequently is noted with local radiculitis, which is due to many causes including herniated lumbar intervertebral disk.

Passive flexion of the neck so that the chin rests on the chest may induce ascension of the spinal cord within the spinal canal. This then puts tension on the various spinal roots, causing excessive pain and indicating disease of particular nerve roots—provided motion of the spinal column was not induced and the patient was relaxed.

With the patient standing with his back toward the examiner, the presence of lordosis, scoliosis, or list affecting the lumbar region is noted. The effect of flexion, hyperextension, and lateral flexion of the trunk on the pelvis is observed.

Psoas muscle spasm usually indicates disease of the psoas muscle or of the lumbar vertebrae and soft tissue adjacent to this muscle. It may be tested with the patient prone and the pelvis firmly pressed against the table with one hand by the examiner. With the other hand grasping the ankle, the leg is moved to the vertical position with the knee flexed at a right angle. The hip is passively hyperextended by lifting up on the ankle. Limitation of motion is produced by involuntary psoas muscle spasm.

Limitation of passive lumbar flexion and resulting pain often accompany disease of the lumbar or lumbosacral articulations. With the patient supine, the examiner grasps one lower extremity with both hands and moves the thigh to a position of maximal flexion. Then he presses firmly downward toward the table and upward toward the patient's head, passively flexing the lumbar spinal column.

Epstein JA: Common errors in the diagnosis of herniation of the intervertebral disc. Indust Med 39:47, 1970.

Rubin P: Cancer of the urogenital tract: Prostatic cancer, advanced and metastatic. JAMA 210:1072, 1969.

Russell ML & others: The cauda equina syndrome of ankylosing spondylitis. Ann Int Med 78:551, 1973.

HERNIATION OF INTERVERTEBRAL DISK

Essentials of Diagnosis

Lumbosacral Disk:

- Back pain aggravated by motion, and pain radiating down the back of the leg and aggravated by coughing or straining.
- Weakness of muscles, decreased sensation, hyporeflexia of leg and foot.
- Sciatic nerve painful to pressure and stretch (straight-leg raising).
- CSF protein may be elevated; myelograms reveal characteristic defect.

Cervical Disk:

- Paroxysmal pains and paresthesias from back of neck radiating into the arms and fingers, usually in distribution of C6, C7, or C8; accentuated by coughing, sneezing, straining.
- Restricted mobility of neck; cervical muscle spasm.
- Paresthesias and pains in fingers, diminished biceps or triceps jerk, weakness or atrophy of forearm and hand muscles.
- Narrowing of vertebral interspace on x-ray; characteristic filling defect or deformity on myelogram.

General Considerations

In most cases rupture or herniation of an intervertebral disk is caused by trauma. Sudden straining with the back in an "odd" position and lifting in the trunk-flexed posture are commonly recognized precipitating causes. The defect may occur immediately after an injury or following an interval of months to years.

The lumbosacral intervertebral disks (L5–S1 or L4–L5) are most commonly affected, producing the clinical picture of sciatica. Herniation occasionally occurs in the cervical region (characterized by cervical radicular complaints); rarely in the thoracic region.

Clinical Findings

A. Symptoms and Signs: These usually depend upon the location and size of the herniated or extruded disk material. Compression of a nerve root by a disk may be confined to a single nerve root; however, several roots may be compressed (eg, cauda equina by disk at L5–S1). Larger cervical and thoracic lesions may even compress the spinal cord and produce symptoms commonly associated with tumors.

1. Lumbosacral disk—In the great majority (over 90%), rupture of the disk occurs at the level of the 4th or 5th lumbar interspace. This is characterized by straightening of the normal lumbar curve, scoliosis toward the side opposite the sciatic pain, limitation of motion of the lumbar spine, impaired straight-leg raising on the painful side, tenderness to palpation in the sciatic notch and along the course of the sciatic nerve, mild weakness of the foot or great toe extensors, impaired perception of pain and touch over the dorsum of the foot and leg (in L5 or S1 distribution), decreased or absent ankle jerk, and radiation of pain along the course of the sciatic nerve to the calf or ankle on coughing, sneezing, or straining.

2. Cervical disk herniation (5–10% of herniated disks)—The cervical disks most commonly involved are between C5–C6 and C6–C7. Paresthesias and pain occur in the upper extremities (hands, forearms, and arms) in the affected cervical root distribution (C6 or C7). Slight weakness and atrophy of the biceps or triceps may be present, with diminution of biceps or triceps jerk. The mobility of the neck is restricted with accentuation of radicular and neck pains by neck motion, coughing, sneezing, or straining. Long tract signs (extensor plantar response, sensory or motor impairment of lower levels, etc) occasionally occur, indicating compression of the spinal cord by the disk.

B. Laboratory Findings: CSF protein may be elevated, and complete or partial CSF block is occasionally demonstrated.

C. X-Ray Findings: Spine x-rays may show loss of normal curvature, scoliosis, and narrowing of the intervertebral disk. A characteristic roentgenologic defect in the subarachnoid space is usually produced by a herniated disk and is readily demonstrable by myelography. Electromyography (EMG) may be of value in localizing the site of a ruptured disk if characteristic denervation potentials can be demonstrated in muscles of a particular root distribution.

Differential Diagnosis

In tumors of the spinal cord the course is progressive, CSF protein is elevated, partial or complete spinal subarachnoid block is present, and the myelographic pattern is distinctive.

In arthritis neurologic findings are usually minimal or absent, and the myelogram is usually negative.

Spinal column anomalies show characteristic x-ray findings, CSF findings are negative, and myelographic changes are dissimilar or absent.

Treatment

A. General Measures:

1. Lumbosacral disk—In the acute phase, bed rest, heat applied locally to the back, salicylate analgesics, and the use of a bed board under the mattress are indicated. Traction to the lower extremities is frequently beneficial. The avoidance of severe physical effort and strain is essential to minimize recurrence of symptoms after the initial episode. Low back belts, braces, or supports may be beneficial. It is important to instruct the patient in the proper methods of bending, lifting (with knees flexed), and carrying (with the object held close to the body).

2. Cervical disk—In acute exacerbations of herniated cervical disks, bed rest with cervical halter traction is indicated. In subacute or mild episodes, intermittent cervical halter traction with various devices may be employed on an outpatient basis or at home. The use of a light collar may be helpful. Local application of heat, diathermy, and similar measures may be of temporary value.

B. Surgical Measures: If the response to conservative measures is poor or recurrences are disabling, diskectomy is indicated. Injection of the enzyme chymopapain into the diseased disk may be effective in relieving pain.

Prognosis

Conservative management with or without traction may bring about improvement to the point of "practical" recovery. Relief of pain usually follows removal of the damaged disk. Reversal of motor dysfunction, muscle atrophy, and skin sensory changes may occur.

Epstein JA, Epstein BS, Lavine LS: Surgical treatment of nerve root compression caused by scoliosis of the lumbar spine. J Neurosurg 41:449, 1974.

Epstein JA & others: Herniated disks of the lumbar spine. JAMA 202:187, 1967.

Fager CA: Results of adequate posterior decompression in the relief of spondylotic cervical myelopathy. J Neurosurg 38:688, 1973.

Jacobs B, Krueger EG, Levy DM: Cervical spondylosis with radiculopathy. JAMA 211:2135, 1970.

Paine KWE, Huang PWH: Lumbar disc syndrome. J Neurosurg 37:75, 1972.

Parkinson D, Shields C: Treatment of protruded intervertebral discs with chymopapain (Discase). J Neurosurg 39:203, 1973.

Petrie JG: Conservative management of lumbar disk protrusion. Postgrad Med 38:654, 1965.

Wiltse LL, Widell EH, Yuan HA: Chymopapain chemonucleolysis in lumbar disk disease. JAMA 231:474, 1975.

INTRACRANIAL TUMORS √

Essentials of Diagnosis

- Headache, personality changes, vomiting.
- Focal neurologic changes, often progressive.
- Increased CSF pressure, papilledema.
- Evidence of space-occupying lesion demonstrable on special examination (EEG, angiogram, pneumogram, cerebroscintigram, echoencephalogram, CAT, etc).

General Considerations

Intracranial tumors account for many admissions to the average neurologic service. Metastatic tumors to the brain arise principally from the lung, breast, gastrointestinal tract, and thyroid. Less frequently, sarcoma, hypernephroma, melanoblastoma, and retinal tumors are the primary sources.

Primary intracranial tumors are unlike the carcinomas and sarcomas found outside the brain in that they rarely metastasize outside the CNS. They may be of congenital origin, eg, dermoids, teratomas, craniopharyngiomas; mesodermal origin, eg, meningiomas, neurinomas, angiomas, and hemangioblastomas; pituitary origin, eg, chromophobe tumors and chromophil tumors; or ectodermal origin, eg, the gliomas.

Gliomas account for 40–50% of intracranial tumors in some series. Depending upon the principal cell types and morphology, gliomas are subclassified into various types (eg, glioblastoma multiforme, astrocytoma, medulloblastoma, astroblastoma, ependymoma, oligodendroglioma). The majority of tumors of the brain in children arise from the cerebellum (medulloblastoma and astrocytoma). In adults, tumors of the cerebral hemispheres are common, particularly astrocytoma and glioblastoma multiforme. Gliomas of the brain in adults are most commonly encountered in the 40–50 year age group.

Clinical Findings

A. Symptoms and Signs: These are commonly divided into manifestations caused by the intracranial mass (headache, vomiting, papilledema) and those resulting from interference with local brain function.

Table 16–5. Frequency of brain tumor types according to age and site.

Age	Cerebral Hemisphere	Intrasellar and Parasellar	Posterior Fossa
Childhood and adolescence	Ependymomas; less commonly, astrocytomas.	Astrocytomas, mixed gliomas, ependymomas.	Astrocytomas, medulloblastomas, ependymomas.
Age 20–40	Meningiomas, astrocytomas; less commonly, metastatic tumors.	Pituitary adenomas; less commonly, meningiomas.	Acoustic neuromas, meningiomas, hemangioblastomas; less commonly, metastatic tumors.
Over age 40	Glioblastoma multiforme, meningiomas, metastatic tumors.	Pituitary adenomas; less commonly, meningiomas.	Metastatic tumors, acoustic neuromas, meningiomas.

Table 16—6. Frequency of major types of brain tumors.

Intracranial Tumors*		Frequency of Occurrence
Gliomas		50%
Glioblastoma multiforme	50%	
Astrocytoma	20%	
Ependymoma	10%	
Medulloblastoma	10%	
Oligodendroglioma	5%	
Mixed	5%	
Meningiomas		20%
Nerve sheath tumors		10%
Metastatic tumors		10%
Congenital tumors		5%
Miscellaneous tumors		5%

*Exclusive of pituitary tumors.

Focal neurologic changes frequently reflect the location of the tumor:

1. Frontal lobe tumor—These tend to produce a disturbed mental state with defective memory, impaired judgment, irritability, mood changes, and facetiousness. Convulsive seizures may occur, as well as loss of speech in left-sided (dominant hemisphere) tumor. Anosmia may occur with tumors at the base of the frontal lobe.

2. Parietal lobe tumor—Sensory and motor abnormalities are common. Motor or sensory focal seizures, contralateral hemiparesis, hyperreflexia, impaired sensory perception, astereognosis, and a positive Babinski toe sign may be present. With a left parietal lobe tumor aphasic components may be demonstrable.

3. Occipital lobe tumor—Visual alterations and seizures preceded by an aura of lights and visual hallucinations are characteristic. Contralateral homonymous hemianopsia, frequently with sparing of the macular area, often occurs. Headache and papilledema may be found.

4. Temporal lobe tumor—Convulsive seizures of the psychomotor type are commonly present, as is aphasia also if the dominant (left) cerebral hemisphere is involved. A contralateral homonymous visual field defect may be demonstrated.

5. Cerebellar tumor—This is characterized by disturbances of equilibrium and coordination, and early development of increased intracranial pressure and papilledema.

B. X-Ray Findings: Skull x-rays, lumbar puncture, pneumograms, electroencephalography, echoencephalogram, cerebroscintigram, and angiography may aid in diagnosis and localization of an intracranial mass. Chest x-ray, gastrointestinal series, urograms, and other studies may be necessary to determine the primary site of a metastatic brain tumor.

Computerized scanning of the brain may reveal details of the brain's internal structure and tissues and outline the area of a brain tumor.

Differential Diagnosis

Differentiate from other disorders which cause increased intracranial pressure or appear to be due to progressive cerebral lesions, eg, intracranial abscess, arachnoiditis, aneurysm, subdural hematoma, and neurosyphilis; and from epilepsy and cerebrovascular accident.

Treatment

A. General Measures: Intravenous hypertonic mannitol or urea will reduce increased intracranial pressure for periods of a few hours and gives welcome relief in the operative and early postoperative phases of treatment. Parenteral corticosteroids may be used to reduce cerebral edema in the preoperative and early postoperative phase. Give dexamethasone, 8–40 mg/day IV or IM. Symptomatic therapy, including the use of analgesics, anticonvulsants, and sedatives as required, is essentially the same as for patients with similar complaints not associated with brain tumors.

B. Specific Measures: In general, treatment consists of surgical removal of the tumor, although gratifying results may be achieved in a small number of selected patients with intensive radiation. Pituitary tumors may be "cured" with x-ray treatment. Medulloblastoma of the cerebellum in children is highly sensitive to an initial course of irradiation, but recurrence is the rule. Radical excision and hemispherectomy is occasionally successful in selected cases.

Prognosis

The outcome in any particular case depends upon the type, size, and location of the tumor. Early diagnosis and proper surgical treatment may be curative in benign tumors (meningiomas, neurinomas) as well as in certain gliomas (especially in frontal and occipital locations).

For the majority of patients with malignant brain tumors, the prognosis is poor.

Ambrose J: Computerized x-ray scanning of the brain. J Neurosurg 40:670, 1974.

Faust DS & others: Radiation therapy in the management of medulloblastoma. Neurology 20:519, 1970.

Fewer D & others: The chemotherapy of brain tumors. JAMA 222:549, 1972.

Geissinger JD, Bucy PC: Astrocytomas of the cerebellum in children. Arch Neurol 24:125, 1971.

Jelsma R, Bucy PC: Glioblastoma multiforme. Arch Neurol 20:161, 1969.

Kistler JP & others: Computerized axial tomography: Clinicopathologic correlation. Neurology 25:201, 1975.

Ojemann RG, Montgomery WW, Weiss AD: Evaluation and surgical treatment of acoustic neurinoma. New England J Med 287:895, 1972.

Olson ME, Chernik NL, Posner JB: Infiltration of leptomeninges by systemic cancer. Arch Neurol 30:122, 1974.

Rubinstein LJ: *Tumors of the Central Nervous System,* Fascicle 6. Armed Forces Institute of Pathology, Washington DC, 1972.

Vannucci RC, Baten M: Cerebral metastatic disease in childhood. Neurology 24:961, 1974.

Weisberg LA: The syndrome of increased intracranial pressure without localizing signs: A reappraisal. Neurology 25:85, 1975.

DEGENERATIVE DISORDERS OF THE CNS

√

MULTIPLE SCLEROSIS
(Disseminated Sclerosis)

Essentials of Diagnosis

- Sudden, transient motor and sensory disturbances; impaired vision.
- Diffuse neurologic signs, with remissions and exacerbations.
- Euphoria (late).
- Onset in early adult life.
- Abnormal colloidal gold curve; increased gamma globulin in CSF.

General Considerations

Multiple sclerosis is characterized by the onset in early adult life of progressive diffuse neurologic disturbances, with irregular fluctuating periods of exacerbation and apparent improvement or quiescence. The etiology is not known; a wide variety of degenerative, toxic, and inflammatory agents and deficiency states have been implicated in various theories of pathogenesis.

Irregular gray patches of degeneration occur in the brain and spinal cord with a predilection for the white matter, varying in size from a few millimeters to several centimeters.

Clinical Findings

A. Symptoms and Signs: The initial attack and subsequent relapses may occur following acute infections, trauma, vaccination, serum injections, pregnancy, or types of somatic stress.

Signs of multiple involvement of the CNS may include slurred speech, intention tremor, nystagmus, retrobulbar neuritis, incontinence, spastic paralysis, pallor of the temporal halves of the optic disks, increased deep tendon reflexes, and bilateral extensor plantar responses. Late in the course of the disease the mental state is characterized by euphoria with little insight into condition or disability. Excited and even maniacal states may occur.

The illness, therefore, is characterized by the fact that (1) the neurologic lesions are widespread and cannot be explained on a single anatomic basis, and (2) the signs and symptoms are subject to repeated exacerbations and remissions.

B. Laboratory Findings: The CSF may show a "first zone" or "second zone" colloidal gold curve.

CSF gamma globulin is likely to be increased. No pathologic alterations in CSF may be noted in some patients.

Differential Diagnosis

Neurosyphilis is classically characterized by Argyll Robertson pupils and positive blood and CSF serology. Posterolateral sclerosis is usually associated with pernicious anemia and achylia, and signs of a posterior and lateral column disorder. Cerebral tumors cause progressive clinical findings, a distinctive EEG, characteristic pneumograms and cerebral angiograms, increased CSF pressure and protein, and a pineal shift in skull x-rays. Friedreich's ataxia is manifested by scoliosis, club foot, absent deep reflexes, and a positive family history. Platybasia, Arnold-Chiari malformation, and cervical spine malformation are differentiated on the basis of skull and cervical x-rays, partial subarachnoid spinal block, and positive myelograms. Tumors of the posterior fossa cause papilledema, increased CSF pressure, and characteristic ventriculograms and vertebral angiograms.

Complications

The hazards of chronic invalidism usually increase the longer the patient survives. The immediate cause of death is usually some intercurrent disease. Infections of the bladder and kidney are common.

Treatment

A. Medical Treatment: There is no specific treatment. Corticosteroids and vasodilators (inhalations of 5–10% CO_2, histamine infusions, amyl nitrite inhalations) have been advocated for treatment of acute relapses, but the results are poor. Therapeutic claims have also been made for tolbutamide, isoniazid, vitamin B_{12}, procaine, blood transfusions, and fat-free diets, but their value has not been established.

B. General Measures: Adequate sleep at night and rest in the afternoon have been found to make patients more comfortable. Avoid sudden changes in temperature (external or internal). Heat makes these patients much worse; cold often improves them temporarily.

Rehabilitation, physical therapy, and psychotherapy are indicated in an attempt to encourage the patient to live with his disability and make the most of whatever assets he still retains.

Prognosis

The course is varied and unpredictable. In almost all cases there is a remission of the initial symptoms; but with each recurrence of a symptom the chances of remission decrease. Early remissions may be remarkably complete; later in the course of the disease remissions tend to be partial. Remissions may last several months to years.

A clinical course of 10–20 years is not uncommon. In one large series, the average survival after onset of symptoms was estimated at 27 years.

Aring CD: Pain in multiple sclerosis. JAMA 223:547, 1973.

Dean G: The multiple sclerosis problem. Sc Am 223:40, July 1970.

Gelenberg AJ, Poskanzer DC: The effect of dantrolene sodium on spasticity in multiple sclerosis. Neurology 23:1313, 1973.

Kolar OJ, Ross AT, Herman JC: Serum and cerebrospinal fluid immunoglobulins in multiple sclerosis. Neurology 20: 1052, 1970.

Kott HS: The treatment of multiple sclerosis. M Clin North America 56:711, 1972.

Kurtzke J: Diagnosis and differential diagnosis of multiple sclerosis. Acta neurol scandinav 46:484, 1970.

Rose AS: Multiple sclerosis: A clinical and theoretical review. J Neurosurg 41:279, 1974.

Rose AS & others: Cooperative study in the evaluation of therapy in multiple sclerosis: ACTH vs placebo. Neurology 20 (part 2):1, 1970.

Schneck S, Claman HN: CSF immunoglobulins in multiple sclerosis and other neurological diseases. Arch Neurol 20:132, 1969.

Sever JL: Perspectives in multiple sclerosis. Neurology 25:486, 1975.

Silberberg D, Lisak R, Zweiman B: Multiple sclerosis unaffected by azathioprine in pilot study. Arch Neurol 28:210, 1973.

PARKINSONISM
(Paralysis Agitans)

Essentials of Diagnosis

- "Pill-rolling" tremor maximal at rest, with fixed facial expression.
- Slow, shuffling, often festinating gait.
- Diminished motor power, rigidity of limb muscles upon passive motion (lead pipe or cogwheel).
- Insidious onset in 50s and 60s with slow progression.

General Considerations

Paralysis agitans is characterized by involuntary tremors, diminished motor power, and rigidity; the mental faculties are usually not affected. Onset is usually in the 50s and 60s. In most cases, a specific etiology cannot be established. The disease occurs as a complication of epidemic encephalitis, and has been known to occur in vascular disorders, neurosyphilis, and following head trauma. Reversible extrapyramidal reactions, including paralysis agitans, with gait and postural abnormalities, rigidity, tremor, salivation, and similar symptoms, may follow the use of tranquilizers such as the phenothiazines. In many cases, however, a precipitating cause is not known, and these are attributed to degeneration of the cells and tracts of the striate bodies, globus pallidus, and substantia nigra.

Clinical Findings

The onset is insidious, with increasing rigidity or tremor (or both). The rate of progression may be slow.

The facial expression may be fixed or less mobile than normal; smiling spreads and disappears slowly. The body movements generally become slower. There may be gradually increasing rigidity with diminished swaying of the arms in walking. The legs may begin to feel stiff and heavy, and excessive effort may be required to lift them from the ground in walking. A stooping posture is common, with the arms at the sides, elbows slightly flexed, and fingers abducted. Intermittent tremor (about 2–6/second) occurs which is worse when the limb is at rest. Tremors frequently are of the pill-rolling type, involving the thumb, index finger, or wrist, and are sometimes associated with a to-and-fro tremor of the head. Emotional disturbances and fatigue are apt to aggravate the tremor.

The limb muscles on passive motion are rigid (lead-pipe or cogwheel). There may be difficulty in getting out of a chair, so that several efforts or attempts to rise are made. Turning is difficult, even when standing or in bed. Movements such as adjusting a tie, buttoning the coat, and brushing the hair ultimately become impossible without assistance. Some patients have a tendency to break into a run or trot (festination gait). The voice tends to become weak, low in volume, and monotonous. Oculogyric crises may occur.

Differential Diagnosis

A. Tremor: Senile tremor is finer and more rapid, and not associated with muscular weakness or rigidity. Hysterical tremor is inconstant, increases when attention is called to the affected part, and decreases when the attention is distracted. Other hysterical symptoms are present also. Familial tremor begins early in life, is increased by voluntary motion, and may remain constant throughout life without other nervous abnormalities. The tremors of hyperthyroidism, toxic tremors (delirium tremens), and those seen in early general paralysis of syphilis are not difficult to distinguish from those of paralysis agitans.

B. Rigidity: In catatonia a fixed, rigid attitude is maintained for long periods and there are associated mental changes. The spasticity which occurs in pyramidal tract disease affects selected muscles, and is greatest at the beginning of passive motion and less as motion proceeds. In multiple arthritis there is a history of pain and evidence of a joint and not a muscle disorder.

Treatment

A. Medical Measures: (See Table 16–7.) Treatment is mainly symptomatic.

1. A number of drugs have been found to be effective in alleviating the symptoms of parkinsonism. These drugs are usually used in combination to obtain the optimal therapeutic result. Combinations such as trihexyphenidyl (Artane) and diphenhydramine (Benadryl) 3 times daily may be used initially. *Caution:* Do not stop drugs abruptly when changing to new ones. The dosage of the new drug should be increased as the other drug is gradually withdrawn.

2. Newer drugs–

a. Levodopa (Dopar, Larodopa) is effective

Table 16—7. Antiparkinsonism drugs.*

Drug	Chief Effect on				Dosage	Precautions and Remarks
	Tremor	Rigidity and Spasms	Akinesia (Weakness)	Oculogyric Crisis		
Trihexyphenidyl (Artane)		●	●	●	1—5 mg 3 times daily, starting at low dosage and slowly increasing. For oculogyric crisis, use 10 mg 3 times daily.	May precipitate acute glaucoma in elderly persons and contraindicated in patients with glaucoma. Blurred vision, dryness of mouth, vertigo, and tachycardia are early toxic symptoms; late symptoms are vomiting, dizziness, mental confusion, and hallucinations. The synthetic drugs are apt to cause more dizziness than the natural alkaloids and are somewhat less potent parasympatholytics.
Biperiden (Akineton)		●		●	2 mg 3—4 times daily.	
Procyclidine (Kemadrin)		●			2.5—5 mg 3 times daily after meals.	
Cycrimine (Pagitane)		●	●	●	1.25—5 mg 3—4 times daily. Dosage may be gradually increased up to the limits of tolerance.	Useful when effects of trihexyphenidyl wear off. Other remarks as for atropine.
Benztropine methanesulfonate (Cogentin)	●	●			0.5 mg 1—2 times daily, increasing by 0.5 mg at intervals of several days to 5 mg daily or toxicity. Often most effective as single dose at bedtime.	Side-effects similar to those of atropine. Best effect by combining with trihexyphenidyl or dextroamphetamine.
Diphenhydramine (Benadryl)	●				50 mg 2—4 times daily.	Reduce dosage if transient drowsiness occurs.
Orphenadrine (Disipal)	●	●			50 mg 3—4 times daily.	
Chlorphenoxamine (Phenoxene)		●			50 mg 3—4 times daily.	Valuable adjunct to other drugs.
Ethopropazine (Parsidol, Lysivane)	●	●			25—30 mg 4 times daily.	May be used in conjunction with other antispasmodic drugs. Drug is related to chlorpromazine; precaution as for this class of drugs.
Dextroamphetamine sulfate (Dexedrine)			●		5 mg morning or noon.	CNS stimulant to be used with caution in cardiac patients.
Levodopa (Dopar, Larodopa, Levopa)	●	●	●		250 mg 3 times daily. Increase to tolerance (4—8 gm daily).	Nausea, vomiting, postural hypotension, choreiform movements.
Amantadine (Symmetrel)	●	●	●		100 mg twice daily.	Jitteriness, insomnia, depression, confusion, hallucinations.

*Modified and reproduced, with permission, from Chusid JG: *Correlative Neuroanatomy & Functional Neurology*, 15th ed. Lange, 1973.

against the akinesia and rigidity of parkinsonism and, to a lesser extent, tremor. Capsules (250 mg) are given 3–4 times daily and increased to tolerance over several weeks or until significant effects are noted. Maximum daily dosage ranges from 4–8 gm. Side-effects—including nausea, vomiting, postural hypotension, cardiac dysrhythmia, and choreiform movements—may respond to adjustment of dosage.

The use of a peripheral decarboxylase inhibitor (carbidopa) in combination with levodopa permits a great reduction in the levodopa dosage required for optimal clinical response. Sinemet is a combination of levodopa and carbidopa recently introduced.

b. Amantadine hydrochloride (Symmetrel)—This antiviral agent for A_2 (Asian) influenza may be effective against akinesia, rigidity, and tremor of parkinsonism. The daily dosage is 200 mg (100 mg twice daily). Side-effects, which may be controlled by adjusting the dosage or concomitant medication, include insomnia, jitteriness, abdominal distress, dizziness, depression, confusion, hallucinations, and livedo reticularis.

B. Surgical Measures: In carefully selected patients, surgical destruction of portions of the globus pallidus or the ventrolateral nucleus of the thalamus has proved highly beneficial.

C. General Measures: Physical therapy should include massage, stretching of muscles, and active exercise when possible. The patient should be taught to exercise daily the muscles most severely affected, especially those of the hands, fingers, wrists, elbows, knees, and neck.

Reassurance and psychologic support are of decided value, stressing the positive aspects of the disease: (1) symptomatic relief with drugs, (2) no impairment of mental faculties, (3) slow progression over many years, and (4) active research and the hope of therapeutic breakthroughs.

Avoid barbiturates. Permit moderate use of alcohol to relax tension. Nonbarbiturate sedatives (eg, meprobamate, not phenothiazines) may be of value.

Prognosis

The disease is usually slowly progressive; the patient may live for many years.

With increased disability, patients are apt to become depressed, anxious, and emotionally disturbed.

Treatment with drugs may produce amelioration of complaints. In selected patients, operative treatment (pallidotomy, thalamotomy) may produce significant improvement of tremor and rigidity. The effect of long-term therapy with newer drugs such as levodopa and amantadine is under current study.

Celesia JJ, Barr AN: Psychoses and other psychiatric manifestations of levodopa therapy. Arch Neurol 23:193, 1970.

Cotzias GC: Levodopa in the treatment of parkinsonism. JAMA 218:1903, 1971.

Mars H: Levodopa, carbidopa and pyridoxine in Parkinson's disease. Arch Neurol 30:444, 1974.

Martin WE & others: Parkinson's disease. Neurology 23:783, 1973.

McDowell FH (editor): Symposium on levodopa in Parkinson's disease. Neurology 22 (part 2):1, 1972.

Pollock M, Hornabrook RW: The prevalence, natural history and dementia of Parkinson's disease. Brain 89:429, 1966.

Schwab RS & others: Amantadine in the treatment of Parkinson's disease. JAMA 208:1168, 1969.

Yahr MD, Duvoisin RC: Drug therapy in parkinsonism. New England J Med 287:20, 1972.

HEPATOLENTICULAR DEGENERATION
(Wilson's Disease)

Wilson's disease is a familial disorder characterized by clinical findings of basal ganglia disease and accompanied by cirrhosis of the liver and usually a greenish-brown corneal pigmentation (Kayser-Fleischer ring). A metabolic disturbance has been implicated because of the increased excretion of copper and amino acids in the urine and the decrease in ceruloplasmin of serum. The cerebellum, cerebral cortex, and other parts of the nervous system may also be affected. The onset of symptoms is insidious, usually between the ages of 11 and 25 years.

Tremors and rigidity are the commonest early symptoms. Tremors are apt to be of the intention or alternating type; bizarre "wing-beating" of the upper extremities is accentuated by extension of these parts. The rigidity resembles paralysis agitans.

Dimercaprol (BAL) has been reported to be effective in removing the excessive copper and presumably impeding the progress of the disease. The clinically useful dose is 2.5 mg/kg IM twice daily in courses of 10–12 days every other month. Penicillamine (Cuprimine) is an effective chelating agent suitable for oral administration, and may far surpass the effect of BAL in increasing excretion of copper. Some of the specific manifestations may be palliated by symptomatic therapy.

The course is progressive, with partial remissions and exacerbations until death occurs (usually within 10 years). The full effect of dimercaprol or penicillamine therapy on the course or longevity has not as yet been determined.

Denny-Brown D: Hepatolenticular degeneration (Wilson's disease): Two different components. New England J Med 270:1149, 1964.

Goldstein NP & others: Wilson's disease (hepatolenticular degeneration). Arch Neurol 24:391, 1971.

Richmond J & others: Hepatolenticular degeneration (Wilson's disease) treated by penicillamine. Brain 87:619, 1964.

Sternlieb I, Scheinberg IH: Pencillamine therapy for hepatolenticular degeneration. JAMA 189:784, 1964.

Sternlieb I, Scheinberg IH: Prevention of Wilson's disease in asymptomatic patients. New England J Med 278:352, 1968.

Symposium on copper metabolism and Wilson's disease. Mayo Clin Proc 49:361, 1974.

CHRONIC PROGRESSIVE (HUNTINGTON'S) CHOREA

Huntington's chorea is a hereditary disease of the basal ganglia and cortex, characterized by the onset in adult life of choreiform movements and mental deterioration. Many cases in America have been traced to 2 brothers who emigrated to Long Island from England. The movements are abrupt and jerky, though less rapid and lightning-like than those of Sydenham's chorea. Any somatic musculature may be involved. The disease is chronically progressive and usually leads to death in about 15 years.

Treatment is symptomatic. Tranquilizers such as reserpine, phenothiazines, or haloperidol are helpful in management.

Bird MT, Paulson GW: The rigid form of Huntington's chorea. Neurology 21:271, 1971.
Duvoisin R: Clinical diagnosis of the dyskinesias. M Clin North America 56:1321, 1972.
Klawans HL, Rubovits R: Central cholinergic-anticholinergic antagonism in Huntington's chorea. Neurology 22:107, 1972.
Klawans H & others: Use of L-dopa in the detection of presymptomatic Huntington's chorea. New England J Med 286:1332, 1972.
Siegel GJ, Mones RJ: Modification of choreiform activity by haloperidol. JAMA 216:675, 1971.
Whittier JR, Heimler A, Korenyi C: The psychiatrist and Huntington's disease. Am J Psychiat 128:1546, 1972.

SYDENHAM'S CHOREA (St. Vitus' Dance)

Essentials of Diagnosis
- Quick, jerky, involuntary, irregular movements of the face, trunk, and extremities.
- Gait and speech often markedly impaired.
- Irritability, restlessness, and emotional instability.
- Mild muscular weakness, hypotonia.
- Associated rheumatic fever or residuals.

General Considerations
Sydenham's chorea is seen mostly in young persons and is characterized by involuntary irregular movements, incoordination of voluntary movements, mild muscle weakness, and emotional disturbance. The disorder is usually (but not always) associated with rheumatic fever and is considered to be one of its sequels; other clinical evidence of rheumatic fever is apt to be present.

Clinical Findings
The patient becomes irritable, excitable, restless, and sleepless. Grimacing, clumsy movements, and stumbling frequently occur. Involuntary dysrhythmic movements of the face, trunk, and extremities occur with varying severity. These are sudden, quick, short, and jerky. Gait and speech may be affected. Voluntary movement and excitement may aggravate the involuntary movements. Affected limbs may be weak and hypotonic.

Clinical evidence of rheumatic fever or rheumatic heart disease is often present, the latter sometimes evident only late in the course of the disease.

Differential Diagnosis
Distinguish from tics or habit spasms, which are usually manifested as facial grimacing with blinking, smacking of lips, and clicking noises, and in which there is no difficulty in articulation, no associated muscle weakness, and no evidence of rheumatic fever; and from Huntington's chorea, which is a progressive hereditary disease of adult life characterized by chorea and mental deterioration and usually leads to death in about 15 years.

Treatment
Corticosteroids and corticotropin may shorten the course and suppress the rheumatic manifestations. Sedatives (such as phenobarbital) or tranquilizers (such as phenothiazines or haloperidol) are helpful in suppressing the involuntary movements of chorea.

Prognosis
The acute phase of chorea usually runs a limited course, with maximum symptoms 2–3 weeks after onset. Gradual recovery occurs in about 2–3 months.

Aron AM, Freeman JM, Carter S: The natural history of Sydenham's chorea. Am J Med 38:83, 1965.
Kurland HD: Symptomatic control of Sydenham's chorea. Internat J Neuropsychiat 1:152, 1965.
Tierney RC & others: Treatment of Sydenham's chorea. Am J Dis child 109:408, 1965.

COMBINED SYSTEM DISEASE (Posterolateral Sclerosis)

Essentials of Diagnosis
- Numbness, "pins and needles," tenderness, weakness, feeling of heaviness of toes, feet, fingers, and hands.
- Stocking and glove distribution of sensory loss; extensor plantar response, hyperreflexia, flexor spasms; flaccid paralysis and hyporeflexia less often; loss of position and vibratory sense.
- Memory defects or psychotic states.
- Associated blood and gastric findings of pernicious anemia.

General Considerations

Posterolateral sclerosis is a progressive degeneration of the posterior and lateral columns of the spinal cord, sometimes with degeneration of the peripheral nerves. The middle and older age groups are most often affected.

Although posterolateral sclerosis is usually associated with pernicious anemia, its severity does not necessarily parallel the degree of anemia, which suggests that the causes of spinal cord and blood changes may not be the same. Degeneration of the spinal cord may develop before clinical manifestations of pernicious anemia.

Clinical Findings

Tingling, numbness, and "pins and needles" sensations in the toes and feet and later in the fingers are the first symptoms. Sensations of swelling, coldness, and wetness of the feet may occur. Weakness of the legs, fatigue, a feeling of heaviness in the feet, and unsteady gait are common. Dyspnea on exertion with recurrent episodes of dizziness may be produced by the anemia; gastric distress may result from achlorhydria.

In the **flaccid** type the involvement is principally of the peripheral nerves, manifested as follows: weakness of the lower extremities (especially of the distal segments), tenderness of the soles and calf muscles, stocking distribution impairment of touch sensibility in the lower extremities up to knee level, loss of appreciation of vibratory sensation, ataxia, a positive Romberg sign, depression or absence of knee and ankle jerks, and extensor plantar responses. In the **spastic** type spinal cord signs, especially of the lateral columns, predominate: increased deep tendon reflexes, clonus and hypertonicity of muscles, and flexor spasms with progressive weakness. Paraplegia in flexion may follow. When sensory losses become more severe, loss of sphincter control and decubiti may occur.

Mental symptoms may also be present, even early in the disease. Apathy, mental dullness, hypomania, paranoid states, hallucinations, disorientation, and memory defects have been reported.

Laboratory findings are as for pernicious anemia.

Differential Diagnosis

The presence of macrocytic anemia and achlorhydria usually makes the diagnosis more certain, but it may be necessary to distinguish from the familial ataxias, tabes dorsalis, multiple sclerosis, myelitis, and spinal compression by tumor.

Treatment

Treat as for pernicious anemia.

Prognosis

With adequate treatment of pernicious anemia, improvement, especially of peripheral nerve involvement, may occur. Little improvement can be expected when the spinal cord is severely affected.

Paresthesias and sensory changes may persist even in those treated intensively, early, and fully.

The prognosis is worse in patients over 60 years of age.

Baker SA, Bogoch A: Subacute combined degeneration of the spinal cord after ileal resection and folic acid administration in Crohn's disease. Neurology 23:40, 1973.

Robertson DM, Dinsdale HB, Campbell RJ: Subacute combined degeneration of the spinal cord. Arch Neurol 24:203, 1971.

Weir DG, Gatenby PBB: Subacute combined degeneration of the cord after partial gastrectomy. Brit MJ 2:1175, 1963.

Wertalik LF & others: Decreased serum B_{12} levels with oral contraceptive use. JAMA 221:1371, 1972.

See also references under Multiple Sclerosis.

DISORDERS OF CRANIAL NERVES

TRIGEMINAL (TRIFACIAL) NEURALGIA
(Tic Douloureux)

Trigeminal neuralgia is characterized by a sudden attack of excruciating pain of short duration along the distribution of the 5th cranial nerve. The attack is often precipitated by stimulation (usually mild) of a "trigger zone" in the area of the pain, and is characterized by recurrent paroxysms of sharp, stabbing pains in the distribution of one or more branches of the nerve. The onset is usually in middle or late life, and the incidence is higher in women. The pain may be described as searing or burning, occurring in lightning-like jabs, lasting only 1–2 minutes or as long as 15 minutes. The frequency of attacks varies from many times daily to several times a month or a year. The patient often tries to immobilize his face during conversation, or attempts to swallow food without chewing in order not to irritate the trigger zone.

Treatment

A. Medical Treatment: Medical treatment includes the following:

1. Carbamazepine (Tegretol)—This tricyclic drug is remarkably effective in relieving and preventing the pain of trigeminal neuralgia. The dose may vary from 0.2–1.2 gm/day. Observe carefully for evidence of serious hematologic and cutaneous reactions.

2. Anticonvulsants, eg, phenytoin sodium (Dilantin), 0.1 gm 4 times daily, may be beneficial in some cases.

3. Massive doses of vitamin B_{12} (1 mg IM daily for 10 days) have been reported to relieve the severe pain.

4. Alcohol injection of the ganglion or the branches of the trigeminal nerve may produce analgesia

and relief from pain for several months or years. Repeated injections may be required at later intervals.

B. Surgical Measures: Surgery may be required if medical treatment gives no relief.

Percutaneous electrocoagulation of the preganglionic rootlets under local anesthesia is an effective and relatively benign mode of treatment of resistant cases of trigeminal neuralgia.

Prognosis

In most cases the paroxysms of pain are present for several weeks or months. Remissions may last from a few days to as long as several months or years. As patients become older, remissions tend to become shorter.

Graham JG, Zilkha KJ: Treatment of trigeminal neuralgia with carbamazepine: A follow-up study. Brit MJ 1:210, 1966.
Henderson WR: Trigeminal neuralgia: The pain and its treatment. Brit MJ 1:7, 1967.
Killian JM, Fromm GH: Carbamazepine in the treatment of neuralgia. Arch Neurol 19:129, 1968.
Onofrio BM: Radiofrequency percutaneous Gasserian ganglion lesions. J Neurosurg 42:132, 1975.
Rushton JG: Medical treatment of trigeminal neuralgia, with a note on the results of alcohol injection. M Clin North America 52:797, 1968.
Sweet WH, Wepsic JA: Controlled thermocoagulation of trigeminal ganglion and rootlets for differential destruction of pain fibers. Part 1. Trigeminal neuralgia. J Neurosurg 40:143, 1974.
Wepsic JA: Tic douloureux: Etiology, refined treatment. New England J Med 288:680, 1973.

BELL'S PALSY
(Peripheral Facial Paralysis)

Bell's palsy is a paralysis of the muscles of one side of the face, sometimes precipitated by exposure, chill, or trauma. It may occur at any age, but is slightly more common in the age group from 20 to 50.

Assure the patient that recovery usually occurs in 2–8 weeks (or up to 1–2 years in older patients). Keep the face warm and avoid further exposure, especially to wind and dust. Protect the eye with a patch if necessary. Support the face with tape or wire anchored at the angle of the mouth and looped about the ear. Electric stimulation (every other day after the 14th day) may be used to help prevent muscle atrophy. Gentle upward massage of the involved muscles for 5–10 minutes 2–3 times daily may help to maintain muscle tone. Heat from an infra-red lamp may hasten recovery.

Prednisone therapy (40 mg daily for 4 days and tapering to 8 mg in 8 days) has been reported to be effective.

In the vast majority of cases, partial or complete recovery occurs. When recovery is partial, contractures may develop on the paralyzed side. Recurrence on the same or the opposite side is occasionally reported.

Adour KK, Wingard J: Idiopathic facial paralysis (Bell's palsy): Factors affecting severity and outcome in 446 patients. Neurology 24:1112, 1974.
Adour KK & others: Prednisone treatment for idiopathic facial paralysis (Bell's palsy). New England J Med 287:1268, 1972.
Conley J: Treatment of facial paralysis. S Clin North America 51:403, 1971.
Hauser WA & others: Incidence and prognosis of Bell's palsy in the population of Rochester, Minn. Mayo Clin Proc 46:258, 1971.
Manning JJ, Adour KK: Facial paralysis in children. Pediatrics 49:102, 1972.
Wilkins RH, Brody IA: Bell's palsy and Bell's phenomenon. Arch Neurol 21:661, 1969.

DISORDERS OF PERIPHERAL NERVES

POLYNEURITIS
(Multiple Neuritis, Peripheral Neuritis, Peripheral Neuropathy)

Essentials of Diagnosis

- Slowly progressive muscular weakness, paresthesias, tenderness, and pain, mostly of distal portions of extremities.
- Stocking and glove hypesthesia or anesthesia, especially for vibratory sense.
- Hyporeflexia or areflexia.
- Muscular wasting of affected parts.

General Considerations

Polyneuritis is a syndrome characterized by widespread sensory and motor disturbances of peripheral nerves. It may appear at any age, although it is most common in young or middle-aged adults, especially in men. In most cases a noninflammatory degeneration of the peripheral nerves is present.

Polyneuritis may be caused by (1) chronic intoxications (eg, alcohol, carbon disulfide, benzene, phosphorus, sulfonamides); (2) infections (eg, meningitis, diphtheria, syphilis, tuberculosis, pneumonia, Guillain-Barré syndrome, mumps); (3) metabolic causes (eg, diabetes mellitus, gout, pregnancy, rheumatism, porphyria, polyarteritis nodosa, lupus erythematosus); (4) nutritional causes (eg, beriberi, vitamin deficiencies, cachectic states); and (5) malignancies.

Clinical Findings

Symptoms usually develop slowly over a period of weeks. Notable exceptions with rapid onset may occur in infections plus alcoholic polyneuritis. Pains, tenderness, paresthesias, weakness and fatigability, and sensory impairment may be present. The pains may be mild or, occasionally, burning and sharp. Muscular weakness is usually greatest in the distal portions of the extremities. Impaired sensory perception, especially of vibration, is frequent; in alcoholic and arsenical polyneuritis, severe and extensive sensory defects may occur. The cutaneous sensory defect may consist of hypesthesia or anesthesia in an irregular stocking or glove distribution.

Tendon reflexes are usually depressed or absent. With paralyzed toes, the plantar response may be absent; with weak abdominal muscles, abdominal skin reflexes may be diminished or absent. Flaccid weakness and muscular atrophy of affected parts may occur, especially in the distal portions of the extremities. Foot drop with associated steppage gait may result.

Trophic changes of the skin of the extremities are manifested by a glossy red skin and impairment of the sweating mechanism. Muscles and nerves may be tender and hypersensitive to pressure and palpation.

Differential Diagnosis

Differentiate from neuritis involving only a single nerve and its distribution; tabes dorsalis, which is not associated with muscular atrophy or nerve tenderness; acute anterior poliomyelitis, with systemic as well as neurologic manifestations; and myositis, in which there is no nerve involvement and usually no sensory or reflex changes.

Treatment

A. Specific Measures: Remove from exposure to toxic agents (eg, alcohol, lead). In lead polyneuritis, calcium disodium edetate (Versenate) may be beneficial. In arsenical polyneuritis, give dimercaprol (BAL).

Give a high caloric diet with liberal use of vitamins, especially B complex. The entire B complex can be administered with thiamine hydrochloride, 15 mg 3–4 times daily orally or parenterally.

B. General Measures: Place the patient at bed rest and forbid use of the affected limb. If a lower extremity is affected, keep a cradle over the foot of the bed to prevent pressure of bed covers. Give analgesics as necessary to control pain. After pain has subsided, massage and passive motion may be of value. Encourage active motion at the same time. Prevent contractures by means of splints and passive stretching.

Prognosis

In most forms of polyneuritis, recovery may occur once the cause has been corrected. In some cases the disorder progresses for weeks, remains stationary for a time, and goes on to slow recovery in 6–12 months. Objective sensory changes usually disappear first, and paralyses later; dysesthesias may persist during recovery.

Dyck PJ: Peripheral neuropathy: Changing concepts, differential diagnosis, and classification. M Clin North America 52:895, 1968.
Gibberd FB: Ophthalmoplegia in acute polyneuritis. Arch Neurol 23:161, 1970.
Howard FM Jr: Peripheral neuropathy as a sign of systemic disease. Postgrad Med 50:107, 1971.
Matthews WB, Howell DA, Hughes RC: Relapsing corticosteroid-dependent polyneuritis. J Neurol Neurosurg Psychiat 33:330, 1970.
Pleasure DE, Lovelace RE, Duvoisin RC: The prognosis of acute polyneuritis. Neurology 18:1143, 1968.
Pleasure DE, Towfighi J: Onion bulb neuropathies. Arch Neurol 26:289, 1972.
Sibley WA: Polyneuritis. M Clin North America 56:1299, 1972.
Toole JM, Parrish ML: Nitrofurantoin polyneuropathy. Neurology 23:554, 1973.
Tsairis P, Dyck PJ, Mulder DW: Natural history of brachial plexus neuropathy. Arch Neurol 27:109, 1972.

LANDRY-GUILLAIN-BARRÉ SYNDROME

In the Landry Guillain-Barré syndrome, patients may often develop polyneuritis a week or 2 after a mild upper respiratory infection or gastroenteritis. Early lower extremity weakness extends within a few days to the upper extremities and face. Facial diplegia, dysphagia, or dysarthria commonly occurs. Weakness of trunk and extremity muscles may be severe; flaccid paraplegia and respiratory muscle weakness requiring a respirator may occur.

Sensory changes usually are not present, but muscle tenderness and nerve sensitivity to pressure may occur. Symptoms may progress over a week to several weeks with variable prognosis. Death may occur due to respiratory failure or intermittent infection within a few weeks after onset. Gradual recovery may take days to weeks; the duration of paralysis in untreated cases is variable.

The cerebrospinal fluid usually shows "albuminocytologic dissociation," especially at the height of the disorder when the total protein may be several hundred mg/100 ml with few or no white cells. Alteration in the immune response of peripheral nerves has been suggested, with hypersensitivity or autoimmune response of nerves leading to demyelination and often a mononuclear inflammatory reaction of nerves. Although good results have been reported after intensive treatment with corticosteroids, many clinicians doubt the effectiveness of such treatment.

Asbury AK, Arnason BG, Adams RD: The inflammatory lesions in idiopathic polyneuritis. Medicine 48:173, 1969.
Eisen A, Humphreys P: The Guillain-Barré syndrome. Arch Neurol 30:438, 1974.
Haymaker W, Kernohan JW: The Landry-Guillain-Barré syndrome. Medicine 28:59, 1949.
Leneman G: The Guillain-Barré syndrome: Definition, etiology, and review of 1100 cases. Arch Int Med 118:139, 1966.
Wisniewski H & others: Landry-Guillain-Barré syndrome. Arch Neurol 21:269, 1969.

PERIPHERAL NERVE INJURIES

Peripheral nerve injuries, ranging from simple contusions causing temporary dysfunction to complete anatomic section causing total cessation of function, may occur with lacerations, bone fractures, crushing injuries, or penetrating wounds. In the acute early phase, associated tissue damage, pain, and other circumstances may interfere with tests of motor or sensory function. Tinel's sign (a tingling sensation in the distribution of an affected nerve) may be elicited after the acute phase by percussion of the nerve or adjacent areas. In some old nerve injuries, trophic changes affecting the nails and skin, as well as painless skin ulcers, may be noted. Electrodiagnostic tests may be helpful in assessing the degree and nature of the neural deficit.

Treatment depends upon many factors, including the time and type of nerve injury, associated defects, and the general condition of the patient. When possible, end-to-end anastomosis of acutely severed nerves should be attempted. In old nerve injuries, good results are possible as long as 1–2 years after injury, when lysis of a scar, resection of a neuroma, nerve transplants, and other surgical procedures may be attempted.

Baker AG, Winegarner FG: Causalgia. Am J Surg 117:690, 1969.

Chase RA: Surgery of the hand. New England J Med 287:1174, 1972.

Chusid JG: Yoga foot drop JAMA 217:827, 1971.

Cracchiolo A III, Marmor L: Peripheral entrapment neuropathies. JAMA 204:431, 1968.

Edshage S: Peripheral nerve injuries: Diagnosis and treatment. New England J Med 278:1431, 1968.

Phalen GS: The carpal tunnel syndrome: Seventeen years' experience in diagnosis and treatment of 654 hands. J Bone Joint Surg 48A:211, 1966.

Sakellarides H: A follow-up study of 172 peripheral nerve injuries in the upper extremity in civilians. J Bone Joint Surg 44A:140, 1962.

NEUROMUSCULAR DISORDERS

The neuromuscular disorders include a number of chronic diseases which are characterized by a progressive weakness and atrophy of certain groups of muscles. It is important to differentiate atrophies from dystrophies: Muscular **atrophies** result from a neural lesion, involving either the cell body or axon of the lower motor neuron; muscular **dystrophies** result from primary disease of the muscle itself.

Aird RB: Disorders of the peripheral motor system. Postgrad Med 40:578, 1966.

Engel WK: Muscle biopsies in neuromuscular disease. P Clin North America 14:963, 1967.

Samaha FJ: Electrodiagnostic studies in neuromuscular disease. New England J Med 285:1244, 1971.

Walton JN: Diseases of muscle. (2 parts.) Abstr World Med 40:1, 81, 1966.

PROGRESSIVE MUSCULAR ATROPHIES
(Motor Neuron Disease)

The progressive muscular atrophies are due to nuclear involvement of the lower motor neuron by progressive lesions. Since the causative agent is usually not known, the classification has been based upon the level of involvement rather than upon etiology. There is no effective treatment.

Aran-Duchenne Atrophy
(Myelopathic Muscular Atrophy)

This is the adult form of progressive spinal muscular atrophy. It is a rare disorder of middle age, starting in the small hand muscles with atrophy and fibrillations and slowly extending to involve the arm, shoulder, and trunk muscles. A degenerative lesion is found in the cervical gray matter of the cord. It may occur as the first stage of an amyotrophic lateral sclerosis (see below).

Werdnig-Hoffman Paralysis

This is a hereditary form of progressive spinal muscular atrophy occurring in infants, starting in the pelvic girdle and thighs and spreading to the extremities. Associated adiposity may produce a pseudohypertrophy.

True Bulbar Palsy

This type is caused by a nuclear involvement of the last 4 or 5 cranial nerves and characterized by twitchings and atrophy of the tongue, palate, and larynx, drooling, dysarthria, dysphagia, and finally respiratory paralysis. True bulbar palsy is usually a manifestation of amyotrophic lateral sclerosis.

Table 16—8. Differential diagnosis of atrophies and dystrophies.

Atrophies	Dystrophies
Generally occur late in life	Usually occur in childhood
Affect distal muscle groups, eg, the small muscles of the hand	Affect the proximal muscle groups, eg, the hip and shoulder girdle
Show fasciculations	No fasciculations
May show spastic phenomena	No spastic phenomena
No familial incidence	Generally familial

Amyotrophic Lateral Sclerosis

This is a combined upper and lower motor neuron lesion which may involve either the spinal or bulbar level, or both. It is a chronic progressive disease of unknown etiology associated with fibrillation and atrophy of the somatic musculature. It is predominantly a disease of middle life, with onset usually between the ages of 40 and 60 years. Degeneration of the motor cells of the spinal cord and brain stem and, to a lesser extent, of the motor cortex may occur, with secondary degeneration of the lateral and ventral portions of the spinal cord. There may be spastic weakness of the trunk and extremities, with associated hyperactive deep reflexes and extensor plantar responses. If the fibers of the bulbar nuclei become involved, pseudobulbar or bulbar paralysis may appear. The initial symptom is often weakness and wasting of the extremities (usually the upper extremities). The course is progressively downhill without remission. The average duration of life from the appearance of the first symptoms is about 3 years.

Neural Form of Peroneal Muscular Atrophy: Charcot-Marie-Tooth Disease

This relatively rare disease is characterized by clubbing of the feet and muscular wasting which begins in the legs and later involves the muscles of the distal portions of the thighs and upper extremities. Atrophy of the leg muscles gives a characteristic "stork-leg" appearance; atrophy usually starts in the intrinsic muscles of the feet and in the peroneal muscles. The onset of symptoms is usually before 20 years of age, but is sometimes delayed until 40 or 50 years. Objective loss of sensation occasionally occurs.

Bobowick AR, Brody JA: Epidemiology of motor neurone disease. New England J Med 288:1047, 1973.

Brody JA & others: Inosiplex and amyotrophic lateral sclerosis. Arch Neurol 30:322, 1974.

Currier RD, Haerer AF: Amyotrophic lateral sclerosis and metallic toxins. Arch Envir Health 17:712, 1968.

Eaton LM & others: Symposium: Amyotrophic lateral sclerosis. Mayo Clin Proc 32:425, 1957.

Edgar AH, Brody JA, Detels R: Amyotrophic lateral sclerosis among native-born and migrant residents. Neurology 23:48, 1973.

Jammes JL: The autonomic nervous system in peroneal muscular atrophy. Arch Neurol 27:213, 1972.

Metcalf CW, Hirano A: Amyotrophic lateral sclerosis. Arch Neurol 24:518, 1971.

Norris FH & others: The administration of guanidine in amyotrophic lateral sclerosis. Neurology 74:721, 1974.

Störtebecker P & others: Vascular and metabolic studies of amyotrophic lateral sclerosis. Neurology 20:1157, 1970.

Yase Y: The pathogenesis of amyotrophic lateral sclerosis. Lancet 2:292, 1972.

PROGRESSIVE MUSCULAR DYSTROPHY

Essentials of Diagnosis

- Onset usually in childhood or at puberty of weakness of the proximal musculature of the extremities.
- Waddling gait and "climbing up" on body to attain upright position.
- Contractures, scoliosis, lordosis, diminished deep tendon reflexes.
- Involved muscle hypertrophic or atrophic.
- Heredofamilial trend.

General Considerations

The most common of the muscular diseases is progressive muscular dystrophy. Three principal types are recognized, depending upon the site of initial muscular involvement and the distribution of apparent hypertrophy and atrophy. In the pseudohypertrophic type (Duchenne), there is enlargement of the calves and sometimes the thighs. In the facioscapulohumeral type (Landouzy-Déjerine), the face and shoulder girdle are involved early. In the limb-girdle type (Erb), the shoulder and pelvic girdle are involved.

The cause is not known. A heredofamilial trend is usually noted. Various types of inheritance may occur: simple dominant, simple recessive, or X-linked recessive.

Clinical Findings

A. Symptoms and Signs:

1. Pseudohypertrophic type (Duchenne)—This type occurs in early youth and is characterized by bulky calf and forearm muscles, which, however, are quite soft as a result of infiltration by fat and fibrous tissue; and progressive atrophy and weakness of the thigh, hip, and back muscles and shoulder girdle. It usually occurs in males and rarely in females, with onset in the first 3 years of life. It is considered to be X-linked and recessive, with a high mutation rate (rarely, autosomal recessive). Symmetric early involvement of the pelvic girdle muscles and, later, of the shoulder girdle muscles occurs. In about 80% of cases there is pseudohypertrophy, particularly of the calf muscles but sometimes of the quadriceps and deltoids. Steady and rapid progression usually leads to inability to walk within 10 years. The gait becomes waddling, and there is difficulty in going up or down stairs. In rising from a recumbent position the patient does so laboriously by "climbing up upon himself." When an effort is made to lift the patient by his armpits, the loose shoulder girdle permits his head to slip through the examiner's hands. Lordosis frequently develops from the weakness of the trunk muscles. Late in the disease the patient becomes too weak to move or support himself. Progressive deformity with muscular contractures, skeletal distortion, and atrophy results. Death from inanition, respiratory infection, or cardiac failure usually occurred in the second decade of life in the past; but with current antibiotic, supportive, and intensive care, patients often reach the middle years.

2. **Facioscapulohumeral type (Landouzy-Déjerine)**—Atrophy begins early in life and affects the muscles of the face, shoulder girdle, and upper arms; the muscles of the forearms are not involved. It occurs in either sex, with onset at any age from childhood until late adult life. It is transmitted usually as an autosomal dominant, occasionally with sex limitation. Abortive cases are common. Initially, the face and shoulder girdle muscles are involved and later the pelvic girdle muscles. Muscular pseudohypertrophy, contractions, and skeletal deformity are the rule. The characteristic facial involvement, with drooping of the eyelids, is known as "myopathic facies" and the thickened overhanging lip as "tapir lip." The weakened shoulder girdle causes "winging" of the scapula. The absence of forearm involvement gives a "Popeye the sailor" appearance. The disease progresses insidiously with prolonged periods of apparent arrest, and most patients survive and remain active to a normal age.

3. **Limb-girdle type (Erb)**—This form of muscular dystrophy involves the shoulder and pelvic girdles. The face is not affected. It occurs in either sex, with onset usually in the second or third decade but occasionally late in the first decade or in middle life. It is usually transmitted as an autosomal recessive characteristic. Primary involvement of either shoulder girdle or pelvic girdle muscle is noted, with spread to the other after a variable period. Muscular pseudohypertrophy occurs uncommonly. Abortive or static cases are uncommon. Variable severity and rate of progression may occur, but severe disability usually is present 20 years after onset. Muscular contractions and skeletal deformity come on late in the course of the disease. Most patients become severely disabled in middle life, and the life span is shortened.

B. Laboratory Findings: Biopsy of muscle may show typical degenerative changes. EMG may show changes characteristic of myopathy. Serum enzymes (creatine phosphokinase, transaminases, aldolase) may be elevated.

Differential Diagnosis

Progressive muscular atrophy develops later in life, beginning distally in the small muscles of the hand. Muscular fibrillation is present.

Dystrophic myotonia involves the sternomastoids, which are rarely affected in other dystrophies, and there is associated myotonia.

Progressive hypertrophic polyneuritis is characterized by distal involvement, sensory changes, and a thickened nerve.

Complications & Sequelae

Contractures commonly occur in the advanced stages. Pes equinus is due to calf muscle contracture.

Respiratory complications, such as pneumonia, are apt to occur. There may be clinical or laboratory evidence of cardiac disease, probably due to intrinsic dystrophy of the myocardium.

Treatment

Supportive measures, physical therapy, and orthopedic devices may give some help and comfort.

Prognosis

The disease is usually progressive and greatly resistant to medical therapy. Patients may continue to show progression for 20—30 years. Patients become progressively weaker, ultimately being confined to chairs or beds.

Jackson CE, Strehler DA: Limb-girdle muscular dystrophy: Clinical manifestations and detection of preclinical disease. Pediatrics 41:495, 1968.

Majora A, Lauberman H: Ocular myopathy. Arch Neurol 20:1, 1969.

McComas AJ & others: Multiple muscle analysis of motor units in muscular dystrophy. Arch Neurol 30:249, 1974.

Pearson CM & others: Skeletal muscle: Basic and clinical aspects and illustrative new diseases. Ann Int Med 67:614, 1967.

Penn AS, Lisak RP, Rowland LP: Muscular dystrophy in young girls. Neurology 20:147, 1970.

MYASTHENIA GRAVIS

Essentials of Diagnosis

- Weakness of the bulbar-innervated musculature, progressing as muscles are used (fatigue).
- Lid ptosis, diplopia, facial weakness; weakness in chewing, swallowing, and speaking.
- Positive neostigmine (Prostigmin) and edrophonium chloride (Tensilon) tests.

General Considerations

This disorder, characterized by marked weakness and fatigability of muscles, is believed to affect the motor apparatus at the myoneural junction. Although almost any muscle in the body may be affected, the disease shows a special affinity for muscles innervated by the bulbar nuclei (face, lips, eyes, tongue, throat, and neck). The cause is essentially unknown, although some investigators consider myasthenia gravis to be a metabolic disorder. Dysfunction at the myoneural junction with rapid splitting and inactivation of acetylcholine has been inferred.

Pathologic examination has failed to demonstrate consistent specific changes in the CNS, peripheral nerves, or muscles. Abnormalities of the thymus gland, including enlargement and tumor formation, have been described in some patients. It has been suggested that myasthenia gravis is an autoimmune disease since multiple auto-antibodies (including antiskeletal muscle antibody) have been found in patient's sera.

Clinical Findings

A. Symptoms and Signs: There is usually pronounced fatigability of muscles, with consequent weakness and paralysis. The muscles innervated by the bulbar nuclei are especially susceptible. Weakness of the extraocular muscles results in diplopia and strabismus. Ptosis of the eyelids may become most apparent late in the day. Speech and swallowing difficulties may be recognized after prolonged exercise of these functions. Difficulty in the use of the tongue and a high-pitched, nasal voice may be present. A snarling, nasal ("myasthenic") smile may be evident.

The disease appears most commonly in women 20–30 years of age.

Other somatic musculature may also be affected, resulting in generalized weakness. Fatigability of the deep tendon reflexes, with increasing diminution in response on repeated tendon tapping, is sometimes demonstrable. After a short rest, a single stimulus may then produce a strong muscle contraction. The Jolly reaction refers to the unusual fatigability of muscle upon repeated electric response, with pronounced capacity to recover after a short rest.

B. Diagnostic Tests:

1. **Neostigmine (Prostigmin) test**—Prompt relief of symptoms (appearing within 10–15 minutes and lasting up to 4 hours) follows the subcutaneous injection of neostigmine methylsulfate, 1.5 mg, in most cases of myasthenia gravis. Atropine sulfate, 0.6 mg, is administered simultaneously to counteract side reactions. Observations are made 30 minutes later. If dysphagia is present, the response to neostigmine may be readily observed fluoroscopically as the patient swallows a thin barium paste.

2. **Edrophonium (Tensilon)**—Edrophonium is a quaternary ammonium salt which exerts a direct stimulant effect on the neuromuscular junction. Intravenous injection of 10 mg edrophonium may relieve weakness within 20–30 seconds. Intramuscular injection of 25–50 mg may produce improvement lasting for several hours. Intravenous injection of 2–3 mg may be used as a test dose to distinguish myasthenic crisis (which improves) from overtreatment intoxication (no change) in myasthenic patients under treatment.

Treatment

A. Emergency Treatment: Sudden inability to swallow or onset of respiratory crises may occur at any time. The patient should always carry 2 ampules of 0.5 mg of neostigmine methylsulfate (Prostigmin), to be given immediately subcut or IM if severe symptoms develop. He should be placed under medical care at once; if additional neostigmine is needed, 1 mg may be given parenterally 2–3 times in 1 hour until an adequate response is obtained.

Progressively and potentially fatal weakness of the muscles of respiration may occur in spite of the administration of increasingly large amounts of neostigmine. A tracheostomy set, oxygen equipment, suction apparatus, and respirator should be available. After tracheostomy is performed, place the patient in a respirator and give oxygen as needed. Withhold neostigmine. Maintain fluid and electrolyte balance during artificial respiration. After a few days, it is usually possible to gradually decrease the time spent in the

respirator. In patients who survive the crisis, remissions may occur, some lasting for several years.

B. General Measures: Acquaint the patient with his disease. Maintain nutrition and health.

C. Specific Measures:

1. Neostigmine bromide, 15 mg orally 4 times a day and increase (up to 180 mg/day) as required.

2. Pyridostigmine bromide (Mestinon), an analogue of neostigmine, is at times more effective in treatment of bulbar muscle weakness. Give 0.6–1.5 gm daily at intervals spaced to provide maximal relief. Long-acting tablets (Mestinon Timespan), 180 mg each, are especially useful at bedtime.

3. Ambenonium chloride (Mytelase) may act twice as long as neostigmine and has fewer side-effects. Start with 5 mg 3 times daily and increase as necessary. The average dose is 5–25 mg 4 times daily.

4. Edrophonium chloride (Tensilon) may relieve weakness. Ten mg IV give relief in 20–30 seconds; 25–50 mg IM give improvement lasting for hours. Two to 3 mg IV may be used as a test dose for patients under treatment to distinguish between myasthenic crisis (improves) and overtreatment (no change).

5. Ephedrine sulfate, 12 mg with each dose of neostigmine, often enhances the action of neostigmine.

6. Potassium has also been found to be of value to supplement neostigmine, but it must be given in nearly toxic doses: 4–6 gm potassium chloride.

7. Side-effects of treatment with anticholinesterase drugs (eg, abdominal cramps, nausea and vomiting) may be ameliorated or prevented by adding atropine or atropine-like drugs to the regimen.

D. X-Ray Therapy: Patients who do not respond satisfactorily to oral medications may be given x-ray therapy (300 R) to the thymus in 10–12 divided doses. Partial remission occurs in about half of patients.

E. Surgical Measures: Beneficial effects have been reported from removal of the thymus gland. In some centers, thymectomy is considered for all patients under 60 years of age who are seriously disabled by myasthenia gravis and are otherwise in good health.

F. Thymoma: For thymoma, the recommended treatment is thymectomy following a 3000 R course of x-ray therapy to the thymus over 3–6 weeks.

G. Corticotropin and Corticosteroids: Encouraging results have been reported with the use of short-term courses of massive amounts of corticotropin (ACTH), long-term periodic corticotropin injections, and long-term oral prednisone (100 mg on alternate days). Long-term alternate-day treatment with high single doses of prednisone has been reported to produce an excellent chemical response, especially in older and male patients. Complications noted with such prednisone therapy include cataracts, hypertension, diabetes mellitus, fluid retention, and osteoporosis.

Management of Newborn Infants of Myasthenic Mothers

Immediately after delivery, children of patients with myasthenia gravis may have severe signs of the disease. Immediate treatment with neostigmine is necessary to preserve life. After a few days the symptoms may disappear, and the child thereafter usually does not suffer from myasthenia.

Prognosis

Spontaneous remissions are common, but relapse is the rule. Pregnancy usually produces amelioration, although exacerbations may also occur.

Myasthenic crisis, with sudden death from apparent respiratory failure, may occur. Survival of crisis may be followed by a remission. Overtreatment with neostigmine may produce muscle weakness simulating myasthenic crisis.

In myasthenic crisis the mortality may be reduced by withdrawing anticholinesterase medications for about 72 hours after onset of respiratory difficulty or arrest and instituting early tracheostomy with positive pressure respiration using a cuffed tracheostomy tube.

Black JT & others: Myasthenia gravis lacking response to cholinergic drugs. Neurology 23:817, 1973.

Brunner NG & others: Corticosteroids in management of severe, generalized myasthenia gravis. Neurology 22:603, 1972.

Cape CA, Utterback RA: Maintenance adrenocorticotropic (ACTH) treatment in myasthenia gravis. Neurology 22:1160, 1972.

Engel WK & others: Myasthenia gravis. Ann Int Med 81:225, 1974.

Fischer KC, Schwartzman RJ: Oral corticosteroids in the treatment of ocular myasthenia gravis. Neurology 24:795, 1974.

Flacke W: Treatment of myasthenia gravis. New England J Med 288:27, 1973.

Osserman KE: Thymectomy for myasthenia gravis. Ann Int Med 69:398, 1968.

Osserman KE & others: Studies in myasthenia gravis: A review of a twenty year experience in over 1200 patients. Mt Sinai J Med 38:497, 1971.

Shapiro SM, Namba T, Grob D: Corticotropin therapy and thymectomy in management of myasthenia gravis. Arch Neurol 24:65, 1971.

Warmolts JR, Engel WK: Benefit from alternate-day prednisone in myasthenia gravis. New England J Med 286:17, 1972.

MYOTONIA CONGENITA
(Thomsen's Disease)

Myotonia congenita is a rare heredofamilial disorder characterized by localized or generalized myotonia. Hypertrophy and hypertonicity of the muscles may occur, rendering them rigid and unyielding. The disease has occurred in 5 successive generations in the family of Dr. Thomsen, who first described it. Although it usually is not serious, the increased muscle stiffness makes it difficult for its victims to enjoy physical activity. Some have periodic attacks of generalized muscular spasm. Typically the disorder is present from birth and there is stiffness and difficulty in relaxation of the entire voluntary musculature. Stiff-

ness is usually accentuated by cold and relieved by exercise, and generalized muscular hypertrophy is common. It is inherited usually as an autosomal dominant characteristic. Quinine has been used successfully in relieving hypertonicity. **Myotonia acquisita** is a form of Thomsen's disease which has its onset late in life.

Bhatt GP, Vijayan N, Dreyfus P: Myotonia: A review of its clinical implications. California Med 114:16, Feb 1971.

MYOTONIA ATROPHICA
(Dystrophia Myotonica; Steinert's Disease, Myotonic Dystrophy)

Myotonia atrophica is a rare heredodegenerative disease of adult life which appears to be a mixture of Thomsen's disease and muscular dystrophy. There is hypertonicity of some muscles, usually of the tongue and the fist-making muscles of the hand, together with atrophy and weakness of the face, jaw muscles, peronei, and others. In both myotonia congenita and myotonia atrophica the patient characteristically grasps an object and then is unable to release his grip immediately. Myotonia, muscle atrophy (especially of face and neck), cataracts, early baldness, testicular atrophy, and evidence of dysfunction of other endocrine glands usually occur. Serum gamma globulin concentration is frequently reduced in myotonic dystrophy (IgG fraction of immunoglobulins) due to increased catabolism of this protein.

Paramyotonia congenita is a relatively rare disorder characterized by myotonia which increases in the presence of cold, intermittent flaccid paresis which is not necessarily dependent upon cold or myotonia, and a hereditary pattern dependent upon a single autosomal dominant gene. It has been suggested that paramyotonia congenita is identical with or closely related to hyperkalemic periodic paralysis.

Bell DB, Smith DW: Myotonic dystrophy in the neonate. J Pediat 81:83, 1972.

Dyken PR, Harper PS: Congenital dystrophia myotonica. Neurology 23:465, 1973.

Jensen HB, Jarnum S: Turnover of IgG and IgM in myotonic dystrophy. Neurology 21:68, 1971.

McComas AJ, Campbell MJ, Sica REP: Electrophysiological study of dystrophia myotonica. J Neurol Neurosurg Psychiat 34:132, 1971.

Thrush DC, Morris CJ, Salmon AV: Paramyotonia congenita: A clinical, histochemical and pathological study. Brain 95:537, 1972.

FAMILIAL PERIODIC PARALYSIS

Hypokalemic periodic paralysis is a rare disorder in which the victim undergoes periodic attacks of flaccid paralysis lasting from a few minutes to several hours. Between attacks he is apparently normal. A severe attack may cause death from respiratory paralysis. A "cadaveric" electric reaction accompanies the attack. Decrease in serum potassium and serum phosphate is associated. Treatment includes oral administration of potassium salts. Attacks in susceptible individuals may be produced by injection of hypertonic glucose, insulin, desoxycorticosterone, or epinephrine, or by water diuresis of excess sodium intake.

During attacks the muscle potassium and sodium are not significantly elevated and the muscle becomes electrically unexcitable. Membrane potentials recorded by microelectrodes within the muscle cell do not disclose hyperpolarization. During attacks increased fluid may be noted in large vacuoles within the endoplasmic reticulum of muscle cells. Accumulation of abnormal glycogen breakdown products in these vacuoles may cause the influx of electrolytes and water into muscle cells to preserve ion balance.

Treatment is with potassium chloride, 5–10 gm orally when diagnosis has been made and then 5 gm 2–4 times daily during acute episodes as needed to prevent weakness or paralysis. In respiratory paralysis, give a prepared solution containing 1 gm potassium chloride in 50–60 ml distilled water very slowly IV. *Caution:* This is a dangerous procedure.

Patients with this disease should avoid high-carbohydrate foods. Routine administration of potassium chloride enteric-coated tablets, 8–12 gm 3 times daily, prevents attacks.

Acetazolamide (Diamox), 250–750 mg daily, has been reported to be effective in preventing attacks.

With treatment, the prognosis is excellent. Death may result from respiratory paralysis, but this is rare.

Adynamia episodica hereditaria, or hyperkalemic periodic paralysis, is a disorder in which an increase in serum potassium accompanies paralytic attacks. Muscle weakness may be provoked in these patients by administration of potassium chloride or by rest after physical exertion. Onset is usually in the first decade. Attacks occur during rest after physical exertion. Mild paresthesias of the limbs usually precede attacks, and if exercise is begun at this stage paralysis may be aborted.

Brooks JE: Hyperkalemic periodic paralysis. Arch Neurol 20:13, 1969.

Campa JF, Sanders DB: Familial hypokalemic periodic paralysis. Arch Neurol 31:110, 1974.

Dyken M, Zeman W, Rusche T: Hypokalemic periodic paralysis. Neurology 19:691, 1969.

Lisak RP & others: Hyperkalemic periodic paralysis and cardiac arrhythmia. Neurology 22:810, 1972.

Meyers KR & others: Periodic muscle weakness, normokalemia and tubular aggregates. Neurology 22:269, 1972.

Streeten DHP, Dalakos TG, Fellerman H: Studies on hyperkalemic periodic paralysis. J Clin Invest 50:142, 1971.

Takagi A & others: Thyrotoxic periodic paralysis. Neurology 23:1008, 1973.

Vroom FQ, Jarrell MA, Maren TH: Acetazolamide treatment of hypokalemic periodic paralysis. Arch Neurol 32:385, 1975.

STIFF-MAN SYNDROME

This is a rare syndrome of tonic muscle rigidity of unknown origin. There are no characteristic histologic changes in muscle. The disorder usually begins with episodic aching and tightness of the axial musculature which over a period of weeks or months becomes constant and spreads to the extremities. Ultimately there is a tight, board-like hardness of most of the limb, trunk, and neck muscles which interferes with voluntary movement. Sudden stimuli may precipitate intensely painful paroxysms of muscle spasm which may last for several minutes. Skeletal abnormalities, including subluxation and spontaneous fractures, are not uncommon. Electromyography reveals persistent tonic contraction, even at rest. Myoneural blocking agents (eg, succinylcholine) and peripheral nerve block abolish the pain and tonicity. Diazepam (Valium) has been used successfully in a few cases. Most victims of this disorder become bedridden invalids.

Gordon EE, Januszko DM, Kaufman L: A critical survey of stiff-man syndrome. Am J Med 42:582, 1967.

Kasparek S, Zibrowski S: Stiff-man syndrome and encephalomyelitis. Arch Neurol 24:22, 1971.

17 . . .
Psychiatric Disorders

James J. Brophy

Psychiatric syndromes have changed over the past 25 years in quality, severity, and frequency, and the practice of psychiatry has changed accordingly. The factors responsible for these changes include the following:

(1) **Cultural:** A change in ethics, customs, and attitudes toward people who deviate from the norm. (2) **Social:** A wider variation of interpersonal behavior, changing technology, and increased education and sophistication. (3) **Family:** A decline of the "extended family," with numerous relatives, and a shift toward the "nuclear family"—a rather isolated unit consisting of parents and children. (4) **Child development:** A function of the schools, preschool care, single parents, less conformity, and greater freedom of choice for the child. (5) **Treatment:** Earlier recognition, newer technics of psychotherapy and behavior therapy, and developments in psychopharmacology.

In the past, by the time most patients were seen by a psychiatrist, the illness was so advanced that the symptoms were well defined and diagnostic entities were well established. The schizophrenics usually were grossly psychotic with unmistakable delusions, hallucinations, and bizarre behavior. These patients are now often treated earlier but with less diagnostic certainty, even though signs and symptoms should be ascertained as accurately as possible. A parallel exists in other specialties of medicine. The pneumonias had a natural course leading to clearly differentiated entities with distinct stages of illness, whereas today the old textbook patterns are less obvious. The terms upper respiratory infection and bronchopneumonia are now used for a wide variety of respiratory problems just as we use terms in mental health in a broad, general way.

Consistent patterns of behavior—which may or may not receive a diagnostic label—are a composite of **biogenetic** characteristics; **developmental** factors, including experience and training; and individual **environmental** circumstances. Most people maintain a fine balance between these forces which allows them to live a relatively stable life.

The balance is often tenuously maintained by basic adjustive technics (also called defense mechanisms), the methods people habitually use in overcoming, avoiding, circumventing, escaping from, or ignoring frustrations and threats. The common ones include the following: (1) **Sublimation,** wherein the drive is turned into a new but useful and more acceptable channel. *Example:* A childish desire to exhibit oneself may be sublimated into a theatrical career. (2) **Repression** is the unconscious purposeful forgetting of urgings or events which would be painful if allowed to become conscious. *Example:* Forgetting well-known dates, etc. (3) **Projection** is the mechanism whereby painful feelings or ideas are projected outward upon persons or things in the environment and felt by the individual as being outside of himself. *Example:* A person with unconscious homosexual impulses feels he must defend himself by assuming that others are making homosexual accusations. (4) **Denial** is used by the individual to treat obvious reality factors as if they did not exist. *Example:* A person realizes that the plumbing is not working properly but does not accept the fact and goes on as if nothing is wrong. (5) **Introjection** (the opposite of projection) is the incorporation by a person of traits that are characteristic of another. *Example:* A depressed person may incorporate the affects and attitudes of another person and so, if he is disliked by the other person, comes to dislike himself. (6) **Regression** is the return to a more infantile level of function. *Example:* Children commonly retreat to a more childish level when siblings are born and demonstrate more immature behavior such as thumb-sucking and bed-wetting. (7) **Undoing** is the mechanism in which a person performs some activity which "undoes" or neutralizes something objectionable that occurred previously. *Example:* A person has a sick mother. Whenever he thinks of her, the thought is immediately replaced by the thought that she is as healthy as any other woman. (8) **Reaction formation** serves to prevent a painful thought from emerging by immediately substituting a pleasant thought. *Example:* A person who cannot acknowledge disliking someone never shows any hostility and always presents a pleasant demeanor. (9) **Isolation** is a separation of the original memory and its affect. *Example:* A beloved wife is killed in a serious accident, yet the husband discusses the details with a complete lack of emotion. (10) **Displacement** is a condition in which not only is the affect connected with a particular person or incident separated from it but the affect is then attached to another. *Example:* The factory worker has problems with his supervisor but cannot vent them at the time. He then goes home and for no apparent reason becomes angry with his wife. **(11) Rationalization** is substitution of an acceptable reason for an unacceptable one. *Example:* A student cannot face studying for an examination and decides that one should be relaxed for examinations, which thus justifies his going to a movie when he should be studying.

When balance of behavior patterns is upset, the results are (1) stress to the individual, producing "neurotic" responses such as anxiety or depression, often accompanied by a disruption of biologic functions such as sleep and appetite; (2) stress to those around the individual, produced by erratic behavior—often called "acting out" or "antisocial behavior"— and incurring the diagnosis of "personality disorder," with the inference that the individual is experiencing little or no anxiety within a rigid maladaptive life style; or (3) a combination of the above, wherein the individual decompensates in relationship to his environment, creating stress to himself and those about him. These conditions are often called "psychoses," "borderline psychoses," or "acute situational reactions," depending on the stress and the adaptive response.

Akiskal HS, McKinney WT: Psychiatry and pseudopsychiatry. Arch Gen Psychiat 28:367, 1973.

Kety S: From rationalization to reason. Am J Psychiat 131:957, 1974.

Romano J: Psychiatry and medicine, 1973. Ann Int Med 79:582, 1973.

Schimel JL & others: Changing styles in psychiatric syndromes: A symposium. Am J Psychiat 130:146, 1973.

PSYCHIATRIC ASSESSMENT

Psychiatric diagnosis rests upon the established principles of history and examination. The assessment must be *complete*. All of the forces contributing to the individual's life situation must be identified, and this can only be done if the examination includes the history, mental status, medical conditions, and pertinent social environmental factors impinging on the individual.

Interview

The manner in which the history is taken is important to its success in eliciting pertinent data. The setting should be quiet, and the patient should be allowed to tell about his problems in an unstructured way without interruption. At some point a statement such as "Tell me about yourself" will be productive. The interviewer should avoid writing, unnecessary direct questioning, and interpretive comments. Long, rambling discussions may be controlled by subtly interjecting questions relevant to the topic, although the patient's digressions sometimes provide important clues to his mental status. The first 5 minutes are the most important part of the interview.

The interviewer should be alert for key words or phrases that can be used to help the patient develop the theme of his difficulties. In the example, "Doctor, I hurt, and when we have the marital problems, things just get worse"—the words "hurt" and "marital problems" are important clues that need amplification when the physician makes his next comment. Nonverbal clues may be as important as words, and one should notice gestures, tones of voice, and facial expressions. Obvious omissions, shying away from painful subjects, and sudden shifts of subject matter give important clues to unconscious as well as conscious material.

Every psychiatric history should cover the following points: (1) complaint, from the patient's viewpoint; (2) the present illness, or the evolution of the complaints; (3) previous disorders and the nature and extent of treatment; (4) the family history—important for genetic aspects and family influences; (5) personal history—childhood development, adolescent adjustment, and adult coping patterns; and (6) current life functioning, with attention to vocational, social, educational, and avocational areas.

It is often essential to obtain additional information from the family. Observing interactions of significant other people with the patient in the context of a family interview may give significant diagnostic information and may even underscore the nature of the problem and suggest a therapeutic approach. An example is the myocardial infarction patient whose wife is afraid of upsetting him, interacts with him in a restrained way, harbors resentment, inadvertently encourages invalidism, and in the long run hinders his convalescence and recovery.

The Mental Status Examination

Observation of the patient and the content of his remarks during the interview constitute the informal part of the mental status examination, ie, that which is obtained indirectly. The remainder of the information comes from direct questioning, which really is intended only to fill in the gaps. The latter is concerned mainly with the sensorium, although much of that information will be obtained indirectly as the patient is interviewed.

The mental status examination includes the following: (1) Appearance: Note bizarre or unusual modes of dress, makeup, etc. (2) Activity and behavior: Gait, gestures, coordination of bodily movements, etc. (3) Affect: Outward manifestation of emotions such as depression, anger, elation, fear, resentment, or lack of emotional response. (4) Mood: Inward feelings, sum of statements, and observable emotional manifestations. (5) Speech: Coherence, spontaneity, articulation, latency of response (the pause before answering), and duration of utterance. (6) Content of thought: Associations, preoccupations, obsessions, depersonalization, delusions, hallucinations, paranoid ideation, anger, fear, or unusual experiences. (7) Sensorium: (a) Orientation to person, place, time, and circumstances; (b) remote and recent memory and recall; (c) calculations, digit retention (forward and backward), serial 7s and 3s; (d) general fund of knowledge (presidents, states, distances, events); (e) abstracting ability, often tested with common proverbs. (8) Judgment regarding common sense problems such as what to do when one runs out of medicine. (9) Insight into the nature and extent of the current difficulty and its ramifications in the patient's life.

The mental status examination is of prime importance in establishing a diagnosis and must be recorded clearly and completely in the chart. It is a graphic summary which can quickly change and can provide valuable clues to diagnosis and treatment. The major headings listed above should be recorded with appropriate comments.

Medical Examination

The examination of a psychiatric patient must include a complete physical examination as well as all necessary laboratory and other special studies.

Special Diagnostic Aids

Many tests and evaluation procedures are available that can be used to support and clarify initial diagnostic impressions.

A. Psychologic Testing: Psychologic testing by a trained psychologist may measure intelligence, provide information about personality, feelings, psychodynamics, and psychopathology, and differentiate psychic problems from organic ones. The place of such tests is similar to that of other tests in medicine—helpful in diagnostic problems but a useless expense when not needed.

1. Objective tests—These tests provide qualitative evaluation compared to standard norms.

a. Intelligence tests—The test usually given is the Wechsler Adult Intelligence Scale (WAIS). Intelligence tests may reveal not only a person's IQ. Performance on nonverbal tests varies noticably with mood disturbance in schizophrenia, other psychoses, or brain disease, whereas performance on verbal tests is fairly stable except when there is damage to the speech areas of the dominant cerebral hemisphere.

b. Minnesota Multiphasic Personality Inventory (MMPI)—This test measures the individual's answers against the response patterns of the general population in the following categories: hypochondriacal, depressive, hysterical, psychopathic, paranoid, psychasthenic, schizophrenic, and hypomanic.

c. Bender Gestalt Test—This test is used to elicit evidence of the perceptive distortions made by persons with organic disorders.

d. Vocational aptitude and interest tests—Several are available and may be used as a source of advice regarding beneficial environmental changes.

2. Projective tests—These tests are unstructured, so that the subject is forced to respond in ways that reflect fantasies and individual modes of adaptation. Conscious and unconscious attitudes may be deduced from the subject's responses. These tests are of very limited usefulness even when done by an expert.

a. Rorschach Psychodiagnostics—This test utilizes 10 inkblots. It requires expert interpretation and is not fully standardized.

b. Thematic Apperception Test (TAT)—This test uses 20 pictures of people in different situations. Interpretation is based on psychoanalytic theory concerning defenses against anxiety feelings and provides a reflection of interpersonal conflicts.

c. Sentence completion tests, Draw-a-Person tests, etc—The dubious value of these tests varies according to the skill of the evaluation.

B. Neurologic Evaluation: Consultation is often necessary and often must include specialized tests such as EEG, echoencephalography, brain scan, cerebral angiography, and pneumoencephalography.

Formulation of the Diagnosis

A psychiatric diagnosis must be based upon positive evidence accumulated by the above technics. It must not be based simply on the exclusion of organic findings.

A thorough psychiatric evaluation has therapeutic as well as diagnostic value, and should be expressed in ways best understood by the patient, family, and other physicians. The problem-oriented medical record is applicable to psychiatric disorders. "Hearing voices" and "fears of radar" are problems understood by the patient who may want access to his record. "Schizophrenia, paranoid type," may be pejorative to the patient and may not help compliance in treatment.

Patient Compliance in Taking Medication

Studies have shown that as many as half of all outpatients fail to take medication as prescribed. This is most apt to be true of patients with chronic illness, and it is a matter of obvious importance in psychiatric patients. Many factors are responsible for inadequate patient compliance, including failure to recognize the need for the medication, carelessness, confusion, unpleasant effects from the medication, denial of illness, delusional beliefs, a false impression of recovery or cure, and inadequate finances. Obviously, noncompliance can lead to serious difficulties.

There are 3 elements to consider in improving compliance:

A. The Physician-Patient Relationship: This implies mutual confidence, clear communication, close follow-up, and ongoing education. Enlisting the aid of individuals close to the patient may be important.

B. Prescription Practices: This includes giving clear verbal and written instructions concerning the amount and timing of dosages, keeping the number of daily doses to a required minimum, and prescribing the least costly effective drugs.

C. Changes in the Patient's Illness: Allowance must be made for the changing status of the patient by modifying the drugs or dosages to meet the individual's varying requirements.

Blackwell B: Drug therapy: Patient compliance. New England J Med 289:249, 1973.

Feighner JP & others: Diagnostic criteria for use in psychiatric research. Arch Gen Psychiat 26:57, 1972.

McLean PD, Miles JE: Evaluation and the problem-oriented record in psychiatry. Arch Gen Psychiat 31:622, 1974.

Moser RH: The first five minutes. JAMA 231:1169, 1975.

Panzetta AF: Toward a scientific psychiatric nosology. Arch Gen Psychiat 30:154, 1974.

Powell RJ: Inadequately written prescriptions. JAMA 226:999, 1973.

Richardson H: The historical approach to the theory of diagnosis. Brit J Psychiat 122:245, 1973.

Simon RJ: Impact of patient history interview on psychiatric diagnosis. Arch Gen Psychiat 24:437, 1971.

Welner A & others: A systematic approach for making a psychiatric diagnosis. Arch Gen Psychiat 31:193, 1974.

TREATMENT APPROACHES

The approaches to treatment of psychiatric patients are, in a broad sense, similar to those in other branches of medicine. For example, the internist treating a patient with heart disease uses not only **medical measures** such as digitalis and pacemakers but also **psychologic** technics in an attempt to change patterns of behavior, **social** and environmental manipulation, and **behavioral** technics, eg, in attempting to modify the marital relationship for his patient's benefit.

The psychiatrist may utilize the same general therapeutic categories (conceptual models), but there is a shift of emphasis in treatment methods and the methods are less explicit. The **medical** approaches used by the psychiatrist include, for example, medications and convulsive therapy. The **psychologic** technics include individual, group, and family therapies. **Social** interventions relate to the patient's environment by means of milieu therapy, partial hospitalization, day care or halfway house placement, etc. **Behavioral** therapy assumes that all behavior is learned behavior and is continued because of positive reinforcement. Therapy is directed toward identifying specific behavior patterns, factors determining such behavior, and ways of modifying it.

Regardless of the methods employed, treatment must be directed toward an objective, ie, **goal-oriented.** This usually involves (1) active patient cooperation; (2) establishing reasonable goals and modifying the goal downward if failure occurs; (3) emphasizing positive behavior (goals) instead of symptom behavior (problems); (4) delineating the method; and (5) setting a deadline.

The physician must resist pressures for prescribed treatment and instantaneous results, either on the part of the patient or those close to him. Beware of demands for a "garage job," in which the family brings the patient to the doctor, tells what is wrong with him, and arranges to "pick up" the repaired item when it is ready. In almost all cases, psychiatric treatment involves the *active participation* of the significant people

in the patient's life. The physician who fails to realize this usually finds that he is prescribing a lot of sedatives and minor tranquilizers and making little therapeutic progress. It takes time to unravel the complex interrelationships between the psyche, the soma, and the sociocultural milieu of the patient. Time must be spent with the patient, and it is often best to schedule fairly frequent appointments of short duration in which active and vigorous therapeutic effort can be exerted by both parties.

All physicians have always treated psychiatric problems and are in an excellent position to meet their patients' emotional needs in an organized and competent way, referring to psychiatrists those patients who represent particularly complex problems. When such a referral is made, it should be conducted like any other referral: in an open manner, with full explanation of the problem to the patient and the referral appointment made while the patient is still in the office.

Lazare A: Hidden conceptual models in clinical psychiatry. New England J Med 228:345, 1973.

Sherman RW: Drugs and the doctor-patient relationship. Arch Int Med 131:604, 1973.

Strauss JS: Diagnostic models and the nature of psychiatric disorder. Arch Gen Psychiat 29:445, 1973.

1. MEDICAL APPROACHES

ANTIPSYCHOTIC TRANQUILIZERS
(Neuroleptics, "Major Tranquilizers")

This group of drugs includes the **phenothiazines, thioxanthenes** (both similar in structure), **butyrophenones, dihydroindolones,** and **dibenzoxazepines.** Table 17–1 lists the drugs in order of increasing milligram potency and decreasing side-effects (with the exception of extrapyranidal symptoms). Thus, chlorpromazine has lower milligram potency and causes more severe side-effects and fewer extrapyramidal complications than fluphenazine.

The only butyrophenone marketed in the USA is haloperidol, which is totally different in structure but very similar in action and extrapyramidal side-effects to the piperazine phenothiazines. Haloperidol has a paucity of autonomic side-effects, markedly lowers hyperactivity and psychotic ideation, and is particularly effective in movement disorders such as those seen in Gilles de la Tourette's syndrome. Molindone is similar in action, side-effects, and safety to the piperazine phenothiazines.

None of the major tranquilizers produce true physical dependency, and they have a wide safety margin between therapeutic and toxic effects.

Table 17—1. Commonly used major tranquilizers.

	Chlor-promazine Ratio	Usual Daily Oral Dose	Usual Daily Maximum Dose*
Phenothiazines			
Chlorpromazine (Thorazine)	1:1	100—200 mg	1 gm
Thioridazine (Mellaril)	1:1	100—200 mg	600 mg
Mesoridazine (Serentil)	1:2	50—100 mg	400 mg
Piperacetazine (Quide)	1:3	30 mg	160 mg
Butaperazine (Repoise)†	1:8	30—50 mg	150 mg
Perphenazine (Trilafon)†	1:10	8—16 mg	48 mg
Trifluoperazine (Stelazine)†	1:20	5—15 mg	40 mg
Fluphenazine (Prolixin, Permitil)†	1:50	2—10 mg	30 mg
Thioxanthenes			
Chlorprothixene (Taractan)	1:1	100—200 mg	600 mg
Thiothixene† (Navane)	1:20	5—20 mg	60 mg
Butyrophenone			
Haloperidol (Haldol)	1:50	2—10 mg	30 mg
Dihydroindolone			
Molindone (Moban)	1:15	50—100 mg	225 mg
Dibenzoxazepine			
Loxapine (Loxitane)	1:10	50—75 mg	250 mg

*Can be higher in some cases.
†Indicates piperazine structure.

Mode of Action

Phenothiazines and thioxanthenes block the uptake of catecholamines at the postsynaptic junction. They also act to decrease amine synthesis and increase adenosine triphosphatase (ATP), creatinine phosphate levels, and phospholipids in the brain. These drugs affect the function of the 3 major integrating systems of the brain: the reticular activating system, the limbic system, and the hypothalamus. One can assume that they decrease extraneous sensory perception, reduce the affective charge of sensation, and lower the somatic response, resulting in a **lower arousal level.**

Clinical Indications

The antipsychotic tranquilizers are used to treat the **schizophrenias, organic brain psychoses, psychotic depression, primary affective (manic depressive) disorders,** and **paranoia.** They may be effective in psychedelic abuse, amphetamine psychosis, and selected cases of delirium. They quickly lower the arousal (activity) level and, perhaps indirectly, gradually improve socialization and thinking. Combinations are not more effective than single drugs but are used when side-effects are a consideration.

Symptoms which are ameliorated by these drugs include hyperactivity, hostility, delusions, hallucinations, negativism, and poor sleep. Individuals with an acute psychosis and good premorbid function respond quite well. Patients with long-standing symptoms and unusual variations often respond poorly.

Phenothiazines and thioxanthenes potentiate the sedative effects of barbiturates. Antacids may impair the absorption of phenothiazines, nearly all of which are highly surface-active, lipophilic, and weakly basic.

Dosage Forms & Patterns

The dosage range is quite broad. For example, chlorpromazine, 25 mg orally at bedtime, may be sufficient for the elderly person with a mild organic brain syndrome, whereas 2500 mg daily may occasionally be used in a young schizophrenic patient. For this reason, it is misleading to depend on static dosage levels. The dosage should be rather low at first. For example, in treating a moderately agitated younger person, give chlorpromazine concentrate, 100 mg orally, and evaluate the effect of the drug over several hours. If there is no or minimal effect, give another 100 mg and gradually increase to a total daily dose adequate to calm the individual without impairing his waking consciousness. It may take several days to arrive at the correct dosage for a given patient.

In the case of a very agitated, destructive patient, oral administration may be supplemented by intramuscular chlorpromazine, 25—50 mg every 2—3 hours as needed. Orthostatic hypotension is the principal side-effect and may be handled by keeping the patient in the recumbent position. Intramuscular administration is 2—3 times as potent as oral and need be used only in patients who are acute management problems. Avoid intravenous use.

Haloperidol, 5 mg IM, is quite effective in the very active patient, particularly in mania, acute delirium, or acute schizophrenic reaction. Observe the response over the next 1—2 hours, and repeat the dose if necessary every several hours until the patient is under control.

The philosophy of administration of these drugs is similar to that which governs the use of insulin in acute diabetic coma. Insulin is given until the glucose level approaches normal. In the acute psychotic patient, the major tranquilizer is given until behavior becomes as near normal as possible. After the acute diabetic situation is resolved, insulin is titrated to maintain a reasonable glucose level, and patients vary widely in their required dosage. After the acute psychiatric situation is resolved, the psychiatric patient will require *only enough medication* to help him maintain reasonable behavior. In the case of the chronic schizophrenic patient—like the brittle diabetic patient—the drugs must be given indefinitely and on a varying dosage schedule related to the patient's needs.

Psychiatric patients—particularly paranoid individuals—often neglect to take their medication. In these cases, the enanthate and decanoate forms of fluphenazine may be given deeply subcutaneously to achieve an effect that will last 10–21 days. A patient who may not take his oral medication will usually come to the physician's office to get his "shot." The usual dose of these long-acting preparations is 25 mg (1 ml) every 2 weeks. The principal side-effects are extrapyramidal reactions, and many physicians give an antiparkinsonism drug prophylactically; it can often be discontinued after 6–10 weeks with little tendency for extrapyramidal symptoms to appear.

In most cases, oral medications are adequate. The elixir is best absorbed; the tablet next best; and the Spansule least well absorbed. The "sustained release" forms of these drugs are expensive and incompletely absorbed, and this form of administration is particularly unsuitable because these drugs are long-lasting. Various factors play a role in the absorption of oral medications. Of particular importance are previous gastrointestinal surgery and concomitant administration of other drugs, eg, antacids.

Divided daily dosages are not necessary after a maintenance dose has been established, and the majority of patients can then be maintained on a single daily dose, usually taken at bedtime. This is particularly appropriate in a case where the sedative effect of the drug is desired for nighttime sleep, thus avoiding undesirable sedative effects during the day. Costs of medication, nursing time, and patient unreliability are reduced when either a single daily dose or a large bedtime/smaller morning dose schedule is utilized.

In the vast majority of cases, one drug from the group is adequate. Antidepressants and sedatives are seldom necessary in combination with the major tranquilizers. If sedation is needed, prescribe one of the sedative phenothiazines for bedtime.

Side-Effects

The sedative effect of these drugs can be used to advantage, and in any case it wears off with time. Arrhythmias, inhibition of ejaculation, and postural hypotension may occur (alpha-adrenergic blocking effect). Agranulocytosis may be detected clinically or with periodic white blood counts. Cholestatic jaundice remits readily and occurs usually in the first 2 months of treatment (as does the agranulocytosis also). Anticholinergic effects include urinary retention, ileus, and closed-angle glaucoma in the elderly.

Photosensitivity and hyperpigmentation are reversible upon discontinuation of the drug. Retinopathy is reported following short-term administration of thioridazine in high doses and lenticular and corneal opacities following long-term administration of chlorpromazine (80% incidence in total dosage greater than 100 gm). These disorders are likewise reversible. The eyes should be examined by an ophthalmologist every 6 months in any patient receiving more than 200 mg of chlorpromazine (or its equivalent) per day.

Metabolic and endocrine effects include weight gain, hyperglycemia, lactation, menstrual problems, male impotence, temperature irregularities, and occasional water intoxication which may be due to inappropriate ADH function, anticholinergic effects, or hypothalamic stimulation. Since phenothiazines increase prolactin release, breast examinations should be done periodically on female patients.

Drug combinations (eg, thioridazine, tricyclic antidepressants, and antiparkinsonism drugs) produce marked anticholinergic effects, often manifested by constipation, paralytic ileus, or urinary retention. Phenothiazines block the antihypertensive effect of guanethidine and may interfere with diphenylhydantoin metabolism.

The seizure threshold is lowered, particularly in older patients taking high dosages. Infrequently, an adverse response occurs. It is characterized by dramatic exacerbations of the psychosis, feelings of terror, and subtle extrapyramidal symptoms. Biperiden, 5 mg IM every 4 hours for several doses, usually relieves the symptoms promptly.

Extrapyramidal effects. (1) Akathisia is the most common extrapyramidal effect and is often mistaken for agitation. It is characterized by motor restlessness and pacing. Antiparkinsonism agents are only partly effective. Decrease the dose or switch to nonpiperazine phenothiazines. Diazepam, 5 mg 3 times daily, is effective in some cases. (2) Acute dystonias usually occur early in treatment and include oculogyric crises. Treatment is with diphenhydramine, 50 mg IV, and benztropine mesylate, 2 mg orally 1–2 times daily, or other antiparkinsonism drugs, all of which are about equal in usefulness. (3) Pseudoparkinsonism is indistinguishable from true parkinsonism, but it occurs later in the course of treatment and responds well to adjustments in dosage and antiparkinsonism drugs, which need not be used prophylactically and often can be discontinued when extrapyramidal symptoms are controlled (usually after 10–12 weeks). (4) Tardive dyskinesias (choreiform and buccal lingual movements) may occur after months or years of therapy, usually in older people, and are usually irreversible. Symptoms are resistant to treatment and often reappear or worsen with cessation of the major tranquilizer. The prevalence ranges from 2–30% of patients receiving long-term major tranquilizers, and no specific treatment has been effective.

American College of Neuropsychopharmacology–FDA Task Force: Neurologic syndromes associated with antipsychotic drug use. New England J Med 289:20, 1973.

Appleton WS: Psychoactive drugs: A usage guide. Dis Nerv System 32:607, 1971.

Ayd FJ Jr: A critical evaluation of molindone (Moban), a new indole derivative neuroleptic. Dis Nerv Syst 35:447, 1974.

Ayd FJ JR: The depot fluphenazines: A reappraisal after 10 years' clinical experience. Am J Psychiat 132:491, 1975.

Ban TA: Haloperidol and the butyrophenones. Psychosomatics 14:286, 1973.

Hollister L: Mental disorders: Antipsychotic and antimanic drugs. New England J Med 286:984, 1972.

Hollister LE & others: Specific indications for different classes of phenothiazines. Arch Gen Psychiat 30:94, 1974.

Kazamatsuri H & others: Therapeutic approaches to tardive dyskinesia: A review of the literature. Arch Gen Psychiat

17:95, 1972.

Man PC, Chen CH: Rapid tranquilization of acutely psychotic patients with intramuscular haloperidol and chlorpromazine. Psychosomatics 14:59, 1973.

Pauling L: On the orthomolecular environment of the mind: Orthomolecular theory. Am J Psychiat 131:1251, 1974.

Van Putten T: The many faces of akathisia. Comprehensive Psychiat 16:43, 1975.

Young DS & others: Effects of drugs on clinical laboratory tests. Clin Chem 18:1041, 1972.

LITHIUM

Lithium carbonate (Eskalith, Lithane, Lithonate) is therapeutically effective in the treatment of primary affective disorders (see The Depressions). It is most effective in the treatment of acute mania and significantly decreases the frequency of relapses into manic episodes. It is possibly helpful in acute depressive episodes but does decrease the frequency of relapse into depressive episodes in bipolar disorders and probably also in unipolar disorders. The precise manner in which lithium exerts its therapeutic effects has yet to be defined, although it probably involves ionic processes at the cell membrane which in turn affect the flow of neurotransmitters mediated by adenylate cyclase or cyclic AMP. There is no conclusive evidence of teratogenicity in humans, but lithium should nonetheless be withheld if possible in the first trimester of pregnancy. Since it freely passes the placental barrier, it should be discontinued prior to delivery, and bottle feeding should be considered since one-half to one-third of the serum level is present in breast milk.

Clinical Indications

Acute mania is the major indication for lithium. Because of the lag period of 4–10 days until therapeutic serum levels of 0.8–1.2 mEq/liter are attained, it is desirable to give an antipsychotic drug initially with the lithium in order to achieve prompt control of the manic symptoms. Haloperidol, 5–50 mg orally daily, can be used and then gradually discontinued over the first week as therapeutic lithium levels are established.

As a prophylactic drug for both mania and depression, lithium significantly decreases attacks in over 50% of cases of bipolar affective disorders. Patients who swing rapidly back and forth between manic and depressive attacks (at least 4 cycles per year) respond poorly to lithium prophylaxis. The prophylactic efficacy of lithium is less well established in unipolar primary affective disorders but is roughly equivalent to that of the antidepressants. Lithium is less effective than antipsychotic drugs in the treatment of schizoaffective schizophrenic disorders and should be used in patients whose problem is probably a primary affective condition and not a schizophrenic episode. Lithium is not effective in alcoholism, barbiturate abuse, hyperkinesis, or obsessive compulsive neurosis.

Dosage Forms & Patterns

Lithium carbonate is available in 300 mg capsules for oral administration 3 times a day. Initially, give 1500–2500 mg daily (approximately 600 mg 3 times a day) in adults and half this dosage in elderly or debilitated patients. Continue this dosage until blood levels—determined 6–8 hours after the last dose—approach the therapeutic level of 0.8–1.2 mEq/liter and titrate the dosage to maintain that serum level. This will usually require about 300 mg of lithium 3 times a day. The drug is absorbed in 1–3 hours, and half of the administered dose is excreted in 24 hours. Close medical supervision and frequent monitoring of serum levels are necessary until therapeutic levels are stable on the same daily dose. Serum levels can then be determined weekly and then monthly in the absence of adverse clinical signs. Serum levels should also be determined when the patient has any clinical condition which may affect sodium levels (eg, influenza or similar disorders which may produce vomiting or diarrhea; anorexia or other situations that can result in decreased food or liquid intake).

Blood levels above 2 mEq/liter are quite serious. Clinical evaluation prior to the institution of lithium therapy should include assessment of kidney, thyroid, and cardiovascular status along with attention to any dietary restrictions such as sodium or any medications such as diuretics.

Side-Effects

A. Early: The early side-effects usually disappear with continued administration. Mild gastrointestinal symptoms may include nausea, vomiting, diarrhea, and abdominal pain. Fine tremors, slight muscle weakness, some degree of somnolence, and moderate polyuria are occasionally present.

B. Lithium Toxicity: Frank toxicity usually occurs at blood levels above 2 mEq/liter and is a function of sodium/lithium balance. The development of toxicity is often insidious and may be the result of some relatively innocuous problem such as influenza or gastrointestinal upset. It may be due to decreased sodium intake for any reasons, or increased sodium loss resulting from diarrhea, dehydration, or the use of diuretics. Lithium overdosage may be accidental or intentional or may occur as a result of poor monitoring. Kidney disease is a major factor in toxic alterations of sodium/lithium balance.

The symptoms of lithium toxicity include severe vomiting, which rapidly worsens the problem as more sodium is lost from the body. Other signs include tremors, marked muscle weakness, slurred speech, ataxia, hyperreflexia, rigidity, seizures, opisthotonos, coma, and death.

C. Other Side-Effects: These include goiter (often euthyroid), occasionally hypothyroidism, changes in the glucose tolerance test toward a diabetic-like curve, occasional precipitation of late-onset diabetes, and infrequent dysarthria in elderly patients. Most of these side-effects subside when lithium is discontinued; when residuals exist, they are usually not serious. Electroencephalographic abnormalities may occur during lithium administration, but they more often represent accentuations of previous abnormalities than specific drug effects on the normal EEG. Patients on long-term lithium therapy frequently demonstrate cogwheel rigidity and occasionally other extrapyramidal signs.

Brenner DL, Fieve RR: Clinical factors in lithium carbonate prophylaxis failure. Arch Gen Psychiat 30:229, 1974.

Prien RF & others: Factors associated with treatment success in lithium carbonate prophylaxis. Arch Gen Psychiat 31:189, 1974.

Prien RF & others: Lithium prophylaxis in recurrent affective illness. Am J Psychiat 131:198, 1974.

Schou M: Lithium in psychiatric therapy and prophylaxis. J Psychiat Res 6:67, 1968.

Singer I, Rotenberg D: Mechanisms of lithium action. New England J Med 289:254, 1973.

Spring GK: Hazards of lithium prophylaxis. Dis Nerv System 35:351, 1974.

Stallone F & others: The use of lithium in affective disorders. 3. A double-blind study of prophylaxis in bipolar illness. Am J Psychiat 130:1006, 1973.

Table 17—2. Commonly used antidepressants.

	Usual Daily Oral Dose	Usual Daily Maximum Oral Dose
Tricyclic compounds		
Imipramine (Tofranil)	50—150 mg	300 mg
Desipramine (Norpramin, Pertofrane)	50—150 mg	300 mg
Nortriptyline (Aventyl)	30—60 mg	100 mg
Amitriptyline (Elavil)	50—150 mg	300 mg
Protriptyline (Vivactil)	15—40 mg	60 mg
Doxepin (Adapin, (Sinequan)	75—150 mg	300 mg
Monoamine oxidase inhibitors (MAOI)		
Tranylcypromine (Parnate)	20—30 mg	30 mg
Phenelzine (Nardil)	45 mg	75 mg

ANTIDEPRESSANTS

There are 2 major groups in this category: the newer **tricyclic compounds** and the older **monoamine oxidase inhibitors (MAOI),** which are used infrequently. (See Table 17—2.) Our discussion will be limited to the tricyclics since, with few exceptions, they are effective in the same group of patients as the MAOI drugs.

The tricyclic antidepressants are almost identical to each other in chemical structure, onset of action, pharmacologic effects, and side-effects. They are similar pharmacologically to the phenothiazine antipsychotic tranquilizers, which are also tricyclic compounds. the tricyclic antidepressants do not produce dependency, but they do have a somewhat narrow margin of safety between therapeutic dosage and overdosage. Combinations with perphenazine or other antipsychotic tranquilizers offer no special advantages.

Clinical Indications

The tricyclic antidepressants are useful in the management of depressions characterized by (1) psychomotor retardation; (2) severe mood disturbance with guilt, hopelessness, and inadequancy; (3) withdrawal from life activities and people; (4) somatic concerns; (5) ruminations; and (6) physical manifestations of emotional problems such as insomnia, constipation, anorexia, and weight loss. Other types of depressions do not generally respond well to antidepressants. Enuresis, narcolepsy, hyperkinetic states, and some cases of phobic anxiety may respond to these drugs.

Dosage Forms & Patterns

These drugs are available for oral and parenteral administration, although the latter route is infrequently used. There is a lag time of several days to several weeks with the oral forms, and individuals vary markedly in plasma concentration (3-fold to 13-fold), even with similar dosages, although there is evidence that a plasma steady state of 50—150 ng/ml is the optimum level. This may partly account for the lag and also for some therapeutic failures. High initial dosages, however, should not be used to overcome the lag because of the hazards of toxicity and suicide.

The dosage should be increased up to 300 mg/day (except protriptyline and nortriptyline) orally over a period of several weeks if depression does not remit on lower doses. The patient should be maintained on the lowest effective dose for as long as the depression continues. If, after adequate trial of the tricyclic antidepressants, the response is not satisfactory, a monoamine oxidase inhibitor or electroconvulsive therapy should be considered.

It is not necessary to give divided doses. A single daily dose at bedtime is effective.

A combination of tricyclic derivatives and MAO inhibitors should be used cautiously (and in that order) only for refractory cases.

Side-Effects

Anticholinergic side-effects include dry mouth, constipation, and exacerbation of prostatic disorders (urinary retention) or glaucoma. Orthostatic hypotension, T wave changes, and cardiac arrhythmias may occur. (Particular caution is required in patients with bundle branch block.) Other side-effects include fine tremors, organic brain syndrome, and occasional psychotic states.

With the exception of doxepin in low dosage, the tricyclic antidepressants antagonize the effects of guanethidine and tend to decrease insulin requirements. Amitriptyline and doxepin have a more pro-nounced sedative effect than the other tricyclics.

Since the margin between therapeutic and toxic doses is narrow, it is of major concern to prescribe nonlethal amounts. Any ingestion of the tricyclics above 1 gm (protriptyline, 200 mg, and nortriptyline, 800 mg) is serious. Disturbances of cardiac rhythm and conduction are most difficult to control. Seizures, bowel and bladder paralysis, and complications of coma—particularly pneumonitis—are common. The tri-cyclics are not dialyzable but do respond to physo-stigmine (the only anticholinesterase agent to pass the blood-brain barrier easily), 1—2 mg IM. Repeat in 15—30 minutes if necessary. Additional doses may be needed in intervals of 30 minutes to 2 hours. A rapid response is virtually diagnostic of poisoning with an anticholinergic agent. Particular caution is required in administering these drugs to patients with a history of respiratory distress, asthma, or cardiac conduction problems. Anticholinergic effects on the esophageal sphincter may contribute to the incidence of hiatus hernia.

See also general references under Antipsychotic Tranquilizers.
Ballin JC: Toxicity of tricyclic antidepressants. JAMA 231:1369, 1975.
Falk MA: Treatment of the depressed outpatient. Postgrad Med 55:77, 1974.
Glassman AJ, Perel JM: The clinical pharmacology of imipra-mine. Arch Gen Psychiat 28:649, 1973.
Granacher RP, Baldessarini RJ: Physostigmine: Its use in acute anticholinergic syndrome with antidepressants and anti-parkinson drugs. Arch Gen Psychiat 32:375, 1975.
Hollister L: Mental disorders: Antianxiety and antidepressant drugs. New England J Med 286:1195, 1972.
Johnson DAW: A study of the use of antidepressant medication in general practice. Brit J Psychiat 125:186, 1974.
Kline NS: Antidepressant medications: A more effective use by general practitioners, family physicians, internists and others. JAMA 227:1158, 1974.
Morris B, Beck AT: The efficacy of antidepressant drugs. Arch Gen Psychiat 30:667, 1974.
Sethna ER: A study of refractory cases of depressive illnesses and their response to combined antidepressant treatment. Brit J Psychiat 124:265, 1974.
Wittenborn JR, Klerman GL (editors): Antidepressants for the individual. Part 1. J Nerv Ment Dis 156:75, 1973.

SEDATIVE-HYPNOTICS
(Antianxiety Agents, Minor Tranquilizers)

The sedatives are a heterogeneous group of drugs which differ in chemical structure but have quite simi-lar pharmacologic and behavioral effects. They are often marketed as "minor tranquilizers" or "anti-anxiety agents," and all have hypnotic properties when given in adequate dosage. They differ mainly in milli-gram potency, dose-response curves, speed of onset, and duration of action. All are general depressants of brain function and decrease anxiety, producing disin-

Table 17—3. Commonly used sedative-hypnotic (minor) tranquilizers.

	Usual Oral Sedative Dose	Usual Oral Hypnotic Dose	Usual Maximum Daily Oral Dose
Barbiturates			
Amobarbital*	30 mg	100 mg	300 mg
Secobarbital†	30 mg	100 mg	300 mg
Phenobarbital	15—30 mg	150 mg	300—400 mg
Pentobarbital†	30 mg	100 mg	300 mg
Nonbarbiturate sedative-hypnotics			
Chloral hydrate†	250 mg	500—1000 mg	2.0 gm
Glutethimide (Doriden)	125 mg	250 mg	500 mg
Paraldehyde†	5—10 ml	20—30 ml	100 ml
Methaqualone (Quaalude, Somnafac, Sopor, Parest)	75 mg	150—300 mg	600 mg
Ethchlorvynol† (Placidyl)	100—200 mg	500 mg	1.0 gm
Methyprylon† (Noludar)	100 mg	300 mg	900 mg
Benzodiazepines			
Diazepam* (Valium)	2—10 mg	20—30 mg	50 mg
Chlordiazepoxide (Librium)	5—25 mg	50—100 mg	75—100 mg
Oxazepam† (Serax)	10 30 mg	30—60 mg	90 mg
Clorazepate (Tranxene)	7.5—15 mg	30 mg	40 mg
Flurazepam† (Dalmane)	15 mg	30 mg	60 mg
Miscellaneous			
Hydroxyzine pamoate (Vistaril)	25—50 mg	100 mg	300 mg
Meprobamate (Equanil, Miltown)	200—400 mg	800 mg	1.2 gm
Doxepin (Adapin, Sinequan)	25 mg	50—100 mg	300 mg

*Intermediate-acting.
†Short-acting.

hibition and a lowering of passive avoidance in suffi-cient dosage. To varying degrees, all have the potential for dependency with tolerance and severe withdrawal symptoms. They are additive to each other and have cross-tolerance and cross-dependence. Some have anti-convulsant and muscle relaxant properties, although muscle relaxation usually occurs in the ataxic dosage range.

Albeit the most expensive, the safest drugs in this group are the benzodiazepines (see Table 17—3). They are usually effective in moderate doses, have a wide margin of safety, are long-acting, and are much less likely to be abused than the other sedatives. In the USA they are more apt to be used in people with complaints referable to a specific organ system or non-specific anxiety than in primary psychiatric problems. In fact, there is no evidence that they are helpful in the major mental illnesses such as psychoses or organic brain syndromes, and their use is frequently associated with worsening of these conditions. All of the benzodiazepines are similar in chemical structure and clinical properties. They vary in milligram potency and duration of action, the latter being a function of lipid solubility and activity of metabolites. Those marketed as minor tranquilizers, such as diazepam, tend to be longer-acting (because of greater lipid solubility and more active metabolites), whereas flurazepam, which is sold as a hypnotic, is shorter-acting (because it is more water-soluble, with inactive metabolites). All have some degree of anticonvulsant activity and produce centrally mediated muscle relaxation in large doses. A major advantage of the benzodiazepines is the fact that they do not stimulate enzyme activity or interfere with most laboratory tests—in contrast to most of the other sedatives, particularly phenobarbital, which stimulate hepatic microsomal enzyme activity.

Clinical Indications

The sedatives are used clinically for the treatment of anxiety, which may be the result of many factors, eg, transient situational problems, acute and chronic stresses of life, chronic medical problems, intractable pain exacerbated by apprehension and depression, and problems which people cannot or will not resolve (unhappy marriages, unsatisfactory jobs, etc). In higher doses these drugs act as hypnotics, and the shorter-acting ones such as secobarbital and flurazepam are more commonly used for this purpose. Whether the indications are anxiety or insomnia, the drugs should be used judiciously and on an "as needed" basis rather than on fixed schedules, which tend to result in tolerance and increased psychologic dependency. There are no clinical indications for sedatives which cannot be met by one of the benzodiazepines. The highly addicting drugs with a narrow margin of safety such as glutethimide, methaqualone, ethchlorvynol, methyprylon, meprobamate, and the barbiturates (with the exception of phenobarbital) should be avoided. Phenobarbital, in addition to its anticonvulsant properties, is a reasonably safe and very cheap sedative but has the aforementioned disadvantage of enzyme stimulation, which markedly reduces its usefulness if any other medications are being used by that patient. While its effect on dicumarol is the most widely known, it increases the catabolism of practically all other drugs including antipsychotics and antidepressants.

Dosage Forms & Patterns (See Table 17—3.)

All of the sedatives may be given orally, and several are available in parenteral form (all of the barbiturates and several of the benzodiazepines). There is evidence that the benzodiazepines are slowly and erratically absorbed when given intramuscularly. The intravenous use of such benzodiazepines as diazepam and chlordiazepoxide produces rapid clinical results but occasional complications of pain and phlebitis. In the average case of anxiety, diazepam, 5—10 mg orally every 4—6 hours as needed, is a reasonable starting regimen. Since people vary widely in their response and since the drugs are long-lasting (the half-life of diazepam and its metabolites is about 30 hours), one must individualize the dosage. Once this is established, an *adequate* dose early in the course of symptom development will be long-lasting and effective and obviate the need for "pill-popping," which contributes to dependency problems.

Side-Effects

The side-effects are mainly behavioral and depend on patient reaction and dosage. As the dosage exceeds the levels necessary for sedation, the side-effects include disinhibition, ataxia, dysarthria, nystagmus, errors of commission (machinery should not be operated until the patient is well stabilized), and excessive sedation, with sleep followed by coma and death if large doses are taken. Bradycardia, hypotension, and respiratory arrest have occurred after the intravenous use of diazepam, but this has usually happened in patients with preexisting cardiopulmonary diseases and is also thought to be related to the propylene glycol solvent.

A serious side-effect of chronic excessive dosage is drug dependency, which may involve tolerance, and physiologic dependency with withdrawal symptoms similar in morbidity and mortality to alcohol withdrawal. Dependency begins in the range of 10 doses per day in the case of barbiturates (eg, ten 100 mg capsules of secobarbital) and the barbiturate-like drugs such as glutethimide and ethchlorvynol. In the case of the benzodiazepines, dependency does not begin until one is in the range of 30 or more doses per day (eg, thirty 10 mg doses of chlordiazepoxide). Duration of usage is also a factor. In the case of the safer drugs, several months of overusage have usually preceded the development of dependency; in the case of the less safe drugs, such as the barbiturates, overusage for a period of weeks may result in a dependent state requiring planned withdrawal.

The sedatives produce cumulative clinical effects with repeated dosage (especially if the patient has not had time to metabolize the previous dose); additive effects when given with other classes of sedatives or alcohol (many "accidental" deaths are the result of concomitant use of sedatives and alcohol); and residual effects after termination of treatment (particularly in the case of drugs which undergo slow biotransformation).

Balter MB, Levine J, Manheimer DI: Cross-national study of the extent of anti-anxiety/sedative drug use. New England J Med 290:769, 1974.

Gardner EA: Implications of psychoactive drug therapy. New England J Med 290:800, 1974.

Greenblatt DJ, Shader RI: Benzodiazepines. New England J Med 291:1011, 1974.

Greenblatt DJ & others: Slow absorption of intramuscular chloridiazepoxide. New England J Med 291:1116, 1974.

Hollister LE: Uses of psychotherapeutic drugs. Ann Int Med 79:88, 1973.

Kales A & others: Chronic hypnotic drug use. JAMA 227:513, 1974.

Katz RL: Drug therapy: Sedatives and tranquilizers. New England J Med 286:757, 1972.

CONVULSIVE THERAPIES

All convulsive therapies are similar in that a grand mal seizure is produced by a chemical (eg, pentylenetetrazol, flurothyl) or by electricity. For electroconvulsive therapy (ECT), the electricity is applied bitemporally or unilaterally on the nondominant side and the patient is medicated with atropine to prevent cardiac arrhythmias, a barbiturate for sedation, and succinylcholine for muscle relaxation. ECT is usually given at a frequency of about 3 times weekly for a "series" of a total of 10–15 seizures. Some administer several seizures at one sitting, with EEG monitoring to determine when the seizure is completed so that the next shock can be delivered.

ECT is safe, fast, and effective in appropriate depressions and is, in the long run, less expensive than prolonged hospitalization. The mode of action is not known. Unilateral ECT causes less memory defect but is less effective, so that more treatments are necessary.

ECT is clinically indicated for depressions of the so-called endogenous type with symptoms of psychomotor retardation, preoccupation with self, ruminations, insomnia, anorexia and weight loss (particularly if suicidal ideation is strong), and for schizophrenic psychoses that do not respond to adequate doses of major tranquilizers. It has been variably successful in a number of other problems such as mania and postcardiotomy psychoses.

Side-effects are limited to memory changes during treatment. Problems such as fractures which used to be direct results of the seizure are prevented with appropriate muscle relaxation.

Abrams R, Taylor MA: Unipolar and bipolar depressive illness: Phenomenology and response to ECT. Arch Gen Psychiat 30:320, 1974.

Bidder TG: Bilateral and unilateral electroconvulsive therapy: A follow-up study and critique. Am J Psychiat 127:737, 1970.

Cohen DB & others: Antidepressant effects of unilateral electric convulsive shock therapy. Arch Gen Psychiat 31:673, 1974.

Murillo LG, Exner JE: The effects of regressive electroconvulsive therapy with process schizophrenics. Am J Psychiat 130:269, 1973.

Stones MJ: Electroconvulsive treatment and short-term memory. Brit J Psychiat 122:59, 1973.

OTHER ORGANIC THERAPIES

Psychosurgery still has a place in selected cases of severe, unremitting anxiety and depression, obsessional neuroses, and, to a lesser degree, some of the schizophrenias. The stereotactic technics that are now being used, including modified bifrontal stereotactic tractotomy, are great improvements over the crude methods of the past.

Electrosleep is currently being studied, but its effectiveness is nonspecific and questionable.

Blumer D: Psychosurgery. Chap 28, pp 470–478, in: *Handbook of Psychiatry,* 3rd ed. Solomon P, Patch VD (editors). Lange, 1974.

Bridges PK & others: A comparative review of patients with obsessional neurosis and depression treated by psychosurgery. Brit J Psychiat 123:663, 1973.

Gilliland IC, Kelly D (editors): Symposium on psychosurgery. Postgrad MJ 49:825, 1973.

Hearst ED & others: Electrosleep therapy. Arch Gen Psychiat 30:463, 1974.

Kelly D & others: Modified leucotomy assessed clinically, physiologically, and psychologically at six weeks and eighteen months. Brit J Psychiat 120:19, 1972.

HOSPITALIZATION

The need for hospital care may range from admission to a medical bed in a general hospital for an acute situational stress reaction to admission to a psychiatric ward in the throes of an acute psychosis. The trend over recent years has been to maintain psychiatric wards in general hospitals in the community, treat patients aggressively, and discharge them promptly to the next appropriate level of treatment—day hospital, halfway house, outpatient therapy, etc.

Hospital care may be indicated when the patient is too sick to care for himself or is a serious threat to himself or others; when observation and diagnostic procedures are necessary; or when specific kinds of treatment such as ECT, complex medication trials, or hospital environment (milieu) are required.

The disadvantages of psychiatric hospitalization include decreased self-confidence by needing hospitalization; the stigma of being a "psychiatric patient"; possible increased dependency and regression; and the expense.

One of the sad commentaries on hospital care of mental patients is the continued segregation of psychiatric from nonpsychiatric patients. Even with more active community treatment, hospital care is still in segregated psychiatric units of general hospitals. Decreased length of hospitalization, acceptance of treatment, and lessening of stigmatization can be accomplished by treating psychiatric patients in regular hospital medical beds. In places where this has been done, there have been few untoward incidents. The major obstacle to be overcome is staff resistance. Ongoing education of the medical and nursing staffs, as well as some selectivity with regard to patients, will help to hasten acceptance of this type of hospitalization.

Crowley TJ & others: Drug and alcohol abuse among psychiatric admissions. Arch Gen Psychiat 30:13, 1974.

Rabiner CJ, Lurie A: The case for psychiatric hospitalization. Am J Psychiat 131:761, 1974.

Reding GR, Maguire B: Nonsegregated acute psychiatric admissions to general hospitals: Continuity of care within the community hospital. New England J Med 289:185, 1973.

Tucker GJ, Maxmen JS: The practice of hospital psychiatry: A formulation. Am J Psychiat 130:887, 1973.

in the past, leaving the individual with distortions of feelings and attitudes which impair his ability to cope with himself and his environment. By discussion of past and present experiences in a framework of free association, the patient "works through" the previous conflicts, thus allowing resolution. The patient transfers the feelings that remain from these past experiences onto the therapist, who assists the patient in resolving his transference feelings and reach self-understanding.

2. PSYCHOLOGIC APPROACHES

INDIVIDUAL THERAPY

Individual therapy involving a therapist and a single patient—the traditional form of psychotherapy—depends principally on verbal interchange to ameliorate or remove psychologic symptoms, promote more adaptive behavioral patterns, and develop emotionally meaningful self-knowledge.

Crisis Therapy

Short-term (weeks); frequency: daily to weekly.

Crisis therapy is offered following a particularly stressful situation and is oriented toward resolution of the crisis, utilizing rapid rapport with the therapist which makes the patient more amenable to try new behaviors. Correlations between antecedents to the crisis and anticipation of situations likely to produce future problems are quickly established. Since in crisis therapy the treatment is given before the emotional conflicts have become established as recurrent symptoms, the goals are relief of symptoms, learning, and prevention in a short, intensive therapeutic procedure.

Eclectic Psychotherapy

Intermediate term (months); frequency: weekly.

This pragmatic type of therapy is usually a combination of approaches, often based on psychoanalytic, behavioral, and common-sense components. The therapist is more active, free associations are little used, and the emphasis is more on the present and the ways in which past experiences are clearly related to past and present behavior. The emphasis is on helping the patient understand and anticipate future problems, and one of the aims of therapy is to support and bolster those defense mechanisms that the patient needs. Medications are frequently used in conjunction with psychotherapy. Family and spouse contacts are used when necessary.

Psychoanalysis

Long-term (years); frequency: daily.

Analytic therapy is based on the assumption that symptoms and maladaptation stem from unresolved conflicts that arrested personality growth at some time

GROUP THERAPY

Group therapy is a form of psychotherapy in which a therapist and 2 or more patients utilize both verbal and nonverbal technics to alter symptoms, particularly those that arise from maladaptive interpersonal behavior patterns.

Types of Group Therapy

A. Family and Couples Therapy: This type of therapy undertakes to examine and modify personal and family modes of interaction which are considered to be the cause of symptoms in one or more members of the family. The family or couple are seen together, since the therapist can see the distortions when the members can be observed interacting. The goal of therapy is not only to relieve symptoms but also to help family members learn new methods to deal with stress in such a way as not to reinforce self-defeating behavior.

B. Individual Group Therapy: The group is composed of unrelated individuals functioning in a "safe laboratory" in which they can learn about their behavior by getting "feedback" from others, observing similar behavior in others, and practicing new modes of behavior. Group therapy is particularly valuable for people who have difficulty in establishing and maintaining relationships.

C. Couples Group Therapy: Composed of 2 or more couples but with the same goals as individual group therapy. It is often enlightening for a couple to recognize their own behavior by observing the behavior of others.

D. Family Group Therapy: Includes 2 or more families. It is not frequently used because it is difficult to monitor the myriad interactions that occur in families, and often the emphasis is on sharing and modeling rather than insight.

Other Approaches to Therapy

There are many forms of therapy, and they vary both in philosophy and technic. Most of the traditional therapies have accepted the assumption that problems arise within the individual and that his symptoms are determined by his particular defense mechanisms. (See p 594.) The newer therapies stress the relationship between the individual, his cultural background, and his environment as a causative factor in symptom production.

The central thesis of **reality therapy** is that people do not act irresponsibly because they are "ill" but that they are ill because they act irresponsibly. The sequence of symptom formation has heretofore been presumed to be as follows: Basic fears originating from childhood (eg, fear of rejection → high expectations of self [which inevitably fail] → feelings of inadequacy and loss of confidence → defensive maneuvers to obtain substitute satisfaction → anxiety when these maneuvers are unsuccessful). Reality therapists believe that if a satisfactory standard of behavior has not been maintained, self-esteem suffers, and that the only way to change this is for the patient to use new responsible patterns of behavior with emphasis on the present and little concern with past events.

The reality therapists believe that the basis for "sick" or irresponsible activity is the parent-child relationship and that the parents' inability to tolerate the child's anger was the reason the child was not taught responsibility. In treatment, the therapist always takes the responsible rather than the expedient course, thus setting the pattern for the patient to behave more responsibly and not face the fear of rejection. Attitudes change after the patient's behavior changes, and such phenomena as understanding, attitudes, and insight do not cause behavioral change. The responsibility for change rests with the patient, and the therapist's function is merely to find ways of behaving that conform to the patient's standards and are consistent with the demands of the real world.

Transactional analysis is based on the premise that everybody still retains (1) vestiges of the child, (2) parental injunctions, and (3) elements of mature behavior. This parent-child-adult substrate varies in proportion, and the therapeutic effort is directed toward increasing the adult behaviors, emphasizing communications which are adult-adult rather than parent-child or adult-child. Many communications are stereotyped and when these serve to avoid meaningful relationships they are called "games." This is a shorthand for identifying behaviors so that patients can identify them, give them up, and substitute more meaningful interactions.

Existential therapy considers the feelings of the patient to be a consequence of existence and a function of the ongoing process of "becoming" or self-actualization. The emphasis is on the freedom to make choices, and the patient's progress toward self-realization depends upon the courage he is able to show in making difficult choices. The patient is helped to realize the futility of protests against past injustices (there is no dwelling on the past) and is expected to use his potential for self-understanding and increased relatedness to his environment.

Although **family therapy** may appear on the surface to be quite different, it is similar to the types of therapy discussed above in that the individual is always considered in the matrix of significant relationships.

The "identified patient"—the family member who has developed symptoms—is considered to be an outward manifestation of the disturbed family interactions. The therapist works with the family as a group, and the emphasis is on the interactions, communications, and dynamics of the unit and not on the disturbance of one particular member. This approach is useful when the disturbance is adversely affecting the family or when the family is contributing to the illness of one of its members. The goal is to find new and more acceptable ways of family functioning.

There are many variations and permutations of both individual and group therapies. **Encounter groups** (also called T groups), sensitivity training groups, or human potential groups have had a phenomenal growth in the past 10 years. They should not take symptomatic or ill individuals as their subject matter but should attempt to increase personal growth and promote interpersonal awareness and trust. Indiscriminate selection of members of these groups has occasionally resulted in a psychiatric casualty—usually a person much more ill than casual observation indicates who cannot tolerate the stress involved.

Some therapies include the use of multiple therapists who may or may not be involved with each other, eg, an individual therapist for one member of a family and the family therapist for all, or an individual therapist for each spouse. Various technics such as hypnosis, relaxation, psychodrama, and role reversal may be used in both individual and group therapy.

Bartolucci G, Drayer CS: An overview of crisis intervention in the emergency rooms of general hospitals. Am J Psychiat 130:953, 1973.

Birk L: Intensive group therapy: An effective behavioral-psychoanalytic method. Am J Psychiat 131:11, 1974.

Cristol AH: Studies of outcome of psychotherapy. Comprehensive Psychiat 13:189, 1972.

Eisler RM: Behavioral technics in family-oriented crisis intervention. Arch Gen Psychiat 28:111, 1972.

Engle GL: Psychoanalysis. JAMA 231:579, 1975.

Frank JD: Psychotherapy: The restoration of morale. Am J Psychiat 131:271, 1974.

Herz MI & others: Individual versus group aftercare treatment. Arch Gen Psychiat 131:808, 1974.

Offenkrantz W, Tobin A: Psychoanalytic psychotherapy. Arch Gen Psychiat 30:593, 1974.

Sloane RB & others: Short-term analytically oriented psychotherapy versus behavior therapy. Am J Psychiat 132:373, 1975.

3. SOCIAL APPROACHES

In contrast to psychologic technics, which deal principally with intrapsychic phenomena, the social approaches to psychiatric treatment attempt to modify attitudes and behavior by altering the **environmental** factors contributing to the patient's maladaptation. The scope of the attempt may range from provision of a therapeutic milieu—eg, in a day hospital or residential community such as Synanon—to minor alterations in school procedures or daily family activities. Various psychologic and behavioral technics may be used within the social approaches.

Part-Time Hospitalization

The patient participates in the hospital milieu either during the day (day hospitals—going home at night), or stays the night (night hospitals—going to work or school during the day), or spends several hours a day in the hospital for up to 5 or 6 days a week (partial day care hospitals).

Self-Help Communities

These are usually sponsored by nongovernmental agencies for the purpose of helping people with a particular type of difficulty. The individual lives-in full time for varying periods and usually continues his affiliation with the group after he leaves. Examples of self-help communities include Synanon (originally organized to help people with narcotics problems), residences for alcoholics, residences for unwed mothers and wayward girls (eg, Door of Hope), Salvation Army, and church-sponsored agencies.

Substitute Homes

Substitute homes provide shelter, a "home-like" environment, and more specific treatment programs to a variable degree and for longer periods of time. Examples of "substitute" homes are foster homes, usually for children; board and care homes, primarily for people who are disabled and unlikely to return to productive function; mental hygiene homes, providing special services for the mentally disabled who are unable to live in board and care homes; family care homes, similar to foster homes but taking adults—usually several at one time; residential treatment centers, taking a number of children and offering fairly intensive treatment programs; and "crash pads," a relatively new approach to short-term residence for young people—often in the process of withdrawing from drugs—who need shelter.

Nonresidential Self-Help Organizations

The following are examples of organizations usually administered by people who have survived similar problems and have banded together to help others cope with the same problem: Alcoholics Anonymous (and Al-Anon, to help families of alcoholics); Recovery Inc., organized and run by people who have had an emotional problem which required hospitalization; Schizophrenics Anonymous; colostomy clubs; mastectomy clubs; the Epilepsy Society; the American Heart Association's Stroke Clubs of America; burn recovery groups; the international by-pass groups for those who have had surgery for obesity; other groups organized to help people deal with practical and psychologic problems of a particular illness; and friendship centers which assist people in their efforts to find specific kinds of help.

Special Professional & Paraprofessional Organizations

Examples of special organizations of this type are Homemaker Service, made up of women who come into the home to help the partially disabled maintain the household; Visiting Nurse Associations, which usually provide more than medical assistance; adult protective services, oriented toward assisting the elderly; Abortion Counseling and Planned Parenthood Services; genetic counseling services; family service agencies, for marriage counseling and family problems; Travelers Aid, for rendering assistance to new residents and transients; legal aid societies; Big Brother, to provide a masculine figure when one is lacking in the family; consumer credit organizations, to help the financially naive organize their financial problems; crisis centers, eg, "free clinics" and county-sponsored satellite clinics; and church-sponsored agencies.

Arthur RA: Social psychiatry: An overview. Am J Psychiat 130:841, 1973.

Dumont MP: Self help treatment programs. Am J Psychiat 131:631, 1974.

Fox, RP: Therapeutic environments. Arch Gen Psychiat 29:514, 1973.

Kiritz S, Moos RH: Physiological effects of social environments. Psychosom Med 36:96, 1974.

Lipowski ZJ: Psychosocial aspects of disease. Ann Int Med 71:1197, 1969.

Weissman MM: The assessment of social adjustment: A review of techniques. Arch Gen Psychiat 32:357, 1975.

4. BEHAVIORAL APPROACHES

Behavior therapy is education and has its foundations in learning theory. The behavior therapist regards his role as that of a teacher who attempts to bring about change. To do so, he must first identify the specific problem and the factors that play a role in precipitating or perpetuating the problem and then attempt to alter those factors such as rewards which support the behavior.

The emphasis of behavior therapy is on "here and now" and **direct** change—to the virtual exclusion of all concern with unconscious conflicts. The goal is to "unlearn" those destructive or unproductive types of behavior that result from faulty learning and to enhance the individual's repertoire of useful social and adaptive skills. Great emphasis is placed on identifying and then obliterating whatever is maintaining the maladaptive behavior.

Whereas **conditioning** is understood by some to be synonymous with a specific type of learning (eg, Pavlov's dogs), behavior therapy is much broader. It includes the relationship with the therapist, utilizes verbal technics to a lesser degree than other therapies, and interprets "behavior" in a broad sense that includes thoughts and feelings.

Many of the technics of behavior therapy require a cooperative effort on the part of a number of people who must all understand and be consistent in their responses to specified behaviors. Thus, a cooperative social setting such as a milieu ward, a Synanon community, or the patient's own home and family is important in implementing many of the following technics.

Technics of Behavior Therapy

A. Modeling: Much learning occurs by imitation. From his earliest years, the individual has modeled his behavior after "significant others" in his life: parents, teachers, peers, employers, public personalities, and historical figures. The therapist makes a conscious effort to serve as a model of particular kinds of behavior which are significant to the patient and within the bounds of his capabilities. This device is particularly useful in people with low self-esteem.

B. Operant Conditioning: The device of operant conditioning is based on the principle that behavior is maintained by the rewards it elicits. Deliberate implementation of various schedules of positive reinforcement (reward) alerts the individual to his behavior and its consequences. Like modeling, operant conditioning is a common procedure in families, and the child soon learns that "good" behavior is rewarded. So-called "token economies" in centers for retarded or autistic patients and those with behavioral problems are effective, particularly where verbal technics have little meaning.

C. Aversive Conditioning: Aversive conditioning is the opposite of operant conditioning but is a less potent shaper of behavior. Undesirable behavior results in an unpleasant consequence (eg, vomiting induced by apomorphine, mild electric or sound shock), whereas satisfactory alternative responses are operantly encouraged. The most common conditions treated by this technic have been enuresis, alcoholism, and homosexuality. The results have been varied, but some successes have been reported, particularly in enuresis.

D. Extinction: Extinction is the process of refusing to reinforce behavior on the theory that behavior cannot be sustained without some sort of reinforcement. Temper tantrums, usually contrived to gain attention of any sort, are "extinguished" in this way. The same is true of noxious attention-getting behaviors such as inappropriate verbal expressions (eg, obscenities).

E. Desensitization: Familiarity lessens anxiety and reduces the tendency to avoid exposure to the feared object, person, or situation. The subject is repeatedly exposed to the feared stimulus (eg, looking at a picture of an elevator when the fear has been riding in elevators) at such a low level of intensity that the fear response is minimal. Exposures are then gradually increased (eg, walking past a real elevator) until the subject is able to tolerate the real experience with markedly reduced fear levels. This technic has been most effective in the treatment of phobias and a variety of situations (such as frigidity or impotence) which engender fears of failure, disapproval, and embarrassment.

F. "Emotive Imagery": Deliberate evocation of mental images that arouse certain feelings can be used as a way of warding off painful emotions resulting from stress-inducing circumstances. Noxious imagery can be used in aversive conditioning and "pleasant thoughts" in operant training. In "mental imagery" desensitization, the phobic or sensitive situation is reproduced in graded quantities and the patient learns to handle minor upsetting imagined situations without anxiety before proceeding to the more difficult ones.

G. "Flooding": Flooding consists of overwhelming the individual, in a safe setting, with anxiety-producing stimuli. The anxiety responses gradually lessen (law of diminishing returns) until extinction occurs. In some ways, flooding is a desensitization technic without the graded approach. It has been used in the treatment of obsessive compulsive patients and those with particular behavior problems such as compulsive hoarding.

H. Role-Playing: In the role-playing technic, patients can practice various types of behaviors in anxiety-producing but "safe" situations. For example, the therapist may assume the role of an angry friend and the patient uses different ways of handling the situation. Role reversal—where the therapist and the patient change roles—then gives the patient a chance to experience the other's feelings and attitudes. Assertive training for inhibited individuals is a variant to help people learn to be more spontaneous and open.

Birk L, Brinkley-Birk AW: Psychoanalysis and behavior therapy. Am J Psychiat 131:499, 1974.

Eisler RM: Shaping components of assertive behavior with instructions and feedback. Am J Psychiat 131:1344, 1974.

Engel BT, Nikoomanesh P, Shuster MM: Operant conditioning of rectosphincteric responses in the treatment of fecal incontinence. New England J Med 290:646, 1974.

Geider MG & others: Specific and nonspecific factors in behavior therapy. Brit J Psychiat 123:445, 1973.

Greenspan SI: The clinical uses of operant learning approaches: Some complex issues. Am J Psychiat 131:852, 1974.

Mathews AM & others: Process variables and the prediction of outcome in behavior therapy. Brit J Psychiat 125:256, 1974.

Rhoads JM, Feather BW: The application of psychodynamics to behavior therapy. Am J Psychiat 131:17, 1974.

Wolpe J & others: The current status of systematic desensitization. Am J Psychiat 130:961, 1973.

COMMON PSYCHIATRIC DISORDERS

SITUATIONAL DISORDERS

Situational reactions are related not so much to the severity of the stress as to the stability of the individual. Some people react hysterically to a mild situational crisis, whereas others seem able to confront the most trying personal experiences with an attitude of imperturbable stoicism.

A diagnosis of transient situational disturbance can be made if psychologic symptoms occur in a previously stable individual following some emotionally traumatic event such as the death of a child, spouse, etc.

Clinical Findings

Symptoms are variable in nature and intensity and may include anxiety, depression (often with agitation), overt anger, guilt, and actual fear. Somatic complaints such as diarrhea, urinary frequency, and incontinence may occur. Physical findings include an anxious appearance, restlessness, hyperventilation, tremulousness, tachycardia, hypertension, dry mouth, and dilated pupils.

Treatment

A. Psychologic: Psychologic measures include crisis therapy, with its emphasis on the immediate problem and helping the patient to reestablish his previous level of functioning. The family should be encouraged to provide support when possible, and several sessions of family therapy may help them to focus on the problem, provide realistic solutions, and anticipate future problems. Family therapy also helps to distribute the problem rather than have one person (the "identified patient") shoulder the problem alone. When marital problems are a major consideration, both the husband and the wife should be seen in joint sessions. Couples therapy, consisting of 4 or 5 couples in a group, is a useful tool when one of the spouses needs support from others with similar problems while initiating changes in the marriage.

B. Medical: Medical treatment is limited to reassurance that the patient's problem is important but that no serious physical problems are present even though some somatic complaints may occur. Mild sedation with sedatives or minor tranquilizers (eg, phenobarbital, 15–30 mg twice a day, or diazepam, 5–10 mg twice a day) may be necessary during the acute phase.

C. Social: Social methods of treatment may involve brief counseling, an emphasis on return to school or job, suggestions about daily routine, and, when necessary, the involvement of outside social agencies such as Homemaker Service or Legal Aid.

Prognosis

Return to satisfactory function after a short period is part of the clinical picture of this syndrome. Resolution may be delayed if other people's responses to the patient's difficulties are thoughtlessly harmful or if the secondary gains appear to the patient to outweigh the advantages of recovery.

Horowitz M: Stress response syndromes. Arch Gen Psychiat 31:768, 1974.

Sifneos PE: *Short Term Psychotherapy and Emotional Crisis.* Harvard Univ Press, 1972.

Walker WR & others: Brief hospitalization on a crisis service: A study of patient and treatment variables. Am J Psychiat 130:896, 1973.

NEUROSES

Essentials of Diagnosis

- Overt anxiety or an overt manifestation of a defense mechanism (such as a phobia) or both.
- No apparent situational basis for the symptoms.
- Overt somatic symptoms, eg, hyperventilation or palpitations.
- Covert somatic symptoms involving a specific organ system, eg, tension headaches.
- Chronic fatigue, irritability, and nervousness.

General Considerations

Anxiety is the common denominator of the neuroses and is the result of a maladaptive attempt to resolve internal conflicts. These conflicts are usually unresolved childhood problems such as dependency, insecurity, hostility, excessive need for affection, concerns about intimacy, and overly strong drives for power and control.

Neuroses have 2 principal components: **psychologic** (tension, fears, difficulty in concentration, apprehension) and **somatic** (tachycardia, palpitations, tremor, sweating, gastrointestinal upset). Sympathomimetic symptoms of anxiety are both a response to a CNS state and a reinforcement of further anxiety. A neurosis can become self-generating since the symptoms reinforce the reaction, causing it to spiral.

The resultant anxiety is handled in different ways (defense mechanisms; see p 594), and this determines the **form** of the neurosis. If the individual has no specific defense mechanisms, the anxiety is free-floating and results in acute anxiety attacks, occasionally becoming chronic. When one or several defense mechanisms are functioning, the consequences are the well-known neurotic problems such as phobias, conversion reactions, dissociative states, obsessions, and compulsions.

Depressions can also be a way of coping with anxiety, and in this context are considered as neurotic manifestations.

Some believe that the neuroses are not a result of unconscious conflicts but are "habits"—persistent patterns of nonadaptive behavior acquired by learning. The "habits," being nonadaptive, are unsatisfactory ways of dealing with life problems—hence the resultant anxiety, which is often handled by the individual. Help is sought only when the anxiety becomes too painful. Exogenous factors such as stimulants (eg, caffeine) must be considered as etiologic or adjunctive factors.

Table 17—4. New nomenclature and code numbers based on APA DSM-II.

I   MENTAL RETARDATION
- ☐ 310.   Borderline
- ☐ 311.   Mild
- ☐ 312.   Moderate
- ☐ 313.   Severe
- ☐ 314.   Profound
- ☐ 315.   Unspecified

With each: Following or associated with
- ☐   .0   Infection or intoxication
- ☐   .1   Trauma or physical agent
- ☐   .2   Disorders of metabolism, growth or nutrition
- ☐   .3   Gross brain disease (postnatal)
- ☐   .4   Unknown prenatal influence
- ☐   .5   Chromosomal abnormality
- ☐   .6   Prematurity
- ☐   .7   Major psychiatric disorder
- ☐   .8   Psycho-social (environmental) deprivation
- ☐   .9   Other condition

II   ORGANIC BRAIN SYNDROMES (OBS)

A   PSYCHOSES

Senile and pre-senile dementia
- ☐ 290.0   Senile dementia
- ☐ 290.1   Pre-senile dementia

Alcoholic psychosis
- ☐ 291.0   Delirium tremens
- ☐ 291.1   Korsakov's psychosis
- ☐ 291.2   Other alcoholic hallucinosis
- ☐ 291.3   Alcohol paranoid state
- ☐ 291.4*   Acute alcohol intoxication*
- ☐ 291.5*   Alcoholic deterioration*
- ☐ 291.6*   Pathological intoxication*
- ☐ 291.9   Other alcoholic psychosis

Psychosis associated with intracranial infection
- ☐ 292.0   General paralysis
- ☐ 292.1   Syphilis of central nervous system
- ☐ 292.2   Epidemic encephalitis
- ☐ 292.3   Other and unspecified encephalitis
- ☐ 292.9   Other intracranial infection

Psychosis associated with other cerebral condition
- ☐ 293.0   Cerebral arteriosclerosis
- ☐ 293.1   Other cerebrovascular disturbance
- ☐ 293.2   Epilepsy
- ☐ 293.3   Intracranial neoplasm
- ☐ 293.4   Degenerative disease of the CNS
- ☐ 293.5   Brain trauma
- ☐ 293.9   Other cerebral condition

Psychosis associated with other physical condition
- ☐ 294.0   Endocrine disorder
- ☐ 294.1   Metabolic and nutritional disorder
- ☐ 294.2   Systemic infection
- ☐ 294.3   Drug or poison intoxication (other than alcohol)
- ☐ 294.4   Childbirth
- ☐ 294.8   Other and unspecified physical condition

B   NON-PSYCHOTIC OBS
- ☐ 309.0   Intracranial infection
- ☐ 309.13*   Alcohol* (simple drunkenness)
- ☐ 309.14*   Other drug, poison or systemic intoxication*
- ☐ 309.2   Brain trauma
- ☐ 309.3   Circulatory disturbance
- ☐ 309.4   Epilepsy
- ☐ 309.5   Disturbance of metabolism, growth, or nutrition
- ☐ 309.6   Senile or pre-senile brain disease
- ☐ 309.7   Intracranial neoplasm
- ☐ 309.8   Degenerative disease of the CNS
- ☐ 309.9   Other physical condition

III   PSYCHOSES NOT ATTRIBUTED TO PHYSICAL CONDITIONS LISTED PREVIOUSLY

Schizophrenia
- ☐ 295.0   Simple
- ☐ 295.1   Hebephrenic
- ☐ 295.2   Catatonic
- ☐ 295.23*   Catatonic type, excited*
- ☐ 295.24*   Catatonic type, withdrawn*
- ☐ 295.3   Paranoid
- ☐ 295.4   Acute schizophrenic episode
- ☐ 295.5   Latent
- ☐ 295.6   Residual
- ☐ 295.7   Schizo-affective
- ☐ 295.73*   Schizo-affective, excited*
- ☐ 295.74*   Schizo-affective, depressed*
- ☐ 295.8*   Childhood*
- ☐ 295.90*   Chronic undifferentiated*
- ☐ 295.99*   Other schizophrenia*

Major affective disorders
- ☐ 296.0   Involutional melancholia
- ☐ 296.1   Manic-depressive illness, manic
- ☐ 296.2   Manic-depressive illness, depressed
- ☐ 296.3   Manic-depressive illness, circular
- ☐ 296.33*   Manic-depressive, circular, manic*
- ☐ 296.34*   Manic-depressive, circular, depressed*
- ☐ 296.8   Other major affective disorder

Paranoid states
- ☐ 297.0   Paranoia
- ☐ 297.1   Involutional paranoid state
- ☐ 297.9   Other paranoid state

Other psychoses
- ☐ 298.0   Psychotic depressive reaction

IV   NEUROSES
- ☐ 300.0   Anxiety
- ☐ 300.1   Hysterical
- ☐ 300.13*   Hysterical, conversion type*
- ☐ 300.14*   Hysterical, dissociative type*
- ☐ 300.2   Phobic
- ☐ 300.3   Obsessive compulsive
- ☐ 300.4   Depressive
- ☐ 300.5   Neurasthenic
- ☐ 300.6   Depersonalization
- ☐ 300.7   Hypochondriacal
- ☐ 300.8   Other neurosis

V   PERSONALITY DISORDERS AND CERTAIN OTHER NON-PSYCHOTIC MENTAL DISORDERS

Personality disorders
- ☐ 301.0   Paranoid
- ☐ 301.1   Cyclothymic
- ☐ 301.2   Schizoid
- ☐ 301.3   Explosive
- ☐ 301.4   Obsessive compulsive
- ☐ 301.5   Hysterical
- ☐ 301.6   Asthenic
- ☐ 301.7   Antisocial
- ☐ 301.81*   Passive-aggressive*
- ☐ 301.82*   Inadequate*
- ☐ 301.89*   Other specified types*

Sexual deviation
- ☐ 302.0   Homosexuality
- ☐ 302.1   Fetishism
- ☐ 302.2   Pedophilia
- ☐ 302.3   Transvestitism
- ☐ 302.4   Exhibitionism
- ☐ 302.5*   Voyeurism*
- ☐ 302.6*   Sadism*
- ☐ 302.7*   Masochism*
- ☐ 302.8   Other sexual deviation

Alcoholism
- ☐ 303.0   Episodic excessive drinking
- ☐ 303.1   Habitual excessive drinking
- ☐ 303.2   Alcohol addiction
- ☐ 303.9   Other alcoholism

Drug dependence
- ☐ 304.0   Opium, opium alkaloids and their derivatives
- ☐ 304.1   Synthetic analgesics with morphine-like effects
- ☐ 304.2   Barbiturates
- ☐ 304.3   Other hypnotics and sedatives or "tranquilizers"
- ☐ 304.4   Cocaine
- ☐ 304.5   Cannabis sativa (hashish, marihuana)
- ☐ 304.6   Other psycho-stimulants
- ☐ 304.7   Hallucinogens
- ☐ 304.8   Other drug dependence

VI   PSYCHOPHYSIOLOGIC DISORDERS
- ☐ 305.0   Skin
- ☐ 305.1   Musculoskeletal
- ☐ 305.2   Respiratory
- ☐ 305.3   Cardiovascular
- ☐ 305.4   Hemic and lymphatic
- ☐ 305.5   Gastro-intestinal
- ☐ 305.6   Genito-urinary
- ☐ 305.7   Endocrine
- ☐ 305.8   Organ of special sense
- ☐ 305.9   Other type

VII   SPECIAL SYMPTOMS
- ☐ 306.0   Speech disturbance
- ☐ 306.1   Specific learning disturbance
- ☐ 306.2   Tic
- ☐ 306.3   Other psychomotor disorder
- ☐ 306.4   Disorders of sleep
- ☐ 306.5   Feeding disturbance
- ☐ 306.6   Enuresis
- ☐ 306.7   Encopresis
- ☐ 306.8   Cephalalgia
- ☐ 306.9   Other special symptom

VIII   TRANSIENT SITUATIONAL DISTURBANCES
- ☐ 307.0*   Adjustment reaction of infancy*
- ☐ 307.1*   Adjustment reaction of childhood*
- ☐ 307.2*   Adjustment reaction of adolescence*
- ☐ 307.3*   Adjustment reaction of adult life*
- ☐ 307.4*   Adjustment reaction of late life*

IX   BEHAVIOR DISORDERS OF CHILDHOOD AND ADOLESCENCE
- ☐ 308.0*   Hyperkinetic reaction*
- ☐ 308.1*   Withdrawing reaction*
- ☐ 308.2*   Overanxious reaction*
- ☐ 308.3*   Runaway reaction*
- ☐ 308.4*   Unsocialized aggressive reaction*
- ☐ 308.5*   Group delinquent reaction*
- ☐ 308.9*   Other reaction*

X   CONDITIONS WITHOUT MANIFEST PSYCHIATRIC DISORDER AND NON-SPECIFIC CONDITIONS

Social maladjustment without manifest psychiatric disorder
- ☐ 316.0*   Marital maladjustment*
- ☐ 316.1*   Social maladjustment*
- ☐ 316.2*   Occupational maladjustment*
- ☐ 316.3*   Dyssocial behavior*
- ☐ 316.9*   Other social maladjustment*

Non-specific conditions
- ☐ 317*   Non-specific conditions*

No mental disorder
- ☐ 318*   No mental disorder*

XI   NON-DIAGNOSTIC TERMS FOR ADMINISTRATIVE USE
- ☐ 319.0*   Diagnosis deferred*
- ☐ 319.1*   Boarder*
- ☐ 319.2*   Experiment only*
- ☐ 319.3*   Other*

*Categories added to ICD-8 for use in U.S. only.

FIFTH DIGIT QUALIFYING PHRASES

Section II	Section III	Section IV through IX	All disorders
☐ .X1 Acute	☐ .X6 Not psychotic now	☐ .X6 Mild	☐ .X5 In remission
☐ .X2 Chronic		☐ .X7 Moderate	
		☐ .X8 Severe	

The treatment approach tends to reflect the philosophic bias of the therapist. Results do not differ significantly among various treatment methods.

Clinical Findings

A. Anxiety: Acute anxiety attacks are characterized by a sudden onset of fear; feelings of tension, restlessness, and breathlessness; a sense of impending doom; hyperventilation; and variable somatic symptoms. There is marked fatigue after the acute attack. Chronic anxiety takes the form of repeated attacks and long-lasting autonomic reactivity (eg, increased blood pressure, perspiration, frequent palpitations). Chronic irritability and fatigue are common.

B. Phobias: Phobic ideation is a mechanism of "displacement" in which the patient has transferred his anxiety from its true object to another that he then proceeds to avoid in order not to feel anxiety—even great terror. However, since phobias are ineffective defense mechanisms, there tends to be an increase in the scope, intensity, and number of phobias.

C. Conversion Reactions: "Conversion" of psychic conflict into physical symptoms in parts of the body innervated by the sensorimotor system (eg, paralysis, aphonia) is a psychiatric defense mechanism that is more common in unsophisticated individuals and in some cultures than others. The term "hysterical conversion" is occasionally used synonymously. The defense mechanisms utilized in this condition are repression (a barring from consciousness) and isolation (a splitting of the affect from the idea). The somatic manifestation that takes the place of anxiety is typically paralysis, and in some instances the organ dysfunction may have symbolic meaning (eg, arm paralysis in marked anger). There is usually a past history of other conversion reactions. Conversion may temporarily "solve the problem." **La belle indifférence** is not a significant characteristic (as commonly believed). Major criteria in diagnosis include a history of conversions, a serious precipitating emotional event, and a temporary "solving of the problem" by the conversion. Hysterical conversions must be differentiated from the hysterical personality (see Personality Disorders) and hysteria.

The history of the term hysteria—not now in the official nomenclature—is in large part the history of psychiatry. The word has been used to mean different things at different times by different people. Today it is most commonly used to denote those individuals, usually women in early to middle adult life, who have many physical complaints, have had polysurgery, and display histrionic behavior. Preoccupation with medical and surgical modalities constitutes a life style which excludes most other activities. This clinical configuration is called Briquet's syndrome, which some clinicians use interchangeably with the term hysteria.

D. Dissociative States: Fugue, amnesia, somnambulism, and multiple personality are the usual dissociative states. The reaction is precipitated by emotional crisis, and although the primary gain is anxiety reduction, secondary gain is a temporary solution of the crisis. The mechanisms include repression and isolation

as well as particularly limited concentration such as seen in hypnotic states. This condition, which is similar in many ways to temporal lobe dysfunction, may last for hours or days.

E. Obsessions and Compulsions: In the obsessive compulsive reaction, the irrational idea or the impulse persistently intrudes into awareness. Obsessions (constantly recurring thoughts such as fears of hitting somebody) and compulsions (repetitive actions such as washing hands many times prior to peeling a potato) are recognized by the individual as absurd and are resisted, but anxiety is alleviated only by ritualistic performance or mechanical impulse or entertainment of the idea. The primary concern of the patient is keeping control of his life situation. These patients are usually predictable, orderly, conscientious, and intelligent.

F. Depressions: See section on depression.

Complications

If unresolved conflicts persist without treatment, a chronic response may become established and permeate the patient's life style. Symptoms characterized by the particular defense, eg, phobias, increase in both scope and type as the pathologic defense mechanism inadequately handles the anxiety.

Treatment

A. Psychologic: Traditional psychotherapy is still the customary way of treating the majority of neuroses. Irrespective of the therapist's philosophic orientation, the relationship with the therapist in individual therapy is anxiety-reducing and effective when the therapy deals with the conflict producing the anxiety. The therapist who can help the patient delineate specific problems and goals is helping the patient find specific alternatives to unproductive or harmful ways of dealing with his problems. When economically feasible, psychoanalysis can be helpful in the neuroses, particularly when the patient is motivated to deal with the past events that have laid the groundwork for the present problem. Other individual approaches such as reality therapy or transactional analysis are particularly helpful when interpersonal relationships are a major factor. Individual group therapy is the treatment of choice when the anxiety is clearly a function of the patient's difficulties in dealing with others, and if these other people are part of the family it is appropriate to include them and initiate family or couple therapy.

Specific technics such as hypnosis and amobarbital interviews are effective in the conversion reactions for relatively quick relief of symptoms. The sooner a conversion is treated, the easier it is to relieve and the less the possibility of secondary gains.

B. Behavioral: Behavioral approaches are widely used in various neurotic problems. Desensitization, by exposing the patient to graded doses of a phobic object or situation, is an effective technic and one that the patient can practice outside of the therapy session. Emotive imagery, wherein the patient imagines the anxiety-provoking situation while at the same time learning to relax, helps to decrease the anxiety when the patient faces the real life situation. Some compulsions are treated by "flooding," ie, saturating the person with the anxiety-producing situation or phobic object. This changes the relationship of the compulsion to the anxiety, and the compulsion is given up since it no longer serves to ward off anxiety. "Modeling" technics are used when anxiety is related to lack of confidence and the patient looks to the therapist as a model of how to handle anxiety-provoking situations. Any of the behavioral technics (see above) can be used in altering the contingencies (precipitating factors or rewards) supporting any anxiety-provoking behavior.

C. Medical: Sedatives and minor tranquilizers may be useful for acute anxiety attacks (eg, chlordiazepoxide, 25–50 mg orally, or oxazepam, 30–60 mg orally) or as an adjunct to some behavioral technics such as desensitization. Doxepin at bedtime is often helpful for sleep and sedation during the following day. Drugs should be avoided as much as possible as a long-term or primary approach to the neuroses. When it is necessary to use sedatives or minor tranquilizers over a prolonged period, their use should be intermittent and not in a fixed dosage schedule. If possible, help the patient to use them only when other technics to relieve anxiety have failed. Low doses of antipsychotic tranquilizers (eg, haloperidol, 1–2 mg daily) can also be used but are of questionable value as sedatives.

D. Social: Social modification may require measures such as family counseling to aid acceptance of the patient's symptoms. Any help in maintaining the social structure is anxiety-alleviating, and work, school, and social activities should be maintained. School counseling and vocational assistance may be provided by specialized professionals, who often need direction from the physician in spelling out the patient's limitations.

Prognosis

The neuroses are usually of long standing and may be quite difficult to treat. Some, such as conversions, will remit quickly, whereas others, such as obsessions and compulsions, tend to be most resistant. All can be relieved to varying degrees with psychotherapy and behavioral technics.

Ackerman SH, Sacher EJ: The lactate theory of anxiety: A review and reevaluation. Psychosom Med 36:69, 1974.

Chodoff P: The diagnosis of hysteria: An overview. Am J Psychiat 131:1073, 1974.

Dyrud J: Treatment of anxiety states. Arch Gen Psychiat 25:298, 1971.

Jonas AD, Jonas DF: The evolutionary mechanisms of neurotic behavior. Am J Psychiat 131:636, 1974.

Kedward HB: The social correlates of chronic neurotic disorder. Social Psychiat 9:91, 1974.

Lewis WC: Hysteria: The consultant's dilemma. Arch Gen Psychiat 30:145, 1974.

Malan DH & others: Psychodynamic changes in untreated neurotic patients. 2. Apparently genuine improvements. Arch Gen Psychiat 32:110, 1975.

Marks I, Lader M: Anxiety states (anxiety neurosis): A review. J Nerv Ment Dis 156:3, 1973.

Razani J: Treatment of phobias by systematic desensitization. Arch Gen Psychiat 30:291, 1974.

Townsend RE & others: A comparison of biofeedback-mediated relaxation and group therapy in the treatment of chronic anxiety. Am J Psychiat 132:598, 1975.

SEXUAL DYSFUNCTION

Essentials of Diagnosis

- Increased or decreased sexual drive.
- Decreased or absent sexual satisfaction.
- Variations in sexual objects and practices.

General Considerations

The development and maintenance of masculinity and femininity is the result of genetic and hormonal factors, the initially assigned sex role, early sex experiences, parental attitudes and child-rearing practices, religious influences, environmental factors (schools, prisons, etc), and, later, positive and negative experiences with persons of the same or opposite sex. Transsexualism, particularly, may be a result of an unusual interplay of many of these factors.

Variations in the search for erotic pleasure embrace a wide range of objects and practices, and whether they are considered pathologic is often a function of cultural mores. The acceptance or rejection of such variations as homosexuality is reflected in the laws of a society and current thinking about whether such variations are pathologic entities, symptoms of other disorders, or simply a matter of individual choice.

Clinical Findings

A. Increased Sexual Drive: Increased libido may be an idiosyncratic characteristic but may also be due to a situational or psychologic disturbance. The presence of highly erotic stimuli, disinhibiting or stimulating drugs (eg, amphetamines), androgens, or certain CNS disorders—particularly lesions of the frontal, temporal, and hypothalamic regions—may be contributing factors.

B. Lack of Sexual Drive: Disinterest in sex may be an individual variation or may be due to preoccupation with other activities, abuse of depressant drugs (eg, sedatives, narcotics), aging, decreased stimulation, chronic debilitating disease, painful diseases, hypogonadism, or biogenetic influences.

C. Frigidity and Impotence: Decreased sexual satisfaction may be relative or absolute. Vaginismus is a conditioned response of reflex spasm of the muscles and not necessarily an avoidance of sex. The woman is frequently orgastic on clitoral stimulation. Frigidity in women (sexual unresponsiveness) is often due to inculcated attitudes or fears but may also be due to a defective personal relationship with the sexual partner or poor technic on his part. Impotence (an erectile disorder) is commonly psychologic, as in anxiety and depression, but is frequently secondary to medical problems such as the pharmacologic effects of alcohol and many drugs, diabetes mellitus, endocrine disorders, physical debility, and neurologic diseases (eg, multiple sclerosis, tabes, and spinal cord disorders).

Premature ejaculation is different from erectile problems and is less a disorder than a matter of the patient not having learned how to delay ejaculation.

D. Variations in the Sexual Object: Homosexual experiences are relatively common, and social and legal attitudes toward homosexuality have changed rather remarkably in recent years. Individuals who have sexual relationships with either sex—so-called **bisexuals**—frequently are homosexuals who have not "come out." This means that the individual is still denying his or her homosexual preference and indulges in heterosexual activity only to prove to himself (herself) and others that he or she is not really homosexual. A strong defense mechanism of denial is evident in this situation. The period of bisexuality often ends when the individual psychologically establishes a sexual preference. Some individuals have an unrestricted desire for sexual expression which never becomes limited by object choice or practices.

Transsexualism is an attempt to deny and reverse the biologic sex and to achieve an opposite gender role identification. The biologic male attempts to assume feminine interests, dress, behavior, anatomy, and total attitude. The converse is true in the biologic female transsexualist. This trend is seen early in childhood, is unremitting, and becomes an obsessive theme, usually with serious attempts to achieve endocrine and surgical intervention.

In **pedophilia**, children are preferred and used as the sexual outlet. Quite frequently, intercourse with an adult is impossible for the pedophiliac—who usually has profound feelings of inadequacy—and potency is achieved only by fondling the child. In some cases there is a basic homosexual orientation, and only male children will be approached.

Incestuous relationships between father and daughter, mother and son, and brother and sister are not usually pedophilia and are often related to marital or family problems and cultural influences. Occasional episodes of **bestiality** (sexual intercourse with an animal) occur under circumstances of deprivation of other outlets and in youthful experimentation. When the habit persists and is the preferred mode, there is usually a severe psychologic disturbance.

Necrophilia (sexual intercourse with a dead body) is a severe aberration, and there are variations wherein parts of a dead body are kept and used as a stimulant to masturbation. This is really a form of **fetishism**, which is a fixation on a part of the body or an article of apparel and serves as a stimulant to masturbation. As in **voyeurism** (sexual gratification by looking at a nude body or a sexual act), there is a replacement of intercourse by the variation.

Visual, tactile, and other sensory accompaniments to intercourse are considered nonpathologic and are not to be confused with variations which replace the act of intercourse.

E. Variations in Sexual Practices: Extragenital copulation (anal or oral) is often a part of foreplay in "normal" heterosexual intercourse. **Exhibitionism**—the exposure of one's body or of the genitals to the opposite sex to stimulate one's own sexual excitement—is also common, and its social and legal acceptance depends in large part upon the setting (eg, indecent exposure versus striptease). **Transvestism** (putting on the garments of the opposite sex) can be a fetish if it creates the sexual excitement necessary for masturbation and orgasm; it can be part of homosexual practice; is invariably present in cases of transsexualism; and occasionally is a foreplay variation in heterosexual activity. **Sadomasochism**—sexual gratification from inflicting or experiencing pain—may be pathologic if it is practiced to an excessive degree. Extreme or bizarre activity, such as bondage, occasionally results in death.

Complications

The major complications are usually conflict with society and its laws. The individual is frequently satisfied with the variations and comes to the physician only on referral by legal authorities or when problems of drive or satisfaction are present.

Treatment

A. Problems of Sexual Drive or Satisfaction:

1. Medical—Medical evaluation must be meticulous. The basic difficulty is often a function of problems of daily living and may not necessarily be due to physical or emotional disorders. The anxiety generated often exacerbates the condition, and particular care and understanding are very important in discussing symptoms such as impotence, frigidity, and altered libido. Careful evaluation of underlying causes (diabetes mellitus, alcohol and other sedative drugs, neurologic disease, etc) is essential. Sedatives and minor tranquilizers (eg, diazepam, 5–10 mg orally) may be given on an as required basis for short periods when anxiety is a major inhibiting factor. Major tranquilizers or antidepressants (Table 17–1) should be used when psychosis or endogenous depression is an underlying factor. It should be remembered, however, that all psychotropic drugs may decrease libido and performance, especially in men.

2. Psychologic—Psychologic intervention is indicated, especially when the problem is rooted in intrapsychic conflicts. Individual therapy can help resolve the conflicts that revolve around inhibitions developed during childhood or adolescence, many of which involve parent-child interactions. Couples therapy is the treatment of choice when the sexual problem is secondary to major marital adjustment problems.

3. Behavioral—Behavioral therapy may be individual, such as desensitization in the case of frigidity; or couple-oriented, wherein the couple are seen together and given specific instructions regarding sexual activities (Masters and Johnson). The goal is to alleviate anxiety due to previous failures and to enhance sexual response in each partner—essentially a process of desensitization and operant conditioning.

4. Social—Social considerations are important in cases where the social structure is inhibiting (eg, if lack of privacy is a problem). Work scheduling, when both partners work different shifts, may be a factor requiring change. Another person residing in the house (eg, a mother-in-law) may be a deterrent to one or both partners.

B. Problems of Variations in Sexual Objects and Practices:

1. Psychologic—Psychologic approaches may be successful if the individual has a desire to change, but this is often not the case. The more recent the onset of the divergent practice, the more effective the treatment. Variations that are of long standing are particularly difficult to modify. Individual psychotherapy has often been helpful in exhibitionism, fetishism, and voyeurism; all are rooted in serious feelings of sexual inadequacy. Pedophilia, which has a similar origin, is much more threatening to society and more difficult to treat. Sadomasochistic practices are intimately bound to aggression and guilt, and in the more serious forms (eg, bondage) occasionally result in death.

In cases where depression is present, treatment can be directed toward the depression and accompanying isolation. Individual group therapy may be the best psychologic approach to the homosexual when change in orientation is desired by the patient. In cases where the homosexual partnership is experiencing adjustment problems, couple therapy is as appropriate as couple therapy of heterosexual couples.

2. Behavioral—Behavioral therapy has been attempted in many cases of homosexuality, but the results have been disappointing. Combined aversion and operant conditioning (eg, induced emesis or electric shock while viewing pictures of nude males and pleasurable stimulation or lack of pain when shown pictures of nude women) have not proved lasting in male homosexuals. Modeling and role-playing can be helpful in voyeurism or fetishism. Inducing a sexual response in the human female herself rather than observing another's experience (voyeurism) tends to lessen anxiety and encourage the patient to attempt the more complicated and anxiety-laden total act. Desensitization is most effective in conditions such as vaginismus. Emotive imagery is useful in lessening anxiety, which may maintain the incomplete variation (eg, fetish) and block an approach to a woman.

3. Social—Social methods of treatment are most useful when the purpose is to help the person adjust to an often hostile society. There are many nonresidential self-help groups such as "gay" clubs and churches which accept the homosexual as he is and assist him to live in a heterosexually oriented society. Family counseling is often necessary to assist family members in accepting the situation and in alleviating their guilt about what role they might have played in creating the problem. Work assistance is necessary since there is a great deal of job discrimination against people with known sexual variations.

4. Medical—Medical treatment is limited to the occasional case of endocrine and surgical management in the carefully evaluated transsexual who is judged to be a suitable candidate for sexual change. Underlying problems amenable to medication (eg, schizophrenia, severe depression) require the appropriate psychotropic drugs.

Prognosis

Problems of sexual drive and satisfaction (eg, frigidity) may respond dramatically to simple technics.

Abel GG, Blanchard EB: The role of fantasy in the treatment of sexual deviation. Arch Gen Psychiat 30:467, 1974.

Ellenberg M: Impotence in diabetes: The neurologic factor. Ann Int Med 75:213, 1971.

Freund K & others: The phobic theory of male homosexuality. Arch Gen Psychiat 31:495, 1974.

Gadpaille WJ: Research into the physiology of maleness and femaleness. Arch Gen Psychiat 26:193, 1972.

Glick BS: Desensitization therapy in impotence and frigidity: A review of the literature and report of a case. Am J Psychiat 132:169, 1975.

Meyer JK & others: Short term treatment of sexual problems: Interim report. Am J Psychiat 132:172, 1975.

Oversey L, Person E: Gender identity and sexual psychopathology in men. J Am Acad Psychoanal 1:53, 1973.

Stoller RJ: Overview: The impact of new advances in sex research on psychoanalytic theory. Am J Psychiat 130:241, 1973.

Stoller RJ: Male transsexualism: Uneasiness. Am J Psychiat 130:536, 1973.

PSYCHOPHYSIOLOGIC DISORDERS

Essentials of Diagnosis

- Symptoms may involve one or more organ systems.
- Subjective complaints exceed objective findings.
- Correlations of symptom development and psychosocial stresses.
- Matrix of biogenetic and developmental patterns.

General Considerations

A major source of diagnostic confusion in medicine has been to assume cause-and-effect relationships when parallel events have been observed. This *post hoc ergo propter hoc* reasoning has been particularly vexing in many situations where the individual exhibits psychosocial distress which could well be secondary to a chronic illness but has been assumed to be primary and causative. An example is the person with a chronic bowel disease who becomes querulous and demanding. Is this a result of problems of coping with a chronic disease, or is it a personality pattern which causes the gastrointestinal problem? There has been no acceptable evidence that a relationship exists between an early psychic event or a personality pattern and any of the so-called psychophysiologic problems such as ulcerative colitis, peptic ulcer, asthma, and essential hypertension.

What does stand out is the undeniable clinical observation that people react differently to illness. Emotional stress often exacerbates or precipitates an acute illness. Vulnerability in one or more organ systems plays a major role in the development of particular symptoms, and the "functional" versus "organic" dichotomy is a hindrance to good treatment.

Clinical Findings

Symptoms or signs may involve any organ system, and demonstrable psychosocial stress often occurs prior to, or coincident with, the development of the symptoms. The symptoms are a reflection of adaptive patterns, coping technics, and reactivity of the particular organ system. There is evidence of long-standing somatic reactivity, often with a history of varying degrees of similar organ system involvement in other members of the family.

Complications

Complications arise mainly in the area of the doctor-patient relationship, wherein the patient tenaciously holds on to symptoms in order to prove that the physician's rejection is in error. The symptoms tend to become set as secondary gain comes into the picture, eg, disability payments. "Doctor shopping" engenders more procedures, which further reinforce the symptoms and present increased risk. Drug dependency frequently ensues as the frustrated physician tries to meet the demands of a frustrated patient. The illness and search for cure become a way of life and totally consume the patient's time and energies to the exclusion of everything else.

The main reason a patient sees the doctor is to be given a diagnosis for his complaint, but closely allied to this is receipt of qualities of reassurance, acceptance, attention, and affection. What can be done specifically to alleviate the complaint is often secondary to the reassurance and support of the physician. Misunderstanding of these priorities adversely affects the doctor-patient relationship. Many patients feel relieved when told after careful examination that there is nothing wrong. Others react quite differently, believing that being told there is nothing wrong means they will receive no care. And this is often true. The doctor prescribes one medicine after another, usually different brands of the same class of tranquilizer. (This type of patient often receives multiple drugs, which is not only a dangerous practice but one that further obscures the diagnosis.) Various tests and procedures are ordered, reinforcing the patient's belief that his problem is purely organic. There is no acknowledgement of the influence of emotional conflicts. In many cases, simple psychotherapeutic approaches by the physician would help the patient. Referral to a psychiatrist is often interpreted by the patient to mean that the physician has "given up." The patient often regards the psychiatrist as someone who is there not to cure him but to "comfort" him or even to "help him to die." In any event, the reactions of the patient are anger at abandonment, fear of the referral, and a continued search for succor.

Treatment

A. Medical: Medical support with careful attention to building a therapeutic doctor-patient relationship is the mainstay of treatment. This is particularly the case with the patient who needs acceptance and reassurance about his symptoms. *It must be accepted that his distress is real.* Diligent attempts should be made to relate symptoms with adverse developments in the patient's life. It may be useful to have the patient keep a meticulous diary, paying particular attention to various pertinent factors evident in the history. There should be regular, frequent, short appointments, and drugs should not be prescribed to replace appointments. One doctor should be the primary physician, and consultants should be used only for evaluation. An emphatic, realistic, optimistic approach must be maintained in the face of the expected ups and downs. Sedatives and minor tranquilizers (chlordiazepoxide, 10–25 mg orally on an as-required schedule) can be used judiciously.

B. Psychologic: Psychologic approaches can be used by the primary physician when it is clear that the patient is ready to make some changes in his life in order to relieve his symptoms. Psychiatric referral is often rejected. Even when it is accepted, the patient's reluctance may foredoom the psychiatrist's efforts to failure. If the primary physician has been working with the patient on psychologic problems related to his physical illness, the groundwork is often laid for successful psychiatric referral. This is often best approached on a "here and now" basis and oriented toward pragmatic changes rather than an exploration of early experiences which the patient frequently fails to relate to his current dicomfort. Individual group therapy with other patients who have similar problems is sometimes of value to improve coping, allow ventilation, and focus on interpersonal adjustment.

C. Behavioral: Behavioral therapy is probably best exemplified by the current efforts in biofeedback technics which have a behavioral basis. In biofeedback, the particular abnormality (eg, increased peristalsis) must be recognized and monitored by the patient and therapist (eg, by an electronic stethoscope to amplify the sounds). This is immediate feedback, and after learning to recognize it the patient can then learn to identify any change he might evoke (eg, a decrease in bowel sounds) and thus become a conscious originator of the feedback instead of a passive recipient. Relief of the symptom operantly conditions the patient to utilize the maneuver that he has come to learn will decrease the symptoms (eg, relaxation causing a decrease in bowel sounds). With emphasis on this type of learning, the patient is able to identify symptoms early and initiate the countermaneuvers, thus decreasing the symptomatic problem.

D. Social: Social endeavors include family, work, and other interpersonal activity. Family members should come for some appointments with the patient so that they can learn how best to live with the patient. Certain "clubs" such as ileostomy clubs provide a climate for encouraging the patient to accept and live with his disabilities. Ongoing communication with the employer is sometimes necessary to encourage his continued interest in the employee over the long term. Employers get as discouraged as physicians in dealing with employees who have chronic problems.

Prognosis

The prognosis is much better if the primary physician is able to deal with the case early before the situation has deteriorated. After the problem has crystallized into chronicity, it is very difficult to effect any change.

Blanchard EB, Young LD: Clinical applications of biofeedback training. Arch Gen Psychiat 30:573, 1974.

Boyar RM & others: Anorexia nervosa: Immaturity of the 24 hour luteinizing hormone secretory pattern. New England J Med 291:861, 1974.

Budzynski TH & others: EMG biofeedback and tension headache: A controlled outcome study. Psychosom Med 35:484, 1973.

Eastwood MR, Trevelyan MH: Relationship between physical and psychiatric disorders. Psychol Med 2:363, 1972.

Henryk-Gutt R, Rees WL: Psychological aspects of migraine. J Psychosom Res 17:141, 1973.

Jenkins CD & others: Prediction of clinical coronary heart disease by a test for the coronary prone behavior pattern. New England J Med 290:1271, 1974.

Kahn AU: Role of counter-conditioning in the treatment of asthma. J Psychosom Res 18:89, 1974.

Mechanic D: Social psychologic factors affecting the presentation of bodily complaints. New England J Med 286:1132, 1972.

Miller NE: Biofeedback evaluation of a new technic. New England J Med 290:684, 1974.

Nemiah JC, Sifneos PE: Psychosomatic illness: A problem in communication. Psychother Psychosom 18:154, 1970.

Rosillo RH: Pain, affects, and progress in physical rehabilitation. J Psychosom Res 17:21, 1973.

PERSONALITY DISORDERS

Essentials of Diagnosis

- Long history dating back to childhood.
- Recurrent maladaptive behavior.
- Minimal anxiety to the person himself.
- Major difficulties with others (society).
- Depression with anxiety when maladaptive behavior fails.

General Considerations

Personality—a hypothetical construct—is the result of the prolonged interaction of an individual with his drives and with outside influences, the sum being the enduring patterns of behavior adopted in order to cope with the environment and which characterize him as an individual. Obviously, the more satisfactory the early development of a person, the stronger the personality development. People who fail to experience and integrate satisfactory early experiences tend to have personality structures which manifest more primitive responses. For example, a person may have a hyperreactive response to a minor slur, such as physically lashing out at another person; or he may overreact to a rejection by perhaps making a suicide attempt in response to rejection by a person with whom he has had little significant involvement.

Lack of a self-identity is characteristic and is manifested by marked dependence on others and a tendency to imitate someone who may be important at a given time. There are repeated attempts to move toward another person, often in this dependent fashion, followed by the inevitable rejections which elicit the overreactive response.

As one study pointed out, an individual is labeled a personality disorder if he is seen in the emergency room at 2:00 a.m. with nothing wrong with him and no interest in treatment. The lack of diagnostic precision in this group is such that the person who acts in an appropriately aggressive way in proper circumstances is said to be "brave." The individual who is always a "doormat" and depends on other people is said to be a "passive-dependent" personality. The person who shows some evidence of aggression is called "passive-aggressive"; and the unfortunate individual who can never seem to do anything well is called an "inadequate personality."

The ambiguity of the term is one of the principal characteristics that perpetuate its use. It implies a developmental maladaption from an early age with subsequent problems of behavior which are repetitive, personally handicapping, and annoying to others. The individual does not learn from his bad experiences and feels little anxiety.

The classification of subtypes depends upon the predominant symptoms and their severity. The most severe disorders—those that bring the patient into greatest conflict with society—tend to be classified as antisocial (psychopathic). From a dynamic viewpoint, the psychopath differs little from the borderline (see p 617).

Classification & Clinical Findings

Paranoid: Defensive, oversensitive, suspicious, hyperalert.—**Cyclothymic:** Wide, inconsistent mood swings, fluctuating between optimistic enthusiasm and pessimistic withdrawal.—**Schizoid:** Shy, introverted, withdrawn, avoiding close relationships.—**Explosive:** Gross verbal and physical outbursts of aggressive behavior without significant provocation.—**Obsessive compulsive:** Rigid thought patterns and persistent ritualized motor behavior with an inability to tolerate uncertainty and lack of control.—**Hysterical:** Dependent, immature, seductive, histrionic, egocentric, vain, emotionally labile.—**Asthenic:** Low energy, lack of enthusiasm, limited capacity for enjoyment, oversensitivity to physical and emotional stress.—**Antisocial:**

Selfish, callous, impulsive, low frustration tolerance, limited loyalty, inability to learn from experience.— **Passive-aggressive**: Stubborn, procrastinating, argumentative, sulking, helpless, clinging, controlling; mostly directed at authority figures.—**Inadequate**: Ineffectual, poor performance, socially inept, lacking in judgment, unable to plan, marginal task performance of all kinds.

Differential Diagnosis

The less severe types tend to show anxiety and depression when pathologic technics fail and can be similar to neurotic problems. The more severe types tend to mimic the major mental illness, eg, the cyclothymic may resemble the manic-depressive and the paranoid may at times be similar to the paranoid schizophrenic.

Treatment

A. Social: Social and milieu environments such as day hospitals, halfway houses, and self-help communities, such as Synanon, utilize peer pressures to modify the self-destructive behavior. The patient with a personality disorder often has failed to profit from experience, and difficulties with authority impair the learning experience. The use of peer relationships and the repetition possible in a structured setting of a helpful community enhances the educational opportunities and increases learning. When one's companions note every flaw in one's character and insist that it be corrected immediately, a powerful learning environment is being created. When problems are detected early, both the school and the home can serve as foci of intensified social pressure to change the behavior, particularly with the use of behavioral technics.

B. Behavioral: The behavioral technics used are principally operant and aversive conditioning. The former simply emphasizes the recognition of acceptable behavior and reinforcing this with praise or other tangible rewards. Aversive responses usually mean punishment, although this can range from ignoring the person to some specific punitive responses such as verbal abuse or mild electric shock. Extinction plays a role in that an attempt is made not to respond to inappropriate behavior, and the lack of response eventually causes the person to abandon that type of behavior. Pouting and tantrum-like responses, for example, diminish quickly when such behavior elicits no reaction.

C. Psychologic: Psychologic intervention is most usefully accomplished in group settings. Individual group therapy is helpful when specific interpersonal behavior needs to be improved (eg, schizoid and inadequate types where involvement with people is markedly impaired). This mode of treatment also has a place with so-called "acting out" patients, ie, those that frequently act in an impulsive and inappropriate way. The peer pressure in the group tends to help structure the patient and act to inhibit some of his rash actions. The group also quickly identifies his types of behavior and helps him to learn to be a better observer

of himself so that he can cope with the antecedents of his unacceptable behavior and thus decrease its frequency. Individual therapy is of limited usefulness even in motivated patients.

D. Medical: Hospitalization in a milieu setting is occasionally indicated, but in most cases treatment can be accomplished in the day treatment center or self-help community. Major tranquilizers may be required for short periods in conditions that have temporarily decompensated into transient psychoses (eg, chlorpromazine, 50 mg orally every 3–4 hours until the patient has quieted down and is regaining contact with reality). In most cases, these drugs are required only for several days and can be discontinued after the patient has regained his previous level of adjustment. Minor tranquilizers (eg, diazepam, 5–10 mg orally several times a day) can be used when a decrease of passive avoidance is desired to allow the patient to learn and practice new kinds of behavior in a therapeutic setting (eg, in the very fearful schizoid patient who passively avoids people and is attempting to learn to interact in a group therapy setting).

Prognosis

Antisocial categories generally have a poor prognosis, whereas persons with mild schizoid or passive-aggressive tendencies have a good prognosis if appropriate treatment is given.

Borriello JF: Patients with acting-out character disorders. Am J Psychother 27:4, 1973.

Crowe RR: An adoption study of antisocial personality. Arch Gen Psychiat 31:785, 1974.

Giovacchini P: Character disorders: Form and structure. Int J Psychoanal 54:153, 1973.

Rioch DMcK: Personality. Arch Gen Psychiat 27:575, 1972.

Slavney PR, McHugh PR: The hysterical personality: A controlled study. Arch Gen Psychiat 30:325, 1974.

Vaillant GE: Sociopathy as a human process. Arch Gen Psychiat 32:178, 1975.

Welner A: Personality Disorder. 2. Followup. Brit J Psychiat 124:359, 1974.

BORDERLINE CONDITIONS*

Essentials of Diagnosis

- Major personality deficits (see Personality Disorders).
- Neurotic manifestations (eg, anxiety, phobias, compulsions).
- Serious problems of interpersonal adjustment, particularly dependency.
- Marked susceptibility to environmental stresses.

*Also called borderline personality organization, borderline personality, pseudoneurotic schizophrenia, latent schizophrenia, hysterical psychosis, "sick hysteric," "as if" personality, borderline syndrome or state, and pseudopsychopathic disorders.

- Occasional psychotic episodes.

General Considerations

The so-called borderline diagnosis (which is not given in official nomenclature) is being used more frequently as the classic psychiatric syndromes appear less prevalent. There is no unanimity of opinion on what constitutes the diagnosis, although most clinicians see it as a stable pathologic personality organization with variable presenting symptoms. In some cases there may be transient psychotic episodes, particularly under stress, whereas in others the initial picture is predominantly neurotic with marked anxiety, phobias, etc. (See Neurotic Disorders.)

The individual with a borderline condition lacks a strong sense of personal identity, passively awaits cues from others, and then imitates and temporarily assumes the characteristics of a person who might be important at a given point in his life. The result is frequent rejection followed by feelings of anger, loneliness, and depression. The absence of sustained relationships increases frustration and hostility, which further alienates people, thus perpetuating the feelings of loneliness and isolation. This leaves the person more vulnerable to stress, which, when sufficiently severe, can cause transient psychotic decompensations.

Clinical Findings

A number of clinical syndromes are subsumed under the borderline category. They usually take their names from the most prominent initial presentation.

Hysterical psychosis refers to the person with a severe hysterical personality disorder (see Personality Disorders) who, under the pressures of a crisis, becomes overwhelmed and unable to respond in a well-organized way. He is unable to deal with reality, shows evidence of a thought disorder with delusions and hallucinations, and manifests volatile affect, depersonalization, and erratic behavior. The symptoms usually last several days to several weeks, though treatment will shorten the course. The erratic behavior can be quite variable and may include asocial activity, sexual misadventures, abuse of alcohol and other drugs, and occasional overt criminal activity.

Pseudoneurotic schizophrenia is most commonly characterized by a total anxiety that is pervasive and leaves no life activities free of tension. Almost all experiences influence this anxiety, usually adversely. In connection with this diffuse anxiety, most other neurotic manifestations are present in varying degrees, including phobias, conversion symptoms, obsessive compulsive mechanisms, depression with poor sleep, anorexia, lack of energy, gastrointestinal symptoms, and palpitations.

Unlike the neurotic patient, who is usually anxious to describe his symptoms carefully, the pseudoneurotic schizophrenic is often nonspecific, refers to generalities, and gives few details. The personality deficits appear in numerous ways, including hysterical features, passivity, marked dependency, and serious difficulties in interpersonal relationships, including sexual maladjustment and drug abuse.

The gross thinking disorders that one sees in classic cases of schizophrenia are not present. Rather, there are impulsive and erratic behavior patterns, some feelings of omnipotence, and occasional, usually short-lived, psychotic episodes which are in response to stress and have 3 characteristic features: hypochondriacal ideae, feelings of depersonalization, and ideas of reference. The patient usually reintegrates quickly to the previous level of adjustment.

"Sick" hysterical personalities, "as if" personalities, and other borderline titles are usually grouped under the heading of **latent schizophrenia,** which is the only term in official nomenclature designated to include the conditions in this section. These patients, like the pseudoneurotic schizophrenic and the patient with hysterical psychosis, have continual difficulties in exerting emotional control; they therefore exhibit chronic severe tension, poor impulse control, recurrent depression, and psychotic decompensation under mild to moderate stress. Inevitably, there are poor interpersonal relationships and the impulsive behavior which frequently involves sexual promiscuity and drug abuse. The cycle is repeated: impulsive behavior, an attempt to establish dependent relationships, a rejection, resultant anger and depression when expectations are not met, a period of isolation (suicide attempts are common during this period), increased stress with occasional psychosis, a fairly quick return to the previous level of marginal adjustment, and then impulsive behavior again.

The 4 factors that commonly stand out are anger as the main affect, the defect in relationships (dependency is very strong), the absence of self-identity, and depressive loneliness.

Complications

A major complication is the difficulty of establishing the appropriate diagnosis, which results in a treatment course that is ineffective or worsens the condition. For example, hospitalization may be necessary during an acute psychotic episode, but behavioral regression is a major danger in the hospital treatment of borderline patients. Another problem is the setting of limits, which is important in borderline patients. If a person is seen in a phase where neurotic signs are prevalent, the therapist may take a nondirective approach, encourage a full range of expression, and unwittingly be a factor in the patient's decompensation.

Many of these patients have seen a succession of psychotherapists, and the repeated failures not only discourage the patient but also tend to result in additional rejection by a therapist, which reinforces the basic problem.

Drug abuse is occasionally a complication of inappropriate treatment. Borderline patients have a tendency to abuse drugs, and the physician may unwittingly contribute to this by prescribing sedatives, particularly since depression and insomnia are frequent complaints. Discriminating use of sedative medications is particularly important, not only because of the drug dependency problem but also because of the relative frequency of impulsive suicide attempts, which usually involve a prescribed sedative-hypnotic drug. Most frequently, this occurs in conjunction with a real or imagined rejection by the physician and is a manifestation of the patient's anger toward him.

Treatment

A. Psychologic: Group psychotherapy can be useful since there is a major problem of poor interpersonal relationships. A setting which can over a long period of time correct some of these problems can offset to some degree the secondary ramifications, ie, rejection, isolation, and anxiety about ability to deal with people. It can provide a supportive arena which can at the same time set limits on behavior. The person learns that there can be satisfying interactions which do not necessarily rely on drugs or on sex-oriented activity. Idealizing or idolizing relationships are handled in the group, thus breaking up the repetitive prior experiences with their inevitable consequences.

Individual psychotherapy of an eclectic nature—with emphasis on the here-and-now and utilization of areas of strength—can occasionally be a valid approach, particularly initially and as a prelude to group therapy. The problems with individual therapy are mentioned in the discussion of complications. Most borderline patients eventually come under the care of a community mental health program which can provide the broad spectrum of treatment required.

B. Medical: Hospitalization is indicated for treatment of the psychotic episode. Often, the structured environment of the hospital alone provides sufficient stabilization, and minimal psychotropic medication can be used. The antipsychotic tranquilizers are the drugs of choice, and the sedating ones such as thioridazine, 100 mg orally every 6—8 hours for a day or so, are usually adequate to bring the patient under control. The dose should then be decreased, and a bedtime dose of 100 mg orally is often sufficient for the next several days, with further decrease and discontinuation as the patient returns to the prepsychotic level of function.

It is seldom necessary to give antipsychotic tranquilizers after an acute psychotic episode has passed. In cases where feelings of depersonalization, mild paranoia, or subtle signs of psychosis persist, the use of a phenothiazine such as perphenazine, 4—8 mg orally at bedtime, is warranted until the symptoms disappear completely (a process that might take several months). The use of sedatives or minor tranquilizers should be very limited because of the potential for abuse and also because of their relative ineffectiveness in these conditions. The depression which is often present rarely responds to antidepressant medications, and these drugs may in fact contribute to a psychotic decompensation.

C. Social: The use of structured environments such as day hospital or therapeutic community settings is effective, and for the more serious cases it is often the only way to avoid chronic hospitalization. The use of psychologic technics such as group therapy within the social setting is desirable. Community social agencies (welfare, vocational rehabilitation, etc) are almost as important to this group as to the schizophrenics, since their lives tend to be chaotic and they frequently lose jobs, require financial assistance, and become involved in erratic behavior which brings them into conflict with society. Early involvement with the appropriate social agency often mitigates stress to the point where the patient does not decompensate and also has fewer symptoms.

D. Behavioral: One of the most important behavioral technics in these cases is modeling. The patient has a lack of identity and is constantly striving to emulate some currently important person. The modeling can be done by others in group therapy, an individual therapist, the personnel in a day care center, or the social worker handling the patient in a welfare case load. The dependency needs of the patient are high; if the physician is the only significant figure, he will find that the demands are too high and all too frequently this type of patient is rejected. It will be recalled that hypochondriacal signs are prominent in this group. Therefore, it is important not to reinforce the somatic symptoms, which can usually be extinguished if the physician assesses the problems, rules out disease, *refrains from giving sedatives,* and works closely with other people involved in the case.

Occasionally, desensitization for specific phobias is useful, but the range of symptoms is so broad that there must be careful evaluation of the specific behavior to be desensitized and concentration limited to that behavior. After the specific behavior improves, another is chosen: The borderline patient has problems in generalizing, so one cannot expect that as one behavior is corrected the patient will improve in other areas. A patient, specific, repetitive approach is usually necessary, with consistent reinforcement of chosen areas until the person has learned the appropriate behavior.

Adler G: Hospital treatment of borderline patients. Am J Psychiat 130:32, 1973.

Chessick RD: Defective ego feeling and the quest for being in the borderline atient. Internat J Psychoanal Psychother 3:73, 1974.

Gunderson JG, Singer MT: Defining borderline patients: An overview. Am J Psychiat 132:1, 1975.

Hoch P, Polatin P: Pseudoneurotic forms of schizophrenia. Psychiat Quart 23:248, 1949.

Hollender MH, Hirsch SJ: Hysterical psychosis. Am J Psychiat 120:1066, 1964.

Kernberg O: Borderline personality organization. J Am Psychoanal A 15:641, 1967.

Lazare A: The hysterical character in psychoanalytic theory. Arch Gen Psychiat 25:131, 1971.

THE SCHIZOPHRENIAS

Essentials of Diagnosis

- Usually a slowly progressive (but may be rapid) withdrawal from reality.
- Inappropriate responses in thinking, speech, and behavior.
- Alternations of mood—flat, euphoric, withdrawn, or depressed—without apparent relationship to circumstances.
- Speech and behavior become irrelevant (circumstantial) or irrational and delusional.

Frequent Additional Signs:

- Depersonalization, in which the patient behaves as if he were a detached observer of his own actions.
- Delusions of grandeur or persecution.
- Religious or sexual preoccupations.
- Logical reasoning becomes difficult.
- Flights of ideas and incoherence take the place of thought.
- Mentation and speech become blocked in emotionally charged situations.
- Auditory hallucinations, stereotyped activity, and ritualistic behavior.
- Disturbances of consciousness, memory, and orientation.

General Considerations

The schizophrenias are a group of syndromes which are the adaptational product of the following variables: (1) **Biogenetic:** A genetic disposition with variable penetrance, probably affecting catecholamine metabolism through a number of poorly understood biochemical mechanisms. The so-called induced psychoses (eg, psychedelic and amphetamine psychoses), along with the most recent twin concordance studies, lend credence to this aspect. (2) **Psychologic:** A result of the childhood and developmental experiences which emphasize family communications and behavior patterns. Social class incidence studies tend to corroborate the findings from various pathogenic environments. (3) **Environmental:** Reflecting the various stresses which the individual withstands to his biologic limits. Studies with sensory deprivation, drugs, and high anxiety indicate that breakdown is a function of the person's ability to withstand stress. Amphetamines and other stimulants used in various "diet pills" *commonly precipitate psychotic symptoms* in schizophrenics who are not known to be clinically ill when the drugs are prescribed.

Classification*

This group includes several categories:

*Other classifications tend to take their names from the predominant features, eg, catatonia. They often change with time, frequently resulting eventually in the type referred to as **chronic undifferentiated**. The categories outlined here are by no means distinct, and features of each of the categories may be evident in a given individual at any one time or at different times.

A. Acute Schizophrenia: Characterized by a precipitous psychotic episode preceded by good adjustment. Remission is prompt, and subsequent reconstitution is adequate to allow return to vocational, educational, and social endeavors. This category tends to overlap with the borderline syndromes. These patients may later be placed in the chronic category if multiple relapses occur.

B. Chronic Schizophrenia: Usually includes longstanding history of chaotic psychic function and social incompetence with evident psychotic symptoms. The age at onset is usually 16–24 years, and 0.5–1% of the population are affected. There may be acute psychosis, but the overall syndrome is that of gradually developing decompensation with a chronic course.

C. Paranoid Schizophrenia: Involves frank delusions of a persecutory nature. Grandiosity underlies paranoia, and the patient is not generally bizarre in his thinking and behavior except when delusional ideation results in suspicious and hyperalert behavior.

D. Schizo-affective Schizophrenia: A diverse group which includes schizophrenics with mood disturbances, disorders which mimic primary affective disorders, and those psychoses that are in early stages and cannot be placed in any of the established categories.

Clinical Findings

A. Primary Symptoms: Bleuler's 4 As, which may not be evident early in the disorder:

1. Disturbances in *a*ffect, either inappropriate or flattened.

2. Loose *a*ssociations, wandering from topic to topic with little relevancy.

3. *A*utistic thinking, or involvement in fantasy material, often completely absorbed in ideas of reference to self.

4. *A*mbivalence, often not quickly apparent but characterized by conflicting and simultaneous positive and negative feelings toward another person.

B. Secondary Symptoms:

1. Erratic behavior, often day-night reversal.

2. Anhedonia, or inability to experience gratification or immersion in life experiences.

3. Anger and frustration, often in reaction to inability to function.

4. Dependence, a part of the boundary problem and the reality problem of being unable to handle the exigencies of life.

5. Depression, with occasional suicide attempts.

6. Pathologic coping devices, or attempts to "explain" what is happening (eg, delusions, hallucinations, preoccupations, and depersonalizations).

7. "Boundary" problems, or inability to separate oneself (both self and body) as a distinct entity from others.

8. Feelings of markedly enhanced or muted sensory awareness.

9. Reports of "racing thoughts."

10. Mental exhaustion.

11. Deficits in focusing attention and concentration.

12. Disturbances in speech perception and word meanings.

Differential Diagnosis

It may be difficult to differentiate schizophrenia from the organic psychoses, eg, exogenous substances such as amphetamines, psychedelics, corticosteroids, and endogenous problems such as thyroid disorders, adrenal and pituitary dysfunction, or neoplastic processes. Primary affective disorders with severe unipolar, withdrawn depressive symptoms or manic-depressive illness are often very difficult to distinguish from the schizo-affective schizophrenias. Hysterical reactions and borderline syndromes at times demonstrate sufficient decompensation to cause diagnostic problems.

Treatment

A. Acute Schizophrenias:

1. Medical—Hospitalization is usually necessary for a short period. Antipsychotics are the treatment of choice during the acute phase (Table 17—1). Chlorpromazine, 50—100 mg orally, or haloperidol, 5 mg orally, can be given on admission and then every 3—4 hours until the patient is calm and has gotten some usually much needed rest. The amount needed daily will vary considerably depending upon the arousal level and the age of the patient. In the patient who refuses oral medication, it may be necessary to use parenteral medication. Chlorpromazine, 25—50 mg IM, or haloperidol, 3—5 mg IM, may be given every 3—4 hours until a favorable response has been achieved. After the first day or so, a daily oral dose can be established, with the major portion administered at bedtime to take advantage of the sedative effect of this drug. As the patient improves, the medication can be decreased, can usually be given in a bedtime dose, and can eventually be discontinued as the patient continues to function well on an outpatient basis. Undertreatment is usually the cause of failure to respond over the first several days of hospitalization. ECT should be considered in those few patients who do not respond to adequate drug treatment. Megavitamin therapy with nicotinic acid, nicotinamide, and ascorbic acid has been extensively investigated over the past years with no demonstrable therapeutic efficacy.

2. Psychologic—Psychologic treatment should be given after the acute crisis has subsided. This consists of individual eclectic therapy, preferably by the same physician who treated the patient initially. The focus is on the "here and now" of the patient's daily concerns and not on his early experiences. There is a major effort to help the person reestablish reality levels and begin again to cope with day-to-day events; little emphasis need be placed on insight at this point. Individual group therapy oriented toward immediate function and acceptance of the patient is often helpful when the patient is able to tolerate interactions with other people. As the condition improves—frequently after discharge from the hospital—the patient is ready for more insight-oriented psychotherapy, either individual or group. It is hoped that improved insight will help the patient recognize antecedents to stress so that they can be avoided. Family or couples therapy may be necessary when the precipitating stress is related to interpersonal problems. This will also help the family to cope with the problem and facilitate therapy.

3. Social—Social inputs, particularly during convalescence, are as important as psychologic treatment. Part-time hospitalization, such as in a day hospital, may be necessary to assist the patient to resume his former life. In some cases, a substitute home will be necessary. The ongoing need for social support varies considerably. Nonresidential self-help groups such as Recovery Inc. are helpful when continued support is necessary. Family counseling is always necessary for specific advice and explanations of what the patient can do and tolerate.

4. Behavioral—Behavioral strategies are usually limited to role-playing and modeling. These assist the patient in reestablishing contacts with the "real world" and practicing appropriate ways to deal with people. Nonacceptance of psychiatric jargon and insistence on appropriate interactions operantly reinforce the desirable behavior and increase its frequency.

B. Chronic Schizophrenias:

1. Medical—Medical treatment is the major ongoing need in this type of illness. Intermittent hospitalization is usually required, and antipsychotics must be given indefinitely. In most cases, the patient should be treated during the acute phase with adequate dosages of a drug such as chlorpromazine or thioridazine—often requiring 500—600 mg orally per day. As the acute illness subsides, the patient frequently no longer needs the sedative drugs and can be gradually switched to a piperazine drug such as perphenazine or fluphenazine. Since many of the patients in this group relapse because they stop taking their medication, an injectable long-acting preparation such as fluphenazine enanthate is helpful when given in dosages of about 25 mg (1 ml) every 2 weeks. Careful attention to medication with appropriate upward adjustment with signs of decompensation can considerably decrease the frequency of hospitalization. It is incumbent on the physician to check the patient periodically for long-term effects of the antipsychotics, eg, tardive dyskinesias (usually evidenced by unusual tongue or snouting movements), pigmentation (check the eyes with a penlight for striate lenticular opacities), cardiac dysfunction (usually evidenced by electrocardiographic changes or arrhythmias), blood dyscrasias (usually a leukopenia occurring in the first several months of treatment), or abnormalities of glucose metabolism (glucose tolerance curve is raised and prolonged).

2. Social—Social methods of treatment are very important in maintaining the maximum level of function and preventing rehospitalization. Part-time hospitalization (day, night, or partial day attendance) is often necessary for prolonged periods to initially substitute for other social involvements and later to facilitate the patient's reintegration into his community. These, like the full-time hospitalization, may be required periodically. Board and care homes may be required in cases of marked disbaility. Nonresidential self-help groups such as Recovery Inc. are often utilized on an indefinite basis and provide a social level of function tolerable to this type of patient. Work agencies (eg, Goodwill Industries Inc.) provide a useful sheltered work situation. Vocational rehabilitation agencies provide assessment and retraining commensurate with the patient's level of function and occasionally can help with job replacement. The family instructions must include a clear discussion of the prognosis to help them plan for their future relationship with the patient. Observations of relatives, patients, and therapists tend to show that the positive interactive effects of drugs and sociotherapy take about 18 months to appear.

3. Behavioral—Behavioral methods are frequently used in hospitals, day or partial care centers, and in the better board and care homes. They include modeling—often in group training—to help reinstitute assertiveness and correct skewed communication patterns. Operant conditioning is often used in "token economies" to reinforce appropriate behaviors. The tokens earned by appropriate activities are used by the patients to pay for desired pastimes, etc, and are intended to simulate the real world, where one must realistically work to get money and defer pleasurable activities until a suitable time. Money is the operant reinforcer for most people, and the tokens have similar reinforcement value.

4. Psychologic—Psychologic therapies are useful only in selected cases. Psychopharmacologic agents are the primary mode of treatment, but psychotherapy can be a valuable adjunct, particularly when its goals are not overly optimistic. Individual therapy is helpful to the patient with specific problems, and family therapy can be particularly helpful when family interactions are playing a role in maintaining aberrant behaviors or when the family needs assistance in dealing with the erratic behavior of the patient.

Prognosis

The prognosis is good in acute schizophrenias for return to a previous level of functioning but is usually poor in chronic schizophrenias. The goals of therapy should be realistic and oriented toward specific living problems.

Arieti S: An overview of schizophrenia from a predominantly psychologic approach. Am J Psychiat 131:241, 1974.

Bleuler M: The long-term course of the schizophrenic psychoses. Psychol Med 4:244, 1974.

Falek A, Moser HM: Classification in schizophrenia. Arch Gen Psychiat 32:59, 1975.

Freedman BJ: The subjective experience of perceptual and cognitive disturbances in schizophrenia. Arch Gen Psychiat 30:333, 1974.

Grinspoon L: Psychotherapy and pharmacotherapy in chronic schizophrenia. Am J Psychiat 124:1645, 1968.

O'Brien CP & others: Group vs. individual psychotherapy with schizophrenics. Arch Gen Psychiat 24:474, 1972.

Paul GL & others: Maintenance psychotropic drugs in the presence of active treatment programs. Arch Gen Psychiat 27:106, 1972.

Pollin W: The pathogenesis of schizophrenia. Arch Gen Psychiat 27:29, 1972.

Wittenborn JR & others: Niacin in the long term treatment of schizophrenia. Arch Gen Psychiat 28:308, 1973.

THE DEPRESSIONS

Essentials of Diagnosis
Present in All Depressions:
- Lowered mood, varying from mild sadness to intense feelings of guilt and hopelessness.
- Difficulty in thinking, including inability to concentrate and lack of decisiveness.
- Loss of interest with diminished involvement in work and recreation.

Present in Severe Depressions:
- Delusions of a hypochondriacal or persecutory nature.
- Depersonalization, including feelings of being apart from reality with total loss of feeling.
- Physical symptoms, eg, anorexia, insomnia, reduced sexual drive, and various somatic complaints.

General Considerations

Depression, like anxiety, is ubiquitous and is a reality of everyday life. It can be a normal reaction to a wide variety of events and must be evaluated as such. When the depression is appropriate to a life event and is not of major magnitude, specific treatment is not necessary. In many cases the patient comes to the physician to find out if the depression is abnormal, and in a significant number of cases all that is needed is to reassure the patient that the depression is not significantly abnormal. Not every depression requires treatment, and the overuse of antidepressant medications is a direct result of the physician's failure to appreciate this.

The whole issue of depression is further confused by the fact that the word is used as an expression of a mood, a symptom, a syndrome, or a disease. Furthermore, the classifications are totally different and do not necessarily relate to each other. So-called neurotic versus psychotic classifications are not well differentiated, and treatment is not predicated on the distinction.

There are 4 basic theoretical models of depression:

(1) The "aggression-turned-inward" construct, which is apparent in many clinical cases of depression but has no substantial proof, although the emergence or expression of anger does at times alleviate the depression.

(2) The "loss" model, which postulates that depression is a reaction to loss of a person, thing, status, self-esteem, or even a habit pattern. This model is often quite evident in everyday life situations, and the

connection between the ·loss and the depressed response is often quite clear.

(3) The "interpersonal relationship" approach, which utilizes behavioral concepts. The person who is depressed may use depression as a means of controlling other people (including doctors). It can be an extension and outgrowth of such simple behavior as pouting, silence, or ignoring something or someone. These ways of coping can grow malignantly as the person expands the reactions to feeling sorry for himself, unloved, and alone. This may temporarily elicit some reassurance or attention from another person, but gradually, like most neurotic patterns, it fails to serve the need and the problem worsens.

(4) The "biogenic amine" hypothesis, which stresses biochemical derangements characterized by a depletion of biogenic amines. The action of reserpine in its physiologic activity and occasional production of depression has been a major support of the hypothesis which requires further investigation.

All 4 factors may be present in a depression, but the classification which follows outlines a practical approach.

Classification

In general, there are 3 major groups of depressions with similar symptoms in each group.

A. Reactive: Depression may occur in reaction to some outside (exogenous) adverse life situation, usually loss of a person by death, divorce, etc; financial reversal; or loss of an established role, such as being needed. Anger and its repression are frequently associated with the loss, which in turn often produces a feeling of guilt. The loss, anger, and guilt are readily apparent as the patient discusses the depression with the physician, who should be particularly alert to these components. Adjectives such as reactive and neurotic (implying anxiety, which is often present in these depressions) are often used in this group of depressions. The symptoms range from mild sadness, anxiety, irritability, worry, and lack of concentration and discouragement to the more severe symptoms of the next group.

B. Primary Affective Disorders: These are *not* in reaction to discernible outside events (endogenous) and are frequently called manic-depressive illness. Twin studies indicate a genetic factor, there being a concordance factor in 57% of monozygotic twins (bipolar, 72%; unipolar, 40%) and 14% in dizygotic twins (both types). These disorders include such descriptions as involutional and postpartum depressions. Multifactorial comparisons show that these patients score higher than others on 3 factors: observed restlessness, retarded movement, and somatic concerns to the point of somatic delusions (psychotic depressions). They also have deep feelings of guilt, loneliness, and hopelessness with a restricted affective range and a loss of interest in daily activities. The problems of anorexia, weight loss, constipation, delusional ideas of sin, guilt, and ill health, and insomnia (particularly early morning awakening) are often present in this group.

There are 2 subtypes of primary affective disorders: **unipolar,** wherein the patient has either recurrent depressions or recurrent manic attacks (the latter is much less common), or **bipolar,** in which both depressive and manic phases are present, frequently alternating, and persisting for variable periods of time. Patients with the unipolar variety tend to be older at onset (often in the 40s), to have fewer attacks, and to have a lower incidence in relatives than patients with the bipolar type, who have peak age at onset of 25 and a high frequency of attacks. The symptoms of the depression are similar in both subtypes.

There are several characteristic features of **mania:** (1) flight of ideas with minimal stimuli; (2) behavior change from quiet and cooperative to excited and aggressive; (3) hyperactivity, including motor, social, and sexual activity; (4) affect with constant elation and anger at any challenge, including a euphoric, expansive mood with grandiosity; (5) easy distractibility; (6) a history of other manic episodes or marked mood swings; and (7) a family history of mood disorder.

Manic patients differ from schizophrenic patients in a number of areas of interpersonal behavior, including projection of responsibility, sensitivity to vulnerable areas in other people, testing of limits, attempts to divide hospital staff, flattering behavior, and ability to evoke anger easily. Understanding these tendencies not only helps in differentiating mania from schizophrenia and schizo-affective disorders but also in dealing realistically with the patient who uses these maneuvers.

C. Secondary to Underlying Disease: Illnesses such as rheumatoid arthritis, hypothyroidism, multiple sclerosis, and chronic heart disease are particularly liable to be associated with depression. Depressions can be associated with other conditions such as organic brain syndromes, schizo-affective schizophrenia, and drug reactions. The classic model of drug-induced depression occurs with reserpine. Various other drugs (eg, contraceptive hormones, corticosteroids, alcohol and other CNS depressants) also produce depression to varying degrees.

Clinical Findings

There is an extremely wide spectrum of symptoms. The depression itself may range from mild sadness to deep gloom. Associated symptoms and signs include psychomotor retardation, somatic concerns or somatic delusions (especially referable to head, heart, and abdomen), restlessness, agitation, withdrawal from social activities, irritability, lack of satisfaction, loss of energy and initiative, preoccupation with self, brooding, ruminations (these repetitive concerns often include body functions), loss of libido, anorexia with resultant weight loss, insomnia (early morning type most serious), hypersomnia (less frequently), constipation, and paranoid ideation. In some instances there may be a feigned but unsuccessful attempt at joviality. Physically the patient may present an appearance ranging from dejection, with bent posture, slow movements, reluctance to speak, and soft voice, to the opposite extreme of agitation.

Differential Diagnosis

Since depression may be a part of any illness—either reactively or as a secondary symptom—careful attention must be given to personal life adjustment problems, the role of medications (eg, reserpine), schizophrenia, and acute or chronic organic brain syndromes.

Complications

The longer the depression continues, the more crystallized it becomes, particularly when there is an element of secondary reinforcement. The most important complication is suicide, which has become a serious medical problem, with approximately 20–60 thousand deaths in the USA each year and up to 50 times as many attempts. Assessment of the actual incidence of suicide is very difficult because of social pressures, reporting variations, uncertainty about accidents (eg, drug overdoses, automobile crashes, falls), and repetition, since about 25% of persons making suicide attempts have made a previous attempt. There are 4 major groups of people who make suicide attempts:

(1) Those who are overwhelmed by problems in living. By far the greatest number fall into this category. There is often great ambivalence; they don't really want to die, but they don't want to go on as before either.

(2) Those who are clearly attempting to control others. This is the blatant attempt of a minor nature in the presence of a significant other person in order to hurt or control that person.

(3) Those with severe depressions. This group would include both exogenous and endogenous conditions and often is a serious attempt that occurs as the person is beginning to improve.

(4) Those with psychotic illness. This person tends to be unpredictable and often successful but is a small percentage of the total.

The immediate goal of psychiatric evaluation is to assess the current suicidal risk and the need for hospitalization versus outpatient management. The intent is less likely to be truly suicidal, for example, if small amounts of poison were ingested or scratching of wrists was superficial; if the act was performed in the presence of others or with early notification of others; or if the attempt was arranged so that early detection would be anticipated.

The patient's current mood status is best evaluated by direct evaluation of his plans and concerns about the future, his own reaction to the attempt, and his thoughts about the reactions of others. The patient's immediate resources should be assessed—people who can be significantly involved, family support, job situation, financial resources, etc.

If hospitalization is not indicated, the physician must formulate and institute a treatment plan or make an adequate referral. The problem is often worsened by the long-term complications of the suicidal attempt, eg, brain damage due to hypoxia; peripheral neuropa-thies due to long periods in one position, causing nerve compressions; and uncorrectable medical or surgical problems such as esophageal strictures and tendon dysfunctions.

Sleep disturbances in the depressions are discussed on p 625.

Treatment of Reactive Depressions

A. Psychologic: Psychologic therapy is often best initiated during crisis situations, since this is the time when people are most amenable to change. The crisis therapy should deal with the crisis, its antecedents, and new ways to deal with similar anticipated problems. When lack of self-confidence, identity problems, and long-term adjustment difficulties are responsible for the depression, individual psychotherapy is oriented toward helping the person change some of these habitual ways of meeting life situations. In many cases, repressed anger and guilt underly the depression. Verbalization and facing these feelings also tend to lessen the depression. When the depression is secondary to serious interpersonal defects, individual group therapy is indicated. Family or couples therapy is warranted in those situations resulting from family or marital dysharmony.

B. Social: Social types of management are particularly important because a frequent consequence of depression is social withdrawal. This in turn exacerbates the emptiness and loneliness resulting in even less social involvement. In more serious cases, day hospitalization is necessary to reinitiate involvement and provide a daily structure of activities. When a specific body loss is involved (eg, mastectomy, colostomy), nonresidential self-help groups of people who have suffered similar losses help the patient deal with the loss. When the loss is material, such agencies as the Red Cross, Legal Aid, and welfare services can be utilized. Work assistance may be necessary, including vocational rehabilitation, when depression is related to loss of self-confidence in the absence of work.

C. Medical: Medical evaluation is necessary to rule out underlying organic disease. It is particularly important to determine whether or not there is a problem of hidden alcoholism or abuse of other drugs. Careful attention is necessary in evaluating prescribed drugs (eg, reserpine, alpha methyldopa) which might be causing mood depression. Minor tranquilizers with low suicide potential (eg, diazepam, 5–10 mg orally every 4–6 hours as indicated) are used when anxiety is a major factor, particularly in crisis situations. Antidepressants are not particularly effective in exogenous depressions, but doxepin is effective in alleviating anxiety and improving sleep when given in bedtime oral doses of 50–100 mg.

D. Behavioral: Behavioral approaches are most valuable in specific conditions which are playing a role in the depression, eg, desensitization is useful in cases where phobias are present. Role-playing can improve assertiveness in patients whose depression is a function of passivity.

Treatment of Primary Affective Disorders

A. Medical: Medical methods are of major importance. Hospitalization with suicidal precautions is required when the patient is suicidal or seriously incapacitated. If the suicide risk is high, ECT should be considered as a treatment of choice. Tricyclic antidepressants (see Table 17–2) are effective and should be used in adequate dosage and given a sufficient period of trial. An example would be imipramine, 100 mg daily to start, increased by 25 mg daily every several days until remission occurs or until 300 mg daily are being given. In resistant cases, a combined tricyclic-MAOI approach can be cautiously attempted. Although lithium is not effective in acute depressions, there is evidence that it decreases the recurrence rate of depressions in primary affective disorders, particularly the bipolar type (mania and depression).

Manic states are treated with haloperidol, 5 mg orally or IM every several hours, until the symptoms subside. At the same time, appropriate laboratory tests are done prior to starting treatment with lithium carbonate. Over a period of about 1 week, haloperidol can be discontinued and lithium blood levels stabilized.

The question of how long one should continue medications has not been satisfactorily answered. In general, the patient should be continued on the smallest amount of tricyclic drug necessary to prevent relapse. This warrants a very gradual reduction in dosage over a period of months until the drug can be stopped. In some patients it will be necessary to maintain them on some antidepressant medication indefinitely.

B. Psychologic: Psychologic therapies are often unnecessary and limited to problem areas which may have exacerbated the depression. These include marked passivity, inability to handle anger, compulsive traits, and excessive use of alcohol and other drugs.

C. Social: Social structuring such as day hospitalization is sometimes important as an alternative to hospitalization when daily supervision is required while the medications are taking effect. This is not adequate for the suicidal patient but is helpful in those patients who are not suicidal but are unable to reinvolve themselves in life activities. Family and work counseling are frequently useful in protracted or recurrent episodes.

D. Behavioral: Behavioral technics, as with the psychologic therapies, are useful mainly in ancillary problem areas.

Prognosis

Exogenous or drug-induced depressions are usually time-limited, and the prognosis with treatment is good if suicide or a pathologic pattern of adjustment does not intervene. Endogenous depressions frequently respond well to effective treatment given *early* and in *adequate* amounts for a reasonable period of time.

Akiskal HS, McKinney WT: Overview of recent research in depression. Arch Gen Psychiat 32:285, 1975.

Allen MG & others: Affective illness in veteran twins: A diagnostic review. Am J Psychiat 131:1234, 1974.

Bostock T, Williams CL: Attempted suicide as an operant be-

havior. Arch Gen Psychiat 31:482, 1974.

Chodoff P: The depressive personality. Arch Gen Psychiat 27:666, 1972.

Kiev A: Prognostic factors in attempted suicide. Am J Psychiat 131:987, 1974.

Klerman GL & others: Treatment of depression by drugs and psychotherapy. Am J Psychiat 131:187, 1974.

Murphy GE: The physician's responsibilities for suicide. (2 parts.) Ann Int Med 82:301, 305, 1975.

Roth M & others: Studies in the classification of affective disorders. Brit J Psychiat 121:147, 1972.

Shopsin B & others: Psychoactive drugs in mania. Arch Gen Psychiat 32:34, 1975.

Vogel GW & others: The effect of REM deprivation on depression. Psychosomatics 14:104, 1973.

Winston F: Oral contraceptives, pyridoxine, and depression. Am J Psychiat 130:1217, 1973.

Woodruff RA: Suicide attempts and psychiatric diagnosis. Dis Nerv System 33:617, 1972.

Zung WWK: From art to science: The diagnosis and treatment of depression. Arch Gen Psychiat 29:328, 1973.

SLEEP DISORDERS

Sleep disturbances occur commonly in psychiatric disorders, particularly in depression. The complaints are difficult to evaluate since approximately 30% of a normal population sample will complain of "insomnia": trouble falling asleep, waking up during the night (the most common), or early final awakening. There are 2 distinct states of sleep as shown on electroencephalographic (EEG) studies: **REM** (rapid eye movement) **sleep**, also called dream sleep, D state sleep, and paradoxical sleep; and **NREM** (nonREM) **sleep**, which is also known as slow wave sleep or S state sleep and is divided into stages 1, 2, 3, and 4. Dreaming occurs in both REM and NREM sleep. There is no clear evidence that REM sleep deprivation is harmful or productive of mental disorder. The stages of NREM sleep have been less well studied because of technical problems in selectively evaluating a particular stage.

Factors contributing to insomnia include (1) situational problems such as transient stress, job pressures, and marital discord; (2) medical disorders which inevitably include pain and physical discomfort; (3) drug-related episodes, including withdrawal from alcohol or sedatives; and (4) psychologic conditions, particularly the major mental illnesses such as schizophrenia and primary affective disorders (see p 623). Schizophrenics vary markedly in the degree of sleep disturbance they endure. In acute episodes the disruption is severe, even to the point of total insomnia. The chronic schizophrenic or the patient in remission often does not have any complaints, and his EEG pattern is not remarkably abnormal. Antipsychotic drugs have a minimal effect on the EEG sleep tracing but are clinically helpful. Sedating phenothiazines such as chlorpromazine given at bedtime obviate the need for sedatives in the schizophrenic with sleep problems.

Sleep disturbance is one of the most common symptoms of primary affective disorders. Many bipolar patients sleep more when they are depressed and less when they are manic. REM sleep is increased and stages 3 and 4 sleep (slow wave) are consistently decreased in the depressive phase. In the manic phase, REM sleep is decreased but there are varying reports on slow wave sleep. Both unipolar and bipolar patients in the depressed phase usually have a decreased total sleep time. The incidence of hypersomnia in depression is low—about 8%. Unfortunately, there is no specific correlation of particular types of depression to clinical type of sleep problem. Antidepressants decrease REM sleep and have varying effects on slow wave sleep. The effect on REM sleep correlates positively with reports that *reductions* in REM sleep tend to parallel *improvement* of the depression. Use of the more sedating tricyclic antidepressants such as amitriptyline, given at bedtime in full dosage, frequently eliminates the need to use a sedative.

In the general population, complaints of sleep disturbance tend to increase with age and level of anxiety, although there is little change in the EEG patterns. Barbiturates and nonbarbiturate sedative-hypnotics such as glutethimide are initially effective and reduce REM sleep slightly, but tolerance develops quickly and there is a return to baseline levels by the end of 1 week. Chronic use of multiple doses of these drugs produces a more marked decrease of both REM and slow wave sleep, with rebound increase of both types of sleep when the drug is withdrawn. For transient sleep difficulties, a sedative such as flurazepam is relatively safe, effective, and not prone to abuse or tolerance.

All of the commonly abused drugs affect sleep. Narcotics substantially reduce REM sleep, but tolerance and a return to normal baseline levels develop in several days. Stimulants effect a moderate reduction in REM sleep and the same quick tolerance. Alcohol and meprobamate are similar to the barbiturates in their effect on sleep. While the proper use of medication may provide symptomatic relief for insomnia over the short term, the clinician must be attuned to the possibility of underlying problems, particularly severe depression. This is of major importance in early and effective treatment since the majority of suicide victims see their physician in the month prior to the suicide and tend to use the drugs prescribed, particularly sedatives, in the suicide act.

Hauri P: Sleep in depression. Psychiat Ann 4:45, 1974.
Kales A & others: Insomnia: An approach to management and treatment. Psychiat Ann 4:28, 1974.
Kay DC: Sleep and some psychoactive drugs. Psychosomatics 14:108, 1973.
Reich L & others: Sleep disturbance in schizophrenia. Arch Gen Psychiat 32:51, 1975.
Vogel GW: A review of REM sleep deprivation. Arch Gen Psychiat 32:749, 1975.

AGGRESSION & VIOLENCE

The many forms of violence preclude satisfactory classification. An arbitrary approach would include 4 categories which are not mutually exclusive: (1) Mass strife involving many people (wars, revolutions, purges). (2) Single incidents of a serious nature involving one or more individuals (mass killings, skyjackings, gang killings). (3) Single incidents by an individual in a serious act which he may or may not have committed before (murder, provoked assault, rape). (4) Repetitive acts of aggression by an individual with no or minimal provocation and of a semiserious nature, often triggered by alcohol or other drugs (wife-beating, reckless driving, child abuse, recurrent brawls).

There may be a demonstrable underlying pathologic process in persons performing aggressive acts. The one that comes most often to the attention of the physician is the last category. It is particularly important to consider any treatable disorders, and these people frequently fall into one of the following diagnostic categories:

(1) Serious family behavior problems with intrafamily physical violence, most commonly involving wife or child. Most cases of child-battering are a result of this sort of intrafamily pathology. Treatment is family therapy, but it is usually not undertaken until an incident occurs that involves the police or the courts. Social sanctions are then brought to bear, and treatment proceeds under a mandate.

(2) Dyscontrol syndrome, which is often unpredictable, is not related to specific provocations, and is frequently a function of the disinhibiting effects of alcohol and other drugs. While there may be no demonstrable CNS dysfunction, a large number of individuals with dyscontrol syndrome report hyperacusis, visual illusions, numbness of extremities, headaches, and drowsiness. EEG abnormalities of a nonspecific nature are common. Treatment must include careful examination for any CNS abnormalities. A trial of anticonvulsant medication (diphenylhydantoin, 300 mg/day) is warranted. Addition of a major tranquilizer (thioridazine, 100—200 mg/day) should be considered if improvement is minimal or does not occur with anticonvulsant therapy alone.

(3) Temporal lobe disorders can result in aggressive behavior, but less than 25% of violence-prone people show definite signs of an organic disturbance, and only a small percentage have temporal lobe dysfunction. Many of these disorders, like dyscontrol syndrome, appear only after ingestion of alcohol or other drugs. In those few cases where temporal lobe dysfunction is demonstrated on EEG, the treatment is anticonvulsant medication (Table 16—1).

(4) Schizophrenic disorders, particularly the paranoid types, are often associated with violent behavior, particularly during acute exacerbations of schizophrenia. The violence is usually related to the patient's delusions and his escalating anxiety and hyperreactivity to incoming sensory stimulation.

Cocozza JJ, Steadman HJ: Some refinements in the measurement and prediction of dangerous behavior. Am J Psychiat 131:1012, 1974.

Gorney R: Interpersonal intensity, competition and synergy: Determinants of achievement, aggression and mental illness. Am J Psychiat 128:436, 1971.

Joseph ED: Aggression redefined: Its adaptational aspects. Psychoanal Quart 42:197, 1973.

Kligman D, Goldberg DA: Temporal lobe epilepsy and aggression. J Nerv Ment Dis 160:324, 1975.

Maletzky BM: The episodic dyscontrol syndrome. Dis Nerv System 34:178, 1973.

Nichol AR & others: The relationship of alcoholism to violent behavior resulting in long-term imprisonment. Brit J Psychiat 123:47, 1973.

DRUG DEPENDENCY

The term drug dependency is used in a broad sense here to include both addictions and habituations. It involves the triad of compulsive drug use referred to as drug addiction, which includes (1) a **psychologic craving** or dependence, and the behavior included in the procurement of the drug ("the life"); (2) **physiologic dependence**, with withdrawal symptoms on discontinuance of the drug; and (3) **tolerance**, ie, the need to increase the dose to obtain the desired effects.

Medical science has been interested in finding the causes and cures of diseases; the public is much more concerned with remedies that will abolish pain, tension, or sleeplessness and which have no effect at all on the cure of disease. The marketplace demands products quite different from those that medical science deems most beneficial in the preservation and prolongation of useful life. In fact, it is one of the tragedies of modern therapeutics that a remedy is expected for every problem. Physicians have put themselves in the untenable position of trying to produce the cures that are demanded. The symptoms run their course and disappear, often regardless of the remedies, but the treatment methods are believed to be effective and thus stimulate a demand for more and better methods. The plethora of prescriptions for sedatives and analgesics attest to this determination of the public to obtain remedies, particularly those stamped with the authority of the prescription pad. As a result, a majority of the population is overmedicated, and the notion that every problem has a pharmacologic cure is perpetuated. This environment contributes to the demand of the younger generation to look for relief in drugs whether they are acquired through legitimate or illigitimate channels.

While detoxification is often required at some point in people who are drug-dependent, this is not necessarily the first nor even the most important approach. The request for detoxification is frequently made by the drug user on the assumption that this is what is expected in exchange for the help he feels he needs. An overemphasis on detoxification gives credence to the dangerous notion that all discomfort, both medical and psychologic, can be relieved by drugs and minimizes the importance of psychologic problems in the development of drug dependency. Detoxification is indicated when there is concrete evidence of physiologic withdrawal (see sections on specific drugs). The drug used should be a long-acting one which produces minimal fluctuations in blood levels from "high" to "low" and is therefore received by the patient as medication rather than "dope."

Bruhn P, Maage N: Intellectual and neuropsychological functions in young men with heavy and long-term drug abuse. Am J Psychiat 132:397, 1975.

Chapel JL: Emergency room treatment of the drug abusing patient. Am J Psychiat 130:257, 1973.

Greaves G: Toward an existential theory of drug dependence. J Nerv Ment Dis 159:263, 1974.

Greenblatt DJ, Shader RI: Drug abuse and the emergency room physician. Am J Psychiat 131:559, 1974.

McBay AJ: Toxicological findings in fatal poisonings. Clin Chem 19:361, 1973.

Wesson DR, Smith DE: A conceptual approach to detoxification. J Psychedelic Drugs 6:161, 1974.

NARCOTIC DEPENDENCY

Essentials of Diagnosis

- High levels of compulsive use, with considerable ancillary behavior involved in "hustling" and "shooting" the drug.
- Tolerance, psychologic, and physical dependence.
- Withdrawal uncomfortable but not life-threatening.
- High drive to obtain the drugs, with associated criminal activity to obtain funds.

General Considerations

The social and economic consequences of narcotic addiction are alarming. The financial loss is estimated to be $1 billion a year in the USA alone.

The principal abused narcotic drug is heroin (metabolized to morphine), which can be obtained from illegal sources. Other common narcotics—which differ from heroin only in milligram potency and duration of action—are, in order of decreasing potency, methadone, morphine, meperidine, and codeine.

Other synthetic congeners include propoxyphene—which is rated somewhere between placebo, aspirin, and codeine—and pentazocine. Pentazocine, along with cyclazocine, is a narcotic antagonist but has agonist properties and produces mild psychotomimetic effects which are transient and dose-related. Thus, it may precipitate withdrawal symptoms in a person addicted to narcotics, but it may also produce physical dependence; and there are reports of withdrawal symptoms when parenteral abuse has been discontinued. The effects of overdosage of all narcotics and chemicals with similar structure, including propoxyphene and pentazocine, are reversed by naloxone. Sudden withdrawal from narcotics is *not* dangerous. There is no mortality rate (unlike alcohol and barbituates) and only a moderate morbidity rate (about the severity of a bout with the "flu"). The addict frequently considers himself to be more "addicted" than he really is, and a withdrawal program is often unnecessary.

The following discussion pertains to heroin, which is quite similar to the other narcotics except for time factors. (In cases of methadone withdrawal, multiply the hours by 4.)

Clinical Findings

A. Mild Intoxication: The symptoms and signs of mild heroin intoxication are analgesia, the "high" which is described as a feeling of euphoria and carefree relaxation, drowsiness, changes in mood, mental clouding, occasional dysphoria with anxiety, frequent nausea, occasional vomiting, miosis, and decreased gastrointestinal function. Tolerance and physical dependence develop with frequent use. The drug may be demonstrated chemically in the urine.

B. Overdosage: Narcotic overdosage causes respiratory depression of all grades of severity up to and including respiratory arrest, nausea and vomiting, deep sleep to coma, pinpoint pupils, peripheral vasodilatation, massive pulmonary edema (possibly secondary to adulterants such as quinine), and EEG changes (increased voltage, lower frequency). The urine is positive for opiates.

C. Symptoms of Withdrawal:

Grade 0: Craving, anxiety (4 hours).

Grade 1: Yawning, lacrimation, rhinorrhea, perspiration (8 hours).

Grade 2: Above plus mydriasis, piloerection, tremors, hot and cold flashes, aching bones and muscles, anorexia (12 hours).

Grade 3: Increased intensity of above plus insomnia, restlessness, and nausea; and increased blood pressure, temperature, respiratory rate and depth, and pulse rate (18–24 hours).

Grade 4: Increased intensity of above plus curled-up position, vomiting, diarrhea, weight loss (about 5 lb daily), spontaneous ejaculation or orgasm, hemoconcentration, leukocytosis, eosinopenia, and hyperglycemia (24–36 hours).

Differential Diagnosis

Mild intoxications and overdoses are difficult to distinguish from other drug reactions without corroborating evidence such as needle tracks on the skin and some fairly reliable history. A narcotic antagonist such as naloxone will immediately help differentiate the narcotic intoxications.

Complications

An abnormal sleep pattern with changes in the amount and distribution of rapid eye movement (REM) sleep may persist for several weeks. Variations in vital signs remain for as long as 4–6 months after withdrawal. The injection of nonsterile material under nonsterile conditions can result in serious infections (including hepatitis) and traumatic insults (eg, hitting an artery, with spasm and gangrene). Pulmonary edema occurs in about 50% of patients. Pneumonia, septic emboli, and alveolar pulmonary block by contaminants are common. Cardiac complications include tachycardia, usually seen with low doses, and bradycardia with high doses.

The annual death rate of narcotic addicts is between 1 and 6%, and half of deaths are due to overdoses. Studies in some specific areas such as the District of Columbia show a recent drop in opiate deaths related to methadone. There were an increasing number of cases in the first 3 years of the present decade and a decreasing number in 1973 and 1974.

Treatment

A. Treatment of Overdosage:

1. Give an antagonist such as naloxone (Narcan), 0.4 mg IV, which acts within 2 minutes but is quickly dissipated and can be repeated at 5- to 10-minute intervals. (Use jugular vein if other veins are not accessible.) The results are so dramatic that if the patient does not respond it can be assumed either that he has taken another drug or that he has taken a combination of drugs with the opiate.

2. Institute supportive medical measures and treat complications.

3. Hospitalize the patient, since the duration of action of the antagonists is much shorter than that of some of the narcotics (eg, methadone). Close observation is necessary for the first 24 hours.

4. Observe for signs of withdrawal, since it is likely that the person is drug-dependent.

B. Treatment of Withdrawal Symptoms:

1. **Medical**—Hospitalize the patient and wait for grade 2 signs to develop (or use naloxone to test for degree of addiction). Give methadone, 10 mg orally. Parenteral use is justified if the patient is vomiting. If signs persist after 2 hours give another 10 mg, and so on until signs are not present. It is rare to have to give more than 40 mg of methadone in 24 hours. Stabilize at the required level (eg, if 40 mg have been required to eliminate signs, give 20 mg every 12 hours the first day). Decrease by 5–10 mg of methadone per 24-hour period, eg, in a patient requiring 20 mg of methadone every 12 hours the first day, the dosage the next day would be 15 mg of methadone every 12 hours. Evaluate carefully for other medical complications, which are quite common.

No other sedative hypnotics or tranquilizers are necessary in the withdrawal stage, and, if used, must be given only for short periods for specific reasons—eg, a sedative the first several nights to ensure restful sleep.

Methadone maintenance programs are used in

chronic recidivism. In the USA, approximately 85,000 people are in methadone maintenance programs. In carefully controlled programs, the dosage is gradually increased to fairly high daily amounts (40—120 mg/24 hours) which satisfy the subject's craving and, because of the tolerance, block the euphoric effects of heroin to a great degree. The methadone maintenance method of managing heroin addiction is controversial since the person remains addicted; however, the addiction is controlled, criminal activity is not necessary to obtain money, and life can revolve around productive activities instead of "hustling" or "pushing" the drug to get money to pay for personal supplies.

2. Social—Self-help communities such as Synanon assist highly motivated narcotic addicts in staying "clean." Substitute homes may be used as "crash pads" for "cold turkey" or sedative-assisted withdrawal. Paraprofessional organizations such as crisis centers provide aid in mitigating withdrawal symptoms and direction for housing and treatment centers. Family counseling should help family members deal realistically with one who is abusing drugs.

3. Behavioral—Aversive conditioning, although frequently tried, is not of lasting value. Modeling technics have been helpful in milieus such as Synanon. Extinction procedures can be tried while the patient is on methadone maintenance, the goal being to disrupt the "ritual" of administration.

4. Psychologic—Eclectic psychotherapy and individual group therapy have had very limited success.

Prognosis

The prognosis for recovery from an overdose is excellent if the patient receives adequate medical care promptly. The response to withdrawal treatment is excellent if the program is structured to prevent drug abuse during withdrawal. The prognosis for long-term abstinence is poor.

Methadone maintenance has been effective in terms of decreasing criminal activities and increasing productive efforts (eg, employment). Long-term results are yet to be evaluated. Use of other drugs (including alcohol and cocaine) while on methadone maintenance is a problem.

Bowden CL, Maddux JF: Methadone maintenance: Myth and reality. Am J Psychiat 129:435, 1972.
Chappel JN: Methadone and chemotherapy in drug addiction. JAMA 228:725, 1974.
Evans LEJ: Treatment of drug overdosage with naloxone, a specific narcotic antagonist. Lancet 1:452, 1973.
Greene MH, Dupont RL: Heroin addiction trends. Am J Psychiat 131:540, 1974.
Kaufman RE, Levy SB: Overdose treatment: Addict folklore and medical reality. JAMA 227:411, 1974.
Primm BJ, Bath PE: Pseudoheroinism. Internat J Addict 8:231, 1973.
Snyder SH: The opiate receptor. Ann Int Med 81:534, 1974.
Stimmel B: The socioeconomics of heroin dependency. New England J Med 287:1275, 1972.
Tenant FS: Complications of propoxyphene abuse. Arch Int Med 132:191, 1973.

Thornton WE, Thornton BP: Narcotic poisoning: A review of the literature. Am J Psychiat 131:867, 1974.
Weisman M & others: Quality of street heroin. New England J Med 289:698, 1973.
Wikler A: Dynamics of drug dependence. Arch Gen Psychiat 28:611, 1973.
Woody GE & others: Depression and anxiety in heroin addicts: A placebo-controlled study of doxepin in combination with methadone. Am J Psychiat 132:447, 1975.

DEPENDENCY ON BARBITURATES, OTHER SEDATIVE-HYPNOTICS, & MINOR TRANQUILIZERS

Essentials of Diagnosis

- Confusion, slurred or incoherent speech, yawning, somnolence, amnesia, ataxia, stupor, coma, respiratory depression, and death.
- Euphoria, excitement, or aggressive behavior may also occur.
- Tolerance, psychologic dependence, and serious physical dependence.
- History often unreliable; any unusual symptoms should alert physician to evaluate for abuse of these drugs.

General Considerations

These drugs are all considered together since they similarly affect behavior and physiology. Since alcohol has considerably greater acceptance and usage and has many long-term physical effects, it will be considered separately. The drugs are all additive to each other, and cross-dependency occurs. Mixed usage is common.

Dependency to the point of addiction varies in each individual, but a useful rule of thumb for the short- and intermediate-acting barbiturates, meprobamate, and the nonbarbiturate sedative hypnotics such as glutethimide, ethchlorvynol, methyprylon, and methaqualone is that 6—8 tablets or capsules of the usual dosage per day represent the lower level of addiction. Levels above this will usually require detoxification.

Addictions are less frequently observed with the longer-acting agents such as phenobarbital, chlordiazepoxide, and the other benzodiazepines. These drugs require large daily amounts (about thirty 10 mg capsules of chlordiazepoxide daily) to produce dependency.

Blood levels and morbidity are related and are of prognostic value. For example, lethal serum levels range upward from 10 mg/100 ml for long-acting barbiturates and from 3 mg/100 ml for short-acting barbiturates.

Clinical Findings

A. Acute Intoxication: Manifestations include drowsiness, sleep, respiratory depression, errors of commission (sometimes resulting in accidents), difficulty in thinking, slowness of speech, impaired memory, narrowed attention range, varying disinhibition, ataxia, nystagmus, and dysarthria. Blood and urine levels of these drugs are important for determining the type and degree of intoxication.

B. Overdosage: Manifested by marked respiratory depression, coma, severe hypotension, decreased gastrointestinal activity, positive Babinski sign, initial pupillary constriction (later dilatation), stupor, shock syndrome, coma, and death. Determination of serum levels is important.

C. Withdrawal: The manifestations of barbiturate withdrawal include restlessness and anxiety (12–16 hours), followed by nausea, vomiting, abdominal cramps, anorexia, twitches (myoclonic muscular contractions or spasmodic jerking of one or more extremities), orthostatic hypotension, tremors, and marked muscular weakness. Increasing irritability (24–36 hours) occurs with exacerbation of the above symptoms. Seizures (early, with danger persisting over the first 2–3 days) are grand mal, with loss of consciousness and postconvulsive stupor. Delirium is accompanied by visual hallucinations, disorientation, paranoid ideation (3–7 days), and occasional "hallucinosis" with paranoid ideation and auditory hallucinations in the presence of a clear sensorium. Longer-acting drugs such as the nonbarbiturate sedative hypnotics and benzodiazepines cause the same withdrawal symptoms, appearing about 24–36 hours later.

Differential Diagnosis

The differential diagnosis includes all other drugs that have depressant qualities and, in the case of delirium, would include a wide variety of different drugs and natural substances such as anticholinergics, jimsonweed, psychedelics, and bromides. The possibility of organic diseases such as diabetic acidosis, insulin reactions, brain disease, and head injury must be considered. Sedative drug reactions must also be differentiated from the primary neuroses and psychoses.

Complications

Complications include pneumonias, infections (when drugs are used parenterally), bullous cutaneous lesions (with barbiturates), renal failure secondary to muscle necrosis in overdoses, peripheral neuropathies related to extended time in pressure positions in overdoses, and results of trauma in all states of acute intoxication.

Treatment

A. Overdoses: See p 628.

B. Withdrawal Reactions:

1. Medical—Evaluate carefully for medical complications. Medical treatment starts with hospitalization since in most cases it is impossible to treat these patients on an outpatient basis. Since all of these drugs are cross-dependent, any of them may be used for the treatment of detoxification. Pentobarbital is often given in oral doses of 200 mg every 4 hours until signs of withdrawal subside. Add up the total given in the first 24 hours and then give that amount over the next 24 hours (one-quarter of the total every 6 hours). Then decrease the 24-hour dose by 100 mg every day until the patient is off medication. If withdrawal signs appear, do not decrease the dose but go back to the last dosage that did not result in withdrawal signs.

Phenobarbital is frequently used instead of pentobarbital (30 mg of phenobarbital are equivalent to 100 mg of pentobarbital). The 24-hour decrease would then be 30 mg of phenobarbital until the patient is off medication.

2. Social—Social measures are important if the patient is to evade the consequences of whatever perpetuating effects may be operative in his environment. Substitute homes and self-help communities such as halfway houses, Salvation Army homes, and crash pads give the patient respite and permit some social planning. Family care homes and residential treatment centers are more desirable approaches but are expensive and limited in number. Crisis centers, "free clinics," and county-sponsored satellite clinics provide some medical care but, more importantly, offer counseling and access to helping social agencies. Family, school, and work counseling play a role in helping the individual regain a place in society and, when possible, utilize the family in helping the person to refrain from continued drug abuse.

3. Behavioral—Behavioral methods such as aversive conditioning have not been shown to be effective except in the improvement of underlying traits which might be playing a role in the drug abuse problem—eg, role-playing is helpful in the passive person to increase assertive behavior.

4. Psychologic—Psychologic treatment has been disappointing. Family or couples therapy is useful in cases where the family or marital disharmony is promoting the drug-taking behavior.

Prognosis

The prognosis for sedative overdosage is good if drug dosage is not massive and if medical care is instituted before hypoxic damage occurs. In cases of withdrawal, the outlook is excellent if the drug abuse can be controlled within the treatment setting. In general, the prognosis for long-term abstinence is poor. There is a high rate of recidivism.

Blumberg AG: Covert drug abuse among voluntary hospitalized psychiatric patients. JAMA 217:1659, 1971.

Bridge TP, Ellinwood EH: Quaalude alley: A one-way street. Am J Psychiat 130:217, 1973.

Gerald MC, Schwirian PM: Nonmedical use of methaqualone. Arch Gen Psychiat 28:627, 1973.

Greenblatt DJ, Schader RI: Meprobamate: A study of irrational drug use. Am J Psychiat 127:1297, 1971.

Smith DE, Wesson DR: Phenobarbital techniques for treatment of barbiturate dependence. Arch Gen Psychiat 24:56, 1971.

Wikler A: Diagnosis and treatment of drug dependence of the barbiturate type. Am J Psychiat 125:758, 1968.

ALCOHOLISM
(Problem Drinking & Alcohol Addiction)

Essentials of Diagnosis
Major Criteria:

- Physiologic dependence as manifested by evidence of a withdrawal syndrome when intake is interrupted.
- Tolerance to the effects of alcohol, wherein a person has high blood levels without gross evidence of intoxication and high daily consumption.
- Evidence of alcohol-associated illnesses, such as alcoholic liver disease, cerebellar degeneration, chronic gastritis, and coagulation disorders.
- Continued drinking despite strong medical and social contraindications and life disruptions.
- Subjective complaints of loss of control over alcohol consumption.

Minor Criteria:

- Alcohol stigmas: Alcohol odor on breath, alcoholic facies, flushed face, tremor, ecchymoses, peripheral neuropathy.
- Laboratory evidence of high blood alcohol levels, liver abnormalities, coagulation defects, EEG abnormalities.
- Surreptitious drinking, repeated attempts at abstinence, or blatantly indiscriminate use of alcohol.
- Unexplained work absences, preference for "livelier" companions, bars, and taverns, frequent automobile accidents, high incidence of erratic behavior.
- Frequent references to drinking behavior, use of alcohol to relieve psychic tension, major family disruptions, and symptoms of depression, isolation, and suicidal preoccupation.

General Considerations

Alcoholism is the biggest health problem after heart disease and cancer; in the USA, alcoholism decreases the life span 10–12 years. Alcohol is involved in approximately 30,000 deaths and one-half million injuries in auto accidents yearly. Along with job absenteeism and medical bills, the yearly costs in the USA are about $25 billion for the 5 billion gallons consumed in 1974—an amount which averages out to about 23 gallons for every man, woman, and child.

Alcoholism is a syndrome consisting of 2 phases: **problem drinking** and **alcohol addiction**. Problem drinking is the repetitive use of alcohol, often to alleviate tension or solve other emotional problems. Alcohol addiction is a true addiction similar to that which occurs following the repeated use of barbiturates or similar drugs. Dependence on other drugs—barbiturates, sedative-hypnotics, minor tranquilizers, etc—is very common. It may occur in an attempt to control

the anxiety generated by heavy alcohol abuse or in the mistaken belief that control by other pharmacologic agents will stop the alcohol abuse.

The most important aspect of medical treatment is to suspect alcoholism early. Particular care should be taken to make the diagnosis when only minor criteria are present, since early recognition results in a much better prognosis. Problem drinking with its attendant symptoms precedes the addiction phase.

Alcoholism should be suspected if alcohol is used to alleviate gastrointestinal pain and in any instance of a gastrointestinal problem, particularly upper or lower gastrointestinal bleeding. In the early phases, sleep is fragmented, with 2–3 hours of sleep, agitation, more alcohol ingestion, and then several more hours of sleep. Physical signs are not present with the exception of an occasional fine eye or hand tremor and suprapatellar hyperreflexia. Alcoholism tends to go unnoticed in its early stages. Suggestive clues are the "green tongue" syndrome from the use of chlorophyll compounds and the so-called chipmunk jaw—facial fullness peculiar to female alcoholics but rarely seen in men. Flushed facies in the male and palmar erythema in the female are early signs. Cigarette burns from falling asleep with lit cigarettes are common.

The form in which alcohol is taken is irrelevant. The person who drinks too much beer is just as much of a problem as the person who drinks hard liquor. Of the alleged 6–10 million alcoholics in the USA, less than 10% are on "skid row," and no economic, social, or ethnic group is immune. The vast majority are working males (about 3:1 male:female incidence), deny the problem, and often don't really believe it is a problem. Usually the spouse, though reluctant to discuss it, is aware of the problem and is deeply concerned. In the later stages, the problem becomes more evident with the emergence of the typical clinical syndromes. Furthermore, the pattern varies enormously. Some alcoholics drink large amounts daily; some are "binge" drinkers; some drink alone and clandestinely; others prefer to drink with friends, usually in local taverns where they can enjoy each other's company. The so-called "social drinker" is suspect particularly when he has a few "quick drinks" before joining friends.

Clinical Findings

A. Acute Intoxication: The signs of alcoholic intoxication are the same as those of overdosage with any other CNS depressant: drowsiness, errors of commission, disinhibition, dysarthria, ataxia, and nystagmus. In severe cases, overdosage is marked by respiratory depression, stupor, shock syndrome, coma, and death. Serious overdoses are frequently due to a combination of alcohol with other sedatives.

B. Withdrawal: There is a wide spectrum of manifestations of alcoholic withdrawal, ranging from anxiety and tremulousness to full-blown delirium tremens. The latter is an acute organic psychosis that is usually manifest within 24–72 hours after the last drink (but may occur up to 7–10 days later) and characterized by mental confusion, tremor, wakefulness, and visual hallucinations (often of snakes, bugs, etc). The acute withdrawal syndrome is often completely unexpected and occurs when the patient has been hospitalized for some unrelated problem and presents as a diagnostic problem. *Suspect alcohol withdrawal in every unexplained delirium.* Seizures occur early in the withdrawal syndrome (the first 24 hours) and are more prevalent in persons who have a history of withdrawal syndromes.

C. Alcoholic Hallucinosis: This syndrome occurs either during heavy drinking or on withdrawal and is characterized by a paranoid psychosis without the tremulousness, confusion, and clouded sensorium seen in withdrawal syndromes. The patient appears normal except for the auditory hallucinations, which are frequently persecutory and may cause the patient to behave aggressively.

D. Chronic Alcoholic Brain Syndromes: These encephalopathies are characterized by increasing erratic behavior, memory and recall problems, and emotional instability—the usual signs of organic brain syndrome due to any cause (see Organic Brain Syndrome, p 638). If confabulation is a prominent symptom, the term Korsakoff's psychosis is used. When eye signs are prominent (oculomotor palsy to ophthalmoplegia) along with the confusional state, the term Wernicke's syndrome is used. The mental symptoms always precede neurologic signs but frequently go unnoticed. Peripheral neuritis occurs in over 50% of these patients, and cerebellar signs occur frequently in the late stages. Some evidence correlates low magnesium levels and the incidence of alcoholic encephalopathies and "alcohol dementia."

Differential Diagnosis

The differential diagnosis of problem drinking is essentially between primary alcoholism (when no other major psychiatric diagnosis exists) and secondary alcoholism, when alcohol is used as self-medication for major underlying psychiatric problems such as schizophrenia or depression. The differentiation is important since the latter group requires treatment for the specific psychiatric problem.

The differential diagnosis of alcoholic withdrawal consists of the possible use of other CNS depressants but is not of serious import since treatment is the same in all cases. Acute alcoholic hallucinosis must be differentiated from other acute paranoid states such as amphetamine psychosis or acute paranoid schizophrenia. An accurate history is the most important differentiating factor. The history is also the most important feature in differentiating chronic organic brain syndromes due to alcohol from other etiologic agents. The form of the brain syndrome is of little help, eg, chronic brain syndromes from lupus erythematosus may be associated with confabulation similar to that resulting from long-standing alcoholism.

Complications

The medical and psychosocial problems of alcoholism are staggering. The central and peripheral nervous system complications include chronic brain syndromes, cerebellar degeneration, and peripheral neuropathies. The effects on the liver not only result in cirrhosis with its direct complications such as liver failure and esophageal varicosities but also in the systemic effects of altered metabolism, protein abnormalities, and coagulation defects.

The loss to industry resulting from alcoholism is particularly disruptive because it mainly affects people 35–55 years old, ie, those who are in the most productive period of their working lives and also the most critical time in family life.

In one large series, 52% of alcoholics were shown to have at least one alcoholic parent. The personal pain caused by alcoholism is reflected in the increased incidence of depression and the increased suicide rates among alcoholics.

Treatment of Problem Drinking

A. Psychologic Treatment: The most important consideration for the physician is to take a nonjudgmental attitude, though this does not mean a passive one. The physician who only sits and listens is actually reinforcing the patient's belief that he is being rejected. There must be an active, nonauthoritarian interest in the problem, with emphasis on the things that can be done. This approach emphasizes the fact that the physician cares and strikes a positive and hopeful note early in treatment.

It is often easier to get information if one phrases the question so that the patient can be more objective, eg, ask the patient what his spouse would say about the drinking pattern if he or she were sitting there. The honesty of the response is often amazing, as if the patient is talking about 2 different people.

Be judicious and tactful. Discuss the problem and allow the patient to come to the point where he discusses the problem of alcoholism. This may take several visits.

Valuable time should not be wasted trying to find out why the patient drinks; come to grips early with the immediate problem of *how to stop the drinking.* This often means early involvement of the spouse and elucidation of specific ways in which he or she can be helpful in stopping the drinking. In fact, if there is a spouse or family, the prognosis is much better, and working with both of the marriage partners—alone or together—should be started immediately.

There is no use going over the past—nothing ever comes of it and the effect simply reinforces the frustration that the patient already feels. Consider what needs to be done immediately and proceed. The psychiatrist should be a consultant and not a dumping ground. To say to a patient, "You have a drinking problem—go see a psychiatrist" is often taken as a rejection and as another excuse to go out and get drunk. Only those patients should be referred who have a serious underlying or associated problem such as psychosis or suicidal ideation. In the case of the remaining large majority, work with them in an active and interested way, using the psychiatrist in a consultation role.

B. Social Methods of Treatment: Get the patient into Alcoholics Anonymous (AA), the spouse into Alanon, and any children aged 12–20 into Alateen. Success is usually proportionate to the utilization of AA, other social agencies, religious counseling, and other resources. The patient should be seen frequently for short periods and charged an appropriate fee. In these early visits the groundwork should be laid for involvement of the family and initiation of the patient and his family into organizations specifically devoted to helping alcoholics and those near to them. The AA member who works with the patient will be a valuable resource for other kinds of support. The biggest obstacle to this early referral is the physician's feeling that the treatment of alcoholism is a hopeless prospect; this makes him reluctant to take the time necessary to arrange the initial contacts.

Do not underestimate the importance of religion, particularly since the alcoholic is often a dependent person who needs a great deal of support. Early enlistment of the help of a concerned clergyman can often provide the turning point for a personal conversion to sobriety.

One of the most important considerations is the job problem; it is usually lost or in jeopardy. In the latter case, some specific recommendations to employers can be offered: (1) Avoid placement in jobs where the alcoholic must be on his own, eg, traveling salesman. (2) Avoid situations where other people depend on the alcoholic worker's performing a job at a specific time. (3) Do not allow the worker to be in constant contact with the public. (4) Use supervision but not surveillance. (5) Keep competition with others to a minimum. (6) Avoid positions which require quick decision-making on important matters.

C. Medical Treatment: Hospitalization is not usually necessary or even desirable at this stage, which is not an acute one. It is sometimes used to dramatize a situation and force the patient to face the problem of alcoholism, but generally it should be used only on medical indications.

When alcohol is being used as self-medication, it is appropriate for a time to change to a more useful medication, eg, a major tranquilizer when there is evidence of an incipient psychosis or a sedative such as clorazepate, 15 mg orally 2–4 times a day, when anxiety is severe.

Because of the many medical complications of alcohol, a complete physical examination with appropriate laboratory tests is mandatory, with special attention to the liver and nervous system.

The medical deterrent drug disulfiram can be of critical importance in helping the alcoholic to make the essential decision that he must *stop drinking*. There should be nothing surreptitious about the use of disulfiram (no slipping the drug into the coffee by the spouse, etc). It should be discussed with the patient with full disclosure of its side-effects, mode of action, and dangers (organic brain syndrome is an infrequent complication). There is no need to put the patient through the discomfort of a trial reaction. The other members of the family should be involved in the discussion and the decision; when possible, it is better to enlist the aid of someone close to the alcoholic who is willing to share his responsibility for taking the medication every day. While this is a source of controversy, the results are much better if the spouse is totally committed to the effort and will make sure the alcoholic gets the drug every day. The initial dosage schedule of disulfiram (after a minimum of 12 hours' abstention from alcohol) is 500 mg/day in a single dose in the morning. This can be decreased to a maintenance dose of 250 mg/day, continued indefinitely. A disulfiram regimen need not interfere with other treatment approaches such as AA.

D. Behavioral Treatment: Conditioning approaches have been used in many settings in the treatment of alcoholism, most commonly as a type of aversion therapy. For example, the patient is given a drink of whisky and then a shot of apomorphine, and proceeds to vomit. In this way a strong association is built up between the vomiting and the drinking. Although this kind of treatment has been successful in some cases, many people do not retain the learned aversive response.

Group behavioral treatment of alcoholism has only been done in experimental settings but demonstrates a leveling-off of drinking while the patients are in the controlled setting. There is no evidence that the gains are sustained outside of the experimental setting.

Simple behavioral responses by significant people around the alcoholic would be of major help if one could teach them the absurdity of many of the "well-meaning" or "nonthinking" responses. Such responses are guaranteed to result in more drinking, eg, sympathy or abuse (both are forms of desired attention by the alcoholic), which is usually elicited by the alcoholic's behavior and psychologically reinforces the guilt and anger, thus producing more drinking. Astute physicians have noted for many years that some families need to have a member who is "sick," inadequate, or a scapegoat, so that a wide variety of family problems can be associated to "father's drinking problem." This helps the family to avoid dealing with problems and also produces in them a sense of helpfulness and adequacy. This in turn is a reinforcement for them to continue to focus on the alcoholic, and the cycle continues.

Treatment of Withdrawal & Hallucinosis

A. Medical Treatment: Alcoholic hallucinosis, which can occur either during or on cessation of a prolonged drinking period, is not a typical withdrawal syndrome and is handled differently. Since the symptoms are primarily those of a psychosis in the presence of a clear sensorium, they are handled like any other psychosis: hospitalization (in most cases) and adequate amounts of a major tranquilizer. Haloperidol, 5 mg orally twice a day for the first day or so, usually ameliorates symptoms quickly, and the drug can be decreased and discontinued over several days as the patient improves. It then becomes necessary to deal with the chronic alcohol abuse, which has been discussed.

Withdrawal symptoms, ranging from a mild syndrome to the severe state usually called delirium tremens, is a medical problem with a morbidity and mortality rate. The patient should be hospitalized and given adequate CNS depressants to counteract the CNS excitability resulting from the sudden cessation of alcohol. Antipsychotic drugs such as chlorpromazine should *not* be used. The choice of the specific depressant is less important than using adequate amounts to bring the patient to a level of moderate sedation, and this will vary from person to person. A common regimen is to use diazepam, 10 mg IV initially and then 5 mg IV every 5 minutes until the patient is calm. Then give the drug orally in a dosage of 5–10 mg every 1–4 hours depending on the clinical need. After stabilization, the required amount of diazepam to maintain a sedated state may be given orally every 8–12 hours. If restlessness, tremulousness, and other signs of withdrawal persist, the dosage is increased until moderate sedation occurs. The dosage is then gradually reduced until withdrawal is complete. This usually requires a week or so of treatment.

Meticulous examination for other medical problems is necessary. Alcoholics commonly have liver disease and associated clotting problems and are also prone to injury—and the combination all too frequently leads to undiagnosed subdural hematoma.

Anticonvulsant drugs are not needed except in the case of a history of seizures, which is customarily treated as a precautionary measure, although there is no clear evidence that this is necessary if adequate doses of sedatives are given. In these situations, diphenylhydantoin can be given in a loading dose—500 mg orally and, several hours later, another 500 mg orally (ie, 1 gm over 4–6 hours). This drug is then continued in a dosage of 300 mg daily.

A general diet should be given, and vitamins in high doses: thiamine, 100 mg 3 times a day; pyridoxine, 100 mg/day; folic acid, 5 mg 3 times a day; and ascorbic acid, 100 mg twice a day. Intravenous glucose solutions should not be given prior to the vitamins. Concurrent administration is satisfactory, and hydration should be meticulously assessed on an ongoing basis.

Chronic brain syndromes secondary to a long history of alcohol intake are not responsive to any specific measures. Attention to the social and environmental care of this type of patient is paramount.

B. Psychologic and Behavior Technics: The comments in the section on problem drinking apply here also; these methods of treatment become the primary consideration after the successful treatment of withdrawal or alcoholic hallucinosis. Psychologic and social measures should be initiated in the hospital shortly before discharge. This increases the possibility of continued posthospitalization treatment.

Bean M: Alcoholics Anonymous: Principles and methods. Psychiat Annals 5:45, 1975.

Criteria Committee, National Council on Alcoholism: Criteria for the diagnosis of alcoholism. Ann Int Med 77:249, 1972.
Favazza AR, Martin P: Chemotherapy of delirium tremens: A survey of physicians' preferences. Am J Psychiat 131:1031, 1974.
Gerrein JR & others: Disulfiram maintenance in outpatient treatment of alcoholism. Arch Gen Psychiat 28:798, 1973.
Gottheil E & others: Alcoholics' patterns of controlled drinking. Am J Psychiat 130:418, 1973.
Overall JE: MMPI personality patterns of alcoholics and narcotic addicts. Quart J Stud Alcohol 34:104, 1973.
Rosenberg CM: Drug maintenance in the outpatient treatment of chronic alcoholism. Arch Gen Psychiat 30:373, 1974.
Sampliner R, Iber FL: Diphenylhydantoin control of alcohol withdrawal seizures. JAMA 230:1430, 1974.
Thompson WL: Diazepam and paraldehyde for treatment of severe delirium tremens: A controlled trial. Ann Int Med 82:175, 1975.

ABUSE OF PSYCHEDELICS

Essentials of Diagnosis

- This is the one class of drugs wherein the hallucinogenic effects are primary: hallucinations, delusions, euphoria, dream-like states, distortion in time, depression, panic or psychosis.
- Used mainly by 2 groups: Those that use drugs indiscriminately and those that are searching for "meaning and identity" in their lives.
- Psychologic dependence develops, but tolerance and physical dependence are not characteristic—although tolerance is seen following daily usage.

General Considerations

About 6000 species of plants are believed to have psychoactive properties. Those currently in use are methylated derivatives of phenylalanine (the precursor of norepinephrine and dopamine) and tryptophan (the precursor of serotonin). Common congeners of phenylalanine are mescaline; 4-methyl-2,5-dimethoxy-alpha-methylphenethylamine (DOM, "STP"); and myristicin. Congeners of tryptophan include lysergic acid diethylamide (LSD), psilocybin, and dimethyltryptamine (DMT).

All of these drugs produce similar behavioral and physiologic effects. They vary in milligram potency and duration of action. The behavior they produce is affected both by the set (ie, the attitude of the user) and the setting (the environment and the people present during use—major factors in compensating for the disintegration of ego boundaries). "Bad trips" are often related to these factors rather than to the particular drug or dosage used. There is no evidence that these drugs have any therapeutic usefulness.

Clinical Findings

A. Acute Intoxication: Sympathomimetic effects are prominent and include mydriasis, tachycardia, hyperreflexia, and increased blood pressure (10—20 minutes). An initial feeling of tension is followed by emotional release such as crying or laughing (1—2 hours). Later, perceptual distortions occur, with visual illusions and hallucinations and a fear of ego disintegration (2—3 hours). Major changes in time sense and overflow and distortion of all perceptions, with mood lability, then occur (3—4 hours). There is a feeling of detachment and a sense of destiny and control (4—6 hours). Occasionally, the acute episode does not remit, and there is a prolonged disintegration of ego function.

B. Chronic Use: Chronic use of these drugs results in memory problems, motivational deficits ("dropping out"), marked passivity, avoidance of competition, and finally gradually decreased use of the drug.

Differential Diagnosis

Amphetamine psychoses, acute schizophrenic episodes, and psychotic organic syndromes all have similarities, but the psychedelic experience is almost unique. A history of ingestion, the relatively clear sensorium, and the obvious organic perceptual changes make the diagnosis. Since there are so many contaminants or substitutes in "street drugs," one is never sure what was taken and the clinical picture may be mixed, usually toward that of a psychotic organic brain syndrome. Phencyclidine ("angel dust," PCP, Sernyl) is a common street drug or component of street drugs. The patient often presents with florid schizophrenic-like symptomatology, usually violently paranoid, delusional, hallucinating, and disoriented. These patients often are misdiagnosed schizophrenics. Recovery often takes a week or so even with high doses of antipsychotics, and reconstitution takes several more days. Chronic schizophrenics may have acute reexacerbations of psychoses for up to 6—8 weeks.

Complications

Erratic behavior under the influence of the drug can lead to injury or death, eg, thinking one is able to fly and leaping from a third-story window. So-called "amotivational syndrome" is thought by some to result after long-term use. It is not known whether the long-term effects on the CNS are reversible.

The incidence of spontaneous abortions and congenital defects in offspring is definitely higher in women with a history of LSD usage. There is no clear evidence that chromosomal damage occurs.

Treatment

A. Acute Intoxication: The victim should be in a protected environment. Use friends or empathic people to "talk him down" by offering sympathetic reassurance, by allaying apprehensions, and by permitting him to ventilate his feelings. This may take several hours.

Psychotropic drugs should not be used unless the victim is intensely upset and out of control since one never really knows what the patient has been taking.

Phenothiazines such as chlorpromazine are effective, but if there are anticholinergic contaminants in the abused drug the side-effects can be dangerous. In serious cases, haloperidol, 5 mg intramuscularly will usually be adequate to achieve control. Then use oral doses of 2 mg every 12 hours. In mild to moderate cases, use a sedative (minor tranquilizer) such as diazepam, 40 mg daily, decreasing the dosage gradually over a period of 1—2 weeks.

B. Chronic Intoxication:

1. Psychologic—Psychologic methods can be effective in patients whose use of psychedelics has been an attempt to gain insight and "understand" themselves. Individual psychotherapy is oriented toward establishing self-identity, gaining insight, crystallizing life goals, and improving interpersonal relationships and growth to deal with life exigencies. Either eclectic or psychoanalytically oriented therapies are appropriate. When identity and interpersonal problems are paramount, individual group therapy provides an arena for the patient to explore the problems, validate conceptions, compare ideas, and receive opinions.

2. Social—Social approaches include counseling for the family, who are often bewildered and afraid; for the drug user whose behavior is erratic; and for the employer, who is annoyed. The self-help communities that provide full-time living facilities and a milieu environment, such as Synanon, can have a positive impact on changing behavior. Substitute homes and treatment centers—including crash pads—are helpful in patients who require environmental change for varying periods of time. Their connections with social agencies facilitate the patient's reintegration into the community, including work, a living situation, and further schooling.

3. Behavioral—Behavioral technics are frequently a part of the social milieus and are effective within those social structures.

4. Medical—Medical treatment is limited to small amounts of major tranquilizers (eg, trifluoperazine, 2—5 mg daily orally) when "flashbacks" occur. (A "flashback" is mental imagery which occurred during the "trip" and recurs later, often triggered by milder drugs such as alcohol or marijuana.) Phencyclidine psychoses will require larger amounts of antipsychotic medication.

Prognosis

The prognosis in acute intoxication is good if the patient is prevented from harming himself or others. In chronic intoxication, the prognosis is guarded depending upon the premorbid personality. The "experimenters" cease using these drugs. Hard-core drug users have a poor prognosis.

Hart JB: Composition of illicit drugs and the use of drug analysis in abuse abatement. J Psychedelic Drugs 5:83, 1972.

Jacobson CB, Berlin CM: Possible reproductive detriment in LSD users. JAMA 222:1367, 1972.

Klepfisz A, Racy J: Homicide and LSD. JAMA 223:429, 1973.

McGlothlin WH, Arnold DO: LSD revisited. Arch Gen Psychiat 24:35, 1971.

Rainey JM, Crowder MK: Prevalence of phencyclidine in street drug preparations. New England J Med 290:466, 1974.

Silverman J: Research with psychedelics. Arch Gen Psychiat 25:498, 1971.

MARIJUANA ABUSE

Essentials of Diagnosis

- Altered time perception, defective memory.
- Usually used in a social setting.
- Psychologic dependence but no tolerance or physical dependence.

General Considerations

Cannabis sativa, a hemp plant, is the source of marijuana, a term used to denote any part of the plant or extract that induces somatic or psychic changes when smoked or ingested. The parts of the plant vary in potency. The resinous exudate of the flowering tops of the female plant (hashish, charas) is most potent, followed by the dried leaves and flowering shoots of the female plant (bhang) and the resinous mass from small leaves of inflorescence (ganja). The least potent parts are the lower branches and the leaves of the female plant and all parts of the male plant.

The active ingredient is tetrahydrocannabinol (THC), which is currently being used in studies to standardize the effects of marijuana, which varies in potency depending on the above constituents and the source of the cannabis plant.

The drug is most potent when inhaled, and it usually takes one or 2 cigarettes to produce the desired "high." Ingestion is much less common. Effects occur in 10–20 minutes after smoking and last 2–3 hours. Cigarettes of good quality contain about 500 mg of marijuana (about 5 mg of THC). As in the case of psychedelics, the "set" and "setting" in which marijuana is used are important factors in drug response. The diverse actions of the drug make pharmacologic classification difficult.

Clinical Findings

With moderate dosage, marijuana produces 2 phases: a mild euphoria followed by sleepiness. In acute marijuana intoxication, the user has an altered time perception, conjunctival injection, loosened emotions, and impaired immediate memory. Psychotomimetic effects occur with high doses. The effects of chronic use have not yet been determined.

Complications

No deaths have been reported, and the studies on long-term physical and mental complications have questionable scientific validity.

Treatment

A. Social: Social and cultural attitudes really determine whether treatment is needed. This is cur-

rently in doubt. "Talking down" is usually all that is necessary in the rare case of hallucinosis associated with marijuana use.

B. Medical: Major tranquilizers may be necessary for the unusual case of high-dosage marijuana intoxication. Sedatives are used for the infrequent acute anxiety reaction that may occur.

C. Psychologic: Psychologic methods of treatment are important only in persons who need to reconcile the use of marijuana with themselves or their families. Some short-term eclectic individual psychotherapy can be helpful in the former and family therapy in the latter.

D. Behavioral: Behavioral technics have no specific role—with the exception of modeling, which can play a part in decision-making about using the drug.

Prognosis

The prognosis is excellent for all but the indiscriminate user, who often combines marijuana with other drugs in chronic usage.

Brill NQ, Christie RL: Marijuana use and psychosocial adaptation. Arch Gen Psychiat 31:713, 1974.

Galanter M & others: Marijuana and social behavior. Arch Gen Psychiat 30:518, 1974.

Hockman JS, Brill NQ: Chronic marijuana use and psycho-social adaptation. Am J Psychiat 130:132, 1973.

Kiplinger GF: Dose-response analysis of the effects of tetrahydrocannabinol in man. Clin Pharmacol Therap 12:650, 1971.

Klonoff H: Marijuana and driving in real life situations. Science 186:317, 1974.

Kupfer DJ & others: A comment on the "amotivational syndrome" in marijuana smokers. Am J Psychiat 130:1319, 1973.

Lieberman CM, Leiberman BW: Marijuana: A medical review. New England J Med 284:88, 1971.

ABUSE OF STIMULANTS

Essentials of Diagnosis

- Stimulants are often associated with antisocial behavior.
- They are often abused in conjunction with other drugs.
- Psychologic dependence and tolerance are high, but there is minimal physical dependence.
- Increased levels of activity, with hyperalertness, insomnia, and anorexia.

General Considerations

The amphetamines ("uppers"–Benzedrine; "speed"–Methedrine) and cocaine are widely abused stimulants. Amphetamines, because of their lower cost, are much more commonly used than cocaine. In 1972, forty companies were marketing amphetamines and amphetamine-like drugs. Abuse unfortunately may start after the drugs have been prescribed as anorexiants in the treatment of obesity, a condition which this group does not significantly alleviate. It is not uncommon to see patients who are taking up to 500 mg (and even 2 gm) of oral amphetamine per day. The intravenous use of methamphetamine in large doses is particularly bad because it magnifies the acute problems, particularly the development of acute disruptive psychosis. Many former speed users revert to intravenous heroin. Other commonly abused stimulants include methylphenidate and phenmetrazine. The FDA is undertaking to control production and distribution of all these drugs, which have little therapeutic use except in treating hyperkinetic children and in proved narcolepsy.

Cocaine is used by sniffing as a "spree" drug. Usage is limited by its high cost and unavailability. It is occasionally administered intravenously but its duration of action, unlike that of speed, is relatively brief.

Clinical Findings

A. Moderate Usage: Moderate exposure results in hyperactivity, stereotyped repetitious behavior, a sense of enhanced physical and mental capacity, a decreased need for sleep, poor appetite, sympathomimetic effects, and possible sexual stimulation and delayed orgasm.

B. High Doses: Chronic high dosages of stimulants can cause suspiciousness and paranoid ideation, bruxism, picking of the face and extremities, preoccupation with one's own thought processes and impaired impulse control, and, later, full-blown paranoid psychosis with clear sensorium.

C. Overdoses: These are most common in neophyte drug users or accidental ingestions. Symptoms include dizziness, tremor, panic, headache, hallucinations, abdominal cramps, and vomiting. Very high doses produce hyperthermia, convulsions, systemic acidosis, and cardiovascular collapse.

D. Withdrawal Symptoms: Withdrawal from stimulants results in prolonged sleep, lassitude, hyperphagia, and some degree of depression lasting several days to several weeks.

Differential Diagnosis

Acute and chronic stimulant abuse cannot be distinguished from paranoid schizophrenia.

Complications

Acute intoxication may result in loss of impulse control, such as antisocial acts or impaired judgment, and acute paranoid psychosis. Problems occur in association with intravenous use, including infections and traumatic complications.

Chronic usage may produce psychotic manifestations with associated behavioral difficulties such as homicide and suicide.

Treatment

A. Medical: Medical hospitalization is necessary when the patient is psychotic or a threat to himself or others. Since there is no physiologic dependence, it is not necessary to gradually decrease the dosage of stimulant; it can be discontinued on admission. The psychosis will gradually resolve, but the process can be helped with the administration of major tranquilizers (eg, chlorpromazine, 50 mg orally) every 4–6 hours until there is less agitation, some sedation, and improved thought processes, the latter usually requiring several days. The major tranquilizers are seldom needed after the first several days. There is frequently a period of depression several days after the patient has "crashed" (come down from the high produced by the stimulants), and the physician must evaluate any suicidal ideation. As in the case of narcotics and any other drug abused by the parenteral route, there should be careful examination for complications such as infectious hepatitis and pulmonary problems. Treatment of severe overdoses begins with control of the hyperthermia by cold packs or ice; diazepam intravenously for the convulsions; and intubation if respiratory functions are impeded.

B. Social: Social assistance is important in all drug abuse problems, but particularly in the stimulant abuser, who frequently has marginal self-control and often desperately needs a structured environment and restraint. Every effort should be made to achieve placement in a self-help community, foster home, or residential treatment center. The ongoing milieu and counseling are usually much more effective than the more formal psychologic treatment. Family counseling is frequently necessary to help the family accept the problem, alleviate their guilt about it, and assist them in encouraging the patient to accept residential treatment. Work and school counseling are also usually necessary.

C. Psychologic: Psychologic methods have been infrequently successful. Group therapy is more successfully used within a milieu or residential setting.

D. Behavioral: Behavioral treatment also is more effective when used within a self-help community or setting which can provide ongoing peer pressure. The contingencies can be controlled, and fellow drug abusers are wise to the "games" of drug use, thus providing direct and effective responses to their fellow users.

Prognosis

Acute situations resolve when the patient is protected from harm, and the acute psychosis resolves with cessation of amphetamine use. Long-term abuse has a more guarded prognosis, although the Scandinavians report that amphetamine usage is self-limiting. The prognosis is poor (or treatment discouraging) in patients who use the intravenous route to take methamphetamine or when there is multiple indiscriminate drug abuse.

Anderson WH & others: Failure of outpatient treatment of drug abuse. 2. Amphetamines, barbiturates, hallucinogens. Am J Psychiat 128:1572, 1972.

Angrist B & others: The antagonism of amphetamine induced

symptomatology by a neuroleptic. Am J Psychiat 131:817, 1974.

Edison GR: Amphetamines: A dangerous illusion. Ann Int Med 74:605, 1971.

Ellinwood EH & others: Evolving behavior in the clinical and experimental amphetamine (model) psychosis. Am J Psychiat 130:1088, 1973.

Greaves G: Sexual disturbance among chronic amphetamine users. J Nerv Ment Dis 155:363, 1972.

Raskind M, Bradford T: Methylphenidate (Ritalin) abuse and methadone maintenance. Dis Nerv System 36:9, 1975.

OVER-THE-COUNTER (OTC) DRUGS

General Considerations

There are 3 principal groups of abused proprietary drugs: (1) atropine-like drugs in combination with sedative and antihistaminic drugs—particularly the common sleeping preparations such as Sominex and Sleepeze—are the most frequently abused drugs that come to the attention of physicians. There are over 600 pharmaceutical preparations containing anticholinergic drugs (in addition to "street drugs" with anticholinergic activity). This is partly because of the tendency of people to take sleeping preparations to relieve anxiety and make suicide attempts. Other sources of this group are jimson weed (the brew is common in prison farms) and the anticholinergic components of various long-acting cold capsules. (2) Bromides are present in Miles Nervine in high concentration and to a lesser degree in Neurosine. (3) Other abused agents such as salicylates, cough syrups such as elixir of terpin hydrate, throat disks containing chloroform, aerosols, airplane glue, and various solvents.

Clinical Findings

In most cases that come to medical attention, a drug-induced organic brain syndrome is present to some degree. This is particularly true of the atropine derivates and bromides. Other findings will relate to the ingested drug.

Treatment

A. Medical: The need for medical treatment depends on the substance abused. Hospitalization is often necessary for evaluation, observation, protection, and specific treatment (eg, administration of chlorides to replace bromides). Physostigmine, 1—2 mg IM and repeated in 30-minute intervals, if necessary, can be helpful in reversing the effects of anticholinergic drugs. Avoid the use of antipsychotics with anticholinergic properties such as thioridazine in the organic brain syndrome. Time and the judicious use of sedatives are adequate. Possible complications (eg, liver or kidney damage with airplane glue or solvents) require careful evaluation. The physician-patient relationship is probably the most important area, since abuse of over-the-counter drugs is frequently a function of patient disappointment in the physician for failing to provide relief. (See Psychophysiologic Disorders, above.) Ignorance is sometimes a factor, and the patient needs clear instructions about what is harmful.

B. Psychologic: Psychologic approaches are directed to any underlying psychiatric or adjustment problems that may be contributing to this type of drug abuse, which often occurs in older people (with the exception of glue-sniffing). Depression is often present and has gone unrecognized and untreated. Families and spouses should be included in the family or couple therapy both to ameliorate underlying problems and to assist the patient in decreasing the drug usage. Crisis therapy is helpful in acute situations and should include other people significant to the patient's problem.

C. Social: Social agencies such as geriatric clubs, recreational groups, and nonresidential self-help groups may provide valuable services since these patients tend to be older, more isolated, and more in need of social supports. Crisis centers are more appropriate for younger patients. In keeping with the idea that drugs are "people substitutes," the older person frequently becomes isolated as a result of death and moving away of friends and associates as well as increasing financial limitations. Welfare departments and church organizations can be helpful in providing financial assistance and social companionship.

El-Yousef MK & others: Reversal of anti-Parkinsonian drug toxicity by physostigmine: A controlled study. Am J Psychiat 130:141, 1973.

Hill JB: Salicylate intoxication. New England J Med 288:1110, 1973.

Ullman KC, Groh RH: Identification and treatment of acute psychotic states secondary to the usage of over the counter sleeping preparations. Am J Psychiat 128:1244, 1972.

•   •   •

ORGANIC BRAIN SYNDROME (OBS)

Essentials of Diagnosis

- Cognitive impairment: disorientation, defective sensation and perception, impairment of capacity for recall and recent memory, impaired thinking and logical reasoning.
- Affective impairment: temperament, mood, emotion.
- Conative impairment: initiative, drive, insight (all introspections).
- History or findings to indicate one or more of the etiologic factors listed below.

General Considerations

Terms that have been used as equivalent to organic brain syndrome include delirium, confusional states, and clouded consciousness. There may or may not be associated psychosis wherein the cognitive impairment proceeds to disordered thinking with delusions and hallucinations, the latter usually being the visual type. All brain syndromes should be considered acute (ie, reversible) until proved otherwise by time; then they are called chronic (ie, irreversible).

Etiology & Classification

There is no relationship between the causes and the manifestations of organic brain syndrome. For example, the OBS of systemic lupus erythematosus can be similar to that from chronic alcohol abuse. When there is evidence of psychotic ideation such as delusions and hallucinations in addition to the essentials of diagnosis, the syndrome is then called **psychotic organic brain syndrome.** When sleeplessness and restlessness are included, the term **delirium** is often used. Thus, a mild organic brain syndrome is often considered to be a mild confusional state, and, at the other end of the spectrum, when psychotic ideation and hyperactivity are included, the term psychotic OBS or delirium is used.

A. Intoxications: Alcohol, barbiturates, other sedatives, bromides, anticholinergic drugs, tranquilizers, antidepressants, pollutants, solvents, a wide variety of over-the-counter and prescribed drugs, and household agricultural and industrial chemicals. (For endogenous metabolic intoxications, see below.)

B. Drug Withdrawal: Alcohol, sedative-hypnotics, and minor tranquilizers.

C. Infections: Acute and chronic infections due to the entire range of microbiologic pathogens.

D. Metabolic Disturbances: Fluid and electrolyte, acid-base, hepatic, kidney, endocrine, pulmonary, other less common problems.

E. Trauma: Subdural hematoma, subarachnoid hemorrhage, intracerebral bleeding, concussion syndrome.

F. Cardiovascular Disorders: Cardiac abnormalities, cerebrovascular spasms and occlusions.

G. Neoplasms: Primary or metastatic lesions of the CNS.

H. Idiopathic Epilepsy: Grand mal and postictal, temporal lobe dysfunction.

I. Collagen and Immunologic Disorders: Lupus erythematosus, immunologic reaction to exogenous substances.

J. Degenerative Diseases: Alzheimer's disease, Pick's disease, multiple sclerosis, parkinsonism.

Clinical Findings

The manifestations are many and varied and include problems with orientation, short or fluctuating attention span, loss of recent memory and recall, impaired judgment, emotional lability, lack of initiative, inability to reason through problems, depression (worse in mild to moderate types), confabulation (not limited to alcohol organic brain syndrome), constriction of intellectual functions, visual hallucinations, and delusions. Physical findings will naturally vary according to the cause. The EEG is often abnormal.

Differential Diagnosis

Patients with nonorganic ("functional") psychoses often remain oriented; the onset is usually gradual; hallucinations are usually auditory rather than visual; and intellectual functions are intact, with good memory and normal EEG.

Patients with nonorganic depressions may be withdrawn and relatively noncommunicative but have intact cognitive functions.

Complications

Chronicity is sometimes a function of early reversal, eg, subdural hematoma, low pressure hydrocephalus. Prompt correction of reversible causes improves recovery of mental function.

Treatment

A. Medical: Provide a pleasant, comfortable, nonthreatening, and physically safe environment with adequate nursing or attendant services. Correct underlying medical problems. Do not overlook any possibility of reversible organic disease. Give major tranquilizers in small doses at first (eg, thioridazine, 25 mg orally at bedtime) and increase according to the need to reduce psychotic ideation or excessive irritability. Bedtime administration obviates the need for sedatives and minor tranquilizers, which often worsen organic brain syndrome.

Failing sensory functions should be supported as necessary with hearing aids, cataract surgery, etc.

B. Social: Substitute home care, board care, or convalescent home care may be most useful when the family is unable to care for the patient. The setting should include familiar people, objects, lights at night, and a simple schedule. Family counseling may help the family to cope and keep the patient at home as long as possible. Volunteer services, including homemakers, visiting nurse, and adult protective services may be required if the patient is left at home.

C. Behavioral: Behavioral technics include operant responses which can be used to induce positive behaviors, eg, paying attention to the patient when he is trying to communicate appropriately, and extinction by ignoring inappropriate responses.

D. Psychologic: Psychologic therapies are not helpful and may make things worse by taxing his limited cognitive resources.

Prognosis

The prognosis is good in acute (reversible) cases; fair in moderate cases; and poor in deteriorated states.

Morse RM, Litin EM: The anatomy of a delirium. Am J Psychiat 128:111, 1971.

Lipowski AJ: Delirium, clouding of consciousness and confusion. J Nerv Ment Dis 145:227, 1967.

GERIATRIC DISORDERS

Essentials of Diagnosis

- Older patients.
- Some degree of organic brain syndrome often present.
- Depression, paranoid ideation, and easy irritability are common.
- High frequency of medical problems.
- Patient is frequently worsened by a wide variety of medications.
- Fear of death is often a major factor.

General Considerations

There are 3 basic factors in the process of aging: biologic, sociologic, and psychologic.

The complex biologic changes depend on inherited characteristics (the best guarantee of long life is to have long-lived parents), nutrition, declining sensory functions such as hearing or vision, disease, trauma, and life style. As a person ages, the CNS becomes less hardy, and relatively minor disorders or combinations of disorders may cause deficits in cognition and affective response. A definite correlation between hearing loss and paranoid ideation exists in the elderly. (See Organic Brain Syndrome, p 638.)

The sociologic factors derive from stresses connected with occupation, family, and community. Any or all of these areas may be disrupted in a general phenomenon of "disengagement" which older people experience as friends die, the children move away, and the surroundings become less familiar. Retirement commonly precipitates a major disruption in a well-established life structure. This is particularly stressful in the person whose compulsive devotion to his job has precluded other interests, so that sudden loss of this outlet leaves a void that is not easily filled.

The psychologic withdrawal of the elderly person is independent of the cultural rejection (the USA tends to be a youth-oriented society). It is frequently related to a loss of self-esteem, which is based on the economic insecurity of older age with its congruent loss of independence, the realization of decreasing physical and mental ability, and the fear of approaching death. One cannot feel very secure with increasing illnesses, decreased earning capacity, and the realization that one must inevitably become more and more dependent on unknown factors. The process of aging is often poorly accepted, and the real or imagined loss of physical attractiveness may have a traumatic impact which the plastic surgeon can only soften for a time. In a culture that stresses physical and sexual attractiveness, it is difficult for most people to accept the change. The real crux of the aging problem is that it requires an awareness of the eventuality of death with appropriate reorganization of one's own life.

Complications

A major complication is often the treatment of a symptom instead of the basic problem, eg, depression is frequently not appreciated as being secondary to organic brain syndrome. Active psychotropic treatment of the depression does not alter the basic problem and may, particularly when antidepressants are used, exacerbate it.

Transient psychoses associated with organic brain syndrome are frequently exacerbated by removing the patient from the environment which has been a strong supportive factor. The older patient has great need for familiar objects and people, and dislocation frequently accelerates a downhill course.

Older persons have greater difficulty in metabolizing drugs. Selection of drug and dosage are important, as well as alertness to untoward drug interactions. Antihistamines are commonly used as soporifics for older persons, and the accompanying drowsiness and ataxia can lead to falls with further complications. Of course, the usual dangers of drug interactions (eg, guanethidine and tricyclics or phenothiazines) and the effects of drugs on the liver with further metabolic derangement must be considered (eg, phenobarbital and its effect on liver enzymes, which increases the catabolism of other drugs). Drug excretion can change in older people, who frequently have liver or kidney dysfunction, and the paradoxic effects of some drugs (eg, barbiturates) are well known. As in the younger patient, the greatest danger probably lies in the use of multiple drugs, and it is not uncommon to see an elderly patient receiving 10 or more medications.

Treatment

A. Social: Socialization, a structured schedule of activities, familiar surroundings, continued achievement, and avoidance of loneliness (probably the most important factor) are some of the major considerations in prevention and amelioration of the psychiatric problems of older age. Isolation must be avoided. Whenever possible, the patient should remain in a familiar setting or return to one for as long as possible. An inexorable downhill trend frequently follows dislocation, with the accompanying disengagement from adaptive activities. The patient can be supported in the primary environment by various agencies which can help avoid a premature change of habits. For patients with disabilities that make it difficult to cope with the problems of living alone, homemaker services can assist in continuing the day-to-day activities of the household; visiting nurses can administer medications and monitor the physical condition of the patient; and geriatric social groups can help maintain socialization and human contacts. In the hospital, attention to the kinds of people placed in the same room is most important. All too often, the 4-bed ward is peopled by 4 withdrawn, nonfunctioning people who provide no stimulation for each other, and the resultant isolation increases the degree of depression; occasionally, a florid psychosis develops. Attention to the proper mixture of active and inactive people can help relieve the loneliness that so often pervades such wards.

B. Medical: Treatment of any reversible components of an organic brain syndrome is obviously the major medical consideration. One commonly over-looked factor is self-medication, frequently with over-the-counter drugs that further impair the patient's al-ready precarious functioning. Careful questioning is necessary to elicit this because of the patient's embarrassment about using a drug not prescribed by a physician. Frequent culprits are bromides and anticholinergic sleeping preparations. Older people tend to have less overall sleep and will respond to careful explanation that this is normal for the age group. Sleep changes and bowel habits require a great deal of attention from the physician since people tend to medicate themselves excessively in response to changes in these physiologic functions. Altered sensory functions, eg, increasing deafness, should be corrected when possible.

Any signs of psychosis, such as paranoid ideation and delusions, respond very well to small amounts of major tranquilizers. Trifluoperazine, 2 mg orally once a day, or fluphenazine, 1–2 mg orally daily, will usually decrease psychotic ideation markedly. If there is associated agitation, haloperidol, 2 mg orally daily, is effective; the dose may be increased as necessary to control symptoms.

For patients who are not psychotic but are excessively irritable and have some loss of impulse control, thioridazine, 50 mg orally at bedtime, helps the patient to sleep and often lasts through the next day. The dosage can be adjusted upward as needed and given in 2 doses: a larger bedtime dose and a smaller morning dose. Since the sedating phenothiazines have more side-effects of the anticholinergic and alpha-adrenergic blocking types, the initial dose should be low and slowly adjusted upward. An alternative drug for this group of patients is haloperidol, 2 mg orally at bedtime and 2 mg in the morning, with dosage adjustments as needed.

The astute use of the major tranquilizers can often maintain the older person in the home environment and delay the traumatic dislocation which usually worsens the patient's condition. Antidepressants and minor tranquilizer-sedatives frequently have a worsening effect and should generally be avoided. The appropriate use of wine and beer is quite rewarding in the hospital and other care facilities as well as at home.

C. Behavioral: The impaired cognitive abilities of the geriatric patient necessitate simple behavioral technics. Positive responses to appropriate behavior encourage the patient to repeat desirable kinds of behavior, and frequent repetition offsets to some degree the defects in recent memory and recall. It also results in participation—a most important element, since there is a tendency in the older population to withdraw, thus increasing isolation and functional decline.

One must be careful not to reinforce and encourage obstreperous behavior by responding to it, thus allowing extinction or at least gradual reduction of inappropriate behavior. At the same time, the obstreperous behavior often represents a nondirective response to frustration and inability to function, and a structured program of activity is necessary (television, occupational therapy, companionship of volunteers, etc).

D. Psychologic: Formal psychologic intervention is of little use in cases of organic brain syndrome. When the problem is depression, loneliness, increasing feelings of uselessness, and a sense of being left out, and—particularly—when death or fear of it is a factor, psychotherapeutic intervention can be effective (see next section).

Assistance in helping the patient accommodate to a changing role and changing commitments can help in readjusting to new goals and viewpoints. The older person steadily loses an important commodity—the future. He often attempts to compensate for this by preoccupation with the past. Involvement with the present and psychotherapy on a "here-and-now" basis can help him to make this adjustment.

Brickner PN: The homebound aged: A medically unreached group. Ann Int Med 82:1, 1975.

Cooper AF & others: Hearing loss in paranoid and affective psychoses of the elderly. Lancet 2:851, 1974.

Goldstein S, Grant A: The psychogeriatric patient in the hospital. Canad MAJ 111:329, 1974.

Krakowski AJ, Langlais, LM: Acute psychiatric emergencies in a geriatric hospital. Psychosomatics 15:72, 1974.

Markson EW: Readjustment to time in old age. Psychiatry 36:37, 1973.

Stotsky BA: Social and clinical issues in geriatric psychiatry. Am J Psychiat 129:117, 1972.

Turner TB: Beer and wine for geriatric patients. JAMA 226:779, 1973.

DEATH & DYING

As Thomas Browne said, "The long habit of living indisposeth us for dying." While we can discuss war, talk glibly about "body counts," and see "The Godfather," it is only when death comes close to us that we really begin to respond to the possibility of our own death.

Death means different things to different people. For some it may represent an escape from unbearable suffering or other difficulties; for others, entrance into a new transcendental life. Death may come as a narcissistic attempt to find lasting fame or importance in martyrdom or heroic adventure; or it may be an atonement for real or imagined guilt or a means of extorting from others posthumously the affection that was not forthcoming during life.

Often the process is more shattering to those whose charge it is to maintain life, and there is a good deal of question about the so-called agony of death. Some observers, including Sir William Osler, take the view that there is no such thing, and the experiences of people who have been resuscitated from cardiac standstill seem to substantiate his view. They describe a sensation of detachment, a final peaceful "letting go," and one is at times impressed with the fact that the dying patient resents his attendants' interference with the process.

How each individual responds to imminent death is not only a function of what death means to that person but also the mechanisms that he uses to deal with problems—and these are usually the same as those that he used throughout life.

An ill person may at first deny that he is concerned with dying and then later admit that he is often afraid to go to sleep because he might not wake up. This is often demonstrated by a need to keep the light on and to call frequently during the night with minor complaints. Some find it necessary to deny impending death to the end. Their families and doctors will often join in the conspiracy of denial, either out of sympathy or for their own reasons. It is important not to force the patient to realize the truth but to allow him the opportunity, *when he is ready,* to discuss and deal with impending death. Frank discussion can mitigate the terror which some patients feel. For many it is a comfort to be actively involved in the process of dying, sharing in the anticipation of death, and making whatever plans may be important.

The reactions of the family are often a combination of pain, anger, sadness, and depression. They react to each other and to the personnel caring for the patient. The staff must be careful not to alienate the family, because this can result in less than optimum care. Some emotional investment in the patient by the staff is proper and inevitable, but it must be handled with insight and professional restraint. An insecure staff member may respond to a patient's death as if it were a professional failure. If the emotional investment is too little, the staff member may seem to be aloof and insensitive, while overconcern may lead to depression and despair, further impairing his capacity to serve as a source of support for the patient and his family in a time of distress.

The physician and staff must be aware of their own anxieties; maintain an appropriate level of involvement (a change of physicians may be necessary when this is impossible); allow for free and ongoing communication between patient, physician, and family; and share as a group—staff and family—the impending and unavoidable loss.

Evans JW: Roles in dying. 2. The family and staff. Psychiat Digest 34:37, 1973.
Hinton J: Talking with people about to die. Brit MJ 3:25, 1974.
Levinson P: Obstacles in the treatment of dying patients. Am J Psychiat 132:28, 1975.
Preston CE: Behavior modification: A therapeutic approach to aging and dying. Postgrad Med 54:64, 1973.
Rachels J: Active and passive euthanasia. New England J Med 292:78, 1975.
Thomas L: Notes of a biology watcher: The long habit. New England J Med 286:825, 1972.

PSYCHIATRIC PROBLEMS ASSOCIATED WITH MEDICAL & SURGICAL DISORDERS

Essentials of Diagnosis

Acute Problems:

- Psychotic organic brain syndrome secondary to the medical or surgical problem, or the effect of the environment (eg, Intensive Care Unit).
- Acute anxiety, often related to ignorance and fear of the immediate problem as well as uncertainty about the future.

Intermediate Problems:

- Depression as a function of the illness or acceptance of the illness, often associated with realistic or fantasied hopelessness about the future.
- Behavioral problems, often related to denial of illness and, in extreme cases, causing the patient to leave the hospital against medical advice.

Recuperative Problems:

- Decreasing cooperation as the patient sees improvement and is not compelled to follow orders closely.
- Readjustment problems with family, job, and society.

General Considerations

A. Short-Term Patients:

1. Postcardiotomy syndrome is usually a transient psychotic organic brain syndrome which is an expression of organic, psychologic, and environmental factors.

2. Intensive care unit psychosis is also a type of psychotic organic brain syndrome which is often related to fear, overstimulation, sleep deprivation, physical discomfort, medication problems (particularly sedatives, analgesics, and other confusional drugs), and metabolic fluctuations.

3. Cardiac care unit—The initial response is anxiety followed by denial, with behavior problems and then depression and increased dependency needs.

4. Pre- and postsurgical anxiety states—Related to ignorance of procedures and fear of surgery, anesthesia, and postsurgical loss.

5. Medical problems—Producing organic brain syndromes (see above).

6. Iatrogenic problems—Medication reactions, complications of diagnostic and treatment procedures, and impersonal and unsympathic staff attitudes.

B. Long-Term Patients: The entire spectrum of psychologic problems may present itself.

1. Tuberculosis services often report a depressive reaction due to the length of hospitalization, separation from family, economic worries, and fears of the future.

2. Orthopedic services frequently must deal with behavior problems such as those that occur when an active young man with high stimulus needs is confined

in a body cast, or relating to the premorbid personality of the patient (eg, accident proneness, drug abuse).

3. Prolonged medical and surgical problems which confine the patient cause increasing irritability and a corresponding staff reaction to the "troublesome patient," with a resultant deterioration in the patient-staff relationship. Burn patients with the acute problems of OBS, the intermediate behavior problems and the ultimate problem of accepting the loss of function and changes in body image are an example of this group. In fact the biggest problem is dealing with the loss whether it be a breast, a limb, or facial disfigurement.

4. Renal dialysis patients and transplant recipients. These patients demonstrate the whole spectrum of problems, particularly resentment at being "tied to the machine."

Clinical Findings

The symptoms that occur in these patients are similar to those discussed in previous sections of this chapter, eg, organic brain syndrome, anxiety, and depression. Behavior problems may include lack of cooperation, increased complaints, demands for medication, sexual approaches to nurses, threats to leave the hospital, and actual signing out against medical recommendations.

Differential Diagnosis

Organic brain syndrome must always be ruled out since it often presents with symptoms resembling anxiety, depression, or psychosis. The schizophrenias may present with any of the above complaints. Personality disorders existing prior to hospitalization often underly the various behavior problems, but particularly the management problems.

Complications

Prolongation of hospitalization causes increased expense, deterioration of patient-staff relationships, and increased probabilities of iatrogenic and legal problems. The possibility of increasing posthospital treatment problems is enhanced.

Treatment

A. Psychotic Organic Brain Syndrome:

1. **Medical**—Medical treatment is discussed in the section on organic brain syndrome (see above).

2. **Social**—Social factors are important since the patient is in a strange setting and requires familiar environmental input. Encourage the family to spend maximum time with the patient. Familiarize the patient with members of the hospital staff and their names, and use the names each time that person sees the patient. Offer repeated clear explanations of the patient's medical problem and procedures and give reasonable reassurances. The selection of patients to occupy the same room is important. A patient with a transient psychosis will do better when the other patients are alert, helpful, and able to exert a reassuring and calming effect.

3. **Psychologic**—Psychologic therapies are not only unwarranted but tend to tax the patient and worsen his condition.

B. Acute Anxiety States:

1. **Psychologic**—Crisis therapy helps the patient understand and cope with the situation. Empathic understanding and explanation assist the development of insight and acceptance. It is appropriate to include important family members, since they can be of major assistance in providing continued empathy and reassurance of an insightful type.

2. **Medical**—Medical measures such as sedatives and minor tranquilizers aid in the transient problem. Diazepam, 5–10 mg orally, or oxazepam, 15–30 mg orally, is usually sufficient to allay anxiety and help the patient tolerate the situation.

C. Depression and Behavior Problems:

1. **Psychologic**—Psychologic treatment should be initiated early at the first signs of depression and behavior problems. The nursing staff and family usually notice this and often respond by hearty superficial reassurance, which frequently worsens the problem. The subject of the depression and underlying concerns should be handled in a sensitive and patient manner. There is no substitute for the primary physician, and time must be taken to deal with the problem. Find out where the patient is in his understanding of the medical problem and what his feelings are about it. He needs adequate ventilation, the knowledge that his physician understands his needs, and the assurance that his physician will stand by him in his illness. Help the patient develop an insightful relationship to past fears and focus on the positive realities of the current situation.

2. **Social**—Social concerns include who is in the room with the patient. Putting a depressed patient in a semiprivate room with a dying patient is obviously detrimental. Most patients relate best with patients of the same racial or ethnic group, particularly if there are language barriers between the patient and staff. Activities are necessary: television, books, occupational therapy, and volunteers should be utilized to fill up the time.

3. **Behavioral**—Behavioral responses can help prevent the development of "invalid" patterns of interactions. The staff, too, operantly respond to appropriate behaviors. (For example, in the case of the patient who has become psychologically dependent on the respirator, visitor time should be increased when the respirator is off in order to decrease the patient's dependence and help him learn to tolerate increasing times off the device.) Inappropriate and childish demands should be ignored as much as possible to allow extinction of immature behavior.

4. **Medical**—Medical treatment has little place in these depressions and behavior problems. Antidepressants are not helpful, and tranquilizers are usually effective only as long as the patient is asleep. When the patient's arousal level is very high, the twice-daily use of a major tranquilizer in small amounts (eg, chlorpromazine, 25–50 mg orally every 12 hours) is help-

ful. The use of beer or wine with meals also improves the ability of patients to tolerate a hospital and its bewildering procedures.

Prognosis

The prognosis is good in all patients that have reversible medical and surgical conditions. It is guarded when there is serious functional loss which impairs vocational, educational, or societal possibilities—especially in the case of progressive and ultimately life-threatening illness.

Asken MJ: Psychoemotional aspects of mastectomy: A review of recent literature. Am J Psychiat 132:56, 1975.

Brightwell DR: Treating obesity with behavior modification. Postgrad Med 55:53, 1974.

Cassem NH, Hackett TP: Psychiatric consultation in a cardiac care unit. Ann Int Med 75:9, 1971.

Cohen F, Lazarus RS: Active coping processes, coping dispositions, and recovery from surgery. Psychosom Med 35:375, 1973.

Craig TJ, Abeloff MD: Psychiatric symptomatology among hospitalized cancer patients. Am J Psychiat 131:1323, 1974.

Estes D, Christian CL: The natural history of systemic lupus erythematosus by prospective analysis. Medicine 50:85, 1971.

Jorgensen JA, Brophy JJ: Psychiatric treatment of severely burned adults. Psychosomatics 14:331, 1973.

Marshall JR: Effective use of a psychiatric consultant on a dialysis unit. Postgrad Med 55:121, 1974.

Mechanic D: Social psychologic factors affecting the presentation of bodily complaints. New England J Med 286:1132, 1972.

Richards DH: A post-hysterectomy syndrome. Lancet 2:983, 1974.

Smith CK & others: Psychiatric disturbance in endocrinologic disease. Psychosom Med 34:69, 1972.

Solow C & others: Psychosocial effects of intestinal by-pass surgery for severe obesity. New England J Med 290:300, 1974.

Stembach RA & others: Aspects of chronic low back pain. Psychosomatics 14:52, 1972.

Surman OS: Usefulness of psychiatric intervention in patients undergoing cardiac surgery. Arch Gen Psychiat 30:830, 1974.

PSYCHIATRIC COMPLICATIONS OF NONPSYCHIATRIC DRUGS

Psychiatric manifestations can occur as adverse effects or side-effects of practically every known therapeutic drug. It is not always easy, however, to determine if psychiatric symptoms arising during drug therapy of patients with physical disorders are due to the drug, based simply upon its known propensity to produce such symptoms. There is always the possibility of predisposing individual psychologic factors, as well as the psychologic and physical effects of the illness itself.

Although even the least noxious of drugs may produce unexpected psychiatric symptoms, there are some commonly used drugs and classes of drugs which, by virtue of the frequency or severity of reactions, deserve special mention:

(1) Anticholinergic drugs: Restlessness, confusion, delirium, paranoid ideation.

(2) Rauwolfia compounds: depression, agitation, paranoid ideation.

(3) Methyldopa: Depression, agitation, delirium.

(4) Digitalis compounds: Drowsiness, confusion, toxic psychosis.

(5) Levodopa: Euphoria, anxiety, toxic psychosis.

(6) Antituberculosis drugs (eg, INH): Insomnia, restlessness, toxic psychosis.

(7) Corticosteroids: Wide spectrum of psychiatric symptoms ranging from euphoria and hypomania to depression.

(8) Antidiabetic drugs: Hypoglycemia, restlessness, confusion, delirium.

18 . . .
Endocrine Disorders

Felix O. Kolb

The Difficulties of Diagnosis of Endocrine Diseases

The diagnosis of endocrine disorders is complicated by the following factors peculiar to these organs:

A. Interrelationships of the Endocrine Glands: Because the endocrine glands are so closely interrelated, the presenting symptoms and signs of any endocrine disorder may represent a secondary disturbance in another gland or even in more than one gland. The diagnostic clue may therefore be in an organ which is secondarily affected by hypofunction or hyperfunction of the gland in question. For example, amenorrhea may be due to an abnormality of the pituitary or adrenal gland rather than due to a primary ovarian lesion.

B. Homeostatic (Compensatory) Mechanisms: A well-balanced system of homeostasis often disguises the existence of a functional change in an endocrine gland, eg, partial pituitary suppression by cortisol administration. Special stress tests are required to clarify the diagnosis. Great strides have been made recently in our knowledge of the organization and control of the endocrine glands and in the messenger systems involved. The importance of prohormones as well as extracellular and intracellular messengers in maintaining homeostasis has been the subject of exciting research (see Rasmussen reference, below).

C. Size of Lesion vs Magnitude of Effect: The metabolic effect of an endocrine disturbance is not necessarily proportionate to the size of the lesion. A small tumor may cause extensive disturbance, whereas a striking enlargement may have no pathologic significance except as a space-occupying lesion.

D. Physiologic vs Pathologic States: The line between a physiologic aberration and a pathologic state may be quite tenuous (eg, physiologic growth spurt vs gigantism). The "target" organ may be unduly sensitive or resistant to usual amounts of hormonal secretion. Many hormones appear to act on target organs by stimulation of cyclic AMP formation; some may act through stimulation of prostaglandins.

E. Deficiencies of Knowledge: Many of the endocrine glands are regulated by neurohumoral factors elaborated in the hypothalamus which control the secretion of the pituitary hormones. Until recently, the diagnosis of disturbances along the pathway of this mechanism was largely beyond the reach of present-day medicine. The recently reported synthesis of TSH- and LH-releasing factors and somatostatin shows promise of future application to diagnosis and treatment (see Schally reference, p 649).

F. Multiple and Nonendocrine Involvement: The increasing number of recognized syndromes of multiple endocrine tumors and autoimmune deficiencies (often familial) and the endocrinopathies associated with nonendocrine gland cancers has complicated the problems of diagnosis. Ectopic production of certain hormones suggests their potential use as quantitative markers in certain diseases.

G. Difficulties of Laboratory Diagnosis: Direct chemical and radioimmunoassays of various hormones in blood and urine are being developed in increasing numbers, but, until they are perfected, less costly and more generally available bedside observations and sensitive indirect procedures are still required to establish the proper diagnosis of most endocrine disorders. Rapid progress has been made in radiologic diagnosis and localization of endocrine tumors.

Bayliss RIS (editor): Investigations of endocrine disorders. Clin Endocrinol Metab 3:423–609, 1974. [Entire issue.]

Besser GM, Mortimer CH: Hypothalamic regulatory hormones: A review. J Clin Path 27:173, 1974.

Catt KJ: ABC of endocrinology. 1. Hormones in general. Lancet 1:763, 1970.

Frohman LA: Clinical neuropharmacology of hypothalamic releasing factors. New England J Med 286:1391, 1972.

Gordan GS, Roof BS: "Humors from tumors": Diagnostic potential of peptides. Ann Int Med 76:501, 1972.

Irvine WJ: Autoimmune mechanisms in endocrine disease. Proc Roy Soc Med 67:499, 1974.

Liddle GW, Hardman JG: Cyclic adenosine monophosphate as a mediator of hormone action. New England J Med 285:560, 1971.

Newsome HH: Multiple endocrine adenomatosis. S Clin North America 54:387, 1974.

Odell WD: Humoral manifestations of nonendocrine neoplasms: Ectopic hormone production. Chap 30, pages 1105–1116, in: Textbook of Endocrinology, 5th ed. Williams RH (editor). Saunders, 1974.

Queener S, Gell NH: Prostaglandins and endocrinology. Pages 7–21 in: Year Book of Endocrinology. Schwartz TB (editor). Year Book, 1974.

Rasmussen H: Organization and control of endocrine systems. Chap 1, pages 1–30, in: Textbook of Endocrinology, 5th ed. Williams RH (editor). Saunders, 1974.

Rees LH, Ratcliffe JG: Ectopic hormone production by non-endocrine tumours. Clin Endocrinol 3:263, 1974.

Snyder N & others: Five families with multiple endocrine adenomatosis. Ann Int Med 76:53, 1972.

Steinbach HL, Minagi H: *The Endocrines: Atlas of Tumor Radiology.* Year Book, 1969.

Weichert RF III: The neural ectodermal origin of the peptide-secreting endocrine glands. Am J Med 49:232, 1970.

COMMON PRESENTING COMPLAINTS

Delayed Growth

Growth delays due to endocrine and metabolic disorders are at times difficult to distinguish from familial or genetic dwarfism. Often there is an association with delayed genital development. Rule out bone diseases and nutritional, metabolic, emotional, and renal disorders which may delay growth. Look for associated stigmas such as polydactylia and webbing. Plotting of the growth rate will demonstrate whether growth has been delayed since birth or only during a specific period in childhood. Hypothyroidism must be excluded, as it is at times subtle and can be diagnosed only by sensitive tests of thyroid function or occasionally by a trial of thyroid therapy. Epiphyseal dysgenesis (stippling) may be the telltale sign of juvenile hypothyroidism. The differentiation of hypopituitarism from delayed adolescence will usually become apparent in adult life. Dwarfing due to isolated lack of pituitary growth hormone has recently been described. Dwarfing is also seen with gonadal dysgenesis in Turner's syndrome and with pseudohypoparathyroidism. A rapid growth spurt with eventual short stature is typical of sexual precocity and of the adrenogenital syndromes. (*Note:* In any problem of growth delay, obtain an accurate determination of bone age and an x-ray of the sella turcica, and measure the skeletal proportions carefully.)

Excessive Growth

Excessive growth may be a familial or racial characteristic or a physiologic event (eg, the growth spurt of puberty) as well as a sign of endocrine disease. If precocious genital development occurs, consider true precocity due to pituitary or hypothalamic disorders, or pseudoprecocious puberty due to excess of adrenal, ovarian, or testicular hormones (often due to tumors). These patients, if not treated rapidly, will eventually be of short stature as a result of premature closure of their epiphyses. Pituitary eosinophilic tumors are rare before puberty; thereafter, they cause pituitary gigantism associated with enlargement of the sella turcica and visual field defects. After closure of the epiphyses acromegalic gigantism will result. A few cases of non-pituitary "cerebral gigantism" have been described. Eunuchoid individuals tend to grow taller, with span exceeding height. Diabetic children are often tall.

Obesity

Although obesity is a common presenting "endocrine" complaint, most cases are due to constitutional factors and excessive food intake. A sudden onset of massive obesity associated with lethargy or polyuria suggests a hypothalamic lesion (rare). While most cases of extreme obesity are associated with delayed puberty, slight excesses of food intake may lead to precocity. Hypothyroidism is usually not associated with marked obesity. In Cushing's disease or syndrome, there is apparent obesity with a characteristic "buffalo hump" and trunk obesity with thin extremities. Striae are common with any type of obesity. They are more often purplish in Cushing's syndrome. Amenorrhea, hypertension, and glycosuria or a diabetic glucose tolerance curve are commonly associated with obesity, and may improve after adequate weight loss. Islet cell adenomas are usually associated with obesity, but these are quite rare. In most instances the obese patient requires increased activity, reduction in caloric intake, and, at times, psychotherapy.

Wasting & Weakness

Pituitary cachexia (Simmonds' disease) is quite rare. Always rule out nonendocrine causes and consider anorexia nervosa and dietary fanaticism before looking for endocrine disturbances. Consider diabetes mellitus, thyrotoxicosis, pheochromocytoma, and Addison's disease if weight loss is progressive.

Abnormal Skin Pigmentation or Color

First consider normal individual, familial, and racial variations. Hyperpigmentation may coexist with depigmentation (vitiligo) in Addison's disease, which must be ruled out by standard tests. Search carefully for pigmentary spots on mucous membranes, gums, and nipples. Differentiate Addison's disease from sprue, hemochromatosis, and argyria. Pregnancy and thyrotoxicosis are at times associated with spotty brown pigmentation, especially over the face (chloasma). A similar type of pigmentation has been seen occasionally with oral contraceptive administration. Other drugs (eg, diethylstilbestrol) will cause localized brown-black pigmentation over the nipples. Brown pigment spots with a ragged border are typical of Albright's syndrome (associated with fibrous dysplasia and precocious sexual development in the female); smooth pigmented nevi are seen in neurofibromatosis. Acanthosis nigricans may be associated with acromegaly and other endocrine tumors. Patients with Cushing's disease usually have a ruddy complexion. Hyperpigmentation, especially after adrenalectomy, suggests a pituitary tumor or, more rarely, an extra-adrenal cancer. Carotenemia with yellowish skin and rosy cheeks is characteristic of primary myxedema. The hypogonadal or hypopituitary patient has a sallow, waxy, and at times yellowish or "fawn" color, and is unable to tan on exposure to sunlight.

Hirsutism

Marked normal variations in the amount of body

hair occur on a racial, familial, or genetic nonendocrine basis. Hirsutism, however, is one of the major presenting complaints of women and may be the first sign of a serious neoplastic disease; if so, it is rarely completely reversible even if the tumor is removed. Hirsutism is of greater significance if it occurs other than at puberty, with pregnancy, or at the menopause, if it is associated with other features of virilization, such as voice changes, balding, or enlargement of the clitoris, and if the onset is sudden. Always investigate the patient's adrenal status and rule out tumor and hyperplasia. Ovarian causes include polycystic ovaries (Stein-Leventhal syndrome), hilar cell tumors, arrhenoblastoma, and theca cell luteinization. As a minimum screening procedure, a urinary 17-ketosteroid determination should be obtained; but the more specific testosterone determinations that are now generally available are of greater diagnostic value. It is important to make certain that the patient has not received androgenic medication or certain drugs (eg, phenytoin).

Change in Appetite

Polyphagia (associated with polydipsia and polyuria) is classically found in uncontrolled diabetes mellitus. However, excessive eating is usually not an endocrine problem but a compulsive personality trait. Only rarely is it due to a hypothalamic lesion, in which case it is associated with somnolence and other signs of the hypothalamic disease, eg, hypogonadism and also congenital abnormalities (Fröhlich's syndrome, Laurence-Moon-Biedl syndrome). Excessive appetite with weight loss is observed in thyrotoxicosis; polyphagia with weight gain may indicate acromegaly or hypoglycemia due to an islet cell adenoma.

Anorexia and nausea associated with weight loss and diarrhea may occur at the onset of addisonian crisis or uncontrolled diabetic acidosis. Anorexia and nausea with constipation are found with any state of hypercalcemia, eg, hyperparathyroidism, and may be indistinguishable from the same symptoms occurring in peptic ulcer (which may coexist with hyperparathyroidism).

Polyuria & Polydipsia

Polyuria, commonly associated with polydipsia, is usually of nonendocrine etiology, due to a habit of drinking excessive water (psychogenic). However, if it is severe and of sudden onset it suggests diabetes mellitus or diabetes insipidus. Diabetes insipidus may develop insidiously or may appear suddenly after head trauma or brain surgery. Always attempt to rule out an organic lesion in or about the posterior pituitary-supraoptic tract. In children one must consider nephrogenic diabetes insipidus and eosinophilic granuloma.

A urine specific gravity over 1.016 virtually rules out diabetes insipidus.

Polyuria and polydipsia are frequently seen in any state of hypercalcemia, such as hyperparathyroidism, and are also part of the syndrome of primary hyperaldosteronism, in which they are typically nocturnal.

Polyuria may occur in renal tubular disorders, such as renal tubular acidosis and Fanconi's syndrome.

Gynecomastia

Enlargement of one or both breasts, usually painless and of rapid onset, is a common finding in adolescent boys. It may also be seen in old men. It is often transient and of little significance. One must differentiate between true glandular enlargement and simple fat pads or ballooning of the areolar tissue. Any painless hard lump, especially if unilateral, may be carcinoma.

True gynecomastia is found in many endocrine and nonendocrine disorders, eg, thyrotoxicosis, liver disease, paraplegia, and adrenal tumors. If associated with small testicles and lack of sperm, it may be part of Klinefelter's syndrome. A buccal smear may indicate a positive chromatin nuclear pattern.

Breast enlargement and tenderness may be due to estrogen therapy but occur also after the administration of androgens, especially to eunuchoid patients. They have been described in heavy marihuana users.

Gynecomastia may be the presenting sign of serious testicular tumors, such as choriocarcinoma, which may be too small to be palpable yet may metastasize widely. It may occur in bronchogenic carcinomas which produce gonadotropic hormones. It has been observed after hemodialysis.

Breast enlargements may be transitory or may persist even after the cause (eg, exogenous estrogen) is removed; plastic surgical removal is often necessary for cosmetic reasons.

Abnormal Lactation

Lactation is a physiologic phenomenon when seen in the newborn ("witch's milk"); it may occur before menstruation or may persist for prolonged periods after recent delivery, and is part of the syndrome of pseudocyesis. It is frequently present in both sexes in acromegaly and, more rarely, in thyrotoxicosis and myxedema. In some patients with amenorrhea with or without small chromophobe adenomas of the pituitary (eg, Chiari-Frommel syndrome), lactation may be so profuse that it is distressing to the patient. It may occur after pituitary stalk section, after thoracoplasty, or even after hysterectomy. Abnormal lactation occurs rarely with estrogen-secreting adrenal tumors and quite rarely with corpus luteum cysts and choriocarcinoma. Some drugs (eg, chlorpromazine) may produce lactation.

Precocious Puberty (in Both Sexes)

Precocious puberty is often a normal variant or a familial trait, but it may indicate serious organic disease. One must differentiate true precocity from pseudoprecocity. At times there is only premature breast development ("thelarche") or only premature appearance of pubic and axillary hair ("adrenarche") with normal subsequent menarche. Hypothalamic lesions, encephalitis, and certain tumors (eg, hamartoma of the tuber cinereum) may cause true sexual precocity. The same is found in girls who have associated fibrous dysplasia of bone and pigment spots (Albright's syndrome). Adrenal hyperplasia or tumor and gonadal tumors usually cause pseudoprecocious puberty with virilization or feminization. Hepatomas may rarely cause isosexual precocity. Reversible precocity with lactation and pituitary enlargement may be seen in juvenile hypothyroidism. The cause must be detected early since almost all children with precocious puberty will eventually be short or even dwarfed as a result of premature closure of the epiphyses, and because many of the responsible tumors are potentially malignant.

Sexual Infantilism & Delayed Puberty

It is often difficult to differentiate between simple functional delay of puberty (often a familial trait) and organic causes for such delays. Any type of gonadal or genetic defect may manifest itself primarily by failure of normal sexual development. Many patients grow to eunuchoid proportions, with span exceeding height. Consider hypothalamic lesions, especially if familial and associated with loss of sense of smell (Kallman's syndrome), craniopharyngioma, pituitary tumors, and defective testes or ovaries, and look for associated stigmas (webbed neck of Turner's syndrome, gynecomastia of Klinefelter's syndrome). Pituitary gonadotropin and urinary steroid excretion studies may help classify these disorders. Determine chromatin sex pattern on a buccal smear or by chromosomal analysis.

Lack of Potency & Libido in Males

Most cases are psychogenic in origin and are not helped by hormone therapy. Occasionally, however, lessening of sex desire or impairment of function may be the presenting sign of pituitary adenoma, Addison's disease, or testicular damage. The earlier in life the deficiency makes its appearance, the more pronounced is loss of libido associated with genital hypoplasia. Diabetes mellitus (especially with neuropathy) and thyrotoxicosis may first become manifest with this complaint. Chronic alcoholism, use of sedative and hypnotic drugs, and, occasionally, CNS lesions may be responsible. Measurement of plasma testosterone and LH may be helpful in differentiating organic and functional states. Be sure to rule out estrogenic or feminizing tumors of the testis or adrenal and search for other signs of feminization, such as gynecomastia. Some patients will benefit from psychotherapy.

Cryptorchism

Failure of descent of the testes is often of great concern to parents, but it is not usually a medical problem since the testes, if present, will descend spontaneously at or shortly after puberty. They may descend after application of heat to the scrotum, as in a warm bath, which demonstrates that they are present and will later descend normally.

There is no agreement about when hormonal therapy should be instituted. If the testes are present,

gonadotropic hormone will bring them down unless a hernia or blockage of the passageway prevents their descent. If there is doubt about whether the testes are present or not, determine urinary or serum gonadotropin levels and obtain a buccal smear to determine the sex chromatin pattern.

Early surgical repair is advisable because intra-abdominal testes may later fail to produce sperm normally and because the incidence of malignancy in intra-abdominal testes is high. Cryptorchism may be associated with hypogonadism or may be part of pseudohermaphroditism.

Bone & Joint Pains & Pathologic Fractures

If the onset is at an early age and if there is a family history of similar disorders, consider osteogenesis imperfecta (look for blue scleras). Bowing of the bone and pseudofractures suggest rickets or osteomalacia, due either to intestinal or, more commonly, renal tubular disorders. If bone pain, bone cysts, and fractures are associated with renal stones, consider hyperparathyroidism. Back pain with involvement of the spine suggests osteoporosis, especially when it occurs after the menopause. Aches and pains in the extremities are suggestive of rickets or osteomalacia. Rule out metastatic tumors, multiple myeloma, and Paget's disease in elderly patients. Differentiate metabolic from nonmetabolic bone disorders. In doubtful cases, bone biopsy is indicated. Bone densitometry measurements are more accurate than x-ray in determining minor mineral losses from the skeleton.

Renal Colic, Gravel & Stone Formation

A metabolic cause must be sought for recurrent stone formation and for kidney stones in children. If there is a family history, cystinuria and uric acid stones must be considered, or renal tubular acidosis with nephrocalcinosis. About 5% of stones are due to hyperparathyroidism, which must be ruled out in every instance of calcium stones. Look for bone disease, especially subperiosteal resorption of the bones of the fingers. Look also for signs of osteomalacia associated with excessive renal loss of calcium. Vitamin D intoxication, sarcoidosis, and excessive intake of milk and alkali must be considered. Any rapid bone breakdown may give rise to renal calcium stones, eg, in Cushing's syndrome. Uric acid stones may occur in patients with gouty arthritis, but often they occur simply because the urinary pH is very acid; they occur also after any type of intensive therapy for leukemia or polycythemia. Idiopathic hypercalciuria is the most common metabolic cause of recurrent calcium stones in males. Primary hyperoxaluria is a rare cause of severe renal calcification and may be associated with deposition of oxalate in soft tissues (oxalosis). Oxalate stones are seen frequently in patients with intestinal disorders (eg, ileitis, shunt procedures for obesity). At times, stones form in a structurally abnormal kidney (eg, medullary sponge kidney). Metabolic causes of renal stones must be corrected early before renal damage due to infection and obstruction occurs, since this may not be reversed upon removal of the initiating factor. The keys to proper diagnosis are careful stone analysis and chemical tests in blood and urine for calcium, phosphate, and uric acid.

Tetany & Muscle Cramps

Mild tetany with paresthesias and muscle cramps is usually due to hyperventilation with alkalosis resulting from an anxiety state. If tetany occurs in children, rule out idiopathic hypoparathyroidism or pseudo-hypoparathyroidism. Look for calcification in the lens, poor teeth, and x-ray evidence of basal ganglia calcification. Consider latent hypoparathyroidism in the post-thyroidectomy patient. Tetany may be the presenting complaint of osteomalacia or rickets or of acute pancreatitis. Neonatal tetany is probably due to the high phosphate content of milk and relative hypoparathyroidism. A similar mechanism has been considered responsible for leg cramps during pregnancy. Neonatal tetany may rarely indicate maternal hyperparathyroidism. Severe hypocalcemic tetany will occasionally produce convulsions and must be differentiated from "idiopathic" epilepsy. Classical signs of tetany are Chvostek's sign and Trousseau's phenomenon. If associated with hypertension, hypokalemia, and polyuria, consider primary hyperaldosteronism. Leg cramps may occur in some diabetic patients. Magnesium deficiency must be considered in tetany unresponsive to calcium.

Mental Changes

Disturbances of mentation are often subtle and may be difficult to recognize, but they may be important indications of underlying endocrine disorders. Nervousness, flushing, and excitability are characteristic of the menopause, hyperthyroidism, and pheochromocytoma. Convulsions with abnormal EEG findings may occur in hypocalcemic tetany or in hypoglycemia, either spontaneously or induced by insulin. Islet cell tumors may cause sudden loss of consciousness, somnolence and prolonged lethargy, or coma. Diabetic acidosis may progress gradually into coma. Hypercalcemia leads to somnolence and lethargy, with marked weakness. Mental confusion may occur in hypopituitarism or Addison's disease or in long-standing myxedema. Confusion, lethargy, and nausea may be the presenting symptoms of water intoxication due to inappropriate or excessive secretion of antidiuretic hormone. Mental deterioration is the rule in long-standing and untreated hypoparathyroidism and hypothyroidism (cretinism). Insomnia and psychosis are part of Cushing's syndrome, either spontaneous or induced. Early detection may prevent permanent brain damage. Mental deficiency may be associated with abnormal excretion of amino acids in the urine (eg, phenylketonuria) and with chromosomal abnormalities.

DISEASES OF THE HYPOTHALAMUS & OF THE PITUITARY GLAND

The function of the pituitary gland is controlled by regulating hormones (factors) produced by the hypothalamus. These releasing and release-inhibiting hormones are relatively simple polypeptides, several of which have been identified and synthesized (Table 18-1). A clinical disorder may be due to lack or excess of a pituitary hormone or, more commonly, to lack of releasing or inhibiting factor of the hypothalamus. Isolated or multiple defects may occur. Accurate radioimmunoassays and stimulation tests have made it possible to classify accurately the location of the defect. The exciting work of Guillemin and Schally in isolating and synthesizing these hypothalamic factors will prove of great value in the control of pituitary functional disorders (eg, of growth, fertility). Since some of these factors, eg, somatostatin, have multiple actions, they show promise for diagnosis and therapy of a variety of disorders (acromegaly, diabetes). It is not true that chromophobe tumors of the pituitary are hormonally inactive. Some have been found to secrete excessive ACTH, growth hormone, prolactin, and thyrotropin. A certain degree of overlap in function has been noted, eg, pituitary enlargement and lactation in juvenile myxedema reversed by the administration of thyroid hormone. Prolactin assays may be most important for the early diagnosis of pituitary lesions.*

*Schwartz TB: What you always wanted to know about prolactin but were afraid to ask. Pages 7-24 in: *Year Book of Endocrinology*. Year Book, 1973.

Table 18-1. The pituitary hormones and their hypothalamic regulatory factors (hormones).*

Hormones	Regulatory Factors (Hormones)
Growth hormone (somatotropin, STH)	Somatotropin-releasing factor (SRF, GH-RH, GH-RF); somatotropin release-inhibiting hormone (SIF, somatostatin)†
Corticotropin (ACTH)†	Corticotropin-releasing factor (CRF or CRH)
Thyrotropin (TSH)	Thyrotropin-releasing hormone (TRF, TRH)†
Follicle-stimulating hormone (FSH)	Gonadotropin-releasing hormone (FSH-RH, GNRH, LRH)
Luteinizing hormone (LH)	LH-RH, LH-RF, LRH†
Prolactin (LTH, mammotropin)	Prolactin-releasing factor (PRF, PRH); prolactin release-inhibiting hormone (PRIH or PIF)
Melanocyte-stimulating hormone	MSH-releasing factor (MRH, MRF); MSH release-inhibiting factor (MRIH, MIF)

*Schally AV & others: Hypothalamic regulatory hormones. Science 179:341, 1973.
†Presently fully identified and synthesized.

Brazeau P, Guillemin R: Somatostatin: Newcomer from the hypothalamus. New England J Med 290:963, 1974.

Gerich JE & others: Effects of somatostatin on plasma glucose and glucagon levels in human diabetes mellitus. New England J Med 291:544, 1974.

Hershman JM: Clinical application of thyrotropin-releasing hormone. New England J Med 290:886, 1974.

Jewelewicz R & others: Clinical studies with gonadotropin-releasing hormone. Bull New York Acad Med 50:1097, 1974.

Meites J: Neuroendocrinology of lactation. J Invest Dermat 63:119, 1974.

Mortimer CH & others: Effects of growth-hormone release-inhibiting hormone on circulating glucagon, insulin, and growth hormone in normal, diabetic, acromegalic, and hypopituitary patients. Lancet 1:697, 1974.

Nelson JC, Kollar DJ, Lewis JE: Growth hormone secretion in pituitary disease. Arch Int Med 133:459, 1974.

PANHYPOPITUITARISM & HYPOPITUITARY CACHEXIA
(Simmonds' Disease)

Essentials of Diagnosis

- Sexual dysfunction; weakness; easy fatigability; lack of resistance to stress, cold, and fasting; axillary and pubic hair loss.
- Low blood pressure; may have visual field defects.
- All low: T_4, ^{131}I uptake, FSH, LH, TSH, urinary 17-ketosteroids and corticosteroids, growth hormone.
- X-ray may reveal sellar lesion.

General Considerations

Hypopituitarism is a relatively rare disorder in which inactivity of the pituitary gland leads to insufficiency of the target organs. All or several of the tropic hormones may be involved. Isolated defects, eg, of the gonadotropins, are not rare. There is also great variation in the severity of the lesions, from those merely involving pathways (hypothalamic lesions) to almost complete destruction of the gland itself. The etiology of this disorder includes circulatory collapse due to hemorrhage following delivery and subsequent pituitary necrosis (Sheehan's syndrome), granulomas, hemochromatosis, cysts and tumors (Rathke's pouch cyst, chromophobe adenoma), surgical hypophysectomy, and functional hypopituitarism as seen in starvation and severe anemia. True pituitary cachexia (Simmonds' disease) is quite rare.

The pituitary tumor may be part of the syndrome of multiple endocrine adenomatosis. Isolated or partial deficiencies of anterior pituitary hormones (eg, FSH, LH, TSH) or their releasing factors may occur (see Odell and Spitz references, below) and may be detected by refined technics.

Clinical Findings

These vary with the degree of pituitary destruction, and are related to the lack of hormones from the "target" endocrine glands.

A. Symptoms and Signs: Weakness, lack of resistance to cold, to infections, and to fasting, and sexual dysfunction (lack of development of primary and secondary sex characteristics, or regression of function) are the most common symptoms. In expanding lesions of the sella, interference with the visual tracts may produce loss of temporal vision, whereas a craniopharyngioma may cause blindness. Short stature is the rule if the onset is during the growth period. Lactation may be seen in both sexes.

In both sexes there is sparseness or loss of axillary and pubic hair, and there may be thinning of the eyebrows and of the head hair, which is often silky.

The skin is almost always dry, with lack of sweating, has a peculiar pallor, and is sallow ("fawn"-colored). Pigmentation is lacking even after exposure to sunlight. Fine wrinkles are seen, and the facies presents a "sleepy appearance."

The heart is small and the blood pressure low. Orthostatic hypotension is often present. Cerebrovascular symptoms or abnormal lactation may occur.

B. Laboratory Findings: The fasting blood sugar is usually low and the glucose tolerance curve flat. The insulin tolerance test (use only 0.05 units/kg IV) shows marked insulin sensitivity and is dangerous in these patients since severe hypoglycemic reactions may occur. The T_4 level is low. Radioactive iodine uptake is low, with a rise following TSH (this does not occur in primary myxedema). Urinary 17-ketosteroids and corticosteroids and plasma cortisol are low but rise slowly after corticotropin administration (this does not occur in primary Addison's disease). Both TSH and corticotropin may have to be given for several days. The metyrapone (Metopirone) test has been used to demonstrate limited pituitary ACTH reserve. Urinary and serum gonadotropins are very low. Anemia is common. Direct assay of growth hormone levels in blood by immunochemical methods, when available, shows low levels with little response to insulin hypoglycemia, to arginine infusion, or to levodopa. ACTH, TSH, LH, and FSH levels are low. The recently synthesized TSH-releasing hormone is a new diagnostic tool to differentiate hypothalamic from pituitary hypothyroidism (see Hershman reference, below). Elevated prolactin levels, not suppressible by levodopa, may be an early finding in chromophobe adenomas.

Measurements of the responses of FSH and LH to LH-releasing hormone and to clomiphene are refined technics to differentiate hypothalamic, pituitary, and primary gonadal deficiency states.

C. X-Ray Findings: X-rays of skull may show a lesion in or above the sella. In growing children, one may find delay in bone age.

D. Eye Examination: Visual field defects (bitemporal hemianopsia) may be present.

Differential Diagnosis

The most difficult problem is differentiation from anorexia nervosa, which may simulate hypopituitarism.

In fact, severe malnutrition may give rise to functional hypopituitarism. By and large, cachexia is far more common in anorexia nervosa, and loss of axillary and pubic hair is rare; at times mild facial and body hirsutism is seen in anorexia nervosa. The 17-ketosteroids are low normal or not as low as in hypopituitarism, and may respond rapidly to corticotropin stimulation, and the gonadotropins are usually present at low levels. Thyroid function tests are least likely to be abnormal in anorexia nervosa. Recently, direct pituitary growth hormone assays have shown high levels in anorexia nervosa and very low levels in hypopituitarism. The response to diet and psychotherapy at times settles the diagnosis.

Primary Addison's disease and primary myxedema are at times difficult to differentiate from pituitary insufficiency, but the response to corticotropin and TSH often helps. Direct radioimmune assay of ACTH and TSH, if available, is a more accurate diagnostic method.

The enlargement of the sella may require pneumoencephalograms to rule out the "empty sella syndrome," where minimal or few endocrine abnormalities are present and radiation or surgery is contraindicated (see Caplan reference, below).

At times hypopituitarism may masquerade as "nephrosis" or as "pernicious anemia."

The severe hypoglycemia after fasting may cause confusion with hyperinsulinism.

The mental changes of hypopituitarism may be mistaken for a primary psychosis.

Complications

In addition to those of the primary lesion (eg, tumor), complications may develop at any time as a result of the patient's inability to cope with minor stressful situations. This may lead to high fever, shock, coma, and death. Sensitivity to thyroid may precipitate an adrenal crisis when thyroid is administered. Corticosteroids may cause psychosis. Rarely, acute hemorrhage may occur in large pituitary tumors with rapid loss of vision, headache, and evidence of acute pituitary failure requiring emergency decompression of the sella. (See Zervas reference, below.)

Treatment

The pituitary lesion, if a tumor, is treated by surgical removal (either through craniotomy or, more recently, through a transsphenoidal approach), x-ray irradiation, or both. Endocrine substitution therapy must be used before, during, and almost always permanently after such procedures.

With the exception of corticotropin, there is no readily available effective pituitary replacement preparation; therapy must therefore be aimed at correcting the end-organ deficiencies. This must be continued throughout life. Almost complete replacement therapy can be carried out with corticosteroids, thyroid, and sex steroids.

A. Corticosteroids: Give hydrocortisone, 20–30 mg orally daily in divided doses. If edema occurs with corticosteroid treatment, prednisolone or dexamethasone (Decadron) is often preferable. Give prednisolone, 5–7.5 mg orally daily in divided doses, or dexamethasone, 0.5–1 mg orally daily in divided doses. Additional amounts of rapid-acting corticosteroids must be given during states of stress, eg, during infection or in preparation for surgery.

B. Thyroid: Thyroid (and insulin) should rarely, if ever, be used in panhypopituitarism unless the patient is receiving corticosteroids. Because of lack of adrenal function, patients may be exceedingly sensitive to these drugs. For this reason one should exercise special care in differentiating primary myxedema from hypopituitarism—often a difficult problem.

Begin with small doses of thyroid, eg, 15–30 mg daily, and gradually increase to tolerance: 60–120 mg are usually adequate. Levothyroxine, 0.1–0.2 mg daily, may be preferred.

C. Sex Hormones:

1. Testosterone or one of the newer anabolic steroids may be used in males and at times also in females, primarily for their tissue building (protein anabolic) effect. For males give one of the longer-acting parenteral testosterone preparations every 3–4 weeks; or methyltestosterone, 10–20 mg orally daily. In females the dosage of these drugs is one-half that for males. If signs of virilizing action appear in the female, the drug should be withdrawn and they will lessen. They do not usually occur if the dose of methyltestosterone is kept under 300 mg/month. Fluoxymesterone may be given in doses of 2–10 mg orally daily. (**Note:** Do not use methyltestosterone for prolonged periods since liver impairment may occur.)

2. Estrogens are useful in the female for their mild anabolic effect, their effect on secondary sex characteristics, and their possible neutralizing effect on androgens. Give diethylstilbestrol, 0.5–1 mg daily orally; ethinyl estradiol, 0.02–0.05 mg daily orally; or conjugated estrogenic substances (eg, Premarin), 0.625–1.25 mg daily orally. Omit treatment for one week each month.

3. Chorionic gonadotropic hormone (APL) in combination with human pituitary FSH or postmenopausal urinary gonadotropin may be used in an attempt to produce fertility.

4. The recently synthesized LH-releasing factor offers a new approach for the diagnosis and treatment of gonadotropin deficiency states (see Roth and Spitz references, below).

Note: Sex hormones, especially estrogens, should be employed cautiously in young patients with panhypopituitarism or the epiphyses will close before maximum growth is achieved. Most androgens, with the possible exception of fluoxymesterone, also share this property—especially when given in large doses.

D. Human Growth Hormone: This hormone is by far the most effective agent for increasing height, but it is available for only a few patients. Human placental lactogen is under investigation as a pituitary growth hormone substitute. A better understanding of growth hormone releasing factors may offer alternative forms of treatment in the future (see VanderLaan reference, below).

E. Other Drugs: Isolated reports have appeared of successful medical treatment using thyroxine, levodopa, and bromocriptine (2-brom-α-ergocryptine) to treat pituitary lesions producing lactation and amenorrhea.

Prognosis

This depends on the primary cause. If it is due to postpartum necrosis (Sheehan's syndrome), partial or even complete recovery may occur. Functional hypopituitarism due to starvation and similar causes may also be corrected. The recent observation that some patients with hypopituitarism may suffer from failure of hypothalamic releasing or inhibiting factors offers hope for simpler therapy in the near future.

If the gland has become permanently destroyed the problem is to replace target hormones, since replacement with pituitary tropic hormones is not yet feasible. It is possible to prolong life if states of stress such as starvation, infection, or trauma are treated with prompt and adequate replacement therapy. If the onset of the disease is in childhood, the patient's ultimate height will be subnormal unless human growth hormone is used. Surgical procedures, eg, hypophysectomy to preserve vision in chromophobe adenomas, are safer since the advent of corticosteroids.

Anorexia nervosa. (Leading article.) Brit MJ 4:183, 1971.

Boyar RMM & others: Anorexia nervosa: Immaturity of the 24 hour luteinizing hormone secretory pattern. New England J Med 291:861, 1974.

Caplan RH, Dobben GD: Endocrine studies in patients with "empty sella syndrome." Arch Int Med 123:611, 1969.

Catt KC: ABC of endocrinology. 2. Pituitary function. Lancet 1:827, 1970.

Coscia AM & others: The effect of synthetic luteinizing hormone-releasing factor on plasma LH levels in pituitary disease. J Clin Endocrinol 38:83, 1974.

Eddy RL & others: Human growth hormone release: Comparison of provocative test procedures. Am J Med 56:179, 1974.

Escamilla RF, Forsham PH: Treatment with human growth hormone for over 8 years: Effects of long-term therapy in a pituitary dwarf. California Med 115:72, Dec 1971.

Espinosa RE, Randall RV: Early symptoms and signs of chromophobe adenoma. M Clin North America 52:827, 1968.

Hershman JM: Clinical application of thyrotropin-releasing hormone. New England J Med 290:886, 1974.

Kolodny HD, Sherman L: Laboratory aids in the diagnosis of pituitary tumors. Ann Clin Lab Sc 4:67, 1974.

Lin T, Tucci JR: Provocative tests of growth hormone release: A comparison of results with seven stimuli. Ann Int Med 80:464, 1974.

Mason AS: Pituitary tumours. Canad J Surg 17:142, 1974.

Matte R & others: Familial hypothalamic hypogonadotropic hypogonadism. Canad MAJ 110:509, 1974.

Moe PJ: Hypopituitary dwarfism: The importance of early therapy. Acta paediat scandinav 57:300, 1968.

Nicholls MG, Espiner EA, Donald RA: Schmidt's syndrome presenting as hypopituitarism. Ann Int Med 80:505, 1974.

Odell WD: Isolated deficiencies of anterior pituitary hormones. JAMA 197:1006, 1966.

Peake GT, Daughaday WH: Disturbances of pituitary function in central nervous system disease. M Clin North America 52:357, 1968.

Ray BS, Patterson RH Jr: Surgical experience with chromophobe adenomas of the pituitary gland. J Neurosurg 34:726, 1971.

Root AW & others: Diagnosis and management of growth retardation with special reference to the problem of hypopituitarism. J Pediat 78:737, 1971.

Roth JC & others: FSH and LH response to luteinizing hormone-releasing factor in prepubertal and pubertal children, adult males and patients with hypogonadotropic and hypergonadotropic hypogonadism. J Clin Endocrinol 35:926, 1972.

Seidensticker JF, Tzagournis M: Anorexia nervosa: Clinical features and long-term follow-up. J Chronic Dis 21:361, 1968.

Sheehan HL, Davis JC: Pituitary necrosis. Brit M Bull 24:59, 1968.

Sheline GE: Treatment of nonfunctioning chromophobe adenomas of the pituitary. Am J Roentgenol 120:553, 1974.

Spitz IM & others: Isolated gonadotropin deficiency. New England J Med 290:10, 1974.

Thorner MO & others: Long-term treatment of galactorrhoea and hypogonadism with bromocriptine. Brit MJ 2:419, 1974.

VanderLaan WP: Changing concepts in the control of growth hormone secretion in man. California Med 115:38, Aug 1971.

VanderLaan WP: Changing concepts of prolactin in man. California Med 118:28, Feb 1973.

Yoshimoto Y & others: Restoration of normal pituitary gonadotropin reserve by administration of luteinizing-hormone-releasing hormone in patients with hypogonadotropic hypogonadism. New England J Med 292:242, 1975.

Zervas NT, Mendelson G: Treatment of acute hemorrhage of pituitary tumours. Lancet 1:604, 1975.

HYPERPITUITARISM
(Eosinophilic Adenoma of the Anterior Pituitary)
GIGANTISM & ACROMEGALY

Essentials of Diagnosis

- Excessive growth of hands (increased glove size), feet (increased shoe size), jaw (protrusion of lower jaw), and internal organs; or gigantism before closure of epiphyses.

- Amenorrhea, headaches, visual field loss, sweating, weakness.

- Elevated serum inorganic phosphorus and BMR; T_4 normal; glycosuria.

- Elevated serum growth hormone with failure to suppress after glucose.

- X-ray: Sellar enlargement and terminal phalangeal "tufting." Increased heel pad.

General Considerations

An excessive amount of growth hormone, presumably due to overactivity of the eosinophilic portion of the anterior lobe of the pituitary, is most often produced by a benign adenoma. The tumor may be small or, rarely, located within the sinuses rather than within the sella. The disease may be associated with adenomas elsewhere, such as in the parathyroids or pancreas. Carcinoid tumors may be associated with acromegaly. If the onset is before closure of the epiphyses, gigantism will result. If the epiphyses have already closed at onset, only overgrowth of soft tissues and terminal skeletal structures (acromegaly) results. At times the disease is transient ("fugitive acromegaly") followed by pituitary insufficiency.

Clinical Findings

A. Symptoms and Signs: Crowding of other hormone-producing cells, especially those concerned with gonadotropic hormones, causes amenorrhea and loss of libido. Production of excessive growth hormone causes doughy enlargement of the hands with spade-like fingers, large feet, jaw, face, tongue, and internal organs, wide spacing of the teeth, and an oily, tough, "furrowed" skin and scalp with multiple fleshy tumors (mollusca). Hoarse voice is common. At times, acanthosis nigricans is present. Pressure of the pituitary tumor causes headache, bitemporal hemianopsia, lethargy, and diplopia. In long-standing cases secondary hormonal changes take place, including diabetes mellitus, goiter, and abnormal lactation. Less commonly, these may be the presenting picture in acromegaly. Excessive sweating may be the most reliable sign of activity of the disease.

B. Laboratory Findings: Serum inorganic phosphorus may be elevated (over 4.5 mg/100 ml) during the active phase of acromegaly. The FSH level is usually low, but it may be normal or even high. Glycosuria and hyperglycemia may be present, and there is resistance to the administration of insulin. Hypercalciuria is common. The BMR may be elevated. The PBI and T_4 may be normal and may not fall after antithyroid medication. 17-Ketosteroids and hydroxycorticosteroids may be high or low, depending upon the stage of the disease. Immunologic assay for growth hormone in blood shows high levels in the active phase of the disease; administration of glucose fails to suppress the serum level (as it does in normal individuals).

C. X-Ray Findings: X-ray of the skull may show a large sella with destroyed clinoids, but a sella of usual size does not rule out the diagnosis. The frontal sinuses may be large. One may also demonstrate thickening of the skull and long bones, with typical overgrowth of vertebral bodies and severe spur formation. Dorsal kyphosis is common. Typical "tufting" of the terminal phalanges of the fingers and toes may be demonstrated, with increase in size of the sesamoid bone. A lateral view of the feet demonstrates increased thickness of the heel pad.

D. Eye Examination: Visual field examination may show bitemporal hemianopsia.

Differential Diagnosis

Hyperpituitarism is to be considered if there is rapid growth or resumption of growth once stopped (eg, change in shoe size or ring size). Suspect the diagnosis also in unexplained amenorrhea, insulin-resistant diabetes mellitus, or goiter with elevated BMR which does not respond to antithyroid drugs. Physiologic spurts of growth and increase in tissue size from exercise, weight gain, or from certain occupations enter into the differential diagnosis. The syndrome of cerebral gigantism with mental retardation and ventricular dilatation but normal growth hormone levels resembles acromegalic gigantism. Myxedema and, rarely, pachydermoperiostitis may resemble acromegaly. Serial photographs are of help in differentiating familial nonendocrine gigantism and facial enlargement. Other conditions causing visceromegaly must be considered (see Sober reference, below).

Complications

Complications include pressure of the tumor on surrounding structures, rupture of the tumor into the brain or sinuses, the complications of diabetes, cardiac enlargement, and cardiac failure. The carpal tunnel syndrome, due to compression of the median nerve at the wrist, may cause disability of the hand. Cord compression due to large intervertebral disks may be seen.

Treatment

The treatment of choice of active tumors without visual field loss used to be pituitary irradiation, with or without the use of sex hormones. If visual fields are markedly reduced, x-ray therapy may be hazardous and surgery is the treatment of choice. The recent finding that conventional x-ray treatment causes a slow fall in growth hormone level favors heavy particle irradiation or surgical hypophysectomy in the future. The simpler cryohypophysectomy has been shown to be an effective and safe procedure. Periodic reassessment of pituitary function after these procedures is advisable. In the "burnt out" case, hormonal replacement as for hypopituitarism is required. Medical treatment of active acromegaly with progesterone and chlorpromazine has been disappointing. The recently synthesized growth hormone release-inhibiting hormone (somatostatin) offers a new approach for the treatment of acromegaly and gigantism (see Yen reference, below). A recent report of medical treatment with bromocriptine (2-brom-a-ergocryptine) offers a novel approach (see Thorner reference), but long-term results must be awaited.

Prognosis

Prognosis depends upon the age at onset and, more particularly, the age at which therapy is begun. Menstrual function may be restored. Severe headaches may persist even after treatment. Secondary tissue and skeletal changes do not respond completely to removal of the tumor. The diabetes may be permanent in spite of adequate pituitary ablation. The patient may succumb to the cardiovascular complications. The tumor may "burn out," causing symptoms of hypopituitarism.

Adams JE & others: Transsphenoidal cryohypophysectomy in acromegaly: Clinical and endocrinological evaluation. J Neurosurg 28:100, 1968.

Aloia JF & others: Treatment of acromegaly. Arch Int Med 131:509, 1973.

Catt KJ: ABC of endocrinology. 3. Growth hormone. Lancet 1:933, 1970.

Dimond RC & others: Chlorpromazine treatment and growth hormones secretory response in acromegaly. J Clin Endocrinol 36:1189, 1973.

Goldfine ID, Lawrence AM: Hypopituitarism in acromegaly. Arch Int Med 130:720, 1972.

Haigler ED: Pituitary gigantism. Arch Int Med 132:588, 1973.

Jacobi JD & others: Pituitary apoplexy in acromegaly followed by partial pituitary insufficiency. Arch Int Med 134:559, 1974.

Kjellberg RN & others: Proton-beam therapy in acromegaly. New England J Med 278:689, 1968.

Lawrence AM, Kirstens H: Progestins in the medical management of active acromegaly. J Clin Endocrinol 30:646, 1970.

Manifestations and treatment of acromegaly. Medical Staff Conference, University of California, San Francisco. California Med 116:57, March 1972.

Martin JB: Neural regulation of growth hormone secretion. New England J Med 288:1384, 1973.

McMillan DE & others: Evaluation of clinical activity of acromegaly by observation of the diurnal variation of serum inorganic phosphate. Metabolism 17:966, 1968.

O'Duffy JD & others: Median neuropathy (carpal-tunnel syndrome) in acromegaly. Ann Int Med 78:379, 1973.

Sober AJ & others: Visceromegaly in acromegaly: Evidence that clinical hepatomegaly or splenomegaly (but not sialomegaly) are manifestations of a second disease. Arch Int Med 134:415, 1974.

Stephenson JN & others: Cerebral gigantism. Pediatrics 41:130, 1968.

Taylor AL & others: Pituitary apoplexy in acromegaly. J Clin Endocrinol 28:1784, 1968.

Thorner MO & others: Bromocriptine treatment of acromegaly. Brit MJ 1:299, 1975.

Wright AD & others: Mortality in acromegaly. Quart J Med 39:1, 1970.

Yen SSC & others: Effect of somatostatin in patients with acromegaly. New England J Med 290:935, 1974.

DIABETES INSIPIDUS

Essentials of Diagnosis

- Polydipsia (4–40 liters/day); excessive polyuria.
- Urine sp gr < 1.006.
- Inability to concentrate urine on fluid restriction. Hyperosmolarity of plasma.
- Vasopressin reduces urine output.

General Considerations

Diabetes insipidus is an uncommon disease of young adults (particularly males) which is characterized by an increase in thirst and the passage of large quantities of urine of a low specific gravity. The urine is otherwise normal. The disease may occur acutely, eg, after head trauma or surgical procedures near the pituitary region, or may be chronic and insidious in onset. It is due to insufficiency of the posterior pituitary or impaired function of the supraoptic pathways which regulate water metabolism. More rarely, it is due to unresponsiveness of the kidney to vasopressin (Pitressin) (nephrogenic diabetes insipidus).

The causes may be classified as follows:

A. Due to Deficiency of Vasopressin:

1. Primary diabetes insipidus, due to a defect inherent in the gland itself (where no organic lesion is demonstrable), may be familial, occurring as a dominant trait; or, more commonly, sporadic or "idiopathic."

2. Secondary diaberes insipidus is due to destruction of the functional unit by trauma, infection (eg, encephalitis, tuberculosis, syphilis), primary tumor or metastatic tumors from the breast or lung (common), vascular accidents (rare), and xanthomatosis (eosinophilic granuloma of Hand-Schüller-Christian disease).

Certain drugs, eg, demeclocycline, may induce diabetes insipidus. Postpartum diabetes insipidus with amenorrhea and galactorrhea has been reported.

B. "Nephrogenic" Diabetes Insipidus: This disorder is due to a defect in the kidney tubules which interferes with water reabsorption and occurs as a sex-linked, recessive trait. Patients with this type of the disease are the so-called "water babies." In adults it may be associated with hyperuricemia. At times this type is acquired, eg, after pyelonephritis, potassium depletion, or amyloidosis. The disease is unresponsive to vasopressin.

Clinical Findings

A. Symptoms and Signs: The outstanding signs and symptoms of the disease are intense thirst, especially with a craving for ice water, and polyuria, the volume of ingested fluid varying from 4–40 liters daily, with correspondingly large urine volumes. Restriction of fluids causes marked weight loss, dehydration, headache, irritability, fatigue, muscular pains, hypothermia, tachycardia, and shock.

B. Laboratory Findings: A polyuria of over 6 liters/day with a specific gravity below 1.006 is highly suggestive of diabetes insipidus, and a specific gravity of 1.015 or higher after fluid restriction rules out the disease. Simple water deprivation with measurement of urine osmolality may be diagnostic. Special tests have been devised to distinguish true diabetes insipidus from psychogenic diabetes insipidus (Hickey-Hare and Carter-Robbins tests). The latter will respond (with reduction in urine flow and increase in urinary specific gravity) to administration of hypertonic (3%) saline solution; true diabetes insipidus does not. Although a positive response tends to rule out true diabetes insipidus, a negative result must be followed by careful prolonged dehydration and measurement of both urine and plasma osmolality and body weight under hospital conditions. Failure to respond to vasopressin (Pitressin) indicates "nephrogenic" diabetes insipidus if the serum calcium and potassium levels are normal. A recently developed radioimmunoassay for arginine vasopressin will facilitate the differential diagnosis of diabetes insipidus and psychogenic polydipsia (see Robertson reference, below).

If true primary diabetes insipidus seems likely on the basis of these tests, search for a possible brain lesion with x-rays of the skull, visual field tests, and encephalograms. Search also for associated bone lesions of xanthomatosis and obtain biopsy for confirmation. Look for a primary tumor in the lung or breast. In nephrogenic diabetes insipidus, rule out pyelonephritis or hydronephrosis.

Differential Diagnosis

The most important differentiation is from the "psychogenic" water habit (see above). Polydipsia and polyuria may also be seen in diabetes mellitus, chronic nephritis, hypokalemia (eg, in primary hyperaldosteronism), and in hypercalcemic states such as hyperparathyroidism. The low fixed specific gravity of the urine in chronic nephritis does not rise after administration of vasopressin. On the other hand, in spite of the inability of patients with diabetes insipidus to concentrate urine, other tests of renal function yield essentially normal results (the NPN may even be below normal).

Complications

If water is not readily available the excessive output of urine will lead to severe dehydration, which rarely proceeds to a state of shock. Insomnia and dysphagia may occur. All the complications of the primary disease may eventually become evident. In patients who also have a disturbed thirst mechanism and who are receiving effective antidiuretic therapy, there is a danger of induced water intoxication.

Treatment

A. Specific Measures: Vasopressin tannate (Pitressin Tannate), 0.5–1 ml in oil IM, is the standard treatment. It is effective for 24–72 hours. It is usually best to administer the drug in the evening so that maximal results can be obtained during sleep. Patients learn to administer the drug themselves, and the dosage is adjusted as necessary. Warn the patient to shake well before filling the syringe. Posterior pituitary snuff inhaled 2–3 times a day may be used and is the most economical form of treatment, but it may be quite irritating and absorption is uncertain. The dose varies from 30–60 mg. Aqueous vasopressin injection is rarely used in continuous treatment because of its short duration of action (1–4 hours). An occasional patient is allergic to animal vasopressin; a synthetic substitute, lysine-8 vasopressin, is available as a nasal spray (lypressin [Diapid]). This form of treatment may be preferred by patients with mild disease. It is free of local side-effects, and water intoxication, which is not unusual with vasopressin tannate in oil, does not occur. A recently synthesized analogue of arginine vasopressin (1-desamino-8-D-arginine vasopressin) is longer-acting

and may become the treatment of choice (see Ward reference, below).

B. Other Measures: Mild cases (or vasopressin-resistant cases) require no treatment other than adequate fluid intake. Hydrochlorothiazide (Hydrodiuril), 50–100 mg/day (with KCl), is of some help in reducing the urine volume of true or nephrogenic diabetes insipidus. Chlorpropamide (Diabinese) has been found to be an effective antidiuretic and may be tried in mild cases or to potentiate the action of vasopressin. After an initial dose of 250 mg twice daily, many patients can be maintained on 125–250 mg daily. Side-effects include nausea, skin allergy, hypoglycemia, and a disulfiram-like reaction to alcohol. Phenformin (DBI) is a less effective antidiuretic agent in doses of 50 mg once or twice daily. Other drugs under investigation are clofibrate, halofenate, and carbamazepine (Tegretol). Solute restriction may be of additional help. Psychotherapy is required for most patients with compulsive water drinking.

C. X-Ray Therapy: This may be used in the treatment of some cases due to tumor (eg, eosinophilic granuloma).

Prognosis

Diabetes insipidus may be latent, especially if there is associated lack of anterior pituitary function; and may be transient, eg, following head trauma. The ultimate prognosis is essentially that of the underlying disorder. Since many cases are associated with organic brain disease, the prognosis is often poor. Surgical correction of the primary brain lesion rarely alters the diabetes insipidus.

If the disease is due to an eosinophilic granuloma of the skull, temporary amelioration or even complete cure may be effected with x-ray therapy.

The prognosis of the "nephrogenic" type is only fair since intercurrent infections are common, especially in infants affected with the disease. The acquired forms of this type may be reversible—eg, if urinary tract infection or obstruction is alleviated.

Bode HH & others: Chlorpropamide for diabetes insipidus with hypodipsia. Am J Med 51:304, 1971.

DeWardener HE: Polyuria. J Chronic Dis 11:199, 1960.

Dousa TP: Cellular action of antidiuretic hormone in nephrogenic diabetes insipidus. Mayo Clin Proc 49:188, 1974.

Ettinger B, Forsham PH: Mechanism of chlorporpamide antidiuresis in diabetes insipidus. J Clin Endocrinol 31:552, 1970.

Gorden P & others: Hyperuricemia: A concomitant of congenital vasopressin-resistant diabetes insipidus in the adult. New England J Med 284:1057, 1971.

Hayek A, Ramirez J: Demeclocycline-induced diabetes insipidus. JAMA 229:676, 1974.

Kimura T & others: Mechanism of carbamazepine (Tegretol)-induced antidiuresis. J Clin Endocrinol 38:356, 1974.

MacVicar AA: Halofenate versus clofibrate in the management of true diabetes insipidus. Canad MAJ 110:1275, 1974.

Merker E, Futterweit W: Postpartum amenorrhea, diabetes insipidus and galactorrhea: Report of a case and review of the literature. Am J Med 56:554, 1974.

Miller M & others: Recognition of partial defects in antidiuretic hormone secretion. Ann Int Med 73:721, 1970.

Mimica N, Wegienka LC, Forsham PH: Lypressin nasal spray. JAMA 203:802, 1968.

Moses AM & others: Mechanism of chlorpropamide-induced antidiuresis in man: Evidence for release of ADH and enhancement of peripheral action. Metabolism 22:59, 1973.

Robertson GL & others: Development and clinical application of a new method for the radioimmunoassay of arginine vasopressin in human plasma. J Clin Invest 52:2340, 1973.

Schwartz IL, Schwartz WB: Symposium on antidiuretic hormones. Am J Med 42:651, 1967.

Ward MK, Fraser TR: DDAVP in treatment of vasopressin-sensitive diabetes insipidus. Brit MJ 3:86, 1974.

INAPPROPRIATE SECRETION OF ANTIDIURETIC HORMONE

This syndrome, which is essentially water intoxication, consists of irritability, lethargy, confusion, and seizures. It may lead to coma and death if not recognized. Laboratory findings include hyponatremia (which usually suggests the diagnosis) and hypoosmolarity of the serum, continued renal excretion of sodium, formation of hyperosmolar urine, and expanded fluid volume. Adrenal and renal function are usually normal.

The disorder is most commonly caused by oat cell bronchogenic carcinoma, but it may also be present in pulmonary tuberculosis, porphyria, acute leukemia, myxedema, and CNS disorders. In children, it may be a complication of pneumoencephalography. It may be induced by chlorpropamide, vincristine, cyclophosphamide, and potassium-depleting diuretics.

Treatment is best accomplished by water restriction, which succeeds if the syndrome is recognized early. In severe cases of hyponatremia, when rapid correction is required, the use of furosemide diuresis with electrolyte replacement may be tried (see Hantman reference, below). Lithium carbonate has been found to be effective in this syndrome, but lithium intoxication may occur (see White reference, below). A search for the primary cause of the disorder must also be undertaken. The prognosis is often poor because of the advanced stage of the syndrome at the time of recognition and the serious primary disorder causing it.

Bartter FL, Schwartz WB: The syndrome of inappropriate secretion of antidiuretic hormone. Am J Med 42:790, 1967.

Bauman G & others: Plasma arginine vasopressin in the syndrome of inappropriate antidiuretic hormone secretion. Am J Med 52:19, 1972.

DeFronzo RA & others: Water intoxication in man after cyclophosphamide therapy: Time, course, and relation to drug activation. Ann Int Med 78:861, 1973.

Fichman MP & others: Diuretic-induced hyponatremia. Ann Int Med 75:853, 1971.

Hantman D & others: Rapid correction of hyponatremia in the syndrome of inappropriate secretion of antidiuretic hormone. Ann Int Med 78:870, 1973.

Mendoza SA, Keller M: Inappropriate secretion of antidiuretic hormone. Western J Med 121:45, 1974.

Vorherr H: Para-endocrine tumor activity with emphasis on ectopic ADH secretion: Genetic, diagnostic, prognostic and therapeutic aspects. Oncology 29:382, 1974.

Weissman PN, Shenkman L, Gregerman RI: Chlorpropamide hyponatremia: Drug-induced inappropriate ADH activity. New England J Med 284:65, 1971.

White MG, Fetner CD: Treatment of the syndrome of inappropriate secretion of antidiuretic hormone with lithium carbonate. New England J Med 292:390, 1975.

DISEASES OF THE THYROID GLAND

Thyroid hormone affects cellular oxidative processes throughout the body. It is normally elaborated within the follicles of the gland by a combination of inorganic iodine, which is trapped by the gland under the influence of pituitary TSH, and tyrosine, forming monoiodotyrosine and diiodotyrosine, which further combine to form thyroxine and triiodothyronine (T_3), the principal hormones of the gland. The "storage" form of the hormone is thyroglobulin, a combination of thyroxine and thyroid globulin, and it is in this colloidal form that the hormone is found within the follicles.

Under the influence of TSH, the active hormones are released from the gland as the need arises. Circulating thyroxine is bound to plasma proteins, primarily thyroxine-binding globulins, and prealbumin. They can be measured as "protein-bound" iodine (PBI) or T_4. High levels of estrogen (eg, in pregnancy or in women taking oral contraceptives) increase the thyroxine-binding globulin levels and thus also the PBI and T_4. The binding can be inhibited by certain compounds, eg, diphenylhydantoin and high doses of aspirin, which lower the PBI and T_4. The free (unbound) levels of circulating hormones regulate TSH release. The physiologic importance of triiodothyronine in clinical disorders is now well established. The availability of synthetic TSH-releasing hormone has been helpful in the evaluation of pituitary reserve and in the diagnosis of both hyper- and hypothyroidism.

The requirements for iodine are minimal (about 20–200 µg/day), but if a true deficiency arises or if the demand for iodine is increased (eg, during puberty), hormone production will be insufficient and circulating levels will be low. This leads to increase in pituitary TSH output, and hyperplasia of the thyroid gland follows.

Thyroid disorders may occur with or without diffuse or nodular enlargement of the gland (goiter). Symptoms may be due to pressure alone or to hyperfunction or hypofunction. A strong genetic predisposition to thyroid disease is being recognized.

Since thyroid hormone affects all vital processes

of the body, the time of onset of a deficiency state is most important in mental and physical development. Prolonged insufficiency which is present since infancy (cretinism) causes irreversible changes. Milder degrees of hypofunction, especially in adults, may go unrecognized or may masquerade as symptoms of disease of another system, eg, menorrhagia. Diagnosis will then depend to a large extent upon laboratory aids, especially the finding of an elevated TSH level.

In any age group, whenever an isolated thyroid nodule is felt which is not associated with hyperfunction or hypofunction—and especially if there is any change in size of the nodule—the possibility of neoplasm must be considered.

Bartuska D: Evolving concepts of the genetics of thyroid disease: A review. Am J Med Sc 266:249, 1973.

Brown J & others: Thyroid physiology in health and disease. Ann Int Med 81:68, 1974.

Catt KJ: ABC of endocrinology. 6. The thyroid gland. Lancet 1:1383, 1970.

Edelman IS: Thyroid thermogenesis. New England J Med 290:1303, 1974.

Gharib H: Triiodothyronine: Physiological and clinical significance. JAMA 227:302, 1974.

Hershman JM: Clinical application of thyrotropin releasing hormone. New England J Med 290:886, 1974.

Hershman JM, Pittman JA: Control of thyrotropin secretion in man. New England J Med 285:997, 1971.

Selenkow HA, Hoffman F (editors): *Diagnosis and Treatment of Common Thyroid Diseases.* Excerpta Medica, International Congress Series No. 227, 1971.

TESTS OF THYROID FUNCTION

The greater availability of the more specific tests of thyroid function has gradually replaced most of the older ones such as the BMR, PBI, BEI, and T_4 by column. The T_4 CPB-MP or T_4(D), or T_4(RIA) combined with the resin uptake of T_3 and measurement of the free thyroxine index (FTI) are most widely used in clinical practice. The recently available TSH(RIA) assay has been of great help in diagnosis.

Protein-Bound Iodine (PBI, "Hormonal Iodine")
Normal: $4-8$ $\mu g/100$ ml serum.

A. Elevated: In hyperthyroidism, thyroiditis, and due to administration of iodides, desiccated thyroid, or thyroxine. Inorganic iodides increase levels for up to 3 weeks; organic iodides (eg, in urograms, cholecystograms) for 6 months or longer; oil-soluble organic iodides (eg, Lipiodol) for months to years. Pregnancy and Enovid or similar preparation raise the PBI due to increased thyroxine-binding protein.

B. Low: Hypothyroidism. Falsely low levels may be due to mercurial diuretics (low for $3-7$ days), urinary loss of protein (eg, in nephrosis), or T_3 (Cytomel) administration.

Butanol-Extractable Iodine (BEI)
Normal: $3-7$ $\mu g/100$ ml.

This test roughly parallels the PBI and is not affected by inorganic iodides. It is, however, raised by organic iodides. A large discrepancy between the PBI and BEI suggests the presence of abnormal iodoproteins, as seen in certain types of goiter.

T_4 by Column
Normal: $3-7.5$ $\mu g/100$ ml.

This test has largely replaced the BEI. It is not affected by inorganic iodides but is elevated by organic iodides and states of increased thyroxine binding.

T_4 CPB-MP or T_4(D)
Normal: $5.3-14.5$ $\mu g/100$ ml.

This is a method of measuring total thyroxine by competitive protein binding or displacement devised by Murphy and Pattee. It is becoming available in most laboratories and is replacing PBI, BEI, and T_4 by column since it is not affected by exogenous iodides. It is, however, affected by states of altered thyroxine binding.

T_4(RIA)
Normal: $5-13$ $\mu g/100$ ml.

This test, which does not require extraction, is gradually replacing the T_4 CPB-MP or T_4(D). It is also affected by states of altered thyroxine binding.

"Free" Thyroxine Determination
Normal: $1.4-3.5$ ng/100 ml.

This test measures the metabolically effective fraction of circulating T_4. It is a difficult test to perform and not generally available.

Radioactive T_3 Uptake of Red Cells or Resin
Normal (varies with methods): Red cells—males, $12-19\%$; females, $13-20\%$. Resin—males, $25-35\%$; females, $24-34\%$. Resin uptake is the preferred test.

This test is not dependent upon exogenous organic or inorganic iodides. It is an indirect measure of thyroxine-binding protein which is of value in certain patients, eg, in pregnancy when the T_4 is falsely high due to increased thyroxine-binding while T_3 uptake is low. In general, T_3 uptake parallels the T_4 except in the rare euthyroid patient with deficient thyroxine-binding protein, where the T_4 is low but the T_3 uptake normal or high. A combination of this test and the T_4 is of greater diagnostic value.

Free Thyroxine Index
Normal: $0.75-2.6$ units if T_4 by column is used; $1.3-5.1$ units if T_4(D) is used with resin T_3 uptake.

This test is a measurement of the product of T_4 and resin T_3 uptake. This corrects for abnormalities of thyroxine binding.

Thyroxine-Binding Globulin (TBG-RIA)
Normal: $2-4.8$ mg/100 ml.

This is a direct and specific test for abnormal

Table 18—2. Typical results of some blood thyroid function tests in various conditions.*
(N = Normal range. ↑ = Elevated. ↓ = Decreased.)

Note: The more direct tests are subject to technical variables. They should be used when the more standard tests do not give decisive information, since many drugs cause interference with these thyroid tests.

	PBI	T_4 Column	T_4 CPB-MP,† T_4(D), T_4(RIA)	T_3 Resin	Cholesterol	Free T_4 Index	RaI (^{131}I) Uptake	Other Useful Tests and Comments
Hyperthyroidism	↑	↑	↑	↑	↓	↑	↑	TSH ↓ LATS ↑
Hypothyroidism	↓	↓	↓	↓	↑	↓	↓	TSH ↑ in primary myxedema, ↓ in pituitary myxedema
Euthyroid, or hypothyroid therapy with: T_4 (1)	↑	↑	↑	↑	N	↑	↓	TSH ↓ with 0.2–0.3 mg
T_3 (2)	↓	↓	↓	↓	N	↓	↓	TSH ↓ with 100 µg
Desiccated thyroid (3)	N	N	N	N	N	N	↓	TSH ↓ with 120–200 mg
Euthyroid following (4) Radiographic contrast dyes	↑	N or ↑	N	N	N	N or ↑	↓	Effects may persist for 2 weeks to years
Pregnancy Hyperthyroid	↑	↑	↑	N or ↑	↓	↑	↑	Effects persist for 6–10 weeks after termination
Euthyroid	↑	↑	↑	↓	N	N	↑	
Hypothyroid	N or ↓	N or ↓	N or ↓	↓	↑	↓	↓	
Birth control pills	↑	↑	↑	↓	N	N	N	TSH normal
Nephrotic syndrome (5)	↓	↓	↓	↑	↑	N	N	Low TP and TBG
Diphenylhydantoin, high doses of salicylates, testosterone	↓	↓	↓	↑	N	N	N	TSH normal
Iodine deficiency	N	N	N	N	N	N	↑	^{131}I ↓ by T_4 or T_3
Iodide ingestion (6)	N or ↑	N	N	N	N	N	↓	^{131}I ↑ with TSH

(1) Therapy with T_4 causes elevated measurements of serum thyroxine because there is no T_3 metabolic effect.

(2) T_3 causes decreased measurements of serum thyroxine because T_4 secretion is depressed or absent. T_3 resin is decreased because of decreased saturation of TBG with T_4.

(3) Assuming normal T_3:T_4 ratio.

(4) Free T_4 index may be increased if measurement for serum T_4 is elevated by contamination.

(5) TBG is lost in this disease, which accounts for decreased serum thyroxine.

(6) Iodides may contaminate PBI by coprecipitation.

*Modified and reproduced, with permission, from Leeper RD: Current Concepts 1:1, 1972. Courtesy of The Upjohn Co., Kalamazoo, Mich.

†Competitive protein binding (Murphy-Pattee).

thyroxine binding and is not affected by alterations in other serum proteins.

T_3 by Radioimmunoassay

Normal: 60–190 ng/ml.

This recently available test is of value in the diagnosis of thyrotoxicosis with normal T_4 values (T_3 thyrotoxicosis) and in some cases of toxic nodular goiter. It may be relatively normal in hypothyroidism.

Radioiodine (^{131}I) Uptake of Thyroid Gland

Normal: 5–35% in 24 hours. The normal range has been lowered in the USA because of increase of dietary intake of iodine. (See Ghahremani reference, below.)

A. Elevated: Thyrotoxicosis, hypofunctioning large goiter, iodine lack; at times, chronic thyroiditis.

B. Low: Administration of iodides (similar to fac-tors raising the PBI), T_4, antithyroid drugs, thyroiditis, myxedema, hypothyroidism.

A scintigram over the gland outlines areas of increased and decreased activity. If the uptake of ^{131}I is blocked, technetium may be used to obtain a scintigram. Suppression of uptake after administration of 100 µg of T_3 daily for several days will determine if the area in the gland is autonomous or TSH-dependent. Administration of TSH for 2 or more days, with increase in ^{131}I uptake over low control levels, indicates the presence of thyroid tissue, and hence shows that low uptake was due to lack of TSH.

Serum Cholesterol

Normal: 150–280 mg/100 ml. This test is nonspecific, as many factors may influence cholesterol level. The absolute level is less significant than the change after institution of therapy.

A. Relatively Elevated: Myxedema. Hypothyroidism.

B. Relatively Low: Thyrotoxicosis (occasionally).

Basal Metabolic Rate (BMR)

(With or without sedation.)

Normal: ± 20%.

A. Elevated:

1. Markedly elevated—Hyperthyroidism, polycythemia, leukemia, pheochromocytoma.

2. Moderately elevated—Hyperthyroidism, anemia, congestive heart failure, Paget's disease, gigantism and acromegaly, malignancy, pregnancy, drugs (eg, caffeine).

3. Slightly elevated—Febrile illnesses (7% per degree F above normal), anxiety.

B. Low: Myxedema (−30% to −60%). Low rates are also found in panhypopituitarism, Addison's disease, anorexia nervosa, chronic debility, starvation, and also at times in nephrosis.

Achilles Tendon Reflex (Photomotograph)

The relaxation time is often prolonged in hypothyroidism, but also in pregnancy, diabetes, etc. It is rapid in hyperthyroidism. Although it lacks specificity for diagnosis, this test may be of value in following response to therapy. Normal range: 240–380 msec.

Serologic Tests

Antibodies against several thyroid constituents may be found in the sera of patients with various types of thyroiditis (especially Hashimoto's disease) and, at times, in adenomatous goiters, in myxedema, and, rarely, in Graves' disease and thyroid carcinoma.

Thyrotropin Immunoassay & Response to TRF

Normal: TSH-RIA less than 10 μU/ml; TRF response: doubling of TSH 90 minutes after administration of 200 μg IM.

Radioimmunoassay of serum TSH is becoming more widely available. TSH elevations may occur in subclinical hypothyroidism (eg, after destructive thyroid treatment), in iodine deficiency goiter, and in some dyshormonogenic goiters. A normal TSH rules out primary hypothyroidism. TSH elevation with nodular goiter usually indicates autoimmune thyroid disease. T_4 treatment is rational in patients with goiter and elevated TSH. After adequate T_4 replacement, patients with myxedema should have undetectable or low TSH levels. A normal TSH response to TRF rules out pituitary hypothyroidism. A prolonged and exaggerated rise in TSH after administration of thyrotropin-releasing factor (TRF) in patients with borderline elevations of TSH may provide further evidence of primary thyroid failure. Patients with hyperthyroidism fail to respond to TRF, and a normal response virtually excludes hyperthyroidism.

Miscellaneous Tests

More sophisticated tests may at times be performed. Many are still mainly research tools. Among them are measurement of free T_4 and thyroid-binding globulin and assay of long-acting thyroid stimulator (LATS) in serum.

Ashkar FS, Abelove WA: Serum thyroxine as an index of thyroid function. Postgrad Med 56:80, 1974.

Beall GN, Solomon DH: LATS and thyroid autoantibodies. Clin Exper Immunol 3:615, 1968.

Braverman LE & others: Pituitary-thyroid responsiveness to intramuscular thyrotropin-releasing hormone based on analyses of serum thyroxine, triiodothyronine and thyrotropin concentrations. New England J Med 292:273, 1975.

Burke G: The thyrotrophin stimulation test. Ann Int Med 69:1127, 1968.

Chopra IJ: A radioimmunoassay for measurement of thyroxine in unextracted serum. J Clin Endocrinol 34:938, 1972.

Dodds WJ, Powell MR: Thyroid scanning with technetium 99m pertechnetate. Radiology 91:27, 1968.

Fisher DA: Advances in the laboratory diagnosis of thyroid disease. (2 parts.) J Pediat 82:1, 187, 1973.

Fleischer N & others: Synthetic thyrotropin releasing factor as a test of pituitary thyrotropin reserve. J Clin Endocrinol 34:617, 1972.

Ghahremani GG & others: New normal values for thyroid uptake of radioactive iodine. JAMA 217:337, 1971.

Havard CWH, Boss M: In vivo tests of thyroid function. Brit MJ 3:678, 1974.

Hershman JM: Clinical applications of thyrotrophin releasing hormone. New England J Med 290:886, 1974.

Howorth PJN, MacLagan NF: Clinical application of serum total-thyroxine estimation, resin uptake, and free-thyroxine index. Lancet 1:224, 1969.

Levy RP & others: Radioimmunoassay of human thyroxine-binding globulin (TBG). J Clin Endocrinol 32:372, 1971.

Males JL: Endocrinology for the clinician. The evaluation of thyroid function. Clin Med 81:9, 1974.

Mayberry WE & others: Radioimmunoassay for human thyrotrophin: Clinical values in patients with normal and abnormal thyroid function. Ann Int Med 74:471, 1971.

Nuki G, Bayliss RIS: The Achilles tendon reflex as an index of thyroid function. Postgrad MJ 44:97, 1968.

Rosenberg IN: Evaluation of thyroid function. New England J Med 286:924, 1972.

Schneider PB: Laboratory examination of the thyroid. 1. In vitro tests. Postgrad Med 56:91, 1974.

Thomson JA & others: Evaluation of discordant laboratory data in patients with thyroid disorders. J Clin Path 21:511, 1968.

Utiger RD: Serum triiodothyronine in man. Ann Rev Med 25:289, 1974.

SIMPLE & NODULAR GOITER

Essentials of Diagnosis

- Enlarged thyroid gland in a patient living in an endemic area.
- No symptoms except those associated with compression by large gland.
- T_4 and serum cholesterol normal; radioactive iodine uptake normal or elevated.
- TSH may be elevated.

General Considerations

Simple goiter is most commonly due to iodine lack, and occurs in endemic areas away from the seacoast. Relative insufficiency of the iodine leads to functional overactivity and hyperplasia of the gland, which becomes filled with colloid poor in iodine. If the deficiency is corrected, the enlargement may subside. In long-standing cases, the goiter persists and is often nodular. Unknown factors other than iodine lack play a role in the genesis of goiter. Simple goiter may occur transiently when there is greater demand for thyroid hormone, eg, with the onset of puberty or during pregnancy. Rarely, goiter may occur in spite of adequate iodine intake when there is interference with formation of thyroid hormones, eg, due to excess intake of certain goitrogenic vegetables (rutabagas, turnips), exposure to thiocyanate, or congenital lack of certain enzyme systems. Goiter is more readily preventable than cured, and is less common since the introduction of iodized salt.

Clinical Findings

A. Symptoms and Signs: The gland is visibly enlarged and palpable. There may be no symptoms, or symptoms may occur as a result of compression of the structures in the neck or chest: wheezing, dysphagia, respiratory embarrassment. (*Note:* Recurrent laryngeal compression is rare.) There may be associated congenital deafness and disorders of taste.

B. Laboratory Findings: The T_4 and serum cholesterol are usually normal. The radioiodine uptake of the gland may be normal or high. Radioactive uptakes over nodules show them to be low in activity (in contrast to toxic nodular goiters).

With special technics it is possible to demonstrate enzymatic defects in thyroid hormone production or abnormal circulating compounds in a considerable number of patients with goiters, especially the familial types. Thyroid autoantibodies may also be demonstrated. The TSH levels may be elevated.

Differential Diagnosis

It may be difficult to differentiate simple goiter from toxic diffuse or nodular goiter, especially in a patient with a great many nervous symptoms. A history of residence in an endemic area, a family history of goiter, or onset during stressful periods of life (eg, puberty or pregnancy) will often help. If nodular, and especially if only a single nodule is present, neoplasm must be considered.

Prevention

With a dietary intake of 100–200 μg of iodine daily, simple goiter should not occur. During times of stress (puberty, pregnancy, and lactation), the upper limits of this dose may be necessary. This amount is provided in 1–2 gm of iodized salt daily. Iodinated oil has recently been introduced in certain areas of the world as a prophylactic agent for goiter.

Treatment

A. Specific Measures:

1. Thyroid–Thyroid, 120–180 mg or more, or levothyroxine, 0.2 mg or more–especially if the goiter is multinodular–appears to be of value in about half of cases. As a guide to therapy, T_4 should be maintained in the high normal range. TSH levels should be suppressed by adequate replacement therapy. Triiodothyronine may be more effective in suppressing large goiters.

2. Iodine therapy (early)–If the enlargement is discovered early, it may disappear completely with adequate iodine administration. Five drops daily of saturated solution of potassium iodide or strong iodine solution (Lugol's solution) in one-half glass water is sufficient. Continue therapy until the gland returns to normal size, and then place the patient on a maintenance dosage or use iodized table salt. Iodized oil injections may be preferable.

3. Iodine therapy (late)–If the enlargement is of long standing iodine therapy as above may be used, but significant regression in the size of the gland should not be expected. *Note:* Thyroid treatment is preferable in most patients with simple goiter. Iodides may induce thyrotoxicosis (see Vagenakis reference, below).

B. Indications for Surgery:

1. Signs of pressure–If signs of local pressure are present which are not helped by medical treatment, the gland should be removed surgically.

2. Potential malignancy–Surgery should be considered for any thyroid gland with a single "cold" (low ^{131}I uptake) nodule, for the chances of a single nodule being malignant are quite high. This is particularly true in younger people and in any case when there is no decrease in size or abnormal growth in spite of thyroid therapy after a period of 3–6 months.

Prognosis

Simple goiter may disappear spontaneously or may become large, causing compression of vital structures. Multinodular goiters of long standing, especially in people over 50 years of age, may become toxic. Whether they ever become malignant is not established.

Astwood EB, Cassidy CE, Aurbach GD: Treatment of goiter and thyroid nodules with thyroid. JAMA 174:459, 1960.

Butterfield IH: Correction of iodine deficiency in New Guinea natives by iodized oil injection. Lancet 2:767, 1965.

Green W & others: Management of the thyroid nodule. JAMA 221:1265, 1972.

Hamburger JI: *Nontoxic Goiter–Concept and Controversy.* Thomas, 1973.

Shimaoka K, Sokal JE: Suppressive therapy of nontoxic goiter. Am J Med 57:576, 1974.

Vagenakis AG & others: Iodide-induced thyrotoxicosis in Boston. New England J Med 287:523, 1972.

Welch CE: Therapy for multinodular goiter. JAMA 195:339, 1966.

Zacharewicz FA: Management of single and multinodular goiter. M Clin North America 52:409, 1968.

HYPOTHYROIDISM

In view of the profound influence exerted on all tissues of the body by thyroid hormone, lack of the hormone may affect virtually all body functions. The degree of severity ranges from mild and unrecognized hypothyroid states to striking myxedema.

A state of hypothyroidism may be due to primary disease of the thyroid gland itself, or lack of pituitary TSH or hypothalamic TRF. A true end-organ insensitivity to normal amounts of circulating hormone has been postulated but is rarely observed. Although gross forms of hypothyroidism, ie, myxedema and cretinism, are readily recognized on clinical grounds alone, the far more common mild forms often escape detection without adequate laboratory facilities.

1. CRETINISM & JUVENILE HYPOTHYROIDISM

Essentials of Diagnosis

- Dwarfism, mental retardation, dry, yellow, cold skin, "pot belly" with umbilical hernia.
- T_4 low; serum cholesterol elevated.
- Delayed bone age; "stippling" of epiphyses.
- TSH elevated.

General Considerations

The causes of cretinism and juvenile hypothyroidism are as follows (after Wilkins):

A. Congenital (Cretinism):

1. Thyroid gland absent or rudimentary (embryonic defect; most cases of sporadic cretinism).

2. Thyroid gland present but defective in hormone secretion, goitrous, or secondarily atrophied. Due to extrinsic factor (deficient iodine, goitrogenic substances [?], in most cases of endemic cretinism); or due to maternal factors (some cases of congenital goiter). Many cases are familial.

B. Acquired (Juvenile Hypothyroidism): Atrophy of the gland or defective function may be due to unknown causes, thyroiditis, or operative removal (lingual thyroid or toxic goiter), or secondary to pituitary deficiency.

Clinical Findings

A. Symptoms and Signs: All degrees of dwarfism may be seen, with delayed skeletal maturation, apathy, physical and mental torpor, dry skin with coarse, dry, brittle hair, constipation, slow teething, poor appetite, large tongue, "pot belly" with umbilical hernia, deep voice, cold extremities and cold sensitivity, and true myxedema of subcutaneous and other tissues. A yellow, carotenemic skin is not infrequent. The thyroid gland is usually not palpable, but a large goiter may be present which may be diffuse or nodular. Sexual development is retarded but maturation eventually oc-

curs. Menometrorrhagia or amenorrhea may be seen in older girls. Rarely, sexual precocity and galactorrhea with pituitary enlargement may occur. Deafness is occasionally associated with goiters. Nephrocalcinosis is a rare finding in cretinism.

B. Laboratory Findings: The BMR is probably the least reliable (especially in infants and children) and the $T_4(D)$ (see above) the most reliable index of thyroid activity; the latter is usually under 3 μg/100 ml. Serum cholesterol is frequently elevated. Radioactive iodine uptake is very low in athyroid individuals, but it may be high in goitrous cretins although the iodine is not bound in the gland and is released. By special technics, abnormal circulating iodine compounds and enzymatic defects in thyroid hormone production and release are demonstrable in some patients. Others show circulating autoantibodies to thyroid constituents. TSH by radioimmunoassay is invariably elevated, and this may be the best screening test where it is readily available, especially in newborns.

C. X-Ray Findings: Delayed skeletal maturation is a constant finding, often with "stippling" of the epiphyses (especially of the femoral head), with flattening; widening of the cortices of the long bones, absence of the cranial sinuses, and delayed dentition may also be noted.

Differential Diagnosis

It is of practical interest to differentiate primary hypothyroidism from pituitary failure because in the latter instance a search for a pituitary lesion must be undertaken. Treatment with thyroid hormone must be instituted cautiously when hypothyroidism is secondary to pituitary failure since it may occasionally precipitate adrenal crisis. Radioiodine uptake studies before and after exogenous TSH administration will often show whether a gland is present or not. TSH assay (when available) generally will help greatly in the differentiation of primary hypothyroidism from pituitary hypothyroidism. True myxedema and hypercholesterolemia are less common with hypopituitarism. Cretinism is most often confused with Down's syndrome, although retarded skeletal development is rare in mongoloid infants. Macroglossia may be due to tumor, eg, lymphangioma. The dry skin of ichthyosis may be misleading. All causes of stunted growth and skeletal development (see above) must be considered as well. Rather than risk the development of full-blown cretinism in the questionable case, a trial of thyroid therapy is reasonable.

Treatment

See Myxedema, below.

Prognosis

The progress and outcome of the disease depend largely upon the duration of thyroid deficiency and the adequacy and persistence of treatment. Since mental development is at stake, it is of utmost importance to start treatment early.

The prognosis for full mental and physical maturation is much better if the onset is later in life. Congenital cretins almost never attain full mental development. Skeletal and sexual maturation, though often retarded, do take place normally under continued thyroid therapy.

By and large, the response to thyroid therapy is gratifying but therapy usually must be maintained throughout life.

De Groot LJ: Current views on formation of thyroid hormones. (3 parts.) New England J Med 272:243, 197, 355, 1965.

Foley TP & others: Successful laboratory screening for congenital hypothyroidism. Lancet 2:77, 1974.

Homoki J & others: Thyroid function in term newborn infants with congenital goiter. Pediatrics 86:753, 1975.

Klein AH & others: Improved prognosis in congenital hypothyroidism treated before age three months. J Pediat 81:912, 1972.

Stanbury JB: Familial goiter. Chap 10 in: *The Metabolic Basis of Inherited Disease,* 3rd ed. Stanbury JB, Wyngaarden JB, Fredrickson DS (editors). McGraw-Hill, 1972.

2. ADULT HYPOTHYROIDISM & MYXEDEMA

Essentials of Diagnosis

- Weakness, fatigue, cold intolerance, constipation, menorrhagia, hoarseness.
- Dry, cold, yellow, puffy skin; scant eyebrows, thick tongue, "water bottle" heart, bradycardia, delayed return of deep tendon reflexes.
- T_4 and radioiodine uptake low.
- Anemia (often macrocytic).
- TSH elevated in primary myxedema.

General Considerations

Primary thyroid deficiency is much more common than secondary hypofunction due to pituitary insufficiency. Primary myxedema occurs after total thyroidectomy, eradication of thyroid by radioactive iodine, ingestion of goitrogens (eg, thiocyanates, rutabagas, lithium carbonate), or chronic thyroiditis. Most cases, however, are due to atrophy of the gland from unknown causes, possibly an autoimmune mechanism. This may also involve other endocrine glands, eg, adrenals, in the same patient (Schmidt's syndrome).

Secondary hypothyroidism may follow destructive lesions of the pituitary gland, eg, chromophobe adenoma or postpartum necrosis (Sheehan's syndrome). It is usually manifested by associated disorders of the adrenals and gonads. Since thyroid hormone is necessary for all glandular functions, primary myxedema may lead to secondary hypofunction of the pituitary, adrenals, and other glands, making diagnosis difficult.

Clinical Findings

These may vary from the rather rare full-blown myxedema to mild states of hypothyroidism, which are far more common and may escape detection unless a high index of suspicion is maintained.

A. Symptoms and Signs:

1. Early—The principal symptoms are weakness, fatigue, cold intolerance, lethargy, dryness of skin, headache, and menorrhagia. Nervousness is a common finding. Physical findings may be few or absent. Outstanding are thin, brittle nails; thinning of hair, which may be coarse; and pallor, with poor turgor of the mucosa. Delayed return of deep tendon reflexes is often found.

2. Late—The principal symptoms are slow speech, absence of sweating, weight gain, constipation, peripheral edema, pallor, hoarseness, aches and pains, dyspnea, anginal pain, deafness, and amenorrhea. Physical findings include puffiness of the face and eyelids, typical carotenemic skin color with rosy cheeks, thinning of the outer halves of the eyebrows, thickening of the tongue, hard pitting edema, and effusions into the pleural, peritoneal, and pericardial cavities. Cardiac enlargement ("myxedema heart") is often due to pericardial effusion. The heart rate is slow; the blood pressure is more often normal than low, and even hypertension may be found which reverses with treatment. Pituitary enlargement and lactation, which may be reversible following thyroid therapy, may occasionally be seen in long-standing hypothyroidism. (*Note:* Obesity is not common in hypothyroidism.)

B. Laboratory Findings: The T_4 is under 3.5 μg/100 ml. Radioiodine uptake is decreased (below 10% in 24 hours), but this test is not always reliable. The radioactive T_3 uptake is usually low. Plasma cholesterol is elevated in primary and, less commonly, in secondary hypothyroidism (fall on thyroid therapy is a sensitive index). Macrocytic anemia may be present. Increase in ^{131}I uptake and T_4 after administration of 10–20 units of thyrotropic hormone (given for several days) suggests secondary hypothyroidism rather than primary myxedema. 17-Ketosteroids may be very low. The radioimmunoassay of TSH is a most useful test since it is consistently elevated in primary hypothyroidism and low in pituitary hypothyroidism.

Differential Diagnosis

Mild hypothyroidism must be considered in all states of neurasthenia, menstrual disorders without grossly demonstrable pelvic disease, unexplained weight gain, and anemia. Myxedema enters into the differential diagnosis of unexplained heart failure which does not respond to digitalis or diuretics, "idiopathic" hyperlipemia, and unexplained ascites. The protein content of myxedematous effusions is high. The thick tongue may be confused with that seen in primary amyloidosis. Pernicious anemia may be suggested by the pallor and the macrocytic type of anemia seen in myxedema. It enters into the differential diagnosis of myasthenic syndromes. (See Takamori reference, below.) Some cases of primary psychosis and cerebral arteriosclerosis or even brain tumors must be differentiated from profound myxedema. (*Note:*

The CSF proteins may be elevated in myxedema.) If laboratory tests are not convincing, response to cautious thyroid administration may establish the true nature of the disorder.

Complications

Complications are mostly cardiac in nature, occurring as a result of advanced coronary artery disease and congestive failure, which may be precipitated by too vigorous thyroid therapy. There is an increased susceptibility to infection: Organic psychoses with paranoid delusions may occur ("myxedema madness"). Rarely, adrenal crisis may be precipitated by thyroid therapy of pituitary myxedema. Hypothyroidism is an accepted cause of infertility, which often responds to thyroid medication.

Caution: Myxedematous patients are unusually sensitive to opiates and may die from average doses.

Refractory hyponatremia may be seen in severe myxedema, possibly due to inappropriate secretion of antidiuretic hormone; however, a defect in distal tubular reabsorption of sodium and water has been recently demonstrated in this disorder. (See Discala reference, below.)

Treatment

A. Specific Therapy: Thyroid or a synthetic preparation is used. The initial dosage varies with the severity of the hypothyroidism.

1. *Caution*—When treating patients with severe myxedema or myxedema heart disease, or elderly patients with hypothyroidism with other associated heart disease, begin with small doses of thyroid, 8–15 mg daily for 1 week, and increase the dose every week by 15 mg daily up to a total of 100–200 mg daily. This dosage should be continued until signs of hypothyroidism have vanished or mild toxic symptoms appear, and the dosage then stabilized to maintain the T_4 at normal levels. An alternative method is the use of small amounts of sodium liothyronine, eg, 5 μg initially with gradual increase to tolerance.

2. Patients with early hypothyroidism may be started with larger doses, 30 mg daily, increasing by 30 mg every week to the limit of tolerance.

3. Maintenance—Each patient's dose must be adjusted to obtain the optimal effect. Most patients require 120–180 mg daily for maintenance. Optimal dosage can be estimated by following the T_4 and TSH levels, but clinical judgment is often the best guide.

4. Levothyroxine sodium (Letter, Synthroid), 0.15–0.3 mg/day, is probably the thyroid drug of choice. Its action is more predictable than that of crude thyroid, T_3, or liotrix. If thyroxine is used, the T_4 should be raised to the high normal level.

5. When a rapid response is necessary, sodium liothyronine (T_3, Cytomel) may be employed. Begin with very low doses because of its speed of action. Begin with 5 μg and increase slowly (see p 714). *Note:* The T_4 cannot be used as a guide to T_3 therapy.

6. Mixtures of T_4 and T_3 in a ratio of 4:1–liotrix (Euthroid, Thyrolar)—have been recently introduced as "complete" replacement therapy (see Smith reference, below).

7. Sodium dextrothyroxine (Choloxin) may be used in cardiac hypothyroid patients who cannot tolerate other thyroid medications, but its value and safety have been questioned recently.

8. **Myxedema coma** is a medical emergency with a high mortality rate. Triiodothyronine, 10–25 μg or more given by stomach tube every 8 hours, or, preferably, levothyroxine sodium (Letter, Synthroid), 200–400 μg IV as a single injection and repeated once in a dose of 100–200 μg in 12 hours, with the addition of hydrocortisone, 100 mg every 8 hours, may be lifesaving. The patient must not be warmed, and adequate pulmonary ventilation must be provided.

9. Suppression of serum TSH will become a useful test of adequate maintenance or replacement therapy in hypothyroidism.

B. Needless Use of Thyroid:

1. Questionable diagnosis—If a patient can tolerate above 200 mg daily of thyroid, the diagnosis of hypothyroidism should be questioned even though some hypothyroid patients require this or larger amounts. Normal individuals and obese and other nonhypothyroid individuals can often tolerate doses up to 300–500 mg daily without changes in BMR or development of toxic symptoms.

2. Nonspecific use of thyroid—The use of thyroid medication as nonspecific stimulating therapy is mentioned only to be condemned. It has been shown that the doses usually employed (100–200 mg) merely suppress the activity of the patient's own gland.

"Metabolic insufficiency" is a questionable entity. The empiric use of thyroid in cases of amenorrhea or infertility warrants further consideration.

Prognosis

The patient may succumb to the complications of the disease if treatment is withheld too long, eg, myxedema coma. With early treatment, striking transformations take place both in appearance and mental function. Return to a normal state is possible, but relapses will occur if treatment is interrupted. On the whole, response to thyroid treatment is most satisfactory in true hypothyroidism, and complete rehabilitation of the patient is possible if treatment is adequate and maintained indefinitely. Chronic maintenance therapy with unduly large doses of thyroid hormone may lead to subtle but important side-effects (eg, bone demineralization).

Becker CE: Coma in myxedema. California Med 110:61, 1969.

Carpenter CCJ & others: Schmidt's syndrome: Thyroid and adrenal insufficiency. Medicine 43:153, 1964.

Cotton GE, Mayberry WE: Suppression of thyrotropin (TSH) in serums of patients with myxedema of varying etiologies treated with thyroid hormones. New England J Med 285:529, 1971.

Discala VA & others: Effects of myxedema on the renal diluting and concentrating mechanism. Am J Med 50:325, 1971.

Lawrence AM & others: The pituitary and primary hypothyroidism. Arch Int Med 132:327, 1973.

Luby E & others: Lithium-carbonate-induced myxedema. JAMA 218:1298, 1971.

Newmark SR, Himathongkam T, Shane JM: Myxedema coma. JAMA 230:884, 1974.

Saben M, Utiger RD: Serum thyroid hormone and thyrotropin concentrations during thyroxine and triiodothyronine therapy. J Clin Endocrinol 39:923, 1974.

Scarpalezos S & others: Neural and muscular manifestations of hypothyroidism. Arch Neurol 29:140, 1973.

Smith RN & others: Controlled clinical trial of combined triiodothyronine and thyroxine in the treatment of hypothyroidism. Lancet 2:145, 1970.

Stock JM, Surks MI, Oppenheimer JH: Replacement dosage of L-thyroxine in hypothyroidism: A reevaluation. New England J Med 290:529, 1974.

Takamori M & others: Myasthenic syndromes in hypothyroidism: Electrophysiological study of neuromuscular transmission and muscle contraction in two patients. Arch Neurol 26:326, 1972.

HYPERTHYROIDISM
(Thyrotoxicosis)

Essentials of Diagnosis

- Weakness, sweating, weight loss, nervousness, loose stools, heat intolerance.
- Tachycardia; warm, thin, soft, moist skin; exophthalmos; stare, tremor.
- Goiter, bruit.
- T_4, radio-T_3 resin uptake, and radioiodine uptake elevated. Failure of suppression by T_3 administration.

General Considerations

Thyrotoxicosis is one of the most common endocrine disorders. Its highest incidence is in women between the ages of 20 and 40. When associated with ocular signs or ocular disturbances and a diffuse goiter, it is called **Graves' disease**. This term, however, is commonly used to mean all forms of hyperthyroidism. Instead of a diffuse goiter, there may be a nodular toxic goiter, or all the metabolic features of thyrotoxicosis may occasionally be present without visible or palpable thyroid enlargement. The latter form is quite common in the elderly patient, who may even lack some of the hypermetabolic signs ("apathetic Graves' disease") but may present with a refractory cardiac illness. Lastly, a poorly understood syndrome of marked eye signs, often without hypermetabolism, may precede, accompany, or follow treatment of thyrotoxicosis, and has been termed hyperexophthalmic Graves' disease, exophthalmic ophthalmoplegia, and malignant (progressive) exophthalmos (infiltrative ophthalmopathy). It has been associated in some instances with the findings of high levels of long-acting thyroid stimulator (LATS), a 7S gamma globulin of extrapituitary origin, although this factor may not be causally related to the disease. LATS is consistently found in the dermopathy ("pretibial myxedema") associated with thyrotoxicosis. Other substances (eg, LATS protector) and evidence for altered cell-mediated immunity have recently been demonstrated in Graves' disease. A rare cause of clinical hyperthyroidism is struma ovarii or hydatidiform mole, although asymptomatic elevation of T_4 may be seen in chorionic tumors, presumably due to ectopic production of TSH.

Clinical Findings

A. Symptoms and Signs: (See Table 18–3.) Restlessness, nervousness, irritability; easy fatigability, especially toward the latter part of the day; and unexplained weight loss in spite of ravenous appetite are often the early features. There is usually excessive sweating and heat intolerance, quick movements with incoordination varying from fine tremulousness to gross tremor. Less commonly, the patient's primary complaint is difficulty in focusing his eyes, pressure from the goiter, diarrhea, or rapid, irregular heart action.

The patient is quick in all motions, including speech. The skin is warm and moist and the hands tremble. A diffuse or nodular goiter may be seen or felt with a thrill or bruit over it. The eyes appear bright, there may be a stare, at times periorbital edema, and commonly lid lag, lack of accommodation, exophthalmos, and even diplopia. The hair and skin are thin and of silky texture. At times there is increased pigmentation of the skin, but vitiligo may also occur. Spider angiomas and gynecomastia are common. Cardiovascular manifestations vary from tachycardia, especially during sleep, to paroxysmal atrial fibrillation and congestive failure of the "high-output" type. At times a harsh pulmonary systolic murmur is heard (Means' murmur). Lymphadenopathy and splenomegaly may be present. Wasting of muscle and bone (osteoporosis)

Table 18–3. Incidence of symptoms and signs observed in 247 patients with thyrotoxicosis.*

Clinical Manifestations	Percent	Clinical Manifestations	Percent
Tachycardia	100	Weakness	70
Goiter†	100	Increased appetite	65
Nervousness	99	Eye complaints	54
Skin changes	97	Swelling of legs	35
Tremor	97	Hyperdefecation (without diarrhea)	33
Hyperhidrosis	91		
Hypersensitivity to heat	89	Diarrhea	23
		Atrial fibrillation	10
Palpitations	89	Splenomegaly	10
Fatigue	88	Gynecomastia	10
Weight loss	85	Anorexia	9
Bruit over thyroid	77	Liver palms	8
Dyspnea	75	Constipation	4
Eye signs	71	Weight gain	2

*Slightly modified and reproduced, with permission, from Williams RH (editor): *Textbook of Endocrinology*, 5th ed. Saunders, 1974.

†Absent in about 3% of patients.

are common features, especially in long-standing thyrotoxicosis. Rarely one finds nausea, vomiting, and even fever and jaundice (in which case the prognosis is poor). Mental changes are common, varying from mild exhilaration to delirium and exhaustion progressing to severe depression.

Associated with severe or malignant exophthalmos is at times a localized, bilateral, hard, nonpitting, symmetric swelling ("pretibial myxedema") over the tibia and dorsum of the feet (infiltrative dermopathy). At times there is clubbing and swelling of the fingers (acropachy). It often subsides spontaneously.

Thyroid "storm," rarely seen today, is an extreme form of thyrotoxicosis, which may occur after iodine refractoriness or thyroid surgery and is manifested by marked delirium, severe tachycardia, vomiting, diarrhea, and dehydration, and often very high fever. The mortality is high.

B. Laboratory Findings: The T_4 level and radioiodine and radio-T_3 uptakes are increased. On rare occasions, the T_4 level may be normal but the serum T_3 elevated ("T_3 thyrotoxicosis"). The radioiodine uptake cannot be suppressed by T_3 administration (see p 657). In toxic nodular goiter, a high radioiodine uptake in the nodule may be diagnostic if combined with elevated T_4 and low TSH levels. Serum cholesterol determinations are low (variable). Postprandial glycosuria is occasionally found. Urinary creatine is increased. Lymphocytosis is common. Urinary and, at times, serum calcium and phosphate are elevated. Serum potassium may be low. Low levels of TSH—and, less consistently, an elevated LATS (long-acting thyroid stimulator) level of unknown source—may be present in the serum or urine, but these tests are not generally available. TSH fails to rise after TRF administration. Increasing evidence for the immunologic basis of thyrotoxicosis is found with refined technics (see Volpe reference, below).

C. X-Ray Findings: Barium swallow may demonstrate low or intrathoracic goiter. Skeletal changes include diffuse demineralization or, at times, resorptive changes (osteitis). Hypertrophic osteoarthropathy with proliferation of periosteal bone may be present, especially in the hands (acropachy).

D. ECG Findings: ECG may show tachycardia, atrial fibrillation, and P and T wave changes.

Differential Diagnosis

The most difficult differentiation is between hyperthyroidism and anxiety neurosis, especially in the menopause. Acute or subacute thyroiditis may present with toxic symptoms, and the gland is usually quite tender. The thyroid antibody test may be positive; T_4 may be elevated, but radioiodine uptake is very low. Exogenous thyroid administration will present the same laboratory features as thyroiditis. A rare chorionic or pituitary tumor may produce the picture of thyrotoxicosis with high levels of TSH. A hypermetabolic state due mainly to overproduction of T_3 has recently been described ("T_3 thyrotoxicosis"; see Sterling reference, below). The T_4 is normal or low

and the radioiodine uptake is normal or moderately elevated but fails to be suppressed by T_3 administration. Serum T_3 is elevated.

Some states of hypermetabolism without thyrotoxicosis, notably severe anemia, leukemia, polycythemia, and malignancy, rarely cause confusion. Pheochromocytoma and acromegaly, however, may be associated with high BMR, with enlargement of the thyroid gland and profuse sweating, and make differentiation difficult.

Cardiac disease (eg, atrial fibrillation, failure) refractory to treatment with digitalis, quinidine, or diuretics suggests the possibility of underlying hyperthyroidism. Other causes of ophthalmoplegia (eg, myasthenia gravis) and exophthalmos (eg, orbital tumor) must be considered. Thyrotoxicosis must also be considered in the differential diagnosis of muscle wasting diseases and diffuse bone atrophy. Hypercalciuria and bone demineralization may resemble hyperparathyroidism. The 2 diseases may be present in the same patient. Diabetes mellitus and Addison's disease may coexist with thyrotoxicosis.

Complications

The ocular and cardiac complications of long-standing thyrotoxicosis are most serious. Severe malnutrition and wasting with cachexia may become irreversible. If jaundice is present, the mortality increases. Periodic paralysis may complicate thyrotoxicosis. Thyroid "storm" (see p 668) is rarely seen but may be fatal. Malignancy rarely accompanies toxic goiter. Complications of treatment for goiter include drug reactions following iodine and thiouracil treatment, hypoparathyroidism and laryngeal palsy from surgical treatment, and progressive exophthalmos. The exophthalmos may progress despite adequate therapy to the point of corneal ulceration and destruction of the globe unless orbital decompression is done. Hypercalcemia and nephrocalcinosis may occur.

Treatment

Treatment is aimed at halting excessive secretion of the thyroid hormone. Several methods are available; the method of choice is still being debated and varies with different patients. The most widely accepted method in the past has been subtotal removal after adequate preparation. There is a greater tendency toward trying long-term medical treatment with antithyroid drugs to achieve remission of the disease and to use radioactive iodine therapy rather than surgical thyroidectomy for thyroid ablation except for large multinodular glands. (*Note:* In this discussion, the term BMR is used in a clinical sense, since laboratory determinations of T_4, T_3, etc have virtually replaced spirometry.)

A. Subtotal Thyroidectomy: Adequate preparation is of the utmost importance. One or 2 drugs are generally necessary for adequate preparation: one of the thiouracil group of drugs alone, or, preferably, a thiouracil plus iodine. Recent reports of the successful use of sympatholytic agents as a mode of preoperative management offer an alternative to the thiouracils. (See Michie reference, below).

1. Thiouracil and similar drugs—Several thiouracil drugs or similar derivatives are available: propylthiouracil, methimazole, and one containing iodine in the molecule, iothiouracil (Itrumil). The modes of action of the first 2 are probably identical; the mode of action of iothiouracil is still not entirely clear, and this drug is of questionable value.

Propylthiouracil has been most widely used and appears to be the least toxic. It is the thiouracil preparation of choice. When given in adequate dosage, propylthiouracil prevents the thyroid gland from transforming inorganic iodine into its organic (hormonal) form. This effect is rapid (within a few hours) and continues as long as the drug is given. As the level of circulating hormone falls, TSH elaboration rises slowly. The BMR and T_4 invariably fall, the rate of fall depending upon the total quantity of previously manufactured hormone available from the gland or in the circulating blood. (More hormone is present if iodine has been given previously.) The average time required for the BMR to return to normal is about 4—8 weeks. If the drug is continued, the BMR will continue to fall until the patient becomes myxedematous.

Preparation is usually continued and surgery deferred until the T_4 and T_3 uptake are normal. There is no need to rush surgery and no danger of "escape" as with iodine. In severe cases, 100—200 mg 4 times daily (spaced as close to every 6 hours as possible) is generally adequate. Larger doses (eg, for patients with very large glands) are occasionally necessary. In milder cases, 100 mg 3 times daily are sufficient, although the larger doses are not necessarily more harmful.

Propylthiouracil appears to be an ideal drug except for 2 disadvantages: the danger of toxic reactions (especially granulocytopenia) and interference with surgery. Toxic reactions to propylthiouracil are rare, however, and could be anticipated if the patient were examined weekly and a weekly or a biweekly blood count taken, but this is rarely feasible. In practice, patients are instructed to watch for fever, sore throat, or rash and to notify their physicians immediately if any of these occurs so that blood count and examination can be performed. If the white count falls below 3000/cu mm or if less than 45% granulocytes are present, therapy should be discontinued. Other rare reactions are drug fever, rash, and jaundice. The second objection is of a technical nature; since the gland may remain hyperplastic and vascular, surgical removal is more difficult. For this reason, combined therapy, using propylthiouracil and iodine, is the method of choice in preparing patients for thyroidectomy (see below).

Methimazole (Tapazole) has a mode of action similar to that of the thiouracils. The average dose is 10—15 mg every 8 hours. The smaller dosage is no guarantee against toxic reactions, especially skin rash, which are more common with this drug than with the thiouracils.

2. Iodine—Iodine is given in daily dosages of 5—10 drops of strong iodine solution (Lugol's solution) or saturated solution of potassium iodide with nonspecific therapy (see below) until the BMR has dropped toward normal, the signs and symptoms have become less marked, and the patient has begun to gain weight. The disadvantages of preparation with iodine are that (1) a few patients may not respond, especially those who have received iodine recently; (2) sensitivity to iodides may be present; (3) if there is too long a wait before surgery, the gland may "escape" and the patient develops a more severe hyperthyroidism than before; and (4) it is generally impossible to reduce the BMR to normal with iodine alone.

3. Combined propylthiouracil-iodine therapy—The advantage of this method is that one obtains the complete inhibition of thyroid secretion with the involuting effect of iodine. This can be done in one of 2 ways:

Propylthiouracil followed by iodine appears at present to be the method of choice. Begin therapy with propylthiouracil; about 10—21 days before surgery is contemplated (when all thyroid tests have returned to normal or low normal range), begin the iodine and *continue* for 1 week after surgery.

Concomitant administration of the 2 drugs from the start in dosages as for the individual drugs, ie, 100—200 mg propylthiouracil 4 times daily and strong iodine solution, 10—15 drops daily. This method is less commonly used and less desirable than sequential administration (outlined above).

Patients who fail to be euthyroid after subtotal thyroidectomy can be re-treated with propylthiouracil or with radioiodine.

B. Continuous Propylthiouracil Therapy (Medical Treatment): Control of hyperthyroidism with propylthiouracil alone, without surgery, is advocated by some. The advantage is that it avoids the risks and postoperative complications of surgery, eg, myxedema, hypoparathyroidism. The disadvantage is the remote possibility of toxic reactions plus the necessity of watching the patient carefully for signs of hypothyroidism. Since the advent of propylthiouracil, it appears that the incidence of toxic reactions is slight.

Begin with 100—200 mg every 6—8 hours and continue until the T_4 and T_3 uptake are normal and all signs and symptoms of the disease have subsided; then place the patient on a maintenance dose of 50—150 mg daily, observing the thyroid function tests periodically to avoid hypothyroidism.

An alternative method is to continue with doses of 50—200 mg every 6—8 hours until the patient becomes hypothyroid and then maintain the T_4 at normal levels with thyroid hormone. (This may be the preferred treatment of exophthalmic goiter.)

The duration of therapy and the recurrence rate with nonsurgical therapy have not been completely worked out. At present it would seem that of the patients kept on propylthiouracil between 6 and 18 months (the dosage slowly decreased), about 50—70% will have no recurrence. Increasing the duration of therapy to about 2 years or more does not increase the "cure" rate. Periodic T_3 suppression tests of ^{131}I uptake after 6 months of therapy may help predict the likelihood of remission of the disease in a given patient. (See Alexander reference, below.) Those having recurrences after cessation of treatment may be treated again with propylthiouracil, with radioiodine, or with surgery.

C. Continuous Iodine Therapy: In the past this method was used in selected cases of mild hyperthyroidism with fair results; however, because of the danger of "escape" and because propylthiouracil is a better drug, iodine should be used only for preoperative preparation. *Note:* Iodide administration to patients rendered euthyroid after treatment of toxic goiter may induce myxedema.

D. Radioactive Iodine (^{131}I): The administration of radioiodine has proved to be an excellent method for destruction of over-functioning thyroid tissue (either diffuse or toxic nodular goiter). The rationale of treatment is that the radioiodine, being concentrated in the thyroid, will destroy the cells that concentrate it. The only objections to date to radioiodine therapy are the possibility of carcinogenesis and the possibility that an early carcinoma which might be removed surgically may remain undetected. For these reasons, the use of radioiodine should generally be limited to older age groups (40 or above); however, the age level is not absolute, and some children may be best treated with radioiodine. *Do not use this drug in pregnant women.* A high incidence of hypothyroidism several years after this form of treatment has recently been recognized, but this has also been found in patients treated in other ways and may be the natural course of the disease. Prolonged follow-up, preferably with T_4 and TSH measurements, is therefore mandatory. There is a greater tendency toward higher-dosage radioiodine ablation of the toxic gland, with subsequent permanent replacement therapy with thyroid hormone, rather than using smaller doses initially, which may require retreatment and may still fail to prevent appearance of myxedema several years later.

E. General Measures:

1. The patient with hyperthyroidism should be at bed rest, especially in severe cases and in preparation for surgery. Mild cases may be treated with propylthiouracil or radioiodine on an ambulatory basis. However, early bed rest hastens recovery.

2. Diet should be high in calories, proteins, and vitamins. Hyperthyroid patients consume great quantities of food, are generally in negative nitrogen and calcium balance, and need the excess foods and vitamins because of their increased metabolic needs. Supplemental vitamin B complex should be given.

3. Sedation—When first seen, these patients are often very nervous. Sedation is always helpful, and large doses, eg, phenobarbital, 30 mg 3—6 times daily, may be necessary.

4. Since many signs resemble the effects of catecholamines, sympathetic blocking agents (reserpine, guanethidine, propranolol) have been recommended. Their use is controversial and should probably be restricted to states of extreme excitability, eg, thyrotoxic storm (see below). Propranolol is especially useful in rapidly controlling tachycardia and cardiac irregularities, but it must be used cautiously in incipient or frank failure. It is especially effective in patients with neuromuscular signs, eg, periodic paralysis or upper motor neuron signs.

F. Treatment of Complications:

1. **Exophthalmos**—The exact cause of exophthalmos in hyperthyroidism is still not known. Although it may be due to excessive secretion of a hormone (EPS?) which is different from TSH or from LATS (long-acting thyroid stimulator), the evidence is still inconclusive. It has been shown that exophthalmos is due to edema and later cellular infiltration of the retrobulbar tissues. Removing the thyroid secretion (extirpation or administration of propylthiouracil) does not necessarily help this condition and may possibly even aggravate it, leading to malignant exophthalmos. It has been suggested that this is because the thyroid secretion exerts an inhibitory effect on the anterior pituitary, and removal of the gland allows the anterior pituitary to secrete more hormones and aggravate the condition. Therefore, it would seem rational to treat exophthalmos by giving thyroid orally. However, since the pituitary TSH levels are usually low in thyrotoxicosis, it is questionable whether such therapy is of use in exophthalmos unless the patient is becoming hypothyroid.

(1) Thyroid—Immediately after surgery, or after the T_4 has returned to normal with propylthiouracil therapy, begin giving thyroid, 100—200 mg daily, or levothyroxine sodium, 0.1—0.3 mg daily. Give a dosage which is adequate to maintain the T_4 at high normal levels. Although it is not always effective, this therapy should be used whenever there is a tendency for progression of the exophthalmos or the presence of hypothyroidism.

(2) Dark glasses, protection from dust, eye shields, tarsorrhaphy, and other measures may be necessary to protect the eyes. Ophthalmologic consultation should be requested.

(3) Corticotropin (ACTH) or corticosteroids in large doses have proved helpful in some cases. They act by reducing the inflammatory reaction in the periorbital tissues. They may also reduce the level of LATS.

(4) Estrogen treatment has been used with some benefit, especially in the postmenopausal age group.

(5) Surgery for malignant exophthalmos—Every patient with exophthalmos should be measured periodically with an exophthalmometer; do not rely upon clinical judgment to determine whether or not exophthalmos is present or progressing. In severe progressive cases, where corneal edema or ulceration, limitation of extraocular muscle movements, and failing vision occur, orbital decompression may be necessary to save the eyesight.

(6) There have been a few encouraging reports on the use of pituitary stalk section or even hypophysectomy with yttrium in severe malignant exophthalmos; however, since EPS and LATS are probably extrapitui-

tary in origin, the rationale of such procedures is questionable. The recently reported cases of hyperthyroidism in the presence of panhypopituitarism (see Krishnamurthy reference, below) make this therapy even more irrational. Orbital irradiation may be helpful (see Donaldson reference, below). Immunosuppressive therapy has also been suggested.

(7) Ultrasonography may become a simple and useful tool for diagnosis and follow-up of thyroidal eye disease (see Werner reference, below).

2. Cardiac complications—A number of cardiac complications are at times associated with hyperthyroidism.

(1) Some degree of tachycardia is almost always found if normal rhythm is present in thyrotoxicosis. This requires only the treatment of the thyrotoxicosis. Reserpine is at times helpful. Phentolamine (Regitine), guanethidine (Ismelin), or propranolol (Inderal) may be preferable drugs.

(2) Congestive failure tends to occur in longstanding thyrotoxicosis, especially in the older age groups. Treatment is the same as for congestive failure due to any cause. Digitalis seems to be effective in congestive failure associated with thyrotoxicosis.

(3) Atrial fibrillation may occur in association with thyrotoxicosis. Treat as any other atrial fibrillation, but do not try to convert the atrial fibrillation in a toxic patient. Most cases will revert to normal rhythm soon after toxicity is removed. However, if fibrillation remains for 2 weeks after surgery or for 2–4 weeks after BMR or other thyroid function tests have returned to normal with propylthiouracil therapy, and if no contraindications are present, one should consider using quinidine to convert to a normal rhythm.

3. "Crisis" or "storm"—Fortunately, this condition is rare with modern therapy. It occurs now mainly in patients inadequately prepared with propylthiouracil and iodine, those with complicating infection, immediately after subtotal thyroidectomy, or, rarely, after ^{131}I therapy. It can occur spontaneously or after any sudden stress in an untreated patient with thyrotoxicosis. It is characterized by high fever, tachycardia, CNS irritability, and delirium. The cause is uncertain, but absolute or relative adrenocortical insufficiency may be a contributing factor. Large doses of the rapidly acting corticosteroids may be lifesaving. Give additional large doses of propylthiouracil by nasogastric tube. Sodium iodide, 1–2 gm IV and repeated every 12–24 hours, has also been advocated. Large doses of corticosteroids, reserpine or guanethidine, or, preferably, propranolol intravenously may be of value. Plasmapheresis has been used in cases not responsive to the above measure (see Ashkar reference, below). Cholestyramine, which binds thyroid hormone in the gut, is an alternative drug. General measures consist of oxygen, cold packs, and sedation.

Prognosis

Thyrotoxicosis is a cyclic disease and may subside spontaneously. More commonly, however, it progresses, especially with recurrent psychic trauma, pregnancy, and other types of stress. The ocular, cardiac, and psychic complications often are more serious than the chronic wasting of tissues and may become irreversible even after treatment. Progressive exophthalmos is perhaps more common after surgical than after "medical" thyroidectomy. Hypoparathyroidism and vocal cord palsy are usually permanent after surgical thyroidectomy. With any form of therapy, unless radical thyroidectomy or large dosage ^{131}I therapy is used, recurrence rates are about 20–30%, especially if thyrotoxicosis is diffuse. With adequate treatment and long-term follow-up, the results are good. It is perhaps wiser to speak of induced remission rather than cure. Post-treatment hypothyroidism is common. It may occur several years after radioactive iodine therapy or subtotal thyroidectomy. Although benign and even malignant thyroid neoplasms may occur following radioiodine treatment, a recent survey shows that the incidence is no greater than after subtotal thyroidectomy (see Dobyns reference, below).

Patients with jaundice and fever have a less favorable prognosis. Thyrotoxic periodic paralysis with hypokalemia—to which males of certain races (Japanese, Chinese) are predisposed—may alter the prognosis. Periorbital swelling and chemosis often precede serious and progressive malignant exophthalmos leading to blindness, and must be watched carefully.

Although it is rare, thyroid storm has the worst prognosis. It is best avoided by careful preoperative preparation of the patient rather than treated once it appears.

Adams DD, Kennedy TH, Stewart RDH: Correlation between long-acting thyroid stimulator protector level and thyroid ^{131}I uptake in thyrotoxicosis. Brit MJ 2:199, 1974.

Alexander WD & others: Prediction of long-term results of antithyroid drug therapy for thyrotoxicosis. J Clin Endocrinol 30:540, 1970.

Ashkar FS & others: Thyroid storm treatment with blood exchange and plasmapheresis. JAMA 214:1275, 1970.

Barnes HV, Gann DS: Choosing thyroidectomy in hyperthyroidism. S Clin North America 54:289, 1974.

Bernard JD & others: Thyrotoxic periodic paralysis in Californians of Mexican and Filipino ancestry. California Med 116:70, Feb 1972.

Braverman LE, Woeber KA, Ingbar SH: Induction of myxedema by iodide in patients euthyroid after treatment of toxic goiter. New England J Med 281:816, 1969.

Brown W & others: Hyperthyroidism due to struma ovarii: Demonstration by radioiodine scan. Acta endocrinol 72:266, 1973.

Conway MJ & others: Thyrotoxicosis and periodic paralysis: Improvement with beta blockade. Ann Int Med 81:332, 1974.

Das G, Krieger M: Treatment of thyrotoxic storm with intravenous administration of propranolol. Ann Int Med 70:985, 1969.

Davis PJ, Davis FB: Hyperthyroidism in patients over the age of 60 years. Medicine 53:161, 1974.

Dillon PT & others: Reserpine in thyrotoxic crisis. New England J Med 283:1020, 1970.

Dobyns BM & others: Malignant and benign neoplasms of the thyroid in patients treated for hyperthyroidism: A report of the cooperative thyrotoxicosis therapy follow-up study. J Clin Endocrinol 38:976, 1974.

Donaldson SS & others: Supervoltage orbital radiotherapy for Graves' disease. J Clin Endocrinol 37:276, 1973.

Dumlao JS: Thyroid storm. Postgrad Med 56:57, 1974.

Hadden DR & others: Propranolol and iodine-131 in the management of thyrotoxicosis. Lancet 2:852, 1968.

Hamburger JI: *Hyperthyroidism–Concept and Controversy.* Thomas, 1972.

Hamilton CR Jr, Adams LC, Maloof F: Hyperthyroidism due to thyrotropin-producing pituitary chromophobe adenoma. New England J Med 283:1077, 1970.

Hayek A, Chapman EM, Crawford JD: Long-term results of ^{131}I treatment of thyrotoxicosis in children. New England J Med 283:949, 1970.

Hershman JM, Higgins HP: Hydatidiform mole: A cause of clinical hyperthyroidism. New England J Med 284:573, 1971.

Hoffenberg R: Aetiology of hyperthyroidism. Brit MJ 3:452, 1974.

Krishnamurthy GT, Blahd WH: Hyperthyroidism in the presence of panhypopituitarism: Thyroid crisis and hypothyroidism following radioiodine treatment. Western J Med 120:491, 1974.

Mestman JH & others: Hyperthyroidism and pregnancy. Arch Int Med 134:434, 1974.

Michie W & others: Beta-blockade and partial thyroidectomy for thyrotoxicosis. Lancet 1:1009, 1974.

Parker JZW, Lawson DH: Death from thyrotoxicosis. Lancet 2:894, 1973.

Resnick JS, Dorman JD, Engel WK: Thyrotoxic periodic paralysis. Am J Med 47:831, 1969.

Roizen M, Becker C: Thyroid storm: A review of cases at University of California, San Francisco. California Med 115:5, Oct 1971.

Rothberg MP & others: Propranolol and hyperthyroidism: Reversal of upper motor neuron signs. JAMA 230:1017, 1974.

Shenkman L & others: Recurrent hyperthyroidism presenting as triiodothyronine toxicosis. Ann Int Med 77:410, 1972.

Sterling K & others: T_3 thyrotoxicosis. JAMA 213:571, 1970.

Symposium on Graves' disease (2nd Keating Symposium). (2 parts.) Mayo Clin Proc 47:783, 897, 1972.

Toft AD & others: Plasma TSH and serum T-4 levels in long-term follow-up of patients treated with ^{131}I for thyrotoxicosis. Brit MJ 3:152, 1974.

Volpe R & others: Peripheral thymus-dependent lymphocytes in Graves' disease and Hashimoto's thyroiditis. New England J Med 288:1313, 1973.

Werner SC, Coleman DJ, Franzen LA: Ultrasonographic evidence of consistent orbital involvement in Graves' disease. New England J Med 290:1447, 1974.

CARCINOMA OF THYROID GLAND

Essentials of Diagnosis

- Painless swelling in region of thyroid, or thyroid nodule not responding to suppression.
- Normal thyroid function tests.
- Past history of irradiation to neck, goiter, or thyroiditis.

General Considerations

Although carcinoma of the thyroid is rarely associated with functional abnormalities, it enters into the differential diagnosis of all types of thyroid lesions. Recent evidence suggests that it may be the end result of long-standing overstimulation of the thyroid gland by pituitary TSH, especially in certain types of goiter and thyroiditis. It is common in all age groups, but especially in patients who have received irradiation therapy to the neck structures (eg, thymus gland). The cell type determines to a large extent the type of therapy required and the prognosis for survival.

Clinical Findings

A. Symptoms and Signs: The principal signs of thyroid cancer are a painless nodule, a hard nodule in an enlarged thyroid gland, so-called lateral aberrant thyroid tissue, or palpable lymph nodes with thyroid enlargement. Signs of pressure or invasion of the neck structures are present in anaplastic or long-standing tumors. A rare patient with medullary carcinoma may present with hypocalcemic tetany due to calcitonin excess.

B. Laboratory Findings: With very few exceptions, all thyroid function tests are normal unless the disease

Table 18–4. Some characteristics of thyroid cancer.

	Papillary	Follicular	Amyloidic Solid	Anaplastic
Incidence*(%)	61	18	6	15
Average age*	42	50	50	57
Females*(%)	70	72	56	56
Deaths due to thyroid cancer*†(%)	6	24	33	98
Invasion: Juxtanodal	+++++	+	++++++	+++
Blood vessels	+	+++	+++	+++++
Distant sites	+	+++	++	++++
Resemblance to thyroid	+	+++	+	±
^{131}I uptake	+	++++	+	0
Degree of malignancy	+	++ to +++	+++	+++++++

*Data based upon 885 cases analyzed by Woolner & others; figures have been rounded to the nearest digit. (After Woolner.)

†Some patients have been followed up to 32 years after diagnosis.

is associated with thyroiditis. The scintigram usually shows a "cold nodule." Serum autoantibodies are sometimes found. Hypocalcemia is only rarely present in medullary carcinoma, but the calcitonin levels are elevated, especially after a calcium infusion (see Deftos reference, below). Calcitonin assay is a reliable clue to silent medullary carcinoma, especially in the familial syndrome, although an occasional extrathyroidal tumor (eg, lung) may also produce calcitonin.

C. X-Ray Findings: Extensive bone and soft tissue metastases (some of which may take up radioiodine) may be demonstrable.

Differential Diagnosis

Since nonmalignant enlargements of the thyroid gland are far more common than carcinoma, it is at times most difficult to establish the diagnosis except by biopsy (which should be an open biopsy rather than needle biopsy). Echography may be helpful in differentiating cystic and solid nodules (see Blum reference, below). The incidence of malignancy is much greater in single than in multinodular lesions, and far greater in nonfunctioning than in functioning nodules. The T_3 suppression test is of some value in differentiating benign from autonomous lesions. The differentiation from chronic thyroiditis is at times most difficult, and the 2 lesions may occur together. Any nonfunctioning lesion in the region of the thyroid which does not decrease in size on thyroid therapy or increases rapidly must be considered carcinoma until proved otherwise.

Table 18–5. Differential diagnosis of thyroid nodules.*

Clinical Evidence	Low Index of Suspicion	High Index of Suspicion
History	Familial history of goiter Residence in area of endemic goiter	Previous therapeutic irradiation of head, neck, or chest Hoarseness
Physical characteristics	Older women Soft nodule Multinodular goiter	Children, young adults; men Solitary, firm, dominant nodule Vocal cord paralysis Enlarged lymph nodes Distant metastatic lesions
Serum factors	High titer of antithyroid antibody	Elevated serum calcitonin
Scanning technics Uptake of ^{131}I Echo scan Thermography Roentgenogram Technetium flow	 "Hot" nodules Cystic lesion Cold Shell-like calcification Avascular	 "Cold" nodule Solid lesion Warm Punctate calcification Vascular
Thyroxine therapy	Regression after 0.3 mg per day for 3 months or more	No regression

*Reproduced, with permission, from Greenspan FS: Thyroid nodules and thyroid cancer. Western J Med 121:359, 1974.

Complications

The complications vary with the type of carcinoma. Papillary tumors invade local structures, such as lymph nodes; follicular tumors metastasize through the blood stream; anaplastic carcinomas invade local structures, causing constriction and nerve palsies, as well as leading to widespread metastases. The complications of radical neck surgery often include permanent hypoparathyroidism, vocal cord palsy, and myxedema.

Medullary carcinoma may be associated with pheochromocytoma and hyperparathyroidism (Sipple's syndrome). Elevated calcitonin levels have been demonstrated in this tumor, although hypocalcemia rarely occurs.

Treatment

Surgical removal, if possible, is the treatment of choice for most thyroid carcinomas. Papillary tumors may respond to thyroid suppressive treatment, which may also be of value in other types (especially after most of the functioning gland has been removed). Some follicular tumors have been treated with radioiodine; metastases may take up radioactive iodine after thyroidectomy or iodide depletion. External irradiation may be useful for local as well as distant metastases. Postoperative myxedema and hypoparathyroidism must be treated in the usual manner.

Recent reports of chemotherapy of inoperable tumors with adriamycin are encouraging, but the drug is fairly toxic (see Gottlieb reference, below).

Prognosis

The prognosis is apparently directly related to the cell type. The anaplastic carcinomas advance rapidly in spite of early diagnosis and treatment, while papillary tumors—in spite of frequent bouts of recurrence—are almost never fatal. Early detection and removal of medullary carcinomas by finding elevated calcitonin levels may lead to a better prognosis. In general, the prognosis is less favorable in elderly patients.

Blum M: Clinical applications of thyroid echography. New England J Med 287:1164, 1972.

Cunliffe WJ & others: A calcitonin-secreting medullary thyroid carcinoma associated with mucosa neuromas, marfanoid features, myopathy, and pigmentation. Am J Med 48:120, 1970.

Deftos LJ: Radioimmunoassay for calcitonin in medullary thyroid carcinoma. JAMA 227:403, 1974.

Geissinger WT & others: Carcinoma of the thyroid. Ann Surg 179:734, 1974.

Goltzman D & others: Calcitonin as a tumor marker in patients with medullary thyroid carcinoma. New England J Med 290:1035, 1974.

Gottlieb JA, Hill CS Jr: Chemotherapy of thyroid cancer with adriamycin: Experience with 30 patients. New England J Med 290:193, 1974.

Greenspan FS: Thyroid nodules and thyroid cancer. Western J Med 121:359, 1974.

Harness JK & others: Differentiated thyroid carcinomas: Treatment of distant metastases. Arch Surg 108:410, 1974.

Keiser HR & others: Sipple's syndrome: Medullary thyroid carcinoma, pheochromocytoma, and parathyroid disease: Studies in a large family. Ann Int Med 78:561, 1973.

Kyriakides G, Sosin H: Anaplastic carcinoma of the thyroid. Ann Surg 179:295, 1974.

Miskin M & others: B-mode ultrasonography in assessment of thyroid gland lesions. Ann Int Med 79:505, 1973.

Rashid AK & others: Mucosal neuroma, pheochromocytoma and medullary thyroid carcinoma: Multiple endocrine neoplasia type 3. Medicine 54:89, 1975.

Silva OL & others: Ectopic secretion of calcitonin by oat-cell carcinoma. New England J Med 290:1122, 1974.

Wilson SM & others: Thyroid carcinoma after irradiation. Arch Surg 100:330, 1971.

Wolfe HJ & others: C-cell hyperplasia preceding medullary thyroid carcinoma. New England J Med 289:437, 1973.

THYROIDITIS

Essentials of Diagnosis

- Painful swelling of thyroid gland, causing pressure symptoms in acute and subacute forms; painless enlargement in chronic.
- Thyroid function tests variable; discrepancy in PBI, T_4, and radioiodine uptake common.
- Serologic autoantibody tests often positive.

General Considerations

Thyroiditis has been more frequently diagnosed in recent years since special serologic tests for thyroid autoantibodies became available. This heterogeneous group can be divided into 2 groups: (1) due to a specific cause (usually infection), and (2) due to unknown, often autoimmune factors. The second is the most common form.

Clinical Findings

A. Symptoms and Signs:

1. Thyroiditis due to specific causes (pyogenic infections, tuberculosis, syphilis)—A rare disorder causing severe pain, tenderness, redness, and fluctuation in the region of the thyroid gland.

2. Nonspecific (?autoimmune) thyroiditis—

a. Acute or subacute nonsuppurative thyroiditis (De Quervain's thyroiditis, granulomatous thyroiditis, giant cell thyroiditis, giant follicular thyroiditis)—An acutely painful enlargement of the thyroid gland, with dysphagia. The pain radiates into the ears. The manifestations may persist for several weeks and may be associated with signs of thyrotoxicosis and malaise. Middle-aged women are most commonly affected. Viral infection has been suggested as the cause.

b. Hashimoto's thyroiditis (struma lymphomatosa, lymphadenoid goiter, chronic lymphocytic thyroiditis)—This is the most common form of thyroiditis, and is seen principally in middle-aged women. Onset of enlargement of the thyroid gland is insidious, with few pressure symptoms. Signs of thyroid dysfunction seldom appear, but in a few cases the disease may progress to myxedema or even to late thyrotoxicosis.

(See Gavras reference, below.) The gland may show marked enlargement.

c. Riedel's thyroiditis (chronic fibrous thyroiditis, Riedel's struma, woody thyroiditis, ligneous thyroiditis, invasive thyroiditis)—This is the rarest form of thyroiditis and is found only in middle-aged women. Enlargement is often asymmetric; the gland is stone hard and adherent to the neck structures, causing signs of compression and invasion, including dysphagia, dyspnea, and hoarseness.

B. Laboratory Findings: The PBI, T_4, and T_3 uptake of red cells or resin are usually markedly elevated in acute and subacute thyroiditis and normal or low in the chronic forms. Radioiodine uptake is characteristically very low in subacute thyroiditis; it may be high in chronic thyroiditis with enlargement of the gland, and low in Riedel's struma. The TSH stimulation test shows lack of response in most forms of thyroiditis. Leukocytosis, elevation of the sedimentation rate, and increase in serum globulins are common in acute and subacute forms. Thyroid autoantibodies are most commonly demonstrable in Hashimoto's thyroiditis but are also found in the other types. The serum TSH level is elevated if inadequate amounts of biologically active thyroid hormones are elaborated by the thyroid gland.

Complications

In the suppurative forms of thyroiditis any of the complications of infection may occur; the subacute and chronic forms of the disease are complicated by the effects of pressure on the neck structures: inanition, dyspnea, and, in Riedel's struma, vocal cord palsy. Many patients remain permanently myxedematous when the disease process subsides. Carcinoma may be associated with chronic thyroiditis and must be considered in the diagnosis of uneven painless enlargements which continue in spite of treatment. Chronic thyroiditis may be associated with Addison's disease (Schmidt's syndrome), thymoma, various collagen diseases, cirrhosis, and gonadal dysgenesis.

Differential Diagnosis

Thyroiditis must be considered in the differential diagnosis of all types of goiters, especially if enlargement is rapid. In the acute or subacute stages it may simulate thyrotoxicosis, and only a careful evaluation of several of the laboratory findings will point to the correct diagnosis. The very low radioiodine uptake in subacute thyroiditis with elevated T_4 and T_3 uptake and a very rapid sedimentation rate is of the greatest help. Chronic thyroiditis, especially if the enlargement is uneven and if there is pressure and invasion of surrounding structures, may resemble carcinoma, and both disorders may be present in the same gland. The subacute and suppurative forms of thyroiditis may resemble any infectious process in or near the neck structures; and the presence of malaise, leukocytosis, and a high sedimentation rate is confusing. The thyroid autoantibody tests have been of help in the diagnosis of chronic thyroiditis, but the tests are not specific and may also be positive in patients with goiters, carcinoma, and occasionally even in thyrotoxicosis. Biopsy may be required for diagnosis.

Treatment

A. Suppurative Thyroiditis: Antibiotics, and surgical drainage when fluctuation is marked.

B. Subacute Thyroiditis: All treatment is empiric, and must be maintained for several weeks since the recurrence rate is high. Corticotropin or corticosteroid treatment is often helpful, especially in the early stages. Salicylates in large doses (6–8 gm/day) may be given for pain. Desiccated thyroid, 120–200 mg (2–3 gr), or thyroxine, 0.2–0.3 mg, may be helpful in shrinking the size of the gland after toxic symptoms have subsided. Low-dosage x-ray therapy (600–1200 R) has been used in the past when other measures have failed, but it is of doubtful value. Propylthiouracil, 100–200 mg every 8 hours, or methimazole, 20–40 mg every 8 hours, may decrease tenderness and toxic symptoms.

Thyroidectomy is rarely required; splitting of the isthmus to relieve pressure and for biopsy is the procedure of choice.

C. Hashimoto's Thyroiditis: Thyroid, thyroxine, or triiodothyronine in full doses may reduce the size of the gland markedly; since the disease will often progress to myxedema, this treatment probably should be continued indefinitely. Corticosteroid treatment often reduces the gland rapidly (this may be of diagnostic help). X-ray therapy, propylthiouracil, and partial thyroidectomy are rarely required.

D. Riedel's struma often requires partial thyroidectomy to relieve pressure; adhesions to surrounding structures make this a difficult operation.

Prognosis

The course of this group of diseases is quite variable. Spontaneous remissions and exacerbations are common in the subacute form, and therapy is nonspecific. The disease process may smolder for weeks. Thyrotoxicosis may occur. The chronic form may be part of a systemic collagen disease (eg, lupus erythematosus, Sjögren's syndrome) with all of the complications of that disease. Recurrent subacute and, more often, chronic thyroiditis lead to permanent destruction of the thyroid gland in a large number of patients and to myxedema. Continuous thyroid replacement therapy, by suppressing TSH, may shrink the gland. It may also lessen the tendency of malignant transformation in chronic thyroiditis.

Colcock BP, Pena O: Diagnosis and treatment of thyroiditis. Postgrad Med 44:83, 1968.

Dawson MA: Thymoma associated with pancytopenia and Hashimoto's thyroiditis. Am J Med 53:406, 1972.

Gavras I, Thomson JA: Late thyrotoxicosis complicating autoimmune thyroiditis. Acta endocrinol 69:41, 1972.

Greene JN: Subacute thyroiditis. Am J Med 51:97, 1971.

Hamburger JI: Subacute thyroiditis: Diagnostic difficulties and simple treatment. J Nuclear Med 15:81, 1974.

Papapetrou PD & others: Long-term treatment of Hashimoto's thyroiditis with thyroxine. Lancet 2:1045, 1972.

Rallison ML & others: Occurrence and natural history of chronic lymphocytic thyroiditis in childhood. J Pediat 86:675, 1975.

Tung KSK, Ramos CV, Deodhar SD: Antithyroid antibodies in juvenile lymphocytic thyroiditis. Am J Clin Path 61:549, 1974.

THE PARATHYROIDS*

HYPOPARATHYROIDISM & PSEUDOHYPOPARATHYROIDISM

Essentials of Diagnosis

- Tetany, carpopedal spasms, stridor and wheezing, muscle and abdominal cramps, urinary frequency, personality changes, mental torpor.
- Positive Chvostek's sign and Trousseau's phenomenon; defective nails and teeth; cataracts.
- Serum calcium low; serum phosphate high; alkaline phosphatase normal; urine calcium (Sulkowitch) negative.
- Basal ganglia calcification on x-ray of skull.

General Considerations

A deficiency of parathyroid hormone is most commonly seen following thyroidectomy or, more rarely, following surgery for parathyroid tumor. Very rarely it follows x-ray irradiation to the neck or massive radioactive iodine administration for cancer of the thyroid. Partial hypoparathyroidism occurs in a significant number of patients after thyroidectomy.

Transient hypoparathyroidism may be seen in the neonatal period, presumably due to a relative underactivity of the parathyroid; or to extraordinary demands on the parathyroids by the intake of cow's milk containing a great deal of phosphate. A similar mechanism may operate in the tetany of pregnancy.

Neonatal tetany may be a manifestation of maternal hyperparathyroidism.

Idiopathic hypoparathyroidism, often associated with candidiasis, may be familial and may be associated with Addison's disease.

Pseudohypoparathyroidism is a genetic defect associated with short stature, round face, obesity, short metacarpals, hypertension, and ectopic bone formation. The parathyroids are present and often hyperplastic, but the renal tubules do not respond to

---

*A useful summary of recent advances in parathyroid disease is contained in Forscher BK, Arnaud CD (editors): Third F. Raymond Keating Jr. Memorial Symposium—Parathyroid hormone, calcitonin and vitamin D: Clinical considerations. (2 parts.) Am J Med 56:743; 57:1, 1974.

the hormone. This resistance may disappear spontaneously or after restoration of serum calcium to normal. Various unusual syndromes have been described which have some features of Albright's original report (Albright's osteodystrophy) but lack others (pseudopseudohypoparathyroidism, pseudohypoparathyroidism type II, pseudo-idiopathic hypoparathyroidism). In some patients, high levels of parathormone lead to osteitis fibrosa, which is reversible with treatment with vitamin D (see Moses reference, below).

Clinical Findings

A. Symptoms and Signs: Acute hypoparathyroidism causes tetany, with muscle cramps, irritability, carpopedal spasm, and convulsions; stridor, wheezing, dyspnea; photophobia and diplopia; abdominal cramps, and urinary frequency. Symptoms of the chronic disease are lethargy, personality changes, anxiety state, blurring of vision due to cataracts, and mental retardation.

Chvostek's sign (facial contraction on tapping the facial nerve near the angle of the jaw) is positive and Trousseau's phenomenon (carpopedal spasm after application of a cuff) is present. Cataracts may occur; the nails may be thin and brittle; the skin dry and scaly, at times with fungus infection (candidiasis) and loss of hair (eyebrows); and deep reflexes may be hyperactive. Choreoathetosis may be found in an occasional patient but is reversible with adequate therapy. Choking of the optic disks is rarely found. Teeth may be defective if the onset of the disease occurs in childhood. Branchial anomalies (eg, cleft palate) may be found. In pseudohypoparathyroidism the fingers and toes are short, with absence of the knuckles of the 4th and 5th fingers on making a fist; ectopic soft tissue calcification may be seen and felt.

B. Laboratory Findings: Serum calcium is low, serum phosphate high, urinary phosphate low (TRP above 95%), urinary calcium low to absent (negative Sulkowitch test), and alkaline phosphatase normal. Alkaline phosphatase may be elevated in pseudohypoparathyroidism. The creatinine clearance is normal. Radioimmunoassayable parathormone level is low or absent in idiopathic or postsurgical hypoparathyroidism but normal or even markedly elevated in pseudohypoparathyroidism.

C. X-Ray Findings: X-rays of the skull may show basal ganglia calcifications; the bones may be denser than normal (in pseudohypoparathyroidism short metacarpals and ectopic bone may be seen, and bones may be demineralized).

D. Other Examinations: Slitlamp examination may show early cataract formation. EEG shows generalized dysrhythmia (partially reversible). ECG may show prolonged Q–T intervals.

Complications

Acute tetany with stridor, especially if associated with vocal cord palsy, may lead to respiratory obstruction requiring tracheostomy. Severe hypocalcemia may lead to cardiac dilatation and failure. The complica-

tions of chronic hypoparathyroidism depend largely upon the duration of the disease and the age at onset. If it starts early in childhood, there may be stunting of growth, malformation of the teeth, and retardation of mental development. There may be associated sprue syndrome, pernicious anemia, and Addison's disease, probably on the basis of an autoimmune mechanism. In pseudohypoparathyroidism, hypothyroidism due to deficiency of thyrotropin is often found. In long-standing cases, cataract formation and calcification in the basal ganglia are seen. Permanent brain damage with convulsions or with psychosis may lead to admission to mental institutions. In addition, there may be complications of overtreatment with calcium and vitamin D, with renal impairment and calcinosis.

Differential Diagnosis

The symptoms of hypocalcemic tetany are most commonly confused with or mistaken for tetany due to metabolic or respiratory alkalosis, in which the serum calcium is normal. Symptoms of anxiety are common in both instances, and fainting is not uncommon in the hyperventilation syndrome. The typical blood and urine findings should differentiate the 2 disorders. This holds true also for less common causes of hypocalcemic tetany, such as rickets and osteomalacia in the early stages. In this condition the serum phosphate is usually low or low normal; rarely high. Confusion might arise with the tetany due to chronic renal failure, in which retention of phosphorus will produce a high serum phosphorus with low serum calcium, but the differentiation should be obvious on clinical grounds (eg, uremia, azotemia).

In primary hyperaldosteronism with tetany (due to alkalosis) there is associated hypertension and hypokalemia with inability to concentrate the urine. Hypomagnesemia must be considered if tetany fails to respond to calcium.

The physical signs of pseudohypoparathyroidism without the abnormal blood chemical findings are seen in certain dysplasias ("pseudopseudohypoparathyroidism").

In order to differentiate true hypoparathyroidism, which responds to parathyroid extract, from pseudohypoparathyroidism, which does not respond, the Ellsworth-Howard test (phosphaturia after administration of 200 units of parathyroid hormone IV) may be performed. The parathyroid hormone resistance has been demonstrated to be due to failure of activation of renal adenylate cyclase with defective excretion of cyclic AMP after administration of parathyroid hormone. High levels of calcitonin have been demonstrated in thyroid tissue of patients with pseudohypoparathyroidism, but thyroidectomy is of little help. Medullary carcinoma of the thyroid is rarely associated with hypocalcemia in spite of excess calcitonin.

At times hypoparathyroidism is misdiagnosed as idiopathic epilepsy, choreoathetosis, or brain tumor (on the basis of brain calcifications, convulsions, choked disks) or, more rarely, as "asthma" (on the basis of stridor and dyspnea). Other causes of cataracts

Table 18—6. Principal findings in the various parathyroid syndromes.*

Syndrome	Low Serum Ca With High Serum P	Serum Alkaline Phosphatase	Cataracts; Calcification of Basal Ganglia	Micro-dactylia; Ectopic Bone	Sub-periosteal Resorption (Osteitis)	Para-thyroid Hyper-plasia	Ellsworth-Howard Test†	PTH Assay
Hypoparathyroidism	+	Normal	+	0	0	0	+	0
Pseudohypoparathyroidism	+	Normal	+	+	0	+	0	Normal or ↑
Pseudopseudohypoparathyroidism	0	Normal	0	+	0	0	+	Normal
Secondary (renal) hyperparathyroidism	+ (NPN↑)	↑	0	0	+	+	±	↑
Pseudohypoparathyroidism with secondary hyperparathyroidism	+ (NPN normal)	↑	±	+	+	+	0	↑

*Modified and reproduced, with permission, from Kolb FO, Steinbach HL: Pseudohypoparathyroidism with secondary hyperparathyroidism and osteitis fibrosa. J Clin Endocrinol 22:68, 1962.
†Responsiveness to parathyroid hormone.

and basal ganglia calcification also enter into the differential diagnosis.

Treatment

A. Emergency Treatment for Acute Attack (Hypoparathyroid Tetany): This usually occurs after surgery and requires immediate treatment. *Note:* Be sure an adequate airway is present.

1. Calcium chloride, 5—10 ml of 10% solution IV slowly until tetany ceases, or calcium gluconate, 10—20 ml of 10% solution IV, may be given. Ten to 50 ml of either solution may be added to 1 liter of 5% glucose in water or saline and administered by slow IV drip. The rate should be so adjusted that hourly determination of urinary calcium (Sulkowitch test) will be positive. *Note:* Do not treat tetany too vigorously, or irreversible tissue calcification will occur.

2. Calcium salts should be given orally as soon as possible to supply 1—2 gm of calcium daily: calcium gluconate, 8 gm 3 times daily; calcium lactate powder, 4—8 gm 3 times daily (some patients prefer tablet form); or calcium chloride, 2—4 gm 3 times daily (as 30% solution). Calcium carbonate is effective in smaller doses than either calcium gluconate or lactate and is better tolerated than calcium chloride. It is the calcium salt of choice at present. OsCal, a preparation of calcium carbonate containing 250 mg calcium, is well tolerated. Dosage is 4—8 tablets/day.

3. Dihydrotachysterol (Hytakerol, AT 10) and calciferol—Give either compound as soon as oral calcium is begun. Begin with 4—10 ml of oily solution of dihydrotachysterol (1.25 mg/ml) orally daily for 2—4 days, reduce dose to 1—2 ml daily for 1—3 weeks, and then determine maintenance requirements. Pure crystalline preparations (eg, Digratyl) in tablets of 0.2 mg are now available. The initial dose is 0.8—2.4 mg daily for several days. Calciferol, 80—160 thousand units (2—4 mg) daily, is just as effective (though slower to act) and probably should be used in most patients.

4. Parathyroid injection, 50—100 units IM or subcut 3—5 times daily as necessary to prevent tetany. Do not use parathyroid hormone for over 1 week. Use only as long as absolutely necessary.

5. Diphenylhydantoin and phenobarbital have recently been shown to control overt and latent tetany without alteration in calcium levels. They may be used as adjuncts in the management of refractory patients.

6. In the future, the more active metabolites of calciferol, 25-hydroxycholecalciferol and 1,25-dihydroxycholecalciferol, will be available for patients refractory to calciferol. (See Russell reference, below.)

B. Maintenance Treatment:

1. High-calcium, low-phosphate diet (omit milk and cheese).

2. Calcium salts (as above except chloride) are continued.

3. Dihydrotachysterol (Hytakerol), 0.5—1 ml daily to maintain blood calcium at normal level. The dose is 0.2—1.8 mg weekly.

4. Calciferol, 40—200 thousand units (1—5 mg) daily, is the drug of choice at present for the majority of patients. In some cases up to 7 or 8 mg of calciferol daily may be needed. Its action is probably similar to that of dihydrotachysterol, and it can certainly be substituted adequately clinically. The initial action of vitamin D appears to be slower. However, the cost to the patient is less than with dihydrotachysterol. It accumulates in the body over prolonged periods, and serum calcium levels should be checked periodically. *Note:* Corticosteroids and sodium phytate (Rencal) are effective antidotes in vitamin D intoxication.

5. Aluminum hydroxide gels may be employed to help lower the serum phosphate level in the initial stages of treatment. They are rarely required for chronic therapy.

Caution: Phenothiazine drugs should be administered with caution in hypoparathyroid patients since they may precipitate dystonic reactions.

Prognosis

The outlook is fair if prompt diagnosis is made and treatment instituted. Some changes (eg, in the EEG) are reversible, but the dental changes, cataracts, and brain calcifications are permanent. They may be in part genetically determined and not related to hypocalcemia per se. Although treatment of the immediate acute attack is simple and effective, long-term therapy is tedious and expensive since a good preparation of parathormone is not available. Adequate control by a fairly intelligent patient is required to avoid undertreatment or overtreatment. Periodic blood chemical evaluation is required since sudden changes in blood levels may call for modification of the treatment schedule. (*Note:* The urinary calcium [Sulkowitch test] is of little value since hypercalciuria, regardless of blood calcium level, may occur with prolonged vitamin D therapy. Sudden appearance of hypercalcemia, especially in children, may be due to associated Addison's disease.)

Unrecognized or late cases may find their way into mental institutions.

Avioli LV: The therapeutic approach to hypoparathyroidism. Am J Med 57:34, 1974.

Blizzard RM & others: The incidence of parathyroid and other antibodies in the sera of patients with idiopathic hypoparathyroidism. Clin Exper Immunol 1:119, 1966.

Bronsky D, Kiamko RT, Waldstein SS: Familial idiopathic hypoparathyroidism. J Clin Endocrinol 28:61, 1968.

Chase LR & others: Pseudohypoparathyroidism: Defective excretion of 3',5'-AMP in response to parathyroid hormone. J Clin Invest 48:1832, 1969.

Chertow BS, Plymate SR, Becker FO: Vitamin-D-resistant idiopathic hypoparathyroidism. Arch Int Med 133:838, 1974.

Fonseca OA, Calverley JR: Neurological manifestations of hypoparathyroidism. Arch Int Med 120:202, 1967.

Frame B & others: Renal resistance to parathyroid hormone with osteitis fibrosa. "Pseudohypohyperparathyroidism." Am J Med 52:311, 1972.

Harrison HE & others: Comparison between crystalline dihydrotachysterol and calciferol in patients requiring pharmacologic vitamin D therapy. New England J Med 276:894, 1967.

Kleeman CR & others: The clinical physiology of calcium homeostasis, parathyroid hormone, and calcitonin. (2 parts.) California Med 114:16, March 1971; 114:19, April 1971.

Kolb FO & others: Primary hypoparathyroidism, Addison's disease and ovarian failure. Page 116 in: *Reproductive Endocrinology*. Irvine WJ (editor). Livingstone, 1970.

Lee JB & others: Parathyroid hormone and thyrocalcitonin in familial pseudohypoparathyroidism. New England J Med 279:1179, 1968.

Miller MJ & others: Branchial anomalies in idiopathic hypoparathyroidism: Branchial dysembryogenesis. Henry Ford Hosp MJ 20:3, 1972.

Mizrahi A & others: Neonatal hypocalcemia: Its causes and treatment. New England J Med 278:1163, 1968.

Moses AM & others: Parathyroid hormone deficiency with Albright's hereditary osteodystrophy. J Clin Endocrinol 39:496, 1974.

Nusynowitz M, Klein M: Pseudoidiopathic hypoparathyroidism. Am J Med 55:677, 1973.

Pak CY & others: Treatment of vitamin D-resistant hypoparathyroidism with 25-hydroxycholecalciferol (25-HCC). Arch Int Med 126:239, 1970.

Parfitt AM: The spectrum of hypoparathyroidism. J Clin Endocrinol 34:152, 1972.

Rodriguez HJ & others: Pseudohypoparathyroidism type II: Restoration of normal renal responsiveness to parathyroid hormone by calcium administration. J Clin Endocrinol 39:693, 1974.

Russell RGG & others: 1,25-Dihydroxycholecalciferol and 1α-hydroxycholecalciferol in hypoparathyroidism. Lancet 2:14, 1974.

Tabaee-Zadeh MJ & others: Kinesiogenic choreoathetosis and idiopathic hypoparathyroidism. New England J Med 286:762, 1972.

Zisman E & others: Studies in pseudohypoparathyroidism: Two new cases with a probably selective deficiency of thyrotropin. Am J Med 46:464, 1969.

HYPERPARATHYROIDISM

Essentials of Diagnosis

- Renal stones, nephrocalcinosis, polyuria, polydipsia, hypertension, uremia, intractable peptic ulcer, constipation.
- Bone pain, cystic lesions, and, rarely, pathologic fractures.
- Serum and urine calcium elevated; urine phosphate high with low to normal serum phosphate; alkaline phosphatase normal to elevated.
- "Band keratopathy" on slitlamp examination of eye.
- X-ray: subperiosteal resorption, loss of lamina dura of teeth, renal parenchymal calcification or stones, bone cysts, chondrocalcinosis.
- Elevated levels of parathyroid hormone.

General Considerations

While primary hyperparathyroidism is a relatively rare disease, it is potentially curable if detected early. Recent surveys suggest that hyperfunction of the parathyroids, often as asymptomatic hypercalcemia, may be present in 0.1% of patients examined. (*Note:* It should always be suspected in obscure bone and renal disease, especially if calculi or nephrocalcinosis are present.) At least 5% of renal stones are associated with this disease.

About 90% of cases of primary hyperparathyroidism are caused by a single adenoma (or, in rare cases, 2 adenomas); 8% are caused by primary hypertrophy and hyperplasia of all 4 glands; and 2% are caused by carcinoma of one gland. Recent findings suggest that chief cell hyperplasia may be more common than previously reported. Multiple adenomas, often familial, of the pancreas and pituitary, thyroid, and adrenal glands may be associated with primary hyperparathyroidism due to tumor or, more commonly, due to hyperplasia of the parathyroids.

Secondary hyperparathyroidism is almost always associated with hyperplasia of all 4 glands, but on rare occasions an autonomous tumor may arise in hyperplastic glands ("tertiary hyperparathyroidism"). It is most commonly seen in chronic renal disease, but is also found in rickets, osteomalacia, and acromegaly.

Hyperparathyroidism causes excessive excretion of calcium and phosphate by the kidneys; this eventually produces either calculus formation within the urinary tract or, less commonly, diffuse parenchymal calcification (nephrocalcinosis). (The 2 types rarely coexist.) If the excessive demands for calcium are met by dietary intake, the bones may not become drained (most common type in the USA). If calcium intake is not adequate, bone disease may occur. Factors other than the calcium intake probably determine whether bone disease will be present in hyperparathyroidism. This may show either diffuse demineralization, pathologic fractures, or cystic bone lesions throughout the skeleton ("osteitis fibrosa cystica").

Clinical Findings

A. Symptoms and Signs: The manifestations of hyperparathyroidism may be divided into those referable to (1) skeletal involvement, (2) renal and urinary tract damage, and (3) hypercalcemia per se. Since the adenomas are small and deeply located, only about 5% of cases of adenoma can be demonstrated by barium swallow displacing the esophagus or by palpation of a mass in the neck. It may be associated with a thyroid adenoma or carcinoma. (*Note:* Some patients have surprisingly few symptoms and the tumors are discovered accidentally by blood chemical findings.)

1. Skeletal manifestations—These may vary from simple back pain, joint pains, painful shins, and similar complaints, to actual pathologic fractures of the spine, ribs, or long bones, with loss of height and progressive kyphosis. At times an epulis of the jaw (actually a "brown tumor") may be the telltale sign of osteitis fibrosa. "Clubbing" of the fingers due to fracture and telescoping of the tips occur more rarely.

2. Urinary tract manifestations—Polyuria and polydipsia occur early in the disease. Sand, gravel, or stones containing calcium oxalate or phosphate may be passed in the urine. Secondary infection and obstruction may cause nephrocalcinosis and renal damage, leading eventually to uremia.

3. Manifestations of hypercalcemia—Thirst, nausea, anorexia, and vomiting are outstanding symptoms. Often one finds a past history of peptic ulcer, with obstruction or even hemorrhage. There may be stubborn constipation, asthenia, anemia, and weight loss. Hypertension is commonly found. Some patients present primarily with neuromuscular disorders such as muscle weakness, easy fatigability, or paresthesias. Depression and psychosis may occur. Of unusual interest is hypermotility of joints. The fingernails and toenails may be unusually strong and thick. Calcium may precipitate in the eyes ("band keratopathy"). In secondary (renal) hyperparathyroidism, calcium also precipitates in the soft tissues, especially around the joints. Recurrent pancreatitis occurs in some patients.

B. Laboratory Findings: Serum calcium is usually high (adjust for serum protein); the serum phosphate is low or normal; the urinary calcium is often high, but at times is normal or low. There is an excessive loss of phosphate in the urine in the presence of low to low normal serum phosphate (low tubular reabsorption of phosphate; TRP below 80–90%); the alkaline phosphatase is elevated only if clinical bone disease is present (in about 25% of cases). The plasma chloride and uric acid levels may be elevated. (In secondary hyperparathyroidism the serum phosphate is high as a result of renal retention, and the calcium is usually low or normal.) Radioimmune assays for parathormone are available to confirm the diagnosis in questionable cases and to establish the diagnosis of "normocalcemic hyperparathyroidism"; however, since the circulating hormone is heterogeneous, there are still great technical problems with any assay procedure (see Arnaud reference, below).

Note: A great number of special tests have been devised to demonstrate abnormal phosphate dynamics in primary hyperparathyroidism. None of these are as consistently reliable as several accurately performed serum calcium determinations, which demonstrate hypercalcemia for which no other cause can be detected. Control of the dietary phosphate is important since high phosphate intake may normalize borderline high serum calcium levels.

C. X-Ray Findings: X-ray rarely demonstrates the tumor on barium swallow; at times, special angiography may demonstrate it. If bone disease is present, one may see diffuse demineralization, subperiosteal resorption of bone (especially in the radial aspects of the fingers), and often loss of the lamina dura of the teeth. There may be cysts throughout the skeleton, mottling of the skull ("salt and pepper appearance"), or pathologic fractures. Articular cartilage calcification (chondrocalcinosis) is commonly found. One may find calculi in the urinary tract or diffuse stippled calcifications in the region of the kidneys (nephrocalcinosis). Soft tissue calcifications around the joints and in the blood vessels may be seen in renal osteitis.

D. Other Examinations: ECG may show a shortened Q–T interval. Slitlamp examination of the eye may show corneal calcification ("band keratopathy").

The localization of parathyroid tumors by selenomethionine scanning, in vivo parathyroid staining, and selective radioimmune assay via venous catheter to localize hyperfunctioning glands is largely experimental at present. Bone densitometry may show loss of trabecular bone not seen on routine x-ray.

Thermography may help locate fair-sized adenomas.

Complications

Although the striking complications are those associated with skeletal damage (eg, pathologic fractures), the serious ones are those referable to renal damage. Urinary tract infection due to stone and obstruction may lead to renal failure and uremia. If the serum calcium level rises rapidly (eg, due to dehydration or salt restriction), "parathyroid poisoning" may occur, with acute cardiac and renal failure and rapid precipitation of calcium throughout the soft tissues (hyperhyperparathyroidism). Peptic ulcer and pancreatitis may be intractable before surgery. Pancreatic islet cell adenoma with hypoglycemia may be associated, or ulcerogenic pancreatic tumor may coexist. Hypertension is frequently found. Reversible changes in glucose tolerance and insulin secretion have been reported. There may be associated hyperthyroidism or thyroid carcinoma. There is also an increased incidence of hyperuricemia and gouty arthritis. Pseudogout may complicate hyperparathyroidism both before and after surgical removal of tumors.

Differential Diagnosis (Tables 18–7 and 18–8.)

If chemical determinations are reliable, the combination of high calcium and low phosphate in the serum, high urinary phosphate and calcium, and normal or high alkaline phosphatase is almost pathognomonic of hyperparathyroidism. Only rarely has this combination been seen in multiple myeloma, metastatic cancer (kidney, bladder, thyroid), and hyperthyroidism. The most common problem is the differentiation of idiopathic hypercalciuria with renal stones from primary hyperparathyroidism with borderline serum calcium levels. If renal damage is present, the typical picture may be obscured, ie, the serum phosphate may not be low. Other causes of hypercalcemia (eg, sarcoidosis, vitamin D intoxication) will respond to the administration of cortisone (cortisone test), which usually does not affect the hypercalcemia of primary hyperparathyroidism. Chlorothiazides may raise the serum calcium level. Hypercalcemia due to hypervitaminosis A must be considered. If bone disease is present, the typical subperiosteal resorption may differentiate osteitis fibrosa from nonmetabolic bone disease (eg, neoplasm) and from osteoporosis. Bone biopsy may at times settle the diagnosis.

Recently, nonmetastasizing carcinomas (eg, of the lung, kidney, or ovary) have been described with blood chemical changes identical with those seen in hyperparathyroidism; these changes are often reversible upon removal or chemotherapy of these tumors, which appear to produce a parathyroid-like humoral agent, possibly a prostaglandin. (See Lafferty and Powell references, below.) If significant hypercalcemia is produced by a disorder other than hyperparathyroidism, the radioimmunoassayable PTH level should be undetectable since the parathyroid glands are suppressed. In actual practice, this is not always the case because of difficulties with the assay and the fact that disorders producing hypercalcemia may coexist with hyperparathyroidism (eg, sarcoidosis, hyperthyroidism, breast carcinoma).

Treatment

A. Surgical Measures: If a parathyroid tumor, the usual cause, is found, it should be removed surgically. The surgeon must be aware that multiple tumors may be present; the tumor may be in the thyroid gland or in an ectopic site, eg, the mediastinum. Hyperplasia of all glands requires removal of 3 glands and subtotal resection of the 4th before cure is assured. Routine radical resection of 3.5 parathyroid glands in all patients with hyperparathyroidism to avoid recurrence, as advocated in some medical centers, is hardly warranted if an experienced neck surgeon manages the patient and if the patient's chemical changes are carefully monitored postoperatively. After surgery the patient may in the course of several hours of days develop tetany (usually transient) as a result of rapid fall of blood calcium even though the calcium level may fall only to the normal or low normal range. *Caution:* Be certain that an adequate airway is present. Therapy is as for hypoparathyroid tetany (see p 674). Prolonged hypocalcemia due to recalcification of the "hungry" skeleton may require large amounts of calcium and vitamin D. Additional magnesium salts may have to be given postoperatively.

B. Fluids: A large fluid intake is necessary so that a diluted urine will be excreted to minimize the formation of calcium phosphate renal stones.

C. Treatment of Hypercalcemia: Force fluids both orally and parenterally (sodium chloride given IV is most helpful); mobilize the patient; reduce calcium intake; and add extra phosphate orally. Cortisone therapy is usually not effective in this type of hypercalcemia. Sodium sulfate and sodium and potassium phosphate as slow intravenous infusions have been used successfully in patients with hypercalcemia but must be used with caution. Furosemide is especially effective (see Suki reference, below); ethacrynic acid may be helpful. Chlorothiazides should not be given. If renal function is impaired, hemodialysis may be lifesaving if only for a short time. Mithramycin effectively reduces the hypercalcemia due to hyperparathyroidism or malignancy, but this drug is quite toxic. Calcitonin (thyrocalcitonin) has been used experimentally in the treatment of hypercalcemia, but its value is uncertain. (*Note:* The patient with hypercalcemia is very sensitive to the toxic effects of digitalis.)

D. Medical Treatment of Mild Hyperparathyroidism: Since this disorder is more frequently recognized by routine chemical screening procedures, a number of elderly patients with relatively mild hypercalcemia and few symptoms are encountered. They are best managed by forcing fluids; avoiding immobilization and chlorothiazides, adding phosphate preparations if renal function is good; and giving estrogenic hormones if postmenopausal. If the patient cannot be followed periodically or becomes symptomatic—eg, passes a stone—neck exploration must be considered.

Prognosis

The disease is usually a chronic progressive one unless treated successfully by surgical removal. There are at times unexplained exacerbations and partial remissions. Completely asymptomatic patients with mild hypercalcemia may be followed by means of serial calcium determinations and treated medically (see above).

Table 18–7. Most common laboratory findings in diseases associated with hypercalcemia.*

	Serum Phosphorus	Serum Alkaline Phosphatase	Blood Urea Nitrogen	Plasma Protein	Urinary Calcium	Renal Phosphorus Clearance	Renal Tubular Reabsorption of Phosphorus	Response to Steroids	Miscellaneous Findings
Malignant tumors Osteolytic metastases	N	N	N	N	↑	N	N	Usually	Visualization of localized bone lesion on x-ray study.
Secretion of parathyroid hormone-like substance	↓ or N	N or ↑	N	N	↑	N or ↑	↓ or N	Sometimes	
Multiple myeloma	N or ↑	N or ↑	↑	↑ (M protein)	↑	N	↓	Usually	Bone marrow abnormality; Bence Jones protein in urine.
Lymphoma or leukemia	N or ↑	N	N or ↑	N or ↑	N or ↑	N	↓ or N	Yes	Bone marrow abnormality.
Hyperparathyroidism†	↓ or N	N or ↑	N	N	N or ↑	↑	↓	Rarely	
Sarcoid	N	N or ↑	N	N (globulin)	N or ↑	↑	↓	Yes	Abnormality on x-ray study of chest; liver disease; lymph node biopsy positive; elevated sedimentation rate.
Vitamin D intoxication	↑	N or ↑	↑	N	↑	↑	↓	Yes	History positive.
Milk-alkali syndrome	N	N	↑	N	N	N	↓ or N	Yes	Alkalosis; rapid improvement after withdrawal of milk and alkali; band keratopathy, calcinosis.
Hyperthyroidism	N	N	N	N	↑	N	N	Sometimes	Protein-bound iodine and ^{131}I uptake abnormal.
Acute bone atrophy (immobilization) Paraplegia	N	N	N	N	↑	N	N	No	
Fracture	N	↑	N	N	↑	N	N	No	
Paget's disease of bone	N	↑↑	N	N	↑	N	N	No	
Adrenal insufficiency	N	N	N or ↑	N or ↑	N	N	↓ or N	Yes	Hyperkalemia, hypotension, etc.
Idiopathic hypercalcemia of infancy	N or ↑	N	↑	N or ↑	N	N	↓ or N	Yes	Characteristic elfin facies; deafness.
(Effects of renal insufficiency)	↑	—	↑	—	↓	↓	↑	—	

*Reproduced, with permission, from Goldsmith RS: Differential diagnosis of hypercalcemia. New England J Med 274:676, 1966.

†Hyperparathyroidism secondary to phosphorus retention in renal insufficiency is probably not associated with hypercalcemia unless glands become autonomous or form adenoma.

Spontaneous cure due to necrosis of the tumor has been reported but is exceedingly rare. The prognosis is directly related to the degree of renal impairment. The bones, in spite of severe cyst formation, deformity, and fracture, will heal completely if a tumor is successfully removed. Once significant renal damage has occurred, however, it progresses even after removal of an adenoma, and life expectancy is materially reduced. Secondary hyperparathyroidism not infrequently results due to irreversible renal impairment. In carcinoma of the parathyroid (rare), the prognosis is not necessarily hopeless. The presence of pancreatitis increases the mortality. If hypercalcemia is severe, the patient may suddenly die in cardiac arrest or may develop irreversible acute renal failure. However, early diagnosis and cure of this disease in an increasing number of patients have led to dramatic metabolic changes and cessation of recurrent renal stones, the most consistent presenting symptom. In some patients, reversal of bizarre neuromuscular disorders (neuropathy, asthenia) occurs. Improvement in mentation is often but not always seen after successful surgery. Prolonged postoperative follow-up must be stressed to ensure that the state of hyperparathyroidism has been reversed. (See Goldsmith & others reference, below).

The distressing bone disease of secondary hyperparathyroidism due to renal failure (renal osteodystrophy) can be partially prevented and treated by careful monitoring of the phosphate and parathormone levels. Resistance to vitamin D can now be overcome by the newer biologically active derivatives, ie, 1,25-dihydroxycholecalciferol and 1α-hydroxycholecalciferol. "Tertiary hyperparathyroidism," ie, hypercalcemia following correction of renal failure, is rarely seen in patients so managed, and parathyroidectomy is rarely required nowadays for this disorder.

Arnaud CD: Parathyroid hormone: Coming of age in clinical medicine. Am J Med 55:577, 1973.

Aurbach GD & others: Hyperparathyroidism: Recent studies. Ann Int Med 79:566, 1973.

Ballard HS, Frame B, Hartsock RJ: Familial multiple endocrine adenoma-peptic ulcer complex. Medicine 43:481, 1964.

Carey RW & others: Massive extraskeletal calcification during phosphate treatment of hypercalcemia. Arch Int Med 122:150, 1968.

Chakmakjian ZH, Bethune JE: Sodium sulfate treatment of hypercalcemia. New England J Med 275:862, 1966.

Christiansen J: Primary hyperparathyroidism and peptic ulcer disease. Scandinav J Gastroent 9:111, 1974.

Coe F & others: Evidence for secondary hyperparathyroidism in idiopathic hypercalciuria. J Clin Invest 52:134, 1973.

Davies DR, Dent CE, Watson L: Tertiary hyperparathyroidism. Brit MJ 3:395, 1968.

Dodds WJ, Steinbach HL: Primary hyperparathyroidism and articular cartilage calcification. Am J Roentgenol 104:884, 1968.

Forscher BK, Arnaud CD (editors): Third F.R. Keating, Jr. Symposium: Parathyroid hormone, calcitonin and vitamin D. Am J Med 56:743, 1974.

Frame B & others: Hypercalcemia and skeletal effects in chronic hypervitaminosis A. Ann Int Med 80:44, 1974.

Gallagher JC, Nordin BE: Treatment with estrogens of primary hyperparathyroidism in postmenopausal women. Lancet 1:503, 1972.

Goldsmith RS, Ingbar SH: Inorganic phosphate treatment of hypercalcemia of diverse etiologies. New England J Med 274:21, 1966.

Goldsmith RE & others: Hyperparathyroidism: Therapy and response with a test for assessment of response. Ann Int Med 75:395, 1971.

Gordan GS: Recent progress in calcium metabolism: Clinical application. California Med 114:28, May 1971.

Haff RC, Armstrong RG: Trends in the current management of primary hyperparathyroidism. Surgery 75:715, 1974.

Holmes EC & others: Parathyroid carcinoma: Collective review. Ann Surg 169:631, 1969.

Keating FR Jr: The clinical problem of primary hyperparathyroidism. M Clin North America 54:511, 1970.

Lafferty FW: Pseudohyperparathyroidism. Medicine 45:247, 1966.

Mallette LE & others: Primary hyperparathyroidism: Clinical and biochemical features. Medicine 53:127, 1974.

Marsden P & others: Familial hyperparathyroidism. Brit MJ 3:87, 1971.

Nathaniels EK & others: Mediastinal parathyroid tumors: A clinical and pathologic study of 84 cases. Ann Surg 171:165, 1970.

Owens MP, Sorock ML, Brown EM: The clinical application of in vivo parathyroid staining. Surgery 64:1049, 1968.

Paterson CR: Drugs for the treatment of hypercalcaemia. Postgrad MJ 50:158, 1974.

Patten BM & others: Neuromuscular disease in primary hyperparathyroidism. Ann Int Med 80:182, 1974.

Petersen P: Psychiatric disorders in primary hyperparathyroidism. J Clin Endocrinol 28:1491, 1968.

Powell D & others: Nonparathyroid humoral hypercalcemia in patients with neoplastic diseases. New England J Med 289:176, 1973.

Raisz LG: The diagnosis of hyperparathyroidism. New England J Med 285:1006, 1971.

Samaan NA & others: Hyperparathyroidism and carcinoid tumor. Ann Int Med 82:205, 1975.

Shieber W & others: Normocalcemic hyperparathyroidism with "normal" parathyroid glands. Arch Surg 103:299, 1971.

Suki WN & others: Acute treatment of hypercalcemia with furosemide. New England J Med 283:836, 1970.

Wasson EC & others: Localization of a parathyroid adenoma by thermography. Western J Med 121:144, 1974.

Yasuda K & others: Glucose tolerance and insulin secretion in patients with parathyroid disorders. New England J Med 292:501, 1975.

METABOLIC BONE DISEASE *

OSTEOMALACIA & RICKETS

Essentials of Diagnosis

- Muscular weakness, listlessness.
- Aching and "bowing" of bones.

*A useful general reference on this subject is Hohl J (editor): Symposium on metabolic bone disease. Orthop Clin North America 3:501, 1972.

Table 18–8.　Differential diagnosis of metabolic and nonmetabolic bone disease.* (TRP = tubular reabsorption of phosphate.)

Disease	Serum					Urine			Comment
	Calcium	Phosphorus	Alkaline Ptase	Urea or Creatinine	Parathyroid Hormone	Calcium	TRP	Hydroxy-proline	
Hyperparathyroidism									
Primary	↑	↓	↑ or N	N or ↑	↑	↑ or N	↓	↑	Phalangeal subperiosteal resorption.
Secondary	↓ or N	↑	↑	↑	↑	N or ↓	↓	↑	
"Tertiary"	↑	N or ↓	↑ or N	↑ or N	↑	↑ or N	↓	↑	Tends to appear after renal transplantation.
Cancer	↑ or N	↑ or N or ↓	↑ or N	↑ or N	↑ or N or ↓	↑	N or ↓	↑	May be abnormal PTH in serum.
Sarcoid	↑ or N	N or ↓	N	↑ or N	↓	↑	N or ↓	↑	Good response to corticosteroids.
Vitamin D intoxication	↑	↑ or N	N	↑ or N	↓	↑	N or ↓	↑	Good response to corticosteroids.
Hyperthyroidism	↑ or N	N or ↑	N	N	N or ↓	↑	N	↑	Serum thyroxine increased.
Acute bone atrophy (immobilization)	↑ or N	↑	N	N	N or ↓	↑	N	↑	
Milk-alkali syndrome	↑	↑ or N	N	↑	N or ↓	N	N or ↓	N or ↑	Alkalosis despite renal insufficiency.
Idiopathic hypercalcemia of infancy	↑	↑ or N	↑	↑	?	↑	N or ↓	↑	"Elfin" facies.
Rickets and osteomalacia									
Vitamin D deficiency	↓	↓	↑	N	↑	↓	↓	N	Irritability, muscular hypotonia.
Vitamin D "refractory"	N	↓	↑	↑ or N	↑ or N	↓	↓	N	Pseudofractures, short stature.
Hypophosphatasia	↑ or N	N	↓	N	?	↑ or N	N	↑	Urinary phosphophosphorylethanol-amine increased; rickets.
Hypoparathyroidism	↓	↑	N	N	↓	↓	↑	N	
Pseudohypoparathyroidism	↓	↑	↑ or N	N	↑ or N	↓	↑	N or ↑	Short ulnar metacarpals.
Pseudopseudohypoparathyroidism	N	N	N	N	N	N	N	N	Short ulnar metacarpals, short stature.
Osteoporosis, idiopathic or senile	N	N	N	N	N	N	N	↑ or N	
Osteogenesis imperfecta	N	N	N or ↑	N	N	N	N	↑ or N	Blue scleras; deafness.
Osteopetrosis	N	N	N	N	N	N or ↓	N	N or ↓	
Paget's disease	N	N	↑	N	N	N	N	↑	Cardiac output increased.
Fibrous dysplasia	N	N	↑ or N	N	N	N	N	↑ or N	Brown spots.

*Modified and reproduced, with permission, from Goldsmith RS: Laboratory aids in the diagnosis of metabolic bone disease. Orthop Clin North America 3:546, 1972.

- Serum calcium low to normal; serum phosphate low; alkaline phosphatase elevated.
- "Pseudofractures" and "washed out" bone on x-ray.

General Considerations

Osteomalacia is the adult form of rickets. It is a condition resulting from a calcium and phosphorus deficiency in the bone. It may be caused by insufficient absorption from the intestine, due either to a lack of calcium alone, or a lack of or resistance to the action of vitamin D. In adults, this form of osteomalacia is almost always found in association with disorders of fat absorption (diarrhea, sprue, pancreatitis, gastrectomy). The other more common variety of osteomalacia is found in association with renal calcium or phosphorus losses ("vitamin D-resistant rickets"). This is often a familial disorder. It is found in tubular disorders, either tubular "leaks" of phosphate and calcium due to failure of reabsorption, or due to excessive losses associated with tubular acidosis (calcium dissolved out of the bone to spare sodium or potassium, or both). There may be associated glycosuria and aminoaciduria (Fanconi's syndrome). Cases of osteomalacia have been described that are due to chronic phosphate depletion from prolonged use of aluminum hydroxide gels and that occur due to long-term anticonvulsant therapy. A rare case of vitamin D-resistant rickets may be due to a mesenchymal tumor.

Almost all forms of osteomalacia are associated with compensatory, secondary hyperparathyroidism, set off by the low calcium level. It is for this reason that most patients will show only slightly low serum calcium levels (compensated osteomalacia). In chronic uremic states a mixed picture of osteomalacia and secondary hyperparathyroidism is seen ("renal osteodystrophy"). Resistance to the action of vitamin D due to failure of its conversion to the biologically active forms, 25-hydroxycholecalciferol and 1,25-dihydroxycholecalciferol, by the liver and kidney, respectively, has recently been demonstrated.

A special form of osteomalacia is the so-called **Milkman's syndrome**, an x-ray diagnosis of multiple, bilaterally symmetric pseudofractures which may represent the shadows of calluses near arterial blood vessels traversing and eroding the soft skeleton. Rickets, which is the counterpart of osteomalacia in the growing child, shows additional features, especially around the epiphyses, which are widened and "moth-eaten" on x-ray. There is also beading of the ribs, Harrison's groove, bowlegs, and disturbances in growth.

In contrast to osteoporosis, where fractures are more common, osteomalacia is more often associated with bowing of bones.

Clinical Findings

A. Symptoms and Signs: Manifestations are variable, ranging from almost none in mild cases to marked muscular weakness and listlessness in advanced cases. There is usually mild aching of the bones, especially of long bones and ribs, and a tendency to bowing. In the very early and acute osteomalacias a rapidly falling calcium level may be associated with clinical tetany, although this is rare. As compensation takes place, tetanic features are absent. In states of deficient absorption, other features of the sprue syndrome, such as glossy tongue or anemia, may be present. A low potassium syndrome with muscular weakness and paralysis may be present with renal tubular disorders.

B. Laboratory Findings: Serum calcium is low or normal, but never high. Serum phosphate is low (may be normal in early stages). The alkaline phosphatase is elevated except in the early phase. Urinary calcium and phosphate are usually low in absorption disorders and high in renal lesions. The intravenous calcium infusion test demonstrates avidity of bone for calcium (80–90% retained) in osteomalacia due to malabsorption. The blood level of 25-hydroxycholecalciferol may be low, but this test is not generally available. There is decrease in bone mass as measured by more sophisticated technics. Laboratory findings of the primary steatorrhea or renal disease may be present. In renal tubular acidosis the serum CO_2 is low and the serum chloride level is elevated; the serum potassium may be very low; the urinary pH is fixed near the alkaline side. Glycosuria and aminoaciduria are found in the Fanconi syndrome.

C. X-Ray Findings: Involvement of the pelvis and long bones, with demineralization and bowing; less often, the spine and skull are involved as well. Fractures are rare except for "pseudofractures." Nephrocalcinosis may be seen in renal tubular acidosis.

D. Bone Biopsy: This may be the only way to make a diagnosis. Undecalcified sections must be used with special staining methods to show undecalcified osteoid and osteoblastic overactivity.

Differential Diagnosis (Table 18–8.)

It is most important to recognize osteomalacia and consider it in the differential diagnosis of bone disease since it is a potentially curable disease. The childhood forms may be mistaken for osteogenesis imperfecta or other nonmetabolic bone disorders.

The acute forms must be differentiated from other forms of tetany. The long-standing disease enters into the differential diagnosis of any metabolic or generalized nonmetabolic bone disease (Table 18–8). The pseudofracture is often the only outstanding sign of latent osteomalacia. Osteoporosis may exist as well, and may obscure the osteomalacia. At times the diagnosis is confirmed by a rise and subsequent fall of the serum alkaline phosphatase after treatment with vitamin D and calcium. Renal tubular acidosis is a cause of nephrocalcinosis and must be considered in the differential diagnosis of kidney calcifications with bone disease such as hyperparathyroidism. Other causes of hypophosphatemia, eg, chronic alcoholism, enter into the differential diagnosis. The joint aches and pains may be mistaken for some form of arthritis. The cachexia suggests malignancy. Bone biopsy (eg, of the rib) with tetracycline labeling or microradiography may establish the diagnosis of latent osteomalacia.

Treatment

A. Specific Measures:

1. **Rickets**—Vitamin D, even in small doses, is specific; 2000–5000 units daily are adequate unless resistance to vitamin D is present.

2. **Adult osteomalacia and renal rickets**—Vitamin D is specific, but very large doses are necessary to overcome the resistance to its calcium absorptive action and to prevent renal loss of phosphate. Give until an effect is noted on the blood calcium. The usual dose is 25–100 thousand units daily. Doses up to 300,000 units or more daily may be necessary, but if the doses are over 100,000 daily, they must be used cautiously with periodic determination of serum and urine calcium; the serum phosphate may remain low.

3. **Pancreatic insufficiency**—Adequate replacement therapy with pancreatic enzyme is of paramount importance; high calcium intake and vitamin K are also of value.

4. **Sprue syndrome**—Folic acid and vitamin B_{12} appear to be of value. A gluten-free diet should be used in patients with gluten sensitivity.

5. **Some rare forms of renal disease**—Treatment is aimed at the altered renal physiology, eg, alkali therapy and potassium replacement in renal tubular acidosis, phosphate therapy, etc.

B. General Measures: High-calcium diet and calcium gluconate or calcium lactate, 4–20 gm daily, or calcium carbonate, 4–8 gm daily. A high-phosphate diet or phosphate salts may be of value in certain types of renal rickets. Magnesium salts may have to be added.

C. Vitamin D Metabolites: In the future, the increasing availability of the biologically active metabolites of calciferol, 25-hydroxycholecalciferol and 1,25-dihydroxycholecalciferol, will help in the treatment of osteomalacia resistant to vitamin D (eg, chronic liver disease and renal failure). The more readily synthesized 1a-hydroxycholecalciferol may prove to be an equally effective substitute (see Chalmers reference, below).

Prognosis

The prognosis is usually excellent in the absorptive disorders if diagnosed early. This does not hold for certain of the vitamin D-resistant forms of osteomalacia or rickets or for Fanconi's syndrome, which respond slowly or not at all unless huge amounts of vitamin D are given. Hypercalcemia may occur as a complication of therapy. In severely refractory cases, parathyroidectomy has improved the prognosis. In the renal forms, the ultimate prognosis is that of the basic kidney disease. Respiratory paralysis due to hypokalemia may prove fatal. The greater availability of the metabolically active metabolites of vitamin D will greatly improve the ultimate outlook in this disorder.

Albright F & others: Osteomalacia and late rickets. Medicine 25:399, 1946.

Arnstein AR & others: Recent progress in osteomalacia and rickets. Ann Int Med 67:1296, 1967.

Avioli L, Haddad JG: Vitamin D: Current concepts. Metabolism 22:507, 1973.

Bordier P & others: Response of adult patients with osteomalacia to treatment with crystalline 1a-hydroxy vitamin D_3. New England J Med 291:866, 1974.

Chalmers TM & others: 1-Alpha-hydroxycholecalciferol as a substitute for the kidney hormone 1,25-dihydroxycholecalciferol in chronic renal failure. Lancet 2:696, 1973.

Coburn JW, Hartenbower DL, Norman AW: Metabolism and action of the hormone vitamin D: Its relation to diseases of calcium homeostasis. Western J Med 121:22, 1974.

DeLuca H: The kidney as an endocrine organ for production of 1,25-dihydroxyvitamin D_3, a calcium-mobilizing hormone. New England J Med 289:359, 1973.

Eddy RL: Metabolic bone disease after gastrectomy. Am J Med 50:442, 1971.

Glorieux FH & others: Use of phosphate and vitamin D to prevent dwarfism and rickets in X-linked hypophosphatemia. New England J Med 287:481, 1972.

Hahn TJ & others: Serum 25-hydroxy calciferol levels and bone mass in children given anticonvulsants. New England J Med 292:550, 1975.

Jaworski ZFG: Pathophysiology, diagnosis and treatment of osteomalacia. Orthop Clin North America 3:623, 1972.

Lotz M, Zisman E, Bartter FC: Phosphorus-depletion syndrome in man. New England J Med 278:409, 1968.

Morris RC Jr & others: Renal acidosis. Kidney Internat 1:322, 1972.

Olefsky J & others: "Tertiary" hyperparathyroidism and apparent "cure" of vitamin D-resistant rickets after removal of ossifying mesenchymal tumor of the pharynx. New England J Med 286:740, 1972.

Paschett JB & others: Effects of 25-hydroxycholecalciferol on urinary electrolyte excretion in hypophosphatemia rickets. Lancet 2:920, 1974.

Sotaniemi A: Radiologic bone changes and hypocalcemia with anticonvulsant therapy in epilepsy. Ann Int Med 77:389, 1972.

Steinbach HL, Noetzli M: Roentgen appearance of the skeleton in osteomalacia and rickets. Am J Roentgenol 91:955, 1964.

Territo MC, Tanaka KR: Hypophosphatemia in chronic alcoholism. Arch Int Med 134:445, 1974.

OSTEOPOROSIS*

Essentials of Diagnosis

- Asymptomatic to severe backache.
- Spontaneous fractures and collapse of vertebrae without spinal cord compression, often discovered "accidentally" on x-ray; loss of height.
- Calcium, phosphorus, and alkaline phosphatase normal.
- Demineralization of spine and pelvis.

General Considerations

Osteoporosis is the most commonly seen meta-

*A recent good general reference on osteoporosis is Nordin BEC (editor): Osteoporosis. Clin Endocrinol Metab 2:153, 1973.

bolic bone disease in the USA. It is characterized by an absolute decrease in the amount of bone present to a level below which it is capable of maintaining the structural integrity of the skeleton. There is a greater loss of trabecular bone than compact bone, accounting for the primary features of the disease, ie, crush fractures of vertebrae, fractures of the neck of the femur, and fractures of the distal end of the radius. Whatever bone is present is normally mineralized. Osteoporosis may be produced secondarily by a number of disorders (see below), but more commonly it is primary and of unknown cause. Since the usual form of the disease is clinically evident in middle life and beyond—and since women are more frequently affected than men—it is often termed "postmenopausal and senile" osteoporosis. The serum calcium, phosphate, and alkaline phosphatase are normal, and the bone formation rate is usually normal whereas the bone resorption rate is increased. The inheritance of low skeletal mass in young adult life (especially in white females), loss of sex hormones at the time of the menopause, the effects of aging, lack of activity, inadequate dietary calcium intake, impaired intestinal calcium absorption, a high phosphate intake, acid ash diet, inappropriate secretion of parathyroid hormone or calcitonin, or some combination of these factors have been considered as possible contributing causes.

Etiology

A. Principal Causes:

1. Lack of activity, eg, immobilization as in paraplegia or rheumatoid arthritis. (Osteoblasts depend upon strains and stresses for proper function.)

2. Lack of estrogens ("postmenopausal osteoporosis"). (Females are deprived of estrogens relatively early in life. About 30% of women over 60 years of age have clinical osteoporosis. Some degree of osteoporosis is almost always present in senility.)

3. More recently a chronic low intake of calcium has been suggested as of etiologic importance. However, the evidence for this is still not conclusive.

4. Intestinal lactase deficiency may be an important factor in elderly patients with osteoporosis. (See Birge reference.)

B. Less Common Causes:

1. Developmental disturbances (eg, osteogenesis imperfecta).

2. Nutritional disturbances (eg, protein starvation and ascorbic acid deficiency).

3. Chronic calcium depletion is claimed by some investigators to cause osteoporosis.

4. Endocrine diseases—Lack of androgens (eunuchoidism, senility in men), hypopituitarism (causes secondary gonadal failure), acromegaly (cause unknown; possibly due to hypogonadism), thyrotoxicosis (not constant; causes excessive catabolism of protein tissue), excessive exogenous or endogenous ACTH or corticosteroids causing catabolism of bone (eg, Cushing's disease), and long-standing uncontrolled diabetes mellitus (rare).

5. Bone marrow disorders—The presence of abnormal cells in the bone marrow, such as in myeloma or leukemia, may prevent osteoblastic activity and cause osteoporosis. This is in addition to the active replacement of the marrow with tumor cells. A bone marrow factor may also play an etiologic role in senile osteoporosis.

6. Prolonged use of heparin may lead to osteoporosis.

7. Idiopathic osteoporosis—The cause is undetermined. It is most common in young men and women but occasionally occurs in older people, and does not respond well to therapy.

8. Idiopathic juvenile osteoporosis is a rare disorder which shows spontaneous remission after puberty.

Clinical Findings

A. Symptoms and Signs: Osteoporosis may first be discovered accidentally on x-ray examination, or may present as backache of varying degrees of severity. On other occasions it presents as a spontaneous fracture or collapse of a vertebra.

B. Laboratory Findings: Serum calcium, phosphate, and alkaline phosphatase are normal. The alkaline phosphatase may be slightly elevated in osteogenesis imperfecta and also in other forms of osteoporosis if there has been a recent fracture. Urinary calcium is high early, normal in chronic forms.

C. X-Ray Findings: X-ray shows compression of vertebrae. The principal areas of demineralization are the spine and pelvis; demineralization is less marked in the skull and extremities. The lamina dura is preserved. Kidney stones may occasionally be seen in acute osteoporosis.

D. Bone densitometry measurements may be helpful in the early detection of bone mineral loss.

Differential Diagnosis (Table 18–8.)

It is important not to confuse this condition with other metabolic bone diseases, especially osteomalacia and hyperparathyroidism; or with myeloma and metastatic bone disease, especially of the breast and uterus, since estrogen therapy may aggravate them (Table 18–8). Bone biopsy may be required, since these conditions may coexist in the postmenopausal patient.

A rare case of hypophosphatasia may appear as "osteoporosis."

Treatment

A. Specific Measures: Specific treatment varies with the cause; combined hormone therapy is usually employed, although its effectiveness has not been proved.

1. Postclimacteric (mostly in females)—Estrogens appear to decrease bone resorption. Before beginning estrogen therapy in a postmenopausal woman, perform a careful pelvic eamination to rule out neoplasm or other abnormality and warn the patient or a relative that vaginal bleeding may occur. Administer estrogen daily except for the first 5–7 calendar days of each month and then repeat the cycle. Any of the following

may be used: (1) Diethylstilbestrol, 0.5–2 mg orally daily as tolerated (may produce nausea). (2) Ethinyl estradiol, 0.02–0.05 mg orally daily as tolerated. (3) Estrone sulfate and conjugated estrogenic substances (Premarin, Amnestrogen, etc) are well tolerated and widely used. The dosage is 1.25–2.5 mg orally daily. The long-acting injectable estrogen preparations may be more reliable.

Testosterone may be used in addition to estorgen for its protein anabolic effect. Give methyltestosterone, 5–10 mg orally daily. Avoid overdosage in females since excessive use may cause the appearance of male secondary sex characteristics. While some of these regress if therapy is stopped, others (eg, hoarseness, hirsutism, clitoral enlargement) may persist. Some of the newer anabolic agents, eg, estradiol valerate and testosterone enanthate (Deladumone), norethandrolone (Nilevar), or methandrostenolone (Dianabol), may be used (see p 722).

2. Old age and idiopathic—As for postclimacteric; both testosterone and estrogens may be used in both males and females. Use with caution in very old people.

3. Patients with malnutrition—Adequate diet is of great importance. However, hormones may be used as above if response to diet alone is poor.

4. Cushing's syndrome—See p 691.

5. Sodium fluoride has recently been tried in refractory osteoporotic patients, but it must be considered still an experimental procedure. Combined with calcium and vitamin D, it appears to enhance bone formation (see Jowsey reference, below).

6. Phosphate supplements may be of value in certain types of osteoporosis (eg, after fracture, myeloma), especially if combined with calcium.

7. Intravenous infusions of calcium have been advocated recently for refractory osteoporosis. This must be considered an experimental procedure and may act by stimulating calcitonin production. Long-term studies have failed to show any beneficial effects of this treatment (see Dudl reference, below).

8. Calcitonin therapy is under investigation but appears to have little effect in arresting osteoporosis. It may be helpful in osteogenesis imperfecta.

B. General Measures: The diet should be high in protein and adequate in calcium (milk and milk products are desirable) and vitamin D. Increased calcium intake by use of supplementary calcium salts (eg, calcium lactate or carbonate), up to 1–2 gm calcium per day, may be warranted. Additional vitamin D (2000–5000 units/day) may be needed if there is associated malabsorption or osteomalacia. Patients should be kept active; bedridden patients should be given active or passive exercises. The spine must be adequately supported (eg, with a Taylor brace), but rigid or excessive immobilization must be avoided.

Prognosis

With proper and prolonged therapy, the prognosis is good for postclimacteric osteoporosis. Spinal involvement is not reversible on x-ray, but progression of the disease is often halted. In general, osteoporosis is a crippling rather than a killing disease, and the prognosis is essentially that of the underlying disorder (eg, Cushing's syndrome). The idiopathic variety does not respond appreciably to any form of therapy except possibly fluoride. Careful periodic records of the patient's height will indicate if the disease has become stabilized. In the future, periodic measurements of bone mass in a given individual with modern technics (eg, bone densitometry) may alert the physician that progressive bone loss is occurring prior to clinical or x-ray evidence of osteoporosis. Measures to prevent progressive resorption of bone may be more effective than treatment of clinical disease.

Birge SJ & others: Osteoporosis, intestinal lactase deficiency and low dietary calcium intake. New England J Med 276:445, 1967.

Dent CE, Friedman M: Idiopathic juvenile osteoporosis. Quart J Med (New Series) 34:177, 1965.

Dudl RJ & others: Evaluation of intravenous calcium as therapy for osteoporosis. Am J Med 55:631, 1973.

Fraser SA & others: Osteoporosis and fractures following thyrotoxicosis. Lancet 1:981, 1971.

Goldsmith RS & others: Effect of phosphate supplements in patients with fractures. Lancet 1:687, 1967.

Griffith GC & others: Heparin osteoporosis. JAMA 193:91, 1965.

Hahn TJ, Boisseau VC, Avioli LV: Effect of chronic corticosteroid administration on diaphyseal and metaphyseal bone mass. J Clin Endocrinol 39:274, 1974.

Harris WH, Heaney RP: Skeletal renewal and metabolic bone disease. (3 parts.) New England J Med 280:3, 253, 303, 1969.

Hossain M, Smith DA, Nordin BEC: Parathyroid activity and postmenopausal osteoporosis. Lancet 1:809, 1970.

Jowsey J & others: Effects of combined therapy with sodium fluoride, vitamin D, and calcium in osteoporosis. Am J Med 53:43, 1972.

Lutwak L, Singer FR, Urist MR: Current concepts of bone metabolism. Ann Int Med 80:630, 1974.

Nordin BEC, MacGregor J, Smith DA: The incidence of osteoporosis in normal women: Its relation to age and the menopause. Quart J Med 35:25, 1966.

Pak CY & others: The treatment of osteoporosis with calcium infusions: Clinical studies. Am J Med 47:7, 1969.

Raisz LG: Physiologic and pharmacologic regulation of bone resorption. New England J Med 282:909, 1970.

Riggs L & others: Treatment for postmenopausal and senile osteoporosis. M Clin North America 56:989, 1972.

Smith DM & others: In vivo measurement of bone mass: Its use in demineralized states such as osteoporosis. JAMA 219:325, 1972.

Spencer H & others: Absorption of calcium in osteoporosis. Am J Med 37:223, 1964.

Villanueva AE & others: Cortical bone dynamics measured by means of tetracycline labeling in 21 cases of osteoporosis. J Lab Clin Invest 68:599, 1966.

NONMETABOLIC BONE DISEASE
(See Table 18–8.)

POLYOSTOTIC FIBROUS DYSPLASIA
(Osteitis Fibrosa Disseminata)

Essentials of Diagnosis

- Painless swelling of involved bone or fracture with minimal trauma.
- Bone cysts or hyperostotic lesions; usually multiple, but occasionally single, in segmental distribution.

General Considerations

Polyostotic fibrous dysplasia is a rare disease which is frequently mistaken for osteitis fibrosa generalisata due to hyperparathyroidism since both are manifested by bone cysts and fractures. Polyostotic fibrous dysplasia is not a metabolic disorder of bone but a congenital dysplasia in which bone and cartilage do not form but remain as fibrous tissue.

Polyostotic fibrous dysplasia with "brown spots" with ragged margins and true precocious puberty in the female is called **Albright's syndrome.** Hyperthyroidism and acromegaly may be present also.

Clinical Findings

A. Symptoms and Signs: The manifestations are painless swelling of the involved bone (usually the skull, upper end of femur, tibia, metartarsals, metacarpals, phalanges, ribs, and pelvis), either singly or in multiple distribution, with cysts or hyperostotic lesions and at times with brown pigmentation of the overlying skin. Involvement is segmental and may be unilateral. True sexual precocity may occur in females, with early development of secondary sex characteristics and rapid skeletal growth.

B. Laboratory Findings: Calcium and phosphorus are normal; the alkaline phosphatase and urinary hydroxyproline may be elevated.

C. X-Ray Findings: X-rays reveal rarefaction and expansion of the affected bones or hyperostosis (especially of base of the skull). Fractures and deformities may also be visible.

Differential Diagnosis (Table 18–8.)

The bone cysts and fractures should by their distribution and skin pigmentation be distinguished from those of hyperparathyroidism and neurofibromatosis. All other types of bone cyst and tumor must be considered also. The hyperostotic lesions of the skull must be distinguished from those of Paget's disease. Biopsy of bone may be required to settle the diagnosis.

Complications

Shortening of the extremity or deformity (eg, shepherd's crook deformity of femur) may follow extensive involvement of bone. The involvement of the orbit may cause proptosis or even blindness. Thyrotoxicosis, Cushing's syndrome, acromegaly, and gynecomastia may be associated features.

Treatment

There is no treatment except for surgical correction of deformities, eg, fractures, expanding cyst in the orbit. Calcitonin has been used in active disease, but the results are not conclusive.

Prognosis

Most lesions heal and the progression is slow. Since precocity is of the isosexual type, girls are susceptible to early pregnancy. They will ultimately be of short stature. On rare occasions sarcomatous transformation of bone occurs.

Bell NH & others: Effect of calcitonin in Paget's disease and polyostotic fibrous dysplasia. J Clin Endocrinol 31:283, 1970.

Benedict P: Endocrine features in Albright's syndrome (fibrous dysplasia of bone). Metabolism 11:30, 1962.

Benedict PH & others: Melanotic macules in Albright's syndrome and in neurofibromatosis. JAMA 205:618, 1968.

Warrick CK: Some aspects of polyostotic fibrous dysplasia: Possible hypothesis to account for associated endocrinologic changes. Clin Radiol 24:125, 1973.

PAGET'S DISEASE
(Osteitis Deformans)

Essentials of Diagnosis

- Often asymptomatic. Bone pain may be the first symptom.
- Kyphosis, bowed tibias, large head, waddling gait, and frequent fractures which vary with location of process.
- Serum calcium and phosphate normal; alkaline phosphatase elevated; urinary hydroxyproline elevated.
- Dense, expanded bones on x-ray.

General Considerations

Paget's disease is a nonmetabolic bone disease of unknown etiology which causes excessive bone destruction and repair, with associated deformities since the repair takes place in an unorganized fashion. Up to 3% of persons over age 50 will show isolated lesions, but clinically important disease is much less common.

Clinical Findings

A. Symptoms and Signs: Often mild or asymptomatic. Deep "bone pain" is usually the first symptom. The bones become soft, leading to bowed tibias, kyphosis, and frequent fractures with slight trauma. The head becomes large, and headaches are a prominent symptom. Increased vascularity over the involved bones causes increased warmth.

B. Laboratory Findings: The blood calcium and

phosphorus are normal, but the alkaline phosphatase is usually markedly elevated. Urinary hydroxyproline and calcium are elevated in active disease.

C. X-Ray Findings: On x-ray the involved bones are expanded and denser than normal. Multiple fissure fractures may be seen in the long bones. The initial lesion may be destructive and radiolucent, especially in the skull ("osteoporosis circumscripta").

D. Bone Scans: Fluoride or technetium pyrophosphate bone scans are helpful in delineating activity of bone lesions (see Khairi reference, below).

Differential Diagnosis

Differentiate from primary bone lesions such as osteogenic sarcoma, multiple myeloma, and fibrous dysplasia and from secondary bone lesions such as metastatic carcinoma and osteitis fibrosa cystica. If serum calcium is elevated, hyperparathyroidism may be present in some patients as well.

Complications

Fractures are frequent and occur with minimal trauma. If immobilization takes place and there is an excessive calcium intake, hypercalcemia and kidney stones may develop. Associated hyperparathyroidism may also be present. Bony overgrowth may impinge on vital structures, especially nerves, causing deafness and blindness. Vertebral collapse may lead to spinal cord compression. Long-standing cases may progress to osteosarcoma. The increased vascularity, acting like multiple arteriovenous fistulas, may give rise to high-output cardiac failure. Rheumatic manifestations and hyperuricemia with acute and chronic joint pain often complicate this disease, especially in joints near involved bone.

Treatment

Mild cases require no treatment.

Supply a high-protein diet with adequate vitamin C intake. A high-calcium intake is desirable also unless the patient is immobilized, in which case calcium must be restricted. Vitamin D, 50,000 units 3 times a week, is helpful in some patients. Anabolic hormones, eg, estradiol valerate and testosterone enanthate (Deladumone), 1–3 ml/month, should be given as for osteoporosis. Corticosteroid treatment relieves pain but aggravates coexisting osteoporosis. Salicylates in large doses have recently been claimed to be useful in combating pain and reducing hypercalciuria. Sodium fluoride has also been tried in refractory cases (see Osteoporosis, p 682). Phosphate therapy may be helpful. Synthetic human and salmon calcitonin and mithramycin have been effective in the treatment of symptomatic and progressive disease. These drugs, as well as the diphosphonates, are experimental agents with great promise. Salmon calcitonin has been recently released as Calcimar for general use.

Prognosis

The prognosis of the mild form is good, but sarcomatous changes (in 1–3%) or renal complications secondary to hypercalciuria (in 10%) alter the prognosis unfavorably. In general, the prognosis is worse the earlier in life the disease starts. Fractures usually heal well. In the severe forms, marked deformity, intractable pain, and cardiac failure are found. The recently introduced therapeutic agents may alter prognosis favorably.

Altman RD & others: Influence of disodium etidronate on clinical and laboratory manifestations of Paget's disease of bone (osteitis deformans). New England J Med 289:1379, 1973.

Barry HC: *Paget's Disease of Bone.* Livingstone, 1969.

Doyle FH & others: Radiological evidence of a dose-related response to long-term treatment of Paget's disease with human calcitonin. Brit J Radiol 47:1, 1974.

Franck WA & others: Rheumatic manifestations of Paget's disease of bone. Am J Med 56:592, 1974.

Goldfield EB: Newer agents in treating Paget's disease of bone. Geriatrics 29:61, 1974.

Goldfield EB & others: Synthetic salmon calcitonin: Treatment of Paget's disease and osteogenesis imperfecta. JAMA 221:1127, 1972.

Guncaga L & others: Diphosphonate treatment of Paget's disease of bone. Hormone Metab Res 6:62, 1974.

Hamilton CR Jr: Effects of synthetic salmon calcitonin in patients with Paget's disease of bone. Am J Med 56:315, 1974.

Khairi MRA & others: Paget's disease of bone (osteitis deformans): Symptomatic lesions and bone scan. Ann Int Med 79:348, 1973.

Kolb FO: Paget's disease. California Med 91:245, 1959.

Lebbin D & others: Outpatient treatment of Paget's disease of bone with mithramycin. Ann Int Med 81:635, 1974.

Russell RGG & others: Diphosphonates in Paget's disease. Lancet 1:894, 1974.

DISEASES OF THE ADRENAL CORTEX

Total destruction of both adrenal cortices is not compatible with human life. The cortex regulates a variety of metabolic processes by means of secretion of some 30 steroid hormones.

The stimulus for release of steroid hormones from the adrenal cortex—with the possible exception of aldosterone—appears to be adrenocorticotropic hormone (ACTH) from the anterior pituitary which, in turn, is under the control of the hypothalamic corticotropin-releasing factor. The plasma free cortisol level regulates ACTH secretion. Aldosterone secretion, in contrast, is principally controlled by volume receptors, angiotensin II, and, possibly, the potassium concentration. Clinical syndromes of adrenal insufficiency or excess may thus be due to primary lesions of the adrenal glands themselves or may be secondary to pituitary disorders. Although the differentiation is often important from the diagnostic standpoint, treatment is usually directed toward the cortical disorder itself, whether primary or secondary. Many of the steroids isolated from the adrenal cortex are not active, and some have more than one action. Transcortin, a globulin, avidly binds cortisol and thus inactivates it. Estrogens increase transcortin levels. An active equilibrium exists between bound and free unbound cortisol. In general, the adrenocortical hormones have 3 types of activity:

(1) **Catabolic (glucocorticoids):** Cortisol and related steroids, the "stress hormones" of the adrenal cortex, are vital for survival. They are glycostatic, and cause gluconeogenesis from protein. They also play a role in potassium and water diuresis. Increased production or administration of large doses causes increased fat deposition in special sites (face, buffalo hump), raises blood pressure, and causes mild hypokalemic alkalosis, eosinopenia, and lymphopenia.

(2) **Electrolyte-regulating (mineralocorticoids):** The principal hormone in this group is aldosterone. Its primary role in retaining sodium and excreting potassium and thus "regulating" the extracellular fluid compartment and the blood pressure. It has minor effects on carbohydrate metabolism.

Most of the clinical features of both adrenal insufficiency and excess can be explained on the basis of the above types of activity. Since mixed pictures occur, however, and since excess of one type of activity may coexist with deficiency of another (eg, congenital adrenal virilism), exact physiologic correlation is difficult. Some phenomena, eg, the pigmentation of adrenal insufficiency, are not yet fully explained, and may be due to a pituitary intermedin or ACTH excess.

(3) **Anabolic (sex steroids):** Dihydroepiandrosterone and related steroids are protein builders and are also virilizing and androgenic, and represent the principal source of androgens in the female. This group also includes adrenal estrogens and progesterone-like steroids, but these are of lesser clinical importance.

Improved chemical and radioimmunoassays of various hormones, stimulation and suppression tests, and refined radiologic procedures have facilitated accurate diagnosis of adrenal disorders.

Catt KJ: ABC of endocrinology. 5. Adrenal cortex. Lancet 1:1275, 1970.

Ganong WF & others: ACTH and the regulation of adrenocortical secretion. New England J Med 290:1006, 1974.

Lieberman L & others: Diagnosis of adrenal disease by visualization of human adrenal glands with [131]I-19-iodocholesterol. New England J Med 285:1387, 1971.

Melby JC: Assessment of adrenocortical function. New England J Med 285:735, 1971.

Singer B: Scientific basis of clinical practice: Adrenal corticosteroids: Physiological considerations. Brit MJ 1:36, 1972.

Smilo RP, Forsham PH: Diagnostic approach to hypofunction and hyperfunction of the adrenal cortex. Postgrad Med 45:146, 1969.

Thorn GW (editor): Symposium on the adrenal cortex. Am J Med 53:529, 1972.

ADRENAL CORTICAL HYPOFUNCTION
(Adrenocortical Insufficiency)

1. ACUTE ADRENAL INSUFFICIENCY
(Adrenal Crisis)

Essentials of Diagnosis
- Onset of weakness, abdominal pain, high fever, confusion, nausea, vomiting, and diarrhea, with infection, or adrenal destruction, or cortisone withdrawal.
- Low blood pressure, dehydration, and increased skin pigmentation.
- Serum sodium low, serum potassium high, blood and urine corticosteroids low.
- Eosinophilia, elevated BUN.

General Considerations

Acute adrenal insufficiency is a true medical emergency caused by sudden marked deprivation or insufficient supply of adrenocortical hormones. Crisis may occur in the course of chronic insufficiency in a known addisonian patient out of control, or it may be the presenting manifestation of adrenal insufficiency. It may be a temporary exhaustion or may go on to permanent insufficiency. Acute crisis is more commonly seen in diseases of the cortex itself than in disorders of the pituitary gland causing secondary adrenocortical hypofunction.

Adrenal crisis may occur in the following situations: (1) Following stress, eg, trauma, surgery, infection, or prolonged fasting in a patient with latent insufficiency. (2) Following sudden withdrawal of adrenocortical hormone after replacement in a patient with chronic insufficiency or in a patient with normal adrenals but with temporary insufficiency due to suppression by exogenous glucocorticoids. (3) Following bilateral adrenalectomy or removal of a functioning adrenal tumor which had suppressed the other adrenal. (4) Following sudden destruction of the pituitary gland (pituitary necrosis), or when thyroid or insulin is given to a patient with panhypopituitarism. (5) Following injury to both adrenals by trauma, hemorrhage, thrombosis, infection, or, rarely, metastatic carcinoma. In overwhelming sepsis (principally meningococcemia), massive bilateral adrenal hemorrhage may occur (Waterhouse-Friderichsen syndrome).

Clinical Findings

A. Symptoms and Signs: The patient complains of headache, lassitude, nausea and vomiting, and often diarrhea. Costovertebral angle pain and tenderness (Rogoff's sign) and confusion or coma may be present. Fever may be 40.6° C (105° F) or more. The blood pressure is low. Other signs include cyanosis, petechiae (especially with meningococcemia), dehydration, abnormal skin pigmentation with sparse axillary hair, and lymphadenopathy.

B. Laboratory Findings: A normal or high eosinophil count in the presence of severe stress due to trauma, infection, and other mechanisms is strongly suggestive of adrenal failure. The blood glucose and serum sodium levels are low. Serum potassium and BUN are high. Hypercalcemia may be present. Blood culture may be positive (usually meningococci). Urinary and blood cortisol levels are very low.

C. ECG Findings: ECG shows decreased voltage.

Differential Diagnosis

This condition must be differentiated from other causes of coma and confusion, such as diabetic coma, cerebrovascular accident, and acute poisoning, and from other causes of high fever. Eosinophilia, which is usually absent in other emergencies, helps in the differentiation. (*Note:* If the diagnosis is suspected, treat with hydrocortisone, 100–300 mg IV, and saline *immediately* without waiting for the results of laboratory tests.)

Complications

Any of the progressive complications of the initiating disease may occur. The complications of treatment or those occurring during the course of treatment are discussed below.

When treatment is instituted, certain complications may be observed. Hyperpyrexia, loss of consciousness, generalized edema with hypertension, and flaccid paralysis due to low potassium has followed excessive use of intravenous fluids and corticosteroids. Psychotic reactions may occur with cortisone therapy.

Treatment

The patient must be treated vigorously and observed constantly until well out of danger. (*Note:* It is better to overtreat rather than to undertreat.)

A. Severe Crisis:

1. Emergency treatment—Institute appropriate antishock measures (see Chapter 1), especially intravenous fluids and plasma, vasopressor drugs, and oxygen. Do not give narcotics or sedatives.

Give hydrocortisone phosphate or hydrocortisone sodium succinate (Solu-Cortef), 100 mg IV immediately and continue intravenous infusions of 50–100 mg every 6 hours for the first day. Give the same amount every 8 hours on the second day and then gradually reduce the dosage every 8 hours.

If hydrocortisone hemisuccinate or hydrocortisone phosphate is not available, give cortisone acetate, 10–25 mg IM in 4 different sites (to a total of 40–100 mg), following with single injections of cortisone, 25–50 mg IM every 6 hours, and gradually lengthen the intervals of administration to 25 mg every 8 hours.

If parenteral hydrocortisone or cortisone is not available, or if the patient is unresponsive, give aqueous adrenocortical extract, 25–50 ml IV immediately and follow with 100–200 ml in 1 liter of saline-dextrose as an IV infusion. This is of doubtful value and is rarely used today.

Give anti-infective agents, eg, as for meningococcal meningitis.

2. Convalescent treatment—When the patient is able to take food by mouth, give oral cortisone, 12.5–25 mg every 6 hours, and reduce dosage to maintenance levels as needed.

B. Moderate Crisis: If the patient's physical condition does not appear to be critical and is not associated with a significant degree of shock, the treatment outlined above may be modified by appropriate reduction in dosage. However, it is generally best to overtreat the patient in moderate crisis during the first 24 hours rather than risk undertreatment.

C. Complications During Treatment: Excessive use of intravenous fluids and corticosteroids may cause generalized edema with hypertension; flaccid paralysis due to potassium depletion and psychotic reactions may occur.

1. Overhydration, usually due to sodium retention, may result in cerebral edema (with unconsciousness or convulsions) or pulmonary edema. Withhold sodium and fluids temporarily and treat for these conditions.

2. Hypokalemia—Flaccid paralysis, with low serum potassium, usually occurring on the 2nd to 4th days of treatment, may be treated with potassium salts.

3. Hyperpyrexia is rare with present treatment methods.

4. For other complications of adrenal steroid therapy (eg, psychotic reactions), see p 718.

Prognosis

Before replacement therapy and antibiotics became available, acute adrenal crisis was often rapidly fatal. Even today, if treatment is not early and vigorous, death occurs in several hours. Once the crisis has passed, the patient must be observed carefully to assess the degree of permanent adrenal insufficiency.

Frawley TF: Treatment of adrenal insufficiency states including Addison's disease. Mod Treat 3:1328, 1966.

2. CHRONIC ADRENOCORTICAL INSUFFICIENCY
(Addison's Disease)

Essentials of Diagnosis

- Weakness, easy fatigability, anorexia; frequent episodes of nausea, vomiting, and diarrhea.
- Sparse axillary hair; increased skin pigmentation of creases, pressure areas, and nipples.
- Hypotension, small heart.
- Serum sodium and chloride and urinary 17-ketosteroids and 17-hydroxycorticosteroids are low. Serum potassium and NPN are elevated. Eosinophilia and lymphocytosis are present.

- Plasma cortisol levels are low to absent and fail to rise after administration of corticotropin.

General Considerations

Addison's disease was a rare disorder before the advent of adrenal surgery for cancer, hypertension, and other disorders. It is characterized by chronic deficiency of hormones concerned with glyconeogenesis and with mineral metabolism, and causes unexplained and often striking skin pigmentation. Electrolyte deficiencies may be the dominant manifestation, and may even be associated with excess of adrenal androgens (see Adrenogenital Syndrome, p 693). If chronic adrenal insufficiency is secondary to pituitary failure (atrophy, necrosis, tumor), lack of glycostasis is more commonly seen than electrolyte deficiencies, and skin pigmentary changes are not encountered. Recently, a rare syndrome of isolated aldosterone lack has been described with persistent hyperkalemia, periodic paralysis, salt wasting, and acidosis. The majority of these patients have hypoaldosteronism on the basis of reduced renin production or release (see Schambelan reference, below).

Tuberculosis accounts today for less than half of cases, and in this form the electrolyte deficiencies are more striking. Idiopathic atrophy accounts for most of the other cases, and in this group hypoglycemia is more striking than the electrolyte changes. There may be associated thyroiditis, hypoparathyroidism, hypogonadism, and candidiasis. An autoimmune mechanism has been postulated for these and other causes of idiopathic atrophy.

Rare causes include metastatic carcinoma (especially of the breast or lung), coccidioidomycosis of the adrenal gland, syphilitic gummas, scleroderma, amyloid disease, and hemochromatosis.

Clinical Findings

A. Symptoms and Signs: The symptoms are weakness and fatigability, anorexia, nausea and vomiting, diarrhea, nervous and mental irritability, and faintness, especially after missing meals. Pigmentary changes consist of diffuse tanning over nonexposed as well as exposed parts or multiple freckles; or accentuation of pigment over pressure points and over the nipples, buttocks, perineum, and recent scars. Black freckles may appear on the mucous membranes of tongue. Seven to 15% of patients have associated vitiligo.

Other findings include hypotension with small heart, hyperplasia of lymphoid tissues, stiffness of the cartilages of the ear (Thorn's sign), scant to absent axillary and pubic hair (especially in females), absence of sweating, severe dental caries, and at times costovertebral angle tenderness.

B. Laboratory Findings: The white count shows moderate neutropenia (about 5000/cu mm), lymphocytosis (35–50%), and a total eosinophil count over 300/cu mm. Hemoconcentration is present. Serum sodium and chloride are low; serum potassium and BUN are elevated. Urinary 17-ketosteroid and 17-hydroxy-

corticosteroid excretion is low. Fasting blood glucose and BMR are low. Hypercalcemia may be present.

Low blood corticosteroids (less than 8 μg/100 ml) are diagnostic.

Adrenal calcification on x-ray may be found in about 10% of cases.

C. Special Tests:

1. The **8-hour intravenous corticotropin** test is the most specific and reliable diagnostic test. It consists of giving 25 units of corticotropin or 0.25 mg of the synthetic cosyntropin (Cortrosyn) in 1000 ml of physiologic saline by IV infusion; in primary Addison's disease the 24-hour urine 17-hydroxycorticosteroid values fail to rise; in adrenal insufficiency secondary to pituitary insufficiency or in patients who have had suppressive corticosteroid therapy, there is a slow, abnormal rise of 17-hydroxycorticosteroid levels, at times only after several days of stimulation. (*Note:* The patient suspected of having Addison's disease can be protected from untoward reactions to ACTH by the administration of 0.1 0.2 mg of 9α-fluorocortisol or 0.5 mg of dexamethasone without materially altering the urinary steroid levels.)

2. A more rapid test is the **plasma cortisol response to ACTH**. Plasma cortisol samples are obtained in the basal state and 30 minutes after IM injection of 25 units of corticotropin or 0.25 mg of cosyntropin (Cortrosyn). If the plasma cortisol does not rise by at least 10 μg/100 ml, the diagnosis of Addison's disease is likely.

3. A simpler, less reliable but rapid test for adrenocortical insufficiency (Perlmutter) is based on simultaneous determination of sodium levels in blood and urine and demonstrates sodium wasting, which is reversible by DOCA administration in Addison's disease but not in salt-losing nephritis.

4. Water excretion tests (Robinson-Kepler-Power or Soffer modification) to demonstrate delayed water diuresis are nonspecific and dangerous.

5. Other tolerance tests are *dangerous and rarely used:* Cutler-Power-Wilder test, prolonged fasting, glucose and insulin tolerance test.

6. Autoimmune antibodies to adrenal tissue may be found in idiopathic adrenal atrophy.

7. Plasma ACTH levels are high in primary adrenal insufficiency.

D. ECG Findings: The ECG shows low voltage and prolonged P–R and Q–T intervals (reversed by cortisone).

E. EEG Findings: Slowing of electrical discharge (reversed by cortisone but not by desoxycorticosterone).

Differential Diagnosis

Differentiate from anorexia nervosa, sprue syndrome, and malignant tumors. Weakness must be differentiated from that due to hyperparathyroidism, hyperthyroid myopathy, and myasthenia gravis; skin pigmentation from that of primary skin diseases, argyria, and hemochromatosis. The serum electrolyte abnormalities may resemble those of salt-losing nephritis and low-sodium states, eg, chronic pulmonary disease with inappropriate secretion of antidiuretic hormone.

Complications

Any of the complications of the underlying disease (eg, tuberculosis) are more likely to occur, and the patient is susceptible to intercurrent infections which may precipitate crisis. Diabetes mellitus and, rarely, thyrotoxicosis may be associated. Thyroiditis, hypoparathyroidism, pernicious anemia, and ovarian failure, probably caused by an autoimmune disorder, may be associated with adrenal failure. Hypercalcemia is most apt to occur in children, especially when the adrenocortical level is suddenly reduced.

The dangers of overzealous treatment as well as inadequate replacement must be guarded against. Psychoses, gastric irritation, and low-potassium syndrome may occur with corticosteroid treatment. Corticosteroid treatment may impair the patient's resistance to tuberculosis, which may spread. Excessive desoxycorticosterone administration is rare today but formerly led to hypertension, edema, anasarca, muscular weakness, and tendon contractures.

Treatment

A. Specific Therapy: Ideal replacement therapy should include a combination of glucocorticoids, mineralocorticoids, and anabolic steroids. In mild cases, cortisone alone—or a combination of cortisone and a mineralocorticoid—is adequate replacement.

1. Cortisone and hydrocortisone are the drugs of choice. Most addisonian patients are well maintained on 25–37.5 mg of cortisone or 20–30 mg of hydrocortisone orally daily in 2–3 divided doses. On this dosage, most of the metabolic abnormalities are corrected. Many patients, however, do not obtain sufficient salt-retaining effect from these drugs and require desoxycorticosterone or fludrocortisone supplementation or extra dietary salt.

2. Fludrocortisone acetate has a potent sodium-retaining effect. The dosage is 0.05–1 mg orally daily or every other day, added to cortisone or hydrocortisone. If postural hypotension occurs, raise the dose. If edema is noted, lower the dose.

3. Desoxycorticosterone acetate controls electrolyte balance, and, since it has no other significant metabolic effect, it must be used in combination with cortisone or hydrocortisone. It is given intramuscularly initially. The usual dose is 1–4 mg IM daily. When the response is adequate, change to desoxycorticosterone trimethylacetate, 25–75 mg IM once monthly (equivalent to 1 mg desoxycorticosterone acetate in oil per day). Alternative forms of therapy are buccal tablets or pellets, but these are rarely used today.

Caution: When using desoxycorticosterone acetate or fludrocortisone, avoid overdosage. Do not place the patient on a low-potassium diet when giving these drugs, for he may develop potassium deficiency.

4. Sodium chloride in large doses (5–20 gm daily) may be used to supplement cortisone therapy instead of desoxycorticosterone acetate or if desoxycorticos-

terone acetate or fludrocortisone is not available.

B. General Measures: Give a high-carbohydrate, high-protein diet. Frequent small feedings tend to be better tolerated than 3 large ones. If replacement therapy is adequate, most patients need no special diets or precautions except to avoid starvation. Prevent exposure to infection and treat all infections immediately and vigorously and raise the dose of cortisone appropriately. Testosterone in the form of methyltestosterone, 10–20 mg daily orally, testosterone propionate in oil, 10–25 mg IM 3 times weekly, or testosterone cypionate (Depo-Testosterone) or enanthate (Delatestryl), 200–400 mg/month, is often helpful for its protein anabolic effect and for the nonspecific feeling of well-being it induces in the debilitated patient. In female patients, smaller amounts (eg, 5 mg of methyltestosterone or 2 mg of fluoxymesterone daily) are adequate. *Note:* All methylated oral androgens may cause liver impairment when used over prolonged periods of time.

C. Treatment of Complications: Treat spread of tuberculosis (especially renal tuberculosis) and intercurrent infections with appropriate measures. The treatment of complications due to inadequate dosage or overdosage of corticosteroids consists of adjusting the dosage or changing the type or mixture of replacement steroids.

Criteria of Adequate Therapy & Overdosage

A. Adequate Therapy:

1. Return of blood pressure to normal (may require up to 3–4 months).

2. Maintenance of normal fasting blood glucose level.

3. Return of serum electrolytes to normal levels.

4. Weight gain (usually due to fluid).

5. Improvement of appetite and strength.

6. Increase in size of heart to normal.

B. Overdosage: Excessive administration of cortisone or desoxycorticosterone acetate must be avoided, especially in patients with cardiac or renal complications.

1. Signs and symptoms of cortisone overdosage are discussed on p 718.

2. Development of dependent edema, or excessive weight gain.

3. Development of hypertension.

4. Increase of diameter of heart above normal.

5. Development of signs of potassium deficiency (weakness followed by loss of muscle power and finally paralysis), especially if the patient is on a low-potassium diet.

Prognosis

With adequate replacement therapy the life expectancy of patients with Addison's disease is markedly prolonged. Active tuberculosis may respond to specific chemotherapy. Withdrawal of treatment or increased demands due to infection, trauma, surgery, or other types of stress may precipitate crisis with a sudden fatal outcome unless large doses of parenteral corticosteroids are employed. Pregnancy may be followed by exacerbation of the disease. Psychotic reactions may interfere with management. Hyperkalemic paralysis is a rare but serious complication if potassium intake is not monitored.

The ultimate prognosis depends largely upon the intelligence of the patient and the availability of medical supervision. A fully active life is now possible for the majority of patients.

Besser GM & others: Immunoreactive corticotrophin levels in adrenocortical insufficiency. Brit MJ 1:374, 1971.

Edmonds M & others: Autoimmune thyroiditis, adrenalitis and oophoritis. Am J Med 54:782, 1973.

Eisenstein AB: Addison's disease: Etiology and relationship to other endocrine disorders. M Clin North America 52:327, 1968.

Irvine WJ, Baines EW: Adrenocortical insufficiency. Clin Endocrinol Metab 1:549, 1972.

Jorgensen H: Hypercalcemia in adrenocortical insufficiency. Acta med scandinav 193:175, 1973.

Mason AS & others: Epidemiological and clinical picture of Addison's disease. Lancet 2:744, 1968.

Perez G & others: Selective hypoaldosteronism with hyperkalemia. Ann Int Med 76:757, 1972.

Schaison G & others: Mineralocorticoid function in 10 cases of Addison's disease. Ann Endocrinologie 31:609, 1970.

Schambelan M & others: Isolated hypoaldosteronism in adults: A renin-deficiency syndrome. New England J Med 287:573, 1972.

ADRENOCORTICAL OVERACTIVITY

Overactivity of the adrenal secretions is caused either by bilateral hyperplasia or by adenoma or, more rarely, carcinoma of one adrenal. The clinical picture will vary with the type of secretion produced, but in general 3 clinical disorders can be differentiated: (1) Cushing's syndrome, in which the glucocorticoids predominate; (2) the adrenogenital syndrome, in which the adrenal androgens predominate (feminizing tumors are rare); and (3) hyperaldosteronism, with electrolyte changes. The clinical picture is most apt to be mixed in cases of malignant tumor and in bilateral hyperplasia. All syndromes of adrenal overactivity are far more common in females than in males.

1. CUSHING'S SYNDROME
(Adrenocortical Hyperfunction)

Essentials of Diagnosis

- Centripetal obesity, easy bruisability, psychosis, hirsutism, purple striae.
- Osteoporosis, hypertension, glycosuria.
- Elevated 17-hydroxycorticosteroids, low serum potassium and chloride, low total eosinophils, and lymphocytopenia.

- Failure of suppression of cortisol secretion by exogenous dexamethasone.
- Special x-ray studies may reveal a tumor or hyperplasia of the adrenals.

General Considerations

This disorder is due to an excess of cortisol elaborated by the adrenal cortex. The adrenal cortex is almost always involved, either by hyperplasia or by adenoma or carcinoma. The primary lesion may be in the pituitary or in the hypothalamus.

Hyperplasia of both adrenal cortices is the most common form (80%). Occult small pituitary adenomas are present in a significant number of these patients. Adenoma of one adrenal (single adenoma) is the next most common form (15%), and this type often constitutes the clearest form of Cushing's syndrome. The opposite adrenal is atrophic.

Carcinoma of the adrenal (5%) is always unilateral and often metastasizes late. A mixed picture with virilization is often present. The opposite gland is atrophic.

Adrenal rest tumors in the ovary rarely cause Cushing's syndrome; they are more commonly associated with virilizing syndromes. Carcinoma of the anterior pituitary is a rare cause of Cushing's disease.

Administration of corticotropin causes adrenal hyperplasia; administration of cortisone causes adrenal atrophy associated with most features of Cushing's syndrome. These effects are partially reversible when medication is withdrawn.

Certain extra-adrenal malignant tumors (eg, bronchogenic oat cell carcinoma) may secrete ACTH or, more rarely, corticotropin-releasing factor and produce severe Cushing's syndrome with bilateral adrenal hyperplasia. Severe hypokalemia and hyperpigmentation are commonly found in this group.

Clinical Findings

A. Symptoms and Signs: Cushing's syndrome or disease causes "moon face" and "buffalo hump," obesity with protuberant abdomen, and thin extremities; a plethoric appearance; oligomenorrhea or amenorrhea (or impotence in the male); weakness, backache, headache; hypertension; mild acne and superficial skin infections; chloasma-like pigmentation (especially on the face), hirsutism (mostly of the lanugo hair over the face and upper trunk, arms, and legs), purple striae (especially around the thighs, breasts, and abdomen), and easy bruisability (eg, hematoma formation following venipuncture). Patients with Cushing's disease or syndrome are less prone than normal people to develop minor colds or allergic disorders. Mental symptoms may range from increased lability of mood to frank psychosis.

B. Laboratory Findings: Glucose tolerance is low, often with glycosuria. The patient is resistant to the action of insulin. Urinary 17-hydroxycorticosteroids and plasma cortisol are high (the latter over 20 μg/100 ml). (*Note:* In patients receiving estrogens—eg, contraceptive pills—the plasma cortisol levels are elevated due to increase in cortisol-binding globulin.) The usual diurnal variation in plasma cortisol levels is absent in Cushing's syndrome. Urinary 17-ketosteroids are often low or normal in Cushing's syndrome due to adenoma; normal or high if the disorder is due to hyperplasia; and very high if due to carcinoma. Total eosinophils are low (under 50/cu mm), lymphocytes are under 20%, and red and white blood cell counts are elevated. Serum CO_2 is high and serum chloride and potassium are low in some cases, especially those associated with malignant tumors.

C. X-Ray Findings: Osteoporosis of the skull, spine, and ribs is common. Nephrolithiasis may be seen. Intravenous urograms or retroperitoneal pneumograms may demonstrate a tumor of the adrenal or bilateral enlargement. X-ray of the sella is usually not helpful since basophilic adenomas are very small, but serial x-rays may demonstrate progressive enlargement (especially after adrenalectomy).

Adrenal angiography or [131]I-19-iodocholesterol scanning may demonstrate small adrenal tumors.

D. ECG Findings: ECG may show signs of hypertension and hypokalemia and a short P–R interval.

E. Special Tests: (*Note:* Exceptions to the following rules are occasionally seen.)

1. Dexamethasone suppression tests—Administration of dexamethasone, 2 mg every 6 hours for 2 days suppresses the activity of hyperplastic adrenals but has no effect on adrenal hyperactivity due to adenoma or carcinoma. A small dose of dexamethasone (0.5 mg every 6 hours for 2 days) will suppress normal adrenals but not hyperplastic adrenals. A rapid screening test for Cushing's syndrome is the administration of 1 mg of dexamethasone at 11:00 p.m. with measurement of the plasma hydroxycorticosteroids the following morning. Patients under stress or those receiving chronic drug therapy may not respond with normal suppression.

2. ACTH stimulation test—The administration of ACTH causes marked hypersecretion of urinary 17-hydroxycorticosteroids and 17-ketosteroids in Cushing's disease or syndrome due to hyperplasia and often also in cases due to adenoma but does not stimulate secretion in cases due to carcinoma.

3. Metyrapone (Metopirone) stimulation test—Failure of corticosteroids to rise after a 4-hour infusion or after an oral dose of 500 mg every hour for 6 doses favors neoplasm rather than hyperplasia.

4. Direct assay of plasma ACTH—This test is not generally available. ACTH is detectable in the plasma in bilateral adrenal hyperplasia but not in adrenal tumors. It is markedly elevated in ectopic tumors producing Cushing's syndrome.

5. The urinary free cortisol test—This test (not generally available) is most specific for the diagnosis of Cushing's syndrome since, unlike the 17-hydroxycorticosteroids, free cortisol is not affected by drugs, obesity, stress, etc. (See Eddy reference, below.)

Differential Diagnosis

The most difficult problem is differentiating true Cushing's syndrome from obesity associated with diabetes mellitus, especially if there are hirsutism and amenorrhea. The distribution of the fat, the virtual absence of virilization, and the laboratory studies often help, but are not infallible. Cushing's syndrome must be differentiated from the adrenogenital syndrome (see below), since the latter may be amenable to medical treatment unless it is caused by tumor. The 2 diseases may coexist. An elderly woman with osteoporosis, diabetes, and mild hirsutism may present a difficult problem in differentiation. Exogenous administration of corticosteroids must be kept in mind.

In rare cases the outstanding manifestation of Cushing's disease or syndrome may be only diabetes, osteoporosis, hypertension, or psychosis. Adrenal disease must be ruled out in patients with these disorders, especially in insulin-resistant diabetes mellitus, since early treatment may be curative. The dexamethasone suppression tests (see above) are most helpful in differentiation.

Complications

The patient may suffer from any of the complications of hypertension, including congestive failure, cerebrovascular accidents, and coronary attacks, or of diabetes. Susceptibility to infections, especially of the skin and urinary tract, is increased. Compression fractures of the osteoporotic spine may cause marked disability. Renal colic may occur. Intractable gastric ulcer may be present. Most serious, perhaps, are the psychotic complications not infrequently observed in this disease. After adrenalectomy, hypercalcemia and pancreatitis may complicate the recovery. Pituitary enlargement (due to chromophobe adenomas) and deepening skin pigmentation have been observed following adrenalectomy for hyperplasia, causing, at times, cranial nerve palsies (Nelson's syndrome).

Treatment

A. Specific Measures:

1. Tumors are removed surgically. Total (preferred) or subtotal resection of both adrenals in patients with diffuse bilateral hyperplasia is the present treatment of choice for rapidly advancing Cushing's syndrome. Adequate preoperative medication and care are of utmost importance. The patient should receive all general measures listed below, plus adequate hormonal supplementation.

If bilateral adrenalectomy is contemplated, give high doses of cortisone, eg, cortisone acetate, 100–300 mg IM, or, preferably, 100–300 mg of Solu-Cortef in divided doses IM or IV, on the day of surgery; continue the IM dosage for 1–2 days after surgery, then gradually decrease the dose and maintain on oral hydrocortisone as for Addison's disease. Because of the danger of precipitating heart failure, care must be taken to avoid excessive fluids and sodium.

In cases of unilateral tumor, the patient is prepared as for total adrenalectomy. After surgery, cortisol as well as corticotropin may be given to stimulate the atrophic gland. Treatment with cortisol may have to be continued for weeks or months since the gland may be slow to recover function.

2. X-ray therapy to the pituitary (either alone or following unilateral adrenalectomy) is the treatment of choice in most milder cases of hyperplasia. It may be tried initially; if not successful, total adrenalectomy must be performed. Partial destruction of the pituitary by other means (proton beam, yttrium implant, cryotherapy) has been attempted. Hypophysectomy may be required for large chromophobe adenomas.

3. Removal of an extra-adrenal malignant tumor producing Cushing's syndrome is rarely feasible but may induce a temporary remission.

4. Chemical treatment by means of adrenocortical inhibitors has been largely unsuccessful. The least toxic of these, mitotane (Lysodren; o,p′DDD), has limited use in inoperable carcinomas. Metyrapone and aminoglutethimide have been used to reduce adrenocortical overactivity, but the results are erratic.

B. General Measures: A high-protein diet should be given, although dietary attempts to correct the negative nitrogen balance are never successful. Testosterone or one of the newer anabolic agents may be of value in reversing the negative nitrogen balance. Potassium chloride administration may replace losses before and after surgery.

Insulin is usually of little value in controlling the glycosuria and hyperglycemia, and is usually unnecessary as the diabetes is quite mild.

Prognosis

This is a chronic disease which is subject to cyclic exacerbations (especially with pregnancy) and rare spontaneous remissions; it is a serious and often fatal disease unless discovered and treated early. A rather rapid course suggests a malignant tumor, but these may be dormant for years.

The best prognosis for eventual recovery is for patients in whom a benign adenoma has been removed and who have survived the postadrenalectomy state of adrenal insufficiency. About 25–50% of patients with bilateral hyperplasia may respond to pituitary irradiation alone or combined with subtotal adrenalectomy.

Complete adrenalectomy necessitates chronic replacement therapy, which is feasible today.

Malignant extra-adrenal tumors are usually rapidly fatal, even after such drastic attempts at treatment as total adrenalectomy.

Baxter JD: Iatrogenic Cushing's syndrome. Western J Med 120:301, 1974.

Cope C, Isard HJ, Wesolowski WE: Selective adrenal phlebography. Radiology 90:1105, 1968.

Eddy RL & others: Cushing's syndrome: A prospective study of diagnostic methods. Am J Med 55:621, 1973.

Egdahl RH: Surgery of the adrenal. New England J Med 278:939, 1968.

Friedman M, Marshall-Jones P, Ross EJ: Cushing's syndrome: Adrenocortical hyperactivity secondary to neoplasms arising outside the pituitary-adrenal system. Quart J Med 35:193, 1966.

Hutter AM Jr, Kayhoe DE: Adrenal cortical carcinoma: Clinical features of 138 patients. Am J Med 41:572, 1966.

Jubiz W & others: Effect of diphenylhydantoin on metabolism of dexamethasone. New England J Med 283:11, 1970.

Liddle GW, Shute AM: The evolution of Cushing's syndrome. Advances Int Med 15:41, 1969.

Liddle GW: Tests of pituitary adrenal suppressibility in the diagnosis of Cushing's syndrome. J Clin Endocrinol 20:1539, 1960.

Minagi H, Steinbach HL: Roentgen aspects of pituitary tumors manifested after bilateral adrenalectomy for Cushing's syndrome. Radiology 90:276, 1968.

Morrow LB & others: Complications of treated Cushing's syndrome. Henry Ford Hosp MJ 21:59, 1973.

Nelson DH & others: ACTH-producing pituitary tumors following adrenalectomy for Cushing's syndrome. Ann Int Med 52:560, 1960.

Nichols T, Nugent CA, Tyler FH: Steroid laboratory tests in the diagnosis of Cushing's syndrome. Am J Med 45:116, 1968.

Orth DN, Liddle GW: Results of treatment of 108 patients with Cushing's syndrome. New England J Med 285:243, 1971.

Rovit RL, Duane TD: Cushing's syndrome and pituitary tumors: Pathophysiology and ocular manifestations of ACTH-secreting pituitary adenomas. Am J Med 46:416, 1969.

Sawin CT: Measurement of plasma cortisol in the diagnosis of Cushing's syndrome. Ann Int Med 68:624, 1968.

Schambelan M: Mineralocorticoid production in hyperadrenocorticism. Am J Med 51:299, 1971.

Sparks L & others: Experience with a rapid oral metyrapone test and the plasma ACTH content in determining the cause of Cushing's syndrome. Metabolism 18:175, 1969.

2. THE ADRENOGENITAL SYNDROME: PREPUBERAL

Essentials of Diagnosis

- Pseudohermaphroditism in females with abnormal urogenital development noted at birth or precocious development early in life. Often familial.

- Enlarged clitoris or phallus, hirsutism, short stature, excessive muscular development, acne, seborrhea.

- 17-Ketosteroids elevated, FSH absent to low, pregnanetriol elevated in usual form.

- Excessive masculinization in males; may be associated with water and electrolyte disturbances, particularly in the neonatal period.

General Considerations

This disorder is produced by androgenic excess, due either to adrenal hyperplasia (often familial) or adrenal tumors, and manifests its virilizing effects by interfering with the normal sexual development of the fetus, infant, or child. The congenital form of the adrenogenital syndrome is due to an inborn error of metabolism with a deficiency of an adrenal enzyme (most commonly 21- or 11β-hydroxylase), resulting in low levels of cortisol with increase in ACTH leading to adrenal hyperplasia; the childhood form, occurring after normal intrauterine development, may be due either to tumor or to hyperplasia. Congenital adrenocortical hyperplasia is rare, often familial, much more common in females, and often associated with an addisonian-like state in male infants. Rarely, congenital virilization is caused by testosterone or progesterone administration to the pregnant mother. Gynecomastia may be the presenting complaint of a feminizing adrenocortical tumor.

Clinical Findings

A. Symptoms and Signs:

1. Congenital adrenocortical hyperplasia—In females, pseudohermaphroditism, enlargement of the clitoris, urogenital sinus formation, and, later, hirsutism are found; in males, phallic enlargement (macrogenitosomia praecox), precocious virilization, and (in infants) an addisonian-like state which may be confused with pyloric stenosis, characterized by nausea and vomiting, dehydration, and electrolyte deficiencies.

2. Adrenogenital syndrome in children—Somatic growth is accelerated; bone age is accelerated with early epiphyseal closure and eventual short stature. Other findings include excessive muscular development ("infant Hercules"), precocious virilization, and in some cases acne and seborrhea. With tumors some clinical features of Cushing's disease may be present. Hypertension may occur.

B. Laboratory Findings: Bone age is advanced on x-ray examination; 17-ketosteroids are elevated for the age. Intravenous urograms, retroperitoneal oxygen studies, or adrenal angiography may demonstrate adrenal pathology. FSH is absent or very low. ACTH stimulation tests and cortisone suppression tests help distinguish normal, hyperplastic, and neoplastic adrenals. Urinary pregnanetriol excretion is elevated in congenital adrenal hyperplasia and in carcinomas. Plasma testosterone is elevated.

Differential Diagnosis

A. In Either Sex: Distinguish from Cushing's syndrome (Table 18–9).

B. In Males: Differentiate from true isosexual precocity, either constitutional or due to hypothalamic or pineal lesions. In this situation the FSH test is positive and the 17-ketosteroids normal or only slightly elevated; the testes are larger than the testes of the adrenogenital boy, and spermatogenesis may occur. The other important condition causing pseudosexual precocity is unilateral or bilateral interstitial tumor of the testis. These are usually palpable within the scrotum. 17-Ketosteroid excretion is not as high in interstitial tumor as in adrenal tumor.

C. In Females: The most important differentiation is from genetic intersexuality (true hermaphrodite with testes, ovotestes, or ovaries). 17-Ketosteroid excretion is normal in intersex, and the chromosomal count on a buccal or vaginal smear helps to establish the diagnosis. Premature appearance of pubic hair may cause confusion, but other stigmas of virilization are not present. Arrhenoblastomas of the ovary do not occur before puberty.

Treatment

Treatment is discussed in the next section.

Prognosis

Males with congenital adrenal hyperplasia, even when treated intensively, often die in infancy of severe fluid and electrolyte loss. Some tumors are malignant and often fatal, but early removal will cause regression of virilization. The use of cortisone in bilateral hyperplasia has been most effective in suppressing adrenal virilization and restoring a normal state with breast development, menses, etc in girls and spermatogenesis in males if started early in life before irreversible changes have occurred. The ultimate prognosis for patients who receive cortisone is not yet known, but in some cases remissions have been sustained for several years even though cortisone is discontinued. Normal pregnancy has occurred after long-term cortisone therapy.

Bongiovanni AM, Root AW: The adrenogenital syndrome. (3 parts.) New England J Med 268:1283, 1342, 1391, 1963.

Brook CGD & others: Experience with long term therapy in congenital adrenal hyperplasia. J Pediat 85:12, 1974.

Gabrilove JL: Feminizing adrenocortical tumors in the male: A review of 52 cases. Medicine 44:37, 1965.

Kenny FM & others: Virilizing tumors of the adrenal cortex. Am J Dis Child 115:445, 1968.

New MI: Congenital adrenal hyperplasia: Symposium on recent clinical advances. P Clin North America 15:395, 1968.

Rappaport R, Cornu G, Royer P: Statural growth in congenital adrenal hyperplasia treated with hydrocortisone. J Pediat 73:760, 1968.

3. ADRENOGENITAL SYNDROME & VIRILIZING DISEASES OF WOMEN

Essentials of Diagnosis

- Menstrual disorders and hirsutism.
- Regression or reversal of primary and second-

Table 18–9. Differentiation of adrenogenital syndrome and Cushing's syndrome.

	Adrenogenital Syndrome	Cushing's Syndrome
Hirsutism	+++	+
Virilism	+++	0
Growth rate	++	*
Muscles	+++	Decr
17-Ketosteroids	+++	+
17-Hydroxy-corticosteroids	N or decr	+++
Pregnanetriol	++	0

*Retarded in children.

ary sex characteristics with balding, hoarse voice, acne, and enlargement of the clitoris.
- Occasionally a palpable pelvic tumor.
- 17-Ketosteroids elevated in adrenal disorders, variable in others.
- Urinary and plasma testosterone elevated.

General Considerations

The diagnosis of virilizing disorders in adult females is more difficult since other sources of abnormal androgens exist, principally the ovaries. There is no interference with formation of the female genital tract or secondary sex characteristics, but rather a regression or sex reversal of varying degree. Although the diagnosis is readily apparent in a complete state of the virilizing syndrome (eg, the adult form of the congenital adrenogenital syndrome), the milder forms, presenting primarily with defeminization or merely excessive hirsutism, may be caused by equally serious adrenal and ovarian disorders such as tumors. A sudden change in amount of hair (other than at puberty, pregnancy, or menopause) is of greater importance than hirsutism which has been present throughout life.

Besides adrenal hyperplasia and tumors, adult female virilization may be caused by the following disorders:

(1) **Ovarian disorders**: Stein-Leventhal syndrome (large, polycystic ovaries, most common), theca luteinization (thecosis ovarii), arrhenoblastoma, hilar cell tumor or hyperplasia, adrenal cell rests, dysgerminoma (rare).

(2) **Hypothalamic-pituitary disorders**: Acromegaly (eosinophilic adenoma), hyperostosis frontalis (Stewart-Morgagni-Morel syndrome).

(3) **Placental causes**: Pregnancy, choriocarcinoma.

(4) **Miscellaneous causes**: True hermaphroditism, thymic tumors, drugs (eg, testosterone).

Clinical Findings

A. Symptoms and Signs: Symptoms include scant menstrual periods or amenorrhea, acne and roughening of the skin, odorous perspiration, and hoarseness or deepening of voice. Hirsutism is present over the face, body, and extremities, with thinning or balding of head hair. Musculature is increased and feminine contours are lost. The breasts and genitalia are atrophied, the clitoris and "Adam's apple" enlarged. A tumor may rarely be palpable on pelvic examination (arrhenoblastoma, polycystic ovaries).

B. Laboratory Findings: Urinary 17-ketosteroid determination is the most important single test in the diagnosis of adrenogenital syndrome. It helps differentiate constitutional hirsutism from adrenal disorders, in which the 17-ketosteroids are significantly elevated. Very high levels favor a diagnosis of adrenal tumor. In arrhenoblastoma or Stein-Leventhal syndrome, 17-ketosteroids may be normal or moderately elevated. The cortisone suppression test may distinguish between adrenal tumors, adrenal hyperplasia, and ovarian lesions. Elevated pregnanetriol levels suggest an adrenal lesion.

The assay of the most potent androgen (testosterone) in the blood has recently become possible and will be the screening procedure of choice for virilized women (see Ettinger references, below).

C. X-Ray Findings: Intravenous urograms, adrenal angiograms, or retroperitoneal pneumograms may reveal an adrenal tumor. Hysterosalpingography may show large ovaries. Pelvic pneumography has been a valuable tool to demonstrate ovarian enlargement.

D. Laparoscopy is often helpful.

Differential Diagnosis

Since hirsutism may be the only sign of adrenal tumor, all of the disorders characterized by excessive hair have to be considered in the differential diagnosis. From the practical standpoint, however, the diagnosis commonly depends upon whether one is dealing simply with racial, familial, or idiopathic hirsutism, where an unusual end-organ sensitivity to endogenous male hormone exists; or whether excessive amounts of male hormone are being produced. In general, if not only hirsutism but also enlargement of the clitoris and deepening of the voice are present (or loss of head hair), and if the onset is rapid, one can assume that a tumor of the adrenal or ovary is present. In these circumstances exploratory operation is mandatory in spite of equivocal laboratory and physical findings. Although virilization is not the rule with Cushing's syndrome, a mixed picture is at times seen in malignant adrenal tumors and, more rarely, in hyperplasia. (See Table 18-9.)

Complications

Aside from the known high incidence of malignancy in tumors causing virilization, the interference with femininity and consequent sterility may be irreversible. Diabetes and obesity may be complicating features. At times mental disorders accompany states of defeminization.

Treatment

When tumor is present, surgical removal is the treatment of choice. In some cases of adrenal hyperplasia, especially starting in infancy, there may be associated manifestations of hypoadrenocorticism (eg, excessive salt and water loss and failure to maintain a fasting blood sugar). This condition is apparently due to a congenital absence of hydroxylating enzymes of the adrenals. The "androgenic" compounds formed have no cortisol activity and are unable to suppress endogenous ACTH; hence the continued adrenal stimulation and large glands. Treatment with corticosteroids has proved valuable in reducing the activity of the glands (apparently by suppressing endogenous ACTH) and in supplying exogenously needed corticosteroids. In adults the drugs of choice appear to be prednisone or prednisolone, 5–15 mg daily orally, or dexamethasone, 0.5–1.5 mg daily orally, in divided doses; use the smallest dose which keeps the 17-ketosteroid, pregnanetriol, and testosterone levels within the normal range.

The response of congenital adrenal hyperplasia to long-term corticosteroid therapy is gratifying, with lessening of virilization and hirsutism and eventually normal cyclic menstruation. Plastic repair (removal of the clitoris and repair of a urogenital sinus) is required. Corticosteroid therapy of milder forms of virilization (eg, simple hirsutism) is less successful. Estrogen therapy may be of some value but must be used in large dosage. A combination of estrogen with nonandrogenic progesterone (eg, Enovid-E) may be used for long-term suppression of ovarian androgens.

Prognosis

The outlook is favorable if a malignant tumor is removed early, since metastasis often occurs late. Cortisone therapy may be of help in hyperplastic lesions. Fertility is often restored.

The ultimate fate of the virilized woman depends not only upon the underlying cause (ie, tumor or hyperplasia), but more particularly upon the age at onset of the virilizing influence and its duration. If virilization is of long standing, restoration of normal femininity or loss of hirsutism is unlikely even though the causative lesion is successfully removed.

Note: Many cases of simple hirsutism in females are not due to a readily demonstrable endocrine disease but to hereditary or racial factors and cannot be treated effectively with systemic medications or surgery. Epilation, preferably by electrolysis, is the treatment of choice.

Ettinger B & others: Plasma testosterone stimulation-suppression: Dynamics in hirsute women. Am J Med 51:170, 1971.

Ettinger B & others: Plasma testosterone stimulation-suppression: Dynamics in hirsute women: Correlation with long-term therapy. Am J Med 54:195, 1973.

Jacobs JP: Hirsutism and benign androgenic hyperplasia of the adrenals. Am J Obst Gynec 101:37, 1968.

Kirschner MA, Jacobs JB: Combined ovarian and adrenal vein catheterization to determine the site(s) of androgen overproduction in hirsute women. J Clin Endocrinol 33:199, 1971.

Lipsett MB & others: Physiological basis of disorders of androgen metabolism. Ann Int Med 68:1327, 1968.

Lipsett M & others: The differential diagnosis of hirsutism and virilism. Arch Int Med 132:616, 1973.

Muller SA: Hirsutism. Am J Med 46:803, 1969.

Nichols T & others: Glucocorticoid suppression of urinary testosterone excretion in patients with idiopathic hirsutism. J Clin Endocrinol 26:79, 1966.

Werk EE & others: Testosterone secreting adrenal adenoma under gonadotropin control. New England J Med 298:767, 1973.

PRIMARY HYPERALDOSTERONISM

Essentials of Diagnosis

- Hypertension, polyuria, polydipsia, muscular weakness, tetany.
- Hypokalemia, hypernatremia, alkalosis, renal damage.
- Elevated urinary aldosterone level and low plasma renin level.
- Tumors usually too small to be visualized by x-ray.

General Considerations

Primary hyperaldosteronism is a relatively rare disorder caused by aldosterone excess. Conn suggested that it may be a common cause of hypertension (20%), but other investigators feel that it accounts for less than 5% of cases. It is more common in females. Four types of primary hyperaldosteronism are recognized: (1) due to adrenocortical adenoma; (2) due to macro- or micronodular cortical hyperplasia; (3) due to adrenocortical hyperplasia with suppressible hyperaldosteronism; and (4) glucocorticoid-suppressible hyperaldosteronism. Edema is rarely seen in primary hyperaldosteronism, but secondary hyperaldosteronism is often found in edematous states such as cardiac failure and hepatic cirrhosis. Since sodium restriction stimulates aldosterone production, low-sodium diets or diuretic agents must be discontinued before the diagnosis can be confirmed with chemical tests.

Clinical Findings

A. Symptoms and Signs: Hypertension (usually benign), muscular weakness (at times with paralysis simulating periodic paralysis), paresthesias with frank tetanic manifestations, headache, polyuria (especially nocturnal), and polydipsia are the outstanding complaints. Edema is rarely present.

B. Laboratory Findings: Low serum potassium, hypernatremia, and alkalosis are pathognomonic of primary hyperaldosteronism, but at times the potassium level is normal. Various degrees of renal damage are manifested by proteinuria, alkaline urine, nephrocalcinosis, and low urine specific gravity unresponsive to vasopressin. If spironolactone, 50–75 mg 4 times daily for 5–8 days, restores serum potassium to normal, suspect hyperaldosteronism. Urinary and plasma aldosterone levels are markedly elevated and plasma renin levels are low.

A diabetic glucose tolerance curve may be seen.

There is resistance to the administration of desoxycorticosterone acetate (20 mg/day for 3 days) with failure to retain fluid and to suppress elevated aldosterone levels.

C. ECG Findings: ECG changes are due to prolonged hypertension and hypokalemia.

D. X-Ray Findings: Cardiac hypertrophy due to hypertension is the only x-ray finding. The tumors are usually too small to be visualized, except by adrenal angiography or [131]I-19-iodocholesterol scanning. These research procedures—as well as plasma aldosterone measurements via a venous catheter—for localization of the lesion may become generally available in the future. (See Horton reference, below.)

E. Other Findings: The plasma volume is increased 30–50% above normal.

Differential Diagnosis

This important reversible cause of hypertension must be considered in the differential diagnosis in any patient who shows muscular weakness and tetanic manifestations; and in the differential diagnosis of periodic paralysis, potassium- and sodium-losing nephritis, nephrogenic diabetes insipidus, and hypercalcemia and hypokalemia (be certain the patient has not been receiving diuretic agents). Excessive ingestion of licorice or laxatives may simulate hyperaldosteronism. The oral contraceptives may raise aldosterone secretion in some patients. Unilateral renal vascular disease producing secondary hyperaldosteronism with severe hypertension must be ruled out. The angiotensin II infusion test, which shows reduced vascular response in this disorder, may be helpful in the differential diagnosis. Plasma renin activity is low in primary hyperaldosteronism and elevated in renal vascular disease. Excessive secretion of deoxycortisol and compound B may produce a similar clinical picture. Low renin levels are found in about 25% of cases of essential hypertension. Their response to diuretics and their prognosis are better than those of patients with hypertension associated with high renin levels. Excess of an as yet unidentified mineralocorticoid is thought to be responsible by some. A rare cause of secondary hyperaldosteronism is juxtaglomerular cell hyperplasia (Bartter's syndrome) or a renin-secreting kidney tumor.

Complications

All of the complications of chronic hypertension are encountered in primary hyperaldosteronism. Progressive renal damage is less reversible than hypertension. The incidence of pyelonephritis and nephrocalcinosis is high.

Treatment

The specific treatment for primary hyperaldosteronism is surgical removal of adenomas or subtotal or total resection of hyperplastic glands if there is failure to respond to spironolactone treatment.

An occasional patient responds to dexamethasone suppression.

Secondary hyperaldosteronism may be treated with the chemical aldosterone antagonist spironolactone, or may respond to unilateral renal artery surgery or nephrectomy.

Prognosis

The hypertension is reversible in about two-thirds of cases, but persists or returns in spite of surgery in the remainder. The renal disease is partially reversible, but once pyelonephritis is established it may continue along its natural course.

The prognosis is much improved by early diagnosis.

Bartter FC: So-called Bartter's syndrome. New England J Med 281:1483, 1969.

Beevers DG & others: The use of spironolactone in the diagnosis and treatment of hypertension associated with mineralo-corticoid excess. Am Heart J 86:404, 1973.

Bravo EL & others: Spironolactone as a non-specific treatment for primary aldosteronism. Circulation 48:491, 1973.

Conn JW, Rovner DR, Cohen EL: Licorice-induced pseudoaldosteronism. JAMA 205:492, 1968.

Conn JW & others: Primary aldosteronism. Arch Int Med 129:417, 1972.

Conn JW & others: Syndrome of hypertension, hyperreninemia and secondary aldosteronism associated with renal juxtaglomerular cell tumor (primary reninism). J Urol 109:349, 1973.

Dunn MJ, Tannen RL: Low-renin hypertension. Kidney Int 5:317, 1974.

Ferriss JB & others: Results of adrenal surgery in patients with hypertension, aldosterone excess and low plasma renin concentration. Brit MJ 1:135, 1975.

George JM & others: The syndrome of primary aldosteronism. Am J Med 48:343, 1970.

Horton R, Flinck E: Diagnosis and localization in primary aldosteronism. Ann Int Med 76:885, 1972.

Jose A, Kaplan NM: Plasma renin activity in the diagnosis of primary aldosteronism. Arch Int Med 123:141, 1969.

Kaplan NN: Adrenal causes of hypertension. Arch Int Med 133:1001, 1974.

Lee MR: Renin-secreting kidney tumors: A rare but remediable cause of serious hypertension. Lancet 2:254, 1971.

Modlinger RS & others: Some observations on the pathogenesis of Bartter's syndrome. New England J Med 289:1022, 1973.

New MI: Dexamethasone-suppressible hyperaldosteronism. J Clin Endocrinol 37:93, 1973.

Peart WS: Renin-angiotensin system. New England J Med 292:302, 1975.

Weinberger MH & others: Hypertension induced by oral contraceptives containing estrogen and gestagen. Ann Int Med 71:891, 1969.

DISEASES OF THE ADRENAL MEDULLA

PHEOCHROMOCYTOMA

Essentials of Diagnosis

- "Spells" or "attacks" of headache, visual blurring, severe sweats, vasomotor changes in a young adult, weight loss.
- Hypertension, often paroxysmal ("spells") but frequently sustained.
- Postural tachycardia and hypotension; cardiac enlargement.
- Elevated BMR with normal T_4; glycosuria, negative cold pressor test; positive provocative (histamine, glucagon) and blocking agent tests (phentolamine).
- Elevated urinary catecholamines or their metabolites.

General Considerations

A not uncommon disease characterized by paroxysmal or sustained hypertension due to a tumor of pheochrome tissue, most commonly located in either or both adrenals (90%) or anywhere along the sympathetic nervous chain, and rarely in such aberrant locations as the thorax, bladder, or brain. About 10% of patients have multiple tumors, and these have a familial tendency. A small percentage becomes malignant and may show functioning metastases. Pheochrome tumors are associated with neurofibromatosis in about 5% of cases (often familial). There may be associated medullary carcinomas of the thyroid, parathyroid adenomas, and neuromas. The tumors, which are more commonly located on the right side, may vary in size and are rarely large enough to be palpable. They contain varying proportions of epinephrine and norepinephrine, with the latter usually predominating (50–90%). Norepinephrine-producing tumors are more likely to cause sustained hypertension; the paroxysmal variety is more common with epinephrine. Pregnancy or trauma is frequently the precipitating event in this disease, which is most common in women between the ages of 20 and 40.

Clinical Findings

A. Symptoms and Signs: Pheochromocytoma is manifested by attacks of severe headache, palpitation or tachycardia, profuse sweating, vasomotor changes (including pallor or flushing of the face or extremities), precordial or abdominal pain, nausea and vomiting, visual disturbances (including blurring or blindness), aphasia and loss of consciousness (rarely), increasing nervousness and irritability, increased appetite, dyspnea, angina, and loss of weight. Physical findings include hypertension, either in attacks or sustained, with cardiac enlargement; postural tachycardia (change of more than 20 beats/minute) and postural hypotension; mild elevation of basal body temperature; abdominal or flank tumor (in about 5%); and, rarely, transient swelling of the thyroid. Retinal hemorrhage or papilledema occurs occasionally.

B. Laboratory Findings: The cold pressor response is negative (blood pressure fall, or a rise of less than 20/15); BMR is elevated; T_4 is normal; and glycosuria or hyperglycemia (or both) may be present. An attack of hypertension may in rare cases be produced by massage of either flank. Blood volume is usually contracted.

C. Special Tests:

1. Provocative test (for use during the normotensive phase)—The histamine test is positive if administration of histamine causes release of medullary hormone and consequent rise in blood pressure. *Caution:* Phentolamine should be on hand in case blood pressure rise is excessive. Tyramine, and especially glucagon, have recently been advocated as safer provocative tests.

2. Blocking agent test (for use during the hypertensive phase)—Administration of phentolamine, 2–5 mg rapidly IV, blocks medullary hormone and causes a fall of blood pressure. (*Note:* The patient should not receive sedatives or antihypertensive drugs for at least 24 hours prior to the test.)

3. Assay of urinary catecholamines on a 24-hour urine specimen—and the simpler test for **3-methoxy-4-hydroxymandelic acid (vanilmandelic acid, VMA)**—are now generally available. The levels of these urinary constituents will be elevated in all cases of sustained and most cases of paroxysmal hypertension due to pheochromocytoma. *Note:* False elevation of catecholamines and of VMA due to interference from dietary products or drugs must be considered.

4. The most reliable test for pheochromocytoma associated with paroxysmal hypertension is direct **assay of epinephrine and norepinephrine** in the blood and urine during or following an attack. High epinephrine levels favor tumor localization within the adrenal gland. Proper collection of specimens is essential. Determination of blood catecholamines via a venous catheter—a research procedure—will help localize ectopic lesions.

5. X-ray visualization of the tumor by intravenous urogram, retroperitoneal oxygen study, or angiography is often successful.

Differential Diagnosis

Pheochromocytoma should always be suspected in any patient with labile hypertension, especially if some of the other features such as hypermetabolism or glycosuria are present in a young person. Because of such symptoms as tachycardia, tremor, palpitation, and high BMR, pheochromocytoma may be confused with thyrotoxicosis. It should be considered in patients with unexplained acute anginal attacks. About 10% are mistakenly treated for diabetes mellitus because of the glycosuria. Pheochromocytoma may also be misdiagnosed as essential hypertension, myocarditis, glomerulonephritis or other renal lesions, toxemia of pregnancy, eclampsia, and psychoneurosis. It rarely masquerades as gastrointestinal hemorrhage and abdominal disorders of an emergency nature. Serotonin-producing tumors may present a similar clinical picture but are quite rare. Conversely, the presence of an abdominal tumor such as aortic aneurysm or renal cyst in a patient with a falsely positive phentolamine test for pheochromocytoma has led to an erroneous diagnosis. Although false-positive tests are not uncommon with pharmacologic agents and may lead to unnecessary explorations, the occasional false-negative test may permit a potentially curable fatal disease to go unrecognized. The availability of urinary catecholamine determination has made the diagnosis much more accurate.

Complications

All of the complications of severe hypertension may be encountered. Hypertensive crises with sudden blindness or cerebrovascular accidents are not uncommon. These may be precipitated by sudden movement, by manipulation during or after pregnancy, by emotional stress or trauma, or during surgical removal of the tumor. Cardiomyopathy may develop.

After removal of the tumor, a state of severe hypotension and shock (resistant to epinephrine and norepinephrine) may ensue with precipitation of renal failure or myocardial infarction. These complications can be avoided by judicious preoperative and operative use of catecholamine blocking agents such as phentolamine and phenoxybenzamine and by the use of blood or plasma to restore blood volume. Hypotension and shock may occur from spontaneous infarction of the tumor.

On rare occasions a patient dies as a result of the complications of diagnostic tests or during surgery.

Some patients have associated medullary thyroid carcinomas or hyperparathyroidism.

There is a high incidence of associated cholelithiasis.

Treatment

Surgical removal of the tumor or tumors is the treatment of choice. This may require exploration of the entire sympathetic chain as well as both adrenals. Administration of phentolamine and blood or plasma before and during surgery and postoperative maintenance with norepinephrine and cortisone have made this type of surgery a great deal safer in recent years. Propranolol (Inderal) is of value in controlling tachycardia and other arrhythmias.

Since there may be multiple tumors, it is essential to recheck urinary catecholamine levels postoperatively.

Long-term treatment with phentolamine is not successful. Recently, oral phenoxybenzamine (Dibenzyline) has been successfully used as chronic treatment in inoperable carcinoma and preoperatively in severely ill patients. Its routine use for 7—10 days or longer prior to surgery allows the blood pressure to stabilize and blood volume to return to normal, thus reducing surgical and postoperative mortality. (*Note:* Monitor blood pressure carefully to avoid severe hypotension.)

Prognosis

The prognosis depends entirely upon how early the diagnosis is made. If the tumor is successfully removed before irreparable damage to the cardiovascular system has occurred, a complete cure is usually achieved. Complete cure (or improvement) may follow removal of a tumor which has been present for many years. Rarely, hypertension persists or returns in spite of successful surgery. Only a small percentage of tumors are malignant.

Before the advent of blocking agents the surgical mortality was as high as 30%, but this is rapidly being reduced.

If after removal of a tumor a satisfactory fall of blood pressure does not occur, always consider the presence of another tumor.

It has been estimated that in the USA alone about 800 deaths a year may be due to unrecognized pheochromocytoma.

Axelrod S, Weinshilboum R: Catecholamines. New England J Med 287:237, 1972.

Batsakis JG & others: Pheochromocytoma of the bladder. Arch Surg 96:254, 1968.

Engleman K, Sjoerdsma A: Chronic medical therapy for pheochromocytoma: A report of four cases. Ann Int Med 61:229, 1964.

Fauvre FM: Cardiomyopathy secondary to pheochromocytoma. California Med 117:58, Oct 1972.

Gitlow SE & others: The biochemical techniques for detecting and establishing the presence of a pheochromocytoma. Am J Cardiol 26:270, 1970.

Gitlow SE & others: Management of patients with pheochromocytoma. Am Heart J 82:557, 1971.

Griffith MI & others: Successful control of pheochromocytoma in pregnancy. JAMA 229:437, 1974.

Lawrence AM: Glucagon provocative test for pheochromocytoma. Ann Int Med 66:1091, 1967.

Rayfield EJ & others: Influence of diet on urinary VMA excretion. JAMA 221:704, 1972.

ReMine WH & others: Current management of pheochromocytoma. Ann Surg 179:740, 1974.

Rossi P, Young IS, Panke WF: Arteriography in pheochromocytoma. JAMA 205:547, 1968.

Sapira JD & others: "Non-pheochromocytoma." JAMA 212:2243, 1970.

Sarosi G, Doe RP: Familial occurrence of parathyroid adenomas, pheochromocytoma, and medullary carcinoma of the thyroid with amyloid stroma (Sipple's syndrome). Ann Int Med 68:1305, 1968.

Schimke RN & others: Pheochromocytoma, medullary thyroid carcinoma and multiple neuromas. New England J Med 279:1, 1968.

Sheps SG, Maher FT: Tests in diagnosis of pheochromocytoma. JAMA 205:895, 1968.

Sjoerdsma A & others: Pheochromocytoma: Current concepts of diagnosis and treatment. Ann Int Med 65:1302, 1966.

Zelch JV, Meaney TF, Belhobek GH: Radiologic approach to the patient with suspected pheochromocytoma. Radiology 111:279, 1974.

DISEASES OF THE PANCREATIC ISLET CELLS*

ISLET CELL FUNCTIONING PANCREATIC TUMORS

The pancreatic islet is composed of 3 types of cells of neural crest origin, each with distinct chemical and microscopic features: the alpha cell, the beta cell, and the nonbeta or delta (or alpha$_1$) cell. Each cell may give rise to benign or malignant neoplasms which are often multiple and usually present with a clinical syndrome related to hypersecretion of a native or ectopic hormonal product. Diagnosis of the tumor depends principally on specific assay of the hormone produced. In malignant insulinoma, an increase in

*Diabetes mellitus and the hypoglycemic states are discussed in Chapter 19.

plasma proinsulin—and, in the Zollinger-Ellison syndrome, "big" gastrin—may be the most specific findings. The exact hormone responsible for the "pancreatic cholera" syndrome remains unknown, but biologically it is secretin-like. Glucagon-secreting alpha cell tumors are the rarest of the functional tumors and present with mild diabetes, migratory erythma, and stomatitis.

In addition to the native hormones, aberrant or ectopic hormones may be secreted by islet cell tumors, including ACTH, melanocyte-stimulating hormone, serotonin, and chorionic gonadotropin, with a variety of clinical syndromes. Islet cell tumors may be part of the syndromes of multiple endocrine adenomatosis type I (with pituitary and parathyroid adenomas) or type II (with medullary thyroid carcinoma and pheochromocytomas).

Direct resection of the tumor (or tumors), which often spreads locally, is the primary form of therapy for all types of islet cell neoplasm except Zollinger-Ellison syndrome, where removal of the end-organ (total gastrectomy) is the treatment of choice. Palliation of functioning malignancies often requires both antihormonal and anticancer chemotherapy. The use of streptozotocin and asparaginase, especially for malignant insulinoma, has produced some encouraging results, although these drugs are quite toxic.

Prognosis in these neoplasms is variable. Long-term survival in spite of widespread metastases has been reported. Earlier diagnosis by hormonal assay may lead to earlier detection and a higher cure rate.

Bhagavan BS & others: Zollinger-Ellison syndrome. Arch Path 98:217, 1974.

Kahn CR & others: Pancreatic cholera: Beneficial effects of treatment with streptozotocin. New England J Med 292:941, 1975.

Mallinson CN & others: A glucagonoma syndrome. Lancet 2:1, 1974.

Schein PS & others: Islet cell tumors: Current concepts and management. Ann Int Med 79:239, 1973.

Schein P & others: Streptozotocin for malignant insulinomas and carcinoid tumor. Arch Int Med 132:555, 1973.

Zollinger RM, Coleman DW: *The Influences of Pancreatic Tumors on the Stomach.* Thomas, 1974.

DISEASES OF THE TESTES*

MALE HYPOGONADISM

Male hypogonadism may be classified according to time of onset, ie, prepuberal, puberal (Klinefelter's syndrome), or postpuberal. Eunuchism implies complete failure of gonadal development; eunuchoidism implies only partial deficiency.

The etiologic diagnosis of hypogonadism (eg, primary or secondary) is usually based on laboratory tests (Table 18–10).

1. PREPUBERAL HYPOGONADISM

The diagnosis of hypogonadism cannot usually be made in boys under the age of 17 or 18 since it is difficult to differentiate from "physiologic" delay of puberty.

Prepuberal hypogonadism is most commonly due to a specific gonadotropic deficiency of the pituitary. It may be familial and associated with anosmia (Kallmann's syndrome). It may also occur as a result of destructive lesions near the pituitary region (eg, suprasellar cyst) or, more rarely, as a result of destruction or malformation of the testes themselves (prepuberal castration).

In cases associated with a complete pituitary defect, the patient is of short stature or fails to grow and mature. Otherwise the patient is strikingly tall due to overgrowth of the long bones. The external genitalia are underdeveloped, the voice is high-pitched, the beard does not grow, and the patient lacks libido and potency and is unable to tan. In adult life he presents a youthful appearance, with obesity (often in girdle distribution), disproportionately long extremities (span

*See also Tumors of the Testis in Chapter 15.

Table 18–10. Laboratory tests in diagnosis of hypogonadism.

Type of Hypogonadism	Urinary or Serum Gonadotropins	Urinary 17-Ketosteroids
Primary testicular failure	"Hypergonadotropic"	
Complete (eg, castration)	Elevated	Low or normal
Partial: Leydig cell failure only	Moderately elevated	Low or normal
Seminiferous tubule failure (eg, Klinefelter's syndrome)	Elevated	Normal or low
Secondary to pituitary failure	"Hypogonadotropic"	
Complete: Panhypopituitarism	Very low	Very low
Partial: Isolated lack of FSH	Very low	Low
Secondary to miscellaneous factors Starvation, anorexia, severe hypothyroidism, etc	Low or low normal	Low to normal

exceeds height), lack of temporal recession of the hairline, and a small Adam's apple. Gynecomastia is occasionally seen (but apparent gynecomastia may be merely fat). The skin is fine-grained, wrinkled, and sallow, especially on the face. The penis is small and the prostate undeveloped. Pubic and axillary hair are scant. The testes may be absent from the scrotum (cryptorchism) or may be in the scrotum but very small. Spermatogenesis does not occur.

Bone age is retarded. Skull x-rays may show a lesion of the sella or above the sella (eg, craniopharyngioma). Anemia may be present. Urinary 17-ketosteroids are low or normal in testicular failure; very low or absent in primary pituitary failure. Urinary FSH is absent in primary pituitary failure, elevated in castration or testicular failure. Plasma testosterone and serum FSH and luteinizing hormone (LH) measurements are more specific than urinary 17-ketosteroids and "FSH" levels respectively.

Determination of the genetic chromosomal type may reveal genetic sex anomalies such as hermaphroditism.

The response to chorionic gonadotropin injections in cases due to pituitary failure will be maturation, rise of urinary 17-ketosteroids, and occasionally descent of cryptorchid testes. (In primary testicular failure, no such response occurs.) Testicular biopsy shows immature tubules and Leydig cells in hypopituitary patients.

Adequate testosterone therapy can make these individuals into apparently normal males except that they usually cannot produce sperm. In order to produce spermatogenesis, a combination of an FSH preparation, eg, human menopausal gonadotropin (Pergonal), with human chorionic gonadotropin (eg, APL) is required. This treatment is expensive and is not generally available. Patients with prepuberal hypogonadism must be placed on testosterone and maintained for life on adequate doses. Long-acting testosterone preparations, 200–300 mg IM every 2–4 weeks, may be employed. An alternative method, oral administration of other androgens, entails all the difficulties and dangers of prolonged oral administration. Dosage varies with different patients, but 10–25 mg of methyltestosterone daily orally is usually adequate to cause and maintain maturation and virilization. There is no great advantage of buccal over oral administration. Fluoxymesterone in doses of 5–10 mg orally may be a better androgen in this age group. (*Note:* Recent reports suggest that there is an association between methylated androgenic anabolic steroid therapy and the development of hepatic injury and hepatocellular carcinoma which may regress after cessation of treatment.) A rare patient with hypogonadotropinism (eg, Prader-Willi syndrome) may respond to clomiphene citrate and achieve normal spermatogenesis. Recent reports demonstrating a dramatic response of FSH and LH to LH-releasing factor seem to locate the defect in isolated hypogonadotropic hypogonadism to the hypothalamus and offer renewed hope for future treatment (see Weinstein reference, below).

Bagheri SA, Boyer JL: Peliosis hepatis associated with androgenic-anabolic steroid therapy: A severe form of hepatic injury. Ann Int Med 81:610, 1974.

Farrell GC & others: Androgen-induced hepatoma. Lancet 1:430, 1975.

Federman DD: The assessment of organ function: The testis. New England J Med 285:901, 1971.

Hamilton CR Jr & others: Hypogonadotropinism in Praeder-Willi syndrome: Induction of puberty and spermatogenesis by clomiphene citrate. Am J Med 52:322, 1972.

Johnson FL & others: Association of androgenic anabolic steroid therapy with development of hepatocellular carcinoma. Lancet 2:1273, 1972.

Sparkes RS, Simpson RW, Paulsen CA: Familial hypogonadotropic hypogonadism with anosmia. Arch Int Med 121:534, 1968.

Weinstein RL, Reitz RE: Pituitary-testicular responsiveness in male hypogonadotropic hypogonadism. J Clin Invest 53:408, 1974.

2. PUBERAL HYPOGONADISM
(Klinefelter's Syndrome)

The outstanding example of this group of diseases is the so-called Klinefelter's syndrome (puberal seminiferous tubule failure). It is a genetic disorder which is recognized at or shortly after puberty. It is at times familial. A similar acquired syndrome has been ascribed to infection. Most commonly there is only failure of the tubules and lack of the testicular estrogenlike hormone, with permanent sterility. The secretory function of the Leydig cells ranges from normal to definite failure. An abnormality in the LH feedback control as well as a disorder in steroidogenesis has recently been demonstrated in Klinefelter's syndrome. Study of the chromosomal pattern shows that the majority of these patients are "chromatin positive." A variant of the syndrome has been reported in hypogonadal males with hypospadias and a "negative" chromatin pattern (Reifenstein's syndrome). A similar picture is at times associated with myotonia dystrophica.

The clinical findings are swelling of the breasts (gynecomastia), sterility, lack of libido and potency (rare), and at times lack of development of body hair, and female escutcheon. Skeleton and muscular development are usually normal. There may be associated mental retardation. The testes are usually small, but are larger than in prepuberal hypogonadism. The penis and prostate are usually normal. The ejaculate usually contains no spermatozoa, although an occasional case with spermatogenesis in a mosaic variant has been described. Urinary 17-ketosteroids are low normal or normal. Urinary and serum FSH is elevated (a most significant finding). Testicular biopsy shows sclerosis of the tubules, nests of Leydig cells, and no spermatozoa. The sex chromatin count is most commonly XXY (rarely, XXXY or "mosaic"), with a chromatin-positive buccal smear. Bone age may be delayed.

All causes of gynecomastia must be differentiated

from Klinefelter's syndrome. The urinary FSH and the testicular biopsy will settle the diagnosis.

No treatment is necessary unless lack of potency is a problem, in which case testosterone should be given as for prepuberal hypogonadism. If gynecomastia is disfiguring, plastic surgical removal is indicated.

Becker KL & others: Klinefelter's syndrome: Clinical and laboratory findings in 50 patients. Arch Int Med 118:314, 1966.

Bowen P & others: Hereditary male pseudohermaphroditism with hypogonadism, hypospadias, and gynecomastia (Reifenstein's syndrome). Ann Int Med 62:252, 1965.

Capell PT & others: Effect of short-term testosterone administration on serum FSH, LH, testosterone: Evidence for selective abnormality in LH control in Klinefelter's syndrome. J Clin Endocrinol 37:752, 1973.

Gordon DL & others: Pathologic testicular findings in Klinefelter's syndrome. Arch Int Med 130:726, 1972.

Laron Z, Hochman IH: Small testes in prepubertal boys with Klinefelter's syndrome. J Clin Endocrinol 32:671, 1971.

Stewart-Bentley M: Leydig cell function in Klinefelter's syndrome. Metabolism 22:875, 1973.

Wershub LP: Hypogonadism in the male. Fertil Steril 15:9, 1964.

3. POSTPUBERAL HYPOGONADISM

Any pituitary lesion (eg, tumor, infection, necrosis) may lead to lack of gonadotropin; often hypogonadism is an early sign. The testes may be damaged by trauma, x-ray irradiation, infection, or in other ways. States of malnutrition, anemia, and similar disorders may lead to functional gonadal underactivity. The male climacteric, although a somewhat disputed syndrome, probably does exist; it makes its appearance about 20 years later than the female menopause.

The symptoms are varying degrees of loss of libido and potency; retardation of hair growth, especially of the face; vasomotor symptoms (flushing, dizziness, chills); lack of aggressiveness and interest; sterility; and muscular aches and back pain. Atrophy or hypoplasia of external genitalia and prostate is rare. The skin of the face is thin, finely wrinkled, and "fawn-colored," and the beard is scant. Hair is absent on the antitragus of the ear (Hamilton's sign). Girdle type obesity and kyphosis of the spine are present.

Urinary 17-ketosteroids are low. Urinary and plasma testosterone levels are low. Urinary and serum FSH or LH may be normal but are low in cases due to pituitary lesions and elevated in true testicular failure. The sperm count is low or spermatozoa may be absent. Bone age is usually normal, but the skeleton may show "epiphysitis," especially of the vertebral column (Scheuermann's disease), and osteoporosis.

True adult hypogonadism must be differentiated from the far more commonly seen psychogenic lack of libido and potency. Recent reports of hormonal differ-

ences in homosexual males must await further evaluation (see Kolodny & Masters reference, below). Confusion may also arise in men who are obese and have a sparse beard and small genitalia but normal sperm counts and urinary FSH ("fertile eunuchs"). These patients may represent examples of end-organ unresponsiveness or isolated lack of luteinizing hormone. The usual form of male infertility is "spermatogenic arrest." The disorder can only be diagnosed by testicular biopsy. Most of these patients have normal gonadotropins and are not benefited by therapy.

Oral methyltestosterone or fluoxymesterone is highly effective. The dosage necessary to control symptoms and to aid in overcoming the protein loss and debility of age is often as low as 5–20 mg daily. This dose may be used for a short period of time to control symptoms or may be continued indefinitely for control of symptoms and for its protein anabolic effect (see warning in Johnson FL reference, p 701). The use of the long-acting testosterones by injection may be more practical for prolonged treatment. Treatment of long-standing hypogonadism with androgens may precipitate anxiety and acute emotional problems which often require concomitant psychotherapy.

Although the existence of a "male menopause" has been suggested in the past, recent evidence of rising levels of LH and falling levels of testosterone in some males past the fifth decade indicates declining testicular function amenable to therapy.

•   •   •

Prognosis of Hypogonadism

If hypogonadism is due to a pituitary lesion, the prognosis is that of the primary disease (eg, tumor, necrosis). The prognosis for restoration of virility is good if testosterone is given. The sooner administration is started, the fewer stigmas of eunuchoidism remain (unless therapy is discontinued).

The prognosis for fertility is usually not good. It is only feasible in instances where the testicular elements are present but are unstimulated due to lack of pituitary tropic hormones. This therapy may become practical with the greater availability of gonadotropin from postmenopausal urine (human menopausal gonadotropins [HMG]). Synthetic LH-releasing factor may offer an effective treatment for hypogonadotropic hypogonadism in the near future.

Minor forms of hypogonadism may require only proper nutrition, thyroid hormone, and general hygienic measures.

Cryptorchism should be corrected surgically early, since the incidence of malignant testicular tumors is higher in ectopic testicles and the chance of ultimate fertility is lessened in long-standing cases.

Crooke AC, Davies AG, Morris R: Treatment of eunuchoidal men with human chorionic gonadotrophin and follicle-stimulating hormone. J Endocrinol 42:441, 1968.

Faiman C & others: "Fertile eunuch" syndrome: Demonstration of isolated luteinizing hormone deficiency by radioimmunoassay technique. Mayo Clin Proc 43:661, 1968.

Huffer V & others: Psychologic studies of adult male patients with sexual infantilism before and after androgen therapy. Ann Int Med 61:255, 1964.

Isurugi K & others: Age related changes in serum LH and FSH levels in normal men. J Clin Endocrinol 39:955, 1974.

Kolodny RC, Masters WH: Hormones and homosexuality. Ann Int Med 79:896, 1973.

London DR: Male infertility. Brit MJ 1:609, 1972.

Meinhard E & others: Testicular biopsy in examination of male infertility. Brit MJ 3:577, 1973.

Money J: Problems in sexual development: Endocrinologic and psychologic aspects. New York J Med 63:2348, 1963.

Rosen SW, Weintraub BD: Monotropic increase in serum FSH correlated with low sperm count in young men with idiopathic oligospermia and aspermia. J Clin Endocrinol 32:410, 1971.

Stearns E & others: Declining testicular function with age. Am J Med 57:761, 1974.

Wilson JD: Recent studies on the mechanism of action of testosterone. New England J Med 287:1284, 1972.

MALE HYPERGONADISM & TESTICULAR TUMORS

In adults, almost all lesions causing male hypergonadism are functioning testicular tumors, which quite frequently are malignant. In children, male hypergonadism may take the form of true precocious puberty, due to pituitary or hypothalamic lesions; or pseudoprecocious puberty, due to lesions of the testes or adrenal glands.

1. PREPUBERAL HYPERGONADISM

The symptoms and signs are premature growth of pubic and axillary hair, beard, and external genitalia and excessive muscular development. In true precocity due to pituitary or hypothalamic lesions the testicles enlarge as well and spermatogenesis occurs. In adrenal virilization or testicular tumor there is testicular atrophy, with or without palpable nodules; spermatogenesis does not take place. In childhood, interstitial cell tumors are the principal testicular tumors to be considered. Bilateral interstitial cell nodules are also seen with adrenal hyperplasia. Cases of hepatoma with true isosexual precocity have been reported.

If the cause of precocity is "constitutional," it is usually a harmless disorder, although the sex activities of these children must be controlled to prevent socially undesirable conceptions. If precocity is due to hypothalamic or pituitary lesions, the prognosis is poor since most of these tumors are not removable. Adrenal tumors and testicular tumors are often malignant.

Most patients with this syndrome who survive into adulthood will be short as a result of premature maturation and closure of their epiphyses.

Table 18–11. Sexual precocity along isosexual pattern.

Types and Causes	Characteristics
Neurogenic Brain tumor Encephalitis Congenital defect with hypothalamic involvement **Pituitary** Idiopathic activation, "constitutional" type	Testes mature normally; spermatogenesis occurs; secondary characteristics normal; sex hormones excreted in normal adult amounts.
Gonadal Interstitial cell tumor of testis	Tumor in one gonad, the other gonad immature or atrophic; spermatogenesis does not occur; sex hormones excreted in excessive amounts.
Adrenal Embryonic hyperplasia or tumor	Testes usually small and immature, occasionally containing aberrant adrenal tissue; no spermatogenesis; often results in adrenocortical insufficiency in males.

Treatment

In cases where the tumor is accessible, surgical removal is the treatment of choice. Bilateral adrenal hyperplasia which causes pseudoprecocious puberty can be successfully treated with cortisone, and normal development and spermatogenesis will occur following treatment. The use of progesterone preparations (eg, Depo-Provera) in the treatment of sexual precocity is under investigation. This treatment may lead to permanent damage to testicular tissue.

Camacho AM & others: Alterations of testicular histology and chromosomes in patients with constitutional precocity treated with medroxyprogesterone acetate. J Clin Endocrinol 34:279, 1972.

Jolly H: *Sexual Precocity.* Thomas, 1955.

Schoen E: Treatment of idiopathic precocious puberty in boys. J Clin Endocrinol 26:363, 1966.

Sigurjonsdottir TJ, Hayles AB: Precocious puberty. Am J Dis Child 115:309, 1968.

2. NEOPLASMS OF THE TESTES IN ADULTS
(Postpuberal Hypergonadism)

Many or most testicular neoplasms are functioning (ie, productive of androgenic or estrogenic hormones), and the majority are highly malignant (Table 18–12). They are at times quite small, and are clini-

Table 18—12. Characteristics of testicular tumors.*

Tumor and Hormone	Clinical Manifestations
Seminoma Elevation of urinary FSH	Onset usually at age 30—50. Tumor radiosensitive. No endocrinologic manifestations.
Teratoma No hormone elaborated except in mixed tumors	May occur in childhood also. No endocrinologic manifestations unless the tumor is of a mixed type. Tumor radioresistant, invasive.
Choriocarcinoma Chorionic gonadotropin elevated. Pregnancy test positive.	Rare. Gynecomastia. Tumor rapidly invasive and metastasizing, radioresistant. Leydig cells overactive due to stimulation by tumor.
Leydig cell 17-Ketosteroids elevated	Very rare. Occurs at any age and causes virilization. At times bilateral, often multiple.
Sertoli cell and tubular adenoma of Pick May elaborate estrogens	Benign tumors, probably developmental rests. Associated with congenital anomalies of genital tract. Rarely feminizing.

*Dean AL: The treatment of testes tumors. J Urol 76:439, 1956.

cally recognized because of their hormonal effects or because of the presence of metastases. In general, once hormonal manifestations have become pronounced, cure by surgical removal is very unlikely. Some tumors are bilateral, eg, interstitial cell tumors. Often a mixed picture is present. Gonadotropin-secreting bronchogenic carcinomas have been recently described (see Faiman reference, below).

The incidence of malignancy in cryptorchism is high.

Treatment

If the diagnosis is made early, surgical removal may be curative; radiotherapy is feasible as a palliative measure in radiosensitive types. Chemotherapy may control the growth of choriocarcinomas.

Faiman C & others: Gonadotropin secretion from a bronchogenic carcinoma. New England J Med 277:1395, 1967.

Kirschner MA, Cohen FB, Jespersen D: Estrogen production and its origin in men with gonadotropin-producing neoplasms. J Clin Endocrinol 39:112, 1974:

MacKenzie AR: Chemotherapy of metastatic testis cancer. Cancer 19:1369, 1966.

Sadoff L & others: New endocrine observations in a male patient with choriocarcinoma. Oncology 29:227, 1974.

Wegienka L, Kolb FO: Hormonal studies of a benign interstitial tumour of the testis producing androstenedione and testosterone. Acta endocrinol 56:481, 1967.

DISEASES OF THE OVARIES*

I. FEMALE HYPOGONADISM

The outstanding symptom of female hypogonadism is amenorrhea (see below). Partial deficiencies, principally corpus luteum failure, may occur which do not always cause amenorrhea but more often produce anovulatory periods or metrorrhagia.

Estrogenic failure has far-reaching effects, especially if it begins early in life (eg, Turner's syndrome).

Primary pituitary disorders are much less common causes of hypogonadism in the female than primary ovarian disorders, and are almost always associated with other signs of pituitary failure.

Ovarian failure starting in early life will lead to delayed closure of the epiphyses and retarded bone age, often resulting in tall stature with long extremities. On the other hand, in ovarian agenesis, dwarfism is the rule (see below). In adult ovarian failure, changes are more subtle, with some regression of secondary sex characteristics. In estrogenic deficiency of long standing in any age group, osteoporosis, especially of the spine, is almost always found since estrogen protects bone against excessive resorption.

A relatively rare form of ovarian failure is seen in states of androgenic excess, usually derived from the adrenal cortex, when estrogens, though present in the body, are suppressed by the presence of large amounts of androgens (see Virilizing Disorders of the Ovary).

AMENORRHEA

Since regular menstruation depends upon normal function of the entire physiologic axis extending from the hypothalamus and pituitary to the ovary and the uterine lining, it is not surprising that menstrual disorders are among the most common presenting complaints of endocrine disease in women. Correct diagnosis depends upon proper evaluation of each component of the axis, and nonendocrine factors must also be considered.

If menstruation is defined as shedding of endometrium which has been stimulated by estrogen or by estrogen and progesterone which are subsequently withdrawn, it is obvious that amenorrhea can occur either when hormones are deficient or lacking (the hypohormonal or ahormonal type) or when these hor-

*General references: (1) Lang WR (editor): Pediatric and adolescent gynecology. Ann New York Acad Sc 142:549, 1967. (2) Swerdloff RS, Odell WD: Gonadotropins: Present concepts in the human. California Med 109:467, 1968. (3) Catt KJ: ABC of endocrinology. 4. Reproductive endocrinology. Lancet 1:1097, 1970.

mones, though present in adequate amounts, are never withdrawn (the continuous hormonal type).

Primary amenorrhea implies that menses have never been established. This diagnosis is not usually made before the age of about 18. Secondary amenorrhea means that menses once established have ceased (temporarily or permanently).

The most common type of hypohormonal amenorrhea is the menopause, or physiologic failure of ovarian function. The most common example of continuous hormonal amenorrhea is that due to pregnancy, when cyclic withdrawal is prevented by the placental secretions. These 2 conditions should always be considered before extensive diagnostic studies are undertaken.

The principal diagnostic aids which are used in the study of amenorrhea are as follows: (1) vaginal smear for estrogen effect; (2) endometrial biopsy; (3) "medical D&C" (see below); (4) BBT determination; (5) urine determinations of 17-ketosteroids, FSH, pregnanediol, and pregnanetriol; (6) culdoscopy and gynecography; (7) chromosomal studies (eg, buccal or vaginal smear); (8) pelvic exploratory operation or laparoscopy, and gonadal biopsy; (9) radioimmune assays of FSH and LH, which are now available for specific diagnosis of certain types of amenorrhea; (10) plasma testosterone assay; (11) skull x-rays for pituitary size; and (12) in young females, bone age.

Baird DT, Fraser IS: Disorders of the hypothalamic-pituitary-ovarian axis. Clin Endocrinol 2:469, 1973.

Dewhurst CJ: Amenorrhea. Brit MJ 1:711, 1971.

Lunenfeld B, Insler V: Classification of amenorrhoeic states and their treatment by ovulation inductions. Clin Endocrinol 3:223, 1974.

Wilson JD & others: Familial incomplete male pseudohermaphroditism, type 2. New England J Med 291:944, 1974.

Wiser WL, Givens JR, Fish SA: Plasma gonadotropin assays in the diagnostic work-up of amenorrhea. Postgrad Med 52:198, 1972.

1. PRIMARY AMENORRHEA

Most cases of primary amenorrhea are of the hypohormonal or ahormonal type. Exact diagnosis is essential to rule out organic lesion along the hypothalamic-pituitary-gonadal axis. The chromosomal sex pattern must be determined in all cases. Pelvic exploration is often required to establish the diagnosis.

The causes are as follows:

(1) **Hypothalamic causes:** Constitutional delay in onset, debility, serious organic illness, lack of LRF.

(2) **Pituitary causes** (with low or absent FSH): Suprasellar cyst, pituitary tumors (eosinophilic adenomas, chromophobe adenomas, basophilic adenomas), isolated lack of pituitary gonadotropins.

(3) **Ovarian causes** (with high FSH): Ovarian agenesis (Turner's syndrome), destruction of ovaries (eg, due to infection or, possibly, autoimmunity), "premenarchal menopause."

(4) **Uterine causes** (usually with normal urinary FSH): Malformations, imperforate hymen, hermaphroditism, unresponsive or atrophic endometrium.

(5) **Miscellaneous causes:** Adrenal virilism, ie, pseudohermaphroditism (with high urinary 17-ketosteroid and pregnanetriol levels), various androgenic tumors. Testicular feminization (with inguinal gonads and blind vagina).

Treatment

Treatment is similar to that of secondary amenorrhea (see below). The underlying organic cause should first be corrected if possible. An abnormal gonad is usually removed surgically, since the incidence of gonadal neoplasm is high. Plastic repair of the vaginal tract is often required. If secondary sex characteristics have not developed, estrogens alone may be of value.

2. SECONDARY AMENORRHEA

Temporary cessation of menses is extremely common and does not require extensive endocrine investigation. In the childbearing age, pregnancy must be ruled out. In women beyond the childbearing age, menopause should be considered first. States of emotional stress, malnutrition, anemia, and similar disorders may be associated with temporary amenorrhea and correction of the primary disorder will usually also reestablish menses. Some women fail to menstruate regularly for prolonged intervals after stopping oral contraceptive pills. Lactation may be associated with amenorrhea, either physiologically or for abnormally prolonged periods after delivery (Chiari-Frommel syndrome).

By the use of the "medical D&C" (see p 725), ie, the administration of progesterone with subsequent withdrawal, these amenorrheas can be arbitrarily divided into amenorrhea with negative D&C and amenorrhea with positive D&C. The former (with the exception of pregnancy) show an atrophic or hypoestrin type of endometrium; the latter show an endometrium of the proliferative type but lacking progesterone.

(1) Secondary amenorrhea with negative medical D&C may be due to the following causes: pregnancy (pregnancy tests positive), menopause (urinary and serum FSH elevated), pituitary tumor, pituitary infarction (Sheehan's syndrome), virilizing syndromes such as arrhenoblastoma, Cushing's disease, Addison's disease, and miscellaneous causes such as anorexia nervosa, profound myxedema, irradiation of the uterine lining, and hysterectomy.

(2) Secondary amenorrhea with positive medical D&C may be due to metropathia hemorrhagica, Stein-Leventhal syndrome, estrogen medication, estrogenic tumors, ie, granulosa cell tumors (rare), hyperthyroidism, and perhaps liver disease.

Some degree of overlap in these 2 groups is sometimes found.

Treatment

The aim of therapy is not only to reestablish menses (although this is valuable for psychologic reasons) but also to attempt to establish the etiology (eg, pituitary tumor) of the amenorrhea and to restore reproductive function.

Treatment depends upon the underlying disease. It is not necessary to treat all cases, especially temporary amenorrhea or irregular menses in unmarried girls or women. These cases usually are corrected spontaneously after marriage or first pregnancy.

In patients whose response to progesterone is normal, the administration of this hormone during the last 10–14 days of each month, orally or parenterally (see p 725), will correct the amenorrhea.

In patients who are unresponsive to progesterone and whose urinary gonadotropin levels are low, treatment of a pituitary lesion may restore menstruation; gonadotropins would appear to be of value, and human pituitary FSH has been used with some success experimentally. This, or FSH from postmenopausal urine in combination with APL, has given good results in secondary amenorrhea. Clomiphene citrate (Clomid) has been extensively and often successfully tried for the treatment of these patients. However, in current clinical practice, estrogen alone or in combination with progesterone is more commonly used. If urinary gonadotropins are high, gonadotropins are of no value; treat with estrogens alone or with estrogens and progesterone. Corticosteroids may restore menstruation in certain virilizing disorders. Wedge resection of the ovaries often restores regular menstruation in the Stein-Leventhal syndrome. The use of LH-releasing hormone is under investigation at present (see Keller reference, below).

General measures include dietary management as required to correct overweight or underweight; psychotherapy in cases due to emotional disturbance; and correction of anemia and any other metabolic abnormality which may be present (eg, mild hypothyroidism).

3. HYPOTHALAMIC AMENORRHEA

Secondary hypothalamic amenorrhea, due to emotional or psychogenic causes is far more common in young women than amenorrhea due to organic causes (except for pregnancy). It is probably mediated by a hypothalamic block of the release of pituitary gonadotropic hormones, especially LH. Pituitary FSH is still produced and is found in normal or low levels in the urine. Since some LH is necessary in the production of estrogen as well as FSH, a state of hypoestrinism with an atrophic endometrium will eventually result. Galactorrhea may be associated with amenorrhea (see Pernoll reference, below).

A history of psychic trauma just preceding the onset of amenorrhea can usually be obtained. The urinary FSH level is normal or low normal, and the 17-ketosteroid level is low normal. Plasma LH is low. Vaginal smear and endometrial biopsy show mild hypoestrin effects. The response to progesterone (medical D&C) is variable. The endometrium responds to cyclic administration of estrogens.

Menses often return spontaneously, after weight gain, or after several induced "cycles." Psychotherapy may be of value. Clomiphene citrate (Clomid) may be tried to reestablish menses. If amenorrhea persists for many years, signs of severe estrogen deficiency will appear and must be treated.

It is most important to recognize this syndrome and not to mistake it for an organic type of amenorrhea with a very different prognosis.

Crooke AC, Tsapoulis AD: Comparison of clomiphene and follicle-stimulating hormone for treatment of anovulation. J Endocrinol 41:ii, May 1968.

Frisch RE, McArthur JW: Menstrual cycles: Fatness as a determinant of minimum weight for height necessary for their maintenance or onset. Science 185:949, 1974.

Keller PJ: Induction of ovulation by synthetic luteinizing hormone-releasing factor in infertile women. Lancet 2:570, 1972.

Kempers RD & others: Induction of ovulation with clomiphene citrate. Obst Gynec 30:699, 1967.

Marshall JC & others: Amenorrhoea in anorexia nervosa: Assessment and treatment with clomiphene citrate. Brit MJ 4:590, 1971.

Pernoll MF: Diagnosis and treatment of galactorrhea. Postgrad Med 49:76, 1971.

Rosenberg E, Nwe TT: Induction of ovulation with human postmenopausal gonadotropin: Experience with 23 patients. Fertil Steril 19:197, 1968.

Shearman RP: Prolonged secondary amenorrhea after oral contraceptive therapy. Lancet 2:64, 1971.

Simmer HH & others: *Testicular Feminization.* Thomas, 1965.

Taymor ML: Gonadotropin therapy. JAMA 203:362, 1968.

TURNER'S SYNDROME
(Primary Ovarian Agenesis, Gonadal Dysgenesis)

Turner's syndrome is a rather rare disorder due to congenital absence of the ovaries and associated with dwarfism and other anomalies. Evidence suggests that in most instances patients with this syndrome lack one of the 2 X chromosomes. A rarer variant shows androgenic tissue in the gonadal remnant with mild virilization.

The principal features include congenital ovarian failure; genital hypoplasia with infantile uterus, vagina, and breasts and primary amenorrhea; scant axillary and pubic hair; short stature, usually between 122–142 cm (48–56 inches); increased carrying angle of arms; webbing of neck (quite common); eye disorders; stocky "shield" chest; cardiovascular disorders, especially coarctation of the aorta, congenital valve defects; osteoporosis and other skeletal anomalies (short metacarpals, exostosis of tibia, etc) with increasing age; and prematurely senile appearance. Nevi are common. Idiopathic edema is seen in infants. There is an increased incidence of autoimmune thyroiditis and diabetes.

Urinary and serum FSH is high, and 17-ketosteroids are low. Bone age is retarded. The chromatin sex pattern most often shows a "negative" buccal smear and XO chromosomal pattern.

Exploratory operation shows a "streak ovary" and, at times, islands of interstitial cells.

The principal disorder to be differentiated is pituitary dwarfism. In this disorder the urinary and serum FSH is low or absent and other signs of pituitary failure are present. The axillary and pubic hair is absent in pituitary dwarfs; although it is scant in Turner's syndrome, it increases with estrogen administration. Other forms of constitutional dwarfism, such as Laurence-Moon-Biedl syndrome, are ruled out by the urinary FSH and lack of stigmas such as polydactylia, and the presence of retinitis pigmentosa and other signs of the disease. The short stature and occasional metacarpal deformities may resemble pseudohypoparathyroidism, but these patients menstruate normally.

With the administration of estrogens some increase in height can be achieved, but this is almost never enough to increase stature significantly; androgens may also promote growth, especially fluoxymesterone in low doses. (See Johansen reference, below.) Some cases respond to pituitary growth hormone.

If untreated, growth will eventually cease since the epiphyses will close spontaneously (though late). The administration of estrogen will develop the breasts and uterus and lead to anovulatory menses upon cyclic withdrawal. *Note:* Endometrial carcinoma has been reported after diethylstilbestrol therapy (see Cutler reference, below). Fertility can never be achieved.

The associated congenital cardiovascular anomalies may cause early death or may require surgical correction (eg, coarctation). Webbing of the neck can be corrected by plastic surgery.

Several variants of this syndrome with different chromosomal patterns have been recently described. "Pure gonadal dysgenesis" has only "streak" gonads without other associated skeletal anomalies. "Mixed" or "atypical" gonadal dysgenesis, a form of hermaphroditism, has a "streak" gonad on one side and an abnormal gonad, prone to neoplasm, on the other side, making prophylactic removal a reasonable procedure.

Cutler BS & others: Endometrial carcinoma after stilbestrol therapy in gonadal dysgenesis. New England J Med 287:628, 1972.

Dmowski WP, Greenblatt RB: Ambiguous external genitalia in the newborn and prepubescent child. JAMA 212:308, 1970.

Donaldson CL & others: Growth hormone studies in Turner's syndrome. J Clin Endocrinol 28:383, 1968.

Doniach D, Roitt IM, Polani PE: Thyroid antibodies and sex-chromosome anomalies. Proc Roy Soc Med 61:278, 1968.

Goldberg MB, Scully AL: Gonadal malignancy in gonadal dysgenesis: Papillary pseudomucinous cystadenocarcinoma in a patient with Turner's syndrome. J Clin Endocrinol 27:341, 1967.

Goldberg MB & others: Gonadal dysgenesis in phenotypic female subjects: A review of eighty-seven cases with cytogenetic studies in fifty-three. Am J Med 45:529, 1968.

Johansen AJ & others: Growth in patients with gonadal dysgenesis receiving fluoxymesterone. J Pediat 75:1015, 1969.

Judd HL & others: Pure gonadal dysgenesis with progressive hirsutism: Demonstration of testosterone production by gonadal streaks. New England J Med 282:881, 1970.

Kallio H: Cytogenetic and clinical study on 100 cases of primary amenorrhea. Acta obst gynec scandinav (Suppl) 24:1, 1973.

Morishima A, Grumbach MM: The interrelationship of sex chromosome constitution and phenotype in the syndrome of gonadal dysgenesis and its variants. Ann New York Acad Sc 155:695, 1968.

Preger L & others: Roentgenographic abnormalities in phenotypic females with gonadal dysgenesis. Am J Roentgenol 104:899, 1968.

Simila S & others: Gonadoblastoma associated with pure gonadal dysgenesis. Clin Pediat 13:177, 1974.

Sohval AR: Hermaphroditism with "atypical" or "mixed" gonadal dysgenesis: Relationship to gonadal neoplasm. Am J Med 36:281, 1964.

Sohval AR: The syndrome of pure gonadal dysgenesis. Am J Med 38:615, 1965.

MENOPAUSAL SYNDROME

Essentials of Diagnosis

- Menstrual irregularities associated with hot flushes and personality changes.
- Age 45–55 years (unless due to surgery or irradiation).
- Hypoestrin vaginal smear, FSH levels elevated; osteoporosis in later years.

General Considerations

The term menopause refers to the permanent or final cessation of menstrual function either as a normal physiologic event or as a result of surgery or ovarian irradiation. In a broader sense the "menopausal syndrome" includes all of the sequelae of permanent cessation of ovarian function, of which the absence of menstruation is only a part.

Most women go through physiologic menopause at about 45–50 years of age, but premature ovarian failure may occur before the age of 30. Early menopause is more common in women who have had an infection or surgical disorder of the genital tract.

The time of onset of the menopause is often a familial trait. Rarely, premature ovarian failure may be part of generalized polyendocrine insufficiency, presumably on an autoimmune basis (see Irvine reference, below). Cyclophosphamide-induced ovarian failure has been reported.

The surgical or x-ray menopause differs from the

natural menopause in its more abrupt onset and the greater severity of manifestations.

The earlier ovarian failure takes place, the more severe are the effects on certain structures, principally the skeleton.

The clinical diagnosis of the menopause is at times difficult, since psychologic factors often overshadow symptoms due to hormonal deficiency. It is also of interest that many women never show any evidence of the menopause, whereas others suffer severely and may even develop psychoses.

Treatment must be directed at the immediate symptoms, but at times—and especially if postmenopausal osteoporosis is present—it must be maintained for prolonged periods.

Although reproductive function ceases, sexual activity past the menopause is not impaired unless psychic factors and misinformation produce an emotional block.

Clinical Findings

A. Symptoms and Signs: Amenorrhea is frequently preceded by menometrorrhagia or oligomenorrhea. Hot flushes are often severe, lasting only a few minutes but recurring frequently. The patient complains of feelings of tension, especially fullness in the head. Weight gain and nervous instability with depression, exhilaration, or lassitude are often present. Various aches and "rheumatic pains" commonly occur. Sexual changes include dyspareunia, loss of libido, or in some cases increased sexual interest. The breasts may be painful. Bladder irritation is common.

There are very few objective findings. Mild hypertension, mild hirsutism, tenderness over the spine, and dry skin with coarsening of the hair may occur.

B. Laboratory Findings: A hypoestrin type vaginal smear and elevated urinary and serum FSH levels are the only laboratory findings, but they may be quite delayed in their appearance.

C. X-Ray Findings: X-ray may show osteoporosis of the spine in later years.

Differential Diagnosis

Since most of the manifestations of the menopausal syndrome are purely subjective, it is often difficult to make an exact diagnosis unless a trial of estrogenic (or androgenic) therapy gives striking relief. The most difficult differentiation is from anxiety states with features of reactive depression. Pheochromocytoma and hyperthyroidism must also be considered. A variety of causes of back pain, including osteoarthritis and rheumatoid arthritis, may be considered in the differentiation from pain due to osteoporosis and menopausal arthralgia. In hypothyroidism menstrual irregularities, emotional changes, and aches and pains are also common. One must make certain that ovarian or uterine neoplasm is not the cause of the menstrual irregularity and back pains.

Complications

The serious complications of the menopause are psychosis and, in long-standing cases, osteoporosis. Diabetes mellitus may appear with the menopause. Senile vaginitis may also occur. The postmenopausal patient is more susceptible to degenerative cardiovascular disease and gout.

Treatment

A. Natural Menopause:

1. Physiologic aspects (estrogen therapy)—If cycles are very irregular and the patient suffers from menopausal symptoms, begin estrogens about 5 days after the onset of the last menstrual period and continue in a cyclic fashion. Give ethinyl estradiol, 0.05 mg, diethylstilbestrol, 0.5–1 mg, or estrone sulfate, 1.25 mg by mouth daily except for the first 5 days of each month. This is simple for patients to remember. In the younger patient who still has an occasional menstrual period, the use of the anovulatory agents may be the preferred treatment and also affords protection against unwanted pregnancies. An occasional patient is even intolerant to physiologic doses of estrogens, responding with painful breasts, fluid retention, etc. Reducing the dosage and the use of diuretics, vitamin B complex, and other measures may be helpful. If spotting or "breakthrough" bleeding occurs, cyclic progesterone therapy may be required. The use of androgens is usually not advisable because of undesirable side-effects (eg, hirsutism, voice changes).

If the patient has become amenorrheal, there is no reason to give estrogens in doses large enough to reinstitute menses but only to control symptoms. This is not always possible.

The duration of therapy has not been standardized and must be adjusted to the individual case. Three months to 1 year usually suffices, but in some cases therapy may have to be continued over prolonged periods.

Because of the anabolic effect of estrogens and because of their known beneficial effects on bone metabolism and on blood vessels, estrogen therapy has been recommended for life for women beyond the menopause. The advisability of this practice remains unsettled. If a patient is on long-term estrogen therapy she should keep an accurate record of her dosage schedule and bleeding. Uterine myomas may increase in size, and endometrial hyperplasia may occur. Whenever bleeding occurs that is not on schedule (during the withdrawal phase), tumor should be suspected. (*Note:* Breast and pelvic examination and vaginal cytologic examination for pelvic malignancy should be done routinely once or twice a year.)

Periodic blood lipid studies should be done in patients receiving long-term estrogen therapy since this treatment may aggravate an underlying lipid disorder. Recent surveys suggest a higher incidence of surgically confirmed gallbladder disease in postmenopausal women on estrogen therapy. The incidence of venous thromboembolic disease or breast tumors was no higher than in untreated controls.

2. Psychologic aspects—Many of the symptoms of the menopause are undoubtedly psychologic. The most common symptom is anxiety, but more severe emotional disorders may occur. The most serious is involutional psychotic reaction or involutional melancholia. Sedative tranquilizers (eg, diazepam) may be of value. Simple explanation and reassurance that their lives need not be changed because of the menopause are adequate in most patients. In more severe cases the aid of a psychiatrist may be necessary.

B. Surgical and X-Ray Menopause: These cases differ from the natural menopause only in the abruptness and severity of the symptoms. It is advisable to help these patients live as normal lives as possible by permanent hormonal replacement therapy. If normal periods cannot be reinstituted but the patient understands that her sexual function will continue unchanged, she usually makes a suitable adjustment. Estrogen therapy is as for natural menopause (see above).

C. Treatment of Complications:

1. **Osteoporosis** is discussed on p 682.

2. **Senile vaginitis**—Give oral diethylstilbestrol or other estrogens daily. Diethylstilbestrol vaginal suppositories containing 1 mg may be used daily for 10–14 days while continuing oral diethylstilbestrol. Dienestrol vaginal cream is often helpful.

Prognosis

Most women pass through the menopause without requiring extensive therapy. A short course of estrogen therapy may alleviate their symptoms. Others, however, require prolonged and intensive therapy. The average duration of symptoms is 2–3 years.

Some patients show severe depression (involutional melancholia or psychotic reaction; see Chapter 17) and even suicidal tendencies.

Consideration has recently been given to long-term replacement therapy with estrogen of postmenopausal females in an attempt to prevent cardiovascular degeneration, osteoporosis, etc. Such a program must be carefully supervised since latent neoplasms of breast and uterus may be stimulated by long-term estrogen therapy.

Boston Collaborative Drug Surveillance Program: Surgically confirmed gallbladder disease, venous thromboembolism, and breast tumors in relation to postmenopausal estrogen therapy. New England J Med 290:15, 1974.

Cohen EJ (editor): Treatment of menopausal problems. Mod Treat 5:543, 1968.

Irvine WJ & others: Immunologic aspects of premature ovarian failure associated with idiopathic Addison's disease. Lancet 2:883, 1968.

Molitch ME & others: Massive hyperlipemia during estrogen therapy. JAMA 227:522, 1974.

Rogers J: Estrogens in menopause and postmenopause. New England J Med 280:364, 1969.

Warne GL & others: Cyclophosphamide-induced ovarian failure. New England J Med 289:1159, 1973.

Wilson RA, Wilson TA: The basic philosophy of estrogen maintenance. J Am Geriatrics Soc 20:521, 1972.

II. FEMALE HYPERGONADISM

Excesses of ovarian hormones are often encountered during the normal reproductive life of women, and most frequently give rise to irregular or excessive menstrual bleeding and, more rarely, to amenorrhea. Excesses before the age of puberty or after the menopause, however, should be thoroughly investigated since the possibility of malignant lesions is great. Estrogenic excess is more common than progesterone excess, which is seen in pregnancy and in chorioepithelioma. Other extra-ovarian sources of estrogens are malignant tumors of the adrenals, which secrete abnormal amounts of estrogens. Since these tumors usually produce excesses of androgens as well, their hyperestrogenic effects are rarely detectable clinically in the female.

Another cause of hyperestrogenism is the ingestion or other use of hormones (eg, in face creams).

PREPUBERAL FEMALE HYPERGONADISM

It is important to differentiate organic lesions of the pituitary-hypothalamic region, which cause true precocious puberty in females, from pseudoprecocity due to granulosa cell tumors and choriocarcinoma. Constitutional true sexual precocity may be partial, consisting only of precocious breast development and early growth of pubic hair, or it may be associated with premature menarche as well. It is often familial. Albright's syndrome causes true precocity with fibrous dysplasia of bone (osteitis fibrosa disseminata) and pigmentary changes of the skin (see Chapter 3).

Granulosa cell tumors of the ovary cause uterine bleeding by virtue of their estrogenic secretions, but they do not cause ovulation and these girls are not fertile. The same is usually true of choriocarcinoma. Both of these tumors are highly malignant.

Simple follicle cysts of the ovary, at times easily palpable, may cause precocity.

Pseudoprecocious puberty may also be caused by ingestion of estrogens. Thiazolsulfone (Promizole) occasionally causes early growth of pubic hair.

The significance of the differentiation between true and pseudoprecocious puberty is that in true precocity ovulatory cycles may occur and the patient must be protected from pregnancy. The most useful guide to the differentiation is the urinary and serum FSH determination. FSH is not present in significant levels in girls before the age of puberty and is absent in pseudoprecocious puberty; whereas girls with true precocious puberty may secrete significant levels of FSH and LH.

The diagnosis of either true or pseudoprecocious puberty is important because many cases are due to tumors which must be found and removed if possible.

Unfortunately, most estrogen-secreting tumors are highly malignant, and tumors of the third ventricle and other lesions near the hypothalamus are quite difficult to remove.

Precocious development of breasts and early onset of menses may cause psychic disturbances, which may be severe. Short stature in adult life is the rule since bone age is advanced and the epiphyses close prematurely. As adults these patients may suffer a great deal from excessive menstrual bleeding, which may cause anemia unless it is checked. Cystic mastitis is a chronic problem, and the incidence of uterine adenofibromas is high. It is not definitely known whether long-standing hyperestrinism causes a higher incidence of breast and genital tract cancer, but it may be a significant aggravating factor.

The only treatment is surgical removal of tumors, but most are malignant and metastasize early. The prognosis for simple constitutional precocity is not so unfavorable, although these girls must be watched to prevent pregnancy. Recent reports on the use of progesterone (Depo-Provera) are encouraging but response is variable (see Rifkind reference, below).

Benedict PH: Sex precocity and polyostotic fibrous dysplasia. Am J Dis Child 111:426, 1966.

Eberlein WR & others: Ovarian tumors and cysts associated with sexual precocity: Report of 3 cases and review of literature. J Pediat 57:484, 1960.

Hahn HB Jr, Hayles AB, Albert A: Medroxyprogesterone and constitutional precocious puberty. Proc Staff Meet Mayo Clin 39:182, 1964.

Kenny FM & others: Radioimmunoassay serum LH and FSH in girls with sexual precocity, premature thelarche and adrenarche. J Clin Endocrinol 29:1272, 1969.

Rifkind AB & others: Suppression of urinary excretion of luteinizing hormone (LH) and follicle stimulating hormone (FSH) by medroxyprogesterone acetate. J Clin Endocrinol 29:506, 1969.

Sigurjonsdottir TJ, Hayles AB: Precocious puberty. Am J Dis Child 115:309, 1968.

ADULT FEMALE HYPERGONADISM

Adult female hypergonadism may be due to estrogenic excess alone or to combined excess of estrogen and progesterone. Estrogenic excess is characterized by menorrhagia or, rarely, amenorrhea. The vaginal smear shows estrogenic excess. Lack of ovulation is demonstrated by the absence of BBT and LH rise. Sterility is the rule. The medical D&C is positive, ie, bleeding starts after a short course of progesterone. Endometrial biopsy shows a proliferative endometrium. The urinary and serum FSH levels are low.

Adult female hyperestrogenism may be caused by (1) states in which ovulation does not occur, leading to "metropathia hemorrhagica" or dysfunctional uterine bleeding; (2) liver disease, which interferes with the catabolism of estrogens; (3) drug administration (eg, estrogen creams or tablets); (4) granulosa cell and

Table 18–13. Hormones elaborated by actively secreting ovarian tumors.

Type	Secretion
Feminizing	
Granulosa	Estrogen +++
Theca cell	Estrogen ++
Luteoma?	Estrogen + and/or progesterone
Virilizing*	
Arrhenoblastoma	Androgen +++
Adrenal rest (lipoid cell)	Androgen ++ and corticosteroids
Hilus cell	Androgen +++
Miscellaneous	
Choriocarcinoma	Gonadotropins ++++ and estrogens; TSH
Dysgerminoma*	Gonadotropins + and androgens?
Gynandroblastoma	Androgens ++ and estrogens +++
Struma ovarii	Thyroxine +

*Most women have complete amenorrhea with negative medical D&C since the endometrium is atrophic.

theca cell tumors (both types are usually present); and (5) Stein-Leventhal syndrome (see below).

Estrogen and progesterone excess often causes amenorrhea without other evidence of hypogonadism. Excess of both hormones may be due to (1) pregnancy, (2) choriocarcinoma or teratoma, (3) luteoma, or (4) malignant adrenal tumors (possibly). Medical D&C is negative. Pregnanediol is found in the urine. Secretory endometrium is demonstrated on biopsy. The urinary FSH level (actually chorionic gonadotropin) may be high and pregnancy tests positive.

Treatment depends upon the cause. Cyclic administration of progesterone, wedge resection of the ovary, or surgical removal of functioning tumors at times restores normal cyclic ovarian function. Recent reports of treatment of functional anovulation with human pituitary or urinary FSH, clomiphene, and LRH (LH-releasing hormone) are encouraging.

The prognosis is that of the underlying disease. Treatment with progesterone alone or with estrogen in cyclic fashion is usually quite effective in temporary disorders of ovulation. Stubborn anovulation may persist, however, after cessation of therapy.

Bagshawe KD: *Choriocarcinoma.* Arnold, 1969.

DeCosta EJ: Ovarian tumors with endocrine activity and related problems. S Clin North America 49:105, 1969.

Felmus LB, Pedowitz P: Clinical malignancy of endocrine tumors of the ovary and dysgerminoma. Obst Gynec 29:344, 1967.

Fox H: Ovarian tumors: Histogenesis and systemic effects. California Med 109:295, 1968.

Rose LI & others: Pure gonadal dysgenesis: Studies of in vitro androgen metabolism. Am J Med 57:957, 1974.

Wolff E & others: Virilizing luteoma of pregnancy. Am J Med 54:229, 1973.

VIRILIZING DISORDERS OF THE OVARY
(See also under Adrenal.)

Stein-Leventhal Syndrome

Stein-Leventhal syndrome occurs only in young women. It is characterized by bilaterally enlarged polycystic ovaries, mild hirsutism, obesity, and oligomenorrhea or amenorrhea. FSH is normal or low, but LH may be elevated; the medical D&C usually produces withdrawal bleeding, estrogen is present, and the urinary 17-ketosteroids are present in high normal amounts. Plasma testosterone values may be elevated. The hirsutism has been shown to be related to abnormal production of testosterone and related compounds by the ovaries and possibly also by the adrenals. Hereditary factors may be involved. Pelvic pneumography is most helpful in demonstrating bilateral enlargement of the ovaries. At operation the enlarged ovaries are found to have many follicles on the surface and are surrounded by a thick capsule ("oyster ovaries").

Wedge resection often restores ovulatory periods and fertility, but hirsutism is not helped by this procedure unless large doses of estrogens are also used. Corticosteroids may be of value. Recently, ovulation followed by pregnancy has been produced by human pituitary or urinary FSH and also by clomiphene. There is danger of rapid enlargement of the ovaries due to cyst formation and rupture if the dosage is not carefully controlled. Multiple pregnancies may occur.

Diffuse Theca Luteinization

This disorder is similar to the Stein-Leventhal syndrome, but many follicles are not found in the ovaries. Hirsutism and often more marked virilization are associated with amenorrhea.

Excessive testosterone and androstenedione production has been demonstrated recently in ovarian slices removed surgically and also in blood and urine in these patients, which may explain the virilization.

There is a greater incidence of endometrial carcinoma in these patients, possibly related to continued estrogen stimulation.

Bardin CW, Hembree WC, Lipsett MB: Suppression of testosterone and androstenedione production rates with dexamethasone in women with idiopathic hirsutism and polycystic ovaries. J Clin Endocrinol 28:1300, 1968.

Cooper HE & others: Hereditary factors in Stein-Leventhal syndrome. Am J Obst Gynec 100:371, 1968.

Ettinger B & others: Plasma testosterone stimulation: Suppression dynamics in hirsute women. Am J Med 51:170, 1971.

Greenblatt RB: *The Hirsute Female.* Thomas, 1963.

Kirschner MA, Bardin CW: Androgen production and metabolism in normal and virilized women. Metabolism 31:667, 1972.

Lipsett MB & others: Physiologic basis of disorders of androgen metabolism. Ann Int Med 68:1327, 1968.

Sherman RP: The enigmatic polycystic ovary. Obst Gynec Surg 21:1, 1966.

Thomas JP: Adrenocortical function in Stein-Leventhal syndrome. J Clin Endocrinol 28:1781, 1968.

Tulchinsky D, Chopra IJ: Estrogen-androgen imbalance in patients with hirsutism and amenorrhea. J Clin Endocrinol 39:164, 1974.

HORMONES & HORMONE-LIKE AGENTS

ANTERIOR PITUITARY & HYPOTHALAMIC HORMONES

All of the anterior pituitary hormones are protein substances and must therefore be administered parenterally to be effective; if taken by mouth, they are digested by the digestive enzymes. In general, with the exception of the growth and lactogenic hormones, whose effects are not mediated directly through other glands, the anterior pituitary hormones appear to have a regulatory function on the other glands of internal secretion. The anterior pituitary in turn is regulated to a great extent by hypothalamic-pituitary humoral "releasing factors."

Several of these hormones have been prepared in "pure" or "almost pure" form: adrenocorticotropin (ACTH, corticotropin), growth, lactogenic (luteotropic), follicle-stimulating (FSH), interstitial cell-stimulating (luteinizing), and thyroid-stimulating (TSH) hormones. There may be other factors in the anterior pituitary, but they have not yet been fully identified. Of the pure preparations, only corticotropin and thyrotropin are at present commercially available. The hypothalamic TSH- and LH-releasing factors and GH release-inhibiting factor (somatostatin) have been isolated recently and synthesized, but they are not as yet generally available.

Corticotropin (ACTH)

Corticotropin has been shown to have remarkable effects in arresting many disease processes which are not satisfactorily influenced by other therapeutic agents. Its effect is principally mediated by the stimulation of the adrenal cortex. Corticotropin is a protein of small molecular size, and certain peptides derived from it have been found to have similar and as marked physiologic effects as the hormone itself.

A. Metabolic Effects in Humans: ACTH in adequate doses in normal human beings produces the following metabolic effects: increased excretion of nitrogen, potassium, and phosphorus; retention of sodium and secondary retention of water; elevation of fasting blood glucose and diabetic glucose tolerance curve; and increased urinary excretion of uric acid, calcium, 17-ketosteroids, and corticosteroids; fall of circulating eosinophils and lymphocytes; and elevation of poly-morphonuclear neutrophils.

B. **Clinical Effects, Uses, and Dosages:** See p 717.

Growth Hormone (GH, STH, Somatotropin)

"Pure" GH has been employed in normal humans, pituitary dwarfs, and panhypopituitary individuals. Only the material prepared from human and possibly monkey pituitary glands has a growth promoting effect in hypopituitary humans. Because the amount of these materials produced is very small, they are available for experimental purposes only. The older crude growth hormone preparations have been of no benefit under controlled experimental conditions.

Lactogenic (Luteotropic) Hormone (Prolactin, Mammotropin)

This hormone has not been employed extensively in human research. Its presence is necessary for the initiation and apparently for the continuation of lactation in breasts which have been prepared for lactation by estrogen and progesterone during pregnancy. Recently, there have been reports of a "growth hormone-like activity" in humans with the use of ovine prolactin.

Follicle-Stimulating Hormone (FSH)

FSH has different actions in male and female. In the female FSH stimulates the development of ovarian follicles. Human FSH combined with chorionic gonadotropin has produced ovulation in patients with amenorrhea. In the male it stimulates the germinal epithelium of the testis to produce spermatozoa. It apparently has no effect on the Leydig cells, hence does not influence testosterone secretion. Human pituitary FSH and FSH from the urine of menopausal women (Pergonal, HMG, menotropins), followed by chorionic gonadotropin, have been used in patients with amenorrhea to induce ovulation. Clomiphene citrate (Clomid), a synthetic analogue of the nonsteroidal estrogen chlorotrianisene (TACE), has been almost equally effective in inducing ovulation.

Interstitial Cell-Stimulating Hormone (ICSH; Luteinizing Hormone)

In the female, ICSH apparently has a dual action, ie, it stimulates the growth of theca lutein cells and transforms the mature follicles into corpora lutea. In the male it stimulates the Leydig cells of the testis to secrete testosterone, and possibly also estrogen.

There is no good commercial pituitary ICSH. Chorionic gonadotropins, which have a similar action, are used clinically.

Thyroid-Stimulating Hormone (TSH, Thyrotropin, Thytropar)

TSH is exceedingly efficient in stimulating the thyroid gland. It has limited clinical usefulness at present; its principal uses are to differentiate pituitary hypothyroidism from primary hypothyroidism or from low radioiodine uptake due to exogenous thyroid hor-mone or iodine. It has also been used in an attempt to "stimulate" metastatic thyroid cancer to take up radioiodine for therapeutic purposes.

The dosage is 5–10 units IM every 12 or 24 hours for 1–3 days. Repeat radioiodine uptake or T_4. If either is increased, primary hypothyroidism is not present.

Note: Allergic and, more rarely, anaphylactic reactions may occur and should be anticipated and promptly treated.

POSTERIOR PITUITARY HORMONES
(See Table 18–14.)

The posterior pituitary hormones are polypeptides composed of 8 amino acids. Their exact chemical structures have been determined and they have recently been synthesized. Like the anterior pituitary hormones they are effective only when administered parenterally, but they can also be absorbed through the nasal mucous membranes (as snuff). They exert 3 actions: They (1) raise blood pressure (pressor action); (2) cause fluid retention without osmotically equivalent sodium retention (antidiuretic action); and (3) cause uterine contractions (oxytocic action).

To date, the antidiuretic and pressor principles have not been fully separated; they may be identical. The oxytocic factor may likewise have some pressor effect.

Clinical Indications

A. **Pressor-Antidiuretic:** The pressor and antidiuretic principle is used primarily for the treatment of diabetes insipidus and to prevent and control abdominal distention.

Table 18–14. Posterior pituitary hormones: Preparations available.

Name	Action	Average Dose
Vasopressin tannate (Pitressin Tannate)	Antidiuretic; pressor	0.3–1 ml IM every 12–72 hours
Vasopressin injection (Pitressin)		0.25–0.5 ml IM every 3–4 hours
Posterior pituitary powder (snuff)		5–20 mg 3–4 times daily
Lypressin (Diapid, lysine-8 vasopressin nasal spray)	Antidiuretic (weak pressor)	1–2 sprays in each nostril 3–5 times daily
Oxytocin injection (Pitocin), synthetic oxytocin (Syntocinon)	Oxytocic	1 ml dissolved in 1 liter saline; give by *slow* continuous IV drip
Nasal spray (Pitocin)		1–2 sprays in each nostril every 4–6 hours

B. Obstetric Use: Oxytocin is employed in obstetrics for induction of uterine contractions, and after delivery to facilitate expulsion of the placenta and control postpartum bleeding.

PITUITARY-LIKE HORMONES ELABORATED BY THE PLACENTA

The most important of the pituitary-like hormones elaborated by the placenta is referred to as "chorionic gonadotropin." Its physiologic action is almost identical with that of ICSH (see above). It has been shown that this hormone apparently functions only if an intact anterior pituitary gland is present. It is of little value by itself in inducing spermatogenesis or ovulation or maintaining a functional corpus luteum, but it may be effective for these purposes if preceded by pituitary or urinary FSH. Many of its alleged effects have been due to the presence of FSH, whose action the presence of chorionic gonadotropin may potentiate.

Placental lactogen (prolactin) is under investigation as a substitute for pituitary growth hormone.

Clinical Indications

In the male, chorionic gonadotropin may induce descent of cryptorchid testes in selected cases and is useful in some types of hypogonadism (although testosterone is generally preferred). In the female, chorionic gonadotropin may aid in inducing ovulation and maintaining corpus luteum in a few selected cases of sterility (if adequate FSH is present). The use of low daily doses of chorionic gonadotropin in the treatment of obesity has no rational basis except for a placebo effect.

Preparations Available

A. Chorionic gonadotropin, derived from the urine of pregnant women, is available commercially under a variety of trade names (eg, APL, Follutein).

B. Equine gonadotropins, derived from the serum of pregnant mares, are also available commercially. This preparation is a mixture of FSH and ICSH. It is not generally recommended because of its marked sensitizing effect and because antihormones are produced by protracted use. Only short courses should be employed.

Average Doses

The usual doses are 200–2000 units IM every day or every other day; 5000–10,000 units IM for several days may be needed to induce ovulation.

THYROID HORMONES

The active principles of the thyroid gland appear to be the iodine-containing amino acids, thyroxine (T_4) and triiodothyronine (T_3). Thyroid hormones act as a general cellular metabolic stimulant with resultant increased oxygen consumption (ie, increased metabolic rate). Their exact mode of action is not known.

Method of Administration

Thyroid hormone, either in the form of thyroglobulin (desiccated thyroid), T_4, or T_3, is effective when taken orally. There is a marked difference in rates of metabolic responses between T_3 and thyroid or T_4. In the case of T_4, little effect is noted after a single dose for about 24 hours, and the maximal effect is not reached for several days. After the medication is stopped there is a slow loss of the effect, depending upon the initial BMR and the level reached during thyroid medication. In general, at least 3–6 weeks must elapse after thyroid medication has been discontinued before one can be reasonably certain that the effects have been dissipated. In the case of T_3, the peak effect is reached in 12–24 hours and the effect is over in about 6–14 days or less.

The dextrorotatory isomers of T_4 (Choloxin) and T_3 exert a less marked "metabolic" effect in the same dosages in which T_4 and T_3 are given. They have been advocated primarily as cholesterol-lowering agents. Their value and safety are questionable. Other analogues—in which such compounds as propionic or acetic acid are substituted for the alanine side chain or in which fewer iodine atoms are incorporated into the molecule—have also been studied.

Clinical Indications

Thyroid hormone is indicated only in thyroid deficiency states. It is not effective and not indicated as a general metabolic stimulant. It has been shown that patients with thyroid deficiencies rarely require over 0.2 gm of desiccated thyroid daily. Patients without deficiency states may tolerate 0.3–0.5 gm or more daily without any clinical effects, although the radioiodine uptake is suppressed. A good general rule is that if a patient requires over 2–3 gr of thyroid daily, his need for thyroid medication should be carefully evaluated. In patients with heart disease, coronary insufficiency or failure may be precipitated by even small amounts of thyroid.

Preparations & Dosages

A. Desiccated Thyroid: This is a good compound for thyroid replacement. The chief difficulty is that the official assay is for iodine content, which may or may not represent active thyroid hormone so that there may be variations in metabolic effect. Pure beef thyroid (Thyrar) is available. Thyroglobulin (Proloid) is more stable in hormonal content. There is no evidence that any of the commercial preparations which contain more or less iodine than the official one are any less "toxic." Replacement therapy may be periodically appraised with T_4 and T_3 uptake determinations, but this may not be reliable because of variable iodine content, and adequacy of replacement must be assessed clinically. The dose is 100–200 mg daily.

Table 18–15. Equivalency of thyroid preparations.

Desiccated Thyroid	Approximate Equivalent In		
	Sodium Levothyroxine (Letter, Synthroid, etc)	Sodium Liothyronine (Cytomel, Trionine)	Liotrix (Euthroid, Thyrolar)
30 mg	0.05 mg	12.5 μg	½
65 mg	0.1 mg	25 μg	1
130 mg	0.2 mg	50 μg	2
200 mg	0.3 mg	75 μg	3

B. Levothyroxine (T$_4$; Synthroid, Letter, Levoid, Titroid): The principal advantage of this compound over desiccated thyroid is its assured constant potency. Because it is about 600 times as potent as thyroid, small changes in dose may lead to toxic levels. Dosage must be appraised by clinical response and by periodic T$_3$ or T$_4$ determinations, which are raised to a higher level by T$_4$ than by desiccated thyroid. One-tenth mg is equivalent to 60 mg of desiccated thyroid. The average dose is 0.15–0.3 mg daily. Tablets of 0.025–0.5 mg are available. This compound is gradually replacing most other preparations for maintenance therapy.

C. Synthroid Injection: 10 ml vial containing 500 μg lyophilized active substance with 10 mg of mannitol. Dilute with 5 ml of sodium chloride just prior to use. For intravenous use in myxedema coma. **Dosage:** 200–400 μg IV on the first day; 100–200 μg IV on the second day.

D. Sodium Liothyronine (T$_3$, Cytomel, Trionine): This preparation has a more rapid action and disappearance of effect than thyroid or thyroxine, and is 3–4 times as calorigenic as T$_4$. Its disadvantage is that the usual thyroid function tests (T$_4$, T$_3$ uptake) cannot be used to determine dosage when this drug is used in replacement therapy. The average maintenance dose is 0.05–0.075 mg daily in divided doses. Available as 5 μg, 25 μg, and 50 μg tablets.

E. Liotrix (Euthroid, Thyrolar): Liotrix, a 4:1 mixture of T$_4$ and T$_3$, is now available as replacement therapy in 4 potencies (Table 18–15). It closely simulates the effects of endogenous thyroid secretion, and its uniform potency should make response predictable. T$_4$ and T$_3$ uptake can be used to follow therapy. These preparations do not appear to be superior to levothyroxine in actual practice.

F. Sodium Dextrothyroxine (Choloxin): Available in 2 mg and 4 mg tablets as a cholesterol-lowering agent. It may also be used as replacement therapy for hypothyroidism in patients with cardiac disease who cannot tolerate other thyroid medications, but its value and safety are questionable.

PARATHYROID HORMONES

Parathyroid hormone is a protein substance derived from parathyroid glands. It is only effective when given parenterally.

Parathyroid hormone has a major effect on calcium and phosphorus and hence bone metabolism. Its effect is to cause an increased renal excretion of phosphorus and a direct decalcification of bone through stimulation of the osteoclasts, leading to mobilization of calcium and phosphorus from bone.

Because of the high cost and general unavailability of parathyroid hormone, 2 other preparations—dihydrotachysterol and vitamin D—are employed in its place. Both of these are sterols and are effective by mouth. Vitamin D, which is less expensive, is almost as effective as dihydrotachysterol, but its action is slower in onset and persists for prolonged periods of time.

Clinical Indications

Parathyroid hormone is indicated only in acute postsurgical hypoparathyroid tetany (after accidental removal of the parathyroid glands) and for special tests (see Ellsworth-Howard test, p 608).

Preparations Available for Treatment of Hypoparathyroidism

A. Parathyroid Injection: The average dose is 50–100 units (0.5–1 ml) in aqueous solution 3–5 times daily IM as indicated.

A single injection of 200 units IV is used for the Ellsworth-Howard test.

B. Dihydrotachysterol (AT 10, Hytakerol, Digratyl): For dosage, see Hypoparathyroidism.

C. Calciferol (Vitamin D$_2$): This preparation has a potency of 40,000 units/mg. The dosage is 1–5 mg daily.

CALCITONIN
(Thyrocalcitonin)

Calcitonin, a calcium-lowering hormone derived from special "C" cells of thyroid and parathyroid glands which decreases bone resorption, has been recently isolated and synthesized from several species. It is highly effective for the treatment of active Paget's disease.

Synthetic salmon calcitonin is now available as Calcimar in vials of 400 Medical Research Council (MRC) units with a separate vial of gelatin diluent. When reconstituted, 0.5 ml contains 100 MRC units. The recommended dosage is 50–100 MRC units daily

IM or subcut. After treatment for 6–12 months, the dose may be reduced to 50 MRC units 3 times a week. (Prior skin sensitivity testing with a dilute solution is required.)

ADRENOCORTICAL HORMONES & THEIR ANTAGONISTS

The hormones of the adrenal cortex are all steroids. To date over 30 different steroids have been isolated and identified from animal adrenal glands or adrenal venous blood. Only a few of these have demonstrable metabolic effects. They can be grouped into (1) glucocorticoids, which are the most important pharmacologic agents; (2) mineralocorticoids, and (3) androgenic and estrogenic steroids.

The question has been raised whether all the steroids apparently isolated from the adrenal cortex are in fact naturally occurring or whether they are artifacts produced in the chemical laboratory. Isolation of hormones from blood obtained by catheterization of renal veins shows that about 90% of the glucocorticoids of the adrenal cortex are 11,17-hydroxycorticosterone (compound F) and about 10% corticosterone (compound B). In general it may be stated that the best demonstration of the effects of adrenocortical hormone or hormones is that seen following corticotropin (ACTH) administration (see below).

Aldosterone, the principal mineralocorticoid, has been isolated from adrenals. This hormone appears to have only sodium- and water-retaining and potassium-losing effects. It is about 20 times as potent as deoxycorticosterone.

Hormones with estrogenic and androgenic effects have also been isolated.

Clinical Effects & Indications

A. Desoxycorticosterone Acetate: The only significant metabolic effects of this hormone are sodium and water retention and increased urinary potassium excretion. In this respect it is about 20 times as potent as cortisone. It has little effect on carbohydrate or protein metabolism.

B. Cortisone Acetate: The principal metabolic effects of cortisone include retention of some sodium and water; increased excretion of nitrogen, potassium, and phosphorus; increased blood glucose and ability to maintain blood glucose levels during fasting in addisonian patients; and return of the EEG pattern to normal in addisonian patients. One of the most important effects is the adrenocortical atrophy which results with prolonged use; this is probably due to endogenous ACTH inhibition and may interfere with the "normal" response of the pituitary-adrenal axis to stress.

For clinical effects and use, see below.

C. Hydrocortisone: This compound is available for oral, intravenous, and local (eg, intra-articular) use. Its actions are similar to those of cortisone and its metabolic effects appear to be identical. It is somewhat more potent than cortisone on a weight basis. Hydrocortisone phosphate (Hydrocortone Phosphate) and hydrocortisone sodium succinate (Solu-Cortef) are also available for intravenous or intramuscular use.

D. Cortisone and Hydrocortisone Analogues: Many modifications have been made in the cortisone-hydrocortisone molecule to decrease side reactions in relationship to therapeutic effect. The only beneficial effects of these modifications have been to decrease the sodium-retaining and potassium-losing effects of the compounds. All of these preparations are more potent on a weight basis than their parent compounds.

E. Fludrocortisone Acetate (Alflorone, Florinef, F-Cortef) and Fluprednisolone: These potent anti-inflammatory drugs have been found useful in Addison's disease and also in dermatologic disorders. They have powerful sodium-retaining as well as glucocorticoid effects. Except in Addison's disease, they must be used locally only; and even with local use their absorption may cause excessive sodium retention.

F. Whole Cortical Extract: A water-soluble extract of the adrenal gland. Although its steroid content (if any) and mode of action are poorly understood, this agent appears to be of value only for an occasional patient who fails to respond to cortisone in the emergency management of adrenal crisis.

G. Mitotane (o,p,DDD, Lysodren): This drug suppresses adrenal steroidogenesis and has been used in the treatment of inoperable adrenal carcinoma. Its toxicity has limited its clinical use.

Preparations Available

A. Desoxycorticosterone Trimethylacetate or Desoxycorticosterone Acetate: Used only for supplementary maintenance in Addison's disease.

1. Desoxycorticosterone trimethylacetate–The most practical and recommended preparation, 25–75 mg IM once a month.

2. Buccal tablets–DOCA is ineffective when swallowed. The dosage is one-half to 2 tablets daily dissolved in the buccal gutter. The drug is almost equally effective in a given dose as when injected.

3. Solution in sesame oil–The dosage is 1–3 mg IM daily for maintenance.

4. Pellets–(Rarely used.) The dosage is one 75 mg pellet for each mg of DOCA required by injection, up to 3 mg/day. If requirements by injection exceed 3 mg, one additional pellet should be implanted (eg, for a requirement of 5 mg/day by injection, implant 6 pellets). The duration of action is 6–8 months.

B. Cortisone (Compound E): See Table 18–16.

C. Hydrocortisone (Compound F): See Table 18–16.

D. Fludrocortisone: See Table 18–16.

E. Prednisone, Prednisolone, and Related Compounds: See Table 18–16.

F. Aldosterone Antagonist: Spironolactone (25 mg tablets), for states of excessive aldosterone production and edema.

G. Hydrocortisone Inhibitor: Metyrapone (250

Table 18–16. Corticotropin (ACTH) and the corticosteroids.

Preparation	Daily Dosage	Remarks	Potency/mg† Compared to Hydrocortisone
Corticotropin (ACTH)* Lyophilized powder	5–200 U	**IV:** Administer in any intravenous fluid by slow drip. For greater effect, give intravenously during entire 24-hour period. May use also for 8–12 hours. Maximal effect obtained by intravenous use of 15–40 U.	
Solution	5–200 U	**Subcut or IM:** Administer in saline every 6 hours. By this route long-acting preparations are usually used (see below). Give 40–200 U.	
Repository injection (gel)	10–200 U	**IM or subcut:** Longer acting than the powder or solution. For maximum effect give every 12 hours. May be used once daily in some patients.	
Cortrophin-Zinc	10–100 U	**IM or subcut:** Duration of action 24 hours.	
Oral Corticosteroids: Cortisone acetate (Cortone, Cortogen)	25–200 mg or more	For maximum effect use every 6 hours or 4 times daily. Rarely used clinically now (sodium retention and potassium excretion) except in Addison's disease.	4/5
Hydrocortisone (Cortef, Cortril, Hydrocortone)	20–200 mg or more	As for cortisone, above.	1
Prednisone (Meticorten, Deltasone, Deltra, Paracort) *and* Prednisolone (Meticortelone, Delta-Cortef, Hydeltra, Paracortol, Prednis, Sterane, Sterolone)	5–20 mg or more (avg, 10–20)	Δ1-Derivative of cortisone and hydrocortisone. Drug of choice; has no significant sodium-retaining effect. Give every 6 hours or 4 times daily. Good economical drugs.	4–5
Meprednisone (Betapar)	4–40 mg (avg, 8–16)	About 20% more potent than prednisone. Available as 4 mg tablet. Less sodium retention and lower cost than prednisone.	5–6
Methylprednisolone (Medrol)	4–40 mg (avg, 8–16)	About 15–25% more potent than prednisone. 16 mg tablets available for alternate day therapy.	5–6
Triamcinolone (Aristocort, Kenacort)	4–40 mg (avg, 8–16)	About the same as methylprednisolone. May produce bizarre effects, eg, nausea, weight loss, dizziness, and vague "toxic" symptoms.	5–6
Dexamethasone (Decadron, Deronil, Gammacorten, Hexadrol, Dexameth)	0.5–10 mg (avg, 1.5–3)	0.75 mg dexamethasone = 5 mg prednisolone. May cause sodium retention, especially at higher levels. No reduction of other side reactions. No advantages over prednisolone.	25–30
Betamethasone (Celestone)	0.6–6 mg (avg, 1.2–2.4)	0.6 mg betamethasone = 5 mg prednisolone. No advantage over prednisolone.	33
Paramethasone (Haldrone)	2–20 mg (avg, 4–8)	2 mg paramethasone = 5 mg prednisolone. No advantage over prednisolone.	10–12
Fluprednisolone (Alphadrol)	1.5–15 mg (avg, 3–5)	1.5 mg fluprednisolone = 5 mg prednisolone. No advantage over prednisolone.	12–15
Fludrocortisone (Florinef, F-Cortef, Alflorone)	0.1–0.3 mg	Used almost entirely in Addison's disease. Potent sodium-retaining effect. Supplements hydrocortisone in Addison's disease. May be useful also as diagnostic tool in adrenal hyperplasia.	20

*Cosyntropin (Cortrosyn), a synthetic corticotropin, is now available. It is used primarily for tests of adrenal function or in patients allergic to animal ACTH. 0.25 mg is equivalent to 25 units of corticotropin.

†To convert to equivalent hydrocortisone dosage, multiply by the potency factor shown. *Note:* If this is greater than 20, the physiologic limits are exceeded.

Table 18—16 (cont'd). Corticotropin (ACTH) and the corticosteroids.

Preparation	Daily Dosage	Remarks
Parenteral Corticosteroids: (1) For IV use only:		
Hydrocortisone IV infusion concentrate	100–200 mg	Most reliable emergency drug in absolute or relative adrenal failure. *Caution:* Must dissolve in at least 500 ml solution.
Parenteral Corticosteroids: (2) For IV or IM use: (Highly soluble. Rapid action and rapid excretion.)		
Hydrocortisone sodium succinate (Solu-Cortef), hydrocortisone 21-phosphate	100–200 mg	Dissolve 1–10 ml or more of solution. May administer in small volume or intravenous fluids. Water-soluble. For emergency use. Active intravenously or intramuscularly. Intramuscular dose must be given every 6 hours for maximum effect.
Prednisolone sodium succinate (Meticortelone Soluble)	50–100 mg	As for hydrocortisone sodium succinate, above, but not used in adrenal insufficiency. Indicated when corticosteroids cannot be taken orally.
Dexamethasone-21-phosphate (Decadron phosphate injection)	8–40 mg	As for prednisolone sodium succinate, above.
Prednisolone-21-phosphate (Hydeltrasol)	40–100 mg	As for prednisolone sodium succinate, above.
Methylprednisolone sodium succinate (Solu-Medrol)	40–120 mg	As for prednisolone sodium succinate, above. Also advocated as retention enemas in ulcerative colitis. Available as 40 mg, 125 mg, 500 mg, and 1000 mg vials with diluent.
Parenteral Corticosteroids: (3) For IM systemic use: (Insoluble. Slowly absorbed and excreted.)		
Cortisone acetate, aqueous suspension	25–200 mg	Intramuscularly only in doses every 12–24 hours. Used as long-acting parenteral corticosteroid, mainly in adrenal insufficiency.
Methylprednisolone acetate	10–80 mg	As hydrocortisone. May be used systemically for anti-inflammatory effect. (Dosage 40–180 mg in single dose.)
Triamcinolone acetonide (Kenalog)	40–80 mg	Intramuscular (40 mg/ml) every 2–4 weeks.
Dexamethasone acetate (Decadron-LA)	4–8 mg	8 mg/ml. Give 0.5–1 ml every 1–3 weeks.

Parenteral Corticosteroids: (4) For local use only intrasynovial, soft tissue): Very insoluble. Many preparations available. (1) Hydrocortisone acetate, 25 mg/ml; (2) hydrocortisone tertiary butyl acetate (Hydrocortone, TBA) 5 ml vials, 25 mg/ml); (3) prednisolone acetate aqueous suspension (Meticortelone) (5 ml vials, 25 mg/ml); (4) prednisolone tertiary butyl acetate (Hydeltra, TBA) (5 ml vials, 20 mg/ml); (5) triamcinolone acetonide (Kenalog) parenteral (5 ml vials, 10 mg/ml); (6) Celestone Solu-span (betamethasone acetate and betamethasone disodium phosphate) (6 mg/ml as sterile aqueous suspension for intramuscular, intrabursal, intra-articular, or intralesional injection), has both local and systemic effects of corticosteroids. (Dosage: 1–2 ml 1–2 times weekly.)

Local Corticosteroids: Almost all of the above steroids, plus others (eg, flurandrenolone [Cordran], fluocinolone acetonide [Synalar], flumethasone pivalate [Locorten], have been incorporated into various vehicles for local application to the skin, eyes, or mucous membranes. They are effective anti-inflammatory agents when so used. At present there appears to be little to choose among them, but marked differences in potency are observed (Table 18–17).

mg tablets or 10 ml ampules of metyrapone ditartrate) for testing of pituitary-adrenal function.

CLINICAL USE OF CORTICOTROPIN (ACTH) & THE CORTICOSTEROIDS

Both pituitary adrenocorticotropin (ACTH), acting by adrenal stimulation, and the C-11-oxygenated adrenal steroids (corticosteroids) have been shown to have profound modifying effects on many disease processes. These effects cannot be explained at present on the basis of the known metabolic and immunologic activities of these compounds.

These agents do not appear to "cure." Their action appears to be a modification of cellular activity or permeability so that "toxins" no longer can affect the cell. When the drug is discontinued, the disease may rapidly recur.

No other hormones or combinations of agents that are available commercially today have the same effects as these substances.

In general these agents are interchangeable, but occasionally a patient will be responsive to one and not to another. Both cause varying degrees of pituitary

Table 18–17. Systemic vs topical activity of corticosteroids. (Hydrocortisone = 1 in potency.)

	Systemic Activity	Topical Activity
Prednisolone	4–5	1–2
Fluprednisolone	8–10	10
Triamcinolone	5	1
Triamcinolone acetonide	5	40
Dexamethasone	30	10
Betamethasone	30	5–10
Betamethasone valerate		50–150
Methylprednisolone	5	5
Fluocinolone acetonide		40–100
Flurandrenolone acetonide		20–50
Fluorometholone	1–2	40

suppression, while the corticosteroids lead to adrenal atrophy after prolonged use as well. They should not be stopped suddenly, and during periods of stress (eg, surgery, trauma) additional amounts of rapidly acting steroids must be provided. Some patients become dependent on corticosteroids, and withdrawal is difficult.

Toxicity & Side Reactions

These agents are potentially very dangerous, but with proper precautions most of these dangers can be avoided. (See below.) Corticosteroids are generally contraindicated during early pregnancy, except in the adrenogenital syndromes.

A. Hyperglycemia and glycosuria (diabetogenic effect) is of major significance in the early or potential diabetic.

B. Marked retention of sodium and water, with subsequent edema, increased blood volume, and hypertension is minimized by the use of the newer agents.

C. Negative nitrogen and calcium balance may occur, with loss of body protein and consequent osteoporosis.

D. Potassium loss may lead to hypokalemic alkalosis.

E. Hirsutism and acne are especially disagreeable in females. Amenorrhea may occur.

F. Cushing's features or facies may develop with prolonged administration.

G. Peptic ulcer may be produced or aggravated.

H. Resistance to infectious agents is lowered.

Technics Employed to Correct or Minimize Dangers

(1) Always reduce the dosage as soon as consistent with the clinical response. Intermittent alternate-day use may be a preferable and safer method of treatment.

(2) During the first 2 weeks of therapy, blood pressure and weight should be carefully observed. Take an initial complete blood count and sedimentation rate and repeat as indicated. Determine the urine glucose; if reducing substances are found in the urine, determine fasting blood glucose. Serum potassium, CO_2, and chloride should be checked occasionally if large doses of these hormones are to be given over a period of more than several days. Eosinophil count or measurement of plasma or urinary steroid levels is indicated if any question of lack of adrenal response to corticotropin arises.

(3) All patients should be on high-protein diets (100 gm or more of protein daily) with adequate calcium intake.

(4) If edema develops, place the patient on a low-sodium diet (200–400 mg of sodium daily). Diuretics may be employed when strict sodium restriction is impossible.

(5) Potassium chloride, as 10% or 20% solution, effervescent tablets, or powder, 3–15 gm daily in divided doses, should be administered if prolonged use or high dosage is employed.

(6) In cases of long-continued administration, anabolic preparations (see p 722) may be used to counteract the negative protein, calcium, and potassium balance. Unfortunately, the distressing osteoporosis cannot be prevented. Sodium fluoride may aid in new bone formation. (See Cass reference, below.)

(7) Do not stop either ACTH or corticosteroids abruptly since sudden withdrawal may cause a severe "rebound" of the disease process or a malignant necrotizing vasculitis. Also remember that cortisone (or hydrocortisone) causes atrophy of the adrenal cortex, probably through endogenous ACTH inhibition; sudden withdrawal may lead to symptoms of Addison's disease.

(8) When treating mild disorders, giving corticosteroids during the daytime only or on alternate days causes less suppression of endogenous ACTH. When discontinuing therapy, withdraw evening dose first.

Contraindications & Special Precautions

A. Stress in Patients Receiving Maintenance Corticosteroids: Patients receiving corticosteroids, especially the oral preparation (or even ACTH), must be carefully watched because suppression of endogenous ACTH interferes with the normal response to stressful situations (eg, surgery or infections). Patients should be warned of this danger, and probably should carry identification cards showing what drug they are taking, the dosage, and the reason for taking it. Whenever such a situation occurs or is about to occur, the dosage of cortisone or hydrocortisone should be increased or parenteral corticosteroids given (or both). If oral cortisone or hydrocortisone can be administered, it must be administered in larger doses at least every 6 hours.

B. Heart Disease: These agents should be used with caution in patients with a damaged myocardium. The increase in extracellular fluid may lead to cardiac decompensation. Always begin with small doses and place the patient on a low-sodium diet.

C. Severe Renal Disease: With the exception of nephrosis, these drugs are probably contraindicated or should be used with extreme caution in patients with major renal damage associated with edema or oliguria.

D. Predisposition to Psychosis: These drugs cause a sense of well-being and euphoria in most persons, but in predisposed patients an acute psychotic reaction may occur. (Insomnia may be the presenting symptom.) In these cases the drug should be stopped or the dosage reduced, and the patient should be carefully observed and protected. Persons have committed suicide under the influence of these drugs.

E. Effect on Thyroid: Over prolonged periods, these drugs may rarely depress thyroid function.

F. Effect on Peptic Ulcer: Active peptic ulcer is a contraindication to the use of these drugs because of the danger of perforation or hemorrhage. These agents also tend to activate ulcers, and should be used only in emergency situations or with optimal anti-ulcer therapy in patients who have a history of peptic ulcer. Acute pancreatitis has been reported as well.

G. Tuberculosis: Active or recently healed tuberculosis is a contraindication to the use of these drugs unless intensive antituberculosis therapy is also carried out. A chest x-ray should be taken before and periodically during treatment with corticosteroids.

H. Infectious Diseases: Because these drugs tend to lower resistance and therefore to promote dissemination of infections, they must be used with extreme caution, even when appropriate antibiotics are being given, in any acute or chronic infection.

I. Bleeding Tendency: A bleeding tendency (eg, ecchymoses) has been reported as a side reaction in patients receiving the newer substituted hormones. Thrombosis may occur, especially on sudden withdrawal or too rapid reduction of dosage.

J. Myopathy: A peculiar steroid myopathy has been reported, especially with the substituted steroids.

K. Fatty Liver: Fatty liver and fat embolism may occur.

L. Ocular Contraindications: These agents apparently stimulate the activity of herpes simplex virus and so are contraindicated for local use in herpes simplex keratitis. Local use in the eye is often complicated by fungal infections of the cornea. Cataract formation has been reported in patients with rheumatoid disorders who are receiving corticosteroids. Increased intraocular pressure and, rarely, pseudotumor cerebri may occur.

M. Diagnostic Errors: Administration of these drugs may interfere with certain immune mechanisms which are of diagnostic value, eg, in skin tests and agglutination tests; they produce leukocytosis and lymphopenia, which may be confusing. The potent substituted corticosteroids (eg, dexamethasone) will suppress the urinary ketosteroids and hydroxycorticosteroid values. The signs and symptoms of infection may be masked by corticosteroid therapy. These drugs may also interfere with normal pain perception (eg, joint pain), which may lead to Charcot-like disintegration of the weight-bearing joints after local or systemic corticosteroid therapy.

Amatruda TT Jr, Hurst MM, D'Esopo NN: Certain endocrine and metabolic facets of the steroid withdrawal syndrome. J Clin Endocrinol 25:1207, 1965.

Berlinger FG: Use and misuse of steroids. Postgrad Med 55:153, 1974.

Cass RM & others: New bone formation in osteoporosis following treatment with sodium fluoride. Arch Int Med 118:111, 1966.

Dale DC & others: Alternate-day prednisone: Leukocyte kinetics and susceptibility to infections. New England J Med 291:1154, 1974.

Daly JR & others: Comparison of effects of long-term corticotrophin and corticosteroid treatment on response of plasma growth hormone, ACTH, and corticosteroid to hypoglycemia. Brit MJ 2:521, 1974.

Hosking D, Chamberlain M: Osteoporosis and long-term corticosteroid therapy. Brit MJ 3:125, 1973.

Jacobsen ME: The rationale of alternate-day corticosteroid therapy. Postgrad Med 49:181, 1974.

Koehler BE & others: The systemic effects of intra-articular corticosteroid. J Rheumatism 1:117, 1974.

Martin MM & others: Intermittent steroid therapy. New England J Med 279:274, 1968.

Melby JC: Systemic corticosteroid therapy: Pharmacology and endocrinologic considerations. Ann Int Med 81:505, 1974.

Rabhan NB: Pituitary-adrenal suppression and Cushing's syndrome after intermittent dexamethasone therapy. Ann Int Med 69:1141, 1968.

Thorn GW, Lauler DP: Clinical therapeutics of adrenal disorders. Am J Med 53:673, 1972.

ADRENAL MEDULLARY HORMONES & ANTAGONISTS OR BLOCKING AGENTS

The adrenal medulla contains 2 closely related hormones, epinephrine (about 80%) and norepinephrine (about 20%). They have different actions, as outlined below.

Since epinephrine may be synthetic or derived from natural sources (usually the latter) and thus contaminated with norepinephrine, the reason for some of the apparently paradoxic physiologic effects of the present preparation becomes clearer.

Epinephrine causes an immediate elevation of blood glucose by inducing glycogenolysis in liver and muscle.

Epinephrine

A. Clinical Uses: Epinephrine is used in a great many clinical disorders, including allergic conditions (eg, bronchial asthma, urticaria, angioneurotic edema); for control of superficial bleeding, especially from mucous membranes; with local anesthetics to slow down absorption; rarely in cardiovascular disorders (eg, Stokes-Adams syndrome, cardiac arrest); and in tests of hepatic glycogen storage.

B. Preparations Available:

1. Epinephrine injection is usually administered subcutaneously but may be given intramuscularly and even intravenously if diluted in 1 liter of solution. The dosage is 0.2—1 ml of 1:1000 solution as indicated.

2. Epinephrine inhalation, 1:100, for inhalation only.

Table 18—18. Effects of epinephrine and norepinephrine.

	Blood Vessels	Cardiac Output	Blood Pressure	Blood Glucose
L-Epinephrine	Vasodilatation (overall) usually	Increased	Elevated (?)	Elevated
L-Norepinephrine (levarterenol)	Vasoconstriction (overall)*	No effect	Elevated	Elevated (one-eighth that due to epinephrine)

*Vasodilator of coronary arteries.

3. Epinephrine in oil injection, 1:500, administered only intramuscularly. Usual dose: 0.2—1 ml.

Levarterenol (Norepinephrine)
   A. Clinical Indications: Levarterenol is used almost exclusively for its vasopressor effect in acute hypotensive states (surgical and nonsurgical shock, central vasomotor depression, and hemorrhage; see Chapter 1), and in the postoperative management of pheochromocytoma.
   B. Preparations Available: Levarterenol bitartrate (Levophed), 0.2% solution containing 1 mg free base/ml (1:1000) in ampules containing 4 ml.
   C. Mode of Administration: Add 4—16 ml of levarterenol (or occasionally more) to 1 liter of any isotonic solution and give intravenously through a Murphy drip bulb. Determine response and then maintain flow at a rate calculated to maintain blood pressure (usual rate, 0.5—1 ml/min). (*Note:* Levarterenol is a very potent drug, and great care must be employed in its use. Do not allow the solution to infiltrate the tissues or slough may result.)

Angiotensin Amide (Hypertensin)
   This octapeptide apparently plays a role in normal blood pressure regulation. It is a potent vasopressor. It may be of use in some cases which are refractory to levarterenol.

Blocking Agents
   A. Alpha-Adrenergic Blocking Agents: These drugs reverse the vasoconstricting effects of epinephrine and norepinephrine.
   1. Phentolamine (Regitine)—Available in 5 mg ampules. Give 5 mg IV for the diagnosis of pheochromocytoma and larger amounts IM or orally for the

preoperative and operative management of pheochromocytoma.
   2. Phenoxybenzamine (Dibenzyline)—Available in 10 mg capsules. The dosage for the chronic treatment of inoperable or malignant pheochromocytoma is 30—60 mg daily.
   B. Beta-Adrenergic Blocking Agents: These drugs reverse the catecholamine-induced vasodilatation and cardiac acceleration. They have been used together with alpha-adrenergic blocking agents in the management of patients with pheochromocytoma and in thyrotoxicosis for the control of cardiac irregularities.
   Propranolol (Inderal) is the only drug of this class now marketed in the USA. It is available for oral administration in tablets containing 10 and 40 mg. The dosage is 10—20 mg 3—4 times a day initially, increasing as necessary up to 40 mg 3—4 times a day.
   An injectable preparation (1 mg/ml) is available for IV administration. The dose is 1—3 mg given *slowly. Note:* Administration is hazardous and must be under ECG control.

HORMONES & HORMONE-LIKE AGENTS AFFECTING BLOOD SUGAR

1. HYPOGLYCEMIC AGENTS

These preparations are discussed in detail in Chapter 19. Tables 18—19 and 18—20 summarize the available compounds and their average doses.

Insulin Preparations
   All preparations are combined with zinc and are

Table 18—19. Characteristics of commercially available insulins.

Type	Appearance	Onset of Action	Duration (Hours)	Buffer	Proteins
Regular crystalline	Clear	Rapid	5—7	None	None
Semi-lente	Turbid	Rapid	12—16	Acetate	None
Globin	Clear	Intermediate	18—24	None	Globin
NPH	Turbid	Intermediate	24—28	Phosphate	Protamine
Lente	Turbid	Intermediate	24—28	Acetate	None
Protamine zinc	Turbid	Prolonged	36+	Phosphate	Protamine
Ultra-lente	Turbid	Prolonged	36+	Acetate	None

Table 18—20. Oral hypoglycemic agents.

	Market Unit (mg)	Usual Times Given Daily	Usual Daily Dose (mg)	Duration of Action (Hours)
Sulfonylurea compounds				
Tolbutamide (Orinase)	500	2	500–3000	6–12
Chlorpropamide (Diabinese)	100, 250	1	100–500	Up to 60
Acetohexamide (Dymelor)	250, 500	1 or 2	250–1500	12–24
Tolazamide (Tolinase)	100, 250	1 or 2	100–500	12–24
Biguanide compounds				
Phenformin (DBI, Meltrol)	25	2–4	50–150	4–6
Phenformin, timed disintegration (DBI-TD, Meltrol-TD)	50* 100*	1 or 2	50–150	8–12

*Capsule. All other preparations are marketed as tablets.

available as 40, 80, and 100 units/ml (U40, U80, U100). Regular insulin is also supplied as 100 and 500 units/ml for the treatment of coma and insulin resistance.

While the standard preparations of insulin are made from a mixture of beef and pork insulin, pure beef insulin, labeled "special," and pure pork insulin, labeled "pork," are available. The latter has a lesser tendency to antibody formation, since it is more like human insulin. Beef insulins are used in patients allergic to pork or who avoid pork for religious reasons.

Fish insulins and desalaninated (dalanated) or purified (single peak or single component) pork insulins are being used experimentally in the management of insulin-resistant diabetes. They will be commercially available soon.

Oral Hypoglycemic Agents
The oral hypoglycemic agents are summarized in Table 18–20.

Tolbutamide (Orinase) Diagnostic
Available as 1 gm powder in vial with 20 ml diluent for intravenous use in the diagnosis of islet cell adenomas and mild diabetes.

2. HYPERGLYCEMIC AGENTS

Glucagon
Glucagon for injection USP is a crystalline polypeptide extracted from the pancreas. It is available as a lyophilized powder, 1 mg with 1 ml diluting solution or 10 mg with 10 ml diluting solution, for intramuscular or intravenous emergency use in hypoglycemic states (eg, insulin reactions). A preparation of zinc

glucagon will become available for the treatment of chronic hypoglycemia.

Diazoxide
Diazoxide, a thiazide compound, has been used successfully in chronic hypoglycemic states. It is still an experimental compound with significant side-effects, including edema, hyperuricemia, and hypertrichosis.

Streptozotocin
Streptozotocin, an antibiotic which selectively destroys pancreatic beta cells, has been used experimentally in inoperable islet cell tumors, but its usefulness is limited by severe renal and hepatic toxicity.

GONADAL HORMONES

MALE SEX HORMONE
(Testosterone)

Of the many steroid hormones which have been isolated from the testis, the most potent androgen is testosterone. It is believed, therefore, that testosterone is "the male sex hormone." Testosterone is responsible for the development of secondary sex characteristics in the male (ie, facial hair, deep voice, development of penis, prostate, and seminal vesicles). Administration of testosterone to the female causes development of male secondary sex characteristics. In the female, the adverse androgenic effects can only be partially overcome by the simultaneous administration of estrogens.

Perhaps of greater importance than its androgenic effect is the protein anabolic (tissue building) effect of testosterone. Testosterone also has mild sodium-, chloride-, and water-retaining effects. It should be used with caution in children to prevent premature closure of the epiphyses.

Free testosterone and testosterone propionate are not effective when swallowed. The only way to administer these agents effectively is parenterally, by intramuscular injection or as implanted pellets. Testosterone preparations which do not occur naturally, eg, methyltestosterone, are effective when swallowed. Methyltestosterone in humans induces a marked creatinuria and has apparently produced jaundice after prolonged administration; otherwise, however, its metabolic and androgenic effects are similar to those of testosterone and testosterone propionate. Testosterone and testosterone propionate, when injected, are partially (about 30–50%) excreted as 17-ketosteroids in the urine. Methyltestosterone is not excreted as 17-ketosteroid. In fact, its administration will result in diminished urinary 17-ketosteroids due to diminished endogenous testosterone production.

Clinical Indications

Testosterone may be indicated in any debilitating disease, in osteoporosis, or in states of delayed growth and development (in both sexes) for its protein anabolic function. It may be of value in large doses in certain refractory anemias. In addition, there are certain uses specific to each sex.

A. Males: Testosterone is used as replacement therapy in failure of endogenous testosterone secretion (eg, eunuchoidism, castration). Its use in impotence, angina pectoris, homosexuality, gynecomastia, and benign prostatic hypertrophy is without benefit.

B. Females: Testosterone is used in women for functional uterine bleeding, endometriosis, dysmenorrhea, premenstrual tension, advanced breast carcinoma, chronic cystic mastitis, and suppression of lactation. The virilizing effects limit the total amount that can be used. While 150–300 mg of testosterone per month are said to be a safe dose, smaller doses may virilize a susceptible patient.

Preparations & Dosages

A. Testosterone (Free): The most common method of administration is in aqueous solution intramuscularly; the dosage is similar to that of testosterone propionate in oil (below). Pellets (rarely used now) may be implanted subcutaneously; the dosage is 4–8 pellets (containing 75 mg each) over 3–4 months.

B. Testosterone Propionate in Oil (Perandren Propionate, Oreton Propionate): The dosage is 10–100 mg IM every 2–3 days.

C. Testosterone Cypionate in Oil (Depo-Testosterone): The duration of action is 2–5 times or more that of testosterone propionate. The dosage is 100–200 mg every 2–3 weeks to 500 mg monthly in a single dose.

D. Testosterone Enanthate in Oil (Delatestryl): The duration of action is comparable to that of testosterone cypionate. The average dose is 200–400 mg IM every 3–4 weeks.

E. Testosterone Phenylacetate (Perandren Phenylacetate): This microcrystalline aqueous suspension for intramuscular use has a prolonged action similar to Depo-Testosterone. It is supplied as 10 ml vials of 50 mg/ml. The average dose is 50–200 mg every 3–5 weeks. It is contraindicated in persons with known sensitivity to procaine.

F. Methyltestosterone (Metandren, Oreton Methyl): Available as tablets of 2, 5, 10, and 25 mg or as linguets of 5 and 10 mg. The dosage is 5–25 mg daily. (*Note:* Do not use in the treatment of thyrotoxicosis, acromegaly, gigantism, or liver disease.)

G. Fluoxymesterone (Halotestin, Ora-Testryl, Ultandren): This drug is a fluoro derivative of methyltestosterone. It is about 2.5 times as potent as the patent drug. Its toxicity is similar to that of methyltestosterone. It may have less effect than other preparations on epiphyseal closure and is therefore the drug of first choice in children, but it must be used cautiously. It is available as tablets of 2, 5, and 10 mg. The dosage is 2–10 mg orally daily.

H. Anabolic Hormones: Several new drugs have been introduced whose relative protein anabolic effects (vs their androgenic effects) are claimed to be greater than those of the other testosterone preparations listed above. These claims have yet to be fully evaluated. Most of them appear to induce BSP retention, and they may have other as yet unrecognized side-effects.

1. Norethandrolone (Nilevar) is given in dosages of 30–50 mg daily orally.

2. Stanolone (Neodrol)—The dosage is 50–150 mg IM once or twice a week.

3. Methandrostenolone (Dianabol)—This drug has a definite androgenic effect in some women at doses of 10–15 mg/day orally, and may cause BSP retention by the liver after prolonged use. The average dose is 5 mg/day.

4. Nandrolone phenpropionate (Durabolin)—The dosage is 25 mg/week or 50–100 mg every 2 weeks IM or subcut. Skin reactions may occur in some patients. Also available is nandrolone decanoate (Deca-Durabolin), 50 mg/ml in oil.

5. Oxymetholone (Anadrol, Adroyd)—The dosage is 2.5 mg orally 3 times daily.

6. Stanozolol (Winstrol), 1–2 mg 3 times daily orally.

7. Ethylestrenol (Maxibolin)—4–8 mg daily as tablets or elixir.

8. Methylandrostenediol (Stenediol)—Tablets and linguets of 10 and 25 mg or suspension of 25 and 50 mg/ml, 10 ml.

9. Dromostanolone propionate (Drolban), 50 mg/ml in oil, is available for palliation of inoperable breast carcinoma in postmenopausal women. The dosage is 100 mg IM 3 times weekly.

10. Calusterone (Methosarb), 50 mg tablets, has been introduced for the treatment of advanced inoperable or metastatic carcinoma of the breast. The usual dose is 200 mg/day orally in divided doses.

Choice of Preparations

In view of the great number of preparations available, it may be difficult to decide which one to use. The physician should choose those preparations which are most economical to the patient and still are effective. The use of short-acting testosterone preparations by repeated injections should be reserved only for those very few conditions in which the patient must be under close observation (preferably in a hospital) or when the dose must be very exact (ie, research). The preparations of choice when both androgenic and anabolic effects are desired are the longer-acting testosterones intramuscularly or subcutaneously. If less androgenicity is desirable one of the newer anabolic agents should be considered, although much more experience will be needed before their true effectiveness has been determined.

Caution: Men receiving testosterone should be observed carefully for prostatic and breast cancer. Recent reports link the prolonged use of methylated oral anabolic androgenic steroids with the development of severe peliosis, hepatitis, and cancer of the liver (see Bagheri and Farrell references, p 701). The virilizing effect of testosterone in women and children may become permanent even after withdrawal of testosterone. Androgenic steroids are contraindicated in pregnant women or women who may become pregnant during the course of therapy since this may virilize the fetus. These hormones alter serum lipids and could conceivably increase susceptibility to atherosclerotic disease.

Wynn V: The anabolic steroids. Practitioner 200:509, 1968.

ESTROGENS

Estrogens control proliferation of endometrium and growth of uterine muscle, changes in vaginal cells (cornification and lowering of vaginal pH below 4.0), and ductal proliferation of breasts. They decrease the rate of bone resorption and have a slight protein anabolic effect and a moderate calcium-, sodium-, and water-retaining effect. They may also have a cholesterol-lowering effect.

Clinical Indications

Estrogens are used in both women and men for the treatment of osteoporosis. In women, estrogen is used as replacement therapy in cases of ovarian failure (eg, menopause). In men, it is used as an adjunct in the treatment of carcinoma of the prostate.

Preparations & Dosages

Many substances have estrogenic activity, including some nonsteroids (eg, diethylstilbestrol, dienestrol, hexestrol). However, only some of the steroids are useful clinically. There is no evidence that any of the estrogens are less "toxic" than others. Toxicity (eg, nausea and vomiting) is usually due to overdosage. Most of the estrogens exert profound physiologic effects in very small doses, and their therapeutic and toxic dosages are quite similar. The physician should familiarize himself with the use of one or 2 preparations and resist the tendency to try out new ones.

There is little need at present to administer estrogens by any but the oral route; absorption in the gastrointestinal tract seems to be complete, and there is no evidence that nausea and vomiting can be minimized by parenteral administration. There is likewise no evidence that the "naturally-occurring" estrogens are any more effective than the synthetic ones, although they may be better tolerated.

Although estrogens apparently play a role in mammary tumors of animals, there is no evidence that they are carcinogenic in humans. Even so, it is advisable to perform periodic breast examinations and Papanicolaou smears in patients receiving prolonged estrogen therapy. Cyclic administration is always preferable when estrogens must be given over long periods.

Caution: Recent reports show the occurrence of adenocarcinoma of the vagina in young women whose mothers were treated with large doses of diethylstilbestrol early in pregnancy. Therefore, this drug should be avoided in pregnant women.

A. Nonsteroid Estrogens:

1. Diethylstilbestrol—A synthetic nonsteroid estrogen; an excellent preparation, and the cheapest available. The dosage is 0.5—1 mg daily orally.

2. Hexestrol, dienestrol, benzestrol, chlorotrianisene (TACE), methallenstril (Vallestril)—These preparations have no advantage over diethylstilbestrol, and are more expensive.

3. Diethylstilbestrol diphosphate (Stilphostrol)—For treatment of prostatic carcinoma; well tolerated in large doses. Dosage is 1 tablet (50 mg) 3 times daily to 4 or more tablets 3 times daily, depending on tolerance.

B. Steroidal Estrogens for Oral Use:

1. Ethinyl estradiol (Estinyl, Feminone, etc)—An excellent synthetic estrogen. The dosage is 0.02—0.05 mg daily orally.

2. Conjugated estrogenic substances (estrone sulfate)—A "natural" estrogen which is well tolerated. The dosage is 0.5—2.5 mg daily orally.

3. Piperazine estrone sulfate (Ogen)—The dose is 1.5—4.5 mg/day.

4. Hormonin—Hormonin # 1 is a mixture of 0.135 mg estriol, 0.3 mg estradiol, and 0.7 mg estrone per tablet. Hormonin # 2 contains double these amounts. The dosage is 1—2 tablets of # 1 or 1 tablet of # 2.

C. Estrogens for Injection:

1. Estrone (Theelin)—Little used at present; the conjugated estrogens listed above are preferred. The dosage is 1 mg 2—3 times weekly or 1000 units daily IM.

2. Estradiol benzoate injection in oil (Progynon and others)—The dosage is 0.5—1 mg every other day IM.

Table 18—21. Oral antifertility drugs available in the USA.

Trade Name	mg	Estrogen	mg	Progestogen
Combination products				
Enovid	0.075	Mestranol	5	Norethynodrel
	0.1	Mestranol	2.5	Norethynodrel (Enovid-E)
	0.15	Mestranol	9.85	Norethynodrel
Norinyl	0.05	Mestranol	1	Norethindrone
Noriday: 21 tablets of Norinyl 1 plus 7 inert tablets				
Norinyl 1+80	0.08	Mestranol	1	Norethindrone
	0.1	Mestranol	2	Norethindrone
Loestrin 1/20 Zorane 1/20	0.02	Ethinyl estradiol	1	Norethindrone acetate
Zorane 1.5/30	0.03	Ethinyl estradiol	1.5	Norethindrone acetate
Lo/Ovral	0.03	Ethinyl estradiol	0.3	Norgestrel
Zorane 1/50	0.05	Ethinyl estradiol	2.5	Norethindrone acetate
Norlestrin and Norlestrin 28	0.05	Ethinyl estradiol	1	Norethindrone acetate
Ortho-Novum	0.05	Mestranol	1	Norethindrone
	0.06	Mestranol	10	Norethindrone
Ortho-Novum 1/50□ 21 or 20	0.05	Mestranol	1	Norethindrone
Ortho-Novum 1/80□ 21	0.08	Mestranol	1	Norethindrone
	0.1	Mestranol	2	Norethindrone
Demulen	0.05	Ethinyl estradiol	1	Ethynodiol diacetate
Ovulen and Ovulen-21	0.1	Mestranol	1	Ethynodiol diacetate
Ovral	0.05	Ethinyl estradiol	0.25	D-Norgestrel
Sequential products				
Oracon	0.1	Ethinyl estradiol	25	Dimethisterone
Ortho-Novum SQ	0.08	Mestranol	2	Norethindrone
Norquen	0.08	Mestranol	2	Norethindrone
Continuous products				
Nor-QD and Micronor	0	0	0.35	Norethindrone

3. Estradiol dipropionate injection (Ovocyclin and others)—This preparation has a slightly longer duration of effect than estradiol benzoate. The dosage is 2—5 mg IM 1—2 times weekly.

4. Estradiol valerate in sesame oil (Delestrogen)—A long-acting estrogen. The dosage is 10—20 mg IM every 2—3 weeks.

5. Estradiol cypionate (Depo-Estradiol)—1 and 5 mg/ml in oil. Long-acting. The dosage is 2—5 mg IM every 3—4 weeks.

6. Conjugated estrogenic substances (estrone sulfate), 2.5 mg daily IM. Premarin IV (20 mg) is a rapid-acting preparation which is given to stop bleeding in menorrhagia.

7. Diethylstilbestrol diphosphate (Stilphostrol), 5 ml ampule containing 0.25 gm, for intravenous use in prostatic carcinoma.

D. Estrogens for Topical Use:

1. Diethylstilbestrol vaginal suppositories, 0.1, 0.25, and 0.5 mg.

2. Dienestrol vaginal cream, 0.01%.

3. Premarin lotion, 1 mg/ml, and cream, 0.625 mg/gm.

PROGESTINS
(Gestagens)

Up to the present time progesterone has had a limited use in clinical medicine. Recently a number of new compounds with progestational activity have been introduced. However, these new compounds also have other actions which are summarized below.

Progesterone leads to the secretory phase of endometrium. In the absence of estrogens it does not have any significant effect on the uterus, ie, the uterus must be stimulated (proliferated) by estrogens before pro-

Table 18—22. Endocrine properties of oral progesterones (currently in clinical use in the USA).*

	Progesta-tional	Estrogenic	Androgenic	Anabolic	Anti-estrogenic	Pregnancy Maintenance
Norethynodrel	+	+	n.d.	0	0	0
Norethindrone	+	0	+	+	+	0
Norethindrone acetate	+	0	+	+	n.d.	0
Dimethisterone	+	0	0	0	n.d.	0
Hydroxyprogesterone caproate (Delalutin)	+	0	0	0	n.d.	+
Medroxyprogesterone acetate (Provera)	+	0	n.d.	0	+	+
Chlormadinone acetate	+	0	0	n.d.	+	+
Ethynodiol diacetate	+	+	+	0	+	0
Dydrogesterone (Duphaston, Gynorest)	+	0	0	0	0	+
Ethisterone	+	0	+	+	n.d.	0

n.d. = Not determined.

*Modified after Greenblatt RB: Medical Science, May 1967.

gesterone can act. Progesterone also causes acinar proliferation of breasts.

Clinical Indications

A. Menstrual Irregularities: Progesterone may be used with estrogens to maintain more "normal" cyclic menstrual function in women who otherwise do not menstruate.

B. "Medical D&C": Progesterone is used to produce the so-called "medical dilatation and curettage," which is actually a test of adequacy of endogenous estrogen production. If withdrawal bleeding does not occur, it may also indicate that the patient is pregnant. The test may be performed in one of 3 ways.

1. Give 10 mg of progesterone IM daily for 5 days. If menstrual bleeding occurs within 2—5 days after stopping, endogenous estrogen production is adequate.

2. Give 20 mg of norethindrone (Norlutin) or medroxyprogesterone (Provera) orally daily for 4—5 days. If menstrual bleeding occurs within 2—3 days, endogenous estrogen production is adequate.

3. Give 250—375 mg of hydroxyprogesterone caproate (Delalutin) IM once. If menstrual bleeding occurs within 10—16 days, endogenous estrogen production is adequate.

C. Obstetric Use: The progestins are used in large doses in some cases of habitual or threatened abortion, eg, hydroxyprogesterone caproate (Delalutin), 500 mg/week IM.

D. Use as Contraceptive: Some of the newer agents are being used effectively as contraceptives; they act by preventing ovulation. These drugs consist of progestational agents combined with various estrogens. They are usually given daily beginning on the 5th day after onset of menses and continued for 20 days; then resumed on the 5th day of the cycle, etc. If breakthrough bleeding occurs, the dose may have to be increased. A small dose of a synthetic progesterone

(norethindrone) used continuously ("the minipill") has been recently introduced as a contraceptive pill. These agents are contraindicated in women with a history of thromboembolism, preexisting genital or breast cancer, liver disease, or cerebrovascular accident.

The principal drugs (and usual dosages) employed for this purpose at present are given in Table 18—21.

The introduction of sequential therapy may provide effective contraception with fewer side-effects. The sequential contraceptives may also provide good estrogen replacement for women near and past the menopause, thus preventing premature osteoporosis, etc.

E. In endometriosis the progestins, at times combined with estrogens, are used continuously in large dosage to induce a state of pseudopregnancy.

F. Precocious Puberty: The progestins have been used recently in children with precocious puberty.

Preparations & Dosages

A. True Progestational Hormones:

1. Progesterone, 5—10 mg daily IM, or 100—200 mg daily orally or IM (for threatened or habitual abortion).

2. Hydroxyprogesterone caproate (Delalutin), 125—250 mg IM every 2 weeks.

3. Ethisterone, 60—100 mg daily orally.

4. Medroxyprogesterone (Provera), 10—30 mg/day orally, or 100 mg IM every 2 weeks (for endometriosis only).

B. Hormones With Progestational (and Other) Activity: See Table 18—22.

Side-Effects of Progesterone & Progesterone Plus Estrogen Treatment

Prolonged progesterone plus estrogen therapy may cause abdominal distention, weight gain, nausea, acne, skin pigmentation, masculinization of a female fetus, and decidual casts ("pseudomalignant changes") of the endometrium. Some of these side-effects may be prevented by lower dosage or sequential therapy (see above). There may be a significant increase in gall-bladder disease. Prolonged amenorrhea may occur after stopping these drugs.

The following adverse reactions have been observed in varying incidence in patients receiving oral contraceptives:

Nausea
Vomiting
Gastrointestinal symptoms
Breakthrough bleeding
Spotting
Change in menstrual flow
Amenorrhea
Edema
Chloasma
Breast changes: tenderness, enlargement, secretion
Loss of scalp hair, hirsutism, and acne
Change in weight (increase or decrease)
Changes in cervical erosion and cervical secretions
Suppression of lactation when given immediately postpartum
Cholestatic jaundice
Erythema multiforme
Erythema nodosum
Hemorrhagic eruption
Migraine
Rash (allergic)
Itching
Rise in blood pressure in susceptible individuals (see Weinberger reference, below)
Mental depression

The following occurrences have been observed in users of oral contraceptives; a cause and effect relationship has not been established uniformly:

Thrombophlebitis
Pulmonary embolism
Ischemic colitis
Neuro-ocular lesions
Carcinogenic potential (see Hertz reference, below)

The following laboratory results may be altered by the use of oral contraceptives:

Bromsulphalein (BSP) retention and results of other hepatic function tests: increased
Coagulation tests: increase in prothrombin, factors VII, VIII, IX, and X
Thyroid function: increase in protein-bound iodine (PBI), butanol extractable iodine (BEI) and T_4, and decrease in T_3 resin uptake values (radioiodine uptake not affected)

Metyrapone test
Pregnanediol determinations
Glucose tolerance test
Blood lipids

Note: A recent report of a possible association of synthetic sex steroids with birth defects (see Janerich reference, below) makes the safety of the use of oral contraceptives as withdrawal-type pregnancy tests doubtful since adequate alternative methods are available. It is prudent to be certain of the absence of pregnancy before starting a woman on oral contraceptives.

Barranco VP, Jones DD: Effect of oral contraceptives on acne. South MJ 67:703, 1974.

Boston Collaborative Drug Surveillance Program: Oral contraceptives and venous thromboembolic disease, surgically confirmed gallbladder disease and breast tumors. Lancet 1:1399, 1973.

Bray GA: Effects of oral contraceptives on carbohydrate metabolism: Oral contraceptive agents. Western J Med 122:33, 1975.

Collaborative Group for the Study of Stroke in Young Women: Oral contraceptives and stroke in young women: Associated risk factors. JAMA 231:718, 1975.

Epstein MT & others: Migraine and reproductive hormones throughout the menstrual cycle. Lancet 1:543, 1975.

Fiser RH: Contraceptives and lipid metabolism: Oral contraceptive agents. Western J Med 122:35, 1975.

Garcia CR, Pincus G: Clinical considerations of oral hormonal control of human fertility. Clin Obst Gynec 7:844, 1964.

Haller J: *Hormonal Contraception.* Geron-X, 1972.

Hertz R: Experimental and clinical aspects of the carcinogenic potential of steroid contraceptives. Internat J Fertil 13:273, 1968.

Janerich DT & others: Oral contraceptives and congenital limb-reduction defects. New England J Med 291:697, 1974.

Lauritzen C: On endocrine effects of oral contraceptives. Acta endocrinol (Suppl) 124:87, 1967.

Northmann BJ & others: Reversible mesenteric vascular occlusion associated with oral contraceptives. Am J Digest Dis 18:361, 1973.

Rose MB: Superior mesenteric vein thrombosis and oral contraceptives. Postgrad MJ 48:430, 1972.

Salhanick HA & others (editors): *Metabolic Effects of Gonadal Hormones and Contraceptive Steroids.* Plenum Press, 1969.

Swerdloff RS: Action and efficacy of systemic contraceptive agents, and introduction of complications: Complications of oral contraceptive agents. Western J Med 122:20, 1975.

Vessey MP & others: Oral contraceptives and breast neoplasia: A retrospective study. Brit MJ 3:719, 1972.

Weinberger MH & others: Hypertension induced by oral contraceptives containing estrogen and gestagen. Ann Int Med 71:891, 1969.

Weinding H, Henry JB: Laboratory test results altered by "the pill." JAMA 229:1762, 1974.

19...
Diabetes Mellitus, Hypoglycemia, & Lipid Disorders

John H. Karam

DIABETES MELLITUS

Classification & Pathogenesis

Clinical diabetes mellitus represents a syndrome with disordered metabolism and inappropriate hyperglycemia due to an absolute deficiency of insulin secretion or to a reduction in its biologic effectiveness. It may result from a number of causes, and at present there is no generally accepted diagnostic classification because the etiologic mechanisms are not clearly understood.

Accumulated experience over the years has made it obvious that insulin plays a key role in regulating blood glucose levels. The development of specific radioimmunoassay technics for measuring circulating insulin levels has provided a means of classifying diabetes mellitus into 2 major types (Table 19–1): (1) hyperglycemia caused by absent or diminished insulin secretion of the pancreatic beta cell in response to glucose (insulinopenic diabetes); and (2) hyperglycemia (in spite of normal or even supernormal insulin secretion in response to glucose) due to impaired response of target organs to insulin (insulinoplethoric diabetes).

A. Insulinopenic (Type I) Diabetes: This represents a pancreatic islet disorder and can be subdivided into at least 2 major subtypes on the basis of clinical severity.

1. A severe form, occurring most commonly in juveniles but also occasionally in adults, especially the nonobese and those who are elderly when hyperglycemia first appears. It is a catabolic disorder in which circulating insulin is virtually absent, and the hyperglycemia fails to respond to all insulinogenic stimuli. Exogenous insulin is therefore required to reverse the catabolic state, prevent ketosis, and bring the blood glucose level down.

2. A milder form occurring predominantly in adults but occasionally in juveniles. Some of these patients are obese, but most are not. Catabolic features are less prominent, and circulating insulin is measurable though often in diminished amounts. The early phase of insulin release is blunted or absent in response to glucose; however, it may often be elicited in response to other insulinogenic stimuli such as acute intravenous administration of sulfonylureas, glucagon, or secretin. Insulin therapy is not usually required to prevent ketosis, and in many cases hyperglycemia responds to oral hypoglycemic agents or, at times, to diet alone.

Insulinopenic diabetes, due to defective pancreatic beta cell function, may be due to many causes. Genetic defects in production of certain macromolecules can interfere with proper insulin synthesis, packaging, or release; or the beta cells may be unable to recognize glucose signals or even to replicate

Table 19–1. Clinical classification of diabetes mellitus syndromes.*

Type	Primary Pathophysiology	Usual Age at Onset	Post-Glucose Plasma or Serum Insulin (μU/ml)†	Treatment
Insulinopenic IA (severe)	Pancreatic beta cell deficiency	Juveniles; nonobese adults	Virtually absent	Insulin, diet
IB (mild to moderate)		Nonobese adults	< 50 at 1 hour	(1) Diet alone. (2) Diet plus oral hypoglycemic agents.
Insulinoplethoric II (mild)	End organ unresponsiveness to insulin action	Obese adults	> 100 at 2 hours	Diet

*Clinical characteristics and treatment not always sharply delineated.
†Normal response is between 50 and 135 μU/ml at 60 minutes and less than 100 μU/ml at 120 minutes after 100 gm oral glucose.

normally. Extrinsic factors that affect beta cell function include damage caused by viruses such as mumps or coxsackie B4 virus; by destructive cytotoxins and antibodies released by sensitized immunocytes; or by autodigestion in the course of an inflammatory disorder involving adjacent exocrine pancreas. In fact, all 3 of these mechanisms could contribute to the development of diabetes after certain viral infections such as mumps, which, in addition to being directly betacytotoxic, also cause exocrine pancreatitis and are potent stimulants of immune responses. An underlying genetic defect in beta cell replication or function may predispose to development of beta cell failure after viral infection.

B. Insulinoplethoric (Type II) Diabetes: This type of diabetes reflects an extrapancreatic disorder and likewise represents a spectrum of disorders. It is characterized by nonketotic, mild diabetes, mainly in adults but occasionally also in children. The primary problem seems to originate outside the pancreas as a result of ineffective insulin action and secondarily affects beta cell function. Hyperplasia of pancreatic beta cells is often present and probably accounts for the normal or exaggerated insulin responses to glucose and other stimuli seen in the milder forms of this disorder. **Obesity** is common in this type of diabetes as a result of excessive caloric intake, possibly facilitated by hunger resulting from mild postprandial hypoglycemia after excess insulin release. In obese patients, insulin insensitivity is correlated with overdistended adipocytes, but liver and muscle cells also resist the deposition of additional glycogen as well as triglycerides in their overfilled storage depots.

Two major mechanisms have been proposed to account for the observed tissue insensitivity to insulin in obesity: Chronic overfeeding may lead to either (1) overdistention of storage depots, with reduced ability to clear nutrients from the circulation; or (2) sustained beta cell stimulation and hyperinsulinism, which in itself induces receptor insensitivity to insulin.

Regardless of the mechanism, a reduction in overfeeding can interrupt the cycle. In the first case, normal tissue sensitivity returns as storage depots become less distended, whereas in the second situation restricted diet would reduce islet stimulation of insulin release, restoring insulin receptor sites and improving tissue sensitivity to insulin. In both cases, reduction of the excessive postprandial insulin release could produce a lessening of hunger.

In addition to obesity, chronic muscle disease (eg, myotonic dystrophy) and liver disease have been associated with carbohydrate intolerance and hyperinsulinism in response to glucose.

Other secondary causes of carbohydrate intolerance include endocrine disorders—often specific endocrine tumors—associated with excess production of growth hormone, glucocorticoids, catecholamines, or glucagon. In all 4 situations, peripheral responsiveness to insulin is impaired. With excess of glucocorticoids, catecholamines, or glucagon, increased hepatic output of glucose is a contributory factor; in the case of cate-

cholamines, decreased insulin release is an additional factor in producing carbohydrate intolerance.

Epidemiologic Considerations

The above comments emphasize the heterogeneity of the disorder termed diabetes mellitus, especially in the adult-onset diabetic. Attempts to define diabetes on the basis of abnormal carbohydrate tolerance alone contributed to much of the confusion and controversy regarding its prevalence, genetic transmission, relationship of complications to control, and recommended therapeutic approaches.

An estimated 4 million people in the USA are known to have diabetes; about 120,000 are children below the age of 15. Information about the epidemiology of mild adult-onset diabetes was a major contribution of the University Group Diabetes Program (UGDP). This study revealed that the vast majority of persons with mild adult-onset diabetes were obese and thus may well have represented a type of diabetes in which tissue insensitivity to insulin was a fundamental pathologic feature; whereas in a smaller group—especially those who were nonobese—the primary cause of carbohydrate intolerance was true beta cell impairment of glucose-induced insulin release. Unfortunately, in the UGDP study, the number of nonobese subjects was too small to permit a valid comparison of the incidence of vascular complications in the obese and nonobese patients.

Clinical Findings

Regardless of whether the primary defect is an absolute (type I) or relative (type II) lack of insulin, features of insulin deficiency may arise. In the severe form of type I, increased catabolism and ketosis occur. The mild form of type I may have many clinical features in common with type II (described above), since the effects of the metabolic derangement may be similar despite wide differences in causes.

A. Symptoms: (See Table 19–2.) The classical symptoms of polyuria, thirst, recurrent blurred vision, paresthesias, and fatigue are manifestations of hyperglycemia and thus are common to both major types of diabetes. Nocturnal enuresis may signal the onset of diabetes in children; likewise, pruritus vulvae and vaginitis are frequent initial complaints of adult fe-

Table 19–2. Clinical features of diabetes.

	Insulino-penic Diabetes	Insulino-plethoric Diabetes
Polyuria and thirst	++	+
Weakness or fatigue	++	+
Polyphagia with weight loss	++	−
Recurrent blurred vision	+	++
Vulvovaginitis or pruritus	+	++
Peripheral neuropathy	+	++
Nocturnal enuresis	++	−
Often asymptomatic	−	++

males with hyperglycemia and glycosuria due to either absolute or relative deficiencies of insulin. Weight loss despite normal or increased appetite is primarily a feature of the insulinopenic variety, whereas weight loss is unusual in diabetics who have normal or increased levels of circulating insulin. Patients with the insulinoplethoric type of diabetes may be relatively asymptomatic and may be detected only after glycosuria or hyperglycemia is noted during a routine examination. Diabetes should be suspected in obese patients, in those with a positive family history of diabetes, in patients presenting with peripheral neuropathy, and in women who have delivered large babies or had polyhydramnios, preeclampsia, or unexplained fetal losses.

B. Physical Signs:

1. Acute diabetes syndrome—In the mild diabetic of either type—or even the moderately severe insulinopenic diabetic—there may be no abnormal physical signs at onset, whereas the patient presenting with the advanced stage of the severe form of insulin deficiency shows apparent weight loss from a combination of dehydration, loss of subcutaneous fat, and muscle wasting.

The mild diabetic is most commonly obese and except for vaginitis in females may have no characteristic physical abnormalities related to diabetes. However, evidence of neuropathy, which is not an uncommon late complication of diabetes, may be apparent early in the disease.

2. Chronic diabetes syndrome—

a. Ocular signs—Premature cataracts and refractive changes occur in the lens. Retinopathy may be of the "background" variety, consisting of microaneurysms, intraretinal hemorrhages, and hard exudates; or of the "proliferative" type, which includes also the formation of new capillaries and duplication of small veins. Complications of proliferative retinopathy include preretinal or vitreous hemorrhage and fibrosis, which can result in retinal detachment and blindness.

b. Cardiovascular signs—Occlusive vascular disease of the lower extremities is a combination of microangiopathy and atherosclerosis of large and medium-sized arteries. It occurs more commonly after age 40, and diabetics have 20 times the incidence of gangrene of the feet than do nondiabetics. If both feet feel cool, a good blood supply might still be present; but if one foot is cooler than the other occlusive arterial disease is usually present in the cooler one.

Hypertension develops with progressive renal involvement, and coronary and cerebral atherosclerosis with all of their sequelae seem to be accelerated in persons with diabetes.

c. Neurologic signs—The general features of peripheral neuropathy are present, usually predominantly sensory in type, with dulled perception of vibration, pain, and temperature, particularly in the lower extremities. However, bilateral atrophy of the first interosseous muscles of the hand is characteristic of diabetic neuropathy. The ankle jerk is often absent, but the knee jerk may be retained. Autonomic neuropathy includes evidence of postural hypotension, decreased cardiovascular responses to Valsalva's maneuver, alternating bouts of diarrhea and constipation, inability to empty the bladder, and impotence. Impotence due to neuropathy differs from the psychogenic variety in that the latter may be intermittent, with erections occurring under special circumstances, whereas diabetic impotence is usually persistent.

d. Skin and mucous membrane signs—Chronic pyogenic infections of the skin may occur, especially in poorly controlled diabetic patients. Likewise, eruptive xanthomas can develop in long-standing uncontrolled cases. An unusual lesion termed "necrobiosis lipoidica diabeticorum" occurs more commonly in females and is usually located over the anterior surfaces of the legs or the dorsal surfaces of the ankles.

"Shin spots" are not uncommon in adult diabetics. They are brownish, rounded, painless atrophic lesions of skin in the pretibial area, found in males more commonly than in females. Candidal infection can produce erythema, edema of intertriginous areas below the breasts, in the axillas, and between the fingers. It causes vulvovaginitis in most chronically uncontrolled diabetic females and is a frequent cause of pruritus.

3. Rare associated disorders—Particularly in males, liver enlargement, "bronzed" skin pigmentation, and loss of body hair may indicate hemochromatosis, while concurrent thyroid disease and adrenal insufficiency with pigmentation may rarely be associated with diabetes, especially in females with the insulinopenic type of diabetes.

C. Laboratory Findings: These involve tests of glucose and ketone bodies in the urine as well as glucose levels in plasma under basal conditions and after glucose administration. In certain circumstances, measurement of circulating levels of insulin as well as other hormones involved in carbohydrate homeostasis, such as glucagon or growth hormone, may be useful. In view of the serious consequences of atherosclerosis in diabetics, estimates of serum cholesterol and triglycerides are essential both in evaluating and controlling the disease. Recently, measurement of the width of the basement membranes of capillaries in skeletal muscle has been advocated as a means of distinguishing "true" genetic diabetes from other disorders of carbohydrate tolerance.

1. Urinalysis—

a. Glycosuria—The Clinitest modification of Benedict's test using 5 drops of urine with 10 drops of water provides a rapid, easy, and semiquantitative estimate of the degree of glycosuria. 0.25% glucose in the urine is required to show a trace reaction (green), and colors progress from yellow through orange until a brick-red color indicates a glucose concentration of 2% or more. When large quantities of glucose are present, the test can be modified so that 2 drops of urine with 10 drops of water will allow estimation of glucose concentrations up to 5% by use of a special color chart.

A more specific and convenient method is the paper strip impregnated with glucose oxidase and a chromogen system (Clinistix, TesTape, Diastix), which is sensitive to as little as 0.1% glucose in urine. A major disadvantage that limits its usefulness in insulin-requiring diabetics is that it fails to estimate the quantity of glycosuria as well as does the more cumbersome Clinitest method, especially since sensitivity of the enzymes may deteriorate with age or exposure to air.

Certain common therapeutic agents interfere with both of these methods. Ascorbic acid, salicylates, methyldopa (Aldomet), and levodopa (Dopar, etc), when taken in large doses, can give positive Clinitest measurements, as can the presence of alkaptonuria, but methods using glucose oxidase give negative results. In fact, these powerful reducing substances, by interfering with the color reaction, may prevent detection of glucose in the urine of diabetics when glucose oxidase paper strips are used. Both of these methods are dependent upon a normal renal threshold for glucose.

b. Ketonuria—Qualitative detection of ketone bodies can be accomplished by nitroprusside tests (Acetest or Ketostix). Although these do not detect the β-hydroxybutyric acid, which lacks a ketone group, the semiquantitative estimation of ketonuria thus obtained is usually adequate for clinical purposes.

2. Blood testing procedures—

a. Methodology and normal fasting glucose—Plasma or serum from venous blood samples may be used and has the advantage over whole blood of providing values for glucose which are independent of hematocrit and which reflect the glucose concentration to which body tissues are exposed. Fluoride anticoagulant in the collecting tube prevents enzymatic glycolysis by blood corpuscles. If serum is used, samples should be refrigerated and separated from corpuscles within an hour after collection. Glucose oxidase and orthotolidine methods are most reliable, with normal values ranging from 60–90 mg/100 ml; serum or plasma methods dependent on reduction of copper or iron give slightly higher values (up to 110 mg/100 ml).

b. Screening tests— Tests on plasma rather than urine are preferable for detection of the unidentified diabetic. A plasma glucose test 2 hours after a standard carbohydrate load represents the most sensitive screening procedure available. Fasting plasma glucose determinations are not recommended for screening because of their insensitivity. However, if elevated above 120 mg/100 ml, they are of great significance.

c. Glucose tolerance tests—If the fasting plasma glucose is over 120 mg/100 ml, further evaluation of the patient with a glucose challenge is seldom necessary. If the screening level of plasma glucose after a glucose load is greater than 120 mg/100 ml, a standardized oral glucose tolerance test should be done. This consists of the administration of 100 gm glucose in 300 ml of water after an overnight fast to subjects who have been receiving at least 150–200 gm of carbohydrate daily for 3 days before the test. For proper evaluation of the test, the subjects should be normally active and free from acute illness. Medications which may impair glucose tolerance include estrogens, contraceptive drugs, glucocorticoids, nicotinic acid, and

diuretics. Blood samples should be obtained hourly for at least 3 hours. The Wilkerson point system as advocated by the USPHS is one of several methods available for interpretation of results. Points are assigned as follows: fasting plasma glucose above 125 mg/100 ml = 1; above 195 mg/100 ml at 1 hour = ½; above 140 mg/100 ml at 2 hours = ½; above 125 mg/100 ml at 3 hours = 1. A total of 2 points or more is considered diagnostic of abnormal carbohydrate tolerance. In these cases, measurement of insulin levels during the first 2 hours may be of use in classifying the patient as well as in selecting therapy.

d. Insulin levels during glucose tolerance test— Serum or plasma is separated within 30 minutes after collection and frozen. Normal insulin levels range from less than 10 to 25 μU/ml in the fasting state and 50–130 μU/ml at 1 hour, and usually return to levels below 100 μU/ml by 2 hours. A value below 50 μU/ml at 1 hour and less than 100 μU/ml at 2 hours in the presence of sustained hyperglycemia implicates insensitivity of beta cells to glucose as the cause of hyperglycemia, whereas levels substantially above 100 μU/ml at these times suggest tissue unresponsiveness to the action of insulin.

3. Capillary morphometry (biopsy of the quadriceps muscle)—The basement membrane of capillaries from skeletal muscle tissue of the quadriceps area is abnormally thickened in all cases of overt spontaneous diabetes in adults with fasting hyperglycemia of 140 mg/100 ml or more but normal in acquired states of carbohydrate intolerance due to pancreatitis, Cushing's syndrome, or pheochromocytoma. This appears to be less useful in diabetic children, being normal in as many as 60% of those below age 18.

Differential Diagnosis

A. Melituria: While melituria reflects hyperglycemia in over 90% of patients, 2 major classes of nondiabetic melituria must be considered.

1. Nondiabetic glycosuria (renal glycosuria)—This is a benign, asymptomatic condition wherein glucose appears in the urine despite a normal amount of glucose in the blood, either basally or during a glucose tolerance test. Its cause may vary from an autosomally transmitted genetic disorder to one associated with dysfunction of the proximal renal tubule (Fanconi's syndrome, chronic renal failure) or merely a consequence of the increased load of glucose presented to the tubules by the elevated glomerular filtration rate during pregnancy. As many as 50% of pregnant women normally have demonstrable sugar in the urine, especially during the third and fourth months. This sugar is practically always glucose except during the late weeks of pregnancy, when lactose may be present.

2. Melituria other than glycosuria— Occasionally, a sugar other than glucose is excreted in the urine. The most common of these is the lactosuria of the late stages of pregnancy and during postpartal lactation; much rarer are other conditions due to inborn errors of metabolism wherein fructose, galactose, or a pentose (L-xylulose) may be excreted in the urine. Testing the urine with paper strips impregnated with glucose oxidase will help differentiate true glycosuria from other meliturias.

B. Hyperglycemia—When hyperglycemia is demonstrated, the diabetic syndrome is present. Causes of hyperglycemia associated with end organ insensitivity to insulin may be included within the syndrome but might be considered distinct from true diabetes mellitus. These include obesity, acromegaly, Cushing's syndrome, liver disease, muscle disorders (myotonic dystrophy), glucagonoma, lipoatrophy, hemochromatosis, and thyrotoxicosis. Pheochromocytoma can induce hyperglycemia by a variety of mechanisms, including end organ resistance, inhibition of insulin release, and hypersecretion of glucagon. Chronic pancreatitis reduces the number of functioning beta cells and can result in a metabolic derangement very similar to that of genetic diabetes mellitus except that a concomitant reduction in pancreatic alpha cells may reduce glucagon secretion despite insulin deficiency, which often raises glucagon levels. An insulin-dependent form of diabetes is occasionally associated with Addison's disease and chronic thyroiditis (Schmidt's syndrome). This occurs particularly in females and probably represents an autoimmune disorder in which there are circulating antibodies to adrenocortical tissue, thyroglobulin, and gastric parietal cells.

Principles of Treatment of Diabetes

Rational therapy of diabetes requires the application of principles derived from current knowledge concerning (1) the nature of the disease and (2) the mechanism of action and the efficacy and the safety of the available treatment regimens (diet, oral hypoglycemic drugs, and insulin). Unfortunately, current knowledge about these matters is not always accurate or complete, and controversy exists about what constitutes the best therapeutic regimen. Fundamental to this controversy is the conflicting evidence about whether microangiopathy is related to the existence and duration of hyperglycemia or whether it reflects a separate, coexisting genetic disorder. Until this conflict is resolved, the therapeutic objective will be to attempt to restore to normal known metabolic derangements in the hope that this approach will impede if not prevent the progression of microvascular disease.

The general principles of therapy emphasized in this chapter will be based on the distinctions outlined in Table 19—1, where hyperglycemia is classified on the basis of its relationship to the amount of insulin released.

In all cases, **diet** will be prescribed individually to meet the needs of each type: caloric restriction in obese patients and regular spaced feedings with a bedtime snack for patients receiving hypoglycemic agents, especially insulin.

Exercise will also be encouraged as an adjunct to diet and insulin replacement in reducing hyperglycemia in the insulinopenic diabetic and to help achieve weight reduction in the insulinoplethoric obese diabetic.

Treatment of the insulinopenic diabetic will be directed toward normalization of the endocrine and metabolic abnormalities. In more severe cases, exogenous insulin replacement will be required, whereas in milder degrees of insulinopenia an attempt to restore endogenous insulin release with sulfonylureas would have the advantage of causing insulin to be released intraportally and would not introduce the immunogenic foreign protein of animal insulin. Potential disadvantages of sulfonylurea therapy will be discussed in the section on safety of oral hypoglycemic agents.

Treatment of insulinoplethoric diabetes will be directed at the cause of insulin insensitivity, eg, weight reduction in cases of obesity and reduction of endocrine hypersecretion in cases of acromegaly or Cushing's syndrome.

A. Available Treatment Regimens:

1. Diet—A proper diet remains a fundamental element of therapy, especially in the nonketotic maturity-onset type. However, in more than half of cases, diabetic patients fail to follow their diet. The reasons for this are varied and include unnecessary complexity of the prescription as well as lack of understanding of the goals by both the patient and the physician. A resurgence of interest in diet therapy for diabetes resulted from the findings of the UGDP report in 1970, which cast doubt on the efficacy and safety of oral hypoglycemic drugs.

Also, the high death toll from cardiovascular disease in diabetics (60—70% as compared to 20—25% in matched nondiabetic populations) created concern and prompted reevaluation of possible atherogenic features of the high cholesterol and high saturated fat ADA diet, which was first recommended in 1949 and has remained unrevised until just recently.

Revised ADA diet. In 1971, certain recommended changes were made in the ADA diet, but as of late 1975 sample menus have not been made available for general use. The new ADA diet again stresses the major goal of caloric restriction as a means of achieving or maintaining ideal weight. The major changes include a restriction of fat intake to 35% or less of the total calories and suggestions that saturated fat be reduced to only one-third of this by substituting poultry, veal, and fish for red meats as a major protein source. At the same time, cholesterol is restricted to less than 300 mg/day. Carbohydrates may be consumed more liberally (as much as 45—50% of total calories) as long as refined and simple sugars are avoided.

Two major observations have been incorporated into the revisions of the ADA diets:

(1) There is no evidence from at least one long-term clinical trial in insulin-requiring diabetics and several short-term trials in maturity-onset diabetics that an increased proportion of dietary carbohydrate causes deterioration of control, especially when the source of carbohydrate is in the form of bread, potatoes, or rice and not simple sugars, and as long as total calories are limited to maintain or achieve ideal weight.

(2) The ADA stresses that—while serum triglyceride elevation conceivably could occur as a result of

increased carbohydrate intake in certain predisposed individuals and should be monitored in all—it is hoped that the restriction of total caloric intake to achieve or maintain ideal weight will not allow enough carbohydrate intake to result in excess production of triglycerides. In fact, in a long-term trial in insulin-treated diabetics, a similar diet containing as much as 64% carbohydrate content did not raise serum triglycerides, whereas serum cholesterol fell below values obtained while on previous standard ADA diets.

Prescribing the diet. In prescribing a diet, it is important to relate dietary objectives to the type of diabetes. In obese patients with mild hyperglycemia, the major goal of diet therapy is weight reduction by caloric restriction. Thus, there is less need in the obese diabetic for exchange lists, emphasis on timing of meals, or periodic snacks, which are so essential in the treatment of insulin-requiring nonobese diabetics.

Because of the prevalence of the obese mild diabetic among the population of diabetics receiving therapy, this type of patient represents the most frequent and thus one of the most important challenges for the physician. It requires an energetic, vigorous program, directed by persons who are aware of the mechanisms by which weight reduction is known to effectively lower hyperglycemia and who are thoroughly convinced of the profoundly beneficial effects of weight control on blood lipid levels as well as on hyperglycemia in obese diabetics. Weight reduction is an elusive goal which can only be achieved by close supervision of the obese patient.

Artificial sweeteners. Diabetic patients who are reluctant to give up the pleasure of the sweet taste of foods may use available products such as saccharin, Aspartame, or cyclamate (if restored by FDA).

2. Oral hypoglycemic drugs—These consist of 2 major types: sulfonylureas and biguanides. Their modes of action are quite different, and considerable controversy exists over their mechanisms of action, therapeutic indications, and especially their safety in long-term use.

a. Sulfonylureas—This group of drugs contains a sulfonic acid-urea nucleus which can be modified by chemical substitutions to produce agents that have similar qualitative actions but differ widely in potency. The mechanism of action of the sulfonylureas—acutely administered—is due to their insulinotropic effect on pancreatic beta cells. However, it remains unclear whether this well-documented acute action can also explain the hypoglycemic effect of sulfonylureas during chronic administration.

To decide which type of diabetic patient should be treated with sulfonylureas requires not only a clear understanding of the metabolic dysfunction in the particular patient but also an accurate appreciation of the mechanism of action of the drug, its efficacy, and its safety for long-term use.

Sulfonylureas are presently not indicated in the juvenile type ketosis-prone insulin-dependent diabetic since they seem to depend on functioning pancreatic beta cells to produce their effect on blood glucose.

However, if extra-beta cell effects are substantiated in man—especially if lowering of pancreatic glucagon is confirmed—their usefulness as an adjunct to insulin therapy would deserve reevaluation.

The type of patient in whom the sulfonylureas seem most appropriate is the nonobese insulinopenic mild maturity-onset diabetic in whom acute administration restores the early phase of insulin release which is refractory to acute glucose stimulation. Use of this group of agents is probably not justified in obese mild diabetics and others with peripheral insensitivity to levels of circulating insulin that are already supernormal and in whom primary emphasis should be on weight reduction.

(1) Tolbutamide (Orinase) is supplied in tablets of 500 mg. It is rapidly oxidized in the liver to an inactive form, and its approximate effect is relatively short (6—10 hours). Tolbutamide is probably best administered in divided doses such as 500 mg before each meal and at bedtime; however, some patients require only 1 or 2 tablets daily. Acute toxic reactions are rare, with skin rashes occurring infrequently. Prolonged hypoglycemia has been reported rarely, mostly in elderly people or in patients receiving certain drugs such as dicumarol, phenylbutazone, or some of the sulfonamides. The latter compounds apparently compete with sulfonylureas for oxidative enzyme systems in the liver, resulting in maintenance of high levels of unmetabolized, active sulfonylureas in the circulation.

(2) Chlorpropamide (Diabinese) is supplied in tablets of 100 and 250 mg. This drug, with a half-life of 32 hours, is slowly metabolized, with approximately 20—30% excreted unchanged in the urine. It can also interact with the above-cited drugs that depend on hepatic oxidative catabolism and is contraindicated in patients with hepatic or renal insufficiency. The average maintenance dose is 250 mg daily, given as a single dose in the morning. Prolonged hypoglycemic reactions are more common than with tolbutamide, particularly in elderly patients, in whom chlorpropamide therapy should be monitored with special care. Doses in excess of 250 mg or 375 mg/day increase the risk of jaundice, which does not occur on the usual dose of 250 mg/day or less. A disulfiram-like reaction may occur when alcohol is ingested.

(3) Acetohexamide (Dymelor) is supplied in tablets of 250 and 500 mg. Its duration of action is about 10—16 hours, being intermediate in action between tolbutamide and chlorpropamide. The usual dose is 0.25—1.5 gm/day in one or 2 doses. Liver metabolism is rapid, but the metabolite produced remains active. Side-effects are similar to those of the other sulfonylurea drugs.

(4) Tolazamide (Tolinase) is supplied in tablets of 100 and 250 mg. It is comparable to chlorpropamide in potency but has a shorter duration of action similar to that of acetohexamide.

(5) Glyburide (Micronase), the newest of these compounds, was recently introduced in Europe but has not yet been approved for use in the USA. Although it is more potent than the other agents, no qualitative differences in action have been documented. Effective dosage varies from 2.5–20 mg; unfamiliarity with its great potency (100 times more potent than tolbutamide) may account for the recorded high incidence of severe hypoglycemic reactions, with occasional fatalities. Special caution is recommended when using this drug, especially in patients with cardiovascular disease or in elderly patients, in whom hypoglycemia carries a special risk.

b. Biguanides—Phenformin (DBI, Meltrol) is the only biguanide available in the USA for clinical use. Since its introduction in 1957, an explanation for its mechanism of action has remained elusive despite considerable investigative effort. Its blood glucose lowering effect does not depend on beta cell stimulation. Glucose is not lowered in normal subjects after an overnight fast, but postprandial blood glucose levels are considerably lower during phenformin administration. Patients with maturity-onset diabetes have considerably less fasting hyperglycemia as well as postprandial hyperglycemia after phenformin; however, hypoglycemia during phenformin therapy is essentially unknown. This agent might therefore be more appropriately termed a "euglycemic" rather than a hypoglycemic agent. Currently proposed mechanisms of action include (1) direct stimulation of glycolysis in peripheral tissues, with increased glucose removal from the blood; (2) reduced hepatic gluconeogenesis; (3) a slowing of glucose absorption from the gastrointestinal tract; and(4) inhibition of plasma glucagon levels.

Phenformin is supplied either in tablets of 25 mg (DBI, Meltrol-25) or as timed-disintegration capsules (DBI-TD, Meltrol-50, Meltrol-100) containing 50 or 100 mg. Side-effects are predominantly gastrointestinal and include anorexia, nausea and vomiting, and diarrhea. These occur rarely when the timed-disintegration capsules are prescribed in the usual dosage of 50 mg daily but increase in frequency with higher dosage. There is probably no reason to use doses greater than 100 mg/day.

Phenformin has been most often prescribed for the patient with refractory obesity whose hyperglycemia is due to ineffective insulin action. It has an insulin-sparing effect through its tendency to reduce postprandial hyperglycemia either by glucose absorption or by a direct effect on the clearance of glucose. Another indication for its use is in certain nonobese adult-onset diabetics in whom sulfonylurea therapy alone is less effective than when combined with phenformin. Until certain questions are resolved concerning long-term safety of phenformin (see below), its use in obese diabetics might best be reserved for those with symptoms such as pruritus or vulvovaginitis—preferably on a short-term basis—until the primary goal of weight reduction is achieved.

3. Insulin—Insulin is indicated for ketosis-prone juvenile-type diabetics as well as for those adult-onset diabetics with insulinopenia who do not respond to diet therapy either alone or combined with oral hypoglycemic drugs. Ideal replacement therapy would provide insulin in a manner comparable to the secretory pattern of normal individuals. It is not possible to completely reproduce the physiologic patterns of insulin secretion with subcutaneous injections of soluble or longer-acting insulin suspensions or combinations of insulins. Even so, with the help of appropriate modifications of diet and exercise, it has been possible to achieve acceptable control of blood glucose using variable mixtures of short- and longer-acting insulins injected twice daily.

a. Insulin preparations—Three principal types of insulins are available: (1) short-acting, with rapid onset of action; (2) intermediate-acting; and (3) long-acting, with slow onset of action. Short-acting insulin (regular insulin) is a crystalline zinc insulin provided in soluble form and thus is dispensed as a clear solution in acid pH. All other commercial insulins have been specially modified to retain more prolonged action and are dispensed as opaque suspensions at neutral pH using either protamine in phosphate buffer (protamine zinc insulin and NPH) or varying concentrations of zinc in acetate buffer (ultralente and semilente). Globin insulin, an intermediate-acting insulin in clear solution, is seldom prescribed in the USA. Likewise, the use of protamine zinc insulin or ultralente preparations is currently decreasing, and almost no indications for their use exist. Present insulin therapy involves no more than 4 insulin preparations:

(1) Regular insulin (crystalline zinc insulin) is a short-acting insulin whose effect appears within 15 minutes after subcutaneous injection and lasts 5–7 hours. It is particularly useful in the treatment of diabetic ketoacidosis and when the insulin requirement is changing rapidly, such as after surgery or during acute infections. When mixed with intermediate forms it apparently retains its rapid action and is useful in providing a rising insulin level during breakfast and supper when administered before these meals.

(2) NPH (new protamine Hagedorn insulin) is a stable mixture of 2 parts crystalline zinc insulin and 1 part protamine zinc insulin. Its onset of action is delayed, and mixing with regular insulin is usually required for proper replacement therapy in insulin-dependent patients. It can be readily mixed with regular insulin to fit the patient's needs and is used for daily replacement therapy in insulin-treated patients. Since its duration often is less than 24 hours, ranging from 18–24 hours, most patients require at least 2 injections daily to maintain a sustained insulin effect.

(3) Lente insulin is a mixture of 30% semilente with 70% ultralente insulin. Its action is essentially identical with that of NPH insulin, and its indications and dosage schedule are similar to NPH for daily insulin replacement.

(4) Semilente insulin has an onset of action that is slower than that of regular insulin but slightly more rapid than either of the intermediate insulins. Its duration of action is 12–16 hours. Semilente can be premixed with lente insulin to provide faster-acting insulin which still retains the more prolonged action of lente insulin.

Most insulins have been prepared in U40 and U80

strengths, but a gradual phasing out of these concentrations is planned now that U100 is widely available and endorsed as the concentration of choice by the ADA. All standard commercial preparations consist of beef insulin, and the Eli Lilly preparations contain as much as 30% pork insulin as well. Recent improvements in purification technics have eliminated contaminating proteins which had molecular weights greater than that of insulin and possessed no insulin-like activity, yet were capable of inducing the production of anti-insulin antibodies in rabbits. This highly purified insulin has been termed **"single peak" insulin** on the basis of its Sephadex gel profile and is currently the form of insulin used commercially in the USA. A further purification step to remove some lower molecular weight impurities has produced a limited supply of insulin without detectable impurity, termed **single component** or **monocomponent insulin.** This has been shown to have very low or no immunogenicity in man during long-term insulin therapy and has been particularly useful in the treatment of insulin allergy and lipodystrophy secondary to insulin injections.

b. Administration of insulin—To reduce confusion and mistakes in insulin administration, all diabetics beginning insulin therapy should receive mixtures of short- and long-acting U100 insulins administered in U100 syringes, although this concentration of insulin is easy to measure with any standard 1 ml syringe. For convenience, plastic disposable syringes are often used, especially for administration away from home. In cases where very low insulin doses are prescribed, as in young children, a specially calibrated 0.35 ml U100 glass syringe is available to facilitate accurate measurement of the dose.

Recent preparations of insulin have been purified to the extent that acid pH is no longer required, and at present all U100 insulin preparations are at neutral pH. Thus, regular insulin can now be mixed with either lente or NPH insulin. When mixing insulin, it is necessary to inject into both bottles a quantity of air equivalent to the volume of insulin to be subsequently withdrawn. It is recommended that the regular insulin be withdrawn first, and then the intermediate insulin. No attempt should be made to mix the insulins in the syringe, and the injection is preferably given immediately after loading the syringe.

Any part of the body covered by loose skin can be used, such as the abdomen, thighs, upper arms, flanks, and upper buttocks. It is important that the site of subcutaneous administration of insulin be rotated so that the same site is not used more often than once every 3 weeks to avoid scarring and consequent variability in insulin absorption. Regular insulin is the only type available for intravenous use.

The more highly purified insulins which have recently become available seem to preserve their potency quite well, so that refrigeration is unnecessary. During travel, reserve supplies of insulin can thus be readily transported for weeks or even months without losing potency as long as they are protected from extremes of heat or cold.

B. Efficacy and Safety of the Hypoglycemic Agents:

1. Cardiovascular mortality—The University Group Diabetes Program (UGDP) reported that the number of deaths due to cardiovascular disease in diabetic patients treated with tolbutamide or with phenformin was excessive compared to either insulin-treated patients or those receiving placebos. Controversy persists about the validity of the conclusions reached by the UGDP because of the heterogeneity of the population studied with its preponderance of obese subjects and certain features of the experimental design such as the use of a fixed dose of oral drug.

A careful statistical reappraisal of the UGDP report has recently been published by the Biometric Society. In regard to cardiovascular mortality from either tolbutamide or phenformin, the Biometric Report concluded that the UGDP report has raised suspicions that cannot be dismissed on the basis of other evidence presently available. This report has prompted the Food and Drug Administration to recommend a special package insert warning that oral hypoglycemic agents may be associated with increased cardiovascular mortality as compared to treatment with diet alone or diet plus insulin. This warning, set in boldface type within a box border, states that these agents should be used in preference to insulin only in patients with maturity-onset diabetes who cannot be controlled by diet alone and only when the advantages in the individual patient justify the potential risk of increased cardiovascular mortality.

2. Lactic acidosis and phenformin therapy—(See p 743.) Hyperlactatemia and lactic acidosis represent a risk of phenformin therapy, especially—and perhaps *only*—when other predisposing factors are present (renal insufficiency in particular).

General Considerations in Treatment of Diabetes

Patients with diabetes can have a full and satisfying life. However, "free" diets and unrestricted activity are still not possible for insulin-requiring diabetics. Until new methods of insulin replacement are developed that provide more normal patterns of insulin delivery in response to metabolic demands, multiple feedings will continue to be recommended and certain occupations potentially hazardous to the patient or others will continue to be prohibited.

Exercise increases the effectiveness of insulin, and moderate exercise is an excellent means of improving utilization of fat and carbohydrate in diabetic patients. A judicious balance of the size and frequency of meals with moderate exercise in a routine manner can often stabilize the insulin dosage in diabetics who tend to slip out of control easily. Strenuous exercise could precipitate hypoglycemia in an unprepared patient, and diabetics must therefore be taught to reduce their insulin dosage in anticipation of strenuous activity or to take supplemental carbohydrate. However, the more knowledgeable the patient is regarding the relationships between caloric intake and expenditure and insulin requirements, the more liberated he can become from the regimentation imposed on him by his disorder.

All diabetic patients must receive adequate instruction on personal hygiene, especially with regard to care of the feet (see p 736), skin, and teeth. All infections—but especially pyogenic infections with fever and toxemia—provoke the release of high levels of insulin antagonists such as glucagon and thus bring about a marked increase in insulin requirements. This is a common precipitating cause of ketosis and acidosis and should be treated promptly· and vigorously. Supplemental regular insulin is often required to correct hyperglycemia during the stress of infection.

Psychologic factors are of great importance in the control of diabetes, particularly when the disease is difficult to stabilize. One reason the diabetic may be particularly sensitive to emotional upset is that alpha cells of diabetics are hyperresponsive to physiologic levels of epinephrine, producing excessive levels of glucagon with consequent hyperglycemia.

Counseling should be directed at avoiding extremes of compulsive rigidity versus self-destructive neglect.

Steps in the Management of the Diabetic Patient

A. Diagnostic Examination: A complete history and physical examination is performed for diagnostic purposes and to rule out the presence of coexisting or complicating disease. Any features of the clinical picture that suggest end organ insensitivity to insulin must be identified. The family history should document not only the incidence of diabetes in other members of the family but also the age at onset, whether it was associated with obesity, and whether insulin was required.

Laboratory work-up should include documentation of the renal threshold for glucose. This is done by carefully instructing the patient to "double void"—a practice that will greatly facilitate future evaluation of control and management. The glucose concentration of this second voided specimen, taken within 30 minutes after emptying the bladder, more closely represents the plasma glucose concentration at the time, so simultaneous measurement of plasma glucose will demonstrate the level at which the tubular maximum for glucose is exceeded.

Baseline values of any observation that may help in the evaluation of future complications should be recorded. These include plasma triglycerides and cholesterol, ECG, chest x-ray, renal function studies, peripheral pulses, and neurologic and ophthalmologic examinations.

B. Patient Education: Since diabetes is a lifelong disorder, education of the patient is probably the most important obligation of the physician who provides initial care. The best persons to manage a disease which is affected so markedly by daily fluctuations in environmental stress, exercise, diet, and infections are the patients themselves and their families. The "curriculum" should include the nature of diabetes and its potential acute and chronic hazards and how they might be recognized early and prevented or treated.

The importance of regular recording of tests for glucose on double-voided urine specimens should be stressed and instructions on proper testing provided. Advice on personal hygiene, including detailed instructions on foot care (see p 736), as well as individual instruction on diet and specific hypoglycemic therapy, should be provided. Patients should be told about community agencies such as Diabetes Association chapters which can serve as a continuing source of instruction.

C. Initial Therapy: Treatment must be individualized on the basis of the type of diabetes and the specific needs of each patient. However, certain general principles of management can be outlined for hyperglycemic states of different types.

1. The obese patient—The most common type of diabetic patient is obese and has hyperglycemia because of insensitivity to normal or elevated circulating levels of insulin (insulinoplethoric diabetes).

a. Weight reduction—Treatment is directed toward achieving weight reduction, and prescribing a diet is only one means to this end. Cure can be achieved by reducing adipose stores, with consequent restoration of tissue sensitivity to insulin. The presence of diabetes with its added risk factors may motivate the obese diabetic to greater effort in correcting his obesity.

b. Hypoglycemic agents—Hypoglycemic agents, including insulin as well as oral hypoglycemic drugs, are not indicated for long-term use in the mild obese diabetic. The weight reduction program can be upset by insulin reactions when insulin therapy is used; it is also possible that administration of insulin to an obese patient who already has excessive circulating levels may have the ill effects of maintaining insulin insensitivity of receptor sites as well as interfering with catabolic mechanisms during caloric deprivation. The obese diabetic who has been previously treated with insulin—often in interrupted fashion—and who requires high doses both to offset excess caloric intake and to overcome tissue insensitivity may develop immune insulin resistance. This not only increases the requirements for exogenous insulin but also impairs the effectiveness of endogenous insulin and may even precipitate ketosis.

The use of oral hypoglycemic agents—especially phenformin—might better be reserved for the moderately severe obese diabetic with severe glycosuria complicated by candidal vulvovaginitis. In such cases, short-term therapy (weeks or months) with phenformin may be indicated until the beneficial effects of simultaneous caloric restriction leading to weight reduction can occur.

2. The nonobese patient—In the nonobese diabetic, mild to severe hyperglycemia is usually due to refractoriness of beta cells to glucose stimulation (insulinopenic diabetes). Treatment depends on whether insulinopenia is severe enough to produce ketoacidosis.

a. Diet therapy—If hyperglycemia is mild, normal metabolic control can occasionally be restored by means of multiple feedings of a diet mildly restricted in calories and devoid of simple sugars. Restriction of saturated fats and cholesterol is also strongly advised.

b. Oral hypoglycemic agents—Unlike obese pa-

Instructions in the Care of the Feet
for Persons With Diabetes Mellitus or Vascular Disturbances

Hygiene of the Feet

(1) Wash feet daily with mild soap and luke-warm water. Dry thoroughly between the toes by pressure. Do not rub vigorously, as this is apt to break the delicate skin.

(2) When feet are thoroughly dry, rub well with vegetable oil to keep them soft, prevent excess friction, remove scales, and prevent dryness. Care must be taken to prevent foot tenderness.

(3) If the feet become too soft and tender, rub them with alcohol about once a week.

(4) When rubbing the feet, always rub upward from the tips of the toes. If varicose veins are present, massage the feet very gently; never massage the legs.

(5) If the toenails are brittle and dry, soften them by soaking for one-half hour each night in lukewarm water containing 1 tbsp of powdered sodium borate (borax) per quart. Follow this by rubbing around the nails with vegetable oil. Clean around the nails with an orangewood stick. If the nails become too long, file them with an emery board. File them straight across, and no shorter than the underlying soft tissues of the toe. Never cut the corners of the nails. (The patient's podiatrist should be told that he has diabetes.)

(6) Wear low-heeled shoes of soft leather which fit the shape of the feet correctly. The shoes should have wide toes that will cause no pressure, fit close in the arch, and grip the heels snugly. Wear new shoes one-half hour only on the first day and increase by 1 hour each day following. Wear thick, warm, loose stockings.

Treatment of Corns & Calluses

(1) Corns and calluses are due to friction and pressure, most often from improperly fitted shoes and stockings. Wear shoes that fit properly and cause no friction or pressure.

(2) To remove excess calluses or corns, soak the feet in lukewarm (not hot) water, using a mild soap, for about 10 minutes, and then rub off the excess tissue with a towel or file. Do not tear it off. Under no circumstances must the skin become irritated.

(3) Do not cut corns or calluses. If they need attention it is safer to see a podiatrist.

(4) Prevent callus formation under the ball of the foot (a) by exercises, such as curling and stretching the toes several times a day; (b) by finishing each step on the toes and not on the ball of the foot; and

(c) by wearing shoes that are not too short and that do not have high heels.

**Aids in Treatment of Impaired
Circulation (Cold Feet)**

(1) Never use tobacco in any form. Tobacco contracts blood vessels and so reduces circulation.

(2) Keep warm. Wear warm stockings and other clothing. Cold contracts blood vessels and reduces circulation.

(3) Do not wear circular garters, which compress blood vessels and reduce blood flow.

(4) Do not sit with the legs crossed. This may compress the leg arteries and shut off the blood supply to the feet.

(5) If the weight of the bedclothes is uncomfortable, place a pillow under the covers at the foot of the bed.

(6) Do not apply any medication to the feet without directions from a physician. Some medicines are too strong for feet with poor circulation.

(7) Do not apply heat in the form of hot water, hot water bottles, or heating pads without a physician's consent. Even moderate heat can injure the skin if circulation is poor.

(8) If the feet are moist or the patient has a tendency to develop athlete's foot, a prophylactic dusting powder should be used on the feet and in shoes and stockings daily. Change shoes and stockings at least daily or oftener.

Treatment of Abrasions of the Skin

(1) Proper first-aid treatment is of the utmost importance even in apparently minor injuries. Consult a physician immediately for any redness, blistering, pain, or swelling. Any break in the skin may become ulcerous or gangrenous unless properly treated by a physician.

(2) Dermatophytosis (athlete's foot), which begins with peeling and itching between the toes or discoloration or thickening of the toenails, should be treated immediately by a physician or podiatrist.

(3) Avoid strong irritating antiseptics such as tincture of iodine.

(4) As soon as possible after any injury, cover the area with sterile gauze, which may be purchased at drugstores. Only fine paper tape or cellulose tape (Scotch Tape) should be used on the skin if adhesive retention of the gauze is required.

(5) Elevate and, as much as possible until recovery, avoid using the foot.

tients with diabetes, nonobese patients with adult-onset diabetes were not represented in the UGDP in sufficient numbers to permit specific conclusions about their increased cardiovascular risk from the use of oral hypoglycemic drugs. When diet therapy is not sufficient to correct hyperglycemia, a trial of sulfonylureas to improve insulin release is often successful. However, in view of the proposed FDA warning, it may be prudent to reserve sulfonylureas for those symptomatic patients with insulinopenia in whom dietary management is unsuccessful and who refuse or are unable to take insulin. In certain of these cases where diet and sulfonylureas achieve only partial improvement in blood glucose, timed-disintegration phenformin, 50 mg, could be added to the regimen. There is no indication for phenformin alone in this group of patients with insulin deficiency.

c. Insulin treatment—If hyperglycemia persists despite diet and oral agents, exogenous insulin must be given, preferably administered in mixtures of regular and intermediate-acting insulins as discussed in the section on insulin administration.

The patient requiring insulin therapy should be initially regulated under conditions of optimal diet and normal daily activities. He should be advised about the benefits of taking 2 injections of insulin mixtures daily and the importance of recording measurements of glucose in double-voided urines at least 4 times a day to assist in regulating the insulin dose until a stable insulin dose is achieved. A typical initial dose schedule in a 70 kg patient taking 2200 Cal divided into 6 or 7 feedings might be 10 units of regular and 10 units of NPH insulin in the morning and 5 units of regular and 5 units of NPH insulin in the evening. The morning urine is a measure of the effectiveness of NPH insulin administered the previous evening; the noon urine reflects the effects of the morning regular insulin; and the 5:00 p.m. and 9:00 p.m. urines represent the effects of the morning NPH and the evening regular insulins, respectively. A properly educated patient might be taught to adjust his own insulin by observing the pattern of glycosuria and correlating it with the approximate duration of action and the time of peak effect after injection of the various insulin preparations (Fig 19–1). Adjustments should be made gradually and preferably not more often than every 3–4 days if possible.

d. Glucagon suppression by somatostatin—The hyperglucagonemia of insulin-requiring diabetics, which contributes significantly to postprandial hyperglycemia, is presumably due to an impaired suppressibility of the diabetic's pancreatic alpha cells by glucose. Somatostatin, a tetradecapeptide originally derived from ovine hypothalami and presently available in synthetic form, has been found to be a potent inhibitor of glucagon release. Its potential therapeutic value when combined with insulin for treatment of the defective "organ of Langerhans," is being intensively studied at present.

Complications of Insulin Therapy

A. Hypoglycemia: Hypoglycemic reactions, the most common complication of insulin therapy, may result from delay in taking a meal or unusual physical exertion. In older diabetics and those taking only longer-acting insulins, autonomic responses are less frequent and the manifestations are mainly from impaired function of the CNS, ie, mental confusion, bizarre behavior, and ultimately coma. More rapid development of hypoglycemia from the effects of regular insulin causes signs of autonomic hyperactivity, both adrenergic (tachycardia, palpitations, sweating, tremulousness) and parasympathetic (nausea, hunger) which may progress to coma and convulsions. All of the manifestations of hypoglycemia are rapidly relieved by glucose administration.

Because of the potential danger of insulin reactions, the diabetic patient should carry packets of table sugar or a candy roll at all times for use at the onset of hypoglycemic symptoms. An ampule of glucagon (1 mg) should be provided to every diabetic receiving insulin therapy, to be injected by family or friends in case of unconsciousness. An identification bracelet, necklace, or card in the wallet or purse should be car-

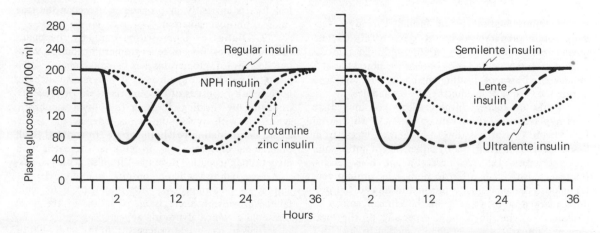

Figure 19–1. Extent and duration of action of various types of insulin (in a fasting diabetic).

I Am a Diabetic and Take Insulin

If I am behaving peculiarly but am conscious and able to swallow, give me sugar or hard candy or orange juice slowly. If I am unconscious, call an ambulance immediately, take me to a physician or a hospital, and notify my physician. *I am not intoxicated.*

My name _____

Address _____

Telephone _____

Physician's name _____

Physician's address _____

Telephone _____

---

ried by every diabetic (see accompanying box).

Treatment of hypoglycemia. All of the manifestations of hypoglycemia are rapidly relieved by glucose administration. In a case of mild hypoglycemia in a patient who is conscious and able to swallow, orange juice, glucose, or any sugar-containing beverage or food may be given. If more severe hypoglycemia has produced unconsciousness or stupor, the treatment of choice is to give 20–50 ml of 50% glucose solution by IV infusion over a period of 2–3 minutes. If intravenous therapy is not available, 1 mg of glucagon injected IM will usually restore the patient to consciousness within 15 minutes to permit ingestion of sugar. Family members should be instructed in how to give glucagon when the need arises. If the patient is stuporous and glucagon is not available, small amounts of honey or syrup can be inserted within the buccal pouch, but in general oral feeding is contraindicated in unconscious patients. Rectal administration of syrup or honey (2 tbsp per pint of warm water) has been effective.

B. Immunopathology of Insulin Therapy: Standard insulin preparations in the USA usually contain bovine insulin. Eli Lilly preparations contain approximately 70% bovine and 30% porcine insulin. At least 5 molecular classes of insulin antibodies are produced during the course of insulin therapy in diabetes.

1. Insulin allergy—Insulin allergy, or immediate type hypersensitivity, is a rare condition in which local or systemic urticaria is due to histamine release from tissue mast cells sensitized by adherence of anti-insulin IgE antibodies. In severe cases, anaphylaxis results. Because sensitivity is often to noninsulin protein contaminants, the new highly purified insulins often produce marked improvement in the clinical course of patients with insulin allergy, especially of the local variety. Similarly, a species change such as to pure beef or pure pork insulin may correct the problem. Anti-

histamines, corticosteroids, and even desensitization may be required, especially for systemic hypersensitivity.

2. Immune insulin resistance—All insulin-treated patients develop a low titer of circulating IgG anti-insulin antibodies which neutralize the action of insulin. In some diabetic patients, principally those with some degree of tissue insensitivity to insulin (such as in the obese) and with a history of interrupted exposure to insulin therapy, a high titer of circulating IgG anti-insulin antibodies develops. This results in extremely high insulin requirements—often more than 200 units daily. This is often a self-limited condition and may clear spontaneously after several months. However, in cases where the circulating antibody is specifically more reactive with beef insulin—a more potent immunogen in man than pork insulin—changing the patient to a less antigenic pork insulin may make possible a dramatic reduction in insulin dosage or at least may shorten the duration of immune resistance. Other forms of therapy include immunosuppression with corticosteroids, and in some adults the foreign insulin can be completely discontinued and the patient maintained on diet along with oral hypoglycemic agents. This is possible only when the circulating antibodies do not effectively bind endogenous (human) insulin.

C. Lipodystrophy at Injection Sites: Atrophy or hypertrophy of subcutaneous fatty tissue leading to disfigurement and scarring may rarely occur at the site of injection. A variety of causes have been suggested, including the acidity or large volume of the insulin used as well as its content of various impurities. This complication has become rarer since the development of highly concentrated, pure insulin preparations of neutral pH. Injection of these preparations directly into the atrophic area often results in restoration of normal contours.

D. Chronic Complications and Prognosis:

1. Diabetic retinopathy—Proliferative retinopathy is a leading cause of blindness in the USA. Photocoagulation—eg, with argon laser beams—to obliterate the abnormal blood vessels is currently the treatment of choice rather than pituitary ablation. A large-scale clinical trial is currently in progress to ascertain the true value of photocoagulation.

2. Diabetic nephropathy—Capillary basement membrane thickening of renal glomeruli produces varying degrees of glomerulosclerosis and renal insufficiency. The clinical syndrome of progressive diabetic nephropathy consists of proteinuria of varying severity occasionally leading to the full-blown nephrotic syndrome with hypoalbuminemia, edema, and an increase in circulating betalipoproteins. In contrast to all other renal disorders, the proteinuria associated with diabetic nephropathy does not diminish with progressive renal failure (patients continue to excrete 10–11 gm/day as creatinine clearance diminishes). As renal failure progresses, there is an elevation in the renal threshold at which glycosuria appears.

Dialysis has been unsuccessful in the treatment of renal failure due to diabetic nephropathy. At present, experience in renal transplantation—especially from related donors—is quite promising and is the treatment of choice in cases where there are no contraindications such as severe cardiovascular disease.

3. Gangrene of the feet in diabetes—The incidence of gangrene of the feet in diabetics is 20 times the incidence in matched controls. The factors responsible for its development are ischemia, peripheral neuropathy, and secondary infection. Ischemia involves small arteries in all cases; however, in as many as one-third of cases of diabetic gangrene, pedal pulses were palpable, indicating sparing of medium-sized and larger arteries. Prevention of foot disease (see p 736) should be emphasized since treatment is difficult once ulceration and gangrene have developed. Amputation of the lower extremities is sometimes required.

Propranolol is contraindicated in patients with ischemic foot ulcers because the drug reduces peripheral blood flow.

4. Diabetic neuropathy—Peripheral and autonomic neuropathy, the 2 most common complications of diabetes, are poorly understood. There is no consistently effective treatment other than optimal control of the diabetes. Ophthalmoplegias inevitably resolve within 6–9 weeks. Diarrhea associated with autonomic neuropathy has occasionally responded to broad spectrum antibiotic therapy, although it often undergoes spontaneous remission. Gastric atony may be so severe as to require gastrojejunal anastomosis. Impotence is usually permanent. Bethanechol (Urecholine) has occasionally improved emptying of the atonic urinary bladder. Mineralocorticoid therapy and pressure suits have reportedly been of some help in patients with orthostatic hypotension occurring as a result of loss of postural reflexes. Diphenylhydantoin in doses of 300–400 mg daily has been recommended for nocturnal pains in the lower extremity but should not be continued if improvement has not occurred after 10 days of therapy.

Prognosis of Diabetes

The effect of diabetic control on the development of complications remains an unresolved controversy. The patient with juvenile-onset insulin-dependent diabetes is at greater risk of developing microangiopathy of the kidneys and retina than the obese diabetic, whose major complications are more apt to be related to disease of the medium-sized and large arteries. Although the quality of control of diabetes most likely plays an important role, complications cannot be attributed solely to poor control.

Until these questions are resolved, the prognosis remains uncertain. A few guidelines, however, are available. In one series of 164 juvenile-onset diabetics with a median age at onset of 9 years, the following outcome was noted after follow-up for 25 years: Out of every 5 diabetics on standard dietary and insulin control, one had died and one was incapacitated with severe proliferative retinopathy and renal failure. However, 2 others were active, contributing members of society despite mild background retinopathy, mild

nephropathy, neuropathy, and some degree of ischemia of the feet, and one was completely free of complications (see Knowles reference).

The period between 10 and 20 years after onset of diabetes seems to be a critical one. If the patient survives this period without fulminating complications, there is a strong likelihood that he will continue to function in reasonably good health. It is clear that the intelligence and motivation of the diabetic patient and his awareness of the potential complications of the disease contribute significantly to the ultimate outcome.

Arello LM & others: The diabetic retinopathy study. Arch Ophth 90:347, 1973.

Bierman E & others: Principles of nutrition and dietary recommendations for patients with diabetes mellitus. Diabetes 20:633, 1971.

Block M & others: Sequential changes in beta-cell function in insulin-treated diabetic patients assessed by C-peptide immunoreactivity. New England J Med 288:1144, 1973.

Bondy PK, Rosenberg LE: *Duncan's Diseases of Metabolism,* 7th ed. 2 vols. Saunders, 1974.

Bray GA & others: The obese diabetic: A symposium on new developments. California Med 119:14, Oct 1973.

Cerasi E, Luft R, Efendic S: Decreased sensitivity of the pancreatic beta cells to glucose in prediabetic and diabetic subjects. Diabetes 21:224, 1972.

Ellenberg M: Impotence in diabetes: The neurologic factor. Ann Int Med 75:213, 1971.

Ellenberg M, Rifkin H: *Diabetes Mellitus: Theory and Practice.* McGraw-Hill, 1970.

Ewing DJ & others: Vascular reflexes in diabetic autonomic neuropathy. Lancet 2:1354, 1973.

Gabbay KH: The sorbitol pathway and the complications of diabetes. New England J Med 288:831, 1973.

Gerich J & others: Effect of somatostatin on plasma glucose and glucagon levels in human diabetes mellitus. New England J Med 291:544, 1974.

Gerich JE, Charles MA, Grodsky GM: Regulation of pancreatic insulin and glucagon secretion. Ann Rev Physiol. In press.

Gilbert JP & others: Report of the Committee for the Assessment of Biometric Aspects of Controlled Trials of Hypoglycemic Agents. JAMA 231:583, 1975.

Karam J, Matin S, Forsham P: Antidiabetic drugs after the University Group Diabetes Program (UGDP). Ann Rev Pharmacol 15:13, 1975.

Karlsson K, Kjellmer I: The outcome of diabetic pregnancies in relation to the mother's blood sugar level. Am J Obst Gynec 111:213, 1972.

Kilo C, Vogler N, Williamson JR: Muscle capillary basement membrane changes related to aging and to diabetes mellitus. Diabetes 21:881, 1972.

Klimt C & others: Standardization of the oral glucose tolerance test. Diabetes 18:299, 1969.

Klimt C & others: The University Group Diabetes Program. Parts 1 and 2. Diabetes 19 (Suppl 2): 747, 1970.

Klimt C & others: The University Group Diabetes Program. Part 5. Evaluation of phenformin therapy. Diabetes 24 (Suppl 1):1, 1975.

Knowles HC Jr: Long-term juvenile diabetes treated with unmeasured diet. Tr A Am Physicians 84:95, 1971.

Levey G, Lasseter K, Palmer R: Sulfonylureas and the heart. Ann Rev Med 25:69, 1974.

Levin M, O'Neal L: *The Diabetic Foot.* Mosby, 1973.

Lieberman P & others: Allergic reactions to insulin. JAMA 215:1106, 1971.

Malins JM: Glucose tolerance and the diabetic population. Postgrad MJ 50 (Suppl 3):529, 1974.

Marble A & others: *Joslin's Diabetes Mellitus*. Lea & Febiger, 1971.

Najarian J & others: Renal transplantation for diabetic glomerulosclerosis. Ann Surg 178:477, 1973.

Oakley WG & others: Long term diabetes. Quart J Med 43:145, 1974.

Oleesky S, Shreeve D, Sutcliffe CH: Brittle diabetes. Quart J Med 43:113, 1974.

Pildes RS: Infants of diabetic mothers. New England J Med 289:902, 1973.

Raskin P & others: Capillary basement membrane width in diabetic children. Am J Med 58:365, 1975.

Rimoin DL: Genetics of diabetes mellitus. Diabetes 16:346, 1967.

Seltzer H: Drug induced hypoglycemia. Diabetes 21:955, 1972.

Siperstein M, Raskin R, Burns H: Electron microscopic quantification of diabetic microangiopathy. Diabetes 22:514, 1973.

Spiro R: Biochemistry of the renal glomerular basement membrane and its alterations in diabetes mellitus. New England J Med 288:1337, 1973.

Steinke J: Management of diabetes mellitus and surgery. New England J Med 282:1472, 1970.

Steinke J, Taylor KW: Viruses and the etiology of diabetes. Diabetes 23:631, 1974.

Takazakura E & others: Onset and progression of diabetic glomerulosclerosis. Diabetes 24:1, 1975.

Tantillo J & others: Immunogenicity of "single peak" beef-pork insulin in diabetic subjects. Diabetes 23:276, 1974.

Unger RH, Orci L: The essential role of glucagon in the pathogenesis of diabetes mellitus. Lancet 1:14, 1975.

West KM: Diet therapy of diabetes: An analysis of failure. Ann Int Med 79:425, 1973.

Williams H, Hutchinson K, Brown GD: Gangrene of the feet in diabetics. Arch Surg 108:609, 1974.

DIABETIC COMA

Coma may be due to a variety of causes not directly related to diabetes, eg, cerebrovascular accidents, alcohol or other drug toxicity, and head trauma. However, certain major causes of coma directly related to diabetes require differentiation: (1) Hypoglycemic coma resulting from excessive doses of insulin or oral hypoglycemic agents. (2) Hyperglycemic coma associated either with severe insulin deficiency (diabetic ketoacidosis) or mild to moderate insulin deficiency (hyperglycemic nonketotic hyperosmolar coma). (3) Lactic acidosis associated with diabetes, particularly when phenformin is administered to patients with renal insufficiency or taken during suicide attempts, and in diabetics stricken with severe infections or cardiovascular collapse.

A careful physical examination is essential to resolve the differential diagnosis. Patients in deep coma from hypoglycemia are generally flaccid and hypothermic and have quiet breathing—in contrast to patients with acidosis, who appear dehydrated and whose respirations are rapid and deep if the pH of arterial blood has dropped to 7.1 or less. The laboratory remains the final arbiter in confirming the diagnosis, but a rapid estimation can be made of blood glucose concentration with paper strips (Dextrostix) and of plasma ketones with either crushed Acetest tablets or Ketostix paper strips.

Alberti K & others: Small doses of intramuscular insulin in the treatment of diabetic "coma." Lancet 2:515, 1973.

Arieff A, Carroll H: Cerebral edema and depression of sensorium in non-ketotic hyperosmolar coma. Diabetes 23:525, 1974.

Arieff A, Carroll H: Nonketotic hyperosmolar coma and the effect of therapy in 37 cases. Medicine 51:73, 1972.

Table 19—3. Laboratory diagnosis of coma in diabetic patients.

	Urine		Plasma		
	Sugar	Acetone	Glucose	Bicarbonate	Acetone
Related to diabetes					
Hypoglycemia	0*	0 or +	Low	Normal	0
Diabetic ketoacidosis	++++	++++	High	Low	++++
Hyperglycemic nonketotic	++++	0	High	Normal or slightly low	0
Lactic acidosis	0 or +	0 or +	Normal or low or high	Low	0 or +
Unrelated to diabetes					
Alcohol or other toxic drugs	0 or +	0 or +	May be low	Normal or low†	0 or +
Cerebrovascular accident or head trauma	+ or 0	0	Often high	Normal	0
Uremia	0 or +	0	High or normal	Low	0 or +

*Leftover urine in bladder might still contain sugar from earlier hyperglycemia.

†Alcohol can elevate plasma lactate as well as ketoacids to reduce pH.

Beigelman P: Severe diabetic ketoacidosis: 482 episodes in 257 patients; experience of 3 years. Diabetes 20:490, 1971.

Beigelman P, Warner NE: Thirty-two fatal cases of severe diabetic ketoacidosis. Diabetes 22:847, 1973.

Felig P: Diabetic ketoacidosis. New England J Med 290:1360, 1974.

Felig P: Insulin: Rates and routes of delivery. New England J Med 291:1031, 1974.

Gerich J, Martin M, Recant L: Clinical and metabolic characteristics of hyperosmolar, nonketotic coma. Diabetes 20:228, 1971.

Gerich JE & others: Prevention of human diabetic ketoacidosis by somatostatin. New England J Med 292:985, 1975.

Lindsey CA, Faloona GR, Unger RH: Plasma glucagon in nonketotic hyperosmolar coma. JAMA 229:1771, 1974.

Oliva P: Lactic acidosis. Am J Med 48:209, 1970.

Soler N & others: Potassium balance during treatment of diabetic ketoacidosis with special reference to the use of bicarbonate. Lancet 2:665, 1972.

Swerdloff R: Atypical diabetic coma. California Med 119:29, Oct 1973.

1. DIABETIC KETOACIDOSIS

Clinical Findings

A. Symptoms and Signs: As opposed to the acute onset of hypoglycemic coma, the appearance of diabetic ketoacidotic coma is usually preceded by a day or more of polyuria and polydipsia associated with marked fatigue, nausea, vomiting, and, finally, mental stupor which can progress to frank neurologic coma. On physical examination, evidence of dehydration in a stuporous patient with rapid deep breathing and a "fruity" odor of acetone on his breath would strongly suggest the diagnosis. Hypotension with tachycardia indicates profound dehydration and salt depletion.

B. Laboratory Findings: 4+ glycosuria and strong ketonuria with hyperglycemia, ketonemia, low arterial blood pH, and low plasma bicarbonate are typical of diabetic ketoacidosis. Serum potassium is usually slightly elevated despite total body potassium depletion resulting from protracted polyuria or vomiting. Lipidemia may be present if the rate of development of ketoacidosis was relatively slow (over several weeks or more of poor control).

Pathophysiology

The 2 major metabolic aberrations of diabetic ketoacidosis are hyperglycemia and ketoacidemia, both due to insulin lack associated with hyperglucagonemia.

A. Hyperglycemia: Hyperglycemia results from increased hepatic production of glucose as well as diminished glucose uptake by peripheral tissues. Hepatic glucose output is a consequence of increased gluconeogenesis resulting from insulinopenia as well as from an associated hyperglucagonemia. Hyperglycemia produces an osmotic overload in the kidney, causing diuresis, with a critical loss of electrolytes in the urine and intracellular dehydration.

B. Ketoacidemia: Ketoacidemia represents the ef-

fect of insulin lack at multiple enzyme loci. Insulin lack associated with elevated levels of growth hormone and glucagon contributes to an increase in lipolysis from adipose tissue and in hepatic ketogenesis. In addition, there is evidence that reduced ketolysis by insulin-deficient peripheral tissues contributes to the ketoacidemia. The only true "keto" acid present is acetoacetic acid, which, along with its by-product acetone, is measured by nitroprusside reagents (Ketostix and Acetest). The sensitivity for acetone, however, is poor, requiring over 10 mM, which is seldom reached in the plasma of ketoacidotic subjects—although this detectable concentration is readily achieved in urine. Thus, in the plasma of ketotic patients, only acetoacetate is measured by these reagents:

Trace reaction $\quad$ = 0.8–2 mM acetoacetate
Moderate reaction = 3–6 mM acetoacetate
Large reaction $\quad$ = 6–10 mM acetoacetate

The more prevalent β-hydroxybutyric acid has no ketone group and is therefore not detected by conventional nitroprusside tests. This takes on special importance with associated circulatory collapse, wherein an increase in lactic acid can shift the redox state to increase β-hydroxybutyric acid at the expense of the readily detectable acetoacetic acid. Bedside diagnostic reagents would then be unreliable, suggesting no ketonemia in cases where β-hydroxybutyric acid is a major factor in producing the acidosis.

Treatment

A. Prevention: Education of diabetic patients to recognize the early symptoms and signs of ketoacidosis has done a great deal to prevent severe acidosis. When heavy ketonuria and glycosuria persist on several successive examinations, supplemental regular insulin should be administered and liquid foods, such as lightly salted tomato juice and broth, should be ingested to replenish fluids and electrolytes. The patient should be instructed to contact his physician if ketonuria persists, and especially if vomiting develops.

If ketosis is severe, the patient should be placed in the hospital for correction of the ketoacidemia as well as the hyperosmolarity, dehydration, and electrolyte depletion with insulin and appropriate solutions of electrolytes.

B. Emergency Measures:

1. Therapeutic flow sheet—One of the most important steps in initiating therapy is to start a flow sheet which lists the time sequence of diagnostic laboratory values in relation to therapeutic maneuvers. Indices of the metabolic defects include urine glucose and ketones and plasma glucose, acetone, bicarbonate, and electrolytes. One physician should be responsible for maintaining this therapeutic flow sheet and prescribing therapy. An indwelling catheter is required in all comatose patients but should be avoided if possible in a fully cooperative diabetic because of the risk of introducing bladder infection. Fluid intake and output should be carefully recorded, and details of the quantity and composition of all fluids and medications should be listed carefully. Gastric intubation and lavage with sodium bicarbonate solution are recommended in the comatose patient. The patient should not receive sedatives or narcotics. Each case must be managed individually depending on the specific deficits present and subsequent responses to initial therapy.

2. Insulin replacement—Only regular insulin should be used initially in all cases of severe ketoacidosis, and it should be given immediately after the diagnosis is established. It acts to rapidly suppress hyperglucagonemia, reverse lipolysis, reduce ketogenesis and gluconeogenesis, and increase tissue uptake of both ketones and glucose. Recent reports suggest that doses of insulin as low as 5–10 units per hour given either by slow intravenous drip or intramuscularly are as effective in most cases as the much higher doses usually recommended. However, there seems to be less danger in using relatively high doses of insulin given both intravenously and subcutaneously as long as the patient is monitored to detect impending hypoglycemia or hypokalemia. Fifty to 100 units of regular insulin can be given intravenously and a similar amount subcutaneously every 2–3 hours. The quantity used does not seem as crucial as its timing, ie, how soon and how frequently it is administered. "Sliding scale" orders are not recommended, and each subsequent dose of insulin for a critically ill patient should be prescribed on the basis of responses of hyperglycemia and ketoacidemia. Rarely, a patient with insulin resistance is encountered, and this requires doubling the insulin dose every 2–4 hours if hyperglycemia does not improve after the first 2 doses of insulin. One must be alert to the danger of anaphylactic shock in resistant patients requiring high doses of insulin if it is given intravenously. Somatostatin's effective inhibition of growth hormone and glucagon secretion may prove to be a valuable adjunct to insulin therapy in the treatment of severe diabetic ketoacidosis.

3. Fluid and electrolyte replacement—In most patients the fluid deficit is 5–10 liters. Initially, normal saline solution is the solution of choice to help reexpand the contracted vascular volume in the dehydrated patient. If the blood glucose is above 500 mg/100 ml, 0.45% saline solution may be used since the water deficit exceeds the sodium loss in uncontrolled diabetes with osmotic diuresis. The use of sodium bicarbonate has been questioned by some on the grounds that it produces rapid potassium shifts and theoretically could reduce dissociation of oxygen from hemoglobin, which has been augmented by the state of acidosis, or may reduce CSF pH. However, these theoretical considerations do not seem too important in the clinical setting, and 1–2 ampules of sodium bicarbonate (44 mEq per 50 ml ampule) added to a bottle of hypotonic saline solution should probably be administered whenever the blood pH is less than 7.1 or blood bicarbonate is below 9 mEq/liter. In the first hour, at least 1 liter of fluid should be infused, and fluid should be given thereafter at a rate of 300–500 ml/hour. When blood glucose falls to less than 250 mg/100 ml,

5% glucose solutions should be used and insulin therapy continued every 2–4 hours until ketonemia has cleared. Glucose administration has the dual advantage of preventing hypoglycemia and also of reducing the likelihood of cerebral edema, which could result from too rapid a decline in hyperglycemia.

4. Potassium and phosphate replacement—Total body potassium loss from polyuria as well as from vomiting may be as high as 200 mEq. However, because of shifts from cells due to the acidosis, *serum* potassium is usually normal or high until after the first few hours of treatment, when acidosis improves and serum potassium returns into cells. Potassium phosphate in doses of 40 mEq/hour should be infused within 3–4 hours after beginning therapy, or sooner if initial serum potassium is inappropriately low. An ECG record can be of help in monitoring the patient and reflecting the state of potassium balance at the time, but it should not replace accurate laboratory measurements. Phosphate is the preferable anion to administer with potassium since severe hypophosphatemia with measurable reduction of oxygen dissociation from hemoglobin is common in ketoacidotic patients treated with insulin. Foods high in potassium content can be prescribed when the patient has recovered sufficiently to initiate oral feedings. (Tomato juice and grapefruit juice contain 14 mEq of potassium per 240 ml, and a medium-sized banana has 10 mEq.)

5. Treatment of associated infection—Appropriate antibiotics should be given if acute bacterial infection, often a precipitating cause, is present.

Prognosis

The frequency of deaths due to diabetic ketoacidosis has been dramatically reduced by improved therapy of young diabetics, but this complication remains a significant risk in the aged and in patients in profound coma in whom treatment has been delayed. Acute myocardial infarction following prolonged hypotension or hemorrhagic pancreatitis precipitating severe ketoacidosis has a high mortality rate. A serious prognostic sign is renal shutdown, and prior kidney dysfunction worsens the prognosis considerably because the kidney plays a key role in compensating for massive shifts of pH and electrolytes. Cerebral edema has been reported to occur rarely as metabolic deficits return to normal. This is best prevented by avoiding sudden reversal of marked hyperglycemia to hypoglycemia since massive fluid shifts into cerebral tissue can occur as a consequence of osmotically active sorbitol and fructose accumulation within neurons during hyperglycemia.

See references on pp 740–741.

2. NONKETOTIC HYPERGLYCEMIC COMA

This second most common form of hyperglycemic coma is characterized by severe hyperglycemia in the absence of significant ketosis, with hyperosmolarity and severe dehydration. It occurs in patients with mild or occult diabetes, and most patients are at least middle-aged to elderly. Underlying renal insufficiency or congestive heart failure is common, and the presence of either worsens the prognosis. A precipitating event is often present such as pneumonia, burns, cerebrovascular accident, or recent operation. Certain drugs such as diphenylhydantoin, diazoxide, glucocorticoids, and diuretics have been implicated in its pathogenesis, as have procedures such as mannitol infusions or peritoneal dialysis.

Pathogenesis

A partial or relative insulin deficiency may initiate the syndrome by reducing glucose utilization of muscle, fat, and liver while inducing hyperglucagonemia and increasing hepatic glucose output. With massive glycosuria, obligatory water loss ensues. If a patient is unable to maintain adequate fluid intake because of an associated acute or chronic illness or has suffered excessive fluid loss such as from burns or therapy with diuretics, marked dehydration results. As plasma volume contracts, renal insufficiency develops, and the resultant limitation of glucose loss leads to increasingly high blood glucose concentrations. A severe hyperosmolarity develops which causes mental confusion and finally coma. It is not clear why ketosis is virtually absent under these conditions of insulin insufficiency, although reduced levels of growth hormone or cortisol may be associated.

Clinical Findings

A. Symptoms and Signs: Onset may be insidious over a period of days or weeks, with weakness, polyuria, and polydipsia. The lack of toxic features of ketoacidosis may retard recognition of the syndrome and delay therapy until dehydration becomes more profound than in ketoacidosis. Reduced intake of fluid is not an uncommon historical feature, either due to inappropriate lack of thirst, gastrointestinal upset, or inaccessibility of fluids to elderly, bedridden patients. Lethargy and confusion develop, progressing to convulsions and deep coma. Physical examination confirms the presence of profound dehydration in a lethargic or comatose patient without Kussmaul respirations.

B. Laboratory Findings: Severe hyperglycemia is present, with blood glucose values ranging from 800–2400 mg/100 ml. In mild cases, where dehydration is less severe, dilutional hyponatremia as well as urinary sodium losses may reduce serum sodium to 120–125 mEq/liter, which protects to some extent against extreme hyperosmolarity. However, once dehydration progresses further, serum sodium can exceed 140 mEq/liter, producing serum osmolarity readings of 330–440 mOsm/kg. Ketosis and acidosis are usually absent or mild. Prerenal azotemia is the rule, with BUN elevations to 90 mg/100 ml being typical.

Treatment

The management of nonketotic hyperglycemic coma differs from that of diabetic ketoacidosis in 3 ways:

(1) Hypotonic saline is preferable to isotonic saline as the initial replacement solution because all patients have marked hyperosmolarity. Because of the severe dehydration, as much as 4–6 liters of 0.45% saline may be required in the first 10 hours. Only if circulatory collapse is present would fluid therapy be initiated with isotonic saline. Once blood glucose is less than 250 mg/100 ml, fluid replacement should include 5% dextrose in either water, 0.45% saline solution, or 0.9% saline solution. An important end point of fluid therapy is to restore urine output to 50 ml/hour or more.

(2) Less insulin is required to reduce the hyperglycemia in nonketotic patients as compared to those with diabetic ketoacidotic coma. An initial dose of only 25 units IV and 25 units subcut of regular insulin is usually quite effective, and subsequent doses need not be greater than 10–25 units subcut every 4 hours in most cases.

(3) With the absence of acidosis, there is no initial hyperkalemia and thus much less potassium is lost in the urine during the initial stages of glycosuria. This results in less severe total potassium depletion than in diabetic ketoacidosis, and less potassium replacement is therefore needed. However, because initial serum potassium is usually not elevated and because it declines rapidly as a result of the sensitivity of the nonketotic patient to insulin, it has been recommended that potassium replacement be initiated earlier than in ketotic patients. Potassium phosphate, 20 mEq/hour, can be given beginning with the initial bottle of fluids administered.

Prognosis

When prompt therapy is instituted, the mortality rate can be reduced from nearly 50% to that related to the severity of coexistent disorders. A BUN in excess of 90 mg/100 ml has a worse prognosis for recovery than a BUN below 50 mg/100 ml, perhaps reflecting the degree of hydration.

See references on pp 740–741.

LACTIC ACIDOSIS

Lactic acidosis is characterized by accumulation of excess lactic acid in the blood. Normally, the principal sources of this acid are the erythrocytes (which lack enzymes for aerobic oxidation), skeletal muscle, skin, and brain. Conversion to glucose and oxidation principally by the liver but also by the kidneys represent the chief pathways for its removal. Overproduction of lactic acid (tissue hypoxia), deficient removal (hepatic failure), or both (circulatory collapse) can cause accumulation of excess lactic acid. Lactic acidosis is not uncommon in any severely ill patient suffering from cardiac decompensation, respiratory or hepatic failure, acute septicemia, acute infarction of lung, bowel, or extremities, leukemia, or terminal metastatic cancer. Hyperlactatemia has been produced by toxic overdoses of phenformin or alcohol. It has been reported with therapeutic doses of phenformin in patients with predisposing factors affecting lactate metabolism or phenformin disposal such as renal dysfunction.

Clinical Findings

A. Symptoms and Signs: The main clinical features of lactic acidosis are marked hyperventilation and mental confusion leading to stupor and coma. When secondary to tissue hypoxia or vascular collapse, the clinical presentation is variable, being that of the prevailing catastrophic illness. However, in the idiopathic or spontaneous variety, the onset is rapid (usually over a few hours), blood pressure is normal, peripheral circulation is good, and there is no cyanosis.

B. Laboratory Findings: Plasma bicarbonate and blood pH are quite low, indicating the presence of severe metabolic acidosis. Ketones are usually absent from plasma and urine or at least not prominent. The first clue may be a high anion gap (serum sodium minus the sum of chloride and bicarbonate anions [in mEq/liter] should be no greater than 15). A higher value indicates the existence of an abnormal compartment of anions. If this cannot be clinically explained by an excess of keto acids (diabetes), inorganic acids (uremia), or anions from drug overdosage (salicylates, methyl alcohol, ethylene glycol), then lactic acidosis is probably the correct diagnosis. The diagnosis is confirmed by demonstrating, in a properly collected sample of blood, a plasma lactic acid concentration of 7 mM/liter or higher (values as high as 30 mM/liter have been reported). Normal plasma values average 1 mM/liter with a normal lactate/pyruvate ratio of 10:1. This ratio is greatly exceeded in lactic acidosis.*

Treatment

Alkalinization with intravenous sodium bicarbonate to keep the pH above 7.2 is the immediate goal of emergency treatment of spontaneous lactic acidosis. Massive doses may be required (as much as 2000 mEq in 24 hours has been used in successfully treated cases). If large volumes of sodium bicarbonate must be given to older patients, hemodialysis may be required to deal with the circulatory overload. Methylene blue, a redox dye, has not been as useful as early reports suggested. If hypoxemia is the precipitating factor, vigorous treatment is indicated.

Prognosis

The mortality rate of spontaneous lactic acidosis approaches 80%. It is slightly lower when lactic acido-

---

*In collecting samples it is essential to rapidly chill and separate the blood to remove red cells, whose continued glycolysis at room temperature is a common source of error in reports of high plasma lactate. Frozen plasma remains stable for subsequent assay.

sis is due to potentially reversible causes such as phenformin, when alkalinization need be maintained only until the drug effect is dissipated. The prognosis in cases induced by hypoxemia is that of the primary disorder that produced the tissue hypoxia.

See references on pp 740–741.

THE HYPOGLYCEMIC STATES

Spontaneous hypoglycemia in adults is of 2 principal types: fasting and postprandial. Fasting hypoglycemia is often subacute or chronic and usually presents with neuroglycopenia as its principal manifestation; postprandial hypoglycemia is relatively acute and is often heralded by symptoms of adrenergic discharge (sweating, palpitations, anxiety, tremulousness).

Differential Diagnosis (See Table 19–4.)

Fasting hypoglycemia may occur in certain endocrine disorders such as hypopituitarism, Addison's disease, or myxedema and in disorders related to liver disease such as acute alcoholism or liver failure. These conditions are usually obvious, with hypoglycemia being only a secondary feature. When hypoglycemia is a primary manifestation developing in adults without apparent endocrine disorders or inborn metabolic diseases from childhood, the principal diagnostic possibilities include (1) hyperinsulinism, either due to pancreatic beta cell tumors or surreptitious administration of insulin (or sulfonylureas); and (2) hypoglycemia due to noninsulin-producing extrapancreatic tumors.

Postprandial (reactive) hypoglycemia may be classified as early (within 2–3 hours after a meal) or late (3–5 hours after eating). Early or alimentary hypoglycemia occurs when there is a rapid discharge of ingested carbohydrate into the small bowel followed by rapid glucose absorption and hyperinsulinism. It

---

Table 19–4. Common causes of hypoglycemia in the absence of clinically obvious endocrine or hepatic disorders.

Fasting hypoglycemia
  Hyperinsulinism
    Pancreatic beta cell tumor
    Surreptitious administration of insulin or sulfonylureas
  Extrapancreatic tumors
Postprandial (reactive) hypoglycemia
  Early hypoglycemia (alimentary)
    Postgastrectomy
    Functional (increased vagal tone)
  Late hypoglycemia (occult diabetes)
    Delayed insulin release due to beta cell dysfunction
  Counterregulatory deficiency
  Idiopathic

may be seen after gastrointestinal surgery, particularly associated with the dumping syndrome after gastrectomy. More commonly, it is functional, and may represent overactivity of the parasympathetic nervous system mediated via the vagus nerve. Rarely, it results from defective counterregulatory responses such as deficiencies of glucagon, cortisol, growth hormone, or autonomic responses.

1. HYPOGLYCEMIA DUE TO PANCREATIC BETA CELL TUMORS

Fasting hypoglycemia in the otherwise healthy adult is most commonly due to an adenoma of the islets of Langerhans. Ninety percent of such tumors are single and benign, but multiple adenomas can occur as well as malignancies with functional metastases. Beta cell hyperplasia as a cause of fasting hypoglycemia is not well documented in adults. Adenomas may be familial and have been found in conjunction with tumors of the parathyroids and pituitary (Wermer's syndrome; multiple endocrine adenomatosis type I).

Clinical Findings

A. Symptoms and Signs: The signs and symptoms are those of subacute or chronic hypoglycemia, which may progress to permanent and irreversible brain damage. Delayed diagnosis has often resulted in prolonged psychiatric care or treatment for psychomotor epilepsy before the true diagnosis was established. In long-standing cases, obesity often results as a consequence of overeating to relieve symptoms.

Whipple's triad is characteristic of hypoglycemia regardless of the cause. It consists of (1) a history of hypoglycemic symptoms, (2) an associated fasting blood glucose of 40 mg/100ml or less, and (3) immediate recovery upon administration of glucose. The hypoglycemic symptoms in insulinoma often develop in the early morning or after missing a meal. Occasionally, they occur after exercise such as jogging or tennis. They typically begin with evidence of CNS glucose lack and can include blurred vision or diplopia, headache, feelings of detachment, slurred speech, and weakness. Personality and mental changes vary from anxiety to psychotic behavior, and neurologic deterioration can result in convulsions or coma. Sweating and palpitations may not occur with subacute hypoglycemia until a profound degree of hypoglycemia develops.

B. Laboratory Findings: Beta cell adenomas do not reduce secretion in the presence of hypoglycemia, and the critical diagnostic test is to demonstrate inappropriately elevated serum insulin levels at a time when hypoglycemia is present. A reliable serum insulin level of 20 μU/ml or more in the presence of blood glucose values below 40 mg/100 ml is diagnostic of inappropriate hyperinsulinism. Other causes of hypoglycemia must be considered, including factitious administration of insulin or sulfonylureas. An elevated circulating pro-

insulin level is characteristic of most beta cell adenomas and does not occur in factitious hyperinsulinism.

C. Diagnostic Tests:

1. Prolonged fasting under hospital supervision is probably the most dependable means of establishing the presence of fasting hypoglycemia, especially in males. In patients with insulinoma, the blood glucose levels often drop below 40 mg/100 ml after an overnight fast. In normal male subjects, the blood glucose does not fall below 55–60 mg/100 ml. In contrast, in premenopausal women who have fasted for only 24 hours, the plasma glucose falls normally to such an extent that it must drop to values lower than 35 mg/100 ml (and to less than 30 mg/100 ml by 36 hours) to be significant. After 36 hours of fasting, premenopausal females normally achieve such low levels of glucose that clinical evaluation of this test for insulinoma becomes quite difficult. If hypoglycemia does not develop in a male patient after 72 hours of fasting terminated with moderate exercise, insulinoma is an unlikely diagnosis.

2. Tolbutamide tolerance testing is hazardous and should be reserved for difficult problem cases in the hands of an experienced physician.

3. Glucose tolerance tests have not been of help in the diagnosis of insulinomas because the variable responsiveness of the adenoma to glucose gives a confusing variety of results. Most adenomas respond poorly to glucose, and a diabetic type of oral glucose tolerance test results. In the rarer tumors that release insulin in response to glucose, more difficulty in maintaining blood glucose can be anticipated at surgery.

4. Leucine and glucagon stimulation tests may produce hyperinsulin responses in some cases of insulinoma. However, they are often equivocal and much less reliable for diagnosis than the prolonged fast.

5. Pancreatic arteriography can occasionally locate tumors preoperatively, but, because of the small size of beta cell adenomas (1 cm or less in most cases), it is often of little help.

Treatment

A. Surgical Treatment: Surgery is the treatment of choice, preferably by an experienced surgeon who is capable of mobilizing the pancreas and exploring adequately the posterior surface of the head and body as well as the tail. In cases where the diagnosis has been established but no adenoma is located, subtotal pancreatectomy is usually indicated, including the entire body and tail of the pancreas. With multiple adenomas, total pancreatectomy may be required. Ten percent glucose in water should be infused during surgery at a rate of 100 ml/hour or even faster, and blood glucose should be monitored.

B. Diet and Chemotherapy: In patients with inoperable functioning islet cell carcinoma or in patients in whom subtotal removal of the pancreas has failed to produce cure, reliance on frequent feedings is necessary. Since most tumors are not responsive to glucose, carbohydrate feedings every 2–3 hours are usually effective in preventing hypoglycemia, although obesity may become a problem. Glucagon should be available for emergency use as indicated in the discussion of treatment of diabetes. Certain drugs such as diazoxide, 300–600 mg/day orally, have been useful with concomitant thiazide diuretic therapy to control sodium retention characteristic of diazoxide. A new drug, streptozotocin, has recently been found to be especially useful in decreasing insulin secretion in islet cell carcinomas, and effective doses have been achieved without the undue renal toxicity that characterized early experience.

Prognosis

When insulinoma is diagnosed early and cured surgically, complete recovery is likely, although brain damage following severe hypoglycemia is not reversible. A significant increase in survival rate has been shown in streptozotocin-treated patients with islet cell carcinoma, with reduction in tumor mass as well as decreased hyperinsulinism.

2. HYPOGLYCEMIA DUE TO EXTRAPANCREATIC TUMORS

These rare causes of hypoglycemia include mesenchymal tumors such as retroperitoneal sarcomas, hepatomas, adrenocortical carcinomas, and miscellaneous epithelial type tumors. The tumors are frequently large and readily palpated or visualized on urograms.

Laboratory diagnosis depends upon fasting hypoglycemia associated with serum insulin levels that are generally below 10 μU/ml. None of these tumors have ever been reported to release immunoreactive insulin, and the mechanism of their hypoglycemic effect remains obscure.

The prognosis for these tumors is generally poor, and surgical removal should be attempted when feasible. Dietary management of the hypoglycemia is the mainstay of medical treatment since diazoxide is usually ineffective.

3. POSTPRANDIAL HYPOGLYCEMIA
(Reactive Hypoglycemia)

Postgastrectomy Alimentary Hypoglycemia

Reactive hypoglycemia following gastrectomy is a consequence of hyperinsulinism resulting from rapid gastric emptying of ingested food which produces overstimulation of vagal reflexes and overproduction of beta-cytotrophic gastrointestinal hormones. Symptoms result from adrenergic hyperactivity in response to the hypoglycemia. Treatment is properly directed at avoiding this sequence of events by more frequent feedings with smaller portions of less rapidly assimilated carbohydrate and more slowly absorbed fat

and protein. In addition, anticholinergic drugs such as propantheline, 15 mg orally 4 times daily, may be useful in reducing vagal overactivity.

Functional Alimentary Hypoglycemia

This syndrome is classified as functional when no postsurgical explanation exists for the presence of early alimentary type reactive hypoglycemia. It is most often associated with chronic fatigue, anxiety, irritability, weakness, poor concentration, decreased libido, headaches, hunger after meals, and tremulousness. However, most patients with these symptoms do not have hypoglycemia; furthermore, even in those who have documented early hypoglycemia, it is likely to be only a secondary manifestation of their nervous imbalance with consequent vagal overactivity causing increased gastric emptying and early hyperinsulinism.

Indiscriminate use and overinterpretation of glucose tolerance tests has led to an unfortunate tendency to overdiagnose functional hypoglycemia. As many as a third or more of *normal* subjects have hypoglycemia with or without symptoms during a 4-hour glucose tolerance test. Accordingly, to increase diagnostic reliability, hypoglycemia should preferably be documented during a spontaneous symptomatic episode accompanying routine daily activity, with clinical improvement following feeding. Personality evaluation suggesting hyperkinetic compulsive behavior in thin, anxious patients, particularly females, supports this diagnosis in patients with a compatible history.

In patients with documented postprandial hypoglycemia on a functional basis, there is no harm and occasional benefit in reducing the proportion of carbohydrate in the diet while increasing the frequency and reducing the size of meals; however, it should not be expected that these maneuvers will cure the neurasthenia, since the reflex response to hypoglycemia is only one component of a generalized primary nervous hyperactivity. Psychiatric counseling and support by the physician and mild sedation should be the mainstays of therapy, with dietary manipulation only an adjunct. Oral anticholinergics have produced benefit in certain advanced cases.

Late Hypoglycemia (Occult Diabetes)

This condition is characterized by a delay in early insulin release from pancreatic beta cells, resulting in initial exaggeration of hyperglycemia during a glucose tolerance test. In response to this hyperglycemia, an exaggerated insulin release produces a late hypoglycemia 4–5 hours after ingestion of glucose. These patients are quite different from those with early hypoglycemia, being more phlegmatic, often obese, and frequently having a family history of diabetes mellitus.

In obese patients, treatment is directed at weight reduction to achieve ideal weight. Like all patients with postprandial hypoglycemia, regardless of cause, these patients often respond to reduced carbohydrate intake with multiple, spaced, small feedings high in protein. They should be considered early diabetics and advised to have periodic medical evaluations.

American Diabetes Association: Special report: Statement on hypoglycemia. Diabetes 22:137, 1973.

Berkovitz S & others: Factitious hypoglycemia: Why not diagnose before laparotomy? Am J Med 51:669, 1971.

Broder L, Carter S: Pancreatic islet cell carcinoma. 1. Clinical features of 52 patients. 2. Results of therapy with streptozotocin in 52 patients. Ann Int Med 79:101, 1973.

Committee of American Diabetes Association: Statement on hypoglycemia. Diabetes 22:137, 1973.

Das Gupta D, Whitehouse F: Significance of the flat oral glucose tolerance test. Postgrad Med 51:55, 1971.

Harrison TS & others: Current surgical management of functioning islet cell tumors of the pancreas. Ann Surg 178:485, 1973.

Hofeldt F & others: Are abnormalities in insulin secretion responsible for reactive hypoglycemia? Diabetes 23:589, 1974.

Karam J: Reactive hypoglycemia: Mechanisms and management. California Med 114:64, May 1971.

Laurent J, Debry G, Floquet J: *Hypoglycemic Tumors.* Excerpta Medica, 1971.

Marks V: Spontaneous hypoglycemia. Brit MJ 1:430, 1972.

Merrimee TJ, Tyson JE: Stabilization of plasma glucose during fasting. New England J Med 291:1275, 1974.

Permutt M & others: Alimentary hypoglycemia in the absence of gastrointestinal surgery. New England J Med 288:1206, 1973.

Schein P & others: Islet cell tumors: Current concepts and management. Ann Int Med 79:239, 1973.

Smith HM (consulting editor): Diazoxide and the treatment of hypoglycemia. Ann New York Acad Sc 150:193, 1968.

Yager J, Young RT: Non-hypoglycemia is an epidemic condition. New England J Med 291:907, 1974.

DISTURBANCES OF LIPID METABOLISM

The principal circulating lipids in man are of 4 types: (1) triglycerides, (2) free cholesterol, (3) cholesteryl esters, and (4) phospholipids. These are transported as spherical macromolecular complexes termed **lipoproteins**, wherein an inner core of hydrophobic lipids (triglycerides and cholesteryl esters) are encased by a membrane of unimolecular thickness consisting of various proteins (apolipoproteins, or simply apoproteins) in association with hydrophilic lipids (free cholesterol and phospholipids).

Classification of Lipoproteins

Specific differences among the various lipoprotein classes involve how much they contain of each of these 4 lipids, which affects their size and density, and the nature of the apoprotein in their membrane. These differences allow classification of lipoproteins on the basis of ultracentrifugal density, with those containing mostly triglyceride being termed **very low density lipoproteins (VLDL)** and those with predominantly cholesterol called **low density lipoproteins (LDL)**; when the total lipid content is slightly less than the weight of protein in the membrane, the density is **high (HDL)**.

When classified on the basis of their mobility on paper electrophoresis, LDL are termed betalipoproteins, VLDL are prebetalipoproteins, and HDL are called alphalipoproteins. These 3 classes of lipoproteins are normally present in fasting sera. A fourth class, normally present only after ingestion of fat, are called chylomicrons. These are of such low density that they float even without centrifugation, and, because of their large size and proportionately low protein content, they fail to migrate on paper electrophoresis, remaining at the origin.

Relationship of Lipoproteinemia to Diabetes

Circulating levels of lipoprotein are often elevated along with glucose in diabetes mellitus. Chylomicrons, which carry ingested fat, and VLDL, which contain triglyceride converted from ingested carbohydrate, are transported in plasma to fat depots where they are cleared by an insulin-dependent lipoprotein lipase. When insulin levels are low (insulinopenic diabetes) or ineffective (insulinoplethoric diabetes), defective glucose removal is associated with impaired removal of VLDL and chylomicrons. Replacement of deficient insulin, or restriction of caloric intake to restore effectiveness of endogenous insulin in obese diabetics, facilitates clearance of these lipoproteins. Their normal end products include a "remnant" particle of very low density which is further hydrolyzed by hepatic lipase to form circulating LDL. LDL are responsible for transporting cholesteryl esters to excretory pathways in the liver. HDL contributes to lipid transport by assisting in activating the lipoprotein lipase as well as in facilitating the removal of cholesterol by activating a circulating enzyme, lecithin-cholesterol acyltransferase (L-CAT), which produces cholesteryl esters for removal by the liver.

Lipoprotein Disorders

An *excess* or *deficiency* of certain lipoproteins can result from primary genetic disorders or may be secondary to acquired metabolic dysfunction. The 5 primary phenotypes described by Fredrickson and coworkers have been recently revised to contain an additional subdivision termed IIB (Table 19–5). This classification, together with their acquired (secondary) counterparts, probably includes the main types of hyperlipidemia seen clinically. These "types" should not be considered disease entities but may be useful for determining the most rational therapy. Until more information becomes available to permit classification on the basis of etiology, the present approach, using paper electrophoresis to define various phenotypes, has been accepted by the World Health Organization.

A. Type I Hyperlipoproteinemia (Hyperchylomicronemia; Bürger-Grütz Disease): This autosomal recessive condition is the rarest form of familial hyperlipoproteinemia and is characterized by massive chylomicronemia when a patient is on a normal diet and complete disappearance a few days after fat is eliminated from the diet. Postheparin lipolytic activity is absent in the serum, indicating that the defect is a deficiency of

Table 19—5. Major categories of primary hyperlipidemia.*

Type	Lipoprotein Abnormalities & Defect	Appearance of Serum†	Cholesterol Elevation‡	Triglyceride Elevation‡	Clinical Presentation	Rule Out
I	Fasting chylomicronemia (due to lipoprotein lipase deficiency). Rare.	Creamy layer over clear infranate	Elevated (to about 10% of triglyceride level)	Often 1000—10,000 or more	Creamy blood, lipemic retina, eruptive xanthomas, hepatosplenomegaly, recurrent abdominal pain; onset in childhood.	Pancreatitis, diabetes.
IIA	Hyperbetalipoproteinemia (lack of a cell surface receptor involved in degrading LDL). Common.	Clear	Usually 300—600 but may be higher	None	Xanthelasma, tendon xanthomas, accelerated atherosclerosis; detectable in childhood.	Hypothyroidism, nephrotic syndrome, hepatic obstruction.
IIB	Mixed lipidemia (both LDL and VLDL elevation). Quite common.	Turbid	Usually 250—600	Usually 200—600	Relatively common. Severe forms are like IIA; milder forms associated with obesity or diabetes.	Same as IIA.
III	Dysbetalipoproteinemia (lipidemia due to excess of remnants; hepatic lipase deficiency?). Rare.	Turbid	Highly variable (from near normal to over 1000)	Highly variable (175—1500 in same patient)	Planar xanthomas, tuberous xanthomas appear in adult. Relatively uncommon. Hyperglycemia, hyperuricemia.	Hepatic disease, diabetes.
IV	Hyperprebetalipoproteinemia (delay in clearance or overproduction of VLDL). Common.	Turbid	300—800	200—5000	Most common, usually in adults. Eruptive xanthomas; accelerated vascular disease, mild glucose intolerance, hyperuricemia.	Nephrotic syndrome, hypothyroidism, glycogen storage disease; oral contraceptives.
V	Mixed lipidemia (both chylomicronemia and VLDL); defects similar to I and IV. Rare.	Creamy layer over turbid infranate	300—1000	Usually 500—10,000 or more	Adulthood mainly; recurrent abdominal pain, eruptive xanthomas, hepatosplenomegaly.	Insulin-deficient diabetes, pancreatitis, alcoholism.

*Modified from Fredrickson, Levy, & others.
†Refrigerated serum overnight at 4° C.
‡mg/100 ml. Normal cholesterol, 150—250 mg/100 ml; triglycerides, < 150 mg/100 ml.

lipoprotein lipase. Lipemia retinalis is seen when serum triglycerides exceed 3000 mg/100 ml. Serum cholesterol is often quite high since it accounts for as much as 10% of the weight of chylomicron particles. Spurious hyponatremia may result from displacement of plasma water by high fat content during routine blood sampling. Pancreatitis is the major hazard, and patients with this disorder may not have accelerated atherosclerosis despite hypercholesterolemia. The diagnosis is suspected in children with recurrent abdominal pain, especially when hepatosplenomegaly is present. Eruptive xanthomas and creamy serum which separates into a creamy supernate and a clear infranate confirm the diagnosis.

Treatment consists of a fat-restricted diet (25—35 gm/day), and the response is usually good.

B. Type IIA (Hyperbetalipoproteinemia): This disorder has recently been shown to result from a defective cell receptor in homozygotes and partially so in heterozygotes, which interferes with clearance of betalipoproteins. This receptor defect also prevents normal feedback inhibition of cholesterol synthesis by betalipoproteins. It is one of the commonest of familial hyperlipoproteinemias and is transmitted as an autosomal dominant, at least in the severe variety. Milder forms may be caused by dietary indiscretion. The major clinical manifestations of this disorder include

an accelerated atherosclerosis, early myocardial infarction, and the presence of tendon xanthomas and xanthelasma. The diagnosis is based on hypercholesterolemia in the presence of clear serum after overnight incubation at 4° C. Dietary restriction of saturated fat and cholesterol is seldom of help in severe cases; more vigorous measures, including oral administration of resins to remove bile salts (cholestyramine or colestipol)—or even jejunoileal bypass surgery—have been reported to reduce serum cholesterol by as much as 50% or more. In mild cases, dietary management may be satisfactory.

C. Type IIB (Mixed Hyperbeta- and Hyperprebetalipoproteinemia): This mixed hyperlipidemia is quite common and often alternates with the IIA pattern in affected relatives. In some cases, hyperlipidemia is particularly sensitive to caloric intake and diet composition and may represent several different disorders. Both the triglyceride/cholesterol ratio and the electrophoretic pattern are indistinguishable from those of type III disease, as is the character of serum turbidity after overnight incubation at 4° C. Ultracentrifugal analysis confirms the diagnosis by showing both an LDL and a VLDL elevation, whereas in type III a "floating beta" particle is obtained.

D. Type III (Hyper-"Remnant"-Lipoproteinemia; Dysbetalipoproteinemia): This rare disorder may result from a defect in hepatic lipoprotein lipase which normally transforms remnant particles into betalipoproteins. Its genetic transmission is not clear, and it is predominantly diagnosed in adults. Patients are often obese and may have tuberous xanthomas, xanthelasma, and accelerated atherosclerosis. Planar xanthomas on the palms have been considered diagnostic. The presence of an abnormal lipoprotein with the electrophoretic mobility of a beta globulin but the flotation characteristics on ultracentrifugation of a VLDL confirms this diagnosis. Treatment is especially gratifying in type III disease. Reduction to ideal weight in the obese patient and maintainance on a low-cholesterol diet may produce dramatic improvement, and total correction of hyperlipoproteinemia may result, especially in response to the addition of clofibrate, 1 gm twice daily, to the dietary regimen.

E. Type IV (Hyperprebetalipoproteinemia): This lipidemia is endogenous as compared to type I and represents a failure in removal of prebetalipoproteins produced by the liver, and possibly the intestine, either in normal amounts or excessively.

Since carbohydrate intake induces this lipoprotein from esterification of endogenous fatty acids, it has been termed carbohydrate-induced hyperlipidemia. It is a common disorder, usually in adults, and often associated with caloric excess. Accelerated coronary artery disease, obesity, hyperuricemia, and eruptive xanthomas occur. Chylomicronemia can occasionally develop, especially if alcohol or fat intake is excessive. A number of secondary disorders such as myxedema, nephrotic syndrome, oral contraceptive hormonal effects, and glycogen storage disease should be ruled out before a primary diagnosis of type IV disease is made. Treatment is directed at weight reduction in the obese, avoiding high-carbohydrate intake and caloric excess. Clofibrate, 1 gm twice daily, is often beneficial.

F. Type V (Mixed Lipidemia): This is a rare disorder wherein excessive prebetalipoproteins and chylomicrons are present. Onset is usually in early adult life and is characterized by recurrent abdominal pain, pancreatitis, hepatosplenomegaly, eruptive xanthomas, and glucose intolerance. The disorder is markedly aggravated by alcohol excess.

Therapy is similar to that for type IV except that fat restriction is necessary as in type I.

Relationship of Lipoproteins to Atheroma
(See Fig 19–2.)

Recent evidence suggests that the arterial wall intima is permeable to small molecular complexes in inverse proportion to their size. In addition, elastin, a component of arterial wall, has a demonstrable affinity for apoprotein B, which is present on all lipoproteins except HDL. Accordingly, small lipoproteins such as HDL, LDL, and certain of the smaller VLDL and remnants enter the intimal walls of arteries, where all except HDL adhere to elastin, which retards their exit and allows their accumulation. This concept would explain why chylomicrons are not considered atherogenic in type I disorders despite severe hypercholes-

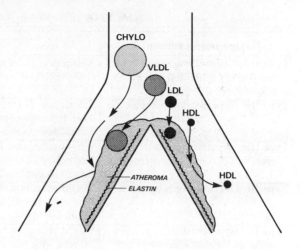

Figure 19–2. Lipoproteins and atheromas.

terolemia and why hypertension or hyperlipidemia, either individually or (especially) in combination, could exaggerate normal atherogenic processes.

General Comments About Therapy

Treatment of the secondary hyperlipoproteinemias consists, where possible, of treatment of the primary disorder such as hypothyroidism, nephrotic syndrome, obstructive jaundice, or estrogen excess from oral contraceptives.

A. Diet Therapy: (Table 19–6.) In primary hyperlipoproteinemia, no one diet is effective in all the lipid transport disorders. Similarly, none of the pharmacologic agents is universally effective. An understanding of lipid transport mechanisms and drug actions has improved the therapeutic approach to the hyperlipidemic patient.

When chylomicrons are elevated, fat intake should be reduced. If insulin-dependent diabetes is present, every effort should be made to restore acceptable diabetes control. When prebetalipoproteins or remnants are excessive, an effort is directed at weight reduction if obesity is present by reducing total calories, especially from carbohydrate and alcohol, to maintain ideal weight. In the presence of hyperbetalipoproteinemia, dietary cholesterol should be reduced to less than 300 mg/day. Reduction of saturated fatty acids in the diet to no more than 10% of the total caloric intake is often beneficial, with a shift of polyunsaturated to saturated fatty acid (Table 19–7) from the usual ratio of 1:5 to 2:1.

B. Hypolipidemic Drugs: Three major classes of drugs are currently in use:

1. Nicotinic acid—Nicotinic acid reduces lipolysis and diminishes production of VLDL. The dosage is 100 mg 3 times daily initially, gradually building up to a level of 3–7 gm/day taken with meals. Cutaneous flushing and pruritus, as well as gastrointestinal upsets, are major side-effects.

Table 19—6. Lipoprotein phenotypes and diet therapy.*

Lipoprotein Pattern	Diet Therapy
Type I: Hyperchylomicronemia with lipoprotein lipase deficiency (fat-induced lipemia)	Restriction of fat to less than 35 gm/day. Supplementation with medium chain triglycerides. Portagen for added calories. Elimination of alcohol.
Type IIa: Hyperbetalipoproteinemia	Calorie and weight control not important. Low cholesterol (< 300 mg/day). P:S ratio (Table 19—7) 2.0 or greater. Total polyunsaturates to be 4 tbsp/day. Avoidance of egg yolks, shrimp, and liver.
Type IIb: Hyperbetalipoprotein-emia and prebetalipoproteinemia	Weight reduction. Low cholesterol (< 300 mg/day). P:S ratio about 2.0. Restriction of carbohydrate as free sugar and concentrated sweets. Restriction of alcohol to 2 servings per day in exchange for serving of bread.
Type III: Dysbetalipoproteinemia	Weight reduction. Balanced diet (carbohydrate 40%, fat 40%, protein 20%). Low cholesterol (< 300 mg/day). P:S ratio not emphasized. Restriction of alcohol as in type IIb.
Type IV: Hyperprebetalipoprotein-emia; endogenous carbohydrate-induced lipemias	Weight reduction to ideal weight. Carbohydrate restriction to 40% of total calories with elimination of concentrated sweets and restriction of alcohol. Substitution of polyunsaturated for saturated fats. Moderate cholesterol restriction (300—500 mg/day).
Type V: Mixed lipidemia (chylomi-crons and prebetalipoproteins)	Weight reduction. Reduction of fat to 30% of total calories, with increase of carbohydrate to 50%. Polyunsaturated fat substituted for saturated. Moderate restriction of cholesterol to 300—500 mg/day. Elimination of alcohol.

*Adapted from Gotto AM & others: Dietary aspects of hyperlipidemia. J Am Dietet A 62:617, 1973.

2. Clofibrate (chlorphenoxyisobutyrate)— Clofibrate has many known effects in the body and both decreases the synthesis of VLDL and increases its catabolism. It is most effective in type III remnant excess but is of value also in disorders with increased VLDL (IIB, IV, V). It may be of some use in LDL excess, but not strikingly so. The dosage is 1.5—2 gm/day. Very few side-effects are known, but myositis has been reported, especially if hypoalbuminemia is present, as in lipidemia associated with nephrotic syndrome. Pharmacokinetic interactions with anticoagulants may occur.

3. Resins to absorb bile acids (cholestyramine, colestipol)—Cholestyramine is an insoluble resin which absorbs bile acids and is thus able to increase cholesterol catabolism and enhance LDL removal. It is not very palatable, and 16—32 gm/day are required in 2—4 divided doses, preferably in orange juice or applesauce. Gastrointestinal side-effects are most common. VLDL excess is not helped and may be aggravated by this therapy.

4. Efficacy and safety—Clofibrate and niacin were evaluated in a national collaborative coronary drug project. Under the particular conditions of the study in a population of males recovering from myocardial infarction, no beneficial effect on mortality rate could be demonstrated for either of these agents as compared to a placebo; in fact, more cardiac arrhythmias were produced.

Table 19—7. Ratio of polyunsaturated to saturated fats (P:S) in certain fats.*

Fat	Fatty Acids (gm/100 gm fat)		P:S Ratio
	Saturated	Polyunsatu-rated	
Vegetable oils			
Safflower	8	72	9.0
Corn	10	53	5.3
Sunflower	12	63	5.3
Soybean	15	52	3.5
Sesame	14	42	3.0
Cottonseed	25	50	2.0
Peanut	18	29	1.6
Olive	11	7	0.6
Palm	45	8	0.2
Cocoa butter	56	2	< 0.1
Coconut	93	1.2	0.01
Animal fats			
Lard	38	10	0.3
Butter	55	3	0.1

*Adapted from: *Fatty Acids in Food Fats.* Home Economics Research Department No. 7, US Department of Agriculture, 1959.

Hypolipoprotein Disorders

A. Tangier Disease (Deficiency of HDL): This autosomal recessive disorder is characterized by low plasma cholesterol, normal or elevated triglyceride levels, and enlargement of the tonsils, with distinctive orange-yellow deposits of cholesteryl esters. Other features include peripheral neuropathy, hepatosplenomegaly, and corneal deposits of lipid. HDL are deficient or absent.

VLDL and chylomicrons may be increased since,

Table 19—8. Low cholesterol, modified fat diets for types IIA, IIB, and III hyperlipoproteinemia.*

Foods to Use	Foods to Avoid	1200 Calories (40% Cal From Unsaturated Fat) Polyunsaturated:Saturated Fat Ratio 2:1	1800 Calories (40% Cal From Unsaturated Fat) Polyunsaturated:Saturated Fat Ratio 2:1
Milk, nonfat	Whole and low-fat milk	2 cups (16 oz) daily	2 cups (16 oz) daily
Fruits (without sugar), fresh, canned, or juices—at least one to be citrus or tomato	Avocado, olives	3 servings daily	3—5 servings daily
Vegetables—at least one to be leafy green or yellow		3 or more servings daily	3 or more servings daily
Breads, cereals, starches, enriched white or whole grain		2—4 servings daily	7 servings daily
Eggs, (with yolks) (250 mg cholesterol per yolk)		Limited to 2 per week (in any form)‡	Limited to 2 per week (in any form)‡
Egg whites		As desired	As desired
Poultry, fish, veal (3 oz cooked per serving)†	Skin and fat on poultry, duck, and goose; shellfish, spare ribs, corned brisket, frankfurters, pan-fried or deep fatfried meats, sausage, luncheon meats, organ meats	9—11 of the main meals per week	9—11 of the main meals per week
Lean beef, lamb, pork, ham, or Canadian bacon (3 oz cooked per serving)	Fat meats, prime cuts, meat drippings and gravies	3—5 servings per week	3—5 servings per week
Fats and oils: Soft margarines (those listing primary ingredient as "liquid oil"), oils such as safflower, soybean, corn, cottonseed, sesame, or sunflower	Butter, cream, hydrogenated shortenings or margarines or cream substitutes	2 tbsp daily	4 tbsp daily
Sugars and sweets: Gelatin dessert, sherbet, fruit ices, angelfood cake, fruit pies made with allowed shortenings	Desserts made with cream, butter, sweet rolls	1 serving per day if substituted for 1 serving bread or cereal	2 servings daily if substituted for 1 serving bread or cereal
Coffee, tea, coffee substitutes, artificial sweeteners, "diet drinks," usweetened gelatin, lemon juice, vinegar, herbs, spices, condiments, fat-free broths or bouillon, sour pickles and relishes		As desired	As desired

*Tables 19—8 and 19—9 adapted from: *Planning Fat-Controlled Meals for 1200 and 1800 Calories.* American Heart Association, 1969; and from Levy R & others: Dietary management of hyperlipoproteinemia. J Am Dietet A 58:406, 1971.
†Poultry, fish, or veal substitutes: 1/2 cup cottage cheese (low fat), 1 cup cooked dried peas or beans, 4 tbsp peanut butter, 1/3 cup nuts (especially walnuts). *Avoid* cheddar type cheeses, hydrogenated nut butters.
‡Eggs (250 mg cholesterol per yolk) are eliminated from the diet when marked cholesterol restriction is desired.

in the absence of HDL, the activation of lipoprotein lipase is reduced (one of the minor HDL apoproteins, apo-Lp-glutamic, is the activator of lipoprotein lipase). Because of its rarity, the prognosis of Tangier disease has not yet been determined, and it may be compatible with a normal life span.

B. Abetalipoproteinemia (Bassen-Kornzweig Syndrome): This rare disorder is characterized by inability to synthesize VLDL or chylomicrons. Accordingly, it presents a malabsorption of fat and is associated with thinness. Acanthocytosis has been found in all cases, and retinitis pigmentosa and ataxia are associated. Growth is often retarded. The diagnosis is confirmed by finding a plasma cholesterol below 80

Table 19–9. Modified fat, controlled carbohydrate, low cholesterol diet
for types IV and V hyperlipoproteinemia.

Foods to Use	Foods to Avoid	1200 Calories (40–50% CHO) Polyunsaturated:Saturated Fat Ratio 1:1	1800 Calories (40–50% CHO) Polyunsaturated:Saturated Fat Ratio 1:1
Milk, nonfat		2 cups (16 oz) daily	3 cups (24 oz) daily
Fruits (without sugar), fresh, canned, or juices—at least one to be citrus or tomato	Avocado, olives	3 servings daily	4 servings daily
Vegetables—at least one to be leafy green or yellow		3 or more servings daily	3 or more servings daily
Breads, cereals, starches, enriched white or whole grain*		3 servings daily	7 servings daily
Eggs (with yolks)†		3 per week	3 per week
Egg whites		As desired	As desired
Cooked lean meats, fish, poultry: Beef, lamb, pork, veal, ham, Canadian bacon‡	Skin and fat on poultry, duck, and goose; shellfish,† fish roe (caviar), pan-fried or deep fatfried meats, marbled or fatty meats, cold cuts or luncheon meats, sausage, frankfurters, corned brisket, spare ribs, organ meats,† gravies	5 oz daily	6 oz daily
Fats and oils: Soft margarines (those listing primary ingredient as "liquid oil"); oils such as safflower, soybean, corn, cottonseed, sesame, or sunflower	Butter, cream, hydrogenated shortenings or margarines, cream substitutes	2 tbsp daily	4 tbsp daily
Sugars and sweets	All desserts, confections, candies made with sugar (white or brown), syrups, honey, jellies, preserves (except as substitutes for bread*)		
Coffee, tea, coffee substitutes, artificial sweeteners, "diet drinks," unsweetened gelatin, lemon juice, vinegar, sour pickles and relishes, herbs, spices, condiments, fat-free broth or bouillon		As desired	As desired

*Substitutes for 1 serving of bread (not to be used more than 3 times a week): 1/3 cup gelatin dessert, 1 tsp honey, jelly, or preserve, 1/4 cut sherbet, 1/2 cup skimmed milk pudding, 1½ inch cube angelfood cake, 1 oz hard sugar candy, 1 oz rum, vodka, whiskey, 1½ oz sweet wine, 2½ oz dry wine, 5 oz beer.
†Substitute for 1 egg yolk (250 mg cholesterol per yolk): 2 oz shellfish, liver or other organ meat.
‡Substitutes for 1 oz meat: 1½ tbsp peanut butter, 1/4 cup low-fat cottage cheese, 1 oz low-fat cheese (less than 2% fat).

mg/100 ml and triglycerides which are lower than in any other disorder and often undetectable. LDL are absent, as are VLDL and chylomicrons. The prognosis is poor, and progressive severe disability with muscular and skeletal deformities results. Fat-restricted diets are necessary, with medium chain triglycerides recommended.

Hypobetalipoproteinemia, either on a genetic basis or acquired secondary to severe malabsorption, has also been described.

Gaucher's Disease

Gaucher's disease is an autosomal recessive disorder due to excess storage of a glucocerebroside in the reticuloendothelial cells. It is due to deficiency of glucuronyl ceramide hydrolase. Proliferation of these abnormal "Gaucher cells" causes progressive hepatomegaly, splenomegaly, neurologic lesions, and skeletal lesions, with bone fracture at the site of the lesions. The disease may have its onset at any age, although onset is usually in childhood. Anemia, jaundice, thrombocytopenia, and increased serum acid phosphatase may also be present. Chemical analysis of tissues for the glycolipid or the deficient enzyme help provide a definitive diagnosis. The course of the disease is variable. In children it usually progresses rapidly, resulting in death in a few months; in older adults, it progresses so slowly that the patient often dies of intercurrent disease.

Treatment is supportive. Splenectomy is indicated only when hypersplenism occurs.

Niemann-Pick Disease (Sphingomyelin Lipidosis)

Niemann-Pick disease is a rare autosomal recessive disorder characterized by the excessive storage of phospholipids, especially sphingomyelin, in the reticuloendothelial system. Manifestations occur early in infancy and consist primarily of hepatosplenomegaly and CNS involvement, with mental retardation and convulsions. Other symptoms and signs include diffuse pulmonary infiltration, cutaneous lesions, a cherry-red macular spot, gastrointestinal bleeding, lymph node enlargement, thrombocytopenia, anemia, and foam cells in hepatic or marrow biopsies. Definitive diagnosis is established only by finding increased levels of sphingomyelin on chemical analysis of tissues.

Treatment is supportive. Death usually occurs during childhood.

Albrink MJ: Dietary and drug treatment of hyperlipidemia in diabetes. Diabetes 23:913, 1974.

Brown M, Goldstein J: Expression of the familial hypercholesterolemia gene in heterozygotes: Mechanism for a dominant disorder in man. Science 185:61, 1974.

Chopra J, Mallick N, Stone MC: Hyperlipoproteinemias in nephrotic syndrome. Lancet 1:317, 1971.

Fredrickson D, Gotto A Jr, Levy R: Familial lipoprotein deficiency (abetalipoproteinemia, Tangier disease). Pages 493–530 in: *The Metabolic Basis of Inherited Disease,* 3rd ed. Stanbury JB, Wyngaarden JB, Fredrickson DS (editors). McGraw-Hill, 1972.

Fredrickson D, Levy R: Familial hyperlipoproteinemia. Pages 545–614 in: *The Metabolic Basis of Inherited Disease,* 3rd ed. Stanbury JB, Wyngaarden JB, Fredrickson DS (editors). McGraw-Hill, 1972.

Goldstein JL, Brown MS: Hyperlipidemia in coronary heart disease: A biochemical genetic approach. J Lab Clin Med 85:15, 1975.

Havel R: Mechanisms of hyperlipoproteinemia. Advances Med Biol 26:57, 1972.

Havel R, Kane J: Drugs and lipid metabolism. Ann Rev Pharmacol 13:287, 1973.

Levy R, Morganroth J, Rifkind B: Treatment of hyperlipidemia. New England J Med 290:1295, 1974.

Miller JD, McCluer R, Kanfer JN: Gaucher's disease: Neurologic disorder in adult siblings. Ann Int Med 78:883, 1973.

Murphy BF: Management of hyperlipidemias. JAMA 230:1683, 1974.

O'Brien JS: Ganglioside storage diseases. New England J Med 284:893, 1971.

Parker F, Short J: Xanthomatosis associated with hyperlipoproteinemia. J Invest Dermat 55:71, 1970.

Philippart M & others: Niemann-Pick disease. Arch Neurol 20:227, 1969.

Smith E, Slater R: Relationship between low density lipoprotein in aortic intima and serum-lipid levels. Lancet 1:463, 1972.

Wilkins RW & others: Clofibrate and niacin in coronary heart disease. JAMA 231:360, 1975.

Yatsu FM: Sphingolipidoses. California Med 114:1, April 1971.

20...
Nutrition; Nutritional & Metabolic Disorders

Milton J. Chatton & Phyllis M. Ullman

Human nutrition in the broad sense involves much more than the traditional concepts derived from the study of nutritional deficiencies. Malnutrition can result from dietary excess or imbalance as well as from deficiency, and may have subtle as well as gross effects. It may be a reflection of biochemical alterations at every level of human nutrition, ranging from variations in the composition of foods through the entire process of ingestion, digestion, absorption, and ultimate utilization by the body at the molecular level. Malnutrition may occur as a result of metabolic requirements which are altered by heredity or disease. Recent data indicate that racial and cultural groups differ greatly not only in their preference for certain foods but also in their ability to tolerate certain foods (eg, dairy products).

Normal human nutrition presupposes the availability of nutrients (proteins, carbohydrates, fats, vitamins, and minerals) adequate to meet the qualitative and quantitative metabolic needs of the body under varying conditions such as growth, development, physical activity, pregnancy and lactation, environmental stress, and illness. Optimal conditions of nutrition unfortunately do not prevail for millions of underprivileged people throughout the world. The world food supply, never evenly distributed in human history for reasons of economics, improvidence, drought, pestilence, ignorance, natural disaster, and conflict, is increasingly threatened by environmental contamination and by a dangerously burgeoning population.

Large scale food production by modern agricultural methods as a means of meeting the needs of the rapidly increasing world population is threatened by the energy crisis. Dwindling fossil fuel supplies threaten to curtail many of the scientific measures for increasing crop yields (eg, fertilizer, pesticides) as well as the production of mechanical equipment for processing and distributing food. At the same time, growing housing and other construction demands are making inroads on available arable land resources.

Rising food costs have accentuated the worldwide food shortage, so that a food crisis exists not only in underdeveloped countries but also for individuals and groups in poverty pockets almost everywhere.

Nutritional deficiencies due to inadequate food supplies may markedly impair the intellectual and physical development and well-being of countless millions who are spared death by actual starvation.

Even if there were an unlimited food supply throughout the world, there would undoubtedly be nutritional problems in otherwise healthy populations arising from defective production, processing, storage, distribution, preservation, contamination, preparation, and serving of foods.

A well-balanced diet (USA) usually consists of 6 basic categories of foods: (1) breads and cereals, (2) vegetables and fruits, (3) meats, (4) dairy products, (5) fats and oils, and (6) sugars (Table 20–1). This diet may be altered by choice or circumstance yet remain nutritionally adequate if the correct combinations and quantity of natural foodstuffs are ingested. Unfortunately, through poverty, ignorance of food selection and preparation, dietary faddism, and confusion regarding the nutritive value of processed foods (eg, frozen foods, dehydrated foods, breakfast cereals, TV dinners), caloric requirements may be met or exceeded without meeting total nutritional needs.

Gaps in our knowledge of some of the precise details of human nutrition are perhaps responsible for the curious dietary philosophies that emerge from time to time. Although not usually harmful (or perhaps even having as yet unrecognized beneficial nutritional value), the use of many of the so-called "health foods," "organic foods," and "natural vitamins" is frequently unsupported by scientific evidence. A rational look at the modern Western diet, however, suggests that it would be advantageous to return to diets which have (1) more vegetable protein and less animal protein, (2) more dietary fiber, (3) less refined sugar, and (4) less total fats. It has been postulated that the disproportionately great increase in certain diseases of industrialized countries—obesity, atherosclerosis, heart disease, diabetes, intestinal disorders, etc—are related in large part to dietary habits.

Harmful effects have been reported from prolonged use of poorly controlled and nutritionally unbalanced medical therapeutic diets (eg, low phenylalanine diet in phenylketonuria).

The criteria for determining the nutritional adequacy of foods, therefore, are subject to continuous reappraisal. The quantity and quality of proteins, fats, carbohydrates, minerals, and vitamins may vary not only with the class of foodstuff but with the specific type and source of food. Furthermore, the roles of food combinations, processed foods, chemical addi-

Table 20—1. Basic food groups: The daily food guide.

Food	Nutrients Provided	Recommended Daily Amounts
Breads and cereals, enriched white or whole grain	Carbohydrate Protein Vitamin B complex	Four or more servings. One serving equals: —1 slice bread —1 oz (1 cup) cereal, ready-to-eat, flake, or puffed —1/2 to 3/4 cup cooked cereal —1/2 to 3/4 cup cooked pastes (macaroni, spaghetti, noodles) —5 saltines, 2 Graham crackers
Fruits and vegetables	Carbohydrate Protein Vitamins A, B complex, C Minerals (iron, calcium, phosphorus, potassium, sodium, and trace elements)	Four or more servings, at least one to be citrus or tomato daily and one to be dark green or deep yellow. One serving equals 1/2 cup vegetable or fruit, one medium orange, apple, or potato, or 1/2 cup (4 oz) juice
Meats (beef, lamb, pork, veal, poultry, game, fish) and eggs	Protein Fat Iron Trace elements Vitamin B complex	Two or more servings. One serving equals: —3 oz cooked, lean, boneless meat or fish (1/4 lb raw) —1/4 chicken or 1/2 cup cooked meat —2 eggs —1 cup cooked dry beans or peas —4 tbsp peanut butter —1/2 cup cottage cheese
Milk and dairy products: Cheese, ice cream, and any product made with milk (whole, low-fat, or nonfat)	Protein Fat Carbohydrate Calcium Riboflavin Vitamin A	Adults: 1—2 cups (8—16 oz) Teenagers: 4 or more cups Children 9—12: 3 or more cups Children under 9: 2—3 cups Pregnant women: 3 or more cups Lactating women: 4 or more cups One serving equals 1 oz cheese, 1/2 cup cottage cheese, 1/2 cup ice cream
Fats and oils: Butter, margarine, cream, oils, salad dressings, avocado, nuts	Fat Vitamins A, D, E	6—12 tsp or more depending upon caloric requirements. At least 1 tbsp oil or margarine daily. One serving equals 2 tbsp cream, 1/8 avocado, 6 small nuts
Sugars, syrups, honey, jellies, etc	Carbohydrate	As needed for caloric requirements

tives, new or unknown micronutrients, and food-drug combinations are receiving deserved attention.

The "biologic value" of the protein contained in various foods depends upon its essential amino acid content. For example, dairy products and eggs contain all of the amino acids and are of high biologic value; meat, poultry, fish, and potatoes have somewhat less biologic value; and cereals, breads, and most root vegetables have only fair biologic value. Proper combination of foods which have only fair protein value, however, may result in apparently adequate protein nutrition.

Qualitative differences in the type of fat in foods may be of importance in nutrition. Comparison of the relatively high content of saturated fats in coconut oil and hydrogenated or solid vegetable shortenings with the high content of polyunsaturated fats in safflower oil and certain other unsaturated vegetable oils pro-

vides an example of qualitative difference in fats which may have a significant application to the dietary prevention and treatment of certain types of hyperlipidemia. Genetic factors play a large role in determining the ability to metabolize fat in several clinical disorders.

Diabetes mellitus is the best known disorder of carbohydrate (and fat) metabolism in which it is important to control the quantity and quality of dietary carbohydrates and lipids. The relationship of sugar to dental caries is reasonably well established. Disaccharide intolerance is a readily treatable form of malabsorption syndrome. Galactosemia and numerous other hereditary disorders of carbohydrate metabolism exist.

There may be a considerable individual variation in the requirement of vitamins for hereditary and acquired reasons. Both markedly decreased and in-

Table 20—2. Nutrient content of foods.*

Food	Average Serving	Protein (gm)	Fat (gm)	Carbo-hydrate (gm)	Calories
Fruits A (unsugared)					
Apples, apricots, berries, grape-fruit, lemons, limes, melons, oranges, peaches, pears, pineapple, tangerines	1/2 cup or 4 oz	0	0	12–15	50–75
Fruits B (unsugared)					
Bananas, fresh figs, grapes, plums	1/2 cup	0	0	20	80
Dried fruit (prunes, apricots, peaches, dates)	1/4 cup				
Vegetables A					
Asparagus, broccoli, brussels sprouts, cabbage, cauliflower, celery, cucumber, eggplant, greens (beet, chard, collard, dandelion, kale, mustard, poke, spinach, turnip), lettuce, mushrooms, okra, parsley, green pepper, radishes, rhubarb, sauerkraut, stringbeans, wax beans, summer squash, tomatoes, watercress	1/2 cup	1–2	0	3–5	16–20
Vegetables B					
Beets, carrots, artichokes, green peas, onions, pumpkin, rutabagas, turnips, winter or yellow squash	1/2 cup	2	0	7–9	35–45
Breads (enriched white or whole grain)					
Bread, cornbread	1 slice	2	1	12–14	65–73
Muffins, biscuits, dinner rolls, buns, pancakes	1				
Waffles	1/2				
Cereals					
Cooked	2/3 cup	2	1	14	65
Dry flaked type	2/3 cup				
Dry puffed type	1 cup				
Shredded wheat	1 biscuit				
Crackers					
Soda or Graham	2 squares	2	1	10	55
Melba toast	4 pieces				
Saltines or Ritz	6				
Ry-Krisp	2				
Oyster	20 (1/2 cup)				
Starches					
Cooked macaroni, noodles, spaghetti, or rice	1/2 cup	3	1	20	100
Corn	1/2 cup or 1 ear	3	1	16–20	85–100
Peas (fresh or frozen)	1/2 cup	4.5		10	58
Potatoes					
Cooked	1 small	3		20	100
Chips	10 (or 1 oz bag)	1	8	10	115
Mashed	1/2 cup	2	4	12	92
Sweet or yams	1/4 cup				
Popcorn (without butter)	1 cup	1		5	25

*From: *Nutritive Value of Foods.* Home & Garden Bulletin No. 72 (revised). US Department of Agriculture, 1970.

Table 20—2 (cont'd). Nutrient content of foods.

Food	Average Serving	Protein (gm)	Fat (gm)	Carbohydrate (gm)	Calories
Soup (canned, undiluted)					
Vegetable or cream style (average)	1/2 cup	3	3–5	10–15	70–120
Milk					
Whole (homogenized)	1 cup (8 oz)	8	10	12	170
Low-fat (2%)	1 cup	8	5	12	125
Nonfat, skimmed, or buttermilk	1 cup	8	0	12	80
Evaporated whole	1/2 cup	8	10	12	170
Powdered skimmed, dry	1/4 cup	8	0	12	80
Yogurt, plain, low-fat	1 cup (8 oz)	8	4	13	125
Meat (medium fat, cooked)					
Beef, ham, lamb, pork, veal	1 oz	7	5	0	73
Liver	1 oz	7	0	0	28
Sausage (pork)	1 oz (2 links)	7	15	0	165
Luncheon (cold cuts)	1 oz	7	10	0	120
Frankfurters (8–9/lb)	1	7	10	0	120
Poultry (cooked)					
Chicken, duck, goose, turkey	1 oz	7	2–5	0	50–75
Fish					
Fin type (cooked)	1 oz	7	2–5	0	50–75
Shellfish					
Clams	5 small	7	0	0	28
Lobster	1 small tail	7	0	0	28
Oysters	5 medium	7	0	2	56
Scallops (12/lb)	1 large	7	0	0	28
Shrimp	5 small	7	0	0	28
Eggs	1	6	6	0	78
Cheese					
American, cheddar, Swiss, blue, processed	1 oz	7	9	1	115
Cheese spreads	1 oz	5	6	2	80
Cottage cheese (creamed)	1/2 cup	16	5	3	130
Cream cheese	1 oz	2	10	0	98
Nuts					
Peanuts (shelled, whole)	25 (1 oz)	8	15	6	190
Peanut butter	1 tbsp (1–2 oz)	4	8	3	95
Almonds, cashews, walnuts	1 oz (8–10 nuts)	5	15	6	180
Pecans	1 oz	2	17	3	190
Fats					
Avocado (4 inch diameter)	1/8	0	4	0	36
Bacon (crisp)	1 strip	2	4	0	45
Butter or margarine	1 tsp or 1/8 inch cut (cube)	0	4	0	36
Cooking fats (shortenings)	1 tsp	0	4	0	36
Cream					
Half and half	2 tbsp	2	4	2	52
Sour	2 tbsp	0	4	2	40
Whipped	1 tbsp	0	5	1	50
Whipped topping (with sugar)	2 tbsp	0	2	2	22
Mayonnaise	1 tsp	0	4	0	36
Salad oils	1 tsp	0	4	0	36
Olives (black or green)	3 medium	0	4	0	36

Table 20—3. Food sources of vitamins.*

Vitamin	Recommended Allowances	Food Sources
Vitamin A activity	Men: 5000 IU/day. Women: 4000 IU/day. Pregnant and lactating women: 5000—6000 IU/day.	Milk, butter, oils, fortified margarines, carotene precursors, carrots, sweet potatoes, apricots, spinach, leafy green vegetables
Vitamin B_1 (thiamine)	1.2—1.4 mg/day. Pregnant and lactating women: 1.5 mg/day.	Enriched white and whole grain breads and cereals, liver, meat, egg yolk, yeast, legumes
Vitamin B_2 (riboflavin)	1.1—1.8 mg/day. Pregnant and lactating women: 1.5—1.9 mg/day.	Milk, meat, liver, eggs, enriched white and whole grain breads and cereals, yeast
Niacin equivalents	13—20 mg/day	Enriched white and whole grain breads and cereals, liver, meat, bran, yeast
Vitamin B_6 (pyridoxine)	2 mg/day. Pregnant and lactating women: 2.5 mg/day.	Bananas, whole grain cereals, chicken, legumes, egg yolk, most dark green leafy vegetables, most fish and shellfish, meats, organ meats, nuts, peanut butter, potatoes, sweet potatoes, prunes, raisins, yeast
Vitamin B_{12} (cyanocobalamin)	3 μg/day. Pregnant and lactating women: 4 μg/day.	Present in foods of animal origin only: liver, kidney, meats, milk, most cheeses, most fish, shellfish, eggs
Folic acid (folacin)	400 μg/day. Pregnant and lactating women: 800 μg/day.	Green leafy vegetables, yeast, organ meats, liver, kidney
Vitamin C (ascorbic acid)	45 mg/day. Pregnant and lactating women: 60 mg/day.	Citrus fruits, tomatoes, parsley, green pepper, radishes; green leafy raw vegetables; melons
Vitamin D	400 IU/day	Butter, fortified margarines and milk, fish liver oils, salt water fish, liver, egg yolk
Vitamin E activity	12—15 IU/day	Vegetable oils, margarines, salad dressings, whole grain cereals, nuts

*From: *Recommended Dietary Allowances,* 8th ed. National Academy of Sciences, 1973; and *Nutritive Value of Foods.* Home & Garden Bulletin No. 72 (revised). US Department of Agriculture, 1970.

Table 20—4. Food sources of minerals.*

Mineral	Recommended Allowances	Food Sources
Calcium	Adults: 0.8 gm/day. Ages 11—18 and pregnant or lactating women: 1.2 gm/day	Milk (1 gm calcium/quart), milk products, cheeses, leafy green vegetables
Phosphorus	Adults: 0.8 gm/day. Ages 11—18 and pregnant or lactating women: 1.2 gm/day	Milk, whole grain cereals, cheeses, legumes, eggs, meat, peanut butter, nuts, liver
Iron	Women: 18 mg.† Men: 10 mg.	Liver, meat, legumes, whole or enriched grains, potatoes, egg yolk, green vegetables, dried fruits
Sodium	100—300 mEq/day or 2.5—7 gm/day	Table salt, seafoods, milk, vegetables, prepared foods
Potassium	50—150 mEq/day or 2—6 gm/day	Meats, cereals, vegetables, legumes, fruits (particularly dried), cream of tartar
Copper	1—2 mg/day	Liver, egg yolk, nuts, legumes, bran, oatmeal
Magnesium	300—450 mg/day	Bananas, whole grain cereals, legumes, milk, nuts, most dark green leafy vegetables
Iodine	100—150 μg/day	Iodized salt, seafoods, vegetables grown in iodine-rich soil
Chlorine	0.5 gm/day	Table salt, seafoods, animal products
Sulfur	Adequate if protein intake is adequate	Protein foods: Meats, fish, poultry, eggs, cheeses, milk
Zinc	15 mg/day	Widespread in foodstuffs
Trace minerals (chromium, cobalt, manganese, molybdenum, selenium)	Minute traces	Leafy green vegetables, whole grains, fruits, legumes, meats, seafoods, organ meats

*From: *Recommended Dietary Allowances,* 8th ed. National Academy of Sciences, 1973; and *Nutritive Value of Foods.* Home & Garden Bulletin No. 72 (revised). US Department of Agriculture, 1970.
†Supplemental iron recommended during pregnancy.

creased physiologic requirements have been described. Periodically, however, there have been proposals to utilize the pharmacologic (rather than physiologic) effect of massive doses of vitamins to prevent or treat clinical disorders which are poorly understood or for which no satisfactory treatment is available. Carefully controlled studies of such hypotheses are necessary, and it should be recognized that large, pharmacologic dosages of some vitamins (eg, vitamins A, D, K, and niacin) are decidedly toxic to man.

Although the roles of iron, cobalt, iodine, and fluoride are well recognized, the roles of zinc, copper, chromium, selenium, and manganese in human nutrition are not so clearly understood. Even more obscure are the metabolic functions of cadmium, strontium, nickel, and molybdenum, which have been the subject of nutritional studies in lower animals. Zinc has been reported to be essential to nucleic acid metabolism and protein synthesis, as well as playing a role in collagen formation, glycolysis, and oxidative phosphorylation. Zinc deficiency has been reported to be associated with dwarfism and hypogonadism. Copper deficiency may result in anemia. Unfortunately, it is difficult to establish firm cause and effect relationships of micronutrient deficiency and human disease on the basis of short-term studies.

The interaction of drugs and dietary factors was perhaps first recognized in the case of chronic alcoholism and vitamin B complex deficiency. It is now known that long-term therapy with many drugs may induce malnutrition through varied mechanisms, including appetite suppression, intestinal malabsorption, altered vitamin synthesis, increased nutritional requirements, and vitamin depletion. Folate deficiency may be caused by chronic alcoholism and by chronic use of oral contraceptives and anticonvulsants. The corticosteroids are known to deplete muscle protein, lower glucose tolerance, and induce osteoporosis. Vitamin K deficiency can be caused by oral antibiotics, especially if the diet is inadequate. It should also be mentioned that certain nutrients can either decrease the effectiveness of drugs (eg, pyridoxine reverses the antiparkinsonism effect of levodopa) or can markedly enhance the toxicity (eg, tyramine-containing substances such as cheese, beer, and red wine can induce hypertensive crises in patients receiving monoamine oxidase inhibitors).

Given an abundant supply of nutritionally adequate food available to all, there remain many factors which can result in malnutrition. Examples are given below.

(1) **Failure to take the proper quantity and quality of foods to meet individual requirements:**
  (a) Psychologic (anorexia nervosa, mental depression, psychosis, individual food eccentricities).
  (b) Psychosocial (dietary fads, "crash diets," reliance on snack foods).
  (c) Cultural (regional or national food habits).
  (d) Educational (ignorance of essentials).

  (e) Inability to obtain, prepare, and serve foods to self (elderly or physically handicapped patients).
  (f) Chronic alcoholism and drug addiction.
  (g) Iatrogenic (protracted use of unbalanced, restrictive, or inadequate therapeutic diets, or use of certain therapeutic drugs).
  (h) Anorexiant drugs (amphetamines).

(2) **Inadequate intake of food because of gastrointestinal disorders:**
  (a) Anorexia following major surgery, especially gastrointestinal surgery.
  (b) Loss of sense of taste or smell.
  (c) Difficulty or inability to swallow food (neurologic or obstructive lesions).
  (d) Pain on ingestion of food (oral, esophageal, or gastric lesions).
  (e) Chronic nausea and vomiting due to any cause.
  (f) Postgastrectomy dumping syndrome.
  (g) Afferent loop (postgastrectomy) pain or vomiting.

(3) **Defective absorption or utilization of food because of gastrointestinal disorders:**
  (a) Chronic diarrhea due to any cause.
  (b) Malabsorption syndromes (postgastrectomy; postsurgical short bowel, with loss of mucosal surface and bile salt depletion; hepatic insufficiency, pancreatic insufficiency, tropical and nontropical sprue, lactase deficiency).
  (c) Protein-losing enteropathy.
  (d) Intestinal parasitism.
  (e) Interference by drugs (eg, mineral oil).

(4) **Increased need for food:**
  (a) Increased physical activity (heavy labor or exercise).
  (b) Chronic febrile states.
  (c) Increased metabolism (hyperthyroidism, ACTH overproduction due to physical stress).
  (d) Abnormal excretion (renal impairment).

(5) **Impaired metabolism of nutrients:**
  (a) Hereditary biochemical disorders ("inborn errors of metabolism").
  (b) Acquired biochemical disorders (liver damage, drugs).

(6) **Interaction of drugs and nutrients.**

The human diet, therefore, must meet the caloric needs and the quantitative and qualitative nutrient requirements of the individual based upon age, weight, physical activity, pregnancy, lactation, and state of health. Special therapeutic diets may be necessary to correct acquired or hereditary nutritional and metabolic abnormalities. In certain instances when patients are unable to take food by mouth, tube feedings or intravenous hyperalimentation may be necessary.

Ahrens RA: Sucrose, hypertension and heart disease: An historical prospective. Am J Clin Nutr 27:403, 1974.

Bayless TM & others: Lactose and milk intolerance: Clinical implications. New England J Med 292:1156, 1975.

Bistrian BR & others: Protein status of general surgical patients. JAMA 230:858, 1974.

Canby TY: Can the world feed its people? National Geographic 148:2, July 1975.

Crosby WH: The iron-enrichment-now brouhaha. JAMA 231:1054, 1975.

Cummings JH: Progsress report: Dietary fibre. Gut 14:69, 1973.

Dunlap WM, James GW, Hume DM: Anemia and neutropenia caused by copper deficiency. Ann Int Med 80:470, 1974.

Faloon WW (editor): Symposium: Drug-nutrient relationship. Am J Clin Nutr 26:104, 1973.

Floch MH (editor): Symposium: The exocrine pancreas in human nutrition. Am J Clin Nutr 26:289, 1973.

Gray GM: Carbohydrate digestion and absorption: Role of the small intestine. New England J Med 292:1225, 1975.

Harper AE, Payne PR, Waterlow JC: Human protein needs. Lancet 1:1518, 1973.

Jukes T: Antibiotics in meat production. JAMA 232:292, 1975.

Jukes T: The organic food myth. JAMA 230:276, 1974.

Mayer J: There's too much humbug on the grocery shelf. Prism 1:31, April 1973.

Mertz W, Cornatzer WE: *Newer Trace Elements in Nutrition.* Dekker, 1972.

Mitchell HS (editor): Recommended dietary allowances up to date: A symposium. J Am Dietet A 64:149, 1974.

Plumley PF, Francis B: Dietary management of diverticular disease. J Am Dietet A 63:527, 1973.

Rosenberg UH, Scrimshaw NS (editors): Symposium on malabsorption and nutrition. Am J Clin Nutr 25:1047, 1972.

Sacks FM & others: Plasma lipids and lipoproteins in vegetarians and controls. New England J Med 292:1148, 1975.

Schlenker ED & others: Nutrition and health of older people. Am J Clin Nutr 26:766, 1973.

Walker ARP: Dietary fibre and the pattern of disease. Ann Int Med 80:663, 1974.

Winick M: Current status of malnutrition in the United States. Am J Trop Med 23:752, 1974.

THERAPEUTIC DIETS*

Special diet therapy should be based upon sound scientific evidence rather than upon myth or tradition. In no aspect of medical therapeutics is there more bias, emotionalism, and inconclusive evidence than in the use of many of the so-called special diets.

There is little evidence to support the value of many classical or traditional diets (eg, Sippy diet for peptic ulcer, low purine diet for gout, low residue diet for ulcerative colitis). There is nothing to substantiate the extravagant claims made for most of the innumerable special diets proposed for the treatment of obesity, and in many instances these diets are nutritionally inadequate. It is not possible to comment individually on the numerous dietary fads which periodically sweep the USA except to state that they are regrettable.

*Diabetic diets and hyperlipidemia diets are discussed in Chapter 19. The low calorie obesity diet is discussed later in this chapter.

On the other hand, there is good clinical and scientific evidence to support the use of special diets for many conditions: low sodium diet for congestive heart failure and arterial hypertension, high potassium diet as an adjunct to corticosteroid therapy, gluten elimination diet in nontropical sprue, disaccharide elimination in disaccharidase deficiency, lactose elimination in lactase deficiency, nutritionally well-balanced and low calorie diet for obesity, controlled carbohydrate diet for diabetes mellitus, and the fat and carbohydrate restrictions in the prevention or treatment of hyperlipidemia. Allergy to certain foods may be very marked in some individuals, and in such instances special nonallergenic diets may be of value. In many instances, however, such "allergies" may be more readily related to psychosocial factors.

Since special therapeutic diets are restrictive, their use should be carefully supervised and they should be discontinued as soon as they are no longer required.

Many special diets are nutritionally unbalanced, monotonous, expensive, difficult to procure, and difficult to adhere to. Consultation and cooperation with a professional dietitian will facilitate optimal use of special diets. The dietitian should be provided with certain information such as the nature of the illness, the type of diet desired by the physician, the total daily amount (in grams) of protein, carbohydrate, and fat, the size and frequency of feedings, the fluid intake desired, the patient's environmental and socioeconomic status, and the expected duration of therapy.

Clear Liquid Diet

This diet relieves thirst and supplies a few calories. It contains only water, sugar, nonresidue protein, and salts. Foods are limited to tea, coffee, broth, strained fruit juices, and carbonated beverages. This diet should be used—for short periods only—for patients with the following conditions: (1) Immediate postoperative status, (2) acute semidebilitation, (3) constricting upper gastrointestinal lesions, and (4) acute gastroenteritis. The diet is administered in 6 small feedings daily.

Full Liquid Diet

This diet does not require chewing and is nutritionally more adequate than the clear liquid diet, but it is still rather deficient in protein, B vitamins, and minerals. In addition to the clear liquid foods, milk, eggnog, plain ice cream, gelatin, soft cereals, puddings, custards, proprietary liquid protein preparations, strained cream soups, and vitamin and mineral supplements are given. The diet is administered in 6 feedings daily as tolerated.

Soft Low Residue Diet

This diet, which is nutritionally adequate, consists of low residue and easily assimilable proteins and carbohydrates. Permitted foods, in addition to those permitted in the liquid diets, include eggs, cottage cheese, ground or tender meat, fish, or chicken, white bread, soda crackers, refined cereals, boiled polished rice, potatoes (without skin), cooked and puréed vegetables, cooked fruits, ripe bananas, applesauce, plain puddings, plain cakes and cookies, marshmallows, and hard candies (melted in mouth).

Avoid corn, potato skins, fibrous vegetables, whole grain or bran cereals, raw fruit, and fried or highly seasoned foods.

Minimum Residue Diet

Indication: Preoperatively, to clear the operative site of any fecal residue; postoperatively, to reduce irritation.

A. Protein: Ground or tender beef, chicken, fish, lamb, liver, veal, crisp bacon, eggs. Avoid milk, milk products, cheeses of all kinds.

B. Carbohydrate: Soda crackers, French bread, melba toast, refined cereals, rice, strained oatmeal, cornflakes, puffed rice, plain cakes and cookies; macaroni, noodles, spaghetti, gelatin desserts, water ices, strained fruit juices, hard candies, marshmallows, sugar, syrup, honey, carbonated beverages, tomato juice.

C. Fat: Butter, margarine, mayonnaise.

D. Other Foods: Beverages such as coffee, tea, Sanka, Postum; salt, vinegar, gravies, spices, and herbs in moderation.

Soft ("Bland") Diet

A. "Classical" or Traditional:

1. Protein—Adequate amounts of lean meats, fish, eggs, cottage cheese, and milk.

2. Fats—Moderate amounts of butter, margarine, cream, and cream cheese (to suppress gastric secretion and motility). Polyunsaturated fats (soft margarines) are recommended in place of saturated types.

3. Carbohydrates—Only potatoes (white or sweet) and applesauce allowed during acute phase.

4. Other foods—Restrict gastric secretagogues and irritants such as alcohol and caffeine (coffee, tea, cocoa, and cola beverages). Chili powder, nutmeg, mustard seeds, cloves, and black pepper should be avoided.

B. Liberal:

1. Protein and fat—As in classical bland diet.

2. Carbohydrates—Fruits, vegetables, and those foods that can be properly chewed and mixed with saliva may be added. Puréed or strained foods are recommended only when dentition is poor.

3. Other foods—Continue restriction of black pepper and control of alcohol, coffee, tea, and cocoa intake.

Note: Meals should be frequent and slowly eaten, with size varied according to individual needs and tolerances.

Low Fat Diet (50–60 gm/day)

Fat and fiber tolerances appear to be very individualized, and no clearcut rationale for any food restriction has been verified. However, the following foods may relieve indigestion or flatulence.

A. Protein: Normal amounts of lean meats, fish, and poultry (with all visible fat removed), eggs as tolerated, low fat or nonfat milk, yogurt, buttermilk, cottage cheese and mild cheddar cheeses, fat-free meat stock, bouillon, or broth.

B. Fats: One to 2 tbsp may be tolerated but may be decreased if weight control is desired. Use butter, margarine, mayonnaise, and oils. Avoid cooking any food in fat.

C. Carbohydrates: Enriched or whole grain breads and cereals; fresh, cooked, canned, or juices of all fruits and most vegetables; soft desserts or those made without added fat.

Avoid or limit intake (according to individual tolerances) of cooked or raw brussels sprouts, broccoli, cauliflower, cabbage, onions, turnips, green peppers, lettuce, radishes, dried peas and beans, nuts, fresh melons, raw apples, chocolate, pastries, and any fried food. Spicy, peppery, and highly seasoned foods may cause discomfort.

D. Beverages: Coffee, tea, fruit juices, carbonated beverages, and decaffeinated beverages may be given. Wine, beer, and alcohol are to be avoided.

Note: Foods should be given in 6 or more small feedings throughout the day.

Low Protein Diet (40–50 gm/day)

A. Protein: Two oz meat, fish, or poultry; 1 cup milk; 1 egg or 1 oz cheese.

B. Carbohydrates: Fruits and juices as desired; cooked and raw vegetables as desired. Three servings of breads and cereals. One serving of potatoes, corn, etc. One serving of dessert. Sugar, hard candies, syrup, or honey as desired.

C. Fats: Butter, margarine, oils, and salad dressings as desired.

D. Salt: Restrict as indicated.

Note: Small, frequent feedings are recommended, with juices and fruits for between-meal snacks.

Low Carbohydrate Diet (100–150 gm/day)

A. Protein: Meat, fish, poultry, cheese, or nuts as desired.

B. Carbohydrates: Breads and cereals, not over 3 servings/day. Unsugared fruits and juices, not over 3 servings/day. Vegetables (raw or cooked), 3–6 servings/day. Starches such as potatoes, rice, or corn, 1 serving/day. No desserts containing sugar; artificially sweetened desserts or beverages in moderation.

C. Fats: Butter, margarine, oils, and salad dressings as desired.

Note: It is recommended that a higher protein intake be taken earlier in the day, with small, frequent feedings of cheese, nuts, etc throughout the day.

High Calorie, High Protein, High Vitamin Diet

Increase caloric value to 25–50% above normal. Increase protein to 90–100 gm/day for adults. Select foods high in vitamin content, especially vitamin B complex. Provide foods in small, frequent feedings (6–8 times/day). Add sugars and fats as tolerated.

A. Protein:

1. Milk—Up to 1 quart/day, as beverage or in or on foods.

2. Eggs—One or more, prepared in any way or added to other foods.

3. Cheeses—All kinds, as meat substitutes, added to sauces or dishes, or as between-meal snacks.

4. Meats, fish, poultry—Two to 3 portions/day (2–3 oz/serving), simply prepared by broiling, roasting, or stewing, or with cream or cheese sauces.

B. Fats: Two to 3 tbsp/day of butter, cream, margarine, mayonnaise, or oils.

C. Carbohydrates:

1. Bread and cereals—Four to 8 servings of any kind, but preferably whole grain or enriched white.

2. Fruits and fruit juices—Four to 6 servings (with added sugar) of any kind, fresh, cooked, or canned.

3. Vegetables—

a. Fresh or raw—Small portions 1–2 times/day with mayonnaise or dressings.

b. Cooked—One or 2 portions/day of green, white, red, or yellow vegetables.

4. Starches—One to 2 servings as potatoes, rice, etc, with added sauces, butter, gravies, or cream or cheese sauces.

5. Soups—Cream style or thick soups as desired.

6. Ice cream, sherbet, custard, pudding, plain cake, fruit dessert, gelatin, or cookies—One to 2 (or more) servings. Brown, white, or maple sugars; jellies, honey, syrups, 2–4 tbsp (or more).

7. Beverages—Coffee and tea in moderation; decaffeinated beverages, Postum, cocoa, eggnog, milk shakes, sweetened carbonated beverages, and fruit juices as desired. Wines and alcohol with discretion. Other milk-containing supplementary foods such as Metrecal, Meritene, Nutrament, or Sustagen can be used for meals or between-meal snacks.

Low Carbohydrate, High Protein, High Fat Diet

Diet may be inadequate in calcium and ascorbic acid.

A. Protein: Meats, fish, poultry, eggs, cheese for meals and between-meal snacks.

B. Fat: Increased use of butter, margarine, mayonnaise, oils, whipping cream, sour cream, cream cheese, and peanut butter (if tolerated).

C. Carbohydrate: Unsugared fresh, frozen, or canned fruits (no juices), fresh, frozen, or canned vegetables, breads, cereals, and starches. Desserts made with sugar substitutes.

Disaccharide Intolerance Diet
(Low Lactose, Sucrose, Maltose, Galactose)

Indication: Those conditions which have been determined to be due to deficiencies of one or more enzymes such as lactase, invertase or sucrase, maltase and isomaltase, and galactase.

In infants, a nonlactose mixture of amino acids such as Nutramigen, a protein hydrolysate, or one of the soybean formulas may be given. In adults, omit all forms of milk, cheese, ice cream, frozen desserts containing milk, milk drinks, white breads and crackers, biscuits, muffins, cream soups, creamed dishes, desserts and prepared foods containing milk, some salad dressings, some cold or luncheon meat products, cream substitutes, candies, some health and geriatric products, and some medications which may use lactose as a bulking agent, filler, or excipient.

Sucrase or invertase deficiency requires the omission of granulated sugar (cane or beet), syrups, jellies, molasses, cakes, cookies, puddings and candies, sorghum, pineapple, carrots, apricots, bananas, dates, melons, oranges, and peas. Some medications such as antibiotic syrups may also contain sucrose.

Isomaltase deficiency may occur in conjunction with invertase deficiency. Germinating cereals, malt, and probably wheat and potatoes should be restricted. Sucrose should also be avoided.

A rare disorder, glucose-galactose malabsorption, requires omission of all sources of sucrose, starch, and lactose. Special formulas and diets need to be devised.

Low Purine Diet

Rigid purine restriction does not significantly reduce the level of serum uric acid, and much better control of hyperuricemia is accomplished with medication. It may occasionally be advisable to limit high purine foods such as organ meats, anchovies, sardines, and dried beans and peas, but the normal well-balanced dietary pattern has been found suitable for most patients. Weight control is recommended, and the patient should be placed upon a decreased caloric diet for gradual weight reduction.

Low Gluten Diet

Eliminates gluten-containing foods such as wheat, oats, rye, barley, and buckwheat.

A. Protein: Meats, fish, poultry, eggs, cheese, and milk as desired. Substitutes such as beans, peas, or nuts may be taken as tolerated.

B. Fat: Butter, margarine, oils, salad dressings, and cream as desired or tolerated.

C. Carbohydrate: Fruits, vegetables, and sugars as desired; desserts such as gelatins, iced milk, and sherbet; cakes, cookies, puddings, or pastries made with corn, rice, potato, or soya starches or flours. (Most commercial or prepared mixes contain flours that should be omitted from this diet.) Breads made from gluten-free wheat starch or special baking mixes such as Paygel, Resource, or those made with corn, rice, potato, soya, or lima bean starches or flours. Cereals: rice, corn, cornflakes, Rice Krispies, corn meal.

D. Other Foods: Condiments, salt, vinegar, spices, and herbs as desired or tolerated.

Sodium Regulated Diets

When prescribing modification of dietary sodium, it is important to take into consideration not only the natural sodium content of foods but also the sodium content of prepared foods, local water supplies, and many types of medication. The need for drastic limitations of dietary sodium nowadays has been obviated for the most part because of the number of effective oral diuretic drugs available. Correction of significant sodium depletion is best accomplished by oral or parenteral sodium chloride preparations.

Sodium Content of Foods

A. High Content: (125–1000 mg and over, or 5.4–43.5 mEq per average serving.) Cheese of all kinds, soda and Graham crackers, condiments, relishes and sauces (soy, Worcestershire, ketchup, chili, barbecue), pickles, olives, cured and canned meats, fish, poultry, commercially prepared desserts, foods made with baking powder or baking soda, buttermilk, sauerkraut, tomato juice, celery, potato chips, snack foods, pretzels, frozen meals or dinners, canned vegetables, canned soups, prepared cereals, frozen peas and lima beans.

B. Medium High Content: (50–125 mg or 2.2–5.4 mEq per average serving.) Commercial breads, butter, margarine, fresh fish and shellfish, milk, fresh meats, poultry, eggs, fresh vegetables, chocolate candies, ice cream, iced milk, sherbet, angel food cake, sponge cake, artichokes, beet greens, turnips, spinach, celery, carrots, beets, chard, and kale.

C. Low Content: (Less than 50 mg or 2.2 mEq per average serving.) All fruits (fresh, frozen, canned, dried), fruit juices, jellies, jams, syrups, honey, sugar (both white and brown), soybean curd, unsalted nuts, hard sugar candies, coffee, oil, tea, sweet or salt-free butter or margarine, herbs, plain gelatin, most fresh vegetables, puffed rice, puffed wheat, shredded wheat, Sugar Pops, nonenriched or quick-cooking cereals such as oatmeal, rolled wheat, cracked wheat, farina, cornmeal, grits, rice, Ralston, Wheatena, or Wheathearts.

Potassium Regulated Diets

When it is necessary to modify the potassium in the diet, one must consider not only the natural potassium content of foods but also the potassium content of special food preparations (eg, salt substitutes, low-salt milk) and certain medications (eg, penicillin G). A high intake is recommended when corticosteroids and certain diuretic drugs are administered.

A. High Content: (300–500 mg or 7.6–12.5 mEq per average serving.) All-Bran, milk of all kinds, yogurt, apricots (fresh and dried), avocados, bananas, dates, melons (casaba and honeydew), oranges (medium to large), peaches (dried), persimmons, raisins, prune juice, cooked chicken, beef, lamb, liver, ham, pork, veal, fish of all kinds, peanuts, pecan halves, artichokes (globe type), cooked dried white or red beans or black-eyed peas, lima beans, beet greens, raw carrots, celery, mushrooms, cooked chard, parsnips, white potatoes, radishes, cooked spinach, sweet potatoes, and raw tomatoes.

B. Medium High Content: (150–300 mg or 3.8–7.7 mEq per average serving.) Fresh and canned peaches, orange juice, cantaloupe, nectarines, plums, watermelon, fresh and cooked asparagus, cabbage, cauliflower, greens, corn, eggplant, onions, rutabagas, squash of all kinds, tomato juice, turnips, shellfish,

cured meats such as corned and dried beef, sausage and luncheon meats, and desserts containing dried raisins and nuts.

C. Low Content: (50–150 mg or 1.28–3.8 mEq per average serving.) Cooked green and wax beans, beets, peas, broccoli, brussels sprouts, carrots, corn, eggplant, mixed vegetables, onions, green peppers, raw lettuce and salad greens, berries of all kinds, bread of all kinds, rolls, buns, hot breads, cheeses of all kinds, cereals (cooked or dry prepared), eggs, canned soups, candies, desserts, and wines.

D. Little or No Content: (Less than 50 mg or 1.28 mEq per average serving.) Beverages such as coffee, beer, gin, rum, vodka, whisky, tea; hard sugar candies, butter, margarine, oils, and shortenings.

Low Calcium Diet
(500–700 mg calcium, 1000–1200 mg phosphorus)
A. Protein:
1. Meat, fish, or poultry. Only 4 oz cooked per day.
2. Eggs—One per day; egg whites as desired.
3. Milk—1 cup (1/2 pint)/day; may use diluted whipping cream as milk substitute.
4. Cheese—Cottage cheese, only 2 oz/day.
Avoid organ meats such as brains, heart, liver, kidney, sweetbreads; sardines, fish roe; game such as pheasant, rabbit, deer; cheddar or other cheeses, milk-containing foods.
B. Fat: Whipping cream, butter, margarine, salad dressings, and oils as desired.
C. Carbohydrate:
1. Fruits—3 to 5 servings daily, including citrus.
2. Vegetables, raw—Salads as desired (see Avoid list).
3. Vegetables, cooked—2 or 3 servings (see Avoid list).
4. Starches—Potatoes and corn, 1 or more servings (see Avoid list).
5. Breads, cereals, and pastes—Enriched white breads, rolls, crackers (see Avoid list), nonenriched farina, cornflakes, corn meal, hominy grits, rice, Rice Krispies, puffed rice, macaroni, spaghetti, noodles.
6. Desserts—Fruit pies, fruit ices, fruit gelatin, puddings made with allowed milk and egg, angel food cake, meringues, shortbreads (see Avoid list), sugar, jellies, honey, sweetened beverages (colas, ginger ale, etc).
Avoid rhubarb, beet greens, chard, collards, mustard greens, spinach, turnip greens, dried beans, peas, lentils, soybeans; whole grain breads, cereals, and crackers; rye bread and all breads made with self-rising flour; oatmeal, brown and wild rice, bran, bran flakes, wheat germ, and any dry cereal not listed above; any milk-containing dessert except as allowed; nuts, peanut butter, chocolate, and cocoa; condiments having a calcium or phosphate base.

High Calcium Diet
Indication: For conditions requiring the intake of over 1 gm calcium per day.

The normal well-balanced diet furnishes 800–1000 mg calcium per day, mostly from milk and cheese. Increasing milk consumption to over 1 quart per day will provide 1150 mg calcium or more. Other foods which will add to the total calcium intake are cheeses, particularly cheddar or American types; leafy green vegetables such as "greens" (dandelion, beet, mustard and turnip, kale), cabbage, broccoli, and brussels sprouts; dried beans and peas, nuts, and milk-containing desserts.

If milk is not well tolerated, calcium gluconate or lactate, 1–2 gm daily, may be used as a supplement.

Diets for Glucose Tolerance Tests

A. 100 gm Carbohydrate Breakfast: Orange juice, 6 oz; cooked or dry, prepared cereal, 1 cup; sugar, 2 tsp; milk, 1/2 cup; bread or toast, 2 slices; margarine or butter, as desired; jelly or honey, 1 tbsp; coffee or tea as desired with 1 tsp sugar.

B. 250 gm Carbohydrate Diet for 5 Days Prior to Test:

1. Morning–Fruit or juice, 1 cup; cereal, 1 cup, or bread, 2 slices; sugar, jelly, or honey, 1 tbsp; milk, 1/2 cup; egg or bacon, as desired; tea or coffee, as desired.

2. Mid-morning–Sweetened carbonated beverage, 1 (6 oz) bottle, or 1 cup fruit juice.

3. Noon–Sandwich made with bread (2 slices) or 1 bun: hamburger, meat, tuna, eggs, cheese, peanut butter, as desired; condiments as desired; milk, 1 glass; ice cream, 1 scoop, or 1 dish (1/2 cup) cornstarch pudding; tea or coffee as desired.

4. Mid-afternoon–Sweetened carbonated beverage, 1 (6 oz) bottle, or 1 small candy bar.

5. Evening–Meat, fish, poultry, eggs, or cheese, as desired; potato, rice, corn, beans, or paste, 1 serving or 1/2 cup; cooked vegetable, 1 or 2 servings; butter or margarine, as desired; salad with dressing, as desired; bread, 1 slice, or 1 biscuit; dessert, 1/6 fruit pie or 1 cupcake or 1 large scoop ice cream or sherbet; tea or coffee, as desired.

Calcium Test Diet
(200 mg calcium, 700 mg phosphorus)

Indication: For diagnosis of hypercalciuria, to be followed for 3 days; in treatment of acute hypercalcemia.

A. Morning: Orange or grapefruit juice, 1/2 cup; cornflakes or Rice Krispies, 3/4 cup; 5 soda crackers or sourdough French bread, 1–2 slices; butter, 3–4 tsp; bacon, 3 strips; sugar and jelly, as desired; coffee or tea made with distilled water.

B. Noon: Broiled, baked, or boiled beef, lamb, veal, or chicken, 3 oz; potato, boiled or baked, 1/2 cup, with butter, 1–2 tsp; tomato, raw, canned, or juice, 1 small or 1/2 cup; 5 soda crackers or 1–2 slices of sourdough French bread; butter, 3 tsp; applesauce, 1/2 cup; coffee or tea made with distilled water.

C. Evening: Broiled, baked, or boiled beef, lamb, veal, or chicken, 3 oz; rice, cooked, 1/2 cup; corn, fresh, frozen, or canned, 1/2 cup; 5 soda crackers or 1–2 slices of sourdough French bread; butter, 5 tsp;

sugar and jelly, as desired; applesauce, 1/2 cup, or banana, 1 small, or 1 peach, fresh or canned; coffee or tea made with distilled water.

D. Between Meals: Distilled water, hard sugar candies, carbonated sweetened beverages.

Avoid all dairy products except butter, including that incorporated in all prepared foods.

Vegetarian Diets

Foodstuffs of vegetable origin constitute most, if not all, of the diet of millions of people throughout the world. For people of the poorer nations, this is a matter of necessity; for a few, the vegetarian diet is one of choice. Strict vegetarians–those living entirely on fruits, vegetables, whole grain cereals, legumes, and nuts–are less numerous than those who also eat dairy products. (lactovegetarians) and those who also eat eggs (ovolactovegetarians). Diets devoid of all animal products–for economic, religious, cultist, or personal reasons–are nutritionally inadequate unless they are varied and provide all of the essential amino acids of proteins, vitamins, and minerals. Clinicians should be aware of the nutritional characteristics of vegetable foodstuffs as it becomes apparent that human beings must rely increasingly on cereal grains, legumes, roots, tubers, and other vegetable sources of food in the not too distant future.

The quantity and quality of protein are of major concern in all diets. Judicious combination of plant protein foods can provide the equivalent nutritional value of high quality animal protein foods. Mixing of dietary cereal grains and legumes has maintained excellent health status for peoples throughout the world, and the supplementary effect of one plant food on another is well established.

Two daily servings of high-protein meat substitutes such as legumes (eg, soybeans, beans, peas, lentils), high-protein nuts (eg, peanuts, almonds, cashews, walnuts), peanut butter, meat analogues (textured vegetable or soy protein products), or dairy products or eggs are recommended. The preschool child in particular needs to be assured of an adequate intake of high-quality protein.

Although protein is of first importance in considering the adequacy of vegetarian diets, other nutrients which may be only marginally present in all-plant diets are calcium, iron, riboflavin, vitamin B_{12}, and, for children not exposed to sunlight, vitamin D.

The greatest risk of inadequacy in an all-plant diet comes from reliance on a single plant food source, eg, from a cereal grain or starchy root crop. Legumes, particularly soybeans, are rich in protein, B vitamins, and iron. Grains are good sources of carbohydrates, proteins, thiamine, iron, and trace minerals. Nuts and other seeds contribute fat, protein, B vitamins, and iron. Dark green, leafy vegetables are sources of calcium, riboflavin, and carotene (vitamin A precursors) and are good supplements to the grains and legumes in the total vegetarian diet.

Since plant foods do not contain vitamin B_{12}, some source needs to be supplied. Milk and eggs are satisfactory sources, but the total vegetarian diet can be supplemented with fortified soybean milk or vitamin B_{12} preparations. Infants also may need supplementary vitamin D, particularly in winter months when exposure to sunlight is limited. Calcium and riboflavin can be obtained from a liberal intake of dark green, leafy vegetables or by consumption of fortified soy milk.

Dietary Fiber

Epidemiologic, clinical, and experimental evidence suggests that removal of fiber (plant constituents which are resistant to digestion by the human gastrointestinal tract) from the diet is directly or indirectly associated with certain diseases which are disproportionately common in industrialized countries of the world. Disorders of the gastrointestinal tract that may be linked to decreased dietary fiber include functional constipation, hiatus hernia, gallbladder disease, appendicitis, diverticulitis, tumors of the colon and rectum, and hemorrhoids; cardiovascular disorders include coronary atherosclerosis, varicose veins, and deep vein thrombosis. These relationships, although conjectural, warrant serious consideration. Therapeutic implications, at least in the case of the mentioned gastrointestinal disorders, seem obvious and have already led to significant modification of older dietary concepts in the treatment of ulcerative colitis, colonic diverticulosis, and so-called spastic constipation. Preventive aspects of diets high in fiber content with regard to the gastrointestinal and cardiovascular disorders are uncertain at present.

The recommended daily fiber food consumption is as follows:

One raw fresh fruit or 1/2 cup of dried fruit (cooked or uncooked).

One cup of raw fresh or lightly cooked fresh vegetables. It is probably more convenient and desirable to eat some combination of several vegetables in smaller amounts each to add up to a cup total. The skins of fruits and vegetables should be eaten if they are edible.

Four to 6 slices of whole wheat bread, corn bread, or rye bread.

Two to 4 tbsp of natural bran or 1/2 cup of All-bran cereal, or a somewhat larger serving of less fibrous cereal (eg, 40% bran or raisin bran).

Snack foods which are good sources of fiber include peanuts, popcorn, graham crackers, raisins, almonds, walnuts, pecans, pumpkin seeds, and sunflower seeds.

Anderson CF & others: Nutritional therapy for adults with renal disease. JAMA 223:68, 1973.

Burkitt DP, Walker ARP, Painter NS: Dietary fiber and disease. JAMA 229:1068, 1974.

Davidson CS: Dietary treatment of hepatic diseases. J Am Dietet A 62:515, 1973.

Ingelfinger FJ (editor): Rationale for diets in gastrointestinal disease. J Am Dietet A 60:473, 1972.

The role of fiber in the diet. Dairy Council Digest 46:1, 1975.

Spiro HM: The rough and the smooth: Some reflections on diet therapy. New England J Med 293:83, 1975.

Vetter L, Shapiro R: An approach to dietary management of the patient with renal disease. J Am Dietet A 66:158, 1975.

TUBE FEEDINGS

There are 2 general types of tube feedings: (1) blended, strained preparations made from common foods, and (2) those with a milk base to which other foods may be added. Commercial preparations are also available.

Tube feedings are employed when the patient is unable or unwilling to take food by mouth. Feedings may be administered through a pliable polyethylene tube passed intranasally and may be kept in place for prolonged periods. In some circumstances, a gastrostomy is necessary.

The tube feeding should supply the patient's requirements for carbohydrate, protein, fat, electrolytes, and water. It must pass through the tube without clogging. The feeding should be as close to the osmolarity of blood plasma as possible.

A person of normal weight needs 15 Calories/lb. However, metabolic demands may necessitate an increase in caloric intake. Protein should make up about 20% of the calories. Carbohydrates (along with electrolytes) give the tube feeding its osmolarity and should be limited to 35–40% of the calories. Fat will provide 30–45% of calories. A suitable concentration is 1 Calorie/ml. An average normal adult requires about 2–2.5 liters of water in 24 hours.

Tube feedings may serve as excellent media for the growth of bacteria and must be refrigerated and not held over 24 hours. To prevent the tube from clogging, each feeding should be followed with a small quantity of water. Measured volumes (150–200 ml) can be given every 2–4 hours.

Caution: (1) Begin with more dilute material and administer slowly.. (2) The best rate is usually 3 liters per 24 hours. (3) Most patients tolerate feedings best when not over 200 ml are given at a time. (4) If foods must be given rapidly, warm to body temperature. (5) If gastric distention is suspected, aspirate with a gastric tube and before each subsequent tube feeding if necessary. (6) Use with care in comatose patients to prevent aspiration. (7) If diarrhea occurs, add 1/2 oz fluid pectin (Certo) to 1 quart of feeding, or liquid antidiarrheal drug in proper dose. (8) Prevent dehydration, hyperosmolality, and azotemia by providing adequate water to allow for the solute load and to permit normal excretion.

Blenderized (Blended) Tube Feeding Formula

The following formula supplies 1 Calorie/ml in a volume of 2500 ml. The nutrient contents are as follows: Protein, 20% or 123 gm; fat, 45% or 123 gm; carbohydrate, 35% or 226 gm; calcium, 1312 mg; phosphorus, 1518 mg; iron, 24 mg; vitamin A, 7582 IU; thiamine, 2.675 mg; riboflavin, 3.746 mg; niacin, 27.91 mg; ascorbic acid, 163 mg; sodium, 2557 mg; potassium, 4159 mg.

Strained oatmeal	10 gm
Dextri-Maltose	50 gm
Instant nonfat dry milk	50 gm
Strained liver	20 gm
Strained beef	568 gm
Strained applesauce	402 gm
Strained green beans	484 gm
Oil	85 ml
Orange juice	200 ml
Milk, homogenized	300 ml
Water	500 ml

Milk Base Tube Feeding Formula

The following formula supplies 1.4 Calorie/ml in a volume of 1500 ml. The nutrient contents are as follows: Protein, 100 gm; fat, 110 gm; carbohydrate, 190 gm; sodium, 3565 mg; potassium, 3900 mg. *Note:* This formula is inadequate in iron.

Homogenized milk	800 ml
Half and half	600 ml
Eggnog powder	100 gm
Instant nonfat dry milk	90 gm
Salt	5.5 gm
Vitamin preparation*	5 ml
Water to 1500 ml	

It has been recommended that pasteurized powdered egg or eggnog powder be substituted for raw egg because of the possibility of salmonella infection. One tbsp (15 gm) powdered egg is equivalent to one egg. Various eggnog powders are available commercially.

It has also been suggested that a milk substitute be used to replace milk in tube-feeding diets for patients who experience gastrointestinal distress (lactose intolerance?) with the conventional milk base diet.

Kark RM: Liquid formula and chemically defined diets: A brief review. J Am Dietet A 64:476, 1974.
Walike BC, Walike JW: Lactose content of tube feeding diets as a cause of diarrhea. Laryngoscope 83:1109, 1973.

INTRAVENOUS HYPERALIMENTATION

When it is not possible to provide adequate nourishment by the normal alimentary route, it may now be possible to meet nutritional needs for extended periods exclusively by intravenous alimentation. This has proved to be effective and even lifesaving in patients with conditions such as severe alimentary disturbances (eg, chronic vomiting or diarrhea, inflammatory intestinal disease, malabsorption, massive resection, pancreatic and enterocutaneous fistulas), acute and chronic renal failure, extensive trauma or burns, or overwhelming infections.

The basic nutrient solution for the average adult consists of 20–25% dextrose, 5% fibrin hydrolysate, 40–50 mEq sodium chloride, 30–40 mEq potassium chloride, and 4–5 mEq magnesium sulfate. Vitamin requirements are added to the solution daily. When intravenous feedings are prolonged for more than 1 month, trace elements may be required.

With careful skin preparation and sterile technic, a catheter is introduced via a subclavian vein and the nutrient solution may be infused into the superior vena cava for long periods if necessary. Patients can be maintained in positive nitrogen balance, with weight gain and clinical improvement over periods up to several months, tiding them over until such time as definitive treatment of the primary medical or surgical problem can be carried out. Clinical application of this new method of nutrition will probably be expanded into practically every medical specialty.

Potential complications of intravenous hyperalimentation include physical injury to structures impinged upon by the catheter (eg, pleura, lungs, blood vessels, brachial plexus, and the heart in the case of subclavian catheterization), local and systemic infection, hypophosphatemia, and hyperosmolar hyperglycemic dehydration. The possibility of such complications can be reduced by proper antiseptic, aseptic, and catheterization technics and careful biochemical monitoring.

Allardyce DB, Groves AC: A comparison of nutritional gains resulting from intravenous and enteral feeding. Surg Gynec Obst 139:179, 1974.
Dudrick SJ, Rhoads JE: New horizons in intravenous feeding. JAMA 215:939, 1971.
Moore FD, Brennan MF: Intravenous feeding. New England J Med 287:862, 1972.
Shils ME: Guidelines for total parenteral nutrition (AMA Council on Foods and Nutrition). JAMA 220:1721, 1972.

VITAMINS & VITAMIN DISORDERS

In illness there may be considerable variation in the body's requirements for vitamins, depending upon age, activity, diet, metabolic rate, and other factors affecting vitamin absorption, utilization, and excretion. Vitamin deficiencies are almost always multiple, although a particular symptom complex may predominate.

Early signs of vitamin deficiency are usually nonspecific, vague, and mild and are easily misinterpreted or missed entirely.

---

*Vitamin supplement contains 2 mg thiamine, 3 mg riboflavin, 30 mg niacin, and 100 mg ascorbic acid.

The "crude" sources containing multiple vitamins are often more effective in therapy than the pure or synthetic preparations; as a rule, only during the more severe phases and in instances of "specific" deficiencies is it necessary to use "pure" vitamins. The use of a "pure" vitamin in the face of a true multiple vitamin deficiency may aggravate rather than alleviate the condition. The treatment of vitamin deficiencies consists of giving an adequate, balanced, high-protein, high-vitamin diet with vitamin supplementation as indicated. In general, it is wise to use vitamins therapeutically in 5–10 times the amounts required for daily maintenance.

Vitamin dependencies, which are of hereditary origin, should be distinguished from the acquired vitamin deficiencies. Almost a dozen vitamin-dependent genetic diseases, involving 6 different vitamins (thiamine, nicotinamide, pyridoxine, vitamin B_{12}, and vitamin D) have been described. The vitamin dependencies do not respond to physiologic replacement therapy but only to large, pharmacologic doses of the needed vitamin. At the other extreme, in the case of at least one vitamin (vitamin D), predisposed patients may react adversely to doses below the recommended prophylactic requirement.

Large doses of some vitamins (eg, vitamins A, D, K, and niacin) are toxic and may cause illness, particularly when continued for long periods. For this reason alone, the current popularity of so-called megavitamin therapy for a variety of imperfectly understood disorders (eg, schizophrenia) is not rational and is potentially hazardous.

Ahmed F & others: Effects of oral contraceptive agents on vitamin nutrition status. Am J Clin Nutr 28:606, 1975.

Graham GG (editor): Johns Hopkins conjoint clinic on vitamins. J Chronic Dis 19:1067, 1966.

Rosenberg LE: Vitamin-dependent genetic disease. Hosp Practice 5:59, 1970.

Scriver CR: Vitamin-responsive inborn errors of metabolism. Metabolism 22:1319, 1973.

Winter SL, Boyer JL: Hepatic toxicity from large doses of vitamin B_3 (nicotinamide). New England J Med 289:1180, 1973.

FAT-SOLUBLE VITAMINS

1. VITAMIN A

Vitamin A is an alcohol of high molecular weight which is stored in the liver. Most of it is derived from conversion of beta-carotene in foods to vitamin A, mainly by the mucosa of the small intestine but also by the liver. It is necessary for normal function and structure of all epithelial cells and for the synthesis of visual purple in the retinal rods (hence for vision in dim light). Carotene only is present in leafy green and yellow fruits and vegetables; vitamin A and, at times, carotene are present in whole milk, butter, eggs, fish, and liver oil. Actually, vitamin A itself is quite rare in foods; therefore, most is derived from carotene-bearing plant sources. The recommended daily allowances for adults are 5000 IU (or USP units) for men, and 4000 IU for women; during pregnancy and lactation, 5000–6000 IU.

Hypovitaminosis A

A. Clinical Findings: Mild or early manifestations consist of dryness of the skin, night blindness, and follicular hyperkeratosis. Severe or late manifestations are xerophthalmia, atrophy and keratinization of the skin, and keratomalacia.

B. Tests for Deficiency: Dark adaptation is impaired. A low serum value (below 20 μg/100 ml) of vitamin A may be found but is not diagnostic. A therapeutic test with 25,000–75,000 IU daily for 4 weeks may be helpful.

C. Treatment: Give oleovitamin A, 15–25 thousand units once or twice daily. If an absorption defect is present, it may be necessary to administer bile salts with the vitamin A or to give the same dosage in oil intramuscularly (50,000 units/ml in sesame oil). Skin lesions or profound malnutrition (eg, kwashiorkor) may require more treatment.

Hypervitaminosis A

This disorder is rare in adults. It may occur in children as a result of excessive ingestion of vitamin A preparations. The minimal toxic adult dose is about 75–100 thousand units daily for 6 months.

A. Clinical Findings: Anorexia, loss of weight, hair loss, hypercalcemia, hyperostosis and periosteal elevation of bone, bony resorption, hepatomegaly, splenomegaly, anemia, skin rash, and CNS manifestations.

B. Tests of Excess: Serum levels of vitamin A over 400 μg/100 ml are found.

C. Treatment: Withdraw the medicinal source.

Frame B & others: Hypercalcemia and skeletal effects in chronic hypervitaminosis A. Ann Int Med 80:44, 1974.

Olson JA: Metabolism and function of vitamin A. Fed Proc 28:1670, 1969.

Roels OA: Vitamin A physiology. JAMA 214:1097, 1970.

2. VITAMIN D

Vitamin D is the generic name for a family of about 10 sterols that have varying degrees of antirachitic potency. The 2 most important of these sterols are ergocalciferol (vitamin D_2) and cholecalciferol (vitamin D_3). The human body can synthesize provitamin D_3 (7-dehydrocholesterol), which can be converted photochemically to vitamin D_3 by ultraviolet irradiation of the skin. Natural sources of vitamin D include liver and viscera of fish, livers of fish-eating animals, egg yolks, and butter.

The daily allowances for adults are not known. For infants and children and for women during pregnancy and lactation—as well as other individuals of both sexes to age 22—the recommended daily allowance is 400 units.

It is the current belief that vitamin D_3 must be transformed in the body to biologically much more active metabolites, 25-hydroxyvitamin D_3 and 1,25-dihydroxyvitamin D_3. These compounds, formed by the sequential hydroxylation of cholecalciferol by the liver and kidneys, are considerably more potent than the parent vitamin.

Vitamin D or its metabolites, together with parathyroid hormone and calcitonin, play an essential hormonal role in calcium homeostasis. The D vitamins maintain normal blood calcium and phosphorus levels by stimulating normal calcium transport in the intestine, mobilizing calcium from and to the bones, and controlling urinary phosphorus excretion.

Impaired metabolism of vitamin D or altered sensitivity of target tissues (intestine and bone) to the vitamin has been described in a wide variety of bone diseases and other disorders associated with abnormal calcium metabolism, eg, malabsorption, liver disease, renal failure, rickets, parathyroid disorders, and sarcoidosis.

There is, therefore, a wide spectrum of responsiveness to vitamin D. Some patients may require more than 50 times the therapeutic dose to correct manifestations of vitamin D deficiency (eg, vitamin D-resistant rickets), whereas others (eg, those with hyperparathyroidism) are hypersensitive even to doses below the recommended requirement.

Hypovitaminosis D

Hypovitaminosis D is usually due to inadequate dietary intake, lack of sunlight, or an intestinal absorption defect (eg, pancreatitis, sprue), and may also be due to biliary cirrhosis.

A. Clinical Findings: Deficiency of vitamin D leads to osteomalacia in children (rickets) or infantile tetany. Some cases of adult osteomalacia appear to be associated with increased requirements of vitamin D.

B. Tests for Deficiency: Serum calcium and phosphorus may be normal or decreased and serum alkaline phosphatase is generally increased. The urinary calcium is usually low.

C. Treatment: See Osteomalacia. Simple dietary increase of vitamin D is relatively ineffective in treating the deficiencies encountered in the malabsorption syndromes and in biliary cirrhosis.

Hypervitaminosis D

This disorder is usually caused by prolonged ingestion of 5–150 thousand units of the drug form daily.

A. Clinical Findings: The manifestations of hypercalcemia are present and may progress to renal damage and metastatic calcification.

B. Tests of Excess: Serum calcium elevation (over 11.5 mg/100 ml) occurs if large doses of vitamin D are taken. (Always consider other causes of hypercalcemia.)

C. Treatment: Withdraw the medicinal source. Complete recovery, although it may be slow, will occur if overtreatment is discontinued in time. Corticosteroids and sodium phytate (Rencal) reverse hypercalciuria due to vitamin D intoxication.

Coburn JW, Hartenbower DL, Norman AW: Metabolism and action of the hormone vitamin D: Its relation to diseases of calcium homeostasis. Western J Med 121:22, 1974.

DeLucca HF: Vitamin D:1973. Am J Med 57:1, 1974.

Palmisano PA: Vitamin D: A reawakening. JAMA 224:1526, 1973.

Shetty KR & others: Protracted vitamin D intoxication. Arch Int Med 135:986, 1975.

3. VITAMIN K

The K vitamins are fat-soluble chemical compounds which are necessary for the synthesis by the liver of blood coagulation factors II (prothrombin), VII, IX, and X. The similarity of the chemical structure of vitamin K to that of coenzyme Q suggests that the K vitamins may also be involved in the oxidative phosphorylation process in cellular mitochondria.

Vitamin K is widely distributed in foods. The naturally occurring form is called vitamin K_1. Vitamin K is also synthesized by microorganisms in the intestines, and, since it differs from K_1 somewhat in chemical structure, is referred to as vitamin K_2. A third form of the vitamin, prepared synthetically, is known as vitamin K_3 (menadione).

The daily allowances of vitamin K are not known, but it is felt that they must be quite small. Vitamin K depletion due to dietary deficiency alone is extremely rare.

Hypovitaminosis K

Hypovitaminosis K may result from biliary obstruction or medical or surgical disorders of the small bowel which interfere with the absorption of fat. Long-term therapy with antibiotics or nonabsorbable sulfonamides which interfere with microorganism synthesis of vitamin K may also cause vitamin K deficiency.

A bleeding tendency or uncontrollable hemorrhage may occur. The coagulation defect may be aggravated by ingestion of drugs that depress prothrombin synthesis (eg, coumarins, salicylates). Prolongation of the prothrombin time as well as abnormal tests for coagulation factors VII, IX, and X may be demonstrated.

Successful treatment of the defective coagulation is dependent upon a functioning hepatic parenchyma, and vitamin K therapy is of no avail if liver disease is severe.

Hypervitaminosis K

Large doses of water-soluble vitamin K (derivatives of K_3; menadione) to infants—particularly premature infants—may cause hemolytic anemia, hyperbilirubinemia, hepatomegaly, and even death. In adults with G6PD deficiency, ordinary doses of menadione or derivatives may cause hemolytic reactions.

Wolf IL, Babior BM: Vitamin K and warfarin: Metabolism, function and interaction. Am J Med 53:261, 1972.

4. VITAMIN E
(Tocopherol)

Vitamin E is a natural antioxidant which plays a role in the normal physiology of animals and probably also of man, although its exact role in man is unclear. It is nontoxic. Anemia due to vitamin E deficiency has been reported in children, especially premature infants being given certain commercial formulas. No well-defined deficiency has been described in adults, although the vitamin is widely held to be a panacea for a great variety of disorders. Recommended daily allowances for adults (based upon the usual range of intake of vitamin E) are 15 IU for males and 12 IU for females, with 15 IU during pregnancy and lactation. Recent data would suggest that the requirement of the vitamin may be related to the polyunsaturated fatty acid content in body tissue.

Bieri JG: Vitamin E. Nutr Rev 33:161, 1975.
Vitamin E: Med Lett Drugs Ther 13:97, 1971.
Williams ML & others: Dietary iron and fat in vitamin E deficiency anemia of infancy. New England J Med 292:887, 1975.
Witting LA: Recommended dietary allowance of vitamin E. Am J Clin Nutr 25:257, 1972.

WATER-SOLUBLE VITAMINS:
VITAMIN B COMPLEX

The members of the vitamin B complex are intimately associated in occurrence in food as well as in function (eg, as coenzymes). As a result of this close interrelationship, it is doubtful that a deficiency of a single B vitamin ever exists except under experimental conditions. Deficiency of a single member of the B complex would probably lead to impaired metabolism of the others. Hence, although certain clinical features may predominate in the absence of a single member of the complex, this does not mean that the deficiency can be entirely corrected by replacing that factor alone. Therefore, "specific therapy" always consists of providing adequate dietary or parenteral sources of all members of the B complex.

1. VITAMIN B₁
(Thiamine Hydrochloride)

Vitamin B_1 is a constituent of the enzyme that decarboxylates the alpha-keto acids (pyruvic acid and alpha-ketoglutaric acid). It is important, therefore, for normal carbohydrate oxidation. Dietary sources are liver, lean pork, kidney, and whole grain cereals. Steaming or exposure to moist heat reduces the thiamine content of foods. The daily dietary allowances are about 1.2–1.4 mg/day.

Hypovitaminosis B₁ (Beriberi)

Hypovitaminosis B_1 results from an inadequate intake due usually to idiosyncrasies of diet or excessive cooking or processing of foods. The increased need for vitamin B_1 during fever, high carbohydrate intake, alcoholism, or thyrotoxicosis may lead to a deficiency.

A. Clinical Findings: Mild or early manifestations consist of vague multiple complaints suggestive of neurasthenia, and include anorexia, formication and muscle cramps, calf tenderness, paresthesias, and hyperactivity followed later by hypoactivity of knee and ankle jerks.

Severe or late manifestations (beriberi) are anorexia, polyneuritis, serous effusions, subcutaneous edema, paralyses (particularly in the extremities), and cardiac insufficiency manifested by tachycardia, dyspnea, edema, and normal or decreased circulation time, elevated venous pressure, and nonspecific ECG changes.

A particularly virulent form of beriberi heart disease, probably associated with metabolic acidosis, is referred to as Shoshin beriberi in the Orient.

B. Treatment: Give thiamine hydrochloride, 20–50 mg orally, IV, or IM daily in divided doses for 2 weeks, and then 10 mg daily orally. Clinical response to thiamine injection within 24–48 hours is one of the best criteria for a diagnosis of thiamine deficiency. An alternative is to give dried yeast tablets (brewer's yeast), 30 gm 3 times daily. Give a well-balanced diet of 2500–4500 Calories/day when tolerated.

Jeffrey FE, Abelman WH: Recovery from proved Shoshin beriberi. Am J Med 50:123, 1971.
Tanphaichitr V & others: Clinical and biochemical studies of adult beriberi. Am J Clin Nutr 23:1017, 1970.
Tomasulo PA, Kater RMH, Iber FL: Impairment of thiamine absorption in alcoholism. Am J Clin Nutr 21:1341, 1968.

2. RIBOFLAVIN (VITAMIN B₂)

Riboflavin serves principally as a coenzyme for hydrogen transfer in the electron transport system of the respiratory chain. It is abundant in milk and milk products, leafy green vegetables, liver, kidneys, and heart. The daily dietary allowances for adults are 1.5–1.8 mg; in pregnancy and lactation, 1.5–2 mg.

Hypovitaminosis B₂ (Ariboflavinosis)

The etiologic factors in ariboflavinosis are similar to those of thiamine deficiency, but inadequate intake of milk is an important contributing factor. The manifestations of deficiency are highly variable and usually occur along with those of thiamine and niacin deficiency, but may occur earlier.

A. Clinical Findings: Mild or early manifestations are oral pallor, superficial fissuring at the angles of the mouth, conjunctivitis and photophobia, lack of vigor, malaise, weakness, and weight loss. Severe or late manifestations consist of cheilosis (fissuring at the angles of the mouth), fissuring of the nares, magenta tongue, moderate edema, anemia, dysphagia, corneal vascularization and circumcorneal injection, and seborrheic dermatitis.

B. Treatment: Give riboflavin, 40–50 mg IV, IM, or orally daily until all symptoms have cleared. An alternative is to give dried yeast tablets (brewer's yeast), 30 gm 3 times daily. A well balanced diet consisting of 2500–4500 Calories/day should be given when tolerated.

Horwitt MK: Nutritional requirements of man, with special reference to riboflavin. Am J Clin Nutr 18:458, 1966.

Rivlin RS: Riboflavin metabolism. New England J Med 283:463, 1970.

3. NICOTINIC ACID (Niacin) & NICOTINAMIDE (Niacinamide)

Niacin and niacinamide function in important enzyme systems concerned with reversible oxidation and reduction by hydrogen transfer. They are present in liver, yeast, meat, whole-grain cereals, and peanuts. Nicotinic acid may be synthesized in the body from tryptophan. Therefore, a high-protein diet virtually assures adequate nicotinic acid. Sixty mg of tryptophan produce 1 mg of nicotinic acid.

The daily allowances for adults are 13–20 mg. Niacin may be used therapeutically as a vasodilating agent for headaches, myalgias, neurologic disorders, and edema of the labyrinth (100 mg or more daily in divided doses). Because niacin decreases the synthesis of low density lipoprotein and lowers serum cholesterol, it has been recommended for the drug treatment of types II, III, IV, and V hyperlipoproteinemia. There is no good evidence that niacin or niacinamide in socalled "megavitamin" dosage is of value in the treatment of schizophrenia. Niacinamide does not possess the vasodilating effect of niacin.

Pellagra

The etiologic factors in deficiency of these components of the B complex are similar to those of thiamine deficiency. Niacin deficiency is the principal but not the only dietary defect in pellagra; low tryptophan content of some foods also plays a role.

A. Clinical Findings: Mild or early manifestations consist of multiple vague complaints, a reddened, roughened skin, and redness and hypertrophy of the papillae of the tongue. Severe or late manifestations are marked roughening of the skin when exposed to light and friction, diarrhea, abdominal distention, scarlet red tongue with atrophy of papillae, stomatitis, depression, mental dullness, rigidity, and peculiar sucking reactions.

B. Treatment: Give nicotinamide (niacinamide), 50–500 mg IV, IM, or orally daily until symptoms subside. Nicotinic acid (niacin) is less often used because of its vasodilating effect; the dosage is similar. Give therapeutic doses of thiamine, riboflavin, and pyridoxine also. An alternative is to give dried yeast tablets (brewer's yeast), 30 gm 3 times daily.

A well balanced diet consisting of 2500–4500 Calories/day and ample proteins should be given when tolerated. Dementia may require constant supervision.

Nicotinic Acid Poisoning

Large oral doses of nicotinic acid may cause flushing and burning of the skin and dizziness, but are usually not harmful. After intravenous administration hypotension may be severe. Anaphylaxis occurs rarely.

Langer T, Levy RI: Effect of nicotinic acid on beta-lipoprotein metabolism. Clin Res 18:458, 1970.

Nicotinic acid in the treatment of schizophrenia. Med Lett Drugs Ther 15:107, 1974.

Prinsloo JG & others: Protein nutrition status in childhood pellagra: Evaluation of nicotinic acid status and creatinine excretion. Am J Clin Nutr 21:98, 1968.

WATER-SOLUBLE VITAMINS: VITAMIN C (Ascorbic Acid)

Vitamin C is concerned with the formation and maintenance of intercellular supporting structures (dentine, cartilage, collagen, bone matrix). Its biochemical action is not clear. It may play a specific role in hydroxylation of proline in collagen, which may be related to connective tissue functioning and wound healing. Vitamin C may also play a role in the body's response to severe stress. Dietary sources include citrus fruits, tomatoes, paprika, bell peppers, and all leafy green vegetables. The ascorbic acid content of foods is markedly decreased by cooking, mincing, air contact, alkalies, and contact with copper utensils. The US recommended allowance for adults is 45 mg daily; for pregnant and lactating women, 60 mg daily.

Ascorbic acid has been used in the treatment of certain poisonings in doses of 0.5 gm or more, but proof of its value is lacking. It is used in dosages up to 200 mg daily orally to promote healing of wounds or ulcers or during recovery from protracted disease (eg, tuberculosis). Pharmacologic megadosages have been recommended for the prevention or palliation of the common cold, but recent studies suggest that massive vitamin C prophylaxis does not result in significantly fewer colds. Recent studies also suggest that large doses of vitamin C are not entirely free of undesirable side-effects.

Hypovitaminosis C (Scurvy)

Scurvy is usually due to inadequate intake of vitamin C but may occur with increased metabolic needs. The disease is seen frequently in formula-fed infants, elderly bachelors and widowers, and food faddists. Vitamin C concentration in tissues has been reported to be decreased in healthy women taking oral contraceptives.

A. Clinical Findings: Mild or early manifestations are edema and hemorrhage of the gingivae, porosity of dentine, and hyperkeratotic hair follicles. Severe or late manifestations consist of severe muscle changes, swelling of the joints, rarefaction of bone, a marked bleeding tendency, extravasation of blood into fascial layers, anemia, loosening or loss of the teeth, and poor wound healing.

B. Tests for Deficiency: Capillary resistance is reduced, and x-rays of the long bones may show typical changes. Epiphyseal changes in children are pathognomonic. There is also a lowering of serum or white cell ascorbic acid levels.

C. Treatment: Give sodium ascorbate injection, 100–500 mg IM, or ascorbic acid, 100–500 mg orally daily, as long as deficiency persists.

Chalmers TC: Effects of ascorbic acid on the common cold: An evaluation of the evidence. Am J Med 58:532, 1975.

Dykes MHM: Ascorbic acid and the common cold: Evaluation of its efficacy and toxicity. JAMA 231:1072, 1975.

Herbert V, Jacob E: Destruction of vitamin B_{12} by ascorbic acid. JAMA 230:241, 1974.

Karlowski TR & others: Ascorbic acid for the common cold: A prophylactic and therapeutic trial. JAMA 231:1038, 1975.

OTHER VITAMINS

Many other vitamins have been described. Some are important in human nutrition and disease; others play an unknown role.

Pyridoxine Hydrochloride

Pyridoxine is important in transamination and decarboxylation of amino acids. Deficiency of the vitamin may result in an anemia with intramedullary hemolysis (see p 285). The recommended daily allowance for adults is about 2 mg/day. It may relieve nervous symptoms and weakness in pellagrins when niacin fails and may relieve glossitis and cheilosis when riboflavin fails. Its role (if any) in human atherosclerosis is uncertain. The therapeutic dosage is 10–50 mg IV or IM daily with other factors of the B complex.

Horrigan D: Pyridoxine-responsive anemia. Blood 42:187, 1973.

Folic Acid

Folic acid seems to be essential for the metabolism of cell nuclear materials. It is effective in the treatment of certain macrocytic anemias and in tropical sprue. The recommended daily allowance for adults is 400 μg daily. In pregnancy this is increased to 800 μg and in lactation to 600 μg.

Body reserves of folate may be rapidly depleted in chronic alcoholism. Folate deficiency has been described in chronic alcoholism and in patients taking oral contraceptives and anticonvulsant drugs.

Eichner ER, Pierce HI, Hillman RS: Folate balance in dietary induced megaloblastic anemia. New England J Med 284:933, 1971.

Herbert V: The five possible causes of all nutrient deficiency illustrated by deficiencies of vitamin B_{12} and folic acid. Am J Clin Nutr 26:77, 1973.

Paine CJ & others: Oral contraceptives, serum folate and hematologic status. JAMA 231:731, 1975.

Cyanocobalamin (Vitamin B_{12})

Vitamin B_{12} is an essential phosphorus- and cobalt-containing material isolated from purified liver extract; it is the effective principle (extrinsic factor), found only in animal food sources, which is lacking in pernicious anemia and certain other disorders of gastrointestinal absorption. Qualitative platelet abnormalities have been reported in cases of severe vitamin B_{12} deficiency. Hyperresponse with thrombosis in such cases may follow vitamin B_{12} therapy. It must be emphasized that vitamin B_{12} deficiency of the body is rarely due to inadequate dietary intake, and often there is no primary intestinal disease. (See Pernicious Anemia.) The recommended daily allowance for adults is 3 μg/day.

Herbert V (editor) & others: Symposium on vitamin B_{12} and folate. Am J Med 48:539, 1970.

Levine PH: A qualitative platelet defect in severe vitamin B_{12} deficiency. Ann Int Med 78:533, 1973.

Lindenbaum J, Pezzimenti JF, Shea N: Small intestinal function in vitamin B_{12} deficiency. Ann Int Med 80:326, 1974.

• • •

OBESITY

Obesity is a complex disorder which may be defined as an increase in weight of over 10% above "normal," due to generalized deposition of fat in the body. "Normal" weight is difficult to determine; clinically, however, the standard age, height, and weight tables are ordinarily used for practical purposes, although they are not always reliable. Body build, musculature, familial tendencies, and socioeconomic factors must be taken into consideration. Social factors have a marked influence on the prevalence of obesity, and situational determinants have a great effect on the eating habits of obese persons. It is important to differentiate weight increase due to depot fat from the increase due to body water or lean body mass. Research technics for evaluating the total body fat are available but are not practical for clinical purposes. The measurement of skinfold thickness (triceps fat fold) has been reported to be a simple and reliable method identifying obesity among individuals in the medium range of body size. About 40–50% of the adult population of the USA are considered to be overweight.

From a metabolic point of view, all obesity has a common cause: intake of more calories than are required for energy metabolism. The reasons for differences in the food intake energy utilizations of various individuals, which make it possible for one person to utilize his calories more "efficiently" than another, are not always known. It has been suggested that there is a more effective absorption of foodstuffs from the gut in obese individuals than in lean subjects. Many clinicians feel that the metabolic changes in obesity are a result of obesity rather than a cause of it. Obese patients have been found to have an increased number of fat cells as well as increased size of fat cells. Weight reduction in obese patients may decrease the size of fat cells, but the total number remains constant.

Although most cases of obesity are due to simple overeating resulting from emotional, familial, metabolic, and genetic factors, a few endocrine and metabolic disorders lead to specific types of obesity (eg, Cushing's syndrome and hypothalamic lesions). Compulsive overeating is similar in some respects to the addiction to tobacco or alcohol. It is particularly difficult to explain the phenomena of fluid retention and fat mobilization and storage.

Hypothyroidism is rarely a cause of obesity.

The association of obesity with increased morbidity and mortality is well known. Hypertension, diabetes mellitus, gallbladder disease, gout, and possibly coronary atherosclerosis are frequently associated with obesity. Obesity presents special hazards in pregnancy and in surgical patients. The psychologic and cosmetic implications of obesity are also significant factors.

An obesity-hypoventilation syndrome ("Pickwickian" syndrome) has been described in extremely obese individuals who show little or no evidence of primary disease of the heart or lungs. It is characterized by somnolence, periodic breathing, cyanosis, hypoxia, hypercapnia, respiratory acidosis, secondary polycythemia, pulmonary hypertension, right ventricular hypertrophy, and heart failure. Patients with the obesity-hypoventilation syndrome apparently have predisposing weak inspiratory muscles and a very low chest wall compliance, so that a critical event which causes transient hypercapnia can initiate the self-perpetuating sequence of cardiopulmonary failure. Weight loss appears to reverse the source of the physiologic disturbances but fails to improve the excessive reduction in chest wall compliance.

Treatment

"Specific" weight-reducing chemical agents and hormones (including the currently popular chorionic gonadotropin), singly or in combination, are either ineffective or hazardous and have no place in the treatment of obesity. Juvenile onset obesity is often very difficult to treat, possibly due to some ill-defined metabolic disorder, and it is important to institute a therapeutic program as early as possible.

A. Diet: Diet is the most important factor in the management of obesity. Preventive education about diet should be started during the formative years, at a time when eating habits are being established. The motivation to reduce caloric intake to normal levels is difficult to achieve in patients with long-standing overeating patterns. Diets which claim to offer easy weight reduction by reliance on certain "special" foods or unusual combinations of foods are not only invalid but may actually be harmful. There are a number of points to consider:

1. Calories–In order to lose weight it is necessary to decrease the intake to below the caloric requirements of the individual. An intake of 500 Calories per day less than the required calories should lead to a weight loss of approximately 1 lb (0.5 kg) a week.

The number of calories per day to prescribe for a patient varies with age, occupation, temperament, and the urgency of the need for weight reduction. A daily caloric intake of 800–1200 Calories is satisfactory for a modest reducing diet.

There is no evidence that adequately supervised rapid weight loss is physically harmful. However, all diets should attempt to maintain nitrogen balance, although this is not always possible. In these markedly restricted diets, ketonuria may appear; it is usually very slight after the first few days, however, and acidosis has never been observed. In addition, since the patients realize they are on a "diet," they often will adhere more willingly when they show rapid weight loss than when the results appear slowly.

2. Proteins–A protein intake of at least 1 gm/kg should be maintained. If it is necessary to add protein to the low-calorie diet, protein hydrolysate or casein (free of carbohydrate and fat) can be used.

3. Carbohydrate and fat–To keep the calories and ketosis down, fats must be decreased. After the protein requirements have been met, the remaining calories may be supplied as half carbohydrate and half fat.

4. Vitamins and minerals–Most reducing diets are likely to be deficient in vitamins but adequate in minerals. Therefore, vitamins should be used to supply the average daily maintenance requirements during the time of weight reduction.

5. Sodium restriction–It has been shown that a normal person on a salt-free diet will lose from 2–3 kg; this reduction is temporary, and the weight will return when salt is added to the diet. The same is true of the obese patient, and, although an apparently dramatic effect can be obtained with salt-free diets, it is of no permanent value.

6. Starvation regimen–Total starvation has again

Table 20—5. Low calorie diets: Foods to be distributed into regular meals during the day.*

	800 Calories	1000 Calories	1200 Calories	1500 Calories
Breads, enriched white or whole grain†	1/2 slice	1 slice	2 slices	3 slices
Fruit, unsugared (1/2 cup)	3 servings	3 servings	3 servings	3 servings
Eggs, any way but fried	One	One	One	One
Fats and oils, butter, margarine, mayonnaise, or oil	None	3 tsp	5 tsp	6 tsp
Milk (nonfat, skimmed, or buttermilk)	2 cups	2 cups	2 cups	2 cups
Meat, fish, or poultry, any way but fried‡	4 oz	5 oz	6 oz	6 oz
Vegetables, raw (salads) (1 serving = 1/2 cup)	2 servings	2 servings	2 servings	2 servings
Vegetables, cooked, green, yellow, or soup (1 serving = 1/2 cup)	2 servings	2 servings	3 servings	3 servings
Starch, potato, etc	None	None	None	1 serving
Artificial sweeteners	As desired	As desired	As desired	As desired

*See also Table 20—2.
†May substitute 1/2 cup cooked cereal or 1 cup dry prepared cereal for 1 slice bread.
‡May substitute 1/2 cup cottage cheese or 3 slices (3 oz) cheddar cheese for 3 oz meat.

been advocated as a weight reduction regimen. Although rapid loss of weight can be achieved by this means, the method may be quite hazardous and must be carried out in a hospital setting with strict supervision. Several deaths have occurred. Total starvation results largely in breakdown of fat, but it may also lead to excessive protein breakdown, fainting due to decrease in extracellular fluid volume because of sodium loss, and other unphysiologic results. Massive weight reduction can result in severe hepatic impairment or even fatal hepatic necrosis. Periodic total fasting to the point of producing ketonemia has seemed to cause accelerated weight loss in patients who fail to lose significantly on 1000 Calorie diets. This accelerated weight loss is spurious, however, and represents fluid loss due to ketonuria.

7. Shunt operation—Jejuno-ileal shunt is being performed on selected patients whose massive obesity (ie, 2—3 times ideal weight) has failed to respond to all conservative measures and is considered to be a hazard to physical, psychologic, and socio-economic well-being. The procedure provides permanent weight reduction and alleviates many of the physiologic abnormalities associated with obesity, but the operation is still largely investigative and should be carried out only by experienced surgeons in medical centers with provision for adequate pre- and postoperative care. Patients must be observed carefully for intestinal malabsorption and fluid and electrolyte disturbances. The long-term effects are not known. Hypocalcemia, renal calculi, severe arthropathy, hepatic steatosis, and, more importantly, hepatic cirrhosis may occur.

B. Medication:

1. Appetite suppressants—Amphetamines and other anorexigenic drugs may be of temporary value in aiding selected patients on reducing regimens by decreasing the appetite and giving a sense of well-being. However, because of their relative long-term ineffi-

ciencies and because of the hazard of drug abuse (in the case of the amphetamines), there has been a significant trend away from the use of these drugs. Despite conflicting opinion regarding the efficacy of appetite suppressing drugs, many physicians do not wish to see them eliminated from medical use—at least in initiation of a weight reduction program.

2. Drugs to speed up metabolism—*Note:* There is no satisfactory drug to speed up metabolism. Thyroid has little or no place in the management of obesity. The low BMR associated with obesity is merely due to the fact that BMR is a measurement of oxygen consumption in terms of body surface area.

Tests which actually measure thyroid function (eg, plasma T_3, T_4) are usually normal in obese patients.

It has been shown that obese people with low BMRs can tolerate 0.2 gm or more of thyroid per day without change in BMR. Prolonged administration of thyroid may suppress the patient's normal thyroid secretion.

There is no scientific evidence to support the hypothesis that human chorionic gonadotropin causes mobilization of the "fat accumulated from overeating" or otherwise exerts a physiologic antiobesity effect.

C. Exercise: Although exercise increases the energy output, extreme exercise is necessary to significantly alter weight. Playing 18 holes of an average game of golf, for instance, raises the total caloric requirements only by about 100—150 Calories. However, increase in activity is an important factor in long-range weight maintenance and for general well-being.

D. Psychologic Factors: Overeating is largely a matter of habit and may be associated with varying degrees of emotional problems. Once significant obesity has been established, many secondary psychologic reactions occur relating to altered body image and changes in interpersonal relationships. Weight reduc-

Table 20–6. Caloric values of common "snack" foods.*

	Amount or Average Serving	Calorie Count		Amount or Average Serving	Calorie Count
Sandwiches			**Candies**		
Hamburger on bun	3 inch patty	500	Chocolate bars		
Peanut butter	2 tsp	370	Plain	1 bar (1¼ oz)	190
Cheese	1½ oz	400	With nuts	1 bar	275
Ham	1½ oz	350	Chocolate covered bar	1 bar	250
Beverages			Chocolate cream, bonbon,		
Carbonated drinks, soda,			fudge	1 piece 1 inch square	90
root beer, etc	6 oz glass	80	Caramels, plain	1 piece ¾ inch cube	35
Cola beverages	12 oz glass (Pepsi)	150	Chocolate nut caramels	1 piece	60
Club soda	8 oz glass	5	**Desserts**		
Chocolate malted milk	10 oz glass (1¼ cups)	450	Pie		
Ginger ale	6 oz glass	60	Fruit (apple, etc)	1/6 pie	560
Tea or coffee, no cream			Custard	1/6 pie	360
or sugar	1 cup	0	Lemon meringue	1/6 pie	470
Tea or coffee, with 2 tbsp			Pumpkin pie with		
cream and 2 tsp sugar	1 cup	90	whipped cream	1/6 pie	460
Alcoholic Drinks			Cake		
Ale	8 oz glass	130	2 layers, iced white	1 serving	345
Beer	8 oz glass	110	Fruit, ¼ inch slice	1 serving	125
Highball (with ginger ale)	8 oz glass	140	**Sweets**		
Manhattan	Average	175	Ice cream		
Martini	Average	160	Vanilla	1/2 cup	195
Old-fashioned	Average	150	Chocolate and other		
Sherry	2 oz glass	60	flavors	1/2 cup	200
Scotch, bourbon, rye	1 oz jigger	80	Milk sherbet	1/2 cup	120
Fruits			Sundaes, small chocolate		
Apple	One 3-inch	90	nut with whipped cream	Average	400
Banana	One 6-inch	100	Ice cream sodas, chocolate	10 oz glass	270
Grapes	30 medium	75	**Late Snacks**		
Orange	One 2¾-inch	80	Cold potato	1/2 medium	65
Pear	One	100	Chicken leg	1 average	88
Salted Nuts			Milk	7 oz glass	140
Almonds	10	130	Mouthful of roast	½ × 2 × 3 inches	130
Cashews	10	60	Piece of cheese	¼ × 2 × 3 inches	120
Peanuts	10	60	Left-over beans	1/2 cup	105
Pecans	10 halves	150	Brownie	¾ × 1¾ × 2¼ inches	300
			Cream puff	4 inch diameter	450

*Modified and reprinted by permission of Smith Kline & French Laboratories.

tion is therefore essential for general psychologic as well as physical well-being. Mildly or moderately obese patients often respond to simple psychologic support, encouragement, dietary management, and situational adjustments. Weight relapses occur frequently and should be dealt with in an understanding manner. Conventional psychotherapy, however, is seldom of lasting value in weight reduction in markedly obese patients. Whatever the cause, the patient must be retrained in his eating habits and educated to understand that once his weight is normal he can easily become obese again by eating more than necessary. Behavior modification therapy and self-help groups of obese patients (similar to AA for alcoholics) are effective for some patients.

Note: Sudden weight reduction in emotionally unstable persons may have severe psychic consequences, eg, anorexia nervosa, psychotic reactions.

Bray GA: Measurement of subcutaneous fat cells from obese patients. Ann Int Med 73:565, 1970.

Bray GA, Bethune JE (editors): *Treatment and Management of Obesity.* Harper & Row, 1974.

Coodley A: Neurosis and obesity. (Correspondence.) JAMA 231:571, 1975.

Council on Foods and Nutrition, AMA: A critique of low-carbohydrate, ketogenic weight reduction regimens. [Dr. Atkins' Diet.] JAMA 224:1415, 1973.

Fikri E: Jejunoileal bypass for morbid obesity: Results and complications in 52 patients. Ann Surg 178:460, 1974.

Garb JR, Stunkard AJ: Effectiveness of a self-help group in obesity control. Arch Int Med 134:716, 1974.

Genuth SM, Castro JH, Vertes V: Weight reduction in obesity by outpatient semistarvation. JAMA 230:987, 1974.

Gwinup G: Effect of exercise alone on the weight of obese women. Arch Int Med 135:676, 1975.

Harger BS, Miller JB, Thomas JC: The caloric cost of running: Its impacts on weight reduction. JAMA 228:482, 1974.

Hirsch J: Jejunoileal shunt for obesity. New England J Med 290:962, 1974.

Holzbach RT & others: Hepatic lipid in morbid obesity: Assessment at and after jejunoileal bypass. New England J Med 290:296, 1974.

Lasagna L: Attitudes toward appetite suppressants: A survey of US physicians. JAMA 225:44, 1973.

Mann GV: The influence of obesity on health. (2 parts.) New England J Med 291:178, 226, 1974.

Moxley RT III, Pozefsky T, Lockwood DH: Protein nutrition and liver disease after jejunoileal bypass for morbid obesity. New England J Med 290:921, 1974.

Nelson RA & others: Physiology and natural history of obesity. JAMA 223:627, 1973.

Rivlin RS: Therapy of obesity with hormones. New England J Med 292:26, 1975.

Rochester DF, Enson Y: Current concepts in the pathogenesis of the obesity-hypoventilation syndrome: Mechanical and circulatory factors. Am J Med 57:402, 1974.

Runcie J, Thomson TJ: Prolonged starvation: A dangerous procedure. Brit MJ 3:432, 1970.

Solow C, Silberfarb PM, Swift K: Psychosocial effects of intestinal bypass surgery for severe obesity. New England J Med 290:300, 1974.

Stunkard AJ, Rush J: Dieting and depression reexamined: A critical review of reports of untoward responses during weight reduction for obesity. Ann Int Med 81:526, 1974.

Tullis IF: Rational diet for mild and grand obesity. JAMA 226:70, 1973.

Vaisrub S: Psychoneurosis and obesity: The hen and egg dilemma. JAMA 230:591, 1974.

ANOREXIA NERVOSA

Anorexia nervosa is a relatively uncommon but serious eating disorder which occurs primarily in females (ratio 7:1) in the second and third decades of life and is manifested by an extreme neurotic aversion to food. The exact cause is not known, but multiple etiologic factors play a role. The illness would appear to have its beginnings in complex psychologic problems—conflicts over sexuality, aggression, and dependency—which at times almost border on the psychotic. The patient may have difficulty with self-identification and may associate food with unacceptable sexual fantasies or even with an unconscious repudiation of sexuality. It is not uncommon for the patient to have a mother who is overly concerned with weight reduction and dietary matters. The patient herself may be overly sensitive about adolescent plumpness.

The relationship between the extreme malnutrition which occurs in anorexia nervosa and certain of the observed and theoretical neuroendocrine abnormalities in the illness has not been clearly established. Disturbance of the "feeding center" in the hypothalamus has been postulated on the basis of experimental studies in animals. There is also a specific defect of cyclic gonadotropin release by the anterior pituitary (sparing other pituitary functions) which results in ovulation failure and decreased estrogen production.

The patient's persistent and morbid refusal to eat adequately, even in the face of real hunger, leads to profound weight loss and emaciation. Every type of deceit will be practiced in order to lose weight, including misrepresentation of food intake, concealment of uneaten food, self-induced vomiting, and surreptitious

purgation. Amenorrhea is a constant manifestation in women of child-bearing age; it may rarely precede weight loss and may persist at times after weight loss has been corrected. Patients complain of intolerance to cold.

Fine downy hair may cover the body and the patient may actually appear hirsute. Axillary and pubic hair is normal. There may be clinical and laboratory evidence of vitamin and mineral deficiencies. Nutritional anemia is common. Gonadotropin and 17-ketosteroid levels may be decreased or normal. Anorexia nervosa must be differentiated from panhypopituitarism (see p 650). Anorexia nervosa should not be confused with what seems to be a common striving, motivated by vanity, for a desirably slender figure.

In the rare instance when anorexia nervosa occurs in males, the clinical picture is similar to that in females, with comparable psychologic problems and deficiency of male gonadal function.

Treatment of anorexia nervosa is difficult and is best carried out by individuals trained and experienced in the care of patients with the illness. The patient should be admitted to the hospital for initial restoration of adequate nutritional status. This requires skilled nursing care and close supervision. The patient should be accompanied during meals and should be encouraged to eat by friendly persuasion and insistence. Punitive attitudes and forced feedings must be avoided since they further aggravate the patient's lack of self-confidence and self-identity. Return of normal body weight is usually accompanied by an improvement of the patient's emotional status and sense of physical well-being. Clomiphene is sometimes useful for reestablishing menstruation. Relapses and remissions are common. Long-term psychotherapy and dietary management are usually required.

If untreated—or if inadequately treated—patients with anorexia nervosa may succumb from inanition, complicating infection, or suicide.

Aro A, Lamberg B-A, Pelkonen R: Dysfunction of the hypothalamic-pituitary axis in anorexia nervosa. (Correspondence.) New England J Med 292:594, 1975.

Boyar RM & others: Anorexia nervosa: Immaturity of 24-hour luteinizing hormone secretory pattern. New England J Med 291:861, 1974.

Bruch H: Perils of behavior modification in treatment of anorexia nervosa. JAMA 230:1419, 1974.

Johanson A: Critical body weight in anorexia nervosa. New England J Med 291:904, 1974.

Maxmen JS, Silberfarb PM, Ferrell RB: Anorexia nervosa: Practical initial management in a general hospital. JAMA 229:801, 1974.

PROTEIN & CALORIE MALNUTRITION

Protein and calorie malnutrition occurs in a clinical continuum ranging from inadequate proteins with adequate calories (kwashiorkor) to inadequate proteins and calories (marasmus). These conditions constitute the most important problems in the nutrition of young children throughout the world.

Kwashiorkor

Kwashiorkor is a nutritional deficiency syndrome which usually occurs in weanling infants (usually 2 years of age or older) at the birth of a sibling but may occur in children of any age, and even in adults. It is attributed primarily to inadequate intake of proteins or perhaps of specific essential amino acids with adequate calories, but mineral and vitamin deficiencies may also play a role. It is prevalent in underprivileged sections of Africa, Asia, southern Europe, and Central and South America, in areas where the protein content of the diet is deficient in amount or of poor quality (vegetable protein). The condition may be precipitated by tropical infections, diarrhea, and extreme heat, which aggravate the nutritional deficiency by curtailing the intake, decreasing the absorption, and increasing the demand. The liver shows the most marked pathologic changes: hepatic enlargement and fatty infiltration which may progress to a condition resembling portal cirrhosis. There is also atrophy of the pancreatic acini with loss of granules followed by fibrosis.

Kwashiorkor is characterized clinically by growth failure, irritability and apathy, skin changes (rash, desquamation, hyperpigmentation or depigmentation, ulceration), cheilosis, stomatitis, conjunctivitis, sparse or depigmented hair, anorexia, vomiting, diarrhea, hepatomegaly, muscular wasting, and edema. Blood changes include anemia, hypoalbuminemia, hyperglobulinemia, and low levels of urea, potassium, cholesterol, alkaline phosphatase, amylase, and lipase.

Prevention of the disease is a combined public health and socioeconomic problem and, in cases where personal or cultural food preferences prejudice the protein intake, a psychologic and educational problem. Treatment consists of supplying an adequate intake of protein (3–4 gm/kg) of high biologic value (eg, milk, eggs, meat, soybeans). Patient and regular administration of skimmed or whole milk will often result in rather prompt recovery if the condition is not too far advanced. If oral feeding is a problem, tube feeding may be necessary. Vitamin supplements may be indicated. Intramuscular injection of the water-soluble palmitate has been recommended in severe vitamin A deficiency. Patients who are dehydrated due to vomiting or diarrhea, especially when critically ill, require appropriate oral or parenteral fluid and electrolyte replacement. Concomitant infections require simultaneous treatment. Whole blood or plasma transfusions may be necessary. During the recovery phase, attention should be paid to total calories as well as high-protein intake.

Kwashiorkor syndromes occur in all degrees of severity, and the rate of recovery with proper treatment varies accordingly. Without treatment, the mortality rate in advanced or complicated cases of this disorder is high.

Marasmus

Marasmus, or total starvation, is characterized by retarded growth, atrophy of tissues, no edema, and skin changes as in kwashiorkor. Subcutaneous fat, however, is minimal or absent. The condition may be caused not only by unavailability of food but also by such factors as prematurity, diarrhea, cystic fibrosis, and mental retardation. Treatment is similar to that for kwashiorkor. *Caution:* Initial feedings of the starving patient should be slow and increased gradually; large quantities of food should be avoided. There must be an adequate intake of calories as well as protein.

Goldsmith GA: Current status of malnutrition in the tropics. Am J Trop Med 23:756, 1974.

Hughes WT & others: Protein-calorie malnutrition. Am J Dis Child 128:44, 1974.

Work TH & others: Tropical problems in nutrition. Ann Int Med 79:901, 1973.

SELECTED HEREDITARY METABOLIC DISEASES*

Garrod's original description of 4 inborn errors of metabolism in 1908 was regarded with interest, but these disorders were largely considered to be rare medical curiosities of little clinical importance. The several hundred hereditary metabolic disorders about which we now have at least some knowledge include common and uncommon, benign and serious diseases, metabolic disturbances involving almost every class of biochemical substance, and diseases of all organs and tissues of the body. Newly recognized metabolic disorders are being reported at a rapid rate (see Chapter 31), and this information has contributed greatly to the study of the molecular biology of humans and animals.

Information about metabolic abnormalities is not only of importance in furthering our understanding of hitherto obscure disease processes, but is fundamental to a proper therapeutic approach to them. Old concepts of hereditary transmission of physical traits simply as dominant or recessive have had to be modified to explain the "asymptomatic carriers" of hereditary traits. Biochemical studies on relatives of patients with hereditary metabolic disorders may reveal deficiencies not clinically manifest. Recognition of the heterozygote carrier may be of extreme value from a eugenic point of view (in preventing potentially incompatible matings) and from the standpoint of the health of the individual (eg, in suggesting special dietary control, appropriate medication, and avoidance of drug idiosyncrasies).

Determination of the genetic basis of metabolic disorders is based on the family history and appro-

*Disturbances of lipid metabolism are discussed in Chapter 19.

priate biochemical studies of the patient and available relatives. Biochemical studies may include the determination of essential blood constituents, abnormal protein molecules, specific enzymes, abnormal metabolites, electrolytes, renal transport mechanisms, and tolerance or restriction tests with food or chemicals.

Several of the hereditary metabolic disorders (eg, diabetes mellitus, hyperlipidemia, gout) as they relate to specific organ systems are discussed in other sections of this book. Some examples of other metabolic disorders that are well known or of unusual interest are included in this chapter. (See also Chapter 31.)

Williams HE: Treatment of metabolic diseases of genetic origin. Ration Drug Ther 8:1, 1974.

ABNORMALITY OF MOLECULAR STRUCTURE OF PROTEIN

Methemoglobinemia

Congenital methemoglobinemia is caused either by a deficiency in the specific enzyme, erythrocyte nucleotide diaphorase, required in conversion of methemoglobin to hemoglobin, or by the presence of an abnormal hemoglobin M. Clinically, it is manifested by a persistent gray cyanosis not associated with cardiac or respiratory abnormality, and by easy fatigability, dyspnea, tachycardia, and dizziness with exertion. The venous blood is brown; the oxygen capacity of arterial blood is reduced, and excessive amounts of methemoglobin are present in the blood.

Continuous administration of methylene blue by mouth, 240 mg daily, will relieve the symptoms and cyanosis in some cases. The prognosis for life is good.

Fialkow PH & others: Mental retardation in methemoglobinemia due to diaphorase deficiency. New England J Med 273:840, 1965.

DISORDERS OF AMINO ACID METABOLISM*

Albinism

Albinism is a rare autosomal recessive disorder associated with the absence of tyrosinase or limitation in the availability of tyrosine in the melanocytes and manifest clinically by the absence of pigment in the

*Frimpter GW: Aminoacidurias due to inherited disorders of metabolism. (2 parts.) New England J Med 289:835, 895, 1973.

Ghadini H: Diagnosis of inborn errors of amino acid metabolism. Am J Dis Child 114:433, 1967.

Menkes JH: Disorders of amino acid metabolism—1971. California Med 115:14, Oct 1971.

skin, hair, and eyes. The skin and hair are white, the irides reddish, and the pupils red. Photophobia, nystagmus, and defective vision may occur.

There is no specific treatment. Patients must avoid exposure to strong sunlight.

Alkaptonuria

Alkaptonuria is a rare metabolic disorder inherited as a recessive trait. It is due to absence from the liver of an enzyme, homogentisate oxidase, which is necessary for the oxidation of homogentisic acid. Absence of the enzyme permits homogentisic acid to be excreted unmetabolized in the urine. Diapers or clothing may be stained with homogentisic acid in the urine. Staining of the cartilage of the nose and ears (ochronosis) may occur in older patients, and ochronosis sometimes causes cartilaginous degeneration of joints and severe arthritis. The urine test for homogentisic acid (with dilute ferric chloride solution) produces a transient deep blue color.

No specific treatment is available.

Brown NK, Smuckler EA: Alkaptonuria and Gilbert's syndrome. Am J Med 48:759, 1970.

Phenylketonuria (Phenylpyruvic Oligophrenia, PKU)

Phenylketonuria is a not uncommon metabolic disorder inherited as a recessive trait. It is due to absence of an enzyme, phenylalanine hydroxylase, which is capable of converting phenylalanine to tyrosine. Phenylalanine accumulates in the blood and the deamination product, phenylpyruvic acid, is excreted in the urine. If untreated, mental retardation and schizoid changes almost invariably occur, frequently to a marked degree. Patients are most often blue-eyed blonds and, because of pigmentary defects, are predisposed to photosensitivity and eczema. Physical development is usually normal. There may be signs of extrapyramidal involvement, with tremor, ataxia, and hypertonicity in two-thirds of cases. Perspiration is usually excessive. Convulsions may occur. Pneumoencephalography may show frontal lobe atrophy. Phenylpyruvic acid may be demonstrated in the urine if a dark green color results when dilute ferric chloride is added to acidified urine. Elevated serum phenylalanine levels (> 20 mg/100 ml) are more definitive, but not every newborn infant with phenylalaninemia has PKU because phenylalaninemia may be transient in nature and may also be found in other, unrelated diseases. The optimum time for initial blood phenylalanine determination is apparently not earlier than 6 days of life and not later than 14 days. Blood phenylalanine may be increased in the absence of positive urine findings.

Since present evidence suggests a positive correlation between biochemical findings of untreated (or delayed treatment of) PKU and mental retardation, early further evaluation by a specialist is necessary to either confirm or disprove the diagnosis. For best results, it is important to start feeding formulas low in phenylalanine before 3 weeks of age. Expert dietary treatment is necessary to maintain normal phenylalanine levels (3–7 mg/100 ml) without causing phenyl-alanine depletion and otherwise seriously disturbing the nutritional status of the infant. Although a careful-ly regulated low-phenylalanine diet should be started in the first few weeks of life to prevent mental retarda-tion, in more established cases such a diet may occa-sionally arrest or improve the condition. Patients with PKU who have not received dietary therapy are rarely normal mentally. Routine testing of newborn infants for PKU is common; large-scale detection programs have been established in many areas of the USA.

Ampola MG: Phenylketonuria and other disorders of amino acid metabolism. P Clin North America 20:507, 1973.

Johnson CF: Phenylketonuria and the obstetrician. Obst Gynec 39:942, 1972.

Strafield B, Holtzman NA: A comparison of the effectiveness of screening for phenylketonuria in the United States, United Kingdom and Ireland. New England J Med 293:118, 1975.

Maple Syrup Urine Disease

Maple syrup urine disease is a recessive familial disorder caused by the absence of amino acid decar-boxylase and resulting in a disorder of metabolism of essential branched-chain amino acids. Symptoms usual-ly appear in the first week of life and consist of spasticity, opisthotonos, irregular respirations, and feeding difficulties. The disease may remain dormant until late childhood and may become apparent due to an episode of infection or trauma. A variant of maple syrup urine disease with intermittent branched-chain ketonuria has been described. The relationship between the CNS changes and the amino acid anomaly is not clear.

The urine has a maple sugar odor and gives char-acteristic positive ferric chloride and 2,4-dinitrophenyl-hydrazine reactions. It is possible to detect a hetero-zygous carrier by means of a leucine "loading" test.

If the disease is detected early, a diet low in branched-chain amino acids (leucine, isoleucine, and valine) may prevent brain damage. A new variant of the disease has been described which responds to thi-amine chloride, 10 mg daily. If detected after severe CNS damage has occurred, death occurs within weeks or months.

Elsas LJ & others: Maple syrup urine disease: Coenzyme func-tion and prenatal monitoring. Metabolism 23:569, 1974.

Goodman SI & others: The treatment of maple syrup urine disease. J Pediat 75:489, 1969.

Scriver CR & others: Thiamine-responsive maple syrup urine disease. Lancet 2:310, 1971.

Homocystinuria

Homocystinuria is a rare hereditary disorder of amino acid metabolism. It is believed to be due to a deficiency of the enzyme cystathionine synthetase in the liver, with resultant deficiency of cysteine in the neonatal period, when the need for cysteine is great. The disorder is characterized clinically by frequent occurrence of mental retardation, dislocation of the lenses, sparse blond hair, long thin extremities with genu valgum, tendency to arterial and venous throm-boses, and emotional disturbances. Plasma homo-cystine and methionine levels are elevated. Urinary excretion of homocystine is increased, and the urine shows a characteristic magenta color on the nitroprus-side test. There are, usually, abnormal EEG findings.

There is no agreement about the best method of treatment. A trial of low-methionine diet with cystine, choline, and folic acid supplementation may be war-ranted. Large doses of pyridoxine (up to 500 mg daily) may be of value.

Freeman JM, Finkelstein JD, Mudd SH: Folate-responsive homocystinuria and "schizophrenia." New England J Med 292:491, 1975.

Shih VE, Efron ML: Pyridoxine unresponsive homocystinuria. New England J Med 283:1206, 1970.

Fanconi's Syndrome

Fanconi's syndrome is a hereditary metabolic dis-order, presumably of multiple causes and associated with multiple defects of the renal transport mecha-nisms. It is manifested clinically by emaciation, dwarf-ism, renal rickets or osteomalacia (resistant to vitamin D in the usual doses), dehydration, hypophosphatemia, spontaneous fractures, polyuria, aminoaciduria, pro-teinuria, and glycosuria. The disorder may not become evident until adult life and should be suspected in any case of spontaneous fracture, glycosuria, and amino-aciduria.

Treatment, which is usually ineffective, consists of giving large doses of vitamin D, alkalinization of the urine with sodium or potassium bicarbonate, and ade-quate hydration. Patients usually die of renal failure.

Efron ML: Aminoaciduria. (2 parts.) New England J Med 272:1058, 1107, 1965.

Hartnup's Disease (H Disease)

Hartnup's disease is a rare genetic defect in the renal transport mechanism for tryptophan. Clinical findings consist of photodermatitis, cerebellar ataxia, mental retardation, renal aminoaciduria, and increased excretion of indole and indican compounds.

Treatment consists of hydration to prevent the formation of renal calculi. Dietary protein restriction and treatment with niacinamide are of questionable value.

Halvorsen K, Halvorsen S: Hartnup's disease. Pediatrics 31:29, 1963.

Leucine Sensitivity Disease

Leucine sensitivity disease is a genetic metabolic disorder characterized by abnormal hypoglycemia and is due to leucine sensitivity. Clinically it is manifest as hypoglycemia, flushing, sweating, and convulsions. It is important to consider leucine sensitivity in infants with hypoglycemia. Sensitivity to the hypoglycemic effects of leucine may also occur in insulinoma and so-called idiopathic hypoglycemia. Intravenous leucine may cause a slight fall in blood sugar in healthy subjects.

No specific treatment is available.

Fajan SS: Current concepts: Leucine-induced hypoglycemia. New England J Med 272:1224, 1965.

DISORDERS OF CARBOHYDRATE METABOLISM

Fructosuria, Essential

Fructosuria is an inborn error of metabolism which is probably due to a deficiency of hepatic fructokinase, resulting in elevated blood levels of fructose and excretion of fructose in the urine. The condition is usually diagnosed on routine urinalysis. The urine sugar test paper reaction utilizing glucose oxidase is negative. However, if the diet contains large quantities of foods rich in fructose and sucrose, a considerable proportion of dietary carbohydrate may be lost.

Froesch ER: Essential fructosuria and hereditary fructose intolerance. In: *The Metabolic Basis of Inherited Disease,* 3rd ed. Stanbury JB, Wyngaarden JB, Fredrickson DS (editors). McGraw-Hill, 1972.

Fructosemia

Hereditary fructose intolerance is a rare inborn error of carbohydrate metabolism due to a deficiency of fructose-1,6-diphosphate aldolase. Fructose intolerance may first be noted when susceptible infants are started on bottle feeding. Gastrointestinal symptoms and hypoglycemic reactions with CNS manifestations may occur, and death may result from inanition or coma. Fructosemia may be chronic and, in addition to the periodic hypoglycemic episodes, there may be hepatosplenomegaly, jaundice, abnormal liver function, fructosuria, and evidence of defective renal transport mechanisms (Fanconi's syndrome).

Prevention is the only treatment. Patients with this hereditary disorder must avoid fructose in any form—fruits, sucrose, sorbitol, or *intravenous fluids which contain fructose* (caution).

Hereditary fructose intolerance. FDA Drug Bull 5:6, June-July 1975.
Levin B & others: Fructosaemia. Am J Med 45:826, 1968.

Galactosemia

Galactosemia is an inborn error of metabolism which is due to a deficiency of the enzyme galactose-1-phosphate uridyl transferase. This enzyme is necessary for the conversion of galactose to glucose. Clinically the disorder becomes manifest soon after birth by feeding problems, vomiting, diarrhea, abdominal distention, hepatomegaly, jaundice, ascites, cataracts, mental retardation, and elevated blood and urine galactose levels. Transferase deficiency can be detected at birth by the enzyme fluorescence spot test on umbilical cord specimens.

Exclusion from the diet of milk and all foods containing galactose and lactose for the first 3 years of life will prevent the above manifestations if instituted immediately and will bring about improvement in those patients in whom symptoms and signs have already appeared.

Tedesco TA & others: The genetic defect in galactosemia. New England J Med 292:737, 1975.

Von Gierke's Disease

Von Gierke's disease is a rare inborn error of metabolism characterized by the excessive deposition of glycogen in the liver and kidney, secondary to a deficiency of the enzyme glucose-6-phosphatase, which is required for the degradation of glycogen to glucose. The disorder becomes manifest in infancy or early childhood by easy fatigability, hepatomegaly (glycogen deposition), and hypoglycemia and ketosis (unavailability of glucose) with resulting shock and convulsions. The serum glucose does not respond to the epinephrine test.

Treatment is directed toward improvement of nutrition and correction of the hypoglycemia by frequent feedings. Corticotropin or the corticosteroids may be of some value. Death usually occurs in infancy or childhood, but if the patient survives this period the symptoms usually lessen as the child grows older.

Hsia DYY: The diagnosis and management of the glycogen storage disease. Am J Clin Path 50:44, 1968.

DISORDERS OF PORPHYRIN METABOLISM

The porphyrins are cyclic compounds containing 4 pyrrole rings which are the precursors of heme and of other important enzymes and pigments. Heme is the complex of iron and porphyrin which unites with the protein globin to form hemoglobin. Disorders of porphyrin metabolism, which may be hereditary or acquired, are due to disturbances in the anabolic sequence of porphyrin metabolism. There has been considerable progress recently in elucidating the nature of the metabolic changes. Several heterogeneous porphyric syndromes are recognized: (1) hereditary porphyrias, either hepatic (hepatogenic) or erythropoietic (congenital); and (2) acquired porphyrinurias, which have in common the excessive excretion of the porphyrins or porphyrin precursors.

Hepatic Porphyrias

The hepatic porphyrias are usually hereditary disorders characterized by excessive production of porphyrins and related compounds by the liver. They become clinically and biochemically manifest only after puberty. Mixed or combined hepatic porphyrias may occur. The porphyric trait, as manifested biochemically, may exist in completely asymptomatic individuals.

A. Acute Intermittent Porphyria: This is the most common type of porphyria. It is an autosomal dominant hereditary disorder and occurs most frequently in women. It is manifested by an extremely wide range of symptoms which can perhaps best be grouped according to nervous system involvement: (1) Autonomic neuropathy: Abdominal colic, nausea, vomiting, constipation or diarrhea, tachycardia, labile blood pressure, sweating, bladder symptoms, and peripheral vascular spasm. (2) Peripheral neuropathy: Flaccid paralysis, muscle and back pain, and cranial nerve palsies. (3) Cortical dysfunction: Psychic disturbances, convulsions, coma. (4) Hypothalamic dysfunction: Inappropriate release of antidiuretic and growth hormones, lactation.

Photosensitivity does not occur. Blood volume decreases by about 20% during attacks. The urine, which contains porphobilinogen, is most often colorless when freshly voided, but may darken on standing or when exposed to ultraviolet light. The modified Ehrlich test of the urine (Watson-Schwartz test) is positive. Type III coproporphyrin and uroporphyrin may be excreted in the urine in large quantities. The decreased activity of erythrocyte uroporphyrinogen I (URO)-synthetase in acute intermittent porphyria can be used for the identification of apparently unaffected carriers. Acute attacks may be precipitated by sulfonamides, anticonvulsants, barbiturates, alcohols, steroids, and many other chemicals, as well as by menses, pregnancy (postpartum), infections, fasting, and psychic trauma.

Treatment is nonspecific. Recent studies have demonstrated that freshly prepared hematin can effectively suppress the hepatic limiting enzyme of porphyrin biosynthesis and produce clinical and chemical remission of acute intermittent porphyria. Phenothiazine drugs given early in the attack may lessen the severity of symptoms purely as a tranquilizer effect. All other drugs or toxins (especially barbiturates and alcohol) must be avoided. A high carbohydrate diet is recommended.

The overall mortality rate is 15–20%. Death usually occurs as a result of motor paralysis during an acute attack. Most patients, however, survive acute attacks, and the prognosis for life is much better than was formerly believed.

B. Porphyria Cutanea Tarda: This purely cutaneous type occurs most commonly in middle-aged persons. Although it is sometimes hereditary, it usually occurs secondary to other liver disorders. The condition is found most commonly in chronic alcoholism but may follow systemic lupus erythematosus and estrogen and iron administration. There is varying photosensitivity of the skin, resulting in eczema, vesicles, and bullae. The hepatic content of porphyrin is greatly increased, and liver function is impaired. Mild jaundice may be present. There is no porphobilinogen in the urine, but uroporphyrin excretion is high and coproporphyrin excretion is low.

Treatment consists of protection of skin from strong light and complete abstinence from alcohol, estrogens, and iron salts. Phlebotomy, with removal of 2500–8500 ml of blood over a period of 3–9 months, has been reported to markedly reduce uroporphyrin excretion associated with a clinical remission in all patients.

Congenital Erythropoietic Porphyria

This is a rare, inherited disorder transmitted as an autosomal recessive trait. It is usually evident from birth and is due to an abnormality of developing normoblasts in the bone marrow which causes increased production of porphyrin. It is characterized by red urine, pink teeth which fluoresce with ultraviolet light, cutaneous photosensitivity with resultant vesicles, bullae, and scarring and pigmentation of the skin, hepatosplenomegaly, and anemia. Porphobilinogen is absent from the urine, but there are large amounts of type I coproporphyrin and uroporphyrin in the feces and urine.

Congenital erythropoietic porphyria must be differentiated from the more recently described erythropoietic protoporphyria. In the latter condition, vesicles and bullae and anemia are rare, and protoporphyrins are increased in the plasma and feces.

Treatment consists of protection against sunlight and ultraviolet light. β-Carotene (Solatene) in high doses (15–180 mg/day) as an oral photoprotective agent has been reported to be a safe and effective method of ameliorating photosensitivity in most patients. Splenectomy may sometimes be of value when hemolysis is present. Few patients in the past have survived beyond 40 years of age.

Acquired (Secondary) Porphyrinurias

Secondary or "symptomatic" porphyrinurias (coproporphyrinurias) may follow poisoning with lead or other heavy metals and many other organic and inorganic poisons. They may also occur in the hemolytic and pernicious anemias, parenchymal liver disease, obstructive jaundice, the collagen diseases, and CNS disorders.

Bloomer JR & others: Blood volume and bilirubin production in acute intermittent porphyria. New England J Med 284:17, 1971.

Marver HS, Schmid R: The porphyrias. In: *The Metabolic Basis of Inherited Disease,* 3rd ed. Stanbury JB, Wyngaarden JB, Fredrickson DS (editors). McGraw-Hill, 1972.

Mathews-Roth MM & others: β-Carotene as an oral photoprotective agent in erythropoietic protoporphyria. JAMA 228:1004, 1974.

Petryka ZJ, Cardinal R, Watson CJ: Effects of hematin on hepatic porphyria. Ann Int Med 83:20, 1975.

OTHER METABOLIC DISORDERS

Cystic Fibrosis (Mucoviscidosis)

Pancreatic cystic fibrosis is a recessive inherited disease causing dysfunction of the exocrine glands of the pancreas, respiratory system, and sweat glands. It usually begins in infancy, and is manifested by steatorrhea, malnutrition, repeated pulmonary infections, bronchitis, viscid sputum, and excessive sodium and chloride loss in the sweat (leading often to heat exhaustion in hot weather or during febrile episodes). Pancreatic enzymes are present in decreased amounts in the stools.

Treatment consists of a high-protein, high-caloric diet, moderate fat restriction, high doses of vitamins (especially vitamin A), and pancreatin to aid digestion. Supplementary salt should be given during hot weather. Both physical and chemical means should be used to decrease viscosity of pulmonary secretions and help in their removal and to provide for adequate ventilation of the lungs. Infections (especially respiratory infections) should be guarded against and treated promptly with antibiotics when they occur. Prophylactic antibiotics are not recommended for patients without pulmonary involvement.

The disease is not curable, but, since its recognition as a disease is only recent, long-term survival figures are not available. Patients with cystic fibrosis are already known to have lived beyond the age of 40.

Berry HK & others: Dietary supplement and nutrition in children with cystic fibrosis. Am J Dis Child 129:165, 1975.
Lieberman J, Rodbard S: Low blood pressure in young adults with cystic fibrosis. Ann Int Med 82:806, 1975.
Moss AJ, Dooley RR, Mickey MR: Cystic fibrosis complicated by heart failure. Western J Med 122:471, 1975.

Primary Hyperoxaluria (Oxalosis)

Primary hyperoxaluria is a rare autosomal recessive hereditary metabolic disease characterized by a continuously high urinary excretion of oxalate (unrelated to dietary intake of oxalate). Two types of hyperoxaluria are now recognized. In the most common type (type I, or glycolic aciduria), excessive amounts of oxalic, glycolic, and glyoxylic acids are excreted in the urine. In type II hyperoxaluria (L-glyceric aciduria), which is due to a different metabolic defect, only oxalic and glyceric acids are excreted in excess in the urine.

Hyperoxaluria is manifested clinically by progressive bilateral calcium oxalate urolithiasis, nephrocalcinosis, and recurrent urinary tract infections. Death usually occurs early as a result of renal failure or hypertension.

There is no specific treatment, although a low-oxalate diet and hydration to increase solubility may be of some help. Pyridoxine, 100–150 mg orally daily, may reduce oxalate excretion. Calcium carbimide, 1 mg/kg orally daily used carefully over a prolonged period, has had limited success. Renal transplantation has been reported to be successful in a patient with renal failure.

Saxon A & others: Renal transplantation in primary hyperoxaluria. Arch Int Med 133:464, 1974.
Solomon CC, Goodman SL, Riley CM: Calcium carbimide in the treatment of primary hyperoxaluria. New England J Med 276:207, 1967.
Williams HE, Smith LH Jr: L-Glyceric aciduria: A new genetic variant of primary oxaluria. New England J Med 278:233, 1968.

Marfan's Syndrome

Marfan's syndrome is an autosomal dominant hereditary disorder of connective tissue, the basic metabolic defect of which remains unknown. Marfan's syndrome may be quite similar to the picture seen in patients with homocystinuria. The disease involves primarily the skeletal system, the cardiovascular system, and the eyes, but there are many other clinical manifestations. These patients are tall and thin. The extremities are long in relation to the trunk: The hands are spider-like (arachnodactyly), with thin, tapered, webbed fingers. Pes planus, pes cavus, and hammer toes may be present. "Tower skull" (long, narrow, and pointed head) and a high palatal arch are common findings. Winging of the scapulas and pigeon or funnel chest may occur. Dislocation of the lens (ectopia lentis), myopia, detached retinas, and other ocular abnormalities may be present. Cardiovascular deformities may include dilatation of the aorta and pulmonic arteries, with resultant valvular insufficiency, dissecting aneurysm, and occasionally atrial septal defect. Serum mucoproteins are low, and urinary excretion of hydroxyproline is increased. Mild, incomplete (atypical) forms of the disease may exist.

Treatment is directed toward cardiovascular complications and is otherwise merely symptomatic and supportive. The mortality rate during infancy is high. Death is usually due to cardiac complications.

Bear ES: Marfan's syndrome with complete heart block and junctional rhythm. JAMA 217:335, 1971.
McKusick VA: *Heritable Disorders of Connective Tissue,* 4th ed. Mosby, 1972.

●   ●   ●

AMYLOIDOSIS

Amyloidosis is a poorly understood disorder of protein metabolism which usually occurs secondary to chronic inflammatory diseases and plasma cell disorders but which may also occur as the so-called "primary" type in patients without apparent preexisting disease. The onset is insidious, and the clinical manifestations may vary widely depending upon the organs or tissues in which the peculiar homogeneous, filamentous glycoprotein (amyloid) substance is deposited extracellularly. There appears to be a relationship between amyloidosis and the various other diseases associated with abnormalities of the serum globulins (eg, multiple myeloma).

Four clinical types of amyloidosis have been described:

(1) Primary systemic amyloidosis, a relatively rare disorder, may occur in hereditary form or as sporadic cases in patients without known preexisting disease. Hereditary amyloidosis is usually transmitted as an autosomal trait. In the case of familial periodic fever, the amyloidosis can rarely be the initial manifestation or it may appear in the late stage of the illness, with renal involvement. Amyloid is deposited chiefly in mesenchymal tissues, with resultant involvement of many organs. Attempts have been made to classify hereditary amyloidosis according to principal organ involvement, ethnic, and genetic data, but there would appear to be overlap. Manifestations are highly variable and may include weakness, fever, weight loss, purpura, macroglossia, lymphadenopathy, abdominal pain, hepatosplenomegaly, congestive heart failure, nephropathy, neuropathy, and abnormality of serum proteins.

(2) Amyloidosis associated with multiple myeloma may be a variation of the primary systemic type, but the relationship is uncertain.

(3) Primary localized (tumor-forming) amyloidosis is a rare disorder involving the skin, thyroid, and upper respiratory tract (eg, the larynx), again in the absence of preexisting disease and without evidence of amyloidosis in other tissues.

(4) Secondary amyloidosis, the most common type, is associated with chronic inflammatory and suppurative disorders. Amyloid is deposited widely in parenchymatous organs. (The liver, spleen, kidneys, and adrenal glands are most frequently involved.) Tuberculosis is the most common predisposing cause, but the condition may also follow rheumatoid arthritis, ulcerative colitis, chronic osteomyelitis, and other chronic wasting and suppurative disorders.

The diagnosis of amyloidosis is based first on a suspicion that it may be present, since clinical manifestations may be varied and atypical. The family medical pedigree may reveal a hereditary origin. Preexisting long-standing infection or debilitating illness should suggest the possibility of its existence. Microscopic examination of biopsy (eg, gingival, renal, rectal) or surgical specimens after suitable staining procedures is diagnostic. It has been reported that fine needle biopsy of subcutaneous abdominal fat is a simple and reliable method for diagnosing secondary systemic amyloidosis. Intravenous injection of Congo red in patients with systemic amyloidosis results in a 90–100% disappearance of the dye within 1 hour (normally, less than 40% is removed).

Treatment of localized amyloid "tumors" is by surgical excision. There is no effective treatment of systemic amyloidosis, and death usually occurs within 1–3 years. Variable effectiveness of corticosteroids has been reported. Treatment of the predisposing disease may cause a temporary remission or slow the progress of the disease, but it is unlikely that the established metabolic process is altered. Early and adequate treatment of pyogenic infections will probably prevent much secondary amyloidosis. Since the advent of antibiotic and other anti-infective drugs for the prompt and effective treatment of infection, the incidence of amyloidosis is expected to decline.

Alexander F, Atkins EL: Familial renal amyloidosis: Case reports, literature review and classification. Am J Med 59:121, 1975.

Amyloidosis. In: *Primer on the Rheumatic Diseases.* JAMA 224 (Suppl):721, 1973.

Cohen HJ & others: Resolution of primary amyloidosis during chemotherapy. Ann Int Med 82:466, 1975.

Franklin EC: The complexity of amyloid. New England J Med 290:512, 1974.

Lowenstein J, Gallo G: Remission of the nephrotic syndrome in renal amyloidosis. New England J Med 282:128, 1970.

Westermark P, Stenkvist B: A new method for the diagnosis of systemic amyloidosis. Arch Int Med 132:522, 1973.

21 . . .
Introduction to Infectious Diseases

Ernest Jawetz & Moses Grossman

Infections can and do involve all human organ systems. In a book organized, as this one is, principally by organ system, many important infectious disease entities are discussed in the chapters devoted to specific anatomic areas. Thus, pneumonias are discussed in Chapter 6, Respiratory Tract & Mediastinum; infective endocarditis in Chapter 7, Heart & Great Vessels; and urinary tract infections in Chapter 15, Genitourinary Tract. Other important infections are described under the heading of the etiologic agent in Chapters 22–27.

In this introductory chapter, we wish to focus on a few broad problems of infectious disease which touch upon many facets of diagnosis and treatment. To minimize duplication, we will refer to other areas of this book for more detailed or supplementary information.

FEVER OF UNDETERMINED ORIGIN (FUO)*

Fever of undetermined origin is defined as an illness of at least 3 weeks' duration with fever over 38° C (100.4° F) as the principal symptom. This "diagnosis" should not be entertained until routine diagnostic procedures, including repeated cultures of blood, tissues, and urine, skin and serologic tests, search for neoplasm or evidence of collagen vascular disease, etc, have failed to permit a specific etiologic diagnosis. Most cases of FUO are eventually found to represent atypical manifestations of common diseases rather than exotic illnesses.

Etiologic Considerations

It is important to proceed systematically in approaching this difficult diagnostic problem. Every effort should be made to identify infectious processes, obscure malignancies, and autoimmune or collagen vascular diseases. Miscellaneous causes constitute a fourth major etiologic category.

A. Infectious Processes: It is well to consider systemic infections and localized infections separately. The former include tuberculosis, disseminated mycoses, infective endocarditis, infectious mononucleosis,

cytomegalovirus infection, toxoplasmosis, brucellosis, salmonellosis, and many other less common diseases.

The most common form of localized infection is an obscure abscess. Liver, spleen, kidney, brain, and bone are organs where an abscess may be difficult to find. Likewise, a collection of pus may form in the peritoneal cavity or in the subdiaphragmatic, subhepatic, paracolonic, or other areas. Cholangitis, urinary tract infection, dental abscess, or a collection of pus in a paranasal sinus may cause prolonged fever before it is identified.

B. Neoplasms: Many malignancies may present with obscure fever as a major symptom. The most common of these are lymphoma and leukemia. Carcinoma of the head of the pancreas, the colon, and other areas may also be associated with fever.

C. Autoimmune Diseases: Juvenile rheumatoid arthritis is an excellent example of a disease in which fever continues for a long time as almost the only symptom. This may occur also in adult rheumatoid arthritis, polyarteritis, and other collagen vascular disorders.

D. Miscellaneous Causes: Many other diseases can cause prolonged fever. Examples are sarcoidosis, other noncaseating granulomas, pulmonary embolization, chronic liver disease, and familial Mediterranean fever.

Approach to Diagnosis

An individual diagnostic plan based on clues obtained by the history and physical examination should be prepared. Tissue biopsy may reveal the diagnosis. Lymph node biopsy is most helpful when there is regional rather than generalized adenopathy. For each biopsy, a careful plan for the study of the tissue should be arranged, eg, touch preparations and special fixatives for histologic examination and culture in several media for *Mycobacterium tuberculosis,* other bacteria, and fungi. Needle biopsy of the liver may be helpful, particularly in miliary tuberculosis. Exploratory laparotomy may be useful when intra-abdominal disease is suspected.

It is most important to diagnose diseases for which effective treatment is available and early institution of therapy may be curative.

With the passage of time, the true cause of fever often becomes apparent; thus, it may be helpful to repeat tests which previously were noncontributory.

*This entity is discussed also in Chapter 1.

About 10% of cases of FUO remain undiagnosed. Therapeutic trials without diagnosis are seldom indicated. There is little benefit in suppressing the fever as such, but doing it may make the patient more comfortable.

Altemeier WA & others: Intra-abdominal abscesses. Am J Surg 125:70, 1973.

Jacoby GA, Swartz MN: Fever of undetermined origin. New England J Med 289:1407, 1973.

Petersdorf RG, Beeson PB: Fever of unexplained origin: Report on 100 cases. Medicine 40:1, 1961.

Pizzo PA & others: Prolonged fever in children: Review of 100 cases. Pediatrics 55:418, 1975.

INFECTIONS IN THE IMMUNODEFICIENT PATIENT

Immunodeficiency may be congenital but more often is due to suppression of the immune system by diseases or drugs. Deficiencies of polymorphonuclear (PMN) cells, T-lymphocytes, or B-lymphocytes tend to predispose the host to infection with different agents. For example, PMN deficiency predisposes to infection with gram-negative or gram-positive bacteria; B-lymphocyte deficiency, infection with extracellular bacteria such as pneumococci and staphylococci; and T-lymphocyte deficiency, infection with intracellular bacteria (mycobacteria, listeria, etc), fungi (candida, aspergillus, etc), protozoa (pneumocystis, etc), and viruses (herpes simplex, etc).

Many opportunistic organisms (ie, organisms which rarely produce invasive infections in an uncompromised host) do not produce disease except in the immunodeficient host. Such hosts are often infected with a number of pathogens simultaneously.

Infections caused by common organisms may present uncommon clinical manifestations. Determination of the specific infecting agents is essential for effective treatment.

Immunodeficient Hosts

Patients deficient in normal immune defenses fall into several groups:

(1) Congenital immune defects of cellular or humoral immunity or a combination of both, eg, Wiskott-Aldrich syndrome. These are usually children.

(2) Patients with malignancy, particularly lymphoreticular malignancy.

(3) Patients receiving immunosuppressive therapy. These include patients with neoplastic disease and those bearing transplants who are receiving corticosteroids or other immunosuppressive drugs.

(4) Patients who have very few PMNs (> 1000/cu mm) or those whose PMNs do not function normally with respect to phagocytosis or the intracellular killing of phagocytosed microorganisms (eg, chronic granulomatous disease).

(5) A larger group of patients who are not classically immunodeficient but whose host defenses are seriously compromised by debilitating illness, surgical or other invasive procedures (eg, intravenous drug abuse or intravenous hyperalimentation), burns, or massive antimicrobial therapy.

Infectious Agents

A. Bacteria: Any bacterium pathogenic for man can infect the immunosuppressed host. Furthermore, noninvasive and nonpathogenic organisms (opportunists) may also cause disease in such cases. Examples include gram-negative bacteria—particularly pseudomonas, serratia, and aeromonas. Many of these come from the hospital environment and are resistant to antimicrobial drugs.

B. Fungi: Candida, aspergillus, cryptococcus, nocardia, and mucor can all cause disease in the immunosuppressed host. Candidiasis (see p 887) is by far the most common and is often found in patients receiving intensive antimicrobial therapy.

C. Viruses: Cytomegalovirus is the most common, but varicella-zoster and herpes simplex viruses are also important. Vaccinia virus may cause serious problems if inadvertently inoculated.

D. Protozoa: *Pneumocystis carinii* (see pp 120 and 862) is an important cause of pneumonia in many immunodeficient patients. It is particularly important to make this diagnosis early because reasonably effective therapy is available. *Toxoplasma gondii* (see p 861) is also important in this group of patients.

Approach to Diagnosis

A systematic approach is necessary, including the following steps:

(1) Review carefully the patient's current immune status, previous antimicrobial therapy, and *all* previous culture reports.

(2) Obtain pertinent cultures for bacteria, fungi, and viruses.

(3) Consider which of the serologic tests for fungal, viral, and protozoal diseases are pertinent.

(4) Consider special diagnostic procedures, eg, lung biopsy or lung puncture or endobronchial brush biopsy to demonstrate pneumocystis.

(5) Consider whether the infection (eg, candidiasis) is superficial or systemic. Therapeutic considerations are quite different in each case.

Approach to Treatment

Caution: It is essential to avoid aggravating the patient's other problems and to avoid gross alterations of the host's normal microbial flora.

Provide general therapeutic measures to improve host defenses, correct electrolyte imbalance, offer adequate caloric intake, etc. Improve the patient's immune status whenever possible. This includes temporary decrease in immunosuppressive drug dosage in transplant patients and modification of chemotherapy in cancer patients.

Granulocyte transfusions may be able to tide the patient over a period of PMN deficiency. Injection of human gamma globulin at regular intervals may compensate for certain B cell deficiencies.

Antimicrobial drug therapy should be specific for the infecting agent and should be lethal for it. Combinations of chemotherapeutic agents may be necessary since multiple infectious agents may be involved.

Note: Many of the drugs used for these infections are seldom used in general practice (eg, pentamidine), and some are quite toxic (eg, amphotericin B). Great care should be exercised in using these agents, and more so when they are used in combination.

Anderson RJ & others: The infectious risk factor in the immunosuppressed host. Am J Med 54:453, 1973.

Gold E: Infections associated with immunologic deficiency diseases. M Clin North America 58:649, 1974.

Klastersky J & others: Therapy with carbenicillin and gentamicin for patients with cancer and severe infections caused by gram-negative rods. Cancer 31:331, 1973.

Remington JS: The compromised host. Hosp Practice 7:59, April 1972.

Walzer PD & others: *Pneumocystis carinii* pneumonia in the US. Ann Int Med 80:83, 1974.

GRAM-NEGATIVE BACTEREMIA & SEPSIS

During the past 2 decades, the frequency and mortality rates of bacteremias due to pneumococci and hemolytic streptococci have greatly diminished while those of bacteremias due to staphylococci have remained about the same. However, bacteremia and sepsis caused by gram-negative bacteria and fungi—especially in hospitals—have increased greatly in incidence and severity during this period. Factors responsible for this shift are larger numbers of debilitated or immunodeficient patients, more extensive surgical procedures, greater use of invasive diagnostic and therapeutic procedures, and the relentless selection pressure of antimicrobial drugs within individual patients and within hospital populations which favors the survival and proliferation of drug-resistant gram-negative bacteria, yeasts, and fungi.

The following are among the most frequent events leading up to gram-negative bacteremia and sepsis:

(1) Urinary tract infection, cystoscopy, catheterization (especially with an indwelling catheter), and urologic surgery.

(2) Tracheostomy, use of respirators with aerosol, use of endotracheal tubes.

(3) Intravenous infusion (plastic catheter needle) without changing site frequently; thrombophlebitis; contaminated solutions; intravenous drug abuse by addicts.

(4) Postsurgical infection, especially during antimicrobial therapy.

(5) Infected burns, wounds; delivery or abortion; perforation of an abdominal viscus.

(6) Severe neutropenia, eg, due to malignancy with or without chemotherapy.

Clinical Findings

A. Symptoms and Signs: The onset might be with a shaking chill followed by an abrupt rise of fever. Alternatively, the patient may only appear flushed and anxious, with moderate temperature elevation. Soon there may be a fall in blood pressure or even frank shock with greatly impaired organ perfusion (kidney, brain, heart), anuria, nitrogen retention, acidosis, circulatory collapse, and death.

Unless the sequence of clinical signs can be reversed early, the mortality rate may be 50% or higher.

B. Laboratory Findings: Initial leukopenia may be present and is often followed by moderate leukocytosis. Proteinuria may precede a drastic reduction in urine volume. There may be evidence of metabolic acidosis or respiratory alkalosis and of disseminated intravascular coagulation (DIC) (see p 315).

Treatment

The consequences of irreversible gram-negative shock are so grave that the clinician must constantly be on guard (see list of predisposing factors, above). Whenever a suspicion of gram-negative bacteremia arises, immediate blood cultures must be taken and a survey of potential sources of infection (catheters, infusions, thrombophlebitis, abscesses) must be carried out. Prompt elimination of these sources is often the most important step in the management of bacteremic shock. Gram-positive bacteremia may occasionally also precipitate shock.

A. Antibiotic Drugs: Suspected or proved gram-negative bacteremia must be promptly and intensively treated with antimicrobial drugs. Selection of the best initial drug depends on the most likely source and type of organisms and on the pattern of drug susceptibility which prevails in a given locality in a given year. In 1975, gentamicin (5 mg/kg/day IM) is the most widely used first drug, sometimes combined with a penicillin (carbenicillin, 30 gm/day IV, or ampicillin, 300 mg/kg/day IV) or a cephalosporin (cephalothin, 12 gm/day IV, or cefazolin, 4 gm/day IM).

B. Management of Shock: (See also discussion in Chapter 1.) Management of bacteremic shock is directed at maintenance of organ perfusion, ventilation, correction of acidosis, and improvement of cardiac function. A central venous pressure (CVP) line is usually placed to monitor maintenance of CVP at 8–12 cm water by various corrective measures. Plasma volume expanders (blood plasma, dextran, electrolyte solutions) are given to maintain organ perfusion and correct the prominent lactic acidosis but avoid pulmonary edema. Cardiac output may be increased by drugs such as isoproterenol (1–2 μg/minute by IV drip) and especially by dopamine. This sympathomimetic amine dilates mesenteric and renal vessels (and thus increases renal blood flow and urine output) in addition to increasing cardiac output if infused in doses of 2–10 μg/kg/minute. Vasoconstrictors such as levarterenol may further restrict organ perfusion and are therefore used sparingly in the early treatment of bacteremic shock. Very large doses of corticosteroids (eg, 2–5 gm hydrocortisone IV) have been administered, but their efficacy remains uncertain. Betamethasone, 1 mg/kg/day IV in 2 doses daily, had no effect on the mortality rate in a controlled study. Heparinization may be considered in DIC.

Prognosis

Persistent gram-negative bacteremia has a high mortality rate—often more than 50%. Bad prognostic signs include hypothermia during bacteremia, severe underlying disease, azotemia, and shock. Failure to drain collections of pus adequately usually interferes with the response to antimicrobial therapy.

Bryant RE & others: Factors affecting mortality of gram-negative rod bacteremia. Arch Int Med 127:120, 1971.

Harris JA, Cobbs, CG: Persistent gram-negative bacteremia. Am J Surg 125:705, 1973.

Martin CM & others: Prevention of gram-negative rod bacteremia associated with indwelling urinary tract catheterization. Page 617 in: *Antimicrobial Agents and Chemotherapy.* American Society of Microbiology, 1973.

ANAEROBIC INFECTIONS*

A large majority of the bacteria which make up the normal human flora are anaerobes. Prominent members of the normal microbial flora of the mouth (anaerobic spirochetes, bacteroides, fusobacteria), the skin (anaerobic diphtheroids), the large bowel (bacteroides, anaerobic streptococci, clostridia), and the female genital tract (bacteroides, anaerobic streptococci, fusobacteria) may produce disease when displaced from their normal sites into tissues or closed body spaces.

Certain characteristics are suggestive of anaerobic infections: (1) They tend to involve mixtures of organisms, frequently several anaerobes. (2) They tend to form closed-space infections, either in discrete abscesses (lung, brain, pleura, peritoneum) or by burrowing through tissue layers. (3) Pus from anaerobic infections often has a foul odor. (4) Septic thrombophlebitis and metastatic suppurative lesions are frequent and often require surgical drainage in addition to antimicrobial therapy. (Most of the important anaerobes except *Bacteroides fragilis* are highly sensitive to penicillin G, but the diminished blood supply which favors proliferation of anaerobes because of reduced tissue oxygenation also interferes with the delivery of antimicrobials to the site of anaerobic infection.) (5) Bacteriologic examination may be negative or may yield only inconsequential aerobes unless rigorous anaerobic culture conditions are used, employing special collection methods and media suitable for fastidious organisms.

The following is a brief listing of important types of infections which are most commonly caused by

*For clostridial infections, see Chapter 23.

anaerobic organisms. Treatment of all of these infections consists of surgical exploration and judicious excision in conjunction with administration of antimicrobial drugs.

Upper Respiratory Tract

Bacteroides melaninogenicus together with anaerobic spirochetes is commonly involved in periodontal infections. These organisms, fusobacteria, and peptostreptococci are responsible for a substantial percentage of cases of chronic sinusitis and probably of peritonsillar abscess, chronic otitis media, and mastoiditis. Hygiene and drainage are usually more important in treatment than antimicrobials, but penicillin G is the drug of choice.

Chest Infections

Aspiration of saliva (which contains 10^8 anaerobic organisms/ml in addition to aerobes) may lead to pneumonitis (aspiration pneumonia), necrotizing pneumonia, lung abscess, and empyema. While polymicrobial infection is the rule, anaerobes—particularly *B melaninogenicus,* fusobacteria, and peptostreptococci—are common etiologic agents. All of these organisms are susceptible to penicillin G and tend to respond to drug treatment combined with surgical drainage when indicated.

Bacteroides fragilis is the cause of about one-fifth of anaerobic chest infections. It is relatively resistant to penicillin but often responds to treatment with clindamycin or chloramphenicol.

Central Nervous System

While anaerobes only rarely produce meningitis, they are a common cause of brain abscess, subdural empyema, or septic CNS thrombophlebitis. The organisms reach the CNS by direct extension from sinusitis, otitis, or mastoiditis or by hematogenous spread from chronic lung infections. Antimicrobial therapy (eg, penicillin, 20 million units IV, and clindamycin, 600 mg IV every 8 hours) against appropriate organisms is an important adjunct to surgical drainage.

Intra-abdominal Infections

In the colon there are up to 10^{11} anaerobes per gram of content—predominantly *B fragilis,* clostridia, and peptostreptococci. These organisms play a central etiologic role in most intra-abdominal abscesses following trauma to the colon, diverticulitis, appendicitis, or perirectal abscess and may also participate in hepatic abscess and cholecystitis, often in association with aerobic coliform bacteria. The gallbladder wall may be infected with clostridia as well. In infections associated with perforation of the lower bowel, penicillin G may be ineffective because of the resistance of *B fragilis;* chloramphenicol, clindamycin, or metronidazole may be the drugs of choice to aid in localization and supplement drainage.

Whereas the normal flora of the upper intestinal tract is more sparse than that of the colon, anaerobes comprise a large portion of it.

Female Genital Tract & Pelvic Infections

The normal flora of the vagina and cervix includes several species of bacteroides, peptostreptococci, lactobacilli, coliform bacteria, and, occasionally, clostridia. These organisms commonly cause genital tract infections and may disseminate from there.

While salpingitis is commonly caused by gonococci, tubo-ovarian and pelvic abscesses are associated with anaerobes in a majority of cases. Postpartum infections may be caused by aerobic streptococci or staphylococci, but in most instances anaerobes are found, and the most severe cases of postpartum or postabortion sepsis are associated with clostridia and bacteroides. These have a high mortality rate, and treatment requires both antimicrobials (penicillin, chloramphenicol, clindamycin) and early hysterectomy.

Bacteremia & Endocarditis*

Anaerobes are probably responsible for 5–10% of cases of bacteremia seen in general hospitals. Most of these originate in the gastrointestinal tract and the female genital tract and—until now—have been associated with a high mortality rate. Endocarditis due to anaerobic and microaerophilic streptococci and bacteroides originate in the same sites. Rigorous anaerobic cultures are essential in patients whose "routine" blood cultures in clinical endocarditis have remained negative in order to identify the causative organism and institute specific and adequate treatment. Most cases of streptococcal endocarditis can be effectively treated with 20–60 million units of penicillin G daily, but optimal therapy of other types of anaerobic bacterial endocarditis must rely on laboratory guidance. Anaerobic corynebacteria (propionibacterium), clostridia, and bacteroides occasionally cause endocarditis. Bacteroides bacteremia may cause disseminated intravascular coagulation (DIC).

Skin & Soft Tissue Infections

Anaerobic infections in the skin and soft tissue usually follow trauma, inadequate blood supply, or surgery and are commonest in areas which can be contaminated by oral or fecal flora. There is often rapidly progressive tissue necrosis and a putrid odor.

Bacterial synergistic gangrene is a painful ulcerating lesion which commonly follows laparotomy performed as part of the management of intra-abdominal infections but produces little fever or systemic toxicity. It is usually caused by a mixture of anaerobic streptococci and *Staphylococcus aureus.* It requires wide excision of the discolored skin and (later) skin grafts, but recovery is the rule.

Synergistic necrotizing cellulitis progresses more rapidly, with high fever and often positive blood cultures for peptostreptococci, bacteroides, and aerobic gram-negative bacteria. It occurs with greatest frequency on the perineum and the lower extremities and is associated with a high mortality rate. Excision of

*See also fuller discussion in Chapter 7.

necrotic tissue must be combined with antimicrobial drugs (eg, gentamicin plus clindamycin) in an effort at early control.

Necrotizing fasciitis is a mixed anaerobic or aerobic infection which rapidly dissects through deep fascial planes and produces severe toxicity with a mortality rate up to 30%. Anaerobic streptococci and *S aureus* are the commonest etiologic organisms. Treatment requires extensive surgical incisions through fascial planes.

Nonclostridial crepitant cellulitis is an infection of subcutaneous or deeper tissues with peptostreptococci and coliform bacteria which leads to gas formation in tissue with minimal toxicity, lack of muscle involvement, and a good prognosis. Improved perfusion, incision and drainage, and antimicrobial drugs (eg, ampicillin) are often successful.

Bartlett JG, Finegold SM: Anaerobic pleuropulmonary infections. Medicine 51:413, 1972.

Bodner SJ & others: Bacteremic bacteroides infections. Ann Int Med 73:537, 1970.

Brewer NS & others: Brain abscess. A review of recent experience. Ann Int Med 82:571, 1975.

Frederick J, Braude AI: Anaerobic infection of the paranasal sinuses. New England J Med 290:135, 1974.

Gorbach SL, Bartlett JG: Anaerobic infections. (3 parts.) New England J Med 290:1177, 1237, 1289, 1974.

Lerner PI: Antimicrobial considerations in anaerobic infections. M Clin North America 58:533, 1974.

Tally FP & others: Treatment of anaerobic infections with metronidazole. Antimicrob Agents Chemother 7:672, 1975.

Thadepalli H & others: Anaerobic infection of the female genital tract. Am J Obst Gynec 117:1034, 1973.

VENEREAL DISEASES

These are infectious diseases transmitted most commonly—or most efficiently—by sexual contact. The frequency of some of these infections (eg, gonorrhea) has increased markedly in recent years as a result of changing patterns of sexual behavior. Others (eg, herpetic and chlamydial genital infections) are only now beginning to be appreciated as important systemic infections with a primarily sexual mode of transmission. Rectal and pharyngeal infections are common in venereal disease as a result of varied sexual practices.

Most of the infectious agents that cause venereal diseases are relatively easily inactivated when exposed to a harsh environment. They are thus particularly suited to transmission by contact with mucous membranes. They may be bacteria (eg, gonococci), spirochetes (syphilis), chlamydiae (LGV), viruses (eg, herpes simplex, hepatitis virus type B, CMV), or protozoa (eg, trichomonas). For most of them, early lesions occur on genitalia or other sexually exposed mucous membranes, but wide dissemination may occur with involvement of tissues and organs which mimic many noninfectious disorders. All venereal diseases have sub-clinical or latent phases which may play an important role in long-term persistence of the infection or in its transmission from infected (but largely asymptomatic) persons to other contacts. Laboratory examinations are of particular importance in the diagnosis of such contagious but asymptomatic patients. Simultaneous infection by several different agents is common.

For each patient, there are one or more sexual contacts who require diagnosis and treatment. Several venereal diseases are reportable to public health authorities. The commonest venereal diseases are gonorrhea, syphilis, condyloma acuminata, chlamydial genital infections, herpesvirus genital infections, trichomoniasis, chancroid, and granuloma inguinale.

Clinical and epidemiologic details and methods of diagnosis and treatment are discussed for each infection separately elsewhere in this book (see Index).

INFECTIONS IN DRUG ADDICTS

The abuse of parenterally administered narcotic drugs has increased enormously. There are an estimated 250 thousand or more narcotic addicts in the USA, mostly in or near large urban centers. Consequently, many physicians and hospitals serving such urban and suburban populations are faced with the diagnosis and treatment of problems that are closely related to drug abuse. Infections are a large part of these problems.

Common Infections That Occur
With Greater Frequency in Drug Users

(1) Skin infections are associated with poor hygiene and multiple needle punctures, commonly due to *S aureus.*

(2) Hepatitis (see p 372) is nearly universal among habitual drug users and is transmissible both by the parenteral and by the fecal-oral route. Many addicts experience hepatitis twice.

(3) Aspiration pneumonia and its complications (lung abscess, empyema, brain abscess) are due to anaerobes, nocardia, and other organisms.

(4) Pulmonary septic emboli may originate in venous thrombi or right-sided endocarditis.

(5) Venereal diseases are not directly related to drug abuse but, for social reasons, occur with greater frequency in population groups which are also involved in drug abuse.

Infections Rare in USA Except in Drug Users

(1) Tetanus: Drug users now form a majority of cases of tetanus in the USA. Tetanus develops most commonly in the unimmunized female addict who injects drugs subcutaneously ("skin-popping").

(2) Malaria: Needle transmission occurs from addicts who acquired the infection in malaria-endemic areas outside of the USA.

(3) Melioidosis: This chronic pulmonary infection caused by *Pseudomonas pseudomallei* is occasionally seen in debilitated drug users.

Infective Endocarditis*

The organisms that cause infective endocarditis in those who use drugs intravenously are most commonly *S aureus,* candida (especially *C parapsilosis*), *Streptococcus faecalis,* and gram-negative bacteria (especially pseudomonas and *Serratia marcescens*).

Involvement of the left side of the heart is somewhat more frequent than involvement of the right side, and infection of more than one valve is not infrequent. Right-sided involvement, especially in the absence of murmurs, is often suggested by manifest pulmonary lesions. The diagnosis must be established by blood culture. Until the etiologic organism is known, treatment must be directed against the most probable organism—especially *S aureus* if the patient suffers from toxic delirium—with petechial rashes in the presence of evidence of drug abuse.

Osteomyelitis†

Osteomyelitis involving vertebral bodies, sternoclavicular joints, and other sites usually results from hematogenous distribution of injected organisms or septic venous thrombi. Pain and fever precede roentgenologic changes by several weeks.

Cherubin CE: Infectious disease problems of narcotic addicts. Arch Int Med 128:309, 1971.

Kaye D: Changes in the spectrum, diagnosis and management of bacterial and fungal endocarditis. M Clin North America 57:941, 1973.

DIAGNOSIS OF VIRAL INFECTIONS

In the diagnosis of viral infections, the current state of clinical knowledge and laboratory technology allows specific identification in the vast majority of cases. Diagnoses such as "viral syndrome," "viral diarrhea," or "flu syndrome" are not helpful.

Some viral illnesses present a clear-cut clinical syndrome (chickenpox, measles, mumps) which identifies the virus involved. Laboratory assistance is required only for confirmation in atypical cases or for the differential diagnosis of 2 syndromes which resemble each other (eg, eczema herpeticum and eczema vaccinatum).

In some instances, the clinical picture has a number of features that are suggestive of viral infection in general but could be caused by any one of a number of viruses. Such a "viral" picture is seen in aseptic meningitis, where the characteristic features are an initial polymorphonuclear pleocytosis in the CSF which then

*See also fuller discussion in Chapter 7.
†See fuller discussion in Chapter 14.

shifts to a preponderance of mononuclear cells, normal CSF glucose, and slight elevation of CSF protein occurring a short time after the period of pleocytosis. It is the nature of the meningeal tissue response to viral invasion that differentiates this syndrome from the very different response to pyogenic bacteria. The viruses involved in aseptic meningitis include mumps and several enteroviruses; the specific viral diagnosis can only be made with laboratory assistance. In the case of the respiratory tract, viral infections also have certain features in common—widespread involvement of the respiratory epithelium with redness and clear nasal secretion, absence of a purulent response—and, if pneumonia is present, it is more apt to be interstitial pneumonia. Measles virus provides a good example of viral respiratory involvement.

Sometimes the statistical predilection of one of the respiratory viruses for an anatomic site allows one to make an "educated guess." For example, respiratory syncytial virus is the most common cause of bronchiolitis, and parainfluenza virus is the most common cause of croup. Once again, however, specific identification of the virus involved can only be made in the laboratory.

At times, accurate diagnosis is of such import to the patient (rubella during pregnancy) or the community (smallpox) that rapid laboratory confirmation of the suspected diagnosis is essential.

The accurate diagnosis of a viral illness requires the close collaboration of the clinician and the laboratory virologist. Knowing which specimens are most likely to be productive, when they should be obtained, and what best to do with them in the laboratory depends on the virologist's understanding of the suspected diagnosis, the timetable of the illness, and the clinician's awareness of laboratory capabilities and limitations.

Laboratory Considerations

There are 3 basic laboratory technics for making a viral diagnosis:

A. Isolation and Identification of the Virus: This requires inoculation of the appropriate specimen into a suitable tissue culture or into a live animal. A variety of technics are then utilized to determine the presence and nature of the particular virus. At times this can be done very simply (eg, in the case of herpes simplex); at times it may be laborious, time-consuming, and expensive (eg, in the case of coxsackievirus). The isolation of virus from a specimen that is normally free of virus (eg, CSF, lung biopsy) or from a pathologic lesion (herpes or varicella vesicle) has great diagnostic significance. However, finding a virus in the nasopharynx or in the stool may denote carriage rather than disease; in this case, additional evidence of a rise in antibody titer will be necessary before a specific diagnosis can be made.

B. Microscopic Methods: This entails the microscopic examination of cells, body fluids, or aspirates to demonstrate either the presence of the virus or of specific cytologic changes peculiar to one virus or a group of viruses (Negri body found in rabies; intracyto-plasmic inclusions in epithelial cells in trachoma or inclusion conjunctivitis). The immunofluorescent methods of identifying antigen in cells with antibody conjugated with fluorescent dye are particularly useful in many viral illnesses (rabies, varicella, variola, herpes, etc). Viruses lead an obligately intracellular existence; therefore, it is better to examine scraped cells rather than exudates or transudates.

C. Serologic Methods: During viral illnesses, specific antibodies develop. The timing of rise in titer and persistence of antibodies varies. A 4-fold rise in antibody titer during the course of the illness is usually considered significant evidence of disease. Since a single serum titer is not particularly helpful, many laboratories will not do the test until paired sera (taken 2–3 weeks apart) are available. It is not practical to do serology tests for a large number of viruses in any patient. Thus, the use of this method requires a specific suspicion of which virus might be involved.

Herrmann EC Jr: The tragedy of viral diagnosis. Postgrad MJ 46:545, 1970.

Lennette EH: Laboratory diagnosis of viral infections: General principles. Am J Clin Path 57:737, 1972.

MISCELLANEOUS RESPIRATORY INFECTIONS

Infections of the respiratory tract are perhaps the most common human ailments. While they are a source of discomfort, disability, and loss of time for most average adults, they are a substantial cause of morbidity and serious illness in young children and in the elderly. As a result of advances in virologic technics, specific associations of certain groups of viruses with certain disease syndromes have been established. Many of these viral infections run their natural course in older children and in adults, without specific treatment and without great risk of bacterial complications. In young infants and in the elderly, or in persons with impaired respiratory tract reserves, bacterial superinfection occurs with some frequency and contributes to both morbidity and mortality.

Several generalizations apply particularly to respiratory viral infections in children. Epithelium of different sites is often involved simultaneously with inflammatory reactions. Thus, there may be coexistent conjunctivitis, otitis, pharyngitis, tracheitis, or bronchitis. Symptoms often point mainly to an anatomic site of principal involvement rather than to a particular etiologic virus. Exceptions, however, exist: rhinoviruses are prominent in the common cold; respiratory syncytial virus is most likely to produce bronchiolitis; and parainfluenza virus tends to produce laryngotracheitis (croup). The incidence of both a specific virus infection and a particular symptom complex is sometimes age-related. Bronchiolitis occurs principally in children under the age of 2. The small diameter of the airway in the very young child predisposes to obstruction, necessitating frequent evaluation of symptoms, signs, and possible therapy. In the elderly individual, emphysema or bronchiectasis similarly contributes to poor ventilation and oxygenation, posing special problems in management.

In the following paragraphs, special entities, their recognition, and therapy are summarized briefly.

Croup (Laryngotracheobronchitis)

This is most commonly a parainfluenza virus infection of small children, with anatomic localization in the subglottal area. It produces hoarseness, a "seal bark" cough, and signs of upper airway obstruction with inspiratory stridor, xiphoid and suprasternal retraction, but no pain on swallowing. Treatment includes hydration, steam inhalation (hot or cold), and alertness to the possibility of complete airway obstruction. Should that emergency occur, intubation or tracheostomy is lifesaving.

Epiglottitis

This is a bacterial infection, usually due to *Haemophilus influenzae*. The epiglottis is markedly swollen and "cherry-red," producing an airway obstruction resembling viral croup but usually in an older child. The patient is often 1–6 years old, febrile, appears toxic, and has pain on swallowing in addition to the "croupy cough." Direct laryngoscopy may result in complete obstruction and must therefore be performed only in a setting where intubation or tracheostomy can be performed immediately and expertly. Such airway maintenance is required in a majority of patients in addition to antimicrobial therapy (currently ampicillin or chloramphenicol—or both—until laboratory results from culture are available).

Bronchiolitis

This viral infection is caused most often by respiratory syncytial virus in children under 2 years of age. It results in a "ball valve" obstruction to expiration at the level of the bronchiole, resembling bronchial asthma in pathophysiology. Clinical signs include low-grade fever, severe tachypnea (up to 100 respirations per minute), an expiratory wheeze, overinflation of lungs, depressed diaphragm, decreased air exchange,

and greatly increased work of breathing. Foreign body aspiration and bronchial asthma may have to be considered in differential diagnosis.

Treatment consists of hydration, humidification of inspired air, and—with rising blood P_{CO_2}—the possible need for ventilatory support.

Common Cold

This familiar syndrome is characterized mainly by nasal obstruction and discharge, sore throat, sneezing, hoarseness, and varying degress of malaise, cough, sinusitis, and otitis. Fever is usually absent in adults but may be present in small children. Rhinoviruses, coronaviruses, parainfluenza viruses, and others may be the etiologic agents. All of these exist in multiple antigenic types, and recurrence of infection after a short interval is common. Secondary bacterial infection is more common in children (15%) than in adults and may produce purulent sinusitis, otitis media, or tracheobronchitis.

Treatment is largely palliative, and its true merits are poorly established. Aspirin (0.6 gm every 4–8 hours in adults) tends to act as an analgesic. Phenylephrine, 0.25% solution as nose drops 4 times daily, or dextroamphetamine (or methamphetamine) inhalers may temporarily relieve nasal congestion. Sedative cough mixtures may suppress the annoying and incapacitating cough at some stages. There is no solid support for the claim that ascorbic acid (1–4 gm daily) can prevent the common cold or markedly alter its severity. Antimicrobial drugs have no place in the management of the common cold unless secondary bacterial infection is unequivocally present. Antihistamines are of value only in allergic or vasomotor rhinitis.

Chanock RM, Parrott RH: Acute respiratory disease of infancy and childhood. Pediatrics 36:21, 1965.

Denny FW: The replete pediatrician and the etiology of lower respiratory tract infections. Pediat Res 3:463, 1969.

Dykes MHM, Meier P: Ascorbic acid and the common cold. JAMA 231:1073, 1975.

Gwaltney JM Jr & others: Rhinovirus infections in an industrial population. New England J Med 275:1261, 1966.

Kendig EL Jr: Pulmonary disorders. In: *Disorders of the Respiratory Tract in Children*, 2nd ed. Vol 1. Kendig EL Jr (editor). Saunders, 1972.

22...
Infectious Diseases: Viral & Rickettsial

Moses Grossman & Ernest Jawetz

VIRAL DISEASES

RUBEOLA
(Measles)

Essentials of Diagnosis

- Prodrome of fever, coryza, cough, conjunctivitis, photophobia, Koplik's spots.
- Rash: brick-red, irregular, maculopapular; onset 3 days after onset of prodrome; face to trunk to extremities.
- Leukopenia.
- Exposure 10–14 days previously.

General Considerations

Measles is an acute systemic viral infection transmitted by inhalation of infective droplets. Its highest age incidence is in young children. One attack confers permanent immunity. Communicability is greatest during the pre-eruptive stage, but continues as long as the rash remains.

Clinical Findings

A. Symptoms and Signs: Fever is often as high as 40–40.6° C (104–105° F). It persists through the prodrome and rash (about 7 days), but may remit briefly at the onset of rash. Malaise may be marked. Coryza resembles that seen with upper respiratory infections (nasal obstruction, sneezing, and sore throat). Cough is persistent and nonproductive. There is conjunctivitis, with redness, swelling, photophobia, and discharge.

Koplik's spots are pathognomonic of measles. They appear about 2 days before the rash and last 1–4 days as tiny "table salt crystals" on the dull red mucous membranes of the cheeks and often on inner conjunctival folds and vaginal mucous membranes. The pharynx is red, and a yellowish exudate may appear on the tonsils. The tongue is coated in the center; the tip and margins are red. Moderate generalized lymphadenopathy is common. Splenomegaly occurs occasionally.

The rash usually appears first on the face and behind the ears 4 days after the onset of symptoms. The initial lesions are pinhead-sized papules which coalesce to form the brick-red, irregular, blotchy maculopapular rash which may further coalesce in severe cases to form an almost uniform erythema on some areas of the body. By the second day the rash begins to coalesce on the face as it appears on the trunk. On the third day the rash is confluent on the trunk, begins to appear on the extremities, and begins to fade on the face. Thereafter, it fades in the order of its appearance. Hyperpigmentation remains in fair-skinned individuals and severe cases. Slight desquamation may follow.

B. Laboratory Findings: Leukopenia is usually present unless secondary bacterial complications exist. Febrile proteinuria is present. Virus can be recovered from nasopharyngeal washings and from blood. A 4-fold rise in serum antibody can substantiate the diagnosis.

Complications

A. CNS Complications: Encephalitis occurs in approximately 1:1000 to 1:2000 cases. Its onset is usually 3–7 days after the rash. Vomiting, convulsions, coma, and a variety of severe neurologic signs and symptoms herald this complication. Treatment is symptomatic and supportive. There is an appreciable mortality rate, and many patients are left with permanent sequelae. Subacute sclerosing panencephalitis (Dawson's) is a very late form of CNS complication, the measles virus acting as a "slow virus" to produce this degenerative CNS disease years after the initial infection.

B. Respiratory Tract Disease: Early in the course of measles, severe viral bronchopneumonia due to measles virus is often present. Secondary bacterial lower respiratory infection, bronchitis, and bronchopneumonia commonly occur later.

C. Secondary Bacterial Infections: Immediately following measles, secondary bacterial infection—particularly cervical adenitis, catarrhal and purulent otitis, and pneumonia—are common.

D. Tuberculosis: Measles produces temporary anergy to the tuberculin skin test; there may be exacerbations in patients with tuberculosis.

Prevention

The use of attenuated live virus vaccine has materially reduced the incidence of measles. It is

791

Table 22—1. Diagnostic features of some acute exanthems.

Disease	Prodromal Signs and Symptoms	Nature of Eruption	Other Diagnostic Features	Laboratory Tests
Measles (rubeola)	3—4 days of fever, coryza, conjunctivitis, and cough.	Maculopapular, brick-red; begins on head and neck; spreads downward. In 5—6 days rash brownish, desquamating.	Koplik's spots on buccal mucosa.	White blood count low. Virus isolation in cell culture. Antibody tests by hemagglutination inhibition and complement fixation or neutralization.
Rubella (German measles)	Little or no prodrome.	Maculopapular, pink; begins on head and neck, spreads downward, fades in 3 days. No desquamation.	Lymphadenopathy, postauricular or occipital.	White blood count normal or low. Serologic tests for immunity and definitive diagnosis (hemagglutination inhibition, complement fixation).
Chickenpox (varicella)	0—1 day of fever, anorexia, headache.	Rapid evolution of macules to papules, vesicles, crusts; all stages simultaneously present; lesions superficial, distribution centripetal.	Lesions on scalp and mucous membranes.	Specialized complement fixation and virus neutralization in tissue culture. Fluorescent antibody test of smear of lesions.
Smallpox (variola)	3 days of fever, severe headache, malaise, chills.	Slow evolution of macules to papules, vesicles, pustules, crusts; all lesions in any area in same stage; lesions deep-seated, distribution centrifugal.		Virus isolation. Serologic tests for immunity. Fluorescent antibody test of smear of lesions.
Scarlet fever	½—2 days of malaise, sore throat, fever, vomiting.	Generalized, punctate, red; prominent on neck, in axilla, groin, skinfolds; circumoral pallor; fine desquamation involves hands and feet.	Strawberry tongue, exudative tonsillitis.	Group A hemolytic streptococci cultures from throat; antistreptolysin O titer rise.
Exanthem subitum	3—4 days of high fever.	As fever falls by crisis, pink maculopapules appear on chest and trunk; fade in 1—3 days.		White blood count low.
Erythema infectiosum	None. Usually in epidemics.	Red, flushed cheeks; circumoral pallor; maculopapules on extremities.	"Slapped face" appearance.	White blood count normal.
Meningococcemia	Hours of fever, vomiting.	Maculopapules, petechiae, purpura.	Meningeal signs, toxicity, shock.	Cultures of blood, CSF. High white blood count.
Rocky Mt. spotted fever	3—4 days of fever, chills, severe headaches.	Maculopapules, petechiae, distribution centrifugal	History of tick bite.	Agglutination (OX19, OX2), complement fixation.
Typhus fevers	3—4 days of fever, chills, severe headaches.	Maculopapules, petechiae, distribution centripetal.	Endemic area, lice.	Agglutination (OX19), complement fixation.
Infectious mononucleosis	Fever, adenopathy, sore throat.	Maculopapular rash resembling rubella, rarely papulovesicular.	Splenomegaly, tonsillar exudate.	Atypical lymphs in blood smears; heterophil agglutination. Mono-spot Test.
Enterovirus infections	1—2 days of fever, malaise.	Maculopapular rash resembling rubella, rarely papulovesicular or petechial.	Aseptic meningitis	Virus isolation from stool or CSF; complement fixation titer rise.
Drug eruptions	Occasionally fever.	Maculopapular rash resembling rubella, rarely papulovesicular.		Eosinophilia.
Eczema herpeticum	None	Vesiculopustular lesions in area of eczema.		Herpes simplex virus isolated in tissue culture; complement fixation. Fluorescent antibody test of smear of lesions.

important to immunize all children. Multiple virus vaccines (measles-mumps-rubella) are available and equally effective. Immunity is lasting, and the complications of vaccination are negligible.

Passive immunity can be provided for exposed susceptible children by administration of gamma globulin (0.1 ml/lb body weight for prevention; 0.02 ml/lb for modification).

Treatment

A. General Measures: Isolate the patient for the week following onset of rash and keep at bed rest until afebrile. Give aspirin, saline eye sponges, vasoconstrictor nose drops, and a sedative cough mixture as necessary.

B. Treatment of Complications: Secondary bacterial infections are treated with appropriate antimicrobial drugs. Postmeasles encephalitis can only be treated symptomatically.

Prognosis

The mortality rate of measles in the USA is 0.2%, but it may be as high as 10% in underdeveloped areas. Deaths are due principally to encephalitis (15% mortality) and bacterial pneumonia.

Barkin RM: Measles mortality: Analysis of the primary cause of death. Am J Dis Child 129:307, 1975.

Bennett DB & others: Failure of vaccinated children to transmit measles. JAMA 224:616, 1973.

Cherry JD & others: Urban measles in the vaccine era: A clinical, epidemiologic, and serologic study. J Pediat 81:217, 1972.

Lerman SJ, Gold E: Measles in children previously vaccinated against measles. JAMA 216:1311, 1971.

EXANTHEM SUBITUM
(Roseola Infantum)

Although this illness is commonly diagnosed in clinical practice, laboratory confirmation is not available since no viral agent has been isolated. The disease has been transmitted by blood filtrates.

The typical clinical picture is sudden development of very high fever (up to 41° C [106° F]) and irritability in a young child (6 months to 3 years). Febrile convulsions occur commonly with the high fever. The physical findings are limited to postoccipital and postauricular lymphadenopathy. Careful examination and urinalysis are essential to rule out other causes of high fever. The febrile state continues for 3 days. As the temperature drops, an evanescent, very transient maculopapular rash appears. The white blood count may be slightly elevated initially, but as the disease progresses leukopenia is invariably present.

Treatment is purely symptomatic. Aspirin and tepid sponges will serve to keep the temperature down. Convulsions are usually very brief but may require anticonvulsant medication.

The prognosis is excellent. There are no reported deaths, and no sequelae occur.

Clemens HH: Exanthem subitum (roseola infantum). J Pediat 26:66, 1945.

Kempe CH & others: Studies on the etiology of exanthem subitum (roseola infantum). J Pediat 37:561, 1950.

RUBELLA
(German Measles)

Essentials of Diagnosis

- No prodrome; mild symptoms (fever, malaise, coryza) coinciding with eruption.
- Posterior cervical and postauricular lymphadenopathy.
- Fine maculopapular rash of 3 days' duration; face to trunk to extremities.
- Leukopenia.
- Exposure 14–21 days previously.
- Arthralgia, particularly in young women.

General Considerations

Rubella is a systemic viral disease transmitted by inhalation of infective droplets. It is only moderately communicable. One attack usually confers permanent immunity. The incubation period is 14–21 days (average, 16 days). The disease is transmissible for 1 week before the rash appears.

The clinical picture of rubella is not characteristic, and the disease is difficult to distinguish from other viral illnesses such as infectious mononucleosis, echovirus infections, and coxsackievirus infections. Definitive diagnosis can only be made by isolating the virus or by serologic means.

The principal importance of rubella lies in the devastating effect this virus has on the fetus in utero, producing teratogenic effects and a continuing congenital infection.

Clinical Findings

A. Symptoms and Signs: Fever and malaise, usually mild, accompanied by tender suboccipital adenitis, may precede the eruption by 1 week. Mild coryza may be present. Joint pain (polyarthritis) occurs in about 25% of adult cases. These symptoms usually subside in less than 7 days.

Posterior cervical and postauricular lymphadenopathy is very common. Erythema of the palate and throat, sometimes blotchy, may be noted. A fine, pink maculopapular rash appears on the face, trunk, and extremities in rapid progression (2–3 days) and fades quickly, usually lasting 1 day in each area. Rubella without rash may be at least as common as the exanthematous disease. Diagnosis depends on epidemiologic evidence of the disease in the community and laboratory confirmation.

B. Laboratory Findings: Leukopenia may be present early and may be followed by an increase in plasma cells. Virus isolation and serologic tests of immunity are available. A rapid rubella virus hemagglutination inhibition test and a fluorescent antibody test are available.

Complications

A. **Complications in Pregnancy**: It is important to know whether an expectant mother has rubella antibodies at the beginning of pregnancy (eg, premarital and prenatal screening).

If a pregnant woman is exposed to a definite or possible case of rubella, an immediate hemagglutination-inhibiting rubella antibody level should be obtained. If antibodies are found, there is no reason for concern. If no antibodies are found, careful clinical and serologic follow-up is essential. If the occurrence of rubella in the expectant mother can be confirmed, therapeutic abortion must be considered. Judgment in this regard is tempered by personal, religious, legal, and other considerations. The risk to the fetus is highest in the first trimester but continues into the second.

B. **Congenital Rubella**: An infant acquiring the infection in utero may be normal at birth but more likely will have a wide variety of manifestations including growth retardation, maculopapular rash, thrombocytopenia, cataracts, deafness, congenital heart defects, organomegaly, and many other manifestations. Viral excretion in the throat and urine persists for many months despite high antibody levels. The diagnosis is confirmed by isolation of the virus. A specific test for IgM rubella antibody is very useful for making this diagnosis in the neonate. Treatment is directed to the many anomalies.

Prevention

Live attenuated rubella virus vaccine should be given to all girls before the menarche. When adult women are immunized, the absence of pregnancy must be established and the absence of antibodies should be established. (In the USA, about 80% of 20-year-old women are immune to rubella.) Birth control must be practiced for at least 3 months after the use of the vaccine. Mild to moderate arthritis involving many joints may follow administration of rubella vaccine.

Treatment

Give aspirin as required for symptomatic relief. Encephalitis and thrombocytopenic purpura can only be treated symptomatically.

Prognosis

Rubella (other than the congenital form) is a mild illness and rarely lasts more than 3–4 days. Congenital rubella, on the other hand, has a high mortality rate, and the congenital defects associated with it require many years of medical and surgical management.

Chin J, Magoffin RL, Lennette EH: The need for routine rubella antibody testing of women. California Med 116:9, March 1972.

Fleet WF & others: Fetal consequences of maternal rubella immunization. JAMA 227:621, 1974.

Grand MG & others: Clinical reactions following rubella vaccination. JAMA 220:1569, 1972.

Judson FN & others: Mandatory premarital rubella serologic testing in Colorado: A preliminary report. JAMA 229:1200, 1974.

Klock LE, Rachelevsky GS: Failure of rubella herd immunity during an epidemic. New England J Med 288:69, 1973.

Krugman S, Katz SL: Rubella immunization: A five-year progress report. New England J Med 290:1375, 1974.

CYTOMEGALOVIRUS DISEASE

Cytomegalovirus disease, once thought to be a rare type of congenital infection which was usually fatal, is now recognized as the cause of several types of disease of which the congenital variety is perhaps the least common.

Cytomegalovirus is isolated easily from the urine and body tissues of acutely ill patients. It can also be isolated from the urine for many months after the acute illness or, in congenital cases, after birth. Characteristic large inclusion bodies are present in the epithelial cells found in the urinary sediment.

Cytomegalovirus infection is particularly likely to occur in immunosuppressed individuals.

Clinical Findings

A. **Congenital Disease**: Rapid onset of jaundice occurs shortly after birth, with hepatosplenomegaly, purpura, hematuria, and signs of encephalitis. Laboratory findings include thrombocytopenia, erythroblastosis, bilirubinemia, and marked lymphocytosis. Downey type abnormal lymphocytes are present in large numbers. Sequelae include intracranial calcifications, microcephaly, mental retardation, convulsive state, and optic atrophy. Although many infections are subclinical, the prognosis is poor in clinical disease. The diagnosis is made by isolation of cytomegalovirus from the urine or by demonstrating IgM antibody in the neonate.

B. **Acute Acquired Cytomegalovirus Disease**: The clinical picture is similar to that of infectious mononucleosis, with sudden onset of fever, malaise, joint pains, and myalgia. Pharyngitis is minimal, and respiratory symptoms are absent. Lymphadenopathy is generalized. The liver is enlarged and often slightly tender. Laboratory findings include the hematologic picture of mononucleosis as well as bilirubinemia. Heterophil antibody does not appear. This infection is common following massive transfusions.

Treatment

There is no specific treatment. Control fever, pain, and convulsions with appropriate drugs. Corticosteroids have been reported to produce amelioration of symptoms. The value of specific antiviral chemotherapy has not been established.

Clizer EE: Cytomegalovirus mononucleosis. JAMA 228:606, 1974.

Dudgeon JA: Cytomegalovirus infection. Arch Dis Childhood 46:581, 1971.

Reynolds DW & others: Maternal cytomegalovirus excretion and perinatal infection. New England J Med 289:1, 1973.

Weller TH: The cytomegaloviruses: Ubiquitous agents with protean clinical manifestations. (2 parts.) New England J Med 285:203, 267, 1971.

VARICELLA (Chickenpox) & HERPES ZOSTER (Shingles)*

Essentials of Diagnosis

- Fever and malaise just before or with eruption.
- Rash: pruritic, centripetal, papular, changing to vesicular, pustular, and finally crusting.
- Leukopenia.
- Exposure 14–20 days previously.

General Considerations

Varicella is a viral disease spread by inhalations of infective droplets or crusts. Most cases occur in children. One attack confers permanent immunity. The incubation period of varicella is 10–20 days (average, 14 days).

Herpes zoster is caused by the same virus and occurs in individuals with a history of chickenpox.

Clinical Findings

A. Varicella:

1. Symptoms and signs—Fever and malaise are usually mild in children and more severe in adults. Itching is characteristic of the eruption. Vesicular lesions, quickly rupturing to form small ulcers, may appear first in the oropharynx. The rash is most prominent on the face, scalp, and trunk, but to a lesser extent commonly involves the extremities (centripetal). Maculopapules change in a few hours to vesicles which quickly become pustular and eventually form crusts. New lesions may erupt for 1–5 days, so that all stages of the eruption are generally present simultaneously. The crusts usually slough in 7–14 days. The vesicles and pustules are superficial, elliptical, and have slightly serrated borders.

The distribution and evolution of varicella distinguish it from herpes zoster and smallpox.

2. Laboratory findings—Leukopenia is common. Multinucleated giant cells may be found in scrapings of the base of the vesicles. Virus isolation is possible.

B. Herpes Zoster: This syndrome is caused by the same virus as varicella. Usually a single, unilateral dermatome is involved. Pain, sometimes very severe, may precede the appearance of the skin lesions. The lesions follow the distribution of a nerve root. Thoracic and lumbar roots are most common, but

cervical roots and the trigeminal nerve may be involved. The skin lesions are similar to those of chickenpox and develop in the same way from maculopapules to vesicles to pustules. Antibody levels are higher and more persistent in zoster than they are in varicella.

Complications

Secondary bacterial infection of the lesions is common and may produce a pitted scar. Cellulitis, erysipelas, and surgical scarlet fever may occur.

Pneumonia of the interstitial type occurs more often in adults. This serious complication may lead to alveolar capillary block, hypoxia, and sometimes death.

Encephalitis occurs infrequently. It tends to exhibit cerebellar signs—ataxia and nystagmus. Most patients recover without sequelae.

Varicella in immunosuppressed patients (eg, children with leukemia receiving antileukemic drugs or children with kidney transplants) is usually very severe and may be fatal.

In immunosuppressed patients, herpes zoster may disseminate, producing skin lesions beyond the dermatome, visceral lesions, and encephalitis. This is a serious, sometimes fatal complication.

Prevention

Active immunization is not available. Zoster hyperimmune globulin is highly effective in prevention, but the supply is limited. Plasma from zoster patients can also be used.

Treatment

A. General Measures: Isolate the patient until primary crusts have disappeared, and keep at bed rest until afebrile. Keep the skin clean by means of frequent tub baths or showers when afebrile. Calamine lotion locally and antihistaminics orally may relieve the pruritus.

B. Treatment of Complications: Secondary bacterial infection of local lesions may be treated with bacitracin-neomycin ointment; if extensive, penicillin intramuscularly may be given. Varicella encephalitis and varicella pneumonia are treated symptomatically. Corticosteroids may have a beneficial effect in the latter. Bacterial pneumonia is treated with appropriate antibiotics.

In the management of varicella and zoster in the immunosuppressed host, cytarabine has not been shown to be effective. Trials with adenine arabinoside are continuing. Zoster immune globulin is not helpful for clinical therapy but only for prevention.

Prognosis

The total duration from onset of symptoms to the disappearance of crusts rarely exceeds 2 weeks. Fatalities are rare except in immunosuppressed patients.

Brunell PA, Gershon AA: Passive immunization against varicella-zoster infections and other modes of therapy. J Infect Dis

127:415, 1973.

Center for Disease Control: Congenital varicella in term infants: Risk reconsidered. J Infect Dis 129:215, 1974.

Judelsohn RG & others: Efficacy of zoster immune globulin. Pediatrics 53:476, 1974.

Stevens DA & others: Adverse effect of cytosine arabinoside on disseminated zoster in a controlled trial. New England J Med 289:873, 1973.

VARIOLA
(Smallpox, Variola Major)

Essentials of Diagnosis

- Severe headache, nausea, fever, and prostration precede eruption by 2–4 days.
- Centrifugal macular rash, changing to papular, vesicular, and pustular; and finally crusting and occasionally hemorrhagic eruptions of similar stage in any given area.
- Leukopenia early; leukocytosis late.
- Exposure 7–21 days previously (usually 10–14 days).

General Considerations

Smallpox is a highly contagious viral disease transmitted by droplets or by contact with infected crusts. All ages are susceptible, depending upon the interval since vaccination. Previous effective vaccination prevents or modifies the disease. Variola major is more virulent than variola minor (alastrim). The incubation period is 7–21 days (average, 12 days).

A worldwide effort is being made by WHO to eradicate smallpox. This has been highly successful in many areas of the world.

Clinical Findings

A. Symptoms and Signs: Fever, usually 38.9–40.6° C (102–105° F) appears 2–4 days before the eruption and may abate temporarily at the beginning of eruption to increase again during the stage of pustule formation. Malaise and prostration are usually marked. Headache and low backache are characteristically severe. Nausea and vomiting, dizziness, and constipation may occur.

Erythematous, hemorrhagic, or morbilliform rashes may occur during the prodromal illness. The rash appears first on the face and scalp, then on the wrists, hands, neck, back, chest, arms, legs, and feet. New lesions appear for 2–3 days. Pink macules rapidly become papules, which become vesicles in about 3 days. On about the 6th day of eruption, the vesicles become pustules; these in turn become crusts on the 11th or 12th day. Marked edema and oozing may occur during the stage of pustule formation. The crusts may persist for a week or longer, especially on the palms and soles. The individual lesions are round and deeply set in the skin, giving a shotty sensation upon palpation. The distribution of the lesions is centrifugal, with lesions densest on the face and distal portions of the extremities. In milder cases the lesions are discrete; in severe cases they may be confluent. The lesions in any given area tend to be in the same stage of evolution.

Lesions on the mucous membranes may precede the exanthem by a short interval.

The initial eruption may be hemorrhagic and accompanied by hemorrhage from mucous membranes. This type is invariably fatal. Delayed hemorrhage (less often fatal) may occur into the vesicles or pustules.

B. Laboratory Findings: Leukopenia may occur during the early stages, succeeded by leukocytosis during the stage of pustule formation. Proteinuria is common. Variola virus grows in many cell cultures and on the chorioallantoic membrane of the embryonated egg.

Complement-fixing and hemagglutination-inhibiting antibodies appear during or after the second week of the disease.

The fluorescent antibody technic may be used for prompt identification of inclusion bodies in material from a pock or cell culture. Immediate identification of a virulent antigen by gel diffusion of vesicle material or crust against hyperimmune specific serum is possible.

Prevention

Immunization with potent vaccinia virus is very effective. Methisazone, 2–4 gm orally daily administered to contacts within 1–2 days after exposure, gives protection against smallpox.

Treatment

A. General Measures: Penicillin may control secondary bacterial invaders during pustulation. Cytarabine has no therapeutic value.

B. Local Measures: Early in the disease, provide good oral hygiene and apply petrolatum or mineral oil swabs to the nares. Gentle cleansing of the skin is advisable. If lesions are confluent and suppurating, treat as pyoderma. Treat itching with antipruritic lotions; restraints and sedation may be necessary.

Prognosis

The crusts usually disappear after 3 weeks. The severity of the illness and mortality depend upon the strain of virus: variola minor, 1%; variola major, 20%. Modified smallpox is rarely fatal.

Kempe CH: Smallpox: Recent developments in selective vaccination and eradication. Am J Trop Med 23:775, 1974.

Mack TM: Smallpox in Europe. J Infect Dis 125:161, 1972.

Monsur KA & others: Treatment of variola major with cytosine arabinoside. J Infect Dis 131:40, 1975.

VACCINIA

Vaccination has undoubtedly been responsible for the virtual elimination of smallpox from the western world. However, recently, the mortality and morbidity of this procedure have outweighed those of the disease itself, at least in the USA and in Europe. For that reason, WHO and USPHS have recommended the discontinuance of routine vaccination in countries where smallpox is no longer endemic. Vaccination is still recommended for hospital workers and for travelers to endemic areas.

Vaccinia is the cutaneous and sometimes general reaction which occurs following the introduction of vaccinia virus in the course of immunization against smallpox. In normal circumstances it consists of a single local lesion at the site of inoculation which undergoes a characteristic evolution depending upon the state of immunity of the patient.

When no local reaction occurs following inoculation, either the vaccine or the technic is at fault. This is not due to immunity.

Types of Reaction

A. Major Reaction: In nonimmune inoculated patients, a papule will appear followed by an umbilicated vesicle which is surrounded by an erythematous area as pustulation occurs. The pustule dries to form a crust. The crust detaches in the ensuing week to leave the characteristic pitted vaccination scar. The sequence of papule to crust takes about 12 days in primary vaccination and about 6 days in revaccination.

Fever and malaise may appear on about the 6th day and persist for 1–2 days. Axillary adenopathy may be present. Viremia occurs regularly; and the virus may be isolated from throat secretions.

B. Equivocal Reaction: Any reaction which does not produce a vesicle and ulcer should be regarded as "equivocal." Such a reaction might represent an allergic reaction to inactive vaccine which does not induce immunity. If an equivocal reaction is observed, the patient should be revaccinated.

Contraindications to Vaccination

The presence of eczema in the patient or a member of his family is a contraindication to vaccination. So is a past history of eczema. Patients with poison oak dermatitis, recent burns, or impetigo should not be vaccinated until after the skin has cleared.

An absolute contraindication to vaccination is any disturbance of immunity—particularly cellular immunity—whether it be congenital or produced by disease or immunosuppressive drugs.

Complications of Vaccination

A. Noninfectious Rashes: Rashes thought to be due to "hypersensitivity" occur frequently about a week after vaccination. The rash may be morbilliform or urticarial, often itches, and may include mucous membrane manifestations.

B. Secondary Bacterial Infections: Streptococcal, staphylococcal, or, very rarely, *Clostridium tetani* infections may occur.

C. Autoinoculation: Autoinoculation may produce satellite lesions resulting from transmission by the patient's or physician's fingers. The most disturbing of these are lesions around the eyelids or conjunctivas. Vaccinial keratitis is much less common but may produce a scar.

D. Generalized Vaccinia: Generalized vaccinia represents a hematogenous spread with few or many lesions throughout the body. The prognosis is excellent.

E. Eczema Vaccinatum: Eczema vaccinatum occurs in persons with generalized dermatoses who themselves are vaccinated or who are exposed to someone with vaccinia. The eruption becomes generalized, particularly in the area of dermatosis; it is associated with high fever and the manifestations of severe systemic disease, and may be fatal. It must be distinguished from generalized herpes simplex infection in persons with dermatoses (Kaposi's varicelliform eruption). An attenuated vaccine appears to result in a lower incidence of eczema vaccinatum.

F. Progressive Primary Vaccinia or Vaccinia Necrosum: This complication occurs in individuals with disturbed cellular immunity. The vaccination lesion progresses inexorably and becomes gangrenous, and metastatic lesions develop. The mortality rate is high.

G. Postvaccinial Encephalitis and Transverse Myelitis: These are very rare complications of vaccination. They occur 7–12 days after vaccination and are essentially not preventable. There is a high mortality rate. Sequelae are common in survivors.

Treatment

No treatment or dressing is required for uncomplicated vaccinia. Secondary infection may be treated with hot compresses and antibiotic ointment or systemic chemotherapy. Generalized vaccinia and eczema vaccinatum should be treated with vaccinia immune globulin, 0.5 ml/kg IM. No specific treatment is available for postvaccinal encephalitis.

Methisazone (Marboran) is effective in some cases of progressive vaccinia and of eczema vaccinatum.

Jaroszynska-Weinberger B: Treatment with methisazone of complications following smallpox vaccination. Arch Dis Childhood 45:573, 1970.

Karzon D: Smallpox vaccination in the United States: The end of an era. J Pediat 81:600, 1972.

Kempe CH & others: Smallpox vaccination of eczema patients with a strain of attenuated live vaccine. Pediatrics 42:980, 1968.

US Public Health Service Advisory Committee on Immunization Practices: Smallpox vaccine. CDC Morbid Mortal Wkly Rep 21 (25) (Suppl):25, June 24, 1972.

MUMPS
(Endemic Parotitis)

Essentials of Diagnosis

- Painful, swollen salivary glands, usually parotid.
- Orchitis, meningoencephalitis, pancreatitis; CSF lymphocytic pleocytosis in meningoencephalitis.
- Exposure 14–21 days previously.

General Considerations

Mumps is a viral disease spread by respiratory droplets which usually produces inflammation of the salivary glands and, less commonly, orchitis, meningoencephalitis, pancreatitis, and oophoritis. Most patients are children. The incubation period is 14–21 days (average 18 days). Infectivity precedes the symptoms by about 1 day, is maximal for 3 days, and then declines until the swelling has disappeared.

Clinical Findings

A. Symptoms and Signs: Fever and malaise are variable but are often minimal in young children. High fever usually accompanies orchitis or meningoencephalitis. Pain and swelling of one or both (75%) of the parotid or other salivary glands occurs, usually in succession 1–3 days apart. Occasionally one gland subsides completely (usually in 7 days or less) before others become involved. Pain and swelling of the testicle (orchitis) occurs in 25% of adult males with mumps. Headache and lethargy suggest meningoencephalitis. Upper abdominal pain, nausea, and vomiting suggest pancreatitis. Lower abdominal pain in females suggests oophoritis.

Tender parotid swelling is the commonest physical finding. Edema is occasionally marked. Swelling and tenderness of the submaxillary and sublingual glands is variable. The orifice of Stensen's duct may be reddened and swollen. Neck stiffness and other signs of meningeal irritation suggest meningoencephalitis. Testicular swelling and tenderness (unilateral in 75%) denote orchitis. Epigastric tenderness suggests pancreatitis. Lower abdominal tenderness and ovarian enlargement may be noted in mumps oophoritis, but the diagnosis is often difficult. Salivary gland involvement must be differentiated from lymph gland involvement in the anterior cervical space.

B. Laboratory Findings: Relative lymphocytosis may be present, but the blood picture is not typical. Serum amylase is commonly elevated with or without pancreatitis. Lymphocytic pleocytosis of the CSF is present in meningoencephalitis, which may be asymptomatic. The diagnosis can be confirmed by isolating mumps virus from saliva or demonstrating a 4-fold rise in complement-fixing antibodies in paired sera.

Differential Diagnosis

Swelling of the parotid gland may be due to causes other than mumps; calculi in the parotid ducts and a reaction to iodides may produce such swelling. Parotitis may also be produced by pyogenic organisms, particularly in debilitated individuals. Swelling of the parotid gland has to be differentiated from inflammation of the lymph nodes which are located more posteriorly and inferiorly than the parotid gland.

Complications

The "complications" of mumps are simply other manifestations of the disease less common than inflammation of the salivary glands. These usually follow the parotitis but may precede it or occur without salivary gland involvement: meningoencephalitis (30%), orchitis (25% of adult males), pancreatitis, oophoritis, thyroiditis, neuritis, and myocarditis.

Aseptic meningitis is common during the course of mumps, often occurs without salivary gland involvement, and is the most common viral meningitis. This is a very benign self-limited illness. Occasionally, however, encephalitis develops. This is associated with cerebral edema, serious neurologic manifestations, and sometimes death.

Prevention

Mumps live virus vaccine is safe and highly effective. It is recommended for routine immunization for children over 1 year of age, either alone or in combination with other virus vaccines. Inactivated vaccine is not recommended. The mumps skin test is not highly reliable in determining immunity. Mumps hyperimmune globulin may be considered for passive protection of certain exposed susceptibles. However, its effectiveness has not been documented in controlled studies.

Treatment

A. General Measures: Isolate the patient until swelling subsides and keep at bed rest during the febrile period. Give aspirin or codeine for analgesia as required, and alkaline aromatic solution mouth washes.

B. Treatment of Complications:

1. Meningoencephalitis—The treatment of aseptic meningitis is purely symptomatic. The management of encephalitis requires attention to cerebral edema, the airway, and maintenance of vital functions.

2. Orchitis—Suspend the scrotum in a suspensory or toweling "bridge" and apply ice bags. Incision of the tunica may be necessary in severe cases. Give codeine or morphine as necessary for pain. Pain can also be relieved by injection of the spermatic cord at the external inguinal ring with 10–20 ml of 1% procaine solution. Reduce inflammatory reaction with hydrocortisone sodium succinate, 100 mg IV, followed by 20 mg orally every 6 hours for 2–3 days.

3. Pancreatitis—Symptomatic relief only, and parenteral fluids if necessary.

4. Oophoritis—Symptomatic treatment only.

Prognosis

The entire course of the infection rarely exceeds

2 weeks. Fatalities (due to encephalitis) are very rare.

Orchitis often makes the patient very uncomfortable but very rarely results in sterility.

Brickman A, Brunell PA: Susceptibility of medical students to mumps: Comparison of serum neutralizing antibody and skin test. Pediatrics 48:447, 1971.

Habel K, Utz JP: Mumps. P Clin North America 7:979, 1960.

Horowitz SD & others: Delayed hypersensitivity after attenuated mumps virus. Pediatrics 45:77, 1970.

Johnstone JA & others: Meningitis and encephalitis associated with mumps infection: A 10-year survey. Arch Dis Childhood 47:647, 1972.

Levitt AP & others: Mumps in a general population. Am J Dis Child 120:134, 1970.

POLIOMYELITIS

Essentials of Diagnosis

- Muscle weakness, headache, stiff neck, fever, nausea, vomiting, sore throat.
- Lower motor neuron lesion (flaccid paralysis) with decreased deep tendon reflexes and muscle wasting.
- CSF shows excess cells. Lymphocytes predominate; rarely more than 500/cu mm.

General Considerations

Poliomyelitis virus is present in throat washings and stools, and infection probably can be acquired by the respiratory droplet route or by ingestion. The incidence of the disease has been sharply reduced since the introduction of effective vaccine. In less than a decade, poliomyelitis has become a rare disease in developed areas of the world.

Three antigenically distinct types of poliomyelitis virus (I, II, and III) are recognized, with no cross-immunity between them.

The incubation period is 5–35 days (usually 7–14 days). Infectivity is maximal during the first week, but excretion of virus in the stools may continue for several weeks. The family or other contacts of diagnosed cases may be "transient carriers" and excrete virus in the absence of symptoms or during the abortive type of infection.

Clinical Findings

A. Symptoms and Signs:

1. Abortive poliomyelitis—The symptoms are fever, headache, vomiting, diarrhea, constipation, and sore throat.

2. Nonparalytic poliomyelitis—Headache, neck, back, and extremity pain; fever, vomiting, abdominal pain, lethargy, and irritability are present. Muscle spasm—spontaneous shortening of the muscle or hyperactive stretch reflex with limitation of extension by pain and contraction—is always present in the extensors of the neck and back, usually present in the hamstring muscles, and variably present in other muscles. Resistance to flexion of the neck is noted after a varying range of free flexion. The patient assumes the "tripod" position upon sitting up, which he usually does by "rolling" to avoid flexing the back. Straight-leg raising is less than 90°. Spasm may be observed when the patient is at rest or may be elicited by putting each muscle through the maximum range of motion. The muscle may be tender to palpation.

3. Paralytic poliomyelitis—Paralysis may occur at any time during the febrile period. In addition to the symptoms of nonparalytic poliomyelitis, tremors and muscle weakness appear. Paresthesias and urinary retention are noted occasionally. Constipation and abdominal distention (ileus) are common. Paralytic poliomyelitis may be divided into 2 forms which may coexist: (1) spinal poliomyelitis, with weakness of the muscles supplied by the spinal nerves; and (2) bulbar poliomyelitis, with weakness of the muscles supplied by the cranial nerves and variable "encephalitis" symptoms. Bulbar symptoms include diplopia (uncommon), facial weakness, dysphagia, dysphonia, nasal voice, weakness of the sternocleidomastoid and trapezius muscles, difficulty in chewing, inability to swallow or expel saliva, and regurgitation of fluids through the nose. The most life-threatening aspect of bulbar poliomyelitis is respiratory paralysis.

Paralysis of the neck flexors is manifested by "neck drop" on lifting the shoulders from the bed. Paralysis of the shoulder girdle often precedes intercostal and diaphragmatic paralysis. Weakness of the intercostal muscles and diaphragm is demonstrated by diminished chest expansion, "rocking horse" respiration with paradoxic movement of the diaphragm, use of accessory muscles, and decreased vital capacity. Cyanosis and stridor may appear later due to hypoxia. Paralysis may quickly become maximal or may progress over a period of several days until the temperature becomes normal.

Deep tendon reflexes are diminished or lost, often asymmetrically, in areas of involvement.

In bulbar poliomyelitis there may be strabismus (rare), facial asymmetry, deviation of jaw on opening, loss of gag reflex, loss of movement of palate and pharyngeal muscles, pooling of secretions in the oropharynx, deviation of tongue, and loss of movement of the vocal cords. In bulbar respiratory involvement, the respirations vary in rate, rhythm, and depth. The patient can usually take deep breaths on command.

Lethargy or coma may be due to encephalitis or hypoxia, most often caused by hypoventilation.

Hypertension, hypotension, and tachycardia may occur. Convulsions are rare.

B. Laboratory Findings: The white count may be normal or mildly elevated. CSF pressure and protein are normal or slightly increased; glucose not decreased; cells usually less than 500/cu mm (predominantly lymphocytes; polymorphonuclears may be elevated at first). CSF is normal in 5% of patients. The virus may be recovered from throat washings (early) and stools (early and late). Neutralizing and complement-fixing antibodies appear during the first or second week of illness.

Differential Diagnosis

Nonparalytic poliomyelitis is very difficult to distinguish from other forms of aseptic meningitis due to other enteroviruses. Muscle tenderness and spasm, if present, point to poliomyelitis. Otherwise, the distinction is made by laboratory means. Acute infectious polyneuritis (Guillain-Barré) and paralysis from a tick bite may initially resemble poliomyelitis but are easily distinguishable on the basis of clinical and laboratory findings.

Complications

Urinary tract infection, atelectasis, pneumonia, myocarditis, and pulmonary edema may occur. Late complications include skeletal and soft tissue deformities, cor pulmonale, osteoporosis, urolithiasis, and chronic colonic distention.

Prevention

Oral live virus vaccine (Sabin) is easily administered, safe, and very effective in providing local gastrointestinal immunity as well as a good level of circulating antibody. It is essential for primary immunization of all infants. The trivalent form of vaccine is preferable. Routine immunization of adults in the USA is not recommended because of the low incidence of the disease. However, adults who are exposed to a case or plan to travel to endemic areas should receive oral poliovaccine. There is no effective passive immunization.

Treatment

A. Early Phase: Special attention must be given to the early detection of cranial nerve involvement, particularly difficulty in swallowing saliva, and to the weakness of muscles of respiration. Perform a brief and cursory muscle check not more than once daily in acute cases. Maintain comfortable but changing positions in a "polio bed": firm mattress, foot board, sponge rubber pads or rolls, sandbags, and light splints.

Hot moist packs (Kenny) may be applied to the extremities or other areas for the relief of pain during the febrile period. Change of position, extremity packs, and analgesic drugs usually suffice to control muscle spasm.

Dehydration and intestinal hypoactivity often lead to fecal impaction. Examine the patient frequently and give sufficient fluids to prevent this.

Bladder weakness may occur with paralysis involving any muscle group, most commonly with paraplegia.

During the early phase and as long as the patient is bedfast, give a neutral ash diet with a maximum of 0.5 gm calcium content daily (no milk or milk products), and maintain fluid intake to ensure an adequate daily output of low specific gravity urine (1.5–2 liters/day for adults). If nasogastric feedings are necessary, use liquid meat baby foods, juices, low-calcium soy-bean milk substitutes, lactose, and vitamins.

B. Severe Cases: In cases of bulbar poliomyelitis or when there is weakness of muscles of respiration, the patient requires intensive care. Attention must be focused on maintaining a clear airway, handling secretions, preventing respiratory infection, and maintaining adequate ventilation. Assisted ventilation and tracheostomy are often required in these patients.

C. Convalescence and Rehabilitation: The principles are to prevent deformity, avoid exercise during the febrile period, and mobilize early; give range of motion exercise and change position frequently during the febrile period; provide early active exercise under skilled direction as soon as feasible. Early bracing and splinting for therapeutic purposes are required to activate the therapy program.

Prognosis

Paralysis may occur or progress during the febrile period (3–10 days). Diffuse mild weakness is more favorable for functional recovery than severe weakness of a few important muscles. Bulbar poliomyelitis (10–20%) is the most serious. The overall mortality rate is 5–10%.

Hopkins CC & others: Surveillance of paralytic poliomyelitis in the US. JAMA 210:694, 1969.

Lepow ML, Nankervis GA, Robbins FC: Immunity after oral poliomyelitis vaccination. JAMA 202:27, 1967.

Weinstein L: Poliomyelitis: A persistent problem. New England J Med 288:370, 1973.

ENCEPHALITIS

Essentials of Diagnosis

- Fever, malaise, stiff neck, sore throat, and nausea and vomiting, progressing to stupor, coma, and convulsions.
- Signs of an upper motor neuron lesion (exaggerated deep tendon reflexes, absent superficial reflexes, pathologic reflexes, spastic paralysis).
- CSF protein and pressure often increased, with lymphocytic pleocytosis.

General Considerations

A. Viral Encephalitis: While arboviruses (Table 22–2) are the principal causes, many other viruses may produce encephalitis. Herpes simplex produces "mass-like" lesions in the temporal lobes. Rabies virus invariably produces encephalitis; mumps virus, poliovirus, and other enteroviruses are infrequent causes.

B. Encephalitis Accompanying Exanthematous Diseases of Childhood: This may occur in the course of measles, varicella, infectious mononucleosis, and rubella.

C. Encephalitis Following Vaccination: Encephalitis may follow use of certain immunizing agents.

Table 22—2. Arbovirus (arthropod-borne) encephalitis.

	Geographic Distribution	Vector; Reservoir	Comment
California encephalitis	Throughout USA	Mosquitoes; small mammals	Mainly in children
Eastern (equine) encephalitis	Eastern part of North, Central, and South America	Mosquitoes; birds, small rodents	Often occurs in horses in the area
St. Louis encephalitis	Western and Central USA, Florida	Mosquitoes; birds (including domestic fowl)	
Venezuelan encephalitis	South America	Mosquitoes	Rare in USA
Western (equine) encephalitis	Throughout western hemisphere	Mosquitoes; birds	Often occurs in horses in the area; particularly affects young children

These include vaccines against smallpox, rabies, pertussis, and others.

D. Toxic Encephalitis: Toxic encephalitis due to drugs, poisons, or bacterial toxins (*Shigella dysenteriae* type 1) may be clinically indistinguishable from infectious encephalitis.

Clinical Findings

A. Symptoms and Signs: The symptoms are fever, malaise, sore throat, nausea and vomiting, lethargy, stupor, coma, and convulsions. Signs include stiff neck, signs of meningeal irritation, tremors, convulsions, cranial nerve palsies, paralysis of extremities, exaggerated deep reflexes, absent superficial reflexes, and pathologic reflexes.

B. Laboratory Findings: The white count is variable. Cerebrospinal fluid pressure and protein content are often increased; glucose is normal; lymphocytic pleocytosis may be present (polymorphonuclears may predominate early in some forms). The virus may sometimes be isolated from blood or, rarely, from cerebrospinal fluid. Serologic tests of blood may be diagnostic in a few specific types of encephalitis.

Differential Diagnosis

Mild forms of encephalitis must be differentiated from aseptic meningitis, lymphocytic choriomeningitis, and nonparalytic poliomyelitis; severe forms from cerebrovascular accidents, brain tumors, brain abscess, and poisoning.

Complications

Bronchial pneumonia, urinary retention and infection, and decubitus ulcers may occur. Late sequelae are mental deterioration, parkinsonism, and epilepsy.

Prevention

Effective measures include vigorous mosquito control and active immunization against childhood infectious diseases.

Treatment

Although specific therapy for the majority of etiologic entities is not available, a variety of treatment measures and procedures may contribute significantly to a more successful outcome. Such measures include reduction of intracranial pressure by the use of mannitol or a urea-invert sugar preparation, the control of convulsions, maintenance of the airway, administration of oxygen, and attention to adequate nutrition during periods of prolonged coma. After 72 hours of conventional intravenous nutrition, a nasogastric tube must be inserted and intestinal feedings begun.

Prevention or early treatment of decubiti, pneumonia, and urinary tract infections is important. Give anticonvulsants as needed.

Several antiviral agents have been used in the specific treatment of viral encephalitis. None of them have been established as being effective.

Prognosis

The prognosis should always be guarded, especially in younger children. Sequelae may become apparent late in the convalescence of what appears to be a successful recovery.

Johnson RT: Neurologic diseases associated with viral infections. Postgrad Med 50:158, 1971.

Olson LC & others: Herpesvirus infections of the human CNS. New England J Med 277:1271, 1967.

Riggs S, Smith DL, Phillips CA: St. Louis encephalitis in adults, Houston, 1964. JAMA 193:284, 1965.

Wilkins RH, Brody IA: Encephalitis lethargica. Arch Neurol 18:324, 1968.

LYMPHOCYTIC CHORIOMENINGITIS

Essentials of Diagnosis

- "Influenza-like" prodrome of fever, chills, malaise, and cough, followed by meningitis with associated stiff neck.

- Kernig's sign, headache, nausea, vomiting, and lethargy.
- CSF: slight increase of protein, lymphocytic pleocytosis (500–1000/cu mm).
- Complement-fixing antibodies within 2 weeks.

General Considerations

Lymphocytic choriomeningitis is a viral infection of the CNS. The reservoir of infection is the infected house mouse, although naturally infected guinea pigs, monkeys, dogs, and swine have been observed. Pet hamsters may be a source of infection. The virus escapes from the infected animal by means of oronasal secretions, urine, and feces, with transmission to man probably through contaminated food and dust. The incubation period is probably 8–13 days to the appearance of systemic manifestations and 15–21 days to the appearance of meningeal symptoms. The disease is not communicable from man to man. Complications are rare.

This disease has not been identified west of the Rocky Mountains. It is principally confined to the eastern seaboard and northeastern states.

Clinical Findings

A. Symptoms and Signs: The prodromal illness is characterized by fever, chills, headache, myalgia, cough, and vomiting; the meningeal phase by headache, nausea and vomiting, and lethargy. Signs of pneumonia are occasionally present during the prodromal phase. During the meningeal phase there may be neck and back stiffness and a positive Kernig sign (meningeal irritation). Severe meningoencephalitis may disturb deep tendon reflexes and may cause paralysis and anesthesia of the skin.

The prodrome may terminate in complete recovery, or meningeal symptoms may appear after a few days of remission.

B. Laboratory Findings: Leukocytosis may be present. CSF lymphocytic pleocytosis (total count is often 500–3000/cu mm) may occur, with slight increase in protein and normal glucose. Complement-fixing antibodies appear during or after the second week. The virus may be recovered from the blood and CSF by mouse inoculation.

Differential Diagnosis

The influenza-like prodrome and latent period before the development of the meningitis helps distinguish this from other aseptic meningitides, meningismus, and bacterial and granulomatous meningitis. A history of exposure to mice is an important diagnostic clue.

Treatment

Treat as for encephalitis.

Prognosis

Fatality is rare. The illness usually lasts 1–2 weeks, although convalescence may be prolonged.

Biggar RJ & others: Lymphocytic choriomeningitis outbreak associated with pet hamsters. JAMA 232:494, 1975.

Maurer FD: Lymphocytic choriomeningitis. J Nat Cancer Inst 20:867, 1958.

DENGUE
(Breakbone Fever, Dandy Fever)

Essentials of Diagnosis

- Sudden onset of high fever, chills, severe aching, headache, sore throat, prostration, and depression.
- Biphasic fever curve: initial phase, 3–4 days; remission, few hours to 2 days; second phase, 1–2 days.
- Rash: maculopapular, scarlatiniform, morbilliform, or petechial; on extremities to torso, occurring during remission or second phase.
- Leukopenia.

General Considerations

Dengue is a viral disease transmitted by the bite of the Aedes mosquito. It is a clinical entity which may be caused by one of several viruses, eg, dengue 1 or 2 or West Nile fever virus. It occurs only in the active mosquito season (warm weather). The incubation period is 3–15 days (usually 5–8 days).

Clinical Findings

A. Symptoms and Signs: Dengue begins with a sudden onset of high fever, chilliness, and severe aching ("breakbone") of the head, back, and extremities, accompanied by sore throat, prostration, and depression. There may be conjunctival redness, and flushing or blotching of the skin. The initial febrile phase lasts 3–4 days, typically but not inevitably followed by a remission of a few hours to 2 days. The skin eruption appears in 80% of cases during the remission or during the second febrile phase, which lasts 1–2 days and is accompanied by similar but usually milder symptoms than in the first phase. The rash may be scarlatiniform, morbilliform, maculopapular, or petechial. It appears first on the dorsum of the hands and feet and spreads to the arms, legs, trunk, and neck but rarely to the face. The rash lasts 2 hours to several days and may be followed by desquamation. Petechial rashes and gastrointestinal hemorrhages occur in a high proportion of cases (mosquito-borne hemorrhagic fever) in Southeast Asia. These probably involve an immunologic reaction (immune complex disease).

Before the rash appears, it is difficult to distinguish dengue from malaria, yellow fever, or influenza. With the appearance of the eruption, which resembles rubella, the diagnosis is usually clear.

B. Laboratory Findings: Leukopenia is characteristic. Thrombocytopenia occurs in the hemorrhagic form of the disease. Virus may be recovered from the blood during the acute phase. Serologic diagnosis must consider the several viruses which can produce this clinical syndrome.

Complications

Depression, pneumonia, iritis, orchitis, and oophoritis are rare complications. Shock occurs in hemorrhagic dengue.

Prevention

Available prophylactic measures include control of mosquitoes by screening and DDT. An effective vaccine has been developed but has not been produced commercially.

Treatment

Treat shock by expanding circulating blood volume. Give salicylates as required for discomfort. Permit gradual restoration of activity during prolonged convalescence.

Prognosis

Fatalities are rare. Convalescence is slow.

Bokisch VA & others: The potential pathogenic role of complement in dengue hemorrhagic shock syndrome. New England J Med 289:996, 1973.

Ehrenkranz NJ: Pandemic dengue in Caribbean countries and the southern United States: Past, present and potential problems. New England J Med 285:1460, 1971.

Halstead SB: Dengue and hemorrhagic fevers of southeast Asia. Yale J Biol Med 37:434, 1965.

COLORADO TICK FEVER

Essentials of Diagnosis

- Fever, chills, myalgia, headache, prostration.
- Leukopenia.
- Second attack of fever after remission lasting 2–3 days.
- Onset 3–6 days following tick bite.

General Considerations

Colorado tick fever is an acute viral infection transmitted by *Dermacentor andersoni* bites. The disease is limited to the western USA and is most prevalent during the tick season (March to August). The incubation period is 3–6 days.

Clinical Findings

A. Symptoms and Signs: The onset of fever (to 38.9–40.6° C [102–105° F]) is abrupt, sometimes with chills. Severe myalgia, headache, photophobia, anorexia, nausea and vomiting, and generalized weakness are prominent symptoms. Abnormal physical findings are limited to an occasional faint rash. Fever continues for 3 days, followed by a remission of 2–3 days and then by a full recrudescence lasting 3–4 days. In an occasional case there may be 2 or 3 bouts of fever.

Influenza, Rocky Mountain spotted fever, and other acute leukopenic fevers must be differentiated.

B. Laboratory Findings: Leukopenia (2000–3000/cu mm) with a shift to the left occurs. Viremia may be demonstrated by inoculation of blood into mice or by fluorescent antibody stain of the patient's red cells (with adsorbed virus). Complement-fixing antibodies appear during the third week after onset.

Complications

Aseptic meningitis or encephalitis occurs rarely. Asthenia may follow.

Treatment

No specific treatment is available. Aspirin or codeine may be given for pain.

Prognosis

The disease is self-limited and benign.

Silver HK, Meiklejohn G, Kempe CH: Colorado tick fever. Am J Dis Child 101:30, 1961.

Spruance SL, Baily A: Colorado tick fever. Arch Int Med 131:288, 1973.

RABIES

Essentials of Diagnosis

- Paresthesia, hydrophobia, aerophobia, rage alternating with calm.
- Convulsions, paralysis, thick tenacious saliva.
- History of animal bite.

General Considerations

Rabies is a viral disease of animals and man, transmitted by infected saliva which gains entry into the body by a bite or an open wound. Bats, skunks, and foxes are extensively infected. Dogs and cats may be infected. Rodents are unlikely to have rabies. The virus gains entry into the salivary glands of dogs 5–7 days before their death from rabies, thus limiting their period of infectivity. The incubation period may range from 10 days to 2 years, but is usually 3–7 weeks. The virus travels in the nerves to the brain, multiplies there, and then migrates along the efferent nerves to the salivary glands.

Rabies is almost uniformly fatal. The most common clinical problem confronting the physician is the management of a patient bitten by an animal. (See Prevention.)

Clinical Findings

A. Symptoms and Signs: There is usually a history of animal bite. Pain appears at the site of the bite, followed by tingling. The skin is quite sensitive to changes of temperature, especially air currents. Attempts at drinking cause extremely painful laryngeal spasm so that the patient refuses to drink (hydrophobia). The patient is restless, and behaves in a peculiar manner. There is muscle spasm, laryngospasm, and extreme excitability. Convulsions occur, and blowing on the back of the patient's neck will often precipitate a convulsion. Large amounts of thick tenacious saliva are present.

B. Laboratory Findings: Biting animals who are apparently well should be kept under observation. Sick or dead animals should be examined for rabies. The diagnosis of rabies in the brain of a rabid animal may be made rapidly by the fluorescent antibody technic.

Prevention

Since the disease is almost always fatal, prevention is the only available approach. Immunization of household dogs and cats and active immunization of persons with an unusual degree of exposure (eg, veterinarians) are important. However, the most important and most common decisions concern handling animal bites.

A. Local Treatment of Animal Bites and Scratches: Thorough and repeated flushing and cleansing of wounds with soap and water is important. If rabies antiserum is to be used, a portion should be infiltrated locally around the wound (after testing for sensitivity to horse serum). Wounds caused by animal bites should not be sutured.

B. The Biting Animal: A dog or cat should be captured, confined, and observed by a veterinarian for 7–10 days. A wild animal, if captured, should be sacrificed and the head shipped on ice to the nearest laboratory qualified to examine the brain for rabies. When the animal cannot be examined, skunks, bats, foxes, and raccoons should be presumed to be rabid. The rabies potential of bites by other animals must be evaluated individually.

C. Postexposure Immunization: The physician must reach a decision based on the recommendations of the USPHS Advisory Committee but should also be influenced by the circumstances of the bite, the extent and location of the wound, the presence of rabies in the region, the type of animal responsible for the bite, etc. Treatment includes both passive antibody and vaccine. The optimal form of passive immunization is human immune rabies globulin (20 IU/kg). Up to 50% of the globulin should be used to infiltrate the wound; the rest is administered intramuscularly. If the human gamma globulin is not available, equine rabies antiserum (40 IU/kg) can be used after appropriate tests for horse serum sensitivity. Duck embryo vaccine is used for active immunization. When hyperimmune globulin or serum is used, 23 doses of duck embryo vaccine should be administered. Local reactions to the vaccine are almost universal, but serious complications are rare.

Treatment

This very severe illness with an almost universally fatal outcome requires skillful intensive care with attention to the airway, maintenance of oxygenation, and control of seizures.

Prognosis

Once the symptoms have appeared, death almost inevitably occurs after 2–3 days as a result of cardiac or respiratory failure or generalized paralysis.

Bhatt DR & others: Human rabies. Am J Dis Child 127:862, 1974.
Corey L, Hattwick MAW: Treatment of persons exposed to rabies. JAMA 232:272, 1975.
Hattwick MA & others: Recovery from rabies: A case report. Ann Int Med 76:931, 1972.
Rubin RM & others: Human rabies immune globulin. JAMA 224:871, 1973.

YELLOW FEVER

Essentials of Diagnosis

- Sudden onset of severe headache, aching in legs, and tachycardia. Later, bradycardia, hypotension, jaundice, hemorrhagic tendency ("coffee-ground" vomitus).
- Proteinuria, leukopenia, bilirubinemia, bilirubinuria.
- Endemic area.

General Considerations

Yellow fever is a viral infection transmitted by the Aedes and jungle mosquitoes. It is endemic to Africa and South America (tropical or subtropical), but epidemics have extended far into the temperate zone during warm seasons. The mosquito transmits the infection by first biting an individual having the disease and then biting a susceptible individual after the virus has multiplied within the mosquito's body. The incubation period in man is 3–6 days.

Clinical Findings

A. Symptoms and Signs:

1. Mild form—Symptoms are malaise, headache, fever, retro-orbital pain, nausea and vomiting, and photophobia. Bradycardia may be present.

2. Severe form—Symptoms are the same as in the mild form, with sudden onset and then severe pains throughout the body, extreme prostration, bleeding into the skin and from the mucous membranes ("coffee-ground" vomitus), oliguria, and jaundice. Signs include tachycardia, erythematous face, and conjunctival redness during the congestive phase, followed by a period of calm (on about the third day) with a normal temperature and then a return of fever, bradycardia, hypotension, jaundice, hemorrhages (gastrointestinal tract, bladder, nose, mouth, subcutaneous), and later delirium. The short course and mildness of the icterus distinguish yellow fever from leptospirosis. The mild form is difficult to distinguish from infectious hepatitis.

B. Laboratory Findings: Leukopenia occurs, although it may not be present at the onset. Proteinuria is present, sometimes as high as 5–6 gm/liter, and disappears completely with recovery. With jaundice there is bilirubinuria and bilirubinemia. The virus may be isolated from the blood by intracerebral mouse inoculation (first 3 days). Antibodies appear during and after the second week.

Differential Diagnosis

It may be difficult to distinguish yellow fever from leptospirosis and other forms of jaundice on clinical evidence alone.

Prevention

Transmission is prevented through mosquito control. Live virus vaccine is highly effective and should be provided for persons living in or traveling to endemic areas. (See Immunization, p 1002.)

Treatment

Treatment consists of giving a liquid diet, limiting food to high-carbohydrate, high-protein liquids as tolerated; intravenous glucose and saline as required; analgesics and sedatives as required; and saline enemas for obstipation.

Prognosis

Mortality is high in the severe form, with death occurring most commonly between the 6th and the 9th days. In survivors the temperature returns to normal by the 7th or 8th day. The prognosis in any individual case should be guarded at the onset, since sudden changes for the worse are common. Hiccup, copious black vomitus, melena, and anuria are unfavorable signs.

Burnet FM: Yellow fever. Chap 25, pp 331–357, in: *Natural History of Infectious Disease*, 3rd ed. Cambridge, 1933.
Yellow fever. WHO Chronicle 26:60, 1972.

INFLUENZA

Essentials of Diagnosis

- Abrupt onset with fever, chills, malaise, cough, coryza, and muscle aches.
- Aching, fever, and prostration out of proportion to catarrhal symptoms.
- Leukopenia.

General Considerations

Influenza is transmitted by the respiratory route. While sporadic cases occur, epidemics and pandemics appear at varying intervals, usually in the fall or winter. Antigenic types A and B produce clinically indistinguishable infections, whereas type C is usually a minor illness. The incubation period is 1–4 days.

It is difficult to diagnose influenza in the absence of a classic epidemic. It resembles many other mild febrile illnesses but is always accompanied by a cough.

Clinical Findings

A. Symptoms and Signs: The onset is usually abrupt, with fever, chills, malaise, muscular aching, substernal soreness, headache, nasal stuffiness, and occasionally nausea. In severe infections the patient may be prostrated. Fever lasts 1–7 days (usually 3–5). Coryza, nonproductive cough, and sore throat are present. Signs include mild pharyngeal injection, flushed face, and conjunctival redness.

B. Laboratory Findings: Leukopenia is common. Proteinuria (due to fever) may be present. The virus may be isolated from the throat washings by inoculation of chick embryo. Complement-fixing and hemagglutination-inhibiting antibodies appear during the second week.

Complications

Influenza causes necrosis of the respiratory epithelium which predisposes to secondary bacterial infections. The most frequent complications are acute sinusitis, otitis media, purulent bronchitis, and pneumonia.

Pneumonia is commonly due to bacterial infection with pneumococci or staphylococci and very rarely to the influenza virus itself.

The circulatory system is not usually involved, but pericarditis, myocarditis, and thrombophlebitis sometimes occur.

Prevention

Polyvalent influenza virus vaccine, 1 ml subcut, or 0.1–0.2 ml intradermally, given twice (1–2 weeks apart), exerts moderate temporary protection. Partial immunity lasts a few months to 1 year. Amantadine hydrochloride (Symmetrel), 200 mg orally daily, markedly reduces the incidence of infection in individuals exposed to influenza A if begun immediately and continued for 10 days. The drug does not prevent other viral diseases.

Treatment

Bed rest to reduce complications is important. Analgesics and a sedative cough mixture may be used. Antibiotics should be reserved for treatment of bacterial complications.

Prognosis

The duration of the uncomplicated illness is 1–7 days, and the prognosis is excellent. Purulent bronchitis and bronchiectasis may result in chronic pulmonary disease and fibrosis which persist throughout life. Most fatalities are due to bacterial pneumonia. Pneumococcal pneumonia is most common, but staphylococcal pneumonia is most serious. In recent epidemics, mortality has been low except in debilitated persons—especially those with severe heart disease.

If the fever persisists more than 4 days, cough becomes productive, or the white count rises about 12,000/cu mm, secondary bacterial infection should be ruled out or verified and treated.

Eickhoff TC: Immunization against influenza, rationale and recommendations. J Infect Dis 123:446, 1971.

Jackson G: Influenza, the present status of chemotherapy. Hosp Practice 6:75, Nov 1971.

Stiver HG & others: Efficacy of "Hong Kong" vaccine in preventing "England" variant influenza A in 1972. New England J Med 289:1267, 1973.

US Public Health Service Advisory Committee on Immunization Practices: Influenza vaccine. CDC Morbid Mortal Wkly Rep 21 (25) (Suppl):10, June 24, 1972.

CAT-SCRATCH FEVER

Essentials of Diagnosis

- A primary infected ulcer or papule-pustule at site of inoculation (30% of cases).
- Regional lymphadenopathy which often suppurates.
- History of scratch by cat at involved area.
- Positive intradermal test.

General Considerations

Cat-scratch fever is an acute infectious disease of unknown cause. It may be transmitted by cats, principally by scratching, although cases have been reported to follow skin pricks by a splinter or thorn. The disease is worldwide in distribution, and appears to be quite common. Children are affected more often than adults.

Clinical Findings

A. Symptoms and Signs: A few days after the scratch, about one-third of cases develop a primary lesion at the site of inoculation. This primary lesion appears as an infected, scabbed ulcer or a papule with a central vesicle or pustule. One to 3 weeks later, symptoms of generalized infection appear (fever, malaise, headache) and the regional lymph nodes become enlarged without evidence of lymphangitis. The nodes may be tender and fixed, with overlying inflammation; or nontender, discrete, and without evidence of surrounding inflammation. Suppuration may occur with the discharge of sterile pus.

Lymph node enlargement must be differentiated from that of lymphoma, tuberculosis, lymphogranuloma venereum, and acute bacterial infection.

B. Laboratory Findings: The sedimentation rate is elevated, the white count is usually normal, and the pus from the nodes is sterile. Intradermal skin testing with antigen prepared from lymph node pus is positive (tuberculin-like reaction) in the majority of cases. Lymph node morphology is fairly characteristic, and a definitive diagnosis can be made by excisional biopsy.

Complications

Encephalitis occurs rarely. Macular or papular rashes and erythema nodosum are occasionally seen.

Treatment

There is no specific treatment. Available anti-microbial drugs are ineffective. Surgical removal of a large node or aspiration of liquid contents usually produces an amelioration of symptoms and fever.

Prognosis

The disease is benign and self-limiting. Symptoms may continue for 5 days to 2 weeks.

Margileth AM: Cat scratch disease: Non-bacterial regional lymphadenitis: The study of 145 patients and a review of the literature. Pediatrics 42:803, 1968.

INFECTIOUS MONONUCLEOSIS

Essentials of Diagnosis

- Fever, sore throat, malaise, lymphadenopathy.
- Frequently splenomegaly, occasionally maculopapular rash.
- Positive sheep cell agglutinins (over 1:100); lymphocytosis with abnormal lymphocytes.
- Hepatitis frequent, and occasionally myocarditis, neuritis, encephalitis.

General Considerations

Infectious mononucleosis is an acute infectious disease due to the Epstein-Barr (EB) herpes virus. It is universal in distribution and may occur at any age, but usually occurs between ages 10 and 35 either in an epidemic form or as sporadic cases. Its mode of transmission is probably by respiratory droplet infection. The incubation period is probably 5–15 days.

Clinical Findings

A. Symptoms and Signs: Symptomatology is varied, but the typical case is represented by fever; discrete, nonsuppurative, slightly painful, moderately enlarged lymph nodes, especially those of the posterior cervical chain; and, in approximately half of cases, splenomegaly. Sore throat is often present, and toxic symptoms (malaise, anorexia, and myalgia) occur frequently in the early phase of the illness. A macular to maculopapular or occasionally petechial rash occurs in less than 50% of cases. Exudative pharyngitis, tonsillitis, or gingivitis may occur.

A common manifestation of infectious mononucleosis is hepatitis with hepatomegaly, nausea, anorexia, and jaundice; CNS involvement with headache, neck stiffness, photophobia, pains of neuritis, and occasionally even Guillain-Barré syndrome; pulmonary involvement with chest pain, dyspnea, and cough, and myocardial involvement with tachycardia and arrhythmias.

The varying symptoms of infectious mononucleosis raise difficult differential diagnostic problems, especially sore throat, hepatitis, rash, and lymphadenopathy.

B. Laboratory Findings: Initially there is a

granulocytopenia followed within 1 week by a lymphocytic leukocytosis. Many lymphocytes are atypical, ie, are larger than normal adult lymphocytes, stain more darkly, and frequently show vacuolization of the cytoplasm and nucleus.

The heterophil test (sheep cell agglutination test) is usually positive but may not become positive until late in the course of the disease (4th week) or may be positive only transiently. A titer over 1:100 is significant. The mononucleosis spot test is easier to perform and more specific, and has replaced the heterophil test in many laboratories. Titer rises in EB virus antibodies can be detected by immunofluorescence and other technics. The STS is falsely positive in less than 10% of cases.

In CNS involvement the CSF may show increase of pressure, abnormal lymphocytes, and protein.

With myocardial involvement the ECG may show abnormal T waves and prolonged P–R intervals.

Liver function tests are commonly abnormal.

Differential Diagnosis

Streptococcal tonsillitis and diphtheria must be considered as other possible causes of exudative tonsillitis or pharyngitis. Rubella and toxoplasmosis may resemble some of the manifestations of infectious mononucleosis.

Complications

These usually consist of secondary throat infections, often streptococcal, and (rarely) rupture of the spleen or hypersplenism.

Treatment

A. General Measures: No specific treatment is available. The patient requires support and reassurance because of the frequent feeling of lassitude and duration of symptoms. Symptomatic relief can be afforded by the administration of aspirin, and hot saline or 30% glucose throat irrigations or gargles 3 or 4 times daily. In severely ill patients, symptomatic relief can be obtained through a short course of corticosteroids. Diagnosis must be well established.

B. Treatment of Complications: Hepatitis, myocarditis, and encephalitis are treated symptomatically. Rupture of the spleen requires emergency splenectomy. Frequent vigorous palpation of the spleen is unwise.

Prognosis

In the uncomplicated case the fever disappears in 10 days, the lymphadenopathy and splenomegaly in 4 weeks. In some cases the illness may linger for 2–3 months.

Death is uncommon; when it does occur it is usually due to splenic rupture or hypersplenic phenomena (severe hemolytic anemia, thrombocytopenia purpura, or encephalitis).

There are usually no sequelae.

Henle W, Henle G: Epstein-Barr virus and infectious mononucleosis. New England J Med 288:263, 1973.

Sawyer RN & others: Prospective studies of a group of Yale University freshmen. 1. Occurrence of infectious mononucleosis. J Infect Dis 123:263, 1971.

Tamir D & others: Infectious mononucleosis and Epstein-Barr virus in childhood. Pediatrics 53:330, 1974.

COXSACKIEVIRUS INFECTIONS

Coxsackievirus infections cause several clinical syndromes. As with other enteroviruses, infections are most common during the summer. Two groups, A and B, are defined by their differing behavior after injection into suckling mice. There are more than 50 serotypes.

Clinical Findings

A. Symptoms and Signs: The clinical syndromes associated with coxsackievirus infection may be described briefly as follows:

1. Summer grippe (Coxsackie A and B)—A febrile illness, principally of children, which lasts 1–4 days; minor symptoms and respiratory tract infection are often present.

2. Herpangina (Coxsackie A2, 4, 5, 6, 7, 10)—Sudden onset of fever, which may be as high as 40.6° C (105° F), sometimes with febrile convulsions; headache, myalgia, vomiting; and sore throat, characterized early by petechiae or papules which become shallow ulcers in about 3 days and then heal.

3. Epidemic pleurodynia (Coxsackie B1, 2, 3, 4, 5)—Sudden onset of recurrent pain in the area of diaphragmatic attachment (lower chest or upper abdomen); fever is often present during attacks of pain; headache, sore throat, malaise, nausea; tenderness, hyperesthesia, and muscle swelling of the involved area; orchitis, pleurisy, and aseptic meningitis may occur. Relapse may occur after recovery.

4. Aseptic meningitis (Coxsackie A2, 4, 7, 9, 10, 16; B viruses)—Fever, headache, nausea, vomiting, stiff neck, drowsiness, CSF lymphocytosis without chemical abnormalities; rarely, muscle paralysis. See also Viral Meningitis.

5. Acute nonspecific pericarditis (Coxsackie B types)—Sudden onset of anterior chest pain, often worse with inspiration and in the supine position; fever, myalgia, headache; pericardial friction rub appears early; pericardial effusion with paradoxic pulse, increased venous pressure, and increase in heart size may appear; ECG and x-ray evidence of pericarditis is often present. One or more relapses may occur.

6. Myocarditis (Coxsackie B3, 4, and others)—Heart failure in the neonatal period may be the result of congenital heart disease due to maternal infection. Adult heart disease may be caused by coxsackievirus group B.

7. Hand, foot, and mouth disease—Coxsackievirus

type 16 and several other types produce an illness characterized by stomatitis and a vesicular rash on the hands and feet. This may take an epidemic form.

B. Laboratory Findings: Routine laboratory studies show no characteristic abnormalities. Neutralizing antibodies appear during convalescence. The virus may be isolated from throat washings or stools inoculated into suckling mice.

Treatment & Prognosis

Treatment is symptomatic. With the exception of myocarditis, all of the syndromes caused by coxsackieviruses are benign and self-limited.

Grist NR, Bell EJ: A six year study of coxsackievirus B infections in heart disease. J Hyg 73:165, 1974.

Novack A & others: A community-wide coxsackievirus A9 outbreak. JAMA 202:862, 1967.

Tindall JP, Callaway JL: Hand, foot and mouth disease: It's more common than you think. Am J Dis Child 124:372, 1972.

ECHOVIRUS INFECTIONS

Echoviruses are enteroviruses which produce several clinical syndromes, particularly in children. Infection is most common during the summer.

Over 20 serotypes have been demonstrated. Types 4, 6, and 9 cause aseptic meningitis, which may be associated with rubelliform rash. Types 9 and 16 cause an exanthematous illness (Boston exanthem) characterized by a sudden onset of fever, nausea, and sore throat, and a rubelliform rash over the face and trunk which persists 1–10 days. Orchitis may occur. Type 18 causes epidemic diarrhea, characterized by a sudden onset of fever and diarrhea in infants. Types 18 and 20 cause common respiratory disease (see Chapter 5). Myocarditis has also been reported.

As is true of the other enterovirus infections also, the diagnosis is best established by correlation of the clinical, epidemiologic, and laboratory evidence. The virus produces cytopathic effects in tissue culture and can be recovered from the feces, throat washings, blood, and CSF. A 4-fold rise in antibody titer signifies systemic infection.

Treatment is purely symptomatic. The prognosis is excellent, although occasional mild paralysis has been reported following CNS infection.

Cherry J: Newer viral exanthems. Advances Pediat 16:233, 1969.

Horstmann DM: Viral exanthems and enanthems. Pediatrics 41:867, 1968.

ADENOVIRUS INFECTIONS

Adenoviruses (there are more than 30 antigenic types) produce a variety of clinical syndromes. These infections are self-limited, and most common among military recruits, although sporadic cases occur in civilian populations. The incubation period is 4–9 days.

There are 5 clinical types of adenovirus infection:

(1) The common cold: Many infections produce rhinitis, pharyngitis, and mild malaise without fever indistinguishable from the symptoms and signs of other infections which produce the common cold syndrome.

(2) Acute undifferentiated respiratory disease, nonstreptococcal exudative pharyngitis: Fever lasts 2–12 days and is accompanied by malaise and myalgia. Sore throat is often manifested by diffuse injection, a patchy exudate, and cervical lymphadenopathy. Cough is sometimes accompanied by rales and x-ray evidence of pneumonitis (primary atypical pneumonia) (especially types 4 and 7 in military recruits). Conjunctivitis is often present.

(3) Pharyngoconjunctival fever: Fever and malaise, conjunctivitis (often unilateral), and mild pharyngitis.

(4) Epidemic keratoconjunctivitis (shipyard eye): Unilateral conjunctival redness, mild pain, and tearing, with a large preauricular lymph node. Keratitis leads to subepithelial opacities (especially type 8).

(5) Acute hemorrhagic cystitis in children: (Often associated with type 11).

Vaccines are not available for general use. Live vaccines containing attenuated type 4 or type 7 have been used in military personnel.

Treatment is symptomatic.

Numazaki Y & others: Acute hemorrhagic cystitis in children. New England J Med 278:700, 1968.

Van der Veen J: The role of adenoviruses in respiratory disease. Am Rev Resp Dis 88:167, 1963.

MISCELLANEOUS VIRAL UPPER RESPIRATORY INFECTIONS
(See Chapter 21.)

ERYTHEMA INFECTIOSUM
(Fifth Disease)

This disease of childhood is presumed to be of viral origin although no virus has been isolated. Clinically, it presents as a fiery red, confluent, edematous, maculopapular rash on the face, giving the appearance of a "slapped cheek." There is usually also a generalized maculopapular rash elsewhere on the body. The child is only mildly ill, with fatigue or malaise. The rash comes and goes but on the whole lasts 7–9 days. The prognosis is excellent, and no treatment is needed.

Ager EA & others: Epidemic erythema infectiosum. New England J Med 275:1326, 1966.

Balfour HH & others: Study of erythema infectiosum: Recovery of rubella virus and ECHO virus 12. Pediatrics 50:285, 1972.

RICKETTSIAL DISEASES (RICKETTSIOSES)

The rickettsioses are a group of febrile diseases caused by infection with rickettsiae. Rickettsiae are obligate intracellular bacteria, most of which (except coxiella of Q fever) are parasites of arthropods. In arthropods, rickettsiae grow in the cells lining the gut, often without harming the host. Human infection results either from the bite of the specific arthropod or from contamination with its feces. In humans, rickettsiae grow principally in endothelial cells of small blood vessels, producing necrosis of cells, thrombosis of vessels, skin rashes, and organ dysfunctions.

Different rickettsiae and their vectors are endemic in different parts of the world, but 2 or more types may coexist in the same geographic area. The clinical picture is variable but usually includes a prodromal stage followed by fever, rash, and prostration. Laboratory diagnosis relies heavily on the nonspecific development of agglutinating antibodies to certain proteus strains (Weil-Felix reaction) and of specific complement-fixing antibodies. Isolation of the organism from the patient is cumbersome and difficult, and is successful only in specialized laboratories.

Prevention & Treatment

Preventive measures are directed at control of the vector, specific immunization when available, and (occasionally) drug chemoprophylaxis. All rickettsiae can be inhibited by tetracyclines or chloramphenicol. All clinical infections respond in some degree to treatment with these drugs. Treatment usually consists of giving either tetracycline hydrochloride or chloramphenicol, 0.5 gm orally every 4–6 hours for 4–10 days (50 mg/kg/day). In seriously ill patients, initial treatment may consist of 1 gm tetracycline hydrochloride or chloramphenicol IV. Supportive measures may include parenteral fluids, sedation, oxygen, and skin care. The vector (louse, tick, mite) must be removed from patients by appropriate measures.

Gear JH: Rickettsial vaccines. Brit M Bull 25:171, 1969.

Woodward TE: An historical account of the rickettsial diseases. J Infect Dis 127:583, 1973.

EPIDEMIC LOUSE-BORNE TYPHUS

Essentials of Diagnosis

- Prodrome of malaise and headache followed by abrupt chills and fever.
- Severe, intractable headaches, prostration, persisting high fever.
- Maculopapular rash appears on the 4th–7th day on the trunk and in the axillas, spreading to the rest of body but sparing the face, palms, and soles.
- Laboratory confirmation by proteus OX19 agglutination and specific complement fixation tests.

General Considerations

Epidemic louse-borne typhus is due to infection with *Rickettsia prowazeki*, a parasite of the body louse, which ultimately kills the louse. Transmission is greatly favored by crowded living conditions, famine, war, or any circumstances that predispose to heavy infestation with lice. When the louse sucks the blood of a person infected with *R prowazeki*, the organism becomes established in the gut of the louse and grows there. When the louse is transmitted to another person (through contact or clothing) and has a blood meal, it defecates simultaneously and the infected feces are rubbed into the itching bite wound. Dry, infectious louse feces may also enter respiratory tract mucous membranes and result in human infection. A deloused and bathed typhus patient is no longer infectious for other humans.

In a person who recovers from clinical or subclinical typhus infection, *R prowazeki* may survive in lymphoid tissues for many years. At times such a person may have recrudescence of disease without exogenous exposure to lice or to the infectious agent. Such a recrudescence (Brill's disease) can serve as a source of infection for lice.

Clinical Findings

A. Symptoms and Signs: Prodromal malaise, cough, headache, and chest pain begin after an incubation period of 10–14 days. There is then an abrupt onset of chills, high fever, and prostration, with "influenzal symptoms" progressing to delirium and stupor. The headache is intractably severe, and the fever is unremitting for many days.

Other findings consist of conjunctivitis, flushed face, rales at the lung bases, and often splenomegaly. A macular rash (which soon becomes papular) appears first in the axillas and then over the trunk, spreading to the extremities but rarely involving the face, palms, or soles. In severely ill patients, the rash becomes hemorrhagic and hypotension becomes marked. There may be renal insufficiency, stupor, and delirium. In spontaneous recovery, improvement begins 13–16 days after onset with rapid drop of fever.

B. Laboratory Findings: The white blood count is variable. Proteinuria and hematuria occur commonly. Serum obtained 5–12 days after onset of symptoms usually shows agglutinating antibodies for proteus OX19 (rarely also OX2)–*R prowazeki* shares antigens with these proteus strains–and specific complement-fixing antibodies with *R prowazeki* antigens. A titer rise is most significant. In primary rickettsial infection, early antibodies are IgM; in recrudescence (Brill's disease), early antibodies are predominantly IgG and the Weil-Felix test is negative.

C. X-Ray Findings: X-rays of the chest may show patchy consolidation.

Differential Diagnosis

The prodromal symptoms and the early febrile stage are not specific enough to permit diagnosis in nonepidemic situations. The rash is usually sufficiently distinctive for diagnosis, but it may be missing in 5–10% of cases and may be difficult to observe in dark-skinned persons. A variety of other acute febrile diseases may have to be considered.

Brill's disease (recrudescent epidemic typhus) has a more gradual onset than primary *R prowazeki* infection, fever and rash are of shorter duration, and the disease is milder and rarely fatal.

Complications

Pneumonia, vasculitis with major vessel obstruction and gangrene, circulatory collapse, myocarditis, and uremia may occur.

Prevention

Prevention consists of louse control with DDT and other insecticides, particularly by applying chemicals to clothing or treating it with heat, and frequent bathing. Immunization with vaccines consisting of inactivated egg-grown *R prowazeki* gives good protection against severe disease but does not prevent infection or mild disease. The usual method is to give 2 injections of 0.5 ml IM 4–6 weeks apart. A booster injection is desirable prior to heavy exposure. Live, attenuated strain vaccine is under investigation.

Treatment

See above.

Prognosis

The prognosis depends greatly upon age and immunization status. In children under age 10, the disease is usually mild. The mortality is 10% in the 2nd and 3rd decades, but may reach 60% in the 6th decade. Active immunization usually changes a potentially serious disease into a relatively mild one, with low or no mortality.

Murray ES & others: Differentiation of 19S and 7S complement-fixing antibodies in primary versus recrudescent typhus. Proc Soc Exper Biol Med 119:291, 1965.

ENDEMIC FLEA-BORNE TYPHUS
(Murine Typhus)

Rickettsia mooseri (R typhi), a parasite of rats, is transmitted from rat to rat through the rat flea (rarely, the rat louse). Man acquires the infection when bitten by an infected flea, which releases infected feces while sucking blood.

Flea typhus resembles Brill's disease (recrudescent epidemic typhus) in that it has a gradual onset and the fever and rash are of shorter duration (6–13 days) and the symptoms less severe than in louse-borne typhus. The rash is maculopapular, concentrated on the trunk, and fades fairly rapidly. Even without antibiotic treatment, flea typhus is a mild disease. Pneumonia or gangrene is rare. Fatalities are rare and limited to the elderly.

Complement-fixing antibodies can be detected in the patient's serum with specific *R mooseri* antigens. The Weil-Felix test reveals agglutinating antibodies for proteus OX19 in rising titer.

Preventive measures are directed at control of rats and their ectoparasites. Insecticides are first applied to rat runs, nests, and colonies, and the rats are then poisoned or trapped. Finally, buildings must be rat proofed. Antibiotic treatment need not be intensive because of the mildness of the natural disease. An experimental vaccine was fairly effective, but it is not commercially available now.

SPOTTED FEVERS
(Tick Typhus)

Tick-borne rickettsial infections occur in many different regions of the world and have been given regional or local names, eg, Rocky Mountain spotted fever in North America, Queensland tick typhus in Australia, boutonneuse fever in Africa. The etiologic agents are all antigenically related to *Rickettsia rickettsi,* and all are transmitted by hard (ixodid) ticks and have cycles in nature which involve dogs, rodents, or other animals. Rickettsiae are often transmitted from one generation of ticks to the next (transovarian transmission) without passage through a vertebrate host. Patients infected with spotted fevers usually develop antibodies to proteus OX19 and OX2 in low titer, in addition to rickettsial complement-fixing antibodies.

Control of spotted fevers involves prevention of tick bites, specific immunization when available, and antibiotic treatment of patients.

1. ROCKY MOUNTAIN SPOTTED FEVER

Essentials of Diagnosis

- History of possible exposure to tick bite in endemic area.
- "Influenzal" prodrome followed by chills, fever, severe headache, widespread aches and pains, restlessness, and prostration—occasionally, delirium and coma.
- Red macular rash appears between the 2nd

and 6th days of fever, first on the wrists and ankles and spreading centrally; it may become petechial.

- Proteus OX19 and OX2 agglutinins appear, as well as specific complement-fixing antibodies.

General Considerations

The etiologic agent, *Rickettsia rickettsi,* is transmitted to man by the bite of the wood tick, *Dermacentor andersoni,* in western USA and by the bite of the dog tick, *Dermacentor variabilis,* in eastern USA. Other hard ticks transmit the rickettsia in the southern USA and in Central and South America and are responsible for transmitting it among rodents, dogs, porcupines, and other animals in nature. Most human cases occur in late spring and summer.

Clinical Findings

A. Symptoms and Signs: Three to 10 days after the bite of an infectious tick there is anorexia, malaise, nausea, headache, and sore throat. This progresses with chills, fever, aches in bones, joints, and muscles, abdominal pain, nausea and vomiting, restlessness, insomnia, and irritability. Delirium, lethargy, stupor, and coma may appear. The face is flushed and the conjunctivas injected. Between days 2 and 6 of fever, a rash appears first on the wrists and ankles, spreading centrally to the arms, legs, and trunk. The rash is initially small, red, and macular but becomes larger and petechial. It spreads for 2–3 days. In some cases there is splenomegaly, hepatomegaly, jaundice, gangrene, myocarditis, or uremia.

B. Laboratory Findings: Leukocytosis, proteinuria, and hematuria are common. Rickettsiae can sometimes be isolated in special laboratories from blood obtained in the first few days of illness. A rise in antibody titer during the second week of illness can be detected by specific complement fixation tests or by the Weil-Felix agglutination test with proteus OX19 and OX2. Antibody response may be suppressed if antimicrobial drugs are given very early.

Differential Diagnosis

The early signs and symptoms of Rocky Mountain spotted fever are shared with many other infections. The rash may be confused with that of measles, typhoid, or meningococcemia. The suspicion of the latter requires blood cultures and CSF examination.

Prevention

Protective clothing, tick-repellent chemicals, and the removal of ticks at frequent intervals are helpful. A vaccine of inactivated *R rickettsi* grown in eggs given IM 3 times at intervals of 1 week offers moderate protection.

Treatment & Prognosis

In mild, untreated cases, fever subsides at the end of the second week. The response to chloramphenicol or tetracycline (see Chapter 28) is prompt if the drugs are started early.

The mortality rate from Rocky Mountain spotted fever varies strikingly with age. In untreated, middle-aged adults it may be 70%; in children, less than 20%.

Hand WL & others: Rocky Mountain spotted fever: A vascular disease. Arch Int Med 125:879, 1970.
McReynolds EW, Shane R: An epidemic of tick-borne typhus in children. Am J Dis Child 126:779, 1973.
Tsianabos T & others: The group-specific antigen of R rickettsi. Appl Microbiol 28:481, 1974.
Vianna NJ, Hinman AR: Rocky Mountain spotted fever on Long Island. Am J Med 51:725, 1971.

2. OTHER SPOTTED FEVERS

Tick-borne rickettsial infections in Africa, Asia, and Australia may resemble Rocky Mountain spotted fever but cover a wide spectrum from very mild to very severe. In many cases, a local lesion develops at the site of the tick bite (eschar), often with painful enlargement of the regional lymph nodes.

RICKETTSIALPOX

Rickettsia akari is a parasite of mice, transmitted by mites *(Allodermanyssus sanguineus).* Upon close contact of mice with men, infected mites may transmit the disease to humans. Rickettsialpox has an incubation period of 7–12 days. The onset is sudden, with chills, fever, headache, photophobia, and disseminated aches and pains. The primary lesion is a red papule which vesicates and forms a black eschar. Two to 4 days after onset of symptoms, a widespread papular eruption appears which becomes vesicular and forms crusts which are shed in about 10 days. Early lesions may resemble those of chickenpox or even smallpox.

Leukopenia and a rise in antibody titer with rickettsial antigen in complement fixation tests are often present. However, the Weil-Felix test is negative.

Treatment with tetracycline produces rapid improvement, but even without treatment the disease is fairly mild and self-limited. Control requires the elimination of mice from human habitations after insecticide has been applied to suppress the mite vectors.

Lackman DB: A review of information on rickettsialpox in the United States. Clin Pediat 2:296, 1963.

SCRUB TYPHUS
(Tsutsugamushi Disease)

Essentials of Diagnosis

- Exposure to mites in endemic area of Southeast Asia and Japan.
- Black eschar at site of bite, with enlarged, tender regional lymph nodes and generalized adenopathy.
- Conjunctivitis and a short-lived macular rash.
- Frequent pneumonitis, encephalitis, and cardiac failure.
- Weil-Felix test positive, with antibody titer rise to proteus OXK.

General Considerations

Scrub typhus is caused by *Rickettsia tsutsugamushi (R orientalis)*, which is principally a parasite of rodents transmitted by mites. The infectious agent can be transmitted from one generation of mites to the next (transovarian transmission) without a vertebrate host. The mites may spend much of their life cycle on vegetation but require a blood meal to complete maturation. At that point, humans coming in contact with infested vegetation are bitten by mite larvae and are infected.

Clinical Findings

A. Symptoms and Signs: After an incubation period of 1–3 weeks, there is a nonspecific prodrome with malaise, chills, severe headache, and backache. At the site of the mite bite a papule develops which vesicates and forms a flat black eschar. The regional draining lymph nodes are enlarged and tender, and there may be generalized adenopathy. Fever rises gradually, and a generalized macular rash appears at the end of the first week of fever. The rash is most marked on the trunk, and may be fleeting or may last for a week. Pneumonitis, encephalitis, and cardiac failure may occur during the second week of fever. The patient appears obtunded, confused, and out of contact with his environment.

B. Laboratory Findings: Blood obtained during the first few days of illness may permit isolation of the rickettsia by mouse inoculation in specialized laboratories. The Weil-Felix test usually shows a rising titer to proteus OXK during the second week of illness. The complement fixation test is often unsatisfactory.

Differential Diagnosis

Leptospirosis, typhoid, dengue, malaria, and other rickettsial infections may have to be considered. When the rash is fleeting and the eschar not evident, laboratory results are the best guide to diagnosis.

Prevention

Efforts must be made in endemic areas to minimize contact between humans and infected mites. Repeated application of long-acting miticides can make endemic areas safe. When this is not possible, insect repellents on clothing and skin provide some protection. For short exposure, chemoprophylaxis with chloramphenicol can prevent the disease but permits infection. No effective vaccines are available at present.

Treatment & Prognosis

Without treatment, fever may subside spontaneously after 2 weeks but the mortality rate may be 10–40%. Early treatment with chloramphenicol or tetracyclines can virtually eliminate deaths.

Berman SJ, Kundin WD: Scrub typhus in Vietnam: Study of 87 cases. Ann Int Med 79:26, 1973.

Sheehy TW & others: Scrub typhus: A comparison of chloramphenicol and tetracycline in its treatment. Arch Int Med 132:77, 1973.

TRENCH FEVER

Trench fever is a self-limited, louse-borne relapsing febrile disease caused by *Rickettsia quintana.* This organism grows extracellularly in the louse intestine and is excreted in feces. Humans are infected when infected louse feces enter defects in skin. No animal reservoir except humans has been demonstrated.

This disease has occurred in epidemic forms during wars in louse-infested troups and civilians, and in endemic form in Central America. Onset is abrupt, with fever lasting 3–5 days, often followed by relapses. The patient becomes weak and complains of severe pain behind the eyes and in the back and legs. Lymphadenopathy and splenomegaly may appear, as well as a transient maculopapular rash. Subclinical infection is frequent, and a carrier state may occur. The differential diagnosis includes dengue, leptospirosis, malaria, relapsing fever, and typhus fever.

R quintana is the only rickettsia which has been grown on artificial media without living cells. The organism can be cultivated on blood agar in 10% fresh blood, and has been recovered from blood cultures of patients. In volunteers, such agar-grown rickettsiae caused typical disease. The Weil-Felix test is negative, but specific complement fixation tests are being developed.

The illness is self-limited and recovery regularly occurs without treatment.

Varela G & others: Trench fever: Propagation of *R quintana* on cell-free medium from blood of patients. Am J Trop Med 18:707, 1969.

Q FEVER

Essentials of Diagnosis

- An acute or chronic febrile illness with

- severe headache, cough, prostration, and abdominal pain.
- Marked pulmonary infiltration on chest films in the presence of relatively slight signs and symptoms.

General Considerations

Coxiella burneti is unique among rickettsiae in that it is usually not transmitted to humans by arthropods but by inhalation of infectious aerosols or ingestion of infected milk. It is a parasite of cattle, sheep, and goats, in which it produces mild or subclinical infection. It is excreted by cows and goats principally through the milk and placenta and from sheep through feces, placenta, and milk. Dry feces and milk, dust contaminated with them, and the tissues of these animals contain large numbers of infectious organisms which are spread by the airborne route. Inhalation of contaminated dust is the main source of human infection. Coxiella in milk is relatively resistant to pasteurization, and infection may occur through drinking infected milk. Spread from one human to another does not occur with significant frequency even in the presence of florid pneumonitis, but fetal infection can occur.

Clinical Findings

A. Symptoms and Signs: After an incubation period of 1–3 weeks, a febrile illness develops with headache, prostration, and muscle pains, occasionally with a nonproductive cough, abdominal pains, or jaundice. Physical signs of pneumonitis are slight. True endocarditis occurs very rarely. The clinical course may be acute or chronic and relapsing.

B. Laboratory Findings: Laboratory examination often shows leukopenia and a diagnostic rise in specific complement-fixing antibodies to coxiella. The Weil-Felix test is negative. Liver function tests occasionally reveal hepatitis. Special laboratories may attempt isolation of the organism from blood.

C. X-Ray Examination: Chest x-ray shows marked pulmonary infiltration.

Differential Diagnosis

Primary atypical pneumonia, viral hepatitis, brucellosis, tuberculosis, psittacosis, and other animal-borne diseases must be considered. The history of exposure to animals or animal dusts or animal tissues (eg, in slaughterhouses) should lead to appropriate specific serologic tests.

Prevention

Prevention must be based on detection of the infection in livestock, reduction of contact with infected animals or dusts contaminated by them, special care during contact with placental tissues, and effective pasteurization of milk.

Treatment & Prognosis

Treatment with tetracyclines can suppress symptoms and shorten the clinical course but does not always eradicate the infection. Even in untreated patients, the mortality rate is negligible.

Fiset P & others: Human fetal infection with *Coxiella burnetii*. Am J Epidem 101:65, 1975.

Schachter J & others: Potential danger of Q fever in a university hospital. J Infect Dis 123:301, 1971.

Wisniewski HJ, Krumbiegel ER: Q fever in Milwaukee. Arch Envir Health 21:58, 1970.

23...
Infectious Diseases: Bacterial

Moses Grossman & Ernest Jawetz

STREPTOCOCCAL SORE THROAT; STREPTOCOCCAL SKIN INFECTIONS

Essentials of Diagnosis

- Abrupt onset of sore throat, fever, malaise, nausea, and headache.
- Throat red and edematous, with or without exudate; cervical nodes tender.
- Scarlatiniform rash or pyoderma or erysipelas.
- Diagnosis confirmed by leukocytosis, throat or skin culture, and rise in antibody titer.

General Considerations

These infections are usually caused by beta-hemolytic group A streptococci. Occasionally, other streptococci are involved, especially group B in neonates. Respiratory infections are transmitted by droplets from patients or carriers. Skin infections may be transmitted by contact or may begin with infections of the throat. If the infecting streptococcus produces erythrogenic toxin and the patient has no preformed antitoxin, scarlet fever may develop (rash, strawberry tongue). The principal importance of group A streptococcal infections lies in their complications (suppuration, rheumatic fever, glomerulonephritis), which are sometimes preventable. The incubation period of streptococcal sore throat is 1–6 days.

Clinical Findings

A. Symptoms and Signs:

1. Streptococcal sore throat—"Strep throat" is characterized by a sudden onset of fever, sore throat, severe pain on swallowing, enlarged and tender cervical lymph nodes, malaise, and nausea. Children may vomit or convulse. The pharynx, soft palate, and tonsils are red and edematous, and there may be a purulent exudate. If scarlet fever rash occurs, the skin is diffusely erythematous, with superimposed fine red papules. The rash is most intense in the groins and axillas, blanches on pressure, and may become petechial. It fades in 2–5 days, leaving a fine desquamation. In scarlet fever, the face is flushed, with circumoral pallor; and the tongue is coated, with protrusion of enlarged red papillae (strawberry tongue).

2. Streptococcal skin lesions—Impetigo begins as a papule which rapidly becomes a vesicle and a pustule with a thick, amber-colored crust. There is little redness, and the crusts appear "stuck on" the skin. Streptococcal pyoderma is often chronic but produces little discomfort. It may become progressive in hot, humid climates.

Streptococci may enter the skin and subcutaneous tissues through abrasions or wounds and may produce progressive erysipelas (fever, chills, rapidly progressive edema and erythema, with a sharp advancing margin) or "surgical scarlet fever"—ie, wound infection with streptococci which produce erythrogenic toxin in a patient without antitoxin, who then develops signs of scarlet fever. Group B streptococci are an important cause of neonatal meningitis and septicemia.

B. Laboratory Findings: Leukocytosis with an increase in polymorphonuclear neutrophils is a regular early finding, and the sedimentation rate may be elevated. The urine often contains protein and a few red cells. Cultures from the throat or from the material under impetigo crusts or wounds yields large numbers of hemolytic group A streptococci (95% inhibited by a bacitracin disk). In 1–3 weeks after onset of infection, there is a rise in antibodies, particularly to streptolysin O (ASO), hyaluronidase, streptokinase, DNase, and other streptococcal antigenic products or constituents. Elevated antibody levels may continue for months after the infection. In pyoderma, antihyaluronidase is the most commonly elevated antibody; in streptococcal respiratory disease, it is antistreptolysin O.

Complications

The suppurative complications of streptococcal sore throat include sinusitis, otitis media, mastoiditis, peritonsillar abscess, and suppuration of cervical lymph nodes, among others. Streptococcal skin infections may lead to bacteremia and sepsis.

The outstanding nonsuppurative complications are rheumatic fever (0.5–3%) and glomerulonephritis (0.2–20%). Rheumatic fever has followed recurrent infections with any type of group A streptococci and begins 1–4 weeks after the onset of streptococcal sore throat. Glomerulonephritis follows a single infection with a nephritogenic strain of streptococcus group A (eg, types 12, 4, 49, 29, and 57), more commonly on the skin than in the throat, and begins 1–3 weeks after the onset of the infection.

Differential Diagnosis

Streptococcal sore throat resembles (and cannot be reliably distinguished clinically from) the pharyngitis caused by adenoviruses, herpesviruses, and occasionally other viruses; infectious mononucleosis with generalized and prominent adenopathy, splenomegaly, abnormal lymphocytes, and a positive serologic (heterophil) test; diphtheria with a more confluent pseudomembrane; candidiasis with white patches of exudate and less erythema; and necrotizing ulcerative gingivostomatitis (NUG, Vincent's fusospirochetal disease), with shallow ulcers in the mouth. The petechial rash of scarlet fever must be distinguished from meningococcemia, and typical scarlet fever rashes resemble sunburn, drug reactions, rubella, and echovirus infections.

Prevention

Benzathine penicillin G, 1.2 million units as a single IM injection every 4 weeks, is the method of choice to prevent reinfection with group A streptococci in persons who have suffered an initial attack of rheumatic fever and are subject to recurrences. Prophylaxis with sulfadiazine, 1 gm orally daily, or penicillin G, 200,000–400,000 units orally daily, is also acceptable but offers less reliable prophylaxis against rheumatic fever recurrences than benzathine penicillin G IM. These regimens are administered continuously for 5 or more years.

There is no definite prophylaxis against glomerulonephritis except the very early eradication of streptococcal infection.

Treatment

A. Specific Measures:

1. Benzathine penicillin G, 2.4 million units IM as a single dose, is optimal. Procaine penicillin G, 300,000 units IM daily for 10 days, is acceptable. Both of these usually abolish the carrier state.

2. Oral penicillin V, 400,000 units 3 times daily, must be taken for 10 days—and this regimen is not easily enforced since the patient becomes asymptomatic in 2–4 days. Penicillin lozenges are worthless. Topical treatment of skin infections is undesirable.

3. Patients hypersensitive to penicillin may be treated with erythromycin, 0.5 gm 4 times daily for 10 days.

B. General Measures: Gargling with warm saline solution provides relief of the sore throat. Bed rest is desirable until the patient is afebrile. Diet may be modified to reduce discomfort, and fluids may be forced during fever. Aspirin provides relief of discomfort.

C. Treatment of Complications: The suppurative complications usually respond promptly to antistreptococcal treatment, and only very rarely is incision and drainage of abscesses needed. Rheumatic fever is best prevented by prompt treatment of severe streptococcal

infections. Its treatment is discussed in Chapter 7.

Very early treatment of streptococcal infections with nephritogenic strains can probably prevent glomerulonephritis. Its treatment is discussed in Chapter 15.

Prognosis

Most streptococcal infections are self-limited. Severe illness or death is rare today except in untreated streptococcal pneumonia or sepsis. Treatment with antimicrobials greatly shortens the course of sore throat, fever, and systemic symptoms. If penicillin or erythromycin in full doses is given for 10 days, group A streptococci will be eliminated. This can prevent rheumatic fever if treatment is started during the first week after infection. Starting treatment even earlier sometimes prevents glomerulonephritis.

Bisno AL & others: Contrasting epidemiology of acute rheumatic fever and acute glomerulonephritis. New England J Med 283:561, 1970.

Dodge WF & others: Poststreptococcal glomerulonephritis: A prospective study. New England J Med 286:273, 1972.

Duma RJ & others: Streptococcal infections. Medicine 48:87, 1969.

Ferrieri P & others: Natural history of impetigo. J Clin Invest 51:2851, 1972.

Howard JB, McCracken GH Jr: The spectrum of group B streptococcal infections in infancy. Am J Dis Child 128:815, 1974.

Shrand HN: Rheumatic fever after streptococcal otitis media. New England J Med 284:221, 1971.

Wannamaker L: Differences between streptococcal infection of the throat and of the skin (2 parts.) New England J Med 282:23, 78, 1970.

Wannamaker LW: Perplexity and precision in the diagnosis of streptococcal pharyngitis. Am J Dis Child 124:352, 1972.

DIPHTHERIA

Essentials of Diagnosis

- Tenacious gray pseudomembrane at portal of entry.
- Sore throat, nasal discharge, hoarseness, malaise, fever.
- Myocarditis, neuritis.
- Smear and culture confirm the diagnosis.

General Considerations

Diphtheria is an acute contagious infection, caused by *Corynebacterium diphtheriae,* which usually attacks the respiratory tract but may involve any mucous membrane or skin wound. The organism usually gains entry through the respiratory tract, and is spread chiefly by respiratory secretions from patients with active disease or healthy carriers. The incubation period is 2–7 days. Myocarditis and late neuritis caused by an exotoxin are also characteristic.

Clinical Findings

A. Symptoms and Signs:

1. Pharyngeal diphtheria—Characteristically, there is a tenacious gray membrane forming from the tonsil onto the pillars and pharyngeal walls, surrounded by a narrow zone of erythema and a wider zone of edema. Early manifestations are mild sore throat, fever, and malaise, rapidly followed by severe signs of toxemia and prostration. Associated edema of the pharynx may add to the respiratory embarrassment and swallowing difficulties.

If myocarditis develops, there is a rapid thready pulse, indistinct heart sounds, cardiac arrhythmia, and, finally, cardiac decompensation with falling blood pressure, hepatic congestion, and associated nausea and vomiting.

In toxic neuritis the cranial nerves are involved first, causing nasal speech, regurgitation of food through the nose, diplopia, strabismus, and inability to swallow, resulting in pooling of saliva and respiratory secretions. The neuritis may progress to involve the intercostal muscles and those of the extremities. Sensory manifestations are much less prominent than motor weakness.

2. Nasal diphtheria—An occasional case will be limited to nasal infection only, producing a serosanguineous discharge with few constitutional symptoms.

3. Laryngeal diphtheria—This form of infection may occur as an extension of pharyngeal disease or separately. The signs and symptoms are those of upper airway obstruction in a progressively more toxic patient.

4. Cutaneous diphtheria—This form of disease occurs more commonly in tropical countries. The lesions resemble impetigo.

B. Laboratory Findings:

Polymorphonuclear leukocytosis may be present. Bacterial culture will confirm the diagnosis. Throat smears are often unreliable. Albuminocytologic dissociation of the CSF is noted in postdiphtheritic neuritis. Proteinuria as a result of toxic nephritis is not uncommon.

C. ECG Findings:

In myocarditis, the ECG may show an arrhythmia, P–R prolongation, heart block, and inversion of the T waves.

Differential Diagnosis

Diphtheria must be differentiated from streptococcal pharyngitis, infectious mononucleosis, adenovirus infection, Vincent's infection, and candidiasis. A presumptive diagnosis of diphtheria must be made on clinical grounds without waiting for laboratory verification since treatment is emergent.

Complications

The most common and most serious complications are myocarditis and toxic neuritis, the latter often producing paralysis of the soft palate and external muscles of the eyes as well as limb muscles.

Prevention

Active immunization with diphtheria toxoid is part of routine childhood immunization (usually in combined form as DTP) with appropriate booster injections.

Adults tend to have severe reactions to the usual childhood toxoid. Therefore, only adsorbed purified "adult type" (Td) toxoid should be used. If this is not available, a test for toxoid sensitivity (Moloney test) should be performed before giving regular toxoid.

Susceptibility to diphtheria can be determined by intradermal injection of 0.1 ml of a solution containing a minute amount of diphtheria toxin (Schick test). Redness and induration of more than 10 mm (72–96 hours after injection) denote absence of circulating antitoxin and thus susceptibility.

Exposed susceptibles should receive a booster dose of toxoid (start active immunization if not previously immune), daily treatment with penicillin by injection, and daily inspection of their throats.

Treatment

A. Specific Measures:

1. Diphtheria antitoxin—Antitoxin must be given in all cases when diphtheria cannot be excluded. The intravenous route is preferable in all but the mildest cases or in patients who are sensitive to horse serum. Conjunctival and skin tests for serum sensitivity should be done in all cases, and desensitization carried out if necessary.

The exact dose of antitoxin is purely empiric: for mild early pharyngeal or laryngeal disease, 20–40 thousand units; for moderate nasopharyngeal disease, 40–60 thousand units; for severe, extensive, or late (3 days or more) disease, 80–100 thousand units.

2. Antimicrobial therapy—Antibiotics are a useful adjunct to antitoxin, suppressing *C diphtheriae* and eliminating hemolytic streptococci, which are frequent secondary invaders. Penicillin and erythromycin are equally effective if given for 7–10 days.

3. Corticosteroids—Corticosteroids have been proposed for 2 clinical settings in diphtheria. An anti-inflammatory dose may be useful in the management of acute, severe laryngeal diphtheria. Additionally, in severe diphtheria, corticosteroids might lessen the incidence of myocarditis.

B. General Measures:

The patient should remain at absolute bed rest for at least 3 weeks until the danger of developing myocarditis has passed.

Give a liquid to soft diet as tolerated, hot saline or 30% glucose throat irrigations 3–4 times daily, and aspirin or codeine as required for relief of pain.

C. Treatment of Complications:

1. Myocarditis—No definitive treatment is known. Oxygen by tent or mask may be needed. Hypertonic glucose solution, 100 ml of 20% solution daily, may be of value. Digitalis and quinidine should be reserved for arrhythmias with rapid ventricular rate. It may be necessary to treat the patient for shock (as outlined in Chapter 1.)

2. Neuritis—Nasal feeding should be attempted if paralysis of deglutition is present. Tracheostomy and the use of a mechanical respirator may be necessary.

Corrective splinting and physical therapy may be of value.

3. **Respiratory tract obstruction**—Croupy cough, stridor, and dyspnea suggest laryngeal obstruction. Suction of membrane and secretions under direct laryngoscopy may help. Intubation or tracheostomy should be performed before the appearance of cyanosis.

4. A chronic skin ulceration due to *C diphtheriae* occurs particularly in warm, humid climates and can be followed by the complications of myocarditis and neuritis. Treatment is required as for pharyngeal disease.

5. Bacterial superinfections producing acute otitis or pneumonitis are discussed in Chapters 5 and 6.

D. Treatment of Carriers: Eradication of organisms from a carrier is difficult. Erythromycin followed by a course of penicillin may be successful. Tonsillectomy is a last resort.

Prognosis

The mortality rate varies between 10 and 30%; it is higher in older persons and when treatment has been delayed. Myocarditis which appears early is often fatal. Disturbances of conduction or the appearance of an arrhythmia implies a poor prognosis. Neuritis is rarely fatal unless respiratory muscle paralysis occurs. Myocarditis and neuritis will subside slowly but completely if the patient survives.

AMA Council on Drugs: Immunologic agents. Pages 863–883 in: *AMA Drug Evaluations,* 2nd ed. American Medical Association, 1973.

Burch GE & others: Diphtheritic myocarditis. Am J Cardiol 21:261, 1968.

McCloskey RV & others: Treatment of diphtheria carriers: Benzathine penicillin, erythromycin, and clindamycin. Ann Int Med 81:788, 1974.

Miller LW & others: Diphtheria immunization: Effect upon carriers and the control of outbreaks. Am J Dis Child 123:197, 1972.

Zalma VL: The Austin, Texas, diphtheria outbreak. JAMA 211:2125, 1970.

PERTUSSIS
(Whooping Cough)

Essentials of Diagnosis

- Paroxysmal cough ending in a high-pitched inspiratory "whoop."
- Two-week prodromal catarrhal stage of malaise, cough, coryza, and anorexia.
- Predominantly in infants under 2 years of age.
- Absolute lymphocytosis.
- Culture confirms diagnosis.

General Considerations

Pertussis is an acute communicable infection of the respiratory tract caused by *Bordetella (Haemophilus) pertussis.* It is transmitted by respiratory droplets from infected individuals. The incubation period is 7–17 days. Infectivity is greatest early in the disease and decreases until the organisms disappear from the nasopharynx (after about 1 month). Infants are most commonly infected; half of all cases occur before 2 years of age.

Clinical Findings

A. Symptoms and Signs: Physical findings are minimal or absent. Fever, if present, is low-grade. Although atypical cases lasting only a few days to a week have been described, the symptoms of classic pertussis last about 6 weeks and are divided into 3 consecutive stages:

1. **Catarrhal stage**—The onset is insidious, with lacrimation, sneezing, coryza, anorexia, malaise, and a hacking night cough which tends to become diurnal.

2. **Paroxysmal stage**—This follows the beginning of the catarrhal stage by 10–14 days, and is characterized by rapid consecutive coughs usually followed by a deep hurried inspiration (whoop). Paroxysms may involve 5–15 coughs before a breath is taken, and may occur up to 50 times in 24 hours. Stimuli such as fright or anger, crying, sneezing, inhalation of irritants, and overdistention of the stomach may produce the paroxysms. The cough is productive of copious amounts of thick mucus. Vomiting is common during the paroxysms.

3. **Convalescent stage**—This stage usually begins 4 weeks after the onset of the illness, and is manifested by a decrease in the frequency and severity of paroxysms of cough.

B. Laboratory Findings: The white count is usually 15–20 thousand/cu mm (rarely, to 50,000), 60–80% lymphocytes. The clinical diagnosis can be confirmed by taking the culture with a nasopharyngeal wire swab and planting it on fresh special media (Bordet-Gengou). A specific immunofluorescent stain of the nasopharyngeal swab may also aid in the diagnosis. The organism is recovered in only 50% or less of clinically diagnosed patients.

Differential Diagnosis

Pertussis must be differentiated from aspiration of a foreign body in children and from viral pneumonia, influenza, and acute bronchitis in older individuals. The lymphocytosis may suggest acute leukemia.

Several types of adenovirus have been shown to produce a clinical picture essentially indistinguishable from that caused by *B pertussis.*

Complications

Asphyxia, the most common complication, occurs most frequently in infants and may lead to convulsions and brain damage. The increased intracranial pressure during a paroxysm may also lead to brain damage by causing cerebral hemorrhage. Pneumonia, atelectasis, interstitial and subcutaneous emphysema, and pneumothorax may occur as a result of damaged respiratory mucosa, inspissated mucus, or increased intrathoracic pressure.

Prevention

Active immunization with pertussis vaccine is recommended for all infants, usually combined with diphtheria and tetanus toxoids (DTP). The newborn derives little or no immunity from his mother. Because of the mildness of the disease in older individuals, neither primary nor booster immunization is recommended after age 4—6 years.

Infants and young children with significant exposure to pertussis should receive antimicrobial prophylaxis (erythromycin or ampicillin). Those previously immunized should receive a booster dose of vaccine. For persons not previously immunized, the administration of 2.5 ml of pertussis immune globulin (human) is recommended.

Treatment

A. Specific Measures:

1. Antibiotics—Give either erythromycin, 50 mg/kg/day orally for 10 days, or ampicillin, 150 mg/kg/day orally for 10 days. Erythromycin has been reported to shorten the course of carriage of the organism more effectively than ampicillin. Antibiotics are of doubtful value at the paroxysmal coughing stage.

2. Hyperimmune gamma globulin, 3—6 ml IM, may hasten recovery, prevent complications, and reduce mortality. It is sometimes recommended for children under 2 years of age.

B. General Measures:

1. Nutrition—Frequent small feedings may be necessary. Re-feed if vomiting occurs shortly after a meal. Parenteral fluids may be used to ensure adequate fluid intake in severe cases.

2. Cough—Sedative and expectorant cough mixtures are of only slight benefit.

3. Nursing care—In very young infants, a paroxysm will often terminate with an apneic spell instead of a whoop. Careful observation, skilled nursing care, and avoidance of stimuli which trigger paroxysms are most important in the young infant.

C. Treatment of Complications: Pneumonia, usually due to secondary invaders, should be treated with erythromycin, ampicillin, or other appropriate antibiotic, depending upon specific bacteriologic diagnosis. Oxygen is often required.

Convulsions may require sedation, 100% oxygen inhalation, lumbar puncture, and anticonvulsive medication.

Prognosis

In children under 1 year of age, the mortality rate until recently was over 20%; this rate has been reduced to 1—2% with antibacterial therapy. Bronchiectasis is a fairly common sequel.

Aftandelians RV, Connor JD: *Bordetella pertussis* serotypes in a whooping cough outbreak. Am J Epidem 99:343, 1974.

Bass JW & others: Antimicrobial treatment of pertussis. J Pediat 75:768, 1969.
Connor JD: Etiologic role of adenovirus in pertussis syndrome. New England J Med 283:390, 1970.
Jamieson WM: Whooping cough. Brit MJ 1:223, 1973.
Linnemann CL Jr & others: Pertussis: Persistent problems. J Pediat 85:589, 1974.

INFECTIONS OF THE CNS

Infections of the CNS can be caused by almost any infectious agent but most commonly are due to pyogenic bacteria, mycobacteria, fungi, spirochetes, and viruses. Certain symptoms and signs are more or less common to all types of CNS infection: headache, fever, sensorial disturbances, neck and back stiffness, positive Kernig and Brudzinski signs, and CSF abnormalities. In patients presenting with these manifestations, the possibility of CNS infection must be considered.

Such an infection constitutes a *medical emergency.* Immediate diagnostic steps must be instituted to establish the specific cause. Normally, these include history, physical examination, blood count, blood culture, lumbar puncture with careful study and culture of the CSF, and a chest film when the patient's condition permits. A nasopharyngeal culture is also helpful. The CSF must be examined for cell count, glucose, and protein, and a smear must be stained for pyogenic bacteria (and acid-fast smear when appropriate) and cultured for pyogenic organisms and for acid-fast organisms and fungi when indicated.

In cases of pyogenic meningitis, *immediate institution of therapy* is essential to prevent death and minimize serious sequelae.

Etiologic Classification

CNS infections can be divided into 3 main categories which usually can be readily distinguished from each other by CSF examination as the first step toward etiologic diagnosis (Table 23—1).

A. Purulent Meningitis: Eg, due to infection with meningococci (40% of cases), pneumococci, streptococci, *Haemophilus influenzae,* staphylococci, and other pyogenic organisms.

B. Granulomatous Meningitis: Eg, due to *Mycobacterium tuberculosis;* coccidioides, cryptococcus, histoplasma, and other fungi; or *Treponema pallidum* (meningovascular syphilis).

C. Aseptic Meningitis: Aseptic meningitis is a much more benign form of meningitis caused principally by viruses, especially mumps virus and the enterovirus group (including coxsackieviruses and echoviruses). Poliovirus was a common cause of aseptic meningitis before the introduction of vaccination. Infectious mononucleosis may be accompanied by aseptic meningitis. Leptospiral infection is usually placed in the aseptic group because of the lymphocytic cellular response and its relatively benign course.

Table 23–1. Typical CSF findings in various CNS diseases.

Type of Infection	Cells/ cu mm	Cell Type*	Pressure	Protein (mg/100 ml)	Glucose† (mg/100 ml)
Purulent meningitis	200–5000	PMN	++++	>100	<40
Granulomatous meningitis	100–500	L‡	+++	>100	<40
Aseptic meningitis	100–700	L‡	N to +	<100	>40
"Neighborhood" reaction §	Variable	Variable	Variable	Variable	>40

*PMN = polymorphonuclear neutrophil; L = lymphocyte; N = normal.
†CSF glucose must be considered in relation to blood glucose. Normally, CSF glucose is 20–30 mg/100 ml lower than blood glucose.
‡PMNs may predominate early.
§May occur in mastoiditis, sinusitis, brain abscess, brain tumor, epidural abscess.

D. Partially Treated Bacterial Meningitis: Bacterial meningitis may present with the same course and some of the same CSF findings as aseptic meningitis following partly effective antimicrobial therapy.

E. "Neighborhood" Reaction: As noted in Table 23–1, this term denotes a purulent infectious process in close proximity to the CNS which spills some of the products of the inflammatory process—pus or protein—into the CSF. Such an infection might be a brain abscess, osteomyelitis of the vertebrae, epidural abscess, etc.

F. Meningitis in the Neonate: In newborn infants, meningitis presents as a totally separate entity. It often accompanies septicemia, is most commonly caused by gram-negative rods (most commonly *Escherichia coli*) or group B beta-hemolytic streptococci, and shows none of the typical signs of meningitis in children or adults. Fever and neck signs are often absent. Instead, the infant shows irritability, lethargy, and anorexia. Antimicrobial therapy is directed to the enteric group of bacteria and the streptococci.

G. Noninfectious Meningeal Irritation: Meningismus, presenting with the classic signs of meningeal irritation with totally normal CSF findings, may occur in the presence of other infections such as pneumonia, shigellosis, etc. Meningeal invasion by neoplastic cells may present not only with physical findings of meningeal irritation but also with increased cells and lowered CSF glucose.

Smith DH & others: Bacterial meningitis: A symposium. Pediatrics 52:586, 1973.

Swartz MN, Dodge PR: Bacterial meningitis: A review of selected aspects. (4 parts.) New England J Med 272:725, 779, 842, 898, 1965.

Wehrle PF & others: Management of acute bacterial meningitis. Pediatrics 44:991, 1969.

Wellman WE: Bacterial meningitis. Postgrad Med 42:7, 1967.

Winkelstein JA: The influence of partial treatment with penicillin on the diagnosis of bacterial meningitis. J Pediat 77:619, 1970.

1. MENINGOCOCCAL MENINGITIS

Essentials of Diagnosis

- Fever, headache, vomiting, confusion, delirium, convulsions.
- Petechial rash of skin and mucous membranes.
- Neck and back stiffness with positive Kernig and Brudzinski signs.
- Purulent spinal fluid with gram-negative intracellular and extracellular organisms.
- Culture of CSF, blood, or petechial aspiration confirms the diagnosis.
- Shock and disseminated intravascular clotting may occur.

General Considerations

Meningococcal meningitis is caused by *Neisseria meningitidis* of group A (the epidemic strain) and groups B and C (the prevalent endemic strains). A large but varying (15–40%) segment of the population are nasopharyngeal carriers of meningococci, but relatively few develop disease. Infection is transmitted by droplets, and many factors probably play a role in determining clinical illness—including prior immunity, physical stress, and immediately antecedent viral infections. The clinical illness may take the form of meningococcemia, a fulminant form of septicemia without meningitis, both meningococcemia and meningitis, or predominantly meningitis.

Clinical Findings

A. Symptoms and Signs: High fever, chills, and headache; back, abdominal, and extremity pains; and nausea and vomiting are present. In severe cases, rapidly developing confusion, delirium, and coma occur. Twitchings or frank convulsions may also be present.

Nuchal and back rigidity are present, with positive Kernig and Brudzinski signs. A petechial rash is found in most cases. Petechiae may vary from pinhead-sized to large ecchymoses or even areas of skin gangrene which may later slough if the patient survives. These petechiae are found in any part of the skin, mucous membranes, or the conjunctivas, but never in the nail beds, and they usually fade in 3—4 days. The increased intracranial pressure will cause the anterior fontanel to bulge (if not closed) and may produce Cheyne-Stokes or Biot's respiration.

Shock due to the effects of endotoxin may be present and is a bad prognostic sign.

B. Laboratory Findings: Leukocytosis is usually marked and occurs very early in the course of the disease. The urine may contain protein, casts, and red cells. Lumbar puncture reveals a cloudy to frankly purulent CSF, with elevated pressure, increased protein, and decreased glucose content. The fluid usually contains more than 1000 cells/cu mm, with polymorphonuclear cells predominating and containing gram-negative intracellular diplococci. The absence of organisms in a gram-stained smear of the CSF sediment does not rule out the diagnosis. The organism is usually demonstrated by smear or culture of the CSF, oropharynx, blood, or aspirated petechiae.

Disseminated intravascular clotting is an important complication of meningococcal infection. Determining factor V, factor VIII activity, reduced platelet count, and elevated fibrin split products can help in establishing this diagnosis.

Differential Diagnosis

Meningococcal meningitis must be differentiated from other meningitides. In small infants the clinical manifestations of meningeal infection may be erroneously diagnosed as upper respiratory infection or other acute infections.

Other bacterial infections (haemophilus, pneumococcus) or echovirus infection may also produce a petechial rash.

Complications

Arthritis, cranial nerve damage (especially the 8th nerve, with resulting deafness), and hydrocephalus may occur as complications. Myocarditis, nephritis, and intravascular coagulation may occur in severe cases.

Prevention

An effective polysaccharide vaccine for groups A and C meningococci is currently in use in the Armed Forces and has reduced the incidence of meningococcus groups A and C infection among military recruits. Its role in civilian practice is not yet established.

Epidemics in closed populations are best controlled by administering antimicrobials that reduce meningococcal carriage. Sulfonamides are not useful because most strains of meningococci are sulfonamide-resistant. Penicillin and ampicillin do not eliminate carriage. Both rifampin and minocycline can eliminate carriage. Rifampin is preferred but permits the emergence of resistant strains. Minocycline has a high incidence of vestibular side-effects.

Exposed household contacts. There is an increased risk to household members, who may be given minocycline or rifampin for 3—4 days. School and work contacts should not be treated. Hospital contacts should be treated only if intensive and intimate expo-sure has occurred, eg, giving mouth-to-mouth resuscitation.

Treatment

A. Specific Measures: Antimicrobial therapy by the intravenous route must be started immediately. If meningococcus is established or strongly suspected as the infectious agent, aqueous penicillin G is the agent of choice (20 million units per 24 hours for adults; 400,000 units/kg/24 hours for children). One-fourth of the dose is given rapidly intravenously and the rest by continuous drip or in divided doses every 4 hours. If the possibility of *Haemophilus influenzae* meningitis has not been ruled out, ampicillin should be used in a dosage of 250 mg/kg/day IV given in 6 divided doses. Cephalosporins are unsuitable for the treatment of meningitis. If the patient is allergic to penicillin, chloramphenicol, 100 mg/kg/day, is the preferred alternative drug. Treatment should be continued for 7—10 days by the intravenous route or until the patient is afebrile for 5 days and has normal CSF glucose and no more than 30—50 cells/cu mm (mostly lymphocytes) in the CSF.

B. General Measures: Hypovolemic shock is the most serious complication of meningococcal infections. Volume expansion with isotonic electrolyte solution is the initial approach while monitoring central venous pressure. Isoproterenol or dopamine is added to the infusion if the patient fails to respond.

Vital signs must be monitored. Ventilatory assistance may be required. If cerebral edema is present—and particularly if herniation of the brain through the foramen magnum is imminent—intravenous mannitol (2 gm/kg) or urea (0.5 gm/kg) may temporarily decrease the intracranial pressure.

Corticosteroids have no established role in the management of meningitis. In the presence of shock and in large amounts, they may potentiate the action of isoproterenol.

Heparinization should be considered if there is clinical or laboratory evidence of intravascular clotting. An initial dose of 50 units/kg IV is given; thereafter, an attempt is made to keep the clotting time at 20—30 minutes.

Prognosis

If the patient survives the first day, the prognosis is excellent. Sequelae are less common than in other forms of purulent meningitis.

Artenstein MS: Meningococcal infections. New England J Med 287:825, 1972.
Fraser DW & others: Trends in meningococcal disease. J Infect Dis 125:443, 1972.
Gotschlich EC: The prevention of epidemiologic meningococcal disease. Am J Med Sc 263:101, 1972.
Jensen WL: Treatment of acute meningococcal infections with penicillin G. Arch Int Med 122:322, 1968.
Kaiser AB & others: Seroepidemiology and chemoprophylaxis of disease due to sulfonamide resistant *Neisseria meningitidis* in a civilian population. J Infect Dis 130:217, 1974.

McGehee WG & others: Intravascular coagulation in fulminant meningococcemia. Ann Int Med 67:250, 1967.

Munford RS & others: Eradication of carriage of *Neisseria meningitidis* in families: A study in Brazil. J Infect Dis 129:644, 1974.

2. PNEUMOCOCCAL, STREPTOCOCCAL, & STAPHYLOCOCCAL MENINGITIS

The symptoms are similar to those of meningococcal meningitis, but a preceding infection is usually present and a focus is often demonstrable in the lungs (pneumococcal), the middle ear, or sinuses. The CSF must be cultured and examined to determine the causative agent.

Specific treatment of pneumococcal and streptococcal meningitis consists of aqueous penicillin, 1 million units IV every 2 hours or by continuous drip.

Staphylococcal meningitis is treated with intravenous methicillin or nafcillin (10–12 gm daily or 300 mg/kg/24 hours) in divided doses. When the organism is definitely penicillin-sensitive, penicillin G is preferred. The duration of therapy must be between 2 and 4 weeks. Complications, including ventriculitis, arachnoiditis, CSF block, and hydrocephalus, are more common in these forms of meningitis than in meningococcal meningitis.

Weiss W & others: Prognostic factors in pneumococcal meningitis. Arch Int Med 120:517, 1967.

3. HAEMOPHILUS INFLUENZAE MENINGITIS

Haemophilus influenzae meningitis occurs most frequently in children under 6 years of age.

Nothing about the onset, symptoms, or signs distinguishes this illness from other purulent meningitides. It may exist for several days as an apparent respiratory infection; however, headache, irritability, fever, malaise, vomiting, unexplained leukocytosis, and some nuchal and back rigidity should suggest meningitis. Lumbar puncture will reveal the gram-negative pleomorphic rods in the purulent spinal fluid smear or culture. Immunofluorescent stains of CSF sediment or culture may provide a rapid specific diagnosis.

It is impossible to distinguish *H influenzae* meningitis from other purulent meningitides on the basis of symptoms and signs. Identification of the specific organism in the CSF establishes the diagnosis.

Prevention

An experimental group b *H influenzae* vaccine has recently been prepared.

Household and hospital contacts require no treatment.

Treatment

A. Specific Measures: The drug of choice is sodium ampicillin, 300 mg/kg/day IV. One-fourth of the dose is given immediately when the diagnosis is made and the remainder in divided doses every 4 hours; intravenous medication must be continued for 10–14 days or until CSF glucose is normal and CSF cells fewer than 30/cu mm. In penicillin allergy, chloramphenicol (100 mg/kg/day) is the drug of choice. Recently, ampicillin-resistant strains of *H influenzae* have appeared in many communities. Such strains produce a penicillinase. If such strains are prevalent, initial treatment consists of both ampicillin and chloramphenicol. The latter is discontinued when ampicillin susceptibility has been established for the isolate in the laboratory.

B. General Measures: The general management is similar to that described above for meningococcal meningitis. Shock is less likely, but subdural effusion and other complications are more common.

Prognosis

The case fatality rate is about 5%. One should aim not only at survival but at prevention of sequelae, including the more subtle forms of CNS damage.

Barrett FF & others: A 12-year review of the antibiotic management of *Hemophilus influenzae* meningitis. J Pediat 81:370, 1972.

Katz SL: Ampicillin resistant *Haemophilus influenzae* type B: A status report. Pediatrics 55:6, 1975.

Robbins JB & others: *Haemophilus influenzae* type B: Disease and immunity in humans. Ann Int Med 78:259, 1973.

Sell SHW & others: Long-term sequelae of *Hemophilus influenzae* meningitis. Pediatrics 49:206, 1972.

Shackleford PG & others: Therapy of *Haemophilus influenzae* meningitis reconsidered. New England J Med 287:634, 1972.

4. TUBERCULOUS MENINGITIS

Essentials of Diagnosis

- Gradual onset of listlessness, irritability, and anorexia.
- Headache, vomiting, coma, convulsions; neck and back rigidity.
- Tuberculous focus may be evident elsewhere.
- CSF shows several hundred lymphocytes, low glucose, and high protein.

General Considerations

Tuberculous meningitis is caused by hematogenous spread of tubercle bacilli from a localized gross or microscopic focus usually in the lungs or the peritracheal, peribronchial, or mesenteric lymph nodes, or it may be a consequence of miliary spread. Its greatest incidence is in children 1–5 years of age.

Clinical Findings

A. Symptoms and Signs: The onset is usually gradual, with listlessness, irritability, anorexia, and fever, followed by headache, vomiting, night cries, convulsions, and coma. In older patients headache and behavioral changes are prominent early symptoms.

Nuchal rigidity, opisthotonos, and paralysis occur as the meningitis progresses. Paralysis of the extraocular muscles is common. Ophthalmoscopic examination may reveal choroid tubercles. General physical examination may reveal evidence of tuberculosis elsewhere. The tuberculin skin test may be negative in miliary tuberculosis.

B. Laboratory Findings: The CSF is frequently yellowish, with increased pressure and 100–500 cells/cu mm (early, polymorphonuclear neutrophils; later, lymphocytes) and decreased glucose content. On standing, the CSF may form a web and pellicle from which organisms may be demonstrated by smear, culture, or guinea pig inoculation. Moderate leukocytosis is common. Chest x-ray often reveals a tuberculous focus.

Differential Diagnosis

Tuberculous meningitis may be confused with any other type of meningitis, but the gradual onset and evidence of tuberculosis elsewhere usually help to clarify the diagnosis.

Other forms of granulomatous meningitis such as fungal meningitis must also be considered.

Complications

After recovery, there may be residual brain damage resulting in motor paralysis, convulsive states, mental impairment, and abnormal behavior. The incidence of these complications increases the longer therapy is withheld.

Prevention

Early identification of tuberculin converters and children with primary tuberculosis and treatment with isoniazid at that stage is the key to preventing tuberculous meningitis.

Treatment

A. Specific Measures: Give isoniazid, 10 mg/kg/day (up to a total of 300 mg/day), rifampin, 600 mg/day, and ethambutol, 15 mg/kg/day. All are given orally, and each can be given as a single daily dose. Treatment should be continued for 18–24 months. In addition, give streptomycin, 1 gm IM daily for 2 weeks, and then continue twice weekly for 60–90 days. Corticosteroid treatment (60 mg prednisone or equivalent daily) should be used initially, continued until improvement is established, and then gradually discontinued.

Caution: Ethambutol rarely causes retinal neuropathy. Visual acuity should be tested monthly with a Snellen chart. Peripheral neuropathy due to isoniazid can be prevented by giving pyridoxine, 50 mg daily orally.

B. General Measures: Treat symptoms as they arise and maintain good nutrition and adequate fluid intake. Treat hyponatremia due to inappropriate ADH secretion which may be present.

Prognosis

The natural course of the untreated disease is death within 6–8 weeks. With early diagnosis and treatment, the recovery rate may reach 90%; if treatment is not instituted until the disease has reached the late stage, the recovery rate is 25–30%. Serious sequelae are the rule.

Lorber J: The results of treatment of 549 cases of tuberculous meningitis. Am Rev Tuberc 69:13, 1954.

Tahernia AC: Tuberculous meningitis: Modern diagnosis, treatment and prognosis, as exemplified in 38 cases in southern Iran. Clin Pediat 6:173, 1967.

SALMONELLOSIS

Salmonellosis includes infection by any of approximately 900 serotypes of salmonellae. Three general clinical patterns are recognized: (1) enteric fever, the best example of which is typhoid fever, due to *Salmonella typhi;* (2) acute gastroenteritis, caused by *S typhimurium* and many other types; and (3) the "septicopyemic" type, characterized by bacteremia and focal lesions and most commonly caused by *S choleraesuis.* Any serotype may cause any of these clinical patterns. All are transmitted by ingestion of the organism in contaminated food or fluid.

1. TYPHOID FEVER

Essentials of Diagnosis

- Gradual onset of malaise, headache, sore throat, cough, and finally "pea-soup" diarrhea or constipation.
- Slow (stepladder) rise of fever to maximum and then slow return to normal.
- Rose spots, relative bradycardia, splenomegaly, and abdominal distention and tenderness.
- Leukopenia; positive blood, stool, and urine culture.
- Elevated or rising specific (Widal) agglutination titers.

General Considerations

Typhoid fever is caused by the gram-negative rod *Salmonella typhi,* which enters the patient via the gastrointestinal tract, where it penetrates the intestinal wall and produces inflammation of the mesenteric lymph nodes and the spleen. Bacteremia occurs, and the infection then localizes principally in the lymphoid tissue of the small intestine (particularly within the 2 feet of the ileocecal valve). Peyer's patches become inflamed and may ulcerate, with a maximum during the third week of the disease. Occasionally the organism may localize in the lungs, gallbladder, kidneys, or CNS, with resulting inflammation. Infection is transmitted by consumption of contaminated food or drink. The sources of most infections are chronic carriers with persistent gallbladder or urinary tract infection. The incubation period is 5–14 days.

Clinical Findings

A. Symptoms and Signs: The onset is usually insidious, but sometimes, especially in children, it may be abrupt, with chills and a sharp rise in temperature. The course of classic untreated typhoid fever can be divided into 3 stages:

1. The prodromal stage—During the period of invasion, the patient gradually begins to feel unwell. Increasing malaise, headache, cough, general body aching, sore throat, and epistaxis are common. Frequently there is abdominal pain, constipation or diarrhea, and vomiting. During this period, the fever ascends in a stepladder fashion, the maximum temperature on each day being slightly higher than on the preceding day. The temperature is generally higher in the evening than in the morning.

2. The fastigium—After about 7–10 days, the fever stabilizes, varying less than 2° F during the day, and the patient becomes quite sick. "Pea-soup" diarrhea or severe constipation, or marked abdominal distention is common. Severe cases develop the "typhoid state," in which the patient lies motionless and unresponsive, with eyes half-shut, appearing wasted and exhausted. He can usually be aroused to carry out simple commands.

3. The stage of defervescence—If the patient survives the severe toxemia of the second stage of the disease and develops no complications, his condition gradually improves. The fever declines in a stepladder fashion to reach normal in 7–10 days. The patient becomes more alert, and his abdominal symptoms disappear. During this stage, relapse may occur as late as 1–2 weeks after the temperature has returned to normal. This relapse is usually milder than the original infection.

During the early prodrome, physical findings are slight. Later, splenomegaly, abdominal distention and tenderness, relative bradycardia, dicrotic pulse, and occasionally meningismus, systolic murmur, and gallop rhythm appear. The rash (rose spots) commonly appears during the second week of the disease. The individual spot, found principally on the trunk, is a pink papule 2–3 mm in diameter which fades on pressure. It disappears over a period of 3–4 days.

B. Laboratory Findings: Blood cultures may be positive in the first week and remain positive for a variable period thereafter. Stools are positive for the organism after the first week of the disease; the urine may be positive at any time.

During the second week of the disease, antibodies begin to appear in the blood and continue to rise in titer until about the end of the third week (Widal test). If an anamnestic response to other infectious diseases or recent vaccination is ruled out, an O (somatic) antibody titer of 1:60 is presumptively diagnostic; a rising titer (as demonstrated by 2 specimens taken approximately a week apart) is diagnostic.

Moderate anemia and leukopenia are the rule.

Differential Diagnosis

This enteric form of infection can be produced by other salmonella species (eg, *Salmonella paratyphi* A, B, C).

Typhoid fever must be distinguished from other prolonged fevers associated with normal or depressed white count. Examples include tuberculosis, viral pneumonia, psittacosis, bacterial endocarditis, brucellosis, and Q fever. *Yersinia enterocolitica* can produce enteritis with fever, diarrhea, vomiting, abdominal pain, and mesenteric adenitis.

Complications

Complications occur in about 30% of untreated cases and account for 75% of all deaths. Intestinal hemorrhage is most likely to occur during the third week and is manifested by a sudden drop in temperature, rise in pulse, and signs of shock followed by dark or fresh blood in the stool. Intestinal perforation is most likely to occur during the third week. Sudden rigor, drop in temperature, and increase in pulse rate, accompanied by abdominal pain and tenderness, may be noted. Less frequent complications include urinary retention, pneumonia, thrombophlebitis, myocarditis, psychosis, cholecystitis, nephritis, spondylitis (typhoid spine), and meningitis.

Prevention

Active immunization should be provided for household members of a typhoid carrier, for travelers to endemic areas, and during an epidemic outbreak.

Typhoid vaccine is administered in 2 injections of 0.5 ml each, subcut, not less than 4 weeks apart. The usual procedure is to revaccinate twice only, with a single injection of 0.5 ml subcut administered at 4-year intervals. (See Immunization Schedules in Appendix.)

Environmental hygiene control requires protection of food and water and adequate waste disposal.

Carriers must be kept under surveillance and not permitted to work as food handlers.

Treatment

A. Specific Measures: Give ampicillin, 100 mg/kg/day IV or 6 gm/day in divided doses every 4 hours by mouth; or chloramphenicol, 1 gm every 6 hours orally until fever disappears and then 0.5 gm every 6 hours for 2 weeks (children, 50 mg/kg/day). Some strains of *S typhi* from Central and South America have acquired resistance to ampicillin or chloramphenicol or both. Sensitivity studies must guide the choice of antibiotic. Infections resistant to both drugs respond to trimethoprim-sulfonamide mixtures.

Table 23–2. Acute bacterial diarrheas and "food poisoning."

Organism	Incubation Period (Hours)	Vomiting	Diarrhea	Fever	Epidemiology	Pathogenesis	Clinical Features
Staphylococcus	1–18	+++	+	–	Staphylococci grow in meats and dairy and bakery products and produce enterotoxin.	Enterotoxin absorbed from gut. Acts on medullary centers.	Abrupt onset, intense vomiting for up to 24 hours, regular recovery in 24–48 hours. Occurs in groups of persons eating the same food. No treatment usually necessary except to restore fluids and electrolytes.
Clostridium perfringens	8–16	±	+++	–	Clostridia grow in rewarmed meat dishes and produce enterotoxin.	Enterotoxin* causes hypersecretion in small intestine.	Abrupt onset of profuse diarrhea; vomiting occasionally. Recovery usual without treatment in 1–4 days. It is sometimes necessary to restore fluids and electrolytes. Many clostridia in cultures of food and feces of patients.
Clostridium botulinum	24–96	±	Rare	–	Clostridia grow in poorly canned or vacuum-packed anaerobic foods and produce toxin.	Toxin absorbed from gut blocks acetylcholine at neuromuscular junction.	Onset of diplopia, dysphagia, dysphonia, other cranial nerve signs, respiratory embarrassment; vomiting infrequent. Treatment requires clear airway, maintenance of ventilation, and intravenous polyvalent botulinus antitoxin (see p 832). Toxin present in food and serum. Mortality rate high.
Escherichia coli (some strains)	24–72	±	++	–	Organisms grow in gut and produce toxin. May also invade superficial epithelium.	Toxin* causes hypersecretion in small intestine ("traveler's diarrhea").	Usually abrupt onset of diarrhea; vomiting rare. A serious infection in neonates, requiring fluid and electrolyte replacement and oral kanamycin. In adults, "traveler's diarrhea" is usually self-limited in 1–3 days. Use diphenoxylate (Lomotil) but no antimicrobials.
Vibrio parahaemolyticus	6–96	+	++	±	Organisms grow in seafood and in gut and produce toxin. May also invade epithelium.	Toxin* causes hypersecretion in small intestine; stools may be bloody.	Abrupt onset of diarrhea in groups consuming the same food, especially crabs and other seafood. Rarely, blood and mucus in stool. Restore fluids and electrolytes if losses are severe. Recovery is usually complete in 1–3 days. Food and stool cultures are positive.
Vibrio cholerae (mild cases)	24–72	+	+++	–	Organisms grow in gut and produce toxin.	Toxin* causes hypersecretion in small intestine.	Abrupt onset of liquid diarrhea in endemic area. Needs prompt replacement of fluids and electrolytes (see p 826). Variable severity. Tetracyclines shorten excretion of vibrios. Stool cultures are positive.
Shigella sp (mild cases)	24–72	±	++	+	Organisms grow in superficial gut epithelium and gut lumen and produce toxin.	Toxin* causes hypersecretion in small intestine; epithelium shed, with pus, mucus, and blood in stools.	Abrupt onset of diarrhea, often with blood and pus in stools, cramps, tenesmus, and lethargy. Stool cultures are positive. Give ampicillin, chloramphenicol, or kanamycin in severe cases. Often mild and self-limited. Restore fluids.
Salmonella sp	8–48	±	++	+	Organisms grow in gut. Do not produce toxin.	Superficial infection of gut; little invasion.	Gradual or abrupt onset of diarrhea and low-grade fever. Replace fluids and electrolytes. Do not give antimicrobials unless systemic dissemination is suspected. Stool cultures are positive. Prolonged carriage is frequent.

*Toxin stimulates adenyl cyclase activity and increases cyclic AMP concentration in gut.

B. General Measures: Prevent decubiti by careful bathing, skin massage, and use of rubber "doughnuts" over pressure areas. Careful oral hygiene is important.

Give a high-caloric, low-residue diet. Hydrocortisone, 100 mg IV every 8 hours, may tide over severely toxic patients.

Parenteral fluids may be necessary to supplement oral intake and maintain urine output. Abdominal distention may be relieved by abdominal stupes. Vasopressin and neostigmine must be used with great caution because of the danger of perforation. Strict stool and urine isolation must be observed.

C. Treatment of Complications: Secondary pneumonia may be treated with antibiotics, depending on the etiologic agent.

Transfusions should be given as required for hemorrhage. If perforation occurs, immediate surgery is required; anticipate and treat shock (see Chapter 1) before it becomes manifest.

D. Treatment of Carriers: Chemotherapy is usually ineffective in abolishing the carrier state. However, a trial of ampicillin first and then chloramphenicol is worthwhile. Cholecystectomy may be effective.

Prognosis

The mortality rate of typhoid fever is about 2% in treated cases. Elderly or debilitated persons are likely to do poorly. The course is milder in children.

With complications, the prognosis is poor. Relapses occur in up to 15% of cases. A residual carrier state frequently persists in spite of chemotherapy.

2. SALMONELLA GASTROENTERITIS

By far the most common form of salmonellosis is acute gastroenteritis. The commonest causative serotypes are *S typhimurium, S derby, S heidelberg, S infantis, S newport,* and *S enteritidis.* The incubation period is 8–48 hours after ingestion of contaminated food or liquid.

Symptoms and signs consist of fever (often with chills), nausea and vomiting, cramping abdominal pain, and diarrhea, which may be bloody. The disease persists over a course of 3–5 days. Differentiation must be made from viral gastroenteritis, food poisoning, shigellosis, amebic dysentery, acute ulcerative colitis, and acute surgical abdominal conditions. Leukocytosis is usually not present. The organisms can be cultured from the stools.

The disease is usually self-limited, but bacteremia with localization in joints or bones may occur, especially in young infants and in patients with sickle cell disease.

Treatment in the uncomplicated case of gastroenteritis is symptomatic only. Antimicrobial therapy may prolong the carriage of salmonellae in the gastrointestinal tract. Young or malnourished infants, severely ill patients, those with sickle cell disease, and those

in whom bacteremia is suspected should be treated with ampicillin (100 mg/kg IV or orally) or chloramphenicol (50–100 mg/kg orally).

3. SEPTICOPYEMIC SALMONELLOSIS

Rarely, salmonella infection may be manifested by prolonged or recurrent fever accompanied by bacteremia and by localization and abscess formation in one or more sites—such as the bones, joints, pleura, pericardium, endocardium, meninges, and lungs. Treatment is as for typhoid fever and should include drainage of accessible lesions.

Aserkoff B, Bennett JV: Effect of therapy in acute salmonellosis on salmonella in feces. New England J Med 281:636, 1969.

Cherubin CE & others: Septicemia with non-typhoid salmonella. Medicine 53:365, 1974.

Fox MD & others: Salmonella surveillance 1970. J Infect Dis 125:196, 1972.

Garcia de Olarte D & others: Treatment of diarrhea in malnourished infants and children: A double-blind study comparing ampicillin and placebo. Am J Dis Child 127:379, 1974.

Gutman LT & others: An outbreak of *Yersinia enterocolitica* enteritis. New England J Med 288:1372, 1973.

Hornick RB & others: Typhoid fever vaccine—yes or no? M Clin North America 51:617, 1967.

Overturf G & others: Antibiotic resistance in typhoid fever. New England M Med 289:463, 1973.

Phillips WE: Ampicillin for chronic typhoid carriers. JAMA 217:913, 1971.

Robertson RP, Wahab MFA, Raasch FO: Evaluation of chloramphenicol and ampicillin in salmonella enteric fever. New England J Med 278:171, 1968.

FOOD POISONING

Food poisoning is a nonspecific term often applied to the syndrome of acute anorexia, nausea, vomiting, or diarrhea which is attributed to food intake, particularly if it afflicts groups of persons and is not accompanied by fever. The actual cause of such acute gastrointestinal upsets might be emotional stress, viral or bacterial infections, food intolerance, or inorganic (eg, sodium nitrite) or organic (eg, mushroom, shellfish) poisons. More specifically, food poisoning may refer to toxins produced by bacteria growing in food (staphylococci, clostridia) or to acute food infections with short incubation periods and a mild course (salmonella gastroenteritis [see above], *Vibrio parahaemolyticus* infection, infection with certain serotypes of *Escherichia coli,* and occasionally shigellosis or cholera). Some prominent features of some of these "food poisonings" are listed in Table 23–2. In general, the diagnosis must be suspected when groups of persons with a common food intake develop acute vomiting or diarrhea. Food and stools must be secured for bacteriologic and toxicologic examination.

Treatment usually consists of replacement of fluids and electrolytes and, very rarely, the management of hypovolemic shock and respiratory embarrassment. If botulism is suspected (see p 832), polyvalent antitoxin must be administered.

Antimicrobial drugs are not indicated unless a specific microbial agent producing progressive systemic involvement can be identified. Antimicrobial drugs may in fact aggravate anorexia and diarrhea and may prolong microbial carriage and excretion.

Note: Iodochlorhydroxyquin (Vioform, Entero-Vioform) is not useful for prophylaxis or treatment of any of these disorders and may be harmful.

Grady GF, Keusch GT: Pathogenesis of bacterial diarrheas. (2 parts.) New England J Med 285:831, 891, 1971.

CHOLERA

Essentials of Diagnosis

- Sudden onset of severe, frequent diarrhea, up to 1 liter/hour.
- The liquid stool (and occasionally vomitus) is gray, turbid, and without fecal odor, blood, or pus (rice water).
- Rapid development of marked dehydration, acidosis, hypokalemia, and hypotension.
- History of sojourn in endemic area or contact with infected person.
- Positive stool cultures and agglutination of vibrios with specific sera.

General Considerations

Cholera is an acute diarrheal disease caused by *Vibrio cholerae* or El Tor vibrios. The latter are currently causing a pandemic. The infection is acquired by the ingestion of food or drink contaminated by feces from cases or carriers containing large numbers of vibrios. The infective dose is near 10^9 vibrios. The vibrios grow in the small intestine (particularly the ileum) and produce a powerful exotoxin. This toxin induces massive hypersecretion of fluids and electrolytes in the gut—presumably by activation of adenylate cyclase, increased production of cyclic adenosine monophosphate, and greatly increased active transport into the gut lumen. This results in massive diarrhea of up to 7 liters/24 hours which is fatal in 50% of patients if untreated. The incubation period is 1–5 days. Only a small minority of exposed persons become ill.

Clinical Findings

A. Symptoms and Signs: The spectrum of severity of illness is very wide. Typical cases have an explosive onset of frequent, watery stools which soon lose all fecal appearance and odor. They are grayish, turbid, and liquid, containing degenerated epithelium and mucus but rarely gross pus or blood. A typical stool may be 7 liters/24 hours containing Na^+, 125 mEq/liter; K^+, 20 mEq/liter; and HCO_3^-, 45 mEq/liter. Vomiting may also occur early. As a result, the patient rapidly becomes markedly dehydrated and acidotic, with sunken eyes, hypotension, subnormal temperature, rapid and shallow breathing, muscle cramps, oliguria, shock, and coma.

B. Laboratory Findings: Blood studies reveal marked hemoconcentration with rising specific gravity of plasma, metabolic acidosis, and often elevation of nonprotein nitrogen. The serum potassium may be normal in spite of severe potassium loss.

The vibrios can be easily grown from the stool—never from blood—and can be identified by agglutination with known specific serum.

Differential Diagnosis

Cholera must be distinguished from other causes of severe diarrhea and dehydration, particularly diarrheas due to shigellae, viruses, *Escherichia coli* enterotoxin, and protozoa in endemic areas.

Prevention

Cholera vaccine gives only limited protection and is of no value in controlling outbreaks. The vaccine is given in 2 injections of 0.5 and 1 ml IM or subcut 1–4 weeks apart. A booster dose of 0.5 ml is given every 6 months when cholera is a hazard. New types of vaccine are being investigated. At present, cholera vaccination is not required for anybody by USA authorities.

In endemic areas, all water, other drinks, food, and utensils must be boiled or avoided. Effective decontamination of excreta is essential, but strict isolation of patients is unnecessary and quarantine is undesirable. In countries with high standards of sanitation and public health, the importation of cholera rarely leads to outbreaks of significant size.

Treatment

Water and electrolyte losses must be restored promptly and continuously, and acidosis must be corrected. Diarrheal loss and hemoconcentration must be measured continuously. In moderately ill patients, it may be possible to provide replacement by oral fluids given in the same volume as that lost. A suitable oral solution contains NaCl, 4 gm/liter; $NaHCO_3$, 4 gm/liter; KCl, 1–2 gm/liter; and glucose, 21 gm/liter. In more severely ill patients or those unable to take fluids by mouth, replacement must be by intravenous fluids. A suitable intravenous solution contains Na^+, 133 mEq/liter; Cl^-, 98 mEq/liter; K^+, 13 mEq/liter; and HCO_3^-, 48 mEq/liter. Initially, this solution is infused at a rate of 50–100 ml/minute until circulating blood volume and blood pressure are restored. It may then be given more slowly to replace lost stool volume. In children, more potassium and less sodium is lost and must be replaced. An older method relied on the degree of hemoconcentration to direct fluid replacement: For every 0.001 increase in plasma specific gravity above 1.025, 4 ml/kg of mixed isotonic sodium lactate and saline (1:2 ratio) were infused.

Tetracycline, 0.5 gm orally every 6 hours for 3—5 days, suppresses vibrio growth in the gut and shortens the time of vibrio excretion.

Whenever cholera is suspected, the Health Department must be notified by telephone.

Prognosis

The untreated disease lasts 3—5 days, with a mortality rate ranging from 20—80%. With prompt and competent treatment, the mortality rate may be reduced to 1%.

Carpenter CCJ: Cholera enterotoxin: Insights into transport processes. Am J Med 50:1, 1971.

Cash RA & others: Response of man to infection with *Vibrio cholerae.* J Infect Dis 129:45, 1974.

Gangarosa EJ: The epidemiology of cholera. Bull New York Acad Med 47:1140, 1971.

Hendrix TR: Pathophysiology of cholera. Bull New York Acad Med 47:1169, 1971.

Phillips RA: Asiatic cholera. Ann Rev Med 19:69, 1968.

BACILLARY DYSENTERY
(Shigellosis)

Essentials of Diagnosis

- Diarrhea, often with blood and mucus.
- Cramps.
- Fever, malaise, prostration, clouded sensorium.
- Pus in stools; organism isolated on stool culture.

General Considerations

Shigella dysentery is a common disease, often self-limited and mild but occasionally serious, particularly in the first 3 years of life. Poor sanitary conditions promote the spread of shigella. *Shigella sonnei* is the leading cause of this illness in the USA, followed by *S flexneri. S dysenteriae* causes the most serious form of the illness. Recently, there has been a rise in strains resistant to multiple antibiotics.

Clinical Findings

A. Symptoms and Signs: The illness usually starts abruptly, with diarrhea, lower abdominal cramps, and tenesmus. The diarrheal stool often is mixed with blood and mucus. Systemic symptoms are fever (in young children, up to 104° F), chills, anorexia and malaise, headache, lethargy, and, in the most severe cases, meningismus, coma, and convulsions. As the illness progresses, the patient becomes progressively weaker and more dehydrated. The abdomen is tender. Sigmoidoscopic examination reveals an inflamed, engorged mucosa with punctate, sometimes large areas of ulceration.

B. Laboratory Findings: The white blood count shows an increase in polymorphonuclear cells with a pronounced shift to the left. The stool shows blood, mucus, and pus. Stool culture is positive for shigellae.

Differential Diagnosis

Bacillary dysentery must be distinguished from salmonella gastroenteritis, enteropathogenic *Escherichia coli* infections, and viral diarrhea. Amebic dysentery may be similar clinically and is diagnosed by finding amebas in the fresh stool specimen. Ulcerative colitis in the adolescent and adult is an important cause of bloody diarrhea.

Complications

Dehydration, acidosis, and electrolyte imbalance occur in infancy. Temporary disaccharidase deficiency may follow the diarrhea. Arthritis is an uncommon complication.

Treatment

A. Specific Measures: Treatment of shock, restoration of circulating blood volume, and renal perfusion are lifesaving in severe cases. The current antimicrobial agent of choice is ampicillin, 100 mg/kg/day orally in 4 divided doses for 5—7 days. The drug should not be continued longer if there is clinical improvement even if stool cultures remain positive. Ampicillin-resistant strains of shigella are increasing in frequency. Tetracycline, chloramphenicol, and kanamycin may also be effective. However, since the majority of cases are mild and self-limited, one cannot justify the use of even mildly toxic antibiotics.

B. General Measures: Parenteral hydration and correction of acidosis and electrolyte disturbances are essential in all moderately or severely ill patients. After the bowel has been at rest for a short time, clear fluids are given for 2—3 days. The diet should then be soft, easily digestible, and given in small frequent feedings, avoiding whole milk and high-residue and fatty foods.

Paregoric provides effective symptomatic relief; atropine sulfate (or tincture of belladonna) is helpful when cramps are severe. Diphenoxylate with atropine (Lomotil) controls moderate diarrhea in adults. The patient should be placed on effective stool isolation precautions both in the hospital and in the home to limit the spread of the infection.

Prognosis

The prognosis is excellent in all but very young or debilitated patients if intravenous rehydration is available. The recent importation of the more virulent *S dysenteriae* from Central America may make this illness a greater threat.

Du Pont HL & others: The response of man to virulent *Shigella flexneri.* J Infect Dis 119:296, 1969.

Grady GF, Keusch GT: Pathogenesis of bacterial diarrheas. (2 parts.) New England J Med 285:831, 891, 1971.

Haltalin KC: Treatment of acute diarrhea in outpatients. Am J Dis Child 124:554, 1972.

Mata LJ & others: Epidemic Shiga bacillus infection in Central America. I. Etiologic investigation in Guatemala, 1969. J Infect Dis 122:170, 1970.

Weissman JB & others: Changing antimicrobial therapy of shigellosis. J Infect Dis 127:611, 1973.

TRAVELER'S DIARRHEA

Whenever a person travels from one country to another, particularly if the change involves a marked difference in climate, social conditions, or sanitation standards and facilities, he is likely to develop diarrhea within 2–10 days. There may be up to 10 or even more loose stools per day, often accompanied by abdominal cramps, nausea, occasionally vomiting, and rarely fever. The stools do not usually contain mucus or blood, and, aside from weakness, dehydration, and occasionally acidosis, there are no systemic manifestations of infection. The illness usually subsides spontaneously within 1–5 days. Rarely, it continues for 2–3 weeks.

Bacteriologic cultures of stools hardly ever reveal salmonellae or shigellae. Contributory causes may at times include unusual food and drink, change in living habits, occasional enteroviral infections, and change in bowel flora. A significant proportion of cases of traveler's diarrhea appears to be caused by acquisition of strains of *Escherichia coli* which produce a potent enterotoxin. This enterotoxin is released by the organisms growing in the small intestine, attaches to ganglioside receptors on intestinal villi, stimulates adenylate cyclase, and increases cyclic adenosine monophosphate concentration in the small intestine. As a result, there is enormous hypersecretion of water and electrolytes into the gut, distention, and massive diarrhea. Special strains of *E coli* which elaborate a heat-labile enterotoxin (LT) and are prevalent in a given environment appear to be particularly responsible. Some individuals do not permit unrestricted multiplication of these organisms; others are perhaps resistant to the LT because of prior exposure.

For most individuals the affliction is short-lived, and its effects may be further reduced by opiates or diphenoxylate with atropine (Lomotil). Antimicrobial drugs generally are not indicated and, indeed, may aggravate the diarrhea. However, no definitive studies on the therapeutic effects of antimicrobials or of peristalsis-slowing agents have been done. In all cases, water and electrolyte balance must be restored.

Gorbach SL & others: Traveller's diarrhea and toxigenic *Escherichia coli*. New England J Med 292:933, 1975.

Merson MH: Toxigenic turista. New England J Med 292:969, 1975.

BRUCELLOSIS

Essentials of Diagnosis

- Insidious onset of easy fatigability, headache, arthralgia, anorexia, sweating, and irritability.
- Intermittent fever, especially at night, which may become chronic and undulant.
- Cervical and axillary lymphadenopathy; hepatosplenomegaly.
- Lymphocytosis, positive blood culture, elevated agglutination titer.

General Considerations

The infection is transmitted from animals to man. *Brucella abortus* (cattle), *B suis* (hogs), and *B melitensis* (goats) are the main agents. Transmission to man occurs by contact with infected meat (slaughterhouse workers), placentae of infected animals (farmers, veterinarians), or ingestion of infected, unpasteurized milk or cheese. Organisms may enter through abraded skin or mucous membranes or via the respiratory tract. The incubation period varies from a few days to several weeks. The disorder may become chronic and persist for years. In the USA, brucellosis is very rare except in midwestern states.

Clinical Findings

A. Symptoms and Signs: The onset may be acute, with fever, chills, and sweats, but often the disease begins so insidiously that it may be weeks before the patient seeks medical care for weakness and exhaustion upon minimal activity. Symptoms also include headache, abdominal pains with anorexia and constipation, and arthralgia, sometimes associated with periarticular swelling but not local heat. The fever may be septic, sustained, low-grade, or even absent but is more often of the intermittent type preceded by chilliness, rising during the evening hours and falling with a sweat (night sweat) in the early morning hours. The chronic form may assume an undulant nature, with periods of normal temperature between acute attacks, and the above symptoms plus emotional instability and weight loss may persist for years, either continuously or intermittently.

Physical findings are minimal. Half of cases have peripheral lymph node enlargement and splenomegaly; hepatomegaly is less common.

B. Laboratory Findings: The white count is usually normal to low, with a relative or absolute lymphocytosis. The organism can be recovered from the blood, CSF, urine, and tissues early in the infection; later, this may be difficult. An agglutination titer greater than 1:100 (and especially a rising titer) supports the diagnosis. A prozone phenomenon (serum agglutinates in high but not in low dilution) is common. IgG antibody indicates active disease, whereas IgM antibody may persist after recovery. The intradermal skin test is of no value. Liver enzyme determinations are often elevated.

Differential Diagnosis

Brucellosis must be differentiated from any acute febrile disease, especially influenza, tularemia, Q fever, and enteric fever. Its chronic form resembles Hodgkin's disease, tuberculosis, and malaria. The chronic form may simulate psychoneurosis, and the latter is sometimes incorrectly called chronic brucellosis.

Complications

The most frequent complications are bone and joint lesions such as spondylitis and suppurative arthritis (usually of a single joint), subacute bacterial endocarditis, encephalitis, and meningitis. Less common complications are pneumonitis with pleural effusion, hepatitis, and cholecystitis. Abortion in humans is no more common with this disease than with any other acute bacterial disease during pregnancy. Pancytopenia is rare.

Prevention

Prevention is by destruction of infected dairy animals, immunization of susceptible animals, and pasteurization of milk and milk products.

Treatment

A. Specific Treatment: Tetracycline, 2 gm orally daily for 21 days, is the treatment of choice. Streptomycin, 0.5 gm IM every 12 hours, is occasionally given at the same time as tetracycline. Relapse may require retreatment. Ampicillin may be effective. Co-trimoxazole (trimethoprim with sulfamethoxazole) has been used effectively in early cases.

B. General Measures: Place the patient at bed rest during the acute febrile stage and maintain adequate nutrition.

Prognosis

In a few cases, brucellosis may remain active for many years as an intermittent illness, but about 75% of patients recover completely within 3–6 months and fewer than 20% have residual disease after 1 year. Treatment has considerably shortened the natural course of the disease. Brucellosis is rarely fatal either in the acute or the chronic form.

Busch LA, Parker RL: Brucellosis in the United States. J Infect Dis 125:289, 1972.

Reddin JL & others: Significance of 7S and macroglobulin agglutinins in human brucellosis. New England J Med 272:1263, 1965.

Street L, Grant WW, Alva JD: Brucellosis in childhood. Pediatrics 55:416, 1975.

Williams E: Brucellosis. Brit MJ 1:791, 1973.

GAS GANGRENE

Essentials of Diagnosis

- Sudden onset of pain and edema in an area of wound contamination.
- Brown to blood-tinged watery exudate, with skin discoloration of surrounding area.
- Gas in the tissue by palpation or x-ray.
- Organisms in culture or smear of exudate.
- Prostration and systemic toxicity.

General Considerations

Gas gangrene or clostridial myositis is produced by entry of one of several clostridia (*Cl perfringens [Cl welchii], Cl novyi, Cl septicum,* etc) into devitalized tissues. They grow and produce toxins under anaerobic conditions, resulting in shock, hemolysis, and myonecrosis. Alpha toxin (lecithinase) is the most potent.

Clinical Findings

A. Symptoms and Signs: The onset is usually sudden, with rapidly increasing pain in the affected area accompanied by a fall in blood pressure, and tachycardia. The temperature may be elevated, but not proportionate to the severity of the inflammation. In the last stages of the disease, severe prostration, stupor, delirium, and coma occur.

The wound becomes swollen, and the surrounding skin is pale as a result of fluid accumulation beneath it. This is followed by a discharge of a brown to blood-tinged, serous, foul-smelling fluid from the wound. As the disease advances, the surrounding tissue changes from pale to dusky and finally becomes deeply discolored with coalescent, red, fluid-filled vesicles. Gas may be palpable in the tissues. In clostridial sepsis, hemolysis and jaundice are common, often complicated by acute renal failure.

B. Laboratory Findings: Gas gangrene is a clinical rather than a bacteriologic diagnosis. Culture of the exudate confirms the diagnosis, and stained smears of the exudate showing the typical gram-positive rods are valuable clues. Neither demonstration of clostridia in the smear from the wound nor the presence of gas is in itself sufficient to make this diagnosis. The clinical picture must be present.

C. X-Ray Findings: X-ray may show gas in the soft tissues spreading along fascial planes.

Differential Diagnosis

Other types of infection can cause gas formation in the tissue, eg, enterobacter and escherichia infections. These organisms produce much more gas than clostridia. Clostridia may produce serious puerperal infection with hemolysis.

Treatment

A. Specific Measures: Give penicillin, 1 million units IM every 3 hours. Polyvalent gas gangrene antitoxin, 20,000 units IV, may be given and repeated every 6–8 hours, although its value is doubtful.

B. Surgical Measures: Adequate surgical debridement and exposure of infected areas is essential. Radical surgical excision may be necessary. Hyperbaric oxygen therapy, if available, may be beneficial when used in conjunction with other measures. A tetanus toxoid booster injection should be given.

Prognosis

Without treatment, the mortality rate is very high.

Altemeier WA, Fullen WD: Prevention and treatment of gas gangrene. JAMA 217:806, 1971.

Davis JC & others: Hyperbaric medicine in US Air Force. JAMA 224:205, 1973.

Pritchard JA, Whalley PJ: Abortion with *Clostridium perfringens* infection. Am J Obst Gynec 111:484, 1971.

ANTHRAX

Anthrax is a disease of sheep, cattle, horses, goats, and swine caused by *Bacillus anthracis,* a gram-positive sporeforming aerobe which is transmissible to man by entry through broken skin or mucous membranes or, less commonly, by inhalation. Human infection is rare. It is most common in farmers, veterinarians, and tannery and wool workers. Several clinical forms have been observed.

Clinical Findings

A. Symptoms and Signs:

1. Cutaneous anthrax ("malignant pustule")—An erythematous papule appears on an exposed area of skin and becomes vesicular, with a purple to black center. The area around the lesion is swollen or edematous and surrounded by vesicles. The center of the lesion finally forms a necrotic eschar and sloughs. Regional adenopathy, variable fever, malaise, headache, and nausea and vomiting may be present. After the eschar sloughs, hematogenous spread and sepsis may occur—at times manifested by shock, cyanosis, sweating, and collapse. Hemorrhagic meningitis may also occur.

Anthrax sepsis sometimes develops without a skin lesion.

2. Pulmonary anthrax ("woolsorter's disease")—This follows the inhalation of spores from hides, bristles, or wool. It is characterized by fever, malaise, headache, dyspnea, and cough; congestion of the nose, throat, and larynx; and auscultatory or x-ray signs of pneumonia. Very rarely, gram-positive sporeforming aerobic bacilli other than *B anthracis* (eg, *B cereus*) can produce a similar disease.

B. Laboratory Findings: The white count may be elevated or low. Sputum or blood culture may be positive for *B anthracis.* Smears of skin lesions show gram-positive encapsulated rods, and cultures should be attempted. Antibodies may be detected by an indirect hemagglutination test.

Treatment

Give penicillin G, 10 million units IV daily; or, in mild, localized cases, tetracycline, 0.5 gm orally every 6 hours.

Prognosis

The prognosis is excellent in the cutaneous form of the disease if treatment is given early. Sepsis and pulmonary anthrax have a grave prognosis. Bacteremia is a very unfavorable sign.

Coorod JD & others: *Bacillus cereus* pneumonia and bacteremia. Am Rev Resp Dis 103:711, 1971.

Lamb R: Anthrax. Brit MJ 1:157, 1973.

TETANUS

Essentials of Diagnosis

- Jaw stiffness followed by spasms of jaw muscles (trismus).
- Stiffness of the neck and other muscles, dysphagia, irritability, hyperreflexia.
- Finally, painful convulsions precipitated by minimal stimuli.
- History of wound and possible contamination.

General Considerations

Tetanus is an acute CNS intoxication caused by fixation in the CNS of a toxin elaborated by the slender, sporeforming, gram-positive, anaerobic bacillus *Clostridium tetani.* The organism is found mainly in the soil and in the feces of animals and humans and enters the body by wound contamination. The infection is most apt to occur in puncture wounds or purulent necrotic lesions, but even the most trivial and relatively clean wound may be inoculated because the organism is universal in distribution. In the newborn, infection often enters through the umbilical cord.

The exotoxin acts on the motor nerve end plates and anterior horn cells of the spinal cord and brain stem. Once the exotoxin is fixed in the tissue, it is doubtful if it can be neutralized. The incubation period is 5 days to 15 weeks (average, 8—12 days).

In the USA today, female heroin users are particularly at risk.

Clinical Findings

A. Symptoms and Signs: Occasionally, the first symptom is pain and tingling at the site of inoculation, followed by spasticity of the group of muscles nearby. This may constitute the entire disease; more frequently, however, the presenting symptoms are stiffness of the jaw, neck stiffness, dysphagia, and irritability. Hyperreflexia develops later, with spasms of the jaw muscles (trismus) or facial muscles and rigidity and spasm of the muscles of the abdomen, neck, and back. Painful tonic convulsions precipitated by minor stimuli are common. Although the patient is awake and alert during the entire course of the illness, during convulsions the glottis and respiratory muscles go into spasm, so that the patient is unable to breathe and cyanosis and asphyxia may ensue. The temperature is only slightly elevated.

B. Laboratory Findings: The diagnosis of tetanus is made clinically. There is usually a polymorphonuclear leukocytosis.

Differential Diagnosis

Tetanus must be differentiated from other types of acute CNS infection. The trismus must be differentiated from that occasionally occurring with the use of phenothiazines. Strychnine poisoning should also be considered.

Complications

Airway obstruction and anoxia are common. Urinary retention and constipation may result from spasm of the sphincters. Respiratory arrest and cardiac failure may occur.

Prevention

Active immunization with tetanus toxoid should be universal. Give 2 injections of 0.5 ml IM, 4–8 weeks apart, with a third approximately 12 months after the second. A booster dose should be administered at the time of injury if more than 5 years have passed since the last booster. To maintain effective protection against tetanus from obscure or trivial injuries, a booster or recall dose of toxoid every 7–10 years is desirable. (See Appendix.)

Passive immunization should be used in nonimmunized individuals and those whose immunization status is uncertain whenever the wound is contaminated, major, or likely to have devitalized tissue. Tetanus immune globulin (human), 250 units IM, is the preferred agent. Tetanus antitoxin (equine or bovine) in a dosage of 3000–5000 units can be used after testing for serum hypersensitivity if tetanus immune globulin is not available. Active immunization with tetanus toxoid should be started concurrently. Table 23–3 provides a guide to normal management.

Adequate debridement of wounds is one of the most important preventive measures. In suspect cases,

benzathine penicillin G, 1.2 million units IM, may be a reasonable preventive measure.

Treatment

A. Specific Measures: Give tetanus immune globulin (human), 5000 units IM; this antitoxin does not cause sensitivity reactions. If tetanus immune globulin is not available, give tetanus antitoxin, 100,000 units IV, after testing for horse serum sensitivity. The value of antitoxin treatment has been questioned.

B. General Measures: Place the patient at bed rest and minimize stimulation. Sedation and anticonvulsant therapy are essential. Experience from areas of high incidence suggests that most convulsions can be eliminated by treatment with chlorpromazine (50–100 mg 4 times daily) or diazepam—combined with a sedative (amobarbital, phenobarbital, or meprobamate). Mild cases of tetanus can be controlled with one or the other rather than both. Only rarely is general curarization required. Other anticonvulsant regimens which have been recommended are as follows: (1) Tribromoethanol, 15–25 mg/kg rectally every 1–4 hours as needed. (2) Amobarbital sodium, 5 mg/kg IM as needed. (3) Paraldehyde, 4–8 ml IV (2–5% solution) may be combined with barbiturates. Penicillin is of value but should not be substituted for antitoxin.

Give intravenous fluids as necessary. Tracheostomy may be required for laryngeal spasm. Assisted respiration is required in conjunction with curarization. Hyperbaric oxygen therapy is of no established value.

Prognosis

The mortality rate is higher in very small children and very old people; with shorter incubation periods; with shorter intervals between onset of symptoms and the first convulsion; and with delay in treatment. If trismus develops early, the prognosis is grave. The overall mortality is about 40%. Contaminated lesions about the head and face are more dangerous than wounds on other parts of the body.

If the patient lives, recovery is complete.

Table 23–3. Guide to tetanus prophylaxis in wound management.*

History of Tetanus Immunization (Doses)	Clean Minor Wounds		All Other Wounds	
	Td	TIG	Td	TIG
Uncertain	Yes	No	Yes	Yes
0–1	Yes	No	Yes	Yes
2	Yes	No	Yes	No[1]
3 or more	No[2]	No	No[3]	No

Td = tetanus toxoid and diphtheria toxoid, adult form. Use only this preparation (Td-adult) in children older than 6 years.
TIG = tetanus immune globulin (human).
[1] Unless wound is more than 24 hours old.
[2] Unless more than 10 years have passed since last dose.
[3] Unless more than 5 years have passed since last dose.
*Recommendations of Public Health Service Advisory Committee on Immunization Practices, MMWR Vol 21, No. 25, 1972.

Adams EB & others: Usefulness of intermittent positive-pressure respiration in the treatment of tetanus. Lancet 2:1176, 1966.
Femi-Pearsö D: Experience with diazepam (Valium) in tetanus. Brit MJ 2:862, 1966.
Peebles TC & others: Tetanus toxoid emergency boosters: A reappraisal. New England J Med 280:575, 1969.
Robles NL, Walski BR, Tella AR: Tetanus prophylaxis and therapy. S Clin North America 48:799, 1968.
Weinstein L: Tetanus. New England J Med 289:1293, 1973.

BOTULISM

Essentials of Diagnosis

- Sudden onset of cranial nerve paralysis, diplopia, dry mouth, dysphagia, dysphonia, and muscle weakness progressing to respiratory paralysis.
- History of recent ingestion of home-canned, smoked, or unusual foods.
- Demonstration of toxin in patient's serum or food.

General Considerations

Botulism is a food poisoning caused by the ingestion of the toxin (usually type A, B, or E) of *Clostridium botulinum,* a strict anaerobic sporeforming bacillus found widespread in soil. Canned, smoked, or vacuum-packed anaerobic foods are involved—particularly home-canned vegetables, smoked meats, and vacuum-packed fish. The toxins block the release of acetylcholine from nerve endings. Clinically, there is early CNS involvement leading to respiratory paralysis. The mortality rate in untreated cases is high. Botulism may follow wound infection.

Clinical Findings

A. Symptoms and Signs: Twelve to 36 hours after ingestion of the toxin, visual disturbances appear, particularly diplopia and loss of power of accommodation. Other symptoms are dry throat and mouth, dysphagia, and dysphonia. There may be nausea and vomiting, particularly with type E. Muscle weakness is prominent and respiration is impaired, but the sensorium remains clear and the temperature is normal. Progressive respiratory paralysis may lead to death unless mechanical assistance is provided.

B. Laboratory Findings: Most routine determinations are within normal limits. Toxin in the patient's serum and in suspected foods may be demonstrated by mouse inoculation and identified with specific antiserum.

Differential Diagnosis

Cranial nerve involvement suggests bulbar poliomyelitis, myasthenia gravis, stroke, infectious neuronitis, or tick paralysis. Nausea and vomiting may suggest intestinal obstruction or other types of food poisoning.

Complications

The dysphagia may cause aspiration pneumonia; such infection and respiratory paralysis are the common causes of death.

Prevention

Home-canned vegetables must be sterilized to destroy spores. Sterilization standards for commercial canned or vacuum-packed foods must be strictly enforced. Boiling any questionable food for 20 minutes can inactivate the toxin, but punctured or swollen cans or jars with defective seals should be discarded. Early

and adequate treatment of wounds prevents wound botulism.

Treatment

As soon as the diagnosis of botulism is suspected, patients should be skin-tested and, if negative, given 2 vials of trivalent A, B, and E botulinus antitoxin. This can be obtained from the Center for Disease Control, Atlanta (telephone 404-633-3311 or 404-633-2176).

Adequate ventilation and oxygenation must be maintained by good respiratory drainage (elevate foot of bed), removal of respiratory obstruction by aspiration or tracheostomy, and mechanical respirator if necessary.

Parenteral fluids or alimentation are given as necessary. Give nothing by mouth while swallowing difficulty persists.

If pneumonitis develops, appropriate antimicrobials are used.

Guanidine hydrochloride, 15–35 mg/kg/day orally, has been used experimentally with occasional benefit.

The removal of unabsorbed toxin from the gut may be attempted if it can be done very soon after ingestion of the suspected toxin. Any remnants of suspected foods must be saved for analysis. Persons who might have eaten the suspected food must be located.

Prognosis

If good ventilation can be maintained and the toxin promptly neutralized, the mortality rate may be substantially lower than the 30–70% which is to be expected in untreated patients. If the patient survives the attack of botulism, there are no neurologic residua.

Koenig MG & others: Type B botulism in man. Am J Med 42:208, 1967.

Merson MH & others: Current trends in botulism in the United States. JAMA 229:1305, 1974.

Werner SB, Chin J: Botulism diagnosis and management. California Med 118:84, May 1973.

TULAREMIA

Essentials of Diagnosis

- Fever, headache, nausea, and prostration.
- Papule progressing to ulcer at site of inoculation.
- Enlarged regional lymph nodes.
- History of contact with rabbits, other rodents, and biting arthropods in endemic area.
- Confirmed by culture of ulcer, lymph node aspirate, or blood.

General Considerations

Tularemia is an infection of wild rodents—particularly rabbits and muskrats—with *Francisella (Pasteurella) tularensis.* It is transmitted from animal to man by contact with animal tissues (eg, trapping muskrats, skinning rabbits), by the bite of certain ticks and biting flies, by the consumption of infected, improperly cooked meat, or by drinking contaminated water. Infection in man often produces a local lesion and widespread organ involvement but may be entirely asymptomatic. The incubation period is 2–10 days.

Clinical Findings

A. Symptoms and Signs: Fever, headache, and nausea begin suddenly, and a local lesion—a papule at the site of inoculation—develops and soon ulcerates. The regional lymph nodes become enlarged and tender and may suppurate. The local lesion may be on the skin of an extremity (ulceroglandular) or in the eye. Pneumonia may develop from hematogenous spread of the organism or may be primary after inhalation of infected aerosols. Following ingestion of infected meat or water, an enteric form (typhoidal) may be manifested by gastroenteritis, stupor, and delirium. In any type of involvement, the spleen may be enlarged and tender and there may be rashes, generalized aches, and prostration. However, asymptomatic infection is not rare.

B. Laboratory Findings: The white blood count is slightly elevated or normal. Culture of blood, an ulcerated lesion, or lymph node aspirate yields the organisms in special culture media early in the illness. A positive agglutination test (more than 1:80) develops in the second week after infection and may persist for several years. A delayed-type skin test (read in 48 hours) becomes positive within a few days after infection; about 50% of patients have a positive skin test when first seen. The skin test (positive = more than 5 mm induration) is highly specific and remains positive longer after infection than the agglutination test.

Differential Diagnosis

Tularemia must be differentiated from rickettsial and meningococcal infections, cat-scratch disease, infectious mononucleosis, and various pneumonias and fungal diseases. Epidemiologic considerations, positive skin tests, and rising agglutination titers are the chief differential points.

Complications

Hematogenous spread to any organ may produce severe problems, particularly meningitis, perisplenitis, pericarditis, and pneumonia.

Treatment

Streptomycin, 0.5 gm IM every 6 hours, together with tetracycline, 0.5 gm orally every 6 hours, is administered until 4–5 days after the patient becomes afebrile. Chloramphenicol may be substituted for tetracycline in the same dosage. Adequate fluid intake is essential, and oxygen may be required. Suppurating lymph nodes may be aspirated but should not be incised during the first week if the process is still localized. Later in the disease, drainage of fluctuant nodes may be needed, and is safe after proper chemotherapy for several days.

Prognosis

The mortality rate of untreated ulceroglandular tularemia is 5%; that of tularemic pneumonia, 30%. Early proper chemotherapy gives a prompt response and eliminates fatalities. Skin tests and agglutination tests suggest that subclinical infection is common in outbreaks of tularemia.

Prevention

Awareness of the risk of infection through contact with potentially infected rodents, biting insects, or water supply is helpful.

Avery FW, Barnett TB: Pulmonary tularemia. Am Rev Resp Dis 95:584, 1967.

Buchanan TM & others: The tularemia skin test. Ann Int Med 74.336, 1971.

Klock LW & others: Tularemia epidemic associated with the deerfly. JAMA 226:149, 1973.

Young LS & others: Tularemia epidemic in Vermont, 1968. New England J Med 280:1253, 1969.

PLAGUE

Essentials of Diagnosis

- Sudden onset of high fever, malaise, muscular pains, and prostration.
- Axillary or inguinal lymphadenitis (bubo).
- Bacteremia, sepsis, and pneumonitis may occur.
- History of exposure to rodents in endemic area.
- Positive smear and culture from bubo and positive blood culture.

General Considerations

Plague is an infection of wild rodents with *Yersinia (Pasteurella) pestis,* a small gram-negative rod. It is transmitted from one rodent to another and from rodent to man by the bites of fleas. Plague bacilli grow in the gut of the flea and obstruct it. When the hungry flea sucks blood, it regurgitates organisms into the bite wound. Feces of fleas may also transmit the infection. If a person develops pneumonia, he can transmit the infection by droplets to other persons. Carriers of pharyngeal plague have been identified in Vietnam. The incubation period is 2–10 days.

Following the flea bite, the organisms spread through the lymphatics to the lymph nodes, which become greatly enlarged (bubo). They may then reach the blood stream to involve all organs. When pneumonia or meningitis develops, the outcome is often fatal.

Clinical Findings

A. Symptoms and Signs: The onset is usually sudden, with high fever, malaise, tachycardia, intense headache, and generalized muscular aches. The patient appears profoundly ill and very anxious. Later, he may become delirious. If pneumonia develops, there is also tachypnea, productive cough, blood-tinged sputum, and cyanosis. Meningeal signs may develop. A pustule or ulcer at the site of inoculation and signs of lymphangitis may occur. Axillary, inguinal, or cervical lymph nodes become enlarged and tender and may eventually suppurate and drain. With hematogenous spread, the patient may rapidly become severely septic and comatose, with purpuric spots (black plague) appearing on the skin.

Primary plague pneumonia results from the inhalation of bacilli in droplets coughed up by another patient with plague pneumonia. This is a fulminant pneumonitis with bloody, frothy sputum and sepsis, and is usually fatal in the unimmunized person unless treatment is started within a few hours of onset.

B. Laboratory Findings: Peripheral white counts range from 12–20 thousand/cu mm. The plague bacillus may be found in smears from aspirates of buboes examined with Gram's or immunofluorescent stain. Cultures from bubo aspirate or pus and blood are positive but may grow slowly. In convalescing patients, an antibody titer rise may be demonstrated by agglutination tests.

C. X-Ray Findings: Pulmonary infiltration in a person suspected of having plague implies a grave prognosis and should lead to strict isolation.

Differential Diagnosis

The lymphadenitis of plague is most commonly mistaken for the lymphadenitis accompanying staphylococcal or streptococcal infections of an extremity, venereal diseases such as lymphogranuloma venereum or syphilis, and tularemia. The systemic manifestations resemble those of enteric or rickettsial fevers, malaria, or influenza. The pneumonia resembles other severe gram-negative or staphylococcal pneumonias or psittacosis.

Prevention

Periodic surveys of rodents and their ectoparasites in endemic areas provide guidelines for the need for extensive rodent and flea control measures. Total eradication of plague from wild rodents in an endemic area is rarely possible.

Drug prophylaxis may provide temporary protection for those exposed to the risk of plague infection, particularly by the respiratory route. Tetracycline, 1 gm daily orally, or sulfisoxazole, 4 gm daily orally, can accomplish this.

Plague vaccines—both live and killed—have been used for many years, but their efficacy is not clearly established. It is believed, however, that the USP formol-killed suspension gives some protection if administered intramuscularly as 2 doses of 0.5 ml each 4 weeks apart, followed by a booster dose of 0.2 ml IM 4–12 weeks after the second dose. For continued exposure, subsequent boosters are given every 6–12 months.

Treatment

Drug therapy must be started promptly when the diagnosis of plague is suspected. Give streptomycin, 1 gm IM, every 6 hours for 2 days and then 0.5 gm IM every 6 hours. Tetracycline, 2 gm daily orally (or parenterally if necessary) is given at the same time. Supportive care may consist of intravenous fluids, pressor drugs, oxygen, and tracheostomy as required.

Prognosis

If the diagnosis can be made and treatment started relatively early, most patients with bubonic plague will recover. In untreated cases, the mortality rate may range from 20–60%. When gross sepsis, pneumonia, and shock supervene, the outlook is poor. Primary pneumonic plague is almost invariably fatal unless treated intensively within hours of onset.

Finegold MJ: Pathogenesis of plague. Am J Med 45:549, 1968.

Meyer KF: Effectiveness of live or killed plague vaccines. Bull WHO 42:653, 1970.

Pan-American Health Organization: *Plague in the Americas.* Science Publication No. 115. Washington DC, 1965.

Reed WP & others: Bubonic plague in the southwestern US. Medicine 49:465, 1970.

LEPROSY

Essentials of Diagnosis

- Pale, anesthetic macular—or nodular and erythematous—skin lesions.
- Superficial nerve thickening with associated sensory changes.
- History of residence in endemic area in childhood.
- Acid-fast bacilli in skin lesions or nasal scrapings, or characteristic histologic nerve changes.

General Considerations

Leprosy is a chronic infectious disease caused by the acid-fast rod *Mycobacterium leprae.* The mode of transmission is unknown but probably involves prolonged exposure in childhood. Only rarely have adults become infected (eg, by tattooing). The disease is endemic in tropical and subtropical Asia, Africa, Central and South America and the Pacific regions, and the southern USA.

Clinical Findings

A. Symptoms and Signs: The onset of leprosy is insidious. The lesions involve the cooler tissues of the body: skin, superficial nerves, nose, pharynx, larynx, eyes, and testicles. The skin lesions may occur as pale, anesthetic macular lesions 1–10 cm in diameter; discrete erythematous, infiltrated nodules 1–5 cm in diameter; or a diffuse skin infiltration. Neurologic disturbances are manifested by nerve infiltration and thickening, with resultant anesthesia, neuritis, paresthesia, trophic ulcers, and bone reabsorption and shortening of digits. In untreated cases, the disfigurement due to the skin infiltration and nerve involvement may be extreme.

The disease is divided clinically and by laboratory tests into 2 distinct types: lepromatous and tuberculoid. In the lepromatous type, the course is progressive and malignant, with nodular skin lesions; slow, symmetric nerve involvement; abundant acid-fast bacilli in the skin lesions, and a negative lepromin skin test. The patient has impaired cellular immunity. In the tuberculoid type, the course is benign and nonprogressive, with macular skin lesions, severe asymmetric nerve involvement of sudden onset with few bacilli present in the lesions; and a positive lepromin skin test. Eye involvement (keratitis and iridocyclitis), nasal ulcers, epistaxis, anemia, and lymphadenopathy may also occur.

B. Laboratory Findings: Laboratory confirmation of leprosy requires the demonstration of acid-fast bacilli in scrapings from involved skin or the nasal septum. Biopsy of an involved, thickened nerve also gives a typical histologic picture.

M leprae has not been grown in culture media, but it multiplies in experimentally injected mouse foot pads.

Differential Diagnosis

The skin lesions of leprosy often resemble those of lupus erythematosus, sarcoidosis, syphilis, erythema nodosum, erythema multiforme, and vitiligo. Nerve involvement, sensory dissociation, and resulting deformity may require differentiation from syringomyelia and scleroderma.

Complications

Intercurrent pulmonary tuberculosis is common in the lepromatous type, probably because of deficient cellular immunity. Amyloidosis may occur with long-standing disease.

Prevention

BCG vaccination is being studied and shows promise as a means of immunizing children. Both dapsone and BCG are being tested for their prophylactic value for family contacts of patients with lepromatous leprosy.

Treatment

Drugs should be given cautiously, with slowly increasing doses, and must be withheld when they induce an exacerbation called "lepra reaction": fever, progressive anemia with or without leukopenia; severe gastrointestinal symptoms, allergic dermatitis, hepatitis, or mental disturbances; or erythema nodosum. It is important, therefore, to observe temperature, blood counts, and biopsy changes in lesions at regular intervals. Corticosteroids are valuable in lepra reactions. The duration of treatment must be guided by progress, preferably as judged by biopsy. Treatment must be continued for several years or indefinitely because recrudescence may occur after cessation of therapy. No isolation procedures are warranted for patients under treatment.

A. Dapsone (DDS) is given orally to adults starting with 25 mg twice weekly and increasing to a maximum of 600 mg weekly. If anemia, fever, jaundice, or granulocytopenia occurs, stop treatment until these changes subside and then start again, or change to another sulfone or give amithiozone (see below).

B. Amithiozone (diphenylthiourea) is given when intolerance to sulfones develops. The dose is 50 mg/day orally, increasing to 200 mg/day.

C. Thalidomide, 100–400 mg orally, is a valuable adjunct (in addition to antileprosy drugs) in the management of the erythema nodosum of lepromatous leprosy. Corticosteroids are less effective.

D. Rifampin is a very effective drug, used for initial treatment in combination with a sulfone. Its high cost limits its use throughout the world.

E. Surgical care of extremities (hands and feet) requires careful consideration.

Prognosis

Untreated lepromatous leprosy is progressive and fatal in 10–20 years. In the tuberculoid type, spontaneous recovery usually occurs in 1–3 years; it may, however, produce crippling deformities.

With treatment, the lepromatous type regresses slowly (over a period of 3–8 years). Recovery from the tuberculoid type is more rapid. Recrudescences are always possible, and it may be safe to assume that the bacilli are never eradicated. Deformities persist after complete recovery and may markedly interfere with function and appearance.

Drutz DJ & others: The continuous bacteremia of lepromatous leprosy. New England J Med 287:159, 1972.

Fasal P, Fasal E, Levy L: Leprosy prophylaxis. JAMA 199:905, 1967.

Pattyn SP: Comments on chemotherapy of leprosy. Leprosy Rev 43:126, 1972.

Sheagren JN & others: Immunologic reactivity in patients with leprosy. Ann Int Med 70:295, 1969.

Shepard CC: Chemotherapy of leprosy. Ann Rev Pharmacol 9:37, 1969.

CHANCROID

Chancroid is an acute, localized venereal disease caused by the short gram-negative bacillus *Haemophilus ducreyi*. Infection occurs by contact during intercourse, although nonvenereal inoculation has occurred in medical personnel through contact with chancroid patients. The incubation period is 3–5 days.

The initial lesion at the site of inoculation is a macule or vesicopustule which soon breaks down to form a painful, soft ulcer with a necrotic base, surrounding erythema, and undermined edges. Multiple lesions—started by autoinoculation—and inguinal adenitis often develop. The adenitis is usually unilateral and consists of tender, matted nodes of moderate size with overlying erythema. The nodal mass softens, becomes fluctuant, and may rupture spontaneously. With lymph node involvement, fever, chills, and malaise may occur.

Culture of material from the lesion in enriched media at 35° C may yield *H ducreyi*. The chancroid skin test may become positive and remain positive for life. Mixed venereal infection is very common.

Balanitis and phimosis are frequent complications. Infection of the ulcer with fusiforms, spirochetes, and other organisms is common.

Chancroid must be differentiated from other venereal infections and pyogenic lesion. The chancre of syphilis is clear and painless with a hard base.

Give either sulfisoxazole, 1 gm orally 4 times daily, or tetracycline, 0.5 gm orally 4 times daily for 1–2 weeks. The drugs are equally effective. Cleansing of ulcerations with soap and water twice daily promotes healing. Fluctuant buboes may be aspirated by needle.

Chancroid usually responds well to treatment. Even without treatment, it usually is self-limited.

Borcherdt K, Hoke AW: Simplified laboratory technique for diagnosis of chancroid. Arch Dermat 102:188, 1970.

Gottlieb SK: Nonspirochetal chancriform ulcer of penis. New England J Med 287:185, 1972.

Kerber RE & others: Treatment of chancroid. Arch Dermat 100:604, 1969.

GONORRHEA

Essentials of Diagnosis

- Purulent urethral discharge, especially in males, with dysuria, yielding positive smear.
- Cervicitis with discharge, or asymptomatic, yielding positive culture.
- Epididymitis, prostatitis, periurethral inflammation, proctitis in male.
- Vaginitis, bartholinitis, salpingitis, proctitis in female.
- Fever, arthritis, skin lesions, conjunctivitis, pharyngitis.
- Gram-negative intracellular diplococci seen in a smear from the male urethra or cultured from any site, particularly the urethra, cervix, and rectum.

General Considerations

Gonorrhea is the most prevalent reportable communicable disease in the USA, with an estimated 2.5 million or more infectious cases annually. It is caused by *Neisseria gonorrhoeae*, a gram-negative diplococcus, typically found inside polymorphonuclear cells. It is most commonly transmitted during any form of sexual activity and has its greatest incidence in the 15- to 29-year-old age group. The incubation period is usually 2–8 days.

Clinical Findings

A. Symptoms and Signs:

1. Men—Initially, there is burning on urination and a serous or milky discharge. One to 3 days later, the urethral pain is more pronounced and the discharge becomes yellow, creamy, and profuse, sometimes blood-tinged. Without treatment, the disorder may regress and become chronic or progress to involve the prostate, epididymis, and periurethral glands with acute, painful inflammation. This in turn becomes chronic, with prostatitis and urethral strictures. Rectal infection is common in homosexual males. Systemic involvement is listed below. Asymptomatic infection is common.

2. Women—Dysuria, frequency, and urgency may occur with a purulent urethral discharge. Vaginitis and cervicitis with inflammation of Skene's and Bartholin's glands are common. Most commonly, however, the infection is asymptomatic, with only slightly increased vaginal discharge and moderate cervicitis on examination. Infection may remain as a chronic cervicitis—the largest reservoir of gonococci in any community. It may progress to involve the uterus and tubes with acute and chronic salpingitis and with ultimate scarring of tubes and sterility. Rectal infection is common both as spread of the organism from the genital tract and as a result of infection by anal coitus. Systemic involvement is listed below.

B. Laboratory Findings: Smears of urethral discharge in men, especially during the first week after onset, usually show typical gram-negative diplococci in the cytoplasm of polymorphonuclear leukocytes. Smears are infrequently positive in women. Cultures are essential in all situations where gonorrhea should be suspected and gonococci cannot be demonstrated in gram-stained smears. This applies particularly to cervical, rectal, pharyngeal, and joint specimens. Specimens of pus or secretions are streaked on a selective medium such as Thayer-Martin or Transgrow. The latter is suitable for transport if a laboratory is not immediately available. The medium must be at room temperature when inoculated and must be incubated at 37° C in a 10% CO_2 atmosphere (closed Transgrow bottle; Thayer-Martin in candle jar). Colonies are identified by oxidase test, Gram's stain, or immunofluorescence. Immunofluorescent stain may also be directly applied to smears of specimens. No good serologic test is available.

Differential Diagnosis

The chief alternatives to acute gonococcal urethritis or cervicitis are nongonococcal urethritis (some caused by chlamydiae; others perhaps by mycoplasmas) and trichomonal and candidal vaginitis and cervicitis. A variety of agents causing salpingitis, pelvic peritonitis, arthritis, proctitis, and skin lesions must also be considered. Reiter's disease (urethritis, conjunctivitis, arthritis) may mimic gonorrhea but may also exist in a patient who has gonorrhea.

Complications

The forms of local extension of the initial infection have been described. Unusual sites of primary infection (eg, the pharynx) must always be considered. Systemic complications follow the dissemination of gonococci from the primary site (eg, genital tract) via the blood stream. Gonococcal bacteremia is associated with intermittent fever, arthralgia, and skin lesions ranging from maculopapular to pustular or hemorrhagic. Rarely, gonococcal endocarditis or meningitis develops. Arthritis and tenosynovitis are common complications, particularly involving the knees, ankles, and wrists. Several joints are commonly involved. Gonococci can be isolated from only a third of arthritides, and cell wall deficient forms in a few additional ones. In the remainder, it is possible that some immune complex disease or hypersensitivity reaction is responsible. Gonococcal arthritis may be accompanied by iritis or conjunctivitis, with negative cultures. The commonest form of eye involvement is the direct inoculation of gonococci into the conjunctival sac. This may occur during passage through an infected birth canal, leading to ophthalmia neonatorum, or by autoinoculation of a person with genital infection. The purulent conjunctivitis may rapidly progress to panophthalmitis and loss of the eye unless treated promptly.

Prevention

Prevention is based on better education, mechanical or chemical prophylaxis, and early diagnosis and treatment. The condom, if properly used, can reduce the risk of infection. Effective drugs taken in therapeutic doses within 24 hours of exposure can abort an infection. The rising drug resistance of gonococci makes the formerly effective regimens of penicillin prophylaxis (taken prior to exposure) less likely to succeed. Intensive search for sex contacts by public health agencies must rely on physician reporting. Contacts are sometimes given full treatment for gonorrhea on epidemiologic grounds, without individual diagnosis, to reduce the reservoir of infection.

Infection of the newborn must be prevented by the instillation of 1% silver nitrate into each conjunctival sac immediately after birth.

Treatment (USPHS recommendations, Feb 1975)

A. Uncomplicated Gonorrhea (Urethral, Cervical, Pharyngeal, Rectal): (For both men and women.) Aqueous procaine penicillin G, 4.8 million units IM injected into 2 or more sites at one visit, together with 1 gm probenecid orally given prior to injections. This treatment can also be effective in aborting syphilis within 2 weeks after infection.

Alternatively, give ampicillin, 3.5 gm orally,

together with probenecid, 1 gm orally, given at one time. *Never* treat gonorrhea with benzathine penicillin G. When a penicillin is not indicated or is ineffective, give tetracycline, 1.5 gm orally stat, then 0.5 gm orally 4 times daily for 4 days (total, 9 gm); or spectinomycin, 4 gm IM in 2 injection sites given at the same time.

B. Follow-Up Treatment: Urethral or rectal specimens must be obtained from men 7 days after completion of treatment. Cervical and rectal specimens must be obtained from women 7–14 days after completion of treatment. Serologic tests for syphilis are required 2 weeks and 2 months later.

C. Treatment of Complications: In general, salpingitis, prostatitis, epididymitis, bacteremia, arthritis, eye infections, and other complications are best treated with penicillin G, 10–20 million units IV daily for 1–2 weeks or longer. Full doses of tetracyclines are probably also effective. Postgonococcal urethritis and chlamydial urethritis can be treated with tetracycline, 0.5 gm orally 4 times daily for 7–10 days. In postgonococcal urethritis, signs and symptoms persist after treatment of presumptive gonococcal urethritis with an adequate drug regimen and no further evidence of gonococci. Gonococcal ophthalmia requires topical as well as systemic penicillin treatment.

Additional supportive treatment is needed for most complications. Prostatitis may be relieved by hot sitz baths or diathermy; acute epididymitis requires bed rest, cold and support to the scrotum, and analgesics. Acute salpingitis requires bed rest during the acute stage, and surgical evaluation if chronic pain and signs of inflammation continue. Aspiration of joints may be necessary to relieve high pressure, to be followed by physical therapy as inflammation subsides.

Prognosis

The regimen given above will cure 90–95% of acute gonococcal infections (mid-1973). However, the steady rise in gonococcal resistance to antimicrobial drugs threatens the efficacy of chemotherapy in the future. In addition, the complications of gonorrhea may cause irreversible damage (urethral stricture, persistent tubo-ovarian abscess, valve destruction in endocarditis, peritoneal adhesions with intestinal obstruction, sterility, etc) which requires surgical treatment.

Follow-up examinations cannot separate failures of chemotherapy from reinfection. The latter occurs at a high rate. In addition, multiple venereal infections from the same exposure are increasingly common. The patient with acute gonorrhea may have undetected syphilis, genital herpes, or chlamydial infection. All of these must be detected by laboratory procedures in repeated follow-up. The recommended parenteral penicillin schedule is probably curative for most cases of coexisting syphilis. Patients treated with other antimicrobials will require additional penicillin treatment if serologic tests for syphilis become positive during 4 months following treatment for gonorrhea.

Handsfield HH & others: Asymptomatic gonorrhea in men. New England J Med 290:117, 1974.

Holmes KH & others: Disseminated gonococcal infection. Ann Int Med 74:979, 1971.

Holmes KH & others: Recovery of *N gonorrhoeae* from "sterile" synovial fluid in gonococcal arthritis. New England J Med 284:318, 1971.

Keisér H & others: Clinical forms of gonococcal arthritis. New England J Med 279:234, 1968.

Schroeter AL, Reynolds G: The rectal culture as a test of cure for gonorrhea in the female. J Infect Dis 125:499, 1972.

Snowe RJ, Wilfert CM: Epidemic reappearance of ophthalmia neonatorum. Pediatrics 51:110, 1973.

Thayer JD, Martin JE: Selective medium for cultivation of *N gonorrhoeae*. Pub Health Rep 79:49, 1965.

Venereal Diseases Branch, Center for Disease Control, USPHS: Recommended treatment schedules for gonorrhea—Feb 1975. Ann Int Med 82:230, 1975.

Webster B (editor): Symposium on venereal diseases. M Clin North America 56:1055, 1972.

GRANULOMA INGUINALE

Granuloma inguinale is a chronic, relapsing, granulomatous anogenital infection due to *Calymmatobacterium (Donovania) granulomatis,* which is related to klebsiella and occurs intracellularly. The pathognomonic cell, found in tissue scrapings or secretions, is large (25–90 μm) and contains intracytoplasmic cysts filled with bodies (Donovan bodies) which stain deeply with Wright's stain.

The incubation period is 8 days to 12 weeks.

The onset is insidious. The lesions occur on the skin or mucous membranes of the genitalia or perineal area. They are relatively painless infiltrated nodules which soon slough. A shallow, sharply demarcated ulcer forms, with a beefy red friable base of granulation tissue. The lesion spreads by contiguity. The advancing border has a characteristic rolled edge of granulation tissue. Large ulcerations which advance up onto the lower abdomen and thighs are not uncommon. Scar formation and healing may occur along one border while the opposite border advances. The process may become indolent and stationary.

The characteristic Donovan bodies are found in scrapings from the ulcer base or on histologic sections. The microorganism may also be cultured on special media. A specific complement fixation test is not widely available.

Superinfection with spirochete-fusiform organisms is not uncommon. The ulcer then becomes purulent, painful, foul-smelling, and extremely difficult to treat. Other venereal diseases may coexist. Rare complications include superimposed malignancy and secondary elephantoid swelling of the genitalia.

Initial treatment consists of tetracycline, 2 gm orally daily for 2 weeks. If the lesion has not regressed satisfactorily, give streptomycin, 0.5 gm IM every 8 hours for 10 days. Ampicillin has also been used.

With antimicrobial therapy, most cases can be cured. In resistant or untreated cases massive extension of the lesion may occur, with resulting anemia, cachexia, and death.

Washing the genitalia with soap and water immediately after intercourse may reduce the likelihood of infection. A serologic test for syphilis must be performed to rule out the existence of this disease.

Lal S & others: Epidemiological and clinical features in 165 cases of granuloma inguinale. Brit J Ven Dis 46:461, 1970.

Thew MA & others: Ampicillin in the treatment of granuloma inguinale. JAMA 210:866, 1969.

BARTONELLOSIS
(Oroya Fever, Carrión's Disease)

Bartonellosis, an acute or chronic infection which occurs in the high Andean valleys of Colombia, Ecuador, and Peru, is caused by a gram-negative, very pleomorphic bacterium (*Bartonella bacilliformis*) which is transmitted to man by the bite of Phlebotomus. The organism is parasitic in man in red cells and cells of the reticuloendothelial system. The initial stage (Oroya fever) exhibits intermittent or remittent fever, malaise, headache, and bone and joint pains. The disease becomes more apparent with the rapid progression of severe macrocytic anemia, hemorrhagic lymph nodes, and hepatosplenomegaly. Masses of organisms fill the cytoplasm of vascular endothelial cells, resulting in occlusion and thrombosis. In favorable cases Oroya fever lasts 2–6 weeks and subsides. In those who survive, the eruptive stage of the disease (verruga peruana) commonly begins 2–8 weeks later. Verruga may also appear in the apparent absence of Oroya fever, possibly because of a mild, subclinical first stage. Multiple miliary and nodular hemangiomas appear in crops, particularly on the face and limbs. The lesions bleed easily, sometimes ulcerate, usually persist for 1–12 months, finally heal without scar formation, and produce little systemic reaction. In early Oroya fever, the organisms are best demonstrated by blood culture. Later, Bartonella organisms appear in red cells in large numbers. The severe macrocytic, hypochromic anemia (hemoglobin as low as 3–5 gm) of Oroya fever is accompanied by jaundice, marked reticulocytosis, and numerous megaloblasts and normoblasts. In verrugous lesions the organisms may be demonstrated in endothelial cells.

Chloramphenicol or a tetracycline, 2 gm daily orally, has been effective in overcoming the infection and reducing the mortality rate. Transfusion may be necessary if the anemia is severe. The Phlebotomus vector should be controlled.

Reynafarje C, Ramos J: The hemolytic anemia of human bartonellosis. Blood 18:562, 1961.

CHLAMYDIAL INFECTIONS*

LYMPHOGRANULOMA VENEREUM

Essentials of Diagnosis

- Evanescent vesicular or ulcerative genital lesion.
- Lymph node enlargement, softening, and suppuration, with draining sinuses.
- Proctitis and rectal stricture in females or homosexual males.
- Systemic, joint, eye, and CNS involvement may occur.
- Positive complement fixation test and sometimes positive skin test.
- Elevated serum globulin.

General Considerations

Lymphogranuloma venereum is an acute and chronic contagious venereal disease caused by an organism of the psittacosis-LGV-trachoma (chlamydia) group. After the genital lesion disappears, the infection spreads to lymph channels and lymph nodes of the genital and rectal areas. The disease is acquired during intercourse or through contact with contaminated exudate from active lesions. The incubation period is 5–21 days. Inapparent infections and latent disease (as shown by skin testing) are not uncommon in promiscuous individuals.

Clinical Findings

A. Symptoms and Signs: In males, the initial vesicular or ulcerative lesion (on the external genitalia) is evanescent and often goes unnoticed. Inguinal buboes appear 1–4 weeks after exposure, are often bilateral, and have a tendency to fuse, soften, and break down to form multiple draining sinuses with extensive scarring. Proctoscopic examination is important for diagnosis and in evaluating therapy. In females, the genital lymph drainage is to the perirectal glands. Early anorectal manifestations are proctitis with tenesmus and bloody purulent discharge; late manifestations are chronic cicatrizing inflammation of the rectal and perirectal tissue. These changes lead to obstipation and rectal stricture and, occasionally, rectovaginal and perianal fistulas. They are also seen in homosexual males.

Systemic invasion may occur, causing fever, arthralgia, arthritis, skin rashes, conjunctivitis, and iritis. Nervous system invasion causes headache and meningeal irritation.

B. Laboratory Findings: The intradermal skin test (Frei test) and the complement fixation test may be

*Trachoma and inclusion conjunctivitis manifest themselves primarily as external eye diseases, but the agents are capable of infecting tissues of the genital tract. For descriptions, see pp 79–81.

positive, but cross-reaction with other chlamydiae occurs. A positive reaction may reflect an old (healed) infection; however, high complement fixation titers usually imply active infection. Skin tests with commercial antigens are sometimes negative even in cases proved by isolation of the agent.

The serum globulin is often greatly elevated, with an inversion of the albumin-globulin ratio. A low-titer false-positive test for syphilis may be present.

Differential Diagnosis

The early lesion of lymphogranuloma venereum must be differentiated from the lesions of syphilis, herpes progenitalis, and chancroid; lymph node involvement must be distinguished from that due to tularemia, tuberculosis, plague, neoplasm, or pyogenic infection; rectal stricture must be differentiated from that due to neoplasm and ulcerative colitis.

Complications

Lymphatic involvement and blocking may cause marked disfiguration of the external genitalia (elephantiasis) as well as extensive scarring. Rectal stricture resists treatment and may require colostomy.

Treatment

A. Specific Therapy: The tetracyclines, 0.25–1 gm orally 4 times daily for 10–20 days, are the antibiotics of choice. Sulfadiazine, 1 gm 3 times daily for 2–3 weeks or longer, has little effect on the chlamydial infection but reduces bacterial complications.

B. Local and General Measures: Place the patient at bed rest, apply warm compresses to buboes, and give analgesics as necessary. Aspirate fluctuant nodes with aseptic care. Extensive plastic operations may be necessary in the chronic anorectal form of the disease. Rectal strictures should be treated by prolonged gentle dilatation, although in extreme cases this may be impossible and colon shunting procedures may be necessary.

Prognosis

Prompt early treatment will cure the disorder and prevent late complications; the longer treatment is delayed, the more difficult it is to eradicate the infection and to reverse the pathologic changes. There may be a higher incidence of rectal carcinoma in persons with anorectal lymphogranuloma venereum.

Abrams AJ: Lymphogranuloma venereum. JAMA 205:59, 1968.
Jawetz E: Chemotherapy of chlamydial infections. Advances Pharmacol 7:253, 1969.
Lassus A & others: Autoimmune serum factors and IgA elevation in lymphogranuloma venereum. Ann Clin Res (Helsinki) 2:51, 1970.
Management of Chancroid, Granuloma Inguinale, and Lymphogranuloma Venereum in General Practice. USPHS Publication No. 255. US Government Printing Office, Washington DC, 1968.

NONGONOCOCCAL URETHRITIS & CERVICITIS

From a portion of males with anterior urethritis and from their female consorts (with or without urethritis or cervicitis), gonococci cannot be isolated. In such patients, there is no improvement with high doses of penicillin, but tetracyclines can often suppress discomfort and discharge. By appropriate laboratory methods, chlamydiae (TRIC agents) of immunologic groups D–J and others can be isolated in 35–50% of cases. These chlamydiae are identical to those causing inclusion conjunctivitis (see p 79), and such patients not infrequently have a follicular conjunctivitis in addition to genital tract involvement. These chlamydiae play an important etiologic role in a high proportion of cases of so-called "nonspecific" or "nongonococcal" urethritis. They do not occur as part of the normal flora. Infection may, however, coexist with gonorrhea and later give rise to "postgonococcal urethritis."

Hilton AL & others: Chlamydia in the female genital tract. Brit J Ven Dis 50:1, 1974.
Holmes KK & others: Etiology of nongonococcal urethritis. New England J Med 292:1199, 1975.
Oriel JD & others: Chlamydial infections of the cervix. Brit J Ven Dis 50:11, 1974.
Oriel JD & others: Infection with chlamydia type A in men with urethritis due to *N gonorrhoeae*. J Infect Dis 131:376, 1975.

PSITTACOSIS
(Ornithosis)

Essentials of Diagnosis

- Fever, chills, malaise, prostration; cough, epistaxis; occasionally, rose spots and splenomegaly.
- Slightly delayed appearance of signs of pneumonitis.
- Isolation of chlamydia or rising titer of complement-fixing antibodies.
- Contact with infected bird (psittacine, pigeons, many others) 7–15 days previously.

General Considerations

Psittacosis is acquired from contact with birds (parrots, parakeets, pigeons, chickens, ducks, and many others). Human-to-human spread is rare. The incubation period is 7–15 days.

Clinical Findings

A. Symptoms and Signs: The onset is usually rapid, with fever, chills, headache, backache, malaise, myalgia, epistaxis, dry cough, and prostration. Signs include those of pneumonitis, alteration of percussion note and breath sounds, and rales. Pulmonary findings may be absent early. Rose spots, splenomegaly, and meningismus are occasionally seen. Delirium, constipation or diarrhea, and abdominal distress may occur. Dyspnea and cyanosis may occur later.

B. Laboratory Findings: The white count is normal or decreased, often with a shift to the left. Proteinuria is frequently present. The organism may be isolated from the blood and sputum by inoculation of mice or cell cultures. Complement-fixing antibodies appear during the second week. Antibody response may be suppressed by early chemotherapy.

C. X-Ray Findings: The x-ray findings in psittacosis are those of central pneumonia which later becomes widespread or migratory. Psittacosis is indistinguishable from viral pneumonias by x-ray.

Differential Diagnosis

This disease can be differentiated from acute viral, mycoplasmal, or rickettsial pneumonias only by the history of contact with potentially infected birds. Rose spots and leukopenia suggest typhoid fever.

Complications

Myocarditis, secondary bacterial pneumonia.

Treatment

Treatment consists of giving tetracycline, 0.5 gm orally every 6 hours or 0.5 gm IV every 12 hours for 10–14 days. Give oxygen and sedation as required.

Prognosis

Psittacosis may vary from a mild respiratory infection (especially in children) to a severe, protracted illness. Mortality with early treatment is very low.

Schaffner W & others: The clinical spectrum of endemic psittacosis. Arch Int Med 119:433, 1967.
Zehmer RB: Human psittacosis in the United States. J Infect Dis 124:622, 1971.

24 . . .
Infectious Diseases: Spirochetal

Harold E. Varmus

SYPHILIS

Syphilis is a complex infectious disease caused by *Treponema pallidum,* a spirochete capable of infecting any organ or tissue in the body. Owing to its protean manifestations, the disease can mimic virtually any known condition and is often called "the great imitator." Transmission occurs most frequently during sexual contact, through minor skin or mucosal lesions; sites of inoculation are usually genital but may be extragential. The organism is extremely sensitive to heat and drying but can survive for days in fluids; therefore, it can be transmitted by blood from infected persons. Syphilis can be transferred via the placenta from mother to fetus after the 5th month of pregnancy (congenital syphilis).

The immunologic response to infection is complex and not well understood, although it provides the basis for most clinical diagnoses. The infection induces the synthesis of a number of antibodies, some of which react specifically with pathogenic treponemes and some with components of normal tissues (see below). If the disease is untreated, sufficient defenses develop to produce a relative resistance to reinfection; however, in most cases these defenses are inadequate to eradicate existing infection and may contribute to tissue destruction in the late stages. Patients treated early in the disease are fully susceptible to reinfection.

The natural history of acquired syphilis is generally divided into 2 major clinical stages: (1) early, or infectious, syphilis and (2) late syphilis. The 2 stages are separated by a symptom-free latent phase during the first part of which (early latency) the infectious stage is liable to recur. Infectious syphilis includes the primary lesions (chancre and regional lymphadenopathy), the secondary lesions (commonly involving skin and mucous membranes, occasionally bone, CNS, or liver), relapsing lesions during early latency, and congenital lesions. The hallmark of these lesions is an abundance of spirochetes; tissue reaction is usually minimal. Late syphilis consists of so-called benign (gummatous) lesions involving skin, bones, and viscera, cardiovascular disease (principally aortitis), and a variety of CNS and ocular syndromes. These forms of syphilis are not contagious. The lesions contain few demonstrable spirochetes, but tissue reactivity (vasculitis, necrosis) is severe and suggestive of hypersensitivity phenomena.

Since 1958 there has been a gradual increase in the frequency of early disease, making syphilis a major public health problem. A particularly high incidence among homosexual males, a high frequency of reinfection of treated persons, and a concomitant dramatic increase in the incidence of gonorrhea are among the noteworthy epidemiologic features. The incidence of congenital syphilis has not risen appreciably. The increase in reported infectious syphilis is undoubtedly accompanied by a rise in latent syphilis following inapparent, undiagnosed, or incompletely treated infectious stages. It is likely that a resurgence of late syphilis will also soon occur. Education of the public about venereal diseases, more responsible case reporting by physicians, more vigorous case finding by public health departments, and more widespread use of serologic screening for syphilis are among the measures that might help control the continued spread of the disease and bring untreated cases to therapy. Attempts to develop a syphilis vaccine have not been successful.

Laboratory Diagnosis

Since the infectious agent for syphilis cannot be cultured in vitro, diagnostic measures are confined principally to serologic testing, direct observation of lesions for spirochetes resembling *T pallidum,* and other examinations (biopsies, lumbar puncture, x-rays) for evidence of tissue damage.

A. Serologic Tests for Syphilis (STS): There are 2 general categories of serologic tests for syphilis: (1) nontreponemal tests which use a component of normal tissue (eg, beef heart cardiolipin) as an antigen to measure nonspecific antibodies (reagin) formed in the blood of patients with syphilis, and (2) treponemal tests which employ live or killed *T pallidum* as antigen to detect antibodies specific for pathogenic treponemes.

1. Nontreponemal antigen tests—Commonly employed nontreponemal antigen tests are of 2 types: (1) flocculation (VDRL, Hinton) and (2) complement fixation (Kolmer, Wassermann). These tests are relatively easy, rapid, and inexpensive to perform and are therefore used primarily for routine screening for syphilis. Quantitative expression of the reactivity of

841

the serum, based upon titration of dilutions of serum, may be valuable in establishing the diagnosis and in evaluating the efficacy of treatment.

The VDRL test (the nontreponemal test in widest use) generally becomes positive 4–6 weeks after infection, or 1–3 weeks after the appearance of the primary lesion; it is almost invariably positive in the secondary stage. The VDRL titer is usually high in secondary syphilis and tends to be lower or even negative in late forms of syphilis, although this is highly variable. A falling titer in treated early syphilis or a falling or stable titer in latent or late syphilis indicates satisfactory therapeutic progress. These serologic tests are not completely specific and must be closely correlated with other clinical and laboratory findings. The tests are positive in patients with nonvenereal treponematoses (see below). More importantly, "false-positive" serologic reactions are frequently encountered in a wide variety of situations including collagen diseases, infectious mononucleosis, malaria, many febrile diseases, leprosy, vaccination, drug addiction, old age, and possibly pregnancy. False-positive reactions are usually of low titer and transient and may be distinguished from true positives by specific treponemal antibody tests.

2. **Treponemal antibody tests**–The fluorescent treponemal antibody absorption (FTA-ABS) test is the most widely employed treponemal test. It measures antibodies capable of reacting with killed *T pallidum* after absorption of the patient's serum with extracts of nonpathogenic treponemes. The FTA-ABS test has now generally replaced the *Treponema pallidum* immobilization (TPI) test, which assays the ability of a patient's serum to immobilize live virulent spirochetes. The FTA-ABS test is at least as specific as and much more sensitive than the TPI test, and it is also easier, cheaper, and safer to perform. It is of value principally in determining whether a positive nontreponemal antigen test is a "false positive" or is indicative of syphilitic disease. Because of its great sensitivity, particularly in the late stages of the disease, it is also of value when there is clinical evidence of syphilis but the routine STS is negative. The test is positive in the majority of patients with primary syphilis and in virtually all patients with secondary disease, and it remains positive permanently in a high percentage of successfully treated patients. False-positive FTA-ABS tests have been occasionally reported in pregnancy, in systemic lupus erythematosus, and in other disorders associated with abnormal globulins.

Final decision about the significance of STS results must be based upon a total clinical appraisal.

B. **Microscopic Examination:** In infectious syphilis, *T pallidum* may be demonstrated by direct dark-field microscopic examination of fresh exudate from lesions or material aspirated from regional lymph nodes. The dark-field examination requires considerable experience and care in the proper collection of specimens and in the identification of pathogenic spirochetes by their characteristic morphology and motility. Repeated examinations may be necessary.

The spirochete is usually not found in any of the late syphilitic lesions by this technic.

An immunofluorescent staining technic for demonstrating *T pallidum* in dried smears of fluid taken from early syphilitic lesions is now available. Slides are fixed and treated with fluorescein-labeled antitreponemal antibody preparations which have been preabsorbed with nonpathogenic treponemes. The slides are then examined for fluorescing spirochetes under an ultraviolet microscope. Because of its relative ease of performance and convenience to physicians, the immunofluorescence technic has replaced dark-field microscopy in most health departments and medical center laboratories.

C. **Spinal Fluid Examination:** The CSF findings in neurosyphilis usually consist of elevation of total protein and gamma globulins, increase in the cell count, and a positive reagin test (STS). False-positive reagin tests rarely occur in the CSF. Improvement of the CSF findings is of great prognostic value. Lumbar puncture is mandatory in all cases discovered beyond the secondary stage, since a positive CSF in the absence of CNS symptoms (asymptomatic neurosyphilis) indicates the need for prolonged penicillin treatment. In a small percentage of cases of CNS syphilis, the CSF is normal.

Treatment

A. **Specific Measures:**

1. **Penicillin**, as benzathine penicillin G or procaine penicillin G with 2% aluminum monostearate (PAM), is the drug of choice for all forms of syphilis and other spirochetal infections. Effective tissue levels must be maintained for several days or weeks because of the spirochete's long generation time. Penicillin is highly effective in early infections and variably effective in the late stages. The principal contraindication is hypersensitivity to the penicillins. The recommended treatment schedules are included below in the discussion of the various forms of syphilis.

2. **Other antibiotic therapy**–Oral tetracyclines and erythromycins are effective in the treatment of syphilis for patients who are sensitive to penicillin or have relapses following one or more courses of penicillin. Tetracycline, 30–40 gm, or erythromycin, 30–40 gm, is given over a period of 10–15 days. Since experience with these antibiotics in the treatment of syphilis is limited, careful follow-up is necessary.

B. **Local Measures (Mucocutaneous Lesions):** Local treatment is usually not necessary. No local antiseptics or other chemicals should be applied to a suspected syphilitic lesion until specimens for microscopy have been obtained.

C. **Public Health Measures:** Patients with infectious syphilis must abstain from sexual activity until rendered noninfectious by antibiotic therapy. All cases of syphilis must be reported to the appropriate public health agency for assistance in identifying and investigating all contacts.

Complications of Specific Therapy

The Jarisch-Herxheimer reaction is ascribed to the

massive destruction of spirochetes by specific treatment and is manifested by fever and aggravation of the existing clinical picture. It is most likely to occur in early syphilis. Treatment is not discontinued unless the symptoms become severe or threaten to be fatal or in the presence of syphilitic laryngitis, auditory neuritis, or labyrinthitis, where such a reaction may cause irreversible damage. This reaction may be prevented or modified by simultaneous administration of corticosteroids. The reaction usually begins within the first 24 hours and subsides spontaneously within the next 24 hours of penicillin treatment.

Follow-Up

Patients who receive treatment for early syphilis should be followed clinically and with periodic quantitative VDRL tests for at least 1 year. Patients with all other types of syphilis should be under similar observation for 2 or more years.

Prevention

Avoidance of sexual contact is the only reliable method of prophylaxis but is an impractical public health measure for obvious reasons.

A. Mechanical: The standard rubber condom is effective but protects covered parts only. The exposed parts should be washed with soap and water as soon after contact as possible. This applies to both sexes.

B. Antibiotic: If there is known exposure to infectious syphilis, abortive penicillin therapy may be used. Give 2.4 million units of procaine penicillin G IM in each buttock once. Treatment of gonococcal infection (and others) with penicillins is probably effective against incubating syphilis in most cases. However, other antimicrobial agents used in the treatment of gonorrhea may be ineffective in aborting preclinical syphilis. In particular, spectinomycin has no demonstrated efficacy in the treatment of spirochetal disease. In view of the increasing use of antibiotics other than penicillin for gonococcal disease, patients treated for gonorrhea should have serologic follow-up tests every 3 months for 1 year (eg, VDRL).

C. Vaccine: An effective vaccine against syphilis is not yet available.

Course & Prognosis

The lesions associated with primary and secondary syphilis are self-limiting and resolve with few or no residua. Late syphilis may be highly destructive and permanently disabling and may lead to death. With treatment, the STS will usually return to negative in early syphilis. In late latent and late syphilis, serofastness is not uncommon even after adequate treatment. In broad terms, if no treatment is given, about one-third of people infected with syphilis will undergo spontaneous cure, about one-third will remain in the latent phase throughout life, and about one-third will develop serious late lesions.

Clark EG, Danbolt N: The Oslo study of the natural course of untreated syphilis. M Clin North America 48:613, 1964.

Idsoe O & others: Penicillin in the treatment of syphilis. Bull WHO 47:1, 1972.
International Union Against the Venereal Diseases and Treponematoses: 27th General Assembly, Venice, May, 1972. Brit J Ven Dis 49:107, 1973.
Krause RM: Workshop on the biology of the treponemes. J Infect Dis 125:332, 1972.
Rosebury T: *Microbes and Morals.* Viking Press, 1971.
Smith JL, Israel CW: Spirochetes in late seronegative syphilis. JAMA 199:980, 1967.
Sparling PF: Diagnosis and treatment of syphilis. New England J Med 284:642, 1971.
Syphilis: A Synopsis. Public Health Services Publication No. 1660. US Government Printing Office, Jan 1968.
Webster B (editor): Symposium on venereal diseases. M Clin North America 56:1055, 1972.

STAGES & TYPES OF SYPHILIS

1. PRIMARY SYPHILIS

This is the stage of invasion and may pass unrecognized. The typical lesion is the chancre at the site or sites of inoculation, most frequently located on the penis, labia, cervix, or anorectal region. Anorectal lesions are especially common among male homosexuals. Occasionally the primary lesion occurs in the oropharynx (lip, tongue, or tonsil), and, rarely, on the breast or finger. The chancre starts as a small erosion 10–90 days (average 3–4 weeks) after inoculation which rapidly develops into a painless superficial ulcer with firm indurated margins and enlargement of regional lymph nodes, which are rubbery, discrete, and nontender. Secondary infection of the chancre is not uncommon and may lead to pain. Healing occurs without treatment, but a scar may form, especially with secondary infection.

The blood STS is usually positive 1–2 weeks after the primary lesion is noted; rising quantitative titers are especially significant when there is a history of previous infection. Immunofluorescent or dark-field microscopy will show organisms in the chancre in over 95% of cases. The spinal fluid is normal at this stage.

The syphilitic chancre may be confused with chancroid, lymphogranuloma venereum, herpes progenitalis, or neoplasm. Any lesion on the genitalia should be considered a possible primary syphilitic lesion.

Treatment

Give benzathine penicillin G, 1.2 million units in each buttock for a total dose of 2.4 million units; or procaine penicillin G with aluminum monostearate in oil (PAM), 2.4 million units IM initially and then 1.2 million units IM every third day to a total of 4.8 million units; or procaine penicillin G, 600,000 units daily IM for 8–10 consecutive days.

2. SECONDARY SYPHILIS

The secondary stage of syphilis usually appears a few weeks (but may appear up to 6 months) after development of the chancre, when sufficient dissemination of *T pallidum* has occurred to produce systemic signs (fever, lymphadenopathy) or infectious lesions at sites distant from the site of inoculation. The most common manifestations are skin and mucosal lesions. The skin lesions are nonpruritic, macular, papular, pustular, or follicular (or combinations of any of these types), although the maculopapular rash is the most common. The skin lesions usually are generalized; involvement of the palms and soles is especially suspicious. Annular lesions simulating ringworm are observed in blacks. Mucous membrane lesions range from ulcers and papules of the lips, mouth, throat, genitalia, and anus ("mucous patches") to a diffuse redness of the pharynx. Both skin and mucous membrane lesions are highly infectious at this stage. Specific lesions—**condylomata lata**—are fused papules on the moist areas of the skin and mucous membranes.

Meningeal, hepatic, renal, bone, and joint invasion with resulting cranial nerve palsies, jaundice, nephrotic syndrome, and periostitis may occur. Alopecia (moth-eaten appearance), iritis, and iridocyclitis may also occur. A transient myocarditis manifested by temporary ECG changes has been noted.

Blood STS is positive in almost all cases. The routine VDRL test is occasionally falsely negative due to extremely high titers of reagin; a quantitative test will be positive at high dilutions of serum. The cutaneous and mucous membrane lesions may show *Treponema pallidum* on microscopic examination. There is usually a transient CSF involvement, with pleocytosis and elevated protein, although only 5% of cases have positive CSF serologic reactions. A transient proteinuria with waxy casts is seen in mild renal involvement. Blood tests may demonstrate hepatic involvement.

The skin lesions may be confused with the infectious exanthems, pityriasis rosea, and drug eruptions. The visceral lesions may suggest nephritis or hepatitis due to other causes. The diffusely red throat may mimic other forms of pharyngitis.

Treatment is as for primary syphilis unless CNS disease is present, in which case treatment is as for neurosyphilis (see below). Isolation of the patient is important.

Sherlock S: The liver in secondary (early) syphilis. New England J Med 284:1437, 1971.

3. RELAPSING SYPHILIS

The lesions of secondary syphilis will heal spontaneously, but secondary syphilis may relapse if undiagnosed or inadequately treated. These relapses may include any of the findings noted under secondary syphilis: skin and mucous membrane, neurologic, ocular, bone, or visceral. Unlike the usual asymptomatic neurologic involvement of secondary syphilis, neurologic relapses may be fulminating, leading to death. Relapse is almost always accompanied by a rising titer in quantitative STS testing; indeed, a rising titer may be the first or only evidence of relapse.

Treatment is as for primary syphilis unless CNS disease is present.

4. LATENT ("HIDDEN") SYPHILIS

Latent syphilis is the clinically quiescent phase during the interval between disappearance of secondary lesions and before the appearance of tertiary symptoms. Early latency is defined as the first 3–5 years after infection during which infectious lesions are likely to recur ("relapsing syphilis"); after 5 years, the patient is said to be in the late latent phase. Transmission to the fetus, however, can probably occur in any phase. There are by definition no clinical manifestations during the latent phase, and the only significant laboratory findings are positive serologic tests. A diagnosis of latent syphilis is justified only when the CSF is entirely negative, x-ray and physical examination shows no evidence of cardiovascular involvement, and false positive tests for syphilis have been ruled out. The latent phase may last from months to a lifetime.

It is important to differentiate latent syphilis from false positive blood tests due to clerical errors, acute fevers, yaws, infectious mononucleosis, malaria, leprosy, leishmaniasis, smallpox vaccination, lymphogranuloma venereum, systemic lupus erythematosus, and other collagen diseases.

Treatment is with benzathine penicillin G, 3 doses of 3 million units at 7-day intervals; procaine penicillin G with aluminum monostearate suspension, 6 doses of 1.2 million units IM at 3-day intervals; or aqueous procaine penicillin G, 12 doses of 600,000 units daily. Only a small percentage of serologic tests will be appreciably altered by treatment with penicillin. The treatment of this stage of the disease is intended to prevent the late sequelae.

Pereyra AJ, Voller RL: A graphic guide for clinical management of latent syphilis. California Med 112:13, May 1970.

5. LATE (TERTIARY) SYPHILIS

This stage may occur at any time after secondary syphilis, even after years of latency. Late lesions probably represent, at least in part, a delayed hypersensitivity reaction of the tissue to the organism and are usually divided into 2 types: (1) A localized gummatous reaction with a relatively rapid onset and generally prompt response to therapy ("benign late syphilis") and (2) diffuse inflammation of a more insidious onset which characteristically involves the CNS and large arteries, is often fatal if untreated, and is at best arrested by treatment. Gummas may involve any area or organ of the body, but most often the skin or long bones. Cardiovascular disease is usually manifest by aortic aneurysm, aortic insufficiency, or aortitis. Various forms of diffuse or localized CNS involvement may occur.

Late syphilis must be differentiated from neoplasms of the skin, liver, lung, stomach, or brain; other forms of meningitis; and primary neurologic lesions.

Treatment is as for latent syphilis. Reversal of positive STS does not usually occur. A second course of penicillin therapy may be given if necessary. There is no known method for reliable eradication of the treponeme from man in the late stages of syphilis. Viable spirochetes are occasionally found in the eyes, in CSF, and elsewhere in "adequately" treated syphilis, but claims for their capacity to cause progressive disease are speculative.

Although almost any tissue and organ may be involved in late syphilis, the following are the most common types of involvement.

Skin

Cutaneous lesions of late syphilis are of 2 varieties: (1) multiple nodular lesions which eventually ulcerate or resolve by forming atrophic, pigmented scars, and (2) solitary gummas which start as painless subcutaneous nodules, enlarge, attach to the overlying skin, and eventually ulcerate.

Mucous Membranes

Late lesions of the mucous membranes are nodular gummas or leukoplakia, highly destructive to the involved tissue.

Skeletal

Bone lesions are destructive, causing periostitis, osteitis, and arthritis with little or no associated redness or swelling but often marked myalgia and myositis of the neighboring muscles. The pain is especially severe at night.

Eyes

Late ocular lesions are gummatous iritis, chorioretinitis, optic atrophy, and cranial nerve palsies, in addition to the lesions of CNS syphilis.

Respiratory System

Respiratory involvement by late syphilis is caused by gummatous infiltrates into the larynx, trachea, and pulmonary parenchyma, producing discrete pulmonary infiltrates. There may be hoarseness, respiratory distress, and wheezing secondary to the gummatous lesion itself or to subsequent stenosis occurring with healing.

Gastrointestinal

Gummas involving the liver produce the usually benign, asymptomatic **hepar lobatum**. Infiltration into the stomach wall causes "leather bottle" stomach with epigastric distress, inability to eat large meals, regurgitation, belching, and weight loss. Occasionally a picture not unlike Laennec's cirrhosis is produced by liver involvement.

Cardiovascular (See also p 228.)

Cardiovascular lesions (10–15% of late syphilitic lesions) are often progressive, disabling, and life-threatening. CNS lesions are often present also. Involvement usually starts as an arteritis in the supracardiac portion of the aorta and progresses to cause one or more of the following: (1) Narrowing of the coronary ostia with resulting decreased coronary circulation, angina, cardiac insufficiency, and acute myocardial infarction. (2) Scarring of the aortic valves, producing aortic insufficiency with its water-hammer pulse, aortic diastolic murmur, frequently aortic systolic murmur, cardiac hypertrophy, and eventually congestive heart failure. (3) Weakness of the wall of the aorta, with saccular aneurysm formation and associated pressure symptoms of dysphagia, hoarseness, brassy cough, back pain (vertebral erosion), and occasionally rupture of the aneurysm. Recurrent respiratory infections are common as a result of pressure on the trachea and bronchi.

Treatment of cardiac problems requires first consideration, after which penicillin G is given as for latent syphilis.

Neurosyphilis

Neurosyphilis (15–20% of late syphilitic lesions; often present with cardiovascular syphilis) is, like cardiovascular syphilis, a progressive, disabling, and life-threatening complication. There are 4 clinical types:

(1) **Asymptomatic neurosyphilis:** Spinal fluid abnormalities (positive spinal fluid STS, increased cell count, occasionally increased protein) without symptoms or signs of neurologic involvement.

(2) **Meningovascular syphilis:** This form is characterized by meningeal involvement or changes in the vascular structures of the brain (or both), producing symptoms of low-grade meningitis (headache, irritability); cranial nerve palsies (basilar meningitis); unequal reflexes; irregular pupils with poor light and accommodation reflexes; and, when large vessels are involved, cerebrovascular accidents. The symptoms of acute meningitis are rare in late syphilis.

(3) **Tabes dorsalis:** This type of neurosyphilis is a chronic progressive degeneration of the parenchyma of the posterior columns of the spinal cord and of the posterior sensory ganglia and nerve roots. The symptoms and signs are those of impairment of proprioception and vibration, Argyll Robertson pupils (which react poorly to light but well to accommodation), and muscular hypotonia and hyporeflexia. Impairment of proprioception results in a wide-based gait and inability to walk in the dark. Paresthesias,

analgesia, or sharp recurrent pains in the muscles of the leg ("shooting" or "lightning" pains) may occur. Crises are also common in tabes: gastric crises, consisting of sharp abdominal pains with nausea and vomiting (simulating an acute abdomen); laryngeal crises, with paroxysmal cough and dyspnea; urethral crises, with painful bladder spasms; and rectal and anal crises. Crises may begin suddenly, last for hours to days, and cease abruptly. Neurogenic bladder with overflow incontinence is also seen. Trophic, painless ulcers may occur over pressure points on the feet. Joint damage may occur as a result of lack of sensory innervation (Charcot joint).

(4) **General paresis:** This is a generalized involvement of the cerebral cortex. The onset of clinical manifestations is insidious. There is usually a decrease in concentrating power, memory loss, dysarthria, tremor of the fingers and lips, irritability, and mild headaches. Most striking is the change of personality; the patient becomes slovenly, irresponsible, confused, and psychotic. Combinations of the various forms of neurosyphilis (especially tabes and paresis) are not uncommon.

Special considerations in treatment of neurosyphilis: It is most important to prevent neurosyphilis by prompt diagnosis, adequate treatment, and follow-up of early syphilis. Examination of all syphilitic patients for evidence of nervous system involvement must be a regular part of the follow-up examination. If neurosyphilis is present, the pretreatment clinical and laboratory evaluation should include detailed neurologic, ocular, psychiatric, and CSF examinations.

Treatment consists of procaine penicillin G, 600,000 units IM daily to a total of 12 million units or more.

All patients must have spinal fluid examinations at 3-month intervals for the first year and every 6 months for the second year following completion of antisyphilis therapy. The adequacy of response is at times difficult to evaluate (especially during a short period of observation), but it may be gauged by clinical improvement and effective and persistent reversal of CSF changes. A second course of penicillin therapy may be given if necessary. Not infrequently, there is progression of neurologic symptoms and signs despite high and prolonged doses of penicillin. It has been postulated that these treatment failures are related to the unexplained persistence of viable *T pallidum* in CNS or ocular lesions in at least some cases.

Yogeswari L, Chacko LW: Persistence of *T pallidum* and its significance in penicillin-treated seropositive late syphilis. Brit J Ven Dis 47:339, 1971.

6. PRENATAL SYPHILIS

All pregnant women should have serologic tests early and late in gestation. Those who have syphilis must receive appropriate treatment without delay. Penicillin dosage schedules as advised for primary and secondary syphilis are satisfactory. When therapy is instituted after the 7th month of gestation in women with untreated early syphilis, larger doses of penicillin are advised. Penicillin prevents congenital syphilis in more than 90% of cases even when syphilis is discovered in the last trimester of pregnancy.

Follow-up must consist of monthly physical examinations and quantitative blood STS until delivery and for a month after delivery. If there is any clinical evidence of relapse, a failure of blood STS titer to fall, or a rise of STS titer, treatment should be repeated.

The infant should be examined for signs of syphilis at birth and again at intervals of 2 or 3 weeks for 4–6 months. If the maternal blood is positive, a positive cord blood STS is of no diagnostic value. However, if the infant's blood is followed serially by quantitative blood STS at 2-week intervals for 4 months, a sustained or rising STS titer indicates a diagnosis of congenital syphilis and a need for treatment. A recent modification of the FTA-ABS test utilizing fluorescein-labeled antihuman IgM allows serologic diagnosis of congenital syphilis when the maternal blood also shows a positive routine FTA-ABS test; this test is not yet widely available.

Alford CA Jr & others: IgM FTA-ABS test in the diagnosis of congenital syphilis. New England J Med 280:1086, 1969.
Mamunes P & others: Early diagnosis of neonatal congenital syphilis: Elevation of a gamma M-fluorescent treponemal antibody test. Am J Dis Child 120:17, 1970.

7. CONGENITAL SYPHILIS

The clinical manifestations of congenital syphilis are quite similar to those of the secondary stage of the acquired form. Skin and mucous membrane lesions, generally highly infectious, are often present at birth or in early infancy. Signs of the disease, however, may be minimal and may be ascribed to minor infections or allergies unless adequate diagnostic measures are taken. Characteristic later stigmas of congenital syphilis include interstitial keratitis, Hutchinson's teeth, 8th nerve deafness (Hutchinson's triad), saddle nose, rhagades, saber shins and other bone changes, hepar lobatum, pneumonia alba, and mental retardation. Any of the tertiary sequelae of the adult disease (CNS, visceral, or cardiovascular) may occur. The STS is usually strongly positive at birth but gradually becomes negative over a period of years. The new IgM FTA-ABS test is usually positive and may help differentiate maternal antibodies from the infant's. Total IgM levels are sometimes elevated.

The newborn is infectious, and suitable precautions must be taken to prevent infection of others.

Early congenital syphilis (< 2 years of age) is treated with 50,000 units/kg of benzathine penicillin G as a single injection; or with a total of 100,000 units/ kg PAM IM given at 2–3 day intervals in divided doses. The treatment of late congenital syphilis is as for late latent syphilis. Neurosyphilis of congenital origin should be treated as the acquired form.

Oppenheimer EH, Hardy JB: Congenital syphilis in the newborn infant. Johns Hopkins Med J 129:63, 1971.

Robinson RCV: Congenital syphilis. Arch Dermat 99:599, 1969.

NONVENEREAL TREPONEMATOSES

A wide variety of treponemal diseases other than syphilis occur endemically in many tropical areas of the world. They are distinguished from disease caused by *T pallidum* by their nonvenereal transmission, relatively high incidence in certain geographic areas and among children, and their tendency to produce less severe visceral manifestations. As in syphilis, organisms can be demonstrated in infectious lesions with dark-field microscopy or immunofluorescence but cannot be cultured in artificial media, the serologic tests for syphilis are positive, the diseases have primary, secondary, and sometimes tertiary stages, and penicillin is the drug of choice. There is evidence that infection with these agents may provide partial immunity to syphilis and vice versa. Treatment with penicillin in doses appropriate to primary syphilis (eg, 1.2–2.4 million units IM of benzathine penicillin G) is generally curative in any stage of the nonvenereal treponematoses. In cases of penicillin hypersensitivity, tetracycline is usually the recommended alternative.

Hume JC: Worldwide problems in the diagnosis of syphilis and other treponematoses. M Clin North America 48:721, 1964.

YAWS
(Frambesia)

Yaws is a contagious disease largely limited to tropical regions which is caused by *Treponema pertenue*. It is characterized by granulomatous lesions of the skin, mucous membranes, and bone. Yaws is rarely fatal, although if untreated it may lead to chronic disability and disfigurement. Yaws is acquired by direct nonvenereal contact, usually in childhood, although it may occur at any age. The "mother yaw," a painless papule which later ulcerates, appears 3–4 weeks after exposure. There is usually associated regional lymphadenopathy. Six to 12 weeks later, similar secondary lesions appear and last for several months or years. Painful ulcerated lesions on the soles are frequent and are called "crab yaws." Late gummatous lesions may occur, with associated tissue destruction involving large areas of skin and subcutaneous tissues. The late effects of yaws, with bone change, shortening of digits, and contractions, may be confused with similar changes occurring in leprosy. CNS, cardiac, or other visceral involvement is rare.

PINTA

Pinta is a nonvenereal spirochetal infection caused by *Treponema carateum*. It occurs endemically in rural areas of Latin America, especially in Mexico, Colombia, and Cuba, and in some areas of the Pacific. A nonulcerative, erythematous primary papule spreads slowly into a papulosquamous plaque showing a variety of color changes (slate, lilac, black). Secondary lesions resemble the primary one and appear within a year after it. These appear successively, new lesions together with older ones; are commonest on the extremities; and later show atrophy and depigmentation. Some cases show pigment changes and atrophic patches on the soles and palms, with or without hyperkeratosis, which are indistinguishable from "crab yaws." Uncommonly, CNS or cardiovascular disease is observed late in the disease.

ENDEMIC SYPHILIS
(Bejel, Skerljevo, Etc)

Endemic syphilis is an acute and chronic infection caused by an organism indistinguishable from *Treponema pallidum*. It has been reported in a number of countries, particularly in the Eastern Mediterranean area, often with local names: bejel in Syria and Iraq; skerljevo in Bosnia; and dichuchwa, njovera, and siti in Africa. Each has local distinctive characters. Moist ulcerated lesions of the skin or oral or nasopharyngeal mucosa are the most common manifestations. Generalized lymphadenopathy and secondary and tertiary bone and skin lesions are also common. Visceral involvement is rare.

MISCELLANEOUS SPIROCHETAL DISEASES

RELAPSING FEVER

Relapsing fever is an acute infectious disease caused by the spirochete *Borrelia recurrentis*. The agent is transmitted by insect vectors from man to man (lice) or from several natural animal reservoirs to man (ticks) when infected insects or their feces are rubbed into the bite puncture wound, excoriated areas of skin, or mucous membranes. The disease is endemic in various parts of the world, including western USA. The incubation period is about 7 days.

Clinical Findings

A. Symptoms and Signs: Relapsing fever is characterized by sudden relapses of fever and a variety of other signs and symptoms occurring at intervals of 1–2 weeks. The relapses duplicate the initial attack but become progressively less severe. It is probable that relapses are due to rapid antigenic variation of the organism in the infected host. Recovery occurs after 2–10 relapses.

Attacks occur abruptly, with fever, chills, tachycardia, nausea and vomiting, myalgia, arthralgia, severe headache, mental changes, and occasionally bronchitis. Hepatomegaly (with or without jaundice) and splenomegaly often appear later. In some cases, an erythematous rash appears early in the course of the disease over the trunk and extremities, followed later by rose-colored spots in the same area. Petechiae may also be present. In severe cases neurologic and psychic manifestations are present at the height of the fever. After 3–10 days the fever falls by crisis. Jaundice, iritis, conjunctivitis, cranial nerve lesions, and hemorrhagic phenomena are more common in the relapses.

B. Laboratory Findings: During the acute episodes, spirochetes may be found in a blood smear stained with Wright's or Giemsa's stain. (Unlike other pathogenic spirochetes, borrelia organisms are visible under the light microscope.) The blood may be injected into a rat and the spirochetes found 3–5 days later in the tail blood. The organism has not been cultured on artificial media. The Weil-Felix test may be positive in a titer of 1:80 or more, and a false positive STS is found in one-third of cases. CSF abnormalities often occur in patients with neurologic signs. Mild anemia and thrombocytopenia may be present, but the white blood cell count is usually normal.

Differential Diagnosis

The manifestations of relapsing fever may be confused with malaria, leptospirosis, meningococcemia, yellow fever, typhus, or rat-bite fever.

Treatment

Treat either with (1) tetracycline drugs, 0.5 gm every 6 hours orally for 7 days; or (2) procaine penicillin G, 600,000 units IM daily for 10 days. Jarisch-Herxheimer reactions may occur, especially when treatment is given in an acute phase. Prevention consists of avoidance or eradication of the arthropod vectors.

Prognosis

The overall mortality rate is usually about 5%. Fatalities are most common in old, debilitated, or very young patients. With treatment, the initial attack is shortened and relapses are largely prevented.

Bryceson AD & others: Louse-borne relapsing fever. Quart J Med 39:129, 1970.

Southern PM, Sanford JP: Relapsing fever. Medicine 48:129, 1969.

RAT-BITE FEVER
(Spirillary Rat-Bite Fever, Sodoku)

Rat-bite fever is an uncommon acute infectious disease caused by *Spirillum minus* and transmitted to man by the bite of a rat. Laboratory workers and inhabitants of slum dwellings are the most susceptible groups in the USA.

Clinical Findings

A. Symptoms and Signs: The original rat bite, unless secondarily infected, heals promptly, but one to several weeks later the site becomes swollen, indurated, and painful, assumes a dusky purplish hue, and may ulcerate. Regional lymphangitis and lymphadenitis, fever, chills, malaise, myalgia, arthralgia, and headache are present. Splenomegaly may occur. A dusky-red, sparse maculopapular rash appears on the trunk and extremities in many cases, and there may be frank arthritis.

After a few days both the local and systemic symptoms subside, only to reappear again in a few days. This relapsing pattern of fever of 24–48 hours alternating with an equal afebrile period becomes established and may persist for weeks. The other features, however, usually recur only during the first few relapses.

B. Laboratory Findings: Leukocytosis is often present, and a blood STS is frequently falsely positive. The organism may be identified in dark-field examination of the ulcer exudate or aspirated lymph node material; more commonly, it is observed after inoculation of a laboratory animal with the patient's exudate or blood. It cannot be cultured in artificial media.

Differential Diagnosis

Rat-bite fever must be distinguished from the rat-bite-induced episodic fever, lymphadenitis, and rash of streptobacillary fever. Reliable differentiation requires an increasing titer of agglutinins against *Streptobacillus moniliformis* or identification of the causative organism. Rat-bite fever may also be distinguished from tularemia and relapsing fever by identification of the causative organism.

Treatment

Treat with procaine penicillin G, 300,000 units IM every 12 hours; or tetracycline drugs, 0.5 gm every 6 hours for 7 days. Give supportive and symptomatic measures as indicated.

Prognosis

The reported mortality rate is about 10%, but this should be markedly reduced by prompt diagnosis and antimicrobial treatment.

Cole JS & others: Rat-bite fever. Ann Int Med 71:979, 1969.
Schwartzman G & others: Repeated recovery of a spirillum by blood culture from two children with prolonged and recurrent fevers. Pediatrics 8:227, 1951.

LEPTOSPIROSIS
(Including Weil's Disease)

Leptospirosis is an acute and often severe infection which frequently affects the liver or other organs and is caused by any of several Leptospira species. The 3 most common species and their reservoirs of infection are: *Lept icterohaemorrhagiae* of rats, *Lept canicola* of dogs, and *Lept pomona* of cattle and swine. Several other species, some as yet unidentified serologically, can also cause the disease, but *Lept icterohaemorrhagiae* causes the most severe illness. The disease is worldwide in distribution, and the incidence is higher than usually supposed. The parasite is often transmitted to man by the ingestion of food and drink contaminated by the urine of the reservoir animal. The organism may also enter through minor skin lesions and probably the conjunctiva as well; and many infections have followed bathing in contaminated pools or streams. The disease is an occupational hazard among sewer workers, rice planters, and farmers. The incubation period is 2–20 days.

Clinical Findings

A. Symptoms and Signs: There is a sudden onset of fever to 39–40° C (102.2–104° F), chills, abdominal pains, vomiting, and myalgia especially of the calf muscles. Extremely severe headache is usually present. The conjunctiva is markedly reddened. The liver may be palpable, and in about 50% of cases (most commonly in *Lept icterohaemorrhagiae* infections) jaundice is present on about the 5th day and may be associated with nephritis. Capillary hemorrhages and purpuric skin lesions may also appear. Meningeal irritation and associated findings of aseptic meningitis may occur. In pretibial fever, patchy erythema occurs on the skin of the lower legs and may be generalized.

Leptospirosis with jaundice must be distinguished from hepatitis, yellow fever, and relapsing fever.

B. Laboratory Findings: The leukocyte count may be normal or as high as 50,000/cu mm, with neutrophils predominating. The urine may contain bile, protein, casts, and red cells. Oliguria is not uncommon, and in severe cases uremia may occur. In cases with meningeal involvement, organisms may be found in the CSF. The organism may be identified by dark-field examination of the patient's blood (during the first 10 days) or by culture on Korthof's medium. The organism may also be isolated from the urine from the 10th day to the 6th week. Specific agglutination titers develop after 7 days and may persist at high levels for many years; specific serologic tests are of particular value in diagnosis of the milder, anicteric forms of the disease.

Complications

Myocarditis, aseptic meningitis, renal failure, and massive hemorrhage are not common but are the usual cause of death. Iridocyclitis may occur.

Treatment

Treat as early as possible (and continue treatment for 6 days) with penicillin, 600,000 units IM every 3 hours for 1 day and then every 6 hours; or with tetracyclines, 0.5 gm every 6 hours. Observe for evidences of renal failure and treat as necessary.

Prognosis

Without jaundice, the disease is almost never fatal. With jaundice, the mortality rate is about 15%.

Berman SJ & others: Sporadic anicteric leptospirosis in South Vietnam. Ann Int Med 79:107, 1973.
Heath CW & others: Leptospirosis in United States. New England J Med 273:857, 1965.
Turner LH: Leptospirosis. Brit MJ 1:537, 1973.

25...
Infectious Diseases: Protozoal

Robert S. Goldsmith

AMEBIASIS

Essentials of Diagnosis

- Recurrent bouts of diarrhea and abdominal cramps, sometimes alternating with constipation.
- Semi-fluid stools containing no pus and only flecks of blood-stained mucus.
- In fulminant cases, bloody exudates and prostration.
- Tenderness and enlargement of the liver is frequent.
- Liver abscess, often without obvious association with dysentery.
- Amebas demonstrable in stools or abscess aspirate. Cysts in stools in quiescent infections. Hematophagous amebas in stools are diagnostic.

General Considerations

Amebiasis is an infection with protean clinical manifestations, almost worldwide in distribution, caused by the protozoon *Entamoeba histolytica.*

Potentially pathogenic amebas may (1) live in the bowel as harmless commensals (asymptomatic amebiasis or carrier state—although some workers insist that they always cause minute lesions)—or, in particular circumstances, they may (2) invade the large bowel wall, causing amebic dysentery, or other viscera (metastatic infection), most commonly the liver (liver abscess). In other words, amebiasis may be asymptomatic, intestinal, or extra-intestinal.

A bacteriophagous "small race," *E hartmanni,* is believed to be generally harmless, unlike the potentially hematophagous and pathogenic "large race." The life cycle of the ameba consists of 2 distinct stages: (1) a cyst (infective) stage, which occurs only in the intestinal lumen and stools; (2) a motile ameba or trophozoite normally living as a commensal in the colon but producing lesions after activation to an invasive phase by, for example, coincident synergistic bacterial or possibly other bowel infections, diet, alterations in the host's physiologic state, or combinations of factors.

Cysts gain entry to man in food and drink contaminated by feces. Trophozoites excyst from each cyst, probably in the region of the ileocecal valve.

They may multiply and live commensally, cysts being passed at irregular intervals. The greatest densities of organisms are at the sites of greatest fecal stasis, ie, the cecum, descending colon, sigmoid, and rectum. During an invasive phase, the trophozoites penetrate the mucosa to produce flask-shaped microabscesses which, by enlargement and coalescence, may produce shallow, undermined ulcers with ragged edges covered by a loose yellow exudate. In fulminating cases the ulceration may be extensive and the bowel quite friable. There is little inflammation, and therefore relatively little fibrosis following healing.

During acute or chronic dysentery, there is frequently some degree of liver tenderness and hepatomegaly. The incidence of liver abscess is not related to the severity of preceding amebic dysentery, and only about one-third of patients give a history of amebic dysentery.

An ameboma (amebic granuloma) is a tumor in the colon, usually in the cecum or sigmoid, caused by local exuberance of granulation tissue or fibrosis, and sometimes by abscess. The same pathologic process may give rise to stricture, most evident in the rectum. As with liver abscess, amebomas and strictures may have no reliable association with active amebic dysentery. Differentiation from carcinoma is important.

Asymptomatic infection (cyst-passers, carrier state) is fairly common. Up to 50% or more of people in endemic areas with poor sanitation may be carriers. Cyst-passers may be convalescents or may have no known relevant history of amebiasis. In some localities many of the cyst-passers may be carrying small races of *E histolytica* of negligible virulence. Confusion with cysts of the nonpathogenic species or subspecies hartmanni is common.

Clinical Findings

A. Symptoms and Signs: The onset is seldom abrupt. (An abrupt onset in amebiasis may signify a concurrent shigella infection.) Increasingly severe diarrhea or moderate dysentery develops over a period of several days, associated with lower abdominal pain or discomfort and tenesmus. The stools (5—10 a day except in fulminating cases, when there may be 20 or more) are brown, semi-fluid, and have a characteristic foul smell, with flecks of blood-stained mucus and, in severe cases, blood and copious mucus. Patients may be afebrile or have irregular and usually low-grade fever.

The acute attack usually subsides spontaneously. Remissions and recurrence follow, sometimes with various abdominal symptoms during remission, leading eventually to severe debility and prostration. Loss of weight becomes notable. Trophozoites are characteristically present in the dysenteric stools; cysts alone are present intermittently during remissions. Amebic ulceration may occur without diarrhea, and severe dysentery may occur in the absence of detectable amebas in the stools.

B. Laboratory Findings: When diarrhea or dysentery is present, the trophozoites may be identified in fresh stools or in tissues obtained from the edges of ulcers at the time of endoscopy. Trophozoites can be found and identified only in fresh stools or stools immediately preserved. Trophozoites are found less frequently in formed stools. If possible, fresh stools should be rushed to the laboratory; otherwise specimens should be preserved in PVA (polyvinyl alcohol) fixative. The trophozoites are large, with a characteristic flowing motility in the warm fresh stool. A few of them will contain ingested red cells (smaller in diameter than free red cells because they are globular in the ameba), and this is pathognomonic provided the trophozoite is not confused with the occasional macrophage also containing red cells. Cysts (in formed stools) and trophozoites must be distinguished from the closely similar *E coli, E hartmanni,* and (occasionally) *E polecki,* as well as from *Iodamoeba bütschlii, Dientamoeba fragilis* (an occasional cause of intestinal disturbance), and *Endolimax nana.* The diagnosis must be positive, and this demands a great deal of skill and experience. In the stool, leukocytes and macrophages are relatively scarce (in contrast to bacillary dysentery) unless there is concomitant bacillary infection, as may be found with varying frequency according to locality. Charcot-Leyden crystals may be present. The white count is elevated, but not to high levels, during the acute attack, and often with hepatic abscess, but there is no eosinophilia.

With liver abscess, material for examination may be obtained by aspiration, although the central markedly necrotic material is usually free from organisms. The appearance is normally characteristic and has been described as resembling "anchovy paste." Divide the aspirated material into a succession of 20–30 ml samples as it is taken, so that the last sample only may be examined. Avoid sending only one large sample.

Specific circulating antibodies may be very useful in the diagnosis of invasive amebiasis (acute intestinal infections or extra-intestinal disease). Useful serologic tests include the indirect hemagglutination, agar diffusion, and complement fixation tests.

Endoscopy may reveal the ulcerative lesions, with intact intervening mucosa. It is very valuable in experienced hands, and should be adopted as a routine.

Differential Diagnosis

Amebic diarrhea or dysentery must be distin-guished from ulcerative colitis, acute nonspecific colitis, and bacillary dysentery. At times amebic dysentery must be distinguished also from schistosomiasis, balantidiasis, regional enteritis, tuberculous enterocolitis, and severe trichuris (whipworm) infection in children.

Complications

Liver abscess is the most common complication of intestinal infection. Amebas from the intestine may rarely travel to and infect the lungs, brain, or skin. Perforation of the bowel may also occasionally take place, and an untreated hepatic abscess may perforate into the adjacent pleural space to produce an effusion and a pneumonitis. The bowel wall in amebic dysentery is quite friable, and surgery is contraindicated. Amebomas usually resolve completely.

Treatment

Amebiasis may present as a severe intestinal infection (dysentery or severe diarrhea), a mild symptomatic intestinal infection, an asymptomatic intestinal infection, or as an ameboma or liver abscess, or in the form of other extra-intestinal infections.

Drugs available for therapy can be classified according to their site of antiamebic action. Luminal amebicides such as diiodohydroxyquin and diloxanide furoate are active against luminal organisms but are ineffective against parasites in the bowel wall or tissues. The parenterally administered tissue amebicides, dehydroemetine and emetine, are effective against parasites in the bowel wall and tissues but not against luminal organisms. Chloroquine, administered orally or parenterally, acts only against organisms in the liver. Antibiotics taken orally are indirect-acting luminal amebicides that exert their effects against bacterial associates of *E histolytica* in the bowel lumen and in the bowel wall but not in other tissues. Given parenterally, antibiotics have little antiamebic activity at any site. Metronidazole is uniquely effective against organisms at 3 sites: the bowel lumen, bowel wall, and tissues.

The following is a partial list of useful antiamebic drugs:

(1) **Tissue amebicides (drugs that act primarily in the bowel wall, liver, and other extra-intestinal tissues):**
   (a) Dehydroemetine, emetine.
   (b) Chloroquine (active principally in liver).
(2) **Luminal amebicides (drugs that act primarily in the bowel lumen):**
   (a) Halogenated hydroxyquinolines: Diiodohydroxyquin, iodochlorhydroxyquin, chiniofon.
   (b) Pentavalent arsenicals: Glycobiarsol carbarsone.
   (c) Alkaloids: Emetine-bismuth-iodide
   (d) Amides: Clefamide, diloxanide furoate.
   (e) Antibiotics (act also in bowel wall): Tetracyclines, paromomycin.
(3) **Tissue and luminal amebicides:** Metronidazole.

Treatment may require the concomitant or sequential use of several drugs. Table 25–1 outlines 2 methods of treatment for each clinical type of amebiasis. No drugs are recommended as safe or effective for chemoprophylaxis.

The recent demonstration that metronidazole is carcinogenic in rodents and mutagenic in bacteria leads to the view that the drug is potentially dangerous to humans as well. The real risk to man is unknown and will probably remain unknown. Therefore, this author concludes that the prudent approach would be to use alternative drugs first, and metronidazole if failures occur. The therapeutic loss using alternative drugs is not in effectiveness but in simplicity of treatment, for no other drug but metronidazole is effective as both a luminal and tissue amebicide. Metronidazole also has fewer side-effects than emetine. Nevertheless, the unknown risk with metronidazole will be worth taking with some patients.

A. Asymptomatic Intestinal Infection: When infection is confined to the bowel lumen, cure may be obtained by use of luminal amebicides alone. Of the many drugs available, none is completely reliable in eradicating the infection. A course of diiodohydroxyquin, alone or with oxytetracycline, is recommended. However, without the additional use of chloroquine, there remains the rare risk of continuing liver infection.

Table 25–1. Treatment of amebiasis.

	Drug(s) of Choice	Alternative Drug(s)
Asymptomatic intestinal infection	Diloxanide furoate,* 500 mg 3 times daily for 10 days, or diiodohydroxyquin, 650 mg 3 times daily for 21 days	As for mild intestinal disease
Mild intestinal infection	(1) Diloxanide furoate,* 500 mg 3 times daily for 10 days or diiodohydroxyquin, 650 mg 3 times daily for 21 days **plus** (2) Oxytetracycline, 250 mg 4 times daily for 10 days, **plus** (3) Chloroquine, 500 mg (salt) twice daily for 2 days and then 250 mg twice daily for 19 days	(1) Metronidazole,† 750 mg 3 times daily for 10 days, **followed by** (2) Diiodohydroxyquin, 650 mg 3 times daily for 21 days
Severe intestinal infection	(1) Emetine, 1 mg/kg subcut or IM (maximum daily dose 65 mg) **or** Dehydroemetine,‡ 1–1.5 mg/kg IM or subcut daily (maximum daily dose 100 mg) Either drug is given for the least number of days necessary to control symptoms (usually 4–6 days) **plus** (2) Oxytetracycline, 250 mg 4 times daily for 10 days, **plus** (3) Diiodohydroxyquin, 650 mg 4 times daily for 21 days, **followed by** (4) Chloroquine, 500 mg (salt) twice daily for 2 days and 250 mg twice daily for 19 days	(1) Metronidazole,† 750 mg 3 times daily for 10 days, **followed by** (2) Diiodohydroxyquin, 650 mg 4 times daily for 21 days
Hepatic abscess	(1) Emetine, 1 mg/kg subcut or IM (maximum daily dose 65 mg) **or** Dehydroemetine,‡ 1–1.5 mg/kg daily IM or subcut for 10 days (maximum total dose, 1 gm) **plus** (2) Chloroquine, 500 mg (salt) twice daily for 2 days and then 250 mg twice daily for 26 days **plus** (3) Diiodohydroxyquin, 650 mg 3 times daily for 21 days	(1) Metronidazole,† 750 mg 3 times daily for 10 days, **followed by** (2) Diiodohydroxyquin, 650 mg 3 times daily for 21 days
Ameboma or extra-intestinal infection	As for hepatic abscess, but not including chloroquine	As for hepatic abscess

*Not approved by the FDA for use in the USA.

†Recent evidence on the possible carcinogenic and mutagenic hazards of metronidazole is summarized in Med Lett Drugs Ther for June 20, 1975 (Vol 17, No. 13, pp 53–54). The Medical Letter consultants conclude that the risk is probably worth taking "in some patients with amebiasis."

‡Available in the USA for investigational use only from the Parasitic Disease Drug Service, Center for Disease Control, Atlanta 30333.

B. Mild Intestinal Infection: In addition to clearing amebas from the bowel lumen, treatment of mild intestinal disease should eradicate trophozoites from the bowel wall and liver. If diloxanide furoate or diiodohydroxyquin is used, concomitant use of oxytetracycline increases cure rates. Chloroquine is added to eradicate trophozoites carried to the liver. If metronidazole is used, a course of diiodohydroxyquin should follow as well.

C. Severe Intestinal Infection: The drug of choice is emetine (or dehydroemetine) given intramuscularly or subcutaneously. Emetine should be used for the minimum number of days (usually 4–6) needed to control severe symptoms. Significant toxicity usually does not occur during this period. Concurrently, the patient is given a full course of oxytetracycline and diiodohydroxyquin. Chloroquine must also be administered to ensure the destruction of trophozoites carried to the liver that are not killed by the short course of emetine.

Metronidazole alone will cure approximately 90% of patients with one course of treatment. To further increase the cure rate, it is suggested that a course of diiodohydroxyquin follow metronidazole.

Bed rest and opiates to control bowel motility are necessary adjuncts in severe amebic dysentery.

D. Hepatic Abscess: Emetine plus chloroquine is as effective as but usually more toxic than metronidazole. Small liver abscesses do not require drainage, but large abscesses should be aspirated with a wide-bore needle under strict aseptic conditions.

Diiodohydroxyquin should be given even when parasites have not been identified in the stool.

E. Ameboma or Extra-intestinal Disease: The drug of choice is emetine, but metronidazole is an alternative drug. Chloroquine does not reach sufficiently high tissue concentrations (except in the liver) to be effective. A simultaneous course of intestinal amebicides should also be given.

Follow-Up Care

A complete follow-up examination consists of study of 6 successive stools (at least 2 following a saline purge) at intervals of a few days. For some patients, sigmoidoscopy and reexamination of stools within 3 months may be indicated.

Prognosis

The mortality rate from untreated amebic dysentery or hepatic abscess may be high. With modern chemotherapy instituted early in the course of the disease, the prognosis is very favorable.

Behrens MM: Optic atrophy in children after diiodohydroxyquin therapy. JAMA 228:693, 1974.
Datta DV, Singh SAK, Chhuttani PN: Treatment of amebic liver abscess with emetine hydrochloride, niridazole, and metronidazole: A controlled clinical trial. Am J Trop Med 23:586, 1974.
Grigsby WP: Surgical treatment of amebiasis. Surg Gynec Obst 128:609, 1969.
Kapoor OP, Joshi VR: Multiple amoebic liver abscesses: A study of 56 cases. J Trop Med 75:4, 1972.
Maddison SE & others: Comparison of intradermal and serologic tests for diagnosis of amebiasis. Am J Trop Med 17:540, 1968.
Oakley GP: The neurotoxicity of the halogenated hydroxyquinolines. JAMA 225:395, 1973.
Powell SJ: Drug therapy of amoebiasis. Bull WHO 40:953, 1969.
Stillman AE, Alvarez V, Grube D: Hepatic amebic abscess: Unresponsiveness to combination of metronidazole and surgical drainage. JAMA 229:71, 1974.
Turner JA & others: Amebiasis: A symposium. California Med 114:44, March 1971.
Voogd CE, Van der Stel JJ, Jacobs JJAA: The mutagenic action of nitroimidazoles. 1. Metronidazole, nimorazole, dimetridazole and ronidazole. Mutat Res 26:483, 1974.
WHO Expert Committee: *Amoebiasis.* WHO Technical Report Series No. 421. World Health Organization, 1969.
Wilmot AJ: *Clinical Amoebiasis.* Blackwell, 1962.
Wolfe MS: Nondysenteric intestinal amebiasis: Treatment with diloxanide furoate. JAMA 224:1601, 1973.
Woodruff AW, Bell JS: Amoebiasis: The evaluation of amoebicides. Tr Roy Soc Trop Med Hyg 61:435, 1967.

AMEBIC MENINGOENCEPHALITIS
(Naegleria Infection)

A free-living amebic organism recently identified as *Naegleria gruberi* has been the causative agent of more than 30 cases of acute purulent meningoencephalitis in Australia, the USA, and Czechoslovakia in recent years. Many patients give a history of swimming in pools or freshwater lakes. The disease is usually fatal; no successful chemotherapy has been devised.

Carter RF: Primary amoebic meningo-encephalitis: Clinical pathological, and epidemiological features of six fatal cases. J Path Bact 96:1, 1968.
Sotelo-Avila C, Taylor FM, Ewing CW: Primary amebic meningoencephalitis in a healthy 7-year-old boy. J Pediat 85:131, 1974.

MALARIA

Essentials of Diagnosis

- Paroxysms (often periodic) of chills, fever, and sweating.
- Splenomegaly, anemia, leukopenia.
- Delirium, coma, convulsions, gastrointestinal disorders, and jaundice.
- Characteristic parasites in erythrocytes, identified in thick or thin blood films.

General Considerations

Four species of ameboid protozoan parasites of the genus *Plasmodium* are responsible for human malaria. Although the infection is generally limited to the tropics and subtropics, large numbers of imported cases occur in the USA. In the tropics, malaria generally disappears at altitudes above 6000 feet. The most common parasites, *P vivax* and *P falciparum,* are found throughout the malaria belt. *P malariae* is also broadly distributed but less common. The 4th parasite, *P ovale,* is rare, but in West Africa it seems to replace *P vivax.* Artificial transmission by blood transfusion or the use of contaminated needles by drug abusers is becoming increasingly important, but in nature infection takes place through the bite of an infected female Anopheles mosquito. The mosquito is the host during the sexual phase of the life cycle; man is the host for the asexual developmental stages. After an infective bite, the first stage of development in man takes place in the liver. Parasites escape from the liver into the blood stream 5½−11 days later. Erythrocytes are invaded, the parasites multiply, and 48 hours later (or 72 in the case of *P malariae*) the red cells rupture, releasing a new crop of parasites. This cycle of invasion, multiplication, and red cell rupture may be repeated many times. Symptoms do not appear until several of these erythrocytic cycles have been completed. The incubation period varies considerably, depending upon the species and strain of parasite, the intensity of the infection, and the immune status of the host. For *P vivax* and *P falciparum* it is usually 10−15 days, but it may be much longer (in some cases even months). The *P malariae* incubation period averages about 28 days. For *P falciparum* only, multiplication is confined to the red cells after the first cycle in liver cells (the pre-erythrocytic stage). Thus, any treatment which eliminates falciparum parasites from the blood stream will cure the infection. Without treatment, the infection will terminate spontaneously in less than 2−3 years (usually 6−8 months). The other 3 species continue to multiply in liver cells long after the initial blood stream invasion. This exoerythrocytic cycle of multiplication coexists with the erythrocytic cycle, and may persist after parasites have apparently disappeared from the blood stream. Cure of *P vivax, P ovale,* and *P malariae* infections requires treatment of parasites in both red cells and liver. Vivax and ovale infections may persist without treatment for as long as 5 years; *P malariae* infections which lasted for 40 years have been recorded.

Clinical Findings

A. Symptoms and Signs: The paroxysms of malaria are closely related to events in the blood stream. The chill, lasting from 15 minutes to an hour, begins as a generation of parasites ruptures their host red cells and escapes into the blood. Nausea, vomiting, and headache are common at this time. The succeeding hot stage, lasting several hours, is accompanied by a spiking fever, sometimes reaching 40° C (104° F) or higher. During this stage the parasites presumably invade new red cells. The third or sweating stage concludes the episode. The fever subsides and the patient frequently falls asleep to awake feeling relatively well. In vivax (benign tertian malaria), ovale, and falciparum (malig-

nant tertian malaria) infections, red cells are ruptured and paroxysms occur every 48 hours. In malariae infections (quartan malaria) the cycle takes 72 hours. In the early stages of infection the cycles are frequently asynchronous and the fever patterns irregular. As the disease progresses, splenomegaly and, to a lesser extent, hepatomegaly appear. *P falciparum* infection is more serious than the others because of the high frequency of severe or fatal complications with which it is associated.

B. Laboratory Findings: The thick blood film, stained with Giemsa's stain or other Romanowsky stains, is the mainstay of malaria diagnosis. The thin film is used primarily for species differentiation after the presence of an infection is detected on a thick film. In all but falciparum infections the number of red cells infected seldom exceeds 2% of the total cells. Very high red cell infection rates may occur with falciparum infection (20−30% or more). For this reason anemia is frequently much more severe in falciparum malaria. The anemia is normocytic, with poikilocytosis and anisocytosis. During paroxysms there may be transient leukocytosis; leukopenia develops subsequently, with a relative increase in large mononuclear cells. During attacks hepatic function tests often become abnormal, but the tests revert to normal with treatment or spontaneous recovery. Hemolytic jaundice may develop in severe infections.

There are no specific blood chemical findings. In *P malariae* infections a form of nephrosis, with protein and casts in the urine, sometimes occurs in children. Severe falciparum infections may cause renal damage.

Differential Diagnosis

Uncomplicated malaria, particularly when modified by partial immunity, must be distinguished from a variety of other causes of fever, splenomegaly, anemia, or hepatomegaly. Some diseases often considered in the diagnosis of malaria in the tropics include genitourinary tract infections, typhoid fever, infectious hepatitis, dengue, kala-azar, influenza, amebic liver abscess, leptospirosis, and relapsing fever. Examination of blood films is essential to differentiate atypical malaria from some of the above.

Complications

Serious complications of malaria occur primarily in falciparum infections, particularly in those persons who have experienced repeated attacks with inadequate treatment. These complications, jointly referred to as pernicious malaria, include cerebral malaria with headache, convulsions, delirium, and coma; hyperpyrexia, closely resembling heat hyperpyrexia; gastrointestinal disorders resembling cholera or acute bacillary dysentery; and algid malaria, which in certain respects resembles acute adrenal insufficiency. Blackwater fever must be considered apart from other falciparum complications. This acute intravascular hemolytic condition develops in patients with longstanding falciparum infections and a history of irregular quinine dosage. The principal findings are profound anemia, jaundice, fever, and hemoglobinuria. The mortality rate may be as high as 30%, primarily due to anuria and uremia.

Treatment

A. **Specific Measures:**

1. **Chloroquine**—Chloroquine is used prophylactically to suppress symptoms of malaria but does not prevent infection. Except for *P falciparum* infections, which are terminated, clinical malaria may ensue after the drug is stopped. Chloroquine is also the drug of choice for terminating acute attacks of malaria, but radical cure occurs only in the case of falciparum malaria. If falciparum malaria does not respond promptly to chloroquine, parasite resistance to this drug must be considered. Although capable of causing ocular toxicity when used in large doses for prolonged periods, chloroquine causes few toxic symptoms when used in the doses given below. Mild headache, pruritus, anorexia, blurring of vision, malaise, and urticaria may occur.

a. **Therapeutic dosage schedule**—Give chloroquine phosphate, 1 gm (salt) as initial dose, 0.5 gm in 6 hours, and 0.5 gm daily for the next 2 days. If the patient cannot absorb the drug rapidly because of vomiting or severe diarrhea, or if he is comatose or has a high parasitic count (100,000/cu mm), chloroquine hydrochloride should be administered IM in an adult dose of 250 mg (salt) depending on body weight. Repeat in 6 hours if necessary, and follow with oral therapy as soon as possible (maximum, 1 gm of salt in 24 hours). It is not necessary to administer this drug intravenously except on rare occasions, since an effective blood level is rapidly attained by the intramuscular route.

b. **Suppressive dosage**—Chloroquine phosphate, 0.5 gm weekly, or the combined tablet of chloroquine, 500 mg (salt), plus primaquine phosphate, 78.9 mg (salt), weekly. Continue either regimen for 8 weeks after the patient has left the endemic area.

2. **Amodiaquine dihydrochloride** is a congener of chloroquine.

a. **Therapeutic dosage schedule**—Give 0.2 gm (base) every 6 hours for 3 doses, then 0.2 gm twice daily for 2 days.

b. **Suppressive dosage**—0.4 gm (base) once weekly and for 8 weeks after the patient has left the endemic area.

3. **Pyrimethamine**, although not recommended for the treatment of acute clinical malaria, is an effective agent for suppressive treatment. Suppressive cure is achieved against *P falciparum* infection and sometimes against *P vivax*. Toxicity is very low at the recommended dosage. Give 25 mg weekly on the same day of each week. For children, give 12.5 mg weekly (may be dissolved in syrup).

4. **Proguanil hydrochloride** is effective for chemosuppression of all forms of malaria. Give 0.1 gm daily or, for partially immune subjects, 0.3 gm once weekly.

5. **Quinine**—If none of the more effective and less

toxic newer agents are available, quinine is still a useful drug in arresting the acute attack of all types of malaria. Quinine in the following dosages may cause "cinchonism" (tinnitus, vertigo, deafness, headache, and visual disturbances) in some individuals. The possibility of blackwater fever arising during or at the cessation of therapy appears to be higher in quinine-treated cases.

Therapeutic dosage schedule: Give quinine sulfate, 0.65 gm 3 times daily orally for 7—10 days; or quinine dihydrochloride, 0.65 gm in 300 ml physiologic saline, glucose-saline mixture, or plasma. *Caution:* Inject intravenously by drip (over at least 30 minutes); repeat in 6 hours if necessary; and give no more than 3 injections in 24 hours. Quinine hydrochloride may also be administered by intravenous drip at the rate of 2 gm in 24 hours. Follow with oral therapy as soon as possible.

6. **Primaquine phosphate**—This drug has been shown to be the most effective agent against the tissue forms of *P vivax, P malariae,* and *P ovale.* It is employed to eliminate tissue parasites rather than to treat the clinical attack. It will prevent relapses in most cases. The patient must be observed carefully. Severe hemolytic reactions occur in some individuals whose red blood cells are deficient in G6PD. Therefore, test for G6PD deficiency before initiating therapy and watch for fall of hemoglobin or reduction in red count.

Dosage for the prevention of relapse is 26 mg (15 mg base) daily in single or divided doses for 14 days. For individuals deficient in G6PD, give primaquine phosphate, 79 mg (45 mg base), and chloroquine phosphate, 0.5 gm weekly, for 8 weeks.

Note: Strains of *P falciparum* resistant to chloroquine and often to many of the other antimalarials have been recorded from Southeast Asia and Latin America. Only in patients from Africa, Indonesia, New Guinea, Asia west of Burma, and Central America north of Panama may it be assumed that falciparum infections will be sensitive to chloroquine and other 4-aminoquinolines. In chloroquine-resistant cases, combine pyrimethamine, 25 mg orally twice daily for 3 days, and either sulfadiazine, 500 mg orally 4 times daily for 5 days, or dapsone, 25 mg orally daily for 28 days, with quinine, 650 mg orally 3 times daily for 14 days. Alternatively, quinine sulfate (650 mg 3 times daily for 3 days) plus a tetracycline (500 mg 4 times daily for 7 days) can be used, or sulformethoxine (single dose of 1 gm) plus pyrimethamine (single dose of 50 mg).

B. **General Measures:** The nonspecific treatment of malaria is similar to that of other acute febrile illnesses. In addition, the WHO 1973 Expert Report suggests the following: "Comatose patients should also receive 3—10 mg of dexamethasone sodium phosphate every 8 hours and 1 unit of dextran 75 every 12 hours to reduce cerebral edema and intravascular sludging, respectively; some workers advocate the use of heparin as an antithrombotic agent, but this compound must be given with caution in the presence of deep jaundice. In some patients with severe falciparum malaria, anuria and consequent nitrogen retention may occur. Dialysis is indicated in these cases if the facilities are available; the same considerations apply to mannitol diuresis. Severe anemia is an indication for blood transfusion."

Prognosis

The uncomplicated and untreated primary attack of vivax, ovale, or falciparum malaria usually lasts 2—4 weeks; that of malariae averages about twice as long (4—8 weeks). Each type of infection may subsequently relapse (once or many times) before the infection terminates spontaneously. Poorly treated or untreated falciparum malaria carries a less favorable prognosis than infections due to the other species because of the tendency to serious complications. When such complications as cerebral malaria and blackwater fever develop, the prognosis is often poor even with treatment. With modern antimalarials the prognosis is good for most malaria infections, even with complications.

Chemotherapy of malaria and resistance to antimalarials. Technical Report Series No. 529, World Health Organization, 1973.

Clyde DF: The problem of drug resistant malaria. Am J Trop Med 21:736, 1972.

Drugs for prevention of malaria. (Editorial.) Brit MJ 3:297, 1974.

Hall AP, Arnold JD, Martin DC: A comparison between the quinine and chloroquine regimens for falciparum malaria in Vietnam. Southeast Asian J Trop Med Public Health 5:128, 1974.

Inter-American Malaria Research Symposium. Am J Trop Med 21:613, 1972.

Maegraith B, Fletcher A: The pathogenesis of mammalian malaria. Advances Parasitol 10:49, 1972.

Neva FA & others: Malaria: Host-defense mechanisms and complications. Ann Int Med 73:295, 1970.

Powell RD: Development of new antimalarial drugs. Am J Trop Med 21:744, 1972.

Walzer PD, Gibson JJ, Schultz MG: Malaria fatalities in the United States. Am J Trop Med 23:328, 1974.

SIMIAN MALARIA IN MAN

Recent work has demonstrated that *Plasmodium knowlesi* of Malaysian macaque monkeys can be transmitted to man in nature; thus a 5th species of plasmodium has been added to those known to cause malaria in man. *P brasilianum* of South and Central American monkeys is morphologically similar to *P malariae* and transmissible to man experimentally. *P cynomolgi* of Southeast Asian macaques is also readily transmissible to man in the laboratory. A naturally acquired *P cynomolgi* infection in man could be mistaken for *P vivax*.

Coatney GR: Simian malarias in man: Facts, implications, and predictions. Am J Trop Med 17:147, 1968.

AFRICAN TRYPANOSOMIASIS
(Sleeping Sickness)

Essentials of Diagnosis

- Inconspicuous local inflammatory reaction (trypanosomal chancre).
- Irregular fever, tachycardia, lymphadenitis, splenomegaly, transient rashes.
- Prolonged course (Gambian trypanosomiasis): Personality changes, headache, apathy, somnolence, tremors, speech and gait disturbances, anorexia, malnutrition, coma.
- Rapid course (Rhodesian trypanosomiasis): Findings as above, but lymph nodes less often enlarged.
- Death may occur before signs of CNS involvement appear.
- Trypanosomes in thick blood films or lymph node aspirates (early stages); CSF with trypanosomes, increased cells and protein (late stages).

General Considerations

Rhodesian and Gambian trypanosomiasis are caused by 2 morphologically similar protozoan parasites, *Trypanosoma rhodesiense* and *T gambiense*, found only as the mature trypanosome form in the blood stream, lymph nodes, myocardium, CSF, and brain. The disease occurs focally throughout tropical Africa. Both trypanosomes are transmitted by the bites of tsetse flies (*Glossina sp*).

Clinical Findings

A. Symptoms and Signs: The trypanosomal chancre, a local inflammatory reaction which appears about 48 hours after the tsetse fly bite, is the first sign of infection. Many patients give no history of such a reaction; in others the lesions are painful or pruritic and persist up to 3 weeks. The second stage, invasion of the blood stream and reticuloendothelial system, usually begins several weeks later. Symptoms may appear at once, particularly in rhodesiense infections, or after several years. An irregular fever pattern with persistent tachycardia is characteristic. Transient rashes, often circinate, and scattered areas of firm edema may appear. There may be delayed sensation to pain with deep hyperesthesia. The spleen is usually enlarged. Enlarged, rubbery, and painless lymph nodes, particularly those of the posterior cervical group (Winterbottom's sign) are commonly found in gambiense infection; lymph nodes are not often enlarged in rhodesiense infection. Signs of myocardial involvement appear early in Rhodesian trypanosomiasis. The patient may succumb to myocarditis before signs of CNS invasion appear. Manifestations of the final CNS stage appear within a few weeks or months of onset in rhodesiense infection. Gambian sleeping sickness differs from the acute and virulent Rhodesian form in that it develops more insidiously, starting 6 months to several years from onset. Personality changes, apathy, and headaches are among the early findings. Tremors, disturbances of speech and gait, mania, somnolence, and anorexia appear late. The patient becomes severely emaciated, and finally comatose. Death often results from secondary infection.

B. Laboratory Findings: Lymph node puncture and examination of fresh and stained aspirates is the method of choice for finding *T gambiense* prior to invasion of the CNS. In early rhodesiense infections blood films will usually reveal a few trypanosomes. In advanced cases lumbar puncture is necessary for diagnosis. The CSF, which is clear, colorless, and under normal pressure, shows increased cells (lymphocytes) and elevated protein. Trypanosomes may be demonstrated in the centrifuged CSF specimen. Serologic tests are of little value in diagnosis.

Other laboratory findings include microcytic anemia, increased sedimentation rate, increased serum globulin, and reduced total serum protein.

Differential Diagnosis

Trypanosomiasis may be mistaken for a variety of other diseases, including malaria, kala-azar, cerebral tumors, encephalitis, and cerebral syphilis. Serologic tests for syphilis may be falsely positive in trypanosomiasis. Malaria, suggested by fever and splenomegaly, may be ruled out by blood examinations; kala-azar, considered because of irregular fever, anemia, splenomegaly, and lymphadenitis, can usually be ruled out clinically without resorting to spleen or marrow puncture. Other CNS conditions are differentiated by neurologic examination and lumbar puncture findings.

Prevention

Excretion of pentamidine isethionate and suramin sodium (see below) from the body is slow. Either drug will prevent infection for a considerable time after injection. A single injection of 0.3–0.7 gm of suramin (IM or IV) will give protection for 6–12 weeks. One IM injection of pentamidine (3 mg/kg) will protect against rhodesiense infection for 2 months and against gambiense infection for 3–6 months.

Treatment

A. Specific Measures: (The following drugs are available only from the Parasitic Disease Drug Service, Center for Disease Control, Atlanta 30333.)

1. Suramin sodium is the drug of choice in the early stages of trypanosomiasis before the CNS is invaded. This organic urea compound is administered intravenously in freshly prepared 10% solution in distilled water. Start treatment with a test dose of 100 mg. For adults, continue with 1 gm doses at 5–7 day intervals to a total of 10 gm. Because of occasional renal toxicity, frequent urinalyses are essential during therapy. Dermatitis and gastrointestinal disturbances are also reported. The drug is contraindicated in renal disease.

2. Pentamidine isethionate is a somewhat less effective alternative to suramin in treating early trypanosomiasis. It is administered as a 2% solution intra-

muscularly. The drug may induce a sudden fall in blood pressure or hypoglycemia if given intravenously. It is contraindicated in renal disease. Administer in doses of 4 mg/kg daily or every other day for 10–15 injections.

3. Tryparsamide, a pentavalent arsenical, has long been used in the treatment of gambiense infections of the CNS. It is much less effective against rhodesiense meningoencephalitis. The drug may cause dermatitis or optic atrophy. Discontinue treatment if eye pain, excessive lacrimation, or photophobia develops. Administer intravenously in a 20% solution in water. The dosage is 20–40 mg/kg, given at weekly intervals to a total course of 10–12 injections. The usual initial dose for adults is 1–1.5 gm; subsequent doses, 2–3 gm. Repeat the course if necessary after a rest period of at least 1 month. A course of suramin or pentamidine should be given simultaneously to remove any parasites remaining in the blood or lymph nodes.

4. Melarsoprol (Mel B; melarsen oxide/BAL) is effective for gambiense and rhodesiense infections of the CNS, but undesirable drug effects are not uncommon. A second course may be given for a relapse, but resistance develops rapidly. Melarsoprol must be given intravenously in 5% solution in propylene glycol. A recently introduced derivative, Mel W, is water-soluble and may be given intramuscularly or subcutaneously. It is necessary to use either suramin sodium or pentamidine isethionate in conjunction with melarsoprol to remove trypanosomes from the blood and lymph nodes. A recommended schedule is 3.6 mg/kg daily for 4 consecutive days, a rest of 7 days, and then a second series of 4 daily doses.

B. General Measures: Good nursing care, treatment of anemia and concurrent infections, and correction of malnutrition are essentials in the management of patients with advanced African trypanosomiasis.

Prognosis

Without treatment, 25–50% of gambiense infections and over 50% of rhodesiense infections are fatal. With treatment, 5–15% of gambiense infections and up to 50% of rhodesiense infections are fatal. Prognosis is considerably more favorable if treatment is started before invasion of the CNS occurs.

Duggan AJ: An approach to clinical problems of Gambian sleeping sickness. J Trop Med 62:268, 1959.

Lumsden WHR: Trypanosomiasis. Brit M Bull 28:34, 1972.

Robertson DHH: The treatment of sleeping sickness (mainly due to *Trypanosoma rhodesiense*) with melarsoprol. Tr Roy Soc Trop Med Hyg 57:176, 1963.

AMERICAN TRYPANOSOMIASIS
(Chagas' Disease)

Essentials of Diagnosis

- Unilateral palpebral and facial edema and conjunctivitis (Romaña's sign).

- Hard, edematous, red, and painful cutaneous nodule (chagoma).
- Intermittent fever, lymphadenitis, hepatomegaly, signs and symptoms of acute or chronic myocarditis or meningoencephalitis.
- Demonstration of trypanosomes in blood smears or by culture, animal inoculation, or complement fixation test.

General Considerations

Chagas' disease is caused by *Trypanosoma cruzi,* a protozoan parasite of the blood and tissues of man and many other vertebrates. *T cruzi* is found in wild animals from southern South America to northern Mexico, Texas, and the southwestern USA. Human infection is less widespread. Many species of reduviid bugs (cone-nosed or kissing bugs) transmit the infection, which results from rubbing infected bug feces, passed during feeding, into the bite wound. In the vertebrate host the trypanosomes first multiply close to the point of entry, assuming a leishmanial form at one stage of their development. They then enter the blood stream and later the heart, brain, and other tissues. Further multiplication causes cellular destruction, inflammation, and fibrosis. In these tissues the parasites again assume a leishmanial form during part of each developmental cycle.

Clinical Findings

A. Symptoms and Signs: The earliest finding in the acute infection is either the chagoma or Romaña's sign. In heavily endemic areas initial infection commonly occurs in childhood. The acute form of the disease may be fatal, particularly in infants and young children. In addition to intermittent fever, local lymphadenitis, and hepatomegaly, there may be splenomegaly, psychologic changes, focal neurologic symptoms, convulsions, tachycardia, cardiac enlargement, arrhythmias, and cardiac failure. Myocardial damage dominates the chronic form of the disease; cases are seen with all types and stages of cardiac disorder. Symptomatic chronic CNS infection is rare; also uncommon are megacolon and megaesophagus, caused by damage to nerve plexuses in the bowel or esophageal wall.

B. Laboratory Findings: Trypanosomes are not usually found in large numbers in the blood except in the early stages of the acute infection. *T rangeli,* a nonpathogenic blood trypanosome also found in man in Central America and northern South America, must not be mistaken for *T cruzi.* In the acute stage trypanosomes may also be found in lymph node aspirates. Blood, or material from lymph nodes, marrow, or spleen, may be cultured on NNN medium or inoculated into laboratory mice or rats. In chronic infections xenodiagnosis, which consists of permitting uninfected reduviids to feed on the patient and then examining them for trypanosomal infection, often establishes the diagnosis. The Machado complement fixation test is of presumptive diagnostic value when positive; it should be used in conjunction with other diagnostic methods.

Differential Diagnosis

The early acute infection, with Romaña's sign, might be confused with trichinosis, but palpebral and facial edema is unilateral, not bilateral, and there is no eosinophilia. The chagoma may be mistaken for any of a variety of tropical skin lesions. Kala-azar resembles Chagas' disease in some respects (intermittent fever, hepatomegaly, splenomegaly), but in the former the spleen is much larger, there are no CNS symptoms, and cardiac symptoms usually appear only after anemia becomes severe. Chronic infection in adults, usually myocardial, is not clinically characteristic. Differentiation from other causes of chronic cardiac disease depends upon positive animal inoculation tests, complement fixation tests, or other laboratory procedures.

Treatment

No drug treatment is established as safe and effective. Bayer 2502 (Lampit) continues under clinical investigation. It is available in the USA only from the Parasitic Disease Drug Service, Center for Disease Control, Atlanta 30333. Primaquine phosphate may also be tried at a dosage of 26.3 mg (salt) for 7–10 days.

Prognosis

Acute infections in infants and young children are often fatal, particularly when the CNS is involved. Adults with chronic cardiac infections also may ultimately succumb to the disease. Mortality rates are not known because infections are often asymptomatic and unrecognized. Other infections, particularly malaria, may seriously complicate the disease.

LEISHMANIASIS

The several types of leishmaniasis are due to species of protozoa related to the trypanosomes and transmitted by sandflies *(Phlebotomus sp),* in which they undergo cyclic development, from animal reservoirs (dogs and rodents). Visceral leishmaniasis (kala-azar) is due to *Leishmania donovani;* cutaneous leishmaniasis of the Old World (Oriental sore) is due to *L tropica.* In the New World, cutaneous leishmaniasis is caused by the *L mexicana* complex of agents, and both cutaneous and mucocutaneous lesions are caused by the *L braziliensis* complex of agents.

Bray RS: Leishmania. Ann Rev Microbiol 28:189, 1974.
Bray RS: Leishmaniasis in the Old World. Brit M Bull 28:39, 1972.
Lainson R, Shaw JJ: Leishmaniasis of the New World: Taxonomic problems. Brit M Bull 28:44, 1972.
Symposium on leishmaniasis. Bull WHO 44:477, 1971.

1. VISCERAL LEISHMANIASIS
(Kala-Azar)

Essentials of Diagnosis

- Irregular fever, insidious and chronic; onset may be acute.
- Progressive and marked splenomegaly and hepatomegaly.
- Progressive anemia, leukopenia, and wasting.
- Progressive darkening of skin, especially on forehead and hands.
- Leishman-Donovan bodies demonstrable in splenic and sternal puncture smears.
- Elevated total proteins due to the IgG fraction of gamma globulins.

General Considerations

Kala-azar is widespread geographically wherever sandfly vectors are found. In each locale the disease has its own peculiar clinical and epidemiologic features. It occurs in the Mediterranean littoral, equatorial Africa, Ethiopia, eastern India, central Asia and China, and South America. Although man is the major reservoir, animal reservoirs such as the dog are important. The incubation period varies from weeks to months. The parasites exist in one form in the body, as oval Leishman-Donovan bodies which parasitize reticuloendothelial cells and lead to their proliferation.

Clinical Findings

A. Symptoms and Signs: The fever is generally mild and is not usually associated with prostration. The characteristic double daily remission may escape detection. The spleen usually enlarges much more than the liver and may be palpable by the second month. Enlargement is painless, steady, and rapid, usually in waves with bouts of fever. At first doughy, the spleen finally becomes large and hard. Wasting occurs without anorexia. Lymphadenopathy may be present.

Post-kala-azar dermal leishmaniasis may appear 1–2 years after apparent cure, especially in India but also in the Sudan and China. This may simulate leprosy as multiple hypopigmented macules or nodules which develop on preexisting lesions. There may even be a degree of leontiasis. They take the form of erythematous patches, often on the face.

B. Laboratory Findings: There is usually progressive gross leukopenia (seldom over 3000/cu mm after the first 1–2 months), with relative or (usually) absolute monocytosis. Nevertheless, an occasional leukocytosis, due to concurrent sepsis, may be confusing. Diagnosis must always be confirmed by demonstrating Leishman-Donovan bodies in blood, sternal marrow, liver, or spleen by stained smears or culture in NNN medium or hamsters. Serologic tests are useful, for they seldom give false-negative results. Some cross-reactions do occur. Diagnosis is supported by an increase in total proteins to and over 10 gm/100 ml, due almost entirely to the IgG fraction of gamma globulin.

Differential Diagnosis

Kala-azar which is of subacute or acute onset resembles enteric fever (but there is no toxemia and Widal's test is negative) or malaria (in which case response to antimalarial therapy may aid the diagnosis, since concomitant malaria parasites may be present in the blood in kala-azar). Many patients present with abdominal enlargement, weakness, and wasting; these patients have irregular fevers and the spleen and liver are palpable, which differentiates this disease from brucellosis. Characteristic double (rarely triple) daily remissions (evening and morning) occur early.

Chronic cases may also be confused with infectious mononucleosis, leukemia, anemias due to other causes, and tuberculosis. Post-kala-azar dermatitis may resemble leprosy.

Treatment

Specific treatment is primarily with pentavalent antimonials, to which cases from India respond best whereas those from the Sudan are most resistant. Children tolerate antimonials well. In all cases resistance to antimonials can develop with inadequate dosage. In addition to antimonials, aromatic diamidines (see below) are powerful agents. They should be preceded by injection of an antihistaminic to minimize reactions. They are less effective for post-kala-azar dermal lesions. Fresh solutions only should be given and ampules stored away from heat. Intravenous injection must be given slowly.

(1) Antimony sodium gluconate, 0.2 gm followed by 0.6 gm daily as 5% solution IM or IV for patients weighing over 30 kg. Continue treatment for 6–10 days. Available in the USA only from the Parasitic Disease Drug Service, Center for Disease Control, Atlanta 30333.

(2) Pentamidine isethionate, 2–4 mg/kg IV or (preferably) IM, daily or on alternate days, up to 15 injections. Available in the USA only from the Parasitic Disease Drug Service, Center for Disease Control, Atlanta 30333.

(3) Stilbamidine isethionate is used only in antimony-resistant cases and must be given with great care because it is unstable and may produce immediate reactions or delayed trigeminal hyperesthesia. The initial adult dose is 25 mg IV daily, increasing by 10–20 mg daily to 2 mg/kg daily. The most that should be given is about 10 injections or a total of about 15 mg/kg.

(4) Ethylstibamine, 0.2 gm initially IV, then 0.3 gm IV daily or every 2 days for 16 doses.

(5) Urea stibamine (carbostibamide), IV in 10 ml water daily, in doses of 0.05, 0.1, 0.15, and subsequently 0.2 gm for about 15 days.

Prognosis

Therapy is effective, but there may be relapses, requiring one or more additional courses of therapy. Keep the patient under observation for at least 6 months. The spleen, blood studies, and body weight should return to normal.

See references above.

Manson-Bahr, PEC: Kala azar. Trop Doctor 3:99, 1973.

Winslow DJ: Visceral leishmaniasis. Page 86 in: *Pathology of Protozoal and Helminthic Diseases.* Marcial-Rojas RA (editor). Williams & Wilkins, 1971.

2. CUTANEOUS LEISHMANIASIS OF THE OLD WORLD
(Oriental Sore)

Oriental sore is widespread throughout the Mediterranean basin, the Near and Middle East, and parts of India. Cutaneous swellings appear about 2–8 weeks after bites of sandflies infected with *Leishmania tropica.* The swellings may ulcerate and discharge pus, or they may remain dry. Dry and moist forms are caused by locally distinct leishmanias.

Lesions tend to heal spontaneously over a period of months to 2 years, but secondary infection may lead to gross extension. Moist ulcerated lesions are covered with a scab and exude purulent material as a result of secondary infection.

Leishmanias cannot be detected in purulent discharge but may be seen in stained scrapings from the cleaned edge of the ulcer. These smears must contain tissue juice.

Single lesions may be cleaned, covered, and left to heal spontaneously. Carbon dioxide snow, infrared therapy, or radiotherapy is often effective. Antibiotics may be required for secondary infections. Antimony sodium gluconate or ethylstibamine as for visceral leishmaniasis may be effective when used for indolent ulcers.

See references above.

Ardehali M: Treatment of cutaneous leishmaniasis with cycloguanil pamoate. Internat J Dermat 13:26, 1974.

Farah FS, Malak JA: Cutaneous leishmaniasis. Arch Dermat 103:467, 1971.

3. AMERICAN CUTANEOUS & MUCOCUTANEOUS (NASO-ORAL) LEISHMANIASIS

Leishmania mexicana is responsible for cutaneous leishmaniasis in Mexico, Central America, and some areas of Brazil. *Leishmania braziliensis* causes lesions ranging from cutaneous ulcers (uta) in Peru to destructive skin ulcers followed by severe naso-oral metastasis (espundia) in many countries of South America.

Espundia is characterized by cutaneous and naso-oral involvement, either by direct extension or, more often, metastatically. The initial lesions on exposed skin, often the ears, take more varied forms than is usual with Oriental sore. Naso-oral involvement may follow healing of initial lesions, even after a considerable interval, or may develop simultaneously. The anterior part of the cartilaginous septum is commonly involved, and there may be gross and hideous erosion, including bone. Regional lymphadenitis is common. Leishman-Donovan bodies may be found in aspirated tissue juice, but the organism grows with difficulty in NNN medium or hamsters. If an injection of a suspension of killed leptomonads produces a fully developed papule in 2–3 days which disappears after a week (positive Montenegro test), the diagnosis is fairly certain. A negative Montenegro test is meaningless.

Specific treatment for *L braziliensis* infections may be combined, if necessary, with local or systemic antibiotics or sulfonamides. Give antimony sodium gluconate, 600 mg IM or IV daily for 6–10 days. If the former drug fails, use amphotericin B, 0.25–1 mg/kg, by slow infusion daily or every 2 days for up to 8 weeks. Single doses containing 350 mg base of cycloguanil pamoate IM are not producing uniformly good results. Ethylstibamine may be given as for visceral leishmaniasis.

The milder forms of solitary nodules and ulcers due to *L mexicana* seldom require treatment. Cycloguanil pamoate, 5 mg/kg as a single repository injection, may be tried to speed healing.

See references above.

Kern F, Pedersen JK: Leishmaniasis in the United States: A report of ten cases in military personnel. JAMA 226:872, 1973.

GIARDIASIS
(Lambliasis)

Giardia lamblia is a cosmopolitan intestinal flagellate protozoon which normally lives in the duodenum or jejunum and is usually of low pathogenicity or nonpathogenic for man. Cysts may be found in large numbers in the stools of asymptomatic persons. In some people, especially children, giardia infections cause irritation of the upper small bowel with resultant acute or chronic diarrhea (often alternating with constipation), mild abdominal cramps, flatulence, abdominal distention, and tenderness. Mucosal invasion may occur, as well as malabsorption and weight loss. The bile ducts and gallbladder may be invaded, perhaps causing a mild cholecystitis. Giardiasis should be sought in troublesome symptoms of dyspepsias, peptic ulcers, or pylorospasm. The distinctive cysts may be found in formed stools, and cysts and trophozoites may be found in liquid stools. However, finding organisms in the stools may be difficult. Sequentially proceed to examination of stools collected after the patient takes a laxative, then to examination of duodenal aspirate, and lastly to duodenal biopsy.

Treatment with quinacrine hydrochloride, 0.1 gm orally 3 times daily for 5–7 days, will result in a 90%

cure rate. Metronidazole is equally effective at a dosage of 0.25 gm 3 times daily for 10 days, but note recently described hazards of this drug as discussed under amebiasis. Either drug may be repeated if necessary. A third alternative is furazolidone, 100 mg 4 times daily for 7 days.

Ament ME: Diagnosis and treatment of giardiasis. J Pediat 80:633, 1972.

Babb RR, Peck OC, Vescia FG: Giardiasis. JAMA 217:1359, 1971.

Bassily S & others: The treatment of *Giardia lamblia* infection with mepacrine, metronidazole and furazolidone. J Trop Med 73:15, 1970.

BALANTIDIASIS

Balantidium coli is a large ciliated intestinal protozoon found throughout the world, particularly in the tropics. Infection results from ingestion of viable cysts from formed stools of humans or swine, the reservoir hosts. In the new host the cyst wall dissolves and the trophozoite may invade the mucosa and submucosa of the large bowel and terminal ileum, causing abscesses and irregularly rounded ulcerations. Many cases are asymptomatic. Chronic recurrent diarrhea, alternating with constipation, is the most common clinical manifestation, but attacks of severe dysentery with bloody mucoid stools, tenesmus, and colic may occur intermittently. Diagnosis is made by finding trophozoites in liquid stools and cysts in formed stools. The treatment of choice is one of the tetracyclines, 2 gm daily in 4 divided doses for 10 days. Carbarsone, diiodohydroxyquin, and iodochlorhydroxyquin have each been effective in a few patients. Asymptomatic infections may terminate spontaneously. In properly treated mild to moderate symptomatic cases, the prognosis is good, but fatalities have occurred in severe infections despite treatment.

Arean VM: Balantidiasis: A review and report of cases. Am J Path 32:1089, 1956.

TOXOPLASMOSIS

The protozoan parasite *Toxoplasma gondii* is found throughout the world in man and in many species of animals and birds. *T gondii* has recently been shown to be a coccidian that exists in 3 infectious forms: The tachyzoite (or endozoite), the proliferative form, is present in large numbers in blood, excreta, and secretions in acute disseminated infections. The cystozoite (or bradyzoite), the resting form, is present within encapsulated cysts, particularly in muscle and nerve tissue, in chronic infections. The oocyst is the form passed only in the feces of cats following their infection by the coccidian intestinal epithelial stages characteristic only of feline toxoplasmosis. The coccidian stages in cats appear to be crucial to the maintenance of the parasite in nature. However, the relative importance of several sources of infection for man remains to be determined, including, particularly, accidental ingestion of oocysts derived from cat feces or the ingestion of encapsulated cysts in raw or undercooked meat.

The clinical patterns of toxoplasmosis can be divided into 4 patterns: acquired toxoplasmosis, congenital infection, retinochoroiditis, and disease in the altered host. In the latter, toxoplasmosis may present as a disseminated disease in patients treated with immunosuppressive drugs or in patients with neoplasms of the lymphatic system. Patients with acquired toxoplasmosis are often asymptomatic but may present with fever, malaise, lymphadenopathy, splenomegaly, and a maculopapular rash. Rarely, severe cases include myocarditis and retinochoroiditis. Congenital transmission occurs only during acute infection, which has been detected in up to 1% of women during pregnancy. Approximately 20–40% of such adult infections are transmitted to the fetus, resulting in some abortions and stillbirths. Signs of congenital toxoplasmosis are present at birth or progress during the first months of life: microcephaly, seizures, mental retardation, hepatosplenomegaly, pneumonitis, rash, fever, retinochoroiditis, and cerebral calcification. The retinochoroiditis form of toxoplasmosis is usually a late manifestation of asymptomatic congenital infection, with symptoms being first noted in the second or third decade of life. The congenital disease is often fatal, and if the infant survives the acute infection, he is likely to be handicapped by serious residual CNS and ocular lesions. The acquired disease is usually asymptomatic or mild, but acute infection in adults may be fatal.

Diagnosis is based on the presence of changing or elevated titers of toxoplasmosis antibodies (which are very specific) and on the isolation of the parasite from infected tissues. Toxoplasma organisms may be directly identified in smears of blood, bone marrow, CSF, or exudates. Inoculation into laboratory animals or serologic tests, including the Sabin-Feldman dye test, the indirect fluorescent antibody test, complement fixation test, and neutralization test are often necessary for diagnosis. In congenital infections, tests should be conducted for IgG and IgM toxoplasmosis antibodies.

Symptomatic acute infections are treated with pyrimethamine, 25 mg daily for 1 month, trisulfapyrimidines, 2–6 gm daily for 1 month, and folinic acid, 6 mg daily for 1 month. Recently, sulfalene and trimethoprim have been found effective. Platelet and white blood cell counts should be carried out twice weekly. Congenital toxoplamosis should be treated whether symptomatic or asymptomatic.

Pregnant women should have their serum examined for toxoplasmosis antibody. Those with negative titers should take precautionary measures to prevent infection—preferably having no further contact with cats and eating no raw meats and no vegetables that are not thoroughly cooked.

Desmonts G, Couvreur J: Congenital toxoplasmosis: A prospective study of 378 pregnancies. New England J Med 290:1110, 1974.

Feldman HA: Toxoplasmosis: An overview. Bull New York Acad Med 50:110, 1974.

Frenkel JK: Pathology and pathogenesis of congenital toxoplasmosis. Bull New York Acad Med 50:182, 1974.

Jacobs L: New knowledge of toxoplasma and toxoplasmosis. Advances Parasitol 11:631, 1973.

O'Connor GR: Manifestations and management of ocular toxoplasmosis. Bull New York Acad Med 50:192, 1974.

Remington JS: Toxoplasmosis in the adult. Bull New York Acad Med 50:211, 1974.

COCCIDIOSIS
(Isosporosis)

Two cosmopolitan intestinal species of coccidia, *Isospora belli* and *I hominis,* are found in man. The infection is usually sporadic, and is most common in the tropics and subtropics, although it has been reported in the USA. Infections result from the ingestion of viable cysts, and it is probable that the protozoa multiply in the intestinal mucosa. Many cases may be asymptomatic. About 1 week after ingestion of viable cysts, mild fever, lassitude, and malaise may appear, followed by mild diarrhea and vague abdominal discomfort. The infection is usually self-limited and symptoms subside within 1–2 weeks, but persistent diarrhea and several deaths have been associated with the infection. Stool concentration technics are usually necessary to find the immature oocysts of *I belli* or the mature sporocysts of *I hominis.* The only treatment necessary is bed rest and a bland diet for a few days.

Brandborg LL & others: Human coccidiosis—a possible cause of malabsorption: The life cycle in small-bowel mucosal biopsies as a diagnostic feature. New England J Med 283:1306, 1970.

Jarpa GA: Coccidiosis humana. Biologica (Santiago) 39:3, 1966.

PNEUMOCYSTIS PNEUMONIA

Pneumocystis pneumonia, an acute interstitial pneumonia characterized by fever, tachypnea, dyspnea, and cyanosis, is a rare disease in the general population but is not uncommon in premature or malnourished infants or the compromised host. Particularly liable to infection are children with primary immune deficiency disorders or adults or children receiving cytotoxic or immunosuppressive drugs. The causative organism is of uncertain classification but is probably a protozoon. The duration of illness is 1–4 weeks, and the fatality rate is high (up to 50%).

Physical signs are slight; there are no diagnostic laboratory tests. Chest x-rays show interstitial pneumonia. The blood gases will usually show hyperventilation with decreased oxygen saturation while the patient is on continuous oxygen, which is consistent with alveolar capillary block syndrome.

Since methods for culturing the organism are not available, diagnosis depends upon identifying the agent in clinical specimens with special stains. The various technics used to obtain histologic materials are relatively unsatisfactory because of poor yields or operative risks. The methods include sputum, tracheal or gastric aspirates, lung biopsy (open, closed, or transbronchoscopic), transthoracic lung aspiration, endobronchial brush biopsy, and bronchopulmonary lavage. The usefulness of serologic studies remains to be determined.

Treatment with pentamidine isethionate (4 mg/kg IM daily for 12–14 days) is effective if started early, but the drug causes side-effects in nearly 50% of patients, including severe renal reactions in some. In the USA the drug is available only from the Parasitic Disease Drug Service, Center for Disease Control, Atlanta 30333. Treatment with pyrimethamine and sulfadiazine may also be tried.

Burke BA, Good RA: *Pneumocystis carinii* infection. Medicine 52:23, 1973.

Drew WL & others: Diagnosis of *Pneumocystis carinii* pneumonia by bronchopulmonary lavage. JAMA 230:713, 1974.

Walzer PD & others: *Pneumocystis carinii* pneumonia in the United States: Epidemiologic, diagnostic, and clinical features. Ann Int Med 80:83, 1974.

26...
Infectious Diseases: Metazoal

Robert S. Goldsmith

TREMATODE (FLUKE) INFECTIONS

SCHISTOSOMIASIS
(Bilharziasis)

Essentials of Diagnosis

- Transient erythematous, pruritic skin rash.
- Fever, malaise, urticaria, eosinophilia, and hepatosplenomegaly.
- Either (1) diarrhea, dysentery, abdominal pain, anorexia, weight loss, splenomegaly, and ascites; or (2) terminal hematuria, urinary frequency, urethral and bladder pain.

General Considerations

Three blood flukes or trematodes are responsible for this worldwide complex of diseases. *Schistosoma mansoni,* the cause of intestinal schistosomiasis, is widespread in Egypt and is common locally in tropical Africa, eastern South America, and the Caribbean (including Puerto Rico but not Cuba). Vesical or urinary schistosomiasis, caused by *S haematobium,* is common in Egypt and in Africa and parts of the Middle East. Asiatic intestinal schistosomiasis, due to *S japonicum* infection, is important in China, Japan, and the Philippines. Various species of snails, the intermediate hosts, are infected by larvae hatched from eggs reaching fresh water in feces or urine. After development, infective larvae (cercariae) leave the snails and penetrate human skin or mucous membranes which come in contact with water. Immature *S mansoni* migrate to branches of the inferior mesenteric veins in the large bowel wall. Here the adults mature, mate, and deposit eggs. Many eggs reach the bowel lumen and are passed in the feces; others lodge in the bowel wall and induce inflammation, fibrosis, ulceration, and granuloma, papilloma, or polyp formation. Eggs may be carried to the liver, where similar changes occur, provoking periportal cirrhosis. Portal hypertension results in splenomegaly and ascites. Eggs may lodge ectopically in the lungs, spinal cord, or other tissues.

S japonicum adults lie in branches of the superior and inferior mesenteric veins in the small and large bowel walls. Eggs are passed in the stool or lodge in the bowel wall, provoking changes similar to those noted above. Because greater numbers of eggs are produced by *S japonicum,* the resulting disease is more extensive and severe. Eggs are frequently carried to the liver (and occasionally to the CNS), and cirrhosis and portal hypertension are common.

The adult *S haematobium* matures in the venous plexuses of the bladder, prostate, and uterus. Eggs are passed in the urine or retained in the tissues, particularly the bladder wall and the female genital organs. In addition to fibrosis, ulceration, and granuloma and papilloma formation, there is often bladder wall calcification, chronic cystitis, pyelitis, or pyelonephritis. Bladder cancer is common in advanced cases in Egypt.

Clinical Findings

A. Symptoms and Signs: The first sign of infection, an itchy, erythematous or petechial rash at sites of penetration of cercariae, lasts about 2–5 days. A second clinical stage occurs 4–5 weeks later as the immature flukes migrate through the blood vessels of various organs. Symptoms at this time are primarily allergic and vary greatly in severity. In addition to fever, urticaria, malaise, and respiratory symptoms, the liver and spleen may be temporarily enlarged. The patient again becomes asymptomatic in 2–8 weeks. The final clinical stage begins 6 months to several years after infection as lesions develop around eggs embedded in the tissues. The course and severity of the disease depend upon the number of adult worms present, the number of eggs produced, and the sites of the lesions they provoke. Diarrhea, dysentery, and abdominal pain are common in the early stages of intestinal infections. Anorexia, weight loss, polypoid intestinal tumors, and signs of portal hypertension and hepatic insufficiency appear as the disease progresses. Death commonly results from intercurrent infection. The symptoms of urinary tract disease (particularly terminal hematuria, frequency, and pain) depend upon the extent of the pathologic changes described above. Ureteral and renal damage may result in fatal uremia, or the patient may die of bladder carcinoma many years after first being infected. Advanced schistosomiasis usually develops only after repeated reinfections.

B. Laboratory Findings: Eosinophilia is common

during the migrations of the immature flukes, but the count usually returns to normal later. Diagnosis depends upon detection of eggs in urine or feces, on biopsy technics, or on serologic and skin tests. Eggs are found in urine by examining the sediment of specimens collected between 9:00 a.m. and 2:00 p.m. or 24-hour urine collections. Eosinophils in the urine should not be mistaken for pus cells. Eggs may be found in stool specimens by direct examination, but some form of concentration is usually necessary and repeated examinations are often needed to find eggs in light infections. *S mansoni* and *S japonicum* infections are often diagnosed by rectal biopsy; biopsy through a cystoscope may confirm the diagnosis of urinary schistosomiasis. Serologic tests become positive a few weeks after infection occurs. The intradermal test produces more false positives as well as false negatives but is often useful as a screening procedure.

Differential Diagnosis

Schistosomiasis mansoni should be considered in all unresponsive gastrointestinal disorders in persons who have been in endemic areas. Early intestinal schistosomiasis may be mistaken for amebiasis, bacillary dysentery, or other causes of diarrhea and dysentery. Later the various causes of portal hypertension or of bowel papillomas and polyps must be considered. Vesical schistosomiasis must be differentiated from other causes of hematuria, prostatic disease, genitourinary tract malignancies, and bacterial infections of the urinary tract.

Complications

Among the many complications of these diseases are transverse myelitis (*S mansoni* eggs in the spinal cord), seizures, optic neuritis, paralysis, mental disorders (*S japonicum* eggs in the brain), liver failure (*S mansoni, S japonicum*), ruptured esophageal varices due to portal hypertension, uremia and bladder neoplasms (*S haematobium*), and chronic pulmonary disease (periarteritis and endarteritis, primarily due to *S mansoni* eggs).

Treatment

A. **General Measures:** For patients with longstanding schistosomiasis and nonreversible lesions, supportive measures, improvements in diet, and corrective surgical procedures are usually more important than specific chemotherapy. Such therapy may even be dangerous in cases with hepatic insufficiency. At best, drugs prevent further progression and the development of complications. Surgical measures include removal of papillomas, polyps, and early carcinoma; splenectomy, portal shunt operations, craniotomy, and other neurosurgical procedures.

B. **Specific Measures:** In less advanced disease drug therapy often causes clinical and parasitologic cure, ie, relief of symptoms and shrinking or elimination of bladder and bowel ulcerations and granulomas. Periodic laboratory follow-up is essential, starting at 3 months and continuing for a year. If ova are not ex-

creted, post-treatment mucosal biopsy should be done. The success of treatment depends upon the demonstration (by various methods) that ova seen are no longer viable or that the number of live ova passed are relatively few in number.

1. **Niridazole,** a nitrothiazole derivative, is an effective oral drug and the drug of first choice for *S mansoni* and *S haematobium* infections and should be tried against *S japonicum.* High cure rates have been achieved on oral doses of 25 mg/kg (maximum, 1.5 gm) daily in 2 divided doses for 7 days. Drug side-effects include occasional nausea, vomiting, anorexia, headache, T wave depression, and possible temporary suppression of spermatogenesis. Deep brown coloration of the urine disappears after treatment. Effects due to destruction of worms and release of foreign proteins may appear after 3–4 days of therapy: tiredness, CNS excitability (rare), and convulsions (very rare). The drug should not be given to patients with advanced schistosomal liver disease and should not be given with isoniazid. Patients should be checked for G6PD deficiency. Available in the USA only from the Parasitic Disease Drug Service, Center for Disease Control, Atlanta 30333.

2. **Sodium antimony dimercaptosuccinate** is an intramuscular preparation with approximately the same side-effects and the same degree of effectiveness as stibophen for *S mansoni* and *S haematobium* infections. Its advantage is the shorter course required. The total dose is 40 mg/kg body weight to be divided into 5 equal injections and given over a period of 2½–5 weeks. If the drug is given at shorter intervals, side-effects are more severe. Available in the USA only from the Parasitic Disease Drug Service, Center for Disease Control, Atlanta 30333.

3. **Stibophen** is less toxic than antimony potassium tartrate and is an alternative drug for *S mansoni* and *S haematobium* infections. Side-effects include gastrointestinal symptoms, headache, weakness, skin rashes, and arthralgia. Adverse reactions are infrequent but are an indication for stopping treatment: progressive proteinuria, fever, precordial pain, hematuria, thrombocytopenia, or hemolytic anemia. Renal, cardiac, and nonschistosomal hepatic disease contraindicate its use. It is supplied in 5 ml ampules of a 6.3% solution. Give 1.5 ml IM as a test dose, then 4 ml IM every weekday (5 days/week) to a total of 40 ml. After 1–2 weeks, the course should be repeated. Stibophen is occasionally effective in *S japonicum* infections in a dosage of 8–10 ml daily for 10 days.

4. **Antimony potassium (or sodium) tartrate (tartar emetic)** is inexpensive and effective but is the most toxic of the antimonial drugs. It is used mainly for *S japonicum* infections. Less toxic drugs are used for the other schistosome species. The patient must be hospitalized and be at bed rest during treatment. The drug is administered intravenously very slowly through a fine needle over a 10-minute period. The initial dose is 8 ml of a freshly prepared 0.5% solution. Subsequent doses of 12, 16, 20, 24, and 28 ml are given on alternate days. Thereafter, continue 28 ml on alternate days

until a total of 360 ml (1.8 gm) has been given. If a second course is required, a few months should elapse before resuming treatment.

Common side-effects include nausea, vomiting, diarrhea, abdominal pain, syncope, tachycardia, dyspnea, paroxysmal coughing, and erythematous rashes. More severe toxic effects include exfoliative dermatitis, toxic liver necrosis, and toxic myocarditis. Cardiac, pulmonary, renal, hepatic, CNS, and febrile diseases are contraindications.

5. Hycanthone, the hydroxymethyl derivative of lucanthone, continues to undergo clinical evaluation for the treatment of schistosomiasis. Its important contribution is its usually high degree of effectiveness in a single IM injection (deep into the gluteus minimus) in a dosage of 3 mg of base per kg (maximum adult dose 200 mg of base). Early confidence in the safety of hycanthone has been shaken by fatalities that have occurred due to acute liver failure and reports of the drug's potential carcinogenic, mutagenic, and teratogenic effects. The drug is not available in the USA.

6. Lucanthone hydrochloride is administered orally and is suitable for treatment only for children under 16. The use of this drug is generally declining. Numerous side-effects include anorexia, nausea, vomiting, dizziness, vertigo, tremors, insomnia, and muscular weakness. The dosage is 15 mg/kg body weight/day divided into 3 doses and given for 7 days. The drug is often curative in *S haematobium* and *S mansoni* infections but is of little value against *S japonicum.*

7. Surgical filtering of *S mansoni* adults from the portal system should be considered whenever splenectomy is contemplated. A single dose of tartar emetic allows most worms to be washed back into the portal venous system, whence they are filtered by tapping the portal vein via the splenic and returning filtered blood to the saphenous vein. Thousands of worms have been removed in this way from a single case.

Prognosis

With treatment the prognosis is good in early and light infections if reinfection does not occur. In advanced disease with extensive involvement of the intestines, liver, bladder, or other organs, the outlook is poor even with treatment.

Clark WD: Acute schistosomiasis in 10 boys. Ann Int Med 73:379, 1970.
Cook JA, Woodstock L, Jordan P: Two-year follow-up of hycanthone-treated schistosomiasis mansoni patients in St. Lucia. Am J Trop Med 23:910, 1974.
Hulbert PB, Bueding E, Hartman PE: Hycanthone analogs: Dissociation of mutagenic effects from antischistosomal effects. Science 186:647, 1974.
Jordan P: Epidemiology and control of schistosomiasis. Brit M Bull 28:55, 1972.
Smith JH, & others: Studies on egg excretion and tissue egg burden in urinary schistosomiasis. Am J Trop Med 23:163, 1974.
Warren KS: The pathology of schistosome infections. Helminthol Abstr 42:592, 1973.
Warren KS & others: Schistosomiasis mansoni in Yemeni in California: Duration of infection, presence of disease, therapeutic management. Am J Trop Med 23:902, 1974.
Winsberg GR & others: Schistosomiasis in Chicago: A study of the Westown Puerto Rican population. Am J Epidem 100:324, 1974.
World Health Organization: Reports on schistosomicidal drugs. 2. Report of a WHO consultant group on the comparative evaluation of new schistosomicidal drugs for use in treatment campaigns. Bol Of Sanit Panam 6:89, 1972.

FASCIOLOPSIASIS

The large intestinal fluke, *Fasciolopsis buski,* is a common parasite of man and pigs in China, Taiwan, Southeast Asia, and India. When eggs shed in stools reach water, they hatch to produce free-swimming larvae which penetrate and develop in the flesh of snails. Cercariae escape from the snails and encyst on various water plants. Man is infected by eating these infected plants, usually water chestnuts or caltrops, uncooked. Adult flukes, mature in about 3 months, live in the small intestine attached to the mucosa or buried in mucous secretions.

After an incubation period of several months, manifestations of gastrointestinal irritation appear in all but light infections. Symptoms in severe infections include cramping epigastric and hypogastric pains, diarrhea, intermittent constipation, anorexia, and nausea. Edema, particularly of the face, and ascites may occur later. Death may result from cachexia or intercurrent infection.

Leukocytosis with moderate eosinophilia is common. The diagnosis depends upon discovery of eggs, or occasionally flukes, in the stools.

Crystalline hexylresorcinol is an effective drug. For adults give 1 gm orally in 0.1–0.2 gm capsules on an empty stomach in the morning. For children, give 0.1 gm/year of age to age 10. A light supper and prepurgation on the previous evening with sodium sulfate is desirable. Two hours after administration, repeat purgation with sodium sulfate. Repeat treatment in 3–4 days. Two courses are usually sufficient; 3 or more may be necessary. For somewhat greater effectiveness administer the drug transduodenally, 1 gm in 20 ml of water. Recently, marketing of hexylresorcinol was discontinued in the USA.

Tetrachlorethylene may be used if hexylresorcinol is not effective or not available. Administer as for hookworm disease. Stilbazium iodide (not available in the USA) has been successfully employed in treatment of children (average weight, 25 kg) in a total dosage of 1800 mg base given in 6 doses orally over 3 days.

In rare cases—particularly in children—heavy infections with severe toxemia have resulted in death in spite of treatment to remove the flukes. With these rare exceptions, the prognosis is good with proper treatment.

Hsieh HC & others: Treatment of *Fasciolopsis buski, Ancylostoma duodenale, Ascaris lumbricoides, Trichuris trichiura,* and *Enterobius vermicularis* infections with stilbazium iodide. J Parasitol 49:425, 1963.

Plaut AG & others: A clinical study of *Fasciolopsis buski* in Thailand. Tr Roy Soc Trop Med Hyg 63:470, 1969.

FASCIOLIASIS

Infection by *Fasciola hepatica,* the sheep liver fluke, results from ingestion of metacercariae on watercress or other aquatic vegetables. It is prevalent in sheep-raising countries, particularly where raw salads are eaten. Light infections may be asymptomatic. During the invasive stage of heavy infections, fever, eosinophilia, and hepatomegaly may be present. During the chronic phase, adult flukes in the liver may be extremely destructive and the patient may present with biliary obstruction.

Diagnosis is made by detecting eggs (which resemble those of fasciolopsiasis) in the feces or in duodenal drainage.

Bithionol, given as for paragonimiasis, is the drug of first choice because of its low toxicity. Fascioliasis may also be treated with emetine hydrochloride, giving 1 mg/kg body weight IM up to a maximum of 65 mg daily for 7 days. Dehydroemetine, if available, is less toxic than emetine. Complete recovery is slow even if all flukes are killed.

D'sa CJ: Human fascioliasis. Proc Roy Soc Med 63:285, 1970.

Knodell RG & others: Fascioliasis: Response to bithionol. California Med 117:72, Dec 1972.

Pantelouris EM: *The Common Liver Fluke.* Oxford Univ Press, 1964.

CLONORCHIASIS

Infection by *Clonorchis sinensis,* the liver fluke, is endemic in parts of Japan, Korea, China, Formosa, and Indochina. Imported cases are seen in the USA. Certain snails are infected as they ingest eggs shed into water in human or animal feces. Larval forms escape from the snails, penetrate the flesh of various fresh water fish, and encyst. Human infection results from eating such fish, either raw or undercooked. In man the ingested parasites excyst in the duodenum and ascend the bile ducts into the bile capillaries where they lodge and mature. The adults remain in the liver throughout their lives, shedding eggs in the bile. Biliary epithelial hyperplasia and fibrosis develop around the worms. In heavy infections eggs may lodge in the liver parenchyma, causing granulomatous reactions.

Most patients harbor few worms and remain permanently free of symptoms from the time of infection.

In some cases, with heavy infection, immature flukes migrating into the biliary capillaries may cause malaise, fever, liver tenderness, and jaundice. These symptoms are transient. With heavy infection symptoms later reappear after the flukes have matured. Progressive liver enlargement, tenderness, and right upper quadrant pain are the common findings. Vague abdominal symptoms, diarrhea, weakness, weight loss, jaundice, tachycardia, and a variety of other findings have been attributed to advanced clonorchiasis.

During the stage of invasion by the immature flukes there is often eosinophilia of 10–40%; later the count usually falls to normal. The diagnosis is established by finding ova in the stools or duodenal aspirate. In advanced disease liver function tests will indicate parenchymal damage.

There is no satisfactory specific drug, and treatment is primarily symptomatic and supportive. Chloroquine phosphate may be tried; although it apparently does not kill the flukes, it often reduces or stops the egg output, and may provide symptomatic relief. The adult dosage is 250 mg of the salt orally 3 times daily for 6 weeks or as long as it is tolerated. Side reactions (nausea, anorexia, headache, pruritus, dizziness) in the first 2 weeks of therapy are common and may require temporary reduction of dosage; later these symptoms usually subside. Bithionol, given as for paragonimiasis, may also be tried.

Clonorchiasis is rarely a fatal disease in itself, but patients with advanced infections and impaired liver function may succumb more readily to other diseases. The prognosis is good for light to moderate infections.

Komiya Y: Clonorchis and clonorchiasis. Pages 53–106 in: *Advances in Parasitology.* Vol 4. Dawes B (editor). Academic Press, 1966.

Strauss WG: Clinical manifestations of clonorchiasis: A controlled study of 105 cases. Am J Trop Med 11:625, 1962.

PARAGONIMIASIS

Paragonimus westermani, the lung fluke, commonly infects man throughout the Far East and locally in West Africa and northern South America. Other mammals may serve as alternate hosts for the adult flukes. Eggs reaching water, either in sputum or feces, hatch in 3–6 weeks. The miracidia penetrate snails and develop, and the emergent cercariae encyst in the tissues of crabs and crayfish. When these crustaceans are eaten raw or pickled—or when crabs are crushed and food vessels or fingers are contaminated by metacercariae that are later ingested—immature flukes excyst in the small intestine and penetrate into the peritoneal cavity. Most migrate through the diaphragm and enter the peripheral lung parenchyma; some may lodge in the peritoneum, the intestinal wall, the liver, or other tissues but usually fail to mature. Rarely, they may migrate to the brain or spinal cord. A capsule of fibrous and inflammatory tissue forms around the parasite as it matures. Later, the capsule swells and ruptures into a bronchiole. Fluid containing eggs, blood, and inflammatory cells is released and expectorated in the sputum.

The infection is asymptomatic until the flukes mature and begin producing eggs. The insidious onset is marked by low-grade fever, cough, or hemoptysis. The cough is dry at first; later it becomes productive of viscous sputum, rusty or blood-flecked. Pleuritic chest pain is common. The condition is chronic and slowly progressive. Dyspnea, signs of bronchitis and bronchiectasis, weakness, malaise, and weight loss are apparent in heavy infections. Many patients with light infections do not appear seriously ill. Parasites in the peritoneal cavity or intestinal wall may cause abdominal pain, diarrhea, or dysentery. Those in the CNS, depending upon their location, may give rise to seizures, palsies, or meningoencephalitis.

Slight leukocytosis and eosinophilia are common. The sputum may contain eosinophils and Charcot-Leyden crystals in addition to blood and eggs. Eggs are more readily demonstrated by examining smears of centrifuged sodium hydroxide-treated sputum sediment. Eggs are also found in stool specimens, particularly after concentration. Skin and complement fixation tests are useful as aids in diagnosis.

Bithionol, 40 mg/kg body weight, should be given on alternate days for 10–15 doses (20–30 days). Full courses of emetine, intramuscularly, followed by chloroquine, have been recommended in the past, but bithionol is now the drug of choice. Side-effects of bithionol, usually mild, are principally diarrhea and nausea. Antibiotics may be necessary to control secondary pulmonary infection. Bithionol is available in the USA only from the Parasitic Disease Drug Service, Center for Disease Control, Atlanta 30333.

Light to moderate infections subside spontaneously in 6–7 years and require little treatment. Heavy infections may be progressive for years and may eventually be fatal.

Higashi K & others: Cerebral paragonimiasis. J Neurosurg 34:515, 1971.
Kim JS: Treatment of *Paragonimus westermani* infections with bithionol. Am J Trop Med 19:940, 1970.
Yokogawa M: Paragonimus and paragonimiasis. Advances Parasitol 7:375, 1969.

CESTODE INFECTIONS

TAPEWORM INFECTIONS
(See also Echinococcosis)

Essentials of Diagnosis
- Finding of segments in clothing or bedding.

- Most infections asymptomatic; occasionally diarrhea or vague abdominal pains.
- Characteristic eggs or segments in the stool.
- Rarely (in cysticercosis), seizures, mental deterioration, signs and symptoms of internal hydrocephalus.

General Considerations

A number of species of adult tapeworms have been recorded as human parasites, but only 6 infect man frequently. *Taenia saginata,* the beef tapeworm, and *T solium,* the pork tapeworm, are cosmopolitan and common. *T solium* is no longer transmitted in the USA. The fish tapeworm, *Diphyllobothrium latum,* is most often found in northern Europe, Japan, and the Great Lakes region of the USA. The dwarf tapeworms, *Hymenolepis nana* and *H diminuta,* are cosmopolitan throughout the tropics and subtropics. The dog tapeworm, *Dipylidium caninum,* is occasionally reported in children in Europe and the Americas.

The adult tapeworm consists of a head (scolex), which is a simple attachment organ, a neck, and a chain of individual segments (proglottids). *H nana* adults are rarely more than 2.5–5 cm long. Beef, pork, and fish tapeworms often exceed 10 feet in length; gravid segments detach themselves from the chain and escape from the host intact, or rupture, releasing eggs in the feces. In the case of *T saginata,* the most common tapeworm found in man in the USA, eggs are expelled from the segments after they pass from the host. The eggs hatch when ingested by cattle, releasing embryos which encyst in muscles as cysticerci. Man is infected by eating undercooked beef containing viable cysticerci. In the human intestine the cysticercus develops into an adult worm.

The life cycle of *T solium* is similar except that the pig is the normal host of the larval stage, and man is infected by eating undercooked pork. However, if he accidentally ingests *T solium* eggs, the larvae find their way to many parts of the body and encyst as cysticerci. Transmission of *T solium* ova may occur from person to person or by autoinfection.

The intermediate hosts of the fish tapeworm are various species of fresh water crustaceans and fish. Eggs passed in human feces are taken up by crustaceans which are in turn eaten by fish. Human infection results from eating raw or poorly cooked fish.

The *H nana* life cycle is unusual in that both larval and adult stages of the worms are found in the human intestine. Adult worms expel infective eggs in the intestinal lumen. Newly hatched larvae invade the mucosa, where they develop for a time before returning to the lumen to mature. *H nana,* requiring no intermediate host, can be transmitted directly from man to man. A similar dwarf tapeworm, *H diminuta,* is a common parasite of rodents. Many arthropods, such as rat fleas, beetles, and cockroaches, serve as intermediate hosts. Man is infected by accidentally swallowing the infected arthropods, usually in cereals or stored products. Multiple dwarf tapeworm infections are the rule, whereas man rarely harbors more than one or 2 of the larger adult tapeworms.

Dipylidium caninum infections generally occur in young children living in close association with infected dogs or cats. Transmission results from swallowing the infected intermediate hosts, fleas or lice.

Spargana, or larval stages of certain tapeworms in frogs, reptiles, birds, and some mammals, may produce a variety of clinical conditions (sparganosis) ranging from local tender swellings (eg, eye) to a form of cutaneous larva migrans. One form is proliferating, invading all soft tissues. Infections are acquired from frog or other meat poultices, eating the raw flesh of small animals, or ingesting infected copepods in water. The diagnosis is usually made after surgical removal, but local physicians will make early diagnoses. Infections in animals are widespread; in humans more local, depending upon individual habits.

Clinical Findings

A. Symptoms and Signs: Adult tapeworms in the human intestine ordinarily cause no symptoms. Occasionally weight loss or vague abdominal complaints may be associated with heavy infections or large worms. Heavy infections with *H nana* may, however, cause diarrhea, abdominal pain, anorexia, weight loss, and nervous disturbances, particularly in children. In 1–2% of those harboring the fish tapeworm, a macrocytic anemia of considerable severity may be found. The anemia may be accompanied by glossitis, lethargy, and signs of nerve damage. In cysticercosis most larval tapeworms lodge in muscles or connective tissues where they remain silent and eventually calcify; in the brain, however, they may cause a wide variety of manifestations. Epileptic seizures, mental deterioration, personality disturbances, and internal hydrocephalus with headache, giddiness, papilledema, and nerve palsies are among the more common consequences of brain involvement.

B. Laboratory Findings: Infection by a beef tapeworm is often discovered by the patient when he finds one or more segments in his clothing or bedding. To determine the species of worm such segments must be flattened between glass slides and examined microscopically. Most tapeworm infections are detected by laboratory examination of stool specimens for eggs and segments. In cysticercosis x-rays often reveal calcified cysticerci in muscles, but those in the CNS rarely calcify and cannot be seen radiologically. When cysticerci lodge in the 4th ventricle the CSF pressure may be abnormal, and the fluid may show increased numbers of mononuclear cells. Skin and complement fixation tests are also available as aids in diagnosis of cysticercosis.

When fish tapeworm macrocytic anemia is discovered, the marrow will be found to be megaloblastic, and hydrochloric acid is usually present in the stomach. This anemia is attributed to the affinity of the worm for dietary vitamin B_{12}.

Differential Diagnosis

Fish tapeworm anemia may mimic pernicious anemia, but the presence of gastric hydrochloric acid and positive stool examinations will establish the diagnosis. Cysticercosis should be considered in all cases of epilepsy in patients who have lived in an endemic area. A search should be made for subcutaneous nodules, and x-ray examination for calcified cysts should be done. Serologic tests may be helpful.

Complications

Pork tapeworm infection may be complicated by cysticercosis if the patient unwittingly contaminates his hands with eggs and transfers them to his mouth. For such a patient, vomiting is also a hazard in that eggs may be propelled up the small intestine into the stomach, where they may hatch.

Treatment

A. Specific Measures:

1. **Niclosamide** is the drug of choice for all tapeworms. Some authorities have recommended quinacrine for *T solium* on the grounds that cysticercosis is theoretically possible after treatment with niclosamide. This hazard is overemphasized since no cases of cysticercosis have been reported after use of niclosamide. However, when the drug is used for *T solium* infection, an effective purge should be given within 1–2 hours after treatment in an attempt to eliminate mature segments before they disintigrate and release ova. Give 4 tablets (2 gm) thoroughly chewed as a single dose for *T saginata, T solium,* and *D latum,* and daily for 5 days for *H nana.* In the case of *H nana* the patient should be re-treated in 3 weeks to kill any worms that have emerged from their larval state in the intestinal villi. The drug should be administered in the morning on an empty stomach. Niclosamide rarely has side-effects and is given to outpatients without prior or post-treatment purges. Niclosamide is available in the USA only from the Parasitic Disease Drug Service, Center for Disease Control, Atlanta 30333.

2. **Paromomycin,** an antibiotic not appreciably absorbed from the gastrointestinal tract, is effective for the treatment of *T solium* and *T saginata* in a dosage of 1 gm 4 times a day for 1 day. The treatment course for *H nana* is 45 mg/kg daily for 5–7 days. Gastrointestinal side-effects are common but not severe.

3. **Quinacrine (mepacrine) hydrochloride** is an alternative but more toxic drug for tapeworms. On the day preceding treatment the patient should have only a liquid diet, with nothing but water or milkless tea or coffee for supper. On the evening before treatment, give a saline purge or a soapsuds enema. On the morning of treatment, withhold breakfast and confine the patient to bed. Give chlorpromazine, phenobarbital, or a similar sedative to prevent vomiting. One hour later, give quinacrine in the range of 0.5 gm for children weighing 40–75 lb to 0.8 gm for adults or children weighing over 100 lb. The dose may be divided to reduce the risk of vomiting, but all of it must be given within about 30 minutes. Administer quinacrine only by duodenal tube for *T solium* infections; for other types of tapeworm infections the duodenal tube may

be used if the patient persistently regurgitates the drug.

Two hours later (2 hours after the last dose, if divided doses are given), repeat the saline purge. No food should be permitted until the bowels move copiously. Side-effects from quinacrine include vomiting, mental changes, and yellowing of the skin. Sodium bicarbonate is given to reduce vomiting.

4. Dichlorophen for 1–2 days is also an effective drug for *T saginata, T solium, D latum,* and *H nana.* Dichlorophen is not available in the USA.

5. Aspidium oleoresin—Use of this drug, which is toxic and frequently contraindicated, is no longer justified for helminths that cause relatively little trouble and are amenable to the newer drugs.

B. Follow-Up Care: If it is preferred that parasitic cure be established immediately, the head (scolex) must be found in post-treatment stools. For quinacrine, stools are examined for several days; for niclosamide, a laxative is given 2 hours after treatment and stools are collected in a preservative for 24 hours. To facilitate examination, toilet paper must be disposed of separately. If no head is found, continue to examine the stools for eggs or proglottids once a month for 6 months.

C. Cysticercosis: No specific treatment is available for cysticercosis. Surgical excision of cerebral cysticerci is rarely helpful. Anticonvulsant drugs are given as for epilepsy.

Prognosis

Because the prognosis is often poor in cerebral cysticercosis, the eradication of a *T solium* infection is a matter of much greater urgency than that of the other tapeworm infections, which are usually benign. With careful treatment, adult tapeworms can be eliminated safely.

Botero D: Paromomycin as effective treatment of Taenia infections. Am J Trop Med 19:234, 1970.

Jopling WH, Woodruff AW: Treatment of tapeworm infections in man. Brit MJ 2:542, 1959.

Pawlowski Z, Schultz MG: Taeniasis and cysticercosis *(Taenia saginata).* Advances Parasitol 10:269, 1972.

ECHINOCOCCOSIS
(Hydatid Disease)

Essentials of Diagnosis

- Cystic tumor of liver, lung, or, rarely, bone, brain, or other organs.
- Allergic manifestations, including urticaria, asthma, pruritus.
- Eosinophilia (5–50%).
- History of close association with dogs in an endemic area.
- Positive complement fixation and skin tests.
- Positive x-ray findings are frequently found.

General Considerations

Human echinococcosis results from parasitism by the larval stage of the small tapeworm, *Echinococcus granulosus.* This tapeworm is found in various hosts throughout the world, but the areas of heaviest human infection are those where sheep are raised, notably South America, Australia, and Greece and other Mediterranean countries. In North America, echinococcosis occurs sporadically in Alaska and northwestern Canada, where Indians and Eskimos are occasionally infected. Endemic foci have recently been reported in California and Utah. The definitive host of the adult worm is usually the domestic dog; other canines, including wolves, foxes, and jackals, are locally important hosts. The sheep is the common host for the larval worm, but cattle, hogs, and, in northwestern North America, caribou and moose may also be infected. Man acquires the infection by ingesting eggs transferred from hand to mouth. The source of eggs is usually the fur of infected dogs. Once swallowed, the eggs liberate embryos which invade the blood stream through the intestinal wall and are carried to the liver. Most larvae are trapped and encyst (as hydatid cysts) in the liver; some may reach the lung, where they develop into pulmonary hydatids; only rarely do larvae reach the brain, bones, skeletal muscles, kidneys, or spleen.

Hydatid cysts are normally unilocular. Multilocular or alveolar cysts are due to infection by *E multilocularis,* mostly in Europe but also in Latin America and Australasia; it might be encountered in man in Alaska and Canada. Man typically is infected from soil or berries, etc, contaminated by eggs from fox feces. Slow growth in the liver provokes intrahepatic portal hypertension with hepatomegaly and no fever. The diagnosis is usually made at autopsy.

Clinical Findings

A. Symptoms and Signs: A liver cyst often remains silent for 5–10 years until it becomes large enough to be palpable or visible as an abdominal swelling. Such cysts rarely produce pressure effects, and cause no symptoms unless they begin to leak or are ruptured. When fluid and hydatid sand does escape from a cyst, pruritus, urticaria, asthma, and other allergic manifestations may appear and the eosinophil count rises. Jaundice and biliary colic with urticaria are a characteristic triad. If the cyst ruptures suddenly, anaphylaxis and even sudden death may occur, or metastases will follow. Pulmonary cysts cause no symptoms (unless leaking occurs) until they become large enough to obstruct the bronchi, causing segmental collapse, or to erode into a bronchus and rupture. Cysts in the brain, symptomatic at a much earlier stage, may cause seizures or symptoms of increased intracranial pressure.

B. Laboratory Findings: When clinical findings, history, and x-ray point to hydatid cyst, the diagnosis can be confirmed with the Casoni intracutaneous test (positive in about 86% of cases) and serologic tests (positive in about 90% of cases). The eosinophil count is usually about 5–20% in asymptomatic cases, but it may go as high as 50% when allergic symptoms are present. X-rays of liver cysts may show calcification of the cyst wall, but this does not mean the cyst is not infective. Diagnosis may occasionally be made by examination of hydatid sand coughed up from a ruptured pulmonary cyst. Because of the danger of leakage or rupture, diagnostic aspiration of suspected hydatid cysts should never be undertaken. The final diagnosis is often made only by examination of cyst contents after surgical removal.

Differential Diagnosis

Hydatid cysts in any site may be mistaken for a variety of malignant and nonmalignant tumors or for abscesses, both bacterial and amebic. In the lung a cyst may be confused with an advanced tubercular lesion. Allergic symptoms arising from cyst leakage may resemble those associated with many other diseases.

Complications

Sudden rupture of a cyst leading to anaphylaxis and sometimes death is the most important complication of echinococcosis. If the patient survives the rupture he still faces the danger of multiple secondary cyst infections arising from seeding of daughter cysts. Segmental lung collapse, secondary infections of cysts, secondary effects of increased intracranial pressure, and severe renal damage due to kidney cysts are other potential complications.

Treatment

The only definitive treatment is surgical removal of the intact cysts, when permitted by their location. Multilocular cysts are usually inoperable. Often, however, the presence of a cyst is only recognized when it begins to leak or when it ruptures. Such an event calls for vigorous treatment of allergic symptoms or emergency management of anaphylactic shock.

Prognosis

Patients may live for years with relatively large hydatid cysts before their condition is diagnosed. Liver and lung cysts often can be removed surgically without great difficulty, but for cysts in sites less accessible to surgery the prognosis is less favorable. It is always grave in secondary echinococcosis and with alveolar cysts. About 15% of patients may eventually die because of the disease or its complications.

Hutchison WF: Serodiagnosis of echinococcus infection. Am J Trop Med 17:752, 1968.

McLoughlin M, Hobbs B: Selective angiography in the diagnosis of hydatid disease of the liver. Canad MAJ 103:1147, 1970.

Saidi F, Nazarian I: Surgical treatment of hydatid cysts by freezing of cyst wall and instillation of 0.5% silver nitrate solution. New England J Med 284:1346, 1971.

Taiana JA: Thoracic hydatid echinococcosis: Diagnosis and treatment. Dis Chest 49:8, 1966.

Williams JF, Adaros HL, Trejos A: Current prevalence and distribution of hydatidosis with special reference to the Americas. Am J Trop Med 20:224, 1971.

Wilson JF, Diddams AC, Rausch RL: Cystic hydatid disease in

Alaska: A review of 101 autochthonous cases of *Echinococcus granulosus* infection. Am Rev Resp Dis 98:1, 1968.

NEMATODE (ROUNDWORM) INFECTIONS

TRICHINOSIS
(Trichiniasis)

Essentials of Diagnosis

- Muscle pains and tenderness, fever, periorbital edema, and splinter hemorrhages.
- Nausea, vomiting, cramps, and diarrhea.
- History of ingestion of raw or improperly cooked pork.
- Eosinophilia (as high as 75%).
- Positive skin test, muscle biopsy, and serologic tests.

General Considerations

Trichinosis is an acute infection caused by the roundworm *Trichinella spiralis.* Although cosmopolitan in distribution, for dietary reasons this parasite is a greater problem in many temperate areas than in the tropics. It is a common parasite of garbage-fed hogs in the USA, and autopsy figures suggest that 10–20% of the human population have been infected at one time or another. Man acquires the infection by eating encysted larvae in raw or undercooked pork, bear, or walrus. In the stomach and duodenum the larvae emerge and rapidly mature. Mating takes place and the female worms burrow into the small intestinal mucosa, producing gastrointestinal symptoms which may be mild or severe depending upon their numbers. The females discharge larvae which migrate in the blood stream to many parts of the body. Larvae reaching striated muscle encyst and remain viable for several years. Calcification of the cysts usually begins within a year. The larvae which do not reach muscle are eventually destroyed. Adult worms and larvae are only rarely found in the stool.

Clinical Findings

A. Symptoms and Signs: The clinical picture varies considerably in severity depending upon the number of larvae disseminated, the tissues invaded, and the general health of the patient; thus the acute disease may be mild or fatal. Gastrointestinal symptoms, if any, usually occur within 2–3 days after eating infected pork. These irritative symptoms are followed a few days later by manifestations of larval migration and muscle invasion including fever, chills, muscle pains and tenderness, difficulty in swallowing and speaking, splinter hemorrhages, periorbital edema,

edema of other dependent parts, urticaria, conjunctival and retinal hemorrhages, and photophobia. Still later, inflammatory reactions around larvae that have failed to reach striated muscle may produce meningitis, encephalitis, myocarditis, pneumonitis, and peripheral and cranial nerve disorders. If the patient survives, the fever usually subsides and recovery begins in the 4th week after onset of symptoms. Vague muscle pains and malaise may persist for several more months.

B. Laboratory Findings: Eosinophilia appears in the 2nd week after onset of symptoms, rises to a maximum of 20–75% in the 3rd or 4th week, and then slowly declines to normal. A delayed reaction to the trichinella skin test (noted only after 12–24 hours) occurs early in the disease (4th to 7th days), while an immediate reaction to the test (noted after 5 minutes) usually occurs from the 3rd week on. The skin test may remain positive up to 7 years after recovery. Precipitation and complement fixation tests become positive in the 2nd or 3rd week of the disease. The precipitation test may remain positive up to 2 years, the complement fixation test up to 9 months. Stool examinations rarely reveal either adult worms or larvae, but encysted larvae may be demonstrated by muscle biopsy (deltoid, biceps, gastrocnemius) in the 3rd to 4th weeks. Chest x-rays during the acute phase may show disseminated or localized infiltrates.

Differential Diagnosis

Mild cases and those with atypical symptoms are often difficult to diagnose. Because of its protean manifestations, trichinosis may resemble many other diseases. Moderate to severe infections with some or all of the most typical signs and symptoms can, however, usually be diagnosed readily. There are often several patients with similar symptomatology at the same time, and this is often the clue that leads to the diagnosis.

Complications

Among the more important complications are secondary bacterial pneumonia, cerebral involvement, pulmonary embolism, and cardiac failure.

Treatment

Treatment is supportive and symptomatic. Severe acute cases require hospitalization and excellent nursing care. Corticotropin (ACTH) and the corticosteroids provide effective relief for the acute symptoms. A reduction of the eosinophil count, disappearance of fever and splinter hemorrhages, and a general improvement in the clinical state of the patient are guides which should be employed to determine the efficacy of treatment. In the acute stage, treat with relatively large doses of either drug for the first 24–48 hours. In the subacute stage, therapy may have to be continued for several days or weeks to prevent recurrence, but give in reduced dosage sufficient to keep symptoms under control. Thiabendazole has been used with reported success to decrease the severity of symptoms in acute trichinosis. Further trials are recommended. An oral dosage of 25 mg/kg body weight twice daily may be given for 2–4 days. Side-effects may occur (see Strongyloidiasis, below).

Prognosis

Death may rarely occur in 2–3 weeks in overwhelming infections; more often, it occurs in 4–8 weeks from a major complication such as cardiac failure or pneumonia.

Clark PS & others: Bear meat trichinosis. Ann Int Med 76:951, 1972.

Gray DF, Morse BS, Phillips WF: Trichinosis with neurological and cardiac involvement. Ann Int Med 57:230, 1962.

Zimmerman WJ, Steele JH, Kagan IG: The changing status of trichiniasis in the US population. Pub Health Rep 83:957, 1968.

TRICHURIASIS
(Trichocephaliasis)

Essentials of Diagnosis

- Most infections are silent; heavy infections may cause abdominal pain, distention, flatulence, and diarrhea.
- Characteristic barrel-shaped eggs observed in the stool.

General Considerations

Trichuris trichiura is a common intestinal parasite of man throughout the world, particularly in the subtropics and tropics. The small slender worms, 30–50 mm in length and often called whipworms, attach themselves to the mucosa of the large intestine, particularly the cecum. The worms cause symptoms only when present in very large numbers. Eggs passed in the feces require 2–4 weeks for larval development after reaching the soil before becoming infective. New infections are acquired by direct ingestion of the infective eggs.

Clinical Findings

A. Symptoms and Signs: Light to moderate infections rarely cause symptoms. Heavy to massive infections (usually 10,000 ova per gram of feces and higher) may be accompanied by a variety of symptoms arising from irritation of the mucosa. Among the most common of these are abdominal pain, tenesmus, diarrhea, distention, flatulence, nausea, vomiting, and weight loss. Heavy infections are most often found in malnourished young children. Blood loss in children may be significant and rectal prolapse and bowel perforation with peritonitis may occur.

B. Laboratory Findings: Detection of whipworm eggs in the stool is essential for diagnosis. Eosinophilia (5–20%) is common with all but light infections, and hypochromic anemia may be present with heavy infections.

Treatment

Patients with asymptomatic light and moderate infections do not require treatment. For those with heavy or symptomatic infections, give mebendazole, 100 mg twice daily for 3 days. Gastrointestinal side-effects from the drug are rare.

If mebendazole is not available, give 1000–1500 ml of 0.2% hexylresorcinol as an enema to be retained for 1 hour. Perianal skin irritation is prevented by the application of a film of petrolatum. Dithiazanine iodide was effective but proved too toxic and has been withdrawn from the market. Thiabendazole should not be used because it is not effective and is potentially toxic.

Jung RC, Beaver PC: Clinical observations of *Trichocephalus trichuris* (whip worm) infestation in children. Pediatrics 8:548, 1951.

Maqbool S, Lawrence D, Katz M: Treatment of trichuriasis with a new drug, mebendazole. J Pediat 86:463, 1975.

Mathan VL, Baker SJ: Whipworm disease. Am J Digest Dis 15:913, 1970.

Wolfe MS, Wershing JM: Mebendazole: Treatment of trichuriasis and ascariasis in Bahamian children. JAMA 230:1408, 1974.

ASCARIASIS

Essentials of Diagnosis

- Pneumonitis with fever, cough, hemoptysis, urticaria, and accompanying eosinophilia.
- Vague abdominal discomfort and colic.
- Inflammatory reactions in organs and tissues invaded by wandering adult worms.
- Characteristic ova in the stool; larvae in the sputum.

General Considerations

Ascaris lumbricoides, a large intestinal roundworm, is the most common of the intestinal helminths of man. It is cosmopolitan in distribution, although it flourishes best in warm, humid climates. In temperate regions it is generally associated with low standards of personal hygiene. The adult worms live in the small intestine. After fertilization, the female produces enormous numbers of characteristic eggs which are carried out to the soil in feces. Under suitable conditions the eggs become infective, containing an active larva, in 2–3 weeks. Man is infected by ingestion of the mature eggs in fecally contaminated food and drink. The eggs hatch in the small intestine, releasing motile larvae which penetrate the wall of the small intestine and reach the right heart via the mesenteric venules and lymphatics. From the heart they move to the lung, burrow through the alveolar walls, and migrate up the bronchial tree into the pharynx, down the esophagus, and back to the small intestine. The larvae mature and female egg production begins about 60–75 days after ingestion of the infective eggs. The large adult worms, 20–40 cm long, may live for a year or more.

Clinical Findings

A. Symptoms and Signs: No symptoms arise from the early migration of the larvae after hatching. In the lung, however, they damage capillary and alveolar walls as they force their way through. Hemorrhage may result from this trauma, and accumulations of leukocytes and serous exudates in and around the airspaces may lead to consolidation. Pneumonitis occasionally develops with heavy infections. Symptoms and signs include fever, cough, hemoptysis, rales, and other evidences of lobular involvement. Eosinophilia is usual at this stage, and urticaria is not uncommon. After passage through the lungs it is believed that (rarely) the larvae may go astray, lodging in the brain, kidney, eye, spinal cord, or skin. Many bizarre symptoms may result from such invasions.

Small numbers of adult worms in the intestine usually produce no symptoms. With heavy infection vague abdominal discomfort and colic may occur, particularly in children. Ascaris infection in childhood can lead to protein and other nutritional deficiencies when a high parasite load is associated with a low protein intake. When the infection is heavy, and particularly if the worms are stimulated by certain oral medications or anesthetics, wandering may occur. Adult worms may be coughed up, vomited, or passed out through the nose. They may also force themselves into the common bile duct, the pancreatic duct, the appendix, diverticula, and other sites. Mechanical blockage and inflammation usually result. With very heavy infestations, masses of worms may cause intestinal obstruction, volvulus, or intussusception; during typhoid fever, bowel perforation may occur. It is important that ascaris infections be cured prior to bowel surgery because the worms have been known to break open suture lines postoperatively.

B. Laboratory Findings: The diagnosis usually depends upon finding the characteristic eggs in stool specimens. Occasionally a spontaneously passed adult worm reveals a previously unsuspected infection. There are no characteristic alterations of the blood picture during the intestinal phase. Skin tests are of no value in diagnosis. During the pulmonary phase there may be eosinophilia, and larvae may occasionally be found in the sputum.

Differential Diagnosis

Ascariasis must be differentiated from allergic disorders such as urticaria, Löffler's syndrome, and asthma. The pneumonitis associated with ascariasis is similar to other types of pneumonitis, especially that occurring with hookworm or strongyloides infection. Ascaris-induced pancreatitis, appendicitis, diverticulitis, etc must be differentiated from other causes of inflammation of these tissues.

Complications & Sequelae

Bacterial pneumonia may be superimposed upon pneumonitis resulting from larval migration. During the migratory stage, allergic manifestations may be severe. Because anesthesia stimulates the worms to become hypermotile, they should be removed in advance for patients undergoing elective surgery.

Treatment

Ascariasis, hookworm, and trichuriasis infections, which often occur together, may be treated simultaneously by mebendazole.

A. Piperazine: Piperazine is the drug of choice. Many brands of syrups and tablets of piperazine citrate or phosphate are available. They occasionally cause headache, dizziness, and visual disturbances and should not be used for patients with hepatic or renal insufficiency or with a history of seizures. Usually, each ml of syrup contains the equivalent of 100 mg piperazine hexahydrate; tablets usually contain 250 or 500 mg. The following daily doses may be given at any time and without special diet or purgation. If necessary, repeat after 1 week.

Up to 30 lb	1 gm	Once daily for 2 con-
30–50 lb	2 gm	secutive days. Heavy
50–100 lb	3 gm	infection may require
Over 100 lb	3.5 gm	3–4 days of treatment.

B. Pyrantel pamoate is a highly effective agent when administered as a single oral dose of 11 mg of base per kg body weight (maximum, 1 gm). Infrequent side-effects include vomiting, diarrhea, headache, rash, and fever. Experience with this drug is still limited.

C. Bephenium Hydroxynaphthoate: Reported cure rates after one dose (5 gm for older children and adults; 2.5 gm for children under 22 kg) vary from 30–82%. However, a 3-day course, as for hookworm infection, can be effective for mixed infections with both parasites.

D. Tetramisole: This new drug is reported to be highly effective as a single oral dose of 2.5mg/kg. It is not available in the USA.

E. Mebendazole: This new broad-spectrum anthelmintic is effective when given in a dosage of 100 mg twice daily for 3 days. Gastrointestinal side-effects are infrequent.

Prognosis

A heavy infection is usually not dangerous as long as the adult worms stay in their normal habitat, but the long list of major complications caused by wandering adults, plus the possibility of intestinal obstruction, requires that such infections be treated as soon as they are recognized.

Bell WJ, Nassif S: Comparison of pyrantel pamoate and piperazine phosphate in the treatment of ascariasis. Am J Trop Med 20:584, 1971.

Piggott J & others: Human ascariasis. Am J Clin Path 53:223, 1970.

Tripathy K & others: Effects of ascaris infections on human nutrition. Am J Trop Med 20:212, 1971.

Wolfe MS, Wershing JM: Mebendazole: Treatment of trichuriasis and ascariasis in Bahamian children. JAMA 230:1408, 1974.

STRONGYLOIDIASIS

Essentials of Diagnosis

- Pruritic dermatitis at sites of penetration of larvae.
- Malaise, cough, urticaria.
- Colicky abdominal pain, flatulence, diarrhea alternating with constipation.
- Eosinophilia; characteristic larvae in fresh stool specimens.

General Considerations

Strongyloidiasis is caused by the roundworm, *Strongyloides stercoralis*. It is common in tropical and subtropical areas throughout the world. In the USA it is prevalent in the southeastern states. The adult female worm burrows into the mucosa of the intestinal villi and lays eggs within the tissues. The duodenum and jejunum are most heavily infected. The eggs develop into rhabditiform larvae which are passed in the feces. The free-living rhabditiform larvae then develop into infective filariform larvae. These larvae penetrate the skin of the next victim, enter the blood stream, and are carried to the lungs where they escape from capillaries into alveoli and ascend the bronchial tree to the glottis. The larvae are then swallowed and carried to the small intestine, where maturation to the adult stage takes place. The time from skin penetration to egg laying by the mature adult is about 4 weeks. The life span of the adult worm may be as much as 5 years.

Autoinfection may occur if the rhabditiform larvae are retained in constipated feces or if there is fecal contamination of the perianal region. Such infection may also occur in the presence of diarrhea. Autoinfection is responsible for the persistence of strongyloidiasis in persons who have left endemic areas.

Clinical Findings

A. Symptoms and Signs: The clinical picture is not distinctive; diagnosis depends upon laboratory demonstration of larvae in the feces. At the points of entry of larvae into the skin there may be linear, erythematous, urticarial wheals that may be intensely pruritic. Papules may develop into vesicles, coalesce, and discharge serous fluid, or they may become hemorrhagic. Vague signs and symptoms during the migratory stage may include malaise, anorexia, fever, and cough. Urticaria is not uncommon. Secondary bacterial pneumonia may be initiated by a heavy larval migration through the lungs. An asymptomatic period of a few weeks usually precedes the gastrointestinal symptoms, of which the most common is localized or diffuse colicky abdominal pain. Diarrhea is common, often alternating with constipation or periods of normal bowel activity. With heavy infection, diarrhea may be persistent and accompanied by malabsorption, lassitude, nausea, vomiting, flatulence, weight loss, and debilitation. Epigastric pain and tenderness may also be present.

A hyperinfection syndrome with strongyloides

has been described as a complication during the course of treatment for other serious diseases, particularly following immunosuppressive therapy or prolonged use of adrenal steroids.

B. Laboratory Findings: During the stage of larval migration there is eosinophilia of 10–50% as well as leukocytosis up to 20,000/cu mm. In the intestinal phase eosinophilia may range from normal to 10%, but the white count is usually normal except in severe acute infections. A mild anemia may be present in this phase. The diagnosis is based on finding the characteristic rhabditiform larvae in a fresh stool specimen or the adult worm or filariform larvae in stools that have been left standing. Eggs are rarely found in the stool even in the case of severe diarrhea. Duodenal intubation or aspiration may be required to establish the diagnosis when larvae are not found in the stools. Duodenal contents are examined directly or after concentration. Larvae are occasionally found in the sputum or urine. Fecal cultivation may produce larvae or free-living adults after about 48 hours. Serologic and intradermal tests are not of diagnostic value, but the complement fixation test for filariasis may often give cross-reactions in patients with strongyloidiasis.

Differential Diagnosis

Because of the varied signs and symptoms at different stages of the infection, diagnosis may be difficult. During the stage of skin invasion, hookworm ground itch and creeping eruption due to *Ancylostoma braziliense* are the conditions which most closely resemble strongyloides ground itch, particularly because of the ankle-foot distribution of the skin lesions. During the later stages of the infection, many causes of transient pneumonitis, urticaria, and gastrointestinal symptoms may have to be considered in the differential diagnosis.

Complications

Larval migration through the lungs may initiate a secondary bacterial pneumonia. Hepatitis, cholecystitis, myocarditis, paralytic ileus, and meningitis may occur with massive infections.

Treatment

In the case of concurrent infection with strongyloides and ascaris or hookworm, which is not uncommon, treat the latter infections first and strongyloidiasis later.

A. Thiabendazole: This is the drug of choice. Give 25 mg/kg body weight orally twice daily for 2–3 days. Side-effects, including headache, weakness, nausea, vomiting, vertigo, and decreased mental alertness, occur in up to 30% of patients and may be severe. These symptoms are lessened if the drug is taken after meals. Crystalluria, leukopenia, and erythema multiforme have been reported and 2 deaths in young children have been associated with the use of the drug.

B. Dithiazanine iodide, although effective, is a potentially toxic drug and has been withdrawn from the market.

Prognosis

Favorable except in massive infections, usually resulting from autoinfection, which may result in intractable diarrhea, severe debilitation, and complications as noted above.

Berkmen YM, Rabinowitz J: Gastrointestinal manifestations of the strongyloidiasis. Am J Roentgenol 115:306, 1972.

Galliard H: Pathogenesis of strongyloides. Helminthol Abstr 36:247, 1967.

Most H & others: The treatment of strongyloides and enterobius infections with thiabendazole. Am J Trop Med 14:379, 1965.

Neefe LI & others: Disseminated strongyloidiasis with cerebral involvement: A complication of corticosteroid therapy. Am J Med 55:832, 1973.

Purtilo DT, Meyers WM, Connor DH: Fatal strongyloidiasis in immunosuppressed patients. Am J Med 56:488, 1974.

Rivera E & others: Hyperinfection syndrome with *Strongyloides stercoralis.* Ann Int Med 72:199, 1970.

ENTEROBIASIS
(Pinworm Infection)

Essentials of Diagnosis

- Perianal pruritus, usually nocturnal, associated with insomnia and restlessness.
- Vague gastrointestinal symptoms.
- Adult worms in stool; eggs on skin of perianal area.

General Considerations

Enterobius vermicularis, a short spindle-shaped roundworm often called the pinworm, is worldwide in distribution and the most common cause of helminthic infection of man in the USA. Man is the only host for the parasite. Children are more often affected than adults. The adult worms inhabit the cecum and adjacent bowel areas, lying with their heads loosely attached to the mucosa. When the fertilized female worms become gravid they migrate down the colon and out onto the skin, where eggs are deposited in large numbers. The females die after oviposition. The eggs become infective in a few hours and may then infect man if transferred to the mouth by inhalation or, more commonly, by hand, food, or drink contamination. The eggs are resistant to household disinfectants and drying, and may remain infective in dust for a considerable time. Retroinfection occasionally occurs when the eggs hatch on the perianal skin and the larvae migrate through the anus into the large intestine. If infective eggs are swallowed they hatch in the duodenum and the larvae migrate down to the cecum, moulting twice en route. The development of a mature ovipositing female from an ingested egg requires about 2 months.

Clinical Findings

A. Symptoms and Signs: The most common and

most important symptom is pruritus of the perianal area, particularly at night. This must be distinguished from similar pruritus due to mycotic infections, allergies, and psychologic disorders. Insomnia, restlessness, enuresis, and irritability are common symptoms, particularly in children. Many mild gastrointestinal symptoms—abdominal pain, nausea, vomiting, diarrhea, anorexia—have also been attributed to enterobiasis, although the association is difficult to prove. It is claimed that these symptoms result from mucosal irritation by the adult worms in the cecum, appendix, and surrounding portions of the bowel.

B. Laboratory Findings: Except for a modest eosinophilia (4–12%), the blood picture is usually normal. The diagnosis depends upon finding adult worms in the stool or eggs on the perianal skin. Eggs are seldom found on stool examination. The most reliable diagnostic technic consists of applying a short strip of sealing cellulose tape (Scotch Tape) to the perianal skin and spreading the tape on a slide for study. Three such preparations made on consecutive mornings before bathing or defecation will establish the diagnosis in about 90% of cases. Five to 7 such examinations are necessary before the diagnosis can be ruled out.

Complications

It has been postulated that the presence of large numbers of worms in the cecum may predispose to appendicitis, but the evidence for this is inconclusive. Female worms occasionally migrate into the vagina, uterus, and fallopian tubes, where they may produce an intense vaginitis. Granulomas rarely occur when worms enter tissue.

Treatment

A. General Measures: All infected members of the family and other close contacts may be treated, since reinfection from nontreated contacts is frequent. Hygienic instruction is of particular importance, eg, careful washing of hands with soap and water after defecation, and again before meals. Fingernails should be kept trimmed close and clean, and the patient should abstain from scratching involved areas and should not put his fingers in his mouth.

B. Specific Measures:

1. Pyrvinium pamoate in syrup, single dose of 5 mg/kg body weight (maximum of 0.25 gm), repeated after 2 weeks. It may cause nausea and vomiting and turns the stools red. A new tablet, with a micronized formulation of pyrvinium particles is reported to be as effective as the suspension.

2. Pyrantel pamoate is an effective oral drug. Its full range of side-effects cannot be assessed until additional experience with the drug becomes available. It is administered in a single oral dose of 11 mg of the base per kg body weight (maximum, 1 gm); repeat after 2 weeks.

3. Mebendazole, a new broad-spectrum anthelmintic, is highly effective when administered as a single 100 mg oral dose, irrespective of body weight. Do not use for children under 2 years of age. Repeat treatment in 2 weeks. Gastrointestinal side-effects are infrequent, but toxicity has not been critically evaluated.

4. Piperazine citrate—Available in syrup containing 100 mg/ml or as tablets of 250 or 500 mg. An alternative drug should be used if a convulsive disorder is present. The dosage for a course of 8 days is as follows:

> Up to 15 lb: 250 mg daily
> 15–30 lb: 250 mg twice daily
> 30–60 lb: 500 mg twice daily
> Over 60 lb: 1 gm twice daily

Prognosis

Although annoying, the infection is benign. Cure is readily attainable with one of several effective drugs, but reinfection is common.

Buchanan RA & others: Pyrvinium pamoate. Clin Pharmacol Therap 16:716, 1974.

Bumbalo TS: Single-dose regimen in treatment of pinworm infection. New York J Med 65:248, 1965.

Mayers CP, Purvis RJ: Manifestations of pinworms. Canad MAJ 103:489, 1970.

Miller MJ & others: Mebendazole: An effective anthelmintic for trichuriasis and enterobiasis. JAMA 230:1412, 1974.

HOOKWORM DISEASE

Essentials of Diagnosis

- Weakness, fatigue, pallor, palpitation, dyspnea associated with a hypochromic, microcytic anemia.
- Diarrhea, flatulence, abdominal discomfort, weight loss.
- Transient episodes of coughing, with sore throat and bloody sputum.
- Pruritic, erythematous, maculopapular or vesicular dermatitis.
- Characteristic eggs in the stool; guaiac-positive stool.

General Considerations

Hookworm disease, widespread in the tropics and subtropics, is caused by *Ancylostoma duodenale* and *Necator americanus.* In the Western Hemisphere necator is the prevailing genus. The adult worms, approximately 1 cm long, attach themselves to the mucosa of the small intestine, where they suck blood and mucosal substances. Symptomatology and pathology are proportionate to the number of worms infecting the patient. A burden of at least 100 worms is necessary to produce anemia and symptoms in an adult. Eggs produced by the female worms are passed in the stool, which must fall on warm, moist soil if larval development is to take place. Infective larvae remain in the soil until they come in contact with human skin. After penetrating the skin, the larvae migrate through the lungs and eventually reach the small intestine, where final development into adult worms takes place.

Clinical Findings

A. Symptoms and Signs: Ground itch, the first manifestation of hookworm infection, is a pruritic erythematous dermatitis, either maculopapular or vesicular, associated with the invasion of infective larvae. Strongyloides infection and creeping eruption caused by nonhuman hookworm species must be considered in the differential diagnosis at this stage. The severity of the dermatitis is a function of the number of invading larvae and the sensitivity of the host. The pulmonary phase of the disease is a transient reaction to larval migration through the lungs. Bloody sputum and cough result from damage caused by larvae breaking into alveoli from small blood vessels. Two or more weeks after the skin invasion, and depending upon the number of worms present, abdominal discomfort, flatulence, diarrhea, and other symptoms of intestinal irritation may appear as worms begin to attach themselves to the mucosa. Anemia appears 10–20 weeks after infection. The severity of the anemia depends upon the worm burden: more than 500 worms are necessary to produce profound anemia. The patient's nutritional status will also influence the severity of the anemia.

B. Laboratory Findings: The diagnosis ultimately depends upon demonstration of characteristic eggs in the stool. This can often be done on microscopic examination, but a better technic is to make thick smears of feces on blotting strips and place them in tubes so that the fecal material is held clear of 1 cm of water in the bottom of the tube. The eggs hatch at room temperature, and identifiable larvae migrate to the water. Larvae may occasionally be discovered in either the stool or sputum. The stool contains occult blood. The severity of the hypochromic microcytic anemia will depend upon the worm burden, which can be estimated by egg counting technics. Eosinophilia is usually present, particularly in the early months of the infection.

Complications

The skin lesions may become secondarily infected. In highly sensitive individuals the allergic reaction to the invading and migrating larvae may be severe. With profound anemia there may be cardiac decompensation with edema and ascites, mental retardation, stunting of growth, and impaired renal function. In heavy infections, hypoproteinemia may also be present. Malabsorption has been described in some cases.

Treatment

A. General Measures: Estimation of the need for treatment should be based on quantitative counts of the eggs in the stools. Light infections require no treatment. Stools should be checked 2 weeks after treatment; if the ova count is still moderate to heavy, a course of the drug should be repeated. If anemia is present, provide a high-protein diet with supplementary iron medication.

If ascariasis and hookworm infections are both present, either give mebendazole for both infections or piperazine first to eradicate ascaris followed by a drug to clear hookworms.

B. Specific Measures:

1. Bephenium hydroxynaphthoate, relatively nontoxic, is a drug of choice for ancylostoma and for mass treatment of children. It may cause nausea and vomiting. Suspend the bitter granules in a flavored vehicle. For ancylostoma, give 5 gm orally twice daily for 1 day, repeating in a few days if necessary. For children weighing less than 22 kg, give half this dose. For necator, the same dose for 3 days may reduce the worm load to acceptable levels. *Do not follow with a purge.*

2. Pyrantel pamoate is a well tolerated and moderately effective new drug for the treatment of hookworm infection. The dosage is 11 mg/kg/day for 3 days.

3. Tetrachlorethylene is a drug of choice for necator and may be used for ancylostoma. *Caution:* Be sure to correct severe anemia before giving this drug. Tetrachlorethylene is contraindicated in patients with alcoholism, chronic gastrointestinal disorders, severe constipation, hepatic disease, and in patients undergoing heavy metal therapy. It is generally recommended that ascarids be removed from the intestinal tract before tetrachlorethylene is used.

Give 30 gm magnesium sulfate in water or 240 ml magnesium citrate solution the night before drug therapy. Eliminate alcohol and fatty foods for 48 hours before medication and give a light evening meal. Give tetrachlorethylene, 0.12 ml/kg body weight (not more than 5 ml) in soluble gelatin capsules containing 1 ml, in the morning on an empty stomach. Side-effects may be reduced by giving the drug at bedtime, also on an empty stomach. Saline purgation following treatment is no longer recommended.

4. Mebendazole, 100 mg twice daily for 3 days, is effective for necator infections and probably for ancylostoma. Gastrointestinal side-effects from the drug are infrequent, although clinical experience is limited.

Prognosis

If the disease is recognized before serious secondary complications appear, the prognosis is favorable. With iron therapy, improved nutrition, and administration of an anthelmintic, complete recovery is the rule. The persistence of a few eggs in the stool of an asymptomatic person who is not anemic is not an indication for repeated treatments.

Roche M, Layrisse M: The nature of "hookworm anemia." Am J Trop Med 15:1032, 1966.

Salem HH & others: Clinical trials with bephenium hydroxynaphthoate against *Ancylostoma duodenale* and other intestinal helminths. J Trop Med 68:21, 1965.

Sato A & others: Anthelmintic activity of pyrantel pamoate against hookworm, *Necator americanus.* Jap J Parasitol 22:331, 1973.

· · ·

VISCERAL LARVA MIGRANS

Infection by the larval dog and cat ascarids, *Toxocara canis* and *T cati,* usually occurs in young children as a result of dirt eating. The larvae, unable to mature in an abnormal host, migrate through the body and lodge in various organs, particularly the lungs, liver, and brain. Because the disease is difficult to diagnose its distribution is not well known, but it is probably cosmopolitan.

Fever, cough, hepatomegaly, and nervous symptoms are the commonest clinical findings. A variety of other symptoms may occur when such organs as the heart, eyes, and kidneys are invaded. Granulomas of the retina may result that resemble retinoblastoma but may only be recognized years after the infection. Other signs and symptoms persist for about 18 months. Many infections are asymptomatic. Eosinophil counts of 30–80% and marked leukocytosis are common. Hyperglobulinemia occurs when the liver is extensively invaded.

Specific diagnosis can only be made by liver biopsy to search for toxocara larvae, but the procedure is seldom justified. Opinions vary on the specificity of available serologic tests.

There is no specific treatment, but thiabendazole should be tried. The cortisones, antibiotics, antihistamines, and analgesics may be needed to provide symptomatic relief. Symptoms may persist for months, but the ultimate prognosis is usually good.

Beaver PC: The nature of visceral larva migrans. J Parasitol 55:3, 1969.

Huntley C, Costas MC, Lyerly A: Visceral larva migrans syndrome: Clinical characteristics and immunologic studies in 51 patients. Pediatrics 36:523, 1965.

Kagan IG: Serologic diagnosis of visceral larva migrans. Clin Pediat 7:508, 1968.

Krupp IM: Hemagglutination test for the detection of antibodies specific for ascaris and toxocara antigens in patients with suspected visceral larva migrans. Am J Trop Med 23:378, 1974.

Woodruff AW: Toxocariasis. Brit MJ 3:663, 1970.

INTESTINAL CAPILLARIASIS

Fatal cases of human infection by the liver parasite *Capillaria hepatica* have been recorded in the past, but the syndrome of intestinal capillariasis recently recognized in the northern Philippines is a new clinical entity. It has also been reported from Thailand. The parasite, *C philippinensis,* is found in the mucosa of the small intestine, especially the jejunum. Infection presents as an intractable diarrhea and many cases have been fatal. A severe protein-losing enteropathy and malabsorption are features of the disease. Adult nematodes and eggs can be found in the stool. Treatment with thiabendazole in a dosage of 12 mg/kg orally twice daily for 30 days has been successful.

Whalen GE & others: Treatment of intestinal capillariasis with thiabendazole, bithionol, and bephenium. Am J Trop Med 20:95, 1971.

FILARIASIS

Essentials of Diagnosis

- Recurrent attacks at irregular intervals of lymphangitis, lymphadenitis, fever, orchitis.
- Hydrocele, chyluria, elephantiasis of legs, arms, genitalia, or breasts.
- Characteristic microfilariae in the blood.
- Eosinophilia; positive skin or complement fixation tests.

General Considerations

Filariasis is caused by infection with one of 2 filarial nematodes, *Wuchereria bancrofti,* and *Brugia malayi.* Infective larvae of *B malayi* are transmitted to man by the bite of certain Mansonia and Anopheles mosquitoes of south India, Ceylon, south China, and southeast Asia. *W bancrofti,* widely distributed in the tropics and subtropics of both hemispheres and on Pacific islands, is transmitted by certain Culex and Aedes mosquitoes. Over months, adult worms mature in or near superficial and deep lymphatics and lymph nodes. Over about 1 year, females produce large numbers of motile larvae (microfilariae), which appear in the peripheral blood. Microfilariae of *W bancrofti* are found in the blood chiefly at night (nocturnal periodicity), except for a nonperiodic variety in the South Pacific. *B malayi* microfilariae are usually nocturnally periodic but may be semi-periodic (present at all times with a slight nocturnal rise). While man is the only vertebrate host for *W bancrofti,* cats, monkeys, and other animals may harbor *B malayi.* Several other species of filarial worms infect man without usually causing important signs or symptoms. The microfilariae of Dipetalonema species (African and South American tropics) and *Mansonella ozzardi* (West Indies and South America) must be differentiated from those of the pathogenic species. Several Dirofilaria species have been reported to occasionally cause signs and symptoms in man, including painful subcutaneous nodules and coin lesions in the lung.

Clinical Findings

A. Symptoms and Signs: The early clinical manifestations are inflammatory; those of the later stages are obstructive. Episodes of fever, with or without inflammation of lymphatics and nodes, occur at irregular intervals in typical early cases. Persistent lymph node enlargement is most common in *B malayi* infections but occurs in some *W bancrofti* endemic areas. Funiculitis and orchitis are common and abscesses may form at sites of lymphatic inflammation. Such episodes may occur intermittently for months or years before the first obstructive signs appear. The number and severity of these attacks, and the extent of the later changes, depends primarily upon the intensity of the infection, which in turn is related to the length of residence in an endemic area. Obstructive phenomena, arising from interference with normal lymphatic flow, include hydrocele, scrotal lymphedema, lymphatic varices, and elephantiasis. Chyluria may result from rupture of distended lymphatics into the urinary tract. In the early stages of elephantiasis the tissues of the affected part are edematous and soft; later, with skin hypertrophy and subcutaneous connective tissue proliferation, the part becomes hard. As the swelling enlarges, sometimes to enormous size, the skin surface folds and fissures. Bancroftian elephantiasis frequently involves the legs and genitalia, less often the arms and breasts; in *B malayi* infections elephantiasis of the legs below the knees is most common and genital structures are rarely affected.

Hydrocele and elephantoid tissue changes in persons residing in endemic areas are usually filarial in origin. Elephantiasis in those who have visited endemic areas only briefly is rarely due to filariasis. Many infections are asymptomatic and detected only by blood examination.

B. Laboratory Findings: Eosinophilia (10–30%, higher with *B malayi*) is usual in the early stages; the count falls, sometimes to normal, as elephantiasis develops. Microfilariae are rare in the blood in the first 2–3 years after infection, abundant as the disease progresses, and again rare in the advanced obstructive stage. Laboratory diagnosis usually requires demonstration of microfilariae, which must be differentiated from the nonpathogenic species. Both day and night blood specimens should be examined for motile larvae and processed by concentration or microfiltration methods. Removal of nodes for diagnosis may further impair drainage from the affected area and is rarely justified. When microfilariae cannot be found, skin testing using an antigen prepared from *Dirofilaria immitis*, and serologic tests may be helpful in diagnostic screening, but false-positive and false-negative reactions occur.

Differential Diagnosis

Diagnosis of the early febrile and inflammatory episodes may be difficult, particularly when the patient has moved away from an endemic area, because attacks of lymphangitis, adenitis, and fever are transitory and microfilariae may be rare in the blood. Filarial funiculitis, orchitis, and epididymitis may suggest gonococcal infection, but there is no urethral discharge in the uncomplicated case. Among the late manifestations, elephantiasis may be confused with hernia, Milroy's disease, multiple lipomatosis, severe congestive heart failure, venous thrombosis, and obstructive lesions of the lymphatics, which may produce nonfilarial elephantiasis of the extremities. The last 3 named can be distinguished readily from filariasis. Multiple lipomas may produce a massive soft lumpy swelling of the proximal part of a limb. In contrast, the filarial lesion starts distally and becomes hard as it enlarges. Milroy's congenital elephantiasis usually involves both legs below the knees. The skin is smooth, there is no eosinophilia, and the patient often has never visited the tropics.

Treatment

A. General Measures: Bed rest is indicated during febrile and local inflammatory episodes. Antibiotics should be given for secondary infections, particularly abscesses over inflamed nodes. Suspensory bandaging is a valuable palliative measure for orchitis, epididymitis, and scrotal lymphedema. Treat mild edema of a limb with rest, elevation, and use of an elastic stocking. Chyluria usually requires no treatment except rest.

B. Surgical Measures: Surgical removal of the elephantoid scrotum, vulva, or breast is relatively easy, and the results are usually satisfactory. Surgery for limb elephantiasis is difficult and the results are often disappointing. Attempt operation only if the swollen limb severely limits the patient's ability to earn a living.

C. Specific Measures: Diethylcarbamazine is the drug of choice. The usual dosage is 2–3 mg of the citrate per kg body weight orally 3 times daily for 14 (sometimes 21) days. Use a single dose on the first day and regulate subsequent dosage to minimize allergic reactions, common early in treatment as microfilariae are killed. The drug itself is nontoxic in usual doses. Microfilariae are rapidly destroyed, but the drug has only a limited action on the adult worms. Since microfilarial relapses often occur 3–12 months after treatment, control of the infection may require several courses over 1–2 years. Drug treatment will not significantly influence the course of advanced filariasis. An important use of the drug is for mass treatment of populations in endemic areas to control transmission.

Prognosis

In early and mild cases the prognosis is good if the patient leaves the endemic area or if transmission in the area is reduced by control measures (mosquito control and drug treatment of human infections).

Ambroise TP: Immunological diagnosis of human filariasis: Present possibilities, difficulties and limitations. Acta trop 31:108, 1974.

Beaver PC, Orihel TC: Human infection with filariae of animals in the United States. Am J Trop Med 14:1010, 1965.

Edeson JFB: Filariasis. Brit M Bull 28:60, 1972.

Hawking F: Advances in filariasis. Tr Roy Soc Trop Med Hyg 59:9, 1965.

Robinson MJ, Viamonte M, Viamonte M Jr: Dirofilariasis: Diagnostic consideration for pulmonary "coin lesions." South MJ 67:461, 1974.

Wijetunge HPA: Clinical manifestations of early bancroftian filariasis. J Trop Med 70:90, 1967.

LOIASIS

Loiasis is a common and distinctive disease of tropical Africa caused by the filarial nematode, *Loa loa.* The intermediate host, Chrysops, a biting fly, carries the infection from man or monkey to man. Infective larvae, introduced by the biting fly, develop into adult worms in about 12 months. It is the adult worms migrating through subcutaneous tissues which cause the symptoms of loiasis, not the larval microfilariae in the blood stream.

Many infected persons remain symptom-free; others develop severe allergic reactions to the infection. The first definite signs of the disease are the appearance of Calabar swelling or the migration of a worm beneath the conjunctiva of the eye. The swelling, which may be painful, is a temporary subcutaneous edematous reaction, often several inches in diameter. The overlying and surrounding skin is often erythematous and pruritic. The swelling may migrate a few inches before disappearing; more often it remains in one place for several days and then subsides. The reaction occurs most frequently on the hands, forearms, and around the eyes, but it may appear anywhere. Some patients experience Calabar swellings at infrequent intervals, others as often as twice a week.

Migrating worms are sometimes visible in subcutaneous tissues, and migration across the eye produces a foreign body sensation, often with considerable irritation. The parasite has also been found in cerebrospinal fluid associated with a meningoencephalitis. Generalized urticaria, edema of a whole limb, extensive erythema, and generalized pruritus have been reported in some patients.

The adult worm may be recovered from the eye or skin (rarely), or microfilariae may be found in daytime blood films (20–30% of patients). Complement fixation and skin tests are often useful in diagnosis. The eosinophil count is elevated, varying between 10–40% or more.

Surgical removal of adult worms is sometimes possible, but the most satisfactory treatment is with diethylcarbamazine, a relatively nontoxic drug which kills both microfilariae and adults. Optimal dosage is 2–3 mg/kg body weight 3 times daily after meals for 14 days. Because allergic reactions (fever, urticaria, rashes, pruritus) are common early in treatment (probably as a result of rapid killing of microfilariae), use only a single dose on the first day of treatment and regulate subsequent dosage according to the patient's reaction. Antihistamine therapy is often helpful early in the course of treatment.

The prognosis is good with treatment. Without treatment, loiasis is annoying and uncomfortable but rarely life-endangering. Fatal encephalitis rarely occurs.

Cahill KM: Other filarial infections of man. New York J Med 63:1551, 1963.

Gordon RM & others: The problem of loiasis in West Africa. Tr Roy Soc Trop Med Hyg 44:11, 1950.

ONCHOCERCIASIS

Man and Simulium black flies are the natural hosts of *Onchocerca volvulus,* a filarial nematode found in many parts of tropical Africa and in localized areas of Central America and northern South America, including southern Mexico, the highlands of Guatemala, and eastern Venezuela. The biting fly introduces infective larvae which develop slowly in the cutaneous and subcutaneous tissues of man. Flies are infected in turn by picking up microfilariae while biting. Adult worms may live for years, frequently in fibrous nodules which develop around one or more of the parasites. Microfilariae, motile and migratory, may be found in the skin, subcutaneous tissues, and lymphatics, and in the conjunctiva and other structures of the eye.

Clinical Findings

A. Symptoms and Signs: Intensity of infection determines the extent and severity of the clinical picture. After an incubation period of several months to 1 year, skin manifestations appear in up to 40% of patients. Localized or generalized pruritus is common, usually causing scratching and skin excoriation. Pigmentary changes, skin thickening, and lichenification may appear later. Erysipeloid or papulovesicular eruptions are sometimes seen. Subcutaneous nodules develop around adult worms; hence they appear at a later stage of the infection. The nodules, usually painless, consist of fibrous tissue surrounding one or many living or dead worms. Common sites are over bony prominences on the trunk, thighs, shoulders, arms, and head. Few patients have more than 3–6 nodules. The most common early ocular finding is a superficial punctate keratitis. Vascular pannus, iritis, and cyclitis are serious later manifestations. While certain retinal changes, atrophic choroiditis, and optic atrophy are seen in patients with onchocerciasis, some investigators doubt that these lesions are actually due to the infection.

B. Laboratory Findings: Eosinophilia of 15–50% is common. Aspiration of nodules will usually reveal microfilariae, and adult worms may be demonstrated in excised nodules. Microfilariae are not found in the blood but can be identified in skin or conjunctival snips or in skin shavings. The snip is performed by tenting the skin with a needle and cutting off a bit of skin above the needle tip. A blood-free shaving may be cut with a razor blade from the top of a ridge of skin firmly pressed between thumb and forefinger. The snip or shaving is examined in a drop of saline under a coverslip on a slide, for many microfilariae emerge from the snip within an hour. Shavings or snips should be taken from several sites over bony prominences of the scapular region, hips, and thighs.

C. Special Examinations: In ocular onchocerciasis, slitlamp examination will usually reveal many microfilariae in the anterior chamber. Complement fixation and skin tests may be of use in screening, but high false-positive reaction rates occur.

Complications

Glaucoma and cataracts arising from iritis and cyclitis may cause blindness. Posterior segment lesions seen in patients with onchocerciasis may also cause blindness.

Treatment

A. Specific Measures:

1. **Diethylcarbamazine** is almost nontoxic and effective against microfilariae but not the adult worms. Give 2–3 mg/kg body weight orally 3 times daily for 14–21 days. To prevent severe allergic symptoms which may be provoked early in therapy as microfilariae are rapidly killed, start treatment with small doses and increase dosage over 3–4 days. When the eyes are involved, particular caution is necessary, starting with a single daily dose of 0.25 mg/kg. Use antihistamines and corticosteroids to control allergic reactions. Cortisone acetate eye drops (1%) are needed to control eye reactions.

2. **Suramin sodium** is effective in eradicating infection by killing the adult worms, but it has the disadvantage of potential renal toxicity (proteinuria, casts, red cells). Renal disease is a contraindication. For adults, give 1 gm of a 10% solution in distilled water IV every 7 days to a total dose of 5–10 gm. Start treatment with a test dose of 0.2 gm. Available in the USA only from the Parasitic Disease Drug Service, Center for Disease Control, Atlanta 30333.

B. **Surgical Measures:** As many nodules as possible should be excised surgically, particularly when nodules are located close to the eyes.

Prognosis

With chemotherapy, progression of all forms of the disease usually can be checked. The prognosis is unfavorable only for those patients seen for the first time with already far-advanced ocular onchoceriasis.

Buck AA (editor): *Onchocerciasis: Pathology and Diagnosis.* World Health Organization 1974.
Duke B, Anderson J: Onchocerciasis and its treatment. Trop Doctor 2:107, 1972.
Nelson GS: Onchocerciasis. Advances Parasitol 8:173, 1970.
Oomen AP: Fatalities after treatment of onchocerciasis with diethylcarbamazine. Tr Roy Soc Trop Med Hyg 63:548, 1969.

DRACUNCULIASIS
(Guinea Worm Infection, Dracunculosis, Dracontiasis)

Dracunculus medinensis is a nematode parasite of man found through northern and central Africa, southern Asia, and northeastern South America. It occurs in the Caribbean but is not seen in the USA except in imported cases. Man is infected by swallowing water containing the infected intermediate host, the crustacean Cyclops, which is common in wells and ponds in the tropics. Larvae escape from the crustacean in the human host and mature in the connective tissues. After mating the male worm dies and the gravid female, now 1 meter or more in length, moves to the surface of the body. The head of the worm reaches the skin surface, a blister develops and ruptures, and the uterus discharges great numbers of larvae whenever the ulcer comes in contact with water. Larval discharge continues intermittently for as long as 3 weeks until the uterus is empty. The female worm then dies and is either extruded or absorbed. In the absence of secondary infection, the ulcer heals in 4–6 weeks following onset.

Clinical Findings

A. **Symptoms and Signs:** Clinical effects are produced only by the female worm. Multiple infections occur, but the usual infection is with a single worm. Several hours before the head appears at the skin surface local erythema and tenderness often develop in the area where emergence is to take place. In some patients there may be systemic symptoms at this time, including urticaria, generalized pruritus, nausea, vomiting, and dyspnea. As the blister forms and ruptures these symptoms subside. The tissues surrounding the ulceration which remains after rupture of the blister frequently become indurated, reddened, and tender; and since 90% of the lesions appear on the leg or foot the patient often must give up walking and work. Uninfected ulcers heal in 4–6 weeks, but secondary infection is so common that the course is often prolonged.

Calcified guinea worms are occasionally revealed as chance findings during x-ray examination of persons in endemic areas.

B. **Laboratory Findings:** When a worm is not visible in the ulcer the diagnosis may be made by detection of larvae in fluid expressed from the moistened ulcer. A skin test is available, but its value as a diagnostic aid is not established. Eosinophilia of about 10% often accompanies the symptoms before blister formation.

Complications

Secondary infection is the rule and may cause development of an abscess which eventually involves deep structures. Ankle and knee joint infection and deformity is a common complication in some areas. If the worm is broken during removal sepsis almost always results, leading to cellulitis, abscess formation, or septicemia.

Treatment

A. **General Measures:** The patient should be at bed rest with the affected part elevated. Cleanse the lesion and control secondary infection with antibiotics.

B. **Specific Measures:** Three drugs are now used which facilitate rapid resolution of symptoms, expulsion or removal of worms, and healing of ulcers. The relative merits of the 3 drugs—metronidazole, niridazole, and thiabendazole—require further controlled clinical trials. Give metronidazole, 750 mg 3 times daily for 10 days, or niridazole, 25 mg/kg in divided doses daily for 7 days, or thiabendazole, 25 mg/kg twice daily for 2 days. The ulcers should be dressed daily and the emerging worms eased out by applying gentle traction to the stick around which they are wound. The extraction process may require several days.

C. **Surgical Removal:** If necessary, following chemotherapy, make multiple incisions under local anesthesia along the worm tract and remove the entire worm carefully. Injection of a contrast medium in the tract followed by x-ray may facilitate locating the worm. Give antihistamines preoperatively to control allergic symptoms arising from manipulation or rupture of the worm.

Kale OO: A controlled field trial of the treatment of dracontiasis with metronidazole and niridazole. Ann Trop Med 68:91, 1974.

Kothari ML & others: Niridazole in dracunculiasis. Am J Trop Med 17:864, 1968.

Muller R: Dracunculus and dracunculiasis. Advances Parasitol 9:73, 1971.

CUTANEOUS LARVA MIGRANS
(Creeping Eruption)

Creeping eruption, prevalent throughout the tropics and subtropics, is caused by the larvae of the dog and cat hookworms, *Ancylostoma braziliense* and *A caninum.* It is a common infection of man in the southeastern USA, particularly where people come in contact with moist sandy soil (beaches, children's sand piles) contaminated by dog or cat feces. The larvae may invade any skin surface, but the hands or feet are usually affected. The larvae may remain active in the skin for several weeks or months, slowly advancing but rarely moving more than a few inches from the penetration site. Eventually, if not killed by treatment, the larvae die and are absorbed.

Soon after invasion of the skin, minute itchy erythematous papules appear at the sites of entry. Two or 3 days later characteristic serpiginous eruptions begin to form as larval migration starts. These intensely pruritic lesions may persist for several months as migration continues. The parasite usually lies slightly ahead of the advancing end of the eruption. Vesiculation and crusting commonly occur in the later stages. About 30% of patients develop transient pulmonary infiltrates and eosinophilia, possibly representing larval migration through the lungs. There are no consistent laboratory findings in most cases.

Simple transient cases usually do not require treatment. The larvae must be killed to provide relief in severe or persistent cases. Thiabendazole, given as for strongyloidiasis, is very effective and the drug of choice. Progression of the lesions and itching are usually stopped within 48 hours. Topically applied thiabendazole cream may also be effective. Antihistamines are helpful in controlling pruritus, and antibiotic ointments may be necessary to treat secondary infections.

Katz R & others: The natural course of creeping eruption and treatment with thiabendazole. Arch Dermat 91:420, 1965.

Stone OJ: Systemic and topical thiabendazole for creeping eruption. Texas Rep Biol Med 27 (Suppl 2):659, 1969.

GNATHOSTOMIASIS

Gnathostomiasis is an infection due to the nematode parasite *Gnathostoma spinigerum,* which is found only in eastern and southern Asia. A single migratory subcutaneous swelling is the most common manifestation. The usually painless swelling, caused by the migrating worm, is firm, pruritic, and variable in size. It may appear anywhere on the body surface, remain in that area for days or weeks, or wander continually. Internal organs, the eye, and the cervix may also be invaded. Occasionally the worm becomes visible under the skin.

Spontaneous pneumothorax, leukorrhea, hematuria, hemoptysis, paroxysmal coughing, and edema of the pharynx with dyspnea have been reported as complications.

A high eosinophilia accompanies the infection. Specific skin-testing antigens are available as a diagnostic aid, but final diagnosis usually rests upon identification of the worm.

Surgical removal of the worm when it appears close to the skin surface is the only effective treatment. Chemotherapy has not proved successful, although symptoms may be relieved by the use of diethylcarbamazine as for filariasis, and thiabendazole should be tried.

Daengsvang S: Human gnathostomiasis in Siam with reference to the method of prevention. J Parasitol 35:116, 1949.

ANGIOSTRONGYLIASIS
(Eosinophilic Meningoencephalitis)

A nematode of rodents, *Angiostrongylus cantonensis,* is recognized as the causative agent of a form of meningoencephalitis now reported from Hawaii, other islands of the Pacific, and the mainland of Southeast Asia. Human infection results from the ingestion of raw slugs, snails, crayfish, or other invertebrates harboring infective larvae. The larvae usually invade the CNS, producing signs and symptoms of meningoencephalitis, including headache, fever, paresthesias, and back and neck stiffness. A characteristic feature is spinal pleocytosis consisting largely of eosinophils. A complement fixation serologic test has been developed. Ocular infection has been reported from Thailand.

No specific drug treatment is available. The illness usually persists for weeks to months and the patient then recovers spontaneously, but fatalities have been reported.

Alicata JE: Present status of *Angiostrongylus cantonensis* infection in man and animals in the tropics. J Trop Med 72:53, 1969.

Tangchai P, Nye SW, Beaver PC: Eosinophilic meningoencephalitis caused by angiostrongyliasis in Thailand: Autopsy report. Am J Trop Med 16:454, 1967.

ARTHROPOD INFECTIONS

MYIASIS

Myiasis is infestation with the larvae of various species of flies. Specific myiases, in which the fly larvae are parasitic, developing only in living flesh (eg, botflies, screw-worm flies), cause the most serious lesions. They are widely distributed (eg, horse, cattle, and sheep botflies), but a few species are prominent in specific geographic areas. In the so-called semispecific myiases, the larvae developing (usually) in decaying flesh may invade wounds or cavities. In intestinal or accidental myiases, the larvae or eggs are ingested or the eggs are laid at the body orifices.

Nasal, oral, ocular, and aural myiases are produced by invasion of these tissues by larvae of the primary screw-worm (*C hominivorax*, warm parts of the western hemisphere), the Old World screw-worm (chrysomyia, oriental and Ethiopian), sheep botfly (*Oestrus ovis*, worldwide), or flesh-flies (*Wohlfahrtia magnifica*, Mediterranean to USSR). Other flies may invade secondarily. There may be extensive tissue destruction.

Intestinal myiasis (various species) is worldwide in distribution, but most cases have been recorded in India. Genitourinary myiasis due to migration of larvae (many species) into the bladder or vagina is rare.

The clinical manifestations are nonspecific, and are ascribable to progressive inflammation, often with great irritation of the affected cavity. Gastrointestinal disturbances may include vomiting and melena, and larvae are commonly passed in the feces spontaneously. In the conjunctival sac or lacrimal duct, the nasal cavity or sinuses, or the oral cavity, larvae may be seen by appropriate methods.

Removal of larvae by irrigation is frequently made more effective by instilling 5–10% chloroform in milk or light vegetable oil for 30 minutes. This is best done after a preliminary lavage. Continue with appropriate treatment to encourage healing. In intestinal myiasis, victims often also harbor one or more species of helminth which should be removed first by appropriate vermifuges.

Ocular Myiasis

Conjunctival infestation with fly larvae occurs frequently in the tropics but is rare in the USA. Several species of flies have been incriminated. Larvae invade the conjunctival sac and produce a nonspecific inflammatory reaction. If they spread throughout the eye and orbit, the inflammatory reaction and eventual necrosis become severe. Destruction of the orbital contents and bony walls of the orbit with invasion of the meninges may occur.

Extreme itching and irritation are the cardinal symptoms. The conjunctiva is red and excoriated. Numerous elongated white larvae are seen, especially in the fornices.

Treatment consists of mechanical removal of the larvae after first instilling cocaine, which has a paralyzing effect upon them. If the larvae can be removed when they are few in number, the course of the disease is automatically terminated. If further infestations are permitted, the prognosis is extremely poor inasmuch as the larvae invade the tissues out of reach of any form of treatment other than exploratory surgery. In such cases, destruction of the bony orbital wall and its contents frequently occurs.

James MT: The flies that cause myiasis in man. Dept Agric Miscell Publ 631, 1947.

27 ...
Infectious Diseases: Mycotic*

Carlyn Halde

COCCIDIOIDOMYCOSIS

Essentials of Diagnosis

- Influenza-like illness with malaise, fever, backache, headache, and cough.
- Pleural pain.
- Arthralgia and periarticular swelling of knees and ankles.
- Erythema nodosum or erythema multiforme.
- Dissemination (rare) may result in meningitis or granulomatous lesions in any or all organs.
- X-ray findings vary widely from pneumonitis to cavitation.
- Positive skin test, serologic tests useful; sporangia containing endospores demonstrable in sputum or tissues.

General Considerations

Coccidioidomycosis should be considered in the diagnosis of any obscure illness in a patient who has lived in or visited an endemic area.

Infection results from the inhalation of arthrospores or mycelial fragments of *Coccidioides immitis*, a fungus which grows in soil in certain arid regions of the southwestern United States, Mexico, and localized areas in Central and South America.

About 60% of infections are subclinical and unrecognized other than by the subsequent development of a positive coccidioidin skin test. In the remaining cases, symptoms may be of severity warranting medical attention. Fewer than 1% show dissemination, but among these patients the mortality rate is high.

Clinical Findings

A. Symptoms and Signs: Symptoms of primary coccidioidomycosis occur in about 40% of infections. These vary from mild to severe and prostrating and resemble those due to viral, bacterial, or other mycotic infections. The onset (after an incubation period of 10–30 days) is usually that of a respiratory tract illness with fever and occasionally chills. Pleural pain is common and usually severe. Muscular ache, backache,

*Superficial mycoses are discussed in Chapter 3.

and headache may be severe. Nasopharyngitis may be followed by bronchitis accompanied by a dry or slightly productive cough. Weakness and anorexia may become marked, leading to prostration. A morbilliform rash may appear 1–2 days after the onset of symptoms.

Arthralgia accompanied by periarticular swellings, often of the knees and ankles, is common. Erythema nodosum may appear 2–20 days after onset of symptoms. Erythema multiforme may appear on the upper extremities, head, or thorax. Breath sounds may become bronchial in nature, especially in the severely ill patient. Persistent pulmonary lesions, varying from cavities and abscesses to parenchymal nodular densities or bronchiectasis, occur in about 5% of diagnosed cases.

About 0.1% of white and 1% of nonwhite patients are unable to localize or control infection due to *C immitis*. Symptoms in progressive coccidioidomycosis depend upon the site of dissemination. Any or all organs may be involved. Pulmonary findings usually become more pronounced, with mediastinal and hilar lymph node enlargement, cough, and increased sputum production. Pulmonary abscesses may rupture into the pleural space, producing an empyema. Extension to bones and skin may take place, and pericardial and myocardial extension is not unusual.

Lesions in the bones are often in the bony prominences and the ends of long bones. The ankle, wrist, and elbow joints are commonly involved. Meningitis occurs in about 25% of disseminated cases. Subcutaneous abscesses and verrucous skin lesions are especially common in fulminating cases. Lymphadenitis may occur and may progress to suppuration. Mediastinal and retroperitoneal abscesses are not uncommon.

B. Laboratory Findings: In primary coccidioidomycosis there may be a moderate leukocytosis and eosinophilia. The sedimentation rate is elevated, returning to normal as the infection subsides. If the sedimentation rate persists or increases, there is a danger of progressive disease. A coccidioidin skin test becomes positive within 1–3 weeks after onset of symptoms. Precipitin antibodies appear in most symptomatic infections but disappear after 1–2 months. Complement-fixing antibodies appear later but persist longer. An initial eosinophilia of 15% or higher together with a persistent rising complement fixation titer is a bad prognostic sign. A rising complement fixation titer may herald dissemination weeks before it is otherwise evident. Demonstrable antibodies in spinal fluid are pathognomonic for coccidioidal meningitis. Spinal fluid findings include increased cell count with lymphocytosis and reduced sugar. Sporangia filled with endospores may be found in clinical specimens. These should be cultured only by trained technicians using safety precautions because of the danger of laboratory infection.

C. X-Ray Findings: X-ray findings vary, but patchy and nodular infiltrations are the most common. Hilar lymphadenopathy may be visible. There may be primary pleural effusion. Thin-walled cavities may appear.

Complications

Pulmonary infiltrations persisting for 6 or more weeks should be suspected of possible progression, especially with increase in area, enlargement of mediastinal and hilar nodes, cavity enlargement, and hemoptysis. Progressive disease is more likely to appear in Negroes, Filipinos, and Mexicans. Pregnant women of any race are also more vulnerable to dissemination.

Treatment

Bed rest is the most important therapeutic measure for the primary infection. This should be continued until there is a complete regression of fever, a normal sedimentation rate, clearing or stabilization of pulmonary radiologic findings, and a lowering of the complement fixation titer. These precautions are especially important for patients in whom the rate of dissemination is high. General symptomatic therapy is given as needed.

There is no specific therapy for patients with disseminated disease. Amphotericin B has proved effective in some patients and should be tried. The drug is suspended in 500 ml of 5% dextrose in distilled water (not saline) and administered IV over a 4-hour period. The adult dose is 0.5–1 mg/kg; however, since this drug has toxic properties (including renal toxicity), therapy should begin with 1 mg/day, increasing by 5 mg increments to 25 mg/day. Continue at this dosage, decreasing with poor tolerance or increasing with poor clinical response. Therapy should be continued to a total dose of 2.5–3 gm. (See p 910 for precautions in the use of this drug.)

The best monitor of renal function is a creatinine clearance test done before treatment and once a week during treatment. Determine the BUN periodically.

Thoracic surgery is indicated for giant, infected, or ruptured cavities. Surgical drainage is also useful for subcutaneous abscesses. Excisional surgery may be used to remove any focus or source of proliferating sporangia. Amphotericin B should be given for 3–4 weeks before and after surgery.

Prognosis

The prognosis is good, but persistent pulmonary cavities may present complications. Nodules, cavities,

and fibrotic residuals may rarely progress after long periods of stability or regression. Before amphotericin B became available the prognosis for disseminated coccidioidomycosis was poor, with a mortality rate approaching 50%.

Bennett JE: Chemotherapy of systemic mycoses. (2 parts.) New England J Med 290:30, 320, 1974.

Fiese MJ: *Coccidioidomycosis.* Thomas, 1958.

Winn WA: Long term study of 300 patients with cavitary-abscess lesions of the lung of coccidioidal origin. Dis Chest 54:268, 1968.

HISTOPLASMOSIS

Essentials of Diagnosis

- Asymptomatic to severe respiratory symptoms with malaise, fever, cough, and chest pain.
- Ulceration of naso- and oropharynx.
- Hepatomegaly, splenomegaly, and lymphadenopathy.
- Anemia and leukopenia.
- Diarrhea in children.
- Positive skin test; positive serologic findings; small budding fungus cells found within reticuloendothelial cells; culture confirms diagnosis.

General Considerations

Histoplasmosis is caused by *Histoplasma capsulatum,* a fungus which has been isolated from soil in endemic areas (central and eastern United States, eastern Canada, Mexico, Central America, South America, Africa, and Southeast Asia). Infection takes place presumably by inhalation of spores or mycelial fragments. These convert into small budding cells which are engulfed by phagocytic cells in the lungs. The organism proliferates and may be carried by the blood to other areas of the body.

Clinical Findings

A. Symptoms and Signs: Most cases of histoplasmosis are asymptomatic or mild and so are unrecognized. Past infection is recognized by the development of a positive histoplasmin skin test and occasionally by pulmonary and splenic calcification. Symptomatic infections may present mild influenza-like characteristics, often lasting 1–4 days. Signs and symptoms of pulmonary involvement are usually absent even in patients who subsequently show areas of calcification on chest x-ray. Moderately severe infections are frequently diagnosed as atypical pneumonia. These patients have fever, cough, and mild chest pain lasting 5–15 days. Physical examination is usually negative. X-ray findings are variable and nonspecific.

Severe infections have been divided into 3 groups: (1) Acute histoplasmosis frequently occurs in epidemics. It is a severe disease with marked prostration, fever, and occasional chest pain, but no particular symptoms relative to the lungs even when x-rays show severe disseminated pneumonitis. The illness may last from 1 week to 6 months, but is almost never fatal. (2) Acute progressive histoplasmosis is usually fatal within 6 weeks or less. Symptoms usually consist of fever, dyspnea, cough, loss of weight, and prostration. Diarrhea is usually present in children. Ulcers of the mucous membranes of the oral pharynx may be present. The liver and spleen are nearly always enlarged, and all the organs of the body are involved. (3) Chronic progressive histoplasmosis may continue for years. It is usually seen in older patients in whom it has been mistaken for tuberculosis. The lungs show chronic progressive changes, often with cavities. The disease closely resembles chronic tuberculosis, and occasionally the patient has both diseases. Chronic histoplasmosis appears to be primarily confined to the lungs, but all organs of the body are involved in the terminal stage.

B. Laboratory Findings: In the moderately to severely ill patient the sedimentation rate is elevated. Leukopenia is present, with a normal differential count or neutropenia. Most patients with progressive disease show a progressive hypochromic anemia. Complement-fixing antibodies can be demonstrated, and a change in titer is of use in prognosis.

Treatment

There is no specific therapy. Bed rest and supportive care are indicated for the primary form. Normal activities should not be resumed until fever has subsided. Resection of lung tissue containing cavities has been useful. Amphotericin B (as for coccidioidomycosis) has proved useful for some patients with progressive histoplasmosis. Some children and adults with milder forms of acute primary or early chronic pulmonary disease respond to sulfadiazine therapy.

Prognosis

The prognosis is excellent for primary pulmonary histoplasmosis; only fair in localized infection; and poor in untreated generalized infection.

Smith JW, Utz JP: Progressive disseminated histoplasmosis. Ann Int Med 76:557, 1972.

Sutliff WD: Histoplasmosis cooperative study. V. Amphotericin B dosage for chronic pulmonary histoplasmosis. Am Rev Resp Dis 105:60, 1972.

Vanek J, Schwartz J: The gamut of histoplasmosis. Am J Med 50:89, 1971.

CRYPTOCOCCOSIS

Cryptococcosis, a chronic disseminated infection which frequently involves the CNS, is caused by *Cryptococcus neoformans*. This is an encapsulated, budding, yeast-like fungus which has been found in soil and in pigeon nests. Human infection is world-wide.

It is believed that most infections are acquired by inhalation. In the lung the infection may remain localized, heal, or disseminate. Upon dissemination lesions may form in any part of the body, but involvement of the CNS is most common and is the usual cause of death. Generalized meningoencephalitis occurs more frequently than localized granuloma in the brain or spinal cord. Solitary localized lesions may develop in the skin and rarely in the bones and other organs.

Cryptococcosis was at one time believed to be invariably fatal, but some cases (especially pulmonary) of spontaneous resolution have been reported. The incidence of fatal cases, on the other hand, is increasing as a result of increased numbers of infections in susceptible debilitated individuals.

In pulmonary cryptococcosis there are no specific signs or symptoms, and many patients are nearly asymptomatic. The patient may present a subacute respiratory infection with low-grade fever, pleural pain, and cough. There may be sputum production. Physical examination usually reveals signs of bronchitis or pulmonary consolidation. X-rays commonly show a solitary, moderately dense infiltration in the lower half of the lung field, with little or no hilar enlargement. More diffuse pneumonic infiltration, also in the lower lung fields, or extensive peribronchial infiltration or miliary lesions, may also occur.

CNS involvement usually presents a history of recent upper respiratory or pulmonary infection. Increasingly painful headache is usually the first and most prominent symptom. Vertigo, nausea, anorexia, ocular disorders, and mental deterioration develop. Nuchal rigidity is present, and Kernig's and Brudzinski's signs are positive. Patellar and Achilles reflexes are often diminished or absent.

Cutaneous lesions are variable in appearance. Acneiform lesions are more commonly seen. These enlarge slowly and ulcerate, often coalescing with other lesions to cover a large area. Bone lesions are painful, and the area is often swollen. Eye involvement may result from direct extension along the subarachnoid space into the optic nerve.

A mild anemia, leukocytosis, and increased sedimentation rate are found. Spinal fluid findings include increased pressure, many white cells (usually lymphocytes), budding encapsulated fungus cells, increased protein and globulin, and decreased sugar and chlorides. The organism is seen in an India ink preparation.

There is no specific therapy for cryptococcosis. Amphotericin B (as for coccidioidomycosis) and flucytosine (Ancobon), 150 mg/kg/day orally, have been successful in some cases. For cryptococcal meningitis, combined therapy must be used to prevent failure due to emergence of flucytosine resistance. Cisternal or Ommaya reservoir (ventricular) amphotericin B therapy has been used. Surgical resection of pulmonary granulomas has been successful.

Lewis JL, Rabinovich S: The wide spectrum of cryptococcal infections. Am J Med 53:315, 1972.

Utz JP: Flucytosine. New England J Med 286:777, 1972.

NORTH AMERICAN BLASTOMYCOSIS

Blastomyces dermatitidis causes this chronic systemic fungus infection. The disease occurs more often in men and in a geographically delimited area of central and eastern United States and Canada. A few cases have been found in Mexico, South America, and Africa.

Mild or asymptomatic cases have not been found. When dissemination takes place, lesions are most frequently seen on the skin, in bones, and in the CNS, although any or all organs of the body may be attacked.

Little is known concerning the mildest pulmonary phase of this disease. Cough, moderate fever, dyspnea, and chest pain are evident in symptomatic patients. These may disappear or may progress to a marked degree with bloody and purulent sputum production, pleurisy, fever, chills, loss of weight, and prostration. Radiologic studies usually reveal massive densities projecting irregularly from the mediastinal nodes, which are markedly enlarged. Raised, verrucous cutaneous lesions which have an abrupt downward sloping border are usually present in disseminated blastomycosis. The surface is covered with miliary pustules. The border extends slowly, leaving a central atrophic scar. In some patients only cutaneous lesions are found. These may persist untreated for long periods, with a gradual decline in the patient's health. Bones—often the ribs and vertebrae—are frequently involved. These lesions appear both destructive and proliferative on x-ray. Symptoms referable to CNS involvement appear in about one-third of cases. The viscera may be invaded, but rarely the gastrointestinal tract.

Laboratory findings usually include leukocytosis, hypochromic anemia, and elevated sedimentation rate. The organism is found in clinical specimens as a 5–20 μm, thick-walled cell which may have a single bud. It grows readily on culture. Complement-fixing antibody titer is variable but useful for prognosis.

There is no specific therapy for blastomycosis. Amphotericin B (as for coccidioidomycosis) appears to be the best drug available for treatment. Surgical procedures may be successful for the removal of cutaneous lesions, persistent cavities, or other localized pulmonary lesions.

Careful follow-up for early evidence of relapse should be made for several years so that amphotericin B therapy may be resumed or instituted in those cases which were initially treated with the less toxic 2-hydroxystilbamidine. Patients whose disease is limited to localized cutaneous lesions have the best prognosis in that they show a better immunologic response to their infection.

Busey JF: Blastomycosis. 3. A comparative study of 2-hydroxy-stilbamidine and amphotericin B therapy. Am Rev Resp Dis 105:812, 1972.

Sarosi GA & others: Clinical features of acute pulmonary blastomycosis. New England J Med 290:540, 1974.

SOUTH AMERICAN BLASTOMYCOSIS
(Paracoccidioidomycosis)

Paracoccidioides brasiliensis infections have been found only in patients who have resided in South or Central America and Mexico.

Ulceration of the naso- and oropharynx is usually the first symptom. Papules ulcerate and enlarge both peripherally and deeper into the subcutaneous tissue. Extensive coalescent ulcerations may eventually result in destruction of the epiglottis, vocal cords, and uvula. Extension to the lips and face may occur. Eating and drinking are extremely painful. Skin lesions, usually on the face, may occur. Variable in appearance, they may have a necrotic central crater with a hard hyperkeratotic border. Lymph node enlargement always follows mucocutaneous lesions, eventually ulcerating and forming permanent draining sinuses. Lymph node enlargement may be the presenting symptom, with subsequent suppuration and rupture through the skin. In some patients gastrointestinal disturbances are first noted. Although the liver and spleen become enlarged, there is a lack of specific gastrointestinal symptoms. Cough, sometimes with sputum, indicates pulmonary involvement, but the signs and symptoms are often mild, even though x-ray findings indicate severe parenchymatous changes in the lungs.

The extensive ulceration of the entire gastrointestinal tract prevents sufficient intake and absorption of food. Most patients become cachectic early. Death usually results from associated malnutrition.

Laboratory findings include elevated sedimentation rate, leukocytosis with a neutrophilia showing a shift to the left, and sometimes eosinophilia and monocytosis. Serologic results are variable. A high titer usually indicates progressive disease; a descending titer is a favorable sign. The fungus is found in clinical specimens as a spherical cell which may have many buds arising from it. Colonial and cellular morphology are typical on culture.

The prognosis for South American blastomycosis has been poor. Amphotericin B (as for coccidioidomycosis) has been used recently with considerable success. Sulfadiazine and triple sulfonamides in daily doses of 2–4 gm have been used for control, and occasional cures have been reported following months or years of therapy. Relapses are frequent when the drug is stopped. Drug toxicity with prolonged high dosage is common. Rest and supportive care are of value in promoting a favorable immunologic response.

Londero AT, Ramos CD: Paracoccidioidomycosis: A clinical and mycologic study of 41 cases in Santa Maria, Brazil. Am J Med 52:771, 1972.

Murray HW & others: Disseminated paracoccidioidomycosis (South American blastomycosis) in the United States. Am J Med 56:209, 1974.

CANDIDIASIS

Candida albicans may be cultured from the mouth, vagina, and feces of about 65% of the population. It is more frequent in debilitated individuals. Thrush, vaginitis, cutaneous lesions (frequently in intertriginous areas), onychia, and paronychia are common. These are discussed elsewhere in this book. Systemic infection is usually found in patients with a history of other pulmonary disorders, diabetes mellitus, or general debilitation, or in those who have undergone prolonged antibiotic therapy. *Candida albicans* is a frequent secondary invader in other types of infection.

Systemic infection is of 2 types. Endocarditis, which almost always affects previously damaged heart valves, usually follows heart surgery or inoculation by contaminated needles or catheters. Splenomegaly and petechiae are usual, and emboli are common. In the other type of systemic infection the kidneys, myocardium, and brain are the usual sites of infection; this type frequently follows antibiotic and glucocorticosteroid therapy for serious debilitating disease. Upper gastrointestinal tract candidiasis is frequently the portal of entry. Splenomegaly and petechiae are rare. Fungiuria is usual in renal disease; however, especially in older persons, Candida organisms can be found in the bladder or as a urethral saprophyte.

It is doubtful if primary bronchial or pulmonary infection occurs. Infection in these areas is nearly always superimposed on other serious underlying disease.

Candida albicans is seen as gram-positive budding cells (2.5–6 μm) and as a pseudomycelium. It grows readily in culture. It is the most common cause of systemic disease, but *C tropicalis* and *Torulopsis glabrata* are not uncommon. Many species may cause endocarditis.

Intravenous administration of amphotericin B (as for coccidioidomycosis) is necessary in serious systemic infections. When combined with flucytosine (Ancobon), 150 mg/kg/day orally, lower doses of this toxic drug may be used and still prevent emergence of resistant organisms. Associated oral, gastrointestinal, and cutaneous lesions should be treated with amphotericin B or nystatin mouthwash, tablets (500,000 units 3 times daily), and lotions. Gentian violet, 1%, in 10–20% alcohol, is also effective for oral, cutaneous, and vaginal lesions. Antibiotic therapy should be discontinued if possible. The correction of underlying factors may be sufficient to control candidiasis without specific therapy. All patients with candidiasis should be carefully examined for diabetes mellitus.

Response to chemotherapy is poor in endocarditis. Valve replacement is usually necessary. In other systemic infections the prognosis is generally good if the underlying predisposing factors are corrected.

Eilard T & others: Treatment of disseminated candidiasis with 5-fluorocytosine. J Infect Dis 130:155, 1974.

Kay JH & others: Surgical treatment of Candida endocarditis. JAMA 203:621, 1968.

Louria DB: Pathogenesis of candidiasis. Pages 417–426 in: *Antimicrobial Agents and Chemotherapy, 1965.* Williams & Wilkins, 1966.

NOCARDIOSIS*

Nocardia asteroides causes pulmonary and systemic nocardiosis. Other species of Nocardia are discussed in the section on mycetoma. The majority of patients with nocardiosis have serious underlying disorders, especially lymphoma, leukemia, and other neoplastic diseases.

Pulmonary involvement usually begins with malaise, loss of weight, fever, and night sweats. Cough and production of purulent sputum are the chief complaints. X-ray shows massive areas of consolidation, usually at the base of both lungs. Small areas of rarefaction caused by abscess formation within these consolidated masses may lead to multiple cavities. The lesions may penetrate to the exterior through the chest wall, invading the ribs. Pleural adhesions are common.

Dissemination may involve any organ. Lesions in the brain or meninges are most frequent, and such dissemination may occur following any minor pulmonary symptoms. Dissemination is common in debilitated patients.

An increased sedimentation rate and leukocytosis with increase in neutrophils are found in systemic nocardiosis. *N asteroides* is usually found as delicate, branching, gram-positive filaments which may be partially acidfast. Identification is made by culture.

Nocardiosis generally responds to sulfisoxazole in a dosage sufficient to maintain a serum level of about 10 mg/100 ml (1–2 gm every 6 hours orally). Sensitivity tests should be used to determine the appropriate antibiotic, which should be administered concurrently in large dosage. Response is slow, and therapy should be continued for months after all clinical manifestations have disappeared. Surgical procedures such as drainage and resection may be imperative.

The prognosis for systemic nocardiosis is poor when diagnosis and therapy are delayed.

Orfanakis MG & others: In vitro studies of the combined effect of ampicillin and sulfonamides on *Nocardia asteroides* and results of therapy in four patients. Antimicrob Agents Chemother 1:215, 1972.

ACTINOMYCOSIS*

Actinomyces israelii and other species of Actinomyces occur in the normal flora of the mouth and

*Included in this chapter by convention since these organisms were thought for many years to be fungi.

tonsillar crypts. They are anaerobic, gram-positive, branching filamentous bacteria (1 μm in diameter) which readily fragment into bacillary forms. In diseased tissue, these filaments are seen as a compact mass called a "sulfur granule." When introduced into traumatized tissue and associated with other anaerobic bacteria, these actinomyces become pathogens. Hard, indurated, granulomatous, suppurative lesions develop which give rise to sinus tracts.

The most common site of infection is the cervicofacial area (about 60% of cases), and infection typically follows extraction of a tooth or other trauma. Lesions may develop in the gastrointestinal tract or lungs following ingestion or aspiration of the fungus from its endogenous source in the mouth.

Cervicofacial actinomycosis develops slowly. The area becomes markedly indurated and the overlying skin becomes reddish or cyanotic. The surface is irregular. Abscesses developing within and eventually draining to the surface persist for long periods. Sulfur granules may be found in the pus. There is usually little pain unless there is marked secondary infection. Trismus indicates that the muscles of mastication are involved. X-ray reveals eventual involvement of the bone with rarefaction as well as some proliferation of the underlying bone.

Abdominal actinomycosis usually causes pain in the ileocecal region, spiking fever and chills, intestinal colic, vomiting, and weight loss. Irregular masses in the ileocecal area or elsewhere in the abdomen may be palpated. Sinuses draining to the exterior may develop. X-ray may reveal the mass or enlarged viscera. Vertebrae and pelvic bones may be invaded.

Thoracic actinomycosis begins with fever, cough, and sputum production. The patient becomes weak, loses weight, may have night sweats and dyspnea. Pleural pain may be present. Dysphagia can result from mediastinal involvement. Multiple sinuses may extend through the chest wall, to the heart, or into the abdominal cavity. Ribs may be involved. X-ray shows massive areas of consolidation, frequently at the bases of the lungs.

The sedimentation rate may be elevated in patients with progressive disease. Anemia and leukocytosis are usually present. The anaerobic, gram-positive organism may be demonstrated as a granule or as scattered branching gram-positive filaments in the pus. Anaerobic culture is necessary to distinguish Actinomyces species from Nocardia species. Specific identification by culture is necessary to avoid confusion with nocardiosis because specific therapy differs radically.

Penicillin G is the drug of choice. Ten to 20 million units are given via a parenteral route for 4–6 weeks. Continue treatment with penicillin V orally. Prolonged massive therapy is necessary in order to push effective levels of the drug into the abscesses where the organism is found. Sulfonamides may be added to the regimen, as well as streptomycin, which will control associated gram-negative organisms. Broadspectrum antibiotics should be considered only if sensitivity tests show that the organism is resistant to penicillin. Immediate amelioration of symptoms or prompt improvement cannot be expected because of the chronic nature of this disease. Therapy should be continued for weeks to months after clinical manifestations have disappeared in order to ensure cure. Surgical procedures such as drainage and resection are of great benefit.

With penicillin and surgery, the prognosis is good. The difficulties of diagnosis, however, may permit extensive destruction of tissue before therapy is started.

Eastridge CE & others: Actinomycosis: A 24-year experience. South MJ 65:839, 1972.

SPOROTRICHOSIS

Sporotrichosis is a chronic fungal infection caused by *Sporothrix schenkii*. It is world-wide in distribution; most patients are people whose occupation brings them in contact with soil, plants, or decaying wood. Infection takes place when the organism is introduced by trauma into the skin, often on the hand, arm, or foot.

The most common form of sporotrichosis begins with a hard, nontender subcutaneous nodule. This later becomes adherent to the overlying skin, ulcerates (chancriform), and may persist for a long time. Within a few days to weeks, similar nodules usually develop along the lymphatics draining this area, and these may ulcerate. The lymphatic vessels become indurated and are easily palpable. The infection usually ceases to spread before the regional lymph nodes are invaded, and blood-borne dissemination is rare. The general health of the patient is not affected. Some patients complain of considerable pain. Skin infection may not spread through the lymphatics but may appear only as warty or papular, scaly lesions which may become pustular.

Pulmonary sporotrichosis presents no characteristic findings. Patients may be asymptomatic although pleural effusion, hilar adenopathy, fibrosis, caseous nodularity, and cavitation have been reported.

Disseminated sporotrichosis presents a picture of multiple, hard subcutaneous nodules scattered over the body. These become soft but rarely rupture spontaneously. Lesions may also develop in the bones, joints, muscles, and viscera.

There are no specific laboratory findings. Cultures are necessary to establish the diagnosis. A skin test with heat-killed vaccine or sporotrichin is positive.

Potassium iodide taken orally in increasing dosage promotes rapid healing, although the drug is not fungicidal. Give as the saturated solution, 5 drops 3 times a day, after meals, increasing by 1 drop per dose until 40 drops 3 times a day are being given. Continue until signs of the active disease have disappeared. The dosage is then decreased by 1 drop per dose until 5 drops are being given, and then is discontinued. Care must be taken to reduce the dosage if signs of iodism appear.

Amphotericin B intravenously (as for coccidioidomycosis) has been effective in systemic infection. Surgery is usually contraindicated except for simple aspiration of secondary nodules.

The prognosis is good for all forms of sporotrichosis except the disseminated type, when decreased natural resistance probably plays a role.

Park CH & others: Cutaneous sporotrichosis. Am J Clin Path 57:23, 1972.

CHROMOBLASTOMYCOSIS

Chromoblastomycosis is a chronic, principally tropical fungal infection caused by several species of closely related fungi having a dark mycelium (Cladosporium [Hormodendrum] spp and Phialophora sp). In nature these fungi grow as filamentous saprophytes in soil and on decaying vegetation.

The disease progresses slowly before the development of clinically characteristic lesions.

Lesions occur most frequently on a lower extremity, but may occur on the hands, arms, and elsewhere. The lesion begins as a papule or ulcer. Over a period of months to years the lesions enlarge to become vegetating, papillomatous, verrucous, elevated nodules with a cauliflower-like appearance or wide-spread dry verrucous plaques. The latter lesions spread peripherally with a raised, verrucous border leaving central atrophic scarring. The surface of the active border contains minute abscesses. Satellite lesions may appear along the lymphatics. There may be extensive secondary bacterial infection with a resulting foul odor. Some patients complain of itching. Elephantiasis may result if there is marked fibrosis and lymph stasis in the limb.

The fungus is seen as brown, thick-walled, spherical, sometimes septate cells in pus. The type of spore formation found in culture determines the species.

Both flucytosine (Ancobon), 150 mg/kg/day orally, and thiabendazole (Mintezol), 25 mg/kg/day orally, have proved effective. Surgical excision and skin grafting may be useful.

The prognosis is favorable if the disease is diagnosed and treated in its early stages.

Bayles MAH: Chromomycosis: Treatment with thiabendazole. Arch Dermat 104:476, 1971.

Mauceri A: Flucytosine: An effective oral treatment for chromomycosis. Arch Dermat 109:873, 1974.

MYCETOMA
(Maduromycosis & Actinomycotic Mycetoma)

Maduromycosis is the term used to describe mycetoma caused by the true fungi. Actinomycotic mycetoma is caused by Nocardia and Streptomyces sp. The many species of causative fungi are found in soil. Organisms are introduced by trauma in barefoot people. Mycetoma may occur on the hand and other parts of the body also. With time, the subcutaneous lesions develop sinuses which drain to the surface as well as deep into muscle and bone. The fungus is compacted into a granule which drains out in the pus.

The disease begins as a papule, nodule, or abscess which over months to years progresses slowly to form multiple abscesses and sinus tracts ramifying deep into the tissue. The entire area becomes indurated, and the skin becomes discolored. Open sinuses or atrophic scars are scattered over its surface. Secondary bacterial infection may result in large open ulcers. When x-rayed, destructive changes are seen in the underlying bone. Extensive fibrosis in the tissue causes elephantiasis. Pain is not a serious complaint until the disease is far advanced.

The fungus occurs as white, yellow, red, or black granules in the tissue or pus. Microscopic examination assists in the diagnosis. The granules of nocardia and streptomyces consist of delicate, gram-positive branching filaments 1 μm in diameter. Maduromycosis caused by the true fungi has granules consisting of hyphae 5 μm in diameter interspersed with large thick-walled chlamydospores.

The prognosis is good for patients with actinomycotic mycetoma since they usually respond well to sulfonamides and sulfones, especially if treated early. Give sulfisoxazole (Gantrisin) or triple sulfonamides, 4–5 gm daily, and increase to 10–12 gm daily if the patient is able to tolerate this dosage. Dapsone (Avlosulfon), 100 mg twice daily after meals, or other sulfones have been reported to be effective. All of these medications must be taken for long periods of time and continued for several months after clinical cure to prevent a relapse. Surgical procedures such as drainage assist greatly in healing.

There is no specific therapy for maduromycosis, and at present the prognosis is poor. Sulfones have been reported to be effective in isolated cases. Surgical excision of early lesions may prevent spread. Amputation is necessary in far-advanced cases.

Zaias N & others: Mycetoma. Arch Dermat 99:215, 1969.

OPPORTUNISTIC FUNGUS INFECTIONS

Debilitating diseases and often the drugs used in their treatment (corticosteroids, antibiotics, antimetabolites), as well as pregnancy and other altered physiologic states, may render a patient susceptible to invasion by many species of fungi which ordinarily are unable to cause disease. These factors may also cause infections due to the pathogenic fungi to be more serious.

The term **phycomycosis** (mucormycosis) is applied to infections caused by members of the genera Mucor, Absidia, Rhizopus, Mortierella, and Basidiobolus. These appear in tissue as broad, branching, nonseptate hyphae which may show a special affinity for blood vessels. Sinus, orbit, brain, lung, and digestive tract infections are often associated with diabetic acidosis. Control of the diabetic condition and antifungal therapy initiated early are essential. Amphotericin B (as for coccidioidomycosis), potassium iodide (as for sporotrichosis), nystatin, and surgery have been successful, but the prognosis is generally poor.

Aspergillosis may be caused by various species of Aspergillus. The colonization of an ectatic bronchus to form a compact mass of mycelium ("fungus ball") is usually associated with some immunity, and the fungus rarely adheres or penetrates the wall of the bronchus. A pulmonary toilet regimen appears as effective as intravenous amphotericin B therapy for patients with aspergillus-colonized cavities. *Aspergillus fumigatus* causes more serious infections. It invades necrotic tissue or pulmonary cavities produced by other causes, sometimes with subsequent radial extension into surrounding tissue and eventual hematogenous dissemination. The prognosis is poor although amphotericin B has been used successfully in some cases.

Aspergillus is recognized in tissue and sputum as dichotomously branched, septate hyphae. Spores may be formed in pulmonary cavities.

Mycotic keratitis has been caused by many species of normally saprophytic fungi. Trauma to the cornea followed by steroid and antibiotic therapy is the predisposing factor in most cases. Prompt withdrawal of corticosteroids, removal of the infected necrotic tissue, and application of fungicidal agents are essential for management.

Burton JR & others: Aspergillosis in four renal transplant recipients: Diagnosis and effective treatment with amphotericin B. Ann Int Med 77:383, 1972.

Hammerman KJ & others: Amphotericin B in the treatment of saprophytic forms of pulmonary aspergillosis. Am Rev Resp Dis 109:57, 1974.

SYSTEMIC ANTIFUNGAL AGENTS*

AMPHOTERICIN B
(Fungizone)

Amphotericin, derived from *Streptomyces nodosus,* is active against a wide variety of fungi causing systemic mycoses and is indicated in severe systemic fungal infections.

This toxic drug is given intravenously in doses rising from 5 mg/day to 25–65 mg/day. (See p 910 for details and precautions.) Fever, nausea, nephrotoxic reactions, and electrolyte disturbances are common side-effects that can be managed to some extent by administering aspirin, corticosteroids, and phenothiazines.

Bennett JE: Chemotherapy of systemic mycoses. (2 parts.) New England J Med 290:30, 320, 1974.

NYSTATIN
(Mycostatin)

Nystatin is used topically in candida infections. See p 910.

*Griseofulvin: See pp 56 and 910.

28 . . .
Anti-infective Chemotherapeutic & Antibiotic Agents

Ernest Jawetz

Some Rules for Antimicrobial Therapy

Antimicrobial drugs are used on a very large scale, and their proper use gives striking therapeutic results. On the other hand, they can create serious complications and should therefore be administered only upon proper indication.

Drugs of choice and second-line drugs are presented in Table 28–4.

The following steps merit consideration in each patient.

A. Etiologic Diagnosis: Formulate an etiologic diagnosis based on clinical observations. Microbial infections are best treated early. Therefore, the physician must attempt to decide on clinical grounds (1) whether the patient has a microbial infection that can probably be influenced by antimicrobial drugs, and (2) the most probable kind of microorganisms causing this type of infection.

B. "Best Guess": Select a specific antimicrobial drug on the basis of past experience (personal or in the literature). Based on a "best guess" about the probable cause of the patient's infection, the physician should choose a drug that is likely to be effective against the suspected microorganism.

C. Laboratory Control: Before beginning antimicrobial drug treatment, obtain meaningful specimens for laboratory examination to determine the causative infectious organism and, if desirable, its susceptibility to antimicrobial drugs.

D. Clinical Response: Based on the clinical response of the patient, evaluate the laboratory reports and consider the desirability of changing the antimicrobial drug regimen. Laboratory results should not automatically overrule clinical judgment. The isolation of an organism that reinforces the initial clinical impression is a useful confirmation. Conversely, laboratory results may contradict the initial clinical impression and may force its reconsideration. If the specimen was obtained from a site which is normally devoid of bacterial flora and not exposed to the external environment (eg, blood, CSF, pleural fluid, joint fluid), the recovery of a microorganism is a significant finding even if the organism recovered is different from the clinically suspected etiologic agent and may force a change in antimicrobial treatment. On the other hand, the isolation of unexpected microorganisms from the respiratory tract, gut, or surface lesions (sites that have a complex flora) must be critically evaluated before drugs are abandoned which were judiciously selected on the basis of an initial "best guess."

E. Drug Sensitivity Tests: Some microorganisms are fairly uniformly susceptible to certain drugs; if such organisms are isolated from the patient, they need not be tested for drug susceptibility. For example, pneumococci, group A hemolytic streptococci, and clostridia respond predictably to penicillin. On the other hand, some kinds of microorganisms (eg, coliform gram-negative rods) are sufficiently variable in their response to warrant drug susceptibility testing whenever they are isolated from a significant specimen.

Antimicrobial drug susceptibility tests (commonly called "disk tests") usually give valuable results. Occasionally there is a marked discrepancy between the results of the test and the clinical response of the patient. The following possible explanations (among others) of such discrepancies may have to be considered:

1. Failure to drain a collection of pus or to remove a foreign body.

2. Failure of a poorly diffusing drug to reach the site of infection (eg, joint cavity, pleural space) or to reach intracellular phagocytized bacteria.

3. Superinfection in the course of prolonged chemotherapy. After suppression of the original infection or of normal flora, a second type of microorganism may establish itself against which the originally selected drug is ineffective.

4. Emergence of drug-resistant mutants from a large microbial population.

5. Participation of 2 or more microorganisms in the infectious process of which only one was originally detected and used for drug selection.

F. Adequate Dosage: To determine whether the proper drug is being used in adequate dosage, a serum assay can be performed. Two days after a drug regimen is established, serum is obtained from the patient 1–2 hours after a drug dose. Dilutions of this serum are set up against the microorganism originally isolated from the patient's infection and the antibacterial activity estimated. If an adequate dose of a proper drug is being employed, the serum should be markedly bactericidal in vitro. In infections limited to the urinary tract, the antibacterial activity of urine can be estimated. In persons with renal insufficiency, the dose or

Table 28–1. Blood levels of some commonly used antibiotics at therapeutic dosages.

	Route	Daily Dose	Expected Concentration per ml Blood or per gm Tissue
Penicillin	IM	0.6–1 million units	1 unit
	Oral	0.6 million units	0.2 unit
Methicillin, nafcillin	IV	6–12 gm	5–30 µg
Cloxacillin, dicloxacillin	Oral	2–4 gm	3–12 µg
Ampicillin	Oral	2–3 gm	3–4 µg
	IV	4–6 gm	10–40 µg
Cephalothin	IV	8–12 gm	10–20 µg
Cefazolin	IM	2–4 gm	8–40 µg
Tetracyclines	Oral	2 gm	6–8 µg
Chloramphenicol	Oral	2 gm	8–10 µg
Erythromycin	Oral	2 gm	0.5–2 µg
Streptomycin	IM	1 gm	10–20 µg
Kanamycin	IM	1 gm	10–15 µg
Gentamicin	IM	0.3 gm	3–6 µg
Vancomycin	IV	2 gm	10–20 µg
Clindamycin	IM	2.4 gm	3–6 µg
Polymyxin B	IV	0.15 gm	1–3 µg
Colistin	IM	0.3 gm	2–5 µg

frequency of administration must be adjusted. This can sometimes be done by reference to dosage nomograms or rules; however, it is best to directly measure the drug level (Table 28–1) in the patient's serum, particularly in the case of drugs that can be oto-, nephro-, or neurotoxic when given at excessive levels.

G. Duration of Antimicrobial Therapy: Generally speaking, effective antimicrobial treatment results in reversal of the clinical and laboratory parameters of active infection and marked clinical improvement within a very few days. Treatment may, however, have to be continued for varying periods to effect cure. A few examples of timing are illustrative:

Streptococcal pharyngitis requires 10 days of effective penicillin levels to eradicate the organism. Acute uncomplicated gonorrhea can be eradicated in males by 24 hours of effective drug levels. Endocarditis caused by viridans streptococci is curable in 3 weeks; that caused by staphylococci usually requires 5–6 weeks of treatment. Little is gained by extending antimicrobial treatment for acute urinary tract infection beyond 10 days. Pneumococcal pneumonia and meningococcal meningitis require penicillin for only 3 days after complete defervescence.

In bacterial meningitis due to *Haemophilus influ-*

Table 28–2. Examples of incompatibilities between antimicrobial drugs and other agents.

Antimicrobial Drug	Other Agent	Results
In vitro incompatibilities when mixed for intravenous administration*		
Amphotericin B	Benzylpenicillin, tetracyclines, aminoglycosides	Precipitate
Cephalosporins	Calcium gluconate or calcium chloride, polymyxin B, erythromycin, tetracyclines	Precipitate
Chloramphenicol	Polymyxin B, tetracyclines, vancomycin, hydrocortisone, B complex vitamins	Precipitate
Gentamicin	Carbenicillin	Inactivation
Methicillin	Any acidic solution, tetracyclines	Inactivation in 6 hours
Nafcillin	Any acidic solution, B complex vitamins	Inactivation in 12 hours
Novobiocin	Aminoglycosides, erythromycins	Insoluble precipitate
Oxacillin	Any acidic solution, B complex vitamins	Inactivation in 12 hours
Penicillin G	Any acidic solution, B complex vitamins, amphotericin B, chloramphenicol, tetracyclines, vancomycin, metaraminol, phenylephrine, carbohydrate at pH > 8.0	Inactivation in 12 hours, precipitate
Polymyxin B	Cephalothin	Precipitate
Tetracyclines	Calcium-containing solutions, amphotericin B, cephalosporins, heparin, hydrocortisone, polymyxin B, chloramphenicol, any divalent cations, iron	Chelation, inactivation, precipitate
Vancomycin	Heparin, penicillins, hydrocortisone, chloramphenicol	Precipitate
Physiologic drug interactions		
Chloramphenicol	Phenytoin, tolbutamide, dicumarol, ethanol	Increased blood concentration of these drugs
Griseofulvin, rifampin	Anticoagulants	Decreased anticoagulant effect
Kanamycin, streptomycin, neomycin, gentamicin, polymyxins	Curare, anticoagulants	Increased curare effect Increased anticoagulant effect
Sulfonamides, chloramphenicol, tetracyclines, nalidixic acid	Anticoagulants	Increased anticoagulant effect (probably due to inhibition of intestinal flora, which produces vitamin K)
Sulfonamides	Sulfonylurea	Hypoglycemia
Sulfonamides (oral)	Methenamine (oral)	Insoluble HCOH-sulfonamide compound in urine

*Many other incompatibilities may occur.

enzae, effective antimicrobial drugs should be continued until the CSF glucose has returned almost to normal. Many months of treatment are required in mycobacterial infections.

To minimize untoward reactions from drugs and the likelihood of superinfection, treatment should be continued only as long as necessary to eradicate the infectious agent.

H. Adverse Reactions: The administration of antimicrobial drugs is commonly associated with untoward reactions. These fall into several groups. (1) Hypersensitivity: The most common hypersensitivity reactions are fever and skin rashes. Hematologic or hepatic disorders and anaphylaxis are rare. (2) Direct toxicity: Most common are nausea, vomiting, and diarrhea. More serious toxic reactions are impairment of renal, hepatic, or hematopoietic functions or damage to the 8th nerve. (3) Suppression of normal microbial flora and "superinfection" by drug-resistant microorgan-

isms, or continued infection with the initial pathogen through the emergence of drug-resistant mutants.

In each case, the physician must evaluate the desirability of continuing a given drug regimen against the risk of discontinuing it. He must evaluate the severity and prognosis of each untoward reaction and choose between continuing a probably offending drug and discontinuing the drug but risking uncontrolled infection. An effective antimicrobial drug regimen which evokes hypersensitivity reactions can sometimes be continued with the simultaneous use of corticosteroids. In the presence of impaired renal function, toxic accumulation of drugs is likely. Therefore, reduction in dosage or frequency of medication is often necessary in renal failure (Table 28–3).

I. Oral Antibiotics: The absorption of oral penicillins, tetracyclines, lincomycins, etc is impaired by food. Therefore, these oral drugs must be given between meals.

Table 28–3. Use of antibiotics in patients with renal failure.

	Principal Mode of Excretion or Detoxification	Approximate Half-Life in Serum		Proposed Dosage Regimen in Renal Failure		Significant Removal of Drug by Dialysis (H = Hemodialysis; P = Peritoneal Dialysis)
		Normal	Renal Failure*	Initial Dose†	Give Half of Initial Dose at Interval of	
Penicillin G	Tubular secretion	0.5 hour	6 hours	6 gm IV	8–12 hours	H, P no
Ampicillin	Tubular secretion	1 hour	8 hours	6 gm IV	8–12 hours	H yes, P no
Carbenicillin	Tubular secretion	1.5 hours	16 hours	4 gm IV	12–18 hours	H yes, P no
Methicillin	Tubular secretion	0.5 hour	6 hours	6 gm IV	8–12 hours	H, P no
Cephalothin	Tubular secretion	0.8 hour	8 hours	4 gm IV	18 hours	H, P yes
Cephalexin	Tubular secretion	1 hour	15 hours	2 gm orally	8–12 hours	H, P yes
Cefazolin	Tubular secretion and glomerular filtration	2 hours	30 hours	2 gm IM	24 hours	H, P no
Streptomycin	Glomerular filtration	2.5 hours	3–4 days	1 gm IM	3–4 days	H, P yes‡
Kanamycin	Glomerular filtration	3 hours	3–4 days	1 gm IM	3–4 days	H, P yes‡
Gentamicin	Glomerular filtration	2.5 hours	2–4 days	3 mg/kg IM	2–3 days	H, P yes‡
Vancomycin	Glomerular filtration	6 hours	6–9 days	1 gm IV	5–8 days	H, P no
Polymyxin B	Glomerular filtration	5 hours	2–3 days	2.5 mg/kg IV	3–4 days	P yes, H no
Colistimethate	Glomerular filtration	3 hours	2–3 days	5 mg/kg IM	3–4 days	P yes, H no
Tetracycline	Glomerular filtration	8 hours	3 days	1 gm orally or 0.5 gm IV	3 days	H, P no
Chloramphenicol	Mainly liver	3 hours	4 hours	1 gm orally or IV	8 hours	H, P poorly
Erythromycin	Mainly liver	1.5 hours	5 hours	1 gm orally or IV	8 hours	H, P poorly
Clindamycin	Glomerular filtration and liver	2.5 hours	4 hours	600 mg IV or IM	8 hours	H, P no

*Considered here to be marked by creatinine clearance of 10 ml/minute or less.
†For a 60 kg adult with a serious systemic infection. The "initial dose" listed is administered as an intravenous infusion over a period of 1–8 hours, or as 2 intramuscular injections during an 8-hour period, or as 2–3 oral doses during the same period.
‡Aminoglycosides are removed irregularly in peritoneal dialysis. Gentamicin is removed 60% in hemodialysis.

J. Intravenous Antibiotics: When an antibiotic must be administered intravenously (eg, for life-threatening infection or for maintenance of very high blood levels), the following cautions should be observed:

(1) Give in neutral solution (pH 7.0–7.2) of isotonic sodium chloride (0.9%) or dextrose (5%) in water.

(2) Give alone without admixture of any other drug in order to avoid chemical and physical incompatibilities (which can occur frequently).

(3) Administer by intermittent (every 2–6 hours) addition to the intravenous infusion to avoid inactivation (by temperature, changing pH, etc) and prolonged vein irritation from high drug concentration, which favors thrombophlebitis.

(4) The infusion site must be changed every 48 hours to reduce the chance of superinfection.

Bauer AW & others: Antibiotic susceptibility testing by a standardized single disc method. Am J Clin Path 45:493, 1966.

Bennett WM & others: A guide to drug therapy in renal failure. JAMA 230:1544, 1974.

Ericsson HM, Sherris JC: Antibiotic sensitivity testing. Acta path microbiol scandinav, Suppl 217, 1971.

Garrod LP, O'Grady F: *Antibiotics and Chemotherapy,* 4th ed. Livingstone, 1974.

Jawetz E: General principles of anti-infective therapy. Chap 48, pp 513–518, in: *Review of Medical Pharmacology,* 4th ed. Meyers FH, Jawetz E, Goldfien A. Lange, 1974.

Weinstein L: Common sense (clinical judgment) in the diagnosis and antibiotic therapy of etiologically undefined infections. P Clin North America 15:141, 1968.

Weinstein L, Dalton AC: Host determinants of response to antimicrobial agents. New England J Med 279:467, 524, 580, 1968.

Ziment I & others: Complications of antibiotic therapy. California Med 117:24, Nov 1972.

PENICILLINS

The penicillins comprise a large group of antimicrobial substances, some of which are natural products of molds and others semisynthetic compounds. They share a common chemical nucleus (6-aminopenicillanic acid) and a common mode of antibacterial action—the inhibition of cell wall mucopeptide (peptidoglycan) synthesis. The penicillins are in 1975 the most important and most widely applicable group of antibacterial drugs. They can be arranged according to several major criteria:

(1) Susceptibility to destruction by penicillinase (ie, hydrolysis by the β-lactamase of bacteria).

(2) Susceptibility to destruction by acid pH (ie, relative stability to gastric acid).

(3) Relative efficacy against gram-positive versus gram-negative bacteria.

Antimicrobial Activity

All penicillins have the same mechanism of anti-

bacterial action. They specifically inhibit the synthesis of bacterial cell walls which contain a complex mucopeptide (peptidoglycan). They inhibit the terminal cross-linking of linear glucopeptides ("transpeptidation") and thus prevent the formation of a rigid cell wall. This leads to lysis of the cell in an isotonic environment and to the formation of "cell wall deficient" forms (L forms, protoplasts) in a hypertonic environment. Most penicillins are much more active against gram-positive than against gram-negative bacteria, probably because of chemical differences in cell wall structure. Penicillins are inactive against bacteria which are not multiplying and thus form no new cell walls ("persisters").

One million units of penicillin G equal 0.6 gm. Other penicillins are prescribed in grams. A blood serum level of 0.01–1 μg/ml penicillin G or ampicillin is lethal for a majority of susceptible microorganisms; methicillin and isoxazolylpenicillins are 2–20% as active.

Resistance

Resistance to penicillins falls into 3 different categories.

(1) Certain bacteria (eg, some staphylococci, gram-negative bacteria) produce enzymes (penicillinases, β-lactamases) which destroy penicillin G, ampicillin, and others. The genetic control of this enzyme resides in a "plasmid" which is transmissible to other bacteria. Clinical penicillin resistance of staphylococci and of gram-negative organisms to ampicillin falls largely into this category.

(2) Certain bacteria are resistant to some penicillins although they do not produce enzymes destroying the drug. Clinical methicillin resistance falls into this category and may be due to cell wall change.

(3) Metabolically inactive organisms which make no new cell wall mucopeptide are temporarily resistant to penicillins. They can act as "persisters" and perpetuate infection during and after penicillin treatment. Cell wall deficient (L) forms are in this category.

Absorption, Distribution, & Excretion

After parenteral administration, absorption of most penicillins is complete and rapid. Because of the irritation and consequent local pain produced by the intramuscular injection of large doses, administration by the intravenous route (continuous infusion, or intermittent addition to a continuous drip) is often preferred. After oral administration, only a portion of the dose is absorbed—from 5–35%, depending upon acid stability, binding to foods, and the presence of buffers. In order to minimize binding to foods, oral penicillins should not be preceded or followed by food for at least 1 hour.

After absorption, penicillins are widely distributed in body fluids and tissues. This varies to some extent with the degree of protein binding exhibited by different penicillins. Penicillin G, methicillin, and ampicillin are moderately protein bound (depending upon the method of measurement, 30–60%), whereas the isoxazolylpenicillins are highly protein bound (90–98%). It is probable that intensive protein binding diminishes the amount of drug available for antibacterial action in vivo and thus delays a therapeutic response. With parenteral doses of 3–6 gm (5–10 million units) per 24 hours of penicillin G, injected by continuous infusion or divided intramuscular injections, average serum levels of the drug reach 1–10 units (0.6–6 μg)/ml. A rough relationship of 6 gm given parenterally per day, yielding serum levels of 1–6 μg/ml, also applies to other penicillins. Naturally, the highly serum bound isoxazolylpenicillins yield, on the average, lower levels of free drug than less strongly bound penicillins.

Special dosage forms of penicillin have been designed for delayed absorption to yield low blood and tissue levels for long periods. The outstanding example is benzathine penicillin G. After a single intramuscular injection of 1.5 gm (2.4 million units), serum levels in excess of 0.03 unit/ml are maintained for 10 days and levels in excess of 0.005 unit/ml for 3 weeks. The latter is sufficient to protect against beta-hemolytic streptococcal infection; the former to treat an established infection with these organisms. Procaine penicillin also has delayed absorption, yielding levels for 24 hours.

In many tissues, penicillin concentrations are equal to those in serum. Lower levels are found in the eye and CNS. However, with active inflammation of the meninges, as in bacterial meningitis, penicillin levels in the CSF exceed 0.2 μg/ml with a daily parenteral dose of 12 gm. Thus, pneumococcal and meningococcal meningitis may be treated with systemic penicillin, and intrathecal injection is contraindicated. Penetration into inflamed joints is likewise sufficient for treatment of infective arthritis caused by susceptible organisms.

Most of the absorbed penicillin is rapidly excreted by the kidneys into the urine; small amounts are excreted by other channels. About 10% of renal excretion is by glomerular filtration and 90% by tubular secretion, to a maximum of about 2 gm/hour in an adult. Tubular secretion can be partially blocked by probenecid (Benemid) to achieve higher systemic levels. Renal clearance is less efficient in the newborn, so that proportionately smaller doses result in higher systemic levels and are maintained longer than in the adult. Individuals with impaired renal function likewise tend to maintain higher penicillin levels longer.

Renal excretion of penicillin results in very high levels in the urine. Thus, systemic daily doses of 6 gm of penicillin may yield urine levels of 500–3000 μg/ml—enough to suppress not only gram-positive but also many gram-negative bacteria in the urine (provided they produce little β-lactamase).

Penicillin is also excreted into sputum and milk to levels of 3–15% of those present in the serum. This is the case in both man and cattle. The presence of penicillin in the milk of cows treated for mastitis presents a problem in allergy.

Indications, Dosages, & Routes of Administration

The penicillins are by far the most effective and the most widely used antimicrobial drugs. All oral penicillins must be given 1 hour away from meal times to reduce binding and acid inactivation. Blood levels of all penicillins can be raised by simultaneous administration of probenecid, 0.5 gm every 6 hours orally (10 mg/kg every 6 hours).

A. Penicillin G: This is the drug of choice for infections caused by gonococci, pneumococci, streptococci, meningococci, non-β-lactamase producing staphylococci, *Treponema pallidum* and many other spirochetes, *Bacillus anthracis* and other gram-positive rods, clostridia, and some listeria and bacteroides.

1. Intramuscular or intravenous—Most of the above-mentioned infections respond to aqueous penicillin G in daily doses of 0.6–5 million units (0.36–3 gm) administered by intermittent IM injection every 4–6 hours. Much larger amounts (6–120 gm daily) can be given by intermittent addition (every 4–6 hours) to an intravenous infusion in serious or complicated infections due to these organisms. Sites for such intravenous administration are subject to thrombophlebitis and superinfection and must be rotated every 2 days and kept scrupulously aseptic. In enterococcal endocarditis, an aminoglycoside is given simultaneously with large doses of penicillin or ampicillin.

2. Oral—Buffered penicillin G (or penicillin V) is indicated only in minor infections (eg, of the respiratory tract or its associated structures) in daily doses of 1–4 gm (1.6–6.4 million units). About one-fifth of the oral dose is absorbed, but oral administration is subject to so many variables that it should not be relied upon in seriously ill patients.

3. Intrathecal—With high serum levels of penicillin, adequate concentrations reach the CNS and CSF for the treatment of CNS infection. Therefore, and because injection of more than 10,000 units of penicillin G into the subdural space may cause convulsions, intrathecal injection has been virtually abandoned.

4. Topical—Penicillins have been applied to skin, wounds, and mucous membranes by compress, ointment, and aerosol. These applications are highly sensitizing and seldom warranted. Rarely, solutions of penicillin (eg, 100,000 units/ml) are instilled into joint or pleural space infected with susceptible organisms.

B. Benzathine Penicillin G: This penicillin is a salt of very low water solubility. It is injected intramuscularly to establish a depot which yields low but prolonged drug levels. A single injection of 2.4 million units IM is satisfactory for treatment of beta-hemolytic streptococcal pharyngitis and perhaps for early syphilis. An injection of 1.2–2.4 million units every 3–4 weeks provides satisfactory prophylaxis for rheumatics against reinfection with group A streptococci. There is no indication for using this drug by mouth. Procaine penicillin G is another repository form for maintaining drug levels for up to 24 hours. For highly susceptible infections, 300–600 thousand units IM are given once daily. For uncomplicated gonorrhea, 4.8 million units of procaine penicillin IM are given once with probenecid, 1 gm orally.

C. Ampicillin, Carbenicillin: These drugs differ from penicillin G in having greater activity against gram-negative bacteria, but, like penicillin G, they are destroyed by penicillinases.

Ampicillin is the drug of current choice for bacterial meningitis in small children, especially meningitis due to *H influenzae;* 250 mg/kg/day are injected IV. Some ampicillin-resistant *H influenzae* are emerging. Ampicillin can be given orally in divided doses, 2–3 gm daily, to treat urinary tract infections with coliform bacteria, enterococci, or *Proteus mirabilis.* It is ineffective against enterobacter and pseudomonas. In salmonella infections, ampicillin, 3–6 gm daily IV or orally, can be effective in suppressing clinical disease (alternative to chloramphenicol in acute typhoid or paratyphoid) and may eliminate salmonellae from some chronic carriers. In malnourished children, ampicillin, 100 mg/kg/day IM, was effective therapy for salmonellosis. Ampicillin is more effective than penicillin G against enterococci and may be used in such infections in combination with an aminoglycoside. Amoxicillin is similar to but better absorbed than ampicillin. Carbenicillin is more active against pseudomonas and proteus, but resistance emerges rapidly. Therefore, a combination of carbenicillin, 12–30 gm/day IV, with gentamicin is suggested in pseudomonas sepsis. Ticarcillin resembles carbenicillin. Hetacillin is converted in vivo to ampicillin and should not be used.

Indanyl carbenicillin, 2–4 gm orally, can be given in urinary tract infections due to some coliforms or pseudomonas.

D. Penicillinase-Resistant Penicillins: Methicillin, oxacillin, cloxacillin, dicloxacillin, nafcillin, and others are relatively resistant to destruction by β-lactamase. The only indication for the use of these drugs is infection by β-lactamase producing staphylococci.

1. Oral–Oxacillin, cloxacillin, dicloxacillin (the isoxazolylpenicillins), or nafcillin may be given in doses of 0.25–0.5 gm every 4–6 hours in mild or localized staphylococcal infections (50–100 mg/kg/day for children). Food must not be given in proximity to these doses because it interferes with absorption.

2. Intravenous–For serious systemic staphylococcal infections, methicillin, 8–12 gm, or nafcillin, 6–12 gm, is administered IV, usually by injecting 1–2 gm during 20–30 minutes every 2 hours into a continuous infusion of 5% dextrose in water or physiologic salt solution. The dose for children is methicillin, 100–300 mg/kg/day, or nafcillin, 50–100 mg/kg/day.

Adverse Effects

The penicillins undoubtedly possess less direct toxicity than any other antibiotics. Most of the serious side-effects are due to hypersensitivity.

A. Allergy: All penicillins are cross-sensitizing and cross-reacting. Any preparation containing penicillin may induce sensitization, including foods or cosmetics. In general, sensitization occurs in direct proportion to the duration and total dose of penicillin received in the past. The responsible antigenic determinants appear to be degradation products of penicillins, particularly penicilloic acid and products of alkaline hydrolysis (minor antigenic determinants) bound to host protein. Skin tests with penicilloyl-polylysine, with minor antigenic determinants, and with undegraded penicillin can identify many hypersensitive individuals. Among positive reactors to skin tests, the incidence of subsequent penicillin reactions is high. Although many persons develop IgG antibodies to antigenic determinants of penicillin, the presence of such antibodies is not correlated with allergic reactivity (except rare hemolytic anemia), and serologic tests have little predictive value. A history of a penicillin reaction in the past is not reliable; however, in such cases the drug should be administered with caution (airway, 0.1% epinephrine in syringe, competent personnel available, intravenous fluids running).

Allergic reactions may occur as typical anaphylactic shock, typical serum sickness type reactions (urticaria, fever, joint swelling, angioneurotic edema, intense pruritus, and respiratory embarrassment occurring 7–12 days after exposure), and a variety of skin rashes, oral lesions, fever, interstitial nephritis, eosinophilia, hemolytic anemia, other hematologic disturbances, and vasculitis. LE cells are sometimes found. The incidence of hypersensitivity to penicillin is estimated to 1–5% among adults in the USA but is negligible in small children. Acute anaphylactic life-threatening reactions are fortunately very rare (0.05%). Ampicillin produces maculopapular skin rashes 10 times more frequently than other penicillins, but some ampicillin rashes are not allergic in origin. Methicillin and other penicillins can induce nephritis with primary tubular lesions, associated with anti-basement membrane antibodies.

Individuals known to be hypersensitive to penicillin can at times tolerate the drug during corticosteroid administration. "Desensitization" with penicillin is rarely warranted.

B. Toxicity: Since the action of penicillin is directed against a unique bacterial structure, the cell wall, it is virtually without effect on animal cells. The toxic effects of penicillin G are due to the direct irritation caused by intramuscular or intravenous injection of exceedingly high concentrations (eg, 1 gm/ml). Such concentrations may cause local pain, induration, thrombophlebitis, or degeneration of an accidentally injected nerve. All penicillins are irritating to the CNS. There is no indication for intrathecal administration at present. In rare cases a patient receiving more than 50 gm of penicillin G daily parenterally has exhibited signs of cerebrocortical irritation, presumably as a result of the passage of unusually large amounts of penicillin into the CNS. With doses of this magnitude, direct cation toxicity (Na^+, K^+) can also occur. Potassium penicillin G contains 1.7 mEq of K^+ per million units (2.8 mEq/gm), and potassium may accumulate in the presence of renal failure. Carbenicillin contains 4.7 mEq of Na^+ per gram—a risk in heart failure.

Large doses of penicillins given orally may lead to gastrointestinal upset, particularly nausea and diarrhea.

Oral therapy may also be accompanied by luxuriant overgrowth of staphylococci, pseudomonas, proteus, or yeasts, which may occasionally cause enteritis. Superinfections in other organ systems may occur with penicillins as with any antibiotic therapy. Methicillin and isoxazolylpenicillins have occasionally caused granulocytopenia, especially in children. Carbenicillin can cause transaminase elevations in serum as well as granulocytopenia. Carbenicillin can also induce hemostatic defects leading to bleeding tendency.

Barrett FF & others: Methicillin-resistant *Staphylococcus aureus* at Boston City Hospital. New England J Med 279:441, 1968.

Border WA & others: Antitubular basement membrane antibodies in methicillin-associated interstitial nephritis. New England J Med 291:381, 1974.

Brown CH & others: The hemostatic defect produced by carbenicillin. New England J Med 291:265, 1974.

Grieco MH: Cross-allergenicity of the penicillins and the cephalosporins. Arch Int Med 119:141, 1967.

Parker CS: Drug allergy. New England J Med 292:511, 732, 957, 1975.

Rudolph AH, Price EV: Penicillin reactions among patients in venereal disease clinics. JAMA 223:499, 1973.

Study group: Prospective study of ampicillin rash. Brit MJ 1:7, 1973.

CEPHALOSPORINS

Cephalosporins are a group of compounds closely related to the penicillins. In place of 6-aminopenicillanic acid, cephalosporins have a nucleus of 7-aminocephalosporanic acid. The mode of action is the same as that of penicillins, there is some (limited) cross-allergenicity, and they are resistant to destruction by β-lactamase. New derivatives are appearing in profusion, but their merits are not well established.

Antimicrobial Activity

Cephalosporins inhibit the synthesis of bacterial cell wall mucopeptide in a fashion analogous to that of penicillins. They are resistant to destruction by β-lactamases, but they can be hydrolyzed by a cephalosporinase produced by certain microorganisms. The cephalosporins are bactericidal in vitro in concentrations of 1–20 μg/ml against most gram-positive microorganisms, except *Streptococcus faecalis*, and in concentrations of 5–30 μg/ml against many gram-negative bacteria, except pseudomonas, herellea, serratia, proteus, and enterobacter. Cephalosporins should not be used in bacterial meningitis. There is at least partial cross-resistance between cephalosporins and β-lactamase resistant penicillins. Thus, methicillin-resistant staphylococci are also resistant to cephalosporins.

Absorption, Distribution, & Excretion

Cephalothin, cephaloridine, cefazolin, and cephapirin are not significantly absorbed from the gut. After parenteral injection, they are distributed widely, and 40–80% of the drugs in serum are protein-bound. Concentrations in synovial fluid, CNS, and CSF are low after parenteral injection. Thus, cephalosporins should not be drugs of choice in meningitis. Excretion of cephalosporins is primarily by tubular secretion into the urine.

Urine levels may reach 200–1000 μg/ml. In the presence of impaired renal function, very high blood and tissue levels of cephalosporins may accumulate and exert toxic effects.

Cephaloglycine, cephalexin, and cephradine are somewhat better absorbed from the gut, and therapeutic urine levels are reached after oral doses. Concentrations in other tissues are marginal.

Indications, Dosages, & Routes of Administration

A. Oral: Cephaloglycine, 0.5 gm 4 times daily orally, yields urine concentrations of 50–500 μg/ml–sufficient for treatment of urinary tract infections due to coliform organisms. Cephalexin, 0.5 gm orally 4 times daily (50 mg/kg/day), can be used in urinary or respiratory tract infections due to susceptible organisms. Cephradine is similar.

B. Intravenous: Cephalothin, 6–12 gm daily (for children, 50–100 mg/kg/day) by continuous drip, gives serum concentrations of 5–20 μg/ml. This is adequate for the treatment of gram-negative bacteremia or staphylococcal sepsis, or as a substitute for penicillin in serious infections caused by susceptible organisms in persons allergic to penicillin (although some cross-hypersensitivity exists). Cephaloridine, 4 gm daily (for children, up to 100 mg/kg/day) IV, gives serum levels of 10–25 μg/ml. Cefazolin, 4 gm daily IV, gives higher levels but is more strongly (85%) protein-bound. The 2 drugs are used for the same indications.

C. Intramuscular: Cephaloridine or cefazolin, 0.5–1 gm IM every 6 hours, is used for the same indications as above in less severely ill patients. Cephalothin is too painful when injected intramuscularly.

Adverse Effects

A. Allergy: Cephalosporins are sensitizing and a variety of hypersensitivity reactions occur, including anaphylaxis, fever, skin rashes, nephritis, granulocytopenia, and hemolytic anemia. The question of cross-allergy between cephalosporins and penicillins remains controversial. However, most persons with documented hypersensitivity to penicillins tolerate cephalosporin treatment without hypersensitivity reaction.

B. Toxicity: Local pain after intramuscular injection, or thrombophlebitis after intravenous injection can occur. Cephaloridine can cause renal damage with tubular necrosis and uremia. Therefore, cefazolin will take its place.

Griffith RS, Black HR: Cephalexin. M Clin North America 54:1229, 1970.

Mandell GL: Cephaloridine. Ann Int Med 79:561, 1973.

Petz LD: Immunologic reactions of humans to cephalosporins. Postgrad MJ 47:64, 1971.

Regamey C & others: Cefazolin vs cephalothin and cephaloridine: A comparison of their clinical pharmacology. Arch Int Med 133:407, 1974.

ERYTHROMYCIN GROUP
(Macrolides)

The erythromycins are a group of closely related compounds characterized by a macrocyclic lactone ring to which sugars are attached. There are several different members of the group.

Erythromycins inhibit protein synthesis and are bacteriostatic or bactericidal for gram-positive organisms—especially pneumococci, streptococci, staphylococci, and corynebacteria—in concentrations of $0.02-2$ $\mu g/ml$. Neisseriae and mycoplasmas are also susceptible. Activity is enhanced at alkaline pH. Resistant mutants occur in microbial populations, including pneumococci and mycoplasmas, and tend to emerge during prolonged treatment. There is complete cross-resistance among all members of the erythromycin group. Absorption of these drugs varies greatly. Basic erythromycins are destroyed by stomach acids. Erythromycin stearate is acid-resistant. The propionyl ester of erythromycin (erythromycin estolate) and the triacetyl ester of oleandomycin are among the best absorbed oral preparations. Oral doses of 2 gm/day result in blood levels of up to 2 $\mu g/ml$, and there is wide distribution of the drug in all tissues except the CNS. Erythromycins are excreted largely in bile; only 5% of the dose is excreted into the urine.

Erythromycins are the drugs of choice in corynebacterial infections (diphtheria, diphtheroid sepsis, erythrasma) and in mycoplasmal pneumonia. They are most useful as substitutes for penicillin in persons with streptococcal and pneumococcal infections who are allergic to penicillin. In rheumatic persons taking penicillin, erythromycin can be given prior to dental procedures as prophylaxis.

Dosages

A. Oral: Erythromycin base, stearate, succinate, or estolate, or troleandomycin, 0.5 gm every 6 hours (for children, 40 mg/kg/day).

B. Intravenous: Erythromycin lactobionate or gluceptate, 0.5 gm every 12 hours.

Adverse Effects

Nausea, vomiting, and diarrhea may occur after oral intake. Erythromycin estolate or triacetyloleandomycin can produce acute cholestatic hepatitis (fever, jaundice, impaired liver function). Most patients recover completely. Upon readministration, the hepatitis promptly recurs. It is probably a hypersensitivity reaction.

Braun P: Hepatotoxicity of erythromycin. J Infect Dis 119:300, 1969.
Breese BB & others: Streptococcal infections of children. Am J Dis Child 128:457, 1974.
Griffith RS, Black HR: Erythromycin. M Clin North America 54:1199, 1970.

TETRACYCLINE GROUP

The tetracyclines are a large group of drugs with common basic chemical structures, antimicrobial activity, and pharmacologic properties. Microorganisms resistant to this group show complete cross-resistance to all tetracyclines.

Antimicrobial Activity

Tetracyclines are inhibitors of protein synthesis and are bacteriostatic for many gram-positive and gram-negative bacteria. They are strongly inhibitory for the growth of mycoplasmas, rickettsiae, chlamydiae (psittacosis-LGV-trachoma agents), and some protozoa (eg, amebas). Equal concentrations of all tetracyclines in blood or tissue have approximately equal antimicrobial activity. Such differences in activity as may be claimed for individual tetracycline drugs are of little practical importance. However, there are great differences in the susceptibility of different strains of a given species of microorganism, and laboratory tests are therefore important. Because of the emergence of resistant strains, tetracyclines have lost some of their former usefulness. Proteus and pseudomonas are regularly resistant; among coliform bacteria, bacteroides, pneumococci, staphylococci, and streptococci, resistant strains are increasingly common.

Absorption, Distribution, & Excretion

Tetracyclines are absorbed somewhat irregularly from the gut. Absorption is limited by the low solubility of the drugs and by chelation with divalent cations, eg, Ca^{++} or Fe^{++}. A large proportion of orally administered tetracycline remains in the gut lumen, modifies intestinal flora, and is excreted in feces. Of the absorbed drug, 40–80% is protein bound in the blood. With full systemic doses (2 gm/day), levels of active drug in serum reach $5-8$ $\mu g/ml$. The drugs are widely distributed in tissues and body fluids, but the levels in CNS, CSF, and joint fluids are only 3–10% of serum levels. Tetracyclines are specifically deposited in growing bones and teeth, bound to calcium. Technetium-labeled tetracycline concentrates in acute myocardial infarcts and can be used as a scan.

Absorbed tetracyclines are excreted mainly in bile and urine. Up to 20% of oral doses may appear in the urine after glomerular filtration. Urine levels may be $5-50$ $\mu g/ml$ or more. With renal failure, doses of tetracyclines must be reduced or intervals between doses increased. Up to 80% of an oral dose appears in the feces.

Demeclocycline, methacycline, minocycline, and doxycycline are well absorbed from the gut but are excreted more slowly than others. This may lead to accumulation and prolonged blood levels. Renal clearance ranges from 9 ml/minute for minocycline to 90 ml/minute for oxytetracycline. Doxycycline does not accumulate greatly in renal failure.

Indications, Dosages, & Routes of Administration

At present, tetracyclines are the drugs of choice in cholera, mycoplasmal pneumonia, infections with chlamydiae (psittacosis-LGV-trachoma), and infections with some rickettsiae. They may be used in various susceptible bacterial infections and in amebiasis. Minocycline is effective chemoprophylaxis of meningococcal disease (200 mg daily for 5 days).

A. Oral: Tetracycline hydrochloride, oxytetracycline, and chlortetracycline are dispensed in 250 mg capsules. Give 0.25–0.5 gm orally every 6 hours (for children, 20–40 mg/kg/day). In acne vulgaris, 0.25 gm once or twice daily for many months is prescribed by dermatologists.

Demeclocycline and methacycline are long-acting tetracyclines available in capsules containing 50 or 150 mg. Give 0.15–0.3 gm orally every 6 hours (for children, 12–20 mg/kg/day). Doxycycline and minocycline are available in capsules containing 50 or 100 mg or as powder for oral suspension. Give doxycycline, 100 mg every 12 hours on the first day and 100 mg/day for maintenance. Give minocycline, 200 mg for the first dose and then 100 mg every 12 hours.

B. Intramuscular or Intravenous: Several tetracyclines (eg, rolitetracycline) are formulated for intramuscular or intravenous injection. Give 0.1–0.5 gm every 6–12 hours in individuals unable to take oral medication (for children, 10–15 mg/kg/day).

C. Topical: Topical tetracycline, 1%, in ointment, can be applied to conjunctival infections.

Adverse Effects

A. Allergy: Hypersensitivity reactions with fever or skin rashes are uncommon.

B. Gastrointestinal Side-Effects: Gastrointestinal side-effects, especially diarrhea, nausea, and anorexia, are common. These can be diminished by reducing the dose or by administering tetracyclines with food or carboxymethylcellulose, but sometimes they force discontinuance of the drug. After a few days of oral use, the gut flora is modified so that drug-resistant bacteria and yeasts become prominent. This may cause functional gut disturbances, anal pruritus, and even enterocolitis with shock and death.

C. Bones and Teeth: Tetracyclines are bound to calcium deposited in growing bones and teeth, causing fluorescence, discoloration, enamel dysplasia, deformity, or growth inhibition. Therefore, tetracyclines should not be given to pregnant women or children under 6 years of age.

D. Liver Damage: Tetracyclines can impair hepatic function or even cause liver necrosis, particularly during pregnancy, in the presence of preexisting liver damage, or with doses of more than 3 gm IV.

E. Kidney Damage: Outdated tetracycline preparations have been implicated in renal tubular acidosis and other forms of renal damage. Tetracyclines may increase BUN when diuretics are administered.

F. Other: Tetracyclines, principally demeclocycline, may induce photosensitization, especially in blonds. Intravenous injection may cause thrombophlebitis, and intramuscular injection may induce local inflammation with pain. Minocycline induces vestibular reactions (dizziness, vertigo, nausea, vomiting) with a frequency of 35–70% after doses of 200–400 mg daily.

Devine LF & others: Minocycline in meningococcal carrier state. Am J Epidem 93:337, 1971.

Hoshiwara I & others: Doxycycline treatment of chronic trachoma. JAMA 224:220, 1973.

Kunin CM: The tetracyclines. P Clin North America 15:43, 1968.

CHLORAMPHENICOL

Chloramphenicol is a potent inhibitor of bacterial protein synthesis which inhibits the growth of many bacteria and rickettsiae in concentrations of 0.5–10 μg/ml. Resistant mutants that produce an enzyme which inactivates the drug are present in most susceptible species. There is no cross-resistance with other drugs.

After oral administration chloramphenicol is rapidly and completely absorbed. Administration of 2 gm/day orally to adults results in blood levels of 10 μg/ml. In children, chloramphenicol palmitate, 50 mg/kg/day orally, is hydrolyzed in the gut to yield free chloramphenicol and gives a blood level of 10 μg/ml. Chloramphenicol succinate, 25–50 mg/kg/day IM or IV, yields free chloramphenicol by hydrolysis and gives blood levels comparable to those achieved by oral administration. After absorption, chloramphenicol is widely distributed to all tissues, including the CNS and CSF. It penetrates cells readily. About 50% of drug in the serum is protein bound. Chloramphenicol is metabolized either by conjugation with glucuronic acid in the liver or by reduction to inactive aryl amines. In hepatic insufficiency, the drug may accumulate to toxic levels. Only 10% of active drug is excreted by glomerular filtration in the urine.

Because of its potential toxicity, chloramphenicol is at present a possible drug of choice only in the following cases: (1) Symptomatic salmonella infection, eg, typhoid fever. (*Note:* In Mexico in 1972, typhoid fever proved to be resistant to chloramphenicol.) (2) *Haemophilus influenzae* meningitis, laryngotracheitis, or pneumonia that does not respond to ampicillin. (3) Occasional gram-negative bacteremia. (4) Severe rickettsial infection. (5) Bacteroides or other anaerobic infections. (6) Meningococcal infection in patients hypersensitive to penicillin. (7) It is occasionally used topically in ophthalmology (0.5% solution).

In serious systemic infection, the dose is 0.5 gm orally every 4–6 hours (for children, 30–50 mg/kg/day) for 7–21 days. Similar amounts are given intravenously.

Adverse Effects

Nausea, vomiting, and diarrhea occur infrequently. The most serious adverse effects pertain to the hematopoietic system. Adults taking chloramphenicol in excess of 50 mg/kg/day regularly exhibit disturbances in red cell maturation after 1–2 weeks of blood levels above 25 μg/ml. There is anemia, rise in serum iron concentration, reticulocytopenia, and the appearance of vacuolated nucleated red cells in the bone marrow. These changes regress when the drug is stopped and are not related to the rare aplastic anemia.

Serious aplastic anemia is a rare consequence of chloramphenicol administration and represents a specific, probably genetically determined individual defect. It is not related to dose or time of intake but is seen more frequently with either prolonged or repeated use. It tends to be irreversible and fatal. It is estimated that fatal aplastic anemia occurs 13 times more frequently after the use of chloramphenicol than as a spontaneous occurrence. Hypoplastic anemia may be followed by the development of leukemia.

Chloramphenicol inhibits the metabolism of certain drugs. Thus, it may prolong the action and raise blood concentration of tolbutamide, diphenylhydantoin, or dicumarol.

Chloramphenicol is specifically toxic for newborns. Because they lack the mechanism for detoxification of the drug in the liver, the drug may accumulate, producing the highly fatal "gray syndrome" with vomiting, flaccidity, hypothermia, and collapse. Chloramphenicol should only rarely be used in infants, and the dose must be limited to less than 50 mg/kg/day in full-term infants and less than 30 mg/kg/day in prematures.

Ingall D, Sherman JD: Chloramphenicol. P Clin North America 15:57, 1968.
Wallerstein RO & others: Statewide study of chloramphenicol therapy and fatal aplastic anemia. JAMA 208:2045, 1969.

AMINOGLYCOSIDES

Aminoglycosides are a group of drugs with similar chemical, antimicrobial, pharmacologic, ototoxic, and nephrotoxic characteristics. Important members are streptomycin, neomycin, kanamycin, gentamicin, and tobramycin. All aminoglycosides inhibit microbial protein synthesis by attaching to the 30S unit of microbial ribosomes, causing progressive breakdown of polysomes, and causing a misreading of the genetic message. All aminoglycosides are much more active at alkaline pH than at acid pH.

1. STREPTOMYCIN

Streptomycin is a product of *Streptomyces griseus*. Dihydrostreptomycin was derived from it by chemical reduction, but it is no longer used because of serious ototoxicity. Streptomycin can be bactericidal for gram-positive and gram-negative bacteria and for *Mycobacterium tuberculosis*. Its antituberculosis activity is described below.

In all bacterial strains there are mutants which are 10–1000 times more resistant to streptomycin than the remainder of the microbial population. These are selected out rapidly in the presence of streptomycin. Treatment with streptomycin for 4–5 days thus results either in eradication of the infecting agent or the emergence of resistant infection which is untreatable with the drug. For this reason, streptomycin is usually employed in combination with another drug to delay the emergence of resistance. Streptomycin may enhance the bactericidal action of penicillins against streptococci, particularly *Streptococcus faecalis*.

Streptomycin is not significantly absorbed from the gut. After intramuscular injection, it is rapidly absorbed and widely distributed in body fluids and tissues except the CNS and CSF. Streptomycin does not penetrate well into living cells. Thus it is only slightly active against intracellular phagocytized bacteria and fails to eradicate those chronic infections in which most organisms are intracellular. With 2 gm given IM daily, serum levels reach 20 μg/ml.

Streptomycin is excreted mainly by glomerular filtration into the urine, where the concentration may be 5–50 times higher than in serum. Activity is enhanced at alkaline pH. In renal failure, excretion of streptomycin is impaired and accumulation to toxic levels occurs unless the dose is greatly reduced and the intervals between injections are lengthened.

Indications & Dosages

The principal indications for streptomycin at present are (1) plague, tularemia; (2) acute brucellosis (used in conjunction with tetracycline); (3) bacterial endocarditis caused by *Streptococcus faecalis* or *S viridans* (used in conjunction with a penicillin); and (4) serious active tuberculosis.

The dose in nontuberculous infections is 0.5 gm IM every 6–12 hours (for children, 20–40 mg/kg/day), depending on severity of the disease.

Adverse Effects

Allergic reactions, including skin rashes and fever, may occur upon prolonged contact with streptomycin, eg, in personnel preparing solutions. The principal side-effects are nephrotoxicity and ototoxicity. Renal damage with nitrogen retention occurs mainly after prolonged high doses or in persons with preexisting impairment of renal function. Damage to the 8th nerve manifests itself mainly by tinnitus, vertigo, ataxia, loss of balance, and occasionally loss of hearing. Chronic vestibular dysfunction is most common after prolonged use of streptomycin. Streptomycin, 2–3 gm/day for 4 weeks, has been used to purposely damage semicircular canal function in the treatment of Ménière's disease.

Streptomycin should not be used concurrently

with other aminoglycosides, and great caution is necessary in persons with impaired renal function.

2. KANAMYCIN

Kanamycin is an aminoglycoside for systemic use in gram-negative sepsis. Kanamycin is bactericidal for many gram-positive (except enterococci) and gram-negative bacteria in concentrations of $1-10$ μg/ml. Activity is enhanced at alkaline pH. Some strains of proteus are susceptible, but pseudomonas and serratia are often resistant. In susceptible bacterial populations, resistant mutants are rare. Kanamycin exhibits complete cross-resistance with neomycin but not with gentamicin.

Kanamycin is not significantly absorbed from the gut. Oral kanamycin can be used like oral neomycin. After intramuscular injection (0.5 gm every $6-12$ hours), serum levels may reach $5-10$ μg/ml. The drug is distributed widely in tissues but does not reach significant concentrations in the CSF, joints, or pleural fluid unless injected locally. Excretion is mainly by glomerular filtration into the urine, where levels of $10-50$ μg/ml are reached, and into the bile. In the presence of renal insufficiency, the drug may accumulate rapidly and reach toxic levels.

Indications & Dosages

The principal indication for systemic kanamycin is bacteremia caused by gram-negative enteric organisms or, occasionally, serious urinary tract infection with enterobacter, proteus, or other "difficult" organisms. The IM dose is 0.5 gm every $6-12$ hours (15 mg/kg/day). In renal failure, the dose is reduced or the interval between injections prolonged (Table 28–3).

Adverse Effects

Like all aminoglycosides, kanamycin is ototoxic and nephrotoxic, but it is believed to be less toxic than neomycin. Proteinuria and nitrogen retention occur commonly during treatment. These responses must be monitored and the dose or frequency of injection adjusted when creatinine clearance falls. In general, these nephrotoxic effects are reversible upon discontinuance of the drug. The auditory portion of the 8th nerve can be selectively and irreversibly damaged by kanamycin. The development of deafness is proportionate to the level of drug and the time of administration, but it can occur unpredictably even after a short course of treatment. Loss of perception of high frequencies in audiograms may be a warning sign. Ototoxicity is a particular risk in patients with impaired kidney function. The sudden absorption of large amounts of kanamycin (or any other aminoglycoside) can lead to respiratory arrest. This has occurred after the instillation of $3-5$ gm of kanamycin (or neomycin) into the peritoneal cavity following bowel surgery. Neostigmine is a specific antidote.

3. NEOMYCIN

Neomycin is analogous in all pharmacologic and antibacterial characteristics to kanamycin. However, it is believed to be more toxic when given parenterally and is therefore used mainly for topical application and for oral administration.

Indications, Dosages, & Routes of Administration

After oral intake, only a minute portion of neomycin is absorbed. Most of the drug remains in the gut lumen and alters intestinal flora. For preoperative reduction of the gut flora, give neomycin, 1 gm orally every $4-6$ hours for $2-3$ days before surgery. In hepatic coma, ammonia intoxication can be reduced by suppressing the coliform flora of the gut with neomycin, 1 gm orally every $6-8$ hours, and limiting the protein intake. Oral neomycin, $50-100$ mg/kg/day, is effective against some enteropathic *Escherichia coli*. To control surface infections of the skin (pyoderma), ointments containing neomycin, $1-5$ mg/gm, are applied several times daily. Solutions containing 10 mg/ml of neomycin can be instilled (up to a total of 0.5 gm/day) into infected joints, pleura, or tissue spaces. Paromomycin (Humatin), a close relative of neomycin, is given in a dosage of 1 gm orally every 6 hours for the treatment of intestinal amebiasis.

Adverse Effects

All topically administered forms of neomycin may produce sensitization. Hypersensitivity reactions occur particularly in the eye and skin after repeated use of neomycin ointments. Topical or oral neomycin rarely produces systemic toxicity. However, oral neomycin alters the intestinal flora and thus predisposes to superinfection. Staphylococcal enterocolitis, occasionally fatal, has followed the use of neomycin for preoperative "bowel sterilization."

4. GENTAMICIN

Gentamicin is an aminoglycoside antibiotic which shares many properties with kanamycin but differs in antimicrobial activity. In concentrations of $0.5-5$ μg/ml, gentamicin is bactericidal not only for staphylococci and coliform organisms but also for many strains of pseudomonas, proteus, and serratia. Enterococci are resistant. Gentamicin is not significantly absorbed after oral intake. After intramuscular injection, gentamicin is rapidly absorbed and widely distributed except into the CNS. Thirty percent of the drug in serum is protein-bound. With doses of $3-7$ mg/kg/day, serum levels reach $3-8$ μg/ml. The half-life is 2 hours. In the presence of renal failure, there is marked accumulation of the drug to toxic levels. Gentamicin is excreted by glomerular filtration into the urine, where levels are $10-100$ times higher than in the serum. Gentamicin activity is greatly enhanced at alkaline pH. Gentamicin may be synergistic with carbenicillin against pseudomonas. However, the 2 drugs cannot be mixed in vitro because they inactivate each other.

Indications, Dosages, & Routes of Administration

Gentamicin is used in severe infections caused by gram-negative bacteria which are likely to be resistant to other, less toxic drugs. Included are sepsis, infected burns, pneumonia and other serious infections due to coliform organisms, klebsiella-enterobacter, proteus, pseudomonas, and serratia. The dosage is 3–5 mg/kg/day IM in 3 equal doses for 7–10 days. In life-threatening infections, 5–8 mg/kg/day have been given. In urinary tract infections caused by these organisms, 0.8–1.2 mg/kg/day is given IM for 10 days or longer. It is necessary to monitor renal, auditory, and vestibular functions and to lengthen the interval between doses if renal function declines (Table 28–3).

For infected burns or skin lesions, creams containing 0.1% gentamicin are used. Such topical use should be restricted to avoid the selection of resistant bacteria in hospitals. In meningitis due to gram-negative bacteria, 1–10 mg gentamicin has been injected daily intrathecally. For endophthalmitis, 10 mg can be injected subconjunctivally.

Renal function must be monitored by repeated creatinine clearance tests. About 2–3% of patients develop vestibular dysfunction (perhaps because of destruction of hair cells), and cases of loss of hearing have been reported in children given 25 mg/kg/day.

Chan RA & others: Gentamicin therapy in renal failure. A nomogram for dosage. Ann Int Med 76:773, 1972.

Finland M (editor): International symposium on gentamicin. J Infect Dis 119:335, 1969.

Holmes RK, Sanford JP: Enzymatic assay for gentamicin. J Infect Dis 129:519, 1974.

Mann CH (editor): Kanamycin: Appraisal after 8 years of clinical application. Ann New York Acad Sc 132:771, 1966.

Riff LJ, Jackson GG: Conditions for gentamicin inactivation by carbenicillin. Arch Int Med 130:887, 1972.

Weinstein L: Streptomycin. Chap 58, pp 1242–1252, in: *The Pharmacological Basis of Therapeutics,* 4th ed. Goodman LS, Gilman A (editors). Macmillan, 1970.

5. SPECTINOMYCIN

This is an aminocyclitol antibiotic (related to aminoglycosides) for intramuscular administration. It is proposed as an alternative to penicillin for the treatment of gonorrhea, and this is its sole indication. Injection of 2 gm into each buttock, just once, produces blood levels of 100 μg/ml. About 5–10% of gonococci are probably resistant, but cure rates of 85% or more have been claimed. There is usually pain at the injection site, and there may be nausea and fever.

POLYMYXINS

The polymyxins are a group of basic polypeptides bactericidal for most gram-negative bacteria except proteus and especially useful against pseudomonas. Only 2 drugs are used: polymyxin B sulfate and colistin (polymyxin E) methanesulfonate.

Polymyxins are not absorbed from the gut. After parenteral injection they are distributed in some tissues but do not reach the CNS, CSF, joints, or ocular tissues unless injected locally. Blood levels usually do not exceed 1–2 μg/ml. Polymyxins are excreted into the urine (colistin more rapidly than polymyxin B), where concentrations of 25–300 μg/ml may be reached. Excretion is impaired in renal insufficiency, so that accumulation to toxic levels can occur unless the dose is drastically reduced and the interval between doses lengthened (Table 28–3).

Indications, Dosages, & Routes of Administration

Polymyxins are indicated in serious infections due to pseudomonas and other gram-negative bacteria which are resistant to other antimicrobial drugs.

A. Intramuscular: The injection of polymyxin B is painful. Therefore, colistimethate, which contains a local anesthetic and is more rapidly excreted in the urine, is given IM, 2.5–5 mg/kg/day, for urinary tract infection.

B. Intravenous: In gram-negative bacterial sepsis, polymyxin B sulfate, 2.5 mg/kg/day, can be injected by continuous IV infusion instead of gentamicin.

C. Intrathecal: In pseudomonas meningitis, give polymyxin B sulfate, 2–10 mg once daily for 2–3 days and then every other day for 2–3 weeks.

D. Topical: Solutions of polymyxin B sulfate, 1 mg/ml, can be applied to infected surfaces, injected into joint spaces, intrapleurally or subconjunctivally, or inhaled as aerosols. Ointments containing 0.5 mg/gm polymyxin B sulfate in a mixture with neomycin or bacitracin are often applied to infected skin lesions. Solutions containing polymyxin B, 20 mg/liter, and neomycin, 40 mg/liter, can be used for continuous irrigation of the bladder with an indwelling catheter and a closed drainage system. Purulent exudates inactivate polymyxins.

Adverse Effects

The toxicities of polymyxin B and colistimethate are similar. With the usual blood levels there are paresthesias, dizziness, flushing, and incoordination. These disappear when the drug has been excreted. With unusually high levels, respiratory arrest and paralysis can occur. Depending upon the dose, all polymyxins are nephrotoxic, producing tubular injury. Proteinuria, hematuria, and cylindruria tend to be reversible, but nitrogen retention or severe electrolyte disturbances may force reduction in dose or discontinuance of the drug. In individuals with preexisting renal insufficiency, kidney function must be monitored (preferably by creatinine clearance) and the dose reduced or the interval between injections increased (Table 28–3).

Hoeprich PH: The polymyxins. M Clin North America 54:1257, 1972.

Ryan KJ & others: Colistimethate toxicity: Report of a fatal case. JAMA 207:2099, 1969.

ANTITUBERCULOSIS DRUGS

Singular problems exist in the treatment of tuberculosis and other mycobacterial infections. They tend to be exceedingly chronic but may give rise to hyperacute lethal complications. The organisms are frequently intracellular, have long periods of metabolic inactivity, and tend to develop resistance to any one drug. Combined drug therapy is often employed to delay the emergence of this resistance. "First line" drugs, often employed together in tuberculous meningitis, miliary dissemination, or severe pulmonary disease, are isoniazid, ethambutol, rifampin, and streptomycin. A series of "second line" drugs will be mentioned only briefly. Most patients become noninfectious within 2–4 weeks after effective drug therapy is instituted.

1. ISONIAZID (INH)

Isoniazid is the hydrazide of isonicotinic acid (INH), the most active antituberculosis drug. INH inhibits most tubercle bacilli in a concentration of 0.2 μg/ml or less. However, most "atypical" mycobacteria are resistant. In susceptible large populations of *Mycobacterium tuberculosis*, INH-resistant mutants occur. Their emergence is delayed in the presence of a second drug. There is no cross-resistance between INH, streptomycin, ethambutol, and rifampin.

INH is well absorbed from the gut and diffuses readily into all tissues, including the CNS, and into living cells. A dose of 8 mg/kg/day results in blood levels of 2 μg/ml or more. The inactivation of INH—particularly its acetylation—is under genetic control. In "rapid inactivators," plasma levels are 0.2 μg/ml or less 6 hours after ingestion of 4 mg/kg INH, whereas in "slow inactivators" plasma levels at that time are 0.8 μg/ml or more. INH and its conjugates are excreted mainly in the urine.

Indications, Dosages, & Routes of Administration
(See also p 127.)

INH is the most widely used drug in tuberculosis. INH should not be given as the sole drug in active tuberculosis. This favors emergence of resistance (up to 20% in some countries). In active, clinically manifest disease, it is given in conjunction with streptomycin, ethambutol, or rifampin. The initial dose is 8–10 mg/kg/day orally (up to 20 mg/kg/day in small children); later, the dosage is reduced to 5–7 mg/kg/day. INH dosage needs to be reduced only in the presence of very severe renal failure.

Children (or young adults) who convert from a negative to a positive tuberculin skin test but who have no evidence of an active lesion may be given 10 mg/kg/day (maximum: 300 mg/day) for 1 year as prophylaxis against the 5–15% risk of meningitis or miliary dissemination. For this "prophylaxis," INH is given as the sole drug. Such INH prophylaxis is also indicated in PPD positive adults who must be immunosuppressed by cancer chemotherapy or for organ transplant.

Toxic reactions to INH include insomnia, restlessness, fever, myalgia, hyperreflexia, and even convulsions and psychotic episodes. Some of these are attributable to a relative pyridoxine deficiency and peripheral neuritis and can be prevented by the administration of pyridoxine, 100 mg/day. Isoniazid can induce hepatitis. Progressive liver damage occurs rarely in patients under age 20; in 1.5% of persons between 30–50 years of age; and in 2.5% of older individuals. The risk of hepatitis is greater in rapid than in slow acetylators of INH and is an important determinant in the prophylactic use of INH. INH can reduce the metabolism of phenytoin, increasing its blood level and toxicity.

Curry FJ: Prophylactic effect of isoniazid in young tuberculin reactors. New England J Med 277:562, 1967.

Lal S & others: Effect of rifampin and isoniazid on liver function. Brit MJ 1:148, 1972.

Maddrey WC, Boitnott JK: Isoniazid hepatitis. Ann Int Med 79:1, 1973.

Wolinsky E: New antituberculosis drugs and concepts of prophylaxis. M Clin North America 58:697, 1974.

2. ETHAMBUTOL

This is a synthetic, water-soluble, heat-stable compound, dispensed as the hydrochloride.

Many strains of *Mycobacterium tuberculosis* are inhibited in vitro by ethambutol, 1–5 μg/ml. The mechanism of action is not known.

Ethambutol is well absorbed from the gut. Following ingestion of 25 mg/kg, a blood level peak of 2–5 μg/ml is reached in 2–4 hours. About 20% of the drug is excreted in feces and 50% in the urine, in unchanged form. Excretion is delayed in renal failure. About 15% of absorbed drug is metabolized by oxidation and conversion to a dicarboxylic acid. In meningitis, ethambutol appears in the CSF.

Resistance to ethambutol emerges fairly rapidly among mycobacteria when the drug is used alone. Therefore, ethambutol is given in combination with other antituberculosis drugs, most commonly INH.

Ethambutol, 15 mg/kg, is usually given as a single daily dose in combination with INH. At times, the dose is 25 mg/kg/day.

Hypersensitivity to ethambutol occurs infrequently. It may cause a rise in the serum uric acid. The commonest side-effects are visual disturbances: reduction in visual acuity, optic neuritis, and perhaps retinal damage occur in some patients receiving ethambutol, 25 mg/kg/day for several months. Most of these changes apparently regress when ethambutol is discontinued. However, periodic visual acuity testing is mandatory during treatment. With doses of 15 mg/kg/day, side-effects are rare.

Doster B & others: Ethambutol in the initial treatment of pulmonary tuberculosis. Am Rev Resp Dis 107:177, 1973.
Place VA & others: Ethambutol in tuberculous meningitis. Am Rev Resp Dis 99:783, 1969.

3. RIFAMPIN

Rifampin is a semisynthetic derivative of rifamycin. Rifampin, 1 μg/ml or less, inhibits many gram-positive cocci, meningococci, and tubercle bacilli in vitro. Gram-negative organisms are often more resistant. Highly resistant mutants occur relatively frequently in susceptible microbial populations. Rifampin is also active against chlamydiae and poxviruses.

Rifampin binds strongly to DNA-dependent bacterial RNA polymerase and thus inhibits RNA synthesis in bacteria and chlamydiae. It blocks a late stage in the assembly of poxviruses. Rifampin penetrates well into phagocytic cells and can kill intracellular organisms.

Rifampin given orally is well absorbed and widely distributed in tissues. It is excreted mainly through the liver and to a lesser extent in the urine. With oral doses of 600 mg, serum levels exceed 5 μg/ml for 4–6 hours, and urine levels may be 10–100 times higher.

In the treatment of tuberculosis, a single oral dose of 600 mg (10–20 mg/kg) is given daily. In order to delay the rapid emergence of resistant microorganisms, combined treatment with ethambutol or another antituberculosis drug is required. Rifampin, 600 mg twice daily for 2 days, can eradicate the meningococcal carrier state, but up to 10% resistant strains may emerge.

In urinary tract infections and in chronic bronchitis, rifampin has not given encouraging results.

Rifampin imparts an orange color to urine and sweat. Occasional adverse effects include rashes, thrombocytopenia, impaired liver function, light chain proteinuria, and some impairment of immune response. Rifampin increases the dose requirement for warfarin in anticoagulation.

Munford RS & others: Eradication of carriage of *Neisseria meningitidis* in families. J Infect Dis 129:644, 1974.
Newman R & others: Rifampin in initial treatment of pulmonary tuberculosis. Am Rev Resp Dis 109:216, 1974.

4. STREPTOMYCIN

The general pharmacologic features and toxicity of streptomycin are described above. Streptomycin, 1–10 μg/ml, is inhibitory and bactericidal for most tubercle bacilli, whereas most "atypical" mycobacteria are resistant. All large populations of tubercle bacilli contain some streptomycin-resistant mutants, which tend to emerge during prolonged treatment with streptomycin alone and result in "treatment resistance" within 2–4 months. This is the main reason why streptomycin is only employed in combination with another antituberculosis drug.

Streptomycin penetrates poorly into cells and exerts its action mainly on extracellular tubercle bacilli. Since at any moment 90% of tubercle bacilli are intracellular and thus unaffected by streptomycin, treatment for many months is required.

For combination therapy in tuberculous meningitis, miliary dissemination, and severe organ tuberculosis, streptomycin is given IM, 1 gm daily (30 mg/kg/day for children) for weeks or months. This is followed by streptomycin, 1 gm IM 2–3 times a week for months or years. In tuberculosis meningitis, intrathecal injections (1–2 mg/kg/day) are sometimes given in addition.

The vestibular dysfunction resulting from prolonged streptomycin treatment results in inability to maintain equilibrium. However, some compensation usually occurs so that patients can function fairly well.

5. ALTERNATIVE DRUGS IN TUBERCULOSIS TREATMENT

The drugs listed alphabetically below are usually considered only in cases of drug resistance (clinical or laboratory) to "first line" drugs and when expert guidance is available to deal with toxic side-effects.

Aminosalicylic acid (PAS), closely related to *p*-aminobenzoic acid, inhibits most tubercle bacilli in concentrations of 1–5 μg/ml but has no effect on other bacteria. Resistant *Mycobacterium tuberculosis* emerges rapidly unless another antituberculosis drug is present.

PAS is readily absorbed from the gut. Doses of 8–12 gm/day orally give blood levels of 10 μg/ml. The drug is widely distributed in tissues (except the CNS) and rapidly excreted into the urine. To avoid crystalluria, the urine should be kept alkaline.

Common side-effects include anorexia, nausea, diarrhea, and epigastric pain. These may be diminished by taking PAS with meals and with antacids, but peptic ulceration may occur. Sodium PAS may be given parenterally. Hypersensitivity reactions include fever, skin rashes, granulocytopenia, lymphadenopathy, and arthralgias.

Capreomycin, 0.5–1.5 gm/day IM, can perhaps

substitute for streptomycin in combined therapy. It is not commercially available. It is nephrotoxic and ototoxic.

Cycloserine, 0.5–1 gm/day orally, has been used alone or with INH. It can induce a variety of CNS dysfunctions and psychotic reactions. These may be controlled by phenytoin, 100 mg/day orally. In smaller doses (15–20 mg/kg/day) it has been used in urinary tract infections.

Ethionamide, 0.5–1 gm/day orally, has been used in combination therapy but produces marked gastric irritation.

Pyrazinamide, 0.75 gm twice daily orally, has been used in combination therapy but may produce serious liver damage.

Viomycin, 2 gm IM every 3 days, can occasionally substitute for streptomycin in combination therapy. It is nephrotoxic and ototoxic.

Ferebee SH: Controlled chemoprophylaxis trials in tuberculosis. Advances Tuberc Res 17:28, 1969.
Rednor DB: Changing concept in treatment of tuberculosis. Chest 61:520, 1972.

SULFONAMIDES & ANTIFOLATE DRUGS

Since the demonstration, in 1935, of the striking antibacterial activity of sulfanilamide, the molecule has been drastically altered in many ways. More than 150 different sulfonamides have been marketed at one time or another, the modifications being designed principally to achieve greater antibacterial activity, a wider antibacterial spectrum, greater solubility, or more prolonged action. Because of their low cost and their relative efficacy in some common bacterial infections, sulfonamides are still used widely in many parts of the world. However, the increasing emergence of sulfonamide resistance (eg, among streptococci, meningococci, and shigellae) and the higher efficacy of other antimicrobial drugs have drastically curtailed the number of specific indications for sulfonamides as drugs of choice. The present indications for the use of these drugs can be summarized as follows:

(1) First (previously untreated) infection of the urinary tract: Many coliform organisms, which are the most common causes of urinary infections, are still susceptible to sulfonamides.

(2) Chlamydial infections of the trachoma-inclusion conjunctivitis-LGV group: Sulfonamides are often as effective as tetracyclines in suppressing clinical activity, and they may be curative in acute infections. However, they often fail to eradicate chronic infection, and they are ineffective in psittacosis.

(3) Parasitic and fungal diseases: In combination with pyrimethamine, sulfonamides are used in toxoplasmosis. In combination with trimethoprim, sulfonamides are sometimes effective in falciparum malaria. Alone or in combination with cycloserine, sulfonamides may be active in nocardiosis.

(4) Bacterial infections: In underdeveloped parts of the world, sulfonamides, because of their availability and low cost, may still be useful for the treatment of pneumococcal or staphylococcal infections; bacterial sinusitis, bronchitis, or otitis media; baciliary (shigella) dysentery; and meningococcal infections. In most developed countries, however, sulfonamides are not the drugs of choice for any of these conditions, and sulfonamide resistance of the respective etiologic organisms is widespread.

(5) Leprosy: Certain sulfones are the drugs of choice in leprosy.

Antimicrobial Activity

The action of sulfonamides is bacteriostatic and is reversible upon removal of the drug or in the presence of an excess of *p*-aminobenzoic acid (PABA). Susceptible microorganisms require extracellular PABA in order to synthesize folic acid, an essential step in the formation of purines. Sulfonamides are structural analogues of PABA, can enter into the reaction in place of PABA competing for the enzyme involved, and can form nonfunctional analogues of folic acid. As a result, further growth of the microorganism is inhibited. Animal cells and some sulfonamide-resistant microorganisms are unable to synthesize folic acid from PABA but depend on exogenous sources of preformed folic acid.

Trimethoprim can inhibit the step in bacterial purine synthesis (dihydrofolic acid reductase) which follows the step blocked by sulfonamides. Trimethoprim plus sulfamethoxazole (co-trimoxazole) can therefore produce sequential blocking of purine synthesis. Such "synergism" has been used in bacterial urinary tract and enteric infection and in malaria. Trimethoprim-resistant coliforms and haemophilus are appearing.

Pharmacologic Properties

The soluble sulfonamides are readily absorbed from the gut, distributed widely in tissues and body fluids, and excreted primarily by glomerular filtration into the urine. Varying amounts of sulfonamides are acetylated by the liver or bound to plasma protein. A portion of the drug in the urine is acetylated, but enough active drug remains in the urine to permit effective treatment of urinary tract infections (usually 10–20 times the concentration present in the blood). In order to be therapeutically effective for systemic therapy, a sulfonamide must achieve a concentration of 8–12 mg/ml of blood. This is accomplished by full systemic doses listed below.

"Long-acting" sulfonamides (eg, sulfamethoxypyridazine, sulfadimethoxine, sulfameter) are readily absorbed after oral intake, but excretion is very slow, resulting in prolonged blood levels. "Intermediate-acting" sulfonamides (eg, sulfamethoxazole) are also excreted relatively slowly. All of these compounds may have a convenience factor but cause a higher incidence of severe toxic reactions.

"Insoluble" sulfonamides (eg, phthalylsulfathiazole) are absorbed only slightly after oral administra-

Table 28—4. Drug selections, 1975—1976.

Suspected or Proved Etiologic Agent	Drug(s) of First Choice	Alternative Drug(s)
Gram-negative cocci		
Gonococcus	Penicillin[1], ampicillin	Tetracycline[2], spectinomycin
Meningococcus	Penicillin[1]	Chloramphenicol
Gram-positive cocci		
Pneumococcus	Penicillin[1]	Erythromycin[3]
Streptococcus, hemolytic groups A, B, C	Penicillin[1]	Erythromycin[3]
Streptococcus viridans	Penicillin[1]	Cephalosporin[4], vancomycin
Staphylococcus, nonpenicillinase-producing	Penicillin[1]	Cephalosporin, vancomycin, lincomycin
Staphylococcus, penicillinase-producing	Penicillinase-resistant penicillin[5]	Cephalosporin, vancomycin, lincomycin
Streptococcus faecalis (enterococcus)	Ampicillin plus aminoglycoside	Penicillin plus gentamicin
Gram-negative rods		
Enterobacter (Aerobacter)	Kanamycin or gentamicin	Chloramphenicol
Bacteroides (except *B fragilis*)	Penicillin[1] or chloramphenicol	Clindamycin
Brucella	Tetracycline plus streptomycin	Streptomycin plus sulfonamide[6]
Escherichia		
E coli sepsis	Kanamycin or gentamicin	Cephalothin, ampicillin
E coli urinary tract infection (first attack)	Sulfonamide[7]	Ampicillin, cephalexin
Haemophilus (meningitis, respiratory infections)	Ampicillin	Chloramphenicol
Klebsiella	Cephalosporin or kanamycin	Gentamicin, chloramphenicol
Mima-Herellea	Kanamycin	Tetracycline, gentamicin
Pasteurella (plague, tularemia)	Streptomycin plus tetracycline	Sulfonamide[6]
Proteus		
P mirabilis	Penicillin or ampicillin	Kanamycin, gentamicin
P vulgaris and other species	Kanamycin or gentamicin	Chloramphenicol
Pseudomonas		
Ps aeruginosa	Gentamicin or polymyxin	Carbenicillin, co-trimoxazole[8]
Ps pseudomallei (melioidosis)	Tetracycline plus sulfonamide	Chloramphenicol
Ps mallei (glanders)	Streptomycin plus tetracycline	
Salmonella	Chloramphenicol or ampicillin	Co-trimoxazole[8]
Serratia	Gentamicin	Co-trimoxazole[8]
Shigella	Ampicillin or chloramphenicol	Tetracycline, kanamycin
Vibrio (cholera)	Tetracycline	Chloramphenicol
Gram-positive rods		
Actinomyces	Penicillin[1]	Tetracycline, sulfonamide
Bacillus (eg, anthrax)	Penicillin[1]	Erythromycin
Clostridium (eg, gas gangrene, tetanus)	Penicillin[1]	Tetracycline, erythromycin
Corynebacterium	Erythromycin	Penicillin, cephalosporin
Listeria	Ampicillin plus aminoglycoside	Tetracycline
Acid-fast rods		
Mycobacterium tuberculosis	INH plus rifampin or ethambutol[9]	Other antituberculosis drugs
Mycobacterium leprae	Dapsone or sulfoxone	Other sulfones, amithiazone
Mycobacteria, atypical	INH plus ethambutol	Rifampin
Nocardia	Sulfonamide[6]	Minocycline, cycloserine
Spirochetes		
Borrelia (relapsing fever)	Tetracycline	Penicillin
Leptospira	Penicillin	Tetracycline
Treponema (syphilis, yaws)	Penicillin	Erythromycin, tetracycline
Mycoplasma	Tetracycline	Erythromycin
Psittacosis-lymphogranuloma-trachoma agents (chlamydiae)	Tetracycline, sulfonamide[6]	Erythromycin, chloramphenicol
Rickettsiae	Tetracycline	Chloramphenicol

[1] Penicillin G is preferred for parenteral injection; penicillin G (buffered) or penicillin V for oral administration. Only highly sensitive microorganisms should be treated with oral penicillin.

[2] All tetracyclines have the same activity against microorganisms and all have comparable therapeutic activity and toxicity. Dosage is determined by the rates of absorption and excretion of different preparations.

[3] Erythromycin estolate and troleandomycin are the best absorbed oral forms.

[4] Cephalothin and cefazolin are the best accepted cephalosporins at present.

[5] Parenteral methicillin, nafcillin, or oxacillin. Oral dicloxacillin or other isoxazolylpenicillin.

[6] Trisulfapyrimidines have the advantage of greater solubility in urine over sulfadiazine for oral administration; sodium sulfadiazine is suitable for intravenous injection in severely ill persons.

[7] For previously untreated urinary tract infection, a highly soluble sulfonamide such as sulfisoxazole or trisulfapyrimidines is the first choice.

[8] Co-trimoxazole is a mixture of 1 part trimethoprim plus 5 parts sulfamethoxazole.

[9] Either or both.

tion and are largely excreted in the feces. Their action is limited to suppression of intestinal flora.

For parenteral (usually intravenous) administration, sodium salts of several sulfonamides are used because of their greater solubility. Their distribution and excretion are similar to those of the orally administered, absorbed sulfonamides. Trimethoprim concentrates by nonionic diffusion in prostatic and vaginal fluids, which are more acidic than serum.

Dosages & Routes of Administration

A. Topical: The application of sulfonamides to skin, wounds, or mucous membranes is undesirable because of the high risk of allergic sensitization or reaction and the low antimicrobial activity. Exceptions are the application of sodium sulfacetamide solution (30%) or ointment (10%) to the conjunctiva, and mafenide acetate cream (Sulfamylon) or silver sulfadiazine to control the flora of the burn wound.

B. Oral: For systemic disease, the soluble, rapidly excreted sulfonamides (eg, sulfadiazine, sulfisoxazole) are given in an initial dose of 2–4 gm (40 mg/kg) followed by a maintenance dose of 0.5–1 gm (20 mg/kg) every 4–6 hours. Trisulfapyrimidines USP may be given in the same total doses. Urine must be kept alkaline.

For urinary tract infections (first attack, not previously treated), trisulfapyrimidines, sulfisoxazole, or another sulfonamide with equally high solubility in urine are given in somewhat lower doses than shown above. Following one course of sulfonamides, resistant organisms usually prevail. Simultaneous administration of sulfamethoxazole, 2 gm/day orally, and trimethoprim, 320 mg/day orally, may be more effective in urinary tract infections than sulfonamide alone.

For "intestinal surgery prophylaxis," insoluble sulfonamides (eg, phthalylsulfathiazole), 8–15 gm/day, are given for 5–7 days before operations on the bowel. Salicylazosulfapyridine, 6 gm/day, has been given in ulcerative colitis. The drug is split in the gut to yield sulfapyridine and salicylate. The latter may have anti-inflammatory action.

"Long-acting" and "intermediate-acting" sulfonamides (eg, sulfamethoxypyridazine, sulfadimethoxine, sulfamethoxazole) can be used in doses of 0.5–1 gm/day (10 mg/kg) for prolonged maintenance therapy (eg, trachoma) or for the treatment of minor infections. These drugs have a significantly higher rate of toxic effects than the "short-acting" sulfonamides.

C. Intravenous: Sodium sulfadiazine can be injected intravenously in 0.5% concentration in 5% dextrose in water or physiologic salt solution in a total dose of 6–8 gm/day (120 mg/kg/day). This is reserved for comatose individuals or those unable to take oral medication.

Adverse Effects

Sulfonamides produce a wide variety of side-effects—due partly to hypersensitivity, partly to direct toxicity—which must be considered whenever unexplained symptoms or signs occur in a patient who may

have received these drugs. Except in the mildest reactions, fluids should be forced, and—if symptoms and signs progressively increase—the drugs should be discontinued. Precautions to prevent complications (below) are important.

A. Systemic Side-Effects: Fever, skin rashes, urticaria; nausea, vomiting, or diarrhea; stomatitis, conjunctivitis, arthritis, exfoliative dermatitis; hematopoietic disturbances, including thrombocytopenia, hemolytic (in G6PD deficiency) or aplastic anemia, granulocytopenia, leukemoid reactions; hepatitis, polyarteritis nodosa, vasculitis, Stevens-Johnson syndrome; psychosis; and many others.

Mafenide application to burns may cause severe pain.

B. Urinary Tract Disturbances: Sulfonamides may precipitate in urine, especially at neutral or acid pH, producing hematuria, crystalluria, or even obstruction. They have also been implicated in various types of nephritis and nephrosis. Sulfonamides and methenamine salts should not be given together.

Precautions in the Use of Sulfonamides

(1) There is cross-allergenicity among all sulfonamides. Obtain a history of past administration or reaction. Observe for possible allergic responses.

(2) Keep the urine volume above 1500 mg/day by forcing fluids. Check urine pH—it should be 7.5 or higher. Give alkali by mouth (sodium bicarbonate or equivalent, 5–15 gm/day). Examine fresh urine for crystals and red cells every 2–4 days.

(3) Check hemoglobin, white blood cell count, and differential count every 3–5 days to detect possible disturbances early.

Ballin JC: Evaluation of silver sulfadiazine for burn therapy. JAMA 230:1184, 1974.

Craig WA, Kunin CM: Trimethoprim-sulfamethoxazole. Ann Int Med 78:491, 1973.

Weinstein L, Madoff MA, Samet CM: The sulfonamides. (2 parts.) New England J Med 263:900, 959, 1960.

SULFONES USED IN
THE TREATMENT OF LEPROSY

A number of drugs closely related to the sulfonamides (eg, dapsone; diaminodiphenylsulfone, DDS) have been used effectively in the long-term treatment of leprosy. The clinical manifestations of both lepromatous and tuberculoid leprosy can often be suppressed by treatment extending over several years.

Absorption, Metabolism, & Excretion

All of the sulfones are well absorbed from the intestinal tract, are distributed widely in all tissues, and tend to be retained in skin, muscle, liver, and kidney. Skin involved by leprosy contains 10 times more drug than normal skin. Sulfones are excreted into the bile and reabsorbed by the intestine. Consequently, blood levels are prolonged. Excretion into the urine is variable and occurs mostly as a glucuronic acid conjugate. Some persons acetylate sulfones slowly and others rapidly, and this requires dosage adjustment.

Adverse Effects

The sulfones may cause any of the side-effects listed above for sulfonamides. Anorexia, nausea, and vomiting are common. Hemolysis, methemoglobinemia, or agranulocytosis may occur.

SPECIALIZED DRUGS AGAINST GRAM-POSITIVE BACTERIA

1. BACITRACIN

This polypeptide antibiotic is selectively active against gram-positive bacteria, including penicillinase-producing staphylococci, in concentrations of 0.1–20 units/ml. Bacitracin is very little absorbed from gut, skin, wounds, or mucous membranes. Topical application results in local effects without significant toxicity. Bacitracin, 500 unit/gm in ointment base, is often combined with polymyxin or neomycin for the suppression of mixed bacterial flora in surface lesions. Systemic administration of bacitracin has been abandoned because of its severe nephrotoxicity.

2. LINCOMYCIN & CLINDAMYCIN

These drugs resemble erythromycin (although different in structure) and are active against gram-positive organisms (except enterococci) in concentrations of 0.5–5 μg/ml. Lincomycin, 0.5 gm orally every 6 hours (30–60 mg/kg/day for children), or clindamycin, 0.15–0.3 gm orally every 6 hours (10–40 mg/kg/day for children) yields serum concentrations of 2–5 μg/ml. The drugs are widely distributed in tissues. Excretion is through bile and urine. The drugs are alternatives to erythromycin as substitutes for penicillin. Clindamycin is effective against most strains of bacteroides and is a drug of choice in anaerobic infections. Seriously ill patients are given clindamycin, 600 mg (20–30 mg/kg/day) IV during a 1 hour period every 8 hours. Success has also been reported in staphylococcal infections, especially osteomyelitis. These drugs are ineffective in meningitis.

Common side-effects are diarrhea, nausea, and skin rashes. Impaired liver function and neutropenia have been noted. If 3–4 gm are given rapidly intravenously, cardiorespiratory arrest may occur. Diarrhea

and colitis associated with clindamycin administration—including some fatal cases—are being reported with increasing frequency.

Bartlett JG & others: Treatment of anaerobic infections with clindamycin. New England J Med 287:1006, 1972.

Gorbach SL, Thadepalli H: Clindamycin in pure and mixed anaerobic infections. Arch Int Med 134:87, 1974.

Tedesco FG & others: Clindamycin-associated colitis: A prospective study. Ann Int Med 81:429, 1974.

3. NOVOBIOCIN

Many gram-positive cocci are inhibited by novobiocin, 1–5 μg/ml, but resistant variants tend to emerge rapidly during treatment. Novobiocin, 0.5 gm orally every 6 hours (30 mg/kg/day for children), yields serum concentrations of 2–5 μg/ml. It is widely distributed in tissues and excreted in urine and feces. It can also be given intramuscularly or intravenously. In the past, a possible indication for novobiocin was infection caused by penicillinase-producing staphylococci. However, many better drugs are now available, so that no clear indication for novobiocin exists.

Skin rashes, drug fever, and granulocytopenia are common side-effects; many others have been observed occasionally.

4. VANCOMYCIN

This drug is bactericidal for most gram-positive organisms, particularly staphylococci and enterococci, in concentrations of 0.5–10 μg/ml. Resistant mutants are rare, and there is no cross-resistance with other antimicrobial drugs. Vancomycin is not absorbed from the gut. It is given orally (3–4 gm/day) only for the treatment of staphylococcal enterocolitis. For systemic effect the drug must be administered intravenously, and for meningitis intrathecally. After intravenous injection of 0.5 gm over a period of 20 minutes, blood levels of 10 μg/ml are maintained for 1–2 hours. Vancomycin is largely excreted into the urine. In the presence of renal insufficiency, marked accumulation may occur and have toxic consequences.

The only indications for vancomycin are serious staphylococcal infection or enterococcal endocarditis untreatable with penicillins. Vancomycin, 0.5 gm, is injected IV over a 20-minute period every 6–8 hours (for children, 20–40 mg/kg/day).

Vancomycin is intensely irritating to tissues. Intramuscular injection or extravasation from intravenous injection sites is very painful. Chills, fever, and thrombophlebitis commonly follow intravenous injection. The drug is both nephrotoxic and ototoxic, and renal function must be monitored.

Friedberg CK & others: Vancomycin therapy for enterococcal and *Streptococcus viridans* endocarditis. Arch Int Med 21:134, 1968.

Wallace JF & others: Oral administration of vancomycin in the treatment of staphylococcal enterocolitis. New England J Med 272:1014, 1965.

URINARY ANTISEPTICS

These drugs exert antimicrobial activity in the urine but have little or no systemic antibacterial effect. Their usefulness is limited to urinary tract infections.

1. NITROFURANTOIN

Nitrofurantoin is bacteriostatic and bactericidal for both gram-positive and gram-negative bacteria in concentrations of 10–500 μg/ml. The activity of nitrofurantoin is greatly enhanced at pH 6.5 or less.

Nitrofurantoin is rapidly absorbed from the gut. The drug is bound so completely to serum protein that no antibacterial effect occurs in the blood. Nitrofurantoin has no systemic antibacterial activity. In kidney tubules, the drug is separated from carrier protein and excreted in urine where concentrations may be 200–400 μg/ml.

The average daily dose in urinary tract infections is 100 mg orally 4 times daily (for children, 5–10 mg/kg/day), taken with food. If oral medication is not feasible, nitrofurantoin can be given by continuous IV infusion, 180–360 mg/day.

Oral nitrofurantoin often causes nausea and vomiting. Hemolytic anemia occurs in G6PD deficiency. Hypersensitivity may produce skin rashes and pulmonary infiltration.

2. NALIDIXIC ACID

This synthetic urinary antiseptic inhibits many gram-negative bacteria in concentrations of 1–50 μg/ml but has no effect on pseudomonas. In susceptible bacterial populations, resistant mutants emerge fairly rapidly.

Nalidixic acid is readily absorbed from the gut. In the blood, virtually all drug is firmly bound to protein. Thus there is no systemic antibacterial action. About 20% of the absorbed drug is excreted in the urine in active form to give urine levels of 10–150 μg/ml, which may produce false-positive tests for glucose.

The dose in urinary tract infections is 1 gm orally 4 times daily (for children, 55 mg/kg/day). Adverse reactions include nausea, vomiting, skin rashes, drowsiness, visual disturbances, and, rarely, increased intracranial pressure with convulsions.

3. METHENAMINE MANDELATE & METHENAMINE HIPPURATE

These are salts of methenamine and mandelic acid or hippuric acid. The action of the drug depends on the liberation of formaldehyde and of acid in the urine. The urinary pH must be below 5.5, and sulfonamides must not be given at the same time. The drug inhibits a variety of different microorganisms except those (eg, proteus) which liberate ammonia from urea and produce strongly alkaline urine. The dosage is 2–6 gm orally daily.

4. ACIDIFYING AGENTS

Urine with a pH below 5.5 tends to be antibacterial. Many substances can acidify urine and thus produce antibacterial activity. Ammonium chloride, ascorbic acid, methionine, and mandelic acid are sometimes used. The dose has to be established for each patient by testing the urine for acid pH with test paper at frequent intervals.

SYSTEMICALLY ACTIVE DRUGS IN URINARY TRACT INFECTIONS

Many antimicrobial drugs are excreted in the urine in very high concentration. For this reason, low and relatively nontoxic amounts of aminoglycosides, polymyxins, and cycloserine (see Antituberculosis Drugs, above) can produce effective urine levels. Many penicillins and cephalosporins and co-trimoxazole can reach very high urine levels and can thus be effective in urinary tract infections.

McGregor RR, Petersdorf RG: Antimicrobial prophylaxis in kidney disease. Postgrad Med 51:105, 1972.

Meyers FH, Jawetz E, Goldfien A: *Review of Medical Pharmacology,* 4th ed. Lange, 1974.

Turck M & others: Relapse and reinfection in chronic bacteriuria. New England J Med 275:70, 1966.

ANTIFUNGAL DRUGS

Most antibacterial substances have no effect on pathogenic fungi. Only a few drugs are known to be therapeutically useful in mycotic infections. Penicillins are used to treat actinomycosis; sulfonamides have been employed in nocardiosis.

1. AMPHOTERICIN B

Amphotericin B, 0.1—0.8 μg/ml, inhibits in vitro several organisms producing systemic mycotic disease in man, including histoplasma, cryptococcus, coccidioides, candida, blastomyces, sporotrichum, and others. Amphotericin B can be used for treatment of these systemic fungal infections. Intrathecal administration is necessary for the treatment of meningitis.

Amphotericin B solutions, 0.1 mg/ml in 500 ml 5% dextrose in water, are given IV by slow infusion. The initial dose is 1—5 mg/day, increasing daily by 5 mg increments until a final dosage of 0.5—1.2 mg/kg/day (25—65 mg/day) is reached. This is usually continued daily or on alternate days for many weeks. In fungal meningitis, amphotericin B, 0.5 mg, is injected intrathecally 3 times weekly; continuous treatment (many weeks) with an Ommaya reservoir is sometimes employed. Relapses of fungal meningitis occur commonly.

Amphotericin B is 85% protein-bound and is little removed by hemodialysis.

The intravenous administration of amphotericin B usually produces chills, fever, vomiting, and headache. Tolerance may be enhanced by temporary lowering of the dose or administration of aspirin, diphenhydramine, phenothiazines, and corticosteroids. Therapeutically active amounts of amphotericin B commonly impair kidney and liver function and produce anemia (impaired iron utilization by bone marrow). Electrolyte disturbances (hypokalemia, distal tubular acidosis), shock, and a variety of neurologic symptoms also occur.

Bennett JE: Chemotherapy of systemic mycoses. (2 parts.) New England J Med 290:30, 320, 1974.
Butler WT: Pharmacology, toxicity and therapeutic usefulness of amphotericin B. JAMA 195:371, 1966.
Medoff G, Kobayashi GS: Amphotericin B. JAMA 232:619, 1975.
Sarosi GA & others: Cryptococcal meningitis: Amphotericin therapy. Ann Int Med 71:1079, 1969.

2. GRISEOFULVIN

Griseofulvin is an antibiotic that can inhibit the growth of some dermatophytes but has no effect on bacteria or on the fungi that cause deep mycoses. Absorption of microsized griseofulvin, 1 gm/day, gives blood levels of 0.5—1.5 μg/ml. The absorbed drug has an affinity for skin and is deposited there, bound to keratin. Thus, it makes keratin resistant to fungal growth and the new growth of hair or nails is first freed of infection. As keratinized structures are shed, they are replaced by uninfected ones. The bulk of ingested griseofulvin is excreted in the feces. Topical application of griseofulvin has little effect.

Oral doses of 0.5—1 gm/day (for children, 15 mg/kg/day) must be given for 6 weeks if only the skin is involved and for 3—6 months or longer if the hair and nails are involved. Griseofulvin is most successful in severe dermatophytosis, particularly if caused by trichophyton or microsporon. Some strains of fungi are resistant.

Side-effects include headache, nausea, diarrhea, photosensitivity, fever, skin rashes, and disturbances of hepatic, nervous, and hematopoietic systems. Griseofulvin increases the metabolism of coumarin so that higher doses of the anticoagulant are needed.

3. NYSTATIN

Nystatin inhibits candida species upon direct contact. The drug is not absorbed from mucous membranes or gut. Nystatin in ointments, suspensions, etc can be applied to buccal or vaginal mucous membranes to suppress a local candida infection. After oral intake of nystatin, candida in the gut is suppressed while the drug is excreted in feces. However, there is no good indication for the use of nystatin orally because increase in gut candida is rarely associated with disease, except in leukemic immunosuppression.

4. FLUCYTOSINE

5-Flucytosine inhibits some candida and cryptococcus strains and some other fungi (eg, torulopsis). Flucytosine is 40% protein-bound and is effectively removed during hemodialysis. Dosages of 3—8 gm daily (150 mg/kg/day) orally have produced good serum (50 μg/ml) and CSF levels and clinical remissions in cases of meningitis or sepsis. Resistant organisms may appear, and toxic effects (bone marrow depression, abnormal liver function, loss of hair) occur. The value of combined use of flucytosine and amphotericin B in candida sepsis has been suggested but not proved.

Hoeprich PD & others: Development of resistance to 5-fluorocytosine in *Candida parapsilosis* during therapy. J Infect Dis 130:112, 1974.
Steer PL & others: 5-Flucytosine: An oral antifungal compound. Ann Int Med 76:15, 1972.

5. MICONAZOLE

Miconazole nitrate is a topical antifungal drug used as a 2% cream in dermatophytosis; it may be more effective than nystatin in vaginal candidiasis. Experimentally, up to 2000 mg/day have been injected IV with equivocal results.

Mandy SJ, Garrott TC: Miconazole treatment for severe derma-tophytoses. JAMA 230:72, 1974.

ANTIMICROBIAL DRUGS USED IN COMBINATION

Indications

Possible reasons for employing 2 or more antimicrobials simultaneously instead of a single drug are as follows:

(1) Prompt treatment in desperately ill patients suspected of having a serious microbial infection. A good guess about the most probable 2 or 3 pathogens is made, and drugs are aimed at those organisms. Before such treatment is started, it is essential that adequate specimens be obtained for identifying the etiologic agent in the laboratory. Gram-negative sepsis is the most important disease in this category at present.

(2) To delay the emergence of microbial mutants resistant to one drug in chronic infections by the use of a second or third non-cross-reacting drug. The most prominent examples are miliary tuberculosis, tuberculous meningitis, and chronic active tuberculosis of an organ with large microbial populations.

(3) Mixed infections, particularly those following massive trauma or those involving vascular structures. Each drug is aimed at an important pathogenic microorganism.

(4) To achieve bactericidal synergism (see below). In a few infections, eg, enterococcal sepsis, a combination of drugs is more likely to eradicate the infection than either drug used alone. Unfortunately, such synergism is unpredictable, and a given drug pair may be synergistic for only a single microbial strain.

Disadvantages

The following disadvantages of using antimicrobial drugs in combinations must always be considered:

(1) The doctor may feel that since he is already giving several drugs he has done all he can for the patient. This attitude leads to relaxation of the effort to establish a specific diagnosis. It may also give a false sense of security.

(2) The more drugs are administered, the greater the chance for drug reactions to occur or for the patient to become sensitized to drugs.

(3) Unnecessarily high cost.

(4) Antimicrobial combinations usually accomplish no more than an effective single drug.

(5) On very rare occasions, one drug may antagonize a second drug given simultaneously. Antagonism resulting in increased morbidity and mortality has been observed mainly in bacterial meningitis when a bacteriostatic drug (eg, tetracycline or chloramphenicol) was given with a bactericidal drug (eg, penicillin or ampicillin). However, antagonism is usually limited by time-dose relationships and is overcome by an excess dose of one of the drugs in the pair and is therefore a very infrequent problem in clinical therapy.

Synergism

Antimicrobial synergism can occur in several types of situations. Synergistic drug combinations must be selected by complex laboratory procedures.

(1) Sequential block of a metabolic microbial pathway by 2 drugs. Sulfonamides inhibit the use of extracellular para-aminobenzoic acid by some microbes for the synthesis of folic acid. Trimethoprim or pyrimethamine inhibits the next metabolic step, the reduction of dihydro- to tetrahydrofolic acid. The simultaneous use of a sulfonamide plus trimethoprim (cotrimoxazole) is effective in some bacterial infections (eg, urinary tract, enteric) and in malaria. Pyrimethamine plus a sulfonamide is used in toxoplasmosis.

(2) One drug may greatly enhance the uptake of a second drug and thereby greatly increase the overall bactericidal effect. Penicillins enhance the uptake of aminoglycosides by enterococci. Thus, a penicillin plus an aminoglycoside may be essential for the eradication of enterococcal (*Streptococcus faecalis*) infections, particularly sepsis or endocarditis. Similarly, carbenicillin plus gentamicin may be synergistic against some strains of pseudomonas.

ANTIMICROBIAL CHEMOPROPHYLAXIS

Anti-infective chemoprophylaxis implies the administration of antimicrobial drugs to prevent infection. In a broader sense, it also includes the use of antimicrobial drugs soon after the acquisition of pathogenic microorganisms (eg, after compound fracture) but before the development of signs of infection.

Useful chemoprophylaxis is limited to the action of a specific drug on a specific organism. An effort to prevent all types of microorganisms in the environment from establishing themselves only selects the most drug-resistant organisms as the cause of a resulting infection. In all proposed uses of prophylactic antimicrobials, the risk of the patient's acquiring an infection must be weighed against the toxicity, cost, inconvenience, and enhanced risk of superinfection resulting from the "prophylactic" drug.

Prophylaxis in Persons of Normal Susceptibility Exposed to a Specific Pathogen

In this category, a specific drug is administered to prevent one specific infection. Outstanding examples are the injection of benzathine penicillin G, 1.2—2.4 million units IM once every 3—4 weeks, to prevent reinfection with group A hemolytic streptococci in rheumatic patients; prevention of meningitis by eradicating the meningococcal carrier state with rifampin, 600 mg orally twice daily for 2 days, or minocycline, 100 mg every 12 hours for 5 days; prevention of syphilis by the injection of benzathine penicillin G, 2.4 million units IM, within 24 hours of exposure; and prevention of clinical rickettsial disease (but not of infection) by the daily ingestion of 1 gm of chloramphenicol or tetracycline during the period of exposure.

Early treatment of an asymptomatic infection is sometimes called "prophylaxis." Thus, administration of isoniazid, 6–10 mg/kg/day (maximum, 300 mg daily) orally for 6–12 months, to an asymptomatic person who converts from a negative to a positive tuberculin skin test may prevent later clinical tuberculosis.

Prophylaxis in Persons of Increased Susceptibility

Certain anatomic or functional abnormalities predispose to serious infections. It may be feasible to prevent or abort such infections by giving a specific drug for short periods. Some important examples are listed below:

A. Heart Disease: Persons with congenital or acquired abnormalities of the heart valves are unusually susceptible to implantation of microorganisms circulating in the blood stream. This bacterial endocarditis can sometimes be prevented if the proper drug can be used during periods of bacteremia. Viridans streptococci enter the blood stream from the upper respiratory tract. Large numbers of these organisms are pushed into the circulation during dental procedures and operations on the mouth or throat. At such times, the increased risk warrants the use of a prophylactic antimicrobial aimed at viridans streptococci, eg, the injection of procaine penicillin G, 600,000 units IM 1–2 hours before the procedure and once daily for 2 days thereafter. In addition, 600,000 units of aqueous penicillin G is injected IM just prior to the procedure. It may be that an aminoglycoside should be given together with penicillin for optimal bactericidal effect. In persons hypersensitive to penicillin or those receiving daily doses of penicillin for prolonged periods (for rheumatic fever prophylaxis), erythromycin, 2 gm daily orally, can be substituted to cover penicillin-resistant viridans streptococci in the throat.

Enterococci cause 5–15% of cases of bacterial endocarditis. They reach the blood stream from the urinary or gastrointestinal tract or from the female genital tract. During surgical procedures in these areas, persons with heart valve abnormalities can be given prophylaxis directed against enterococci, eg, penicillin G, 5 million units, plus gentamicin, 3 mg/kg IM daily, beginning on the day of surgery and continuing for 3 days.

During and after cardiac catheterization, blood cultures may be positive in 10–20% of patients. Many of these persons also have fever, but very few acquire endocarditis. Prophylactic antimicrobials do not appear to influence these events.

B. Respiratory Tract Disease: Persons with functional and anatomic abnormalities of the respiratory tract—eg emphysema or bronchiectasis—are subject to attacks of "recurrent chronic bronchitis." This is a recurrent bacterial infection, often precipitated by acute viral infections and resulting in respiratory decompensation. The most common organisms are pneumococci and *Haemophilus influenzae.* Chemoprophylaxis consists of giving tetracycline or ampicillin, 1 gm daily orally, during the "respiratory disease season." This is successful only in patients who are not hospitalized; otherwise, superinfection with pseudomonas, proteus, or yeasts is common. Similar prophylaxis of bacterial infection has been applied to children with mucoviscidosis who are not hospitalized. In spite of this, such children contract complicating infections caused by pseudomonas and staphylococci.

C. Recurrent Urinary Tract Infection: In some women recurrent urinary tract infection (eg, postcoital cystitis) can be prevented for months by daily use of co-trimoxazole. Eventually, however, superinfection with resistant organisms occurs.

D. Chronic Diseases and Immunosuppressive Therapy: Persons with chronic disease ("visceral angiitis," collagen vascular diseases) or with organ transplants who are receiving massive doses of corticosteroids and immunosuppressive drugs are especially susceptible to microbial infections. There is, however, no sound approach to antimicrobial prophylaxis because administration of any drug or drug group regularly leads to superinfection with drug-resistant organisms.

Prophylaxis in Surgery

Several well-controlled studies have established that the overall incidence of postoperative infections is not diminished by the administration of antimicrobials during or after surgery in "clean" elective procedures. In compound fractures, penetrating wounds of body cavities, operation on a ruptured abdominal viscus, and other "contaminated" procedures, antimicrobial drugs are often aimed at the organisms most likely to produce serious infections. A penicillin and an aminoglycoside or a cephalosporin are often administered in such situations. This approach does not significantly alter the incidence of wound infections, but it may diminish the incidence of major bacteremia or life-threatening systemic infections. However, it must be accepted that general antimicrobial prophylaxis to protect against any and all types of postoperative infection does not exist.

Before elective operations on the lower intestinal tract, it has been customary to reduce the bowel flora by the preoperative oral administration of either an insoluble sulfonamide (phthalylsulfathiazole) or neomycin-kanamycin. It is assumed that the reduction in numbers of intestinal bacteria will reduce the hazard of peritoneal infection after accidental contamination with bowel contents. Oral insoluble drugs suppress the bowel flora only transiently and partially. The lowest number of bacteria are present within 2–3 days after starting neomycin, 1 gm every 4–6 hours. Soon thereafter, bacterial numbers rise and the composition of the bowel flora changes. It is probable that the skill of the surgeon and strict aseptic technic are far more important than the "prophylaxis" in preventing peritoneal infection. Preoperative oral neomycin may lead to implantation of neomycin-resistant staphylococci in the bowel and predisposes to the development of staphylococcal enterocolitis with high morbidity and mortality.

In cardiovascular surgery, endothelial damage predisposes to infection, particularly endocarditis due to viridans streptococci. When penicillin G is given for 5 days postoperatively, this complication is virtually unknown, although endocarditis and pericarditis due to staphylococci and gram-negative bacteria may develop. Specific drugs directed against staphylococci (methicillin) or pseudomonas (polymyxin) prevent infection by these particular bacteria but favor the selection of other resistant microorganisms (serratia, fungi).

In other surgical procedures, it has been proposed that the administration of a cephalosporin in full dosage for just 12 hours may reduce the chance of postoperative infection. While the efficacy of such "prophylaxis" is not fully established, at least it minimizes the risk of selecting highly resistant organisms.

The organism most frequently producing deep infection of the operative site in orthopedic surgery is *Staphylococcus aureus*. Administration of a specific antistaphylococcal drug can have a prophylactic effect.

Topical antimicrobials are sometimes used to prevent local infections. Application of bacitracin-neomycin-polymyxin or gentamicin creams to skin sites of intravenous needles, tubes, or catheters may delay infection of the site but should never be an alternative to the every-48-hour rotation of such puncture sites. For the prevention of urinary tract infection in the presence of an indwelling catheter, only sterile, closed drainage systems must be employed. Incorporation of neomycin-polymyxin solutions into such drainage systems may further delay the growth of bacteria.

Barnett JA, Sanford JP: Bacterial shock. JAMA 209:1514, 1969.

Ericson C & others: Cloxacillin in the prophylaxis of postoperative infections of the hip. J Bone Joint Surg 55A:808, 1973.

Harding GKH, Ronald AR: A controlled study of antimicrobial prophylaxis in women. New England J Med 291:597, 1974.

Hunt TK & others: Antibiotics in surgery. Arch Surg 110:148, 1975.

Johnstone FRC: Infection on a surgical service: Present incidence compared with that of 1957. Am J Surg 120:192, 1970.

Macgregor RR, Petersdorf RG: Antimicrobial prophylaxis in kidney disease. Postgrad Med 51:105, 1972.

McGowan JE, Finland M: Usage of antibiotics in hospitals: Effects of requiring justification. J Infect Dis 130:165, 1974.

ANTIVIRAL CHEMOTHERAPY

Several compounds can influence viral replication and the development of viral disease.

Amantadine hydrochloride, 200 mg orally daily for 2–3 days before and 6–7 days after influenza A infection, reduces the incidence and severity of symptoms. The most marked untoward effects are insomnia, dizziness, and ataxia. Amantadine may accumulate in renal insufficiency, with increased toxicity.

Isoquinolines. Several substituted isoquinolines have antiviral activity against influenza B, influenza A_2, rhinoviruses, and other agents both in vitro and in experimentally infected volunteers. Their clinical use in spontaneous viral infections is not yet established.

Idoxuridine, 0.1% solution or 0.5% ointment, can be applied topically every 2 hours to acute dendritic herpetic keratitis to enhance healing. It is also used, with corticosteroids, for stromal disciform lesions of the cornea to reduce the chance of acute epithelial herpes. It may have some toxic effects on the cornea and should probably not be used for more than 2–3 weeks. Intravenous injection of idoxuridine (100–400 mg/kg over a period of 5 days, not to exceed 30 gm) has been proposed for herpetic encephalitis, but the results of this treatment have been discouraging.

Cytarabine also inhibits DNA viruses. It has been applied topically in herpetic keratitis due to idoxuridine-resistant virus. Cytarabine, 0.3–2 mg/kg as a single daily dose IV for 5 days, has been given in disseminated herpes simplex and in disseminated zoster with doubtful benefit. Adenine arabinoside is currently under test, with some encouraging results.

Methisazone can inhibit the growth of smallpox virus in man if administered to exposed persons within 1–2 days after exposure. Methisazone, 2–4 gm daily orally (for children, 100 mg/kg/day), gives striking protection against the development of clinical smallpox and permits an asymptomatic, immunizing infection. It can also inhibit the growth of vaccinia virus and is used for the treatment of complications of smallpox vaccination (eg, progressive vaccinia). The most pronounced toxic effect is profuse vomiting.

Photodynamic inactivation is a form of topical treatment of superficial herpes lesions of the mucous membranes and skin. Vesicular lesions are unroofed, painted with 0.1% proflavine or neutral red, and exposed to 15 watts of white light for 15 minutes. This exposure is repeated 6–8 hours later. The dye binds to viral DNA and, upon exposure to light, the virus is inactivated. Some controlled studies suggest that this treatment speeds healing of individual lesions and reduces the frequency of recurrences. However, there is experimental evidence that such treatment can induce neoplastic changes in cells. The magnitude of the benefits and risks has not been defined.

Ch'ien LT & others: Effect of adenine arabinoside on severe *Herpesvirus hominis.* J Infect Dis 128:658, 1973.

Felber TD & others: Photodynamic inactivation of herpes simplex: Report of a clinical trial. JAMA 223:289, 1973.

Gurwith MJ, Harman CE, Merigan TC: Approach to diagnosis and treatment of herpes simplex encephalitis: Report of 2 cases. California Med 115:63, Dec 1971.

Myers MG & others: Failure of neutral-red photodynamic inactivation in recurrent herpes simplex virus infections. New England J Med 293:945, 1975.

29...
Disorders Due to Physical Agents

Milton J. Chatton

DISORDERS DUE TO COLD

Body response to low temperatures may be either quantitative or qualitative. Severe systemic hypothermia can develop in normal individuals during exposure to cold weather. Debilitated patients have a lower degree of tolerance to cold. Some persons have a familial or acquired hypersensitivity to cold and may develop urticaria upon even limited exposure to a cold wind. Actual immersion in cold water may result in severe systemic symptoms, including shock. In many patients, cold hypersensitivity is an autosomal dominant hereditary disorder. Familial cold urticaria, manifested as a burning sensation of the skin occurring about 30 minutes after exposure to cold, does not seem to be a true urticarial disorder. In some patients, however, cold urticaria may be due to an underlying disease (eg, collagen disease, lymphoma, multiple myeloma) associated with cryoglobulinemia, which often results in purpura, Raynaud's phenomenon, and leg ulceration. Cold urticaria may also be associated with cold hemoglobinuria (see Table 9–3) as a complication of syphilis or for unknown reasons. The diagnosis of cold urticaria can usually be confirmed by application of an ice cube to the skin.

Accidental systemic hypothermia may result from exposure to prolonged or extreme cold. This is considerably more serious when there is altered homeostasis due to associated debility or disease, in which case hypothermia may follow exposure even to ordinary temperatures. Body temperature in accidental hypothermia may range from 25–35° C (77–95° F). Otherwise physically healthy patients with acute toxic reactions to drugs (eg, alcohol) or severe psychiatric disorders usually respond to passive rewarming. Patients with severe organic illness require rapid, active, internal rewarming and treatment of arrhythmia and shock, but the chances of recovery are poor.

In the normal individual, exposure to cold produces immediate localized vasoconstriction followed by generalized vasoconstriction. When the skin temperature falls to 25° C (77° F), tissue metabolism is slowed but the demand for oxygen is greater than the slowed circulation can supply and the area becomes cyanotic. At 15° C (59° F), tissue metabolism is markedly decreased and the dissociation of oxyhemoglobin is reduced, which gives a pink, well oxygenated appearance to the skin. Tissue survival at this temperature is slight. Tissue death may be caused by ischemia and thromboses in the smaller vessels or by actual freezing. Freezing (frostbite) does not occur until the skin temperature drops to −10 to −4° C (14–24.8° F) or even lower, depending on such factors as wind, mobility, venous stasis, malnutrition, and occlusive arterial disease.

Prevention of Cold Injury

"Keep warm, keep moving, and keep dry." Individuals should wear warm, dry clothing, preferably several layers, with a windproof outer garment. Wet clothing, socks, and shoes should be removed as soon as possible and replaced with dry ones. Extra socks, mittens, and insoles should always be carried in a pack when in cold or icy areas. Cramped positions, constricting clothing, and prolonged dependency of the feet are to be avoided. Exercising arms, legs, fingers, and toes to maintain circulation is essential. Avoiding wet and muddy ground and keeping sheltered from wind are important. Good nutrition and skin cleanliness are necessary. Tobacco and alcohol should be avoided when the danger of frostbite is present.

Burch GE, Giles TD: Cold hypersensitivity. Arch Int Med 134:663, 1974.

Hudson LD, Conn RD: Accidental hypothermia: Associated diagnoses and prognosis in a common problem. JAMA 227:37, 1974.

CHILBLAIN
(Pernio)

Chilblains are red, itching skin lesions, usually on the extremities, caused by exposure to cold without actual freezing of the tissues. They may be associated with edema or blistering and are aggravated by warmth. With continued exposure, ulcerative or hemorrhagic lesions may appear and progress to scarring, fibrosis, and atrophy.

Treatment consists of elevating the affected part

slightly and allowing it to warm gradually at room temperature. Do not rub or massage injured tissues or apply ice or heat. Protect the area from trauma and secondary infection.

Hilton PE, Anderson PC: Cutaneous effects of cold exposure. Missouri Med 70:23, Jan 1973.

FROSTBITE

Frostbite is injury of the superficial tissues due to freezing; it may be divided into 3 grades of severity: (1) **First degree:** freezing without blistering or peeling; (2) **second degree:** freezing with blistering or peeling; and (3) **third degree:** freezing with death of skin and perhaps the deeper tissues.

In mild cases the symptoms are numbness, prickling, and itching. With increasing severity there may be paresthesia and stiffness. Thawing causes tenderness and burning pain. The skin is white or yellow, loses its elasticity, and becomes immobile. Edema, blisters, necrosis, and gangrene may appear.

Treatment

A. Immediate Treatment:

1. Rewarming—The value of rewarming has not been conclusively established since patients are seldom seen while the tissues are still frozen. Superficial frostbite (frostnip) of extremities in the field can be treated by firm, steady pressure (without rubbing), by placing fingers in the armpits, and, in the case of the toes or heels, by removing footwear, drying feet, rewarming, and covering with adequate dry socks or other protective footwear. Rapid thawing at temperatures slightly above body heat may significantly decrease tissue necrosis. It has been suggested that rewarming is best accomplished by immersing the frozen portion of the body for several minutes in water heated to 40.5° C (105° F) *(not warmer)*. After thawing has occurred and the part has returned to normal temperature (usually in 30–90 minutes, discontinue external heat. Do not permit the patient to walk on thawed feet or toes since this is likely to cause serious tissue destruction. Never permit rewarming by exercise or thawing by rubbing with snow or ice-water. The patient's whole body temperature should be maintained by wrapping him in a blanket to keep him warm (not hot).

2. Protection of the part—Avoid trauma, eg, pressure or friction. Physical therapy is contraindicated in the early stage. Keep the patient at bed rest with the affected parts elevated and uncovered at room temperature. Do not apply casts, dressings, or bandages.

3. Anti-infective measures—Prevention of infection after the rewarming process is of great importance. Protect skin blebs from physical contact. Local infections may be treated with mild soaks. Prophylactic antibiotics are probably advisable. If ulceration has occurred, antitetanus immunization is warranted.

4. Anticoagulants—If anticoagulants are to be of

value they must be given within 24 hours after thawing. Rapid-acting heparin sodium to prolong the clotting time for about 1 week may be useful in preventing secondary thromboses in surrounding areas.

B. Follow-Up Care: Gentle progressive physical therapy to promote circulation is important as the healing process occurs. Buerger's exercises should be instituted as soon as tolerated.

C. Surgery: Immediate regional sympathectomy has been reported to protect against early and late sequelae of frostbite. In general, other surgical intervention is to be avoided. *Amputation should not be considered until it is definitely established that the tissues are dead.* Tissue necrosis (even with black eschar formation) may be quite superficial and the underlying skin may heal well spontaneously.

Knize DM & others: Prognostic factors in the management of frostbite. J Trauma 9:749, 1969.
Paton BC: The patient who came in from the cold. Emergency Med 2:12, Nov 1970.

IMMERSION SYNDROME
(Immersion Foot or Trench Foot)

Immersion foot (or hand) is caused by prolonged immersion in cool or cold water or mud. The affected parts are first cold and anesthetic; become hot with intense burning and shooting pains during the hyperemic period; and pale or cyanotic with diminished pulsations during the vasospastic period; later followed by blistering, swelling, redness, heat, ecchymoses, hemorrhage, or gangrene and secondary complications such as lymphangitis, cellulitis, and thrombophlebitis.

Treatment is best instituted during stage of reactive hyperemia. Immediate treatment consists of protecting the extremities from trauma and secondary infection and gradual rewarming by exposure to cool air (not ice or heat). Do not massage or moisten the skin or immerse the part in water. Bed rest is required until all ulcers have healed. Keep the affected parts elevated to aid in removal of edema fluid, and protect pressure sites (eg, heels) with pillows. Penicillin should be used if infection develops.

Later treatment is as for Buerger's disease.

Keatinge WR: *Survival in Cold Water: The Physiology and Treatment of Immersion Hypothermia and of Drowning.* Davis, 1969.

DISORDERS DUE TO HEAT

Exposure to excessive heat results in prompt peripheral vasodilatation, increased cardiac output, and sweating. The resultant circulatory instability may lead to syncope if the patient remains erect and immobile, but muscular activity usually prevents syncope.

Fluid loss through sweating may amount to 3–4 liters/hour with heavy work at high temperatures. The salt content of sweat increases to 0.2–0.5% with rising temperatures.

Acclimatization usually results after 8–10 days of exposure to high temperatures; but even a fully acclimatized person may suffer a disorder in the event of excessive fatigue, severe infection, alcohol intoxication, use of belladonna-like drugs, or failure to maintain hydration, salt intake, or caloric intake. Elderly or obese persons and those with chronic debilitating diseases are most susceptible to disorders due to sustained climatic heat. Breakdown may be due to circulatory failure or failure of the sweating mechanism. Cessation of sweating may indicate impending stroke or collapse.

Prevention of Disorders Due to Heat

Avoid unnecessary exposure to heat and maintain adequate fluid and salt intake, using 0.1% saline as drinking water or salt tablets and water. Activity should be increased slowly until acclimatized. Clothing should be loose-fitting (preferably white) and permeable to moisture. Avoid alcoholic indulgence, excessive fatigue, and infections. Maintain good nutrition.

Knochel JP: Environmental heat illness: An eclectic review. Arch Int Med 133:841, 1974.

HEAT EXHAUSTION
(Heat Prostration)

Heat exhaustion is due to inadequacy or collapse of the peripheral circulation secondary to salt depletion and dehydration. The condition usually occurs in patients with underlying cardiac, cerebral, or systemic disease. The symptoms are weakness, dizziness, stupor, and headache, with or without muscle cramps. The skin is cool and pale and there is profuse perspiration, oliguria, tachycardia, and hypotension. Mental confusion and muscular incoordination may occur. Laboratory studies reveal hemoconcentration and salt depletion.

Place the patient at rest in a cool place, elevate feet, and massage his legs. Unless the patient is in danger of cardiac failure, give sodium chloride, 0.1% solution, by mouth, or physiologic saline, 1000–2000 ml IV. Treat shock when present (see Chapter 1). Avoid immediate reexposure to heat.

Ansari A, Burch GE: Influence of hot environments on the cardiovascular system. Arch Int Med 123:371, 1969.
Knochel JP, Dotin LN, Hamburger RJ: Heat stress, exercise and muscle injury: Effects on urate metabolism and renal function. Ann Int Med 81:321, 1974.

HEAT STROKE
(Sunstroke)

Heat stroke is a rare disorder but a medical emergency characterized by sudden loss of consciousness and by failure of the heat-regulating mechanism as manifested by high fever and cessation of sweating. The condition often afflicts the elderly, alcoholics, the physically exhausted, or persons with cardiovascular or debilitating disease. There may be premonitory headache, dizziness, nausea, convulsions, and visual disturbances. The skin is hot, flushed, and dry; the pulse rapid, irregular, and weak; and the blood pressure low. The rectal temperature may be as high as 42–44° C (107.6–111.2° F). Hydration and salt content of the body are normal.

Treatment is aimed first at reducing high temperature. Place the patient in a shady, cool place and remove his clothing. Cool by fanning after sprinkling with water. As soon as possible, immerse the patient in cold water or use ice packs or ice-water enemas. Do not lower the rectal temperature below 39° C (102.2° F) too rapidly. Massage the extremities vigorously to maintain circulation. Repeated small doses of chlorpromazine intravenously may be required to control delirium and shivering and to make treatment more tolerable for the conscious patient. Maintain an adequate airway and administer oxygen to combat hypoxia. Systemic heparin may be given for disseminated intravascular coagulation. Do not use dextran. Sedatives are to be avoided unless the patient is having convulsions, since they further disturb the heat-regulating mechanism. Give physiologic saline solution, 1000 ml *very slowly* IV. Observe for systemic infection and give appropriate treatment. Isoproterenol (but not vasopressors) may be necessary for the treatment of shock (see Chapter 1).

Patients with heat stroke should avoid immediate reexposure to heat. Hypersensitivity to high temperatures may remain for a considerable time. It may be expedient to move to a more moderate climate in order to prevent a further episode of heat stroke.

Clowes GHA Jr, O'Donnell TF Jr: Heat stroke. New England J Med 291:564, 1974.
Medical Staff Conference: Heat Stroke. Western J Med 121:305, 1974.
Perchick JS, Winkelstein A, Shadduck RK: Disseminated intravascular coagulation in heat stroke. JAMA 231:480, 1975.

HEAT CRAMPS

Heat cramps are painful spasms of the involuntary muscles of the abdomen and extremities, due primarily to salt depletion. The skin is moist and cool, and muscle twitchings may be present. The temperature is normal or only slightly increased. Laboratory studies reveal hemoconcentration and low serum sodium.

Sodium chloride, 1 gm every one-half to 1 hour with large amounts of water, or physiologic saline solution by mouth or intravenously, usually relieves the attack promptly. Place the patient in a cool place and massage sore muscles gently. Rest should be continued for 1–3 days depending upon the severity of the attack.

Layzer RB, Rowland LP: Cramps. New England J Med 285:31, 1971.

BURNS

Burns may be caused by a wide variety of agents, including flame, hot water, steam, chemicals, electricity, or radiation. The general principles of management are about the same in all types. There is considerable difference of opinion about what constitutes the optimal type of treatment for burns.

Evaluation of the Patient

A. General Condition of the Patient: Treatment and prognosis depend upon the severity of the burns, the time elapsed before proper treatment, the age of the patient (outlook is less favorable in elderly patients), and whether or not there are complicating medical disorders (eg, diabetes, cardiovascular, and renal disease). Inhalation of smoke and fumes can cause serious respiratory obstruction or pulmonary edema. Shock may appear quite early, and if not treated promptly can progress rapidly to stupor, coma, and death. Shock should be anticipated in all patients with burns involving more than 15–20% of the body surface area.

B. Depth or Degree of Burns:

1. First degree–Erythema without blistering.

2. Second degree–Erythema with blistering.

3. Third degree–Destruction of full thickness of skin and often of deeper tissues.

C. Estimate of Extent of Burn: The amount of body surface burned and the depth of the burn determine the fluid losses. The "rule of nines" is a useful means of estimating the percentage of total body surface involved by second or third degree burns of specific skin areas (see Fig 29–1). The extent of burn is commonly overestimated. Second and third degree burns of over 15–20% of total body surface (10% in children and the elderly) usually cause marked fluid loss which results in burn shock. Burn mortality is markedly influenced by the depth and extent of the burn and the age of the patient. Burns of over 50% of body surface are frequently fatal, especially in children and the older age group.

D. Clinical Observations: Vital signs (pulse, temperature, respiration, and blood pressure) should be recorded hourly for the first 24 hours and at appropriate intervals thereafter. The general status of the patient should be carefully evaluated frequently; observe especially for evidence of shock, infection, or respiratory embarrassment. Fluid intake and output must be carefully recorded.

E. Special Laboratory Examinations: In severe burns, determine the hematocrit repeatedly as a guide to fluid therapy. Blood typing and cross-matching should be done in preparation for whole blood transfusion if needed.

F. The Critically Burned Patient: Patients with critical burns should be transported to a specialized burn center in a general hospital as soon as possible—preferably within 48 hours. Artz has categorized critical burns as follows:

(1) Second degree burns over more than 30% of body surface.

(2) Third degree burns of face, hands, feet, or over more than 10% of body surface.

(3) Burns complicated by respiratory tract injury, major soft-tissue injury, or fractures.

(4) Electrical injury.

Symptoms of Fluid Deficiency in Burns

Very close attention to clinical signs and symptoms is of great importance, particularly during the first 24 hours after the burn has occurred. Excessive thirst, vomiting, restlessness, disorientation, and mania—together with increase in pulse rate, decrease in

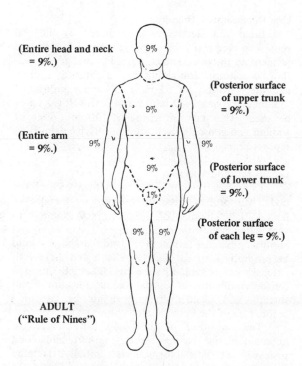

(Entire head and neck = 9%.)

9%

(Posterior surface of upper trunk = 9%.)

9%

(Entire arm = 9%.)

9%   9%

9%

(Posterior surface of lower trunk = 9%.)

1%

(Posterior surface of each leg = 9%.)

9%   9%

ADULT
("Rule of Nines")

Figure 29–1. Estimation of body surface area in burns. (Reproduced, with permission, from Wilson JL [editor]: *Handbook of Surgery,* 5th ed. Lange, 1973.)

blood pressure, collapsed veins, and oliguria—are indications that fluid losses have exceeded the rate of fluid replacement. During this critical early phase the adequacy of treatment is best judged by the urinary output, which should ideally be 30–50 ml/hour. If the rate of urinary excretion is below these suggested volumes, it is important to exclude acute renal insufficiency as a cause of the oliguria before increasing the fluid intake.

Urine volumes greater than 100 ml/hour indicate that too much fluid has been given, but after 48 hours the urinary output is completely unreliable as a guide to therapy. In part this is due to the release of nitrogenous wastes from the burned tissues, which act as diuretics; in addition, electrolyte deficits may force compensatory elimination of water, as in the developing phase of a low-salt syndrome. Under these conditions, therapy is guided almost exclusively by clinical signs and symptoms, using enough fluid to maintain normal turgor of the unburned skin, fullness of the veins, and moisture of the oral mucosa. The quantities of fluid required may be surprisingly large. However, care must be taken to avoid simple overhydration with edema of the unburned tissues or water intoxication, which may lead to coma or death.

Fluid may be administered to the acute burn patient intravenously or by mouth. Severely burned patients often vomit when given significant amounts of oral fluids and usually require intravenous therapy. However, the oral route of fluid administration is preferred and oral should be substituted for intravenous fluids as soon as possible.

Intravenous Replacement Therapy

The objective of fluid therapy in acute burns is to maintain adequate tissue perfusion as indicated by blood pressure, pulse, urine output, acid-base balance, and the clinical state of consciousness and hydration of the patient. The volume of fluid required can be calculated initially in a variety of ways (eg, Evans, Brooke, and Baxter formulas) provided the replacement program is adjusted in accordance with the *clinical evaluation and response of the patient*. With this principle in mind, the following formula can be used to make a preliminary estimate of fluid needs:

During the first 24 hours after a severe burn (the period of maximal loss), give 1 ml of plasma and 1 ml of balanced electrolyte solution (eg, lactated Ringer's injection USP) for each 1% of body surface burned and each kg of body weight. In addition, adults require 1000–2000 ml of balanced electrolyte solution to replace insensible loss.

Example: 70 kg man with a 40% burn.

1. Plasma: $1 \times 70 \times 40 =$ 2800 ml
2. Electrolyte solution: $1 \times 70 \times 40 =$ 2800 ml
3. Insensible loss (electrolyte solution) =   1400 ml

Total fluids first 24 hours: 7000 ml
During second 24 hours, give half this amount.

If more than 50% of the body surface is burned, calculations should be based on only 50% involvement. In no case should more than 10,000 ml of fluid be given in the first 24-hour period. In fact, 100 ml/kg body weight is usually sufficient as a maximum. Excess fluid in the early post-burn period serves to increase the amount of edema formation and exerts little or no effect on blood volume. For this reason, the hematocrit may remain elevated during the first day and fluid intake should not be increased with a view to restoring the hematocrit rapidly to normal.

Experience shows that an electrolyte solution such as lactated Ringer's can usually be substituted for plasma in the above formula in burns of less than 35–40% of body surface.

Acidosis is frequently present and may be corrected by administration of 0.5 mEq of $NaHCO_3$/kg body weight per mEq/liter decrease in plasma bicarbonate. Isotonic $NaHCO_3$ solution containing the calculated mEq of $NaHCO_3$ required for treatment of the acidosis can be substituted for an equivalent volume of balanced electrolyte solution in the fluid replacement formula. After the first few days, potassium loss is usually marked, making it advisable to give about 100 mEq potassium ion per day intravenously or by mouth.

Destruction of erythrocytes occurs in deep burns, but blood replacement is rarely required early in the post-burn period. Later, 3–5 days after the burn, transfusion of whole blood or packed red cells may be used to correct a reduced red cell mass.

Oral Replacement Therapy

Fluid and electrolyte replacement by the oral route can frequently be employed, alone or as a supplement to the intravenous route. For oral administration, a solution containing 5.5 gm/liter of sodium chloride (93 mEq Na^+/93 mEq Cl^-) and 4 gm/liter of sodium bicarbonate (47 mEq Na^+/47 mEq HCO_3^-) may be used. This mixture contains 140 mEq/liter of sodium and is usually well tolerated if given slowly as repeated sips.

Guides to Fluid Therapy

Patients with burns over more than 25% of the body will probably require intravenous therapy—at least initially—because of their tendency to vomit. In such patients an intravenous catheter for infusion and an inlying bladder catheter for bladder drainage should be promptly inserted. Elderly patients and those with extensive burns should have a jugular catheter inserted for determination of central venous pressure. Fluid therapy and bladder drainage should be instituted before care of the burn wound is begun.

The objectives of fluid administration are to maintain plasma volume, urinary output, and blood pressure at satisfactory levels. Initially, lactated Ringer's solution is administered rapidly during the first 2 hours until a urinary output of 30–50 ml/hour is established. Plasma may then be administered simultaneously with the electrolyte solution, the rate being determined by the volume of fluid required to maintain the urinary output. Central venous pressure is monitored to avoid circulatory overloading, especially in elderly patients or when there is pre-existing cardiovascular disease.

When urinary output lags below the optimum of 30–50 ml/hour, the rate of administration of the electrolyte solution may be doubled and the urinary response noted. Hypotension as a cause of the oliguria must be ruled out; plasma must be administered rapidly if hypotension occurs or is suspected. If urinary output remains low in spite of satisfactory venous and arterial pressure and a presumably adequate fluid intake, it may be helpful to administer mannitol as a diuretic.

The hematocrit rises in severe burns and may reach 60–65%. Adequate fluid therapy will control the rising hematocrit, but it is unnecessary and unwise to push fluids during the first 24–48 hours with the primary objective of lowering the hematocrit. It will come down spontaneously as edema fluid is returned to the circulation from the burn site. The most important parameters to observe in following the burn patient are the urinary output, the central venous and arterial blood pressures, and the clinical condition. Determination of pH and electrolyte values on blood and urine will serve as a guide to the adjustment of the electrolyte composition of the intravenous fluids. In respiratory tract burns, arterial pH, Pa_{CO_2}, and Pa_{O_2} aid in early detection and management of respiratory insufficiency.

EARLY CARE OF THE BURN WOUND

First Aid

Immersion of small or minor burned areas in cold water for one-half hour immediately after the burn, if feasible, will relieve pain and reduce cell damage.

A. First degree burns require no treatment.

B. Minor second degree burns may be washed with bland soap and water. Large blebs should be punctured aseptically but not removed. The wound is then covered with sterile petrolatum gauze and a pressure dressing. Change the dressing every 5–8 days. Healing usually takes about 2 weeks.

C. Severe burns should not be washed, greased, powdered, or painted with medication of any kind. Wrap the burned area in clean towels or sheets and transfer the patient to a hospital immediately.

Surgical Measures in Severe Burns

A. Control pain, which is usually marked, with morphine sulfate, 10–15 mg IV or IM, or other narcotic. General anesthesia is unnecessary for the initial cleansing and dressing of severe burns if a narcotic is used and procedures are done gently.

B. Treatment of Burned Area: The primary objectives are to prevent infection and promote early wound closure. Aseptic technic is essential. Wear cap, mask, sterile gown, and gloves when dressing burns. Sterile linen, instruments, and dressings are required. Cleanse burn and surrounding area with bland or hexachlorophene soap and sterile warm water. Wash gently with gauze sponges. Remove grease or oil with ether or benzene. Debride carefully. Remove only loose and necrotic tissue. Puncture blebs aseptically and leave them in place as protective coverings.

1. Closed treatment–Apply petrolatum gauze and a pressure dressing. Place a single layer of petrolatum (or Xeroform) gauze smoothly over the burn, cover this with soft pads or other absorbent dressings, and secure firmly in place with stockinet or elastic or gauze bandage.

A variation of the closed technic consists of application to the burned areas of gauze roller bandages kept saturated with 0.5% silver nitrate solution. Dressings are changed daily. This method of burn treatment has not been widely used and may involve a hazard of systemic toxicity and sodium depletion.

2. Exposure treatment–In this form of treatment, no dressings or medications are applied to the burn after cleansing and debridement. On exposure to air a coagulum of serum seals the burn wound. This is the preferred method of treating burns of the head, neck, genitalia, and perineum. It is also suitable for limited burns on one side of the trunk or extremity. In mass casualities it may be necessary to treat the burns in this manner. The patient is placed on clean sheets. He must be turned frequently when burns encircle the body in order to avoid maceration. If infection occurs beneath the coagulum, it should be removed and warm saline compresses applied to the area.

C. Prevention of Infection: Reliance is placed on thorough cleansing of the burn and on aseptic dressing technics. Prophylactic antibiotics are rarely used. Cultures are obtained from exudates, and specific antibiotics chosen on the basis of sensitivity studies when signs of infection appear. Thorough but gentle daily bathing of the patient, followed by applications, during the day, of mafenide (Sulfamylon), a sulfonamide derivative, is reported to control surface infection when used in conjunction with the exposure method of treatment.

Gentamicin, 0.1% ointment, is an excellent topical application, but the expense of therapy will necessarily limit its use. Gentamicin is effective against many strains of pseudomonas as well as some gram-negative bacilli. Since resistance to the antibiotic may occur, it has been recommended that this topical preparation be restricted to patients with severe burns. Patients being treated with topical gentamicin should be isolated from other patients to prevent spread of possible resistant strains.

Silver sulfadiazine (Silvadene) is an effective topical cream with a wide antibacterial spectrum. It is painless to apply and the emergence of resistant organisms is not common, but it is doubtful if silver sulfadiazine is superior to other anti-infective agents in improving patient survival statistics.

Immunization against tetanus should be given during the first 24 hours in all major burns.

Burns of Specific Anatomic Areas

(1) **Respiratory tract burns** should be suspected in burns of the head and neck and when burns are sustained in a closed space. Inhalation of flame or hot gases produces severe tracheobronchitis and pneumonitis. Obstructive laryngeal edema may develop rapidly, preceded by stridor, copious respiratory tract secretions, dyspnea, and cyanosis. Tracheostomy should be done without delay if there is significant obstruction or retained secretions. Oxygen, humidification, and intravenous corticosteroids may be required. Pulmonary edema is treated by careful fluid restriction, diuretics, anticongestive drugs, and positive pressure ventilation. In cases of respiratory tract burns (when pneumonia is suspected), give penicillin until sputum cultures can be obtained and a specific antibiotic chosen.

(2) **Head and neck burns** are treated by exposure (see above). They are often less deep than suspected initially, and rapid healing is favored by the great vascularity of the region. Early grafting of eyelid burns is important to avoid ectropion and corneal ulceration due to exposure.

(3) **Hand burns** must be carefully cleansed and the fingers dressed individually with petrolatum gauze. Remove rings. Immobilize the entire hand in the position of function by pressure dressings and splints. Soon after the first redressing, which is done 5–8 days after the burn, areas of third degree burn should be excised in a bloodless field (using a pneumatic tourniquet) and a skin graft applied in order to obtain the earliest possible restoration of function.

(4) **Joints** should be maintained in optimal position and all third degree involvement grafted early to avoid disabling contractures.

(5) **Perineum and genitalia burns** are left exposed and cleansed with soap and water when they become soiled with feces or urine. An inlying Foley catheter for constant drainage of the bladder may be advisable in genital burns.

LATER CARE OF THE BURN WOUND

Redressing & Reevaluation

Observe strict aseptic technic in all burn dressings. Remove the original burn dressing down to the petrolatum gauze after 5–8 days. The depth and extent of the burn can be accurately determined at this time. Second degree burns require only reapplication of the pressure dressing and should heal in about 2 weeks. Third degree burns require special management.

Treatment of Third Degree Burns

A. **Removal of Slough:** The necrotic surface of a third degree burn usually does not separate for many weeks. Significant areas of slough or necrosis should therefore be removed in the operating room under general anesthesia 10–14 days after the burn if the patient's general condition allows. Burns of the face permit more conservative debridement since slough separates rapidly in this region.

B. **Skin Grafting:** Early skin grafting (preferably within the first few weeks following the burn) is essential to avoid chronic sepsis, malnutrition, and scar contractures. Skin grafting should be started as soon after removal of slough as possible. The denuded granulating surface should be firm and bright red, with a minimum of exudate. Warm saline dressings (changed several times daily) may be of assistance in the preparation of the burn wound for skin grafting. Homografts or heterografts, when used as temporary cover of the burn wound, may minimize fluid loss and infection while the patient is being prepared for autografting.

C. **Control of Infection:** Signs of infection include rising temperature, tachycardia, general toxicity, local pain and tenderness, and increased drainage. Pockets of pus trapped beneath slough must be sought and liberated by debridement. Warm saline dressings (changed several times daily) are applied to infected areas. Cultures are taken and antibiotic chosen by sensitivity studies. Prolonged antibiotic therapy is not necessary if drainage and dressings are adequate. Skin grafts will not survive in the presence of a virulent, invasive infection, but grafting should be done as soon as the infection is under control. A daily tub bath in warm water with soap may be helpful in cleaning up a chronically septic burn. Bland ointment dressings can be soaked off relatively painlessly in the tub and reapplied after the bath. Continuous dressings soaked repeatedly with 0.5% silver nitrate solution between daily tub baths are an effective means of controlling surface infection.

General Supportive Measures

Chronic infection, exudative loss of protein, catabolic response to stress, and anorexia and depression caused by pain and toxemia can produce rapid nutritional depletion in the severely burned patient. The anemia that is often present is usually the result of hemolysis at the time of burning with subsequent inhibition of erythropoiesis by infection. The most effective supportive measures are a high-caloric, high-protein intake at the outset of therapy, vitamin supplements, and blood transfusions to keep the hemoglobin above 12 gm/100 ml.

The excretion of potassium is high during the acute phase of burns and may remain elevated for several weeks. In addition, a poor food intake at this time will prevent adequate replacement of potassium. Beginning on the third or fourth day of treatment, give potassium chloride, 3–4 gm orally (not in tablet form) in fruit juice or broth 3 times a day, until a full normal diet is taken.

Curling's ulcer, which may become evident in 5–10 days after the burn, requires treatment as for peptic ulcer due to any cause.

Since the badly burned patient is subject to multiple and severe stresses, his emotional responses may be so marked as to interfere with treatment. The clinician must provide the necessary support, explanation, and reassurance to alleviate the patient's distress in order to enhance recovery and prevent serious psychiatric complications.

Andreasen NJC & others: Management of emotional reactions in seriously burned adults. New England J Med 286:65, 1972.

Artz CP: Burns: From first aid to skin graft. Drug Therapy 5:127, April 1975.

Artz CP, Moncrief JA: *The Treatment of Burns.* Saunders, 1969.

Ballin JC: Evaluation of a new topical agent for burn therapy: Silver sulfadiazine (Silvadene). JAMA 230:1184, 1974.

Baxter CR, Marvin JA, Curreri PW: Early management of thermal burns. Postgrad Med 55:131, 1974.

Czaja AJ, McAlhany JC, Pruitt BA Jr: Acute duodenitis and duodenal ulceration after burns. JAMA 232:621, 1975.

Hinton P & others: Blood volume changes and transfusion requirements of burned patients after the shock phase of therapy. Lancet 1:913, 1972.

Hutcher N, Haynes BW Jr: The Evans formula revisited. J Trauma 12:453, 1972.

MacArthur JD, Moore FD: Epidemiology of burns: The burn-prone patient. JAMA 231:259, 1975.

Moncrief JA: Burns. New England J Med 288:444, 1973.

Waisbren BA, Stern M, Collentine GE: Methods of burn treatment: Comparison by probit analysis. JAMA 231:255, 1975.

Walsh WA & others: Gasoline immersion burns. New England J Med 291:830, 1975.

DROWNING

Drowning is the 4th leading cause of accidental death in the USA. The number of deaths due to drowning could undoubtedly be significantly reduced if adequate preventive and first aid instruction programs were instituted. Swimming instruction should be given to as many people as possible at an early age. Private swimming pools should be properly enclosed, public pools should have trained life-guards, and hazardous swimming areas should be properly posted. As many individuals as possible should be taught the proper technic of artificial respiration. Compulsory teaching of artificial respiration to school children has been suggested. Swimmers should be cautioned against hyperventilation as a means of prolonging underwater swimming because of the possibility of inducing unconsciousness.

Spontaneous recovery usually occurs in victims of near drowning. If the victim is not breathing, clear the pharynx with the fingers and institute immediate artificial respiration by fully extending the victim's head and blowing intermittently through his mouth or nose (see Appendix). (Attempts to "drain water" from the victim are of doubtful value and may waste valuable time.) The prone position is not superior to the supine position with respect to drainage of water from the lungs. If intermittent positive pressure equipment is available, administration of 100% oxygen may be of considerable value. Mouth-to-mouth respiration should never be delayed or discontinued during transportation of the patient or in attempting to procure oxygen apparatus, airways, a defibrillator, or other equipment. Artificial respiration should be continued as long as the heart is still beating, no matter how weakly. If carotid pulsations cease, give simultaneous artificial ventilation and external cardiac massage (see Appendix). Summon an emergency vehicle for transportation to a hospital. Do not interrupt resuscitation for even a few seconds. Because metabolic acidosis is almost a constant finding, it is recommended that all patients be given sodium bicarbonate, 1 mEq/kg body weight IV, as soon as possible. Additional bicarbonate should be given as required.

Since fresh water is hypotonic and salt water is hypertonic, the pathophysiology of drowning in the 2 circumstances has been held to be sufficiently different—at least in theory—that different treatment rationales have been proposed. Actually, clinical experience has failed to support significant therapeutic differences. Pulmonary resuscitation is essential for each.

In fresh water drowning, asphyxia, metabolic acidosis, ventricular fibrillation, reflex pulmonary hypertension, hemodilution, hypervolemia, hemolysis, and hyponatremia occur. Treatment includes cardiopulmonary resuscitation and correction of circulatory changes, blood hemolysis, and electrolyte imbalance. The pneumonitis due to fresh water aspiration may be improved by the administration of corticosteroids.

In salt water drowning, the pathologic findings consist of asphyxia, metabolic acidosis, pulmonary edema, hemoconcentration, hypovolemia, hypoproteinemia, and hypernatremia. Acute renal failure may occur. Cardiopulmonary resuscitation and correction of plasma and electrolyte deficiencies may be required.

When near drowning occurs in chlorinated fresh water, the most serious problem appears to be pulmonary edema and resultant hypoxia and metabolic acidosis. Hemolysis also occurs but may be less severe and slower in onset than when pure fresh water is aspirated. Treatment is directed primarily at the pulmonary edema, aspiration pneumonitis, and hypoxia.

Careful monitoring of cardiorespiratory function, measurement of urine output, and serial determination of blood gases and electrolytes are required. Supportive measures to correct hypoxia and acid-base, electrolyte, and circulatory disturbances should be continued until the victim is clearly out of danger.

Prophylactic antibiotics have been suggested for the prevention of aspiration pneumonia.

Grausz H, Amend WJC Jr, Early LE: Acute renal failure complicating submersion in sea water. JAMA 217:207, 1971.

Modell JH: *The Pathophysiology and Treatment of Drowning and Near-Drowning.* Thomas, 1971.

Pace NL: Positive end-expiratory pressure (PEEP) in treating salt water near-drowning. Western J Med 122:165, 1975.

ELECTRIC SHOCK

The possibility of life-threatening electrical injury exists in all electrified areas—home, school, industry, agriculture, recreation, and even in hospitals. Electric shock may result from carelessness, ignorance, faulty appliances and equipment, or from an act of nature—lightning. Dry skin provides a high-resistance barrier to ordinary levels of external electric current. Skin moistened with water, sweat, saline solution, or urine, however, has greatly reduced resistance to electric current. The effect of electric current may be purely a local unpleasant tingling or a painful sensation. The amount and type of current, the duration and area of exposure, and the pathway of the current through the body determine the degree of damage. When the heart is a component of the electrical pathway (circuit), the effect may be lethal.

Direct current is much less dangerous than alternating current. Alternating current of high voltage with very high cycles may be less dangerous than a low voltage with low cycles. With alternating currents of 25–300 cycles, low voltages (below 220) tend to produce ventricular fibrillation; high voltages (over 1000), respiratory failure; intermediate voltages (220–1000), both. Domestic house current of 110 volts with low cycles (about 60 cycles per second) is, accordingly, dangerous to the heart since it may cause ventricular fibrillation.

Electric burns are of 3 distinct types: flash (arcing) burns, flame (clotting) burns, and the direct heating effect of tissues by the electric current. The latter lesions are usually sharply demarcated, round or oval, painless gray areas with inflammatory reaction. Little happens to them for several weeks; sloughing then occurs slowly over a fairly wide area. Electric shock may produce momentary or prolonged loss of consciousness. With recovery there may be muscular pain, fatigue, headache, and nervous irritability. The physical signs vary according to the action of the current. With ventricular fibrillation, no heart sounds or pulse can be found and the patient is unconscious. The respirations continue for a few minutes, becoming exaggerated as asphyxia occurs and then ceasing as death intervenes. With respiratory failure, respirations are absent and the patient is unconscious; the pulse can be felt, but there is a marked fall in blood pressure and the skin is cold and cyanotic. Electric shock may be a hazard in routine hospital equipment which is usually considered to be harmless (eg, electrocardiographs, suction machines, electrically operated beds, x-ray units). Proper installation, utilization, and maintenance by qualified personnel should minimize this hazard. Battery operated devices provide the maximum protection from accidental electric shock. Electrochemical cutaneous burns have been reported with direct current voltages as low as 3 volts.

Treatment

A. Emergency Measures: Free the victim from the current at once. This may be done in many ways, but the rescuer must protect himself. Turn off the power, sever the wire with a dry wooden-handled axe, make a proper ground to divert the current, or drag the victim carefully away by means of dry clothing or a leather belt.

Institute cardiopulmonary resuscitation immediately (see Appendix) if breathing is depressed or absent, and continue until spontaneous breathing and cardiac function return or rigor mortis sets in.

B. Hospital Measures: Hospitalize the patient when revived and observe for shock, sudden cardiac dilatation, secondary hemorrhage, acidosis, or myoglobinuria.

Perform lumbar puncture cautiously if signs of increased intracranial pressure are noted.

Treat tissue burns conservatively. The direction and extent of tissue injury may not be apparent for weeks. Infection is usually not a problem early. Patience and delay are important in treatment; allow granulation tissue to be well established before attempting surgery. Hemorrhage may occur late and may be severe.

The unpredictable damage to deep tissues in electric burns makes it difficult to assess the fluid requirements for patients who are in shock.

Prognosis

Complications may occur in almost every part of the body. The most common cause of death in those who survive the original electric shock is systemic infection.

Hartford CE & others: Electrical injury. J Trauma 11:331, 1971.

Kay NRM, Boswick JA Jr: The management of electrical injuries of the extremities. S Clin North America 53:1459, 1973.

Starmer CF, McIntosh HD, Whalen RE: Electrical hazards and cardiovascular function. New England J Med 284:181, 1971.

IRRADIATION REACTIONS

The effects of radiation may develop during or after the course of therapeutic x-ray or radium administration or after any exposure to ionizing radiation (eg, x-rays, neutrons, gamma rays, alpha or beta particles). The harmful effects of radiation are determined by the degree of exposure, which in turn depends not only upon the quantity of radiation delivered to the body but also the type of radiation, which tissues of the body are exposed, and the duration of exposure. Three hundred to 500 R (400–600 rads) of x-ray or gamma radiation applied to the entire body at one time would probably be fatal. (For purposes of comparison, a routine chest x-ray delivers about 0.3 R.) Tolerance to radiation is difficult to define and there is no firm basis for evaluating radiation effects for all types and levels of irradiation. The maximum permissible daily occupational total body exposure for radiation workers has been established at 5 rem/year (multiplied by number of years of age > 18) by the Federal Radiation Council (May, 1960).

Behrens CF, King ER (editors): *Atomic Medicine,* 5th ed. Williams & Wilkins, 1969.
Lawrence JH: *Recent Advances in Nuclear Medicine.* Grune & Stratton, 1971.

ACUTE (IMMEDIATE) RADIATION EFFECTS ON NORMAL TISSUES

Clinical Findings

A. Injury to Skin and Mucous Membranes: Irradiation causes erythema, epilation, destruction of fingernails, or epidermolysis, depending upon the dose.

B. Injury to Deep Structures:

1. Hematopoietic tissues—Injury to the bone marrow may cause diminished production of blood elements. Lymphocytes are most sensitive, polymorphonuclear leukocytes next most sensitive, and erythrocytes least sensitive. Damage to the blood-forming organs may vary from transient depression of one or more blood elements to complete destruction.

2. Cardiovascular—Pericarditis with effusion or constrictive carditis may occur after a period of many months. Myocarditis is less common. Smaller vessels (the capillaries and arterioles) are more readily damaged than larger blood vessels. If injury is mild, recovery occurs.

3. Gonads—In males, small single doses of radiation (200–300 R) cause aspermatogenesis and larger doses (600–800 R) may cause sterility. In females, single doses of 200 R may cause temporary cessation of menses and 500–800 R may cause permanent castration. Moderate to heavy radiation of the embryo in utero results in injury to the fetus or in embryonic death and abortion.

4. Respiratory tract—High or repeated moderate doses of radiation may cause pneumonitis, often delayed for weeks or months.

5. The salivary glands may be depressed by radiation, but relatively large doses may be required.

6. Mouth, pharynx, esophagus, and stomach—Mucositis with edema and painful swallowing of food may occur within hours or days after onset of radiation. Gastric secretion may be temporarily (occasion-ally permanently) inhibited by moderately high doses of radiation.

7. Intestines—Inflammation and ulceration may follow moderately large doses of radiation.

8. Endocrine glands and viscera—Hepatitis and nephritis may be delayed effects of therapeutic radiation. The normal thyroid, pituitary, pancreas, adrenals, and bladder are relatively resistant to low or moderate doses of radiation.

9. The brain and spinal cord may be damaged by high doses of radiation because of impaired blood supply.

10. Peripheral and autonomic nerves are highly resistant to radiation.

C. Systemic Reaction (Radiation Sickness): The basic mechanisms of radiation sickness are not known. Anorexia, nausea, vomiting, weakness, exhaustion, lassitude, and in some cases prostration may occur, singly or in combination. Radiation sickness associated with x-ray therapy is most likely to occur when the therapy is given in large dosage to large areas over the abdomen, less often when given over the thorax, and rarely when therapy is given over the extremities. With protracted therapy, this complication is rarely significant. The patient's psychologic reaction to his illness or to the treatment plays an important role in aggravating or minimizing such effect.

Prevention

Persons handling radiation sources can minimize exposure to radiation by recognizing the importance of time, distance, and of shielding. Areas housing x-ray and nuclear materials must be properly shielded. Untrained or poorly trained personnel should not be permitted to work with x-ray and nuclear radiation. Any unnecessary exposures, diagnostic or therapeutic, should be avoided. X-ray equipment should be periodically checked for reliability of output, and proper filters should be employed. When feasible, it is advisable to shield the gonads, especially of young persons. Fluoroscopic examination should be performed as rapidly as possible, using an optimal combination of beam characteristics and filtration; the tube-to-table distance should be at least 45 cm (18 inches), and the beam size should be kept to a minimum required by the examination. Special protective clothing may be necessary to protect against contamination with radioisotopes. In the event of accidental contamination, removal of all clothing and vigorous bathing with soap and water should be followed by careful instrument (Geiger counter) check for localization of ionizing radiation.

Active research is being conducted on the use of pharmacologic radioprotectant agents (eg, glycine, alloxan, polyethylene), but no safe and effective drugs are as yet available for this purpose.

Treatment

There is no specific treatment for the biologic effects of ionizing radiation. The success of treatment of local radiation effects will depend upon the extent, degree, and location of tissue injury. Treatment is supportive and symptomatic.

A systemic radiation reaction following radiation therapy (radiation sickness) is preferably prevented, but when it does occur it is treated symptomatically and supportively. No truly effective antinauseant drug is available for the distressing nausea that frequently occurs. Dimenhydrinate, 100 mg, or perphenazine, 4–8 mg, 1 hour before and 1 hour and 4 hours after radiation therapy—or 4 times daily—may be of value. Whole blood transfusions may be necessary if anemia is present. Transfusion of marrow cells has been employed recently. Disturbances of fluid or electrolyte balance require appropriate treatment. Antibiotics may be of use in the event of secondary infection.

Bloomer WD, Hellman S: Normal tissue responses to radiation therapy. New England J Med 293:80, 1975.

DELAYED (CHRONIC) EFFECTS OF EXCESSIVE DOSES OF IONIZING RADIATION

Clinical Findings

A. Somatic Effects: Skin scarring, atrophy, and telangiectases, obliterative endarteritis, pulmonary fibrosis, intestinal stenosis, and other late effects may occur.

Cataracts may occur following irradiation of the lens.

Leukemia may occur, perhaps only in susceptible individuals, many years following radiation. Under the usual conditions of radiation therapy this is rare; the incidence of cataracts in properly protected radiation workers should be about the same as in the general population.

The incidence of neoplastic disease is increased in persons exposed to large amounts of radiation, particularly in areas of heavy damage.

Microcephaly and other congenital abnormalities may occur in children exposed in utero, especially if the fetus was exposed during the first 4 months of pregnancy.

Life-shortening may be one of the late consequences of accidental or therapeutic exposure to radiation. In the case of atom bomb survivors, however, the tumor-independent life-shortening effect has so far been equivocal.

B. Genetic Effects: Alteration of the sex ratio at birth (fewer males than females) suggests genetic damage. The incidence of congenital abnormalities, stillbirths, and neonatal deaths when conception occurs after termination of radiation exposure is apparently not increased.

Anderson RE: Longevity in radiated human populations, with particular reference to the atomic bomb survivors. Am J Med 55:643, 1973.

Gofman JW, Tamplin AR: Radiation, cancer, and environmental health. Hosp Practice 5:91, Oct 1970.

Maynard CD: Clinical Nuclear Medicine. Lea & Febiger, 1969.

Norwood WD: Atomic power safety: A common sense approach. JAMA 221:1392, 1972.

Parker LN & others: Thyroid carcinoma after exposure to atomic radiation. Ann Int Med 80:600, 1974.

Vaughn JM: The Effects of Radiation on the Human Skeleton. Oxford, 1973.

• • •

DECOMPRESSION SICKNESS (Caisson Disease, Bends)

Decompression sickness has long been known as an occupational hazard of professional divers who are involved in deep-water exploration, rescue, salvage, or construction, and professional divers and their surface supporting teams are familiar with the prevention, recognition, and treatment of this disease. In recent years the sport of scuba (self-contained underwater breathing apparatus) diving has become very popular, and a large number of untrained individuals are exposed to, but unfamiliar with, the hazards of decompression sickness.

At low depths the greatly increased pressure (eg, at 30 meters [100 feet] the pressure is 4 times greater than at the surface) compresses the respiratory gases into the blood and other tissues. During ascent from depths greater than 9 meters (30 feet), gases dissolved in the blood and other tissues escape as the external pressure decreases. The appearance of symptoms is dependent upon the depth and duration of submersion, the degree of physical exertion, the age, weight, and physical condition of the diver, and the rate of ascent. The size and number of the gas bubbles (notably nitrogen) escaping from the tissues are dependent upon the difference between the atmospheric pressure and the partial pressure of the gas dissolved in the tissues. It is the release of gas bubbles, and particularly the location of their release, which determines the symptoms.

Decompression sickness may also occur in rapid ascents from sea level to high altitudes when there is no adequate pressurizing protection.

The onset of symptoms occurs within 30 minutes in half of cases and almost invariably within 6 hours. Symptoms, which are highly variable, include pain (largely in the joints), pruritic rash, visual disturbances, weakness or paralysis, dizziness or vertigo, headache, dyspnea, paresthesias, aphasia, and coma.

Early recognition and prompt treatment are extremely important. Continuous administration of oxygen is indicated as a first aid measure, whether or not cyanosis is present. Aspirin may be given for pain, but narcotics should be used very cautiously since they may obscure the patient's response to recompression. Rapid transportation to a treatment facility for recompression is necessary not only to relieve symptoms but to prevent permanent impairment. The physician should be familiar with the nearest recompression center. The local public health department or nearest naval facility should be able to provide such information. The importance of treating plasma deficit has been recently emphasized. Hypothermia may also be indicated.

Lambertson CJ & others: Symposium on undersea-aerospace medicine: Modern aspects of treatment of decompression sickness. Aerospace Med 39:1055, 1968.

Miles S: *Underwater Medicine,* 3rd ed. Lippincott, 1969.

Sanford JP: Medical aspects of recreational skin and scuba diving. Ann Rev Med 25:401, 1974.

MOUNTAIN SICKNESS

Modern, rapid means of transportation have increased the number of unacclimatized individuals who are exposed to the effects of high altitude. Lack of sufficient time for acclimatization, increased physical activity, and varying degrees of health may be responsible for the acute and chronic disturbances which result from hypoxia at altitudes of greater than 2000 meters (6560 feet). Marked individual differences in tolerance to hypoxia exist.

Acute Mountain Sickness

Initial manifestations include dizziness, headache, lassitude, drowsiness, chilliness, nausea and vomiting, facial pallor, dyspnea, and cyanosis. Later, there is facial flushing, irritability, difficulty in concentrating, vertigo, tinnitus, visual (retinal hemorrhages may occur) and auditory disturbances, anorexia, insomnia, increased dyspnea and weakness on exertion, increased headaches (due to cerebral edema), palpitations, tachycardia, Cheyne-Stokes breathing, and weight loss. Voluntary, periodic hyperventilation may relieve symptoms. In most individuals, symptoms clear within 24–48 hours, but in some instances, if the symptoms are sufficiently persistent or severe, return to lower altitudes is required. Administration of oxygen will often relieve acute symptoms. Judicious use of sedatives may be of value for some adults with irritability and insomnia. Preventive measures include adequate rest and sleep the day before travel, reduced food intake, and avoidance of alcohol, tobacco, and unnecessary physical activity during travel.

Acute High-Altitude Pulmonary Edema

This serious complication usually occurs at levels above 3000 meters (9840 feet). Early symptoms of pulmonary edema may appear within 6–36 hours after arrival at a high-altitude area—dry, incessant cough, dyspnea at rest, and substernal oppression. Later, wheezing, orthopnea, and hemoptysis may occur. Physical findings include tachycardia, mild fever, tachypnea, cyanosis, and rales and rhonchi. The patient may become confused or even comatose, and the entire clinical picture may resemble severe pneumonia. Microthrombi are often seen in the pulmonary capillaries. The white count is often slightly elevated, but the blood sedimentation rate is usually normal. Chest x-ray findings vary from irregular patchy exudate in one lung to nodular densities bilaterally or with transient prominence of the central pulmonary arteries. Transient, nonspecific ECG changes, occasionally showing right ventricular strain, may occur. Pulmonary arterial blood pressure is elevated, whereas pulmonary wedge pressure is normal. Treatment consists of bed rest in the semi-Fowler position and continuous oxygen administration by tent or mask at 6–8 liters/hour. Subjective discomfort is relieved within 30 minutes to 2 hours, and recovery is usually complete within 2–3 days. If treatment facilities are not available and safe transportation is feasible, the patient should be moved to lower altitudes as soon as possible. If response to oxygen is not complete, or if oxygen is not available, rapid intravenous digitalization has been recommended. Improvement of overall gas exchange by the use of diuretic drugs has been reported. If bacterial pneumonia exists, appropriate antibiotic therapy should be given.

Preventive measures include education of prospective mountaineers regarding the possibility of serious pulmonary edema; optimal physical conditioning before travel; gradual ascent to permit acclimatization; a period of rest and inactivity for 1–2 days after arrival at high altitudes; prompt medical attention if respiratory symptoms develop; and, in the case of individuals with a history of high-altitude pulmonary edema, routine hospitalization with special observation for tachycardia and cough. Mountaineering parties at levels of 3000 meters (9840 feet) or greater, if hospital facilities are not available, should carry a supply of oxygen and equipment sufficient for several days. Persons with symptomatic cardiac or pulmonary disease should avoid high altitudes.

Subacute Mountain Sickness

This occurs most frequently in unacclimatized individuals and at altitudes above 4500 meters (14,760 feet). Symptoms, which are probably due to CNS anoxia without associated alveolar hyperventilation, are similar to but more persistent and severe than those of acute mountain sickness. There are additional problems of dehydration, skin dryness, and pruritus. The hematocrit may be elevated, and there may be ECG and chest x-ray evidence of right ventricular hypertrophy. Treatment consists of rest, oxygen administration, and return to lower altitudes.

Chronic Mountain Sickness

This uncommon condition, which is encountered in individuals living in high-altitude communities for prolonged periods, is difficult to differentiate clinically from chronic pulmonary disease. The disorder is characterized by somnolence, mental depression, cyanosis, clubbing of fingers, polycythemia (hematocrit often >

75%), signs of right ventricular failure, ECG evidence of right axis deviation and right atrial and ventricular hypertrophy, and x-ray evidence of right heart enlargement and central pulmonary vessel prominence. There is no x-ray evidence of structural pulmonary disease. Pulmonary function tests usually disclose alveolar hypoventilation and elevated CO_2 tension but fail to reveal defective oxygen transport. There is a diminished respiratory response to CO_2. Almost complete disappearance of all abnormalities eventually occurs when the patient returns to sea level.

Hussey HH: Effects of high altitude on the eyes. JAMA 232:1270, 1975.

Lenfant C, Sullivan K: Adaptation to high altitudes. New England J Med 284:1298, 1971.

Wilson R: Acute high-altitude illness in mountaineers and problems of rescue. Ann Int Med 78:421, 1973.

MEDICAL EFFECTS OF AIR TRAVEL & SELECTION OF PATIENTS FOR AIR TRAVEL

The decision about whether or not it is advisable for a patient to travel by air depends not only upon the nature and severity of the illness but also upon such factors as the duration of flight, the altitude to be flown, pressurization, the availability of supplementary oxygen and other medical supplies, the presence of attending physicians and trained nursing attendants, and other special considerations. Medical hazards or complications of modern air travel are remarkably uncommon; unless there is some specific contraindication, air transportation may actually be the best means of moving patients. The Air Transport Association of America defines an incapacitated passenger as "one who is suffering from a physical or mental disability and who, because of such disability or the effect of the flight on the disability, is incapable of self-care; would endanger the health or safety of such person or other passengers or airline employees; or would cause discomfort or annoyance of other passengers."

Cardiovascular Disease

A. Cardiac Decompensation: Patients in congestive failure should not fly until they are compensated by appropriate treatment, or unless they are in a pressurized plane with 100% oxygen therapy available during the entire flight.

B. Compensated Valvular or Other Heart Disease: Patients should not fly over 2400–2800 meters (7870–9180 feet) unless aircraft is pressurized and oxygen is administered at altitudes approaching or above 2400 meters.

C. Acute Myocardial Infarction, Convalescent and Asymptomatic: At least 6–8 weeks of convalescence are recommended even for asymptomatic patients if flying is contemplated. Ambulatory, stabilized, and compensated patients tolerate air travel well. Oxygen should be available.

D. Angina Pectoris: Air travel is inadvisable for patients with severe angina. In mild to moderate cases of angina, air travel may be permitted, especially in pressurized planes. Oxygen should be available.

Respiratory Disease

A. Nasopharyngeal Disorders: Nasal allergies and infections predispose to development of aerotitis. Chewing gum, nasal decongestants, and appropriate anti-infective treatment may prevent aerotitis.

B. Asthma: Patients with mild asthma can travel without difficulty. Patients with status asthmaticus should not be permitted to fly.

C. Pneumonia: Unless there is marked impairment of pulmonary function, pneumonia patients may fly if oxygen is available.

D. Tuberculosis: Patients with active, communicable tuberculosis or pneumothorax should not be permitted to travel by air.

E. Other Pulmonary Disorders: Patients may be flown safely unless there is marked impairment of pulmonary function.

Anemia

If hemoglobin is less than 8–9 gm/100 ml, oxygen should be available. Patients with severe anemia should not travel until hemoglobin has been raised to a reasonable level. Patients with sickle cell anemia appear to be particularly vulnerable.

Diabetes Mellitus

Diabetics who do not need insulin or who can administer their own insulin during flight may fly safely. "Brittle" diabetics who are subject to frequent episodes of hypoglycemia should be in optimal control before flying and should carry sugar or candy in case hypoglycemic reactions occur.

Contagious Diseases

Patients with contagious diseases are not permitted to travel by scheduled passenger airlines at any time.

Patients With Surgical Problems

Patients convalescing from thoracic or abdominal surgery should not fly until 10 days after surgery, and then only if their wound is healed and there is no drainage.

Colostomy patients may be permitted to travel by air providing they are nonodorous and colostomy bags are emptied before flight.

Patients with large hernias, unsupported by a truss or binder, should not be permitted to fly in nonpressurized aircraft because of an increased danger of strangulation.

Postsurgical or post-traumatic eye cases require pressurized cabins and oxygen therapy to avoid retinal damage due to hypoxia.

Psychiatric Disorders

Severely psychotic, agitated, or disturbed patients should not be permitted to fly on scheduled airlines even when accompanied by a medical attendant.

Extremely nervous or apprehensive patients may travel by air if they receive adequate sedatives or tranquilizers before and during flight.

Motion Sickness

Patients subject to motion sickness should receive sedatives or antihistamines (eg, dimenhydrinate or meclizine), 50 mg 4 times daily, before and during the flight. Small meals of easily digested food before and during flight may reduce the tendency to nausea and vomiting.

Pregnancy

Pregnant women may be permitted to fly during the first 8 months of pregnancy unless there is a history of habitual abortion or premature birth. During the 9th month of pregnancy a statement must be furnished that delivery is not due within 72 hours of destination time. Infants less than 1 week old should not be flown at high altitudes or for long distances.

Moylan JA Jr, Pruitt BA Jr: Aeromedical transportation. JAMA 224:1271, 1973.

Wolf CR: Aerotitis in air travel. California Med 117:10, Nov 1972.

30 . . .
Poisons

Robert H. Dreisbach

DIAGNOSIS OF POISONING

The diagnosis of poisoning, when not obvious, depends in great measure upon considering the possibility that poisoning has occurred. Once the physician includes poisoning in his differential diagnosis, he will be more likely to take the necessary steps to confirm or reject this possibility.

In general, the steps leading to a diagnosis of poisoning are as follows:

(1) Question the patient or his relatives or co-workers carefully concerning the presence of poisons in the environment.

(2) Take a careful history and perform a complete physical examination. The history is likely to be unreliable, especially in suicidal poisoning.

(3) Take samples for laboratory evaluation of damage to specific organs and to confirm or rule out exposure to specific poisons. Gastric contents usually have the highest concentration of poison and can be used to indicate the possibility but not the seriousness of poisoning.

Cases of poisoning generally fall into 3 specific categories: (1) exposure to a known poison, (2) exposure to an unknown substance which may be a poison, and (3) disease of undetermined etiology in which poisoning must be considered as part of the differential diagnosis. For further information on the diagnosis and treatment of poisoning, consult the books listed in the bibliography (p 956).

EXPOSURE TO KNOWN POISONS

In most cases of poisoning, the agent responsible is known and the physician's only problem is to determine whether the degree of exposure is sufficient to require more than emergency or first aid treatment. The exact quantity of poison absorbed by the patient will probably not be known, but the physician may be able to estimate the greatest amount which the patient could have absorbed by examining the container from which the poison was obtained and comparing the missing quantity with the known fatal dose. Reported minimum lethal doses are useful indications of the relative hazards of poisonous substances, but the fatal dose may vary greatly. If the poison is known to have caused serious or fatal poisoning, treatment for exposure to any quantity must be vigorous.

EXPOSURE TO SUBSTANCES WHICH MAY BE POISONOUS

If a patient has been exposed to a substance whose ingredients are not known, the physician must identify the contents without delay. The following sources are suggested for identifying the contents of trade-named mixtures.

Call Poison Information Center

Obtain the telephone number of the nearest Poison Information Center from the local medical society (or use the number listed below). Make certain that 24-hour service is available. Poison information centers are in most cases able to identify the ingredients of trade-named mixtures, give some estimate of their toxicity, and suggest the necessary treatment.

Altanta	(404) 659—1212
Chicago	(312) 942—5969
Denver	(303) 893—7771
Kansas City, Missouri	(816) 421—8060
Los Angeles	(213) 664—2121
Memphis	(901) 525—3005
New Orleans	(504) 899—3409
New York	(212) 340—4495
San Francisco	(415) 431—2800
Seattle	(206) 634—5252

Books

Since available proprietary mixtures number in the hundreds of thousands, it is impractical to include all of these names in a single reference work. However, a number of books are useful in determining the contents of mixtures and should be available to every physician:

1. Frear DEH: *Pesticide Handbook—Entoma* (annual publication). College Science Publishers. (Lists 7700 pesticide mixtures.)

2. Gleason MN, Gosselin RE, Hodge HC, Smith RP: *Clinical Toxicology of Commercial Products,* 3rd ed. Williams & Wilkins, 1969. (Lists ingredients of about 17,000 household products.)

3. *The Merck Index,* 8th ed. Merck, 1968.

4. *American Drug Index* (annual). Lippincott.

5. *Physician's Desk Reference* (annual publication). Medical Economics, Inc. (Tablet and capsule identification guide.)

6. Dreisbach RH: *Handbook of Poisoning: Diagnosis & Treatment,* 8th ed. Lange, 1974. (Lists 6000 poisons and trade-named mixtures.)

7. Hayes WJ: *Clinical Handbook on Economic Poisons.* US Public Health Service Publ No. 476. Government Printing Office, 1963.

8. Griffenhagen GB (editor): *Handbook of Non-Prescription Drugs* (annual publication). American Pharmaceutical Association.

9. Berg GL (editor): *Farm Chemical Handbook* (annual publication). Meister.

The Manufacturer or His Local Representative

Another way to identify the contents of a substance is to telephone the manufacturer or his representative. He should have information concerning the type of toxic hazard to be expected from the material in question and will know what treatment should be given.

DIFFERENTIAL DIAGNOSIS OF DISEASES WHICH MAY BE THE RESULT OF POISONING

In any disease state of questionable etiology, poisoning by one or more substances must be considered as part of the differential diagnosis. For example, the high incidence of cases of lead poisoning which have been discovered in a few medical centers in recent years indicates that many cases must go unrecognized. Some of these patients had symptoms for more than a year and had been seen by several physicians before the diagnosis was made. Admittedly, the diagnosis of lead poisoning is difficult, but the possibility of this disorder must be considered before the necessary steps to confirm the diagnosis can be taken. The most important confirmatory steps in any case of poisoning are the discovery of a source of the poison and a history of exposure to it.

Intentional self-administration of drugs or chemicals for suicidal, "mind-altering," or therapeutic purposes should be included as possible sources of poisoning. The patient may not admit such use until the physician can find suggestive evidence, either by laboratory examination of blood, urine, or gastric content or by other means. The willingness of some individuals to ingest or inject substances without knowing what they are causes frequent bizarre episodes. Street drugs are sometimes adulterated with potent agents, including strychnine, with fatal results.

In making the differential diagnosis of a disease which may be the result of poisoning, the number of poisons which must be considered in any particular case can be reduced by classifying exposure possibilities. A convenient classification based on exposure consists of the following groups: (1) household, (2) medicinal, (3) industrial, (4) agricultural, and (5) natural.

The following tabular presentation is intended to supplement a careful inquiry to elicit intentional ingestion of drugs or chemicals.

HISTORY & PHYSICAL EXAMINATION

Symptom History

A. **General Health:**
1. **Weight loss**—Any chronic poisoning, but especially lead, arsenic, dinitrophenol, thyroid, mercury, and chlorinated hydrocarbons.
2. **Asthenia**—Lead, arsenic, mercury, chlorinated organic compounds.
3. **Loss of appetite**—Trinitrotoluene.

B. **Head and CNS:**
1. **Delirium, hallucinations**—Alcohol, antihistamines, atropine and related drugs, camphorated oil, lead, marihuana, cocaine, amphetamines, bromides, quinacrine, salicylates, phenylbutazone, methyl bromide, pesticides.
2. **Depression, drowsiness, coma**—Barbiturates or other hypnotics, alcohol, solvents, antihistamines, pesticides, atropine or related drugs, cationic detergents, lead, opium and opium derivatives, paraldehyde, cyanides, carbon monoxide, phenol, salicylates, chlorpromazine, akee.
3. **Muscular twitchings and convulsions**—Pesticides, strychnine, camphor, atropine, cyanides, ethylene glycol, nicotine, black widow spider.
4. **Headache**—Nitrites, hydralazine, trinitrotoluene.

C. **Eyes:**
1. **Blurred vision**—Atropine, pesticides, cocaine, solvents, dinitrophenol, nicotine, methyl alcohol.
2. **Colored vision**—Santonin, aspidium, digitalis.
3. **Double vision**—Alcohol, barbiturates, nicotine, phosphate ester insecticides.

D. **Ears:**
1. **Tinnitus**—Quinine, salicylates, quinidine.
2. **Deafness or disturbances of equilibrium**—Streptomycin, dihydrostreptomycin, quinine, neomycin, gentamicin.

E. **Nose:**
1. **Anosmia**—Phenol nose-drops, chromium.
2. **Fetor nasalis**—Chromium.

F. **Mouth:**
1. **Loosening of teeth**—Mercury, lead, phosphorus.
2. **Painful teeth**—Phosphorus, mercury, bismuth.
3. **Dry mouth**—Atropine and related drugs.
4. **Salivation**—Lead, mercury, bismuth, thallium, phosphate ester insecticides, other heavy metals.

G. **Cardiorespiratory System:**
1. **Respiratory difficulty, including dyspnea on exertion and chest pain**—Insecticides, salicylates, botulism, nickel carbonyl, black widow spider, scorpion, shellfish, fish, physostigmine, pneumoconioses, cyanide, carbon monoxide, atropine, strychnine.
2. **Palpitation**—Nitrites, sympathomimetics.
3. **Cough**—Smoke, dust, silica, beryllium.

H. **Gastrointestinal System:**
1. **Vomiting, diarrhea, abdominal pain**—Caused by almost all poisons, particularly detergents, corrosives, metals, phenols, solvents, cold wave neutralizer, food poisoning.
2. **Jaundice**—Chlorinated compounds, arsenic, chromates, cinchophen, mushrooms, phenothiazines, sulfonamides, chlorpromazine, ethylene chlorhydrin, trinitrotoluene, aniline.
3. **Blood in stools**—Warfarin, corrosives, iron, salicylates.

I. **Genitourinary:**
1. **Anuria**—Mercurials, sulfonamides, carbon tetrachloride, formaldehyde, phosphorus, ethylene chlorhydrin, turpentine, oxalic acid, chlordane, castor bean, jequirity bean, trinitrotoluene.
2. **Polyuria**—Lead.
3. **Menstrual irregularities**—Estrogens, lead, bismuth, mercurials, other heavy metals.
4. **Color of urine**—Warfarin (red), fava beans (red), hepatotoxins (orange).

J. **Neuromuscular System:**
1. **Muscular weakness or paralysis**—Lead, arsenic, botulism, poison hemlock, organic mercurials, thallium, tri-orthocresyl phosphate, pesticides, shellfish.
2. **Muscle fasciculations**—Organophosphates, nicotine, black widow spider, scorpion.

K. **Endocrine System:**
1. **Libido decreased**—Lead, mercury, other heavy metals, sedatives and hypnotics.
2. **Breast enlargement**—Estrogens.

L. **Anemia:** Lead, benzene, chloramphenicol.

Physical Examination
A. **General:**
1. **Blood pressure fall**—Nitrites, veratrum, cold wave neutralizer, acetanilid, chlorpromazine, quinine, volatile oils, aconite, disulfiram, iron salts, methyl bromide, arsine, phosphine, nickel carbonyl, stibine.
2. **Blood pressure rise**—Epinephrine or substitutes, veratrum, ergot, cortisone, vanadium, lead, nicotine.
3. **Tachycardia**—Potassium bromate.
4. **Bradycardia**—Veratrum, zygadenus.
5. **Fever**—Dinitrophenol or other nitrophenols, jimson weed, atropine, boric acid.
6. **Hypothermia**—Akee.

B. **Skin:**
1. **Cyanosis in the absence of respiratory depression or shock**—Methemoglobinemia from aniline, nitrobenzene, acetanilid, phenacetin, nitrate from well water or food, bismuth subnitrate, cloth-marking ink (aniline), chloramine-T.
2. **Dryness**—Atropine and related compounds.
3. **Increased perspiration**—Alcohol, aspirin, arsenic, fluorides, insulin, mercuric chloride, organophosphates, pilocarpine.
4. **Corrosion or destruction**—Acids or alkalies, permanganate.
5. **Jaundice from liver injury**—Chlorinated compounds, arsenic, chromates, cinchophen, neocinchophen, mushrooms, phenothiazines, and sulfonamides.
6. **Jaundice from hemolysis**—Aniline, nitrobenzene, pamaquine, pentaquine, primaquine, benzene, castor beans, jequirity beans, fava beans, phosphine, arsine, nickel carbonyl.
7. **Redness**—Carbon monoxide, cyanide.
8. **Staining of skin**—Iodine (black), nitric acid (yellow), silver nitrate (blue-black).
9. **Rash**—Bromides, sulfonamides, antibiotics, poison oak, salicylates, trinitrotoluene, chromium, gold salts, chlorinated compounds.
10. **Loss of hair**—Thallium, arsenic, sulfides.

C. **Eyes:**
1. **Dilated pupil**—Atropine and related drugs, cocaine, nicotine, solvents, amphetamines, hallucinogens, depressants.
2. **Contracted pupils**—Morphine, cholinergic drugs, phenothiazines, organophosphates.
3. **Pigmented scleras**—Quinacrine, santonin, jaundice from hemolysis or liver damage.
4. **Pallor of optic disk**—Quinine, nicotine, carbon disulfide.

D. **Perforated Nasal Septum:** Chromium, cocaine.

E. **Mouth:**
1. **Black line on gum or gingival inflammation**—Lead, mercury, arsenic, bismuth.
2. **Salivation**—Organophosphates, mercury, mushrooms.
3. **Breath odor**—Recognizable as such (alcohol, ether, paraldehyde, phenols and cresols, sulfides), garlic odor (arsenic, parathion, phosphorus), bitter almonds (cyanides).

F. **Lungs:**
1. **Wheezing**—Organophosphates, cholinergics, mushrooms.
2. **Decreased vital capacity**—Silica, beryllium dusts, other dusts.
3. **Rapid respirations**—Cyanide, atropine, cocaine, carbon monoxide, carbon dioxide.

4. **Slow respirations**—Cyanide, carbon monoxide, barbiturates, morphine, botulism, aconite, magnesium.
5. **Pulmonary edema**—Metal fumes, hydrogen sulfide, methyl bromide, methyl chloride.

G. **Central Nervous System:** Mental deterioration may occur as a result of poisoning due to alcohols, thallium, lead, mercury.

H. **Muscles:**
1. **Muscle weakness or paralysis (may be limited to a single muscle or muscle group)**—Lead, arsenic, botulism, poison hemlock, organic mercurials, tri-orthocresyl phosphate, carbon disulfide, insecticides.
2. **Muscle twitching**—Pesticides, nicotine, manganese, shellfish.

LABORATORY EXAMINATION

Simplified Laboratory Tests

A. Phenistix Test: A Phenistix test on fresh urine can be used to indicate the possibility of salicylate or phenothiazine tranquilizer ingestion. A positive test should be followed by quantitative determination of the serum salicylate level.

B. Salicylates in Urine: To 5 ml of acidified urine add 10% tincture ferric chloride drop-by-drop until precipitation ceases. A purple color indicates a positive test. (Boiling the urine eliminates diacetic acid, which also gives a positive test.)

C. Blood Bromide: The La Motte Chemical Company, Towson, Baltimore, Maryland 21204, has available a simplified procedure for determining blood bromide levels. The test is performed by adding gold chloride reagent to 2 ml of deproteinized blood serum. The resulting color reaction is compared with a known bromide standard until a color match is obtained.

D. Urine Bromide and Iodine: To 10 ml of urine add a few drops of fuming nitric acid and 5 ml of chloroform; mix gently and let stand 3 minutes. The chloroform settles to the bottom and takes on a pink to violet color in the presence of iodides or a yellow color in the presence of bromides. A positive test is not an indication of poisoning but only of absorption of bromide.

E. Urine Phenothiazine Tranquilizers: Add 1 ml of a test solution containing 5 parts 5% ferric chloride, 45 parts 20% perchloric acid, and 50 parts 50% nitric acid to 1 ml of urine. A pink to red-purple color develops immediately that is proportionate to the daily dose of drug. All colors appearing after 10 seconds should be disregarded.

F. Iron in Gastric Contents: Dilute gastric contents or vomitus with sufficient water to make the specimen fluid. Filter and test the filtrate with 1 ml of 10% potassium ferricyanide solution. An intense blue color indicates the presence of ferrous salts. Repeat the test with 10% potassium ferrocyanide solution, which gives a similar blue color with ferric salts.

Special Examinations

Special chemical examinations for lead or other heavy metals, insecticides, cholinesterase, depressants, tranquilizers, alkaloids, etc, may be necessary in the differential diagnosis of poisoning. The following laboratories are suggested for the performance of such analyses. It is wise to make prior arrangements with the laboratory to make certain that they will accept samples for analyses.

(1) County coroner's laboratory—Metals, blood alcohol, barbiturates, alkaloids.

(2) City, county, or state police laboratory—Blood alcohol, barbiturates, other poisons.

(3) State toxicologist's office—As under (1). Analyses in connection with criminal poisonings.

(4) Federal Bureau of Investigation Laboratory, Washington, DC (only through local police).

(5) State departments of public health will usually perform analyses relating only to cases of occupational poisoning: insecticides, metals.

(6) County hospital laboratory—Lead, barbiturates, alkaloids, blood alcohol.

(7) Private laboratories—Metals, barbiturates.

(8) Technical Development Laboratory, United States Public Health Service, PO Box 769, Savannah, Georgia—Insecticides in blood, body fat, blood cholinesterase. (Send weighed, frozen sample, with patient identification and history. Specify pesticide.)

Decker WJ, Treuting JJ: Spot tests for rapid diagnosis of poisoning. Clin Toxicol 4:89, 1971.

PRINCIPLES OF TREATMENT OF POISONING
(See also First Aid Measures, p 932.)

In the emergency treatment of any poisoning in which the toxin has been taken by mouth, the following general procedures should be carried out: (1) Support vital functions. Maintain airway and respiration. Combat shock, collapse, and specific manifestations as they arise. (2) Give antidote. (3) Remove poison by emesis, lavage, catharsis, or diuresis as soon as possible.

Removal of Poison

Caution: Do not use stomach tubes or emetics in poisonings due to corrosive agents; gastric perforation may result.

A. Adsorption: Activated charcoal is effective for adsorbing almost all poisons. Ten to 15 gm should be administered for each 1 gm of poison. Nuchar C (West Virginia Pulp and Paper Co), Darco G60 (Atlas), and Norit A (American Norit Co) are suitable products. Prepare ahead several 500 ml polyethylene bottles, each containing 50 gm charcoal. For use, add 400 ml

---

First Aid Measures in Poisoning

The following summary is provided for the physician's use in giving instructions for first aid treatment in response to an emergency inquiry. With the exceptions noted under Ingested Poison, any of these procedures can be carried out by laymen.

Ingested Poison

Lay persons should not attempt treatment if the patient is convulsing or unconscious. If the patient has ingested corrosives (acid or alkali) or petroleum products (kerosene, gasoline, paint thinner, lighter fluid, etc), the procedures described in paragraph 3 below should not be used.

1. Have the patient drink one of the following to dilute the poison and slow absorption: milk, beaten eggs, a suspension of flour, starch, or mashed potatoes in water, or water.
2. Give activated charcoal if available.
3. Stimulate vomiting by rubbing the pharynx and the back of the tongue with a finger or spoon handle. If vomiting cannot be started in this way, give 15 ml (½ oz) syrup of ipecac in ½ glass of water.
4. Conserve body warmth by applying blankets. Avoid external heat.

Inhaled Poisons

1. Carry the victim to fresh air immediately; loosen tight clothing.
2. Give artificial respiration by direct inflation (see p 1026) if respiration is depressed. Remove any objects from the patient's mouth, hold his chin up, tilt his head back as far as possible, and blow into his mouth or nose until his chest rises. Repeat 10–15 times/ minute. Obtain a resuscitator from the police department, fire department, or medical supply service company to facilitate oxygen administration.

Skin Contamination

1. Drench skin with water in tub or shower.
2. Direct a stream of water onto the skin while removing the patient's clothing.
3. Do not use chemical antidotes.

Eye Contamination

1. Holding the lids apart, wash the eye for 5 minutes with running water at eye fountain or with gentle stream of water from a hose or tap.
2. Do not use chemical antidotes.

Snake, Insect, or Arachnid Bite

1. Immobilize patient immediately.
2. Give specific antiserum as soon as possible.
3. If the patient must be moved, carry him on a stretcher as gently as possible.
4. Incision and suction will remove up to 10% of injected snake venom in the first half hour.

Injected Poisons (Overdosage of Drugs)

1. Make the patient lie down.
2. Apply a rubber band tourniquet (1 X 24 inches) proximal to the injection. The pulse should not disappear in vessels beyond the tourniquet, nor should a throbbing sensation be felt by the patient. Loosen tourniquet for 1 minute in every 15.

Identification of Unknown Toxic Agent

The following information is useful in attempting to identify a toxic agent. It should be available when you call your Poison Information Center.

1. Physical state (solid, liquid, gas).
2. Odor.
3. Trade-name.
4. Use.
5. Presence of poison label.
6. Inflammability warning.

---

distilled water and shake. Give orally or use as lavage fluid.

B. Emesis: This is the quickest and most effective way to evacuate gastric contents.

1. Indications—For removal of poison in cooperative patients and for promptness, since emesis can be done in the home in the first few minutes after poisoning.

2. Contraindications—(1) Drowsy or unconscious patients or after kerosene ingestion (danger of aspiration of stomach contents). (2) Ingestion of corrosive poisons or convulsants.

3. Technic—Introduce a finger into the throat, or give an emetic and follow with copious quantities of warm water. The most useful preparation is syrup of ipecac, 15 ml, and repeat in 20 minutes if necessary. Ipecac is not effective after charcoal, and is a depressant if retained.

C. Gastric Aspiration and Lavage:

1. Indications—(1) Removal of excess of noncorrosive poisons which may later be absorbed from the gastrointestinal tract. (2) Removal of CNS depressant poisons when vomiting does not occur (vomiting center paralyzed). (3) For collection and examination of gastric contents for identification of poison. (4) For convenient administration of antidotes.

2. Contraindications—(1) Corrosion of tissues by poison. (2) Struggling, delirious, stuporous, or comatose patients. (3) Kerosene or other hydrocarbons. Danger of aspiration pneumonia is reduced by tracheal intubation.

3. Technic—Gently insert a lubricated, soft but noncollapsible stomach tube through the mouth or nose into the stomach. Aspirate stomach and save contents separately; then lavage repeatedly with 50–100 ml quantities of fluid. Always remove excess lavage fluid.

Collect and save washings in clean containers for toxicologic examination when indicated. In forensic cases, seal with sealing wax and place in a locked refrigerator; deliver to toxicologist personally and get a signed receipt. If facilities for refrigeration are lacking, preserve the specimen with equal quantities of 95% alcohol.

4. Gastric lavage fluids—(1) Warm tap water or 1% salt solution. (2) Activated charcoal: Use 50 gm in 400 ml water and stir until completely wet. The suspension should have a slightly thickened consistency. (3) Thin soluble starch paste. (4) Sodium bicarbonate, 1%. (5) Sodium thiosulfate, 1%.

Inactivation by Demulcents

Demulcents precipitate metals and also help to limit the absorption of many poisons. These bland agents are also soothing to inflamed mucous membranes. Use the whites of 3 or 4 eggs beaten in 500 ml of milk or water, skimmed milk, or thin flour or starch solution (boiled, if possible). Follow with gastric lavage.

Supportive & Symptomatic Measures

The victim of acute poisoning must be kept under close observation in order to anticipate the immediate and delayed complications of the poisoning. Suicidal patients may need special surveillance and should be seen by a psychiatrist.

A. Circulatory Failure:

1. Shock (see p 2)—The principal measures include recumbent position, warmth, and blood and parenteral fluids.

2. Cardiac failure (see p 213)—The principal measures include rest, oxygen, and digitalis.

3. Pulmonary edema—Give 40% oxygen by mask. If pulmonary edema is due to gaseous irritants, give aminophylline, 0.5 gm IV, to relieve associated bronchial constriction. The oxygen should be given at slightly increased pressure by means of a mask with an adjustable exit valve. The oxygen concentration should not exceed 40% to avoid lung injury.

B. Respiratory Abnormalities:

1. Respiratory obstruction—Correct by oropharyngeal airway, intratracheal intubation, or tracheostomy.

2. Respiratory depression—Remove from toxic atmosphere. Administer artificial respiration as needed. A resuscitator or other means of automatic ventilation requires constant supervision. Stimulants (analeptic drugs) are of no value for poisoning with depressant drugs.

3. Hypostatic pneumonia—The principal measures include antibiotics and intratracheal aspiration as needed.

C. CNS Involvement:

1. CNS excitement—Use anticonvulsant drugs: Give diazepam (Valium), 10 mg IV. Maintain respiration.

2. CNS depression—Maintain respiration.

D. Agranulocytosis: In the presence of fever, sore throat, or other signs of infection, give penicillin, 1 million units daily, or a broad-spectrum antibiotic in maximum doses until infection is controlled. Give repeated transfusions of fresh blood or white cells. Isolate patient.

E. Methemoglobinemia: Give 100% oxygen by mask, and methylene blue, 5–25 ml of 1% solution slowly IV.

Increased Drug Excretion

A. Diuretics: Osmotic diuretics (eg, mannitol, urea, hypertonic glucose) or saluretic agents (eg, ethacrynic acid, furosemide) may increase drug excretion in cases of serious poisoning with drugs primarily excreted by the kidney (eg, salicylates and phenobarbital). Osmotic diuretics may also relieve cerebral edema (eg, in lead poisoning). Forced diuresis requires an adequate osmotic load and appropriate parenteral fluids and is not without hazard. Basic drugs (eg, amphetamines, strychnine) are best excreted by maintaining an acid urine. Weakly acidic drugs (eg, salicylates, phenobarbital) are best excreted with an alkaline urine. Contraindications to osmotic diuresis include renal insufficiency, pulmonary edema, cardiac insufficiency, and persistent severe hypotension despite adequate fluid replacement.

B. Dialysis: Early enthusiasm for treating acute poisoning of all types with peritoneal dialysis or hemodialysis has been tempered by 2 decades of clinical experience and better appreciation of the dangers. Assuming that technical and professional resources are available for prompt and safe dialysis, the indications for it can now be summarized as follows: (1) Known or suspected potentially lethal amounts of a dialyzable drug (Table 30–1). (2) Poisoning with deep coma, apnea, severe hypotension, fluid and electrolyte or acid-base disturbance, or extreme body temperature changes which cannot be corrected by conventional measures. (3) Poisoning in patients with severe renal, cardiac, pulmonary, or hepatic disease, and poisoning in patients who are pregnant.

Careful observation and treatment of the patient are required before, during, and after dialysis. Constant monitoring of vital signs, central venous pressure, and frequent laboratory determinations of fluids, electrolytes, and blood gases are required.

Peritoneal dialysis will continue to be the principal method of dialysis employed for acute poisonings not requiring maximally rapid dialysis.

Dialysis should usually augment rather than be used in lieu of well established emergency and supportive measures.

Knepshield JH & others: Dialysis of poisons and drugs: Annual review. Tr Am Soc Artific Int Organs 19:590, 1973.

Manes M, Mann JT Jr: Easily swallowed formulations of antidote charcoals. Clin Toxicol 7:355, 1974.

Picchioni AL, Chin L, Laird HE: Activated charcoal preparations: Relative antidotal efficacy. Clin Toxicol 7:97, 1974.

Vale JA & others: Use of charcoal haemoperfusion in the management of severely poisoned patients. Brit MJ 1:5, 1975.

Table 30–1. Toxic agents for which peritoneal dialysis or hemodialysis may be indicated.*

Sedative-hypnotics	Other metals
Alcohols	Calcium
Chloral hydrate	Lithium
Ethanol	Magnesium
Ethchlorvynol	Potassium
Ethylene glycol	
Methanol	**Halides**
Barbiturates	Bromides
Carbamates	Fluorides
Ethinamate	Iodides
Meprobamate	
Paraldehyde	**Alkaloids**
	Quinidine
Nonnarcotic analgesics	Quinine
Acetaminophen	Strychnine
Aspirin	
Methyl salicylate	**Miscellaneous**
Phenacetin	Anilines
	Antibiotics
Amphetamines	Borates
	Boric acid
Heavy metals	Carbon tetrachloride
Arsenicals	Chlorates
Arsine	Dichromate
Arsenic (after	Isoniazid
dimercaprol)	Mushroom
Iron (after deferoxamine)	Nitrobenzenes
Lead (after edetate)	Nitrofurantoin
Mercury (after	Phenytoin
dimercaprol)	Thiocyanates

*Dialysis has *not* proved especially useful for the following compounds:

Amitriptyline	Hallucinogens
Anticholinergics	Heroin
Atropine	Imipramine
Antidepressants	Methaqualone
Antihistamines	Methyprylon
Chlordiazepoxide	Nortriptyline
Diazepam	Oxazepam
Digitalis	Phenelzine
Diphenoxylate	Phenothiazines
Glutethimide	Propoxyphene

TREATMENT OF COMMON SPECIFIC POISONINGS (ALPHABETICAL ORDER)

ACIDS, CORROSIVE

The strong mineral acids exert primarily a local corrosive effect on the skin or mucous membranes. In severe burns, circulatory collapse may result. Symptoms include severe pain in the throat and upper gastrointestinal tract, marked thirst, bloody vomitus; difficulty in swallowing, breathing, and speaking; discoloration and destruction of skin and mucous membranes in and around the mouth; and shock.

The MLD is 1 ml of concentrated acid.

Inhalation of volatile acids, fumes, or gases such as chlorine, fluorine, bromine, or iodine cause severe irritation of the throat and chest with paroxysmal coughing and inhibition of respiration, followed by pulmonary edema.

Treatment

A. Ingested: Dilute immediately by giving 200 ml of milk of magnesia, aluminum hydroxide gel, milk, or water to drink; give beaten eggs (at least 12) as a demulcent. Pass a nasogastric tube gently and lavage with 2–4 liters of milk of magnesia in 100 ml portions. Leave the tube in place until the extent of the injury is known. Do not give bicarbonate or carbonates.

Relieve pain and treat shock. Administer corticosteroids.

B. Skin Contact: Flood with water for 15 minutes. Use no chemical antidotes; the heat of the reaction may cause additional injury. Relieve pain and treat shock.

C. Eye Contact: Flood with water for 5 minutes, holding the eyelids open. Relieve pain by use of local anesthetic agent.

D. Inhalation: Remove from further exposure to fumes or gas. Treat pulmonary edema.

Jones FL: Chlorine exposure from mixing household cleaners. JAMA 222:1312, 1972.

ALCOHOL, ETHYL

Beverages containing ethyl alcohol have been widely used and abused throughout history. Although the acute and chronic toxic effects of alcohol are principally on the nervous and gastrointestinal systems, it may be seen from Table 30–2 that many other parts of the body are also susceptible to the potentially harmful effects of this agent.

The principal manifestation of ethyl alcohol poisoning is CNS depression and gastric irritation, with

Table 30—2. Toxicity of alcohol.

Psychoneurologic syndromes
Acute alcoholism
Intoxication, excitement, coma
Withdrawal syndromes
Hallucinosis, convulsions, delirium tremens
Nutritional syndromes
Wernicke-Korsakoff syndrome, pellagra

Gastrointestinal syndromes
Acute and chronic gastritis, malabsorption syndrome, fatty liver, cirrhosis, acute and chronic pancreatitis

Hematologic syndromes
Anemia due to acute or chronic blood loss
Cytoplasmic vacuolization of erythroid precursors
Megaloblastic marrow alterations (inhibition of folate metabolism) with anemia
Sideroblastic marrow abnormalities
Stomatocytic erythrocyte changes
Hemolytic anemia, thrombocytopenia
Defective granulocyte mobilization

Neuromuscular syndromes
Peripheral polyneuropathy
Acute and chronic alcoholic myopathy

Cardiovascular syndromes
Alcoholic cardiomyopathy

Metabolic syndromes
Lactic acidosis, hypoglycemia, hypomagnesemia, hypouricemia, hyperlipidemia

Conditions aggravated by alcohol
Traumatic encephalopathy, epilepsy, Hodgkin's disease, porphyria, peptic ulcer

Drugs which contraindicate concomitant use of alcohol
Disulfiram, sedatives, hypnotics, tranquilizers, phenformin

---

nausea and vomiting. Hypoglycemia is indicated by hypothermia, conjugate deviation of the eyes, extensor rigidity, positive Babinski reflexes, and trismus. Other manifestations include convulsions, fever to 40—42° C (104—107.6° F), and cerebral edema with severe head ache.

Differentiate from depressant poisoning, head injury, mental disorders, and insulin hypoglycemia.

The MLD is 300 ml.

Treatment of Acute Alcoholic Intoxication*

A. Emergency Measures: Remove unabsorbed alcohol by gastric lavage with tap water. Instill 4 gm of sodium bicarbonate.

B. General Measures: (Similar to those for barbiturate poisoning.)

1. Maintain the airway and respiration and keep the patient warm.

2. If the patient is comatose and areflexic, treat as for barbiturate poisoning.

3. Give glucose orally or IV for hypoglycemia.

4. For intractable retching or acute alcoholic excitation, give diazepam (Valium), 10 mg IV.

Demakis JG & others: The natural course of alcoholic cardiomyopathy. Ann Int Med 80:293, 1974.

Eichner ER: The hematologic disorders of alcoholism. Am J Med 54:621, 1973.

Jones KL & others: Pattern of malformation in offspring of chronic alcoholic mothers. Lancet 1:1267, 1973.

Korsten MA & others: High blood acetaldehyde after ethanol administration. New England J Med 292:386, 1975.

*See also discussion of alcoholism in Chapter 17.

Parker BM: The effects of ethyl alcohol on the heart. JAMA 228:741, 1974.

Thompson WL & others: Diazepam and paraldehyde for treatment of severe delirium tremens. Ann Int Med 82:175, 1975.

ALCOHOL, METHYL

Methyl alcohol is a CNS depressant which produces specific damage to the retinal cells and metabolic acidosis. The MLD is 30—60 ml. Symptoms include headache, abdominal pain, dyspnea, nausea, vomiting, and blindness. Examination reveals flush or cyanosis, excitement or depression, delirium, coma, and convulsions. The presence of methanol in the urine is diagnostic.

Treatment

Lavage well with 1—2% sodium bicarbonate solution. Keep the patient in a dark room. Check CO_2 combining power. Give intravenous fluids to combat metabolic acidosis, and sodium bicarbonate, 5—15 gm orally every 2—3 hours. Give ethyl alcohol, 5% solution, 5 ml/kg orally or IV every 2 hours for 3—4 days, to block the metabolism of methyl alcohol until it is excreted. Maintain blood ethanol at 1 mg/ml. Administration of insulin plus glucose has also been suggested. Dialysis is useful.

Hussey HH: Methanol poisoning. JAMA 229:1335, 1974.

Keyvan-Larijarni H, Tannenberg AM: Methanol intoxications:

Comparison of peritoneal dialysis and hemodialysis treatment. Arch Int Med 134:293, 1974.

Tephly TR, Watkins WD, Goodman JI: The biochemical toxicology of methanol. Essays in Toxicol 5:149, 1974.

ALKALIES

The strong alkalies are common ingredients of household cleaning compounds and may be detected by their "soapy" texture. Clinitest tablets are also a source. They exert a local corrosive effect on mucous membranes and may produce circulatory failure. Symptoms include burning pain in the upper gastrointestinal tract, nausea, vomiting, and difficulty in swallowing and breathing. Examination reveals destruction and edema of the affected skin and mucous membranes, and bloody vomitus and stools.

The MLD is 1 gm.

Treatment

A. Ingested: Immediate esophagoscopy in order to irrigate injured areas directly with 1% acetic acid until neutralized and to evaluate the extent of damage is the treatment of choice. Dilute immediately with 500 ml of dilute vinegar (1 part vinegar to 4 parts water) or citrus juice.

Relieve pain and treat shock.

Corticosteroids help prevent esophageal strictures or stenosis. The suggested drug for ages 1–4 is prednisolone, 10–15 mg 4 times a day, for about 2 weeks.

B. Skin Contact: Wash with running water until the skin no longer feels soapy. Relieve pain and treat shock.

C. Eye Contact: Wash with water continuously for 15 minutes, holding the lids open. Relieve pain. Have the eye examined by an ophthalmologist to determine the extent of damage.

Berenson MM, Temple AR: Detergent ingestion: Unique experience of a family. Clin Toxicol 7:25, 1974.

Feldman M, Iben AB, Hurley EJ: Corrosive injury to oropharynx and esophagus. California Med 118:6, Jan 1973.

Sperling HV, Wheeler MJ: An unusual complication of lye ingestion. JAMA 228:871, 1974.

ANTICOAGULANTS

Dicumarol, ethyl biscoumacetate, phenindione, and warfarin are used medically to inhibit the clotting mechanism by inhibiting prothrombin formation in the liver. Abnormal bleeding occurs only after prolonged administration. The MLD of dicumarol and warfarin is 0.1 gm; of phenindione, 0.2 gm; of ethyl biscoumacetate, 0.6 gm. The pathologic findings consist of numerous gross and microscopic hemorrhages.

Clinical Findings

A. Symptoms and Signs: The principal manifestation of poisoning with the anticoagulants is bleeding: hemoptysis, hematuria, bloody stools, hemorrhages into organs, widespread bruising, and bleeding into joint spaces. Phenindione may also cause jaundice, hepatomegaly, skin rash, and agranulocytosis.

B. Laboratory Findings: The prothrombin concentration is lowered after administration of coumarin and indandione anticoagulants. Gross or microscopic hematuria may be present. The red cell count may also be reduced. The white count may be decreased after phenindione administration.

Treatment

A. Emergency Measures: Discontinue the drug at the first sign of bleeding. If ingestion of more than 10 times a daily therapeutic dose is discovered within 2 hours, remove by gastric lavage and catharsis.

B. General Measures: Give phytonadione, 5–10 mg orally. For more rapid effect, give 10–40 mg slowly IV as the diluted emulsion. Give transfusions of fresh blood, fresh plasma, or fresh frozen plasma if hemorrhage is severe. Absolute bed rest must be maintained to prevent further hemorrhages.

Coon WW, Willis PW III: Hemorrhagic complications of anticoagulant therapy. Arch Int Med 133:386, 1974.

O'Reilly RA: Interaction of sodium warfarin and disulfiram (Antabuse®) in man. Ann Int Med 78:73, 1973.

Pettifor JM, Benson R: Congenital malformations associated with the administration of oral anticoagulants during pregnancy. J Pediat 96:463, 1975.

Soloway HB: Drug-induced bleeding. Am J Clin Path 61:622, 1974.

ARSENIC

Arsenic is found in pesticides and industrial chemicals. Symptoms of poisoning usually appear within 1 hour after ingestion but may be delayed as long as 12 hours. They include abdominal pain, difficulty in swallowing, persistent vomiting, diarrhea, urinary suppression, and skeletal muscle cramps. Later findings are severe thirst and shock. In chronic poisoning, symptoms can be vague.

The MLD is 0.1 gm.

Treatment

A. Emergency Measures: Induce vomiting. Follow with 500 ml of milk. Lavage with 2–4 liters of warm tap water, 200 ml at a time. Treat shock.

B. Antidote: Give dimercaprol injection (BAL), 10% solution in oil. The side-effects include nausea, vomiting, headache, generalized aches, and burning sensations around the head and face. These usually subside in 30 minutes. Either ephedrine, 25 mg orally, or an antihistamine such as diphenhydramine, 25–50 mg orally, will reduce the side-effects if given 30 minutes before dimercaprol.

1. Severe poisoning—Give IM, 3 mg/kg for each injection (1.8 ml/60 kg). **First and second days**: One injection every 4 hours day and night. **Third day**: One injection every 6 hours. **Fourth to 14th day**: One injection twice a day until recovery is complete.

2. Mild poisoning—2.5 mg/kg/dose (1.5 ml/60 kg). **First and second days**: One injection every 4 hours for 4 doses. **Third day**: One injection twice a day. **Fourth and subsequent days**: One injection once or twice a day for 10 days or until recovery is complete.

C. General Measures: Relieve pain and treat diarrhea. Hemodialysis will speed the removal of arsenic combined with dimercaprol.

Martin DW Jr, Woeber KA: Arsenic poisoning. California Med 118:13, Mar 1973.

Rosenberg HG: Systemic arterial disease and chronic arsenicism in infants. Arch Path 97:360, 1974.

Yeh S: Skin cancer in chronic arsenicism. Human Path 4:469, 1973.

BARBITURATES & OTHER DEPRESSANTS
(Sedative-Hypnotics & Tranquilizers)

The barbiturates are among the most common offenders in accidental as well as suicidal poisoning. Other (or multiple) sedative-hypnotic drugs—particularly alcohol—may be involved. Obtain data on the drug and its dosage and time of ingestion from the patient, relatives, friends, or attending physician when possible.

Symptoms of mild poisoning consist of drowsiness, mental confusion, and headache. There may be euphoria or irritability. Moderate or severe poisoning causes delirium, stupor, shallow and slow respirations, circulatory collapse, cold clammy skin, cyanosis, pulmonary edema, dilated and nonreacting pupils, hyporeflexia, coma, and death.

The MLD is 0.5—2 gm. The lethal serum level in unsupported patients who have taken short-acting barbiturates is about 3.5 mg/100 ml; and with long-acting barbiturates, the lethal level is about 8 mg/100 ml. The analytical method must be specific for unmetabolized drug.

Treatment

Note: The critical factor in the management of barbiturate poisoning is constant medical and nursing attendance to maintain physiologic responses until the danger of respiratory failure and circulatory depression has passed.

A. Mild Poisoning: Induce vomiting and give symptomatic and supportive nursing care. Keep the patient under observation until he is out of danger. Place suicidal patients under psychiatric care.

B. Moderate or Marked Poisoning: Most patients will survive even days of unconsciousness if the airway is kept open (may require tracheostomy) and if artificial respiration is maintained with a tank respirator,

IPPB, or other mechanical ventilating apparatus. Oxygen concentration must not exceed 40%. The patient should be hospitalized, and antishock measures instituted. Examine the patient and record the following at intervals of 1—4 hours (or oftener if the patient's condition is very poor): temperature, pulse, respiration, and blood pressure; mental status or state of consciousness, skin color (cyanosis or pallor), lung bases (pulmonary edema), reflexes (corneal, pupillary, gag, patellar), and sensation (response to pain).

1. Airway—Aspirate mucus, pull tongue forward, and insert oropharyngeal airway. Intratracheal or tracheostomy intubation and mechanical assistance to respiration with constant supervision may be required. Serial determination of blood gases is of great value.

2. Lavage with 2—4 liters of warm tap water, preferably containing activated charcoal. This is of doubtful value and may be dangerous if done after the patient has become drowsy or comatose. *Caution:* The danger of aspiration pneumonia is great in stuporous or comatose patients.

3. Excretion of phenobarbital can be increased by alkalinization of the urine. If renal function is adequate, give sodium lactate or sodium bicarbonate orally or intravenously.

4. Insert an indwelling catheter and save urine for toxicologic quantitation.

5. Parenteral fluids—Monitor central venous pressure. Serum sodium should also be monitored in order to control the sodium content of parenteral fluids. If cardiac failure is absent and renal function is adequate, give 1 liter of 0.45% sodium chloride solution and 1—2 liters of 5% dextrose solution IV daily to maintain a urine output of 1—1.5 liters/day. Unless fluid loss has been excessive, restrict fluids to 2—3 liters during the first 24 hours to reduce danger of pulmonary edema. In phenobarbital overdosage, if renal function is adequate, give up to 100 ml/kg of fluid daily, one-third as 30% urea, one-third as 10% invert sugar in distilled water, and one-third as 0.145 M sodium bicarbonate (1.2%), plus 5 mEq/liter of potassium chloride. The amount of fluids should not exceed insensible losses (800—1000 ml/24 hours) plus the urine output. In the event of shock, give plasma or other fluids intravenously in order to maintain a satisfactory blood pressure. (See treatment of shock, p 4.)

6. CNS stimulants (analeptics or convulsant drugs) are contraindicated. They do not shorten the duration of effect of poisoning and, if convulsions occur, postconvulsive depression will add to the severity of barbiturate depression. Hyperthermia and cardiac arrhythmias are also dangers.

7. Hemodialysis or peritoneal dialysis is indicated in severe cases when the necessary equipment and trained personnel are available. This is usually reserved for patients with hepatic or renal diseases. Dialysis is of doubtful value in glutethimide poisoning.

Brown SS, Goenechea S: Methaqualone: Metabolism, kinetic, and clinical pharmacologic observations. Clin Pharmacol Therap 14:314, 1973.

Eisar EV, LaBocki NL, Pinckney L: Chlorpheniramine-dependent cytopenia. JAMA 231:735, 1975.

Hansen AR & others: Glutethimide poisoning: A metabolite contributes to morbidity and mortality. New England J Med 292:250, 1975.

Hooshmand, H: Toxic effects of anticonvulsants: General principles. Pediatrics 53:551, 1974.

Lansky LL: An unusual case of childhood chloral hydrate poisoning. Am J Dis Child 127:275, 1974.

Locket S: Clinical toxicology. 6. Poisoning by the barbiturates and a variety of hypnotics and sedatives. Practitioner 210:836, 1973.

Myers RR, Stockard JJ: Neurologic and electroencephalographic correlates in glutethimide intoxication. Clin Pharmacol Therap 17:212, 1975.

BELLADONNA DERIVATIVES
(Atropine & Scopolamine)

The belladonna alkaloids are parasympathetic depressants with variable CNS effects. The patient complains of dryness of the mouth, thirst, difficulty in swallowing, and blurring of vision. The physical signs include dilated pupils, flushed skin, tachycardia, fever, delirium, delusions, paralysis, stupor, and a rash on the face, neck, and upper trunk.

The MLD of atropine is 2–10 mg.

Treatment

Remove the poison by lavage and catharsis, and counteract excitement.

A. Emergency Measures: Induce vomiting and lavage with 2–4 liters of water, preferably containing activated charcoal. Follow lavage with sodium sulfate, 30 gm in 200 ml of water.

B. General Measures: Short-acting barbiturates such as secobarbital, 0.1 gm by mouth, may be used if the patient is excitable. Treat respiratory difficulty as for barbiturate poisoning. Alcohol or cold water sponge baths are indicated to control high temperatures. Maintain blood pressure. Give physostigmine salicylate, 1–2 mg IM, to reverse the central and peripheral effects of atropine.

Rumack BH, Temple AR: Lomotil® poisoning. Pediatrics 53:495, 1974.

BROMIDES

Bromides are CNS depressants still found in hypnotic and anticonvulsant preparations. Acute poisoning is rare. The symptoms include anorexia, constipation, drowsiness, apathy, and hallucinations. The physical examination reveals dermatitis, conjunctivitis, foul breath, furred tongue, sordes, unequal pupils, ataxia, abnormal reflexes (often bizarre), toxic psychosis, delirium, and coma.

The MLD is 10 gm or more.

Treatment

A. Emergency Measures: Lavage copiously with saline to remove unabsorbed bromides and later to remove those excreted into the stomach. Follow with sodium sulfate, 30 gm in 200 ml of water for catharsis.

B. General Measures: Give sodium chloride in addition to the regular dietary salt intake: (1) 1000 ml of physiologic saline IV or rectally once or twice daily; or (2) 1–2 gm as salt tablets every 4 hours orally. Continue until the blood bromide level is below 50 mg/100 ml.

Force fluids to 4 liters daily.

Diuretics will aid excretion of bromide.

Pleasure JR, Blackburn MG: Neonatal bromide intoxication. Pediatrics 55:503, 1975.

Torosian G, Finger KF, Stewart RB: Hazards of bromides in proprietary medication. Am J Hosp Pharm 30:716, 1973.

CARBON MONOXIDE

Carbon monoxide poisoning results from unvented or inadequately vented combustion devices. Voluntary inhalation of carbon monoxide in exhaust fumes is often used for suicidal purposes. The gas exerts its toxic effect by combining with hemoglobin to form a relatively stable compound (carboxyhemoglobin) which secondarily causes tissue anoxia. Manifestations are headache, faintness, giddiness, tinnitus, vomiting, vertigo, loss of memory, fainting, collapse, paralysis, and unconsciousness. Skin color varies from normal (more than half) to flushed, cyanotic, or, uncommonly, cherry-pink. Blisters and bullous lesions also occur. Subclinical toxicity has been reported in dense traffic situations. Persistent neurologic complications are common.

Treatment

Remove the patient from the toxic atmosphere. Loosen his clothing and keep him warm and at rest. Give artificial respiration with 100% oxygen for at least 1 hour. Give 50 ml of 50% glucose IV for cerebral edema as needed. Maintain body warmth and blood pressure. Reduce hyperthermia by cooling applications.

Boqusz M & others: A comparison of two types of carbon monoxide poisoning. Arch Toxicol 33:141, 1975.

Sammons JH, Coleman RL: Fire fighters' occupational exposure to carbon monoxide. J Occup Med 16:543, 1974.

Sone S & others: Pulmonary manifestations in acute carbon monoxide poisoning. Am J Roentgenol 120:865, 1974.

CARBON TETRACHLORIDE

Carbon tetrachloride is a local irritant and cellular poison which when ingested, inhaled, or absorbed through the skin may severely damage the heart, liver, and kidneys. The effects are increased by ingestion of alcohol. Manifestations include headache, hiccup, nausea, vomiting, diarrhea, abdominal pain, drowsiness, visual disturbances, neuritis, and intoxication. Early signs are jaundice, liver tenderness, oliguria, and uremia. Nephrosis and cirrhosis may occur later.

The MLD is 3 ml.

Treatment

A. Emergency Measures: Remove the patient from exposure and keep him recumbent and warm. For poisoning due to ingestion, lavage copiously with tap water, and give sodium sulfate, 30 gm, in 200 ml of water. Do not give stimulants.

B. General Measures: Give inhalations of 100% oxygen by mask for 1 hour and artificial respiration if respirations are depressed. Treat cardiac, hepatic, and renal complications symptomatically. Do not give alcoholic beverages or stimulants. Maintain urine output at 4 liters daily by osmotic diuresis if renal function is normal.

Jones CC: Carbon tetrachloride poisoning: Report of a case. Texas Med 69:86, 1973.

CHLORINATED INSECTICIDES
(Chlorophenothane [DDT], Lindane, Toxaphene, Chlordane, Aldrin, Endrin)

DDT and other chlorinated insecticides are CNS stimulants which can cause poisoning by ingestion, inhalation, or direct contact. The MLD is about 20 gm for DDT, 3 gm for lindane, 2 gm for toxaphene, 1 gm for chlordane, and less than 1 gm for endrin and aldrin. Poisoning following ingestion of DDT solution usually results from the organic solvent, whereas fatalities from the other chlorinated insecticides have resulted from the insecticide alone. The manifestations of poisoning are tired and aching limbs, nervous irritability, mental sluggishness, muscle twitchings, convulsions, and coma.

Treatment

A. Emergency Measures: (Avoid epinephrine, which may cause ventricular fibrillation.) Give activated charcoal at once if available, lavage with large quantities of warm tap water, and give sodium sulfate, 30 gm in 200 ml of water as cathartic.

B. General Measures: Pentobarbital sodium, 0.1 gm orally, may be sufficient to calm the patient. For convulsions give amobarbital sodium, 0.25–0.5 gm as fresh 10% solution slowly IV or IM. Maintain the airway and give oxygen. Avoid stimulants.

Dudley AW Jr, Thapar NT: Fatal human ingestion of 2,4-D: A common herbicide. Arch Path 94:270, 1972.
Mayersdorf A, Israeli R: Toxic effects of chlorinated hydrocarbon insecticides. Arch Envir Health 28:159, 1974.
Morgan DP, Roan CC: Liver function in workers having high tissue stores of chlorinated hydrocarbon pesticides. Arch Envir Health 29:14, 1974.

CYANIDES: HYDROCYANIC ACID
(Prussic Acid, Rat Poison, Cyanogas, Cyanogen)

Hydrocyanic acid and the cyanides cause death by inactivation of the respiratory enzyme, preventing utilization of oxygen by the tissues. The clinical combination of cyanosis, asphyxia, and the odor of bitter almonds on the breath is diagnostic. Respiration is first stimulated and later depressed. A marked drop in blood pressure may occur.

The MLD is 0.05 gm.

Treatment

A. Emergency Measures: *Act quickly.* Use nitrites to form methemoglobin, which combines with cyanide to form nontoxic cyanmethemoglobin. Then give thiosulfates to convert the cyanide released by dissociation of cyanmethemoglobin to thiocyanate.

1. Poisoning by inhalation—Place patient in open air in recumbent position. Remove contaminated clothing. Give artificial respiration.

2. Poisoning by ingestion—Induce vomiting immediately with a finger down the patient's throat. Do not wait until lavage tube has arrived; death may occur within a few minutes.

3. Give amyl nitrite inhalations for 15–30 seconds every 2 minutes.

B. Antidote: Administration of antidotes must be based on hemoglobin level. At 14 gm/100 ml hemoglobin, give 0.39 ml/kg of 3% sodium nitrite IV and 1.95 ml/kg of 25% sodium thiosulfate IV. At lower hemoglobin levels, reduce dosage in exact proportion. Further administration should not exceed 40% methemoglobinemia. Inject sodium nitrite over 10–15 minutes and monitor blood pressure during administration.

C. General Measures: Combat shock and give 100% oxygen by forced ventilation.

Berlin CM Jr: The treatment of cyanide poisoning in children. Pediatrics 46:793, 1970.
Renner G: Biochemische Reaktionen der Blausäure als grundlagen der Therapie der Blausäure vergiftung. Deutsch Med Woch 99:1693, 1974.

DIGITALIS

Because digitalis, digitoxin, and related drugs have a prolonged action, poisoning is most likely to occur when large doses are given to patients who have previously received digitalis drugs. Digitalizing doses should therefore be given only to patients who have not received digitalis for at least 1 week.

Clinical Findings

The principal manifestations of digitalis poisoning are vomiting and irregular pulse. Other signs include anorexia, nausea, diarrhea, yellow vision, delirium, slow pulse, fall of blood pressure, and ventricular fibrillation. The ECG may show lengthened P–R interval, heart block, ventricular extrasystoles, ventricular tachycardia, and a depressed ST segment.

The MLD of digitalis is 3 gm; of digitoxin, 3 mg.

Treatment

A. Emergency Measures: Delay absorption by giving tap water, milk, or activated charcoal and then remove by gastric lavage or emesis followed by catharsis. Do not give epinephrine or other stimulants. These may induce ventricular fibrillation.

B. General Measures: Give potassium chloride, 2 gm dissolved in water, every hour orally; or 0.3% in 5% dextrose slowly IV during ECG monitoring until the ECG shows improvement or evidence of potassium intoxication. Serum potassium must be determined prior to and during potassium administration. Ventricular defibrillation and ventricular pacing may be required.

Beller GA & others: Correlation of serum magnesium levels and cardiac digitalis intoxications. Am J Cardiol 33:225, 1974.

Bertler A, Gustafson A, Redfors A: Massive digoxin intoxication: Report of 2 cases with pharmacokinetic correlations. Acta med scandinav 194:245, 1973.

Smith TW: Digitalis toxicity: Epidemiology and clinical use of serum concentration measurements. Am J Med 58:470, 1975.

Steentoft A: Fatal digitalis poisoning. Acta pharmacol 32:353, 1973.

FLUORIDES SOLUBLE IN WATER
(Insect Powders)

Symptoms include vomiting, diarrhea, salivation; shallow, rapid, and difficult respirations; convulsive seizures; rapid pulse; coma, and cyanosis. Interference with calcium metabolism causes severe damage to the vital centers and may result in death due to respiratory failure.

The MLD is 1 gm.

Treatment

A. Emergency Measures: Lavage with lime water; 1% calcium chloride, calcium lactate, or calcium gluconate; or large quantities of milk to form insoluble calcium fluoride. Give calcium gluconate, 10%, 10–20 ml IV; or calcium chloride, 5%, 10–20 ml IV for convulsions. Give sodium sulfate, 30 gm, in 200 ml of water as cathartic, and egg whites in milk as demulcent.

B. General Measures: Treat shock and give supportive measures.

Abukurah AR & others: Acute sodium fluoride poisoning. JAMA 222:816, 1972.

Burke WJ, Hoegg UR, Phillips RE: Systemic fluoride poisoning resulting from fluoride skin burn. J Occup Med 15:39, 1973.

IODINE

The clinical features of iodine poisoning include a characteristic stain of the mouth and odor of the breath, yellow or bluish vomitus, pain and burning in the pharynx and esophagus, marked thirst, diarrhea (stools may be bloody), weakness, dizziness, syncope, and convulsions.

The MLD is 2 gm.

Treatment

A. Emergency Measures: Give 15 gm cornstarch or flour in 500 ml of water or, if available, 250 ml of 1% sodium thiosulfate in water. Follow with an emetic or remove by lavage with sodium thiosulfate solution, 1%, and repeat until evidence of iodine has disappeared from the gastric contents. Then give demulcents, eg, milk or barley water.

B. General Measures: Maintain blood pressure and respiration.

IRON POISONING

Iron salts are used extensively as antianemic agents in a large number of prescription and over-the-counter "blood tonic" drugs. They are responsible for many instances of mild to severe acute poisoning as well as chronic poisoning.

Acute poisoning is manifested by lethargy, nausea, vomiting, tarry stools, diarrhea, fast and weak pulse, hypotension, dehydration, acidosis, and coma within ½–1 hour following ingestion of iron salts. If this is not fatal, the symptoms may clear in a few hours and the patient may be asymptomatic for 12–24 hours. Symptoms then return, with cyanosis, pulmonary edema, shock, convulsions, anuria, hyperthermia, and death in coma within 24–48 hours. The MLD is 5–10 gm. Late sequelae include hepatic failure and pyloric stenosis.

Chronic poisoning may follow prolonged excess dosage of parenteral iron, causing exogenous hemosiderosis with damage to the liver and pancreas.

Treatment

In patients not in shock or coma, induce emesis with syrup of ipecac if the patient has not vomited.

Follow with gastric lavage using 5% sodium dihydrogen phosphate (half-strength Fleet's Enema solution) until clear. Leave 50 ml of 1.5% sodium dihydrogen phosphate solution in the stomach at the end of lavage. Draw blood for hemoglobin, white count, serum iron, total iron-binding capacity, electrolyte concentrations, blood typing, and rapid serum iron test (Fischer test; see reference below). The Fischer test can be performed in the emergency room to determine the potential seriousness of iron absorption. Start an infusion of isotonic saline or dextrose solution to correct electrolyte disturbance and dehydration.

If the Fischer test indicates the presence of unbound serum iron—or in the presence of signs of systemic iron toxicity—give deferoxamine mesylate (Desferal), 80 mg/kg IV over 8 hours, while blood pressure is monitored to avoid deferoxamine hypotension. Repeat deferoxamine after 12 hours if symptoms and iron determination warrant. Deferoxamine is contraindicated in patients with severe renal disease or anuria.

Treat shock by appropriate fluids and transfusion (see p 4).

Fischer DS: A method for the rapid detection of acute iron toxicity. Clin Chem 13:6, 1967.

Horak E, Sunderman FW: An accurate spectrophotometric method for serum iron and iron-binding capacity without deproteinization or centrifugation. Ann Clin Lab Sci 4:87, 1974.

Wallack MK, Winkelstein A: Acute iron intoxication in an adult. JAMA 229:1333, 1974.

Yeh YY, Zee P: Micromethod for determining total iron-binding capacity by flameless atomic absorption spectrophotometry. Clin Chem 20:360, 1974.

KEROSENE & RELATED COMPOUNDS
(Petroleum Ether, Charcoal Lighter Fluid, Paint Thinner, Benzine, Gasoline, Etc)

Kerosene poisoning results from ingestion. Gasoline or other volatile hydrocarbons can also cause poisoning by inhalation. Ingestion is especially dangerous because aspiration leads to pulmonary irritation for the reason that intratracheal toxicity is 100 times as great as oral toxicity. Acute manifestations are vomiting, pulmonary edema, bronchial pneumonia, vertigo, muscular incoordination, weak and irregular pulse, neuropathy, twitchings, and convulsions. Chronic poisoning causes also headache, drowsiness, dim vision, cold and numb hands, weakness, loss of memory, loss of weight, tachycardia, mental dullness or confusion, sores in the mouth, dermatoses, and anemia.

The MLD is 10–50 ml.

Treatment

Remove the patient to fresh air. Since aspiration during vomiting is a great danger, use of lavage or emesis induced by syrup of ipecac is controversial. Removal of ingested hydrocarbon is only suggested if the amount exceeds 1 ml/kg. If lavage is done, take extreme care to prevent aspiration. Use warm saline and leave 60 ml salad oil in stomach. Follow with sodium sulfate, 30 gm in 200 ml of water. Give prednisolone, 2–10 mg every 6 hours orally to reduce the pulmonary reaction. Watch closely for 3–4 days for symptoms of respiratory involvement. Treat pulmonary edema by positive pressure oxygen administration. Oxygen concentration should not exceed 40%. If fever occurs, give antibiotics.

Cohen S: Glue-sniffing. JAMA 231:653, 1975.

Daffner RH, Jimenez JP: The double gastric fluid level in kerosene poisoning. Radiology 106:383, 1973.

Gwinn AL, Lee FA: Pneumatocele formation following hydrocarbon pneumonitis. Am J Dis Child 127:875, 1974.

LEAD

Lead poisoning may occur by ingestion or by inhalation of lead dust or fumes. Poisoning is manifested by a metallic taste, anorexia, irritability, apathy, abdominal colic, vomiting, diarrhea, constipation, headache, leg cramps, black stools (lead sulfide), oliguria, stupor, convulsions, palsies, and coma. Chronic lead poisoning causes variable involvement of the CNS, the blood-forming organs, and the gastrointestinal tract.

Diagnostic laboratory tests include blood lead (> 80 μg/100 ml), urine coproporphyrin (> 500 μg/liter), urine δ-aminolevulinic acid (> 13 mg/liter), x-ray of abdomen (radiopaque paint), and x-ray of long bones (lead line).

The MLD is 0.5 gm of absorbed lead.

Treatment
A. Acute Poisoning:

1. Establish adequate urine flow (0.5–1 ml/minute). Give dextrose in water (10%, 10–20 ml/kg body weight) over 1–2 hours, or mannitol solution (20%) at a rate of 1 ml/minute until 10 ml/kg have been given. Daily urine output should be 350–500 ml/sq M.

2. Control convulsions with paraldehyde. Diazepam can be used initially, but barbiturates are best saved for long-term control of convulsions after the acute phase is under control.

3. For symptomatic children, including those with lead encephalopathy, give BAL (dimercaprol) and EDTA (calcium disodium edetate) as follows: Begin first with BAL, 4 mg/kg IM, and repeat every 4 hours for 5 days (30 doses). Four hours after the first BAL injection, give EDTA, 12.5 mg/kg (20% solution, with 0.5% procaine added) IM, in a different site from BAL. Repeat every 4 hours for 5 days (30 doses). If symptoms have not improved by the 4th day, extend treatment to 7 days (42 doses each of both BAL and

EDTA). If blood lead is still above 80 μg/100 ml 14 days later, repeat the 5-day course of both drugs.

4. For asymptomatic children, if blood lead is above 100 μg/100 ml, give a 5-day course of BAL-EDTA as above. If blood lead is below this level, give EDTA intramuscularly alone every 6 hours for 5-day course (20 injections).

5. For adults with encephalopathy, painful neuropathy, or abdominal symptoms, give BAL-EDTA intramuscularly as above or, if the patient is BAL-intolerant, give 50 mg/kg EDTA IV as 0.5% solution over not less than 8 hours.

6. Follow-up therapy (all cases)—Give penicillamine (Cuprimine) orally daily in 2 doses one-half hour before meals. The daily dosage is 30–40 mg/kg for children and 500–750 mg for adults. Therapy should be continued for 1–2 months for adults and for 3–6 months for children. Do not give oral therapy if ingestion of lead is possible. Blood lead should be below 60 μg/100 ml at the end of treatment.

B. Chronic Poisoning: Remove permanently from exposure and give an adequate diet with vitamin supplements. Courses of oral penicillamine as for acute poisoning may be employed, especially when hematologic complications have occurred.

Beattie AD & others: Role of chronic low-level lead exposure in aetiology of mental retardation. Lancet 1:589, 1975.

Chisholm JJ Jr: Chelation therapy in children with subclinical plumbism. Pediatrics 53:441, 1974.

De la Burdé B, Shapiro IM: Dental lead, blood lead, and pica in urban children. Arch Envir Health 30:281, 1975.

Klein R: The pediatrician and the prevention of lead poisoning in children. P Clin North America 21:277, 1974.

Kubasik NP, Volosin MT: Heavy metal poisoning: Clinical aspects and laboratory analysis. Am J Med Technol 39:443, 1973.

Landrigan PJ & others: Epidemic lead absorption near an ore smelter. New England J Med 292:123, 1975.

National Institute of Environmental Health Sciences: Conference on low level lead toxicity. Environ Health Perspective 7:1, May 1974.

MERCURY

Acute poisoning (by ingestion or inhalation) is manifested by a metallic taste, salivation, thirst, a burning sensation in the throat, discoloration and edema of oral mucous membranes, abdominal pain, vomiting, bloody diarrhea, anuria, and shock. Chronic poisoning causes weakness, ataxia, intention tremors, irritability, depression, and muscle cramps. Chronic intoxication in children may be a cause of acrodynia.

The MLD is about 70 mg of mercury bichloride.

Treatment

A. Acute Poisoning: Give whites of eggs beaten with water or skimmed milk as precipitant; dimercaprol (BAL) at once as for arsenic poisoning; and sodium sulfate, 30 gm in 200 ml of water as cathartic. Maintain fluid output with 1000 ml of physiologic saline solution intravenously at once and repeat as necessary. Treat oliguria and anuria if they occur. Hemodialysis can be used to speed the removal of mercury combined with dimercaprol.

B. Chronic Poisoning: Remove from exposure.

Joselow MM, Louria DB, Browder AM: Mercurialism: Environmental and occupational aspects. Ann Int Med 76:119, 1972.

Massachusetts Department of Public Health: Mercury and hazards of vacuum cleaning. New England J Med 292:369, 1975.

Nagi NA, Yassin AK: Organic mercury poisoning in children. J Trop Med 77:128, 1974.

Ramel C: The mercury problem: A trigger for environmental pollution control. Mutat Res 26:341, 1974.

Valsamis MP, Mancall E: Toxic cerebellar degeneration (mercury). Human Path 4:513, 1973.

Wands RJ & others: Chronic inorganic mercury poisoning due to laxative abuse: A clinical and ultrastructural study. Am J Med 57:92, 1974.

MORPHINE & OTHER NARCOTIC ANALGESICS

Morphine acts primarily on the CNS, causing depression and narcosis. The manifestations of poisoning with morphine and its substitutes, heroin, meperidine, propoxyphene, and methadone, are headache, nausea, excitement, depression, pin-point pupils, slow respirations, apnea, rapid and feeble pulse, shock, and coma.

The MLD is 65 mg in susceptible individuals.

Treatment

As an antidote for overdosage, give naloxone hydrochloride, 0.005 mg/kg IV. Naloxone is free of depressant effects on the respiration and has a longer duration of action than either nalorphine or levallorphan. It is effective against pentazocine, for which nalorphine and levallorphan are contraindicated. Repeat injection of the antagonist only as necessary to maintain the response to stimuli. If effective increase in pulmonary ventilation is not achieved with the first dose, the dose may be repeated every 15 minutes until respirations return to normal and the patient responds to stimuli.

Maintain adequate ventilation with artificial respiration, using oxygen if necessary.

Huber DH & others: Heroin-overdose deaths in Atlanta. JAMA 228:319, 1974.

Lee KD, Lovejoy FH, Haddow JE: Childhood methadone intoxication. Clin Pediat 13:66, 1974.

Lovejoy FH, Mitchell AA, Goldman P: The management of propoxyphene poisoning. J Pediat 85:98, 1974.

Mauer SM & others: Hemodialysis in an infant with propoxyphene intoxication. Clin Pharmacol Ther 17:88, 1975.

Oh SJ, Rollins JL, Lewis I: Pentazocine-induced fibrous myopathy. JAMA 231:271, 1975.

MUSHROOMS

The Amanita genus of mushrooms accounts for almost all cases of fungus poisoning in the United States. *Amanita muscaria* poisoning, of rapid onset, often responds promptly to atropine if treatment is given early, whereas poisoning by *A phalloides* is more often of slow onset and many symptoms do not respond to atropine. (See Table 30–3.)

Lampe KF: Mushroom poisoning in the young child. Pediatrics 2:83, 1973.

Bartter FC: Thioctic acid and mushroom poisoning. (Correspondence.) Science 187:216, 1975.

Paaso B, Harrison DC: A new look at an old problem: Mushroom poisoning—clinical presentations and new therapeutic approaches. Am J Med 58:505, 1975.

OXALIC ACID

Oxalic acid, a component of bleaching powder, is a corrosive which also precipitates ionized calcium. Poisoning is manifested by burning in the mouth and throat, violent abdominal pains, bloody vomitus, dyspnea, tremors, oliguria, and circulatory collapse.

The MLD is 4 gm.

Treatment

A. Emergency Measures: Give at once one of the following to precipitate as insoluble calcium oxalate: (1) Calcium lactate or other calcium salt, 30 gm in 200 ml of water; or (2) large amounts of milk. Give whites of eggs beaten in milk as demulcent.

B. General Measures: Give calcium gluconate or calcium lactate, 10 ml of 10% solution IV, and calcium orally, 1–2 gm 4 times daily. Institute supportive measures as required.

PHENOLS & DERIVATIVES

The phenols are present in carbolic acid, lysol, cresol, and creosote. Hexachlorophene—2,2′-methylenebis (3,4,6-trichlorophenol)—is a widely used antiseptic (pHisoHex, etc). They are local corrosives and also have marked systemic effects (after oral or dermal absorption) on the nervous and circulatory systems. Manifestations include burning in the upper gastrointestinal tract, thirst, nausea and vomiting, erosions of mucous membranes, dark vomitus, oliguria, muscle spasms, circulatory collapse, and respiratory failure.

The MLD is 2 gm. Hexachlorophene orally (250 mg/kg) was fatal to a child.

Treatment

A. Ingestion: Delay absorption by giving tap water, milk, or activated charcoal and then remove by repeated gastric lavage with tap water or by inducing vomiting. Then give castor oil, 60 ml, followed by sodium sulfate, 30 gm, in 200 ml of water. Do not give

Table 30–3. Mushroom poisoning.

	Amanita Muscaria	*Amanita Phalloides, A Brunnescens, A Verna*
Pharmacologic action	Muscarinic or atropine-like effects.	Direct toxic action on almost all cells, especially the liver, heart, and kidneys.
Onset	Sudden (1–2 hours).	Delayed (12–24 hours).
Symptoms and signs	Confusion, excitement, thirst, nausea and vomiting, diarrhea, wheezing, salivation, slow pulse, small pupils (muscarine), dilated pupils (atropine), tremors, weakness, collapse, and even death.	Confusion, depression, headache, convulsions, coma, nausea and vomiting, bloody vomitus and stools, painful enlargement of liver, jaundice, oliguria, pulmonary edema.
Treatment	(1) Remove gastrointestinal contents by emesis and lavage followed by catharsis. (2) Antidote: Atropine sulfate, 1–2 mg subcut, and repeat every 30 minutes as needed if signs of muscarine intoxication occur. (3) Give barbiturate sedatives for excitement. (4) Force fluids by oral and parenteral routes. (5) Treat shock.	(1) Give thioctic acid, 300 mg IV daily over the entire 24 hours. (2) Relieve pain with narcotics as needed. (3) Maintain blood sugar with 4–5 liters of 5% dextrose solution every 24 hours if renal function is adequate. (4) Treat shock. (5) Institute hemodialysis immediately.

mineral oil and do not use alcohol for lavage. Give supportive measures as outlined on p 933.

B. External Burns: Wash with rubbing alcohol and then soap and water. Remove contaminated clothing.

Henry LD, Di Maio JJM: A fatal case of hexachlorophene poisoning. Military Med 139:41, 1974.

Kimbrough RD: Review of recent evidence of toxic effects of hexachlorophene. Pediatrics 13:391, 1973.

Lundell E, Nordman R: A case of infantile poisoning by topical applications of Castellani's solution. Ann Clin Res 5:404, 1973.

Trout ME: Hexachlorophene in perspective. J Clin Pharmacol 13:451, 1973.

PHENOTHIAZINE TRANQUILIZERS
(Chlorpromazine, Promazine, Prochlorperazine, Etc)

Chlorpromazine and related drugs are synthetic chemicals derived in most instances from phenothiazine. They are used as antiemetics and psychic inhibitors and as potentiators of analgesic and hypnotic drugs.

The acute fatal dose for these compounds appears to be above 50 mg/kg. Fatal poisoning from ingestion of approximately 75 mg/kg of chlorpromazine has been reported.

Clinical Findings

A. Symptoms and Signs: Minimum doses induce drowsiness and mild hypotension in as many as 50% of patients. Larger doses cause drowsiness, severe postural hypotension, tachycardia, dryness of the mouth, nausea, ataxia, anorexia, nasal congestion, fever, constipation, tremor, blurring of vision, stiffness of muscles, and coma. Intravenous injection of solutions containing more than 25 mg/ml of these drugs causes thrombophlebitis and cellulitis in a small number of patients.

Prolonged administration may cause leukopenia or agranulocytosis, jaundice, and generalized maculopapular eruptions; overdosage causes a syndrome similar to paralysis agitans, with spasmodic contractions of the face and neck muscles, extensor rigidity of the back muscles, carpopedal spasm, motor restlessness, salivation, and convulsions.

B. Laboratory Findings:

1. Liver function tests indicate the presence of obstructive jaundice.

2. Urine—Phenothiazine compounds in urine acidified with dilute nitric acid can be detected by the addition of a few drops of tincture of ferric chloride. A violet color results.

Treatment

Remove overdoses by gastric lavage or emesis. For severe hypotension, shock treatment may be necessary. Avoid the use of pressor drugs. Control convulsions cautiously with pentobarbital. Avoid other depressant drugs.

For intolerable extrapyramidal signs (ataxia, etc), give antiparkinsonism drugs such as benztropine, 0.05–0.1 mg/kg IM, followed by oral administration of the same dose up to 4 times daily. In the presence of fever, sore throat, pulmonary congestion, or other signs of infection, give penicillin, 1 million units daily, or a broad-spectrum antibiotic in maximum doses until infection is controlled. No measures have been helpful for jaundice other than discontinuing the drug.

Crane GE: Clinical psychopharmacology in its 20th year: Late, unanticipated effects of neuroleptics may limit their use in psychiatry. Science 181:124, 1973.

Joubert PH, Olivier JA: Fatal suicidal ingestion of thioridazine. Clin Toxicol 7:133, 1974.

Kiloh LG, Smith JS, Williams SE: Antiparkinson drugs as causal agents in tardive dyskinesia. MJ Australia 2:591, 1973.

Peele R, Von Loetzen IS: Phenothiazine deaths: A critical review. Am J Psychiat 130:306, 1973.

PHOSPHATES, ORGANIC
(Pesticide Sprays: Parathion, TEPP, Malathion, Thimet, Phosdrin, Systox, HETP, EPN, OMPA, Etc)

Inhalation, skin absorption, or ingestion of organic phosphorus causes marked depression of cholinesterase, resulting in continuous and excessive stimulation of the parasympathetic nervous system. Manifestations of acute poisoning appear within hours after exposure and include headache, sweating, salivation, lacrimation, vomiting, diarrhea, muscular twitchings, convulsions, dyspnea, and blurred vision. Pulse and blood pressure can be extremely variable. Contracted pupils with the above symptoms and signs and a history of exposure during the past 24 hours warrant therapy.

The MLD is 0.02–1 gm.

Treatment

A. Emergency Measures: Maintain airway and give artificial respiration. If the material has been ingested, remove poison by inducing vomiting or gastric lavage with tap water. Remove from the skin (especially the hair and under the fingernails) by washing copiously. Emergency care personnel must use care to avoid contamination. Counteract parasympathetic stimulation by giving atropine sulfate, 2 mg IM every 3–8 minutes until symptoms are relieved or signs of atropinization (dilated pupils, dry mouth) appear. Repeat as necessary to maintain complete atropinization. As much as 12 mg of atropine has been given safely in the first 2 hours. Give pralidoxime (Protopam)—only after complete atropinization—1 gm slowly IV in aqueous solution. Repeat after 30 minutes if respiration does not improve.

B. General Measures: Give 40% oxygen under positive pressure if pulmonary edema or respiratory difficulty appears. Prolonged artificial respiration may be necessary. Take a blood sample for determination of red cell cholinesterase levels. (This is of no practical value in immediate diagnosis or treatment of the acute episode, but aids in confirmation of the diagnosis.)

Gehlbach SH, Williams WA: Pesticide containers. Arch Envir Health 30:49, 1975.

Sidell FR: Soman and sarin: Clinical manifestations and treatment of accidental poisoning by organophosphates. Clin Toxicol 7:1, 1974.

Sim VM: Anticholinesterase poisoning. Am Family Physician 9:146, 1974.

PHOSPHORUS, INORGANIC
(Rat Paste, Fireworks, Matches)

Phosphorus poisoning may result from contact, ingestion, or inhalation. Phosphorus is a local irritant and systemic toxin which acts on the liver, kidneys, muscles, bones, and cardiovascular system. Toxicity is manifested early by a garlic taste, pain in the upper gastrointestinal tract, vomiting, and diarrhea. Other symptoms and signs are headache, pleuritis, extreme weakness, jaundice, oliguria, petechiae, prostration, and cardiovascular collapse.

The MLD is 50 mg.

Treatment

A. Emergency Measures: Lavage with 5–10 liters of tap water or induce emesis with 0.5–1 liter volumes at least 3 times. Give sodium sulfate, 30 gm in 200 ml of water; and liquid petrolatum, 120 ml. (No other oils may be used.) Give whites of eggs beaten in milk as demulcent.

B. General Measures: Observe carefully for several days, and treat as for acute hepatitis if signs of jaundice or liver involvement appear.

Winek CL, Collom WD, Fusia EP: Yellow phosphorus ingestions: Three fatal poisonings. Clin Toxicol 6:541, 1973.

SALICYLATE POISONING

Salicylate poisoning is most commonly caused by aspirin ingestion. Effects include acid-base disturbances, hypoprothrombinemia, hyperthermia, and gastroenteritis. The acid-base disturbances are the most dangerous. Respiratory alkalosis appears first, followed by metabolic acidosis. Severe poisoning is associated with initial serum salicylate levels above 100 mg/100 ml. A half-time of disappearance of 24 hours can be used to estimate the initial level.

Salicylates stimulate the respiratory center, producing hyperpnea, CO_2 loss, a falling serum CO_2 content, a normal or high arterial blood pH; this combination represents respiratory alkalosis. In an effort to compensate, the kidneys excrete increased amounts of bicarbonate, potassium, and sodium, but retain chloride. The chief dangers during this stage are hypokalemia and dehydration. Salicylates also interfere with carbohydrate metabolism, which results in the formation of fixed acids, probably ketones.

When the patient is first seen he may be in alkalosis or acidosis. Diagnosis and treatment are dependent upon determination of serum CO_2 content, potassium, sodium and chloride, and arterial pH. The urine is unreliable as an indication of acidosis or alkalosis.

The clinical picture includes a history of salicylate ingestion, hyperpnea, flushed face, hyperthermia, tinnitus, abdominal pain, vomiting, dehydration, spontaneous bleeding, twitchings, convulsions, pulmonary edema, uremia, and coma. Salicylates may give a false-positive ketonuria and glycosuria, or true ketonuria and glycosuria may be present. The Phenistix or ferric chloride test aids in diagnosis of salicylate ingestion (see p 931).

The MLD is 5–10 gm.

Treatment

A. Emergency Measures: Empty the stomach by giving ipecac or other emetic. If emesis is not thorough, aspirate the gastric contents without using additional fluids, and then lavage with 2–4 liters of warm tap water containing activated charcoal. Follow with saline catharsis. Treat shock with whole blood or plasma transfusion.

B. General Measures: Salicylate poisoning can only be treated adequately with knowledge of the blood pH, serum sodium, and serum CO_2 content or CO_2 combining power. Hydration in the first hour should begin with 400 ml/sq meter of IV fluid prepared as follows: To each 100 ml of 5% dextrose, add 5 mEq of sodium chloride (1.7 ml of 3 mEq/ml) and 2.5 mEq of sodium bicarbonate (2.8 ml of 7.5%). After the first hour, the same solution can be continued at one-third the initial rate until urine flow begins, dehydration is corrected, or evidence of renal insufficiency appears (rising BUN). After urine flow is established, up to 50% of the sodium in the above solution can be replaced by potassium (use 3 mEq/ml solution) depending on the measured potassium deficit. Treat profound acidosis with sodium bicarbonate, 7.5% solution (44.6 mEq/50 ml), 3–5 mEq/kg orally or IV, diluted in 5% dextrose over 2–4 hours. Maintenance of alkaline urine greatly speeds the excretion of salicylates but is difficult and dangerous in seriously ill infants. Further adjustment of sodium and potassium in fluids should be based on serum sodium and potassium determinations.

Phytonadione, 50 mg IV, should be given once for hypoprothrombinemia. Whole blood cell or platelet transfusion is recommended for thrombocytopenia. Peritoneal dialysis or an artificial kidney may be lifesaving for critically ill patients with a high serum salicylate concentration or renal insufficiency.

Reduce fever with cold water (10° C) sponge baths.

Boston Collaborative Drug Surveillance Program: Aspirin use in patients with major upper gastrointestinal bleeding and peptic-ulcer disease. New England J Med 290:1158, 1974.

Buchanan N, Rabinowitz L: Infantile salicylism: A reappraisal. J Pediat 84:391, 1974.

Crout JE, Hepburn B, Ritts RE: Suppression of lymphocyte transformation after aspirin ingestion. New England J Med 292:221, 1975.

Hoon JR: Bleeding gastritis induced by long-term release aspirin. JAMA 229:841, 1974.

Seaman WE, Ishak KG, Plotz PH: Aspirin-induced hepatotoxicity in patients with systemic lupus erythematosis. Ann Int Med 80:1, 1974.

Wolfe JD & others: Aspirin hepatitis. Ann Int Med 80:74, 1974.

SNAKE (& GILA MONSTER) BITES

The venom of poisonous snakes and lizards may be predominantly neurotoxic or predominantly hemotoxic (cytolytic). Neurotoxins cause respiratory paralysis; hemotoxins cause hemorrhage due to hemolysis and destruction of the endothelial lining of the blood vessels. The manifestations are local pain, thirst, profuse perspiration, nausea, vomiting, stimulation followed by depression, local redness, swelling, extravasation of blood, and collapse.

Treatment

A. Emergency Measures: Immobilize the patient and the bitten part immediately. Avoid manipulation of the bitten area. Use of tourniquet and incision and suction will remove up to 10% of venom if done in the first 30 minutes but is dangerous after hemorrhagic venoms. Incision should be 1/8 inch deep and 1/4 inch long in the area of the bite. Use extreme caution on hands and fingers to avoid damage to underlying structures. If a tourniquet is used, it should remain in place until specific antiserum has been administered. Do not give alcoholic beverages or stimulants. Give specific antiserum intravenously after testing for serum sensitivity with 0.02 ml of 1:100 dilution of antiserum in 0.9% saline. (Follow printed instructions.) Carry the patient to a car and transport him to a hospital or other medical facility for definitive treatment. Maintain blood pressure by giving blood transfusions. Cortisone or substitutes in large doses will relieve symptoms temporarily but may not reduce the mortality rate. Corticosteroids should not be given if the patient is receiving antiserum. If marked swelling occurs in an extremity, with indication of nerve compression, relieve pressure in fascial spaces by incision.

B. General Measures: Give plenty of warm fluids. Use barbiturates as necessary for sedation.

Hasiba U & others: Disseminated intravascular coagulation-like syndrome after envenomation by the snake *Crotalus horridus horridus*. New England J Med 292:505, 1975.

Huang TT & others: The excisional therapy in the management of snake bite. Ann Surg 179:598, 1974.

Minton SA: *Venom Diseases*. Thomas, 1974.

SPIDER BITES & SCORPION STINGS

The toxin of the less venomous species of spiders and scorpions causes only local pain, redness, and swelling. That of the more venomous species, including black widow spiders (*Latrodectus mactans*), causes generalized muscular pains, convulsions, nausea and vomiting, variable CNS involvement, and shock.

Treatment

A. Emergency Measures: As for snake bite (see above), except that incision and suction are probably useless. If absorption has occurred, give calcium gluconate, 10%, 10 ml IV or IM, or mephenesin, 10–30 ml of 2% IV and repeat as necessary. Patients under 14 years of age should receive specific antiserum. Corticosteroids may be of value in severe cases.

B. General Measures: Hot baths are of value for relief of pain. For local pain with no systemic involvement apply cold compresses. Give adequate sedation and institute supportive measures as indicated. Early excision of the necrotic lesion of the brown spider bite has been recommended.

Auer AI, Hershey FB: Surgery for necrotic bites of the brown spider. Arch Surg 108:612, 1974.

Santhanakrishnan BR, Raju VB: Management of scorpion sting in children. J Trop Med 77:133, 1974.

STRYCHNINE

Strychnine poisoning may result from ingestion or injection. The manifestations are convulsions, opisthotonos, dyspnea, foaming at the mouth, and asphyxia.

Treatment

A. Emergency Measures: Keep the patient quiet in a darkened room. Control convulsions with succinylcholine and give artificial respiration and oxygen. Give diazepam, 10 mg IV, and repeat every 30 minutes. If possible, lavage gently with activated charcoal before symptoms appear. Do not lavage after twitching or convulsions have appeared unless succinylcholine is being given.

B. General Measures: Inhalation of ether or chloroform may be used to quiet the patient.

Sgaragli GP, Mannaioni PF: Pharmacokinetic observations on a case of massive strychnine poisoning. Clin Toxicol 6:533, 1973.

WASP, BEE, YELLOW JACKET, & HORNET STINGS

Stings of these common insects, although locally painful, usually cause only mild symptoms of brief duration. Local cold compresses, application of baking soda solution, and oral salicylates or antihistamines are sufficient treatment. Multiple stings may cause a shock-like reaction with hemoglobinuria. Sensitive individuals may develop an acute allergic or even fatal anaphylactic response after a single sting.

Treatment

A. Emergency Measures: Give epinephrine hydrochloride, 1:1000 solution, 0.2–0.5 ml subcut or IM; and then diphenhydramine hydrochloride, 5–20 mg slowly IV. Treat shock.

B. General Measures: Give corticosteroids intramuscularly to support shock therapy.

Lichtenstein LM, Valentine MD, Sobotka AK: Venom treatment in anaphylactic sensitivity to Hymenoptera sting. New England J Med 290:1223, 1974.

Mueller HL, Schmid WH, Rubinsztain R: Stinging insect hypersensitivity. Pediatrics 55:530, 1975.

PSYCHOTOMIMETIC AGENTS

Classification

1. LSD (lysergic acid diethylamide): Semisynthetic, from ergot.

2. DMT (dimethyltryptamine): Synthetic and from a South American plant (*Piptadenia peregrina*).

3. DET (diethyltryptamine): Synthetic.

4. "STP," DOM (2,5-dimethoxy-4-methylamphetamine): Synthetic.

5. Marihuana: One active principle is tetrahydrocannabinol. From the Indian hemp plant (*Cannabis sativa*).

6. Mescaline (3,4,5-trimethoxyphenethylamine): Synthetic; also from peyote, a cactus (mescal, *Lophophora williamsii*).

7. Psilocybin and psilocin: Derivatives of 4-hydroxytryptamine. Synthetic; also from a mushroom (*Psilocybe mexicana*).

8. Bufotenine (dimethyl serotonin): Synthetic; also from *Piptadenia peregrina, Amanita muscaria,* and the skin of a toad (*Bufo marinus*).

9. Ibogaine: Alkaloid from the plant *Tabernanthe iboga.*

10. Harmine and harmaline: From plants (*Peganum harmala* and *Banisteria caapi*).

11. Ditran and phencyclidine (PCP, Sernylan): Synthetic.

12. Amphetamine and related drugs: See below.

13. MDA (methylene dioxyamphetamine): Synthetic.

14. Cocaine: From the leaves of the plant *Erythroxylon coca.*

15. Volatile hydrocarbons: Gasoline, toluene.

Clinical Findings

Manifestations requiring medical intervention are hyperexcitability, uncontrollability, ataxia, hypertension or hypotension, coma, and prolonged psychotic states. Some of these agents are suspected of causing permanent cerebral damage.

Treatment

Give chlorpromazine, 0.5–2 mg/kg IM, to control the acute phase. (In STP poisoning and possibly after LSD, the combination is reported to be hazardous.) Treat coma as for barbiturate poisoning. The phencyclidine psychotic state may require 2 weeks of restricted sensory input.

Campbell AMG & others: Cerebral atrophy in young cannabis smokers. Lancet 2:1219, 1971. [See also correspondence in 1:202, 1972.]

Drug Dependence. Excerpta Medica (monthly).

Eastman JW, Cohen SM: Hypertensive crisis and death associated with phencyclidine poisoning. JAMA 231:1270, 1975.

Klepfisz A, Racy J: Homicide and LSD. JAMA 223:429, 1973.

Klock JC, Boerner U, Becker CE: Coma, hyperthermia and bleeding associated with massive LSD overdose: Report of eight cases. Western J Med 120:183, 1974.

Nahas GG: *Marihuana: Deceptive Weed.* Raven Press, 1973.

National Clearinghouse for Drug Abuse Information: Reports on most of above drugs.

Sadow RL: LSD, alcohol and homicide. JAMA 225:1123, 1973.

Stein JI: Phencyclidine induced psychosis: The need to avoid unnecessary sensory influx. Mil Med 138:590, 1973.

TREATMENT OF LESS COMMON SPECIFIC POISONINGS (ALPHABETICAL ORDER)

Acetaldehyde (Industrial)

Inhalation of vapors causes severe irritation of mucous membranes with coughing, pulmonary edema, followed by narcosis. Ingestion causes narcosis and respiratory failure. The MLD in adults is about 5 gm.

Remove from exposure or remove ingested poison by gastric lavage or emesis followed by catharsis. Give oxygen for respiratory difficulty. Treat pulmonary edema.

Aconite (Liniment)

Manifestations are burning followed by numbness and tingling of the mouth, throat, and hands; blurred vision; weak pulse; fall of blood pressure; shallow respirations; convulsions; and respiratory or cardiac failure. The MLD is 1 gm of aconite or 2 mg of aconitine.

Remove ingested poison by gastric lavage or emesis followed by catharsis. Give artificial respiration or oxygen as necessary. Give digitalis to counteract cardiac depression. Treat convulsions. Give atropine, 1 mg to prevent vagal slowing of the heart.

Akee (Tree)

Manifestations are abdominal discomfort, vomiting, convulsions, coma, hypothermia, and fall of blood pressure. Jaundice may appear during the recovery phase.

Remove ingested akee by gastric lavage or emesis followed by catharsis. Control convulsions. Give carbohydrates as 5% glucose intravenously or as sugar dissolved in fruit juice orally to protect from liver damage.

Aminopyrine, Antipyrine, Phenylbutazone
(Analgesics)

Manifestations are dizziness, cyanosis, coma, and convulsions. Prolonged administration causes epigastric pain, urticaria, leukopenia, liver damage, exfoliative dermatitis, gastric or duodenal erosion, adrenal necrosis. The MLD is 5—30 gm.

Treat acute poisoning as for salicylates. Treat chronic poisoning by discontinuing drug.

Amitriptyline, Doxepin, Desipramine, Imipramine, Nortriptyline, Protriptyline
(Tricyclic antidepressants)

Overdoses cause anxiety, agitation, delirium, tachycardia, convulsions, hypotension, pyrexia, heart block and other arrhythmias, dilated pupils, and coma.

Remove ingested drug by gastric lavage, emesis, and catharsis. Control convulsions with diazepam (Valium), 0.2 mg/kg IV. Maintain respiration.

Goel KM, Shanks RA: Amitriptyline and imipramine poisoning in children. Brit MJ 1:261, 1974.

Greenblatt DJ, Koch-Weser J, Shader RI: Multiple complications and death following protriptyline overdose. JAMA 229:5506, 1974.

Amphetamine, Methamphetamine, Dextroamphetamine, and Ephedrine (Sympathomimetics)

Manifestations are tachycardia, dilated pupils, blurred vision, spasms, convulsions, gasping respirations, cardiac arrhythmias, psychosis, and respiratory failure. The blood pressure is elevated initially but below normal later. The MLD is 120 mg.

Remove ingested drug by emesis or gastric lavage followed by catharsis. Give artificial respiration if cyanosis is present. Maintain blood pressure in cardiovascular collapse by the administration of fluids. Give chlorpromazine, 1 mg/kg IM; give half that amount if these drugs have been taken with sedative-hypnotics.

Van Hoof F, Heyndrickx A, Timperman J: Report of a human fatality due to amphetamine. Arch Toxicol 32:307, 1974.

Aniline (Industrial or cloth-marking ink)

Manifestations are cyanosis, shallow respirations, fall of blood pressure, convulsions, and coma. Blood methemoglobin, as determined photometrically, may reach 60% or more of total hemoglobin. The MLD is 1 gm.

Remove aniline from skin by washing thoroughly with soap and water or, if ingested, remove by emesis, gastric lavage, and catharsis. Give fluids and oxygen if respiration is shallow or if there is evidence of air hunger. As antidote for methemoglobinemia give methylene blue, 10—50 ml of 1% solution IV.

Antimony (Paint)

Manifestations are severe diarrhea with mucus followed by blood, hemorrhagic nephritis, and hepatitis. The MLD is 100 mg.

Remove ingested poison by gastric lavage, emesis, and catharsis. Treat as for arsenic poisoning.

Arsine (Industrial)
(See also Arsenic, p 936.)

Manifestations are pyrexia, cough, abdominal pain, hemolytic anemia, hemoglobinuria, anuria, methemoglobinemia, and diarrhea.

Alkalinize urine as for fava bean poisoning. Give blood transfusions if anemia is severe. Treat anuria.

Barium (Rodenticide)

Manifestations are tightness of the muscles of the face and neck, fibrillary muscular tremors, weakness, difficulty in breathing, irregularity of the heart, convulsions, and cardiac and respiratory failure. The MLD is 1 gm.

Give 10 ml of 10% sodium sulfate slowly IV and repeat every 15 minutes until symptoms subside. Give 30 gm sodium sulfate in 200 ml of water orally or by gastric tube and repeat in 1 hour.

Benzene (Solvent)

Manifestations are visual blurring, tremors, shallow and rapid respiration, ventricular irregularities, unconsciousness, and convulsions. Repeated exposure results in aplastic anemia and abnormal bleeding. The MAC is 35 ppm.

Remove patient from contaminated air and give artificial respiration with oxygen. Treat ingested poison as for gasoline poisoning.

Beryllium (Industrial)

Manifestations include acute pneumonitis; chest pain, bronchial spasm, fever, dyspnea, cough, and cyanosis. Right heart failure may occur. Pulmonary granulomatosis with weight loss and marked dyspnea may occur years after initial exposure. X-ray examination reveals diffuse increase in density of the lung fields or snowstorm appearance. No degree of exposure is safe.

Place the patient at complete bed rest and administer 60% oxygen by mask for cyanosis. EDTA has been suggested. The administration of corticosteroid or related drugs gives symptomatic relief but is not curative.

Bleaching Solutions (Household)

Clorox, Purex, Sani-clor, etc cause irritation and corrosion of mucous membranes with edema of the pharynx and larynx. Perforation of the esophagus or stomach is rare. The MLD is 15 ml.

Remove ingested solution by gastric lavage or emesis, using a solution of milk of magnesia or, preferably, sodium thiosulfate, 30—50 gm/liter, or milk. After emesis or lavage, give a cathartic consisting of sodium sulfate, 30 gm, and sodium thiosulfate, 10 gm, in 250 ml of milk or water. *Caution:* Do not use acid antidotes. Treat as for sodium hydroxide poisoning.

Boric Acid (Antiseptic)

Manifestations from ingestion or skin application are fever, anuria, and flushing followed by desquamation, lethargy, and convulsions. The MLD is 5—15 gm.

Remove ingested boric acid by emesis or gastric lavage followed by catharsis. Maintain urine output by giving liquids orally or, in the presence of vomiting, by giving 5% dextrose intravenously. Control convulsions by the cautious administration of ether. Remove circulating boric acid by peritoneal dialysis or with an artificial kidney. Treat anuria as for mercury poisoning.

Bromates (Cold wave neutralizer)

Manifestations are vomiting, abdominal pains, oliguria, coma, convulsions, fall of blood pressure, hematuria, and proteinuria. The MLD is 4 gm.

Remove poison by gastric lavage, emesis, and catharsis. Give sodium thiosulfate, 1—5 gm IV as a 10% solution. Treat shock by administration of repeated small blood transfusions.

Cadmium (Metal plating)

Ingestion causes diarrhea, vomiting, muscular aches, salivation, and abdominal pain. Inhalation causes shortness of breath, pain in the chest, foamy or bloody sputum, muscular aches. Chronic exposure produces, in addition, anemia, and x-ray examination indicates lung consolidation. A sulfosalicylic acid precipitable protein is present in the urine. The MLD is about 10 mg.

Treat pulmonary edema and give calcium edathamil. Remove ingested poison by emesis or gastric lavage followed by catharsis.

Caffeine, Aminophylline (Stimulants)

Manifestations are sudden collapse and cardiac arrest within 1—2 minutes after intravenous or rectal administration, and convulsions. The MLD is 1 gm.

Give oxygen by artificial respiration with forced ventilation, maintain blood pressure, remove rectally administered aminophylline by enema, and control convulsions as for strychnine poisoning.

Camphor (Stimulant)

Manifestations are a feeling of tension, dizziness, irrational behavior, rigidity, tachycardia, twitching of the facial muscles, and generalized convulsions. The MLD is 1 gm.

Remove ingested poison by gastric lavage or emesis followed by catharsis. Control convulsions.

Cantharidin (Irritant)

Manifestations are severe vomiting, diarrhea, fall of blood pressure, hematuria, and death in respiratory failure or uremia. The MLD is 10 mg.

Remove ingested poison by gastric lavage or emesis followed by catharsis. Treat cardiovascular collapse by blood transfusions and intravenous saline. Treat anuria.

Castor Beans (Plant)

Manifestations are vomiting, diarrhea, severe abdominal pain, cyanosis, circulatory collapse, and oliguria. Urine may show protein, casts, red blood cells, and hemoglobin. The MLD is 1 bean.

Remove ingested beans by gastric lavage or emesis followed by catharsis. Maintain blood pressure by blood transfusions. Alkalinize urine by giving 5—15 gm of sodium bicarbonate daily to prevent precipitation of hemoglobin or hemoglobin products in the kidneys. Treat anuria.

Chloramine-T (Disinfectant)

Manifestations are cyanosis, frothing at the mouth, and respiratory failure within a few minutes to 1 hour after ingestion. The MLD is 0.5 gm.

Remove ingested chloramine-T by gastric lavage or emesis followed by catharsis. Give antidotes as for cyanide poisoning.

Chlorates (Disinfectant)

Manifestations are cyanosis, hemolysis, anuria, and convulsions. The MLD is 15 gm. Laboratory findings include methemoglobinemia, anemia of the hemolytic type, and elevation of serum potassium.

Remove ingested chlorate by gastric lavage or emesis followed by catharsis. Treat methemoglobinemia with methylene blue. Force fluids to 2—4 liters daily to remove chlorate if urine output is adequate.

Chlorinated Hydrocarbons

For volatile chlorinated hydrocarbons, see Carbon Tetrachloride; for nonvolatile chlorinated hydrocarbons, see Chlorophenothane (DDT).

Chlorinated Naphthalene (Insulator)

The principal manifestation is a papular, acneform eruption which progresses to pustule formation. Jaundice, enlargement of the liver, and weakness also occur. Impairment of hepatic cell function is revealed by appropriate tests.

Treat liver damage as outlined under carbon tetrachloride poisoning.

Chromium & Chromate (Rustproofing)

Ingestion causes abdominal pain, vomiting, shock, and oliguria or anuria. Skin contact leads to incapacitating eczematous dermatitis and ulceration. Ulceration and perforation of the nasal septum also occur.

Acute hepatitis has been observed. Examination of the urine reveals proteinuria and hematuria. The MLD of soluble chromate is 5 gm.

Remove ingested chromate by gastric lavage, emesis, and catharsis. Treat oliguria and liver damage.

Cocaine (Local anesthetic)

Manifestations are restlessness, excitability, hallucinations, irregular respirations, convulsions, and circulatory failure. The MLD is 30 mg.

Remove the drug from the skin or mucous membranes by washing with tap water or normal saline. Remove ingested cocaine by gastric lavage or emesis followed by catharsis. Limit absorption from an injection site by a tourniquet or ice pack. Control convulsions by giving thiopental sodium. Prevent hypoxia by the administration of oxygen.

Colchicine (Gout remedy)

Manifestations are burning in the throat, watery to bloody diarrhea, cardiovascular collapse, and oliguria. The MLD is 6 mg.

Remove ingested poison by emesis or gastric lavage followed by catharsis. Give oxygen for respiratory difficulty. Treat oliguria.

Croton Oil (Irritant)

Manifestations are burning pain in the mouth and stomach, tenesmus, watery or bloody diarrhea, fall of blood pressure, and coma. The MLD is 1 gm.

Remove ingested croton oil by gastric lavage or emesis followed by saline catharsis. Treat shock. Maintain hydration by giving fluids orally or intravenously. Relieve pain with morphine sulfate, 10 mg.

Detergents (Soaps, detergents, and antiseptics.)

A. Cationic Detergents: These include the antiseptics of the quaternary ammonium type (Zephiran, Diaperene, Phemerol). Manifestations are severe vomiting, shock, convulsions, and death within 1–4 hours. The MLD is 1–3 gm.

Remove unabsorbed detergent by emesis or gastric lavage. Ordinary face soap is an effective antidote for unabsorbed cationic detergent but is not effective against the systemic effects. Treat respiratory embarrassment or shock with appropriate supportive measures. Short-acting barbiturates should be used to control convulsions.

B. Anionic or Nonionic Detergents: These compounds, which are present in general laundry detergents and dishwashing solutions, are less toxic than the cationic detergents. Certain laundry compounds and electric dishwasher detergents may contain alkalies, however, and their ingestion requires immediate treatment for caustic poisoning. Poisoning with certain phosphate additives to some detergents requires treatment with parenteral calcium.

Dinitrophenol (Insecticide)

Manifestations are fever, prostration, thirst, excessive perspiration, difficulty in breathing, muscular tremors, and coma. Cataracts occur after repeated ingestion. The MLD is 100 mg.

Remove ingested poison by emesis, gastric lavage, and catharsis. If the body temperature is elevated, reduce to normal by immersion in cold water or by applying cold packs.

Dioxane (Solvent)

Prolonged exposure may lead to kidney and liver damage and pulmonary edema.

Remove from further exposure and treat symptomatically.

Disulfiram (Antabuse) Plus Alcohol
(Alcohol sensitizer)

Manifestations are flushing, sweating, tachycardia, fall of blood pressure, cardiac arrhythmias, air hunger, and cardiac pain.

Give artificial respiration with oxygen, and ephedrine, 25 mg subcut to maintain normal blood pressure.

Ergotamine (Migraine remedy)

Manifestations are rise or fall of blood pressure, weak pulse, convulsions, and loss of consciousness. Prolonged administration causes numbness and coldness of the extremities, tingling, pain in the chest, gangrene of the fingers and toes, contractions of the facial muscles, and convulsions. The maximum safe dose is 6 mg/day.

Remove ingested drug by emesis or gastric lavage followed by catharsis. Treat convulsions as for strychnine poisoning.

Estrogens (Female sex hormones)

Manifestations are excessive vaginal bleeding and enlargement of the breasts. Discontinue further administration.

Ethylene Chlorohydrin (Fumigant)

Manifestations are abdominal pain, excitability, delirium, respiratory slowing, fall of blood pressure, twitching of muscles, cyanosis, and coma with respiratory and circulatory failure. The MLD is 5 ml.

Remove from further exposure and remove ingested poison by emesis, gastric lavage, and catharsis. Treat as for methyl bromide poisoning.

Ethylene Glycol (Anti-freeze)

The initial symptoms in massive dosage (over 100 ml in a single dose) are those of alcoholic intoxication. These symptoms then progress to stupor, anuria, and unconsciousness with convulsions. Smaller amounts (10–30 ml) result in anuria beginning 24–72 hours after ingestion. The urine may show calcium oxalate crystals, protein, red cells, and casts.

Remove ingested glycol by gastric lavage or emesis and catharsis. Give calcium gluconate, 10 ml of 10% solution IV, to precipitate oxalate. Give artificial respiration, using oxygen for depressed respiration. In the absence of renal impairment, force fluids to 4 liters or more daily to increase excretion of glycol. Give ethyl alcohol as in methyl alcohol poisoning. Treat uremia as for carbon tetrachloride poisoning. Dialysis is useful.

Fava Beans (Plant)

Manifestations are fever, jaundice, dark urine, oliguria, and pallor. The urine may show presence of hemoglobin.

Give blood transfusions until anemia is corrected. Alkalinize urine with 5–15 gm of sodium bicarbonate every 4 hours to prevent the precipitation of hemoglobin in the kidneys. In the presence of normal kidney function, maintain urine output by giving 2–4 liters of fluid daily orally or IV. Give cortisone, 25–100 mg daily. Treat anuria.

Fish Poisoning

Manifestations are vomiting and muscular weakness progressing to paralysis, abdominal pain, and convulsions.

Remove ingested fish by gastric lavage or emesis followed by catharsis. Maintain adequate airway or give artificial respiration. Treat convulsions.

Fluoroacetate (Rodenticide)

Symptoms begin within minutes to hours with vomiting, excitability, convulsions, irregularity of the heart, and depression of respiration. The fatal dose is estimated to be 50–100 mg.

Remove ingested poison by emesis, gastric lavage, and catharsis. Control convulsions as for strychnine poisoning. Monoacetin (commercial 60% glycerol monoacetate) has been suggested as an antidote. The dosage is 0.1–0.5 ml/kg diluted in 5 parts of saline solution IV.

Food Poisoning: Bacterial

Manifestations are nausea, vomiting, diarrhea, and weakness progressing for 12–24 hours. Abdominal pain may be severe. Fever, shock, and dehydration occur rarely.

Remove toxin from gastrointestinal tract by gastric lavage or emesis. If diarrhea is not present, a saline cathartic may be given. Give nothing by mouth until vomiting has subsided. Then give oral fluids as tolerated for 12–24 hours before beginning a regular diet. If vomiting and diarrhea are severe, maintain fluid balance by giving 5% dextrose in saline intravenously. Give codeine phosphate, 30 mg orally or subcut, or paregoric, 4–12 ml after each bowel movement. Give atropine sulfate, 1 mg subcut, if gastrointestinal hyperactivity persists. Give bismuth subcarbonate, 1 gm after each bowel movement.

Food Poisoning: Nitrites

Manifestations are flushing of the skin, vomiting, dizziness, marked fall of blood pressure, cyanosis, and respiratory paralysis. The MLD is 2 gm.

Remove ingested poison by gastric lavage or emesis followed by catharsis. Maintain blood pressure by the injection of epinephrine, 1 ml of 1:1000 solution subcut, or levarterenol. Treat methemoglobinemia by

the administration of methylene blue, 5–25 ml of 1% solution slowly IV.

Formaldehyde (Disinfectant)

Manifestations are severe abdominal pain followed by cardiovascular collapse, loss of consciousness, anuria, and circulatory failure. The MLD is 60 ml.

Remove ingested poison by gastric lavage or emesis followed by catharsis, preferably with 1% ammonium carbonate solution. Treat shock by administration of fluids.

Gold Salts (Antirheumatic)

Manifestations are skin rash, itching, eruptions, metallic taste, hepatitis, granulocytopenia, and aplastic anemia. Give dimercaprol (BAL).

Hydralazine (Hypotensive)

Manifestations are fever, diffuse erythematous facial dermatitis, lymph gland enlargement, splenomegaly, arthralgia, and simulated disseminated lupus erythematosus.

Discontinue further use at the first indication of joint involvement or rash. Give aspirin, 1–3 gm daily, or cortisone, 50–150 mg daily, until symptoms regress.

Hydrogen Sulfide & Carbon Disulfide (Fumigants)

Manifestations are painful conjunctivitis, appearance of a halo around lights, anosmia, pulmonary edema, restlessness, blurred vision, unconsciousness, and paralysis of respiration. Prolonged exposure causes persistent low blood pressure, impaired gait and balance, memory loss, mental depression, and parkinsonian tremor. The MAC is 20 ppm.

Remove from further exposure. Treat pulmonary edema.

Hydroquinone (Photo developer)

Repeated exposure will produce skin sensitivity reactions. Ingestion of 10 gm will cause symptoms similar to those due to phenol poisoning. Treat as for phenol poisoning.

Ipecac, Emetine (Emetics)

Manifestations are fatigue, dyspnea, tachycardia, low blood pressure, unconsciousness, and death from heart failure. The ECG reveals depressed T waves and arrhythmias. The MLD of emetine is 1 gm.

Remove ingested poison by gastric lavage or emesis followed by catharsis. Cautious digitalization may be helpful for myocardial weakness.

Iproniazid, Isocarboxazid, Pheniprazine, Nialamide, Phenelzine (Stimulants)

Overdoses cause ataxia, stupor, excitement, fall of blood pressure, tachycardia, and convulsions. Repeated administration may cause weakness, hallucinations, mania, urine retention, liver injury with nausea, and vomiting. The MLD is 5 gm.

Remove ingested drug by gastric lavage, emesis,

and catharsis. Give artificial respiration if respiration is depressed. Maintain blood pressure. Do not give stimulants. Discontinue administration at the first appearance of jaundice. Treat liver impairment as for carbon tetrachloride poisoning.

Larkspur (Liniment)

Manifestations are tingling and burning sensations of the mouth and skin, vomiting, diarrhea, fall of blood pressure, weak pulse, and convulsions.

Remove by gastric lavage or emesis followed by saline catharsis. Give atropine, 2 mg subcut. Give artificial respiration. Maintain blood pressure.

Magnesium Salts (Cathartic)

Manifestations are watery diarrhea, gastrointestinal irritation, vomiting, tenesmus, collapse, flaccid paralysis, and, in the presence of impaired renal function, severe fall of blood pressure. The MLD is 30–60 gm.

Dilute orally or rectally administered magnesium sulfate by giving tap water. Give artificial respiration if necessary. Give calcium gluconate, 10 ml of 10% solution IV slowly, as a specific antidote.

Manganese (Industrial)

Ingestion causes lethargy, edema, and symptoms of extrapyramidal tract lesions. Inhalation causes bronchitis, pneumonia, and liver enlargement. Signs of parkinsonism also occur. Hepatic cell function tests may be impaired. The MAC is 6 mg/cu mm.

Remove from further exposure. Give EDTA.

Meprobamate (Sedative)

Manifestations are drowsiness and incoordination progressing to coma with cyanosis and respiratory depression. The MLD is 12 gm.

Remove ingested drug by gastric lavage or emesis followed by catharsis. Use resuscitative measures as for barbiturates if respiratory depression is present.

Metal Fumes (Industrial)

Inhalation of zinc oxide or other metal fumes causes fever, chills, muscular aches, and weakness. Pulmonary edema may follow.

Treat pulmonary edema. Bed rest and administration of analgesics will ordinarily relieve generalized symptoms.

Metaldehyde (Snail bait)

Manifestations are severe vomiting, abdominal pains, temperature elevation, muscular rigidity, convulsions, coma, and death from respiratory failure up to 48 hours after ingestion. The MLD for adults is about 5 gm.

Treat as for acetaldehyde poisoning, but note that snail bait commonly also contains arsenic.

Methenamine (Urinary antiseptic)

Manifestations are skin rash, kidney and bladder irritation, hematuria, and vomiting.

Discontinue further administration.

Methyl Bromide & Methyl Chloride (Fumigants)

Manifestations are dizziness, drowsiness, fall of blood pressure, coma, convulsions, and pulmonary edema after a latent period of 1–4 hours.

Treat convulsions as for strychnine poisoning. Treat pulmonary edema by administering 60% oxygen by face mask. Humidify inspired oxygen by using 20% ethyl alcohol in humidifier or nebulizer.

Methyl Sulfate (Industrial)

Ingestion or contact causes corrosion equivalent to that from sulfuric acid. Vapor exposure causes irritation and erythema of the eyes, pulmonary edema, proteinuria, and hematuria. The MLD for adults is about 1 gm.

Treat as for corrosive acid poisoning.

Methysergide Maleate (Sansert) (Migraine remedy)

Methysergide, which has been effectively employed in the prevention of migraine attacks, may cause hazardous fibrotic disorders involving primarily the retroperitoneal areas (retroperitoneal fibrosis) but also suggestive fibrotic changes affecting the aorta, heart valves, and lungs. Manifestations may include chest pain, dyspnea, fever, pleural effusion; pain in the back, abdomen, and pelvis; hydronephrosis, renal insufficiency, intermittent claudication, and edema of the lower extremities.

Cessation of methysergide therapy results in partial or complete remission of the disorder. Surgical removal of adhesions may be necessary.

Metol (Photo developer)

Repeated exposure may cause skin sensitivity reactions characterized by weeping and crusting. Ingestion may cause methemoglobinemia with cyanosis similar to that from antipyrine.

Remove from further exposure. Treat ingestion as for antipyrine.

Naphthalene (Moth balls)

Manifestations are diarrhea, oliguria, anemia, jaundice, pain on urination, and anuria. The MLD for adults is about 2 gm.

Remove ingested naphthalene by gastric lavage or emesis followed by catharsis. Alkalinize urine by giving sodium bicarbonate, 5 gm orally every 4 hours or as necessary to maintain alkaline urine. Give repeated small blood transfusions until hemoglobin is 60–80% of normal.

Naphthol (Industrial)

Acute poisoning is the same as that with phenol. Prolonged contact may cause bladder tumors, hemolytic anemia, and cataracts. Addition of ferric chloride to acidified urine gives a violet or blue color indicating the presence of a phenolic compound. The MLD is 2 gm.

Treat as for phenol poisoning.

Naphthylamine (Industrial)

Repeated exposure may cause skin sensitivity reactions with weeping and crusting. Exposure to large amounts may cause methemoglobinemia with cyanosis.

Remove from further exposure. Treat cyanosis as for aniline poisoning.

Nickel Carbonyl (Industrial)

Immediate symptoms are cough, dizziness, and weakness. Delayed reactions are characterized by dyspnea, cyanosis, rapid pulse, and respiratory embarrassment. The MAC is 1 ppm.

Treat cyanosis and dyspnea by giving 100% oxygen by mask. Treat pulmonary edema. Give sodium diethyldithiocarbamate, 50–100 mg/kg orally or IM.

Nicotine (Tobacco)

Manifestations are respiratory stimulation, nausea, diarrhea, tachycardia, elevation of blood pressure, salivation, and, with large doses, rapid progression to prostration, convulsions, respiratory slowing, cardiac irregularity, and coma. The fatal dose of pure nicotine is about 1 mg/kg. The MLD of tobacco is 5 gm.

Remove nicotine from skin by scrubbing or, if ingested, remove by thorough gastric lavage. Inject hexamethonium chloride, 25–50 mg subcut. Repeat each hour until blood pressure falls to normal. Treat convulsions as for strychnine poisoning.

Pamaquine (Anthelmintic)

Hemolytic anemia and methemoglobinemia occur most commonly in Negroes. Gastric distress and weakness occur after large doses.

Reduce dosage or discontinue drug. Treat hemolytic anemia by the administration of sodium bicarbonate to alkalinize the urine and prevent the precipitation of acid hematin. Give blood transfusions if anemia is severe.

Paraldehyde (Hypnotic)

Manifestations are deep sleep with ordinary doses and respiratory or cardiac depression occasionally with doses over 10 ml.

Treat as for acetaldehyde or barbiturate poisoning.

Pentylenetetrazol (Stimulant)

Manifestations are increased respiration, twitching, convulsions, and respiratory failure beginning within minutes after administration. The MLD by the intravenous route is 1 gm.

Treat as for strychnine poisoning.

Permanganate (Antiseptic)

Ingestion of solid or concentrated permanganate causes laryngeal edema, necrosis of oral mucosa, slow pulse, and cardiovascular collapse. Anuria may occur. The MLD is 10 gm.

Remove ingested poison by gastric lavage or emesis followed by catharsis. Treat shock and anuria.

Phenacetin & Acetanilid (Analgesics)

Acute poisoning is similar to that due to salicylates. Prolonged administration leads to renal impairment, cyanosis, hemolytic anemia, and skin eruptions. The MLD is 5–20 gm.

Treat as for salicylate poisoning. Treat methemoglobinemia by giving methylene blue, 5–25 ml of 1% solution slowly IV.

Phenolphthalein (Laxative)

Manifestations are erythematous, itching skin rash, or purging, collapse, and fall of blood pressure.

Prevent further use. Treat blood pressure fall by administration of fluids.

Physostigmine, Neostigmine, & Related Drugs (Parasympathomimetics)

Manifestations are tremors, marked peristalsis, involuntary defecation and urination, pin-point pupils, difficult breathing, convulsions and severe respiratory difficulty. The MLD is 6 mg.

Give atropine sulfate, 2 mg IV or IM every 2–4 hours as necessary to relieve respiratory difficulty and other symptoms.

Picrotoxin (Stimulant)

Manifestations are increased respiration, twitching, convulsions, and respiratory failure, beginning 20 minutes to 1 hour after exposure and persisting up to 24 hours. The MLD is 20 mg.

Remove ingested poison by gastric lavage or emesis followed by catharsis in the absence of convulsions. Treat convulsions as for strychnine poisoning.

Poison Hemlock (Plant)

Manifestations are gradually increasing muscular weakness followed by paralysis with respiratory failure. Proteinuria also occurs.

Treat respiratory failure by artificial respiration with oxygen. Remove ingested poison by gastric lavage or emesis followed by catharsis.

Poison Ivy, Poison Oak (Plants)

Local effects begin after a delay of hours to days and include itching, swelling, vesiculation, generalized edema, proteinuria, and microscopic hematuria.

Minimize skin contamination by washing with strong soap and water. Remove ingested plant material by gastric lavage or emesis followed by saline catharsis. Treat exudative stage by exposure to air or with wet dressings of aluminum acetate, 1%. Generalized reactions may be treated with cortisone or related steroids to relieve symptoms.

Procaine (Local anesthetic)

Manifestations are dizziness, weakness, fall of blood pressure, muscular tremors, convulsions, and cardiovascular collapse. The MLD is 1 gm.

Treat as for cocaine poisoning.

Propylthiouracil (Antithyroid)

Manifestations are skin rash, urticaria, joint pains, fever, and leukopenia.

Treat agranulocytosis by the administration of large doses of penicillin or broad-spectrum antibiotics to control intercurrent infections.

Quinidine (Antifibrillatory)

Manifestations are tinnitus, diarrhea, dizziness, severe fall of blood pressure with disappearance of pulse, respiratory failure, thrombocytopenic purpura after prolonged use, urticaria, and anaphylactoid reactions. The ECG may show widening of QRS complex, lengthened Q–T interval, premature ventricular beats, and lengthened P–R interval. The MLD is 1 gm.

Remove ingested drug by gastric lavage or emesis followed by catharsis. Raise blood pressure by intravenous saline or blood transfusions or with levarterenol. The administration of sixth-molar sodium lactate solution intravenously is said to reduce the cardiotoxic effects of quinidine.

Quinine, Quinacrine, Chloroquine (Antimalarials)

Manifestations are progressive tinnitus, blurring of vision, weakness, fall of blood pressure, anuria, and cardiac irregularities. Repeated ingestion of quinine causes visual loss associated with pallor of optic disks, narrowing of retinal vessels, and papilledema. Quinacrine causes hepatitis, aplastic anemia, psychosis, and jaundice. Chloroquine causes dizziness and blurred vision. The urine may show red cells, protein, and casts. The MLD is 1 gm.

Remove ingested drug by gastric lavage or emesis followed by catharsis. Treat shock. Give 2–4 liters of fluids daily to promote renal excretion. Treat anuria.

Rauwolfia (Antihypertensive)

Manifestations are diarrhea, nasal stuffiness, cardiac pain, extrasystoles, congestive failure, tremors, and emotional depression.

Discontinue further administration.

Shellfish

Manifestations are numbness and tingling of lips, tongue, face, and extremities, respiratory weakness or paralysis, and convulsions.

Remove ingested shellfish by gastric lavage or emesis followed by catharsis. Give artificial respiration with oxygen, and maintain blood pressure.

Silver Nitrate (Antiseptic)

Silver nitrate is a protein precipitant. Poisoning is manifested by nausea, vomiting, diarrhea, bloody stools, blue discoloration about the mouth, and shock.

Lavage with saline solution to precipitate silver chloride. Give whites of eggs beaten in milk as demulcent, and sodium sulfate, 30 gm in 200 ml of water as cathartic. Institute supportive measures.

Dimercaprol (BAL) has not proved effective.

Stibine (Industrial)

Manifestations are weakness, jaundice, anemia, and weak pulse. The MAC is 0.1 ppm.

Treat by blood transfusion and alkalinization of the urine.

Streptomycin (Antituberculosis)

Manifestations are 8th nerve injury with tinnitus, deafness, loss of sense of balance, and vertigo.

Discontinue administration at the first sign of 8th nerve injury.

Sulfonamides (Antibacterial)

Manifestations are skin eruptions, fever, hematuria, and oliguria or anuria with azotemia. The urine shows crystals, red cells, and protein.

If kidney function is normal, force fluids to 4 liters daily to speed excretion of sulfonamides. Treat anuria.

Talc (Dusting powder)

Prolonged inhalation causes fine fibrosis of the lungs and calcification of the pericardium.

Remove from further exposure. Treat as for silicosis.

Tetrachloroethane (Solvent)

Manifestations are irritation of the eyes and nose, headache, nausea, abdominal pain, jaundice, and anuria. Hepatic cell impairment may be revealed by appropriate tests. The urine may show proteins, red cells, or casts. The MLD is 1 gm.

Treat as for carbon tetrachloride poisoning.

Thallium (Rodenticide)

Thallium poisoning is characterized by slow onset of ataxia, pains and paresthesias of the extremities, bilateral ptosis, loss of hair, fever, and abdominal pains. Progression of poisoning is indicated by lethargy, jumbled speech, tremors, convulsions and cyanosis, pulmonary edema and respiratory difficulty. The MLD is 1 gm.

Remove ingested poison by emesis, gastric lavage, and catharsis. The administration of Prussian blue has been suggested. Maintain urine output at 1 liter or more daily unless renal insufficiency appears, in which contingency only sufficient fluid to replace losses is given. Maintain blood pressure.

Stevens W & others: Eleven cases of thallium intoxication treated with Prussian blue. Int J Clin Pharmacol 10:1, 1974.

Thanite (Insecticide)

Manifestations are respiratory difficulty and convulsions.

Remove ingested poison by emesis or gastric lavage. Treat convulsions as for strychnine poisoning.

Thiocyanates (Insecticides)

Manifestations are disorientation, weakness, low

blood pressure, psychotic behavior, and convulsions. The fatal serum level of thiocyanate is 20 mg/100 ml.

Remove ingested thiocyanate by gastric lavage or emesis followed by catharsis. Give 2–4 liters of fluid orally or IV daily to maintain adequate urine output. Remove thiocyanate by peritoneal dialysis or by hemodialysis if necessary.

Thioglycollate (Cold wave)

Repeated application to the skin may cause sensitivity dermatitis with edema, itching, burning, and rash.

Discontinue use.

Thyroid (Medicinal)

Manifestations are fever, tachycardia, hypertension, and cardiovascular collapse at doses of 0.3 gm/kg.

Maintain normal body temperature and force fluids. Digitalize if cardiac weakness is present.

Trichloroethylene (Solvent)

Manifestations are dizziness, headache, excitement, loss of consciousness. Irregular pulse may occur. The MLD is 5 ml.

Remove patient to fresh air and give artificial respiration. Do not give epinephrine or other stimulants.

Trinitrotoluene (Explosive)

Manifestations are jaundice, dermatitis, cyanosis, pallor, loss of appetite, and oliguria or anuria. The liver may be enlarged or atrophic. Hepatic cell injury may be revealed by appropriate tests. The MLD is 1 gm.

Remove from skin by thorough washing with soap and water. Remove swallowed trinitrotoluene by gastric lavage or emesis and catharsis. Protect liver by giving 10 ml of 10% calcium gluconate IV 3 times daily and a high-carbohydrate and high-calcium diet, including at least 1 quart of skimmed milk daily. Give vitamin D in high doses daily.

Tri-orthocresyl Phosphate (Plasticizer)

After 1–30 days' delay, weakness of the distal muscles develops, with foot drop, wrist drop, and loss of plantar reflex. Death may occur from respiratory muscle paralysis. The MLD for adults is about 5 gm.

Remove by gastric lavage or emesis followed by catharsis. Maintain respiration if necessary by tank respirator.

Veratrum, Zygadenus (Plants)

Manifestations are nausea, severe vomiting, muscular weakness, slow pulse, and low blood pressure. Excessive amounts may cause marked rise in blood pressure.

Remove ingested poison by gastric lavage or emesis followed by catharsis. Atropine, 2 mg subcut, will block the reflex fall of blood pressure and the bradycardia. Elevation of blood pressure is treated by the administration of phentolamine hydrochloride, 25 mg subcut repeated every 4 hours.

Volatile Anesthetics: Ether, Chloroform, Halothane, Divinyl Ether, Cyclopropane, Ethyl Chloride, Ethylene, Nitrous Oxide

Manifestations are excitement, unconsciousness, depression and paralysis of respiration. Cardiac irregularities occur with cyclopropane, chloroform, and halothane. Severe fall of blood pressure or cardiac arrest may also occur. The MLD is 1–30 ml.

Remove volatile anesthetic by artificial respiration. Maintain blood pressure by intravenous saline, blood transfusions, and levarterenol. Prevent hypoxia by administering oxygen.

Volatile Oils: Turpentine, Pine Oil, Menthol, Absinthe, Savin, Pennyroyal, Eucalyptus

Manifestations are vomiting, diarrhea, unconsciousness, shallow respiration, hematuria, and convulsions. The MLD is 15 gm.

Give 60–120 ml of liquid petrolatum or castor oil and then remove oils by gastric lavage, taking care to prevent aspiration. Follow with a saline cathartic. Give artificial respiration if necessary. If kidney function is normal, give fluids, 2–4 liters daily, after the danger of pulmonary edema has passed.

Zinc Stearate (Dusting powder)

Inhalation causes fever, dyspnea, cyanosis, and bronchial pneumonia.

Give penicillin, 1 million units IM daily, or a broad-spectrum antibiotic to prevent bronchial pneumonia.

Zinc Sulfate (Astringent)

Manifestations are burning pain in the mouth and throat, vomiting, diarrhea, anuria, and cardiovascular collapse. The MLD is 30 gm.

Give milk or starch drinks to dilute the poison and remove by gastric lavage. Replace fluid loss with 5% dextrose in saline. Relieve pain by giving morphine sulfate, 10 mg.

* * *

AIR POLLUTION

There is considerable evidence that the present levels of atmospheric contaminants which exist in many larger urban areas are sufficient to cause discomfort or significantly impair health. Air pollution is increasing, and it is presumed that the associated health hazard will also increase. Toxicologic and epidemiologic studies suggest that the noxious nature of the atmosphere is usually due to a complex mixture of pollutants and to meteorologic factors.

It is difficult to identify the irritant or toxic potential of single pollutants in the urban atmosphere. The large number of organic and inorganic compounds found in urban air may vary considerably according to the nature, source, and volume of emitted pollutants (eg, industrial processes, automotive exhaust, domestic heating and incineration) and climatic influences (eg, temperature, sunshine, humidity, barometric pressure, wind currents).

Air pollutants are usually divided into 2 broad classes: (1) particulates (smoke, dust, ash, mists, and fumes which exist in the atmosphere in either a solid or liquid state) and (2) gases (eg, carbon monoxide, sulfur oxides, hydrogen sulfide, nitrogen oxides, and carbon compounds—particularly those reacting in the atmosphere to form photochemical smog).

Air pollution is not believed to be the cause of specific illnesses which may result in death, but it may seriously aggravate preexisting respiratory and cardiac conditions. The irritating effects of air pollution on the eye and upper respiratory tract are well known. Inhalation of irritant materials may interfere with lung function, aggravating chronic bronchitis, chronic constrictive ventilatory disease, pulmonary emphysema, and bronchial asthma. Carbon monoxide can interfere with oxygen delivery to the heart and to the brain—perhaps a critical factor in patients with coronary artery disease or in police and motorists in city traffic whose mental functioning is impaired by cerebral hypoxia. The par-

ticulate fraction contains a number of carcinogenic substances, and these could play a part in the rapidly changing incidence of different cancers.

The ill effects of atmospheric pollution are most obvious during acute episodes of unusually high pollution. Marked increases in the incidence of illnesses and deaths due to cardiorespiratory damage were reported in the Meuse Valley in Belgium in 1930, in Donora, Pennsylvania, in 1948, and in London in 1952 and 1962.

The insidious long-term toxic potential of exposure to single or multiple air pollutants is not known.

Ayers SM, Evans RG, Buehler ME: Air polution: A major public health problem. CRC Crit Rev Clin Lab Sci 3:1, 1972.

Bailey WC & others: Silico-mycobacteria disease in sand blasters. Am Rev Resp Dis 110:115, 1974.

Cohen AA & others: Symptom reporting during recent publicized and unpublicized air pollution episodes. Am J Pub Health 54:442, 1974.

Lange ES: Bronchitis, emphysema and air. Am J Roentgenol 120:924, 1974.

Lebowitz MD & others: Effect of air pollution and weather on lung function in exercising children and adolescents. Am Rev Resp Dis 109:262, 1974.

●   ●   ●

General Bibliography

Arena JM: The peril in plants. Emergency Med 6:221, 1974.

Burston GR: *Self-poisoning.* Lloyd-Luke, 1970.

Dreisbach RH: *Handbook of Poisoning: Diagnosis & Treatment.* 8th ed. Lange, 1974.

Goodman LS, Gilman A (editors): *The Pharmacological basis of Therapeutics,* 4th ed. Macmillan, 1970.

Hamilton A, Hardy HL: *Industrial Toxicology,* 3rd ed. Publishing Sciences Group, 1974.

Hardin JW, Arena JM: *Human Poisoning From Native and Cultivated Plants.* Duke Univ Press, 1969.

Lampe KF, Fagerström R: *Plant Toxicity and Dermatitis: A Manual for Physicians.* Williams & Wilkins, 1968.

Martin EW: *Hazards of Medication.* Lippincott, 1971.

Meyers FH, Jawetz E, Goldfein A: *A Review of Medical Pharmacology,* 4th ed. Lange, 1974.

National Clearinghouse for Poison Control Centers: Bulletin and information cards. (Monthly.)

Schlosser L: Review of the (toxicological) literature—1973. Arch Toxikol 31:279, 1974.

Seminar on childhood poisoning. Paediatrician 2:2, 1973.

US National Institute of Occupational Safety and Health: *Toxic Substances List.* US Government Printing Office, 1974.

Selected References on Adverse Reactions to Drugs

Adverse Reactions. A monthly report of adverse reactions to drugs and therapeutic devices by the Adverse Reactions Branch, Food and Drug Administration, US Department of Health, Education, and Welfare, Washington, DC.

Adverse Reactions Titles. Excerpta Medica (monthly bibliography).

Clin-Alert. A weekly to fortnightly serial publication of all adverse drug reactions reported in the international medical literature. Science Editors, Inc., Louisville, Kentucky.

FDA Clinical Experience Abstracts. Food and Drug Administration (monthly).

FDA Drug Bulletin. Food and Drug Administration (monthly).

The Medical Letter on Drugs and Therapeutics. A fortnightly periodical presenting brief, current clinical evaluations of drugs, including adverse reactions. Therapeutic Information, Inc., New York, New York.

Meyler L: *Side Effects of Drugs.* Excerpta Medica. (7 vols.)

Meyler L, Peck HM (editors): *Drug-Induced Diseases.* Excerpta Medica. (4 vols.)

Moser RH: *Diseases of Medical Progress: Present Status.* Abstracts of published adverse reactions to drugs appearing monthly in Clinical Pharmacology and Therapeutics.

31...
Medical Genetics

Margaret S. Kosek

The rapid advance of the science of genetics in recent years has so many applications to clinical medicine that a knowledge of basic genetic principles is now a necessity for diagnostic purposes. Many cases of mental retardation, infertility, dwarfism, habitual abortion, and multiple congenital anomalies are associated with specific chromosomal defects. Cells of certain tumors have an abnormal chromosomal composition, in some instances a specific one. Many of the metabolic disorders are hereditary, and even in the case of some drug reactions the problem lies not only with the drug but also with the patient who has inherited an enzymatic defect which prevents normal detoxification. Future genetic investigation promises to increase our understanding of the causes and the mechanisms of individual responses to disease.

GENERAL CONSIDERATIONS

Inherited characteristics are carried from generation to generation by the **chromosome**, a complex protein structure in the nucleus of the cell. Man normally has 46 chromosomes, which are arranged in 23 pairs. One of these pairs determines the sex of the individual; these are the **sex chromosomes**, which are designated as XX (female) and XY (male). The remaining 22 pairs are called **autosomes** (not sex determiners). Pairs of autosomes are **homologous**, ie, each member of a pair has the same configuration and genetic material as the other member of the pair. The sex chromosomes, on the other hand, are **heterologous**, ie, the X chromosome differs both in size and total function from the Y chromosome.

The X chromosome is roughly 5 times the size of the Y chromosome. Both the X and Y chromosomes have a genetic as well as sex determining aspect, but the genetic information is more extensive on the X chromosome. With the Y chromosome, the genetic information is so limited that it has only been recently discovered.

GENES

Chromosomes are composed of thousands of **genes**, which are the basic units of heredity. It is the gene which is the information area for the transmission of an inherited trait. The genes are arranged in a linear fashion on the chromosomes. The exact location of a gene on a chromosome is its **locus**. Each chromosome has thousands of loci arranged in a definite manner, and the number and arrangement of genes on homologous chromosomes are identical. Genes which occupy homologous loci are **alleles**, or partner genes. Each individual, therefore, has 2 of each kind of gene, one on each pair of chromosomes.

Although genes usually remain stable from generation to generation, it is possible for them to undergo a change, or **mutation**, and thereby to transmit a new or altered trait. This change will then be transmitted to future generations. Mutation may occur spontaneously or may be induced by such environmental factors as radiation, medication, or viral infections. Both advanced maternal and paternal age favor mutation. With women, trisomy 21 is the classic example. With men over 30, fresh gene mutation accounts for sporadic cases of achondroplasia, hemophilia A, and Marfan's syndrome.

Jones KL & others: Older paternal age and fresh gene mutation: Data on additional disorders. J Pediat 86:84, 1975.

THE CHEMICAL BASIS OF HEREDITY (THE GENETIC CODE)

Chromosomes are composed of many deoxyribonucleic acid (DNA) molecules, each of which is a gene. DNA has 2 functions. First, it is able to synthesize or **replicate** itself, thereby assuring the integrity of hereditary transmission to future generations. Second, the sequential order of the bases (cytosine, guanine, adenine, thymine) of DNA acts as the **genetic code** that determines the development and metabolism of cells. DNA accomplishes this by directing the synthesis of ribonucleic acid (RNA). RNA, by its base sequence, determines the amino acid composition of proteins, and this in turn determines the function of proteins. The location of these proteins (which include the enzymes) determines the function of cells.

MODES OF INHERITANCE

1. MENDELIAN (AUTOSOMAL) INHERITANCE

The essential definitions of modes of inheritance can be illustrated by studying the inheritance of a **single** characteristic carried by only **one** gene and not influenced by environmental factors.

Syndactyly (webbed fingers or toes) is a clinical example of this. Fig 31−1 illustrates a family tree with the abnormality. The gene for syndactyly is represented as **D** and the gene for normal interdigital spaces as **d**.

Each parent is represented by 2 genes, each of which they received from their mother and father, respectively. Their genetic constitution has arbitrarily been designated Dd. The male parent (Dd) will be able to produce sperm that are either D or d. The female parent will be able to produce ova that are either D or d. The possible offspring are DD, Dd or dd.

If we examine the parents and offspring for the presence of syndactyly, we find it in both parents (Dd and Dd) and 3 (DD, Dd, Dd) of the 4 offspring. Since these people have the same physical characteristic, ie, syndactyly, they are said to have the same **phenotype**. Their genetic composition, or **genotype**, is different, for it may be either Dd or DD. The genotype, therefore, may be the same as the phenotype, but it does not have to be. Since syndactyly is present if D is one gene of a pair of genes (Dd) as well as both genes (DD), it is a **dominant** trait. Normal digital spaces (d) are present only if d is on both genes (dd) and is a **recessive** trait. If an individual's genetic constitution for syndactyly contains similar genes (DD, dd), the person is a **homozygote**; if it contains dissimilar genes (Dd), the person is a **heterozygote**.

In addition to dominant and recessive inheritance, an **intermediate** inheritance may also occur. Hemoglobin S disease is an example of this. The S homozygote has sickle cell anemia; the S heterozygote has sickle cell trait; and the patient without S is normal.

Inheritance is either **autosomal** or **X-linked (sex-linked)** depending on the chromosomal location of the gene. In investigating family trees for genetic disease, certain inheritance patterns with distinct features become evident. **Autosomal dominant inheritance** (Fig 31−1) has 3 criteria: (1) every affected person has an affected parent; (2) every affected person who marries a normal person has a 1:2 chance of having each offspring identified; and (3) every normal child of an affected person will have normal offspring. With **autosomal recessive inheritance**, the following characteristics are present: The vast majority of affected persons have parents who are normal in all outward appearances. In affected families, each child has a 1:4 chance of having a genetic defect. When an affected person and a normal person marry, their offspring will be normal in most cases. If their offspring is affected, the "normal" parent is a heterozygote. When 2 affected parents marry, all their children will be affected. Lastly, the rarer the defect, the more likely it is that there is consanguinity in the family tree.

With **X-linked recessive inheritance**, there are 2 main characteristics: the defect is carried by women and exhibited by men, and affected men can pass the disease only through their daughters. Hemophilia is an important clinical example of this (Fig 31−2). The female with her 2 X chromosomes must have the gene for hemophilia present in each X chromosome to have this recessive disease. Since the frequency of this gene in the population is low, the chances of 2 affected X

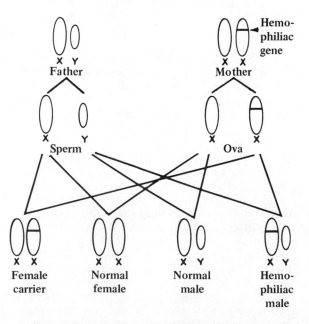

Figure 31−2. The inheritance of hemophilia from a female carrier, illustrating "mother-to-son" inheritance of X-linked recessive disease.

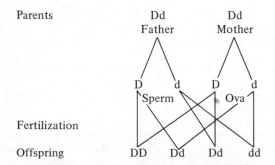

Figure 31−1. Mode of inheritance of syndactyly.

chromosomes occurring together, although possible, is highly unlikely. Therefore, hemophilia is very rare in females. Males, with their XY chromosome composition, need the hemophilia gene present only on one chromosome (the X) to have it expressed clinically, for there is no homologous locus in the Y chromosome to neutralize the effect of the hemophiliac gene. Since the Y chromosome had to come from the father, the affected X chromosome was from the mother, thereby giving the "mother-to-son" inheritance pattern. In the case of **X-linked dominant inheritance**, no fully dominant X-linked gene has been discovered in humans.

Genes do not always have an "all or none" action. A certain number of offspring may fail to show expression of a gene even though the gene may be a dominant or homozygous recessive. **Penetrance** is the statistical concept that refers to the frequency with which a gene or genotype is morphologically manifest in the offspring. A comparable term, **expressivity**, refers to the degree of phenotypic expression of a trait (ie, forme fruste vs full expression). These variables make genetic analysis far more difficult.

The genetic disorders carried by a single gene have been most completely studied. They frequently have a characteristic somatic or biochemical defect that can be readily traced in many generations. On the whole, these genetic disorders are rare. It is much more difficult to determine the mode of inheritance of the common diseases of possible genetic background (eg, arteriosclerosis) because the disease may be the result not only of genetic constitution but also of environmental factors (eg, diet).

Some Diseases With Known Modes of Inheritance

AD = Autosomal dominant
AR = Autosomal recessive
XD = X-linked (sex-linked) dominant
XR = X-linked (sex-linked) recessive

Central Nervous System
A. Diffuse cerebral sclerosis (Pelizaeus-Merzbacher type): XD?, XR?
B. Diffuse cerebral sclerosis (Sholz type): XD?, XR?
C. Lowe's ocular cerebral renal disease: XR
D. Retinoblastoma: AD

Digestive System
A. Cystic fibrosis of the pancreas: AR
B. Hyperbilirubinemia:
 1. Congenital nonhemolytic jaundice with kernicterus (Crigler-Najjar): AR
 2. Familial nonhemolytic jaundice (Gilbert's disease): AD
 3. Chronic idiopathic jaundice (Dubin-Johnson): Probably AD
 4. Chronic familial nonhemolytic jaundice (Rotor's syndrome): AD

Genitourinary System
A. Cystinosis: AR
B. Cystinuria: AR
C. Fanconi's syndrome (infantile and adult): AR
D. Hartnup disease: AR
E. Nephrogenic diabetes insipidus: XR
F. Renal glycosuria: AD
G. Vitamin D-resistant rickets: XD

Skin
A. Albinism: AR
B. Anhidrotic ectodermal dysplasia: AR?
C. Xeroderma pigmentosum: AR

Hematologic System
A. Cell Disorders:
 1. Congenital nonspherocytic hemolytic anemia (pyruvate kinase deficiency): AR
 2. Sickle cell disease (homozygous hemoglobin S): AD
 3. Sickle cell trait (heterozygous hemoglobin S): AD
 4. Spherocytosis: AD
 5. Thalassemia major (homozygous): AD
 6. Thalassemia minor (heterozygous): AD
B. Plasma Disorders:
 1. Congenital agammaglobulinemia: XR
 2. Congenital afibrinogenemia: AR
 3. Hemophilia A (AHG deficiency): XR
 4. Hemophilia B (PTC deficiency): XR
 5. Hemophilia C (PTA deficiency): AD
 6. Deficiency of Hageman factor (factor XII): AR
 7. Deficiency of labile factor (factor V, plasma accelerator globulin, plasma AC globulin): AR
 8. Deficiency of stabile factor (factor VII, serum prothrombin conversion accelerator, SPCA): AR
 9. Deficiency of Stuart-Prower factor (factor X): AR
 10. Von Willebrand's disease (factor VIII deficiency): AD

Musculoskeletal System
A. Severe generalized familial muscular dystrophy (Duchenne's pseudohypertrophic muscular dystrophy): XR
B. Muscular dystrophy (facioscapulohumeral syndrome of Landouzy-Dejerine): AD
C. Progressive dystrophia ophthalmoplegica: AD
D. Myotonia atrophica: AD
E. Progressive muscular dystrophy (tardive type of Becker): XR
F. Charcot-Marie-Tooth peroneal muscular atrophy: AD, AR
G. Pseudohypoparathyroidism: XR
H. Periodic paralysis:
 1. Hyperkalemic: AD
 2. Hypokalemic: AD
 3. Normokalemic: AD

Endocrine System

A. Pituitary:
   1. Pituitary diabetes insipidus: AD
B. Thyroid:
   1. Familial cretinism with goiter—
      a. Iodide trapping defect: AR
      b. Iodide organification defect: AR?, AD?
      c. Iodotyrosyl coupling defect: AR?
      d. Deiodinase defect: AR
      e. Abnormal serum iodoprotein: AR
C. Adrenal:
   1. Congenital virilizing adrenal hyperplasia: AR

Metabolic Disorders

A. Carbohydrate:
   1. Idiopathic spontaneous hypoglycemia: AR
   2. Diabetes mellitus: AR
   3. Galactosemia: AR
   4. Glycogen storage disease (types 1, 2, 3, 4, 5, 6) (Von Gierke's disease): AR
   5. Gargoylism (lipochondrodystrophy) (Hurler's disease): AR, XR
   6. Hyperoxaluria: AR
   7. Hereditary fructose intolerance and essential fructosuria: AR
   8. Hereditary lactose intolerance: AR
   9. Hereditary disaccharide intolerance: AR
   10. Monosaccharide malabsorption: AR
   11. Mucopolysaccharidoses—
      a. Type 1. Hurler's disease: AR
      b. Type 2. Hurler's disease: XR
      c. Type 3. Sanfilippo syndrome (heparitinuria): AR
      d. Type 4. Morquio's disease: AR
      e. Type 5. Scheie's syndrome: AR
B. Fat:
   1. Idiopathic hyperlipemia (Bürger-Grütz disease): AR
   2. Familial high density lipoprotein disease (Tangier disease): AR
   3. Abetalipoproteinemia (acanthocytosis): AR
   4. Primary hypercholesterolemia: AD
   5. Gaucher's disease (cerebroside lipidosis): AR, AD
   6. Niemann-Pick disease (sphingomyelin lipidosis): AR
   7. Tay-Sachs disease (infantile amaurotic idiocy): AR
   8. Vogt-Spielmeyer disease (juvenile amaurotic idiocy): AR
   9. Metachromatic leukodystrophy (sulfatide lipidosis): AR
   10. Fabry's disease (glycolipid lipidosis): XR
C. Protein:
   1. Amino acids—
      a. Argininosuccinic aciduria: AR
      b. β-Aminoisobutyric aciduria: AR
      c. Citrullinemia: AR
      d. Cystathioninemia: AR
      e. Glucoglycinuria: AD
      f. Glycinuria: AR

g. Histidinemia: AR
h. Homocystinuria: AR
i. Hydroxykynureninuria: AR
j. Hydroxyprolinemia: AR
k. Hyperlysinemia: AR
l. Hyperprolinemia: AR
m. Hypervalinemia: AR
n. Isovaleric acidemia: AR
o. Maple syrup urine disease: AR
p. Phenylketonuria: AR
q. Tryptophanuria: AD (?)
r. Tyrosinosis: AR
   2. Porphyrias—
      a. Congenital erythropoietic porphyria: AR
      b. Erythropoietic porphyria: AR
      c. Acute intermittent porphyria: AD
      d. Porphyria cutanea tarda hereditaria: AD
   3. Other—
      a. Hypophosphatasia: AR
      b. Deficiency of pseudocholinesterase: AR
      c. Deficiency of glucose-6-phosphate dehydrogenase: XD
      d. Acatalasia: AR
      e. Alkaptonuria: AR
      f. Congenital methemoglobinemia: AR
      g. Hyperuricemia: AD
      h. Hereditary orotic aciduria: AR
D. Minerals:
   1. Hepatolenticular degeneration (Wilson's disease): AR
   2. Hemochromatosis: AD, AR

McKusick VA: *Mendelian Inheritance in Man: Catalogs of Autosomal Dominant, Autosomal Recessive and X-linked Phenotypes,* 4th ed. John Hopkins Univ Press, 1975.

2. POLYGENIC INHERITANCE

The study of **single** common malformations of man reveals an increased incidence of these defects in monozygotic twins and in family studies. This suggests that the effects of many genes (polygenic) in specific combinations is the probable explanation, since they are seen in people whose genetic structure would be the most similar.

Some examples are shown below:

Defect	Risk of Recurrence of Defect in Siblings Born Subsequently to Unaffected Parents
Cleft lip (with or without cleft palate)	4.9%
Cleft palate alone	2.0%
Clubfoot	2–8%
Anencephaly	3.4%
Meningomyelocele	4.8%
Dislocation of the hip	3.5%
Pyloric stenosis	3.2%

CYTOGENETICS

Cytogenetics is the study of the chromosomal structure of cells. Because of the constancy of chromosomal number and morphology, classification of chromosomes is possible. The basic characteristics of chromosomes are (1) total length, (2) position of the centromere, (3) the length of the arms, and (4) the presence or absence of satellites.

The 2 halves of the chromosome are called **chromatids.** A palely staining cross-over point or primary constriction called the **centromere** (centrosome) divides the chromosome into 2 arm lengths. Chromosomes are described according to the position of the centromere. If the centromere is at the middle of the chromosome, it is a **metacentric** chromosome; if near the middle of the chromosome, it is **submetracentric;** and if near the end of the chromosome, it is **acrocentric.** On some chromosomes there is a secondary constriction. The chromosomal material distal to this constriction is called a **satellite.**

In the Denver classification, chromosomes are arranged in 7 groups according to descending total length: group A (chromosomes 1–3); group B (chromosomes 4, 5); group C (chromosomes 6–12); group D (chromosomes 13–15); group E (chromosomes 16–18); group F (chromosomes 19, 20); and group G (chromosomes 21, 22). The X chromosome is in group C and the Y chromosome is in group G. Four new staining technics disclose banded regions on each chromosome (Fig 31–13) which are unique and allow absolute identification of the chromosome. These banded patterns vary with the stain and produce complementary rather than redundant information.

The chromosomal analysis is recorded by a uniform system of notation. First, there is the total chromosome count, followed by the sex chromosomes, and then any abnormalities thereafter. The autosomes are all designated by their number (1–22), and, if the autosomes cannot be identified, the involved chromosome group is identified by its letter (A–G). A plus (+) or minus (–) sign indicates, respectively, a gain or loss of chromosomal material. The letter *p* represents the short arm of the chromosome and the letter *q* represents the long arm. Other common symbols are *i* for isochromosome; *r* for ring chromosome; *s* for satellite; *t* for translocation; *inv* for inversion; *mar* for marker; *[:]* for chromosomal break; *[::]* for chromosomal break and join; and *end* for endoreduplication. *Examples:* The normal male is 46,XY; a girl with Down's syndrome is 47,XX,21(+); a boy with cri du chat syndrome is 46,XY,5p(–).

The Paris Conference has added the classification of the newly discovered banded patterns of the chromosomes. The short and long arms of each chromosome are divided into regions which are numbered outward from the centromere. Within each region, the bands now recognized are also numbered from proximal to distal so that 4p21 is chromosome 4, short arm, region 2, band 1. (See Fig 31–13.)

Dubrillaux B, Lejeune J: New techniques in the study of human chromosomes: Methods and applications. Advances Human Genet 5:119, 1975.

Paris Conference: Standardization in human cytogenetics. Birth Defects 8:1, 1971.

Methods of Cellular Division

Cells divide in one of 2 ways: by **mitosis** (Fig 31–3) or by **meiosis** (Fig 31–6). In mitosis a mother cell divides longitudinally to produce 2 daughter cells of exactly the same chromosomal number and composition as the mother cell. This type of cellular division

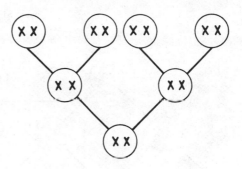

Figure 31–3. Normal mitoses (female).

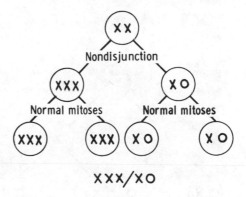

Figure 31–4. Formation of mosaic with 2 stem cells.

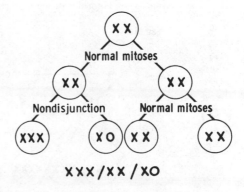

Figure 31–5. Formation of mosaic with 3 stem cells.

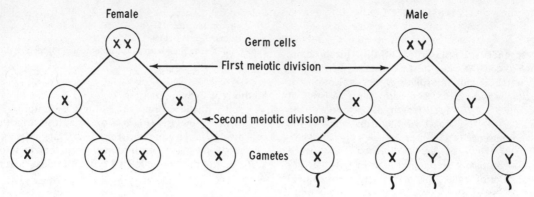

Figure 31—6. Normal meiosis.

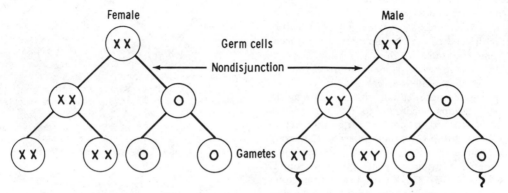

Figure 31—7. Formation of abnormal gametes by nondisjunction in first meiotic division.

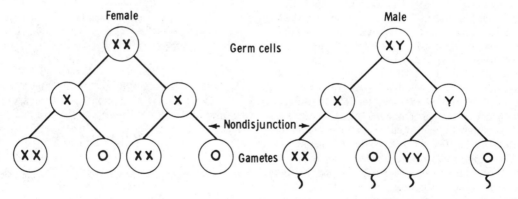

Figure 31—8. Formation of abnormal gametes by nondisjunction in second meiotic division.

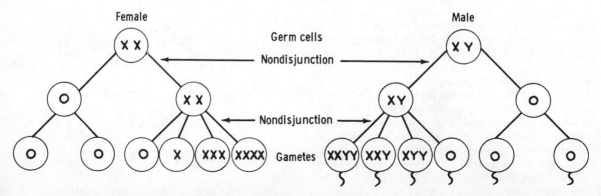

Figure 31—9. Formation of abnormal gametes by nondisjunction in first and second meiotic division.

is purely multiplicative (1 cell → 2 cells → 4 cells → 8 cells, etc). Meiosis occurs in the ovary or testis and involves 2 separate steps. The first step is **reduction-division**, in which the germ cell with a **diploid (2n)** number of chromosomes (46) produces 2 cells with a **haploid (n)** number of chromosomes (23). During this step chromosomal material is exchanged between like chromosomes, thereby accounting for the random distribution of maternal and paternal genes. The second step is **equational division**, in which 4 daughter cells with a haploid number of chromosomes are formed by longitudinal division of the chromosomes produced in the first step of meiotic division. In the male, the 4 haploid cells are sperm. In the female, one of the 4 haploid cells is large and matures to form an ovum. The other 3 haploid cells are small cells called polar bodies, and undergo spontaneous degeneration.

TYPES OF CHROMOSOMAL ABNORMALITIES

Chromosomal abnormalities can be those of number, structure, or a combination of both. They affect the autosomes as well as the sex chromosomes. Often they are associated with such factors as advanced parental age, radiation exposure, certain viral infections, and membership in a family with multiple cytogenetic defects. Once produced, these abnormalities are capable of perpetuating themsleves.

Abnormalities of Morphology

A. Nondisjunction: (See Figs 31–3 to 31–9.) Nondisjunction is failure of a chromatid pair to separate in a dividing cell. If it occurs in either the first or second divisions of meiosis, this results in gametes with abnormal chromosomal patterns. If it occurs in mitosis, **mosaic** patterns occur, ie, one area of an organism will have one genetic pattern and another area of the same organism another genetic pattern.

In medical practice, patients with a mosaic genetic constitution present an incomplete and variable clinical picture with features of each of the genetic syndromes represented in the mosaic.

B. Translocation: (See Fig 31–10.) In translocation there is an exchange of chromosomal material between 2 nonhomologous chromosomes.

C. Deletion: In deletion there is a loss of chromosomal material due to breakage of a chromatid during cell division.

D. Duplication: If breakage occurs in a chromatid during cell division, the broken portion may realign itself so that many loci are duplicated on one chromosome and are entirely absent from the other member of the pair of chromosomes.

E. Occurrence of Isochromosomes: An isochromosome is a chromosome in which the arms on either side of the centromere have the same genetic material in the same order.

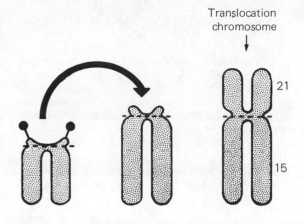

Figure 31–10. Diagrammatic representation of chromosomes 21 and 15 to show how one kind of translocation chromosome probably forms. A normal chromosome 21 is shown at left; the part above the stippled line breaks off (and is lost) as the translocation chromosome forms. A normal chromosome 15 is shown in the center; again the part above the stippled line breaks off and is lost. The abnormal translocation chromosome is shown being formed by end-to-end fusion of parts (below the stippled line) of chromosomes 21 and 15. (Redrawn and reproduced, with permission, from Moore KL: Human chromosomes: Review article. Canad MAJ 88:1071, 1963.)

F. Inversion: Inversion occurs if, after fracture of a chromatid, the fragment reattaches itself to the same chromosome in an upside down manner. The same genetic material is present but is distributed in a different order.

Abnormalities of Chromosomal Number (Aneuploidy)

A. Monosomy: (Chromosomal number is 45.) In monosomy, only one member of a pair of chromosomes is present. *Example:* Stillborns, monosomy 21–22.

B. Trisomy: (Chromosomal number is 47.) Trisomy is caused by nondisjunction of a chromosome pair during the first meiotic division, with the result that 3 chromosomes are present instead of the usual 2. *Example:* Trisomy 13; 18; 21.

C. Polysomy: (Chromosomal number is 48 or more.) Polysomy occurs when one chromosome is represented 4 or more times. *Example:* XXXXY.

D. Complex Aneuploidy: In complex aneuploidy, 2 or more chromosomes have an abnormal variation in number; the structure of these chromosomes is normal. *Example:* Trisomy 21 and XXX in the same patient.

METHODS OF STUDY
OF CHROMOSOMAL ABNORMALITIES

Several laboratory tests are available for the study of patients with known or suspected chromosomal aberrations: (1) the study of cells for the presence of sex chromatin bodies (Barr bodies) in their nuclei; and (2) chromosomal analysis, which includes specific identification of chromosomes as well as their total number. The first test is easily obtainable, relatively inexpensive, and used for screening tests. The chromosome count is a reliable but expensive test which at present can only be done by highly trained personnel in medical centers.

Sex Chromatin Analysis (See Fig 31–11.)

A. The X Chromosome: The sex chromatin (Barr) body is a solid, well defined planoconvex mass, approximately 1 μm in diameter, which is near or at the inner surface of the nuclear membrane. It is visible by light microscopy and, with proper staining, can be identified in all tissues of the body. The most frequent source of specimens for study is in the desquamated cells—buccal, vaginal, and amniotic. The sex chromatin body represents the heterochromatic X chromosome. The number of these chromatin bodies in a cell is one less than the number of X chromosomes in that cell. Females have an incidence of 40–60% and are "chromatin positive." Males do not possess the sex chromatin bodies and are therefore "chromatin negative." For an unknown reason, sex chromatin bodies are diminished in the first few days of life and during treatment with corticotropin, corticosteroids, testosterone, and progesterone. Diethylstilbestrol, on the other hand, causes a significant increase in sex chromatin bodies. The sex chromatin can be seen in the trophoblast at the 12th day, and in the embryo itself at the 16th day. Analysis of amniotic cells for sex chromatin can predict the sex of the unborn child.

B. The Y Chromosome: Quinacrine mustard (QM), a fluorescent material, binds itself to chromo-

Table 31–1. Sex chromosome abnormalities.*

Phenotype	Sex Chromatin	Sex Chromosome	Chromosome Number	Clinical Picture
Female	Positive	XX	46	Normal female.
Female	Few smaller than normal Barr bodies (7%)	Xx (partial deletion)	46	Streak gonads. No secondary sex characteristics. Amenorrheic.
Female	Negative	XO	45	Turner's syndrome.
Female	Positive for 2 Barr bodies	XXX	47	Usually normally appearing female with mental retardation. Occasional menstrual disturbances and absence of secondary sex characteristics.
Female	Positive for 3 Barr bodies	XXXX	48	Normal female with mental retardation.
Female	Positive for 4 Barr bodies	XXXXX	49	Mental retardation with mongoloid facies and simian palmar crease. Skeletal defects similar to those of 49,XXXXY.
Hermaphrodite	Positive	XX	46	Variable phenotype. Both testicular and ovarian tissue in gonads.
Male	Negative	XY	46	Normal male.
Male	Positive for 1 Barr body	XXY	47	Klinefelter's syndrome.
Male	Negative	XYY	47	Undescended testes, ± mental retardation, irregularity of teeth. Tall (> 6 feet). Radioulnar synostosis.
Male	Negative	XYYY	48	Mild psychomotor retardation, inguinal hernia, undescended testes, pulmonary stenosis, simian lines, dental dysplasia.
Male	Positive for 1 Barr body	XXYY	48	Klinefelter's syndrome.
Male	Positive for 2 Barr bodies	XXXY	48	Klinefelter's with more mental retardation and testicular atrophy.
Male	Positive for 3 Barr bodies	XXXXY	49	Mental retardation, hypoplastic external genitals, and skeletal defects. Facies suggestive of Down's syndrome.

*Normal male and normal female included for comparison.

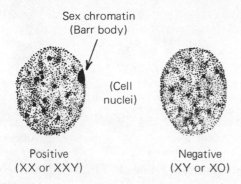

Sex chromatin
(Barr body)

(Cell
nuclei)

Positive
(XX or XXY)

Negative
(XY or XO)

Figure 31–11. Normal chromatin pattern. (Redrawn and reproduced, with permission, from Eggen RR: Cytogenetics: Review of newest advances in a new field of clinical pathology. Am J Clin Path 39:3, 1963.)

somal DNA and gives each chromosome a characteristic pattern. Since the fluorescence of the distal portion of the Y chromosome is characteristically the brightest, it can be reliably and easily identified. This is true in the dividing cell as well as in the interphase cell. In the interphase cell, the distal portion of the Y chromosome is seen as a single fluorescent body (the F body, or the "male chromatin body") in 25–50% of the cells. In XYY individuals, 2 of these fluorescent bodies are seen. This technic is applicable to all cells of the body.

Chromosomal Analysis

Chromosome analyses are done by growing cells of a biopsy in tissue culture, chemically inhibiting their mitoses at a specific phase (metaphase), and then sorting and counting the chromosomes. Specimens are

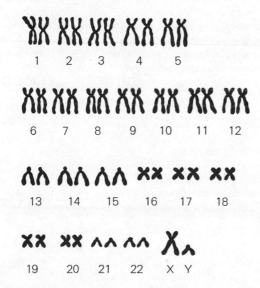

Figure 31–12. Karyotype of normal male with routine staining technic. (Reproduced, with permission, from Krupp MA & others: *Physicians's Handbook,* 17th ed. Lange, 1973.)

most often taken from the peripheral blood, bone marrow, skin, and testes. A statistically significant number of cells must be counted. The results of these analyses appear in the literature as the **karyotype**, which is a drawing or photograph of a systematized array of chromosomes of a single cell (Fig 31–13).

The present indications for this highly technical procedure are as follows: (1) Patients with malformations consistent with autosomal trisomy or deletion syndromes. (2) Parents of patients with a trisomy syndrome if the mother is younger than 30 years of age or if there are other similarly affected siblings. (3) Parents of all children with Down's syndrome who are found to be of the translocation or mosaic type. (4) Patients with an abnormality on sex chromatin analysis. (5) Children who are grossly retarded physically or mentally, especially if there are associated anomalies. (6) All cases of intersex. (7) All females with evidence of Turner's syndrome, whether they are chromatin positive or chromatin negative. (8) All males with Klinefelter's disease, whether they are chromatin positive or chromatin negative. (9) Tall males (over 6 feet) with behavioral disorders.

PRENATAL DIAGNOSIS

In the last 5 years, great strides have been made in prenatal diagnosis, enabling the genetic counselor to make definitive statements for a specific pregnancy in a selected number of inherited diseases. **Ultrasonic scanning,** a safe procedure, can make the diagnosis of intrauterine anencephaly or polycystic kidneys. **X-ray** of the fetus may disclose gross skeletal malformations as well as bony malformations known to be associated with specific diseases. In **amniography** and **fetography,** contrast medium is placed in the amniotic fluid to permit diagnosis of soft tissue malformations as well as some gastrointestinal tract anomalies. **Fetoscopy,** performed with an endoscope introduced into the uterus, can diagnose gross anomalies, but the risk of postprocedure abortion is great.

Amniocentesis is by far the most frequent procedure for prenatal diagnosis. In the 12th–16th week of pregnancy, 10–30 ml of amniotic fluid are removed by a transabdominal approach. The amniotic fluid is used for chemical analysis and the amniotic cells are cultured for cytogenetic and enzymatic analysis. The physician can now diagnose about 60 metabolic disorders, since a specific enzyme disorder has been shown to exist in each (Table 31–2). In addition, chromosomal analysis allows for specific syndrome identification as well as fetal sex identification for families who have known X-linked recessive diseases.

The indications for amniocentesis are as follows:

(1) **Advanced maternal age:** Example: Down's syndrome. The risk of Down's syndrome increases from 1:2000 live births at maternal age 20, to 1:300 at age 35, to 1:100 at age 40, and to 1:40 at age 45.

Table 31–2. Inherited disorders detected in utero.

Disease	Antenatal Diagnosis	Disease	Antenatal Diagnosis
Acatalasemia	Feasible	Metachromatic leukodystrophy	Yes
Anencephaly	Yes	Methylene tetrahydrofolate deficiency	Feasible
Argininosuccinicaciduria	Feasible	Methylmalonic aciduria (B_{12} unrespon-	Feasible
Citrullinemia	Feasible	sive)	
Congenital adrenal hyperplasia	Yes, but late	Methylmalonic aciduria (B_{12} responsive)	Yes
	in pregnancy	Mucopolysaccharidosis, type 1 (Hurler's	Yes
Congenital erythropoietic porphyria	Feasible	syndrome)	
Cystinosis	Feasible	Mucopolysaccharidosis, type 2 (Hunter's	Yes
Fabry's disease	Yes	syndrome, severe form)	
Farber's disease	Feasible (?)	Mucopolysaccharidosis, type 2 (Hunter's	Feasible
Fucosidosis	Feasible	syndrome, mild form)	
Galactosemia	Yes	Mucopolysaccharidosis, type 3 (Sanfilippo	Feasible
Gaucher's disease, adult type (1)	Yes	A syndrome)	
Gaucher's disease, acute type (2)	Yes	Mucopolysaccharidosis, type 3 (Sanfilippo	Feasible
Gaucher's disease, juvenile type (3)	Uncertain	B syndrome)	
Glycogen storage disease, type 2	Yes	Mucopolysaccharidosis, type 4 (Morquio's	Feasible (?)
Glycogen storage disease, type 3	Feasible	disease)	
Glycogen storage disease, type 4	Feasible	Mucopolysaccharidosis, type 5 (Scheie's	Feasible
GM_1 gangliosidosis, type 1 (general-	Yes	syndrome)	
ized) (visceral Tay-Sachs)		Mucopolysaccharidosis, type 6 (Maroteaux-	Feasible (?)
GM_1 gangliosidosis, type 2 (juvenile)	Yes	Lamy syndrome)	
GM_2 gangliosidosis, type 1 (Tay-Sachs)	Yes	Orotic aciduria	Feasible
GM_2 gangliosidosis, type 2 (Sandhoff's	Feasible	Phenylketonuria	Feasible (?)
disease)		Phosphohexose isomerase deficiency	Feasible
GM_2 gangliosidosis type 3 (juvenile)	Feasible	Pyruvate decarboxylase deficiency	Feasible
Homocystinuria	Feasible	Refsum's syndrome	Feasible
Hyperammonemia, type 1	Feasible (?)	Sickle cell anemia	Feasible
Hyperammonemia, type 2	Feasible	Sphingomyelin lipidosis, type A (Niemann-	Yes
Hyperargininemia	Feasible	Pick disease) (acute neuronopathic type)	
Hyperglycinemia	Feasible	Sphingomyelin lipidosis, type B (no CNS	Feasible
Hyperlysinemia (persistent)	Feasible (?)	involvement, chronic form)	
Hypervalinemia	Feasible	Sphingomyelin lipidosis, type C (CNS	Feasible (?)
Intermittent branched chain ketonuria	Feasible	involvement, subacute form)	
Isovaleric acidemia	Feasible	Sphingomyelin lipidosis, type D (Nova	Uncertain
Krabbe's disease	Yes	Scotian form)	
Lactosyl ceramidosis	Feasible	Spina bifida	Yes
Lesch-Nyhan syndrome	Yes	Testicular feminization	Feasible
Lysosomal acid phosphatase deficiency	Yes	Thalassemia	Feasible
Mannosidosis	Feasible	Wolman's disease	Feasible
Maple syrup urine disease	Yes	Xeroderma pigmentosum	Feasible

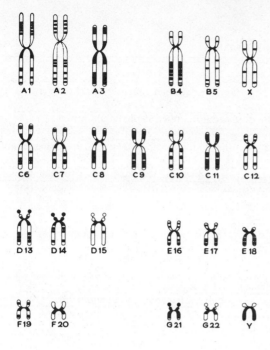

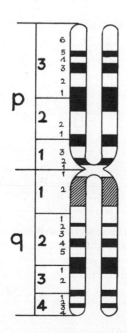

Figure 31—13. *Top:* Karyotype of normal male with new Giemsa technic. Demonstrates specific banding pattern of chromosomes. (Redrawn and reproduced, with permission, from Drets ME, Shaw MW: Specific banding patterns of human chromosomes. Proc Nat Acad Sc USA 68:2073, 1971.) *Bottom:* Chromosome No. 1. The numbers identify the regions and banded areas designated by the Paris Conference. All chromosomes are comparably identified. (Redrawn from: Paris Conference on Standardization in Human Genetics. Birth Defects 8:1, 1971.)

(2) Carrier of X-linked disease: *Examples:* Hemophilia A, Duchenne's muscular dystrophy. Males fetuses have a 50% chance of being affected and could be aborted if that is the parents' wish.

(3) Biochemical disease: *Example:* Tay-Sachs disease. Enzymatic studies on cultured amniotic fluid cells identify over 60 inborn errors of metabolism (Table 31—2). Before these complicated studies are undertaken, it should be established that both parents are heterozygotes.

(4) Parental chromosomal abnormality: *Example:* Translocation carrier of Down's syndrome. There is an up to 20% risk that the fetus has one of the chromosomal abnormalities.

(5) Previous trisomy: *Example:* A pregnancy—either abortus, stillbirth, or live fetus—had a proved trisomy 21. The risk of recurrence is about 1%.

(6) Open neural tube defects: *Examples:* Anencephaly, meningomyelocele. Amniotic fluid protein markers are present in fetal neural tube defects. Alpha-fetoprotein measurement was the initial protein marker but has been criticized because it lacks specificity and because the gestational age of the fetus must be known accurately. Recently, FDP (fibrin/fibrinogen degradation products), which have a constant level throughout normal pregnancy, have been shown to be elevated with fetal neural tube defects.

In several thousand reported cases, the morbidity of amniocentesis is approximately 1%. For the mother, the problem is infection and bleeding. Maternal blood group sensitization is avoided by giving RhoGam to an Rh-negative mother whose mate is Rh-positive. For the fetus, the risk is abortion, puncture, and possibly induced malformation.

Canadian guidelines for antenatal diagnosis of genetic disease: A joint statement. Canad MAJ 111:183, 1974.

Gardner L: Genetically expressed abnormalities in the fetus. Clin Obst Gynec 17:171, 1974.

Kaback MM, O'Brien JS: Tay-Sachs: Prototype for prevention of genetic disease. Hosp Practice 8:107, 1973.

Laurence KM: Fetal malformations and abnormalities. Lancet 2:939, 1974.

Nadler HL: Prenatal diagnosis of inborn defects: A status report. Hosp Practice 10:41, 1975.

Purdie DW & others: Raised amniotic fluid FDP in fetal neural-tube anomalies. Lancet 1:1013, 1975.

CHROMOSOMAL DISORDERS

Frequency

Chromosomal anomalies occur surprisingly often. In studies of spontaneous abortions, one-third of cases have chromosomal anomalies, the most frequent of which are trisomy 18, triploidy, and 45XO. With live births, trisomy of the sex chromosomes is most frequent. The XXX genotype is 1 per 1000 female births

Table 31–3. Autosomal disorders.

Chromosome Defect	Signs
1q+	Peaked nose, micrognathia; long, tapering fingers; congenital heart disease, small or absent thymus
4p+	Severe psychomotor and growth retardation, microcephaly, abnormal facies, abnormal vertebrae and pelvis
4p – (Wolf's syndrome)	Severe growth and mental retardation, midline scalp defects, seizures, abnormal facies, hypospadias
4q+	Low birth weight, mental retardation, hypotonia, early closure of fontanels
5p – (cri du chat syndrome)	Microcephaly, cat-like cry, abnormal facies, low birth weight, abnormal dermatoglyphics
5q –	Long-standing aregenerative macrocytic anemia
7q+	Low birth weight, mental retardation, fuzzy hair, wide fontanels, abnormal facies, bony abnormalities such as kyphoscoliosis, dislocated hip
8+ (trisomy 8)	Mild mental retardation, concomitant strabismus, skeletal defects of ribs and vertebrae
8p+	Small hands with short 5th fingers and dysplastic toenails
8q –	Mental retardation, limited joint mobility, rib and vertebral anomalies
9p+	Mental retardation, moderate microcephaly, brachycephaly, abnormal facies, hypoplasia of phalanges, abnormal dermatoglyphics
9p –	Mental retardation, hypertonia, abnormal facies, congenital heart disease
t(9q+:22q –) (Philadelphia chromosome)	Associated with chronic myelogenous leukemia
9+ (trisomy 9)	Microcephaly, abnormal facies, small penis, undescended testes, long flexed fingers, severe congenital heart disease
10q+	Severe psychomotor and growth retardation, abnormal facies, abnormalities of digits (webbing, wide spacing)
11p+	Mental retardation, hypotonia, abnormal facies, strabismus
11q+	Mental retardation, low birth weight, abnormal facies, congenital heart disease, renal disease
13+ (trisomy 13; trisomy D; Patau's syndrome)	Severe mental retardation, congenital heart disease; cerebral malformations, especially olfactory bulbs; abnormal facies, low birth weight
13q+d	Psychomotor retardation, microcephaly, abnormal facies, delayed and abnormal dentition, increased fetal hemoglobin
13q –	Microcephaly, psychomotor retardation, eye and ear defects, hypoplastic or absent thumbs, genitourinary anomalies
14q+	Mental retardation, failure to thrive, seizures, microcephaly, abnormal facies
15q+	Severe psychomotor retardation with normal growth, strabismus, hypotonia, seizures, abnormal facies
18+ (trisomy 18; trisomy E; Edward's syndrome)	Severe mental retardation, long narrow skull with prominent occiput, congenital heart disease, flexion deformities of fingers, abnormal facies, low birth weight
21+ (trisomy 21; Down's syndrome; mongolism)	Mental retardation, brachycephaly, prominent epicanthic folds, Brushfield spots, poor nasal bridge development, congenital heart disease, hypermobility of joints
21q – (G I deletion syndrome, antimongolism)	Mental and growth retardation, microcephaly, antimongoloid slant to palpebral fissures, hypertonia, abnormal facies, skeletal defects
22q+ (cat eye syndrome)	Coloboma (cat eye), anal atresia, severe psychomotor retardation, congenital heart disease
22+ (trisomy 22)	Mental and growth retardation, microcephaly, abnormal facies, abnormal thumbs
22q – (G II deletion syndrome)	Mental retardation with microcephaly, hypotonia, abnormal facies, syndactyly of fingers
Monosomy 22	Moderate mental retardation, antimongoloid slant of eyes, spade hands, abnormal facies

and the XXY is 2 per 1000 male births. Down's syndrome (trisomy 21) is the most frequent autosomal anomaly. Its incidence is 1 per 2000 if the mother is 25 and 1 per 100 if the mother is 40 or over. Trisomy 13 and 18 are 0.3 and 0.2 per 1000 live births, respectively.

Chromosomal studies done on abortuses, still-births, and tissues of infants who die in the neonatal period can provide valuable information for explaining habitual abortions, monitoring a subsequent pregnancy, and furnishing genetic counseling.

Carr DH: Cytogenetic aspects of induced and spontaneous abortions. Clin Obst Gynec 15:203, 1972.

DISORDERS DUE TO ABNORMALITIES OF THE X & Y CHROMOSOMES

Most disorders of the sex chromosomes (Table 31–1) are compatible with life and do not display marked phenotypic abnormalities. With the exception of Turner's syndrome (XO), these disorders are due to an excess number of sex chromosomes. Both the multiple X and multiple Y syndromes have diverse clinical features. These include (singly or in combination) such problems as mental retardation, sterility, abnormal sex characteristics, and skeletal anomalies. The more the number of X or Y chromosomes, the greater the disability. Abnormal stature may also be associated with the sex chromosomes, since patients with Turner's syndrome are usually under 5 feet tall and those with a multiple Y syndrome are over 6 feet tall. Nonspecific behavioral disorders are more common than expected in the multiple Y syndromes. This is the only clearly identified relationship between chromosomal defects and psychiatry.

At present, there are far more patients with known multiple X syndromes than with multiple Y syndromes. This may only reflect the fact that screening procedures for the X chromosomes have been available over 10 years whereas methods of screening for the Y chromosome have been available for only a few years.

The **Lyon hypothesis** states that for patients with multiple X chromosome constitutions (including the normal female), only one X chromosome is genetically active and capable of transmitting its information; the others became genetically inactive early in embryonic formation by an unknown mechanism. The same is suspected to be true for the multiple Y chromosome states, but there is no evidence to support this as yet.

Smith DW: *Recognizable Patterns of Human Malformation.* Saunders, 1970. [Vol 7 in series of *Major Problems in Clinical Pediatrics.*]
What becomes of the XYY male? (Editorial.) Lancet 2:1297, 1974.

AUTOSOMAL DISORDERS

Although autosomes far outnumber sex chromosomes, very few disorders were attributed to autosomal aberrations until recent staining technics revealed a characteristic pattern for each autosome. Initially, patients with clinically identifiable syndromes—trisomy 13, 18, and 21—demonstrated severe growth and mental retardation in addition to multiple congenital defects and died early. As more cases were found, it was apparent that the physical appearance became less characteristic with survival beyond the first few months. Now, with the use of banding technics, hundreds of case reports are available describing partial deletions and partial trisomies for almost every chromosome. Identifiable cases include those with mental retardation and minor congenital anomalies as well as those with normal intelligence and minor defects, previously described as variations of normal. The ages of patients now range from newborns to 50 years.

With this knowledge, there can be a correlation of an autosomal defect and clinical findings. For example, chromosome 13 now accounts for 7 separate clinical entities, allowing the construction of a phenotypic map resulting from trisomy or deletion of a small amount of genetic material (Fig 31–14).

In addition, identification of carriers of balanced translocations allows genetic counseling and prenatal diagnosis to prevent recurrences.

The most prevalent autosomal disorder is Down's syndrome or mongolism. Ninety-five percent of cases are due to trisomy 21 and the remaining 5% are due to translocations of 15/21, 21/21, and 22/21 types. The trisomy 21 cases have an increasing frequency with advancing maternal age. The translocation cases account for the carrier state of Down's syndrome, for familial Down's syndrome, and for the occurrence of Down's syndrome in younger mothers. Physical examination cannot distinguish between trisomy and translocation Down's syndrome.

Lewandowski RC Jr, Yunis JJ: New chromosomal syndromes. Am J Dis Child 129:515, 1975.
Smith DW, Wilson AA: *The Child with Down's Syndrome (Mongolism): Cause, Characteristics and Acceptance.* Saunders, 1973.
Van Den Berghe & others: Distinct hematologic disorder with deletion of long arm of the No. 5 chromosome. Nature 251:437, 1974.

CANCER

Studies of cancer patients indicate that genetic factors play a role in only a small percentage of cases. With carcinoma of the stomach, breast, colon, prostate, and endometrium, a hereditary factor with a site-specific basis is operating, for relatives of a patient with these malignancies have a 3-fold higher risk of

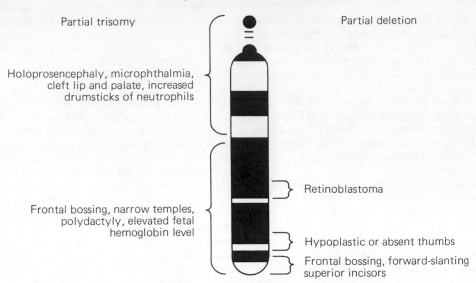

Partial trisomy   Partial deletion

Holoprosencephaly, microphthalmia,
cleft lip and palate, increased
drumsticks of neutrophils

Retinoblastoma

Frontal bossing, narrow temples,
polydactyly, elevated fetal
hemoglobin level

Hypoplastic or absent thumbs

Frontal bossing, forward-slanting
superior incisors

Figure 31—14. Provisional phenotypic map of chromosome 13. (Redrawn and reproduced, with permission, from Lewandowski RC Jr, Yunis JJ: New chromosomal syndromes. Am J Dis Child 129:515, 1975.)

having the same malignancy. Only rarely do the mendelian laws of inheritance appear. In general, the majority of cases of cancer are of unknown cause.

Chromosomes & Malignancy

A. **Chromosome Breakage Syndromes:** Six inherited diseases—Bloom's syndrome, Fanconi's anemia, ataxia-telangiectasia, glutathione reductase deficiency, Kostmann's agranulocytosis, and pernicious anemia—have a tendency to chromosomal breakage and rearrangement in vitro. In addition, each of these diseases has a relatively high incidence of neoplasia, primarily leukemia and lymphoma. At this time, the role of chromosomal breakage in the production of malignancy is speculative.

B. **Leukemia:** Trisomy 21 is the only cytogenetic disease with a clear-cut relationship to leukemia. Children with trisomy 21 have a 20-fold increased risk of developing acute leukemia.

Chromosomal studies of leukemia reveal many abnormalities, but only in the case of chronic myelogenous leukemia and possibly acute myelogenous leukemia are the findings consistent and significant. In acute leukemias, about 50% of reported cases subjected to cytogenetic study have chromosomal abnormalities. These are usually aneuploidy and mainly diploidy. No specific chromosome or group of chromosomes is involved. In a given case, the chromosomal defect persists for the duration of the disease; if it disappears with remission, the same defect recurs with reappearance of leukemia. The Christchurch (Ch) chromosome, initially implicated in chronic lymphocytic leukemia, is now recognized as a family marker chromosome.

In **chronic myelogenous leukemia (CML),** many patients have an abnormal chromosome (Ph or Phil-

adelphia) in their leukemic cells in the peripheral blood and bone marrow—in the preleukemic stage as well as before and after treatment. In 1973, Rowley discovered that the Ph chromosome was a translocation between chromosomes 22 and 9. More recently, the translocation was also found between chromosomes 22 and 2, 19, and homologous 22, without apparent difference in clinical or hematologic pattern or in the course of the disease. The bulk of CML cases, however, are translocations between chromosomes 22 and 9. At present, patients with chronic myelogenous leukemia can be divided into 2 groups on the basis of the Philadelphia chromosome. Those that have the defect (Ph-positive) have clinical and hematologic features of typical chronic myelogenous leukemia, respond rapidly to chemotherapy, and are easily controlled therapeutically. They have an equal sex distribution, a median age of 48, and a longer survival than the Ph-negative patients. The Ph-negative patients are clinically and hematologically heterogenous. They are predominantly males with a median age of 66. They respond poorly to treatment and die in the first year of their disease. Although the Ph chromosome appears to have this prognostic and therapeutic value, the exact significance of its presence is not known.

In 1973, Sandberg and his coworkers studied a group of patients with **acute myelogenous leukemia (AML)** for a relationship between their chromosomal studies and their prognosis. No specific chromosomal abnormality was present. If, however, the patient had one or more normal metaphases in one bone marrow examination, it was extremely important, for it meant that the patient was capable of repopulating his marrow with normal cellular elements after treatment of his AML. A patient with no normal metaphases may respond to treatment initially but have a poor clinical course, presumably due to an inability to repopulate his marrow. In the marrow examination, the presence of one normal metaphase was more important than the percentage of normal metaphases.

C. Lymphoma: Lymphomas resemble other solid tumors in having no characteristic karyotype. Most chromosome counts are in the hyperploid range. Spiers found a deletion of the short and long arms of chromosome E17—18 in a few cases of Hodgkin's disease, follicular lymphoma, and reticulum cell sarcoma. This defect is called the Melbourne chromosome, and a relationship to the tumors is suggested.

D. Dysgenetic Gonad: A recent survey of the clinical literature reveals that patients with gonadal dysgenesis of any type have a 25% risk of malignancy in their gonads if their karyotype contains a Y chromosome. No specific malignancy was found, but a gonadoblastoma was the most common type.

E. Solid Tumors: The presence of nuclear hyperchromatism and abnormal mitotic figures in tumor cells has led to chromosomal analysis of solid malignant tumors. No consistent chromosomal pattern occurs in any type of malignant tumor, but certain generalities emerge from these studies.

1. Abnormalities in chromosomal number and structure—The chromosomal count is usually greater than 46 and is most often polyploidy or near polyploidy, ie, a multiple of the haploid number 23. Most of the additional number of chromosomes fit into the known chromosomal groups. Occasionally an abnormally shaped chromosome (ring, etc) called a "marker" is present and is able to perpetuate itself. The latter probably arises from abnormal chromosomal breakage and union.

2. Wide scatter of the chromosome count—Unlike normal tissue, tumor tissue shows a wide scatter of the chromosomal count around the modal chromosome number. The modal number is not specific for any particular tumor.

3. One of 2 stemline cells is present in each tumor—Stemline cells are cells with identical numerical or structural features that represent the largest percentage of the cell population. These stemline cells remain constant for a given tumor and are not altered by treatment. The chromosomal structure of tumor cells of malignant effusions and metastases is usually the same as that of the parent tumor. Interestingly, another tumor of the same pathologic diagnosis may have different stemline cells.

Baikie AG: Chronic granulocytic leukemia. Australian MJ 2:12, 1974.

German J: *Chromosomes and Cancer.* Wiley, 1974.

Gunz FW & others: Relevance of the cytogenetic status in acute leukemia in adults. J Nat Cancer Inst 50:55, 1973.

The Philadelphia chromosome and chronic myelocytic leukemia (CML): Still a complex relationship? (Editorial.) Acta med scandinav 196:353, 1974.

Sakurai M, Sandberg AA: Prognosis of acute myeloblastic leukemia: Chromosomal correlation. Blood 41:93, 1973.

Schellhas HF: Malignant potential of the dysgenetic gonad. Obst Gynec 44:298, 1974.

Schroeder TM, Kurth R: Spontaneous chromosomal breakage and high incidence of leukemia in inherited disease: Analytical review. Blood 37:96, 1971.

CHROMOSOMES & IONIZING RADIATION

The major problem of ionizing radiation is not the danger of lethal doses but of small doses that allow the cells to multiply after permanent alteration of their genetic material.

Detectable chromosomal changes occur after diagnostic and therapeutic x-ray as well as with beta and gamma radiation (^{131}I, ^{32}P). These usually persist for a few hours to several weeks. In vitro studies reveal a direct relationship between the dose of ionizing radiation and the number of chromosomal abnormalities.

Newcombe HB: The genetic effects of ionizing radiation. Advances Genet 16:239, 1971.

VIRUSES, CHEMICALS, & CHROMOSOMES

For more than half a century, viruses and chemicals have been known to induce chromosomal aberrations in plants and animals. Only in the past decade have human chromosomal defects been proved to be caused by these agents. The measles, chickenpox, hepatitis, and rubella viruses may cause chromosomal aberrations in the leukocytes which may persist for several months after the clinical illness. Drugs such as ozone, analogous and intermediary metabolites of nucleic acids, and alkylating agents have deleterious effects on chromosomes. A study of workers exposed to the leukemogen benzene reveals an increased amount of structural chromosomal abnormalities in their peripheral blood cells. Recently, patients receiving azathioprine or those taking oral contraceptives have been shown to have an increased incidence of chromosomal breaks.

It is hoped that these new findings will add to our understanding of "spontaneous" chromosomal changes as well as chemical carcinogenesis.

Hunter T & others: Azathioprine in rheumatoid arthritis: A long-term follow-up study. Arthritis Rheum 18:15, 1975.

Littlefield LG & others: Chromosomal breakage studies in lymphocytes from normal women, pregnant women, and women taking oral contraceptives. Am J Obst Gynec 121:976, 1975.

Shaw MW: Chromosome mutations in man. Pages 81—97 in: *Mutagenic Effects of Environmental Contaminants.* Sutton HE, Harris MI. Academic Press, 1972.

The susceptibility of the fetus and child to chemical pollutants. (Conference.) Pediatrics 53 (Suppl 2):777—860, 1974.

GENETIC COUNSELING

With our new scientific tools for the detection of genetic disease by amniocentesis and biochemical identification of heterozygotes, the clinician will face the problem of transmitting this information to his patient in a meaningful manner. The National Foundation has a list of genetic counseling centers where adequately trained personnel can assist with or perform this function.

In undertaking genetic counseling, the physician needs the following specific information: (1) An accurate diagnosis, since closely related disorders—especially biochemical defects—may have a markedly different prognosis and mode of inheritance. (2) A detailed family history with an accurate pedigree showing the affected and nonaffected members. (3) A knowledge of the behavior of the disorder from the literature. With this information at hand, the risk of recurrence can be estimated.

In informing the family of the chances of recurrence, the counselor must use terms and analogies the parents can understand. The parents must be aware of the range of possible defects involved. Only with this information can the parents decide whether or not to have more children.

An aspect of counseling that is frequently neglected is the extension of counseling to other members of the family. This involves not only informing and instructing high-risk relatives but also reassuring low-risk relatives.

Bergsma D (editor): Contemporary genetic counselling. Birth Defects 19:1, 1973.

Bergsma D (editor): *International Directory of Genetic Services,* 4th ed. Birth Defects Series. The National Foundation, New York, 1974.

Fraser FC: Genetic counselling. Am J Human Genet 26:636, 1974.

32...
Malignant Disorders

Sydney E. Salmon

Although neoplastic disorders have been discussed in the context of the organ system of their origin elsewhere in this book, certain general features of malignancy as a systemic disease which have relevance to a variety of neoplasms require special emphasis. These features include (1) unusual symptoms and syndromes which may be important in the diagnosis and management of cancer, (2) the diagnosis and treatment of emergency problems and complications of malignancy, (3) cancer chemotherapy for advanced disease, and (4) adjuvant chemotherapy for micrometastases of primary cancers.

THE PARANEOPLASTIC SYNDROMES

The clinical manifestations of malignancy usually appear to be due to pressure effects of local tumor growth or to infiltration or metastatic deposition of tumor cells in a variety of organs in the body, or to certain systemic symptoms. Except in the case of functioning tumors such as those of the endocrine glands, systemic symptoms of malignancies usually are not specific and often consist of weakness, anorexia, and weight loss. In the paraneoplastic syndromes ("beyond tumor growth"), rather bizarre symptoms and signs may occur, producing clinical findings resembling those of primary endocrine, metabolic, hematologic, or neuromuscular disorders. At present, the possible mechanisms for such effects can be classed in 3 groups: (1) effects initiated by a tumor product (eg, carcinoid syndrome), (2) effects of destruction of normal tissues by tumor (eg, hypercalcemia with osteolytic skeletal metastases), and (3) effects due to unknown mechanisms (eg, osteoarthropathy with bronchogenic carcinoma). In some of the paraneoplastic syndromes associated with ectopic hormone production, tumor tissue itself has been found to contain and secrete the hormone which produces the syndrome.

The paraneoplastic syndromes are of considerable clinical importance for the following reasons:

(1) They sometimes accompany relatively limited neoplastic growth and may provide the clinician with an early clue to the presence of certain types of cancer. In some cases, early diagnosis may favorably affect the prognosis.

(2) The pathologic (metabolic or toxic) effects of the syndrome may constitute a more urgent hazard to the patient's life than the underlying malignancy (eg, hypercalcemia, hyponatremia) and may respond to treatment even though the underlying neoplasm does not.

(3) Effective treatment of the tumor should be accompanied by resolution of the paraneoplastic syndrome, and, conversely, recurrence of the cancer may be heralded by return of the systemic symptoms.

Not all endocrine or metabolic syndromes associated with cancer are necessarily "paraneoplastic." In some instances, the secretory product or syndrome results from the continuation of function of the normal precursor cell type which became malignant. In these instances, the function of the tumor cell may be a normal one exaggerated enormously in magnitude (eg, adrenal carcinoma, insulinoma, and carcinoid syndrome) by the increased number of functioning cells. Although the details of the mechanism of some metabolic effects are not known, in some instances the identical symptom complex (eg, hypercalcemia) may be induced by entirely different mechanisms. Hypercalcemia may in some instances be due to secretions of parathyroid hormone, an osteoclast-activating factor, or other hormone secretion by the tumor or to direct invasion of the skeleton by metastases of the tumor. In still other cases, the mechanism of hypercalcemia remains obscure. In each of these situations, effective treatment of the malignancy is usually associated with normalization of the serum calcium, although nonspecific supportive measures may also be of benefit.

Frequently reported paraneoplastic syndromes and endocrine secretions associated with certain functional malignancies are summarized in Table 32–1. Although this list is not complete, it indicates the variety of syndromes and abnormalities which have been described. The pathophysiologic explanation for many of these abnormalities remains unclear; however, recognition of such associations can be quite useful.

A major monograph on this subject is cited below.

Hall TC (editor): Paraneoplastic syndromes. Ann New York Acad Sc 230:1–577, 1974. (Entire issue.)

Table 32—1. Paraneoplastic syndromes and certain endocrine secretions associated with cancer.

Hormone Excess or Syndrome	Broncho-genic Carcinoma	Breast Carcinoma	Renal Carcinoma	Adrenal Carcinoma	Hepatoma	Multiple Myeloma	Lymphoma	Thymoma	Prostatic Carcinoma	Pancreatic Carcinoma	Chorio-carcinoma
Hypercalcemia	++	++++	++	++	+	++++	+	+	++	+	+
Cushing's syndrome	+++		+	+++				++	+	++	
Inappropriate ADH secretion	+++						+			+	
Hypoglycemia				+	++		+				
Gonadotropins	+				+						++++
Thyrotropin											+++
Polycythemia			+++	+	++						
Erythroid aplasia								++			
Fever			+++		++		+++	++		+	
Neuromyopathy	++	+						++	+	+	
Dermatomyositis	++	+								+	
Coagulopathy	+	++			+	+			+++	+++	
Thrombophlebitis			+						+	+++	
Immunologic deficiency						+++	+++	+++			

DIAGNOSIS & TREATMENT OF EMERGENCIES & COMPLICATIONS OF MALIGNANT DISEASE

Malignancies are chronic diseases, but acute emergency complications do develop. Such complications may be due either to local accumulations of tumor, as in spinal cord compression, superior vena cava syndrome, and malignant effusions; or to more generalized, systemic effects of cancer, as in hypercalcemia, septicemia and opportunistic infections, disseminated intravascular coagulation, hyperuricemia, and carcinoid syndrome. Although some of these acute problems arise in nonmalignant disorders, their severity and treatment are often somewhat different. Obviously, the acute complications of neoplastic disease must be treated even if the underlying malignancy is incurable. Indeed, one of the most important aspects of management of the patient with advanced cancer is the recognition and effective treatment of such acute problems.

Relatively few complications of malignancy are true emergencies—ie, it is not often essential to institute antineoplastic therapy within minutes. However, they should be recognized and treated promptly. Complications which may require true emergency management include hypercalcemia, severe hyperuricemia, severe carcinoid symptoms, and rapidly forming effusions in the pericardium or pleural space.

SPINAL CORD COMPRESSION

Spinal cord compression due to tumor is manifested by progressive weakness and sensory changes in the lower extremities, back pain, and blockage of contrast material as shown by myelography. It occurs as a complication of lymphoma or multiple myeloma, carcinomas of the lung, prostate, breast, and colon, and certain other neoplasms. Back pain at the level of the lesion occurs in 80% of cases. Since involvement is usually extradural, a mixture of nerve root and spinal cord symptoms often develops.

The initial findings of impending cord compression may be quite subtle, and this possibility should always be considered when patients with malignancy develop unexplained weakness of the lower extremities or back pain. Prompt diagnosis and therapy are essential if paraplegia, quadriplegia, or other types of permanent residual or spinal cord damage are to be prevented. Once paralysis develops, it is usually irreversible. Conversely, patients who are treated promptly may have complete return of function and may respond favorably to subsequent therapy of the malignancy.

The management of spinal cord compression often requires prompt intervention by a team of specialists: The patient's primary physician or a medical oncologist should coordinate the diagnostic and therapeutic program with the help of the radiologist, radiotherapist, and neurosurgeon. When the symptoms and the results of the neurologic examination are consistent with a diagnosis of cord compression, an emergency myelogram should be performed, usually by a neurosurgeon, who then also follows the patient in case decompression laminectomy becomes necessary. If a block is demonstrated on myelography, the contrast medium is often left in the spinal canal, so that alleviation of the block can subsequently be demonstrated on follow-up x-rays after treatment.

Emergency treatment consists of (1) mechlorethamine (nitrogen mustard, Mustargen), freshly mixed, 0.4 mg/kg IV; (2) prednisone, 60 mg/day orally for 5–7 days, with subsequent tapering; and (3) radiotherapy to the involved area, usually initiated within 24 hours and continued to tolerance in a relatively short intensive course.

If treatment is begun promptly, decompression laminectomy is rarely indicated except in patients with extremely rapid progression of signs and symptoms. Patients must be followed closely, as occasional patients may require surgical intervention.

When the block is relieved, the flow of contrast in the remainder of the canal should be assessed, as blocks due to tumor (especially lymphoma) often are multiple.

Once the cord problem has subsided, systemic chemotherapy for the malignancy is indicated.

SUPERIOR VENA CAVA SYNDROME

Superior vena cava syndrome is a potentially fatal complication of bronchogenic carcinoma, occasional lymphomas, and certain other neoplasms which metastasize to the mediastinum. It is characterized by brawny edema and flushing of the head and neck and dilated neck and arm veins. Partial syndromes may result from subclavian vein obstruction. The onset of symptoms is acute or subacute. Venous pressure in the upper extremities is increased, and bilateral brachial venography or sodium pertechnetate Tc 99m scanning demonstrates a block to the flow of contrast material into the right heart as well as large collateral veins. The patient is often in a state of low cardiac output and is at risk of sudden death from cardiovascular collapse. Although the underlying carcinoma is usually incurable when the syndrome develops, emergency therapy for this complication can provide effective palliation for 6 months or more and is not necessarily a terminal event. Since this complication may be rapidly fatal, treatment should be initiated within hours of recognition. Treatment is sometimes indicated even when the diagnosis of cancer has not been confirmed histologically since the syndrome is almost always due to cancer and thoracotomy or mediastinoscopy may lead to death. In such unproved cases of cancer, the block should be unequivocally demonstrated angiographically, and other signs of tumor should be present on chest x-ray as well.

Emergency treatment consists of (1) administration of freshly mixed mechlorethamine, 0.4 mg/kg IV, to initiate tumor shrinkage; (2) intravenous injection of a potent parenteral diuretic (eg, ethacrynic acid) to relieve the edematous component of vena caval compression; and (3) mediastinal irradiation, starting within 24 hours, with a treatment plan designed to give a high daily dose but a short total course of therapy to rapidly shrink the local tumor even further. Intensive combined therapy will reverse the process in up to 90% of patients. In patients with a subacute presentation, radiation therapy alone usually suffices.

The ultimate prognosis depends on the nature of the primary neoplasm. Even in bronchogenic carcinoma, occasional patients have slowly growing tumors which may not cause further symptoms for considerable periods of time.

MALIGNANT EFFUSIONS

The development of effusions in closed compartments such as the pleural, pericardial, and peritoneal spaces presents significant diagnostic and therapeutic problems in patients with advanced neoplasms. Most malignant effusions are not acute emergencies, but they can be if they accumulate unusually rapidly or occur in the pericardial space. Although direct involvement (thickening) of the serous surface with tumor appears to be the most frequent initiating factor in such cases, not all effusions in cancer patients are malignant. Benign processes such as congestive heart failure, pulmonary embolus, trauma, and infection (eg, tuberculosis) may be responsible, mimicking the effects of a neoplasm. Bloody effusions are usually malignant but occasionally are due to embolus with infarction or trauma. Chylous effusions may be associated with thoracic duct obstruction or may result from mediastinal lymph node enlargement in lymphoma. Cytology or cell block of the fluid—or hook needle biopsy (eg, with the Cope pleural biopsy needle)—should be used to prove that the effusion is truly neoplastic before local therapy is used to prevent recurrence. Pericardial effusions should be tapped with continuous ECG monitoring with a V lead attached to the pericardiocentesis needle so that the epicardium will be detected should it be contacted.

The management of malignant effusions should be appropriate to the severity of involvement. Effusions due to lung, ovarian, and breast carcinoma often require more than simple drainage. In other neoplasms, simple drainage is sometimes sufficient, especially if it coincides with the initiation of effective systemic chemotherapy. Drainage of a large pleural effusion can be accomplished rapidly and with relative safety with a closed system using a disposable phlebotomy set which is connected to a vacuum phlebotomy bottle after the needle has been passed through the skin of the thorax. Thoracentesis performed in this fashion requires very little manipulation of the patient and prevents the problems of inadvertent pneumothorax associated with multiple changes of a stopcock connected to a syringe. Nonetheless, post-tap films are indicated after thoracentesis to assess the results and to rule out pneumothorax.

Recurrent effusions which do not respond to repeated taps may often be controlled by instillation of either mechlorethamine or quinacrine. Mechlorethamine injection will eliminate or suppress an effusion in two-thirds of patients with effusions due to carcinoma. The alkylating agent thiotepa appears to be preferable for suppression of ascites since it produces less local pain and discomfort in the peritoneum than do the other agents.

The procedure is as follows: Most of the pleural, ascitic, or pericardial fluid is withdrawn. While a free flow of fluid is still present, mechlorethamine is instilled into the cavity. The dose employed is 0.4 mg/kg, or a total dose of 20–30 mg in the usual patient. The solution should be freshly mixed at the time of injection to avoid hydrolysis prior to administration. After the drug is injected and the needle withdrawn, the patient is placed in a variety of positions in order to distribute the drug throughout the cavity. On the following day, the remaining fluid is withdrawn from the body cavity. Inasmuch as mechlorethamine and triethylenethiophosphoramide are absorbed systemically from the cavity, this treatment is not advised for patients who already have significant pancytopenia or bone marrow depression due to prior chemotherapy. In such cases, quinacrine is substituted for the alkylating agent inasmuch as it does not produce hematopoietic depression. Quinacrine is usually administered into the cavity in a dose of 200 mg/day for 5 days, with daily drainage of residual fluid.

Nausea and vomiting commonly follow the instillation of mechlorethamine but can often be controlled with prophylactic administration of an antiemetic prior to the procedure and at intervals afterward. Pleural pain and fever may occur after intracavitary administration of either alkylating agents or quinacrine but are more common with the latter compound. Narcotic analgesics are indicated for pain during the acute period; however, the need for these usually abates within several days. Once a pleural space or other potential space has been effectively sealed with such drug treatments, recurrent effusion is usually not a problem.

Dollinger MR, Krakoff IH, Karnofsky DA: Quinacrine (Atabrine) in the treatment of neoplastic effusions. Ann Int Med 66:249, 1967.

HYPERCALCEMIA

Hypercalcemia secondary to malignancy is a fairly common medical emergency. It is particularly frequent in breast carcinoma and multiple myeloma but occurs also with a variety of other cancers, all of which need not metastasize to bone to initiate the syndrome. The typical findings consist of anorexia, nausea, vomiting, constipation, muscular weakness and hyporeflexia; confusion, psychosis, tremor, lethargy, and elevated serum calcium. However, a wide range of symptom complexes may be observed, and sometimes the only abnormal finding will be an elevated serum calcium. ECG often shows a shortening of the Q–T interval. When the serum calcium rises above 12 mg/100 ml, sudden death due to cardiac arrhythmia or asystole may occur. The tragic medical and social consequences of untreated hypercalcemia are best illustrated in the instance of the young mother with breast cancer who dies of unrecognized hypercalcemia. Inasmuch as the underlying cancer can often be palliated for many years after an episode of hypercalcemia, this complication of malignancy need not indicate a poor prognosis and should be treated as a medical emergency.

In the absence of signs or symptoms of hypercalcemia, an elevated serum calcium should be repeated immediately to exclude the possibility of laboratory error.

Emergency treatment for hypercalcemia due to malignancy consists of (1) intravenous fluids, 3–4 liters/day (including saline infusions); (2) low-calcium diet; (3) prednisone, 60–80 mg/day orally for 4–5 days, followed by tapering; (4) intravenous administration of a potent diuretic (eg, ethacrynic acid) once saline infusion has been initiated; and (5) for severe hypercalcemia (greater than 15 mg/100 ml) or refractory cases, mithramycin (Mithracin), 25 μg/kg IV every other day for 2–4 doses. Although mithramycin therapy is often effective in relieving hypercalcemia and can be used less frequently for chronic management, the drug has significant toxicities, including a potential hemorrhagic syndrome. In most instances, however, only several doses are required, and these complications are unlikely to occur. Mithramycin therapy should therefore be considered as part of the initial management of severe hypercalcemia and as an adjunctive agent in milder cases.

If alternative therapy is needed for refractory cases, intravenous 8–10 hour infusions of isotonic sodium sulfate, once daily for 1 or 2 days, will often reduce the serum calcium very rapidly. Patients treated with sodium sulfate will receive extremely large sodium loads with this treatment inasmuch as the isotonic solution used for infusion contains 38.9 gm of sodium sulfate per liter and up to 3 liters have been given. Such treatment, although effective, may induce hypernatremia, and the patient's condition must be such that a sodium load can be tolerated. Patients with uremia may be made worse, and the serum sodium may climb to 160 mEq/liter. Patients with cardiac disease who are susceptible to congestive failure may be pushed into overt heart failure. Thus, there is no standard dosage, and the patient must be both carefully selected and closely watched. Sodium phosphate infusions are not advisable since they are associated with extreme danger of metastatic calcification in addition to the hypernatremic effects.

Once the acute hypercalcemic episode has been treated, it is usually appropriate to begin systemic chemotherapy. In the instance of breast cancer, hypercalcemia may appear as a "flare" after initiation of estrogen therapy. In most instances, it is advisable to discontinue the estrogen and change to a different form of chemotherapy. If chronic hypercalcemia persists—even if only to a moderate degree—the patient should be treated with small doses of prednisone or oral sodium phosphate supplements (1–2 gm/day) and encouraged to maintain a high fluid intake in the hope of preventing renal damage. When phosphate is used, if no alternative source of phosphate is available, disposable Fleet's Phospho-Soda enemas can be given orally. (*Caution:* Excessive dosage will lead to diarrhea.) Chronic hypercalcemia which is refractory to the above measures can sometimes be managed with once-weekly mithramycin injections, 25 μg/kg IV. In most instances, when the malignancy responds to chemotherapy, hypercalcemia subsides.

Chakmakian ZH, Bethune JE: Sodium sulfate treatment of hypercalcemia. New England J Med 275:862, 1966.
Perlia CP & others: Mithramycin in the treatment of hypercalcemia. Cancer 25:389, 1970.

HYPERURICEMIA & ACUTE URATE NEPHROPATHY

Increased blood levels of uric acid are often observed in patients with neoplasms who are receiving cancer chemotherapy. In this circumstance, hyperuricemia should more appropriately be viewed as a preventable complication rather than an acute emergency, inasmuch as uric acid formation can be inhibited prophylactically. At present, hematologic neoplasms such as leukemia, lymphoma, and myeloma most frequently present the problem of hyperuricemia after therapy, but hyperuricemia may occur with any form of malignancy which undergoes rapid destruction and release of nucleic acid constituents, and in some instances prophylaxis will not have been given. Less commonly, certain rapidly proliferating neoplasms with a high nucleic acid turnover (eg, acute leukemia) may be present with hyperuricemia even in the absence

of prior chemotherapy. If the patient is also receiving a thiazide diuretic, the problem may be compounded by decreased urate excretion. Routine follow-up of patients receiving cancer chemotherapy should include measurements of serum uric acid and creatinine as well as complete blood counts. Rapid elevation of the serum uric acid concentration usually does not produce gouty arthritis in these patients but does present the danger of acute urate nephropathy. In this form of acute renal failure, uric acid crystallizes in the distal tubules, the collecting ducts, and the renal parenchyma. The danger of uric acid nephropathy is present when the serum urate concentration is above 15 mg/100 ml, and in some instances it may rise to as high as 80 mg/100 ml.

Prophylactic therapy consists of the administration of allopurinol, 100 mg 3 times daily, starting 1 day prior to the initiation of chemotherapy. Administration of allopurinol inhibits xanthine oxidase and prevents conversion of the highly soluble hypoxanthine and xanthine to the relatively insoluble uric acid. Patients who are to receive mercaptopurine or azathioprine for cancer chemotherapy should have its dose reduced to 25–35% of the usual dose if they are also receiving allopurinol, inasmuch as the latter drug potentiates both the effects and toxicity of mercaptopurine.

Emergency therapy for established severe hyperuricemia consists of (1) hydration with 3–4 liters of fluid per day; (2) alkalinization of the urine with 6–8 gm of sodium bicarbonate per day (in order to enhance urate solubility); (3) allopurinol, 200 mg 4 times daily orally; and (4) in severe cases, with serum urate levels above 25–30 mg/100 ml, emergency hemodialysis or peritoneal dialysis. *Caution:* Once the uropathy is established, items 1–3 are in fact dangerous until some means of getting rid of excess fluid is assured.

Since patients who suffer from this complication are often in the process of entering a stage of complete remission of the neoplasm, the prognosis is good if renal damage can be prevented.

BACTERIAL SEPSIS IN CANCER PATIENTS

Many patients with disseminated neoplasms have increased susceptibility to infection. In some instances this results from impaired host defense mechanisms (eg, acute leukemia, Hodgkin's disease, multiple myeloma, chronic lymphocytic leukemia); in other patients it results from the myelosuppressive and immunosuppressive effects of cancer chemotherapy or a combination of these factors. In patients with acute leukemia and in those with granulocytopenia (less than 600 granulocytes per cu mm), infection is a medical emergency. Although fever alone does not prove the presence of infection, in these patients as well as in patients with multiple myeloma or chronic lymphocytic leukemia fever is virtually pathognomonic of infection. While infections in patients with myeloma or chronic leukemia are often due to sensitive organisms, patients with leukemia or pancytopenia are far less fortunate, as resistant gram-negative organisms are more often responsible. Appropriate cultures (eg, blood, sputum, urine, CSF) should always be obtained prior to initiation of therapy; however, one usually cannot await the results of these studies before initiating bactericidal antibiotic therapy. The results of Gram stains may be quite rewarding if they clearly show a predominant organism in the sputum, urine, or CSF.

Emergency Treatment

In the absence of granulocytopenia and in nonleukemic patients, the empirical combination of cephalosporin and gentamicin has proved exceedingly useful for patients with acute bacteremia. Therapy with combinations of this nature must be given judiciously, as they are of very broad spectrum; they should always be replaced by the most appropriate antibiotics as soon as culture data become available. The combination of cephalosporin and kanamycin is ineffective against pseudomonas infection. In the current era of intensive chemotherapy of cancer, bacteremic infection with pseudomonas is now the most frequent infection in granulocytopenic patients and is all too often fulminant and fatal within 72 hours. Recent observations suggest that prompt institution of combination therapy with gentamicin and carbenicillin offers the best chance of curing pseudomonas bacteremia in cancer patients. Because of drug interactions, these 2 compounds cannot be mixed but must be administered separately. This combination is of lesser efficacy against *Escherichia coli* sepsis and should not be used for that purpose. Initial treatment of febrile patients with acute leukemia and granulocytopenia should consist of 3 drugs: cephalothin, gentamicin, and carbenicillin. If a causative organism is isolated, the combination is replaced with the best agent or agents; otherwise, the combination is continued until the infection has resolved.

Granulocyte transfusions have recently been proved to have significant value in the treatment of granulocytopenic cancer patients with sepsis; however, until recently, the complex procurement procedures limited their availability. Untreated patients with chronic myelogenous leukemia (CML) can serve as excellent granulocyte donors for cancer patients with granulocytopenia. Although collection is ideally carried out with a blood cell separator, simple leukapheresis technics may also be of value with CML donors. Use of normal donors requires use of a blood cell separator or filtration-leukapheresis device. Optimal use of normal granulocyte transfusion appears to require at least 4 daily transfusions (in addition to antibiotics) to localize infection.

Schimpff S & others: Empiric therapy with carbenicillin and gentamicin for febrile patients with cancer and granulocytopenia. New England J Med 284:1061, 1971.

CARCINOID SYNDROME

Although tumors of argentaffin cells are rare and usually slow-growing, they synthesize and secrete a variety of vasoactive materials including serotonin, histamine, catecholamines, and vasoactive peptides. These substances are capable of initiating acute severe vascular changes which may be fatal.

Carcinoid tumors usually arise from either the ileum, the stomach, or the bronchus, and tend to metastasize relatively early, even though they may grow at an indolent pace.

The manifestations of carcinoid syndrome include facial flushing, edema of the head and neck (especially severe with bronchial carcinoid), abdominal cramps and diarrhea, asthmatic symptoms, cardiac lesions (pulmonary or tricuspid stenosis or insufficiency), telangiectases, and increased urinary 5-hydroxyindoleacetic acid (5-HIAA). Acute and particularly severe symptoms occur in patients with bronchial carcinoids and usually begin with a period of disorientation and tremulousness followed by fever and flushing episodes which may last 3 or 4 days. Hypotension and pulmonary edema have also been observed. Even a small coin lesion on chest x-ray may be capable of producing the entire syndrome and may not be recognized until after the diagnosis of carcinoid has been established biochemically. The biochemical diagnosis should be sought in all patients with such symptoms, even if the responsible tumor cannot be located. A qualitative test for urinary 5-HIAA is positive in most instances and indicates that the patient is probably secreting 25–30 mg of 5-HIAA per day. False negatives may occur in patients receiving phenothiazines, and false positives have been observed after ingestion of serotonin-rich foods such as bananas or walnuts or in patients taking cough syrups containing glycerol guaiacolate. Ideally, the patient should be taken off all drugs for several days prior to the urine collection.

A provocative test for the induction of the flush can be performed by injecting 5 μg of epinephrine (0.5 ml of 1:1000 solution diluted 100 times) IV. If positive, the facial flush and some dyspnea usually appear within several minutes.

Emergency therapy is indicated in patients with bronchial carcinoids and prolonged flushing episodes and consists of the administration of prednisone, 15–30 mg orally daily. This treatment has a dramatic effect and is usually continued for prolonged periods. The flushing itself may well be due to kinins rather than serotonin, and corticosteroids often do not change the effects of other mediators of the syndrome. These other manifestations may require additional treatment. The abdominal cramps and diarrhea can usually be managed with tincture of opium or diphenoxylate with atropine (Lomotil), alone or in combination with an antiserotonin agent such as methysergide maleate.

Phenothiazines may also be of some benefit in relieving the symptoms of flushing.

Patients with intestinal carcinoids may do satisfactorily for 10–15 years with supportive therapy, and in these instances cancer chemotherapy may not always be indicated. Because of the more aggressive symptomatology of the bronchial lesions, if they cannot be resected or have metastasized, chemotherapy with an alkylating agent should also be considered.

Melmon KL: The endocrinologic manifestations of the carcinoid tumor. Chap 17, pp 1161–1180, in: *Textbook of Endocrinology,* 4th ed. Williams RH (editor). Saunders, 1968.
Saterlee WG, Serpick A, Bianchine JR: The carcinoid syndrome: Chronic treatment with para-chlorophenylalanine. Ann Int Med 72:919, 1970.

CANCER CHEMOTHERAPY

Administration of cytotoxic drugs and hormones has become a highly specialized and increasingly effective means of treating advanced cancer patients with a variety of malignancies. Treatment is optimally directed by a medical oncologist or cancer chemotherapist who either provides primary care for such patients or serves as a consultant to the patient's family physician. The aim of this section is to provide the nonspecialist with useful information about the types of advanced cancer which are likely to respond to currently available chemotherapeutic agents, about the pharmacology and toxicity of the agents, and to assist in the evaluation of response to treatment.

Cancer chemotherapy is usually curative in advanced stages of choriocarcinoma in women and in Burkitt's lymphoma; occasionally in certain testicular tumors; and in some cases of acute leukemia. Hodgkin's disease, diffuse histiocytic lymphoma, insulinoma, and certain other tumors. Combined with surgery and irradiation, chemotherapy also increases the cure rate in Wilms's tumor, and initial data (as discussed below) suggest that a similar approach may provide long-term disease control in early breast cancer, osteogenic sarcoma, and other neoplasms. Chemotherapeutic management, in most instances with combination chemotherapy, provides significant palliation of symptoms along with prolongation of survival in many children with acute leukemia, Ewing's sarcoma, retinoblastoma, rhabdomyosarcoma, adults with Hodgkin's disease, non-Hodgkin's lymphomas, mycosis fungoides, multiple myeloma, macroglobulinemia, carcinomas of the breast, endometrium, and prostate, or oat cell carcinoma of the lung. Patients with carcinoma of the colon or larynx or the chronic leukemias also achieve some relief of symptoms with treatment, although significant prolongation of survival has yet to be demonstrated. Until recently, no effective therapy was available for most patients with sarcoma. This picture is improving with the use of doxorubicin (Adriamycin) and several other drugs. Present therapy is usually unsuccessful in most cases of cancer of the lung, kidney, or pancreas.

A summary of malignancies responsive to chemotherapy and the current treatment of choice is offered in Table 32–2. In some instances (eg, Hodgkin's disease), optimal therapy may require a combination of therapeutic modalities, eg, radiation therapy plus chemotherapy rather than chemotherapy alone. All patients with stage I or II Hodgkin's disease should receive radiation therapy. Table 32–3 outlines the currently used dosage schedules and the toxicities of the cancer chemotherapeutic agents. The dosage schedules given are for single agent therapy. Combination therapy, as is now used in advanced Hodgkin's disease, testicular tumors, and certain other neoplasms, requires downward modifications of the dosage shown—otherwise, the combined toxicity would be prohibitive. Such combination therapy should be attempted only by specialists who have adequate supportive services available (eg, platelet transfusions) for use as necessary. Nonspecific immunotherapy with BCG may prove to be a useful adjunct in treatment of acute leukemia and melanoma, but its role in cancer therapy has yet to be defined. Although preliminary studies are encouraging and suggest prolongation of remission duration, the use of nonspecific immunotherapy with BCG is still investigational.

MECHANISMS OF ACTION OF CANCER CHEMOTHERAPEUTIC AGENTS

Although the primary emphasis of this chapter is on the empirical applications of cancer chemotherapy, a brief note must be made of the cytokinetics and mechanisms of drug action inasmuch as the field of medical oncology has now progressed into the era of "enlightened empiricism." At the clinical level of detectability of tumors, growth characteristics vary considerably between tumors of different histologies or tissue of origin. One such distinction is in the "growth fraction"—the percentage of tumor cells that are proliferating at any given time in a tumor. The leukemias, certain lymphomas, and genital tract tumors have relatively high growth fractions and, as a result, are susceptible to treatment with drugs that have specific toxicity for proliferating cells. Drugs that have selective toxicity for proliferating cells include cytarabine, mercaptopurine, thioguanine, methotrexate, fluorouracil, azacytadine, vincristine, vinblastine, bleomycin, and certain steroid hormones. These drugs are therefore classed as **cell cycle specific (CCS)** agents, and their utility has proved to be greatest in tumors with high growth fractions such as those mentioned above. Cytarabine is an excellent example of a drug with selective toxicity during just one phase of the cell cycle, that of DNA synthesis (the "S phase"), and its current use is virtually limited to the management of acute leukemia, where it has had a major beneficial effect.

Table 32—2. Malignancies responsive to chemotherapy.

Diagnosis	Current Treatment of Choice	Other Valuable Agents
Acute lymphocytic leukemia	Induction: Vincristine plus prednisone Remission maintenance: Mercaptopurine, methotrexate, and cyclophosphamide in various combinations	Asparaginase,* daunorubicin,* BCNU (carmustine),* cytarabine, allopurinol,† craniospinal radiation therapy, BCG*
Acute myelocytic and myelomonocytic leukemia	Combination chemotherapy: Doxorubicin, vincristine, cytarabine, prednisone	Methotrexate, thioguanine, mercaptopurine, daunorubicin, allopurinol,† BCG,* azacytadine*
Chronic myelocytic leukemia	Busulfan	Vincristine, mercaptopurine, hydroxyurea, melphalan, cytarabine, allopurinol†
Chronic lymphocytic leukemia	Chlorambucil and prednisone (if indicated)	Vincristine, androgens,† allopurinol,† doxorubicin
Hodgkin's disease	Combination chemotherapy: Mechlorethamine, vincristine, procarbazine, prednisone, bleomycin ("MOPP-bleo")	Vinblastine, doxorubicin, BCNU (carmustine),* dacarbazine, VP-16,* VM-26*
Non-Hodgkin's lymphomas	Combination chemotherapy: Cyclophosphamide, doxorubicin, vincristine, prednisone	Bleomycin, CCNU, BCNU, VP-16,* VM-26*
Multiple myeloma	Melphalan plus prednisone	Cyclophosphamide, vincristine, BCNU (carmustine),* doxorubicin, androgens†
Macroglobulinemia	Chlorambucil	
Polycythemia vera	Busulfan, chlorambucil, or cyclophosphamide	
Carcinoma of lung	Cyclophosphamide or other alkylating agents	Methotrexate, doxorubicin, quinacrine,† hexamethylmelamine*
"Head and neck" carcinomas	Methotrexate, bleomycin	Hydroxyurea, fluorouracil
Carcinoma of endometrium	Doxorubicin plus cyclophosphamide	Progestins
Carcinoma of ovary	Doxorubicin plus cyclophosphamide, melphalan	Fluorouracil, vincristine, hexamethylmelamine*
Breast carcinoma	(1) Combination chemotherapy or melphalan if lymph nodes are positive at mastectomy. (2) Combination chemotherapy ("D/C" or "CMF"); hormonal manipulation for late recurrence	Cyclophosphamide, doxorubicin, vincristine, methotrexate, fluorouracil, quinacrine,† prednisone†
Choriocarcinoma (trophoblastic neoplasms)	Methotrexate, alone or in combination with vincristine and dactinomycin	Vinblastine, mercaptopurine, chlorambucil
Carcinoma of testis	Combination therapy: Vinblastine, bleomycin	Methotrexate, dactinomycin, mithramycin, doxorubicin, cyclophosphamide
Carcinoma of prostate	Estrogens	Doxorubicin, prednisone†
Wilms's tumor (children)	Dactinomycin after surgery and radiation therapy	Vincristine, methotrexate, cyclophosphamide
Neuroblastoma	Cyclophosphamide plus doxorubicin and vincristine	Dactinomycin, daunorubicin,* doxorubicin
Carcinoma of adrenal	Mitotane (o,p'DDD, Lysodren)	
Carcinoma of colon	Fluorouracil plus methyl-CCNU*	Cyclophosphamide, mitomycin C
Carcinoid	Cyclophosphamide	Dactinomycin, methysergide†
Insulinoma	Streptozotocin*	
Osteogenic sarcoma	Doxorubicin or methotrexate with citrovorum rescue initiated after amputation	Cyclophosphamide
Miscellaneous sarcomas	Doxorubicin plus dacarbazine	Methotrexate, dactinomycin, cyclophosphamide, vincristine
Melanoma	Dacarbazine (DTIC), BCG*	BCNU (carmustine),* hydroxyurea

*Investigational agent. Treatment available through qualified investigators and centers authorized by National Cancer Institute and Cooperative Oncology Groups.
†Supportive agent, not oncolytic.

A second major group of drugs is classed as **cell cycle nonspecific (CCNS)** agents. Most of these drugs act by complexing with cellular DNA and are capable of doing this whether cells are proliferating or not. Examples are the alkylating agents (eg, mechlorethamine, cyclophosphamide, melphalan, BCNU, etc) and antibiotics such as dactinomycin, doxorubicin, and mitomycin. Such drugs are useful in the treatment of a variety of so-called "solid tumors," which generally have low growth fractions at the clinical phase of disease; but they also are quite useful in high growth fraction tumors. Tumor kinetics are far from static, however, and our strategy of approach in cancer chemotherapy is now undergoing radical revision to maximally exploit our knowledge of cytokinetics, pharmacokinetics, selective cell line sensitivity, etc.

For example, drugs that have had the greatest value in man are those that produce a fractional kill of at least 5–6 logs (100,000-fold to 1 million-fold reduction in tumor cell number) in animal tumor systems. Because patients with human tumors present with $10^{10}–10^{12}$ tumor cells, use of effective combination chemotherapy should be given serious consideration after a major reduction in the body burden of tumor is first accomplished with surgery or irradiation. Under such circumstances, the growth fraction of the tumor may increase and the fraction of tumor cells susceptible to a cell cycle specific agent may also increase and make the tumor more susceptible to treatment.

ADJUVANT CHEMOTHERAPY FOR MICROMETASTASES

The most important role for effective cancer chemotherapy is undoubtedly as an "adjuvant" to initial or "primary field" treatment with other methods of treatment such as surgery or radiation therapy. Failures with primary field therapy are due principally to occult micrometastases outside the primary field. These distant micrometastases are usually present in patients with one or more positive lymph nodes at the time of surgery (eg, in breast cancer) and in patients with tumors having a known propensity for early hematogenous spread (eg, osteogenic sarcoma, Wilms's tumor). The risk of recurrent or metastatic disease in such patients can be extremely high (80%). Only systemic therapy can adequately attack micrometastases. Chemotherapeutic regimens which are at least moderately effective against advanced cancer may have curative potential (at the right dosage and schedule) when combined with primary therapy such as surgery. Recent studies show prolongation of disease-free survival in patients with osteogenic sarcoma or breast cancer who receive adjuvant chemotherapy. In osteogenic sarcoma, methotrexate with citrovorum (folinic acid) rescue, doxorubicin alone, and doxorubicin in combination with other drugs have proved effective. In breast cancer, women with positive lymph nodes at the

time of mastectomy have benefited from combination chemotherapy (both pre- and post-menopausal age groups), or single agent chemotherapy with melphalan (premenopausal only). Useful combination chemotherapy regimens for adjuvant therapy for breast cancer include "CMF" (cyclophosphamide-methotrexate-fluorouracil) and "D/C" (doxorubicin-cyclophosphamide). The end results obtained with combination chemotherapy will probably prove superior to results obtained with single agents because combination chemotherapy has a greater tumor cell "log kill." Adjuvant chemotherapy should definitely be considered as part of standard and indicated therapy in the patient groups discussed above. Other areas of current investigation include adjuvant chemotherapy for "Dukes C" colon cancer (fluorouracil alone or in combination with methyl-CCNU or BCG) and in testicular (vinblastine and bleomycin) and gynecologic neoplasms (various drugs). Thus, adjuvant chemotherapy (with curative intent) should now be given serious consideration for every patient who undergoes primary surgical staging and therapy and is found to have a stage and histologic type of cancer known to be associated with a high risk of micrometastasis. This policy is particularly germane to those tumor types for which palliative chemotherapy has already been developed and been shown to be effective in advanced stages of the disease.

Bonadonna G & others: Adjuvant study with combination chemotherapy in operable breast cancer. Proc Am Soc Clin Oncol 16:254, 1975.

Cortes EP & others: Amputation and Adriamycin in primary osteosarcoma. New England J Med 291:998, 1974.

Fisher B & others: L-Phenylalanine mustard (L-PAM) in the management of primary breast cancer: A report of early findings. New England J Med 292:117, 1975.

Jaffe N & others: Adjuvant methotrexate and citrovorum-factor treatment of osteogenic sarcoma. New England J Med 291:994, 1974.

TOXICITY & DOSE MODIFICATION OF CHEMOTHERAPEUTIC AGENTS

A number of cancer chemotherapeutic agents have cytotoxic effects on rapidly proliferating normal cells in the bone marrow, mucosa, and skin. Still other drugs such as the vinca alkaloids produce neuropathy, and the hormones often have psychic effects. Acute and chronic toxicities of the various drugs are summarized in Table 32–3. Early recognition of significant toxicity is important to make certain that the ratio of benefit to toxic effects of treatment remains favorable. Appropriate dose modification usually minimizes these side-effects, so that therapy can be continued with relative safety.

Bone Marrow Toxicity

Depression of the bone marrow is usually the

Table 32–3. Dosage and toxicity of cancer chemotherapeutic agents.

Chemotherapeutic Agent	Usual Adult Dosage	Acute Toxicity	Delayed Toxicity
Alkylating agents			
Mechlorethamine (nitrogen mustard, HN2, Mustargen)	0.4 mg/kg IV in single or divided doses.	Nausea and vomiting	Moderate depression of peripheral blood count. Excessive
Chlorambucil (Leukeran)	0.1–0.2 mg/kg/day orally; 6–12 mg/day.	None	doses produce severe bone marrow depression with leuko-
Cyclophosphamide	3.5–5 mg/kg/day orally for 10 days; 1 gm/sq m IV as single dose every 3–4 weeks.	Nausea and vomiting	penia, thrombocytopenia, and bleeding. Alopecia and hemorrhagic cystitis are peculiar toxicities of cyclophosphamide
Melphalan (Alkeran)	0.25 mg/kg/day orally for 4 days every 6 weeks.	None	(p 984), while Busulfan occasionally causes pigmentation
Thiotepa	0.2 mg/kg IV for 5 days.	None	and several other unusual toxicities (p 985).
Busulfan (Myleran)	2–8 mg/day orally; 150–250 mg/course.	None	
Structural analogues or antimetabolites			
Methotrexate (amethopterin, MTX)	2.5–5 mg/day orally; 15 mg intrathecally weekly or every other week for 4 doses. 20–25 mg IM twice weekly is well tolerated and may be preferable.	None	Oral and gastrointestinal tract ulceration, bone marrow depression, leukopenia, thrombocytopenia.
Mercaptopurine (Purinethol, 6-MP)	2.5 mg/kg/day orally.	None	Usually well tolerated. Larger dosages may cause bone marrow depression.
Thioguanine (6-TG)	2 mg/kg/day orally.	None	Usually well tolerated. Larger dosages may cause bone marrow depression.
Fluorouracil (5-FU)	15 mg/kg/day IV for 3–5 days, or 15 mg/kg weekly for at least 6 weeks..	None	Nausea, oral and gastrointestinal ulceration, bone marrow depression.
Cytarabine (Ara-C, Cytosar)	100 mg/sq m/day for 5–10 days given by continuous IV infusion, or in divided doses subcut or IV every 8 hours.	None	Nausea and vomiting, bone marrow depression, megaloblastosis, leukopenia, thrombocytopenia.
Hormonal agents			
Androgens			
Testosterone propionate	100 mg IM 3 times weekly.	None	Fluid retention, masculinization. There is a 10% incidence of cholestatic jaundice with fluoxymesterone.
Fluoxymesterone (Halotestin)	10–20 mg/day orally.	None	
Calusterone (Methosarb)	200 mg/day orally in divided doses.	None	None.
Estrogens			
Diethylstilbestrol	1–5 mg 3 times a day orally.	Occasional nausea and vomiting	Fluid retention, feminization, uterine bleeding.
Ethinyl estradiol (Estinyl)	3 mg/day orally.	None	
Progestins			
Hydroxyprogesterone caproate (Delalutin)	1 gm IM twice weekly.	None	Occasional fluid retention.
Medroxyprogesterone (Provera)	100–200 mg/day orally; 200–600 mg orally twice weekly.	None	
Adrenocorticosteroids			
Prednisone	20–100 mg/day orally or, when effective, 50–100 mg every other day orally as single dose.	None	Fluid retention, hypertension, diabetes, increased susceptibility to infection, "moon facies," osteoporosis.

Table 32—3 (cont'd). Dosage and toxicity of cancer chemotherapeutic agents.

Chemotherapeutic Agent	Usual Adult Dosage	Acute Toxicity	Delayed Toxicity
Miscellaneous drugs			
Vinblastine (Velban)	0.1–0.2 mg/kg IV weekly.	Nausea and vomiting	Alopecia, loss of reflexes, bone marrow depression.
Vincristine (Oncovin)	1.5 mg/sq m with a maximum of 2 mg IV weekly.	None	Areflexia, muscular weakness, peripheral neuritis, paralytic ileus, mild bone marrow depression (p 984).
Dactinomycin (actinomycin D, Cosmegen)	0.01 mg/kg/day IV for 5 days, or 0.04 mg/kg IV weekly.	Nausea and vomiting	Stomatitis, gastrointestinal tract upset, alopecia, bone marrow depression.
Mithramycin (Mithracin)	0.05 mg/kg IV every other day for 4 doses.	Nausea and vomiting, diarrhea	Bone marrow depression, hemorrhagic syndrome, hypocalcemia.
Doxorubicin (Adriamycin)	40–75 mg/sq m IV every 3 weeks. Total dose must not be above 525 mg/sq m.	Nausea and vomiting	Alopecia, myelosuppression, mucositis, myocarditis (p 985).
BCNU (carmustine)	80 mg/sq m IV every 6 weeks.	Nausea and vomiting	Bone marrow depression.
Procarbazine (N-methylhydrazine, Matulane)	50–300 mg/day orally.	Nausea and vomiting	Bone marrow depression, mental depression, monoamine oxidase inhibition.
Dacarbazine (dimethyl triazeno imidazole carboxamide, DTIC)	250 mg/sq m/day for 5 days every 3 weeks.	Anorexia, nausea, vomiting	Bone marrow depression.
Mitomycin (Mutamycin)	0.05 mg/kg/day for 10 days with repeat after 28 days (2 day interruption may be necessary after day 5).	Fever, anorexia, nausea, vomiting	Bone marrow depression.
Bleomycin (Blenoxane)	15 units/sq m IV twice weekly to a total of 200–300 units (lower doses in Hodgkin's disease).	Allergic and hypotensive reactions	Fever, dermatitis, pulmonary fibrosis (p 984).
Mitotane (o,p′DDD, Lysodren)	6–12 gm/day orally.	Nausea and vomiting	Dermatitis, diarrhea, mental depression, muscle tremors.
Supportive agents			
Allopurinol (Zyloprim)	300–800 mg/day orally for prevention or relief of hyperuricemia.	None	Usually none. Enhances effects and toxicity of mercaptopurine when used in combination.
Quinacrine (Atabrine)	100–200 mg/day by intracavitary injection for 6 days.	Local pain and fever	None.
Immunostimulant			
BCG	6×10^8 viable organisms applied by scarification every 2–4 weeks.	Fever	Local inflammation, occasional systemic BCG disease (p 985).

most significant limiting toxicity in cancer chemotherapy.

Commonly used short-acting drugs which affect the bone marrow are the oral alkylating agents (eg, cyclophosphamide, melphalan, chlorambucil), procarbazine, mercaptopurine, methotrexate, vinblastine, fluorouracil, dactinomycin, and doxorubicin. In general, it is preferable to use alkylating agents in intensive "pulse" courses every 3–4 weeks rather than to administer in continuous daily schedules. This allows for complete hematologic (and immunologic) recovery between courses rather than leaving the patient continuously suppressed with a cytotoxic agent. This approach reduces side-effects and does not reduce therapeutic efficacy. The standard dosage schedules which produce tumor responses with these agents often do induce some bone marrow depression. In such instances, if the drug is not discontinued or its dosage reduced, severe bone marrow aplasia can develop and may result in pancytopenia, bleeding, or infection. Simple guidelines to therapy can usually prevent severe marrow depression.

Table 32—4. Scheme for dose modification of cancer chemotherapeutic agents.

White Count (/cu mm)	Platelet Count (/cu mm)	Suggested Drug Dosage (% of full dose)
> 5000	> 100,000	100%
4000—5000		75%
3000—4000	75,000—100,000	50%
2000—3000	50,000—75,000	25%
< 2000	< 50,000	0%

Complete blood counts (white blood counts, differential, hematocrit or hemoglobin, and platelet count) should be obtained frequently. With long-term chemotherapy, counts should be obtained initially at weekly intervals; the frequency of counts may be reduced only after the patient's sensitivity to the drug can be well predicted (eg, 3—4 months) and cumulative toxicity excluded.

In patients with normal blood counts, drugs should usually be started at their full dosage and tapered if need be, rather than starting at a lower dose and escalating the dose to hematologic tolerance. When the dose is escalated, toxicity often cannot be adequately anticipated, especially if it is cumulative, and marrow depression is often more severe.

Drug dosage can usually be tapered on a fixed schedule as a function of the peripheral white blood count or platelet count (or both). In this fashion, smooth titration control of drug administration can usually be attained for oral alkylating agents or antimetabolites. A scheme for dose modifications is shown in Table 32—4. Alternatively, the interval between drug courses can be lengthened, thereby permitting more complete hematologic recovery.

Drugs with delayed hematologic toxicities do not always fit into such a simple scheme, and in general they should only be administered by specialists who are quite familiar with specific toxicities. Drugs which require more special precautions regarding toxicity include doxorubicin, mitomycin, busulfan, cytarabine, bleomycin, and mithramycin, as well as the investigational agents BCNU (1,3-bis[2-chloroethyl]-1-nitrosourea, carmustine), CCNU, methyl-CCNU, and daunorubicin.

Gastrointestinal & Skin Toxicity

Since antimetabolites such as methotrexate and fluorouracil act only on rapidly proliferating cells, they damage the cells of mucosal surfaces such as the gastrointestinal tract. Methotrexate has similar effects on the skin. These toxicities are at times more significant than those which have occurred in the bone marrow, and they should be looked for routinely when these agents are used.

Erythema of the buccal mucosa is an early sign of mucosal toxicity. If therapy is continued beyond this point, oral ulceration will develop. In general, it is wise to discontinue therapy at the time of appearance of early oral ulceration. This finding usually heralds the appearance of similar but potentially more serious ulceration at other sites lower in the gastrointestinal tract. Therapy can usually be reinstituted when the oral ulcer heals (within 1 week to 10 days). The dose of drug used may need to be modified downward at this point, with titration to an acceptable level of effect on the mucosa.

Miscellaneous Drug-Specific Toxicities

The toxicities of individual drugs have been summarized in Table 32—3; however, several of these warrant additional mention since they occur with frequently administered agents, and special measures are often indicated.

A. Cyclophosphamide-Induced Hemorrhagic Cystitis: Metabolic products of cyclophosphamide which retain cytotoxic activity are excreted into the urine. Some patients appear to metabolize more of the drug to these active excretory products; if their urine is concentrated, severe bladder damage may result. In general, it is wise to advise patients receiving cyclophosphamide to maintain a large fluid intake. Early symptoms include dysuria and frequency despite the absence of bacteriuria. Such symptoms develop in about 20% of patients who receive the drug. Should microscopic hematuria develop, it is advisable to stop the drug temporarily or switch to a different alkylating agent, increase fluid intake, and administer a urinary analgesic such as phenazopyridine. With severe cystitis, large segments of bladder mucosa may be shed and the patient may have prolonged gross hematuria. Such patients should be observed for signs of urinary obstruction and may require cystoscopy for removal of obstructing blood clots. Patients whose tumors respond to cyclophosphamide who develop severe cystitis should stop taking all drugs until the syndrome clears and should then be given different alkylating agents (eg, chlorambucil, melphalan, mechlorethamine), which lack this toxicity, as they are likely to be equally effective against the tumor.

B. Vincristine Neuropathy: Neuropathy is a toxic side-effect which is peculiar to the vinca alkaloid drugs and is particularly observed with vincristine. The peripheral neuropathy can be sensory, motor, autonomic, or a combination of these effects. In its mildest form it consists of paresthesias ("pins and needles") of the fingers and toes. Occasional patients develop acute jaw or throat pain after vincristine therapy. This may be a form of trigeminal neuralgia. With continued vincristine therapy, the paresthesias extend to the proximal interphalangeal joints, hyporeflexia appears in the lower extremities, and significant weakness develops in the quadriceps muscle group. At this point, it is wise to discontinue vincristine therapy until the neuropathy has subsided somewhat. A useful means of judging whether the peripheral motor neuropathy is significant enough to warrant stopping treatment is to have the patient attempt to do deep knee bends or get up out of a chair without using his arms.

Constipation is the most common symptom of the autonomic neuropathy which occurs with vincristine therapy. This symptom should always be dealt with prophylactically, ie, patients receiving vincristine should be started on stool softeners and mild cathartics when therapy is instituted. If this potential complication is neglected, severe impaction may result in association with an atonic bowel.

More serious autonomic involvement can lead to acute intestinal obstruction with signs indistinguishable from those of an acute abdomen. Bladder neuropathies are uncommon but may be severe.

These 2 complications are absolute contraindications to continued vincristine therapy.

C. Methotrexate Toxicity and "Citrovorum Rescue": In addition to standard uses of methotrexate for chemotherapy, this drug is finding increasing use in a very high dosage which, if given without an antidote, would lead to fatal bone marrow or epithelial toxicity. It is now recognized that the bone marrow toxicity of methotrexate can be completely reversed by early administration of citrovorum factor (folinic acid, Leucovorin). If an overdose of methotrexate is administered accidentally, folinic acid therapy should be initiated as soon as possible, preferably within 1 hour. Intravenous infusion should be employed for large overdosages, inasmuch as it is generally advisable to give folinic acid in amounts equal to the weight of the methotrexate administered. Up to 75 mg should be given in the first 12 hours, followed by 12 mg IM every 4 hours for 6 doses.

Intentional high-dosage methotrexate therapy with citrovorum rescue should only be considered for patients with extremely good renal function. Daily monitoring of the serum creatinine is mandatory because methotrexate metabolism is slowed by renal insufficiency and high-dosage methotrexate can in itself induce renal injury. Use of this approach remains somewhat controversial in the management of osteosarcoma and certain other tumors, principally because of the considerable toxicities which may occur if renal function becomes impaired. When this form of therapy is used, folinic acid therapy should probably be initiated within 4 hours of the methotrexate dose and continued for 3 days.

D. Busulfan Toxicity: The alkylating agent busulfan, which is frequently used for treatment of chronic myelogenous leukemia, has curious delayed toxicities, including (1) increased skin pigmentation, (2) a wasting syndrome reminiscent of adrenal insufficiency, and (3) progressive pulmonary fibrosis. Patients who develop either of the latter 2 problems should be taken off busulfan and switched to a different drug (eg, melphalan) when additional therapy is needed. The pigmentary changes are innocuous, and will usually regress slowly after treatment is discontinued; in this instance, change to a different compound is optional.

E. Bleomycin Toxicity: This antibiotic has found increasing application in cancer chemotherapy in view of its striking effects on squamous cell carcinomas, Hodgkin's disease, non-Hodgkin's lymphomas, and testicular tumors. Bleomycin produces edema of the interphalangeal joints and hardening of the palmar and plantar skin, as well as sometimes also inducing an anaphylactic or serum sickness-like reaction, or a serious or fatal pulmonary fibrotic reaction (seen especially in elderly patients receiving a total dose of over 300 units). If nonproductive cough, dyspnea, and pulmonary infiltrates develop, discontinue the drug and institute antibiotic and high-dose corticosteroid therapy. Fever alone or with chills is an infrequent complication of bleomycin treatment and does not constitute an absolute contraindication to continued treatment. The fever may be avoided by prednisone administration at the time of injection. Moreover, fever alone is not predictive of the pulmonary toxicity. About 1% of patients (especially those with lymphoma) may have a severe or even fatal hypotensive reaction after their initial dose of bleomycin. In order to identify such patients, it is wise to administer a test dose of 5 mg (5 units) of bleomycin first with adequate monitoring and emergency facilities available should they be needed. Patients exhibiting a hypotensive reaction should not receive further bleomycin therapy.

F. Doxorubicin-Induced Myocarditis: The anthracycline antibiotics doxorubicin and daunomycin both have a delayed cardiac toxicity. The problem is greater with adriamycin because it appears likely that this drug will have a major role in the treatment of sarcomas, breast cancer, lymphomas, and certain other solid tumors. Recent studies of left ventricular function indicate that some reversible changes in cardiac dynamics occur in most patients by the time they have received 300 mg/sq m. Serial echocardiographic measurements can detect these abnormalities. Echocardiographic measurement of the "left ventricular ejection fraction" appears most useful in this regard. Doxorubicin should not be used in elderly patients with significant intrinsic cardiac disease, and no patient should receive a total dose in excess of 550 mg/sq m. Patients who have had prior chest or mediastinal radiotherapy may be more prone to develop doxorubicin heart disease. ECGs should be obtained serially. The development of S–T and T wave abnormalities, changes in the systolic time interval, or the appearance of a high resting pulse may herald the appearance of cardiac toxicity. Unfortunately, toxicity may be irreversible or fatal at high dosage levels. At lower dosages (eg, 350 mg/sq m), the symptoms and signs of cardiac failure generally respond well to digitalis, diuretics, and cessation of doxorubicin therapy.

G. Reactions to BCG: BCG is a viable preparation of a strain of *Mycobacterium bovis* which has been used as a nonspecific immunostimulant in various adjuvant trials and in chemoimmunotherapy. Its use in cancer therapy should still be considered investigational. Because of its widespread use, a comment must be made about its toxicities, most of which are attributable to its being a viable, antigenic bacterium. Fever commonly is associated with its application by scarification. Although intradermal injection of tumor nodules (eg, melanoma) with BCG has also been used, this route of administration is more hazardous and has been associated with acute anaphylaxis and disseminated intravascular coagulation. Systemic BCG disease is an occasional complication of BCG treatment by any route of administration, and is manifest as recurrent fever and hepatic dysfunction. The systemic disorder should be promptly treated with antituberculosis therapy (see Chapter 6) and usually responds quickly.

Frei E & others: New approaches to cancer chemotherapy with methotrexate. New England J Med 292:845, 1975.

Proceedings of the High-Dose Methotrexate Meeting. Cancer Chemother Rep 6 (part 3):1–82, 1975.

EVALUATION OF TUMOR RESPONSE

Inasmuch as cancer chemotherapy can induce clinical improvement, significant toxicity, or both, it is extremely important to critically assess the beneficial effects of treatment to determine that the net effect is favorable. The most valuable signs to follow during therapy include the following:

A. Tumor Size: Demonstration of significant shrinkage in tumor size on physical examination, chest film or other x-ray, or special scanning procedure such as bone scanning (breast, prostate cancer) or scanning with ^{111}In-bleomycin (many tumors).

B. Marker Substances: Significant decrease in the quantity of a tumor product or marker substance which reflects the amount of tumor in the body. Examples of such markers include the paraproteins in the serum or urine in multiple myeloma and macroglobulinemia, chorionic gonadotropin in choriocarcinoma and testicular tumors, urinary steroids in adrenal carcinoma and paraneoplastic Cushing's syndrome, and 5-hydroxyindoleacetic acid in carcinoid syndrome. Secreted tumor antigens are becoming of increasing importance with the recent recognition of alpha$_1$ fetoprotein in hepatoma, in teratoembryonal carcinoma, and in occasional cases of gastric carcinoma and the carcinoembryonic antigen in carcinomas of the colon, lungs, and breast. Technics for measurement of these 2 fetal proteins are now generally available. Two polyamines, spermidine and putrescine, also appear to have value in predicting the efficacy of cancer chemotherapy.

C. Organ Function: Normalization of function of organs which were previously impaired as a result of the presence of a tumor is a useful indicator of drug effectiveness. Examples of such improvement include the normalization of liver function (eg, increased serum albumin) in patients known to have liver metastases and improvement in neurologic findings in patients with cerebral metastases. Disappearance of the signs and symptoms of the paraneoplastic syndromes often falls in this general category and can be taken as indication of tumor response.

D. General Well Being and Performance Status: A valuable sign of clinical improvement is the general well being of the patient. Although this finding is a combination of subjective and objective factors and may be subject to placebo effects, it nonetheless serves as an obvious and useful sign of clinical improvement and can be used in reassessment of some of the objective observations listed above. Factors included in the assessment of general well being include improved appetite and weight gain and increased "performance status" (eg, ambulatory versus bedridden). Evaluation of factors such as activity status has the advantage of summarizing beneficial and toxic effects of chemotherapy and enables the physician to judge whether the net effect of chemotherapy is worthwhile palliation.

33...

Immunologic Disorders

Samuel Strober & Hugh O. McDevitt

A wide variety of diseases in man are now known to be associated with disorders of the immune response. Recent studies of immunoglobulin structure and function and of the cellular basis of immunity have resulted in a better understanding of these disorders. This chapter is designed to provide an approach to the patient with immunologic disease by outlining some of the advances that have significant clinical application. A discussion of immunologic deficiency disorders, HL-A-linked diseases, autoimmunity, and the gammopathies will illustrate the practical uses of current concepts and technics in clinical immunology.

IMMUNOGLOBULIN STRUCTURE & FUNCTION

The basic unit of all immunoglobulin molecules consists of 4 polypeptide chains linked by disulfide bonds. There are 2 identical heavy chains (molecular weight 53–75 thousand) and 2 identical light chains (molecular weight about 23,000). Both heavy and light chains have a C-terminal constant (C) region (constant amino acid sequence within a class or type) and an N-terminal variable (V) region, with considerable variation in amino acid sequence from molecule to molecule. The V regions of heavy and light chains together form the antibody combining site which is responsible for the specific interaction with antigen. A schematic diagram of the basic immunoglobulin molecule is shown in Fig 33–1.

The class of heavy chain and the type of light chain are determined by the amino acid sequence in the constant region in the case of heavy chains, and in both the constant and variable regions in the case of light chains. Five classes of heavy chains have been identified (γ, a, μ, δ, and ϵ) and 2 types of light chains (κ and λ). Either type of light chain can be associated with each of the heavy chain classes. Approximately 70% of human immunoglobulin molecules carry κ light chains and 30% carry λ light chains.

Immunoglobulin Classes

A. Immunoglobulin M (IgM): IgM is made up of 5 identical basic immunoglobulin units. Each unit has a μ heavy chain and a κ or λ light chain. These units are connected to each other by disulfide bond bridges and a small polypeptide known as J chain. The molecular weight of IgM is about 900,000, and the sedimentation coefficient is 19S. The IgM molecule is found predominantly in the intravascular compartment and does not cross the placenta.

B. Immunoglobulin A (IgA): IgA is present in high concentrations in the blood and in seromucous secretions such as saliva, colostrum, tears, and secretions of the bronchi and the gastrointestinal tract. IgA found in the serum is a single basic immunoglobulin unit with a heavy chains. Exocrine or secretory IgA is made up of 2 basic units connected to each other by J chain. A 60,000 molecular weight molecule called transport-piece or T-piece is attached to the Fc portion. The latter molecule is necessary for the transportation of IgA molecules into the lumens of exocrine glands. Secretory IgA appears to play an important role in host defense mechanisms against viral and bacterial infections. IgA does not cross the placenta.

C. Immunoglobulin G (IgG): IgG is a single basic immunoglobulin unit with γ heavy chains and comprises about 85% of total serum immunoglobulins. Its molecular weight is approximately 150,000, and its sedimentation coefficient is 7S. IgG is distributed in the extracellular fluid and crosses the placenta. Both IgG and IgM molecules bind complement via a receptor present in the constant region of the γ and μ heavy chains.

D. Immunoglobulin E (IgE): IgE is present in the serum in very low concentrations as a single basic immunoglobulin unit with ϵ heavy chains. Approximately 50% of patients with allergic diseases have increased serum IgE levels. IgE is a skin-sensitizing or reaginic antibody by virtue of a mast cell attachment site present on the constant region of the ϵ heavy chain. The specific interaction between antigen and IgE bound to the surface of mast cells results in the release of inflammatory mast cell products such as histamine and serotonin. A wheal and flare reaction or severe bronchospasm may be precipitated by such interactions in the tissues of the skin or lungs, respectively.

E. Immunoglobulin D (IgD): IgD is present in the serum in very low concentrations as a single basic immunoglobulin unit with δ heavy chains. The role of IgD is not yet known.

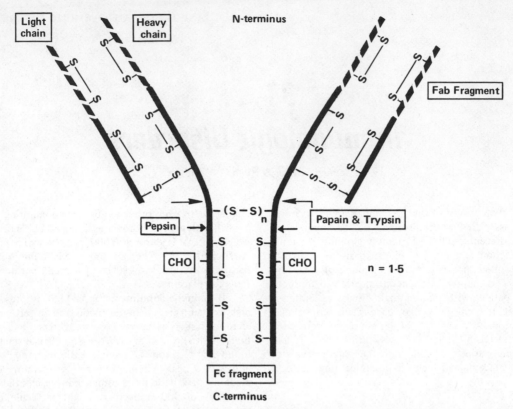

Figure 33—1. Structure of immunoglobulins. Electron microscopic studies have demonstrated that immunoglobulin molecules are Y-shaped. Solid lines indicate regions of constant amino acid sequences; broken lines indicate variable regions. Note symmetry in structure of molecule. One intrachain disulfide loop recurs for every 110–120 amino acid residues along heavy and light chains; about 60 residues are contained within each loop. From 1–5 inter-heavy chain disulfide bonds are present in each molecule depending on subclass of heavy chain. Points of cleavage of heavy chains by the proteolytic enzymes papain, trypsin, and pepsin, in relation to the inter-heavy chain disulfide bonds, are indicated. (Reproduced, with permission, from Freedman SO [editor]: *Clinical Immunology.* Harper, 1971.)

Franklin EC, Fragione B: Immunoglobulins. Ann Rev Med 20:155, 1969.
Natvig JB, Kunkel HG: Human immunoglobulins: Classes, subclasses, genetic variants, and idiotypes. Advances Immun 16:1, 1973.

CELLULAR BASIS OF IMMUNE RESPONSES

Development of T & B Lymphocytes

Lymphocytes are able to interact with antigens and initiate the immune responses of vertebrates. In avian species, 2 lines of lymphocytes have been identified: one derived from the thymus and the other from the bursa of Fabricius. The thymus-derived cells are involved in cellular immune responses; the bursa-derived cells are involved in humoral antibody responses. The lymphocytes of mammalian species can also be divided into 2 cell lines: T lymphocytes, which are analogous to the thymus-derived cells in birds; and B lymphocytes, which are analogous to the bursa-derived cells.

Both T and B lymphocytes are derived from precursor cells in the marrow. In the case of T lymphocytes, the precursor cells migrate to the thymus, where they develop some of the functional and cell surface characteristics of mature T cells. Thereafter, the cells migrate to the T-dependent areas of the peripheral lymphoid tissues (paracortical areas of lymph nodes and periarteriolar sheath of the spleen), and enter the pool of long-lived lymphocytes which recirculate from the blood to the lymph. Some maturation of T cells may occur in the peripheral tissues under the influence of a thymic humoral hormone (thymosin).

Two sequences of B cell maturation are now recognized: antigen-independent and antigen-dependent maturation. Antigen-independent maturation includes those stages of B cell development from precursor cells in the marrow through the virgin B cell (a cell which has not been exposed to antigen previously) found in the peripheral lymphoid tissues. Several developmental stages occur in the marrow, and others occur following migration to the solid lymphoid tissues in the periphery. The production and maturation of virgin B cells is an ongoing process even in adult animals. Antigen-dependent maturation occurs following the interaction of antigen with virgin B cells. Memory B cells and antibody-forming cells (plasma cells) are the final products of this developmental sequence. Many of the memory B cells are long-lived and recirculate from the blood to the lymph. Mature B cells in the periphery are found predominantly in the thymus-independent areas (primary follicles and germinal centers) of the lymph nodes and spleen.

Subpopulations of T Cells

T lymphocytes are heterogeneous with respect to their cell surface features and functional characteristics. At least 3 subpopulations of T cells are now recognized.

A. Helper or Cooperator Cells: These cells help to amplify the production of antibody-forming cells from B lymphocytes after interaction with antigen. The precise mechanism by which T cells cooperate with B cells is not clear.

B. Cytotoxic or Killer T Cells: These cells are generated after mature T cells interact with certain antigens such as those present on the surface of foreign cells. These cells are responsible for organ graft rejection and for cell-mediated killing of foreign cells in vitro.

C. Suppressor T Cells: These cells suppress rather than amplify the formation of antibody-forming cells from B lymphocytes. Suppressor T cells are regarded as regulatory cells which modulate humoral antibody formation. Alterations in these cells may play an important role in those disease entities in which there is an overproduction (systemic lupus erythematosus or autoimmune thyroiditis) or an underproduction (common variable agammaglobulinemia) of immunoglobulin. The mechanism of action of suppressor cells has not yet been elucidated.

Other Cells Involved in Immune Responses

A. Macrophages: Macrophages are involved in the initial ingestion and processing of some antigens (especially particulate substances) before interaction with lymphocytes. They are thought to play an important role in allowing T and B lymphocytes to cooperate in the induction of humoral antibody responses. In addition, they appear to be effector cells for certain types of tumor immunity in that they can kill tumor cells in vitro.

B. K Cells: These cells are thought to be lymphocytic (nonphagocytic) in origin but are not directly linked to the T or B cell lineage. They are capable of killing a foreign cell in vitro after they have been incubated with antibodies specifically directed against the foreign cells (antibody-dependent cell-mediated immunity). K cells may play an important role in effector mechanisms in tumor immunity.

Good RA: Structure-function relations in the lymphoid system. Clin Immunobiol 1:1, 1972.

MECHANISMS OF AUTOIMMUNE DISEASE

Cell-Mediated Autoimmunity

Certain autoimmune diseases are mediated by T cells which have become specifically immunized to autologous tissues. Cytotoxic or killer T cells generated by this aberrant immune response attack and injure specific organs in the absence of serum autoantibodies. Autoimmune allergic encephalomyelitis and lymphocytic choriomeningitis are 2 examples of T cell-mediated autoimmune disease in animals.

Humoral Antibody-Mediated Autoimmunity

Several autoimmune diseases have been shown to be caused by humoral autoantibody in the absence of cell-mediated autoimmunity. The autoimmune hemolytic anemias, idiopathic thrombocytopenia, and Goodpasture's syndrome appear to be mediated solely by autoantibodies directed against autologous cell membrane constituents. In these diseases, antibody attaches to cell membranes, fixes complement, and thereby causes severe injury to the cell.

Immune Complex Disease

In this group of diseases (systemic lupus erythematosus, rheumatoid arthritis, some drug-induced hemolytic anemias and thrombocytopenias), autologous tissues are injured as "innocent bystanders." Autoantibodies are not directed against cellular components of the target organ but rather against autologous or heterologous antigens in the serum. The resultant antigen-antibody complexes bind nonspecifically to autologous membranes (eg, glomerular basement membrane) and fix complement. Fixation and subsequent activation of complement components produce a local inflammatory response which results in tissue injury.

Samter M (editor): *Immunological Diseases,* 2nd ed. Vol 1. Little, Brown, 1971.

GENETIC CONTROL OF THE IMMUNE RESPONSE

In recent years it has become apparent that the ability to mount a specific immune response is under direct control by genes other than those which are the structural genes for the immunoglobulin light and heavy chains. The former genes are closely associated on the same chromosome with the structural genes for the major transplantation antigens. The major transplantation antigens are the cell surface glycoproteins (found on all tissues of the body) which elicit the strongest transplantation rejection reaction when tissues are exchanged between 2 members of a particular species. In man, this genetic region has been designated the *human leukocyte antigen (HL-A)* complex because these antigens were first detected on peripheral blood lymphocytes.

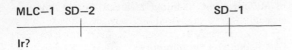

Figure 33–2. Genetic map of major histocompatibility complex in man. Genetic loci of the serologically determined antigens (SD-1, SD-2), mixed lymphocyte culture antigens (MLC-1), and immune response genes (Ir) are shown.

The major transplantation antigens in man are detected by serologic technics and have been given the designation *serologically detectable first and second locus,* or *SD-1* and *SD-2* antigens. A schematic diagram of the human leukocyte antigen genetic complex is given in Fig 33–2. Each of these genes has many different alleles in the population. Thus, there are more than 10 distinct forms of the SD-1 gene and 20 distinct forms of the SD-2 gene. Since a given individual receives one SD-1 and one SD-2 gene from each parent, the number of possible combinations of transplantation antigens in a particular individual is very large, explaining the great difficulty in identifying 2 individuals in the random population who are identical for the major transplantation antigens. (There are undoubtedly a large number of minor transplantation antigens which have not yet been identified in man.)

An additional set of genes, closely linked to SD-2, determines the structure of a series of cell surface glycoproteins which are found predominantly on the surface of B lymphocytes and some T lymphocytes. These antigens were originally detected by their ability to stimulate the mixed lymphocyte culture reaction. This is a proliferative reaction which occurs when lymphocytes from 2 unrelated individuals are cultured together in vitro. Extensive analysis has shown that, in man, genetic differences on other chromosomes do not lead to mixed lymphocyte culture stimulation. This is due primarily to genes in the HL-A complex which map to the left of SD-2 and have been given the name of the *mixed lymphocyte culture* genes, or MLC genes.

A genetic region determining the structure of the mixed lymphocyte culture antigens and mapping within the major transplantation antigen complex of the mouse was identified several years ago. At the same time, it became apparent that a series of genes determining the ability to mount a specific immune response to a given antigen or antigenic determinant also mapped in the same region. The latter genes determining the ability to respond well or poorly to a particular antigen have been given the designation of immune response or *Ir* genes. Specific Ir genes have been identified in the mouse and rat controlling the ability to mount a strong or weak immune response to a wide variety of synthetic polypeptides, native proteins, viruses, thyroglobulin, and basic encephalitogenic proteins. In both man and monkey, the evidence indicates that Ir genes controlling immune responses to antigens such as ragweed allergen are closely linked to the major

transplantation antigen gene complex. Presumably, in man these Ir genes will map in the same region as the genes determining the structure of MLC antigens (Fig 33–2).

While the exact mechanism of action of Ir genes is not yet known, it is clear that they affect the ability to recognize foreign antigens and to initiate the development of cellular and humoral immunity to these antigens. Genes with such a strong effect on specific immune responsiveness might be expected to have major effects on resistance or susceptibility to a wide variety of infectious, neoplastic, and autoimmune diseases.

This appears to be the case. Although methods are not yet available for Ir genotyping in man, methods are available for HL-A typing and for typing for particular MLC antigens in man, and such typing procedures have revealed extraordinarily strong associations between these genes and particular human diseases.

Benacerraf B, McDevitt HO: Histocompatibility linked immune response genes. Science 175:273, 1972.

Moller G (editor): HL-A and disease. Transplant Rev 22:1, 1975.

CLINICAL IMMUNOLOGY LABORATORY TESTS

Procedures for Testing Cell-Mediated Immunity or T Cell Function

A. Skin Testing: Cell-mediated immunity can be assessed qualitatively by evaluating skin reactivity following intradermal injection of a battery of antigens to which humans are frequently sensitized (ie, streptokinase, streptodornase, PPD, trichophyton, dermatophyton, or candida). Skin painting with dinitrochlorobenzene (DNCB) is helpful if there is doubt about prior exposure to any of the above antigens since DNCB functions as both the sensitizing and the "test" antigen. Anergy or lack of skin reactivity to all of these substances indicates a marked depression of cell-mediated immunity.

B. In Vitro Stimulation of Peripheral Blood Lymphocytes With Phytohemagglutinin (PHA) or Allogeneic Lymphocytes (Mixed Lymphocyte Culture, MLC): T but not B lymphocytes are transformed to blast cells upon short-term incubation with PHA or allogeneic lymphocytes in vitro. Quantitative determinations of blast transformation can be made by following the cellular uptake of ^{3}H-thymidine introduced into the culture medium. The in vitro uptake of ^{3}H-thymidine by human peripheral blood lymphocytes serves as an indicator of T cell function and correlates well with the manifestations of cell-mediated immunity as measured by skin reactivity.

Procedures for Measuring Humoral Immunity or B Cell Function

There are 4 methods of assessing humoral immunity: (1) Quantitative and qualitative determinations of serum immunoglobulins; (2) determination of isohemagglutinin and febrile agglutinin titers; (3) determination of antibody titers following primary or booster immunization with tetanus toxoid, diphtheria toxoid (Schick test), and pertussis vaccines; and (4) determination of the percentage of peripheral blood lymphocytes bearing surface immunoglobulins by im-

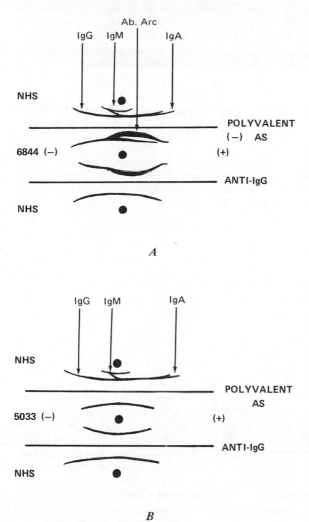

A

B

Figure 33—3. *A:* Immunoelectrophoretic pattern of a monoclonal immunoglobulin (myeloma protein). *Top:* Normal human serum (NHS) run against a polyvalent antiserum (polyvalent AS). *Middle:* Serum from patient with IgG myeloma protein run against polyvalent AS and specific anti-γ heavy chain (anti-IgG) antisera. *Bottom:* NHS run against anti-IgG. This myeloma protein formed a dense arc when run against a specific anti-κ chain antiserum. No arc developed with anti-λ chain antiserum. *B:* Electrophoretic pattern of agammaglobulinemia. *Top:* NHS run against polyvalent AS. *Middle:* Serum from patient with agammaglobulinemia run against polyvalent AS and anti-IgG. *Bottom:* NHS run against anti-IgG. (Reproduced, with permission, from DHEW Publication No. [HSM] 72—1802: *Radial Imunodiffusion Test and the Immunoelectrophoresis Test for Qualitation and Quantitation of Immunoglobulins.* US department of Health, Education, and Welfare, January, 1972.)

munofluorescent staining technics. Serum immunoglobulins can be measured in 2 ways as follows:

A. Immunoelectrophoresis: Immunoelectrophoresis is most useful as a screening device for semiquantitative estimates of the amounts of IgG, IgA, or IgM in the serum or urine and for identifying abnormal immunoglobulin molecules such as myeloma (M) proteins. The absence of certain immunoglobulin classes or the presence of abnormal immunoglobulin molecules in concentrations too low to be detected by serum electrophoresis will be readily apparent on immunoelectrophoresis.

The immunoelectrophoresis plate is made up of a gel material. Long troughs and a circular well are cut into the gel as shown in Fig 33—3. Serum or concentrated urine is placed in the well. An electric charge is applied to the longitudinal ends of the plate, and an anti-whole human serum antiserum, usually developed in goats or horses, is then placed in the trough. As the human serum and goat or horse reagents diffuse through the gel, precipitin arcs are formed which identify the various protein constituents of human serum. The major serum immunoglobulin classes have characteristic arcs which are shown in Fig 33—3. The density of each arc is a measure of the amount of immunoglobulin present. Abnormal immunoglobulins such as myeloma (M) proteins form a sharp arc which merges with the normal immunoglobulin arc of the same class. Once an abnormal immunoglobulin or immunoglobulin fragment (ie, light chain) is found in the serum or urine, further characterization with respect to the heavy chain class and light chain type should be performed using class- or type-specific antisera (Fig 33—3).

B. Quantitative Immunoglobulin Determinations; Radial Diffusion Technic: Quantitative determinations of the serum IgG, IgA, and IgM levels can be carried out quickly in the clinical laboratory using the radial diffusion technic. Circular wells are cut in a gel plate impregnated with a specific goat or horse antiserum directed against a single human immunoglobulin class. A circular precipitin ring will form after the human serum proteins placed in the well diffuse through the gel. The radius or diameter of the precipitin ring is proportionate to the concentration of serum immunoglobulin. The precise immunoglobulin level is determined by comparing the diameter of the unknown serum to that of a standard containing known levels of immunoglobulins. Quantitative immunoglobulin measurements do not differentiate between normal and abnormal immunoglobulin molecules as does the immunoelectrophoresis procedure. The normal serum concentrations of the 3 major immunoglobulin classes are as follows:

IgG 711—1536 mg/100 ml (92—207 UI/ml)
IgA   59—489 mg/100 ml (54—268 IU/ml)
IgM   37—212 mg/100 ml (69—287 IU/ml)

TECHNICS FOR IDENTIFICATION
OF HUMAN T & B CELLS

B Cells

Cell surface characteristics found on B but not T cells include the following: (1) easily detectable surface immunoglobulin, (2) a receptor for complement (C'3), and (3) a receptor for the Fc portion of immunoglobulins which have been aggregated or complexed with antigen.

Surface immunoglobulin is commonly detected by direct fluorescence staining of live cell suspensions with fluorescein-conjugated heterologous antisera directed against human immunoglobulin. The receptor for complement is identified by incubating suspensions of live lymphocytes in vitro with sheep red blood cells coated with antibody and complement. The sensitized red cells adhere to the surface of the lymphocytes via the complement receptor and form rosettes which are identified under the light microscope. The receptor for aggregated immunoglobulin is identified by incubating lymphocytes in vitro with fluorescein-labeled IgG aggregates.

T Cells

Methods currently used to identify peripheral T lymphocytes in man depend upon the presence of surface markers which are shared by human thymocytes and the absence of surface markers associated with B cells. T cell markers include T cell–specific surface antigens identified by heterologous antisera and a surface receptor which binds sheep red blood cells. The heterologous antisera have been used in both immunofluorescent staining and in vitro cytotoxicity assays. The receptor for sheep red blood cells is detected by incubating live suspensions of human lymphocytes in vitro with sheep red blood cells and monitoring the formation of spontaneous rosettes under the light microscope. Approximately 75% of human peripheral blood lymphocytes are T cells and 25% are B cells.

INTERPRETATION OF RESULTS
OF T & B CELL TYPING

Immunodeficiency Diseases

Thymic hypoplasia is associated with a marked decrease in the percentage and absolute number of T cells in the peripheral blood. On the other hand, the absence of B cells in the blood is frequently found in X-linked agammaglobulinemia. Typing of peripheral blood T and B cells can help to establish the diagnosis of the above diseases in early childhood.

Lymphoproliferative Diseases

The presence of a marked increase in the percentage and absolute count of peripheral blood lymphocytes which bear immunoglobulin of a single heavy chain class and light chain type represents a monoclonal proliferation of cells. Almost all patients with chronic lymphocytic leukemia and non-Hodgkin's lymphoma with blood involvement show this picture. On the other hand, lymphocytosis secondary to viral or bacterial infection is associated with a normal percentage of B cells and the usual distribution of immunoglobulin classes on the cell surface.

A marked decrease in the percentage of B cells in the peripheral blood (> 5%) is seen in some cases of multiple myeloma but not in benign monoclonal gammopathy. This may provide a diagnostic tool for differentiating these disease states in the future.

TESTS FOR AUTOANTIBODIES ASSOCIATED
WITH AUTOIMMUNE DISEASES

Assays for autoantibodies are similar to those used for detection of antibodies to heterologous antigens. Four of the more commonly used methods are discussed below:

Tanned Red Blood Cell Hemagglutination

Red cells (human, sheep, etc) are incubated with tannic acid, so that the cell surface becomes "sticky." The tanned cells are subsequently incubated with the specific antigen (eg, thyroglobulin), which is absorbed to the cell surface. The antigen-coated cells are suspended in the unknown serum, and antibody is detected by red cell agglutination. Antigen-coated latex particles are substituted for red cells in the latex fixation test.

Radioimmune Precipitation

Specific antigen (eg, DNA) is radiolabeled, usually by iodination (^{125}I) or tritiation (^{3}H). Labeled antigen is incubated with the unknown serum to allow antigen-antibody complexes to form. Complexes are then precipitated by the addition of ammonium sulfate or anti-immunoglobulin. The amount of radioactivity in the supernatant or precipitate is related to the amount of antigen bound by specific antibody in the unknown serum.

Immunofluorescence Microscopy

This technic is most frequently used for detection of antinuclear antibody. Frozen sections of mouse liver are cut and placed on glass slides. Unknown serum is placed over the sections and washed away. A fluorescein-conjugated rabbit anti–human immunoglobulin is applied thereafter and washed. Antinuclear antibody specifically binds to the mouse cell nucleus, and the fluorescein conjugate binds to the human antibody. Fluorescence of the cell nucleus observed by fluorescence microscopy indicates a positive test.

Complement Fixation

Specific antigen, unknown serum, and complement are incubated together. Sheep red blood cells

Table 33–1. Some autoimmune diseases
and their associated antibodies.

Autoimmune Disease	Associated Autoantibodies
Autoimmune hemolytic anemia	Anti–blood group substance antibody
Autoimmune thyroiditis	Antithyroglobulin antibody
Chronic active hepatitis	Anti–smooth muscle, anticytoplasmic, antinuclear, anti-immunoglobulin (rheumatoid factor) antibody
Goodpasture's syndrome	Anti–basement membrane antibody
Idiopathic thrombocytopenic purpura	Antiplatelet antibody
Pemphigoid	Anti–basement membrane antibody
Pemphigus vulgaris	Anti-intercellular antibody
Pernicious anemia	Anti–parietal cell, anti–intrinsic factor antibody
Polymyositis	Antinuclear antibody
Primary biliary cirrhosis	Antimitochondrial antibody, antinuclear antibody
Rheumatoid arthritis	Anti-immunoglobulin (rheumatoid factor), antinuclear antibody
Scleroderma	Antinuclear antibody
Sjögren's syndrome	Anti-immunoglobulin, anti–salivary gland, antinuclear antibody
Systemic lupus erythematosus	Antinuclear, anti-DNA, anti-ENA (extractable nuclear antigen), anti-immunoglobulin, antilymphocyte, anti–red blood cell antibody

coated with anti-sheep cell antibody are subsequently added to the reaction mixture for 30 minutes at 37° C. Lysis of sheep cells indicates that complement is present (attaches to sheep cell surface). Lack of lysis indicates that complement has been consumed by the interaction of antibody in the unknown serum with the specific antigen. Lack of lysis is therefore interpreted as a positive test for the presence of specific antibody.

A list of autoimmune diseases and frequently associated autoantibodies is shown in Table 33–1. Many of the autoantibodies are not specific for a single disease entity (eg, antinuclear antibody, rheumatoid factor). Tests for the latter autoantibodies are best used as screening procedures in that a negative result makes the diagnosis of certain autoimmune diseases unlikely. For example, a negative antinuclear antibody test makes the diagnosis of systemic lupus erythematosus unlikely, since this antibody is detected in the serum of more than 95% of lupus patients.

HL-A & MLC TYPING

Serologic methods for detecting HL-A antigens have taken advantage of the fact that the mother, when pregnant, frequently makes antibodies to the paternal transplantation antigens possessed and released by the developing fetus. By screening a large number of pregnancy sera and using these sera to test lympho-

cytes isolated from the peripheral blood of a large number of normal human donors, it is possible to build up a panel of sera from several different donors which react, for example, with the same 25% of lymphocytes from a large number of randomly selected normal donors. Such a panel of antisera can then be defined as detecting the same human leukocyte antigen. In a similar manner, a second set of sera may define another antigen. By testing with a large number of pregnancy sera and screening a large number of donors, it has become possible over the years to build up panels of antisera which identify more than 10 distinct, "private" antigenic specificities at the SD-1 locus and more than 20 distinct antigenic specificities at the SD-2 locus.

As it is routinely done, HL-A typing involves placing a microdroplet of tissue culture medium containing 1000–2000 peripheral blood lymphocytes from the patient to be tested in a series of wells under mineral oil. Antisera detecting a particular antigenic specificity are then injected into separate wells along with the lymphocytes. From 3–5 antisera for each antigenic specificity, or a total of 100–150 antisera, are tested against each donor's lymphocytes. After a brief period of incubation, a source of complement (normal rabbit serum) is added, and after further incubation the cells are scored microscopically for percentage of killing. If all the cells are killed by antibody and complement, the reaction is said to be 4+. If fewer than 25% are killed, it is scored as 0 or 1+. By scoring the reaction of the patient's lymphocytes with the panels of antisera defining each transplantation antigen specificity and comparing the results with those of lymphocytes of known transplantation antigen type, an unequivocal assignment of transplantation antigen type can be achieved for 95–98% of a random sample of Caucasian donors. There are wide population variations in distribution of HL-A antigens—eg, between the black and white populations. In addition, Oriental populations contain new HL-A antigens which have not yet been fully characterized and identified.

Mixed lymphocyte culture typing is a much more extensive process. Because antibodies to define MLC antigens are not yet available (although they are in the mouse, and soon will be in man), MLC typing necessarily requires culturing the patient's lymphocytes with irradiated stimulator lymphocytes from a panel of individuals who are known to be homozygous at the MLC locus. (These MLC homozygous individuals are identified by extensive population screening studies.) The x-irradiated stimulator lymphocytes and the patient lymphocytes are co-cultured in tissue culture medium for 4 days. Then, for an additional 18 hours, the culture is pulsed with tritiated thymidine. If the patient shares MLC antigens with the particular stimulator lymphocyte being tested, his lymphocytes will not respond and will take up very little of the tritiated thymidine. If the patient does not possess the same MLC antigen as the stimulator lymphocytes, his lymphocytes will recognize the MLC antigens on the stimulator lymphocytes and will begin to proliferate briskly. This rapid proliferation is assessed by the uptake of tritiated thymidine during the last 18 hours of the period of co-culture. Results can be expressed either as increase in counts per minute over background, or as a stimulation index of the amount of tritiated thymidine incorporated in the test culture divided by the background incorporation level.

MLC typing is a laborious and costly procedure, and it is hoped that it will soon be replaced by serologic methods for detecting the MLC antigens on lymphocytes. Because some diseases show much stronger associations with particular MLC antigens than they do with the HL-A antigens themselves, MLC typing is already valuable in certain clinical situations and is likely to become more so as the technics for typing become simpler, more reliable, and more precise.

Vyas GN & others (editors): *Laboratory Diagnosis of Immunologic Disorders.* Grune & Stratton, 1975.

GAMMOPATHIES

The gammopathies include those disease entities in which there is a disproportionate proliferation of a single clone of antibody-forming cells which produce a homogeneous heavy chain, light chain, or complete immunoglobulin molecule. The amino acid sequence of the variable (V) regions is fixed, and only one type (κ or λ) of light chain is produced.

Benign Monoclonal Gammopathy

The diagnosis is made upon finding a homogeneous (monoclonal) immunoglobulin (with either κ or λ chains but not both) in immunoelectrophoresis of the serum of an otherwise normal individual. Screening of large populations in Sweden shows that the incidence of homogeneous immunoglobulins in the serum increases with age and may approach 3% in individuals 70 years of age or older. Follow-up studies show that a small percentage of apparently normal persons with a homogeneous serum immunoglobulin will go on to develop multiple myeloma. Parameters that suggest a favorable prognosis in "benign" monoclonal gammopathy include the following: (1) concentration of homogeneous immunoglobulin < 1 gm/100 ml, (2) no significant increase in the concentration of the homogeneous immunoglobulin from the time of diagnosis, (3) no decrease in the concentration of normal immunoglobulins, (4) absence of a homogeneous light chain in the urine (Bence Jones proteinuria), (5) normal hematocrit and serum albumin concentration.

Multiple Myeloma

This disease is characterized by the spread of neoplastic plasma cells throughout the bone marrow. Rarely, a single extraosseous plasmacytoma may be found. Anemia, hypercalcemia, increased susceptibility to infection, and bone pain are frequent findings. Certain diagnosis depends upon the presence of the following: (1) x-ray findings of osteolytic lesions or diffuse osteoporosis, (2) presence of a homogeneous serum immunoglobulin (myeloma protein) or a single type of light chain in the urine (Bence Jones proteinuria), (3) finding of an abnormal plasma cell infiltrate in the bone marrow biopsy.

Waldenström's Macroglobulinemia

Waldenström's macroglobulinemia is characterized by a proliferation of abnormal lymphoid cells which have the features of both lymphocytic and plasmacytic lines. These cells secrete a homogeneous macroglobulin (IgM) which is easily detected and characterized by immunoelectrophoresis. Bence Jones proteinuria is present in 10% of cases. Clinical manifestations frequently depend upon the physicochemical characteristics of the macroglobulin. Raynaud's phenomenon and peripheral vascular occlusions are associated with cold-insoluble proteins (cryoglobulins). Retinal hemorrhages, visual impairment, and transient neurologic deficits are not uncommon with high-viscosity serum. Bleeding diatheses and hemolytic anemia can occur when the macroglobulin complexes with coagulation factors or binds to the surface of red blood cells.

Primary Amyloidosis

Idiopathic or primary amyloidosis is commonly associated with increased plasmacytosis in the bone marrow or lymphoid tissues, a homogeneous serum immunoglobulin or Bence Jones proteinuria, and decreased levels of normal serum immunoglobulins. Recent evidence indicates that—at least in some cases—amyloid is made up of many identical variable (V) regions which are strung together to form a long polypeptide chain. These findings closely link primary amyloidosis with the gammopathies. The "primary" distribution pattern of amyloid infiltrates includes the heart, tongue, gastrointestinal tract, ligaments, and peripheral nerves, with sparing of the parenchymal organs such as the spleen, liver, and kidneys.

Heavy Chain Disease (a, γ, & μ)

These are rare disorders in which the abnormal serum and urine protein is a part of a homogeneous a, γ, or μ heavy chain. The clinical presentation is more typical of lymphoma than multiple myeloma, and there are no destructive bone lesions. Alpha chain disease is frequently associated with severe diarrhea and infiltration of the lamina propria of the small intestine with abnormal plasma cells.

Franklin EC, Zucker-Franklin D: Current concepts of amyloid. Advances Immun 15:249, 1972.

Ossermann EF: Multiple myeloma and related plasma cell dyscrasias. Pages 520–547 in: *Immunological Diseases,* 2nd ed. Samter M (editor). Little Brown, 1971.

IMMUNOLOGIC DEFICIENCY DISEASES

The immunologic deficiency diseases include congenital and acquired disorders of humoral immunity (B cell function) or cell-mediated immunity (T cell function). The most recent classification of immunodeficiency disorders recommended by WHO is shown below:

Infantile X-linked agammaglobulinemia (see below)
Selective immunoglobulin deficiency (see below)
Transient hypogammaglobulinemia of infancy
X-linked immunodeficiency with hyper-IgM
Thymic hypoplasia (pharyngeal pouch syndrome, DiGeorge's syndrome) (see below)
Immunodeficiency with normal serum globulins or hyperimmunoglobulinemia
Immunodeficiency with ataxia-telangiectasia (see below)
Immunodeficiency with thrombocytopenia and eczema (Wiskott-Aldrich syndrome) (see below)
Immunodeficiency with thymoma
Immunodeficiency with generalized hematopoietic hypoplasia
Severe combined immunodeficiency (see below):
  (1) With dysostosis
  (2) With adenosine deaminase deficiency
Variable immunodeficiency (common, largely unclassified) (see below)

Cooper MD & others: Developmental defects of T and B cell lines in humans. Transplant Rev 16:51, 1973.
Cooper MD & others: Meeting report of the Second International Workshop on Primary Immunodeficiency Disease in Man. Clin Immunol Immunopathol 2:416, 1974.

INFANTILE X-LINKED AGAMMAGLOBULINEMIA

This hereditary disorder results in a deficit in B cell function with essentially intact T cell function.

Clinical Findings
The diagnosis is based on the low IgG levels in serum, an X-linked pattern of heredity, intact cell-mediated immunity, and the absence of plasma cells in biopsy specimens of regional lymph nodes draining the site of recent antigenic stimulation such as DTP vaccine.
A. Symptoms and Signs: There are no symptoms during the first 9 months of life (probably due to presence of maternal antibody). During the second year, the infant shows increased susceptibility to pyogenic

infections (gram-positive organisms) and *Haemophilus influenzae,* resulting in recurrent furunculosis, pneumonia, and meningitis. There is normal susceptibility to viral exanthematous infections such as rubella, measles, chickenpox, and varicella. Other characteristic findings are chronic sinusitis, bronchiectasis, and arthritis of the large joints which has the appearance of rheumatoid arthritis.
B. Laboratory Findings: IgG levels in the serum are less than 100 mg/100 ml, serum IgA and IgM levels are less than 1% of normal, and isohemagglutinins are low or absent. The Schick test is positive, and antitoxin titers do not rise after vaccination with DTP vaccine. The peripheral lymphocyte count and skin reactivity to candida antigen, PPD, and DNCB are normal. There are no immunoglobulin-staining lymphocytes in the peripheral blood in most cases.

Treatment
Recurrent bacterial infections can be prevented by the administration of gamma globulin for an indefinite period of time. The gamma globulin is usually administered intramuscularly. The usual loading dose is 300 mg gamma globulin (~ 1.8 ml) per kg body weight in 3 equally divided injections. Thereafter, monthly injections of 0.6 ml/kg body weight are given to maintain an IgG level of at least 200 mg/100 ml.

THYMIC HYPOPLASIA (DiGeorge's Syndrome)

DiGeorge's syndrome is a failure of embryogenesis of the third and fourth pharyngeal pouches. This results in aplasia of the parathyroid and thymus glands. The syndrome presents as a pure T cell functional deficiency with intact B cell function.

Clinical Findings
A. Symptoms and Signs: The major manifestations are neonatal tetany, hypertelorism, and increased susceptibility to viral, fungal, and bacterial infections. Infections are frequently lethal.
B. Laboratory Findings: Serum immunoglobulin levels are normal. The humoral antibody response may be low or normal depending on the antigen used for immunization. (A low response is thought to be due to lack of T helper cells.) Skin reactivity to intradermal injections of candida antigen or skin painting with DNCB is markedly depressed, as is blastogenesis of peripheral blood lymphocytes upon incubation with PHA or with allogeneic lymphocytes. Serum calcium and the peripheral lymphocyte count are low. Biopsy of lymph nodes shows normal germinal center formation but marked deficits in the thymus-dependent or paracortical areas. There are no T cells in peripheral blood.

Treatment
Transplantation of fetal thymic tissue has been

successful in reversing the deficits in cell-mediated immunity and raising the peripheral lymphocyte count to normal. The thymus-dependent areas of the lymph nodes of such transplant recipients are also repopulated.

SEVERE COMBINED IMMUNODEFICIENCY

Both T and B cell function are markedly decreased in this entity, which is inherited in an autosomal recessive or X-linked pattern. A sporadic appearance in families also occurs. Dysostosis and adenosine deaminase deficiency are associated with severe combined immunodeficiency in some cases.

Clinical Findings
A. Symptoms and Signs: Increased susceptibility to infection is noted at 3–6 months of age. Death usually occurs within 2 years. The period of infancy is marked by watery diarrhea, usually associated with salmonella or enteropathic *Escherichia coli* infections. Pulmonary infections, usually with pseudomonas and *Pneumocystis carinii,* are common, as is candidiasis affecting the mouth and diaper areas. Common viral exanthems such as chickenpox and measles are often lethal.

B. Laboratory Findings: Serum immunoglobulin levels are usually less than 1% of normal, and antibodies do not form in response to vaccinations such as DTP. The peripheral lymphocyte count is less than 2000/cu mm. Decreased delayed hypersensitivity is manifested by lack of skin reactivity to painting with DNCB or intradermal injection with candida antigen. Lymph node biopsy shows no lymphocytes, plasma cells, or lymphoid follicles.

Treatment
Passive administration of gamma globulin is ineffective. Bone marrow transplantation has been successful in several cases, but the complications of graft vs host or secondary disease prevent its widespread use.

IMMUNODEFICIENCY WITH THROMBOCYTOPENIA & ECZEMA (Wiskott-Aldrich Syndrome)

This disorder is characterized by eczema, thrombocytopenia, and recurrent bacterial and viral infections. Inheritance is X-linked, and affected individuals rarely survive more than 10 years. There appears to be a combined T and B cell functional deficit. IgM levels are low and isohemagglutinins absent, but IgG and IgA levels are normal. Cell-mediated immunity is impaired as measured by decreased skin reactivity to common fungal antigens and decreased response to PHA stimulation in vitro.

IMMUNODEFICIENCY WITH ATAXIA-TELANGIECTASIA

The clinical presentation of ataxia-telangiectasia begins in infancy with ataxia and choreoathetoid movements. Telangiectasia of the conjunctiva, face, arms, and eyelids is first noted 5–10 years later. Chronic sinusitis and respiratory infections follow, and death due to intercurrent pulmonary infection or lymphoreticular neoplasm occurs in the second or third decade. Approximately 80% of affected individuals lack serum and secretory IgA. In addition, there is a marked deficit in T cell function associated with a hypoplastic or dysplastic thymus gland. The disease is inherited in an autosomal recessive pattern.

VARIABLE IMMUNODEFICIENCY

Primary Acquired Agammaglobulinemia
Onset is in adulthood with increased susceptibility to pyogenic infections; recurrent sinusitis and pneumonia progressing to bronchiectasis; sprue-like syndrome with diarrhea, steatorrhea, malabsorption, and protein-losing enteropathy; and hepatosplenomegaly.

There is no arthritis of the type associated with congenital agammaglobulinemia. Autoimmune diseases are common. Laboratory study discloses serum IgG levels usually less than 500 mg/100 ml; serum IgA and IgM levels are below the lower limits of normal, but this is variable. Lymph node biopsy shows marked reduction in plasma cells. Noncaseating granulomas are frequently found in the spleen, liver, lungs, or skin.

Recent evidence suggests that suppressor T cells inhibit B cells from producing antibody-forming cells in certain cases of adult-onset agammaglobulinemia. The absolute B cell count in the peripheral blood in these cases is normal. Although therapy at present is similar to that of congenital agammaglobulinemia, newer therapeutic goals may include elimination of suppressor T cells.

Immunodeficiency Associated With Sarcoidosis
The immunodeficiency associated with sarcoidosis is characterized by a partial deficit in T cell function with intact B cell function. Patients with sarcoidosis show a greater incidence (50%) of nonreactivity to intradermal injections of common antigens (candida, mumps, PPD) as compared to controls. However, complete lack of skin reactivity to a battery of skin tests is infrequent. In addition, reactivity is dependent upon the immunogenicity (potency) of the antigenic stimulus. For example, negative reactions may occur after skin painting with DNCB, but skin painting with poison ivy extract regularly elicits a positive reaction. A similarly positive reaction to PPD is usually noted during active infection with *Mycobacterium tuberculosis* but is frequently absent after vaccination with BCG.

Serum immunoglobulin levels are normal or high, and specific antibody formation is generally intact.

Immunodeficiency Associated with Hodgkin's Disease

A moderate to severe deficit in T cell function with intact B cell function is frequently found in Hodgkin's disease. Only 10–20% of patients with Hodgkin's disease show skin reactivity to mumps, candida, or trichophyton antigen as compared to 70–90% of controls. Lack of reactivity to DNCB is also common. Many patients show depressed responses to in vitro stimulation of peripheral blood lymphocytes with PHA. Serum immunoglobulins are normal, and specific antibody formation is intact except in agonal cases.

The clinical significance of depressed cell-mediated immunity in Hodgkin's disease is difficult to evaluate since most patients are treated with potent immunosuppressive agents. Nevertheless, frequent infections with herpes zoster and cryptococcus are probably related to immunodeficiency associated with the underlying disease.

Table 33–2. Mechanisms of injury in common types of autoimmune disease.

Mechanism of Tissue Injury	Disease and Target Tissue
Immune complex disease	Systemic lupus erythematosus: Glomerulonephritis secondary to attachmentof anti-DNA-DNA immune complexes and complement to glomerular basement membrane. Rheumatoid arthritis: Arthritis secondary to fixation of complement by anti-IgG-IgG immune complexes in joint fluid and synovial linings.

(Similar mechanisms may be involved in poststreptococcal glomerulonephritis, hypocomplementemic nephritis, and polyarteritis nodosa.)

Mechanism of Tissue Injury	Disease and Target Tissue
Cell-mediated (T cell) immune injury	Autoimmune thyroiditis: Thyroiditis secondary to direct tissue injury by autoimmunized killer T cells. Polymyositis: Myositis secondary to direct injury of skeletal muscle fibers by killer T cells.
Humoral antibody–mediated immune injury	Goodpasture's syndrome: Glomerulonephritis secondary to attachment of anti-basement membrane antibody and complement to glomerular basement membrane. Autoimmune hemolytic anemia: Hemolysis secondary to attachment of antibodies to red blood cells and subsequent removal by spleen or intravascular complement-dependent lysis.

(Similar mechanisms may be involved in systemic lupus erythematosus, idiopathic thrombocytopenic purpura, Sjögren's syndrome, and pernicious anemia.)

SELECTIVE IMMUNOGLOBULIN DEFICIENCY

Absence of serum IgA with normal levels of IgG and IgM is found in a small percentage of normal individuals. Occasionally, a sprue-like syndrome with steatorrhea has been associated with an isolated IgA deficit. Treatment with commercial gamma globulin (Cohn fraction II) is ineffective since IgA and IgM are not present in this preparation. Frequent infusions of plasma (containing IgA) are hazardous since anti-IgA antibodies may develop, resulting in systemic anaphylaxis or serum sickness.

AUTOIMMUNE DISEASES

The diagnosis and treatment of specific autoimmune diseases are described elsewhere in this volume according to the diseased target organ or tissue. Mechanisms of tissue injury which are common to some of these diseases are listed in Table 33–2. Autoantibodies associated with certain autoimmune diseases do not appear to be implicated in the pathogenesis of tissue injury but are thought instead to be by-products of the injury (eg, autoimmune thyroiditis and antithyroglobulin antibody).

ASSOCIATIONS BETWEEN HL-A AND MLC ANTIGENS AND SPECIFIC DISEASE ENTITIES

Table 33–3 is a partial list of some of the stronger and more interesting associations between HL-A and specific diseases. These associations range from the very strong association between HL-A 27 and those rheumatic syndromes in which sacroiliitis and spondylitis play a prominent part (ankylosing spondylitis, Reiter's disease, and psoriatic spondylitis as well as spondylitis associated with ulcerative colitis and regional enteritis) to those associations which, while statistically significant, are very weak, such as the association between HL-A 7 and multiple sclerosis. Thus, the association between HL-A 27 and ankylosing spondylitis is such that 90% of patients with this disease possess the 27 antigen while only 4–7% of the control population carries the same antigen. On the other hand, in multiple sclerosis, 36% of the patients are HL-A 7 positive, while the same antigen is found in 25% of normal controls. The strong association between HL-A 27 and ankylosing spondylitis is already proving of diagnostic v8lue in many clinical situations in which a young individual, particularly a male, develops peripheral arthritis which is seronegative and there is no evident spondylitis. However, the association between HL-A 7 and multiple sclerosis is not strong enough to be of any diagnostic value.

Table 33–3. HL-A and disease associations.

Disease	HL-A Antigen	Frequency in Patients (%)	Frequency in Controls (%)
Ankylosing spondylitis	27	90	7
Reiter's disease	27	76	6
Acute anterior uveitis	27	55	8
Psoriasis	13	18	4
	17	29	8
	16	15	5
Graves' disease	8	47	21
Celiac disease (gluten-sensitive enteropathy)	8	78	24
Dermatitis herpetiformis	8	62	27
Myasthenia gravis	8	52	24
Systemic lupus erythematosus	15	33	8
Multiple sclerosis	3	36	25
	7	36	25
Acute lymphatic leukemia	2	63	37
Hodgkin's disease	4c(5)	25	16
	1	39	32
	8	26	22
Chronic hepatitis	8	68	18
Ragweed hay fever			
Ra 5 sensitivity	7	50	19
Allergen E sensitivity	Multiple (in family studies)		

Table 33–4. Association of HL-A and rheumatic diseases.

Disease	HL-A Antigen	Controls (%)	Patients, (%)
Ankylosing spondylitis	27	4–7	90
Reiter's disease	27	4–7	76
Acute anterior uveitis	27	4–7	60
Psoriatic arthritis			
With sacroiliitis	27	4–7	35
Without sacroiliitis	27	4–7	18
Chronic inflammatory bowel disease			
With spondylitis	27	6	67
Without spondylitis	27	6	...
Juvenile rheumatoid arthritis	27	6	39–42
Yersinia enterocolitica arthritis	27	14	88
Systemic lupus erythematosus (white)	15	8	36
Systemic lupus erythematosus (black)	5	15	40–50
Rheumatoid arthritis	"Ra"	8	60–70

Many of the other diseases listed in Table 33–3 show strong but not complete associations between HL-A and diseases, eg, myasthenia gravis. Some of these diseases show a stronger association with a particular MLC type than they do with the HL-A antigens. Thus, in multiple sclerosis, MLC type 7a (which is frequently found on the same chromosome with HL-A antigen 7) is very strongly associated with multiple sclerosis. In Denmark, where the most extensive studies have been done, 70% of patients with multiple sclerosis possess the MLC-7a antigens, while only 30–40% possess HL-A 7. Since MLC-7a is found in only 14–15% of the control population, this association reaches the level of diagnostic significance and usefulness in individual patient diagnosis. A similar association between MLC-8a and myasthenia gravis has also been found.

Table 33–4 lists the associations between HL-A and MLC and the rheumatic diseases. In addition to the very strong association between HL-A W27 and many different types of rheumatic disease, it is important to note that in recent work one particular MLC type, so far only given the designation "Ra," is found in 50–70% of patients with rheumatoid arthritis, although it is only present in 8–10% of a normal control population. Thus, rheumatoid arthritis also appears to

be a disease which shows a very strong association with a particular MLC type, although no association has yet been detected with a particular HL-A antigen.

The mechanism responsible for all of these associations between HL-A and particular diseases is not yet known. While it is frequently assumed that these associations reflect the action of a specific immune response (Ir) gene, this has not yet been proved for any human disease and for only one animal model (ie, autoimmune thyroiditis in the mouse). While other mechanisms may be involved, it seems clear that as typing methods improve these associations will prove to be of increasing diagnostic and prognostic value.

Bergsma D, McKusick V (editors): *Immunologic Deficiency Diseases in Man.* (National Foundation–March of Dimes original article series.) Williams & Wilkins, 1974.

Blaese RM & others: The Wiskott-Aldrich syndrome: A disorder with a possible defect in antigen processing or recognition. Lancet 1:1056, 1968.

Bobrove AM & others: Quantitation of T and B lymphocytes and cellular immune function in Hodgkin's disease. Cancer 36:169, 1975.

Peterson RDA, Cooper MD, Good RA: Lymphoid tissue abnormalities associated with ataxia-telangectasia. Am J Med 41:342, 1966.

Samter M (editor):*Immunologic Diseases.* Vol 2. Little, Brown, 1971.

Svejgaard A & others: HL-A and disease associations: A survey. Transplant Rev 22:1, 1975.

Waldmann TA & others: Role of suppressor T cells in pathogenesis of common variable hypogammaglobulinemia. Lancet 2:609, 1974.

Appendix

The Problem-Oriented Record (POR) 999

Medical Recommendations for Foreign Travel 1000

Recommended Schedule for Active Immunization & Skin Testing of Children 1001

Recommended Immunization of Adults for Travel 1002

Hypersensitivity Tests & Desensitization 1003

Chemical Constituents of Blood & Body Fluids 1003

Normal Values 1018

Conversion Tables 1021

Nomograms for Determination of Body Surface Area 1023

Abbreviations 1024

Schedules of Controlled Drugs 1025

Heart-Lung Resuscitation 1026

THE PROBLEM-ORIENTED RECORD (POR)

The Weed system of problem-oriented record-keeping offers a systematic and efficient method of recording the diagnosis, treatment, and follow-up care of patients.

The patient's complete medical history, physical findings, and initial laboratory findings provide the information (data base) which enables the physician to define and enumerate the significant clinical problems (complete problem list) that require solution. These "problems" may be partially or definitely diagnosed diseases, psychosocial difficulties, or significant but unexplained symptoms or physical and laboratory findings. The problems are numbered at the outset in logical priorities; all further diagnostic and therapeutic plans and progress notes are identically numbered. Thus it is possible to follow the status of each problem—resolved or unresolved—at any given time. Progress notes are recorded both in narrative form and on flow sheets.

The Weed system is valuable as an educational device for the physician in training, and it may also be useful to the more experienced clinician in establishing diagnostic and therapeutic priorities and evaluating results of therapy. As with the conventional source-oriented record, the problem-oriented record requires valid observations and adequate language to record the observations.

The system lends itself well to peer review and to computer use for quality control and data compilation for medical research.

All clinicians should be familiar with the Weed system and some of the current references dealing with its advantages and limitations.

Feinstein AR: The problems of the "problem-oriented medical record." Ann Int Med 78:751, 1973.

Fletcher RH: Auditing problem-oriented records and traditional records. New England J Med 290:829, 1974.

Goldfinger SE: The problem-oriented record: A critique from a believer. New England J Med 288:606, 1973.

Hirsch EO: A problem-and-objective-oriented approach to patient-care evaluation. New England J Med 292:1348, 1975.

Hurst JW, Walker HK: *The Problem-Oriented System.* Medcom, 1974.

Problem-oriented medical records. Lancet 1:295, 1972.

Weed LL: *Medical Records, Medical Education and Patient Care: The Problem-Oriented Record as a Basic Tool.* Year Book, 1970.

MEDICAL RECOMMENDATIONS FOR FOREIGN TRAVEL

Medical advice for the traveler will naturally vary with the geographic destination, the length and nature of the trip, the mode of travel, the health of the patient, special local health hazards, and the adequacy of medical resources in the areas to be visited. When contemplating foreign travel, it is always advisable to plan well ahead (ie, about 2 months, especially for required inoculations).

A thorough current physical examination is advisable not only for health reasons but also for certification of freedom from physical, mental, or communicable disease, which may be required in certain countries. A current dental examination and needed dental care are recommended prior to travel.

Patients should be advised about the necessity for avoiding physical exhaustion and dietary and alcohol excesses and of the possible physiologic effect of rapid changes in time zones.

Special local conditions of the foreign area which must be considered—especially when they vary considerably from those at home—include extremes of temperature, altitude, endemic or epidemic diseases, transportation facilities, living accommodations, and the quality of food and water supplies. Language barriers may pose a difficulty if medical problems arise.

Organizations or agencies which provide various types of general or special services for travelers include the following:

Organization	Services
1. Health departments (local and state) or travel agencies.	Information regarding health precautions and required inoculations.
2. American embassies or consulates in foreign countries.	Advice regarding local physicians, hospitals, and general health problems.
3. Medical Passport Foundation, 35 East Sixty-Ninth St., New York 10021.	Detailed health form, including recent laboratory reports and ECG tracings, provided by traveler's physician (nominal fee).
4. Medic Alert Foundation International, Turlock, CA 95380	Metal medical identification emblems. Twenty-four-hour international collect call medical information (nominal fee).
5. International Associations for Medical Assistance to Travelers (IAMAT), 745 Fifth Ave., New York 10022	Information regarding well trained English-speaking physicians in over 50 countries (no fee).
6. Intermedic, 777 Third Ave., New York 10017	Information regarding well trained English-speaking physicians in over 50 countries (no fee).

Active Immunization Against Infectious Diseases

Every individual, child or adult, should be adequately immunized against infectious diseases. The schedule of administration, dose, and recommended method of choice vary with each product and change often. Always consult the manufacturer's package insert and follow its recommendations.

The schedule for active immunizations in childhood (Table 1) is adapted from: *Report,* 16th ed, by the Committee on Control of Infectious Diseases, American Academy of Pediatrics, 1970.

Regularly Prescribed Medications

The traveler should take along a sufficient quantity of chronically required nonperishable medications, needles, syringes, etc to cover his entire trip plus an adequate reserve supply in case of delays, loss, or breakage. Although the same drugs are available in most countries, they frequently have unfamiliar names, may require prescriptions from local physicians, and may be of variable quality. Some drugs available in foreign countries have not yet been admitted to the American market. Unfamiliar nonprescription (over-the-counter) drugs are especially to be avoided.

Patients with chronic illness which requires treatment (eg, diabetes mellitus, heart disease) should be given a concise statement of their condition and treatment regimen which can be shown to a physician in case of need. A medical identification tag, bracelet, or card (eg, diabetes mellitus, drug allergy) should be carried. Advise patients that insulin preparations are preferably refrigerated to maintain full potency. If this is not possible during travel, the insulin should be protected against warming or freezing. Advance inquiry about the availability of the prescribed type of insulin and facilities for refrigeration is essential. Travel agents and consular representatives can provide the names of physicians or hospitals in the vicinity.

Contingency Drugs & Supplies

A. Systemic Anti-infectives: If exposure to infectious and parasitic diseases (eg, malaria) is a prominent risk in the areas to be visited, appropriate drugs should be carried with instructions for use.

B. Local Anti-infectives and Protectives: Topical anti-infective ointments (eg, bacitracin, neomycin) and adhesive bandages are all that is necessary for minor cuts and abrasions. Prevent sunburn with protective lotions or creams. Use dusting powder for moist areas of the body in humid climates, especially in socks.

C. Antinauseants: Any of several motion sickness remedies can be used. The best results are achieved when these preparations are taken one-half hour before departure.

D. Antacids: For minor gastric upsets due to overindulgence or unfamiliar foods.

Table 1. Recommended schedule for active immunization and skin testing of children.

Age	Product Administered	Test Recommended
2–3 months	DTP[1] Oral poliovaccine[2], trivalent	
3–4 months	DTP	
4–5 months	DTP Oral poliovaccine, trivalent	
10–12 months		Tuberculin test
12 months	Measles vaccine[3]	
15–19 months	DTP Oral poliovaccine, trivalent	
3–4 years	DTP Rubella vaccine[5]	Tuberculin test[4]
6 years	TD[6] Oral poliovaccine, trivalent	Tuberculin test[4]
8–10 years	Mumps vaccine[7]	Tuberculin test[4]
12–14 years	TD	Tuberculin test

[1] **DTP:** Toxoids of diphtheria and tetanus, alum-precipitated or aluminum hydroxide absorbed, combined with pertussis bacterial antigen. Suitable for young children. Three doses of 0.5 ml IM at intervals of 4–8 weeks. Fourth injection of 0.5 ml IM given about 1 year later.

[2] **Oral live poliomyelitis virus vaccine:** Trivalent (types 1, 2, and 3 combined) is preferred. Trivalent given 3 times at intervals of 6–8 weeks and then as a booster 1 year later. Inactive (Salk type) trivalent vaccine is available but not recommended.

[3] **Live measles virus vaccine,** 0.5 ml IM. When using attenuated (Edmonston) strain, give human gamma globulin, 0.01 ml/lb, injected into the opposite arm at the same time, to lessen the reaction to the vaccine. This is not advised with "further attenuated" (Schwarz) strain. Inactivated measles vaccine should not be used. At 1 year of age, combined live attenuated measles-mumps-rubella vaccine may be given (see notes 5 and 7).

[4] The frequency with which **tuberculin tests** are administered depends on the risk of exposure, ie, the prevalence of tuberculosis in the population group.

[5] **Rubella live virus vaccine (attenuated)** may be given between age 1 year and puberty. Administration to adolescent girls is preferred by some. The entire contents of a single-dose vaccine vial, reconstituted from the lyophilized state, are injected subcutaneously. The vaccine must *not* be given to women who are pregnant or are likely to become pregnant within 3 months of vaccination. Adult women must also be warned that there is a 40% likelihood of developing arthralgias and arthritis (presumably self-limited) within 4 weeks of vaccination. Reinfection with wild-type virus can occur in vaccinated persons.

[6] **Tetanus toxoid** and **diphtheria toxoid,** purified, suitable for adults, given to adults every 7–10 years.

[7] **Live mumps virus vaccine (attenuated),** 0.5 ml IM.

E. Antidiarrheal Precautions:

1. **Preventive**—Minor gastrointestinal disturbances are usually physiologic responses to changing time-tables and habits. If water is of doubtful purity, use halogen or iodine preparations as directed below.

2. **Therapeutic**—Diphenoxylate (Lomotil), 2.5 mg following each liquid bowel movement, or 3–4 times daily as needed. Give codeine, 30 mg, for severe diarrhea, severe cramps, or tenesmus.

F. Sedatives*: Sedative-hypnotic drugs can be used for very nervous, anxious patients who are fearful of flying, or for sleep.

G. Analgesics: Aspirin for headache or moderate pain. If codeine is carried as an antidiarrheal agent, it can be used if a stronger analgesic is required.* An anesthetic ointment may be useful for burns or pruritus.

H. Eyeglasses: Either a prescription or an extra pair of glasses should be carried.

I. Dentures: If dentures are required, spare dentures should be carried.

J. A supply of commercial handwashing packets should be carried.

K. Insect Repellents: These may not only provide comfort against annoying insects but may prevent serious diseases transmitted by insects. Dimethylphthalate and many proprietary preparations are available (eg, Off, 612). Apply repeatedly to exposed skin. Long-sleeved clothing and full-length trousers are required in areas where there are many insects.

Food & Water Safety

A. Water Purification: A dropper bottle filled with ordinary household sodium hypochlorite bleaching solution (eg, Clorox, Purex) can be used to make water safer for drinking. One drop to 1 glass of water will serve for water that is not grossly contaminated. Allow to stand for 15 minutes before drinking. Muddy

*All medications should be carried in their originally prescribed and properly labeled containers—especially sedatives, hypnotics, and narcotics. Sedatives, hypnotics, and narcotics should not be carried in large quantities. It is advisable for the attending physician to provide a written prescription or statement describing the need for all medication and hypodermic syringes (eg, for diabetics). (Harper SB: Letter to Editor. JAMA 221:715, 1972.)

water or water containing organic material should be filtered or allowed to clarify for several hours and decanted into a clean glass. Two drops of sodium hypochlorite solution are then added. Allow to stand for 15 minutes before drinking.

Globaline, an iodine compound, may be used to purify drinking water. It is available in tablet form. Add 1 tablet per pint of water and let stand at least 3 minutes. It may cause a brown precipitate.

Precautions: Water, ice, or soft drinks of doubtful purity should not be used. Bottled or pure water should be used for drinking and brushing teeth.

B. Food Safety: Unless in an area with high sanitary standards, it is generally inadvisable to eat local raw fruits and vegetables and raw fish or shellfish. Hot foods, thoroughly cooked (especially in the case of pork), are the safest; avoid stews and chopped meats when questionable. Dairy products which require pasteurization, as well as all meats or other proteins, may be dangerous if not kept under refrigeration.

C. Swimming Safety: Water may not be safe for swimming purposes in either natural water resources or in swimming pools in certain areas. It is best to check with responsible local health authorities.

Barrett-Connor E: Advice to travelers. Western J Med 123:22, 1975.

Drugs purchased abroad: Caution to travelers. Med Lett Drugs Ther 15:48, 1973.

Gorbach S & others: Traveler's diarrhea and toxigenic *Escherichia coli.* New England J Med 292:933, 1975.

Physician's Guide to Medical Advice for Overseas Travelers. American Medical Association, 1975.

Ramras DG: Immunizations and prophylaxis for foreign travelers. California Med 118:92, May 1973.

Rowland HAK: Going abroad. Brit MJ 1:639, 1972.

RECOMMENDED IMMUNIZATION OF ADULTS FOR TRAVEL

Every adult, whether traveling or not, must be immunized with tetanus toxoid. Purified toxoid "for adult use" must be used to avoid reactions. Every adult should also receive primary vaccination for poliomyelitis (oral live trivalent vaccine) and for diphtheria (use purified toxoid "for adult use"). Every traveler must fulfill the immunization requirements of the health authorities of different countries. These are listed in *Immunization Information for International Travel,* USPHS, Division of Foreign Quarantine, 7915 Eastern Ave., Silver Spring, Maryland 20910.

The following are suggestions for travel in different parts of the world.

Tetanus

Booster injection of 0.5 ml tetanus toxoid, for adult use, every 7–10 years, assuming completion of primary immunization. (All countries.)

Smallpox

Vaccination or revaccination with live smallpox vaccine (vaccinia virus) by multiple pressure method is recommended for travelers to all smallpox endemic areas. WHO certificate requires registration of batch number of vaccine. The physician should ascertain a "take" by observing vesicle formation after administration of either liquid or freeze-dried effective vaccine. (Some countries.)

Typhoid

Suspension of killed *Salmonella typhi.* For primary immunization, inject 0.5 ml subcut (0.25 ml for children under 10 years) twice at an interval of 4–6 weeks. For booster, inject 0.5 ml subcut (or 0.1 ml intradermally) every 3 years. (Some countries.)

Paratyphoid vaccines are not recommended and are probably ineffective at present.

Yellow Fever

Live attenuated yellow fever virus, 0.5 ml subcut. WHO certificate requires registration of batch number of vaccine. Vaccination available in USA only at approved centers. Vaccination must be repeated at intervals of 10 years or less. (Africa, South America.)

Cholera

Suspension of killed vibrios, including prevalent antigenic types. Two injections of 0.5 and 1 ml are given IM 4–6 weeks apart. This must be followed by 0.5 ml booster injections every 6 months during periods of possible exposure. Protection depends largely on booster doses. WHO certificate is valid for 6 months only. (Middle Eastern countries, Asia, occasionally others.)

Plague

Suspension of killed plague bacilli given IM, 2 injections of 0.5 ml each, 4–6 weeks apart, and a third injection 6 months later. (Asia, occasionally South America and others.)

Typhus

Suspension of egg-grown inactivated typhus rickettsiae given subcut, 2 injections of 0.5 ml each, 4–6 weeks apart. Booster doses of 0.5 ml every 6 months may be necessary. (Southeastern Europe, Africa, South America.)

Hepatitis

No active immunization available. Temporary passive immunity may be induced by the IM injection of human gamma globulin, 0.02 ml/kg every 2–3 months, or 0.1 ml/kg every 6 months. Recommended for all parts of the world where environmental sanitation is poor and the risk of exposure to infectious hepatitis high through contaminated food and water and contact with infected persons.

Advisory Committee on Immunization Practices: *Recommendations.* USPHS Publication No. (HSM) 72-8154, 1972.

Committee on Control of Infectious Diseases: *Report,* 16th ed. American Academy of Pediatrics, 1970.

Immunization Information for International Travel. USPHS, Division of Foreign Quarantine, 7915 Eastern Ave., Silver Spring, Maryland 20910.

Peebles TC & others: Tetanus toxoid emergency boosters: A reappraisal. New England J Med 280:575, 1969.

Tahernia AC: Diphtheria: Still lethal. Clin Pediat 8:508, 1969.

Woodson RD & others: Hepatitis prophylaxis abroad. JAMA 209:1053, 1969.

HYPERSENSITIVITY TESTS & DESENSITIZATION

Tests for Hypersensitivity

Before injecting antitoxin or similar material derived from animal sources, always perform the following tests for hypersensitivity. If both tests are negative, desensitization is not necessary and a full dose of the antitoxin may be given. If one or both of the tests are positive, desensitization is necessary.

A. Intradermal Test: Inject 0.1 ml of a 1:10 dilution of the antitoxin intradermally on the flexor surface of the forearm. A large wheal and surrounding areola appearing within 5–20 minutes constitute a positive test.

B. Conjunctival Test: Instill 1 drop of a 1:10 dilution of the antitoxin into the conjunctival sac of one eye as a test dose and 1 drop of physiologic saline into the other eye as a control. Conjunctival redness, itching, and lacrimation appearing within 5–20 minutes in the test eye constitute a positive test.

Desensitization

A. Precautionary Measures:

1. If extreme hypersensitivity is suspected, it is advisable to have desensitization performed by one who is experienced in dealing with such problems.

2. An antihistaminic drug should be administered before beginning desensitization in order to lessen any reaction that might occur.

3. Epinephrine, 0.5–1 ml of 1:1000 solution, must be ready for immediate administration.

B. Desensitization Method: The following plan may be used in desensitization. Give doses of antitoxin intramuscularly at 30-minute intervals and observe closely for reactions.

1st dose: 0.1 ml (1:10 dilution)
2nd dose: 0.2 ml (1:10 dilution)
3rd dose: 0.5 ml (1:10 dilution)
4th dose: 0.1 ml (undiluted)
5th dose: 0.2 ml (undiluted)
6th dose: 0.5 ml (undiluted)
7th dose: 1 ml (undiluted)
8th and subsequent doses: 1 ml (undiluted) every 30 minutes until the total amount of antitoxin is given.

Treatment of Reactions

A. Mild: If a mild reaction occurs, drop back to the next lower dose and continue with desensitization. If a severe reaction occurs, administer epinephrine (see below) and discontinue the antitoxin unless treatment is urgently needed. If desensitization is imperative, continue slowly, increasing the dosage of the antitoxin more gradually.

B. Severe: If manifestations of a severe reaction appear, give 0.5–1 ml of 1:1000 epinephrine subcut at once. The symptoms include urticaria, angioneurotic edema, dyspnea, coughing, choking, and shock. Observe the patient closely and repeat epinephrine as necessary (see p 12).

Corticosteroids may be used (eg, hydrocortisone, 100 mg IV), but their effect begins only after 18 hours.

Brown EA: The conjunctival test (2 parts.) Ann Allergy 20:608, 674, 1962.

Hartman MM: Capabilities and limitations of major drug groups in allergy: The role within current theories. Ann Allergy 27:164, 1969.

Samter M & others: Answers to questions on allergic emergencies. Hosp Med 4:61, 1968.

Sherman WB: *Hypersensitivity: Mechanism and Management.* Saunders, 1968.

CHEMICAL CONSTITUENTS OF BLOOD & BODY FLUIDS

Interpretation of Laboratory Tests

Normal values are those that fall within 2 standard deviations from the mean value for the normal population. This normal range encompasses 95% of the population. Many factors may affect values and influence the normal range; by the same token, various factors may produce values that are normal under the prevailing conditions but outside the 95% limits determined under other circumstances. These factors include age, race, sex, environment, posture, and diurnal and other cyclic variations. (See Tables 2 and 3.)

Normal values vary with the method employed, the laboratory, and conditions of collection and preservation of specimens. With increasing awareness of the proper application of laboratory control of performance and of method, variations in normal values occur less frequently. The normal values established by individual laboratories should be clearly expressed to ensure proper interpretation by the physician.

Interpretation of laboratory results must always be related to the condition of the patient. A low value may be the result of deficit or of dilution of the substance measured, eg, low serum sodium. Deviation from normal may be associated with a specific disease or with some drug consumed by the subject—eg, gout and treatment with chlorothiazides or with antineoplastic agents are associated with elevated serum uric acid concentrations. (See Tables 5 and 6.)

Values may be influenced by the method of collection of the specimen. Inaccurate collection of a 24-hour urine specimen, variations in concentration of the randomly collected urine specimen, hemolysis in a blood sample, addition of an inappropriate anticoagulant, and contaminated glassware or other apparatus are examples of causes of erroneous results.

Note: Whenever an unusual or abnormal result is obtained, all possible sources of error must be considered before responding with therapy based on the laboratory report. Laboratory medicine is a specialty, and experts in the field should be consulted whenever results are unusual or in doubt.

Validity of Laboratory Tests*

The clinical value of a test is related to its specificity and sensitivity and the incidence of the disease in the population tested.

Specificity means percentage of negative results among people who do not have the disease. The test for phenylketonuria is highly specific: 99.9% of normal individuals give a negative result. In contrast, the CEA (carcinoembryonic antigen) test for carcinoma of the colon has a variable specificity: about 3% of nonsmoking individuals give a false positive result (97% specificity), whereas in smokers 20% give positive results (80% specificity). The overlap of serum thyroxine levels between hyperthyroid patients and those on oral contraceptives or those who are pregnant is an example of a change in specificity from that prevailing in a different set of individuals.

Sensitivity means percentage of positive results in patients with the disease. The test for phenylketonuria is highly sensitive: a positive result is obtained in all who have the disease (100% sensitivity). The CEA test has low specificity: only 72% of those with carcinoma of the colon provide a positive result when the disease is extensive and only 20% are positive with early disease. Lower sensitivity occurs in the early stages of many diseases—in contrast to the higher sensitivity in well-established disease.

The predictive value of a positive test defines the percentage of positive results that are true positives. This is related fundamentally to the incidence of the disease. In a group of patients on a urology service, the incidence of renal disease is higher than in the general population and the serum creatinine level will have a higher predictive value in that group than for the general population.

Tables 2 and 3 indicate the different predictive values of a test with high specificity (95%) and high sensitivity (95%) when the incidence of the disease is 10% and 1% in a population of 10,000 subjects.

*This section is an abridged version of an article by Krieg AF, Gambino R, Galen RS: Why are clinical laboratory tests performed? When are they valid? JAMA 233:76, 1975. Reprinted from the Journal of the American Medical Association. Copyright 1975. American Medical Association.

Table 2. Data for disease with 10% incidence. (Sensitivity and specificity, 95%.)

Subjects	Number With Positive Test	Number With Negative Test
1000 diseased	950	50
9000 nondiseased	450	8550
Total	**1400**	**8600**

Table 3. Data for disease with 1% incidence. (Sensitivity and specificity, 95%.)

Subjects	Number With Positive Test	Number With Negative Test
100 diseased	95	5
9900 nondiseased	495	9405
Total	**590**	**9410**

Table 4. Effect of incidence on predictive value of positive result.

Prevalence (%)	Predictive Value of a Positive Result (%)
0.1	2
1.0	16
2.0	28
5.0	50
10.0	68
50.0	95

Table 4 shows the effect of incidence on the predictive value of a test with 95% sensitivity and 95% specificity.

Before ordering a test, attempt to determine whether test sensitivity, specificity, and predictive value are adequate to provide useful information. To be useful, the result should influence diagnosis, prognosis, or therapy; lead to a better understanding of the disease process; and benefit the patient.

Effect of Meals & Posture on Concentration of Substances in Blood

A. Meals: The usual normal values for blood tests have been determined by assay of "fasting" specimens collected after 8–12 hours of abstinence from food. With few exceptions, water is usually permitted as desired.

Few routine tests are altered from usual fasting values if blood is drawn 3–4 hours after breakfast. When blood is drawn 3–4 hours after lunch, values are more likely to vary from those of the true fasting state (ie, as much as +31% for glutamic-oxaloacetic transaminase [GOT], −5% for lactate dehydrogenase, and lesser variations for other substances). Valid measurement of triglyceride in serum or plasma requires abstinence from food for 10–14 hours.

Table 5. Drugs interfering directly with chemical tests.*

Many drugs and metabolites react with ferric chloride and affect tests for ketone bodies, phenylpyruvic acid, homogentisic acid, and melanogen. Dyes (eg, methylene blue, phenazopyridine, BSP, phenolsulfon-phthalein, indigocarmine, indocyanine green, azure A) color plasma and urine; they affect most colorimetric procedures. Some drugs act as indicators (eg, phenolphthalein, vegetable laxatives) and affect tests carried out at a particular pH.

Test	Drug	Effect†	Cause
Bilirubin	Caffeine, theophylline	−	Color reaction depressed
BSP	Dyes (eg, phenazopyridine)	+	Interfering color
Calcium	Edathamil (EDTA)	−	Interferes with dye-binding methods; no effect on flame methods
Chloride	Bromide	+	Reacts like chloride
Cholesterol	Bromide	+	Enhances color when iron reagent used
Glucose	Dextran	+	Copper complex in copper reduction methods
Iron	Intravenous iron-dextran	+	Total iron increased
Iron-binding capacity (unsaturated)	Intravenous iron-dextran	−	Available transferrin saturated
Protein	Dextran	−	Hemodilution
Quinidine	Triamterene	+	Interfering fluorescence
Uric acid	Ascorbic acid, theophylline	+	Phosphotungstic acid reduced
Urine			
Catecholamines	Erythromycin, methyldopa, tetracyclines, quinine, quinidine, salicylates, hydralazine, B vitamins (high dose)	+	Interfering fluorescence
Chloride	Bromide	+	Reacts like chloride
Creatinine	Nitrofuran derivatives	+	React with color reagent
Glucose	Some vaginal powders	+	Contain glucose: urine contaminated
(Benedict's test)	Drugs excreted as glucuronates	+	Reduce Benedict's reagent
	Salicylates	+	Excreted as salicyluric acid
	Ascorbic acid (high doses)	+	Reduces Benedict's reagent
	Chloral hydrate	+	Metabolites reduce
	Nitrofuran derivatives	+	Metabolites reduce
	Cephalothin	+	Black-brown color
5-HIAA	Phenothiazines	−	Inhibit color reaction
	Mephenesin, methocarbamol	+	Similar color reaction
17-OH steroids, 17-Ketogenic steroids,	Meprobamate, phenothiazines, spironolactone, penicillin G	+	Increases absorbance of final reaction mixture
17-Ketosteroids	Cortisone	+	Measured as part of steroid in sample
		+	Mainly 17-OH and 17-KGS
Pregnanediol	Mandelamine	+	Unknown
Protein	Tolbutamide	+	Metabolite precipitated by salicylsulfonic acid and by heat and acetic acid
Phenolsulfonphthalein	Dyes and BSP	+	Interfering colors
Uric acid	Theophylline, ascorbic acid	+	Phosphotungstic acid reduced
Vanilmandelic acid	Mandelamine	+	Similar color

*Modified and reproduced, with permission, from Lubran M: The effects of drugs on laboratory values. M Clin North America 53:211, 1969.

†+ indicates a false-positive or enhanced effect; − a false-negative or diminished effect.

Table 6. Drugs affecting prothrombin time (Quick one-stage test) of patients on anticoagulant therapy with coumarin or phenindione derivatives.*

Prothrombin Time Increased By	Prothrombin Time Decreased By
ACTH	Antihistamines
Alcohol (in large amounts)	Barbiturates
Amidopyrin	Corticosteroids
Aminosalicylic acid	Digitalis (in cardiac failure)
Anabolic steroids (eg, norethandrolone)	Diuretics
Benziodarone	Glutethimide
Broad-spectrum antibiotics (eg, tetracyclines)	Griseofulvin
Chloral hydrate	Meprobamate
Cholestyramine	Mineral oil
Clofibrate	Oral contraceptives
Diazoxide	Rifampin
Diphenylhydantoin	Vitamin K (in polyvitamin preparations and
Heparin	some diets)
Hydroxyzine	Xanthines (eg, caffeine)
Indomethacin	
Mefenamic acid	
Methylthiouracil, propylthiouracil	
Oral sulfonamides	
Phenylbutazone, oxyphenbutazone	
Phenyramidol	
Quinine, quinidine	
Salicylates (in excess of 1 gm per day)	
Thyroid hormones	
D-Thyroxine	

*Modified and reproduced, with permission, from Lubran M: The effects of drugs on laboratory values. M Clin North America 53:211, 1969.

B. Posture: Plasma volume measured in a person who has been supine for several hours is 12–15% greater than in a person who has been up and about or standing for an hour or so. It follows that measurements performed on blood obtained after the subject has been lying down for an hour or more will yield lower values than when blood has been obtained after the same subject has been upright. An intermediate change apparently occurs with sitting.

Values in the same subject change when position changes from supine to standing as follows: increase in total protein, albumin, calcium, potassium, phosphate, cholesterol, triglyceride, glutamic-oxaloacetic transaminase (GOT), the phosphatases, total thyroxine, and hematocrit, erythrocyte count, and hemoglobin. The greatest change occurs in concentration of total protein and enzymes (+11%) and calcium (+3 to +4%). In a series of studies, change from the upright to the supine position resulted in the following decreases: total protein, −0.5 gm; albumin, −0.4 to −0.6 gm; calcium, −0.4 mg; cholesterol, −10 to −25 mg; total thyroxine −0.8 to −1.8 μg; hematocrit, −4 to −9%, reflecting hemodilution as interstitial fluid reentered the circulation.

A tourniquet applied for 1 minute instead of 3 minutes produced the following changes in reported values: total protein, +5%; iron, +6.7%; cholesterol, +5%; glutamic-oxaloacetic transaminase, +9.3%; and bilirubin, +8.4%. Decreases were observed for potassium, −6%; and creatinine, −2.3%.

SI Units *(Système International d'Unités)*

A "coherent" system of measurement has been under development by an international organization designated the General Conference of Weights and Measures. An adaptation has been tentatively recommended by the Commission on Quantities and Units of the Section on Clinical Chemistry, International Union of Pure and Applied Chemistry. SI units are in use in some European countries, and the conversion to SI will continue if the system proves to be helpful in understanding physiologic mechanisms.

Eight fundamental measurable properties of matter (with authorized abbreviations shown in parentheses) were selected for clinical use:*

length: metre (m)
mass: kilogram (kg)
amount of substance: mole (mol)
time: second (s)
thermodynamic temperature: kelvin (K)

*Note to the reader: The "British" spellings metre and litre should be accepted as part of the SI vocabulary. The British (or French) gramme, kilogramme, etc are spelled gram, kilogram, etc in all of the American (USA) discussions of these matters the editors have seen. In giving SI measurements in the following pages, gram will be abbreviated g although we have used gm in the surrounding text. In giving traditional measurements, the American spelling of liter will be used.

electric current: ampere (A)
luminous intensity: candela (cd)
catalytic activity: katal (kat)

Derived from these are the following measurable properties:

mass concentration: kilogram/litre (k/l)
mass fraction: kilogram/kilogram (k/k)
volume fraction: litre/litre (l/l)
volume: cubic metre (m^3); for clinical use, the unit will be the litre (l)
substance concentration: mole/litre (mol/l)
molality: mole/kilogram (mol/kg)
mole fraction: mole/mole (mol/mol)
pressure: pascal = newton/m^2 (Pa)

Decimal factors are as follows:

Number	Name	Symbol
10^{12}	tera	T
10^9	giga	G
10^6	mega	M
10^3	kilo	k
10^2	hecto	h
10^1	deca	da
10^{-1}	deci	d
10^{-2}	centi	c
10^{-3}	milli	m
10^{-6}	micro	μ
10^{-9}	nano	n
10^{-12}	pico	p
10^{-15}	femto	f
10^{-18}	atto	a

In anticipation that the SI system may be adopted in the next several years, values are reported here in the traditional units with equivalent SI units following in parentheses.

COMMON CLINICAL VALUES IN TRADITIONAL & SI MEASUREMENTS

Albumin, Serum: See Protein, serum.

Aldolase, Serum: Normal (varies with method): 4–14 units/ml (Bruns). Males, < 33 units; females, < 19 units (Warburg and Christian).
   A. Precautions: Serum should be separated promptly. If there is to be any delay in the determination, the serum should be frozen.
   B. Physiologic Basis: Aldolase, also known as zymohexase, splits fructose-1,6-diphosphate to yield dihydroxyacetone phosphate and glyceraldehyde-3-phosphate. Because it is present in higher concentration in tissue cells than in serum, destruction of tissue results in elevation of serum concentration.

C. Interpretation: Elevated levels in serum occur in myocardial infarction, muscular dystrophies, hemolytic anemia, metastatic prostatic carcinoma, leukemia, acute pancreatitis, and acute hepatitis. In obstructive jaundice or cirrhosis of the liver, serum aldolase is normal or only slightly elevated.

Ammonia, Blood: Normal (Conway): 80–110 μg/100 ml whole blood. (SI: 47–65 μmol/l.)
   A. Precautions: Do not use anticoagulants containing ammonia. Suitable anticoagulants include potassium oxalate, EDTA, and heparin that is ammonia-free. The determination should be done immediately after drawing blood. If the blood is kept in an ice-water bath it may be held for up to 1 hour.
   B. Physiologic Basis: Ammonia present in the blood is derived from 2 principal sources: (1) In the large intestine, putrefactive action of bacteria on nitrogenous materials releases significant quantities of ammonia. (2) In the process of protein metabolism, ammonia is liberated. Ammonia entering the portal vein or the systemic circulation is rapidly converted to urea in the liver. Liver insufficiency may result in an increase in blood ammonia concentration, especially if protein consumption is high or if there is bleeding into the bowel.
   C. Interpretation: Blood ammonia is elevated in hepatic insufficiency or with liver by-pass in the form of a portacaval shunt, particularly if protein intake is high or if there is bleeding into the bowel.
   D. Drug Effects on Laboratory Results: Elevated by methicillin, ammonia cycle resins, chlorthalidone, spironolactone. Decreased by monoamine oxidase inhibitors, oral antimicrobial agents.

Amylase, Serum: Normal (varies with method): 80–180 Somogyi units/100 ml serum. (One Somogyi unit equals amount of enzyme which will produce 1 mg of reducing sugar from starch at pH 7.2.) 0.8–3.2 IU/liter.
   A. Precautions: If storage for more than 1 hour is necessary, blood or serum must be refrigerated.
   B. Physiologic Basis: Normally, small amounts of amylase (diastase), molecular weight about 50,000, originating in the pancreas and salivary glands, are present in the blood. Inflammatory disease of these glands or obstruction of their ducts results in regurgitation of large amounts of enzyme into the blood and increased excretion via the kidney.
   C. Interpretation:
   1. **Elevated** in acute pancreatitis, obstruction of pancreatic ducts (carcinoma, stone, stricture, duct sphincter spasm after morphine), mumps, occasionally in the presence of renal insufficiency, occasionally in diabetic acidosis, and occasionally with inflammation of the pancreas from a perforating peptic ulcer. Rarely, combination of amylase with an immunoglobulin produces elevated serum amylase activity (macroamylasemia) because the large molecular complex (molecular weight at least 160,000) is not filtered by the glomerulus.

2. Decreased in hepatitis, acute and chronic; pancreatic insufficiency, and occasionally in toxemia of pregnancy.

D. Drug Effects on Laboratory Results: Elevated by morphine, codeine, meperidine, methacholine, pancreozymin, sodium diatrizoate, cyproheptadine, perhaps by pentazocine, thiazide diuretics. Pancreatitis may be induced by indomethacin, furosemide, chlorthalidone, ethacrynic acid, corticosteroids, histamine, salicylates, and tetracyclines. Decreased by barbiturate poisoning.

Amylase, Urine: Normal: Varies with method. 40–250 Somogyi units/hour.

A. Precautions: If the determination is delayed more than 1 hour after collecting the specimen, urine must be refrigerated.

B. Physiologic Basis: See Amylase, Serum. If renal function is adequate, amylase is rapidly excreted in the urine. A timed urine specimen (ie, 2, 6, or 24 hours) should be collected and the rate of excretion determined.

C. Interpretation: Elevation of the concentration of amylase in the urine occurs in the same situations in which serum amylase concentration is elevated. Urinary amylase concentration remains elevated for up to 7 days after serum amylase levels have returned to normal following an attack of pancreatitis. Thus the determination of urinary amylase may be useful if the patient is seen late in the course of an attack of pancreatitis. An elevated serum amylase with normal or low urine amylase excretory rate may be seen in the presence of renal insufficiency.

Bicarbonate, Serum or Plasma (measured as CO_2 content): Normal: 24–48 mEq/liter or 55–65 vol%. (SI: 24–48 mmol/l.)

A. Precautions: Plasma or serum is preferably drawn under oil and handled anaerobically.

B. Physiologic Basis: Bicarbonate-carbonic acid buffer is one of the most important buffer systems in maintaining normal pH of body fluids. Bicarbonate and pH determinations on plasma serve as a basis for assessing "acid-base balance."

C. Interpretation:

1. Elevated in—

(a) Metabolic alkalosis (arterial blood pH increased) due to ingestion of large quantities of sodium bicarbonate, protracted vomiting of acid gastric juice, accompanying potassium deficit.

(b) Respiratory acidosis (arterial blood pH decreased) due to inadequate elimination of CO_2 (leading to elevated P_{CO_2}) because of pulmonary emphysema, poor diffusion in alveolar membrane disease, heart failure with pulmonary congestion or edema, ventilatory failure due to any cause, including oversedation, narcotics, or inadequate artificial respiration.

2. Decreased in—

(a) Metabolic acidosis (arterial blood pH decreased) due to diabetic ketosis, starvation, persistent diarrhea, renal insufficiency, ingestion of excess acidi-

fying salts, or salicylate intoxication.

(b) Respiratory alkalosis (arterial blood pH increased) due to hyperventilation (decreased P_{CO_2}).

Bilirubin, Serum: Normal: Direct (glucuronide), 0.1–0.4 mg/100 ml. Indirect (unconjugated), 0.2–0.7 mg/100 ml. (SI: direct, up to 7 μmol/l; indirect, up to 12 μmol/l.)

A. Precautions: The fasting state is preferred to avoid turbidity of serum. For optimal stability of stored serum, samples should be frozen and stored in the dark.

B. Physiologic Basis: Destruction of hemoglobin yields bilirubin, which is conjugated in the liver to the diglucuronide and excreted in the bile. Bilirubin accumulates in the plasma when liver insufficiency exists, biliary obstruction is present, or the rate of hemolysis increases. Rarely, abnormalities of enzyme systems involved in bilirubin metabolism in the liver (eg, absence of glucuronyl transferase) result in abnormal bilirubin concentrations.

C. Interpretation:

1. Direct and indirect forms of serum bilirubin are elevated in acute or chronic hepatitis, biliary tract obstruction (cholangiolar, hepatic, or common ducts), toxic reactions to many drugs, chemicals, and toxins, and Dubin-Johnson and Rotor's syndromes.

2. Indirect serum bilirubin is elevated in hemolytic diseases or reactions and absence or deficiency of glucuronyl transferase, as in Gilbert's disease and Crigler-Najjar syndrome.

3. Direct and total bilirubin can be significantly elevated in normal and jaundiced subjects by fasting 24–48 hours (in some instances even 12 hours) or by prolonged caloric restriction.

D. Drug Effects on Laboratory Results: Elevated by acetaminophen, chlordiazepoxide, novobiocin, acetohexamide. Many drugs produce impairment of liver function.

Calcium, Serum: Normal 8.5–10.5 mg/100 ml or 4.2–5.2 mEq/liter. (Ionized, 4.2–5.2 mg/100 ml or 2.1–2.6 mEq/liter.) (SI: total, 2.1–2.6 mmol/l; ionized, 1.05–1.3 mmol/l.)

A. Precautions: Glassware must be free of calcium. The patient should be fasting. Serum should be promptly separated from the clot.

B. Physiologic Basis: Endocrine, renal, gastrointestinal, and nutritional factors normally provide for precise regulation of calcium concentration in plasma and other body fluids. Since some calcium is bound to plasma protein, especially albumin, determination of the plasma albumin concentration is necessary before the clinical significance of abnormal serum calcium levels can be interpreted accurately.

C. Interpretation:

1. **Elevated** in hyperparathyroidism, secretion of parathyroid-like hormone by malignant tumors, vitamin D excess, milk-alkali syndrome, osteolytic disease such as multiple myeloma, invasion of bone by metastatic cancer; Paget's disease of bone, Boeck's sarcoid,

and immobilization. Occasionally elevated with hyperthyroidism and with ingestion of thiazide drugs.

2. Decreased in hypoparathyroidism, vitamin D deficiency (rickets, osteomalacia), renal insufficiency, hypoproteinemia, malabsorption syndrome (sprue, ileitis, celiac disease, pancreatic insufficiency), severe pancreatitis with pancreatic necrosis, and pseudohypoparathyroidism.

Calcium, Urine, Daily Excretion: Ordinarily there is a moderate continuous urinary calcium excretion of 50–150 mg/24 hours, depending upon the intake. (SI: 1.2–3.7 mmol/day.)

A. Procedure: The patient should remain on a diet free of milk or cheese for 3 days prior to testing; for quantitative testing, a neutral ash diet containing about 150 mg calcium per day is given for 3 days. Quantitative calcium excretion studies may be made on a carefully timed 24–hour urine specimen. The screening procedure with the Sulkowitch reagent is simple and useful.

B. Interpretation: On the quantitative diet a normal person excretes 125± 50 mg (1.8–4.4 mmol) of calcium per 24 hours. Normally, a slight (1+) cloud reaction (Sulkowitch) occurs if milk and cheese are not present in the diet. In hyperparathyroidism, the urinary calcium excretion usually exceeds 200 mg/24 hours (5 mmol/day). Urinary calcium excretion is almost always elevated when serum calcium is high.

Carbon Dioxide Combining Power, Serum or Plasma: Normal: 24–29 mEq/liter or 55–75 vol%. (SI: 24–29 mmol/l.)

Plasma or serum CO_2 combining power is elevated or decreased in the same clinical circumstances as plasma or serum bicarbonate. Anaerobic handling of the specimen is not necessary. The method is the same as for bicarbonate determination except that the serum or plasma is exposed to an "alveolar" air concentration of CO_2 (ie, 40–50 mm Hg [SI: 5.3–6.7 kPa] partial pressure or 5–6% CO_2) prior to the determination.

See Bicarbonate, above, for interpretation.

Ceruloplasmin and Copper, Serum: Normal: Ceruloplasmin, 27–37 mg/100 ml (SI: 1.8–3.3 μmol/l); copper, 70–200 μg/100 ml (SI: 11–31 μmol/l).

A. Precautions: None.

B. Physiologic Basis: About 5% of serum copper is loosely bound to albumin and 95% to ceruloplasmin, an oxidase enzyme that is an $alpha_2$ globulin with a blue color. In Wilson's disease, serum copper and ceruloplasmin are low and urinary levels of copper are high.

C. Interpretation:

1. Elevated in pregnancy, hyperthyroidism, infection, aplastic anemia, acute leukemia, Hodgkin's disease, cirrhosis of the liver, and with use of oral contraceptives.

2. Decreased in Wilson's disease and accompanied by increased urinary excretion of copper, malabsorption, nephrosis.

Chloride, Serum or Plasma: Normal: 96–106 mEq/liter or 340–375 mg/100 ml. (SI: 96–106 mmol/l.)

A. Precautions: Determination on whole blood yields lower results than those obtained using serum or plasma as the specimen. Always use serum or plasma.

B. Physiologic Basis: Chloride is the principal inorganic anion of the extracellular fluid. It is important in maintenance of acid-base balance even though it exerts no buffer action. When chloride as HCl or NH_4Cl is lost, alkalosis follows; when chloride is retained or ingested, acidosis follows. Chloride (with sodium) plays an important role in control of osmolarity of body fluids.

C. Interpretation:

1. Elevated in renal insufficiency (when Cl intake exceeds excretion), nephrosis (occasionally), renal tubular acidosis, ureterosigmoid anastomosis (reabsorption from urine in gut), dehydration (water deficit), and overtreatment with saline solution.

2. Decreased in gastrointestinal disease with loss of gastric and intestinal fluids (vomiting of acid gastric juice, diarrhea, gastrointestinal suction), renal insufficiency (with salt deprivation), overtreatment with diuretics, chronic respiratory acidosis (emphysema), diabetic acidosis, excessive sweating, adrenal insufficiency (NaCl loss), hyperadrenocorticism (chronic K^+ loss), and metabolic alkalosis (NaHCO₃ ingestion; K^+ deficit).

Chloride, Urine:

Urine chloride content varies with dietary intake, acid-base balance, endocrine "balance," body stores of other electrolytes, and water balance. Relationships and responses are so variable and complex that there is little clinical value in urine chloride determinations other than in balance studies.

Cholesterol, Plasma or Serum: Normal: 150–280 mg/100 ml. (SI: 3.9–7.2 mmol/l.)

A. Precautions: The fasting state is preferred.

B. Physiologic Basis: Cholesterol concentrations are determined by metabolic functions which are influenced by heredity, nutrition, endocrine function, and integrity of vital organs such as the liver and kidney. Cholesterol metabolism is intimately associated with lipid metabolism.

C. Interpretation:

1. Elevated in familial hypercholesterolemia (xanthomatosis), hypothyroidism, poorly controlled diabetes mellitus, nephrotic syndrome, chronic hepatitis, biliary cirrhosis, obstructive jaundice, hypoproteinemia (idiopathic, with nephrosis or chronic hepatitis), and lipidemia (idiopathic, familial).

2. Decreased in acute hepatitis and Gaucher's disease, occasionally in hyperthyroidism, acute infections, anemia, malnutrition.

D. Drug Effects on Laboratory Results: Elevated by bromides, anabolic agents, trimethadione, oral contraceptives. Decreased by cholestyramine resin, haloperidol, nicotinic acid, salicylates, thyroid hormone, estrogens, clofibrate, chlorpropamide, phenformin, kanamycin, neomycin, phenyramidol.

Cholesterol Esters, Plasma or Serum: Normal: 65–75% of total serum or plasma cholesterol.

    A. Precautions: None.

    B. Physiologic Basis: Cholesterol is esterified in the intestinal mucosa and in the liver. Cholesterol exists in plasma or serum as the free form (25–33% of total) and as the ester (67–75% of total). In the presence of acute hepatic insufficiency (as in acute hepatitis), the concentration of esters is reduced.

    C. Interpretation:

    1. Elevated along with cholesterol in absence of hyperbilirubinemia (see Cholesterol, above). The ratio of ester/total cholesterol under these circumstances is normal. With hyperbilirubinemia, absolute values may be elevated, but not in the same proportion as total cholesterol, so that the ester/total cholesterol ratio is less than 65%.

    2. Decreased in acute hepatitis. Cholesterol esters may be decreased also in chronic hepatitis and chronic biliary obstruction; in these situations the decrease in cholesterol ester exceeds the decrease in total cholesterol, which results in an ester/total cholesterol ratio of less than 65%.

Creatine Phosphokinase (CPK), Serum: Normal: Varies with method. 10–50 IU/liter.

    A. Precautions: The enzyme is unstable, and the red cell content inhibits enzyme activity. Serum must be removed from the clot promptly. If assay cannot be done soon after drawing blood, serum must be frozen.

    B. Physiologic Basis: CPK splits creatine phosphate in the presence of ADP to yield creatine + ATP. Skeletal and heart muscle and brain are rich in the enzyme.

    C. Interpretation: Normal values vary with the method.

    1. Elevated in the presence of muscle damage such as with myocardial infarction, trauma to muscle, muscular dystrophies, polymyositis, severe muscular exertion, hypothyroidism, and cerebral infarction (necrosis). Following myocardial infarction, serum CPK concentration increases rapidly (within 3–5 hours), and remains elevated for a shorter time after the episode (2 or 3 days) than does GOT or LDH.

    2. Not elevated in pulmonary infarction or parenchymal liver disease.

Creatine Phosphokinase Isoenzymes, Serum: See Table 7.

Table 7. Creatine phosphokinase isoenzymes.

Isoenzyme	Normal Levels
(Fastest) Fraction 1, BB	Absent to small amount
Fraction 2, MB	Absent to trace
(Slowest) Fraction 3, MM	Major fraction

    A. Precautions: As for CPK, above.

    B. Physiologic Basis: CPK consists of 3 proteins separable by electrophoresis. Skeletal muscle is characterized by isoenzyme MM, myocardium by isoenzyme MB, and brain by isoenzyme BB.

    C. Interpretation: When CPK is elevated because of myocardial damage, there may be an increase in fraction 2, MB. If there is trauma to skeletal muscle or heavy physical exertion, fraction 3, MM, will be elevated. A large amount of fraction 1, BB, may appear following brain damage. Experience has not been extensive enough to define the specificity of changes in various diseases.

Creatine, Urine (24 Hours): Normal: See Table 8.

Table 8. Urine creatine and creatinine, normal values (24 hours).*

	Creatine	Creatinine
Newborn	4.5 mg/kg	10 mg/kg
1–7 months	8.1 mg/kg	12.8 mg/kg
2–3 years	7.9 mg/kg	12.1 mg/kg
4–4½ years	4.5 mg/kg	14.6 mg/kg
9–9½ years	2.5 mg/kg	18.1 mg/kg
11–14 years	2.7 mg/kg	20.1 mg/kg
Adult male	0–50 mg	25 mg/kg
Adult female	0–100 mg	21 mg/kg

*SI factors: creatine, mg/day × 0.0076 = mmol/day; creatinine, mg/day × 0.0088 = mmol/day.

    A. Precautions: Collection of the 24-hour specimen must be accurate. The specimen may be refrigerated or preserved with 10 ml of toluene or 10 ml of 5% thymol in chloroform.

    B. Physiologic Basis: Creatine is an important constituent of muscle, brain, and blood; in the form of creatine phosphate it serves as a source of high-energy phosphate. Normally, small amounts of creatine are excreted in the urine, but in states of elevated catabolism and in the presence of muscular dystrophies, the rate of excretion is increased.

    C. Interpretation:

    1. Elevated in muscular dystrophies such as progressive muscular dystrophy, myotonia atrophica, and myasthenia gravis; muscle wasting, as in acute poliomyelitis, amyotrophic lateral sclerosis, and myositis manifested by muscle wasting; starvation and cachectic states, hyperthyroidism, and febrile diseases.

    2. Decreased in hypothyroidism, amyotonia congenita, and renal insufficiency.

Creatinine, Plasma or Serum: Normal 0.7–1.5 mg/100 ml. (SI: 60–130 μmol/l.)

    A. Precautions: Other materials than creatinine may react to give falsely high results.

    B. Physiologic Basis: Creatinine, which is derived from creatine, is excreted by filtration through the glomeruli of the kidney. Endogenous creatinine is apparently not excreted by renal tubules. Retention of creatinine is thus an index of glomerular insufficiency. Creatinine clearance closely approximates the inulin clearance and is an acceptable measure of filtration rate.

C. Interpretation: Creatinine is elevated in acute or chronic renal insufficiency, urinary tract obstruction, and impairment of renal function induced by some drugs. Values of less than 0.7 mg/100 ml are of no known significance.

D. Drug Effects on Laboratory Results: Elevated by ascorbic acid, barbiturates, sulfobromophthalein, methyldopa, and phenolsulfonphthalein, all of which interfere with the determination of the alkaline picrate method (Jaffe reaction).

Creatinine, Urine: See Table 8 for normal values.

Glucose, Plasma, Serum: Normal: Fasting "true" glucose, 65–110 mg/100 ml. (SI: 3.6–6.1 mmol/l.) Because of the difference in glucose concentration in erythrocytes and plasma, whole blood concentrations will vary depending on the hematocrit.

A. Precautions: If determination is delayed beyond 1 hour, sodium fluoride, about 3 mg/ml blood, should be added to the specimen. The filtrates may be refrigerated for up to 24 hours. Errors in interpretation may occur if the patient has eaten sugar or received glucose solution parenterally just prior to the collection of what is thought to be a "fasting" specimen. Determination of serum or plasma concentration is preferred over whole blood.

B. Physiologic Basis: The glucose concentration in extracellular fluid is normally closely regulated, with the result that a source of energy is available to tissues and no glucose is excreted in the urine. Hyperglycemia and hypoglycemia are nonspecific signs of abnormal glucose metabolism.

C. Interpretation:

1. Elevated in diabetes mellitus, hyperthyroidism, adrenocortical hyperactivity (cortical excess), hyperpituitarism, and hepatic disease (occasionally).

2. Decreased in hyperinsulinism, adrenal insufficiency, hypopituitarism, hepatic insufficiency (occasionally), functional hypoglycemia, and by hypoglycemic agents.

D. Drug Effects on Laboratory Results: Elevated by corticosteroids, chlorthalidone, thiazide diuretics, furosemide, ethacrynic acid, triamterene, indomethacin, oral contraceptives (estrogen-progestin combinations), isoniazid, nicotinic acid (large doses), phenothiazines, and paraldehyde. Decreased by acetaminophen, phenacetin, cyproheptadine, pargyline, and propranolol.

Protein-Bound Iodine (PBI)

In most areas of the world, measurement of T_4 has replaced PBI and BEI in the assessment of thyroid function. Consult local laboratory for values. For further discussion, see p 1014.

Iron, Serum: Normal: 50–175 µg/100 ml. (SI: 9–31.3 µmol/l.)

A. Precautions: Syringes and needles must be iron-free. Hemolysis of blood must be avoided. The serum must be free of hemoglobin.

B. Physiologic Basis: Iron concentration in the plasma is determined by several factors, including absorption from the intestine, storage in intestine, liver, spleen, and marrow, breakdown or loss of hemoglobin, and synthesis of new hemoglobin.

C. Interpretation:

1. Elevated in hemochromatosis, hemosiderosis (multiple transfusions, excess iron administration), hemolytic disease, pernicious anemia, hypoplastic anemias, often in viral hepatitis. Spuriously elevated if patient has received parenteral iron during the 2–3 months prior to determination.

2. Decreased in iron deficiency with infections, nephrosis, and chronic renal insufficiency, and during periods of active hematopoiesis.

Iron-Binding Capacity, Serum: Normal: Total 250–410 µg/100 ml. (SI: 44.8–73.4 µmol/l.) Percent saturation, 20–55%.

A. Precautions: None.

B. Physiologic Basis: Iron is transported as a complex of the metal-binding globulin transferrin or siderophilin. Normally, this transport protein carries an amount of iron which represents about 30–40% of its capacity to combine with iron. Thus the "unsaturated" iron-binding capacity is normally 60–70% of the total capacity.

C. Interpretation of Unsaturated Iron-Binding Capacity:

1. Elevated in the presence of low serum iron or iron deficiency anemia, acute or chronic blood loss, pregnancy, acute hepatitis, and ingestion of oral contraceptive drugs.

2. Decreased in the presence of high serum iron, hemochromatosis, hemosiderosis, hemolytic disease, pernicious anemia, acute and chronic infections, cirrhosis of the liver, uremia, and malignancy.

Lactate Dehydrogenase, Serum, Serous Fluids, Spinal Fluid, Urine: Normal: Serum, 200–450 units (Wroblewski), 60–100 units (Wacker), 90–200 IU/liter. Serous fluids, lower than serum. Spinal fluid, 15–75 units (Wroblewski); 6.3–30 IU/liter. Urine, less than 8300 units/8 hours (Wroblewski).

A. Precautions: Any degree of hemolysis must be avoided because the concentration of LDH within red blood cells is 100 times that in normal serum. Heparin and oxalate may inhibit enzyme activity.

B. Physiologic Basis: LDH catalyzes the interconversion of lactate and pyruvate in the presence of NADH or $NADH_2$. It is distributed generally in body cells and fluids.

C. Interpretation: Elevated in all conditions accompanied by tissue necrosis, particularly those involving acute injury of the heart, red cells, kidney, skeletal muscle, liver, lung, and skin. Marked elevations accompany hemolytic anemias, and the anemias of vitamin B_{12} and folate deficiency, and polycythemia rubra vera. The course of rise in concentration over 3–4 days followed by a slow decline during the following 5–7 days may be helpful in confirming the presence of a myocardial infarction; however, pulmonary infarction, neoplastic disease, and megaloblastic anemia must be excluded. Although elevated during the acute phase of infectious hepatitis, enzyme activity is seldom increased in chronic liver disease.

Lactate Dehydrogenase Isoenzymes, Serum: Normal serum levels are as shown in Table 9.

Table 9. Lactate dehydrogenase isoenzymes.

	Isoenzyme	Percentage of Total (and Range)
(Fastest)	1 (a_1)	28 (15–30)
	2 (a_2)	36 (22–50)
	3 (β)	23 (15–30)
	4 (γ_1)	6 (0–15)
(Slowest)	5 (γ_2)	6 (0–15)

A. **Precautions:** As for LDH (see above).

B. **Physiologic Basis:** LDH consists of 5 separable proteins, each made of tetramers of 2 types or subunits, H and M. The 5 isoenzymes can be distinguished by kinetics, electrophoresis, chromatography, and immunologic characteristics. By electrophoretic separation, the mobility of the isoenzymes corresponds to serum proteins α_1, α_2, β, γ_1, and γ_2. These are usually numbered 1 (fastest moving), 2, 3, 4, and 5 (slowest moving). Isoenzyme 1 is present in high concentrations in heart muscle (tetramer H H H H) and in erythrocytes and kidney cortex; isoenzyme 5 in skeletal muscle (tetramer M M M M) and liver.

C. **Interpretation:** In myocardial infarction, the α isoenzymes are elevated–particularly LDH 1–to yield a ratio of LDH 1:2 of > 1.0. Similar α isoenzyme elevations occur in renal cortex infarction and with hemolytic anemias.

LDH 5 and 4 are relatively increased in the presence of acute hepatitis, acute muscle injury, dermatomyositis, and muscular dystrophies.

D. **Drug Effects on Laboratory Results:** Decreased by clofibrate.

Lipase, Serum: Normal: 0.2–1.5 units.

A. **Precautions:** None. The specimen may be refrigerated up to 24 hours prior to the determination.

B. **Physiologic Basis:** A low concentration of fat-splitting enzyme is present in circulating blood. In the presence of pancreatitis, pancreatic lipase is released into the circulation in higher concentrations, which persist, as a rule, for a longer period than does the elevated concentration of amylase.

C. **Interpretation:** Serum lipase is elevated in acute or exacerbated pancreatitis and in obstruction of pancreatic ducts by stone or neoplasm.

Magnesium, Serum: Normal: 1.5–2.5 mEq/liter. (1.8–3 mg/100 ml.) (SI: 0.8–1.3 mmol/l.)

A. **Precautions:** None.

B. **Physiologic Basis:** Magnesium is primarily an intracellular electrolyte. In extracellular fluid it affects neuromuscular irritability and response. Magnesium deficit may exist with little or no change in extracellular fluid concentrations. Low magnesium levels in plasma have been associated with tetany, weakness, disorientation, and somnolence.

C. **Interpretation:**

1. **Elevated** in renal insufficiency and in overtreatment with magnesium salts.

2. **Decreased** in chronic diarrhea, acute loss of enteric fluids, starvation, chronic alcoholism, chronic hepatitis, hepatic insufficiency, and excessive renal loss. May be decreased in and contribute to persistent hypocalcemia of hypoparathyroidism (especially after surgery for hyperparathyroidism) and when large doses of vitamin D and calcium are being administered.

Nonprotein Nitrogen (NPN), Blood, Plasma, or Serum: Normal: 15–35 mg/100 ml.

A. **Precautions:** See Urea, below.

B. **Physiologic Basis and Interpretation:** See Urea, below, and Creatinine, above.

Phosphatase, Acid, Serum: Normal: Bodansky units, 0.5–2; King-Armstrong, 1–5; Gutman, 0.5–2; Shinowara, 0–1.1; Bessey-Lowry, 0.1–0.63. Females: 0.2–9.5 IU/liter. Males: 0.5–11 IU/liter.

A. **Precautions:** Avoid hemolysis of the specimen, which releases erythrocyte phosphatase to give factitiously high results. Serum may be refrigerated 24–48 hours prior to determination.

B. **Physiologic Basis:** Phosphatase active at pH 4.9 is present in high concentrations in the prostate gland and in erythrocytes. In the presence of carcinoma of the prostate which has gone beyond the capsule of the gland or has metastasized, serum acid phosphatase concentration is increased.

C. **Interpretation:** Increased in carcinoma of the prostate, metastatic or invasive beyond the capsule of the gland, and occasionally in acute myelocytic leukemia.

Phosphatase, Alkaline, Serum: Normal: Bodansky, 2–5 units; King-Armstrong, 5–13 units; Gutman, 3–10 units; Shinowara, 2.2–8.6 units; Bessey-Lowry, children, 2.8–6.7 units; Bessey-Lowry, adults, 0.8–2.3 units. 30–85 IU/liter.

A. **Precautions:** Serum may be kept in refrigerator 24–48 hours, but values may increase slightly (10%). The specimen will deteriorate if not refrigerated. Do not use fluoride or oxalate.

B. **Physiologic Basis:** Alkaline phosphatase is present in high concentration in growing bone, in bile, and in the placenta. The phosphatase in serum consists of a mixture of isoenzymes not yet clearly defined. It appears that the enzyme of hepatic origin is resistant to heat; that of osseous origin is sensitive to heat. The isoenzymes may be separated by electrophoresis; liver alkaline phosphatase migrates faster than bone and placental alkaline phosphatase, which migrate together.

C. **Interpretation:**

1. **Elevated in—**

a. Children (normal growth of bone).

b. Osteoblastic bone disease—Hyperparathyroidism, rickets and osteomalacia, neoplastic bone disease (osteosarcoma, metastatic neoplasms), ossification as in myositis ossificans, Paget's disease (osteitis deformans), and Boeck's sarcoid.

c. Hepatic duct or cholangiolar obstruction due to stone, stricture, or neoplasm.

d. Hepatic disease resulting from drugs such as chlorpromazine, methyltestosterone.

e. Pregnancy.

f. With no clinical correlate to account for a high enzyme level in the serum, an indication of the source of the increased concentration may be obtained by measuring activity before and after heating the serum at 56° C for 10 minutes.

Bone: residual activity < 25% of control.

Hepatic: residual activity > 35% of control.

Placental: more resistant than hepatic.

"Normal" or "mixed": residual activity 25—30% of control.

2. **Decreased** in hypothyroidism and in growth retardation in children.

D. **Drug Effects on Laboratory Results:** Elevated by acetohexamide, tolazamide, tolbutamide, chlorpropamide, allopurinol, sulfobromophthalein, carbamazepine, cephaloridine, furosemide, methyldopa, phenothiazine, and oral contraceptives (estrogen-progestin combinations).

Phosphorus, Inorganic, Serum: Normal: Children, 4—7 mg/100 ml. (SI: 1.3—2.3 mmol/l.) Adults, 3—4.5 mg/100 ml. (SI: 1—1.5 mmol/l.)

A. **Precautions:** Glassware cleaned with phosphate cleaners must be thoroughly rinsed. The fasting state is necessary to avoid postprandial depression of phosphate associated with glucose transport and metabolism.

B. **Physiologic Basis:** The concentration of inorganic phosphate in circulating plasma is influenced by parathyroid gland function, intestinal absorption, renal function, bone metabolism, and nutrition.

C. **Interpretation:**

1. **Increased** in renal insufficiency, hypoparathyroidism, and hypervitaminosis D.

2. **Decreased** in hyperparathyroidism, hypovitaminosis D (rickets, osteomalacia), malabsorption syndrome (steatorrhea), ingestion of antacids which bind phosphate in the gut, starvation or cachexia, chronic alcoholism (especially with liver disease), hyperalimentation with phosphate-poor solutions, carbohydrate administration (especially intravenously), renal tubular

defects, use of thiazide diuretics, acid-base disturbances, diabetic ketoacidosis (especially during recovery), genetic hypophosphatemia, and occasionally during pregnancy and with hypothyroidism.

Potassium, Serum or Plasma: Normal: 3.5—5 mEq/liter; 14—20 mg/100 ml. (SI: 3.5—5 mmol/l.)

A. **Precautions:** Avoid hemolysis, which releases erythrocyte potassium. Serum must be separated promptly from the clot or plasma from the red cell mass to prevent erythrocyte potassium loss.

B. **Physiologic Basis:** Potassium concentration in plasma determines the state of neuromuscular and muscular irritability. Elevated or decreased concentrations of potassium impair the capability of muscle tissue to contract.

C. **Interpretation:**

1. **Increased** in renal insufficiency (especially in the presence of increased rate of protein or tissue breakdown); adrenal insufficiency; and too rapid administration of potassium salts, especially intravenously and with spironolactone.

2. **Decreased in—**

a. Inadequate intake (starvation).

b. Inadequate absorption or unusual enteric losses—Vomiting, diarrhea, or malabsorption syndrome.

c. Unusual renal loss—Secondary to hyperadrenocorticism (especially hyperaldosteronism) and to adrenocorticosteroid therapy, metabolic alkalosis, use of diuretics such as chlorothiazide and its derivatives and the mercurials, and renal tubular defects such as the De Toni-Fanconi syndrome and renal tubular acidosis.

d. Abnormal redistribution between extracellular and intracellular fluids—Familial periodic paralysis, testosterone administration.

D. **Drug Effects on Laboratory Results:** Elevated by triamterene, phenformin. Decreased by degraded tetracycline, phenothiazines, and sodium polystyrenesulfonate resin.

Proteins, Serum or Plasma (Includes Fibrinogen): Normal: See Interpretation, below.

A. **Precautions:** Serum or plasma must be free of hemolysis. Since fibrinogen is removed in the process of coagulation of the blood, fibrinogen determinations cannot be done on serum.

B. **Physiologic Basis:** Concentration of protein determines colloidal osmotic pressure of plasma. The concentration of protein in plasma is influenced by the nutritional state, hepatic function, renal function, occurrence of disease such as multiple myeloma, and metabolic errors. Variations in the fractions of plasma proteins may signify specific disease.

C. **Interpretation:**

1. **Total protein, serum—**Normal: 6—8 gm/100 ml. (SI: 60—80 g/l.) See albumin and globulin fractions, below.

2. **Albumin, serum or plasma—**Normal: 3.5—5.5 gm/100 ml. (SI: 35—55 g/l.)

a. **Elevated** in dehydration, shock, hemoconcentration, administration of large quantities of concen-

Table 10. Protein fractions as determined by electrophoresis.

	Percentage of Total Protein
Albumin	52—68
α_1 globulin	2.4—4.4
α_2 globulin	6.1—10.1
β globulin	8.5—14.5
γ globulin	10—21

Table 11. Gamma globulins by immunoelectrophoresis.

IgA	90—450 mg/100 ml
IgG	700—1500 mg/100 ml
IgM	40—250 mg/100 ml
IgD	0.3—40 mg/100 ml
IgE	0.006—0.16 mg/100 ml

Table 12. Some constituents of globulins.

Globulin	Representative Constituents
a_1	Thyroxine-binding globulin Transcortin Glycoprotein Lipoprotein Antitrypsin
a_2	Haptoglobin Glycoprotein Macroglobulin Ceruloplasmin
β	Transferrin Lipoprotein Glycoprotein
γ	γG γD γM γE γA

trated albumin "solution" intravenously.

b. **Decreased** in malnutrition, malabsorption syndrome, acute or chronic glomerulonephritis, nephrosis, acute or chronic hepatic insufficiency, neoplastic diseases, and leukemia.

3. **Globulin, serum or plasma**—Normal: 1.5—3 gm/100 ml. (SI: 15—30 g/l.)

a. **Elevated** in hepatic disease, infectious hepatitis, cirrhosis of the liver, biliary cirrhosis, and hemochromatosis; disseminated lupus erythematosus; acute or chronic infectious diseases, particularly lymphogranuloma venereum, typhus, leishmaniasis, schistosomiasis, and malaria; multiple myeloma; and Boeck's sarcoid.

b. **Decreased** in malnutrition, congenital agammaglobulinemia, acquired hypogammaglobulinemia, and lymphatic leukemia.

4. **Fibrinogen, plasma**—Normal: 0.2—0.6 gm/100 ml. (SI: 5.9—17.6 μmol/l.)

a. **Elevated** in glomerulonephritis, nephrosis (occasionally), and infectious diseases.

b. **Decreased** in disseminated intravascular coagulation (accidents of pregnancy including placental ablation, amniotic fluid embolism, violent labor, meningococcal meningitis, metastatic carcinoma of the prostate and occasionally of other organs, and leukemia), acute and chronic hepatic insufficiency, and congenital fibrinogenopenia.

Sodium, Serum or Plasma: Normal: 136—145 mEq/liter. (SI: 136—145 mmol/l.)

A. **Precautions**: Glassware must be completely clean.

B. **Physiologic Basis**: Sodium constitutes 140 of the 155 mEq of cation in plasma. With its associated anions it provides the bulk of osmotically active solute in the plasma, thus affecting the distribution of body water significantly. A shift of sodium into cells or a loss of sodium from the body results in a decrease of extracellular fluid volume with consequent effect on circulation, renal function, and nervous system function.

C. **Interpretation**:

1. **Increased** in dehydration (water deficit), CNS trauma or disease, and due to hyperaldosteronism or to corticosterone or corticosteroid excess.

2. **Decreased** in adrenal insufficiency; renal insufficiency, especially with inadequate sodium intake; renal tubular acidosis; as a physiologic response to trauma or burns (sodium shift into cells); unusual losses via the gastrointestinal tract, as in acute or chronic diarrhea, intestinal obstruction or fistula, and in unusual sweating with inadequate sodium replacement. In some patients with edema associated with cardiac or renal disease, serum sodium concentration is low even though total body sodium content is greater than normal; water retention (excess ADH) and abnormal distribution of sodium between intracellular and extracellular fluid contribute to this paradoxical situation. Hyperglycemia occasionally results in shift of intracellular water to the extracellular space, producing a dilutional hyponatremia.

Thyroxine (T_4), Total, Serum: Normal: Radioimmunoassay (RIA), 5—14 μg/100 ml (SI: 64—180 nmol/l); competitive binding protein (CPB) (Murphy-Pattee), 4—11 μg/100 ml. (SI: 51—142 nmol/l.)

A. **Precautions**: None.

B. **Physiologic Basis**: The total thyroxine level does not necessarily reflect the physiologic hormonal effect of thyroxine. Levels of thyroxine vary with the concentration of the carrier proteins (thyroxine-binding globulin and prealbumin), which are readily altered by physiologic conditions such as pregnancy and by a variety of diseases and drugs. Any interpretation of the significance of total T_4 depends upon knowing the concentration of carrier protein either from direct measurement or from the result of the erythrocyte or resin uptake of triiodothyronine (T_3)

(see below). It is the concentration of free T_4 and of T_3 that determines hormonal activity.

C. Interpretation:

1. **Elevated** in hyperthyroidism, at times with active thyroiditis, acromegaly, and with elevation of thyroxine-binding proteins.

2. **Decreased** in hypothyroidism (primary or secondary) and with decreased thyroxine-binding proteins.

D. **Drug Effects on Laboratory Results:** Increased by ingestion of excess thyroid hormone T_4. A variety of drugs alter concentration of thyroxine-binding proteins (see below), with parallel changes in total T_4 concentration. Decreased by ingestion of T_3 which inhibits thyrotropin secretion with resultant decrease in T_4 secretion and concentration. T_4 synthesis may be decreased by aminosalicylic acid, corticosteroids, lithium, the thiouracils, methimazole, and sulfonamides. Total T_4 concentration may be reduced because of displacement from carrier protein-binding sites by aspirin, chlorpropamide, phenytoin, halofenate, and tolbutamide. Cholestyramine may reduce T_4 concentration by interfering with its enterohepatic circulation.

Thyroxine, Free, Serum (FT_4): Normal (equilibrium dialysis): $0.8-2.4$ ng/100 ml. (SI: $0.01-0.03$ nmol/l.) May be estimated from measurement of total thyroxine and resin T_3 uptake.

A. **Precautions:** None.

B. **Physiologic Basis:** The metabolic activity of T_4 is related to the concentration of free T_4. T_4 is apparently largely converted to T_3 in peripheral tissue cells. (T_3 is secreted by the thyroid gland as well.) There is evidence that both T_4 and T_3 are active hormones.

C. **Interpretation:**

1. **Elevated** in hyperthyroidism and at times with active thyroiditis.

2. **Decreased** in hypothyroidism.

D. **Drug Effects on Laboratory Results:** Elevated by ingestion of excess thyroid hormone T_4. Decreased by T_3, thiouracils, and methimazole.

Thyroxine-Binding Globulin (TBG), Serum: Normal (radioimmunoassay): $2-4.8$ mg/100 ml.

A. **Precautions:** None.

B. **Physiologic Basis:** TBG is the principal carrier protein for T_4 and T_3 in the plasma. Variations in concentration of TBG are accompanied by corresponding variations in concentration of T_4 with intrinsic adjustments that maintain the physiologically active free hormones at proper concentration for euthyroid function. The inherited abnormalities of TBG concentration appear to be X-linked.

C. **Interpretation:**

1. **Elevated** in pregnancy, in infectious hepatitis, and in hereditary increase in TBG concentration.

2. **Decreased** in major depleting illness with hypoproteinemia (globulin), nephrotic syndrome, cirrhosis of the liver, active acromegaly, estrogen deficiency, and hereditary TBG deficiency.

D. **Drug Effects on Laboratory Results:** TBG or binding capacity increased by estrogens and progestins, including oral contraceptives, chlormadinone, perphenazine, and clofibrate. Decreased by androgen, anabolic steroids, cortisol, prednisone, corticotropin, and oxymetholone.

Triiodothyronine Uptake: Resin (RT_3U) or Thyroxine-Binding Globulin (TBG Assessment): Normal: RT_3U, as percentage of uptake of ^{125}I-T_3 by resin, $25-36\%$; TBG assessment, as ratio of binding of ^{125}I-T_3 by TBG in the test serum/normal serum, $0.85-1.15$.

A. **Precautions:** None.

B. **Physiologic Basis:** When serum thyroxine-binding proteins are normal, more TBG binding sites will be occupied by T_4 in T_4 hyperthyroidism and fewer binding sites will be occupied in hypothyroidism. ^{125}I-labeled-T_3 added to serum along with a secondary binder (resin, charcoal, talc, etc) is partitioned between TBG and the binder. The binder is separated from the serum and the radioactivity of the binder is measured for the RT_3U test and of the serum for the TBG assessment. Since the resin takes up the non-TBG bound radioactive T_3, its activity varies inversely with the numbers of available TBG sites, ie, RT_3U is increased if TBG is more nearly saturated by T_4 and decreased if TBG is less well saturated by T_4. The radioactive T_3 bound by TBG is measured directly in the serum assay, thus providing a direct measure of sites not occupied by T_4.

C. **Interpretation:**

1. RT_3U is increased and TBG assessment is decreased when available TBG sites are decreased, as in hyperthyroidism, active acromegaly, nephrotic syndrome, severe hepatic cirrhosis, and hereditary deficiency of TBG.

2. RT_3U is decreased and TBG assessment is increased when available TBG sites are increased, as in hypothyroidism, the newborn, infectious hepatitis, and hereditary increase in TBG.

D. **Drug Effects on Laboratory Results:** RT_3U is elevated and TBG assessment is decreased by excess T_4, androgens, anabolic steroids, corticosteroids, corticotropin, anticoagulant therapy (heparin and warfarin), oxymetholone, phenytoin, phenylbutazone, and large doses of salicylate. RT_3U is decreased and TBG assessment is elevated by T_3 therapy, estrogens, and progestins, including oral contraceptives; and by thiouracils, chlormadinone, perphenazine, and clofibrate.

Thyroxine Index: Estimation of Free Thyroxine or Calculation of "Corrected" T_4 From Values for Total T_4 and RT_3U or TBG Assessment: Normal (varies with method):

$$\text{Free thyroxine index} = RT_3U \text{ (in \%)} \times TT_4 \text{ in } \mu g/100 \text{ ml}$$

$$\text{Free thyroxine index} = \frac{TT_4 \text{ in } \mu g/100 \text{ ml}}{\text{TBG assessment ratio}}$$

A. Precautions: None.

B. Physiologic Basis: This calculation yields a value for TT_4 corrected for altered TBG concentration. The concentration of free thyroxine (FT_4) per se depends on the equilibrium among FT_4, T_4 bound to thyroxine-binding proteins (T_4-TBP), and unbound sites of TBP according to the ratio (T_4-TBP/TBP). (T_4-TBP) is essentially the same as total T_4; therefore, $FT_4 \propto (TT_4)/(\text{TBG assessment})$ or $FT_4 \propto (TT_4)(RT_3U)$. The corrected TT_4 is thus an index from which FT_4 can be derived.

Transaminase Enzyme Tests, Serum or Serous Fluid: Normal: SGOT, 5–40 units (6–25 IU/liter). SGPT, 5–35 units (3–26 IU/liter).

A. Precautions: None.

B. Physiologic Basis: Glutamic-oxaloacetic transaminase (aspartate aminotransferase), glutamic-pyruvic transaminase (alanine aminotransferase), and lactic dehydrogenase are all intracellular enzymes involved in amino acid or carbohydrate metabolism. The enzymes are present in high concentrations in muscle, liver, and brain. Elevations of concentrations of these enzymes in the blood indicate necrosis or disease, especially of these tissues.

C. Interpretation:

1. **Elevated** in myocardial infarction; acute infections or toxic hepatitis; cirrhosis of the liver; liver neoplasm, metastatic or primary; and in transudates associated with neoplastic involvement of serous cavities. SGOT is elevated in muscular dystrophy, dermatomyositis, and paroxysmal myoglobinuria.

2. **Decreased** with pyridoxine (B_6) deficiency (often a result of repeated hemodialysis) and pregnancy.

D. **Drug Effects on Laboratory Results:** Elevated by a host of drugs, including anabolic steroids, androgens, clofibrate, erythromycin (especially estolate) and other antibiotics, isoniazid, methotrexate, methyldopa, phenothiazines, oral contraceptives, salicylates, acetaminophen, phenacetin, indomethacin, acetohexamide, allopurinol, dicumarol, carbamazepine, chlordiazepoxide, desipramine, imipramine, codeine, morphine, meperidine, tolazamide, propranolol, guanethidine, pyridoxine, and drugs that produce spasm of the sphincter of Oddi.

Triglycerides, Serum: Normal: < 165 mg/100 ml. (SI: < 1.65 g/l.)

A. Precautions: Subject must be in a fasting state (preferably for at least 16 hours). The determination may be delayed if the serum is promptly separated from the clot and refrigerated.

B. Physiologic Basis: Dietary fat is hydrolyzed in the small intestine, absorbed and resynthesized by the mucosal cells, and secreted into lacteals in the form of chylomicrons. Triglycerides in the chylomicrons are cleared from the blood by tissue lipoprotein lipase (mainly adipose tissue) and the split products absorbed and stored. Free fatty acids derived mainly from adipose tissue are precursors of the endogenous triglycerides produced by the liver. Transport of endogenous triglycerides is in association with β lipoproteins, the very low density lipoproteins. (For further details, see Chapter 19.) In order to assure measurement of endogenous triglycerides, blood must be drawn in the postabsorptive state.

C. Interpretation: The concentration of triglycerides, cholesterol, and the lipoprotein fractions (very low density, low density, and high density) are interpreted collectively. Disturbances in normal relationships of these lipid moieties may be primary or secondary.

1. **Elevated (hyperlipoproteinemia)**–

a. Primary–Type I hyperlipoproteinemia (exogenous hyperlipidemia), type II hyperbetalipoproteinemia, type III broad beta hyperlipoproteinemia, type IV hyperlipoproteinemia (endogenous hyperlipidemia), and type V hyperlipoproteinemia (mixed hyperlipidemia).

b. Secondary–Hypothyroidism, diabetes mellitus, nephrotic syndrome, chronic alcoholism with fatty liver, ingestion of contraceptive steroids, biliary obstruction, stress.

2. **Decreased (hypolipoproteinemia)**–

a. Primary–Tangier disease (a-lipoprotein deficiency), abetalipoproteinemia, and a few rare, poorly defined syndromes.

b. Secondary–Malnutrition, malabsorption, and occasionally with parenchymal liver disease.

Urea Nitrogen & Urea, Blood, Plasma, or Serum: Normal: BUN, 8–25 mg/100 ml (SI: 2.9–8.9 mmol/l). Urea, 21–53 mg/100 ml (SI: 3.5–9 mmol/l).

A. Precautions: *Do not use* ammonium oxalate or "double oxalate" as anticoagulant, for the ammonia will be measured as urea. Do not use too much oxalate, for it will impair urease activity.

B. Physiologic Basis: Urea, an end-product of protein metabolism, is excreted by the kidney. In the glomerular filtrate the urea concentration is the same as in the plasma. Tubular reabsorption of urea varies inversely with rate of urine flow. Thus urea is a less useful measure of glomerular filtration than is creatinine, which is not reabsorbed. BUN varies directly with protein intake and inversely with the rate of excretion of urea.

C. Interpretation:

1. **Elevated in**–

a. Renal insufficiency–Nephritis, acute and chronic; acute renal failure (tubular necrosis), urinary tract obstruction.

b. Increased nitrogen metabolism associated with diminished renal blood flow or impaired renal function–Dehydration from any cause, gastrointestinal bleeding (combination of increased protein absorption from digestion of blood, plus decreased renal blood flow).

c. Decreased renal blood flow–Shock, adrenal insufficiency, occasionally congestive heart failure.

2. **Decreased in** hepatic failure, nephrosis not complicated by renal insufficiency, and cachexia.

D. Drug Effects on Laboratory Results: Elevated by many antibiotics that impair renal function, guanethidine, methyldopa, indomethacin, isoniazid, propranolol, and potent diuretics (decreased blood volume and renal blood flow).

Uric Acid, Serum or Plasma: Normal: Males, 3–8 mg/100 ml (SI: 0.18–0.48 mmol/l); females, 1.5–6 mg/100 ml (SI: 0.09–0.36 mmol/l).

A. Precautions: If plasma is used, lithium oxalate should be used as the anticoagulant; potassium oxalate may interfere with the determination.

B. Physiologic Basis: Uric acid, an end-product of nucleoprotein metabolism, is excreted by the kidney. Gout, a genetically transmitted metabolic error, is characterized by an increased plasma or serum uric acid concentration, an increase in total body uric acid, and deposition of uric acid in tissues. An increase in uric acid concentration in plasma and serum may accompany increased nucleoprotein catabolism (blood dyscrasias, therapy with antileukemic drugs), thiazide diuretics, or decreased renal excretion.

C. Interpretation:

1. Elevated in gout, toxemia of pregnancy (eclampsia), leukemia, polycythemia, therapy with antileukemic drugs and a variety of other agents, renal insufficiency, glycogen storage disease (type I), Lesch-Nyhan syndrome (X-linked hypoxanthine-guanine phosphoribosyltransferase deficit), and Down's syndrome. The incidence of hyperuricemia is greater in Filipinos than in whites.

2. Decreased in acute hepatitis (occasionally), treatment with allopurinol, probenecid.

D. Drug Effects on Laboratory Results: Elevated by salicylates (low doses), thiazide diuretics, ethacrynic acid, spironolactone, furosemide, triamterene, and ascorbic acid. Decreased by salicylates (large doses), methyldopa, clofibrate, phenylbutazone, cinchophen, sulfinpyrazone, and phenothiazines.

Uric Acid, Urine: Normal: 350–600 mg/24 hours on a standard purine-free diet. (SI: 2.1–3.6 mmol/day.) Normal urinary uric acid/creatinine ratio for adults is 0.21–0.59; maximum of 0.75 for 24-hour urine while on purine-free diet.

A. Precautions: Diet should be free of high-purine foods prior to and during 24-hour urine collection. Strenuous activity may be associated with elevated purine excretion.

B. Physiologic Basis: Elevated serum uric acid may result from overproduction or diminished excretion.

C. Interpretation:

1. Elevated renal excretion occurs in about 25–30% of cases of gout due to increased purine synthesis. Excess uric acid synthesis and excretion are associated with myeloproliferative disorders. Lesch-Nyhan syndrome (hypoxanthine-guanine phosphoribosyltransferase deficit) and some cases of glycogen storage disease are associated with uricosuria.

2. Decreased in renal insufficiency, in some cases of glycogen storage disease (type I), and in any metabolic defect producing lacticacidemia or β-hydroxybutyricacidemia. Salicylates in doses of less than 2–3 gm/day often produce renal retention of uric acid.

• • •

General Bibliography

Castleman B, McNeely BU (editors): Normal laboratory values: Case records of the Massachusetts General Hospital. New England J Med 290:39, 1974.

Constantino NV, Kabat HF: Drug-induced modifications of laboratory test values. Am J Hosp Pharm 30:24, 1973.

Hansten PD: *Drug Interactions: Clinical Significance of Drug-Drug Interactions and Drug Effects on Clinical Laboratory Results.* Lea & Febiger, 1971.

Henry RJ: *Clinical Chemistry: Principles and Technics,* 2nd ed. Hoeber, 1974.

Lubran M: The effects of drugs on laboratory values. M Clin North America 53:211, 1969.

Meyers FH, Jawetz E, Goldfien A: *Review of Medical Pharmacology,* 4th ed. Lange, 1974.

Schwartz MK: Interference in diagnostic biochemical procedures. Advances Clin Chem 16:1, 1973.

Tietz NW: *Fundamentals of Clinical Chemistry.* Saunders, 1970.

Winston S: Collection and preservation of specimens. Pp 1–17 in: *Standard Methods of Clinical Chemistry.* Vol 5. Academic Press, 1965.

Wirth WA, Thompson RL: The effect of various conditions and substances on the results of laboratory procedures. Am J Clin Path 43:579, 1965.

Young DS: "Normal laboratory values." (Case records of the Massachusetts General Hospital) in SI units. New England J Med 292:795, 1975.

Young DS: Standardized reporting of laboratory data: The desirability of using SI units. New England J Med 290:368, 1974.

Young DS & others: Drug interference with clinical laboratory tests. Clin Chem 18:1041, 1972.

NORMAL VALUES

HEMATOLOGY

Bleeding time: 1–7 minutes (Ivy).

Cellular measurements of red cells: Average diameter = 7.3 μm (5.5–8.8 μm).
Mean corpuscular volume (MCV): 82–98 fl.
Mean corpuscular hemoglobin (MCH): 27–33 pg.
Mean corpuscular hemoglobin concentration (MCHC): 31–35%.
Color, saturation, and volume indices: 1 (0.9–1.1)

Clot retraction: Begins in 1–3 hours; complete in 24 hours.

Coagulation time (Lee-White): At 37° C, 6–12 minutes; at room temperature, 10–18 minutes.

Fragility of red cells: Begins at 0.45–0.38% NaCl; complete at 0.36–0.3% NaCl.

Hematocrit (PCV): Men, 40–52%; women, 37–47%.

Hemoglobin [B]: Men, 14–18 gm/100 ml; women, 12–16 gm/100 ml. (Serum hemoglobin: 2–3 mg/100 ml.)

Platelets: 200–400 thousand/μl.*

Prothrombin [P]: 75–125%.

Red blood count (RBC): Men, 4.5–6.2 million/μl*; women, 4–5.5 million/μl.*

Reticulocytes: 0.5–1.5% of red cells.

Sedimentation rate: Less than 20 mm/hour (Westergren); 0–10 mm/hour (Wintrobe).

White blood count (WBC) and differential: 5–10 thousand/μl.*

Myelocytes	0 %
Juvenile neutrophils	0 %
Band neutrophils	0–5 %
Segmented neutrophils	40–60%
Lymphocytes	20–40%
Eosinophils	1–3 %
Basophils	0–1 %
Monocytes	4–8 %

*The microliter (μl, 10^{-6} liter) has replaced the cubic millimeter in SI terminology. This change has not yet been made in the body of this book.

BLOOD (B), PLASMA (P), OR SERUM (S): CHEMICAL CONSTITUENTS

Below are listed the specimen used, the amount of blood [B], plasma [P], or serum [S] needed to provide an adequate specimen, the fasting state, and the normal values. Values vary with the procedure employed.

Acetone bodies: [P, 2 ml] 0.3–2 mg/100 ml.

Aldolase: [S, 4 ml] 4–14 units/ml (Bruns). Men, < 33 units; women, < 19 units (Warburg and Christian).

Amino acid nitrogen: [P, 2 ml fasting] 3–5.5 mg/100 ml.

Ammonia*: [B, 2 ml] 80–110 μg/100 ml.

Amylase: [S, 2 ml] 80–180 units/100 ml (Somogyi). 0.8–3.2 IU/liter.

a_1-Antitrypsin: [S, 1 ml] 210–500 mg/100 ml.

Ascorbic acid: [P, 7 ml] 0.4–1.5 mg/100 ml.

Base, total serum: [S, 2 ml] 145–160 mEq/liter.

Bicarbonate: [S, 2 ml] 24–28 mEq/liter.

Bilirubin: [S, 3 ml] (Van den Bergh test.) Direct, 0.1–0.4 mg/100 ml. Indirect, 0.2–0.7 mg/100 ml.

Calcium: [S, 2 ml fasting] 8.5–10.5 mg/100 ml; 4.2–5.2 mEq/liter (varies with protein concentration).

Calcium, ionized: [S, 1 ml] 4.25–5.25 mg/100 ml.

CO_2 combining power: [S or P, 1 ml] 55–75 vol%.

CO_2 content: [S or P, 1 ml] 24–29 mEq/liter; 55–65 vol%.

Carotenoids: [S, 2 ml fasting] 50–300 μg/100 ml.

Ceruloplasmin: [S, 2 ml] 23–50 mg/100 ml.

Chloride: [S, 1 ml] 96–106 mEq/liter; 340–375 mg/100 ml (as chloride).

Cholesterol: [S, 1 ml] 150–280 mg/100 ml.

Cholesterol esters: [S, 1 ml] 50–65% of total cholesterol.

Complement: [S, 5 ml] C3 100–190 mg/100 ml; C4 20–60 mg/100 ml.

*Do not use anticoagulant containing ammonium oxalate.

Copper: [S, 5 ml] 70−133 μg/100 ml.

Cortisol: [P] 4−18 μg/100 ml (circadian variation).

Creatine phosphokinase: [S, 3 ml] 0−4.5 units (Hughes). 10−50 IU/liter. Varies with method.

Creatinine: [B or S, 1 ml] 0.7−1.5 mg/100 ml.

Folic acid: [S, 4 ml] > 5−24 ng/ml.

Glucose (Folin): [B, 0.1−1 ml fasting] 80−120 mg/100 ml.

Glucose (true): [B, 0.1−1 ml fasting] 65−110 mg/100 ml.

Glucose tolerance: See p 722.

Iron: [S, 2 ml] 50−175 μg/100 ml.

Iron-binding capacity, total: [S, 2 ml] 250−410 μg/100 ml. Percent saturation: 20−25%.

Lactate dehydrogenase (SLDH): [S, 2 ml] 215−540 units (Wroblewski). 90−200 IU/liter.

Lactic acid: [B, 2 ml in iodoacetate] 0.44−1.8 mM/liter; 4−16 mg/100 ml.

Lipase: [S, 2 ml] 0.2−1.5 units (ml of 0.1 N NaOH).

Lipids, total: [S] 500−600 mg/100 ml.

Magnesium: [S, 2 ml] 1.5−2.5 mEq/liter. (1.8−3 mg/100 ml).

Nonprotein nitrogen (NPN)*: [S or B, 1 ml] 15−35 mg/100 ml.

Norepinephrine: [P] < 0.5 μg/liter.

Osmolality: [S, 5 ml] 285−295 mOsm/kg water.

Oxygen:
  Capacity: [B, 5 ml] 16−24 vol% (varies with hemoglobin concentration).
  Arterial content: [B, 5 ml] 15−23 vol% (varies with hemoglobin concentration).
  Arterial % saturation: 94−100% of capacity.
  Arterial P_{O_2} (Pa_{O_2}): 80−100 mm Hg (sea level).

Pa_{CO_2}: [Arterial blood, 5 ml] 35−45 mm Hg.

pH (reaction): [P (arterial), 1 ml] 7.35−7.45.

Phosphatase, acid: [S, 2 ml] 1−5 units (King-Armstrong), 0.5−2 units (Bodansky), 0.5−2 units (Gutman), 0−1.1 units (Shinowara), 0.1−0.63 units (Bessey-Lowry). Females: 0.2−9.5 IU/liter. Males: 0.5−11 IU/liter.

Phosphatase, alkaline: [S, 2 ml] 5−13 units (King-Armstrong), 2−4.5 units (Bodansky), 3−10 units (Gutman), 2.2−8.6 units (Shinowara). Adults, 0.8−2.3 units (Bessey-Lowry); children, 2.8−6.7 units (Bessey-Lowry). Adults, 30−85 IU/liter.

Phospholipid: [S, 2 ml] 145−200 mg/100 ml.

Phosphorus, inorganic: [S, 1 ml fasting] 3−4.5 mg/100 ml (children, 4−7 mg); 1−1.5 mM/liter.

Potassium: [S, 1 ml] 3.5−5 mEq/liter; 14−20 mg/100 ml.

Protein:
  Total: [S, 1 ml] 6−8 gm/100 ml.
  Albumin: [S, 1 ml] 3.5−5.5 gm/100 ml.
  Globulin: [S] 1.5−3 mg/100 ml.
  Fibrinogen: [P, 1 ml] 0.2−0.6 gm/100 ml.
  Separation by electrophoresis: See Table 10.

Prothrombin clotting time: [P, 2 ml] By control.

Pyruvic acid: [B, 2 ml] 0.07−0.22 mM/liter; 0.6−2 mg/100 ml.

Serotonin: [B] 0.05−0.2 μg/ml.

Sodium: [S, 1 ml] 136−145 mEq/liter; 310−340 mg/100 ml (as Na).

Specific gravity: [B, 0.1 ml] 1.056 (varies with hemoglobin and protein concentration).
  [S, 0.1 ml] 1.0254−1.0288 (varies with protein concentration).

Sulfate: [P or S, 2 ml] 0.5−1.5 mEq/liter.

Transaminases: [S, 2 ml]
  Glutamic-oxaloacetic (SGOT), 5−40 units; 6−25 IU/liter at 30° C.
  Glutamic-pyruvic (SGPT), 5−35 units; 3−26 IU/liter at 30° C.

Transferrin: [S, 2 ml] 200−400 mg/100 ml.

Triglycerides: [S, 1 ml] < 165 mg/100 ml. (5.4 mEq/liter).

Urea nitrogen*: [S or B, 1 ml] 8−25 mg/100 ml.

Uric acid: [S, 1 ml] 3−8 mg/100 ml.

Vitamin B_{12}: [S, 2 ml] > 100 pg ml.

Volume, blood (Evans blue dye method): Adults, 2990−6980 ml. Women, 46.3−85.5 ml/kg; men, 66.2−97.7 ml/kg.

Zinc: [S, 3 ml] 65−145 μg/ml.

---

* Do not use anticoagulant containing ammonium oxalate.

*Do not use anticoagulant containing ammonium oxalate.

HORMONES, SERUM, OR PLASMA

Pituitary:
Growth (HGH): [S, 3 ml] Adults, 1–10 ng/ml (by RIA).
Thyroid-stimulating (TSH): [S, 3 ml] < 15 μU/ml.
Follicle-stimulating hormone (FSH): [S, 2 ml] prepuberal, 2–12 mIU/ml; adult, 6–30 mIU/ml; castrate or postmenopausal, 30–200 mIU/ml (by RIA).
Luteinizing hormone (LH): [S, 2 ml] Prepuberal, 2–12 mIU/ml; adult, 6–30 mIU/ml.
Corticotropin (ACTH): [P, 3 ml] Late afternoon, < 3 ng/100 ml (by RIA).

Adrenal:
Aldosterone: [P] Supine, normal salt intake, 2–9 ng/100 ml.
Cortisol: [S, 2 ml] 8 a.m., 7–18 μg/100 ml; 5 p.m., 2–9 μg/100 ml.

Epinephrine: [P] < 0.1 μg/liter.

Thyroid:
Thyroxine, free (FT_4): [S, 6 ml] 0.8–2.4 ng/100 ml.
Thyroxine, total (TT_4): [S, 3 ml] 4–11 μg/100 ml T_4 (by CPB); 5–14 μg/100 ml (by RIA).
Thyroxine-binding globulin: [S, 4 ml] 2–4.8 mg/100 ml.
Triiodothyronine: [S, 2 ml] 80–220 ng/100 ml.
Triiodothyronine uptake (RT_3U): [S, 3 ml] 25–36%; as TBG assessment, 0.85–1.15.

Parathyroid: Parathyroid hormone levels vary with method and antibody.

Islets:
Insulin [S, 1 ml] 4–25 μU/ml.

Stomach:
Gastrin: [S, 2 ml, special handling] Up to 200 pg/ml.

Kidney:
Renin activity: [P, 2 ml, special handling] Supine, normal sodium intake, 1–3 ng/ml/hour; standing or while on low sodium diet or diuretics, 3–6 ng/ml/hour.

Gonad:
Testosterone: [S, 4 ml] Prepuberal, < 100 ng/100 ml; adult males, 300–1000 ng/100 ml; adult female, 20–80 ng/100 ml; luteal phase, up to 120 ng/100 ml.
Estradiol (E_2), RIA: [S, 5 ml, special handling] Male 12–34 pg/ml; female, menstrual cycle 1–10 days, 24–68 pg/ml; 11–20 days, 50–186 pg/ml; 21–30 days, 73–149 pg/ml.
Progesterone, RIA: [S, 2 ml] Follicular phase, 20–150 ng/100 ml; luteal phase, 300–2400 ng/100 ml; pregnancy, > 2400 ng/100 ml; males, 15–150 ng/100 ml.

Placenta:
Estriol (E_3), RIA: [S, 2 ml] Male and nonpregnant female, < 0.2 μg/100 ml.
Chorionic gonadotropin: [S, 2 ml] Normal male and nonpregnant female, none detected.

NORMAL CSF VALUES

Appearance: Clear and colorless.

Chlorides (as NaCl): 700–750 mg/100 ml; 120–130 mEq/liter.

Globulin: 0–6 mg/100 ml.

Glucose: 50–85 mg/100 ml.

Cells: Adults, 0–5 mononuclears/μl.* Infants, 0–20 mononuclears/μl.*

Pressure (reclining): Newborn, 30–80 mm water. Children, 50–100 mm water. Adults, 70–200 mm water (avg = 125).

Proteins, total: 20–45 mg/100 ml in lumbar CSF.

Specific gravity: 1.003–1.008.

RENAL FUNCTION TESTS

p-Aminohippurate (PAH) clearance (RPF): Men, 560–830 ml/minute; women, 490–700 ml/minute.
Creatinine clearance, endogenous (GFR): Approximates inulin clearance (see below).

Filtration fraction (FF): Men, 17–21%; women, 17–23%. (FF = GFR/RPF.)

Inulin clearance (GFR): Men, 110–150 ml/minute; women, 105–132 ml/minute (corrected to 1.73 square meters surface area).

Maximal glucose reabsorptive capacity (Tm_G): Men, 300–450 mg/minute; women, 250–350 mg/minute.

Maximal PAH excretory capacity (Tm_{PAH}): 80–90 mg/minute.

Phenolsulfonphthalein (PSP, phenol red): Administer 1

*See note on p 1018.

ml IV. In first 15 minutes, 25% or more should be excreted; in 30 minutes, 40% or more; in 2 hours, 55% or more.

Specific gravity of urine: 1.003–1.030.

Urea clearance (C_u): Standard, 40–65 ml/minute; maximal, 60–100 ml/minute.

MISCELLANEOUS NORMAL VALUES

Addis urine sediment count: Maximum values/24 hours are as follows:
Red cells, 1 million
White and epithelial cells, 2 million
Casts, 100 thousand
Protein, 30 mg

Aldosterone, urinary: 2–26 µg/24 hours; varies with sodium and potassium intake.

Catecholamines, urine: < 10 µg epinephrine; < 100 µg norepinephrine; varies with method.

Congo red test: [S] More than 60% retention in serum after 1 hour.

Fecal fat: Less than 30% dry weight.

Follicle-stimulating hormone (FSH), urinary: Before puberty, less than 5 mouse units/24 hours; after puberty, 5–50 mouse units/24 hours; after menopause, up to 150 mouse units/24 hours.

11,17-Hydroxycorticoids, urinary: Men, 4–12 mg/24 hours; women, 4–8 mg/24 hours. Varies with method used.

Insulin tolerance: [B] Glucose level decreases to half of fasting level in 20–30 minutes; returns to fasting level in 90–120 minutes.

17-Ketosteroids, urinary: Under 8 years, 0–2 mg/24 hours; adolescents, 2–20 mg/24 hours. Men, 10–20 mg/24 hours; women, 5–15 mg/24 hours. Varies with method used.

Lead, urine: 0–0.12 mg/24 hours.

Urobilinogen, fecal: 40–280 mg/24 hours.

Urobilinogen, urine: 0–4 mg/24 hours.

Vanillylmandelic acid (VMA), urine: Up to 7 mg/24 hours.

. . .

Fahrenheit/Celsius Temperature Conversion

F°	C°	F°	C°
90	32.2	100	37.8
91	32.8	101	38.3
92	33.3	102	38.9
93	33.9	103	39.4
94	34.4	104	40.0
95	35.0	105	40.6
96	35.6	106	41.1
97	36.1	107	41.7
98	36.7	108	42.2
99	37.2	109	42.8

Milliequivalent Conversion Factors

mEq/liter of:	Divide mg/100 ml or vol% by:
Calcium	2.0
Chloride (from Cl)	3.5
(from NaCl)	5.85
CO_2 combining power	2.222
Magnesium	1.2
Phosphorus	3.1 (mM)
Potassium	3.9
Sodium	2.3

Apothecary Equivalents

Metric		Approximate Apothecary Equivalents		Metric		Approximate Apothecary Equivalents	
30	gm	1	oz	25	mg	3/8	gr
6	gm	90	gr	20	mg	1/3	gr
5	gm	75	gr	15	mg	1/4	gr
4	gm	60	gr	12	mg	1/5	gr
3	gm	45	gr	10	mg	1/6	gr
2	gm	30	gr	8	mg	1/8	gr
1.5	gm	22	gr	6	mg	1/10	gr
1	gm	15	gr	5	mg	1/12	gr
0.75	gm	12	gr	4	mg	1/15	gr
0.6	gm	10	gr	3	mg	1/20	gr
0.5	gm	7½	gr	2	mg	1/30	gr
0.4	gm	6	gr	1.5	mg	1/40	gr
0.3	gm	5	gr	1.2	mg	1/50	gr
0.25	gm	4	gr	1	mg	1/60	gr
0.2	gm	3	gr	0.8	mg	1/80	gr
0.15	gm	2½	gr	0.6	mg	1/100	gr
0.12	gm	2	gr	0.5	mg	1/120	gr
0.1	gm	1½	gr	0.4	mg	1/150	gr
75	mg	1¼	gr	0.3	mg	1/200	gr
60	mg	1	gr	0.25	mg	1/250	gr
50	mg	3/4	gr	0.2	mg	1/300	gr
40	mg	2/3	gr	0.15	mg	1/400	gr
30	mg	1/2	gr	0.12	mg	1/500	gr
				0.1	mg	1/600	gr

Desirable Weights (Pounds)

Men (Age 25 and Over)					Women (Age 25 and Over)				
Height* Feet	Inches	Small Frame	Medium Frame	Large Frame	Height† Feet	Inches	Small Frame	Medium Frame	Large Frame
5	2	112–120	118–129	126–141	4	10	92– 98	96–107	104–119
5	3	115–123	121–133	129–144	4	11	94–101	98–110	106–122
5	4	118–126	124–136	132–148	5	0	96–104	101–113	109–125
5	5	121–129	127–139	135–152	5	1	99–107	104–116	112–128
5	6	124–133	130–143	138–156	5	2	102–110	107–119	115–131
5	7	128–137	134–147	142–161	5	3	105–113	110–122	118–134
5	8	132–141	138–152	147–166	5	4	108–116	113–126	121–138
5	9	136–145	142–156	151–170	5	5	111–119	116–130	125–142
5	10	140–150	146–160	155–174	5	6	114–123	120–135	129–146
5	11	144–154	150–165	159–179	5	7	118–127	124–139	133–150
6	0	148–158	154–170	164–184	5	8	121–131	128–143	137–154
6	1	152–162	158–175	168–189	5	9	126–135	132–147	141–158
6	2	156–167	162–180	173–194	5	10	130–140	136–151	145–163
6	3	160–171	167–185	178–199	5	11	134–144	140–155	149–168
6	4	164–175	172–190	182–204	6	0	138–148	144–159	153–173

*With shoes with 1-inch heels.

*For women between 18 and 25, subtract 1 lb for each year under 25.
†With shoes with 2-inch heels.

*This table was derived primarily from data on the Build and Blood Pressure Study, 1959, Society of Actuaries. A useful discussion is presented in Seltzer CC, Mayer J: How representative are the weights of insured men and women? JAMA 201:221, 1967.

Pounds to Kilograms
(1 kg = 2.2 lb; 1 lb = 0.45 kg)

lb	kg	lb	kg	lb	kg	lb	kg	lb	kg
5	2.3	50	22.7	95	43.1	140	63.5	185	83.9
10	4.5	55	25.0	100	45.4	145	65.8	190	86.2
15	6.8	60	27.2	105	47.6	150	68.0	195	88.5
20	9.1	65	29.5	110	49.9	155	70.3	200	90.7
25	11.3	70	31.7	115	52.2	160	72.6	205	93.0
30	13.6	75	34.0	120	54.4	165	74.8	210	95.3
35	15.9	80	36.3	125	56.7	170	77.1	215	97.5
40	18.1	85	38.6	130	58.9	175	79.4	220	99.8
45	20.4	90	40.8	135	61.2	180	81.6		

Feet and Inches to Centimeters
(1 cm = 0.39 in; 1 in = 2.54 cm)

ft	in	cm	ft	in	cm	ft	in	cm	ft	in	cm	ft	in	cm
0	6	15.2	2	4	71.1	3	4	101.6	4	4	132.0	5	4	162.6
1	0	30.5	2	5	73.6	3	5	104.1	4	5	134.6	5	5	165.1
1	6	45.7	2	6	76.1	3	6	106.6	4	6	137.1	5	6	167.6
1	7	48.3	2	7	78.7	3	7	109.2	4	7	139.6	5	7	170.2
1	8	50.8	2	8	81.2	3	8	111.7	4	8	142.2	5	8	172.7
1	9	53.3	2	9	83.8	3	9	114.2	4	9	144.7	5	9	175.3
1	10	55.9	2	10	86.3	3	10	116.8	4	10	147.3	5	10	177.8
1	11	58.4	2	11	88.8	3	11	119.3	4	11	149.8	5	11	180.3
2	0	61.0	3	0	91.4	4	0	121.9	5	0	152.4	6	0	182.9
2	1	63.5	3	1	93.9	4	1	124.4	5	1	154.9	6	1	185.4
2	2	66.0	3	2	96.4	4	2	127.0	5	2	157.5	6	2	188.0
2	3	68.6	3	3	99.0	4	3	129.5	5	3	160.0	6	3	190.5

ABBREVIATIONS

Ab, antibody
ACD, anterior chest diameter
ADH, antidiuretic hormone
Ag, antigen
A/G ratio, albumin-globulin ratio
AHF, antihemophilic factor
AHG, antihemophilic globulin
ASO, arteriosclerosis obliterans
A-V, arteriovenous
AV, atrioventricular
B cells, "bursa"-dependent (ie, thymus-independent) lymphocytes
BAL, British anti-Lewisite (dimercaprol)
BBB, bundle branch block (R or L)
BCG, bacillus Calmette-Guérin; ballistocardiograph
BEI, butanol-extractable iodine
BLB, Boothby-Lovelace-Bulbulian (oxygen mask)
BMR, basal metabolic rate
BSP, Bromsulphalein
BUN, blood urea nitrogen
C, complement
CBC, complete blood count
CNS, central nervous system
COPD, chronic obstructive pulmonary disease
CPK, creatine phosphokinase
CSF, cerebrospinal fluid
CVA, cerebrovascular accident
CVP, central venous pressure
D&C, dilatation and curettage
DNA, deoxyribonucleic acid
DTP, diphtheria-tetanus-pertussis
ECG, electrocardiogram
ECW, extracellular water
EDTA, calcium disodium edetate
EEG, electroencephalogram
EFA, essential fatty acids
EMG, electromyogram
ESR, erythrocyte sedimentation rate
EST, electroshock therapy
fl, femtoliter (10^{-15} liter, formerly cu μ, cubic micron)
FSH, follicle-stimulating hormone
FTA, fluorescent treponemal antibody
FUO, fever of undetermined origin
GFR, glomerular filtration rate
G6PD, glucose-6-phosphate dehydrogenase
GTT, glucose tolerance test
Hct, hematocrit
Hgb, hemoglobin
HL-A, histocompatibility locus-A
ICS, intercostal space

ICSH, interstitial cell-stimulating hormone
ICU, intensive care unit
ICW, intracellular water
IDU, 5-iodo-2-deoxyuridine (idoxuridine)
Ig, immunoglobulin
INH, isonicotinic acid hydrazide (isoniazid)
IPPB, intermittent positive pressure breathing
ISW, interstitial water
IU, international unit
IUCD, intrauterine contraceptive device
IVP, intravenous pyelogram
kg, kilogram (10^3 gm)
LATS, long-acting thyroid stimulator
LBBB, left bundle branch block
LDH, lactic acid dehydrogenase
LE, lupus erythematosus
LSD, lysergic acid diethylamide
LVH, left ventricular hypertrophy
M, molar
MAC, maximum allowable concentration
mcg, μg, microgram (10^{-6} gm)
MCH, mean corpuscular hemoglobin
MCHC, mean corpuscular hemoglobin concentration
MCL, midcostal line
MCV, mean corpuscular volume
mEq, milliequivalent
mg, milligram (10^{-3} gm)
μl, microliter (formerly cu mm, cubic millimeter)
MLD, minimum lethal dose
μm, micrometer (formerly μ, micron)
mM, millimols
mOsm, milliosmols
ng, nanogram (10^{-9} gm)
nm, nanometer (10^{-9} m)
NPH, neutral protamine Hagedorn (isophane insulin)
NPN, nonprotein nitrogen
OT, old tuberculin
PA, posteroanterior
PABA, para-aminobenzoic acid
Pa_{CO_2}, arterial CO_2 tension
Pa_{O_2}, arterial O_2 tension
PAS, para-aminosalicylic acid
PBI, protein-bound iodine
P_{CO_2}, carbon dioxide partial pressure
PCV, packed cell volume

PEEP, positive end-expiratory pressure
pg, picogram (10^{-12} gm, formerly $\gamma\gamma$ or $\mu\mu$g, micromicrogram)
PGH, pituitary growth hormone
pHa, arterial pH
PID, pelvic inflammatory disease
pK, dissociation constant
PKU, phenylketonuria
PMI, point of maximal impulse
PMN, polymorphonuclear neutrophil
PPD, purified protein derivative (of tuberculin)
ppm, parts per million
PSP, phenolsulfonphthalein
PT, prothrombin time
PTA, plasma thromboplastin antecedent
PTC, plasma thromboplastin component
PTT, partial thromboplastin time
PZI, protamine zinc insulin
R, roentgen
RA, right atrium
RBBB, right bundle branch block
RBC, red blood count
RDS, respiratory distress syndrome
RNA, ribonucleic acid
RPF, renal plasma flow
RVH, right ventricular hypertrophy
SA, sinoatrial
SBE, subacute bacterial endocarditis
SGOT, serum glutamic-oxaloacetic transaminase
SGPT, serum glutamic-pyruvic transaminase
SI, *Système International d'Unités*
SLE, systemic lupus erythematosus
STS, serologic test for syphilis
T cells, thymus-dependent lymphocytes
TBW, total body water
$TCID_{50}$, 1/50 of the tissue culture immunizing dose
THAM, tromethamine with sodium and potassium chloride
TIBC, total iron-binding capacity
TPI, *Treponema pallidum* immobilization
TSH, thyroid-stimulating hormone
VDRL, Venereal Disease Research Laboratories
VMA, vanillylmandelic acid
vol%, volumes percent
WBC, white blood count
WBPTT, whole blood partial thromboplastin time

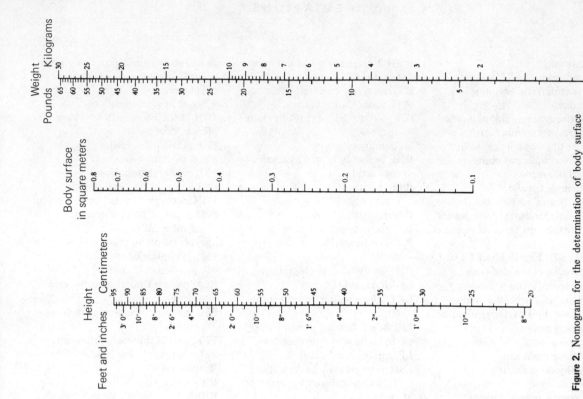

Figure 2. Nomogram for the determination of body surface area of children. (Reproduced, with permission, from DuBois: *Basal Metabolism in Health and Disease.* Lea & Febiger, 1936.)

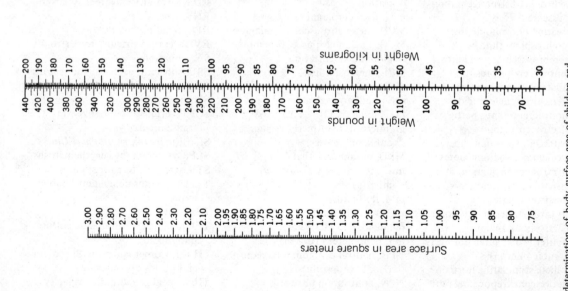

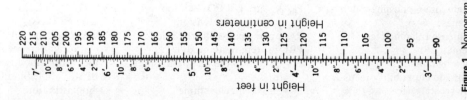

Figure 1. Nomogram for the determination of body surface area of children and adults. (Reproduced, with permission, from Boothby & Sandiford: Boston MSJ 185:337, 1921.)

Table 13. Schedules of controlled drugs.*

Schedule I: (All nonresearch use forbidden.)

Narcotics: Heroin and many nonmarketed synthetic narcotics

Hallucinogens:

LSD

MDA, STP, DMT, DET, mescaline, peyote, bufotenine, ibogaine, psilocybin

Marihuana, tetrahydrocannabinols

Schedule II: (No telephoned prescriptions, no refills.)

Narcotics:

Opium

Opium alkaloids and derived phenanthrene alkaloids: Morphine, codeine, hydromorphone (Dilaudid), oxymorphone (Numorphan), oxycodone (dihydrohydroxycodeinone, a component of Percodan)

Designated synthetic drugs: Meperidine (Demerol), alphaprodine (Nisentil), anileridine (Leritine), methadone, levorphanol (Levo-Dromoran), phenazocine (Prinadol)

Stimulants:

Coca leaves and cocaine

Amphetamine

Dextroamphetamine

Methamphetamine

Phenmetrazine (Preludin)

Methylphenidate (Ritalin)

Above in mixtures with other controlled or uncontrolled drugs (Dexamyl, Eskatrol)

Depressants:

Amobarbital

Pentobarbital

Secobarbital

Mixtures of above (eg, Tuinal)

Methaqualone

Schedule III: (Prescription must be rewritten after 6 months or 5 refills.)

Narcotics: The following opiates in combination with one or more active nonnarcotic ingredients, provided the amount does not exceed that shown:

Codeine and dihydrocodeine: Not to exceed 1800 mg/100 ml or 90 mg/tablet or other dose unit

Dihydrocodeinone (hydrocodone and in Hycodan): Not to exceed 300 mg/100 ml or 15 mg/tablet

Opium: 500 mg/100 ml, or 25 mg/5 ml, or other dosage unit (paregoric)

Narcotic antagonist: Nalorphine

Depressants:

Schedule II barbiturates in mixtures with noncontrolled drugs or in suppository dose form

Butabarbital (Butisol)

Glutethimide (Doriden)

Methyprylon (Noludar)

Stimulants:

Benzphetamine (Didrex)

Chlorphentermine (Pre-Sate)

Diethylpropion (Tenuate)

Mazindol (Sanorex)

Phendimetrazine

Schedule IV: (Prescription must be rewritten after 6 months or 5 refills. Differs from Schedule III in penalties for illegal possession.)

Stimulants:

Phentermine

Fenfluramine (Pondimin)

Depressants:

Chloral hydrate

Chlordiazepoxide (Librium)

Clonazepam (Clonopin)

Clorazepate (Tranxene)

Diazepam (Valium)

Ethchlorvynol (Placidyl)

Ethinamate (Valmid)

Flurazepam (Dalmane)

Meprobamate

Methylphenobarbital (Mebaral)

Oxazepam (Serax)

Paraldehyde

Phenobarbital

Schedule V: (As any other [nonnarcotic] prescription drug; may also be dispensed without prescription unless additional state regulations apply.)

Narcotics: The following drugs in combination with other active, nonnarcotic ingredients and provided the amount per 100 ml or 100 gm does not exceed that shown:

Codeine: 200 mg

Dihydrocodeine: 100 mg

Ethylmorphine: 100 mg

Diphenoxylate (not more than 2.5 mg and not less than 0.025 mg of atropine per dosage unit, as in Lomotil)

*Modified and reproduced, with permission, from Meyers FH, Jawetz E, Goldfien A: *Review of Medical Pharmacology,* 4th ed. Lange, 1974.

HEART-LUNG RESUSCITATION
(Modified after Safar.)

Phase I: First Aid (Emergency Oxygenation of the Brain)

Must be instituted within 3–4 minutes for optimal effectiveness and to minimize the possibility of permanent brain damage. Time is a crucial factor.

Step 1: Place patient supine on a firm surface (not a bed). A 4 × 6′ plywood sheet to be placed under the bed patient should be available in emergency care centers.

Step 2: Tilt head far backward by lifting up the patient's neck and pressing down on the forehead and maintain in this hyperextended position. Keep mandible displaced forward by pulling strongly at the angle of the jaw. (See diagrams, p 1009, for alternative methods.)

If Victim is Not Breathing:

Step 3: Clear mouth and pharynx of mucus, blood, vomitus, or foreign material.

Step 4: Separate lips and teeth to open oral airway.

Step 5: If steps 2–4 fail to open airway, forcibly blow air through mouth (keeping nose closed) or nose (keeping mouth closed) and inflate the lungs 3–5 times. Watch for chest movement. If this fails to clear the airway immediately, roll the patient to his side and deliver a sharp blow between the shoulder blades. If this measure also fails and if pharyngeal or tracheal tubes are available, use them without delay. Tracheostomy may be necessary.

Step 6: Feel the carotid or femoral artery for pulsations.

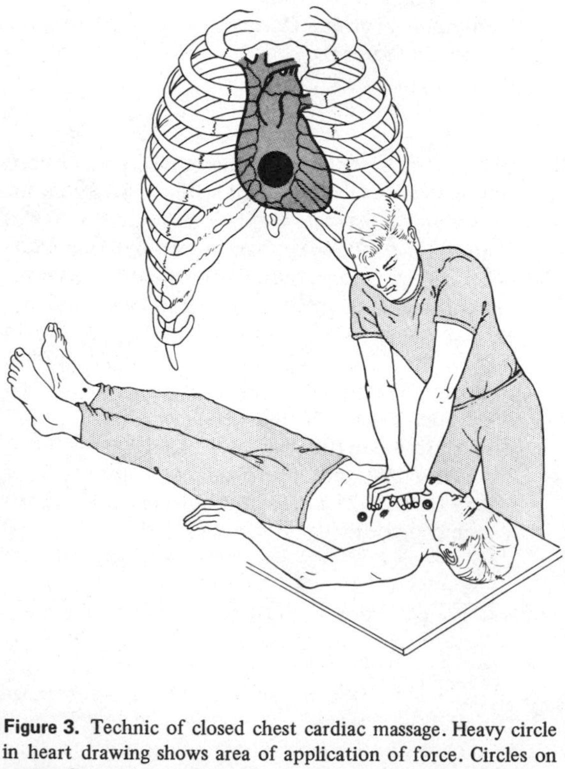

a. If Carotid or Femoral Pulsations Are Present:

Give lung inflation by mouth-to-mouth breathing (keeping patient's nostrils closed) or mouth-to-nose breathing (keeping patient's mouth closed) 12–15 times per minute—allowing about 2 seconds for inspiration and 3 seconds for expiration—until spontaneous respirations return. Continue as long as the pulses remain palpable and previously dilated pupils remain constricted. Bag-mask technics for lung inflation should be reserved for experts. If pulsations cease, follow directions as in 6b, below.

b. If Carotid or Femoral Pulsations Are Absent:

Deliver a single, sharp, quick blow of the fist to the midportion of the sternum (precordial thump) in case of witnessed cardiac arrest or in the monitored patient. If response (return of pulsations) is not immediate, begin external cardiac compression *without delay*. Alternate cardiac compression (closed heart massage) and pulmonary ventilation (as in 6a, above). Place the heel of one hand on the lower third of the sternum just above the level of the xiphoid. With the heel of the other hand on top of it, apply firm vertical pressure sufficient to force the sternum about 1½–2 inches (4–5 cm) downward (less in children) about once every second (60–80 per minute). For children, use only one hand; for babies, use only 2 fingers of one hand, compressing 80–100 times per minute. After 15 sternal compressions, alternate with 2 quick, deep lung inflations. Repeat and continue this alternating procedure until it is possible to obtain additional assistance and more definitive care. If 2 operators are available, pause after every 5th compression while partner gives 1 mouth-to-mouth inflation. Check carotid pulse after 1 minute and every 5 minutes thereafter. Check pupils periodically. Pupils that remain widely dilated are an indication of cerebral hypoxia and brain damage. Resuscitation must be continuous during transportation to the hospital.

Figure 3. Technic of closed chest cardiac massage. Heavy circle in heart drawing shows area of application of force. Circles on supine figure show points of application of electrodes for defibrillation.

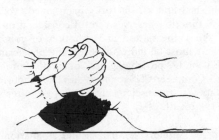
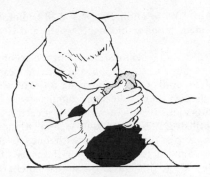

Figure 4. *Method A:* Clear mouth and throat. Place patient supine. Pull strongly forward at angle of mandible. Close patient's nose with your cheek. Gauze (as shown) or airway may be used but is not necessary.

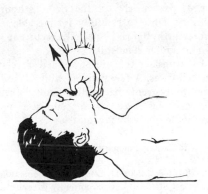
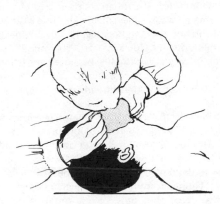

Figure 5. *Method B:* Clear mouth and throat. Place patient supine. Insert left thumb between patient's teeth, grasp mandible firmly in midline, and draw it forward (upward) so that the lower teeth are leading. Close patient's nose with right hand. Gauze (as shown) or airway may be used but is not necessary.

Phase II: Restoration of Spontaneous Circulation

Until spontaneous respiration and circulation are restored, there must be no interruption of artificial ventilation and cardiac massage while steps 7–13 (below) are being carried out. Three basic questions must be considered at this point:

(1) What is the underlying cause, and is it correctable?

(2) What is the nature of the cardiac arrest?

(3) What further measures will be necessary? The physician must plan upon the assistance of trained hospital personnel,* an ECG, a defibrillator, and emergency drugs.

Step 7: If a spontaneous effective heartbeat is not restored after 1–2 minutes of cardiac compres-

*In the hospital a physician able to intubate the trachea will quickly visualize the larynx, suck out all foreign material, pass a large cuffed endotracheal tube, and attach the airway to an oxygen-powered mechanical breathing device for prolonged artificial ventilation and administration of 100% oxygen. Serial arterial blood gas, pH, and bicarbonate determinations are important. Continuous cardiac monitoring is required.

sion, have an assistant give epinephrine (adrenaline), 0.5–1 mg (0.5–1 ml of 1:1000 aqueous solution) diluted to 10 ml IV every 5 minutes as indicated. Epinephrine may be given by the intracardiac route by experienced operators if necessary.

Step 8: Promote venous return and combat shock; elevation of the legs, intravenous fluids, tourniquets on the extremities, and vasoactive drugs (eg, levarterenol) may be of value. (See Chapter 1.)

Step 9: If the victim is pulseless for more than 5 minutes, give sodium bicarbonate solution, 1 mEq/kg as a 5 or 7.5% solution rapidly IV to combat metabolic acidosis. Repeat every 10 minutes as indicated until, but not after, effective spontaneous circulation is restored.

Step 10: If pulsations still do not return, determine the type of "cardiac arrest" by ECG: (1) Asystole, (2) shock (electrical activity without effective mechanical contraction), or (3) ventricular fibrillation. In case of asystole and shock, continue artificial respiration and external cardiac compression, epinephrine, and sodium bicarbonate. Give also calcium chloride, 5–10 ml (0.5–1 gm) of 10% solution IV every 5–10 minutes as indicated. Monitor blood pH, gases, and electrolytes.

Step 11: If ECG demonstrates ventricular fibrillation, maintain respiration and external cardiac massage until just before giving an external defibrillating shock. Become familiar with the manufacturer's recommendations for each type of defibrillator. A 200–400 watt-second DC shock is given across the heart, eg, with one electrode firmly applied to the skin over the apex of the heart and the other over the sternal notch. (If an AC defibrillator is used, 440–1000 volts AC are given for 0.1–0.25 second.) Monitor with ECG. If cardiac function is not restored, resume external massage and repeat 3 or more shocks at intervals of 1–3 minutes. If cardiac action is reestablished but remains weak, give calcium chloride as above. If fibrillation persists or recurs, give lidocaine hydrochloride (Xylocaine), 50–100 mg IV and repeat if necessary. It may be necessary in such cases also to use a pacemaker to capture or override the abnormal rhythm. In some instances of cardiac arrest with electrical sinus bradycardia (with a heart rate of < 60/minute when associated with CVP or systolic blood pressure < 90 mm (HG) or cardiac arrest with sinus bradycardia associated with high degree of AV block, atropine sulfate, 0.4–0.6 mg IV, may be of value.

Step 12: Thoracotomy and open heart massage may be considered (but only in a hospital) if cardiac function fails to return after all of the above measures have been used for a period of 25–30 minutes.

Step 13: If cardiac, pulmonary, and CNS functions are restored, the patient should be carefully observed for shock and complications of the precipitating cause.

Phase III: Follow-Up Measures

When cardiac and pulmonary function have been reestablished and satisfactorily maintained, evaluation of CNS function deserves careful consideration. Decisions about the nature and duration of subsequent treatment must be individualized. The physician must decide if he is "prolonging life" or simply "prolonging dying." Complete CNS recovery has been reported in a few patients unconscious up to a week after appropriate treatment.

Step 14: Support ventilation and circulation. Treat any other complications that might arise. Do not overlook the possibility of complications of external cardiac massage (eg, broken ribs, ruptured viscera).

Step 15: Meticulous postresuscitation care is required, particularly for the first 48 hours after recovery. Observe carefully for possible multiple cardiac arrhythmias, especially recurrent fibrillation or cardiac standstill.

Step 16: Consider the use of assisted circulation in selected cases. A few patients who cannot be salvaged by conventional cardiopulmonary resuscitation may be saved by the addition of partial cardiopulmonary bypass measures.

Goldberg AH: Cardiopulmonary arrest. New England J Med 290:381, 1974.

Green HL, Hieb GE, Schatz IJ: Electronic equipment in critical care areas: Status of devices currently in use. Circulation 43:A101, 1971.

Jude JR, Nagel EL: Cardiopulmonary resuscitation 1970. Mod Concepts Cardiovas Dis 39:133, 1970.

Standards for cardiopulmonary resuscitation (CPR) and emergency cardiac care (ECC). JAMA 227:833, 1974.

Stephenson HE, Jr: *Cardiac Arrest and Resuscitation,* 4th ed. Mosby, 1974.

Index

Aarane, **113**
Abbreviations, 1023
Abdominal
  angina, 352
  aorta, aneurysms of, 245
  distention, 118
  pain in pregnancy, 453
ABE, 174
Abetalipoproteinemia, 751
ABO incompatibility, 317
Abortion, 460
  habitual, 462
  therapeutic, 463
    complications in, 463
Abrasions, corneal, 77
Abscess
  anal, 369
  brain, 572
  breast, 414
  hepatic, 852
  lung, 123
  nasal septal, 96
  parapharyngeal, 102
  periapical, 329
  peritonsillar, 101
  retropharyngeal, 102
  of teeth, 329
Absorbable gelatin sponge, 71
Acanthocytes, 293
Acantholysis, 37
Acanthosis nigricans, 646
Acatalasemia, 966
Accelerated conduction syndrome, 212
Acetaldehyde poisoning, 947
Acetaminophen, 9
Acetanilid, 953
Acetazolamide, 83, 217, 240, 563, 564
Acetest, 730
Acetic acid douches, 422
Acetohexamide, 721, 732
Acetone bodies, normal values, 1018
Acetyldigitoxin, 236
Acetylsalicylic acid. See Aspirin.
Achalasia of esophagus, 333
Achilles tendon reflex as test of thy-
  roid function, 659
Achlorhydria, 347, 348, 585
Acid-base
  balance, treatment of, in shock, 7
  disturbances, diagnostic approach,
    26–30
Acidemia, isovaleric, 966
Acid-fast rods, drug selections for, 906
Acidifying
  agents, 909
  salts, 242
Acidosis
  lactic, 23
  metabolic, 22
  renal tubular, 538

Acidosis (cont'd)
  respiratory, 22
Acids, corrosive, poisoning due to, 934
Aciduria
  glycolic and L-glyceric, 781
  methylmalonic, 966
  orotic, 966
Acne
  bacillus, 46
  lotion, 72
  vulgaris, 45
Aconite poisoning, 947
Acrisorcin cream, 61, 74
Acromegaly, 652
Acropachy, 665
ACT, 266
ACTH, 711, 716
  clinical use of, 715
  direct assay of plasma, 692
  stimulation test, 692
Actidil, 14
Actinic
  keratitis, 77
  keratosis, 65
Actinomyces israelii, 887
Actinomycin D, 549, 980, 983
Actinomycosis, 887
Actinomycotic mycetoma, 889
Activated clotting time, 266
Acylanid, 235, 236
Adams-Stokes syndrome, 211
Adapin, 601, 602
Addiction, drug, and infection, 788
Addison's disease, 688
Addis urine sediment test, normal
  values, 1020
Ademol, 239
Adenine arabinoside, 913
Adenitis, mesenteric, 358
Adenocarcinoma
  of kidney, 548
  of small intestine, 350
Adenoma
  bronchial, 131
  eosinophilic, of anterior pituitary, 652
  parathyroid, 674
  of small intestine, 351
Adenomatosis, pulmonary, 132
Adenomyomatosis of gallbladder, 389
Adenomyosis, 429
Adenotonsillectomy, 101
Adenovirus infections, 808
Adhesive absorbent bandage, 56
ADH, inappropriate secretion of, 656
  974
Adjuvant chemotherapy for micrometas-
  tases, 981
Adrenal
  carcinoma, 974, 980
  cortex, diseases of, **686–697**

Adrenal (cont'd)
  cortical
    extract, 715
    hypofunction, 687
  crisis, 687
  hyperplasia, congenital, 966
  hormone, normal values, 1020
  insufficiency, 678, 688
    acute, 687
  medulla, diseases of, **697–699**
  medullary hormones, antagonists, and
    blocking agents, **719–720**
Adrenalectomy in treatment of breast
  cancer, 408
Adrenalin, 6
Adrenergic
  beta receptor blockade, 241
  drugs used in hypotensive states, 6
Adrenocortical
  failure, treatment of, in shock, 7
  hormones, 715
  hyperfunction, 691
  hypofunction, 687
  insufficiency, **687–691**
  overactivity, 691
Adrenogenital syndrome, 693, 694
  prepuberal, 693
Adriamycin, 980, 983
Adroyd, 722
Adson's test, 566
Adynamia episodica hereditaria, 593
Adynamic ileus, 354
Aedes mosquito, 802, 804
Aerophagia, 324
Aerosol therapy and aerosolized drug
  therapy, 140
Aerotitis, 926
Affective disorders, primary, treat-
  ment of, 625
Afferent loop syndrome, 347
Agammaglobulinemia
  primary acquired, 996
  X-linked, 992
    infantile, 995
Agglutination inhibition test for
  pregnancy, 450
Aggression and violence, 626
Agnogenic myeloid metaplasia, 300
Agranulocytosis, 306
AHF, 309
  concentrate, 310, 317
AID, 443
"Aid-to-Psoriasis" suit, 44
AIH, 443
Air
  block, 150
  pollution, 955
  sickness. See Motion sickness.
  travel, selection of patients for, 926
Airway obstruction, causes of, 104

Akee poisoning, 948
Akineton, 582
Akrinol, 61
Alastrim, 796
Albinism, 677, **777**
Albright's
    osteodystrophy, 673
    syndrome, 685
Albumin
    normal values, 1019
    serum, 1007
        or plasma, 1013
Alcohol
    addiction, 631
    dementia, 632
    ethyl, poisoning due to, 934
    methyl, poisoning due to, 935
    toxicity of, 935
Alcoholic
    hallucinosis, 632
    withdrawal, 631
Alcoholics Anonymous, 633
Alcoholism, 631
Aldactone, 219, 239, **240**, 696, 715
Aldolase, serum, 1007, 1018
Aldomet, 183
Aldosterone
    antagonist, 240
    normal values, urinary, 1021
Aldosteronism, primary, 179
Aldrich's syndrome, 312
Aldrin, 939
Alflorone, 715, 716
ALG, 529
Alimentary hypoglycemia, functional, 746
Alkali poisoning, 936
Alkalosis
    hypochloremic, 222
    metabolic, 23
    respiratory, 22
Alkaptonuria, 777
Alkeran, 982
Alkylating agents
    in cancer chemotherapy, 980
    in multiple myeloma, 300
Alleles, 957
Allergic
    alveolitis, extrinsic, 116
    conjunctivitis, 80
    diseases, classification of, 12
    disorders, drugs used in, 14
    reactions, systemic, 12
    rhinitis, 97
Allergy to fungi, 60
Allodermanyssus sanguineus, 811
Allopurinol, **547**, 977, 980, 983
Alopecia, 67
    areata, 68
    drug-induced, 68
    idiopathic, 68
    totalis, 68
    universalis, 68
Alphadrol, 716
Alphaprodine, 11
Alpha thalassemia, 291
Aluminum
    acetate ointment, 74
    hydroxide gel, 343
    subacetate solution, 71
Alveolar
    cell carcinoma, 132
    proteinosis, 132

Alveolar-arterial oxygen gradient, 138
Alveolar-capillary block syndrome, 141
Alveolitis, allergic, extrinsic, 116
Amantadine, 582
    hydrochloride, 583, 805, 913
Amaurosis fugax, 252
Amblyopia ex anopsia, 85
    first stage, 85
Amebas
    large race, 850
    life cycle, 850
    small race, 850
Amebiasis, 850
    liver abscess due to, 851
    treatment of, 852
Amebic
    dysentery, 850, 851
    granuloma, 850
    liver abscess, 850, 851
    meningoencephalitis, 853
Amebicides, tissue and luminal, 851
Ameboma, 850, 851, 852
Amenorrhea, 450, 695, **704**
Amethopterin, 982
Amicar, 310
Amino acid(s)
    branched-chain, 778
    metabolism, disorders of, 777
    nitrogen, normal values, 1018
Aminoaciduria, 537
Aminocaproic acid, 310
Aminoglutethimide, 693
Aminoglycoside(s), 900
    and penicillin, combined, 176
p-Aminohippurate clearance, normal
        values, 1020
Aminophylline, 137, 196, 239
    poisoning, 949
Aminopyrine poisoning, 948
Aminosalicylic acid, 127, **904**
Amitriptyline, 601
    poisoning due to, 948
AML, 970
Amniography, 965
Ammonia
    blood, 1007
    normal values, 1018
    production of, in distal tubule, 20
Ammonium chloride, 242, 909
Amnesia, retrograde, 573
Amniocentesis, 965
Amobarbital, 602
Amodiaquine dihydrochloride, 855
Amphetamines, 636
    poisoning, 948
Amphotericin B, 884, 885, 886, 887, 889,
        890, 910
    lotion, 72
Ampicillin, 894, 896
Amputation
    in Buerger's disease, 257
    for gangrene, 250
Amylase
    normal values, 1018
    serum, 1007
    urine, 1008
Amyl nitrite, 190, 239
    pearl, 239
Amyloidosis, 298, **781**
    primary, 994
Amyotrophic lateral sclerosis, 589
Anabolic hormones, 687, **722**

Anaerobic infections, 786
Anahist, 14
Anal
    abscess, 369
    condylomas, 369
    fissure, 369
    incontinence, 370
Analgesic(s)
    narcotic, 10
    nephropathy, 535
    nonnarcotic, 9
    poisoning due to, 942
Anaphylactic
    reactions, 12
    shock, 12, 896
Anaphylactoid purpura, 313
Ancobon, 887
Ancylostoma duodenale, 875
Androgen(s), **721**, 980, 982
    therapy for breast cancer, 407
Androgenic steroids for aplastic anemia,
        277
Anemia(s), **273–293**
    addisonian, 275
    and air travel, 926
    aplastic, **276**, 460
    of azotemia, 293
    of cancer, 293
    of cirrhosis, 292
    drug-induced, 284
    folic acid deficiency, 459
    hemolytic, **279–285**
        acquired, 279
        acute, 282
        of cirrhosis, 293
        congenital, 281
        hereditary nonspherocytic, micro-
            angiopathic, 285
    of infection, 293
    with intramedullary hemolysis, 285
    iron deficiency, 273, 459
    of lead poisoning, 278
    megaloblastic
        nutritional, 276
        of pregnancy, 276, 459
    myelophthisic, 293
    of myxedema, 278
    pernicious, **275**, 276, 993
        of pregnancy, 459
    pyridoxine responsive, 285
    refractory normoblastic, 285
    secondary, 292
    sickle cell, 286, 460, 966
    sideroachrestic, 274, 285, 290
Anencephaly, 960, 966
Anesthetics
    local, in eye, precautions in use of, 87
    volatile, poisoning due to, 955
Aneuploidy, 963
Aneurysm(s)
    of abdominal aorta, 245
    aortic, 228
    of descending aorta, 150
    dissecting, 195
        of aorta, 244
    femoral, 246
    intracranial, 570
    popliteal, 246
    saccular, 243
    of thoracic aorta, 243
    ventricular, 196
Angel dust, 635

Angina
abdominal, 352
Ludwig's, 102
pectoris, 187
prevention of, 190
propranolol in, 241
preinfarction, 192
unstable, 192
Angiography, coronary, 189
Angioma
cerebral, 571
of small intestine, 351
Angioneurotic edema, 47
Angiostrongyliasis, 881
Angiostrongylus cantonensis, 881
Angiotensin
amide, 720
II infusion test, 697
Angle-closure glaucoma, 76
Anhydron, 239
Anileridine, 11
Aniline poisoning, 948
Anions, 15, 17
Ankle swelling in pregnancy, 452
Ankylosing spondylitis, **489**, 998
Anorexia nervosa, 651, 775
Ansolysen, 183, 185
Antabuse and alcohol, effects of, 950
Antacids, 343
Antenatal visits in high-risk pregnancy,
467
Anterior chest wall syndrome, 189
Anthracosis, 114
Anthralin, 44
Anthrax, 830
Antianxiety agents, 602
Anti-arrhythmic activity, propranolol
in, 241
Antibacterial therapy in pneumonia, 117
Antibiotic(s)
agents, **891–913**
powder, topical, 71
in renal failure, 893
Antibodies, antinuclear, test, 50
Antibody-forming cells, 989
Antibody-mediated autoimmunity,
humoral, 989
Anticancer chemotherapy, 409, **979–986**
Anticholinergic drugs in treatment of
ulcer, 343
Anticoagulant(s)
circulating, 317
inhibitors of, 310
oral, 267
poisoning due to, 936
therapy, 196, 567
in thrombophlebitis, 266
Anticonvulsants, 562, 564
Antidepressants, 601
Antidiarrheal agents, 324
Antidiuretic hormone, inappropriate
secretion of, 656, 974
Antifertility drugs, oral, 724
Antifolate drugs, 905
Antifungal agents, **890,** 909
Anti-GBM
disease, 523
nephritis, 526
Antigenic determinants, minor, 896
Antigens, 12
mixed lymphocyte culture, 990
Antihemophilic factor, 309

Antihistamines, 14
Anti-infective agents, **891–913**
Antilymphocytic globulin, 529
Antimalarials in arthritis, 482
Antimetabolites in cancer chemo-
therapy, 980
Antimicrobial
drugs
combination, **911–913**
and other agents, incompatibil-
ities between, 892
therapy
duration of, 892
rules for, 891
in shock, 8
Antimongolism, 968
Antimony
dimercaptosuccinate, sodium, 864
poisoning, 948
potassium tartrate, 864
sodium gluconate, 859
Antinuclear antibody test, 50
Antiparkinsonism drugs, 582
Antipruritic drugs, systemic, 33
Antipsychotics, 597
Antipyretic drugs, 2
Antipyrine poisoning, 948
Antiseborrheic shampoo, 74
Antiseptics, urinary, 909
Antiserum, snakebite, 946
Antisocial personality, 616
Antispasmodic drugs in treatment of
ulcer, 343
Antistreptolysin O titer, 163
Antithyroid drugs, 455
Antituberculosis drugs, 903
primary, 127
Antitumor chemotherapy, 465
Antiviral chemotherapy, 913
Anus
carcinoma of, squamous cell, 370
diseases of, **368–370**
Anxiety, 611
Aorta
abdominal, aneurysms of, 245
coarctation of, 157, 179
descending, aneurysm of, 150
diseases of, **243–247**
dissecting aneurysms of, 244
occlusive disease of, 247
thoracic, aneurysms of, 243
Aortic
aneurysms, 228
dissection, acute, 244
insufficiency, 166, 167, 168, **172**
stenosis, 166, 167, 171
Aortitis, 228
APC, 9
Aphasia, treatment of, in hemiplegia,
570
Aphthous ulcer, 330
APL, 651, 713
Aplasia
erythroid, 974
pure red cell, 278
Aplastic
anemia, **276,** 460
crisis, 279, 282
Apothecary equivalents, 1021
Appendiceal abscess, 359
Appendicitis, 357
in pregnancy, 474

Appetite
change in, 647
suppressants, 773
Apresoline, 183
Ara-C, 295, 982
Arachnid bite, 63, 932, **946**
Arachnodactyly, 781
Aramine, 6
Aran-Duchenne atrophy, 588
ARDS, 137
ARF, 137
Artane, 582
Arfonad, 185
Argininosuccinicaciduria, 966
Argyll Robertson pupil, 153
Ariboflavinosis, 770
Aristocort, 716
Arrhenoblastoma, 695
of ovary, 437
Arrhythmia(s)
cardiac, 199, 201
sinus, 201
Arsenical(s)
melanosis, 65
pentavalent, 851
Arsenic poisoning, 936
Arsine poisoning, 948
Arterial
disease(s)
degenerative and inflammatory,
243
in diabetic patients, 250
embolism, 254
insufficiency to intestine, 253
occlusion, acute, 254
thrombosis, acute, 255
Arteriolar nephrosclerosis, 532
Arteriosclerosis, 243
Arteriosclerotic
heart disease, 187
occlusive disease, **247–258**
Arteritis
giant cell, 258
idiopathic, of Takayasu, 258
temporal, 258, 488
Arthritic joints, general principles in
physical management of, 500
Arthritis, 163
acute infections, 493
assistive devices in, 501
braces in, 500
degenerative, 512
exercise in, 500
gonorrheal, 511
gouty, 496
hypertrophic, 512
and inflammatory intestinal diseases, 491
patient, examination of, 477
and psoriasis, 491
pyogenic, chronic, 495
rheumatoid, **479,** 993
conservative management, 480
and salmonella osteomyelitis, 504
in sarcoidosis, 499
splints in, 500
syphilitic, 509
tophaceous, chronic, 498
Arthrodesis, 501
Arthropathy
neurogenic, 493
neurotrophic, 509

Arthroplasty, 501
Arthropod(s)
  infection, 882
  skin lesions due to, 63
Arthropod-borne encephalitis, 801
Artificial
  insemination, 443
  respiration, **1026—1028**
Arvin, 267
Asbestosis, 114
Ascariasis, 872
Ascaris lumbricoides, 872
Ascites, 28
Ascorbic acid, 758, **770,** 1018
  in treatment of common cold, 79p
Aseptic meningitis, 807
"As if" personality, 617
Asparaginase, 980
Aspartane, 732
Aspergillosis, 890
Aspergillus fumigatus, 113
Aspidium oleoresin, 869
Aspiration pneumonia, 121
Aspirin, 9
  in arthritis, 481
  poisoning, 945
Asthenic personality, 616
Asthma, 111
  treatment of, 112
Asthmatic bronchitis, chronic, 226
Astiban, 864
Asymptomatic
  infection, early treatment of, 912
  neurosyphilis, 845
AT, 674, 714
Atabrine, 868, 983
Ataxia-telangiectasia, 970
  immunodeficiency with, 996
Atelectasis, pulmonary, 133
Atheroma and lipoproteins, relation-
    ship between, 749
Athlete's foot, 59
Atomic irradiation, sickness due to,
    922—924
Atopic
  asthma, 111
  dermatitis, 37
Atresia, tricuspid, 161
Atrial
  fibrillation, 205, 668
    chronic, 205
    paroxysmal, 205
  flutter, 206
    chronic, 206
    paroxysmal, 206
  premature beats, 203
  septal defect, 155, 158
  tachycardia, paroxysmal, 203
Atrioventricular conduction system, 209
Atroph(ies)
  and dystrophies, differential diag-
      nosis of, 588
  muscular, 588, 589
  Sudeck's, 262
Atropine
  poisoning, 938
Atypical pneumonia, primary, 121
Audiometric tests, 88
Auricular. See Atrial.
Auscultation, cardiac, 154
Autoimmune disease(s), 997
  and associated antibodies, 993

Autoimmune disease(s) (cont'd)
  and FUO, 783
  mechanisms of, 989
    injury in, 997
  tests for autoantibodies associ-
      ated with, 992
Autoimmunity
  cell-mediated, 989
  humoral antibody-mediated, 989
Autosomal
  disorders, 969
  inheritance, 958
Autosomes, 957
Aversive conditioning, 608
Azacytadine, 979, 980
Azaribine, 44
Azotemia, anemia of, 293

B
  cell(s)
    function, procedures for measur-
        ing, 990
    maturation, 988
    technics for identification of, 992
  lymphocytes, 988
  and T lymphocytes, 988
Bacillary dysentery, 827
Bacillus
  cereus, 830
  subtilis, 115
Bacitracin, 908
Backache
  gynecologic, 441
  in pregnancy, 451
Back pain, low, 576
Bacteremia
  and endocarditis, 787
  and sepsis, gram-negative, 785
Bacteremic shock, 785
Bacterial
  diarrhea, acute, and food poisoning,
      824
  diseases, **814—840**
  endocarditis, prophylaxis for, 913
  infections, **814—840**
  pneumonias, 119
  sepsis and cancer, 977
  synergistic gangrene, 787
Bacteriuria, 540
Bacteroides pneumonia, 120
Bad trip, 634
BAL, 583, 936, 941, 942
Balantidiasis, 861
Balantidium coli, 861
Baldness, 67
  male pattern, 68
Band keratopathy, 675, 676
BAO, 345
Barber's itch, 53
Barbiturates, 602
  dependency on, 629
  poisoning, 937
Barium poisoning, 948
Barr body, 964, 965
Barrett's esophagus, 336
Bartholin's duct and gland, cyst and
    abscess of, 423
Bartonellosis, 838
Basal
  body temperature, 444
  cell carcinomas, 65

Basal (cont'd)
  metabolic rate, 659
Base, total serum, 1018
BaSon test, 266
Bassen-Kornzweig syndrome (abeta-
    lipoproteinemia), 751
Battey organism, 129
Bauxite pneumoconiosis, 114
BBT, 444
BCG, 980
  as anticancer drug, 980, 983
  immunotherapy, 983
  reactions to, 985
  vaccination, 126
BCNU, 980, 983
Beau's lines, 69
Bedbugs, 63
Bedsores, 55
Bee stings, 947
Behavior therapy, technics of, in psy-
    chiatry, 608
BEI test, 657
Bejel, 847
Belladonna
  poisoning, 938
  preparations, 343
Bell's palsy, 586
Benadryl, 14, 582
Bence Jones
  myeloma, 298
  proteinuria, 298
Bender Gestalt Test, 596
Bendroflumethiazide, 239
Bends, 924
Benedict's test, drugs interfering
    with, 1005
Benisone gel, 74
Benzagel, 46
Benzathine penicillin G, 895
Benzedrine, 636
Benzene poisoning, 948
Benzodiazepines, 602
Benzoic acid and salicylic acid
    ointment, 74
Benzoin, compound, 74
Benzoyl peroxide, 46
Benzthiazide, 239
Benztropine methanesulfonate, 582
Benzyl benzoate, 62
Bephenium hydroxynaphthoate, 873, 876
Beriberi, 769
  heart, 229
  Shoshin, 769
Berlock hyperpigmentation, 67
Berylliosis, 114
Beryllium poisoning, 948
Bestiality, 613
Beta-adrenergic blocking agents, 720
Betamethasone, 716, 717
  benzoate gel, 74
  valerate, 44
Betapar, 716
Beta receptor blockade, adrenergic, 241
Betazole, 275
Bicarbonate
  reabsorption, defects of, 538
  serum or plasma, 1008
Biguanide(s), 733
  compounds, 720
Bile
  acids, resins to absorb, 750
  reflux, 347

Bilharziasis, 863
Biliary
  cirrhosis, 384
  stricture, 392
  tract
    carcinoma of, 393
    diseases of, 370
Bilirubin
  normal values, 1018
  serum, 1008
  test, drugs interfering with, 1005
Biopsy
  in breast cancer, 402
  renal, 522
Biperiden, 582
Biphenyls, polychlorinated, as tera-
    togens, 455
Bird mites, 64
Bisacodyl, 323
Bisexuality, 613
Bismuth
  hydroxide, 325
  magma, 325
  and paregoric, 325
  subcarbonate, 325
Bithionol, 866, 867
Black
  eye, 77
  widow spider bites, 63, 946
Blackfan-Diamond syndrome, 279
Blacklight lamps, 44
Blackwater fever, 854
Bladder
  cancer, 863
  pain, 521
  tumors of, 549
Bland diet, 761
Blastomyces dermatitidis, 509, 886
Blastomycosis
  North American, 886
    of bones and joints, 508
  South American, 886
Bleaching solutions, poisoning due to, 949
Bleeding
  breakthrough, 445
  disorders, **307–318**
    differential diagnosis of, 309
    transfusions in, 319
  gastrointestinal, massive, 326
  intracranial, 568
  in peptic ulcer, 342
  postpartum, 466
  rectal. See specific causes, particu-
    larly ulcerative colitis, polyposis,
    cancer, fissure, hemorrhoids.
  subarachnoid, 570
  third trimester, 466
  time, normal values, 1018
  uterine, abnormal, 417
  vaginal, postmenopausal, 418
  vitreous, 79
Blended tube feeding formula, 765
Blenoxane, 980, **983,** 985
Bleomycin, 980, **983,** 985
Blepharitis, 82
Blindness, night, 767
Block
  atrioventricular
    complete, 211
    partial, 210
    second degree, 210
    third degree, 210

Block (cont'd)
  bundle branch, 209
  heart, complete, 211
  sino-atrial, 209
Blocking agent test, 698
Blood
  ammonia, 1007
  and body fluids, chemical constituents
    of, **1003–1017**
  cast, 524
  coagulation of, 307
  diseases of, **273–320**
  effect of meals and posture on con-
    centration of substances in, 1004
  fresh, 318
  glucose, 1011
  levels of antibiotics, 892
  spitting or coughing of, 107
  sugar, hormones and hormone-like
    agents affecting, 720
  transfusions, **318–320**
  urea nitrogen, normal values, 1019
  vessels, diseases of, **243–272**
  volume, normal values, 1019
Bloom's syndrome, 970
Blurred vision, 75
BMR, 659
Bockhart's impetigo, 53
Body
  fluid(s), 15
    compartments, 16
  ringworm, 57
  surface area
    estimation of in burns, 917
    nomograms, 1022
  temperature, 1
  water, 15
    total, 15
    volume and distribution of, 15
Boeck's sarcoid, 142
Boerhaave's syndrome, 321
Boils, 54
Bone(s)
  atrophy, acute, 678, 680
  brittle, 517
  cancer, 680
  densitometry, 683
  disease, **502–520**
    metabolic, **679–684**
    nonmetabolic, **685–686**
  marrow
    toxicity, 981
    transplantation, 278
  pain, 648
  tumors
    primary, **518–519**
    and tumor-like lesions, **516–517**
Bones and joints
  coccidioidomycosis of, 508
  cryptococcosis of, 508
  disorders of, **502–520**
  histoplasmosis of, 508
  infections of, **502–511**
    mycotic, 507
  North American blastomycosis of,
    509
  syphilis of, 509
  tuberculosis of, 510
Borderline conditions in psychiatry,
    617
Boric acid poisoning, 949
Borrelia recurrentis, 848

Borrmann classification of gastric
    carcinoma, 347
Botflies, 882
Botulism, 832
Bowen's disease, 65
Braces in arthritis, 500
Bradycardia, sinus, 203
Brain
  abscess, 572
  scan, computerized, 579
  tumor(s), **578–579**
    frequency of types, 578, 579
Brasivol, 46
Braxton Hicks contractions, 454
Breakbone fever, 802
Breakthrough bleeding, 445
Breast
  abscess, 414
  cancer
    female, **399,** 974, 980
      advanced, hypercalcemia in, 410
      biopsy in, 402
      causes of, 400
      choice of primary treatment
        for, 404
      clinical staging of, 403
      curative treatment for, 403
      palliative treatment for, 405
      TNM system of staging of, 403
    male, 411
  cystic mastitis of, chronic, 412
  diseases of, **399–414**
  fibroadenoma of, 413
  soreness in pregnancy, 452
Breath, bad, 321
Brenner tumor of ovary, 435
Brill's disease, 809
Briquet's syndrome, 611
Brittle bones, 517
Bromate poisoning, 949
Bromide(s), 562
  poisoning, 938
Brompheniramine, 14
Bronchi
  disorders of, **107–111**
  foreign bodies in, 104, 105
  inflammation of, 107
Bronchial
  adenoma, 131
  asthma, 111
  narrowing, 106
Bronchiectasis, 109
Bronchiolar carcinoma, 132
Bronchiolitis, 790
Bronchitis, 107
  acute, 96
  chronic asthmatic, 226
Bronchodilators
  aerosolized, 138
  oral, 140
Bronchogenic
  carcinoma, **130,** 974
    gonadotropin-secreting, 704
  cyst, 150
Bronchopneumonia, 120
Bronchospasm, relief of, 137
Brown tumor, 676
Brucella osteomyelitis, 505
Brucellosis, 828
Brufen, 10
Brugia malayi, 877
BSP test, drugs interfering with, 1005

Buerger's disease, 256
Buffalo hump, 691
Bufotenine, 947
Bulbar palsy, 588
Bundle
    branch block, 209
    of His electrograms, 206
Bürger-Grütz disease, 747
Burn(s), **917–921**
    critical, classification of, 917
    edema in, 27
    electric, 922
    estimation of body surface area, 917
    fluid problems in, 917, 918
    shock, 3
    third degree, 920
    wound
        early care of, 919
        later care of, 920
Burow's solution, 71, 91
Burr cells, 285
Bursa-derived cells, 988
Bursitis, 499
Busulfan, 296, 980, 982
    toxicity, 985
Butanol-extractable iodine test, 657
Butaperazine, 598
Butazolidin, 9, 269
Butterfly pattern or rash, 49
Butyrophenone, 598

Cachexia, hypopituitary, **650**
Cadaveric electric reaction, 593
Cadmium poisoning, 949
Cafergot, 559
Caffeine poisoning, 949
Caisson disease, 924
Calamine lotion, 72
Calcareous tendinitis, scapulohumeral, 514
Calciferol, 674, 714
Calcimar, 686, 714
Calcitonin, 677
    synthetic salmon, 686, 714
Calcium, 24
    absorption, defects of, 537
    carbimide, 781
    carbonate, 343
    chloride, 674
    diet
        high, 755
        low, 763
        test, 764
    disodium edetate, 278, 587, 941
    food sources of, 758
    infusion test, 681
    in renal stone formation, 545
    salts, 674
    serum, 1008
        normal values, 1018
    test, drugs interfering with, 1005
    urine, 1009
Calculi
    renal, 545
    urinary, **545–548**
California encephalitis, 801
Callosities, 49
Calluses, 49
    treatment of, 736
Calorie(s)
    diet, low, 773

Calorie(s) (cont'd)
    malnutrition, 774
    in snack foods, 774
Calusterone, 722, 982
Camphor poisoning, 949
Cancer. See also specific types.
    anemia of, 293
    bacterial sepsis and, 977
    breast
        female, 399
        male, 411
    chemotherapeutic agents
        dose modification of, 984
        mechanisms of action of, 979
        toxicity and dose modification 981, 982
    chemotherapy, **979–986**
    genetic aspects of, 969
Candida albicans, **60**, 61, 115, 421, **887**
Candidal onychomycosis, 60
Candidiasis, 887
    cutaneous, 61
    oral, 331
Canker sore, 330
Cannabis sativa, 635
Cantharidin poisoning, 949
Capillariasis, intestinal, 877
Capillary morphometry, 730
Capreomycin, 904
Capsebon, 45
Capsulitis, adhesive, 513
Carbamazepine, 10, 562
Carbarsone, 851
Carbenicillin, 177, **896**
Carbohydrate
    diet, low, 761
    metabolism, disorders of, 779
Carbolfuchsin, 62, 270
    solution, Castellani's, 39, 49
Carbolic acid poisoning, 943
Carbon
    dioxide
        combining power, 1009, 1018
        monoxide poisoning, 938
        tetrachloride poisoning, 939
Carbonic anhydrase inhibitors, 240
Carbostibamide, 859
Carbuncles, 54
Carcinoid, 980
    syndrome, 978
    tumors of small intestine, 350
Carcinoma. See specific types.
Cardiac. See also Heart.
    arrest, treatment of, **1025–1028**
    arrhythmias, 198, 201
        in pneumonia, 119
    disorders, treatment of, in shock, 7
    enlargement in common valve lesions, 168
    failure, **213–220**
        electrolyte disturbances in, 222
        high-output, **222**, 686
        in myocardial infarction, 196
        refractory, 221
        vasodilators in treatment of, 219
    hypertrophy, idiopathic, 230
    massage, 209, 1026
        closed chest, 1026
    patient
        and pregnancy, 233
        and surgery, 232
    tamponade, 224

Cardiac (cont'd)
    tumors, primary, 232
Cardilate, 239
Cardiogenic shock, 196
Cardiomyopath(ies), 229
    hypertrophic, 242
Cardiopulmonary bypass, 1028
Cardiovascular
    disease
        and air travel, 926
        diagnosis, 152
        hypertensive, 178
        syphilitic, 228
    drugs, **233–242**
    manifestations of tertiary syphilis, 845
Cardioversion, 203, 204, 238
Carditis, rheumatic, 162
Cardrase, 240
Caries, 328
Carmustine, 980, 983
Carotenoids, normal values, 1018
Carotid sinus syncope, 556
Carpal tunnel syndrome, **515**, 653
Carrión's disease, 838
Carter-Robbins test, 654
Caruncle, urethral, 423
Cascara sagrada, 323
Casoni intracutaneous test, 869
Castellani's
    carbolfuchsin solution, 39, 49
    paint, 62, 270
Castor bean poisoning, 949
Castration, female, in treatment of breast cancer, 408
Cataract, 84
Catecholamines, urinary, 181, 698
    normal values, 1021
    test for, drugs interfering with, 1005
Caterpillars, urticating, 64
Cat eye syndrome, 968
Cathartic colitis, 325
Catheterization, venous, short-term, 268
Cations, 15, 16, 17
Cat-scratch fever, 806
Causalgia, **261**, 514
CCNU, 980
CCK, 389
Cedilanid, 236
Cedilanid-D, 236
Cefazolin, 893, 897
Celestone, 716, 717
Celiac
    disease, 998
    sprue, 355
    and superior mesenteric artery disease, 253
Cell-mediated
    autoimmunity, 989
    immunity tests, 990
Cellular
    basis of immune responses, 988
    division, 962
Cellulitis, 55
    of floor of mouth, 102
    nonclostridial crepitant, 787
    orbital, 79
    synergistic necrotizing, 787
Cellulose phosphate in prevention of renal stones, 546
Celontin, 562, 564

Central nervous system
 defects, congenital, **565–566**
 disorders
  degenerative, **580–585**
  traumatic, **573–578**
  vascular, **566–572**
 infections of, 818
Centromere, 961
Cephalalgia, histaminic, 559
Cephalexin, 897
Cephaloglycine, 897
Cephaloridine, 897
Cephalosporins, 897
Cephalothin, 176, 897
Ceramidosis, lactosyl, 966
Cercariae, 863
Cerclage, Shirodkar, 461
Cerebellar tumor, 579
Cerebral
 angioma, 571
 edema, 573
 ischemia, transient, 566
Cerebrospinal fluid findings in CNS
  diseases, 819
Cerebrovascular
 accidents, 195, 566
  recovery and convalescence after,
   569
 disease, occlusive, 251
 disorders, diagnosis of, 568
Ceruloplasmin
 normal values, 1018
 serum, 1009
Cerumen, impacted, 90
Cervical
 carcinoma, 424
 disk herniation, 577
 polyps, 428
 rib syndrome, 565
 spine, osteoarthritis of, 512
 spondylosis, 512
Cervicitis, 422
 nongonococcal, 840
Cervicobrachial pain
 intrathoracic origin of, 516
 syndromes, **512–516**
Cervix
 cancer of, staging of, 425
 uterine, carcinoma of, 424
Cestode infections, **867–870**
Chagas' disease, 857
Chagoma, 858
Chalazion, 82
Chancre, syphilitic, 843
Chancroid, 835
Charcoal, activated, 931
Charcot joint, 493, 509, 565
Charcot-Marie-Tooth disease, 589
Cheilitis, chronic angular, 331
Chemical(s)
 and chromosomes, 971
 peritonitis, 397
Chemoprophylaxis, antimicrobial, 911
Chemosurgery, 66
Chemotherapeutic agents, **891–913**
 cancer, dose modification of, 984
Chemotherapy
 as adjunct to radical mastectomy, 405
 adjuvant, for micrometastases, 981
 antiviral, 913
 for breast cancer, 409
 cancer, **979–986**

Chemotherapy (cont'd)
 combination
  in Hodgkin's disease, 302
  in malignant melanoma, 304
 malignancies responsive to, 980
Chest pain, **106**, 152
 noncardiac causes, 152
Chiari-Frommel syndrome, 705
Chickenpox, 792, 795
 diagnostic features of, 792
 in pregnancy, 472
Chiggers, 64
Chigoes, 64
Chilblain, 914
Chiniofon, 851
Chlamydiae, pneumonia due to, 122
Chlamydial
 conjunctivitis, 79
 infections, **839–840**, 905
Chloasma, 67
Chlomophene. See Clomiphene.
Chloral hydrate, 602
Chlorambucil, 297, 302, 980, 982
Chloramine-T poisoning, 949
Chloramphenicol, 899
Chlorate poisoning, 949
Chlordane, 939
Chlordiazepoxide, 563, 602
Chloride(s), 242
 normal values, 1018
 serum, 1009
 test, drugs interfering with, 1005
 urine, 1009
Chlorinated
 hydrocarbon poisoning, 949
 insecticides, poisoning due to, 939
 naphthalene, poisoning due to, 949
Chlorine, food sources of, 758
Chlorisondamine chloride, 183
Chlormadinone acetate, 725
Chlormerodrin, 240
Chloroform poisoning, 955
Chlorophenothane poisoning, 939
Chloroquine, 50, 852, 853, 855
 in arthritis, 482
 poisoning, 954
Chlorothiazide, 182, 239
Chlorotrianisene, 723
Chlorpheniramine, 14
Chlorphenoxamine, 582
Chlorphenoxyisobutyrate, 750
Chlorpromazine, 598
 poisoning, 944
Chlorpropamide, 721, 732
Chlorprothixene, 598
Chlortetracycline, 899
Chlorthalidone, 239
Chlor-Trimeton, 14
Cholangitis, 387
 primary sclerosing, 393
Cholecystitis
 acute, 387
  in pregnancy, 473
 chronic, 389
Cholecystokinin, 389
Choledocholithiasis, **390**, 473
Cholelithiasis, 388
Cholera, 826
 immunization, 1002
Cholestasis, benign intermittent, 378
Cholesterol
 esters, 1010

Cholesterol
 esters (cont'd)
  normal values, 1018
 serum, 658
 test, drugs interfering with, 1005
Cholesterolosis, 388
Cholestyramine, 750
Choloxin, 663, 714
Chondroblastoma, 519
Chondrocalcinosis and pseudogout, 499
Chondromyxoid fibroma, 518
Chondrosarcoma, 518
Chorea
 Huntington's, 584
 Sydenham's, 162, 584
Choriocarcinoma (chorio-epithelioma),
  464, 704, 974, 980
Choriomeningitis, lymphocytic, 801
Chorionic gonadotropin, 418, 651, 713
 normal values, 1020
Chorioretinitis, 81
Christmas disease, 309
Chromate poisoning, 949
Chromatids, 961
Chromatin-positive patients, 701
Chromium poisoning, 949
Chromoblastomycosis, 889
Chromosomal
 abnormalities
  methods of study, 964
  quinacrine mustard test for, 964
  types of, 963
 analysis, 965
 notation system, 965
Chromosome(s), 957
 breakage syndromes, 970
 deletions, 963
 Denver classification of, 961
 disorders, **967–972**
 duplication of, 963
 inversion of, 963
 and ionizing radiation, 971
 and malignancy, 970
 nondisjunction, 963
 sex, 957
 translocation, 963
 viruses, chemicals, and, 971
Chromosome 13, phenotypic map of, 970
Chrysarobin, 74
Chrysotherapy in arthritis, 481
Chvostek's sign, 672, 673
Chylomicronemia, fasting, 748
Cinchonism, 238
Cineangiocardiography, coronary, 189,
  152
Circulating anticoagulants, 317
Circulatory
 eczema, 39
 shock, 2
Cirrhosis
 anemia of, 292
 biliary, 384
  primary, 993
 nodular, 381
Cisternal reservoir administration of
  amphotericin B, 885
Citrovorum rescue, 985
Citrullinemia, 966
Clantis lotion, 46
Clark test, 418, 427
Classical bland diet, 761
Classification, psychiatric, 610

Claudication, intermittent, 250
Clefamide, 851
Cleft
  lip, 960
  palate, 960
Click(s)
  heart, 154
  syndrome, 170
Clindamycin, 893, 908
Clinitest, 730
Clofibrate, 750
Clomid, 418, 443, 706, 712
Clomiphene citrate, 418, 443, 706, 712
Clonorchiasis, 866
Clonorchis sinensis, 866
Clorazepate, 602
Clostridial food poisoning, 824
Clot retraction, normal values, 1018
Clotrimazole, 74
Clotting time, activated, 266
Clouding, vitreous, 75
Cloxacillin, 896
Clubbing of fingers, 69
Clubfoot, 960
Cluster headaches, 559
Clutton's joints, 509
CMF, 980, 981
CML, 970, 978
CNS, infections of, 818
^{60}Co, 426
CO_2
  combining power, normal values,
    1018
    serum or plasma, 1009
  content, 1018
  tension, arterial, 108
Coagulation
  disseminated intravascular, 315
  factors, 307
    vitamin K in, 768
  mechanisms, 307
  problems, diagnosis of, 308
  time, normal values, 1018
Coagulopathy, 974
  consumption, 312
Coal tar lotion, 72
COAP, 295
Coarctation of aorta, 157, 179
Cobaltous chloride, 277
Cocaine, 636
  poisoning, 950
Coccidioides immitis, 883
Coccidioidin skin test, 883
Coccidioidomycosis, 883
  of bones and joints, 507
Coccidiosis, 861
Cocoa butter, 73
Codeine, 11
Cogentin, 582
Coitus, painful, 440
Colace, 323
Colchicine, 9, 497
  poisoning, 950
Cold
  feet, treatment of, 736
  common, 96, 790, 808
  disorders due to, **914–915**
  hemoglobinuria, 283
  injury, prevention of, 914
  sore, 50, 331
Colestipol, 750
Colistin, 902

Colitis
  functional (spastic), 325
  granulomatous, 363
  ulcerative, 361
Collagen diseases, **478–501**
Collapse therapy in tuberculosis, 128
Colon
  cancer of, 366, 980
    in pregnancy, 472
  diseases of, **361–367**
  irritable, 325
  polyps, 365
  toxic dilatation of, 363
Colonic obstruction, 366
Colorado tick fever, 803
Colostomy
  care of, 367
  patients and air travel, 926
Coma, 553
  diabetic, 740
  in diabetic patients, laboratory
    diagnosis of, 740
  myxedema, 663
  nonketotic hyperglycemic, 742
Combined system disease, 584
Combining power, CO_2, 1009, 1018
Common
  cold, 96, 808
  respiratory disease, 96
Complement fixation test, 992
  for syphilis, 841
Compliance, effective, 138
Compound
  B, 715
  F, 715
Compulsions, 611
Computerized brain scan, 579
Concentration
  hydrogen ion, 21
    altered, clinical states of, **22–23**
  solute, 15, 18
Conditioning therapies, 601
Condom, 46
Conduction
  disturbances of, **209–212**
  prolonged, 210
Conductive deafness, 89, 90
Condyloma, anal, 369
Condylomata lata, 844
Congestive heart failure. See Cardiac
    failure.
Congo red test, 782
  normal values, 1021
Conjunctival
  discharge, 75
  foreign body, 76
  lacerations, 79
  test for hypersensitivity, 1003
Conjunctivitis, 79
  acute, 75
  allergic, 80
  bacterial, 79, 80
  chlamydial, 80
  chemical, 78
  fungal, 80
  gonococcal, 78
  inclusion, 80, 840
  leptothrix, 80
  parasitic, 80
  silver nitrate, 80
  viral, 79
Connective tissue diseases, **478–501**

Consciousness, disorders of, **553–555**
Constipation, 322
  in pregnancy, 452
  in vincristine therapy, 985
Consumption coagulopathy, 315
Contagious disease and air travel, 926
Contraception, 444
Contraceptives, oral
  and acne vulgaris, 44
  contraindications to, 446
  effectiveness of, 446
  effects of, 445
  hormone-related side-effects of, 445
  oncology and, 446
  selection of, 446
Contrecoup injury, 573
Contusions, eye, 77
Conversion
  reactions, 611
  to sinus rhythm, 238
  tables, 1021, 1023
Convulsions, febrile, 561
Convulsive
  disorders, **560–564**
  therapies, 604
Coombs test, 279, 280, 281
Cooperator cells, 989
COPD, 1024
Copper
  food sources of, 758
  normal values, 1009, 1019
Coproporphyrin
  type
    I, 780
    III, 780
  in urine, 780
Coproporphyrinurias, 780
Copulation, extragenital, 613
Cordran, 717
Cornea, fungal overgrowth of, 87
Corneal
  abrasions, 77
  foreign body, 76, 87
  lacerations, 79
  trauma or infection, 75
  ulcer, 77
Corns, 49
  treatment of, 736
Coronary
  angiography, 189
  artery disease, 187
  cineangiography, 152
  heart disease, surgery for, 191
  insufficiency, 192
Cor pulmonale, chronic, 226
Corpus
  luteum cysts of ovaries, 435
  of uterus, cancer of, 427
Corrigan's pulse, 172
Cortef, 716
Cortical extract, whole, 715
Corticosteroid(s), 497, 716, 717
  in arthritis, 482
  for breast cancer, 407
  clinical use of, 717
  in chronic respiratory failure, 140
  in leukemia, 298
  local, 717
  oral, 716
  parenteral, 717
  in rheumatic fever, 164
  for shock, 7

Corticosteroid(s) (cont'd)
  topical, potentiation of, 33
Corticosterone, 715
Corticotropin, 711, 715, 716, **717**
  test, 689
Cortisol
  free, urinary, 692
  normal values, 1019
Cortisone(s)
  acetate, 715, 716, 717
  clinical use of, 717
Cortogen, 716
Cortone, 716
Cortril, 716
Cortrophin-Zinc, 716
Cortrosyn, 689, 716
Corynebacterium acnes, 46
Cosmegen, 983
Cosmetic disfiguration in skin dis-
  orders, 33
Cosyntropin, 689, 716
Co-trimoxazole, 542, 905
Cotton wool exudates, 180
Cough, 106
  in tuberculosis, 128
Coumadin, 266, 267
Counseling, genetic, 972
Countershock, direct current
  in atrial fibrillation, 205
  in paroxysmal ventricular tachy-
    cardia, 207
Cover test, 85
Coxiella burneti, 813
Coxsackievirus infections, 807
CPK
  isoenzymes, 1010
  serum, 1010, 1019
  urine, 1010
Crab(s), 63
  yaws, 847
Cramps
  heat, 916
  leg, in pregnancy, 453
  muscle, 249, 649
Cranial nerve(s)
  disorders of, **585–586**
  paralysis, 575
Creatine phosphokinase
  isoenzymes, 1010
  serum, 1010, 1019
  urine, 1010
Creatinine
  clearance, endogenous, normal values,
    1020
  serum, 1010
    normal values, 1019
  urine, 1010
    test for, drugs interfering with,
      1005
Creeping eruption, 881
C region, 987
Creosote (cresol) poisoning, 943
Crepitant cellulitis, nonclostridial,
  787
Cretinism, 661
CRF, 139
Cricothyrotomy, 104
Cri du chat syndrome, 968
Crigler-Najjar syndrome, 378
Crisis therapy, 605
Crohn's
  disease, 349

Crohn's (cont'd)
  granulomatosis, 363
Crotamiton, 62, 64
Croton oil poisoning, 950
Croup, 790
Cryoglobulinemia, 300
Cryoglobulins, 259
Cryohypophysectomy, 653
Cryoprecipitate, 310
Cryosurgery, 66, 84
Cryptitis, 368
Cryptococcosis, 885
  of bones and joints, 508
Cryptorchism, 648, 702
CSF
  findings in CNS diseases, 819
  normal values, 1020
C-terminal constant region, 987
Cumertilin, 240
C_u, normal values, 1020
Cuprimine, 583, 942
Cushing's syndrome, 179, 691, 974
  differentiation from adrenogenital
    syndrome, 694
Cutler-Power-Wilder test, 689
Cyanide poisoning, 939
Cyanocobalamin, 276, 758, 771
Cyanogas poisoning, 939
Cyanogen poisoning, 939
Cyanosis, 107, 154
  in congenital heart disease, 155
  peripheral, 154
Cyclamate, 732
Cyclophosphamide, 295, 298, 299, 302,
  980, 982
Cyclophosphamide-induced hemorrhagic
  cystitis, 984
Cyclopropane poisoning, 955
Cycloserine, 905, 909
Cyclothiazide, 239
Cyclothymic personality, 616
Cycrimine, 582
Cystadenoma(s), 436
  of ovary, 436
  pseudomucinous, 436
  serous, 436
Cystic
  disease
    medullary, 537
    of renal medulla, 537
  duct syndromes, 389
  fibrosis, 781
  mastitis of breast, chronic, 412
Cysticercosis, 867, 868, 869
Cystine stones, 547
Cystinosis, 966
Cystinuria, 546, 547
  congenital, 537
Cystitis, hemorrhagic
  acute, 808
  cyclophosphamide-induced, 984
Cystocele, 430
Cystosarcoma phyllodes, 413
Cysts
  esophageal, 335
  ovarian
    corpus luteum, 435
    endometrial, 435
    follicle, 434
    retention, 434
    theca lutein, 435
Cytarabine, 295, 913, 980, 982

Cytogenetics, 961
Cytologic examination, vaginal, 425
Cytomegalovirus disease, 794
Cytomel, 663, 714
Cytosar, 295, 913, 980, 982
Cytosine arabinoside, 913
Cytotoxic
  drugs
    in arthritis, 482
    and hormones, 982
  T cells, 989
Cytoxan, 295, 298, 299, 302

Dacarbazine, 980, 983
Dacryocystitis, 82
Dactinomycin, 549, 980, 983
Dalmane, 602
Dandruff, 45
Dandy fever, 802
Dane particle, 372
Daranide, 240
Daraprim, 855, 861
Daunorubicin, 980
DBI, 721, 733
DBI-TD, 721
D&C
  medical, 705, 706, **725**
  surgical, **448**, 461
D/C, 980, 981
DC countershock, synchronized, 205
DDT poisoning, 939
Deafness, 88
  classification of, 88
  sensorineural and conductive, dif-
    ferentiation of, 89
Death and dying, 641
Decadron, 716, 717
Deca-Durabolin, 277, 722
Decompression sickness, 924
Decubitus ulcers, 55
Defense mechanisms in disturbed behavior,
  594
Deferoxamine, 383
Defibrillation, 1028
Defibrination syndrome, 309, 315
Degenerative
  disorders of CNS, **580–585**
  and inflammatory venous disease,
    262–271
Dehydration, treatment of, in shock, 7
Dehydroemetine, 852
Deladumone, 476
Delalutin, 417, 725, 982
Delatest, 277
Delatestryl, 277, 418, 722
Delestrogen, 417, 724
Deletions, chromosome, 963
Delfen, 447
Delta-Cortef, 716
Deltasone, 716
Deltra, 716
Deluteval-2X, 429
Demeclocycline, 899
Dementia, alcohol, 632
Demons-Meigs syndrome, 435
Demulcents in poisoning, 933
Demulen, 724
Dengue, 802
Denial, 594
Dental decay, 328
Dentinogenesis imperfecta, 517

Depo-Estradiol, 724
Depolarization of heart, 208
Depo-Provera, 429
Depo-Testosterone, 722
Depressants, poisoning due to, 937
Depression, 622
  theoretical models of, 622
DeQuervain's thyroiditis, 671
Dermabrasion, 46
Dermacentor
  andersoni, 803, 811
  variabilis, 811
Dermatitis
  actinica, 42
  acute, subacute, or chronic, 35
  atopic, 37
  circulatory, 39
  contact, 34
  exfoliative, 33, 41
  herpetiformis, 998
  medicamentosa, 40
  overtreatment of, 33
  seborrheic, 45
  stasis, 39
  venenata, 34
Dermatomyositis, 487, 974
Dermatophytid, 60
Dermatophytosis, 59
Dermatoses, 34–50
  stages of, rules of topical treat-
    ment of, 32
Dermoid cysts, 436
Deronil, 716
Descensus, uterine, 432
Desensitization, 97, **1003**
  phobic, 608
Desferal, 383
Desipramine, 601
  poisoning due to, 948
Desquamative interstitial pneumonia, 142
Desquamex gel, 46
Desirable weight tables, 1023
Deslanoside, 235, 236
Desonide cream, 74
Desoxycorticosterone
  acetate, 690, 715
  trimethylacetate, 715
Desoxyn, 563
DET, 947
Detergents, poisoning due to, 950
De Toni-Fanconi-Debré syndrome, 537
Detoxification, drug, 627
Devegan, 421
Dexameth, 716
Dexamethasone, 554, 579, 716, 717
  suppression test, 692
Dexedrine, 563, 582
Dextran, 5
Dextroamphetamine
  poisoning, 948
  sulfate, 563, 582
Dextrothyroxine, sodium, 663, 714
DHE, 559
Diabetes
  insipidus, 647, 654
    nephrogenic, 654, 655
    psychogenic, 655
    renal, 538
  mellitus, 727
    and air travel, 926
    arterial disease and, 250
    gangrene of feet in, 739

Diabetes
  mellitus (cont'd)
    insulinopenic, 727
    insulinoplethoric, 727, 735
    and lipoproteinemia, relation-
      ship between, 747
    occult, 746
    and pregnancy, 469
  syndrome
    acute, 729
    chronic, 729
Diabetic
  coma, 740
  ketoacidosis, 741
  ketosis, 27
  nephropathy, 738
  neuropathy, 729, 739
  retinopathy, 729, 738
Diabinese, 721, 732
Dialysis, 933
  extracorporeal, 528
  peritoneal, in heart failure, 220
Diamox, 217, 240, 563, 564
Dianabol, 277, 722
Diaphragmatic hernia, 337
Diaphragm, cervical, and jelly, 447
Diapid, 655, 712
Diarrhea, 324, 824, 825, 827
  traveler's, 828
Diastolic murmurs, 154
Diazepam, 563, 602
Diazoxide, 721
Dibenzoxazepines, 597
Dibenzyline, 242, 699, 720
DIC, 315
Dichlorphenamide, 240
Dicloxacillin, 896
Dicumarol, 266, 936
Dicurin Procaine, 240
Dienestrol, 723
  vaginal cream, 421
Diet(s)
  basic foods, 755
  bland, 761
  calcium test, 764
  in congestive heart failure, 217
  in diabetes, 731
  disaccharide intolerance, 762
  and drugs, interaction 759
  in duodenal ulcer, 342
  for glucose tolerance tests, 764
  high
    calcium, 764
    calorie, protein, and vitamin, 761
  low
    calcium, 763
    calorie, 773
    carbohydrate, 761
    cholesterol, modified fat, 751
    fat, 761
    gluten, 762
    protein, 761
    purine, 762
    sodium, 184, 218, 219
  minimum residue, 761
  modified fat, controlled carbohydrate,
    low cholesterol, 752
  and nutrition, **754–766**
  therapeutic, 760
  vegetarian, 764
Dietary fiber, 765
Diethylcarbamazine, 878, **880**, 881

Diethylstilbestrol, 407, 723, 982
  diphosphate, 723
  vaginal suppository, 421
Diethyltryptamine, 947
DiGeorge's syndrome, 995
Digitalis, 198, **233**
  in congestive heart failure, 217
  determination, radioimmunoassay for,
    234
  oral administration of, 237
  poisoning, 939
  preparations, choice of, 235, 236
  toxicity, 234
Digitoxin, 235, 236
  poisoning, 939
Digoxin, 235, 236
Digratyl, 674, 714
Dihydroepiandrosterone, 687
Dihydroergotamine, 559
Dihydroindolones, 597
Dihydrotachysterol, 674, 714
Diiodohydroxyquin, 851, 852, 861
Dilantin, 208, 562, 564
Dilatation and curettage
  medical, 705, 706, **725**
  surgical, **448**, 461
  in therapeutic abortion, 462
Dilation, pupillary, 87
Diloxanide furoate, 851, 852, 853
Dilutional hyponatremia, 21
Dilution syndrome, 18
Dimercaprol, 583, 936, 941, 942
Dimetane, 14
Dimethisterone, 725
2,5-Dimethoxy-4-methylamphetamine, 947
Dimethylphthalate, 1001
Dimethyl serotonin, 947
Dimethyl triazeno imidazole carboxamide,
  983
Dimethyltryptamine, 634, 947
Dinitrophenol poisoning, 950
Dioctyl sodium sulfosuccinate, 323
Dioxane poisoning, 950
Diphenhydramine, 14, 581, 582
  in arsenic poisoning, 936
Diphenoxylate, 325, 1001
Diphenylhydantoin. See Phenytoin.
Diphtheria, 875
  toxoid, 1001
Diphtheria-tetanus-pertussis immuniza-
  tion, 1001
Diphyllobothrium latum, 867
Diplopia, 76
Dipylidium caninum, 867
Dirofilaria immitis, 878
Disaccharidase deficiency, 356
Disaccharide intolerance diet, 762
Disengagement phenomenon, 640
Disipal, 582
Disk
  sensitivity study, 504
  tests, 891
Displacement, 594
Dissecting aneurysms of aorta, 244
Dissection, aortic, acute, 244
Disseminated intravascular coagulation,
  315
Dissociative states, 611
Distributive shock, 3, 4
Disulfiram poisoning, 950
Disulfonamide diuretics, 239
Dithiazanine iodide, 874

Ditran, 947
Diuretic(s), 239, 933
  in congestive heart failure, 217
  mercurial, 240
  oral, 182, 239
  phase of acute renal failure, 533
  for shock, 7
  thiazide, 239
    in prevention of renal stones, 546
Diuril, 182, 239
Diverticular disease of colon, 364
Diverticulitis, 364
  Meckel's, 351
Diverticulosis, 364
Diverticulum
  Meckel's, 351
  urethral, 424
Divinyl ether poisoning, 955
Dizziness, 557
DMT, 634, 947
DOCA, 689, 715
DOM, 634, 947
Donath-Landsteiner test, 282
Dopa, 66
Dopamine hydrochloride, 6
Dopar, 581, 582
Doppler ultrasound technic, 252
Douches, acetic acid, 422
Down's syndrome, 661, 968, 969
Doxepin, 601, 602
  poisoning due to, 948
Doxinate, 323
Doxorubicin, 980, 983
Doxorubicin-induced myocarditis, 985
Doxycycline, 899
Dracontiasis, 880
Dracunculiasis, 880
Dracunculosis, 880
Dracunculus medinensis, 880
Draw-a-Person test, 596
Dream sleep, 625
Dressings, wet, 71
Drolban, 722
Dromostanolone propionate, 722
Drowning, 921
Drug(s)
  addicts and infections, 788
  affecting prothrombin time, 1006
  in cancer chemotherapy, 980, 982, 983
  controlled, schedule of, 1025
  dependency, **627–638**
  detoxification, 627
  and diet, interaction of, 759
  effect on intrauterine and newborn
    patient, 455
  eruption(s), 40
    diagnostic features of, 792
    interfering with chemical tests,
      1005
  teratogenic and fetotoxic, 455
  therapy, aerosolized, 140
DSM-II, 610
D state sleep, 625
DTIC, 980, 983
DTP, 816, 1024
  immunization, 1001
Dubin-Johnson-Sprinz-Nelson syndrome,
  378
Duchenne muscular dystrophy, 589
Ductus arteriosus, patent, 155, 159
Dulcolax, 323
Dumping syndrome, 346

Duodenal ulcer, 341
  hemorrhage due to, 342
  penetration of, 342
  perforation of, 342
Duodenoscopy, 342
Duphaston, 725
Durabolin, 722
Dura-Testosterone, 277
Dwarfism, 706
Dydrogesterone, 725
Dying and death, 641
Dymelor, 721, 732
Dyrenium, 239, 240
Dysbetalipoproteinemia, 748
Dyscontrol syndrome, 626
Dysentery
  amebic, 850
  bacillary, 827
Dysgenetic gonad, 971
Dysgerminoma, 438
Dysmenorrhea, 419
  primary, 419
Dyspareunia, 440
Dyspepsia, functional, 325
Dysplasia
  mammary, 412
  polyostotic fibrous, 685
Dyspnea, 106, 152
  exertional, 152, 215
  paroxysmal nocturnal, 152, 215
Dystrophia myotonica, 592
Dystroph(ies), 588
  and atrophies, differential diagno-
    sis of, 588
  myotonic, 592
  post-traumatic sympathetic, 261
  progressive muscular, 589
  reflex sympathetic, 514
Dysuria, 521

EACA, 310
Ear, diseases of, **88–95**
  external, **90–91**
  inner, **94–95**
  middle, **91–94**
Eastern equine encephalitis, 801
EB virus, 806
Echinococcosis, 869
Echinococcus
  granulosus, 869
  multilocularis, 869
Echocardiography, 152
  in mitral insufficiency, 170
Echography, thyroid, 670
Echovirus infections, 808
Eclampsia, 457
Ecolid, 183
ECT, 604
Ecthyma, 53
Ectopia lentis, 781
Ectopic
  kidney, 539
  pregnancy, 455
Ectropion, 82
Eczema, 37
  circulatory, 39
  herpeticum, 38, 51, 792
    diagnostic features of, 792
  and thrombocytopenia, immunodeficiency
    with, 996
  vaccinatum, 38, 797

Edecrin, 183, 219, 221, 239
Edema, 153
  angioneurotic, 47
  cerebral, 573
  pulmonary, acute, 221
Edrophonium test, 591
EDTA, 941
Edward's syndrome, 968
Effective compliance, 138
Effusion(s)
  malignant, 975
  pleural, 145
Ehrlich test, 780
Eisenmenger's syndrome, 160, 161
Ejaculation, premature, 613
Elavil, 601
Elbow, tennis, 515
Electric
  burns, 922
  countershock, **208**, 1028
  shock, 922
Electrocoagulation, percutaneous, 586
Electroconvulsive therapy, 604
Electrograms, His bundle, 206
Electrolyte(s), 15
  concentrates, 29
    examples of, 29
  disturbances in cardiac failure, 222
  and fluids
    diagnostic approach to disturbances
      of, **26–30**
    disorders of, **15–31**
      pharmacologic activity, **21–26**
    physiology of, 16
    preparations, oral, 30
Electrolyte-regulating mineralocorti-
  coids, 687
Electronystagmography, 89
Electroshock. See Electroconvulsive
  therapy.
Electrosleep, 604
Electrosurgery for skin tumors, 66
Elephantiasis, Milroy's congenital,
  878
Elipten, 693
Elliptocytosis, hereditary, 282
Ellsworth-Howard test, 673
Embolism
  cerebral, 568
  pulmonary, acute, 195
Emboli, thrombotic, 144
Embryoma of kidney, 549
Embryonal tumor, 551
Emesis in poisoning, 932
Emetine, 852
  poisoning, 951
Emetine-bismuth-iodide, 851
Emko, 447
Emotional headache, 558
Emotive imagery, 608
Emphysema, chronic pulmonary, 135
Empty sella syndrome, 651
Empyema, 123
  pleural, 147
Emulsion(s), 72
  base, 73
  sun screen, 72
Encephalitis, **800**, 801
  postvaccinial, 797
  postvaricella, 795
  toxic, 801
  viral, 800

Encephalopath(ies)
  alcoholic, 632
  hypertensive, 525
Enchondroma, 518
Encounter groups, 606
Endemic syphilis, 847
Endocarditis
  and bacteremia, 787
  infective, 174, 788
Endocrine
  ablation, therapeutic, in treatment
     of female breast cancer, 408
  disorders, **645–726**
    difficulties of diagnosis of, 645
    secretions associated with cancer, 974
Endometrial ovarian cysts, 435
Endometriosis, 429
Endometrium, uterine, carcinoma of,
  427, 980
Endomyocardial diseases, 229
Endrin poisoning, 939
Enduron, 239
Enema(s), 323
  oil retention, 323
  saline, 323
  soapsuds, 323
  tap water, 323
ENG, 89
Enovid, 417, 429, 444, 450, 724
Enovid-E, 429
Entamoeba histolytica, 850
Enteritis, regional, 349
Enterobiasis, 874
Enterobius vermicularis, 874
Enterocele, 431
Enterocolitis
  pseudomembranous, 357
  regional, 349
  tuberculous, 360
Enterovirus infections, diagnostic
    features of, 792
Entropion, 82
Enuresis, 521
Environmental control, 140
Eosinophilia
  pulmonary infiltrations with, 113
  in schistosomiasis, 863
Eosinophilic
  adenoma, 652
  granuloma of bone, 304
  meningoencephalitis, 881
Ephedrine poisoning, 948
Ephelides, 65, 67
Epicondylalgia, 515
Epicondylitis, 515
Epidemic
  parotitis, 798
  pleurodynia, 807
Epidermophyton, 59, 60
Epiglottitis, 790
Epilepsia partialis continua, 561
Epileps(ies), **560–564**, 574
  drugs used in, 562
  international classification of, 561
Epileptic seizures, international
    classification of, 561
Epinephrine, 6, 719
  normal values, 1019, 1020
Epiphyseal giant cell tumor, 519
Epiphysitis, 509
Epistaxis, 99
EPN poisoning, 944

EPS, 667
Epstein-Barr virus, 806
Equanil, 563, 602
Equational division of chromosomes, 963
Equine gonadotropins, 713
Erb type muscular dystrophy, 590
Ergonovine maleate, 466
Ergotamine, 259
  with caffeine, 559
  poisoning, 950
  tartrate, 559
Ergotrate, 466
Eruption, drug, 40, 792
Erysipelas, 55
Erysipeloid, 55
Erysipelothrix rhusiopathiae, 55
Erythema
  infectiosum, 808
    diagnostic features of, 792
  marginatum, 162
  multiforme, 36
  nodosum, 35
  solare, 42
Erythermalgia, 260
Erythroblastosis fetalis, 474
  tooth discoloration due to, 328
Erythrocyte casts, 524
Erythroid aplasia, 974
Erythrol tetranitrate, 239
Erythromelalgia, 260
Erythromycin, 176, **898**
  estolate, 898
  gluceptate, 898
  lactobionate, 898
Erythropoiesis, ineffective, 285
Erythropoietic porphyria, congenital,
  780, 966
Escherichia coli food poisoning, 824
Esidrix, 239
Eskalith, 600
Esophageal
  cysts, 335
  diverticulosis, 335
  ring, lower, 334
  webs, 334
Esophagitis
  acute corrosive, 340
  reflux, 336
Esophagogastroduodenoscopy, fiberoptic,
  326
Esophagus
  Barrett's, 336
  benign
    neoplasms of, 338
    stricture of, 337
  carcinoma of, 339
  diseases of, **333–339**
  foreign bodies in, 104, 105
  leiomyoma of, 150
Esotropia, 85
Estinyl, 723, 982
Estradiol
  benzoate, 723
  cypionate, 724
  dipropionate, 724
  normal values, 1020
  valerate, 417, 724
Estriol, normal values, 1020
Estrogen(s), **723**, 980, 982
  poisoning, 950
  therapy for breast cancer, 406
  topical, 824

Estrogenic substances, conjugated, 724
Estrogen-progesterone test for preg-
  nancy, 450
Estrone, 723
Ethacrynic acid, 183, 219, 221, 240
Ethambutol, 127, **903**
Ethchlorvynol, 602
Ether poisoning, 955
Ethinyl estradiol, 723, 724, 982
Ethionamide, 905
Ethisterone, 725
Ethopropazine, 582
Ethosuximide, 562, 564
Ethotoin, 562
Ethoxzolamide, 83, 240
Ethyl
  alcohol poisoning, 935
  chloride poisoning, 955
Ethylene, 955
  chlorohydrin poisoning, 950
  glycol poisoning, 950
Ethylestrenol, 722
Ethylstibamine, 859
Ethynodiol diacetate, 725
Eurax, 62, 64
Euthroid, 663, 714
Ewing's sarcoma, 519
Exanthem(s)
  acute, 792
    diagnostic features of, 792
  subitum, 792, 793
    diagnostic features of, 792
Exanthematous diseases in pregnancy,
  472
Excision, local, in breast cancer, 404
Exercise
  in arthritis, 500
  test, 189
Exfoliative dermatitis, 41
Exhaustion, heat, 916
Exhibitionism, 613
Existential therapy, 606
Exna, 239
Exophthalmic ophthalmoplegia, 664
Exophthalmos, 664, 667
  malignant (progressive), 664
Exotropia, 85
Expectoration, 106
Explosive personality, 616
Expressivity, 959
External cardiac massage, 1026
Extinction, 608
Extracorporeal dialysis, 528
Extrinsic asthma, 111
Eye
  bandages, 86
  complications in tertiary syphilis,
    844
  disorders of, **75–87**
    technics of treatment, 86
  fungal overgrowth of, 87
  infections, principles of treatment,
    86
  medications, contaminated, 87
  myiasis of, 882
  pain, 75
  patients, postsurgical or post-trau-
    matic, and air travel, 926
  strain, 75
  tumors of, 82
  warm compresses to, 87
Eyelids, granulated, 82

Fabry's disease, 966
Facial
    nerve paralysis, 93
    paralysis, peripheral, 586
Facioscapulohumeral muscular dystrophy, 590
Factor IX complex, 310
Factorate, 310
Failure
    left ventricular, 215
    right ventricular, 216
Fainting, 555
    in pregnancy, 451
Fallot, tetralogy of, 160
    propranolol in, 242
Familial
    Mediterranean fever, 398
    periodic paralysis, 592
Family
    planning, 444
    therapy, 605
Fanconi's
    anemia, 970
    syndrome, 538, 681, **778**
Farber's disease, 966
Fasciitis, necrotizing, 787
Fascioliasis, 866
Fasciolopsiasis, 865
Fasciolopsis buski, 865
Fasting
    in relation to blood tests, 1004
    test, prolonged, 689
Fat(s)
    bodies, oval, 530
    diet, low, 761
    necrosis, 413
    ratio of polyunsaturated to saturated, 750
Fatigue
    exertional, 216
    in heart disease, 152
Fatty liver, 381
Fava bean poisoning, 951
F body, 965
F-Cortef, 715, 716
Febrile convulsions, 561
Fecal
    fat, normal values, 1021
    impaction, 323
Feedings, tube, 765
Feet, care of, in diabetes mellitus and vascular disorders, 736
Felty's syndrome, 292
Feminization, testicular, 966
Feminone, 723
Femoral
    aneurysms, 246
    artery, occlusive disease of, 248
Fern test, 442
Ferric chloride test, 777
Ferrous salts, 274
Fetography, 965
Fetoscopy, 965
Fetotoxic drugs, 455
Fetus, effects of maternal medications on, 455
FEV, 108
FEV$_1$, 107
Fever(s), 1, 974. See also specific types.
    clinical classification of causes of, 2
    complicating leukemia, 295
    factitious or false, 2

Fever(s) (cont'd)
    hay, 112
    periodic, 398
    Q, 812
    rat-bite, 848
    relapsing, 848
    Rocky Mountain spotted, 810
    sore, 50
    spotted, **810-811**
    trench, 812
    of undetermined origin, **1**, 783
FF, normal values, 1020
Fiber, dietary, 765
Fiberoptic esophagogastroduodenoscopy, 326
Fibrillation
    atrial, 205
    ventricular, 209, 1028
Fibrin monomer, 315
Fibrinogen, 315, 316
    deficiency, 309
    serum or plasma, normal values, 1013, 1019
    uptake test, 265
Fibrinous pleurisy, 145
Fibroadenoma of breast, 413
Fibro-AHG, 310
Fibroid tumor, 428
Fibroma(s)
    chondromyxoid, 518
    of ovary, 435
Fibromyoma, 428
Fibrosarcoma, 518
Fibrosis
    cystic, 781
    pulmonary, 141
Fibrous dysplasia, 680
Fifth disease, 808
Filariasis, 877
Filariform larvae, 873
Filtration fraction, normal values, 1020
Fireworks, poisoning due to, 945
Fischer test, 941
Fish poisoning, 951
Fissure-in-ano, 369
Fistula-in-ano, 369
Fi test, 315
Flagyl, 421, 861
Flashback, 634
Flatulence, 324
Fleas, 64
Flea-borne typhus, endemic, 810
Flocculation test for syphilis, 841
Flooding as psychiatric therapy, 608
Floppy valve syndrome, 170
Floraquin, 421
Florinef, 715, 716
Flucytosine, 508, 910
Fludrocortisone acetate, 690, 715, 716
Fluid(s)
    body, 15
        compartments of, 16
    deficiency in burns, 917
    and electrolytes
        deficits, 27
        diagnostic approach to disturbances of, 26-30
        disorders of, 15-31
            summary of clinical approach, 28
        maintenance of, 26
        pharmacologic activity of, 21-26
    losses, 17

Fluid(s)
    losses (cont'd)
        gastrointestinal, 27
    parenteral, daily maintenance rations, 26
    therapy for shock, 5
Fluke(s)
    blood, 863
    infections, **863-867**
    intestinal, 865
    liver, 866
        sheep, 866
    lung, 866
Flumethasone, 717
Flumethiazide, 239
Fluocinolone, 40, 44, 74
    acetonide, 38, 72, 717
Fluocinonide gel, 74
Fluorescein paper strips, 87
Fluorescent treponemal antibody absorption test, 842
Fluoride poisoning, 940
Fluoroacetate poisoning, 951
9a-Fluorocortisol, 689
Fluorouracil, 66, 980, 982
Fluoxymesterone, 277, 702, 722, 982
Fluphenazine, 598
Fluprednisolone, 715, 716
Flurandrenolone, 717
Flurazepam, 602
Flurobate gel, 74
Flurothyl, 604
Flutter
    atrial, 206
    ventricular, 209
Foam, spermatocidal, 447
Folacin, 758
Folic acid, 276, 758, 771, 1019
    deficiency, 276, 293
        anemia, 459
Folinic acid, 276
Follicle cysts of ovaries, 434
Follicle-stimulating hormone, 712
Follicular
    hyperkeratosis, 767
    lymphoma, giant, 303
Folliculitis, 53
Follutein, 713
Food(s)
    basic diet, 755
    nutrient content of, 756, 757
    organic and health, 754
    poisoning, **825,** 951
        and acute bacterial diarrhea, 824
        bacterial, 951
        clostridial, 824
        E coli, 824
        salmonella, 824
        shigella, 824
        staphylococcal, 824
        vibrio, 824
    safety in foreign travel, 1002
    snack, calories, 774
    sources of
        minerals, 758
        vitamins, 758
Foot
    athlete's, 59
    care, instructions, 736
    circulatory insufficiency of, 250
    infections, ulcers, and gangrene of, 250
    occlusive disease in, 249

Forced expiratory volume, 108
Foreign
    bod(ies)
        in air and food passages, **104-105**
        bronchial, 105
        corneal, removal of, 87
        esophageal, 104, 105
        intraocular, 77
        ocular, 76
    travel, medical recommendations for,
        1000-1002
Formaldehyde poisoning, 951
Fostex, 45, 46
Fostril Hc, 46
Fracture(s)
    bone, 678
    pathologic, 648, 676
Fragilitas ossium, 517
Frambesia, 847
Freckle(s), 65, 67
    Hutchinson's, 65
Freon, 46
Friction rub, 223
Friedländer's bacillus, 119
Frigidity, 612
Fröhlich's syndrome, 647
Frontal lobe tumors, 579
Frostbite, 915
Fructosemia, 779
Fructosuria, 779
FSH, 712
    normal values, 1021
FTA-ABS test, 842
FT₄, normal values, 1015
5-FU, 66, 982
Fucosidosis, 966
Functional alimentary hypoglycemia,
    746
Fundal cancer, 427
Fungal
    conjunctivitis, 80
    diseases, **883-890**
    overgrowth in eye, 87
Fungicidal agents, 60
Fungizone, 887
    lotion, 72
Fungus infections
    opportunistic, 889
    of skeletal system, 508
FUO, **1**, 783
Furacin, 423
Furazolidone-nifuroxime, 421, 423
Furosemide, 183, 219, 239
Furunculosis, 54

Galactorrhea, 706
Galactosemia, 779, 966
Gallbladder
    adenomyomatosis of, 389
    carcinoma of, 393
    gangrene of, 387
    strawberry, 388
Galleries of mites, 62
Gallstones, 388
Gamma benzene hexachloride, 62
Gammacorten, 716
Gammopath(ies), 994
    monoclonal, benign, 994
Ganglioneuroma, 150
Ganglionic blocking agents, 183
Gangliosidosis, 966

Gangrene
    bacterial synergistic, 787
    of gallbladder, 387
Gas gangrene, 829
Gasoline poisoning, 941
Gastric
    acid in pernicious anemia, 275
    aspiration and lavage in poisoning,
        932
    ulcer, 345
Gastrin, normal values, 1020
Gastritis
    acute, 340
        corrosive, 340
    chronic, 340
Gastroenteritis
    acute, 358
    salmonella, 825
Gastrointestinal
    disease
        as cause of fever, 2
        fluid loss in, 28
    disorders, psychologic, 325
    fluid losses, volume and electrolyte
        content of, 28
    hemorrhage, massive upper, 326
    manifestations of tertiary syphilis,
        835
    toxicity of cancer chemotherapeutic
        agents, 984
    tract, diseases of, **321-370**
Gaucher cells, 753
Gaucher's disease, 752, 966
G I deletion syndrome, 968
G II deletion syndrome, 968
Gelfoam, 56
Gels, 74
Gemonil, 562
Genes, 957
Genetic(s)
    code, 957
    control of immune response, 989
    counseling, 972
    disorders detected in utero, 966
    medical, **957-972**
Genitourinary tract
    disorders of, **521-552**
    roentgenographic examination of, 522
Gentamicin, 176, 892, 900, **901**
    topical application of, 919
Gentian violet, 62, 74, 887
Geriatric disorders, 640
German measles, 792, 793
    diagnostic features of, 792
Gestagens, 724
Gexane, 62
GFR, 522
    normal values, 1020
Giant
    cell
        arteritis, 258
        tumor, 519
            epiphyseal, 519
        follicular lymphoma, 303
    hives, 47
Giardia lamblia, 860
Giardiasis, 860
Giemsa's stain, 854
Gigantism, 652
    nonpituitary cerebral, 646
Gila monster bites, 946
Gilbert's syndrome, 378

Gilchrist's disease, 509
Gingival pigmentation, 332
Gingivitis, necrotizing ulcerating, 329
Gingivostomatitis, herpetic, 330
Gitaligin, 235, 236
Gitalin, 235, 236
Glanzmann's
    disease, 312
    thrombasthenia, 309
Glaucoma
    acute, 75, 76
    chronic, 83
Globaline, 1002
Globulin
    normal values, 1020
    serum, 1014
β-Globulins by electrophoresis, 1014
Glomerular
    basement membrane, 523, 526
    filtration rate, 522
Glomerulonephritis, 522
    chronic, 525
    hypocomplementemic, 530
    idiopathic rapidly progressive, 527
    latent, 526
    membranoproliferative, 530
    in pregnancy, 469
    prognosis in, 525
Glossina, 856
Glossitis, 332
Glossodynia, 332
Glossopyrosis, 332
Glucagon, 721
    suppression by somatostatin, 737
Glucocorticoids, 687
Glucose
    absorption, defects of, 538
    blood, 1011
    fasting, in diabetes, 730
    normal values, 1020
    and phosphate absorption, defects
        of, 538
    plasma or serum, 1011
    reabsorptive capacity, maximal, nor-
        mal values, 1020
    test, drugs inferfering with, 1005
    tolerance tests, 689, 730, 764
Glucose-galactose malabsorption, 762
Glucose-6-phosphate dehydrogenase,
    282, 284, 855
    deficiency, **284**, 907
Glutamic-oxaloacetic transaminase, nor-
    mal values, 1016, 1019
Glutamic-pyruvic transaminase, normal
    values, 1016, 1019
Glutathione reductase deficiency,
    970
Gluten diet, low, 762
Glyburide, 732
L-Glyceric aciduria, 781
Glycerol in glaucoma, 76
Glyceryl trinitrate, 188, 190, 239
Glycobiarsol, 851
Glycogen storage disease, 966
Glycolic aciduria, 781
Glycosuria, 729
    nondiabetic, 730
    renal, 538, 730
Glycopyrrolate, 48
Glycosuric rickets, 538
Gnathostoma spinigerum, 881
Gnathostomiasis, 881

Goiter
  lymphadenoid, 671
  nodular, 659
  simple, 659
Gold salts
  in arthritis, 481
  poisoning, 951
Gonadal
  dysgenesis, 706
  hormones, **721–726**
    normal values, 1020
Gonad, dysgenetic, 971
Gonadotropin(s), 974
  chorionic, 418, 651, 713
    normal values, 1020
  equine, 713
  human menopausal, 443
  urinary, in hypogonadism, 700
Gonococcal conjunctivitis, 78
Gonorrhea, 836
  as complication in pregnancy, 470
Gonorrheal
  arthritis, 511
  vaginitis, 421
Goodpasture's syndrome, 116, 526, 993
Gout, **496**, 546
Gouty arthritis, 496
G6PD, 282, 284, 855
  deficiency, 284, 907
Gram-negative cocci and rods, drug
    selections for, 906
Gram-positive
  bacteria, specialized drugs against,
    908
  cocci and rods, drug selections
    for, 906
Grand mal, 560
Granulated eyelids, 82
Granuloma
  of bone, 304
  inguinale, 370, 838
Granulomatosis, Crohn's, 363
  Wegener's, 116, 143, 489
Granulomatous colitis, 363
Granulosa cell tumor, 438
Gravel formation, 648
Graves' disease, **664**, 998
  hyperexophthalmic, 664
Gravindex test for pregnancy, 450
Grippe, 96
  summer, 807
Griseofulvin, 56, 910
Gris-Peg, 57
Group therapy, types of, 605
Growing pains, 163
Growth
  delayed, 646
  excessive, 646
  hormone, 712
Guanethidine, 183, 185
Guillotine amputation, 251
Guinea worm infection, 880
Gumma
  formation, 509
  of testicle, 552
Gynecologic
  backache, 441
    causes of, 441
  disorders, **415–449**
Gynecomastia, 414, **647**, 701
Gynergen, 559
Gynorest, 725

Haemophilus
  influenzae, 107, 494, 790, 995
    meningitis, 821
    pneumonia, 119
  vaginalis vaginitis, 421
Hair disorders, 66
Hairy cell leukemia, 303
Haldol, 598
Haldrone, 716
Halitosis, 321
Hallucinosis, alcoholic, 632
Haloperidol, 598
Halotestin, **722**, 982
Halothane poisoning, 955
Ham's test, 282
Hand, foot, and mouth disease, 807
Hand-Schüller-Christian disease, 305
Haptoglobins, 281, 282
Harmaline, 947
Harmine, 947
Harrison's groove, 681
Hartnup's disease, 778
Hashimoto's thyroiditis, 671, 672
Hay fever, 97, 112
HB Ag, 320
HB$_C$Ab, 372
HB$_S$Ag, 372, 375
HCO$_3^-$, 108
H disease, 778
HDL, 747
Head
  injury, 573
  louse, 63
  and neck tumors, 980
Headache(s), **557–560**
  associated with specific entities, 557
  cluster, 559
  histaminic, 559
  lumbar puncture, 558
  due to meningeal involvement, 558
  migraine, 558
  due to musculoskeletal involvement,
    560
  as ocular symptom, 75
  in pregnancy, 452
  sinus, 98
  tension, 560
Heaf test, 124
Hearing loss, 88
  and paranoid ideation, 640
Heart
  block, 211
    complete, 211
    incomplete, 210
  boot-shaped, 160
  disease(s), **152–242**
    acquired, **161–200**
    arteriosclerotic, 187
    asymptomatic valvular, manage-
      ment of, 165
    congenital, **155–161**
      pulmonary hypertension in, 161
    coronary, surgery for, 192
    functional and therapeutic classi-
      fication of, 155
    ischemic, 187
      prevention of, 187
    nonspecific manifestations of,
      152–155
    in pregnancy, 469
    pulmonary, 226
    rheumatic, 165, 166, 167

Heart
  diseases (cont'd)
    signs of, 153
  enlargement of, in common valve
    lesions, 168
  failure, **213–222**
  murmurs, sounds, and clicks, 154
  physiologic load imposed on, by preg-
    nancy, 233
  radioisotope scanning of, 152, 167
  rupture of, 196
  sounds, 154
Heartburn, 321, 337
Heart-lung resuscitation, 1026
Heat
  cramps, 916
  disorders due to, **915–917**
  exhaustion, 916
  prostration, 916
  rash, 48
  stroke, 916
Heavy chain(s), 987
  diseases, 298, 994
Heinz bodies, 282, 284
Helper cells, 989
Hemagglutination
  inhibition test for pregnancy, 450
  test, red blood cell, 992
Hemangioma, 65
Hematemesis, 326
Hematinic agents, 481
Hematocrit, normal values, 1018
Hematology, normal values in, 1018
Hematopoietic hypoplasia, generalized,
    with immunodeficiency, 995
Hematoma
  of nasal septum, 96
  subdural, 574
Hemianopsia, care of, in hemiplegia,
    570
Hemiplegia, rehabilitation of patients
    with, 569
  special problems in, 570
Hemlock poisoning, 953
Hemochromatosis, 384
Hemodialysis, 534, 536
Hemofil, 310
Hemoglobin(s)
  A, 286
  A$_2$, 286
  abnormal, 285
  F, 286
  fetal, hereditary persistence of, 289
  H disease, 291
  normal values, 1018
  S, 286
  S-C disease, 289
  sickle, 286
Hemoglobinopathies, **286**, 287
Hemoglobinuria, paroxysmal, 283
  nocturnal, 283
Hemolysis test, sucrose, 283
Hemolytic
  anemia(s), **279–285**
    autoimmune, 993
  disease of newborn, 474
  transfusion reaction, 319
Hemolytic-uremic syndrome, 532
Hemopericardium, 225
Hemophilia, 309
  genetic aspects of, 958
  vascular, 314

Hemoptysis, 107
Hemorrhage. See also Bleeding.
  complicating leukemia, 295
  extradural, 574
  gastrointestinal
    blood replacement in, 327
    emergency operation, indications
      for, 327
    massive upper, 326
    medical measures in, 327
  intracerebral, 568
  subarachnoid, 568, 574
  in tuberculosis, 128
Hemorrhagic
  cystitis, cyclophosphamide-induced,
    984
  disorders, **307–318**
  pancreatitis, acute, 393
Hemorrhoids, 368
  in pregnancy, 452
Hemothorax, 147
Henoch-Schönlein syndrome, 313
Heparin, 254
Hepar lobatum, 845
Hepatic
  abscess, 852, 853
    pyogenic, 386
  dysfunction, constitutional, 378
  porphyrias, 779
Hepatitis
  alcoholic, 376
  cholangiolitic, 374
  chronic, 375, 998
    active, 375, 993
    persistent, 375
  fulminant, 374
  infectious, 372
    and serum, differentiating fea-
      tures of, 372
    variants of, 374
  long incubation period, 372
  lupoid type, 375
  post-transfusion, 320
  short incubation period, 372
  temporary passive immunization for,
    1002
  viral, 372
Hepatocellular jaundice, 371
Hepatolenticular degeneration, 537,
  583
Hepatoma, 974
Hereditary hemorrhagic telangiectasia,
  313
Heredity, chemical basis of, 957
Hernia
  and air travel, 926
  diaphragmatic, 337
  hiatus, 337
  in pregnancy, 473
Herniation of intervertebral disk, 577
Herpangina, 807
Herpes
  genitalis, 471
  labialis, 331
  simplex, 50
    disseminated, 51
    keratitis, 78
    photodynamic inactivation in
      treatment of, 913
    virus, 38
  zoster, 51, **795**
Herpetic stomatitis, 330

Herplex, 913
Heterografts in burn treatment, 920
Heterophil test, 807
HETP poisoning, 944
Hexadrol, 716
Hexamethonium, 183
Hexamethylmelamine, 980
Hexestrol, 723
Hexetidine gel, 421
Hexylresorcinol, 865
5-HIAA, 351
Hiatus hernia, 337
Hiccup, 322
Hickey-Hare test, 654
High
  calcium diet, 763
  calorie, protein, and vitamin diet,
    761
  output failure, 222
High-risk pregnancy, 467
Hinton test, 841
Hip dislocation, congenital, 960
Hippocratic nails, 69
Hirschsprung's disease, 364
Hirsutism, 68, 646
His bundle electrograms, 206
His-Purkinje-ventricular impulses, 206
Histadyl, 14
Histalog, 275
Histamine test, 698
  for pheochromocytoma, 181
Histaminic cephalalgia, 559
Histiocytosis, 304
  X, 304
Histocompatibility complex, genetic
  map of, 990
Histoplasma capsulatum, 508, 884
Histoplasmin skin test, 884
Histoplasmosis, 884
  of bones and joints, 508
Hives, 47
HL-A
  antigens and specific disease entities,
    associations between, 997
  complex, 989
  and disease associations, 998
  and rheumatic diseases, associ-
    ation of, 998
  typing, 993
HL-A 7, 997
HL-A W27, 997
HMG, 443, 702
Hoarseness, 103
Hodgkin's disease, 150, **301**, 980, 998
  immunodeficiency associated with,
    980, 997
  staging of, 302
Homocystinuria, 778, 966
Homogentisate oxidase, 777
Homogentisic acid, 777
Homografts in burn treatment, 920
Homosexuality, 613
Hookworm disease, 875
Hordeolum, 82
Hormonal
  contraception, 445
  iodine test, 657
Hormone(s)
  adrenal medullary, and antagonists
    or blocking agents, **719–720**
  adrenocortical, and their antago-
    nists, **715–719**

Hormones (cont'd)
  affecting blood sugar, **720–721**
  anterior pituitary-like, **711–712**
  gonadal, **721–726**
  and hormone-like agents, **711–726**
  male sex, **721–723**
  parathyroid, 714
  pituitary-like elaborated by
    placenta, 713
  posterior-pituitary, 712
  serum or plasma, normal values, 1020
  steroid, in cancer chemotherapy, 980
  therapy for breast cancer, 405
  thyroid, **713–714**
Hormonin, 723
Horner's syndrome, 130, 565
Hornet stings, 947
Horseshoe kidney, 539
Horton's cephalalgia, 559
Housemaid's knee, 499
HSV, 330
Human
  growth hormone, 651
  leukocyte antigen complex, 989
Humatin, 901
Humoral
  antibody-mediated autoimmunity,
    989
  immunity, procedures for measuring,
    990
Hunter's syndrome, 966
Huntington's chorea, 584
Hurler's syndrome, 966
Hutchinson's freckle, 65
Hyaluronate, mucin clot tests for, 477
Hycanthone, 865
Hydroxyurea, 980
Hydatid
  cysts, 869
  disease, 869
Hydatidiform mole, 464
Hydeltra, 716, 717
Hydeltrasol, 717
Hydralazine, 183
  poisoning, 951
Hydrarthrosis, intermittent, 495
Hydrochlorothiazide, 239
Hydrocortisone, 715, 716, **717**, 718
  ointment or cream, 74
  21-phosphate, 717
  sodium succinate, 688, 717
Hydrocortone, 716, 717
Hydrocyanic acid poisoning, 939
Hydrodiuril, 239
Hydroflumethiazide, 239
Hydrogen
  ion(s)
    concentration, 20, 21
      altered, clinical states of, **22–24**
    in renal tubule, 20
    secretion, defects of, 538
    sulfide poisoning, 951
Hydromorphone, 11
Hydromox, 239
Hydronephrosis, 539
Hydropericardium, 225
Hydrophilic ointment, 73
Hydrophobia, 803
Hydroquinone poisoning, 951
Hydrothorax, 147
Hydroxychloroquine, 50
25-Hydroxycholecalciferol, 681

11,17-Hydroxycorticoids, urinary, normal values, 1021
11,17-Hydroxycorticosterone, 715
5-Hydroxyindoleacetic acid, 351
Hydroxyprogesterone caproate, 417, 725, 982
Hydroxyquinolines, halogenated, 851
Hydroxyzine pamoate, 602
Hygroton, 239
Hykinone, 317
Hymenectomy, 440
Hymenolepis
 diminuta, 867
 nana, 867
Hyperaldosteronism, 696, 697
Hyperalimentation, intravenous, 766
Hyperammonemia, 966
Hyperargininemia, 966
Hyperbetalipoproteinemia, 748
Hyperbilirubinemic states, 378
Hypercalcemia, **25**, 676, 767, 974, **976**
 in advanced breast cancer, 410
 idiopathic, 680
  of infancy, 678
 laboratory findings in diseases associated with, 678
Hypercalciuria, idiopathic, 538
Hypercapnia, 22
Hyperemesis gravidarum, 454
Hyperglycemia in diabetic keto-acidosis, 741
Hyperglycemic agents, 721
Hyperglycinemia, 966
Hypergonadism
 female, 709, 710
 male, 703
Hyperimmunoglobulinemia, 995
Hyperkalemia, 23
Hyperkeratosis, follicular, 767
Hyperlipidemia, primary, major categories of, 748
Hyperlipoproteinemia, 747
Hyperlysinemia, 966
Hypermagnesemia, 26
Hypermenorrhea, 417
Hypermetabolism, 665
Hypernatremia, 19
Hypernephroma, 548
Hyperosmolality, 19
Hyperostosis, 685
 frontalis, 695
Hyperoxaluria, primary, 781
Hyperparathyroidism, 545, 674, 680
 primary, 675
  in renal stone formation, 545
 secondary, 674, 676
 tertiary, 676, 679
Hyperphosphatemia, 537
Hyperpigmentation
 Berlock, 67
 of skin, 67
Hyperpituitarism, 652
Hyperplasia, adrenal, congenital, 966
Hyperprebetalipoproteinemia, 748, 749
Hyper-"remnant"-lipoproteinemia, 748
Hypersensitivity
 disorders, 12
 reactions, 12
 tests, 1003
Hypersplenism, 291
Hypertensin, 720
Hypertension, **178**, 696

Hypertension (cont'd)
 essential, 178, 179
 malignant, 179
 portal, 863, 864
 primary, 178
 propranolol in, 241
 pulmonary, in congenital heart disease, 161
 renal, 179
 secondary, 179
Hypertensive
 cardiovascular disease, 178
 crises, acute, 184
 encephalopathy, 525
 vascular disease, 178
Hyperthermia, 575
Hyperthyroidism, 658, **664**, 678, 680
Hypertonic solutions, intra-amniotic injection of, in therapeutic abortion, 463
Hypertrophic
 cardiomyopathy, 231, 242
 scars, 69
Hypertrophy, idiopathic cardiac, 230
Hypertropia, 85
Hyperuricemia, 496, **977**
 complicating leukemia, 296
Hypervalinemia, 966
Hyperventilation, 22
Hypervitaminosis
 A, 767
 D, 768
 K, 768
Hypesthesia, stocking and glove, in polyneuritis, 586
Hyphema, 77
Hypocalcemia, 25, 537, 673
Hypochloremic alkalosis, 222
Hypocomplementemic glomerulonephritis, 530
Hypogammaglobulinemia, transient, of infancy, 995
Hypoglycemia, 738, 974
 alimentary, 746
 common causes of, 744
 due to
  extrapancreatic tumors, 746
  pancreatic beta cell tumors, 745
 functional alimentary, 746
 late, 746
 postprandial, 746
 reactive, 746
Hypoglycemic
 agents, 720
  oral, 721, 732
 states, 744
Hypogonadism
 female, 704
 laboratory diagnosis of, 700
 male, 700
 postpuberal, 702
 prepuberal, 700
 prognosis of, 702
 puberal, 701
Hypokalemia, 24, 222
Hypokalemic periodic paralysis, 592
Hypolipidemic drugs, 749
Hypolipoprotein disorders, 750
Hypomagnesemia, 26
Hyponatremia, 19
 dilutional, 21
Hypoparathyroidism, 672, 680

Hypoparathyroidism (cont'd)
 pseudo-idiopathic, 673
Hypophosphatasia, 680
Hypophysectomy in treatment of breast cancer, 408
Hypopituitary cachexia, 650
Hypoplasia, thymic, 992, 995
Hypostatic pneumonia, 120
Hypotension, 555
 in cardiac failure, 197
Hypotensive
 drugs, 181, 182
 states, adrenergic drugs used in, 6
Hypothalamic
 amenorrhea, 706
 hormones, 711
Hypothalamus, disorders of, **649-656**
Hypothyroidism, 658, 661, 662
 adult, 662
 juvenile, 661
 primary, 662
 secondary, 662
Hypotropia, 85
Hypoventilation and obesity, 140
Hypovitaminosis
 A, 767
 B₁, 769
 B₂, 770
 C, 771
 D, 768
 K, 768
Hypoxia, treatment of, in shock, 7
Hypsarhythmia, 563
Hysterectomy, 449
Hysterical
 personality, 616
 psychosis, 617
Hysterosalpingography, 442
Hytakerol, 674, 714

Ibogaine, 947
Ibuprofen, 10, 482
Ichthammol, 270
Ichthyol, 270
ICSH, 712
ICW, 16, 17
Idoxuridine, 78, 913
IgA, 987
IgD, 987
IgE, 987
IgG, 987
IgM, 987
IHSS, 231
Ileitis, regional, 349
Ileocolitis, granulomatous, 349
Ileus, adynamic or paralytic, 354
 in pregnancy, 473
Iliac arteries, occlusive disease of, 247
Imipramine, 601
 poisoning due to, 948
Immersion
 foot, 915
 syndrome, 915
Immobilization, 678
Immune
 complex disease, 522, 989
 response(s)
  cellular basis of, 988
  genes, 990
  genetic control of, 989

Immunity
    humoral, procedures for measuring, 990
    tests, cell-mediated, 990
Immunization
    of adults for travel, 1002
    of children, 1001
Immunoblastic lymphadenopathy, 304
Immunodeficiency
    associated with
        Hodgkin's disease, 997
        sarcoidosis, 996
    with ataxia-telangiectasia, 996
    diseases determined by cell typing, 992
    disorders, classification of, 995
    with generalized hematopoietic hypoplasia, 995
    and infections, 784
    severe combined, 996
    with thrombocytopenia and eczema, 996
    with thymoma, 995
    variable, 996
    X-linked, with hyper-IgM, 995
Immunodeficient hosts, 784
Immunoelectrophoresis, 991
Immunofluorescence microscopy, 992
Immunoglobulin(s)
    A, 987
    classes, 987
    D, 987
    deficiency, selective, 997
    determinations, quantitative, 991
    E, 987
    G, 987
    M, 987
    molecules, basic unit of, 987
    monoclonal, immunoelectrophoretic pattern of, 991
    structure of, 988
        and function, 987
Immunologic
    deficiency, 974
        diseases, 995–998
    disorders, 987–998
    reactions, lung diseases due to, 111
Immunology, clinical laboratory tests for, 990
Immunostimulant therapy, 983
Immunosuppressive
    drugs in nephrotic syndrome, 531
    therapy, chronic diseases and, 912
Impetigo, 53, 814
    Bockhart's, 53
    neonatorum, 53
Impotence, 612
Inadequate personality, 617
Incest, 613
Inclusion conjunctivitis, 80, 840
Incontinence
    anal, 370
    urinary, 521
        stress, 521
Incontinentia pigmenti, 66
Inderal, 160, 171, 190, 204, 241, 699, 720
Indigestion
    chronic, 389
    nervous, 325
Indoklon, 604
Indomethacin, 10, 497
    in arthritis, 482

Infant, effects of maternal medications on, 455
Infantilism, sexual, 648
Infarction
    intestinal, 352
    myocardial, 193
Infection(s)
    anaerobic, 786
    asymptomatic, early treatment of, 912
    mycotic, of bones and joints, 507
    ocular, 86
    treatment of, in shock, 7
Infectious
    diseases, 791–890
        immunization against, 1001, 1002
        introductory discussion of, 783–789
    mononucleosis, 792, 806
        diagnostic features of, 792
Infective endocarditis, 174
Infertility, 441, 663
    female, 442
    male, 443
Inflamed eye, differential diagnosis of, 75
Inflammatory
    carcinoma of breast, 401
    and degenerative venous disease, 262–271
    headache, 558
Influenza, 805
    pneumonia due to, 122
Ingested poison, 932
INH, 126, 127, 903
Inhaled poison, 932
Inheritance
    mendelian (autosomal), 958
    modes of, 958
    polygenic, 960
    X-linked, 959
Insect
    bite, 63, 932
    powder, poisoning due to, 940
    repellent for traveling, 1001
Insecticides, chlorinated, poisoning due to, 939
Insemination, artificial, 443
Insomnia, 625
Insufficiency
    adrenocortical, 687
        chronic, 688
    aortic, 166, 167, 168, 172
    mitral, 166, 167, 168, 169
    tricuspid, 166, 167, 173
Insufflation, tubal, in infertility, 442
Insulin, 720
    allergy, 738
    normal values, 1020
    preparations, 733
    resistance, immune, 738
    single
        component, 721
        peak, 721
    therapy
        complications of, 737
        immunopathology of, 738
    tolerance
        normal values, 1021
        test, 689
Insulinoma, 980
Insulinopenic diabetes, 727
Insulinoplethoric diabetes, 727, 735
Intelligence tests, 596

Intermediate coronary syndrome, 192
Intermittent positive pressure breathing, 227
Interstitial
    cell stimulating hormone, 712
    nephritis, 535
    pancreatitis, acute, 393
    pneumonia
        desquamative, 142
        idiopathic, 142
    water, 15
Interstitium, diseases of, 532
Intertrigo, 48
Intervertebral disk, herniation of, 577
Intestinal
    arthritis, 491
    capillariasis, 877
    infarction, 352
    obstruction, functional, 354
    polyposis, multiple, 351
Intestine, small, tumors of, 350
Intoxication, water, 533
Intra-amniotic injection of hypertonic solutions in therapeutic abortion, 463
Intracellular water, 16, 17
Intracranial
    aneurysm, 570
    bleeding, 568
    tumors, 578–579
Intradermal test for hypersensitivity, 1003
Intraocular foreign body, 77
Intrauterine contraceptive device, 447
Intravascular coagulation, disseminated, 315
Intravenous hyperalimentation, 766
Intrinsic
    asthma, 111
    factor, 275
Introjection, 594
Intropin, 6
Inulin clearance, 522, 594, 1020
Inversine, 183
Invertase deficiency, 762
Iodide ingestion, 658
Iodinated oil, 660
Iodine, 666
    butanol-extractable, 657
    deficiency, 658
    food sources of, 758
    poisoning, 940
    protein-bound, 657, 1011
    radioactive, 667
    test, hormonal, 657
    in thyroid disease, 660, 666
Iodochlorhydroxyquin, 851
5-Iodo-2-deoxyuridine, 78
Ionizing radiation, 924
Ipecac poisoning, 951
IPPB, 138, 140, 227
Iproniazid poisoning, 951
Ir genes, 990
Iridodialysis, 77
Iridocyclitis, 81
Iritis, 75, 81
Iron
    deficiency anemia, 273, 459
    food sources of, 758
    in gastric contents, 931
    normal values, 1011, 1019
    oral preparations, 274

Iron (cont'd)
parenteral preparations, 274
poisoning, 940
test, drugs interfering with, 1005
Iron-binding capacity
normal values, 1011, 1019
test, drugs interfering with, 1005
Iron-dextran injection, 274
Irradiation
reactions, **922—925**
supervoltage, in breast cancer, 404
Irritable colon, 325
Ischemia, mesenteric vascular, chronic, 352
Ischemic heart disease, prevention of, 187
Islet cell
functioning pancreatic tumors, 699
tumor of pancreas, 344
Ismelin, 183, 185
Isocarboxazid poisoning, 951
Isochromosomes, 963
Isolation, 594
Isomaltase deficiency, 762
Isoniazid, 126, 127, **903**
Isoproterenol, 6, 219, 241
Isoquinolines, 913
Isordil, 239
Isosexual precocious puberty, 415
Isosorbide dinitrate, 239
Isosporosis, 862
Isotope renography, 253
Isovaleric acidemia, 966
Isoxazolylpenicillins, 895
ISW, 17
Itching, 33
IUCD, 447
IUDR, 78
Ivy, poison, 953

Jacksonian epilepsy, 561
Jaffe reaction, 1010
Jarisch-Herxheimer reaction, 842
Jaundice, 370
congenital hemolytic, 281
familial chronic idiopathic, 378
recurrent, of pregnancy, 379
Jejunal ulcer, 346
Jellies, contraceptive, 447
Jiggers, 64
Jock itch, 58
Joint(s). See also Bone and Joint Diseases.
Charcot, 565
disease, degenerative, 492
fluid, 477, 478
pain, 648
replacement in arthritis, 501
Junctional
rhythm, atrioventricular, 206
tachycardia, atrioventricular, 206

Kala-azar, 859
Kallman's syndrome, 648, 700
Kanamycin, 176, 901
Kaon, 30
Kaopectate, 325
Kaposi's varicelliform eruption, 38, 51
Karyotypes, 965, 967
Kayexalate, 24, 30
Kayser-Fleischer ring, 537, 583

K cells, 989
Kegel exercises, 439
Keith-Wagener classification of retinal changes, 180
Keloids, 69
Kemadrin, 582
Kenacort, 716
Kenalog, 717
Kenny packs, 800
Keralyt Gel, 49
Keratitis, 77, 78
Keratoacanthomas, 65
Keratoconjunctivitis, epidemic, 808
Keratolytic agents, 52
Keratopathy, band, 675, 676
Kerion, 57
Kerosene poisoning, 941
Ketoacidemia in diabetic ketoacidosis, 741
Ketoacidosis, diabetic, 741
Ketonuria, 730
intermittent branched chain, 966
Ketosis, diabetic, 27
17-Ketosteroids, urinary
in hypogonadism, 700
normal values, 1021
test for, drugs interfering with, 1005
Ketostix, 730
K gluconate, 30
Kidney(s)
adenocarcinoma of, 548
cystic diseases of, 536
disorders of, **522—539**
ectopic, 539
embryoma of, 549
horseshoe, 539
polycystic, 536
stones, 496, 545
structural defects of, 536
Kiesselbach's area, 99
Killer T cells, 989
Kissing bugs, 858
Klebsiella pneumonia, 119
Klinefelter's syndrome, 701, 964
Kolmer test, 841
Koplik's spots, 791
Kostmann's agranulocytosis, 970
Krabbe's disease, 966
K-triplex, 30
Kveim reaction, 142
Kwashiorkor, 776
KW classification, 180
Kwell, 62

La belle indifférence, 611
Laboratory tests, validity, 1004
Labyrinthine tests, 88
Labyrinthitis, 95
Lacerations, ocular, 79
β-Lactamase, 894
Lactase deficiency, 683
Lactate dehydrogenase, 1011, 1019
Lactation, 446
abnormal, 647
and breast cancer, 399
suppression of, 475
Lactic
acid
dehydrogenase in myocardial infarction, 194
normal values, 1019

Lactic (cont'd)
acidosis, **23**, 743
and phenformin therapy, 734
Lactogen, human placental, 651, 713
Lactogenic hormone, 712
Lactosyl ceramidosis, 966
Lambliasis, 860
Lampit, 858
Lanatoside C, 235, 236
Landouzy-Déjerine muscular dystrophy, 590
Landry-Guillain-Barré syndrome, 587
Lanolin, 73
Lanoxin, 235, 236
Larkspur poisoning, 952
Larodopa, 581, 582
Larva migrans
cutaneous, 868, **881**
visceral, 877
Laryngitis, 102, 103
Laryngotracheobronchitis, 790
Larynx
carcinoma of, 980
diseases of, **102—104**
foreign bodies in, 104, 105
tumors of, 103
Laser in retinal detachment, 84
Lash operation, 462
Lasix, 183, 219, 239
Lassar's paste, 73
Latex test, 315
Latrodectus mactans, 63, 946
LATS, 659, 664, 665
Laurence-Moon-Biedl syndrome, 647, 707
Laxatives, 323
L-CAT, 747
LDH in myocardial infarction, 195
LDL, 747
Lead
poisoning, 780, 941
anemia of, 278
urine, normal values, 1021
Lecithin-cholesterol acyltransferase, 747
Left ventricular filling pressure, 219
Leg
cramps in pregnancy, 453
occlusive disease in, 249
Leiomyoma(s)
of esophagus, 150
of small intestine, 351
Leishman-Donovan bodies, 859
Leishmaniasis, 858, 859, 860
Lens, dislocation of, 781
Lentigines, 67
Leprosy, **834**, 905
sulfones in treatment of, 907
Leptospirosis, 849
Leptothrix conjunctivitis, 80
Lesch-Nyhan syndrome, 966
Letter, 663, 714
Letterer-Siwe disease, 305
Leucine sensitivity disease, 778
Leucovorin, 276
Leukapheresis, 978
Leukemia(s), **294—298**, 980
acute, 294
lymphatic, 998
monocytic, 304
treatment of complications, 295
chronic
lymphatic, 297

Leukemia(s)
  chronic (cont')
    lymphocytic, 992
    myelocytic, 296
  genetics in, 970
  hairy cell, 303
Leukeran, 982
Leukoderma, 67
Leukodystrophy, metachromatic, 966
Leukoplakia, 65, 331, 333
Leukorrhea, 420
  differential diagnosis of causes of,
    421
Levamine, 452
Levarterenol, 6, 720
Levodopa, 581, 582
Levoid, 714
Levophed, 6, **720**
Levorphanol, 11
Levothyroxine sodium, 663, 667, 714
Leydig cell tumor, 704
L forms, 894
Libido, lack of, 648
Librium, 563, 602
Lichen
  planopilaris, 67
  planus, 43
  simplex chronicus, 39
Lid(s)
  granulated, 82
  lacerations of, 79
  papillomas of, 82
  verrucae of, 82
Lidocaine in cardiac arrhythmias, 198,
    208
Ligation, tubal, 464
Light
  chains, 987
  sensitivity, polymorphous, 42
Limb-girdle type muscular dystrophy,
    590
Lincomycin, 908
  in infective endocarditis, 176
Lindane poisoning, 939
Liotrix, 663, 714
Lipase, serum, 1012, 1019
Lipid(s)
  metabolism, disturbances of, 747
  normal values, 1019
Lipidemia, mixed, 748, 749
Lipidosis, sphingomyelin, 753, 966
Lipodystrophy
  at insulin injection sites, 738
  intestinal, 356
Lipoid
  cell tumor, virilizing, 437
  pneumonia, 122
Lipomas of small intestine, 351
Lipoprotein(s), 747
  and atheroma, relationship between,
    749
  phenotypes and diet therapy, 750
Lipoproteinemia and diabetes, relation-
    ship between, 747
Lippes loop, 447
Liquid diet, 760
Listeria, 906
Lithane, 600
Lithium carbonate, 600
Lithonate, 600
Little's area, 99
Livedo reticularis, 260

Liver
  abscess, due to amebiasis, 850, 851, 853
  disease(s), 370
    drug- and toxin-induced, 379
  fatty, 381
  fluke, 866
  injury, comparison of various features
    in different forms of, 373
  neoplasms of, 386
  scans, 371
Loa loa, 879
Locorten, 717
Loestrin, 724
Loiasis, 879
Lomidine, 857
Lomotil, 325
Long-acting thyroid stimulator, 659,
    664, 665
Lo/Ovral, 724
Lotions, 72
Lotrimin, 74
Louse, pubic, head, or body, 63
Louse-borne typhus, epidemic, 809
Low
  back pain, 576
  calcium diet, 763
  calorie diet, 773
  carbohydrate diet, 761
  cholesterol diet, 751, 752
  fat diet, 761
  gluten diet, 762
  protein diet, 761
  purine diet, 762
  sodium
    diets, 184, 221
    syndrome, 222
Low-resistance shock, 3, 4
Lown-Ganong-Levine syndrome, 213
Loxapine, 598
Loxitane, 598
Loxosceles, 63
LSD, 634, 947
Lucanthone hydrochloride, 865
Ludwig's angina, 102
Lugol's solution, 666
Lumbosacral disk herniation, 577
Lumpectomy, 404
Lung(s)
  abscess, 123
  carcinoma of, 980
  diseases due to immunologic reac-
    tions, 111
  disorders of, **111–116**
  infections of, **116–129**
  pump, 134
  shock, 134
Lupoid type hepatitis, 375
Lupus erythematosus
  discoid, 49
  systemic, 483, 993, 998
Luteinizing hormone, 712
Luteotropic hormone, 712
LVFP, 219
Lymphadenitis, 271
  acute mesenteric, 360
  cervical, 129
Lymphadenopathy, immunoblastic, 304
Lymphangitis, 271
Lymphatic(s)
  channels, diseases of, **271–272**
  diseases of, **243–272**
  leukemia, acute, 294, 998

Lymphedema, 272
Lymphocyte(s)
  B and T, development of, 988
  culture antigens, mixed, 990
Lymphocytic
  choriomeningitis, 801
  leukemia, 980
    chronic, 992
Lymphogranuloma venereum, 370, **839**
Lymphoma, 150, 678, 974
  giant follicular, 303
  malignant, 303
  non-Hodgkin's, 992
  of small intestine, 351
Lymphoproliferative diseases deter-
    mined by cell typing, 992
Lymphosarcoma, 150
Lyon hypothesis, 969
Lypressin, 655, 712
Lysergic acid diethylamide, 634, 947
Lysine monohydrochloride, 217, 242
Lysine-8 vasopressin, 712
Lysivane, 582
Lysodren, 693, 715, 980, 983
Lysol poisoning, 943
Lysosomal acid phosphatase deficiency,
    966

MacDonald operation, 462
Machado complement fixation test, 858
Macroamylasemia, 1007
Macrogenitosomia praecox, 694
Macroglobulinemia, 300, 980
  Waldenström's, 994
Macrolides, 898
Macrophages, 989
MAD, 896
Maduromycosis, 889
Mafenide, 907, 919
Magnesia magma, 323
Magnesium, 25
  food sources of, 758
  normal values, 1019
  oxide, 343
  salts, poisoning, 952
  serum, 1012
  sulfate soaks, 71
Malabsorption
  glucose-galactose, 762
  syndrome, 355
Malaria, 853
  algid, 854
  benign tertian, 854
  cerebral, 854
  malignant tertian, 854
  quartan, 854
  simian, in man, 856
Malassezia furfur, 61
Malathion poisoning, 944
Male
  chromatin body, 965
  hypergonadism, 703
  hypogonadism, 700, 701
  sex hormone, 721
Malignancies responsive to chemo-
    therapy, 980
Malignant
  disorders, **973–986**
  effusions, 975
  hypertension, 179
  lymphoma, 303

Malignant (cont'd)
  melanoma, 65, 66
  pustule, 830
Mallory-Weiss syndrome, 321, 326
Mammotropin, 712
Malnutrition
  factors resulting in, 759
  protein and calorie, 774
Mammary dysplasia, 412
Mammography, 402
Mandelic acid, 909
Manganese poisoning, 952
Mannitol, 36
  in glaucoma, 76
  hexanitrate, 239
Mammosidosis, 966
Mantoux test, 124
MAO, 345
MAOI, 601
Maple syrup urine disease, 778, 966
Marasmus, 776
Marboran, 797, 913
Marfan's syndrome, 155, **781**
Marginal ulcer, 346
Marie-Strümpell disease, 81, 489
Marihuana, 947
  abuse, 635
Maroteaux-Lamy syndrome, 966
Marrow toxicity, bone, 981
Mastectomy
  radical
    chemotherapy as adjunct to, 405
    complications of, 410
    extended, 404
    modified, 404
    radiotherapy as adjunct to, 405
    standard, 403
    survival rate, 403
  simple, 404
Masters-Allen syndrome, 441
Mastitis
  of breast, cystic, chronic, 412
  puerperal, 476
Mastoiditis, 93
Matches, poisoning due to, 945
Matulane, 983
Maxibolin, 722
Maximal
  expiratory flow rate, 108
  voluntary ventilation, 108
May-Hegglin anomaly, 312
MCHC, normal values, 1018
MCH, normal values, 1018
MCV, normal values, 1018
MDA, toxicity of, 947
Mean corpuscular
  hemoglobin, 1018
  volume, 1018
Means' murmur, 664
Measles, 791
  German, **792**, 793
  in pregnancy, 472
  vaccine, 1001
Measures and weights, new nomenclature
  for, 1006
Mebendazole, 873, 874, 876
Mebaral, **562**, 564
Mecamylamine, 183
Mechlorethamine, 302, 975, 980, 982
Meckel's diverticulitis, 351
Mediastinal tumor(s), 149
  differential diagnosis of, 150

Mediastinitis, 151
Mediastinum, diseases of, **149–151**
Medical
  conditions complicating pregnancy,
    469
  D&C, 705, 725
  recommendations for foreign travel,
    1000–1002
Mediterranean fever, familial, 398
Medrol, 716
Medroxyprogesterone acetate, 417, 725,
    982
Medulla, adrenal, diseases of, **697–699**
Medullary
  cystic disease, 537
  reticulosis, hystiocytic, 304
MEFR, 108
Megacolon
  congenital, 364
  toxic, 363
Megaloblastic anemia, 276, 459
Megaloureter, 539
Meiosis, 961, 962
Mel
  B, 857
  W, 857
Melanoma, malignant, 65, 66
Melanosis, arsenical, 66
Melarsoprol, 857
Melasma, 67
Melbourne chromosome, 971
Melena, 326
Melituria, 730
Mellaril, 598
Melphalan, 297, 300, 980, 982
Meltrol, 721, 733
Meltrol-TD, 721
Membranoproliferative glomerulonephritis,
    530
Menadione sodium bisulfite, 317
Menarche, 416
Mendelian inheritance, 958
Ménière's
  disease, 90, 94
  syndrome, 557
Meningeal irritation, noninfectious, 819
Meningismus, 819
Meningitis
  aseptic, 807, 818
  granulomatous, 818
  Haemophilus influenzae, 821
  meningococcal, 819
  in neonates, 819
  pneumococcal, 821
  purulent, 818
  staphylococcal, 821
  streptococcal, 821
  tuberculous, 821
Meningococcal meningitis, 819
Meningococcemia, 792
Meningoencephalitis
  amebic, 853
  mumps, 798
Meningomyelocele, 960
Meningovascular syphilis, 845
Menopausal syndrome, 707
Menopause, 416
Menorrhagia, 417
Menstruation, 416
Mental
  changes in endocrine disorders, 649
  status examination, 595

Meperidine, 11
Mephenytoin, **562**, 564
Mephobarbital, **562**, 564
Mephyton, 317
Meprednisone, 716
Meprobamate, 563, 602
  poisoning, 952
Meralluride, 240
Mercaptomerin, 240
Mercaptopurine, 295, 297, 980, 982
Mercuhydrin, 240
Mercumatilin, 240
Mercurial diuretics, 240
Mercurophylline, 240
Mercury
  organic, as teratogen, 455
  poisoning, 942
Mercuzanthin, 240
Merethoxylline procaine, 240
Mersalyl, 240
Mesantoin, **562**, 564
Mescaline, 634, 947
Mesenteric
  adenitis, 358
  artery, superior, disease of, 253
  vascular
    insufficiency, 352
    occlusion, 352
Mesonephroma of ovary, 437
Mesoridazine, 598
Mestranol, 724
Metabolic
  acidosis, 22
  alkalosis, 23
  diseases
    bone, **679–684**
    hereditary, **776–780**
  disorders, **777–782**
  headache, 558
Metacercariae, 866
Metachromatic leukodystrophy, 966
Metahydrin, 239
Metaldehyde poisoning, 952
Metal fumes, poisoning due to, 952
Metamine, 239
Metamucil, 323
Metandren, 722
Metaphysitis, 509
Metaraminol for shock, 6
Metazoal diseases, **863–882**
Methacycline, 899
Methadone, 11, 628
  maintenance programs, 628
Methallenestril, 723
Methamphetamine, 563, 637, 948
Methandrostenolone, 277, 722
Methanesulfonate, 948
Methapyrilene, 14
Methaqualone, 602
Metharbital, 562
Methazolamide, 240
Methedrine, 636
Methemalbumin, 319
Methemoglobinemia, 777
Methenamine
  hippurate, 909
  mandelate, 909
  poisoning, 952
Methicillin, 176, 894, 897
Methimazole, 666
Methionine, 909
Methisazone, 796, 797, 913

Methium, 183
Methosarb, 722, 982
Methotrexate, 465, 980, 982, 985
Methoxsalen, 67
Methsuximide, 562, 564
Methyclothiazide, 239
Methyl
    alcohol poisoning, 935
    bromide poisoning, 952
    chloride poisoning, 952
    sulfate poisoning, 952
Methylandrostenediol, 722
Methyldopa, 182, 183
Methylene
    blue, 933
    dioxyamphetamine, toxicity of, 947
    tetrahydrofolate deficiency, 966
N-Methylhydrazine, 983
Methylmalonic aciduria, 966
Methylphenidate, 637
Methylprednisolone, 716, 717
Methyltestosterone, 722
Methyprylon, 602
Methysergide maleate, 559
    retroperitoneal fibrosis due to, 952
Meticortelone, 716, 717
Meticorten, 716
Metol poisoning, 952
Metopirone, 650
    stimulation test, 692
Metronidazole, 421, 851, 852, 861
    possible carcinogenicity of, 852
Metrorrhagia, 417
Metyrapone, 650
    stimulation test, 692
MicaTin, 58, 59, 74
Miconazole, 58, 59, 74, 910
Microfilariae, 878
Micrometastases, adjuvant chemo-
        therapy for, 981
Micronase, 732
Micronor, 444, 724
Microscopy, immunofluorescence, 992
Microspherocytes, 285
Microsporum, 57
Middle ear diseases of, **91–92**
Migraine, 558
Miliaria, 48
Milk
    and alkalies, excessive intake of, 545
    base tube feeding formula, 766
    of bismuth, 325
    of magnesia, 323
Milk-alkali syndrome, 678, 680
Milkman's syndrome, 681
Milliequivalent
    conversion factors, 1021
    weights, 16
Milontin, 562
Milroy's congenital elephantiasis, 878
Miltown, 563, 602
Mineral(s)
    food sources of, 758
    oil, 323
Minimum residue diet, 761
Minipill, 444, 446, 725
Minnesota Multiphasic Personality
        Inventory, 596
Minocycline, 899
Minoxidil, 184
Minute ventilation, 138
Miracil D, 865

Mites, 62, 64
Mithracin, 976, 983
Mithramycin, 976, 980, 983
Mitomycin, 981, 983
Mitosis, 961
Mitotane, 693, 715, 983
Mitral
    insufficiency, 165, 166, 167, **168**
    stenosis, **165**, 166, 167, 168
Mittelschmerz, 417
Mixed lymphocyte culture antigens, 990
MLC
    antigens, 990
        and specific disease entities,
            associations between, 997
    typing, 993
MMPI, 596
Moban, 598
Modeling, 608
Mohs technic, 66
Molar weights, 16
Molecular structure of protein, abnor-
        mality of, 777
Mole, hydatidiform, 464
Molindone, 598
Mongolian spots, 66
Mongolism, 968, 969
Moniliasis. See Candidiasis.
Monk's cowl, 38
Monoamine oxidase inhibitors, 601
Monoclonal
    gammopathy, benign, 994
    immunoglobulin, immunoelectro-
        phoretic pattern of, 991
    spike, 299
Monocytic leukemia, acute, 304
Mononucleosis, infectious, 792, 806
Monosomy, 963, 968
Monsel's solution, 52
Montenegro's test, 860
Moon face, 691
MOPP, 302
MOPP-Bleo, 980
Morning sickness, 454
Morphine, 11
    poisoning, 942
Morquio's disease, 966
Mosaic, 961, 963
Mosquito
    Aedes, 802, 804
    jungle, 804
Motion sickness, 557
    and air travel, 926
Motor neuron disease, 588
Motrin, 10, 482
Mountain sickness, 925
Mouth
    cancer, 333
    cellulitis of floor of, 102
    diseases of, **328–333**
Mouth-to-mouth breathing, 1027
6-MP, 982
MTX, 982
Mucin clot tests for hyaluronate, 477
Mucopolysaccharidosis, 966
Mucormycosis, 889
Mucous colitis, 325
Mucoviscidosis, 781
Multiple
    myeloma, 298, 519, 678, 974, 980, 994
    neuritis, 586
    sclerosis, 580, 998

Mumps, 798
    meningoencephalitis, 798
    oophoritis, 798
    orchitis, 798
    pancreatitis, 798
    thyroiditis, 798
    virus vaccine, 1001
Murine typhus, 810
Murmur(s)
    cardiac, 154
    in cardiovascular lesions, 168
    diastolic, 154
    ejection, 154
    machinery, 159
    Means', 654
    regurgitant, 154
    systolic, 154
Muscle cramps, 249, 649
Muscular
    atrophies, 588, **589**
    dystroph(ies), 588, **589**
        pseudohypertrophic, 589
Musculoskeletal headache, 560
Mushroom poisoning, 943
Mustargen, 975, 982
Mutamycin, 983
Mutation, 957
MVO_2, 197
MVV, 108
Myasthenia gravis, 590, 998
Mycetoma, 889
Mycobacteria, atypical, 906
    pulmonary disease due to, 129
Mycobacterium tuberculosis, 124, 510,
        543, 783
Mycoplasmal
    infections, drug selections for, 906
    pneumonia, 121
Mycosis fungoides, 304
Mycostatin, 71, 890
    mouth rinses, 331
Mycotic
    diseases, **883–890**
    infections
        of bones and joints, 507
        of skin, **56–62**
Myelitis, transverse, 797, 864
Myeloblastic leukemia, acute, treat-
        ment of, 295
Myelocytic leukemia, 980
Myelofibrosis, 277, 300
Myeloma
    Bence Jones, 298
    multiple, 298, 519, 678, 974, 980, 994
    plasma cell, 519
Myelomatosis, 536
Myelopathic muscular atrophy, 588
Myeloproliferative disease, 546
Myelosclerosis, 300
Myiasis, 882
Myleran, 982
Myocardial
    damage in trypanosomiasis, 857
    disease, primary, 229
    infarction, 193
        painless, 194
        premature or impending, 192
    oxygen consumption, 197
Myocarditis, 807
    acute and chronic, 229
    doxorubicin-induced, 985
    in trypanosomiasis, 856

Myocardium, diseases of, **226—231**
Myoma of uterus, 428
Myotonia, 592
Myotonic dystrophy, 592
Myringoplasty, 90
Myristicin, 634
Mysoline, **562**, 564
Myxedema, 662
  coma, 663
  madness, 663
  pretibial, 664

Naegleria infection, 853
Nafcillin, 896
Naffziger's syndrome, 565
Nail disorders, 69
Nalidixic acid, 909
Nalline, 942
Nandrolone, 277, 722
Naphthalene
  chlorinated, poisoning due to, 949
  poisoning, 952
Naphthol poisoning, 952
Naphthylamine poisoning, 953
Naqua, 239
Narcolepsy, 554
Narcotic(s)
  dependency, 627
  poisoning, 942
Nardil, 601
Nasal
  septum
    abscess of, 96
    hematoma of, 96
  tumors, 99
  vestibulitis, 95
Naso-oral leishmaniasis, 860
Naturetin, 239
Nausea, 321
Navane, 598
Necator americanus, 875
Necrophilia, 613
Necrosis
  fat, 413
  piecemeal, 375
  renal papillary, 535
Necrotizing
  cellulitis, synergistic, 787
  fasciitis, 787
Negatan, 426
"Neighborhood" reaction, 819
Nelson's syndrome, 692
Nematodal infections, **870—882**
Neo-Antergan, 14
Neodrol, 722
Neohetramine, 14
Neohydrin, 240
Neomycin, 71, 900, 901
Neoplasms. See specific types.
  and FUO, 783
Neoplastic disorders, **973—986**
Neostigmine
  poisoning, 953
  test, 591
Neo-Synephrine, 6
Nephritis
  hereditary chronic, 536
  interstitial, 535
Nephrocalcinosis, 538, **545**
Nephropathy
  analgesic, 535

Nephropathy (cont'd)
  diabetic, 738
  gouty, 496
  uric acid, 535, 977
Nephroptosis, 539
Nephrosclerosis, arteriolar, 532
Nephrosis, 530
Nephrotic syndrome, 530
Neptazane, 240
Nerve deafness, 89, 90
Nervous
  indigestion, 325
  system, disorders of, **553—593**
Neuralgia
  post-zoster, 52
  trigeminal, 585
Neuritis, 586
Neuroblastoma, 150, 980
Neurodermatitis, localized, 39
Neurofibroma, 150
Neurofibromatosis, 698
Neurogenic arthropathy, 493
Neuroleptics, 597
Neurologic evaluation of psychiatric
  patients, 596
Neuromuscular disorders, **588—593**
Neuromyopathy, 974
Neuropathy
  diabetic, 729, 738
  peripheral, 586
  vincristine, 984
Neuroses, 609
  intestinal, 325
Neurosyphilis, 845
Neurotic patients and air travel, 927
Neurotrophic arthropathy, 509
Nevi, 65, 66
Newborn, hemolytic disease of, 474
Niacin, 758, 770
Niacinamide, 770
Nialamide poisoning, 951
Nickel carbonyl poisoning, 953
Niclosamide, 868
Nicotinamide, 770
Nicotine poisoning, 953
Nicotinic acid, 749, 770
  in nerve deafness, 90
  poisoning, 770
Niemann-Pick disease, **753**, 966
Night blindness, 767
Nikolsky's sign, 37
Nilevar, 722
Nilodin, 865
Nipple discharge, differential diagno-
  sis of, 413
Niridazole, 864
Nitranitol, 239
Nitrates, 238
  long-acting, 190, 239
Nitrites, 238
  poisoning, 951
Nitrofurantoin, 909
Nitrofurazone, 423
Nitrogen
  liquid, 52
  mustard, 299, 302, 975, 982
  nonprotein, 1012
Nitroglycerin, 188, 190, 239
Nitromersol, 74
Nitrous oxide poisoning, 955
Nocardiosis, 887
Nocturia, 216

Nodal
  rhythm, 206
  tachycardia, atrioventricular, 206
Nodular cirrhosis, 381
Noise as factor in nerve deafness, 90
Noludar, 602
Nomograms, body surface area, 1024
Nonclostridial crepitant cellulitis, 787
Nongonococcal urethritis and cervicitis,
  840
Nongranulomatous uveitis, 81
Non-Hodgkin's lymphomas, 980, 992
Nonketotic hyperglycemic coma, 742
Nonmetabolic bone disease, **685—686**
Nonphotochromogens, 129
Nonprotein nitrogen, 1012, 1019
Nonpsychiatric drugs, psychiatric com-
  plications of, 644
Nonrapid eye movement sleep, 625
Nonrheumatic mitral insufficiency, 170
Nontreponemal tests for syphilis, 841
Nonvenereal treponematoses, 847
Norepinephrine, 6, 241, **720**
  effects of, 720
  normal values, 1019
  for shock, 6
Norethandrolone, 722
Norethindrone, 417, 446, 725
  test for pregnancy, 450
Norethynodrel, 725
  test for pregnancy, 450
Noriday, 724
Norinyl, 446, 724
Norinyl 1+80, 724
Norit A, 931
Norlestrin, 429, 446, 724
Norlutin, 417, 725
Norpramin, 601
Nor-QD, 445, 724
Norquen, 724
North American blastomycosis, 509, 886
Nortriptyline, poisoning due to, 948
Nosebleed, 99
Nose, diseases of, **95—100**
Novobiocin, 892, 908
NPN, normal values, 1019
NREM sleep, 625
N-terminal variable region, 987
Nuchar C, 931
Nucleotide diaphorase, 777
Nutramigen, 762
Nutrient content of foods, 756, 757
Nutrition
  human, **754—766**
  intravenous hyperalimentation in, 766
  tube feedings in, 765
Nystatin, 71, 331, 887, 890, 910

Oak, poison, 953
Obesity, 646, **771**
  in diabetes, 728
  and hypoventilation, 140
Obesity-hypoventilation syndrome, 772
Objective tests, 596
OBS, 638
Obsessions, 611
Obsessive compulsive personality, 616
Obstetric(s), **450—476**
Obstruction
  colonic, 366
  functional intestinal, 354

Obstruction (cont')
  organic intestinal, 353
  due to ulcer
    peptic, 342
    surgery for, 344
Obstructive uropathy, 536
Occipital lobe tumor, 579
Occlusion, arterial, acute, 254
Occlusive disease
  of aorta and iliac arteries, 247
  cerebrovascular, 251
  of femoral and popliteal arteries, 248
  in lower leg and foot, 249
Ochronosis, 777
Ocular
  disorders, precautions in manage-
    ment of, 87
  emergencies, **76–79**
  infections, treatment of, 86
  lacerations, 79
  myiasis, 882
  pain, 75
Ogen, 723
Ogino, contraception method of, 444
Oil
  iodinated, 660
  volatile, poisoning due to, 955
Oily lotion, 72
Ointment(s), 74
  bases, 73
Oliguric phase of acute renal failure,
    534
Olive oil, 323
Ommaya reservoir, 885
OMPA poisoning, 944
Onchocerciasis, 879
Oncovin, 983
Onycholysis, 69
Onychomycosis, candidal, 60
o,p'DDD, 693, 715, 980, 983
Open-angle glaucoma, 83
Operant conditioning, 608
Ophthalmia
  neonatorum, 80
  sympathetic, 78
Ophthalmoplegia, exophthalmic, 664
Opportunistic infections, fungal, 889
Orabase, 330
Oracon, 444, 724
Oral
  cancer, 333
  contraceptives, 444
    contraindications to, 446
    effects of, 445
    hormone-related side-effects of,
      445
Ora-Testryl, 713
Orbital cellulitis, 79
Orchitis, mumps, 798
Oretic, 239
Oreton, 722
Organic
  brain syndrome, 638
    in hemiplegia, 570
  therapies, 604
Oriental sore, 858, 860
Orinase, 721, 732
Ornithosis, 840
  pneumonia due to, 122
Orotic aciduria, 966
Oroya fever, 838
Orphenadrine, 582

Ortho-Novum, 444, 724
  SQ, 724
Ortho-para'DDD, 693, 715, 980, 983
Orthopnea, 106, 152, 215
Orthostatic hypotension, 555
OsCal, 674
Osmolality, 1019
Osmolarity, 19
Osmotic fragility, 281
Osteitis
  deformans, 685
  fibrosa
    cystica, 676
    disseminata, 685
  syphilitic, 509
Osteoarthritis, 492
  of cervical spine, 512
Osteoarthropathy, pulmonary, 107
Osteoclastoma, 519
Osteodystrophy
  Albright's, 673
  renal, 679, 681
Osteogenesis imperfecta, 517, 680, 683
Osteogenic sarcoma, 518, 980
Osteolytic metastases, 678
Osteoma, osteoid, 518
Osteomalacia, 679
  and rickets, 680
Osteomyelitis, 502, 788
  acute pyogenic, 502
  brucella, 505
  chronic pyogenic, 506
  salmonella, 504
    and arthritis, 504
Osteoperiostitis, 509
Osteopetrosis, 680
Osteoporosis, 681, **682**
  circumscripta, 686
  idiopathic or senile, 680
Osteopsathyrosis, 517
Ostium
  primum defect, 158
  secundum defect, 158
OTC drugs, abuse of, 638
O_2 tension, arterial, 108
Otitis, 89, 91, 92, 93
Otorrhagia, 573
Otorrhea, 575
Otosclerosis, 90
Ototoxic drugs, 89
Ouabain, 236
Ovalocytosis, 282
Ovarian
  agenesis, primary, 706
  cancer, secondary, 439
  cysts, 435
  fibromas, 435
  tumors, **434–439**
    hormones elaborated by, 710
    in pregnancy, 472
Ovariectomy, 448
Ovar(ies)
  carcinoma of, 980
  diseases of, **704–711**
  oyster, 437, 711
  streak, 707
  virilizing disorders of, 711
Overdosage of drugs, 932
Overhydration, 18
Over-the-counter drugs, abuse of, 638
Ovocyclin, 724
Ovral, 724

Ovulation
  hormonal suppression of, 444
  induction of, in infertility, 442
Ovulen, 724
Ovulen-21, 724
Oxacillin, 896
Oxalate stones, 546
Oxalic acid poisoning, 943
Oxalosis, 781
Oxaluria, 546
Oxazepam, 602
Oxsoralen, 67
Oxycodone, 11
Oxygen
  administration, 137
  blood, normal values, 1019
  gradient, alveolar-arterial, 138
  therapy in chronic respiratory
    failure, 139
Oxymetholone, 277, 722
Oxymorphone, 11
Oxyphenbutazone, 9, 497
Oxytetracycline, 899
Oxytocin injection, 712
Oxyuriasis of intestine. See Enterobiasis.

^{32}P, **296, 306**
Pacemaker, artificial, 211
Pa_{CO_2}, 108
Paget's
  carcinoma, 401
  disease, 680, 685
    of bone, 678
    of skin, 65
Pagitane, 582
PAH clearance, normal values, 1020
Pain, 8
  abdominal, in pregnancy, 453
  anginal, as precursor of myocardial
    infarction, 194
  chest, 106, 153
  low back, 576
  in myocardial infarction, 193
  pelvic, 440
  pleuritic, 118
  as symptom of genitourinary tract
    disease, 521
  syndromes, cervicobrachial, **512–516**
Paint thinner poisoning, 941
Palindromic rheumatism, 495
Palpitation, 153
Palsy
  Bell's, 586
  bulbar, 588
Pamaquine poisoning, 953
Pancoast's syndrome, 130
Pancreas
  carcinoma
    of body and tail of, 397
    of head of, 396
  diseases of, **393–397**
  islet cell tumor of, 344
Pancreatic
  carcinoma, 974
  fibrosis, 781
  tumors
    beta cell, hypoglycemia due to, 745
    islet cell functioning, 699
Pancreatitis
  acute, 393
  chronic relapsing, 395

Pancytopenia, 276
Panhypopituitarism, 650
Pa_{O_2}, 108
PAP, 138
  syndrome, 121
Papanicolaou examination, 425
Papaverine, 254
Papilledema, 180
Papillitis
  anal, 368
  chronic lingual, 332
Papilloma of lids, 82
Para-aminobenzoic acid, 42, 905
Para-aminosalicylic acid, 904
Parabromdylamine, 14
Paracentesis, 220, 224
Paracoccidioides brasiliensis, 886
Paracoccidioidomycosis, 886
Paracort, 716
Paracortol, 716
Paradione, 562, 564
Paradoxic pulse, 224
  sleep, 625
Paragonimiasis, 866
Paraldehyde, 602
  poisoning, 953
Paralysis
  agitans, 581
  cranial nerve, 575
  familial periodic, 592
  hypokalemic periodic, 592
  peripheral facial, 586
  rehabilitation in, 569
  Werdnig-Hoffmann, 588
Paramethadione, 562, 564
Paramethasone, 716
Paramyotonia congenita, 592
Paraneoplastic syndromes, **973–974**
Paranoid personality, 616
Parapharyngeal abscess, 102
Paraplegia, 678
Parasympatholytic drugs in treatment
  of ulcer, 343
Parathion poisoning, 944
Parathyroid(s), **672–679**
  adenoma, 675
  dysfunction in pregnancy, 471
  hormone, 673, **714**
    normal values, 1020
  injection, 674, 714
  poisoning, 677
  syndromes, principal findings in, 674
  tetany, 673
Paregoric, 325
Parenteral
  fluids, daily maintenance rations, 26
  infusion, solutions for, 29
Parest, 602
Parietal lobe tumors, 579
Parkinsonism, 581
Parnate, 601
Paromomycin, 851, 868, 901
Parotitis, endemic, 798
Paroxysmal
  atrial tachycardia, 203
  labyrinthine vertigo, 94
  nocturnal hemoglobinuria, 283
  ventricular tachycardia, 207
Parrot's nodes, 509
Parsidol, 582
PAS, 127
Passive-aggressive personality, 617

Patau's syndrome, 968
Patch test, 124
Patent ductus arteriosus, 155, **159**
Pathologic fractures, 648
Patient compliance in taking medica-
  tion, 596
PBI, 657, 1011
P_{CO_2}, 1019
PCP, 635
PCV, normal values, 1018
Peak airway pressure, 138
Pectin-kaolin compounds, 325
Pediculosis, 63
Pedophilia, 613
PEEP, 139
Peganone, 562
Pellagra, 770
Pelvic
  inflammatory disease, 433
  pain, psychogenic, 440
Pemphigoid, 993
Pemphigus, 37, 993
Penetrance, 959
Penicillamine, 537, 547, 583, 942
Penicillin(s), **894,** 909
  allergy, 896
Penicillinase, 894
Pentaerythritol tetranitrate, 190, 239
Pentamidine isethionate, 857, 859
Pentazocine, 10
Pentobarbital, 601
Pentolinium tartrate, 183, 185
Pentylenetetrazol, 604
  poisoning, 953
Peppermint, spirit of, 324
Peptic
  esophagitis, 336
  ulcer, 341
Peptidoglycan, 894
Perandren, 722
Percodan, 11
Pergonal, 443, 701, 702, 712
Periadenitis, 330
Periampullary area, carcinoma of, 396
Periapical abscess, 329
Periarteritis nodosa, 486
Periarthritis, scapulohumeral, 513
Pericardial cysts, 150
Pericarditis
  acute, 195, 223
    nonspecific, 807
  chronic constrictive, 225
  with effusion, 224
  infectious, 223
  inflammatory, 223
  rheumatic, 161, 225
  tuberculous, 225
  viral, 223
Pericardium, diseases of, **223–226**
Periodic
  disease, 398
  paralysis, familial, 592
Periodontal disease, 329
Periostitis, 509
Peripheral nerves, disorders of, **586–588**
Peritoneal dialysis in heart failure, 220
Peritonitis, 28
  acute, **397–398**
  benign paroxysmal, 398
Peritonsillar abscess, 101
Peritrate, 190, 239
Perlmutter test, 689

Permanganate poisoning, 953
Permitil, 598
Pernox, 46
Pernicious
  anemia, 275, 276, 970, 993
    of pregnancy, 459
  vomiting of pregnancy, 454
Pernio, 914
Peroneal
  artery, occlusive disease of, 249
  muscular atrophy, 589
Perphenazine, 598
Persisters, 894
Personality disorders, 616
Pertofrane, 601
Pertussis, 817
Pesticides, poisoning due to, 944
Petit mal, 561, 564
Petrolatum, 73
  liquid, 323
Petroleum ether poisoning, 941
Peutz-Jeghers syndrome, 351
Phacoemulsification, 85
Phacofragmentation, 85
pH of arterial blood, 108
Pharyngitis, simple, 100
Pharyngoconjunctival fever, 808
Pharynx, diseases of, **100–102**
Phenacemide, 562, 564
Phenacetin poisoning, 953
Phenazocine, 11
Phencyclidine, 635, 947
Phenelzine, 601
  poisoning, 951
Phenergan, 14
Phenformin, 721, 733
Phenindione
  derivatives, 936
  poisoning, 934
Pheniprazine, poisoning due to, 951
Phenmetrazine, 637
Phenobarbital, 562, 564, 602
Phenol
  poisoning, 943
  red, normal values, 1020
Phenolphthalein poisoning, 953
Phenolsulfonphthalein
  normal values, 1020
  test, urine, drugs interfering with, 1005
Phenothiazine(s), 598
  poisoning, 944
  in urine, 931
Phenoxene, 582
Phenoxybenzamine, 242, 699, 720
Phensuximide, 562, 564
Phentolamine, 181, 242, 699, 720
  test, 698
Phenurone, 562, 564
Phenylalanine hydroxylase, 777
Phenylbutazone, 9, 269, 497
  in arthritis, 482
  poisoning, 948
Phenylephrine, 6, 241
Phenylketonuria, 777, 966
Phenylpyruvic oligophrenia, 777
Phenytoin sodium, 208, 562, 564
Pheochromocytoma, 179, 697
  propranolol in, 241
  tests for, 181
Philadelphia chromosome, 968
Phlebography, 265
Phlebotomus, 858

Phlebotomy, 306
Phlegmasia cerulea dolens, 268
pH, normal values, 1019
Phobias, 611
Phoria, 85
Phosdrin poisoning, 944
Phosphatase, acid and alkaline
    normal values, 1019
    serum, 551, 1012
Phosphate(s)
    absorption, defects of, 538
    organic, poisoning due to, 944
Phosphohexose isomerase deficiency, 966
Phospholipid, normal values, 1019
Phosphorus
    absorption defects of, 537
    food sources of, 758
    inorganic
        normal values, 1019
        poisoning, 945
        serum, 1013
Photocoagulation in retinal detach-
    ment, 84
Photochromogens, 129
Photodermatitis, 42
Photodynamic inactivation in treat-
    ment of herpes simplex, 913
Photophobia, 75
Photosensitivity, 780
Phthirus pubis, 63
Phycomycosis, 889
Physical
    agents, disorders due to, **914–927**
    therapy in chronic respiratory
        failure, 140
Physostigmine poisoning, 953
Phytonadione, 317
Pickwickian syndrome, 216, 772
Picrotoxin poisoning, 953
PID, 433
Piebaldism, 66
Piecemeal necrosis, 375
PIE syndrome, 113
Pigmentary disorders, 66
Pigmentation
    abnormal skin, 646
    of gingivas, 332
Pill, contraceptive, 444
Pilocarpine, 83, 332
Piminodine, 11
Pinguecula, 81
Pinta, 847
Pinworm infection, 874
Piperacetazine, 598
Piperazine, 873, 875
    estrone sulfate, 723
Pitocin, 712
Pitressin, 327, 654, 655, 712
Pituitary
    gland, diseases of, **649–656**
    hormone(s)
        anterior, 711
        assay, 674
        normal values, 1020
        posterior, 712
Pituitary-like hormones, placental, 713
Pityriasis rosea, 44
PKU, 777
Placenta
    pituitary-like hormones of, 713
    premature separation of, 466
    previa, 466

Placidyl, 602
Plague, 833
    immunization, 1002
Plantar wart, 52
Plasma, 318
    bicarbonate, 108
    cell(s), 989
        in multiple myeloma, 298
        myeloma, 519
    fresh frozen, 310, 319
    or serum albumin for shock, 5
Plasmodium, 853
Platelet(s)
    defects, 312, 313
    normal values, 1018
Platelet-ADP release dysfunction, 313
Pleura, diseases of, **145–149**
Pleural
    effusion, 145
    empyema, 147
    space, rupture of pus into, 123
Pleurisy, fibrinous, 145
Pleuritic pain, 118
Pleurodynia, epidemic, 807
Plummer-Vinson syndrome, 274
Pneumococcal
    corneal ulcer, 78
    meningitis, 821
    pneumonia, 117
Pneumoconioses, 114
Pneumocystis pneumonia, 120, 862
Pneumomediastinum, 149
Pneumonia(s), **116–123**
    desquamative interstitial, 142
    idiopathic interstitial, 141
Pneumoperitoneum, 128
Pneumothorax, 128
    spontaneous, 147
    tension, 148
    traumatic, 149
Podophyllin, 52, 369
Poison(s). See also specific types.
    eye contamination, 932
    hemlock, 953
    history and physical examination, 929
    identification of, 928
    Information Center, 928
    injected, 932
    ivy, 34, 953
    oak, 953
    removal of, 932
    skin contamination, 932
Poisoning, **928–956**. See also specific
    types.
Poliomyelitis, 799
    virus vaccine, 1001
Pollution, air, 955
Polyarteritis nodosa, 486
Polycystic
    kidneys, 536
    ovarian syndrome, 437
Polycythemia, **107**, 227, 548, 974
    vera, 305, 980
Polydipsia, 647
Polygenic inheritance, 960
Polymenorrhea, 417
Polymorphous light eruption, 42
Polymyalgia rheumatica, 488
Polymyositis, 487, 993
Polymyxins, 902
Polyneuritis, 586
Polyostotic fibrous dysplasia, 685

Polyposis, multiple intestinal, 351
Polyps
    cervical, 428
    colonic, 365
    intestinal, 365
    rectal, 365
Polyserositis, recurrent, 398
Polysomy, 963
Polythiazide, 239
Polyunsaturated and saturated fats in
    certain fats, ratio of, 750
Polyuria, 647, 655
Polyvalent influenza virus vaccine, 805
Pomeroy method, 464
Popliteal
    aneurysms, 246
    artery, occlusive disease of, 248
POR, 999
Pork insulin, 721
Porphyria(s)
    acute, 780
    cutanea tarda, 780
    erythropoietic, 780
        congenital, 966
    hepatic, 779
Porphyrin metabolism, disorders of, 779
Porphyrinurias, acquired, 780
Postcholecystectomy cystic duct syn-
    dromes, 389
Posterior pituitary
    hormones, 712
    powder, 712
    snuff, 655, 712
Posterolateral sclerosis, 580, **584**
Postganglionic blocking agents, 183, 184
Postgastrectomy syndrome, 346
Postmeasles encephalitis, 793
Postmenopausal
    osteoporosis, 683
    vaginal bleeding, 418
Postnasal pack, 99
Postoperative patient and air travel, 926
Postpartum hemorrhage, 466
Postphlebitic syndrome, 269
Postprandial hypoglycemia, 746
Postpuberal hypergonadism, 703
Poststreptococcal glomerulonephritis, 523
Post-tracheostomy care, 104
Post-traumatic
    cerebral syndrome, 574
    sympathetic dystrophy, 261
Postural hypotension, 555
Posture in relation to blood tests, 1006
Post-zoster neuralgia, 52
Potassium, **23–25**
    chloride, 207
    deficiency, 690
    depletion, 239
    food sources of, 758
    gluconate, 30
    intoxication, 533
    iodide, 888
    normal values, 1019
    permanganate, 71
    regulated diet, 763
    secretion, excess, 538
    serum, 1013
        and ECG, 24
    wastage syndrome, 538
Potency, lack of, 648
Powders for skin diseases, 71
PPD-S, 124

Precholecystectomy cystic duct syndromes, 389
Precocious puberty, 647, 685, 703
  isosexual, 415, 703
Prednis, 716
Prednisolone, 716, 717
Prednisolone-21-phosphate, 717
Prednisone, 295, 716, 980, 983
Preeclampsia, 458
Preeclampsia-eclampsia, 457
Preexcitation, ventricular, 212
Pregnancy
  and air travel, 927
  anemia of, 459
  in cardiac patients, 233
  and diabetic patients, 469
  diagnosis, 450
  ectopic, 455
  high-risk, 467
  immunodiagnostic tests, 450
  manifestations of, 450
  medical complications in, 469
  minor discomforts of, 451
  ovarian tumors in, 472
  physiologic load imposed on heart, 233
  surgical complications in, 472
  tests, 450
  toxemia of, 457
  vomiting of, 454
Pregnanediol test, urine, drugs interfering with, 1005
Pregnosticon, 450
Preludin, 637
Premarin, 421, 723, 724
Premature
  beats
    atrial, 203
    ventricular, 207
  ejaculation, 613
  labor, prevention of, 475
Premenstrual tension syndrome, 419
Prepuberal hypergonadism, 703, 709
Pressure sore, 55
Primaquine phosphate, 855
Primidone, **562**, 564
Problem drinking, 631
Problem-oriented record, 999
Procainamide, 240
Procaine poisoning, 953
Procarbazine, 980, 983
Prochlorperazine poisoning, 944
Procyclidine, 582
Profilate, 310
Progestational hormones, 725
Progesterone(s), 417, **725**
  normal values, 1020
  test, 450
Progestins, **724**, 982
Progestogens, endocrine properties of, 725
Proglottids, 867
Progressive muscular
  atrophies, 588
  dystrophy, 589
Proguanil hydrochloride, 855
Progynon, 723
Projection, 594
Projective tests, 596
Prolactin, 712, 713
Prolapse, uterine, 432
Prolixin, 598
Promazine poisoning, 944

Promethazine, 14
Pronestyl, 240
Prophylaxis, antimicrobial, 911
Propion Gel, 421
Propionic acid gel, 421
Proplex, 310
Propoxyphene, 10
Propranolol, 160, 171, 183, 184, 190, 204, 241
Propylthiouracil, 666
  poisoning, 954
Prostaglandins, 463
Prostatic
  carcinoma, 551, 974, 980
  hyperplasia, benign, 550
Prostatism, 550, 551
Prostatitis, 544
Prostigmin test, 591
Prostration, heat, 916
Protein(s)
  bound iodine, 657, 1011
  fractions by electrophoresis, 1014
  malnutrition, 775
  normal values, 1019
  serum or plasma, 1013
  test, drugs interfering with, 1005
  total, 1013
Protein-bound iodine, 657
  normal values, 1019
  test, 657
Protein-losing enteropathy, 357
Proteinosis, alveolar, 132
Proteinuria, Bence Jones, 298
Proteus pneumonia, 119
Prothrombin
  clotting time
    drugs affecting, 1006
    normal values, 1019
  complex
    deficiency, 309, 316
    disorders, acquired, 316
  depressant drugs, 267
Proton beam, 693
Protoplasts, 894
Protozoal diseases, **850-862**
Protriptyline, 601
  poisoning due to, 948
Provera, 417, 725, 982
Pruritus, 33
  ani and vulvae, 48
Prussic acid poisoning, 939
Pseudocausalgia, 515
Pseudocyst, 394
Pseudofractures, 679, 681
Pseudogout and chondrocalcinosis, 499
Pseudohemophilia, 314
Pseudohypertrophic muscular dystrophy, 589
Pseudohypoparathyroidism, 537, **672**, 680
Pseudo-idiopathic hypoparathyroidism, 673
Pseudomembranous enterocolitis, 357
Pseudomonas
  corneal ulcer, 78
  pneumonia, 119
Pseudoneurotic schizophrenia, 617
Pseudo-obstruction, intestinal, 354
Pseudoprecocious puberty, 415
Pseudopseudohypoparathyroidism, 673, 680
Pseudopsychopathic disorders, 617

Psilocin poisoning, 947
Psilocybin, 634
  poisoning, 947
Psittacosis, 840
  pneumonia due to, 122
Psittacosis-lymphogranuloma-trachoma
  agents, drug selections for, 906
Psoriasis, **43**, 998
  and arthritis, 491
PSP, normal values, 1020
Psychedelics, abuse of, 634
Psychiatric
  assessment, 595
  complaints, 594
  complications of nonpsychiatric
    drugs, 644
  conditions, classification of, 610
  disorders, **594-644**
    behavioral approaches, 601
    common, **608-625**
    medical approaches, 597
    psychologic approaches, 605
    social approaches, 606
    treatment approaches, **597-608**
  hospitalization, 604
  interview, 595
  patient, medical examination, 596
  problems associated with medical and
    surgical disorders, 642
Psychiatry, 605
Psychoanalysis, 605
Psychogenic pelvic pain, 440
Psychologic
  gastrointestinal disorders, 325
  testing, 596
Psychomotor seizures, 563
Psychophysiologic disorders, 614
Psychosurgery, 604
Psychotic patients and air travel, 927
Psychotomimetic agents, poisoning due
  to, 947
Psyllium hydrophilic mucilloid, 323
Pterygium, 81
PTT, 309, 310
Puberty
  delayed, 648, 700
  precocious, 647, 685, 703
    isosexual, 415
Puerperal mastitis, 476
Pulmonary
  adenomatosis, 132
  atelectasis, 133
  edema, acute, 221
    of extrinsic origin, 141
    high-altitude, 925
  embolism, 265
  emphysema, chronic, 135
  fibrosis, 141
  function tests, 108
  heart disease, 226
  hypertension in congenital heart
    disease, 161
  infiltrations with eosinophilia, 113
  osteoarthropathy, 107
  stenosis, 157
  thromboembolism, 143
  tuberculosis, 124
  vasculitis, 116
Pulse
  deficit, 205
  paradoxic, 224
Pulseless disease, 258

Pump lung, 134
Pupillary dilation, 87
Pure red cell aplasia, 278
Purified protein derivative, 124
Purine diet, low, 762
Purinethol, 295, 982
Purpura, **311–314**
Pyelonephritis, 539
Pylephlebitis, 359
Pyloric stenosis, 960
Pylorospasm, 325
Pyoderma, 32, 51
Pyrantel pamoate, 873, 875, 876
Pyrazinamide, 905
Pyribenzamine, 14
Pyridoxine, 758, 771
    responsive anemias, 285
Pyrilamine, 14
Pyrimethamine, 855
Pyronil, 14
Pyrosis, 321, 337
Pyrrobutamine, 14
Pyruvate decarboxylase deficiency, 966
Pyruvic acid, normal values, 1019
Pyrvinium pamoate, 875

Q fever, 812
    pneumonia due to, 122
QM, 964
Quaalude, 602
Quadriceps muscle, biopsy of, 730
Quide, 598
Quinacrine, 860, 868, 983
    mustard test for chromosomal
        abnormalities, 964
    poisoning, 954
Quinethazone, 239
Quinidine, 204, 237
    poisoning, 954
    test, drugs interfering with, 1005
Quinine, 855
    poisoning, 954
Quinolor compound ointment, 46
Quinsy, 101

Rabies, 803
    globulin, human immune, 804
Radial diffusion technic of immuno-
        globulin determination, 991
Radiation
    acute, effects of on normal tissues,
        922
    ionizing
        and chromosomes, 971
        delayed effects of, 924
    sickness, 923
Radioactive
    iodine therapy in hyperthyroidism,
        667
    T₃ uptake of red cells or resin,
        test for, 657
Radioimmune precipitation test, 992
Radioimmunoassay for digitalis deter-
        mination, 234
Radioiodine uptake of thyroid gland,
        658
Radioisotope scanning of heart, 167
Radionuclide scanning in breast
        cancer, 401
Radiophosphorus, 296, 306

Radiotherapy
    as adjunct to radical mastectomy, 405
    for breast cancer, 405
Ragweed hay fever, 998
Rapid eye movement sleep, 625
Rash, heat, 48
Rat
    paste, poisoning due to, 945
    poison, 939
Rat-bite fever, 848
Rate, cardiac, disturbances of, **201–209**
Rathke's pouch cyst, 650
Rationalization, 595
Raudixin, 183
Rauwolfia, 183
    poisoning, 954
Raynaud's disease and phenomenon, 259
RBC, normal values, 1018
Reabsorption, bicarbonate, defects of,
        538
Reaction formation, 594
Reactive
    depressions, treatment of, 624
    hypoglycemia, 746
Reality therapy, 606
Rectocele, 431
Rectum
    cancer of, 366
        in pregnancy, 472
    diseases of, **361–367**
    polyps of, 365
Red
    blood count, 1018
    cell(s)
        aplasia, pure, 278
        cellular measurements, 1018
        fragility, normal values, 1018
        survival, 281, 282
    eye, differential diagnosis of, 75
Red-bugs, 64
Reduction-division, 963
Reduviid bugs, 858
Reflux esophagitis, 336
Refractive error, 75
Refsum's syndrome, 966
Regional enteritis, 349
Regitine, 181, 242, 698, 720
Regression, 594
Rehabilitation of patients with stroke
        or hemiplegia, 569
Reifenstein's syndrome, 701
Reiter's
    disease, 998
    syndrome, 492
Relapsing fever, 848
REM sleep, 625
Renal
    agenesis, 539
    biopsy, 522
    carcinoma, 974
    colic, 648
    diabetes insipidus, 538
    diseases, hereditary, **536–539**
    failure
        acute, 532
        antibiotics in, 893
    function tests, 521, 1020
    glycosuria, 538, 730
    insufficiency, 678
        chronic, 527
    medulla, cystic disease of, 537
    osteodystrophy, 529, 679, 681

Renal (cont'd)
    papillary necrosis, 535
    pelvis, tumors of, 549
    plasma flow, 522
    radiography, 522
    stone(s), 496, **545**
    transplant, 528
    tubular
        acidosis, 538
        defects, 537, 538
        function, multiple defects of, 537
        necrosis, 533
    tubule(s)
        diseases of, 532
        hydrogen ions in, 20
Rendu-Osler-Weber disease, 313
Renese, 239
Renin
    activity, normal, 1020
    renal vein, 179, 253
Repoise, 598
Repression, 594
Reptilase, 267
Reserpine, 183
Respiration, artificial, **1026–1028**
Respiratory
    acidosis, 22
    alkalosis, 22
    assistance, **1026–1028**
    disease
        acute undifferentiated, 808
        and air travel, 926
        common, 96
        distress syndrome, 134
    failure
        acute, 137
        chronic, 139
    system, diseases of, **106–151**
    tract infections, 789
Resulin, 46
Resuscitation, artificial (heart-lung),
        1026–1028
Retention cysts, 434
Reticulocytes, 1018
Reticuloendotheliosis, leukemic, 303
Reticulosis, histiocytic medullary, 304
Retin A, 46
Retina, detachment of, 84
Retinopathy, diabetic, 729, 738
Retropharyngeal abscess, 102
Rezamid, 46
Rhabditiform larvae, 873
Rheumatic
    disorders, **477–501**
    fever, 161
        prevention of recurrence of, 163
    heart disease, 165
    pericarditis, 162, 225
    valvulitis, inactive, 165
Rheumatism, palindromic, 495
Rheumatoid
    arthritis, 479, 993
    spondylitis, 489
Rh incompatibility, 319
Rhinitis, allergic, 97
Rhinorrhea, 575
RhoGAM, 474
Rhₒ(D) immune globulin, 474
Rhus toxin, 35
Rhythm
    method, 444
    nodal or junctional, 206

Rhythm (cont'd)
and rate, cardiac, disturbances of, **201–208**
Rib(s)
beading of, 681
cervical, 565
notching, 181
Riboflavin, 758, 769
Rickets, **679**, 768
glycosuric, 538
and osteomalacia, 680
vitamin D-resistant, 537
Rickettsiae, **809–812**
pneumonia due to, 122
Rickettsial
diseases, **809–813**
infections, drug selections for, 906
Rickettsialpox, 811
Riedel's struma (thyroiditis), 671
Rifampin, 127, 904
Ringworm, 57
Rinne test, 89
Ritalin, 637
Robinson-Kepler-Power test, 689
Rocky Mountain spotted fever, 810
diagnostic features of, 792
pneumonia due to, 122
Role-playing, 608
Romaña's sign, 857
Romanowsky's stain, 854
Rorschach psychodiagnostics, 596
Roseola infantum, 793
Rose-water ointment, 73
Rotor's syndrome, 379
Rouleau formation, 298
Roundworm infections, **870–876**
RPF, 522
normal values, 1020
RT$_3$U, normal values, 1015
Rubella, 792, 793
congenital, 794
diagnostic features of, 792
in pregnancy, 472
virus vaccine, live, 794, 1001
Rubeola, 791, 792
pneumonia due to, 122
Rubin test, 442
Rule of nines, 917

Saber shin, **509**
Saccharin, 732
Saccular aneurysm, 243
Sadomasochism, 613
Saf-T-Coil, 447
St. Louis encephalitis, 801
St. Vitus' dance, 584
Salbutamol, 113
Salicylamide, 9
Salicylate(s), 9
in arthritis, 481
poisoning, 945
Salmonella
gastroenteritis, 825
osteomyelitis, 504
and arthritis, 504
typhi, 504
Salmonellosis, 822
food poisoning, 824
septicopyemic, 825
Salpingitis, 433

Salt(s)
depletion and heat cramps, 916
equivalent values, 30
Saluron, 239
Salyrgan, 240
Sandhoff's disease, 966
Sanfilippo syndrome, 966
Sansert, 559, 952
Saphenous veins, varicosities of, 262
Sarcoid, 678
Boeck's, 142
of bone, 680
Sarcoidosis, 142
arthritis in, 499
immunodeficiency associated with, 966
Sarcoma, 980
Ewing's, 519
osteogenic, 518, 980
reticulum cell, 304
of small bowel, 351
Sarcoptes scabiei, 62
Satellite, 961
SBE, 174, 175
Scabies, 62
Scalenus anticus syndrome, 565
Scalp, ringworm of, 57
Scanning, radionuclide, 401
Scapulocostal syndrome, 514
Scapulohumeral
calcareous tendinitis, 514
periarthritis, 513
Scarlet fever, 792
surgical, 814
Scars, hypertrophic, 69
Schatzki's ring, 334
S/C hemoglobin disease, 287, **288**
Schiller test, 425
Schilling test, 275, 276
Schistosomiasis, 863
Schizoid personality, 616
Schizophrenia, 617, 620, 626
Schmidt's syndrome, 662, 671
Scholtz regimen, 38
Scleral lacerations, 79
Scleroderma, 487, 993
Sclerosis
amyotrophic lateral, 589
disseminated, 580
multiple, 998
posterolateral, 584
progressive systemic, 487
Sclerotherapy, compression, 263
Scolex, 867
Scopolamine poisoning, 938
Scorpion stings, 946
Scotochromogens, 129
Scratch-itch cycle, 39
Screw-worm flies, 882
Scrub typhus, 812
Scuba diving, hazards of, 924
Scurvy, 771
SD-1, 990
SD-2, 990
Seasickness, 557
Sebical shampoo, 45, 74
Sebizon, 45
Seborrheic dermatitis, 45
Sebulex, 45, 74
Secobarbital, 602
Sedative-hypnotics, 602
dependency on, 629
poisoning due to, 937

Sedimentation rate, 1018
Seizures, epileptic, 560
Selenium sulfide, 45
Sella syndrome, empty, 651
Selsun, 45, 74
Semikon, 14
Seminiferous tubule failure, 701
Seminoma, 551, 704
Senile
keratoses, 65
vaginitis, 709
Sensitivity tests, drug, 891
Sensitization due to ocular medications, 87
Sentence completion tests, 596
Sepsis and bacteremia, gram-negative, 785
Septal defect
atrial, 158
ventricular, 159
Septectomy, ventricular, 230
Septic arthritis, 493
Septicopyemic salmonellosis, 825
Septum, nasal, hematoma and abscess of, 96
Sequential pill, 444
Serax, 602
Serentil, 597
Sernyl, 635, 947
Serologic tests for syphilis, 841
Serotonin, 1019
Serous cystadenomas, 436
Serpiginous ulcer, 78
Serratia pneumonia, 119
Sertoli cell tumor, 704
Serum
acid phosphatase, 1012
albumin, 1007
alkaline phosphatase, 1012
amylase, 1007
bilirubin, 1008
calcium, 1008
chloride, 1009
cholesterol, 1009
esters, 1010
creatinine, 1010
globulin, 1014
iron, 1011
iron-binding capacity, 1011
lactic acid dehydrogenase in myocardial infarction, 194, 1012
lipase, 1012
magnesium, 1012
phosphorus, inorganic, 1013
sickness-like reactions, 13
sodium, 1014
transaminase, 1016
uric acid, 1017
Sex
chromatin, 964
count in hypogonadism, 701
chromosome(s), 957
abnormalities, 964
Sexual
drive, 612
dysfunction, 612
infantilism, 648
object, variations in, 613
precocity, 647, 703
Sézary's syndrome, 304
SGOT, 195, 371, 1016, 1019
SGPT, 371, 1016, 1019

Sheehan's syndrome, 650
Sheep cell agglutination test, 807
Shellfish poisoning, 954
Shigella dysentery, 824
Shigellosis, 827
Shingles, 51, 795
Shipyard eye, 808
Shirodkar operation, 462
Shock
  anaphylactic, 12, 896
  bacteremic, 785
  cardiogenic, 3, 196
  impending, in pancreatitis, 394
  lung, 134
  syndrome, 2–8
Shohl's solution, 545
Shoshin beriberi, 769
Shoulder, frozen, 513
Shoulder-hand syndrome, 196, **516**
Sialadenitis, 331
Sicca syndrome, 488
Sick
  hysteric, 617
  sinus syndrome, 203
Sickle cell
  anemia, **286**, 460, 966
  disease, modes of inheritance of,
    958
  trait, 288
    modes of inheritance of, 958
Sickledex, 287
Sickness, sleeping, 856
Sideroachrestic anemias, 274, **285**, 290
Sideroblasts, ringed, 285
Siderosis, 114
Silicosis, 114, 115
Silo-filler's disease, 132
Silvadene, 919
Silver nitrate, 71, 74, 426
  conjunctivitis, 80
  poisoning, 954
Simian malaria in man, 856
Simmond's disease, 650
Sims-Huhner test, 442
Sinequan, 601, 602
Singultus, 322
Sino-atrial block, 209
Sinograms, 506
Sinus
  arrhythmia, 202
  bradycardia, 203
  infection, 97
  rhythm, conversion to, 238
  tachycardia, 153, **202**
Sinusitis, 98
Sipple's syndrome, 670
Situational disorders, 608
SI units, 1006
Sjögren's syndrome, 488, 993
Skerljevo, 847
Skin
  and appendages, diseases of, **32–74**
  bacterial infections of, **53–56**
  fungal infections of, **56–62**
  infections, 787
    streptococcal, 814
  manifestations in syphilis, 845
  parasitic infestations of, **62–64**
  pigmentation, abnormal, 646
  test(s)
    for children, 1001
    tuberculin, 124

Skin (cont'd)
  toxicity of cancer chemotherapeutic
    agents, 984
  tumors of, **64–66**
  viral infections of, **50–52**
Skipped beat, 153
SLDH, 1011, 1019
SLE, 483
Sleep disorders, 625
Sleeping sickness, 856
Slow wave sleep, 625
Small intestine, tumors of, 350
Smallpox, 792, **796**
  in pregnancy, 472
  vaccination, 1022
Snack foods, calories in, 774
Snake bite(s), 932
  poisoning, 946
Soaks, 71
Sodium
  antimony gluconate, 859
    dimercaptosuccinate, 864
  bicarbonate, 71
  chloride, 71
  content of foods, 763
  dextrothyroxine, 663, 714
  fluoride, 686
  food sources of, 758
  levothyroxine, 663, 667, 714
  liothyronine, 663, 714
  metabisulfite test, 287
  normal values, 1019
  phosphate, 323
  regulated diet, 762
  salicylate, 164
  sulfacetamide, 54
  sulfate for hypercalcemia, 976
  thiosulfate, 74
  wasting, 689
Sodoku, 848
Soft
  diet, 761
  soap liniment, 74
  tissue infections, 787
Solatene, 780
Solu-Cortef, 688, 717
Solu-Medrol, 717
Solute concentration, 15, **18**
Somatostatin, 645, 742
Somatotropin, 712
Somnafac, 602
Sonography, 522
Sopor, 602
Sore, Oriental, 858
Sparganosis, 868
Specific gravity, 1019, 1020
Spectinomycin, 902
Speed, 636
Spermatocidal foam, 447
Spermatogenic arrest, 702
Spherocytosis, hereditary, 281
Sphincter(s)
  care of, in hemiplegia, 570
  of Oddi, 396
Sphingomyelin lipidosis, 753, 966
Spider bites, 63, 932, **946**
Spike, monoclonal, 299
Spina bifida, 966
Spinal cord compression, 974
Spine, cervical, osteoarthritis of, 512
Spirillary rat-bite fever, 848
Spirillum minus, 848

Spirochetal infections, **841–849**
  drug selections for, 906
Spironolactone, 219, 239, **240**, 696
Splenectomy, 280, 292
  in aplastic anemia, 276
Splenomegaly, 292
Splinter hemorrhages, 153
Splints in arthritis, 500
Spondylitis
  ankylosing, 489, 998
    Marie-Strümpell, 81
  rheumatoid, 489
Spondylosis, cervical, 512
Sponge kidney, 537
Spoon nails, 69
Sporotrichosis, 888
Spots before the eyes, 75
Spotted fevers, 810
Sprue, 355
Sputum, characteristics of, 106
Squamous cell
  carcinoma, 65
  epithelioma, intraepidermal, 65
S state sleep, 625
Stanolone, 722
Staphylococcal
  food poisoning, **824**, 825
  meningitis, 821
  pneumonia, 120
Staphylococci, 53
Starch lotion, 72
Starvation in obesity, 772
Stasis
  dermatitis, 39, 269
  eczema, 39
  ulcer, 269
Status
  asthmaticus, 112
  epilepticus, 561
Steatorrhea, idiopathic, 355
Steinert's disease, 592
Stein-Leventhal syndrome, **437**, 695, **711**
Stelazine, 598
Stenediol, 722
Stenosis
  aortic 166, 167, 168, **171**
  idiopathic hypertrophic subaortic,
    propranolol in, 242
  mitral, 165, 166, 167, **168**
  pulmonary, 155, 156
  pyloric, 960
  tricuspid, 166, 167, **173**
Sterane, 716
Sterilization, 464
Sterisil, 421
Steroid(s), 687
  therapy, local, eye, 87
Sterolone, 716
Stevens-Johnson syndrome, 36
Stewart-Morgagni-Morel syndrome, 695
STH, 712
S-thalassemia, 289
Stibine poisoning, 954
Stiff-man syndrome, 593
Stilbamidine, 859
Stilbazium iodide, 865
Stilphostrol, 723
Stimulants, abuse of, 636
Stokes-Adams syndrome, 211
Stomach
  diseases of, **339–349**
  "leather bottle," 845

Stomal ulcer, 346
Stomatitis
  herpetic, 330
  ulcerative, 330
Stones, urinary, **545–548**, 648
Stork-leg, 589
Stoxil, 913
STP, 634, 947
Strabismus, 85
"Strep throat," 814
Streptococcal
  meningitis, 821
  pneumonia, 119
  skin infections, 814
  sore throat, 814
Streptococci, beta-hemolytic, 55
Streptomycin, 126, 127, **900**, 904
  toxicity, 954
Streptozotocin, 721
Stress incontinence, urinary, 439
Strictures, benign anorectal, 369
Stridor, 673
Stroke(s), 251, **566**
  heat, 916
  recovery and convalescence after, 569
Strongyloidiasis, 873
Struma lymphomatosa, 671
Strychnine poisoning, 946
STS, 807, 841
Stupor, 553
Sty, 82
Subaortic stenosis, 230
Subarachnoid hemorrhages, 568, **570**, 574
Subclavian steal syndrome, 513
Subendocardial fibroelastosis, 229
Sublimation, 594
Sucrase deficiency, 762
Sucrose hemolysis test, 283
Sudden death due to acute myocardial
  infarction, 195
Sudeck's atrophy, 262
Sulfadiazine, 907
Sulfadimethoxine, 907
Sulfameter, 905
Sulfamethoxypyridazine, 905
Sulfamylon, 907, 919
Sulfate, plasma or serum, normal
  values, 1019
Sulfisoxazole, 907
Sulfonamide(s), 905
  precautions in use of, 907
  toxicity, 954
Sulfones in treatment of leprosy, 907
Sulfonylurea compounds, 721, 732
Sulforcin, 46
Sulfur
  food sources of, 758
  granule, 888
Sulfur-salicylic acid ointment, 74
Sulkowitch test, 672, 674
Sultrin cream, 421
Summer grippe, 807
Sunburn, 42
Sunlamps, 44
Sun-screens, 72, 74
Sunstroke, 916
Superior vena cava syndrome, 975
Suppressor T cells, 989
Suramin sodium, 857, 880
Surface
  area nomograms, 1022
  body, estimation of in burns, 917

Surgery
  and cardiac patients, 232
  during pregnancy, 472
Sweeteners, artificial, 732
Swimming safety in foreign travel, 1002
Sycosis vulgaris, 53
Sydenham's chorea, 162, **584**
Symmetrel, 582, 583, 805, 913
Sympathetic ophthalmia, 78
Symptoms, general, **1–14**
Synanon, 607
Syncope, **555–557**
Syndactyly, genetic aspects of, 958
Synergism, antimicrobial, 911
Synkayvite, 317
Synovectomy, 501
Synovial fluid examination, 477
Synthroid, 663, 667, 713
Syntocinon, 712
Syphilis, **841–847**
  of bones and joints, 509
  and cardiovascular disease, 228
  in pregnancy, 469
Syringobulbia, 565
Syringomyelia, 565
Système International d'Unités, 1006
Systemic lupus erythematosus, 483
Systoles, premature ventricular, 153
Systox poisoning, 944

T

and B cells, 988
cell(s), 989, 990
  technics for identification of, 992
  groups, 606
T_3, 656, 663, 665, 713, 714
  by radioimmunoassay, 658
  thyrotoxicosis, 665
T_4, 656, 657, 713, 714
  normal values, 1014
T & A, 101
Tabes dorsalis, 845
TACE, 723
Tachycardia
  nodal or junctional, 206
  paroxysmal, 153
    atrial, 203
    ventricular, 207
  sinus, 153, **202**
Tachycardia-bradycardia, 203
Taenia, 867
Takayasu, idiopathic arteritis of, 258
Talc poisoning, 954
Tamponade, cardiac, 224
Tangier disease, 750
TAO, 256
Tapazole, 666
Tapeworm infections, 867
Taractan, 598
Target
  cells, 288
  lesions, 36
Tar lotion, coal, 72
Tartar emetic, 864
TAT, 596
Tay-Sachs disease, 966
Technetium, 658
Teeth
  abscess of, 329
  discolored, 328
Tegretol, 562

Telangiectasia, hereditary hemorrhagic,
  313
Teldrin, 14
Telogen effluvium, 68
Temperature(s)
  body, 1
  Fahrenheit/Celsius conversion, 1021
Temporal
  arteritis, 258, 488
  lobe
    disorders, 626
    tumor, 579
Tendinitis, 499
  scapulohumeral, calcareous, 514
Tendon rupture, 501
Tensilon, 591
TEPP poisoning, 944
Teratogenic drugs, 455
Teratoid tumors of ovary, 436
Teratoma, 150, 704
Terbutaline, 113
Testes
  carcinoma of, 980
  diseases of, **700–704**
  neoplasms of, 703
  tumors of, **551**, 704
Testicle, gumma of, 589
Testicular
  failure, primary, 700
  feminization, 966
Testosterone, 721, 723
  enanthate, 277, 418, 722
  normal values, 1020
  propionate, 982
Tests, chemical, drugs interfering
  with, 1005
Tetanus, 830
  immunization, 1002
Tetany, 649, 673
  hypoparathyroid, 674
  in pregnancy, 471
Tetrachlorethylene, 865
Tetrachloroethane poisoning, 954
Tetracycline(s), 176, 898
  tooth discoloration due to, 328
Tetrahydrocannabinol, 636
Tetralogy of Fallot, 160
  propranolol in, 241
Tetramisole, 873
6-TG, 982
Thalassemia, 290, 291, 966
Thallium poisoning, 954
Thanite poisoning, 954
THC, 636
Theca
  cell tumors, 438
  lutein cysts of ovaries, 435
  luteinization, 711
Theelin, 723
Thematic apperception test, 596
Thenylene, 14
Theobroma oil, 73
Thiabendazole, 874
Thiamine, 758, 769
Thiazide(s), 182, **239**
  diuretics in prevention of stones, 546
Thimet poisoning, 944
Thiocyanate poisoning, 954
Thiodiazine diuretics, 239
Thioglycollate poisoning, 955
Thioguanine, 980, 982
Thiomerin, 240

Thioridazine, 598
Thiotepa, 550, 976, 982
Thiothixene, 598
Thiouracil drugs, 666
Thioxanthenes, 598
Thomsen's disease, 592
Thonzylamine, 14
Thoracentesis in pleural effusion, 146
Thoracic
    aorta, aneurysms of, 243
    outlet syndrome, 512, 565
Thorazine, 598
Throat, sore, streptococcal, 814
Thrombasthenia, 309, 312
Thromboangiitis obliterans, 256
Thrombocytopenia and eczema, immuno-
        deficiency with, 996
Thrombocytopenic purpura, 309, 311
    idiopathic, 993
    thrombotic, 314
Thromboembolism, pulmonary, 143
Thrombophlebitis, 268, 974
Thromboplastin time, partial, 309
    whole blood, 266
Thrombosis
    arterial, acute, 255
    cerebral, 566, 568
Thrombotic thrombocytopenic purpura,
        314
Thrombo-Wellco, 315
Thrush, 331, 887
Thymic hypoplasia, 992, 995
Thymoma, 150, 591, 974
    immunodeficiency with, 995
Thymus, 150
Thymus-derived cells, 988
Thyrar, 713
Thyroglobulin, 713
Thyroid
    cancer, 669
    crisis, 668
    desiccated, 713, 714
    drugs, poisoning due to, 954
    function tests, 657, 658
    gland, diseases of, 656–672
    hormone, 713
        normal values, 1020
    needless use of, 663
    nodules, 670
    storm, 665, 668
    substernal, 150
Thyroid-binding globulin test, 659
Thyroid-stimulating hormone, 659, 712
Thyroidectomy, 665
Thyroiditis, 671, 672
    autoimmune, 993
Thyrolar, 659, 714
Thyrotoxicosis, 664
    in pregnancy, 471
    T_3, 665
Thyrotropin, 712, 974
    immunoassay, 659
Thyrotropin-releasing factor, 659
Thyroxine, 713
    determination, free, 657
    index, 657, 1015
    normal values, 1014, 1015
Thyroxine-binding globulin
    normal values, 1015
    test, 657
Tibial artery, occlusive disease, 249
Tic douloureux, 585

Tick(s), 64
    typhus, 810
Tietze's syndrome, 106
Tinctures, 74
Tinea, 57–61
Tine test, 124
Tinnitus, 95
Titroid, 714
Tm_G, normal values, 1020
TNM system of staging of breast
        cancer, 403
Tobramycin, 900
Tocopherol, 769
Tofranil, 601
Tolazamide, 721, 732
Tolbutamide, 721, 732
Tolinase, 721, 732
Tolnaftate, 72
Tonsillitis, 100, 101
Tooth discoloration, 328
Topocide, 62, 72
Torulosis, 508
Toxaphene poisoning, 939
Toxemia of pregnancy, 457
Toxic
    agents, peritoneal dialysis or hemo-
        dialysis for, 934
    delirium in pneumonia, 118
    dilatation of colon, 363
    megacolon, 363
Toxicity
    bleomycin, 985
    busulfan, 985
    of cancer chemotherapeutic agents,
        984
    methotrexate, 985
Toxocara, 877
Toxoplasmosis, 861
TPI test, 842
Tracheobronchitis, 96
Tracheostomy, 104
Trachoma, 80, 840
Tranexamic acid, 47
Tranquilizers
    antipsychotic, poisoning due to,
        937
    major, 597
    minor, 602
        dependency on, 629
Transactional analysis, 606
Transaminase(s)
    normal values, 1019
    serum, 1016
Transfusion(s), 318–320
Transplantation
    bone marrow, 278
    kidney, 528
Transsexualism, 613
Transvestism, 613
Tranxene, 602
Tranylcypromine, 601
Traumatic
    diseases of CNS, 573–578
    headache, 558
Traveler's diarrhea, 828
Trematode infections, 863–867
Tremor, pill-rolling, 581
Trench
    fever, 812
    foot, 915
    mouth, 329
Trendelenburg's test, 262

Treponema
    carateum, 847
    pallidum, 509, 841, 847
        immobilization test, 842
    pertenue, 847
Treponematoses, nonvenereal, 847
Tretinoin, 46
TRF, 659
Triamcinolone, 74, 716, 717
    acetonide, 38, 40, 44, 50, 60, 717
Triamterene, 239, 240
Triazure, 44
TRIC agent, 840
Trichinella skin test, 871
Trichiniasis, 870
Trichinosis, 870
Trichlormethiazide, 239
Trichloroethylene poisoning, 955
Trichocephaliasis, 871
Trichomonas vaginalis vaginitis, 421
Trichophyton, 57, 59, 60
Trichosel medium, 420
Trichotillomania, 68
Trichuriasis, 871
Tricofuron, 421, 423
Tricuspid
    atresia, 161
    insufficiency, 166, 167, 173
    stenosis, 166, 167, 173
Tricyclic antidepressants, 601
Tridione, 562, 564
Trifacial neuralgia, 585
Trifluoperazine, 598
Trigeminal neuralgia, 585
Trigger zone in tic douloureux, 585
Triglycerides, normal values, 1016, 1019
Trihexyphenidyl, 582
Triiodothyronine, 713
    by radioimmunoassay, 658
    uptake, resin, normal values, 1015
Trilafon, 598
Trimethadione, 562, 564
Trimethaphan, 185
Trimethoprim/sulfamethoxazole, 542
Trinitrotoluene poisoning, 955
Trionine, 714
Tri-orthocresyl phosphate poisoning, 955
Tripelennamine, 14
Triprolidine, 14
Triprolidine, 14
Trisomy, 963, 967, 968
Trisulfapyrimidines, 907
Troleandomycin, 898
Trolnitrate phosphate, 239
Trophoblastic neoplasms, 980
Tropia, 85
Tropical sprue, 355
Trypanosomal chancre, 856
Trypanosomiasis, 856, 857
Tryparsamide, 857
Tryptophan, transport mechanism of, 778
TSH, 712
    serum, 659
Tsutsugamushi disease, 812
Tubal
    insufflation in infertility, 442
    ligation, 464
Tube feedings, 765
Tuberculin tests, 124, 1001
Tuberculosis
    of bones and joints, 510
    intestinal, 360
    pericarditis, 224, 225

Tuberculosis (cont'd)
  in pregnancy, 469
  pulmonary, 124
  treatment, alternative drugs in, 904
  of urinary tract, 543
Tuberculous meningitis, 821
Tubular
  adenoma of Pick, 704
  transport, 532
Tubule
  distal, anomalies of, 538
  necrosis, renal, 533
  proximal, anomalies of, 537
Tularemia, 832
Tumor(s)
  of bladder, 549
  bone, primary; **518–519**
  brain, frequency of types, 578, 579
  Brenner, 435
  embryonal, 551
  frontal lobe, 579
  of genitourinary tract, **548–552**
  granulosa cell, 438
  intracranial, **578–579**
  larynx, 103
  mediastinal, 149, 150
  nasal, 99
  occipital lobe, 579
  ovarian, 434
  parietal lobe, 579
  of renal pelvis, 549
  response, evaluations of , 986
  of skin, **64–66**
  of small intestine, 350
  temporal lobe, 579
  teratoid, 436
  testicular, 551, 703, 704
  theca cell, 438
  and tumor-like lesions of bone,
    516–517
  of ureter, 549
  virilizing lipoid cell, 437
Tungiasis, 64
Tuning fork tests, 88
Turner's syndrome, 155, 706, 964
Tween-80, 124
Tympanites, 324
Tympanoplasty, 90
Typhoid
  fever, 822
  immunization, 1002
Typhus
  endemic flea-borne, 810
  epidemic louse-borne, 809
  fevers, 792
  immunization, 1002
  murine, 810
  pneumonia due to, 122
  scrub, 812
  tick, 810
Tyramine provocative test, 698
Tyrosinase, 777
Tzanck test, 37, 51

UGDP, 728, 734
Ulcer(s)
  aphthous, 330
  corneal, 77
  decubitus, 55
  duodenal, 341
  gastric, 345

Ulcer(s) (cont'd)
  jejunal, 346
  marginal, 346
  peptic, 341
  serpiginous, 78
  stasis, 269
  stomal, 346
Ulceration in chronic venous insuffi-
    ciency, 270
Ultandren, 722
Ultrasonic scanning, 965
Ultrasound, 152, 167
  echocardiography, 152
  in urinary tract examination, 522
Ultraviolet keratitis, 77
UML-491, 559
Underarm lotion, 72
Undoing, 594
Universal joint syndrome, 441
University Group Diabetes Program, 728,
    734
Upper respiratory diseases, miscel-
    laneous viral, 808
"Uppers," 636
Urate nephropathy, acute, 977
Urea
  blood, 1016
    normal values, 1021
  clearance, 1021
  in glaucoma, 76
  intravenous, 554
  stibamine, 859
Uremia, **527**, 534
Ureteral stone, 474, 547
Ureter, tumors of, 549
Urethral
  caruncle, 423
  diverticulum, 424
Urethritis, nongonococcal, 840
Uric acid
  nephropathy, 535
  normal values, 1017, 1019
  stones, 546
  test, drugs interfering with, 1005
Urinalysis, 521
Urinary
  antiseptics, 909
  follicle-stimulating hormone, 1021
  incontinence, 521
  stones, **545–548**
  stress incontinence, 439
  symptoms, 521
    in pregnancy, 451
  tract infections, **539–545**
    in pregnancy, 470
Urine
  amylase, 1008
  calcium, 1009
  characteristics of, 521
  chloride, 1009
  creatine, 1010
  creatinine, 1010
  examination of, 540
  tests, drugs interfering with, 1005
  vanillylmandelic acid, 1021
Urobilinogen, fecal, 1021
Uropathy, obstructive, 536
Uroporphyrin, urine, 780
Urticaria, 47
Uterine
  bleeding, 416
  lacerations, 466

Uterine (cont'd)
  prolapse, 432
Uterotubal insufflation, 442
Uterus
  carcinoma of, 427
  malposition of, 432
  myoma of, 428
  prolapse of, 432
  tipped, 432
UTI, 539
Uveitis, 81
  acute anterior, 75, 998
  sympathetic, 78

Vaccination, BCG, 126
Vaccine
  influenza, 805
  mumps virus, 1001
  poliomyelitis, 1001
  rabies, 804
    duck embryo, 804
  rubella virus, live, 794, 1001
  smallpox, 1002
  typhus, 1002
  yellow fever, 1002
Vaccinia, 797
  necrosum, 797
  pneumonia due to, 122
Vagal stimulation, 204
Vaginal
  bleeding, postmenopausal, 418
  cytology, 425
  discharge, white, 420
  smears, 417
Vaginismus, 612
Vaginitis, 421
Valium, 563, 602
Vallestril, 723
Valvulitis, rheumatic, inactive, 165
Vancomycin, 908
Vanillylmandelic acid, 181, 698, 1021
  test, urine, drugs interfering with,
    1005
Varicella, 51, 792, **795**
  pneumonia due to, 122
Varicose veins, 262, 453
Variola, 122, 792, **796**
Vascular
  diseases of CNS, **566–571**
  headache, 558
  hemophilia, 309, **314**
  malformation, 568
  shock, 3, 4
Vasculitis, pulmonary, 116
Vasoactive drugs for shock, 6
Vasodepressor syncope, 555
Vasodilators, 260
  in treatment of cardiac failure, 219
Vasomotor
  disorders traumatically induced, 261
  shock, 3, 4
Vasopressin, 327, 654, 712
Vasospastic disorders, **259–261**
Vasovagal syncope, 555
VC test, 108
VDRL test, 841
Vegetarian diet, 764
Veins
  thrombophlebitis of, 264, 268
  varicose, 262
Velban, 983

Vena cava obstruction, superior, 270
Venereal disease, generalizations concerning, 787
Venesection, 220, 306
Venezuelan encephalitis, 801
Venous
    catheterization, short-term, 268
    disease, degenerative and inflammatory, 262–270
    insufficiency, chronic, 265, 268
    pressure, 216
Ventilation, minute, 138
Ventilators, mechanical, 138
Ventilatory assistance, weaning in, 139
Ventricular
    flutter and fibrillation, 209
    preexcitation, 212
    premature beats, 207
    septal defect, 155, 159
    tachycardia, paroxysmal, 207
Veratrum poisoning, 955
Verrucae, **52**, 65, 82
Versenate, 587
Vertigo, **555–557**
    paroxysmal labyrinthine, 94
Vesical stone, 547
Vestibulitis, nasal, 95
Vibrio food poisoning, 824
Vinblastine, 302, 980, 983
Vincent's infection, 329
Vincristine, 295, 983
    neuropathy, 984
Vineberg procedure, 193
Vioform, 49, 851
Violence and aggression, 626
Viomycin, 905
Viral diseases, **791–808**
Virilizing diseases, 437, 694, 711
Viruses and chromosomes, 971
Visceral larva migrans, 877
Vision
    blurred, 75
    double, 76
    tests for children, 85
Vistaril, 602
Vital capacity test, 108
Vitamin(s)
    A, 758, 767
    B$_1$, 758, 769
    B$_2$, 758, 769
    B$_6$, 758
    B$_{12}$, 275, 276, 758, 771
    B complex, 769
    C, 758, 770
        and common respiratory disease, 96
    D, 674, 678, 682, 758, 767
        deficiency, 680
        intoxication, 678, 680
    D-resistant rickets, 681
    D$_2$, 714
    diet, high, 761
    disorders, **766–771**
    E, 758, 769
    fat-soluble, **767–769**

Vitamin(s) (cont'd)
    food sources of, 758
    K, 317, **768**
    water-soluble, **769–771**
Vitiligo, 66, 646
Vitreous
    hemorrhage, 79
    opacities, 75
Vivactil, 601
VLDL, 747
VM-26, 980
VMA, 698, 1021
Vocational aptitude and interest tests, 596
Volatile
    anesthetics, poisoning, 955
    oils, poisoning, 955
Vollmer test, 124
Volume, water, 17
Vomiting, 321
    of pregnancy, 454
Von Gierke's disease, 779
Von Willebrand's disease, 314
Voyeurism, 613
VP-16, 980
V region, 987

Waldenström's macroglobulinemia, 994
Walthard cell rests, 435
Warfarin, 266, 267
Warts, **51**, 65, 82
Wasp stings, 947
Wasserman test, 841
Wasting, 646
Water
    absorption, defects of, 538
    babies, 654
    body, 15, 16
    deficit, 17
    disturbances of, diagnosis, **26–30**
    excess, 17, 18
    interstitial and intracellular, 16
    intoxication, 533
    loss, 17
    purification in foreign travel, 1001
Waterhouse-Friderichsen syndrome, 315, 687
Watson-Ehrlich reaction, 278
Watson-Schwartz test, 780
Weakness, 646
Weaver's bottom, 499
Weber test, 89
Weed system, 999
Weeping dermatitis, acute, 35
Wegener's
    granulomatosis, 116, 143
    syndrome, 489
Weight(s)
    and measures, new nomenclature for, 1006
    molar and milliequivalent, 16
    tables, 1023
Weil's disease, 849
Werdnig-Hoffman paralysis, 588

Western equine encephalitis, 801
Wet dressings, 71
Wheezing, 106
Whipple's disease, 356
Whipworm infestation, 871
White blood count, normal values, 1018
Whitfield's ointment and solution, 74
Whole blood
    partial thromboplastin time, 1024
    for shock, 5
Whooping cough, 817
Wickham's striae, 43
Wilms's tumor, **549**, 980
Wilson's disease, 385, **583**
Wing-beating of arms, 583
Winstrol, 722
Winterbottom's sign, 856
Wiskott-Aldrich syndrome, 312, **996**
Witch's milk, 647
Withdrawal
    in alcohol dependency, 631
    in barbiturate dependency, 630
    in narcotic dependency, 627
Wolff-Parkinson-White syndrome, 212
Wolf's syndrome, 968
Wolman's disease, 966
Wood's light, 56
Wool fat, 73
Woolsorter's disease, 830
Wuchereria bancrofti, 877

Xanthines, 239
X chromosome, 957
Xenodiagnosis, 858
Xeroderma pigmentosum, 966
Xeroradiography, 402
X-linked inheritance, 958
X, Y chromosome disorders, 969
Xylocaine in arrhythmias, 198, 208

Yaws, 847
Y chromosome, 957
Yellow
    fever, 804
        vaccination, 1002
    jacket stings, 947
Yersinia enterocolitica infection, 823
Yomesan, 868
Yttrium implant, 693

Zarontin, 562, 564
Zenker's diverticula, 335
ZIG, 52
Zinc
    oxide ointment and paste, 73
    poisoning, 955
Zollinger-Ellison syndrome, 341, 344
Zoster, herpes, 51
Zoster-immune globulin, 52
Zygadenus poisoning, 955
Zyloprim, 547, 983